Principles and Practice of Pediatric Surgery

Principles and Practice of Pediatric Surgery

Volume 2

EDITORS

Keith T. Oldham, MD

Professor and Chief, Division of Pediatric Surgery, Medical College of Wisconsin
Marie Z. Uihlein Chair and Surgeon-in-Chief
Children's Hospital of Wisconsin, Milwaukee, Wisconsin

Paul M. Colombani, MD

Robert Garrett Professor of Pediatric Surgery, Professor of Surgery, Pediatrics and Oncology
Chief, Division of Pediatric Surgery, The John Hopkins University School of Medicine
Children's Surgeon-in-Charge, The Johns Hopkins Hospital, Baltimore, Maryland

Robert P. Foglia, MD

Associate Professor of Surgery and Pediatrics, Department of Surgery
Division of Pediatric Surgery, Washington University School of Medicine
Surgeon-in-Chief, Department of Surgery, St. Louis Children's Hospital, St. Louis, Missouri

Michael A. Skinner, MD

Associate Professor and Chief, Division of Pediatric Surgery
Duke University Medical Center, Durham, North Carolina

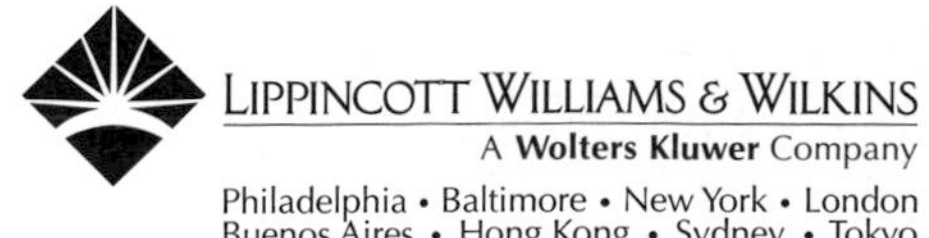

LIPPINCOTT WILLIAMS & WILKINS
A Wolters Kluwer Company
Philadelphia • Baltimore • New York • London
Buenos Aires • Hong Kong • Sydney • Tokyo

Acquisitions Editor: Brian Brown
Managing Editor: Michelle M. LaPlante
Project Manager: Fran Gunning
Manufacturing Manager: Ben Rivera
Marketing Manager: Adam Glazer
Production Services: TechBooks
Compositor: TechBooks
Printer: Maple Press

530 Walnut Street
Philadelphia, PA 19106 USA
LWW.com

Printed in the USA

Library of Congress Cataloging-in-Publication Data

Principles and practice of pediatric surgery / editors, Keith T. Oldham . . . [et al.].
p. ; cm.
Includes bibliographical references and index.
ISBN 0-7817-4290-0 (alk. paper)
1. Children—Surgery. I. Oldham, Keith T.
[DNLM: 1. Surgical Procedures, Operative—methods—Child. 2. Surgical Procedures, Operative—methods—Infant. WO 925 P9566 2005]
RD137.P875 2005
617.9′8—dc22

2004023430

Care has been taken to confirm the accuracy of the information presented and to describe generally accepted practices. However, the authors, editors, and publisher are not responsible for errors or omissions or for any consequences from application of the information in this book and make no warranty, expressed or implied, with respect to the currency, completeness, or accuracy of the contents of the publication. Application of this information in a particular situation remains the professional responsibility of the practitioner.

The authors, editors, and publisher have exerted every effort to ensure that drug selection and dosage set forth in this text are in accordance with current recommendations and practice at the time of publication. However, in view of ongoing research, changes in government regulations, and the constant flow of information relating to drug therapy and drug reactions, the reader is urged to check the package insert for each drug for any change in indications and dosage and for added warnings and precautions. This is particularly important when the recommended agent is a new or infrequently employed drug.

Some drugs and medical devices presented in this publication have Food and Drug Administration (FDA) clearance for limited use in restricted research settings. It is the responsibility of the health care provider to ascertain the FDA status of each drug or device planned for use in their clinical practice.

10 9 8 7 6 5 4 3 2 1

We wish to dedicate this effort to our parents:

Richard and Gladys Oldham
Louis and Phyllis Colombani
Peter and Elda Foglia
Rodney and Patsy Skinner

Our commitment, like yours, is to foster learning and idealism in those we teach.

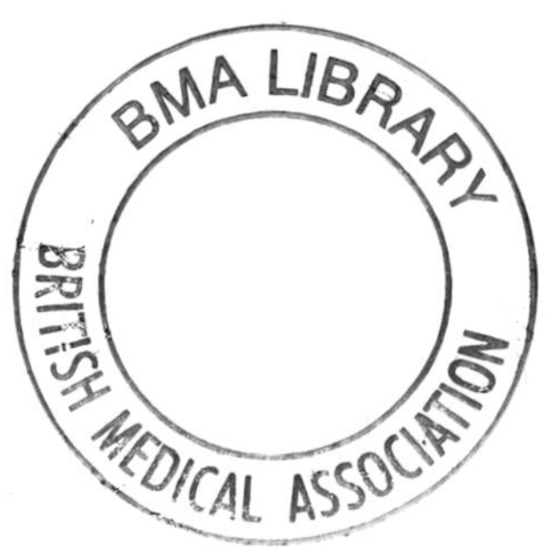

CONTRIBUTORS LIST

E. Stanton Adkins, III, MD
Assistant Professor
Department of Pediatrics and Surgery
University of South Carolina School of Medicine
Attending Surgeon
Department of Surgery
Palmetto Health Children's Hospital
Columbia, South Carolina

John J. Aiken, MD
Associate Professor
Department of Surgery/Pediatric Surgery
Childen's Hospital of Wisconsin
Milwaukee, Wisconsin

Craig T. Albanese, MD
Professor, Surgery, Pediatrics and Obstetrics and Gynecology
Chief, Division of Pediatric Surgery
Stanford University Medical Center
Director of Surgical Services
Lucile Packard Children's Hospital
Stanford, California

Sharma Anshuman, MD
Assistant Professor
Department of Anesthesiology
Washington University School of Medicine
Director, Department of Pediatric Cardiac Anesthesia
St. Louis Children's Hospital
St. Louis, Missouri

Robert J. Arceci, MD, PhD
Director of the Division of Pediatric Oncology
King Fahd Professor of Pediatric Oncology
Professor of Oncology
Professor of Pediatrics
The Sidney Kimmel Comprehensive Cancer Center at Johns Hopkins
Bunting Blaustein Cancer Research Building
Baltimore, Maryland

Richard G. Azizkhan, MD
Surgeon-in-Chief
Lester W. Martin Chair of Pediatric Surgery
Cincinnati Children's Hospital Medical Center
Professor of Surgery and Pediatrics
University of Cincinnati School of Medicine
Cincinnati, Ohio

Kristin Baird, MD
Sidney Kimmel Cancer Comprehensive Cancer Center
Johns Hopkins University School of Medicine
Baltimore, Maryland

Edward M. Barksdale, Jr., MD
Associate Professor
Department of Surgery
University of Pittsburgh
Attending Surgeon
Department of Pediatric Surgery
Children's Hospital of Pittsburgh
Pittsburgh, Pennsylvania

Françoise Baylis, PhD
Professor
Dalhousie Medical School
Department of Bioethics
Halifax, Nova Scotia
Canada

Spencer W. Beasley, MD
Consultant Paediatric Surgeon
Christchurch Hospital
Christchurch
New Zealand

Stuart Berger, MD
Professor, Department of Pediatrics
Medical College of Wisconsin
Director, Herma Heart Center
Children's Hospital of Wisconsin
Milwaukee, Wisconsin

David A. Bloom, MD
Associate Dean, Medical School Administration
Professor, Urology Surgery
University of Michigan
Department of Urology
Ann Arbor, Michigan

Mary L. Brandt, MD
Professor of Surgery
Michael E. DeBakey Department of Surgery
Baylor College of Medicine
Houston, Texas

Melanie L. Brown, MD
Attending Physician
Department of Pediatrics
The University of Chicago
Pritzker School of Medicine
Chicago, Illinois

Pamela I. Brown, MD, PhD
Clinical Assistant Professor
Department of Pediatrics-Gastroenterology
University of Michigan
C.S. Mott Children's Hospital
Ann Arbor, Michigan

Kristina A. Bryant, MD
Assistant Professor
Department of Pediatrics
University of Louisville
Louisville, Kentucky

Kristina N. Bryowsky, Pharm D, BCPS
Clinical Pharmacist, NICU
Department of Pharmacy
St. Louis Children's Hospital
St. Louis, Missouri

Imad F. Btaiche, PharmD, BCNSP
Clinical Assistant Professor
College of Pharmacy
University of Michigan
Ann Arbor, Michigan

Terry L. Buchmiller-Crair, MD
Assistant Professor of Surgery
Children's Hospital of New York Presbyterian
Weill Medical College of Cornell University
New York, New York

Rebecca H. Buckley, MD
Professor
Division of Pediatric Allergy and Immunology
Duke University Medical Center
Durham, North Carolina

Andrew I.M. Campbell, MD
Clinical Fellow
Department of Cardiothoracic Surgery
Children's Hospital of Philadelphia
Philadelphia, Pennsylvania

Donna A. Caniano, MD
Professor of Surgery and Pediatrics
Department of Surgery
Ohio State University College of Medicine and Public Health
Surgeon-in-Chief
Children's Hospital
Columbus, Ohio

Michael G. Caty, MD
Associate Professor of Surgery and Pediatrics
Chief, Division of Pediatric Surgery
State University of New York at Buffalo
Buffalo, New York
Surgeon-in-Chief
Division of Pediatric Surgery
Women and Children's Hospital of Buffalo
Buffalo, New York

Allen R. Chen, MD, PhD, MHS
Assistant Professor
Oncology Center
Johns Hopkins Hospital
Baltimore, Maryland

Christine J. Cheng, MD
Assistant Professor
Division of Plastic and Reconstructive Surgery
Washington University School of Medicine
Attending Physician
St. Louis Children's Hospital
St. Louis, Missouri

Robert E. Cilley, MD
Professor of Surgery
Division of Pediatric Surgery
Department of Surgery
Penn State College of Medicine
Milton S. Hershey Medical Center
Hershey, Pennsylvania

F. Sessions Cole, MD
Park J. White, MD, Professor of Pediatrics
Vice Chairman, Department of Pediatrics
Director, Division of Newborn Medicine
Acting Director, Division of Allergy and Pulmonary Medicine
Department of Pediatrics
Washington University School of Medicine
St. Louis Children's Hospital
St. Louis, Missouri

Paul M. Colombani, MD
Robert Garrett Professor of Pediatric Surgery
Professor of Surgery, Pediatrics and Oncology
Chief, Division of Pediatric Surgery
Johns Hopkins University School of Medicine
Children's Surgeon-in-Charge
Johns Hopkins Hospital
Baltimore, Maryland

Arthur Cooper, MD, MS
Professor of Clinical Surgery
Columbia University College of Physicians and Surgeons
Director of Trauma and Pediatric Surgical Services
Columbia University Affiliation
Harlem Hospital Center
New York, New York

Timothy M. Crombleholme, MD
Professor of Surgery and Developmental Biology
Department of Surgery
University of Cincinnati College of Medicine
Director, Cincinnati Center for Fetal Diagnosis and Treatment
The Center for Molecular Fetal Therapy
Division of General, Thoracic and Fetal Surgery
Cincinnati Children's Hospital Medical Center
Cincinnati, Ohio

Andrew M. Davidoff, MD
Associate Professor, Department of Surgery
St. Jude Children's Research Hospital and University of Tennessee Health Science Center
Memphis, Tennessee

Jeffrey Dawson, MD
Associate Professor
Department of Pediatrics
Washington University School of Medicine
Attending Neonatologist
Division of Newborn Medicine
St. Louis Children's Hospital
St. Louis, Missouri

Antonio De Maio, PhD
Associate Professor
Department of Pediatric Surgery
Johns Hopkins University
Johns Hopkins Hospital
Baltimore, Maryland

William R. DeFoor, MD
Assistant Professor of Surgery
Division of Pediatric Surgery
Division of Pediatric Urology
Children's Hospital Medical Center of Cincinnati
Cincinnati, Ohio

Patrick A. Dillon, MD
Assistant Professor of Surgery and Pediatrics
Washington University School of Medicine
St. Louis Children's Hospital
St. Louis, Missouri

Peter W. Dillon, MD
Professor of Surgery and Pediatrics
Department of Surgery
Division of Pediatric Surgery
Penn State College of Medicine
Director of Surgical Services
Penn State Children's Hospital
Milton S. Hershey Medical Center
Hershey, Pennsylvania

Daniel P. Doody, MD
Department of Pediatric Surgery
Massachusetts General Hospital
Boston, Massachusetts

George T. Drugas, MD
Associate Professor of Surgery and Pediatrics
University of Rochester School of Medicine and Dentistry
Rochester, New York

Craig DuFresne, MD
Aesthetic, Plastic and Reconstructive Surgery
Chevy Chase, Maryland

Martin R. Eichelberger, MD
Director of Emergency Trauma Services
Children's National Medical Center
Washington, District of Columbia

Richard A. Falcone, Jr., MD
Assistant Professor
Division of Pediatric and Thoracic Surgery
Cincinnati Children's Hospital Medical Center
Department of Surgery
University of Cincinnati College of Medicine
Cincinnati, Ohio

Mary E. Fallat, MD
Professor of Surgery
Department of Surgery
Division of Pediatric Surgery
University of Louisville
Director of Trauma Services
Department of Pediatric Surgery
Kosair Children's Hospital
Louisville, Kentucky

Anne C. Fischer, MD, PhD
Assistant Professor and Attending Surgeon
Department of Surgery
Division of Pediatric Surgery
Johns Hopkins University
Johns Hopkins Hospital
Baltimore, Maryland

Steven J. Fishman, MD
Assistant Professor
Department of Surgery
Harvard Medical School
Assistant in Surgery
Department of Surgery
Children's Hospital
Boston, Massachusetts

Alan W. Flake, MD
Professor, Department of Surgery
University of Pennsylvania
Director, Children's Institute for Surgical Sciences
Children's Hospital of Philadelphia
Philadelphia, Pennsylvania

Robert P. Foglia, MD
Associate Professor of Surgery and Pediatrics
Department of Surgery
Division of Pediatric Surgery
Washington University School of Medicine
Surgeon-in-Chief
Department of Surgery
St. Louis Children's Hospital
St. Louis, Missouri

Henri R. Ford, MD
Professor, Pediatric Surgery
University of Pittsburgh
Chief, Pediatric Surgery
Children's Hospital of Pittsburgh
Pittsburgh, Pennsylvania

John W. Foreman, MD
Professor of Pediatric Nephrology
Department of Pediatrics
Duke University Medical Center
Durham, North Carolina

Dominic Frimberger, MD
Research Fellow
Department of Urology
Johns Hopkins University School of Medicine
Baltimore, Maryland

Karen S. Frush, MD
Associate Clinical Professor of Pediatrics
Department of Pediatrics
Chief Medical Director of Children's Services
Duke University Hospital and Health System
Durham, North Carolina

Herbert Edgar Fuchs, MD
Associate Professor of Surgery
Duke Unversity
Head of Pediatric Neurosurgical Services
Department of Surgery
Duke University Medical Center
Durham, North Carolina

Victor Garcia, MD
Professor of Surgery and Pediatrics
University of Cincinnati
Cincinnati, Ohio

John P. Gearhart, MD
Professor and Director of Pediatric Urology
Johns Hopkins Children's Center
Baltimore, Maryland

James D. Geiger, MD
Associate Professor of Surgery
University of Michigan
C.S. Mott Children's Hospital
Ann Arbor, Michigan

Claudia Gerard, MD
Clinical Instructor
Division of Neonatology
Sierra Vista Hospital
San Luis Obispo, California

B. Robert Gibson, MD
Clinical Assistant Instructor
Department of Surgery
State University of New York at Buffalo
Buffalo, New York

George K. Gittes, MD
Associate Professor
Department of Surgery
University of Missouri at Kansas City
Director, Surgical Research
Children's Mercy Hospital
Kansas City, Missouri

Arun K. Gosain, MD
Professor
Department of Plastic and Reconstructive Surgery
Medical College of Wisconsin
Milwaukee, Wisconsin

Arin K. Greene, MD
Division of Plastic Surgery
Harvard Medical School
Brigham and Women's Hospital
Boston, Massachusetts

Philip C. Guzzetta, Jr., MD
Professor of Surgery and Pediatrics
George Washington University School of Medicine
Attending Pediatric Surgeon
Children's National Medical Center
Washington, District of Columbia

Ada Hamosh, MD, MPH
Associate Professor, Pediatrics
McKusick-Nathans Institute of
Genetics Medicine
Johns Hopkins Hospital
Baltimore, Maryland

Aaron Hamvas, MD
Professor of Pediatrics
Division of Newborn Medicine
Medical Director, NICU
St. Louis Children's Hospital
St. Louis, Missouri

Sherrie M. Hauft, MD
Assistant Professor of Pediatrics
Departments of Pediatrics
and Newborn Medicine
Washington University School of Medicine
St. Louis, Missouri

Kurt F. Heiss, MD
Associate Professor of Surgery
Departments of Surgery and Pediatrics
Emory University School of Medicine
Emory Children's Center
Atlanta, Georgia

Michael A. Helmrath, MD
Assistant Professor of Surgery
Baylor College of Medicine
Texas Children's Hospital Care Center
Houston, Texas

Alan W. Hemming, MD, MSC
Associate Professor of Surgery
Department of Surgery
University of Florida
Director of Hepatobiliary Surgery
Division of Transplantation
Shands at University of Florida
Gainesville, Florida

Barry A. Hicks, MD
Associate Professor of Surgery and Pediatrics
University of Texas-Southwestern School of Medicine
Director, Pediatric Trauma Program
Children's Medical Center of Dallas
Dallas, Texas

Meghan A. Higman, MD
Assistant Professor
Departments of Pediatrics and Oncology
Sidney Kimmel Comprehensive Cancer Center at
Johns Hopkins Bunting-Blaustein Cancer
Baltimore, Maryland

Ronald B. Hirschl, MD
Professor
Department of Surgery
University of Michigan Health System
Department of Surgery
C.S. Mott Children's Hospital
Ann Arbor, Michigan

Gary E. Hirshberg, MD
Associate Professor of Anesthesiology
and Pediatrics
Department of Anesthesiology
Division of Pediatric Anesthesiology
Washington University School of Medicine
Anesthesiologist-in-Chief
Department of Anesthesiology
St. Louis Children's Hospital
St. Louis, Missouri

Jeff C. Hoehner, MD, PhD
Assistant Professor of Surgery
Pediatric Surgery
Johns Hopkins University School of Medicine
Johns Hopkins Hospital
Baltimore, Maryland

George W. Holcomb, III, MD, MBA
Katharine B. Richardson Professor of Surgery
Children's Mercy Hospital
Surgeon-in-Chief
Children's Mercy Hospital
Kansas City, Missouri

Thomas H. Inge, MD
Assistant Professor of Surgery and Pediatrics
Surgical Director, Comprehensive Weight Management
Center
Division of Pediatric General and
Thoracic Surgery
Cincinnati Children's Hospital Medical Center
Cincinnati, Ohio

Thomas Jaksic, MD, PhD
Associate Professor of Surgery
Harvard Medical School
Children's Hospital Boston
Boston, Massachusetts

Patrick J. Javid, MD
Research Fellow
Department of Surgery
Children's Hospital Boston
Boston, Massachusetts

M. Barry Jones, MD
Assistant Professor of Anesthesiology
Department of Anesthesiology
Washington University School of Medicine
Director of Pain Management
Departments of Pediatric Anesthesiology and Pain Management
St. Louis Children's Hospital
St. Louis, Missouri

Madelyn Kahana, MD
Professor
University of Chicago Children's Hospital
Pediatric Care Center
Chicago, Illinois

Alex A. Kane, MD
Assistant Professor of Plastic and Reconstructive Surgery
Washington University School of Medicine
St. Louis Children's Hospital
St. Louis, Missouri

Bruce A. Kaufman, MD
Professor of Neurosurgery
Medical College of Wisconsin
Chief, Pediatric Neurosurgery
Children's Hospital of Wisconsin
Milwaukee, Wisconsin

Michael A. Keating, MD
Clinical Professor of Urology in Surgery
University of South Florida School of Medicine
Medical Director, Spina Bifida Clinic
Department of Surgery
Division of Urology
Nemours Children's Clinic Orlando
Orlando, Florida

Sundeep G. Keswani, MD
Post-Doctoral Research Fellow
The Center for Molecular Fetal Therapy
Division of General, Thoracic, and Fetal Surgery
Cincinnati Children's Hospital Medical Center
Cincinnati, Ohio

Karen M. Kling, MD
Assistant Professor of Surgery
Department of Pediatric Surgery
Johns Hopkins University School of Medicine
Department of Pediatric Surgery
Johns Hopkins Hospital
Baltimore, Maryland

David N. Korones, MD
Associate Professor
Pediatric M&D Hematology/Oncology
University of Rochester
Rochester, New York

Subra Kugathasan, MD
Associate Professor of Pediatrics
Medical College of Wisconsin
Medical Director, Inflammatory Bowel Disease Program
Division of Pediatric Gastroenterology
Children's Hospital of Wisconsin
Milwaukee, Wisconsin

Dave R. Lal, MD
Fellow in Pediatric Surgical Oncology
Department of Surgery
Memorial Sloan-Kettering Cancer Center
New York, New York

Kevin P. Lally, MD
Chief, Division of Pediatric Surgery
University of Texas Health Sciences Center
Houston, Texas

Jacob C. Langer, MD
Professor of Surgery
University of Toronto
Chief, Pediatric General Surgery
Hospital for Sick Children, Toronto
Toronto, Ontario
Canada

Max R. Langham, Jr., MD
Professor of Surgery
Department of Surgery
University of Florida
Attending Surgeon and Director of Pediatric Liver Transplantation
Department of Surgery
Shands Childrens' Hospital
Gainesville, Florida

Michael P. LaQuaglia, MD
Professor, Department of Surgery
Weill-Cornell University Medical School
Chief of Pediatric Surgery
Memorial Sloan-Kettering Cancer Center
New York, New York

Marc A. Levitt, MD
Assistant Professor
Department of Pediatric Surgery
Schneider Children's Hospital
Long Island Jewish Medical Center
Professor of Surgery and Pediatrics
Albert Einstein College of Medicine
New Hyde Park, New York

Anna Lijowska, MD
Resident
Children's Hospital St. Louis
St. Louis, Missouri

Lori Luchtman-Jones, MD
Assistant Professor of Pediatrics
Washington University School of Medicine
Director, Hematology Laboratory
St. Louis Children's Hospital
St. Louis, Missouri

Ross T. Lyon, MD
Associate Professor of Surgery
Weill-Cornell Medical College
Division of Vascular Surgery
New York Presbyterian Hospital
New York Weill-Cornell Medical Center
New York, New York

David K. Magnuson, MD
Assistant Professor
Department of Surgery
Case Western Reserve University
Division Chief, Pediatric Surgery
University Hospital Health System
Rainbow Babies and Children's Hospital
Cleveland, Ohio

Paul N. Manson, MD
Professor, Surgery-Plastic Surgery
Johns Hopkins Outpatient Center
Baltimore, Maryland

Jeffrey L. Marsh, MD
Chief, Pediatric Plastic Surgery
Director, Cleft Lip/Palate and Craniofacial
Deformities Center
St. John's Mercy Medical Center
St. Louis, Missouri

Amit Mathur, MBBS, MD
Assistant Professor of Pediatrics
Associate Medical Director, NICU
Washington University School of Medicine
Department of Pediatrics
Division of Newborn Medicine
St. Louis Children's Hospital
St. Louis, Missouri

Eugene D. McGahren, III, MD
Associate Professor
Department of Medicine-Surgery
University of Virginia Health System
Charlottesville, Virginia

Milissa A. McKee, MD
Assistant Professor of Surgery
and Pediatrics
Yale University School of Medicine
New Haven, Connecticut

John J. Meehan, Jr., MD
Assistant Professor of Surgery
University of Iowa Health Care
Iowa City, Iowa

Sheilendra S. Mehta, MD
Pediatric Surgery Research Fellow
Pediatric Surgery Department
Children's Mercy Hospital
Kansas City, Missouri

Rebecka L. Meyers, MD
Chief, Division of Pediatric Surgery
Associate Professor
Departments of Surgery and Pediatrics
University of Utah School of Medicine
Primary Children's Medical Center
Salt Lake City, Utah

Robert K. Minkes, MD
Chief, Section of Pediatric Surgery
Associate Professor
Department of Surgery
Louisiana University School of Medicine
Director of Pediatric Surgical Education
Head, Pediatric Surgery
Department of Surgery
Children's Hospital of New Orleans
New Orleans, Louisiana

Sally E. Mitchell, MD
Associate Professor of Radiology, Surgery, and Pediatrics
Director, Interventional Pediatrics Associates

Director, Interventional Radiology
Johns Hopkins Medical Institutions
Baltimore, Maryland

David P. Mooney, MD
Trauma Department
Children's Hospital of Boston
Boston, Massachusetts

R. Lawrence Moss, MD
Associate Professor and Chief, Section of Pediatric Surgery
Yale University School of Medicine
New Haven, Connecticut
Surgeon-in-Chief
Yale University Children's Hospital
New Haven, Connecticut

Cheryl A. Muszynski, MD
Associate Professor of Neurosurgery
Medical College of Wisconsin
Staff Physician
Pediatric Neurosurgery
Children's Hospital of Wisconsin
Milwaukee, Wisconsin

George B. Mychaliska, MD
Assistant Professor of Surgery and Pediatrics
Department of Surgery
Washington University School of Medicine
Attending Pediatric Surgeon
Department of Surgery
St. Louis Children's Hospital
St. Louis, Missouri

Evan P. Nadler, MD
Assistant Professor of Surgery
New York University School of Medicine
New York, New York

John Noseworthy, MD
Associate Professor of Surgery
Mayo Medical School
Professor of Surgery
Thomas Jefferson University
Medical Chief of Development
Nemours Foundation
Jacksonville, Florida

Jed G. Nuchtern, MD
Associate Professor
Department of Surgery
Baylor College of Medicine
Staff Surgeon
Department of Pediatric Surgery
Texas Children's Hospital
Houston, Texas

Steven Ognibene, MD
Chief Resident in General Surgery
University of Rochester School of Medicine and Dentistry
Rochester, New York

Keith T. Oldham, MD
Professor and Chief
Division of Pediatric Surgery
Medical College of Wisconsin
Marie Z. Uihlein Chair and Surgeon-in-Chief
Children's Hospital of Wisconsin
Milwaukee, Wisconsin

Daniel J. Ostlie, MD
Director of Trauma/Critical Care
Children's Mercy Hospitals and Clinics
Assistant Professor of Surgery
University of Missouri at Kansas City School of Medicine
Kansas City, Missouri

Charles N. Paidas, MD
Associate Professor
Department of Surgery
Johns Hopkins University School of Medicine
Associate Professor
Department of Pediatric Surgery
Johns Hopkins Hospital
Baltimore, Maryland

Walter Pegoli, Jr., MD
Associate Professor of Surgery and Pediatrics
Section Chief
Pediatric Surgery
University of Rochester School of Medicine and Dentistry
Rochester, New York

Alberto Peña, MD
Chief, Pediatric Surgery
Schneider Children's Hospital
Long Island Jewish Medical Center
Professor of Surgery and Pediatrics
Albert Einstein College of Medicine
New Hyde Park, New York

Craig A. Peters, MD
Associate Professor
Harvard Medical School
Boston Children's Hospital
Boston, Massachusetts

Heidi J. Pinkerton, MD
Division of Pediatric Surgery
Children's Hospital of Wisconsin
Milwaukee, Wisconsin

David Pinkstaff, MD
Senior Resident
Department of Urology
Mayo Clinic Jacksonville
Jacksonville, Florida

Shawn J. Rangel, MD
Section of Pediatric Surgery
Yale University School of Medicine
New Haven, Connecticut

Sonja A. Rasmussen, MD, MS
Associate Director for Science
Division of Birth Defects and Developmental Disabilities
National Center on Birth Defects and Developmental Disabilities
Atlanta, Georgia

Pramod P. Reddy, MD
Assistant Professor of Pediatric Urology
Cincinnati Children's Hospital and Medical Center
Cincinnati, Ohio

Michael X. Repka, MD
Professor
Department of Ophthalmology and Pediatrics
Johns Hopkins University School of Medicine
Johns Hopkins Hospital
Baltimore, Maryland

Frederick J. Rescorla, MD
Professor of Surgery
Department of Surgery
Indiana University School of Medicine
Staff Surgeon
Pediatric Surgery
JW Riley Hospital for Children
Indianapolis, Indiana

Jorge Reyes, MD
Professor of Surgery and Division Chief
Transplant Division
University of Washington Medical Center
Seattle, Washington

Henry E. Rice, MD
Assistant Professor
Division of Pediatric Surgery
Duke University Medical Center
Durham, North Carolina

Mark A. Rich, MD
Clinical Associate Professor of Urology in Surgery
University of South Florida School of Medicine
Division Chief
Department of Surgery
Division of Urology
Nemours Children's Clinic - Orlando
Orlando, Florida

Bradley M. Rodgers, MD
Professor of Surgery and Pediatrics
University of Virginia Health System
Chief, Pediatric Surgery
University of Virginia Health System
Charlottesville, Virginia

Austin S. Rose, MD
Assistant Professor
Department of Otolaryngology Head and Neck Surgery
University of North Carolina
Chapel Hill, North Carolina

Joan L. Rosenbaum, MD
Associate Professor of Pediatrics
St. Louis Children's Hospital
St. Louis, Missouri

David Rowe, MD
Department of Plastic Surgery
Medical College of Wisconsin
Milwaukee, Wisconsin

Anthony D. Sandler, MD
Chair, Division of Pediatric Surgery
Associate Professor of Surgery
University of Iowa Health Care
Iowa City, Iowa

Thomas T. Sato, MD
Associate Professor
Surgery (Pediatric Surgery)
Medical College of Wisconsin
Staff Surgeon
Children's Hospital of Wisconsin
Milwaukee, Wisconsin

Robert S. Sawin, MD
Associate Professor
University of Washington
Surgeon in Chief
Children's Hospital and Regional Medical Center
Seattle, Washington

Cindy L. Schwartz, MD
Associate Professor
Department of Oncology and Pediatrics
Johns Hopkins University School of Medicine
Associate Director of Clinic Programs
Department of Pediatric Oncology
The Sidney Kimmel Comprehensive Cancer Center at Johns Hopkins
Baltimore, Maryland

Marshall Z. Schwartz, MD
Professor of Surgery and Pediatrics
Thomas Jefferson University
Philadelphia, Pennsylvania

Robert C. Shamberger, MD
Robert E. Gross Professor of Surgery
Harvard Medical School
Chief of Surgery
Children's Hospital
Boston, Massachusetts

Curtis A. Sheldon, MD
Professor of Surgery
Cincinnati Children's Hospital Medical Center
Cincinnati, Ohio

Robert L. Sheridan, MD
Assistant Chief of Staff
Shriners Hospital for Children
Boston, Massachusetts

Joel Shilyansky, MD
Assistant Professor
Department of Pediatric Surgery
Medical College of Wisconsin
Children's Hospital of Wisconsin
Milwaukee, Wisconsin

Nicholas A. Shorter, MD
Professor and Chief
Division of Pediatric Surgery
SUNY-Downstate Medical Center
Brooklyn, New York

Lesley Simpson, MD
Sidney Kimmel Cancer Comprehensive Cancer Center
Johns Hopkins University School of Medicine
Baltimore, Maryland

Michael A. Skinner, MD
Associate Professor and Chief
Division of Pediatric Surgery
Duke University Medical Center
Durham, North Carolina

Paul D. Sponseller, MD, MBA
Professor
Orthopaedic Surgery
Johns Hopkins University
Head, Orthopedic Surgery
Johns Hopkins Hospital
Baltimore, Maryland

Thomas L. Spray, MD
Chief, Division of Cardiothoracic Surgery
Children's Hospital of Philadelphia
Director of the Pediatric Heart and Heart/Lung Transplantation Program and Professor of Surgery at the University of Pennsylvania School of Medicine
Division of Cardiothoracic Surgery
Children's Hospital of Philadelphia
Philadelphia, Pennsylvania

Paul T. Stockmann, MD
Assistant Professor of Surgery
Wayne State University
Children's Hospital of Michigan
Detroit, Michigan

Mark D. Stringer, MS, FRCS
Consultant Paediatric Hepatobiliary/Transplant Surgeon and Reader in Paediatric Surgery
Children's Liver and GI Unit
St. James's University Hospital
Leeds, United Kingdom

Steven Stylianos, MD
Associate Professor of Surgery and Pediatrics
Columbia University College of Physicians and Surgeons
Director, Regional Pediatric Trauma Program
Children's Hospital of New York
New York, New York

Karl Sylvester, MD
Assistant Professor, Surgery
Stanford University Medical Center
Lucile Packard Children's Hospital
Stanford, California

Edward P. Tagge, MD
Professor and Chief, Division of Pediatric Surgery
Medical University of South Carolina
Charleston, South Carolina

Derya U. Tagge, MD
Assistant Professor
Department of Surgery
Medical University of South Carolina
Charleston, South Carolina

Daniel H. Teitelbaum, MD
Professor of Surgery
Section of Pediatric Surgery
Department of Surgery
University of Michigan Health System
Ann Arbor, Michigan

Patrick B. Thomas, MD
Department of Surgery
Medical University of South Carolina
Charleston, South Carolina

Ronald G. Tompkins, MD, ScD
John F. Burke Professor of Surgery
Department of Surgery
Harvard Medical School
Chief of Staff
Shriners Hospitals for Children
Boston, Massachusetts

Thomas F. Tracy, Jr., MD
Professor
Department of Surgery and Pediatrics
Brown Medical School
Pediatric Surgeon in Chief
Hasbro Children's Hospital
Providence, Rhode Island

William R. Treem, MD
Professor
Division of Pediatric Gastroenterology
and Nutrition
Duke University Medical Center
Durham, North Carolina

Anthony P. Tufaro, DDS, MD
Assistant Professor
Department of Surgery
Division of Plastic and Reconstructive Surgery
Johns Hopkins University
Attending Surgeon
Department of Surgery
Division of Plastic and Reconstructive
Surgery
Johns Hopkins Hospital
Baltimore, Maryland

David W. Tuggle, MD
Professor of Surgery
Vice-Chairman of the Department of Surgery
Chief, Section of Pediatric Surgery
Paula Milburn Miller/Children's Medical Research
Institute Chair in Pediatric Surgery
Oklahoma City, Oklahoma

David E. Tunkel, MD
Director of Pediatric Otolaryngology
Associate Professor of Otolaryngology-Head and Neck
Surgery and Pediatrics
Department of Otolaryngolology-Head and
Neck Surgery
Johns Hopkins University School of Medicine
Baltimore, Maryland

James S. Tweddell, MD
Professor and Chief
Division of Cardiothoracic Surgery
Department of Surgery
Medical College of Wisconsin
Chief, Cardiothoracic Surgery
Children's Hospital of Wisconsin
Milwaukee, Wisconsin

Martin H. Ulshen, MD
Professor of Pediatric Gastroenterology
and Nutrition
Duke University Medical Center
Durham, North Carolina

Jeffrey S. Upperman, MD
Assistant Professor of Surgery
Department of Pediatric Surgery
Children's Hospital of Pittsburgh
Pittsburgh, Pennsylvania

Craig A. Vander Kolk, MD
Associate Professor of Plastic Surgery
and Assistant Professor of Pediatrics
Johns Hopkins University School of Medicine
Johns Hopkins Outpatient Center
Baltimore, Maryland

Virginia L. Vega, MD
Research Fellow
Department of Surgery-General
Division of Pediatric Surgery
Johns Hopkins University School of Medicine
Baltimore, Maryland

John H.T. Waldhausen, MD
Associate Professor
Department of Surgery
University of Washington
Director of Surgical Education
Department of Surgery
Children's Hospital and Regional
Medical Center
Seattle, Washington

Sonya R. Walker, MD
Department of Surgery
University of Pittsburgh
School of Medicine
Division of Pediatric Surgery
Children's Hospital of Pittsburgh
Pittsburgh, Pennsylvania

Julian Wan, MD
Clinical Associate Professor
Department of Urology
University of Michigan
Ann Arbor, Michigan

Brad W. Warner, MD
Professor of Surgery
University of Cincinnati
College of Medicine
Attending Surgeon
Department of Pediatric Surgery
Cincinnati Children's Hospital Medical Center
Cincinnati, Ohio

Bryan C. Weidner, MD
Assistant Professor
Department of Surgery
Division of Pediatric Surgery
University of Alabama at Birmingham
Attending Surgeon
Department of Pediatric Surgery
Children's Hospital
Birmingham, Alabama

Karen Wickline, MD
Associate Professor of Pediatrics
Director, Newborn Medicine
Follow-Up Program
Division of Newborn Medicine
Department of Pediatrics
Washington University School of Medicine
St. Louis Children's Hospital
St. Louis, Missouri

John S. Wiener, MD
Associate Professor
Department of Surgery
Assistant Professor
Department of Pediatrics
Duke University
Head
Section of Pediatric Urology
Duke University Medical Center
Durham, North Carolina

Delbert R. Wigfall, MD
Associate Clinical Professor of Pediatrics
Director of Pediatric Dialysis
Department of Pediatrics
Division of Nephrology
Duke Children's Hospital and Health Center
Durham, North Carolina

Holly L. Williams, MD
Chief of Pediatric Surgery
Kaiser, Oakland California
Associate Clinical Professor of Surgery
University of California, San Francisco
San Francisco, California

Gordon Worley, MD
Associate Clinical Professor
Developmental Medicine and Pediatric Rehabilitation
Duke University Medical Center
Durham, North Carolina

Quira Zeidan, MD
Division of Pediatric Surgery
Johns Hopkins University School of Medicine
Baltimore, Maryland

PREFACE

In the preface to the text that preceded this edition, we predicted that the pace of change in the clinical practice of pediatric surgery, and in our understanding of the scientific principles that are the basis for that practice, would soon render the text obsolete. That expectation was more predictable than prescient, and it has clearly come to pass. During the intervening years, important basic science advances in pharmacology, immunology, genetics, embryology, developmental biology, and other relevant areas were reported almost daily. Virtually every knowledgeable physician and scientist anticipates that this process will continue, perhaps accelerating further. The trend is similar in clinical practice. Although the rate of real change is arguably slower, it is undoubtedly substantial. Minimally invasive surgical techniques or their derivatives are now employed for many, perhaps most, major intracavitary procedures in infants and children. Now routine are minimally invasive complex procedures such as laparoscopic pullthrough for imperforate anus and Hirschsprung's disease, among others, while repair of tracheoesophageal fistula, portoenterostomy for biliary atresia, and other procedures requiring a high level of surgical precision are more and more feasible. Robotic technology is now in place in a number of major children's centers around the world, and this too will be an engine for change.

Since the original version of this text was published in 1997, serious effort has been invested in the development of rigorous clinical research tools to improve medical and surgical practice and to quantify outcomes. Evidence-based decision making and demonstrable quality are now demanded from the public, payors, and other health care providers in a way not imagined even a few years ago. Emerging problems require new surgical approaches. For example, the field of bariatric surgery as it relates to children and adolescents has developed of necessity in the last several years, driven by a stunning worldwide obesity epidemic and a host of attendant comorbidities now affecting the young. Each of these individual areas, and many others, receive explicit and detailed new attention in this text, either in the form of entirely new or substantially revised chapters.

In planning this textbook, the editors made the decision to emphasize the various clinical practice issues that define contemporary pediatric surgery. This decision reflects the reality that pediatric surgery is fundamentally a clinical science. Our intent is to transmit the information necessary for surgeons, pediatricians and other physicians, allied health professionals, and students to learn of and engage knowledgeably in its practice. We believe that we have substantially strengthened the text with regard to its utility as a daily reference tool for those involved in the care of surgical problems in infants and children. However, we have labored diligently to maintain the unique and rigorous examination of relevant scientific principles that distinguished the original effort. We have also continued a successful effort to enlist contributors who are active surgical scientists and innovators in their areas of interest. With this commitment in mind, we are very pleased to welcome Michael Skinner, MD from Duke University to our editorial group. As before, this effort has yielded a group of contributors who are somewhat earlier in their careers than the norm for this type of endeavor, but who we believe represent present and future leaders in pediatric surgery. We believe the result is a unique reference text that accurately reflects contemporary pediatric surgical practice and affords a critical and reasoned view of relevant basic and clinical science.

Keith T. Oldham, MD
Professor and Chief
Division of Pediatric Surgery
Medical College of Wisconsin
Marie Z. Uihlein Chair and
Surgeon in Chief
Children's Hospital of Wisconsin

ACKNOWLEDGMENTS

We have been fortunate as editors to benefit from the abundant talents and considerable effort of many individuals in the production of this text. Most importantly, we wish to thank our contributors, leaders all in the field of pediatric surgery, for their generosity in time and effort.

We thank as well the many individuals at Lippincott Williams & Wilkins who have seen this text through conception, gestation and now delivery. Without the efforts of Michelle LaPlante, Senior Managing Editor, we would not have reached our objective. As in the past, we have been fortunate to enjoy the considerable artistic talents of Holly Fischer and her dedication to our work. Lastly, we wish to acknowledge the essential administrative support of Teresa Hauser, Mary Artley, Linda Brockman, and Laura Cornelius. Their collective contributions of gracious tenacity and fine editorial assistance bring us now to successful completion in this effort.

CONTENTS

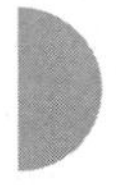

Chapter 58

Congenital Diaphragmatic Hernia

Kevin P. Lally

INTRODUCTION

Congenital diaphragmatic hernia (CDH) is a rare congenital anomaly characterized by a defect in diaphragm development with subsequent herniation of abdominal contents into the thorax. The two most prevalent types are herniation anteriorly in the diaphragm (Morgagni hernia) and posterolateral (Bochdalek-type) hernias. The incidence of posterolateral CDH has been reported from between 1 in 2,000 and 1 in 5,000 live births (1). The true incidence is higher because some fetuses with severe multiple anomalies, including CDH, do not survive to birth because the pregnancy is spontaneously aborted. Many of the fetuses who survive to delivery have significant lung hypoplasia and other anomalies. The lung hypoplasia and associated anomalies lead to a high mortality and long-term morbidity. In addition to the high inherent mortality (CDH accounts for more than 1% of total infant mortality in the United States), CDH ranks among the more costly of correctable conditions, with an estimated cost per new case of $250,000, and an overall estimated yearly cost of $264,000,000 in the United States (1995 dollars) (2).

The relative rarity of CDH prevents the conduct of well-designed clinical studies at single centers. As a result, the management of CDH has evolved through several eras, each based largely on retrospective reviews from centers with varying numbers of patients. In the past few years, a number of centers have collaborated to collect multiinstitutional data on CDH. More recently, these multiinstitutional data from more than 1,000 neonates have been used to categorize patients into low- and high-risk groups (3). This may allow for better comparisons between centers and potentially for stratification of patients for future studies.

Kevin P. Lally: Division of Pediatric Surgery, University of Texas Health Sciences Center, Houston, Texas 77030.

History

Riverius recorded the first congenital diaphragmatic hernia in 1679 (4). A posterolateral defect was shown at autopsy of an infant who died in 1701 by Holt. Morgagni described several types of diaphragmatic hernia in 1761, including the anterior hernia defect now associated eponymously with him. There were scattered reports of CDH in the nineteenth century, including one by Victor Bochdalek, who described two infants with posterolateral defects found at autopsy. This posterolateral diaphragmatic defect is now known as a Bochdalek hernia. Although there were some attempts at repair of this defect throughout the late nineteenth and early twentieth century, the first successful repair of a posterolateral CDH in a child was reported by Heidenhain in 1905. Hedblom first suggested that early intervention and reduction of the hernia might improve survival and proposed the paradigm that visceral herniation and lung compression led to pulmonary hypoplasia (5). In 1940, Ladd and Gross reported 9 of 16 survivors, and in 1946, Gross reported the first survivor repaired at less than 24 hours of age (6). Operative mortality for neonates was high during this time, and many surgeons recommended delaying repair until the child was older; however, regardless of management, most of these infants succumbed from respiratory failure. Gross recommended that repair should not be delayed and that it should occur immediately. This policy led to attempts at earlier repair with the intent of relieving a tension effect of the intestines in the thorax. By the 1980s, CDH was considered one of the most urgent of surgical emergencies. Survival at that time was quoted at around 50%, despite advances in neonatal critical care. These data were misleading, however, because many patients were now surviving transfer to tertiary facilities, whereas they would have died in the past. During the 1980s and 1990s, there were many advances in neonatal respiratory care, including the availability of extracorporeal membrane oxygenation (ECMO), high-frequency oscillation, surfactant, and inhaled nitric oxide (NO). Although all these therapies have been used in infants with CDH, as discussed here, evidence of effectiveness has been lacking for many.

Diaphragm and Lung Development

The posterolateral defect in the diaphragm was originally believed to represent a failure of the pleuroperitoneal canal to close, but more recent information supports a different concept. Greer and others showed that the problem may arise within the pleuroperitoneal fold which gives rise to the diaphragm (7). Using an animal model, Babiuk et al. found no evidence that the musculature for the diaphragm originates from the septum transversum or the lateral body wall. Rather, cellular muscle precursors migrate from cervical somites and populate the diaphragm (8). The mesenchymal substrate that forms the diaphragm likely originates from the somatopleure. Knockout mice for c-met receptors (which bind HGF/SF, a chemoattractant for guiding muscle precursor cells) show formation of an amuscular diaphragm.

Much of critical organogenesis in the fetus occurs during the same time period as diaphragm development. Cardiac and lung formation occur during the third and fourth weeks of gestation. Lung development is discussed elsewhere (see Chapter 11), but the major components of the conducting airways have developed by the sixteenth week of gestation. Development of respiratory bronchioles and alveoli continues until well after birth. Lung development in infants with CDH is impaired early enough in gestation that there is a smaller number of bronchial divisions and alveoli. Some researchers have suggested that the primary problem in patients with CDH is pulmonary hypoplasia with secondary diaphragm maldevelopment (9). The etiology of the lung hypoplasia is unclear at this time; however, a number of the genes responsible for lung development have altered expression in a murine model of CDH (10). Alveolar growth and pulmonary vasculature are linked. The importance of this observation is that the pulmonary vasculature in infants with CDH is also abnormal. There is clear evidence of a smaller vascular tree as well as abnormal muscularization of the arterioles in the gas-exchanging portions (respiratory bronchioles and distal airways) of the lung. This likely contributes to the significant pulmonary hypertension seen clinically in these patients.

During the eighth to tenth week of gestation, the developing extracoelonic intestine normally returns to the abdomen. With return of the bowel, a defect in the diaphragm allows the intestine to enter the thorax. The pulmonary hypoplasia demonstrable in animal models of CDH can be modulated, depending on the timing and amount of intestine herniated into the thorax. This observation may be relevant in infants with CDH because patients with a large anatomic defect have a significantly higher morbidity and mortality rate compared with infants with a small defect (11).

As mentioned previously, critical organogenesis occurs during the same general time frame as CDH development. This includes cardiac development and is consistent with the clinical observation that 20% to 25% of infants with CDH have associated congenital heart disease. It is unclear whether there is a specific field defect in the mesoderm in some of these patients or whether the defects occur as a result of a teratogen (10). The defects may range from a smaller than average left ventricle to a variety of major anomalies, including hypoplastic left heart. Presence of significant cardiac anomalies, is associated with a much worse survival in patients with CDH (12).

Posterolateral Hernia

Diagnosis

Classically, infants with CDH present in respiratory distress either at birth or within the first few hours of life. Currently, between 40% and 60% of infants with CDH are diagnosed prenatally (13).

The diagnosis of congenital diaphragmatic hernia is suspected when the prenatal ultrasound demonstrates the heart in an abnormal location and fluid-filled loops of bowel are visualized in the thorax (Fig. 58-1). The diagnosis can be confused with a cystic adenomatoid malformation of the lung, and a fetal magnetic resonance imaging may be helpful to distinguish the two (14) (Fig. 58-2).

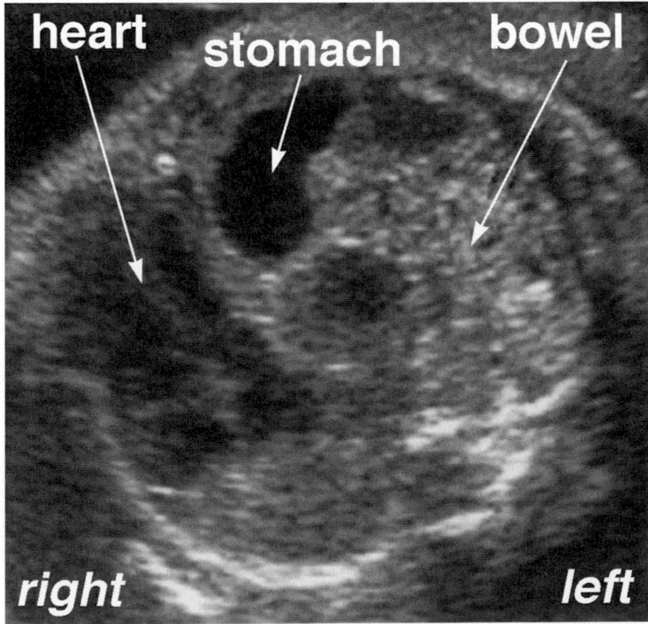

FIGURE 58-1. Prenatal ultrasound of a fetus with diaphragmatic hernia. At the level of the four-chamber heart view, the stomach and bowel can be clearly visualized.

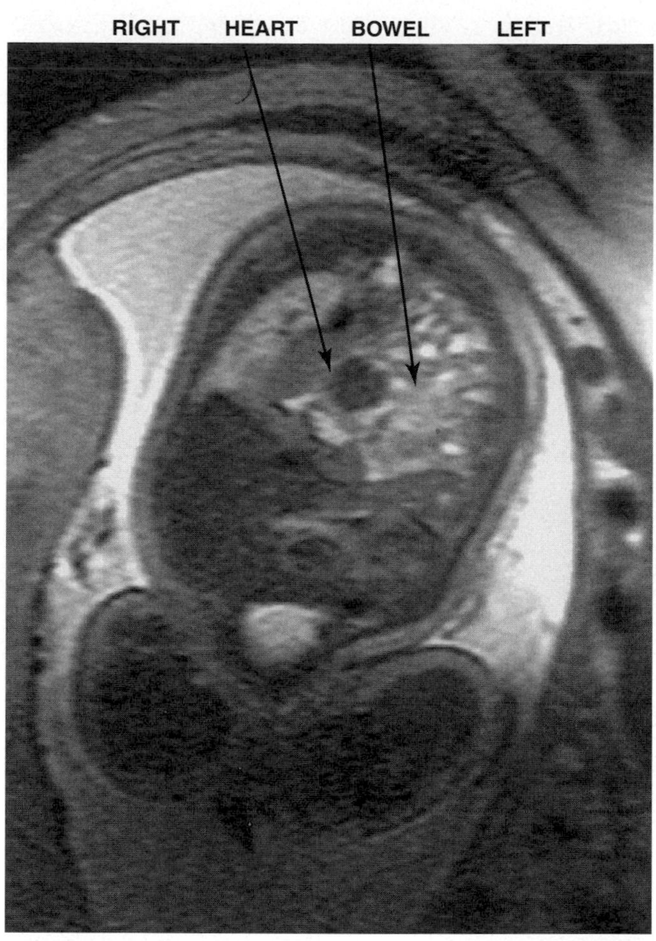

FIGURE 58-2. Prenatal MRI of a fetus with a left-sided diaphragmatic hernia. The heart can be seen pushed to the right, and the bowel is in the left thorax.

In infants who present at or after delivery, respiratory distress may be due to underlying pulmonary hypoplasia or from compression, over hours or occasionally days, of the lung from gas-filled loops of bowel. The infant will often have a scaphoid abdomen (Fig. 58-3). A chest radiograph will usually show gas-filled loops of bowel in the chest with a shift of the heart away from the side of the defect side (Fig. 58-4). Eighty percent of infants with CDH have a left-sided defect, and 19% right, but whether left or right, the heart is shifted to the contralateral side. One percent of patients have bilateral herniae. The prognosis for these patients is much worse than for those with unilateral hernia (15). There may be bowel sounds in the chest, and the cardiac exam will show the shift of the heart to the side opposite the hernia. As for prenatal diagnosis, there can occasionally be confusion with a cystic adenomatoid malformation of the lung in newborns. Location of the nasogastric tube in the thorax on radiograph or an upper gastrointestinal contrast study will aid in confirming the diagnosis.

The majority of infants with CDH will develop symptoms within the first 24 hours of life, although symptoms can be manifest at older ages and sometimes even at several months of age or later. Infants presenting with symptoms later may have feeding difficulty, respiratory problems, or bowel obstruction from an incarcerated hernia. In older patients, an upper gastrointestinal contrast study is often of value in establishing the diagnosis (16).

MANAGEMENT

Prenatal Management

Because a large number of infants with CDH are now diagnosed in utero, the option to treat the patient before delivery is available. CDH has a significant mortality rate and long-term morbidity, and this mortality rate has spurred the hope that in utero intervention may improve outcome. One of the difficulties in evaluating the risks and benefits of prenatal intervention is the inability to determine

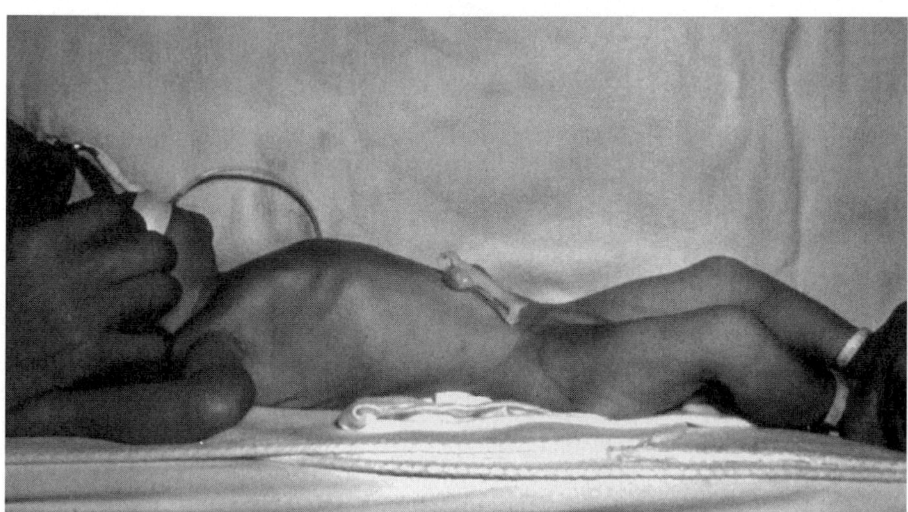

FIGURE 58-3. A newborn with a congenital diaphragmatic hernia. Note the scaphoid abdomen.

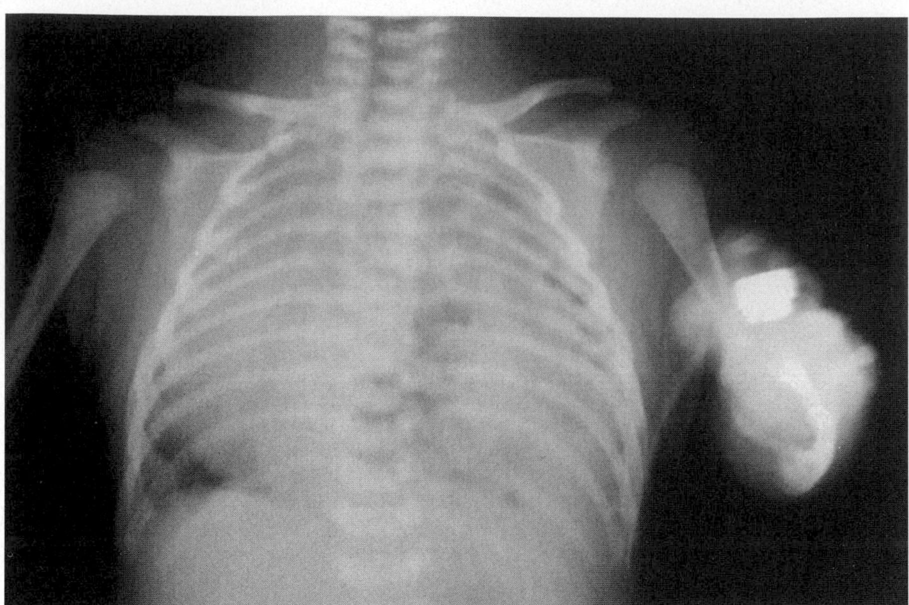

FIGURE 58-4. A chest radiograph of a newborn with a left-sided CDH. The heart can be seen shifted to the right and there are multiple air filled bowel loops in the left chest.

which fetus is at the highest risk of death. Use of the ratio of lung to head or lung to thorax size, and even blood flow velocity as determined by ultrasound have been suggested (17,18). None of these has been validated in a large series at present, and many are observer dependent. At present, the problem of correctly stratifying a heterogenous group of patients and offering prenatal therapy to the selected high-risk fetus has not been resolved. Suggested methods to treat the fetus have included both medical and surgical approaches.

Medical Therapy

Experimental models of CDH have suggested that the lungs of affected animals are immature in a number of ways. One observation that has led clinicians to attempt therapeutic intervention is that both rodent and sheep in models of CDH appear to be surfactant deficient (19,20). Suen and colleagues showed decreased levels of disaturated phosphatidylcholine, total lung DNA, and total lung protein, all indicative of lung immaturity. In animals with CDH, antenatal glucocorticoid administration has been shown to increase heart size, increase surfactant protein synthesis and endothelin receptor levels, increase total lung protein synthesis, and upregulate peptide growth factor gene expression (21–23).

The use of glucocorticoids in humans followed these reports in the hope that the fetus would increase intrinsic surfactant production. Despite the clear benefits of antenatal corticosteroids in animal models, there are many known potential adverse effects in humans (24). Because corticosteroids are widely used in obstetric practice for fetuses at risk of preterm delivery, their use in mothers carrying a fetus with CDH has been embraced in a number of institutions. However, there are at present no clinical data that show clear benefit from the use of antenatal corticosteroids in humans with regard to CDH. A case series of three surviving patients using a very prolonged course of antenatal steroids has been published (25). These data are anecdotal, and the use of prenatal corticosteroids to improve outcome in fetuses with CDH should be considered unproven at present. Other agents, such as thyrotropin-releasing hormone, have been shown to influence lung development in animal models of CDH (26). None have been studied clinically, and there are no accepted indications for their use in patients.

Fetal Surgical Therapy

Reports showing a poor outcome for fetuses diagnosed with CDH, as well as the high infant mortality seen in the 1980s, prompted a search for an approach to correct the malformation in utero. The concept of correction during a period of in utero support at a point where subsequent lung development could occur, was and is theoretically attractive. The first reported successful repair of a fetal CDH was by Harrison and colleagues in 1990 (27). Although in utero repair is possible for fetuses without a herniated liver, there has been no significant difference in mortality between an in utero open repair group and a conventionally treated group. When the liver was herniated into the chest, in utero operative reduction resulted in acute obstruction of umbilical venous flow and fetal death. Interest in the open antenatal surgical approach to CDH waned after a series of poor outcomes, and this approach was abandoned (28). A major concern that has been noted previously, is difficulty in correctly stratifying high- versus low-risk fetuses (29). This is recently reviewed (30).

With the observation that spontaneously occurring laryngeal atresia was associated with lung hypertrophy, Wilson and colleagues devised a series of studies that showed that tracheal ligation in experimental fetal animals resulted in larger and more mature lungs at birth (31). In an attempt to use this information in fetal intervention relevant to CDH, a technique known as PLUG (plug the lung until it grows) was developed (32). A series of reports followed, with varying modifications on how to safely and transiently occlude the trachea without significant long-term damage (33). Although human CDH survivors have been reported using this approach, concerns that tracheal occlusion may delay pulmonary maturation, a lack of controlled trials, and the risks of preterm labor continue to limit fetal intervention. A federally funded randomized trial of tracheal occlusion was halted early as outcomes in the fetal treatment group were not superior to conventional therapy following delivery. Despite a large literature on the topic, fetal intervention (both medical and surgical) has not been proven to benefit fetuses with CDH and, currently, there are no indications for fetal intervention in patients with CDH.

Postnatal Management

Prenatal diagnosis of CDH enables the medical team to be present at delivery for those infants and, most important, allows prenatal parental counseling. Known CDH patients should clearly be delivered at an institution that has the necessary equipment and personnel to offer contemporary management of most of the problem. Infants with respiratory distress should be treated initially with endotracheal intubation. Keeping inspiratory pressures low is a priority because even a short duration of high-pressure ventilation can cause lung injury (34). Management options for these patients encompass a number of different modalities, and there is no consensus on a single best approach. Many questions exist regarding the benefit and appropriateness of new techniques and therapies. Some of the issues in the management of CDH include best ventilator strategies, high-frequency oscillatory ventilation (HFOV), inhaled NO, exogenous surfactant, and ECMO.

Ventilator Strategy

Mechanical ventilation is the initial therapy for infants with respiratory failure from CDH. With the advent of neonatal mechanical ventilation in the 1960s, many CDH infants with previously fatal respiratory failure were surviving long enough to undergo surgical repair. As a result, the mortality of CDH climbed during that time due to an increase in both the number of patients undergoing operation and the severity of illness in those patients. At the onset, the goal of mechanical ventilation was adequate oxygen delivery. As understanding of perinatal physiology grew, the critical importance of pulmonary hypertension and right-to-left ductal shunting was appreciated. Boix-Ochoa first reported that differences in pre- and postductal pH and $Paco_2$ could be used to differentiate between survivors and nonsurvivors (35). Rudolf and Yuan then showed that the neonatal pulmonary vascular system was sensitive to changes in $Paco_2$ and pH. Drummond and others demonstrated that by increasing pH and decreasing $Paco_2$, ductal shunting could be reversed (36). Despite limited number of patients in this report, this resulted in the era where hyperventilation was widely used as the primary ventilator strategy for CDH patients. However, the high ventilator rates and inspiratory pressures caused significant barotrauma. This strategy persisted until Wung and others demonstrated that much of the mortality in CDH infants was, in fact, due to ventilator-induced lung injury (37). During this period, it was shown that lung injury and mortality were reduced in neonates who met ECMO criteria and thus had a period of "lung rest" while supported on ELMO. From the 1990s and onward, ventilation strategy in most centers has focused on minimizing barotrauma by allowing spontaneous ventilation with minimal set respiratory rates, the use of pressure-limited ventilation, tolerance of high $Paco_2$, minimal sedation, and avoidance of paralysis. The goal of ventilator support is to afford adequate hemoglobin saturation with oxygen and to maintain an acceptable arterial pH. Using this concept of permissive hypercapnia, several authors have reported survival rates approaching 90% (38–40).

High-Frequency Oscillation

HFOV has been used in patients with CDH since it was first introduced in the 1980s. The concept is to avoid high inspiratory pressures while providing effective ventilation. How HFOV is used, however, is quite important. Paranka and colleagues showed that HFOV was of little benefit when used in a high-pressure lung recruitment strategy in patients with CDH (41). Others, however, have shown that when used as the initial mode of therapy, HFOV can be an effective mode of ventilatory support in CDH (42–43). In those centers that use HFOV as initial therapy, hyperventilation and high mean airway pressures are avoided. More recently, HFOV has also been used as a second-line or "failure" therapy in infants not effectively managed with conventional ventilation (44). The use of HFOV in this setting is typically at mean airway pressures of 14 to 16 cm H_2O and amplitudes of less than 45 mm Hg. Importantly, when used in these patients, the strategy is not one of lung recruitment because the hypoplastic lungs do not have a population of recruitable alveoli, rather the goal is simply adequate gas exchange.

The optimal mode of ventilation for patients with CDH is not clear. However, regardless of the choice, management strategies designed to limit lung distention and inspiratory pressures appear to be the most effective.

Nitric Oxide and Pulmonary Hypertension

Persistent pulmonary hypertension (PPHN) remains a significant problem in infants with CDH. Multiple factors, including decreased cross-sectional area of the pulmonary arteries due to lung hypoplasia, increased medial thickness of the pulmonary arteries, adventitial thickening, blunted oxygen-induced vasodilation, and increased endothelin-A receptor expression, are believed to contribute to the pulmonary hypertension seen with CDH (45–46).

NO, originally identified as endothelial-derived relaxing factor, is a potent vasodilator including within the pulmonary circulation. Therefore, it has been an agent of considerable interest in CDH patients. NO improves oxygen saturation in neonates with respiratory failure secondary to PPHN, decreases the need for ECMO, and is widely used in term neonates with respiratory failure (47,48). When inhaled NO first became available for clinical use, there was hope that this would prove useful in patients with CDH. There were encouraging anecdotal reports and even some more recent reports suggesting benefit (49). Unfortunately, results from several randomized trials in the subgroup of patients with CDH have been poor to date. When used as the initial therapy for infants with CDH and severe respiratory failure, NO does not improve overall survival or reduce the need for ECMO (48).

As survival for infants with CDH has improved steadily, it has been increasingly recognized that pulmonary hypertension is an important component of the ongoing pathophysiology in these infants. In some infants, the pulmonary hypertension adversely affects right heart function and some level of afterload reduction can assist in patient management. It is possible that NO or other selective pulmonary vasodilators may be useful in patients with CDH, either for management of heart failure early on or for management of PPHN later in their hospital course. Involvement and close collaboration with cardiologists and the use of real-time echocardiography to assist in management of the PPHN has been suggested to be beneficial by some authors (44). Drugs that serve as NO donors may also prove to be helpful in management of cardiac dysfunction and the long-term pulmonary hypertension because this may last for months or longer in some infants with CDH (50).

Surfactant

Animal models of CDH have shown that the lungs of affected animals are surfactant deficient (20,51). Surfactant phospholipids and apoprotein SP-A are decreased in rats with nitrofen-induced CDH; however, the synthetic capacity to produce surfactant is equal to controls in these experiments. Immunohistochemistry reveals surfactant to reside in intracellular granules in CDH lungs from these rats versus a uniform distribution on the alveolar surface in control normal lungs. Surfactant deficiency can be ameliorated by a number of methods in animals, including the use of vitamin A and prenatal corticosteroids (52,53).

There are some data to suggest that the lungs of human infants with CDH may be relatively surfactant deficient (54,55). Given this observation, other authors reported the use of exogenous surfactant in infants with CDH in small case reports (56,57). However, other groups more recently showed that the surfactant pool in infants with CDH is not different when compared with controls (58,59). Despite the paucity of supportive data, the use of surfactant in infants with CDH has been incorporated into the treatment protocols for patients with CDH at a number of centers (19,60). More recently, data from the CDH registry have shown no benefit with the use of exogenous surfactant, and indeed suggest diminished rates of survival in some patients receiving surfactant (61). Use of exogenous surfactant in infants with CDH has not been studied in a controlled clinical trial. Therefore, at present, use of exogenous surfactant should be avoided in term infants with CDH unless in the context of a clinical trial.

Surfactant use has also been proposed for infants with CDH while on ECMO. Lotze et al. conducted a randomized trial examining this question and could not demonstrate benefit; however, the sample size was small (54). Colby reported CDH registry data on surfactant use in patients on ECMO and was also unable to show benefit (62). Given these findings, there is no current indication for routine surfactant use in infants with CDH on ECMO.

Extracorporeal Membrane Oxygenation

The first report of the use of ECMO for an infant with CDH was by German and colleagues in 1977. Since then, more than 5,000 infants with CDH have been treated with ECMO support. Most early patients treated with ECMO likely had significant ventilator-induced lung injury. Selection criteria for ECMO were (and are) widely divergent (63). Initially, use of ECMO was restricted to patients meeting specific criteria similar to those for infants with other causes of respiratory failure. However, the etiology of the respiratory failure in this patient population is clearly quite different; hence, different selection criteria may be appropriate in patients with CDH. Use of ECMO began to evolve as surgeons recognized that CDH infants represented a physiologic rather than anatomic emergency and began to defer operative repair from the time of birth, sometimes for several weeks. With this approach, infants who require escalating therapy are stabilized with ECMO first. The large majority of patients (more than 90%) with CDH who are treated with ECMO are now placed on ECMO prior to repair (64). The timing of repair once a patient is placed on ECMO varies, and there are no published comparative data supporting either early or late repair on ECMO, or repair after ECMO. The criteria for use of ECMO are those of a patient who is clinically deteriorating and requires a level of mechanical ventilation that is associated with a high risk of lung injury (peak inspiratory pressure > 25 mm Hg or failing HFOV). These do vary from center to center and ECMO is often a clinically based decision.

All infants with CDH treated with ECMO were initially placed on venoarterial ECMO. Broader use of venovenous ECMO led to its application in CDH patients. There are a number of series that have demonstrated most patients with CDH treated with ECMO can be effectively treated with venovenous ECMO (65). The use of ECMO varies widely among those centers that offer it, but the overall survival for CDH infants who require ECMO is approximately 55% and has not changed appreciably since ECMO was first introduced (66). Survival does appear better in infants treated with ECMO who are delivered later in gestation when compared with those delivered earlier in gestation (67). Although ECMO has become a standard therapy for infants with CDH, its use in infants with CDH has not been studied in a specific large randomized trial. Indeed, several centers have more recently reported survival rates approaching 90% without the use of ECMO and with no patient selection (44).

Lung Distention

In 1993, Wilson and colleagues showed that occlusion of the trachea in lambs with experimentally induced CDH leads to significant lung growth (31). CDH animals treated with tracheal occlusion had normal-appearing lungs with normal function and a significant improvement in survival compared with control CDH animals (68). The potential implications for infants with CDH were attractive, and these studies led to a proliferation of work on tracheal occlusion and CDH in animal models and in humans.

Investigators demonstrated that tracheal occlusion can lead to surfactant deficiency in animals so treated. This surfactant deficiency is not changed by reversing the occlusion, but can be altered by administering antenatal corticosteroids (69). Other studies showed that relatively short duration tracheal occlusion in the fetal lamb can lead to significant lung growth and that tracheal occlusion later in gestation can preserve type II pneumocytes (70). Some investigators have used this model to examine accelerated lung growth and have shown that tracheal occlusion results in lung growth in the rat model of nitrofen-induced CDH and in sheep (71).

Several groups have explored the concept that tracheal occlusion could be used in human fetuses; however, as mentioned previously, this approach has not proven clinically useful to date. Nobuhara and colleagues evaluated the mechanisms of the lung growth after tracheal occlusion and showed that this was a pressure related phenomenon that could be used in animals model after birth (72). This observation prompted interest in attempting lung distension in patients with CDH postnatally. Several investigators have reported preliminary results demonstrating improvement of lung function and evidence of lung growth in high-risk infants on ECMO (73,74). Although it is an exciting concept that postnatal lung growth might be inducible lung distension has not been studied in a randomized trial or using specific, established selection criteria. Whether this will have any future clinical application requires further study.

Surgical Management

Timing of Operation

In 1946, Gross reported the first correction of a CDH in a newborn less than 24 hours of age. The concept behind the recommendation of urgent operation was that the distended intestine within the thorax could create a tension phenomenon similar to a tension pneumothorax. By emergently relieving this problem, it was believed that the ipsilateral lung could then expand and would function better in terms of gas exchange. Importantly, however, most of the patients in the earlier series had survived for hours or days before developing symptoms. With the advent of advanced ability to care for the critically ill newborn in the 1960s and 1970s, increasingly sicker patients survived transfer to a referral center. Despite a changing patient population, emergent operation was still used in most institutions throughout the 1980s. In the late 1980s, some reports were published that suggested that a period of delay prior to operation was beneficial. These studies showed that survival was not adversely affected by waiting. Two small, randomized trials of delayed operation were completed. Both showed no difference in outcome between early and late repair groups (75). Although delayed operation has now become widely accepted, it remains unclear how to select the optimal time for repair of the defect (76). Some repair the diaphragmatic defect when the patient is weaning from mechanical ventilation; others wait until there is echocardiographic evidence that the pulmonary hypertension has resolved. Our approach is to repair the defect when the patient requires 50% F_{IO_2} or less and has been weaning from mechanical ventilation. Optimally, the pulmonary hypertension will have resolved, but this can take months in some patients.

Operative Approach

Once a decision has been made to proceed with correction of the defect, the most common approach is through a subcostal incision on the side of the defect. Frequently, the spleen, small intestine, and large intestine are herniated through the defect (Fig. 58-5). Once the hernia is reduced, the edges of the diaphragm should be clearly identified. This often involves unrolling and dissecting the posterior-medial diaphragm edge just cephalad to the

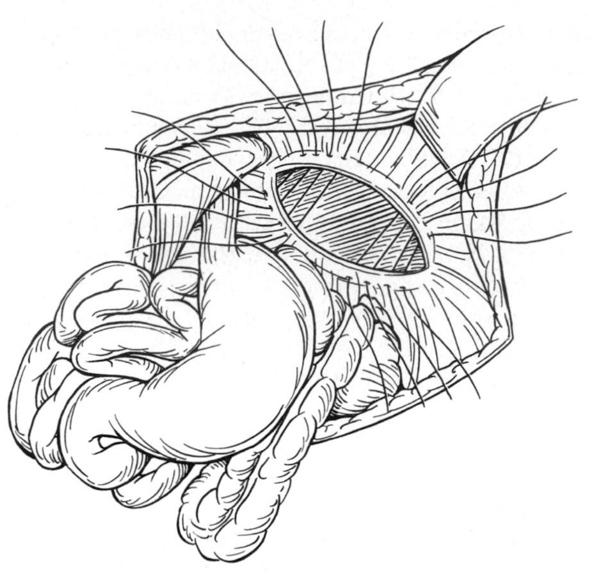

FIGURE 58-5. Primary repair of a left sided hernia. The posterior diaphragm rim has been unrolled and sutures placed around the defect.

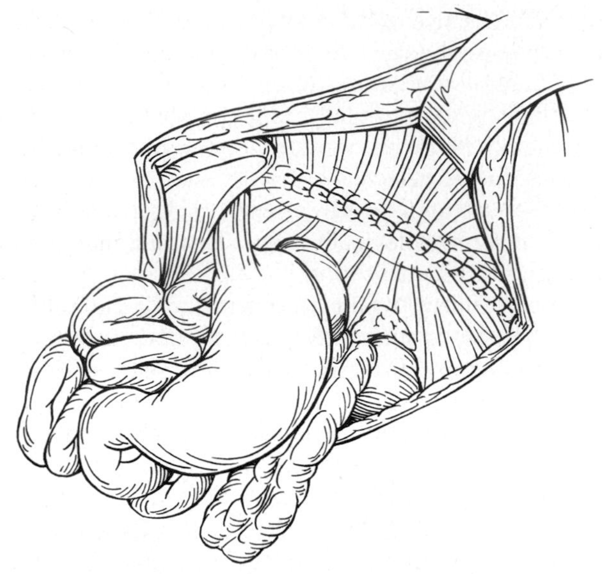

FIGURE 58-7. Appearance of the left diaphragm after a primary repair.

ipsilateral adrenal gland. Interrupted nonabsorbable sutures are usually used in a primary repair. Simple interrupted, mattress sutures, and pledgetted sutures have all been used with success (Figs. 58-6 and 58-7). Although a primary repair of the defect is optimal, excessive tension should be avoided if at all possible. A transthoracic approach to repair is used by some surgeons; however, on the left side, most use a transabdominal approach. Repair of the defect through a chest incision can be very useful in patients with a large, right-sided defect. This can make reduction of the liver easier than trying to reduce it from within the abdomen.

Patch repair of the defect should be used liberally. Just more than one-half of the patients with CDH who undergo operation have a patch used in the repair in contemporary practice (76). The optimal patch material for this defect is unknown. Although polytetrafluoroethylene is the most widely used, it does not grow with the patient and thus there may be a high recurrence rate. Newer materials, such as acellular human dermis and patch material derived from porcine intestine, have been used and may prove effective, but there are no published data on long-term follow-up. A variety of experimental approaches have been described, including the use of bioengineered

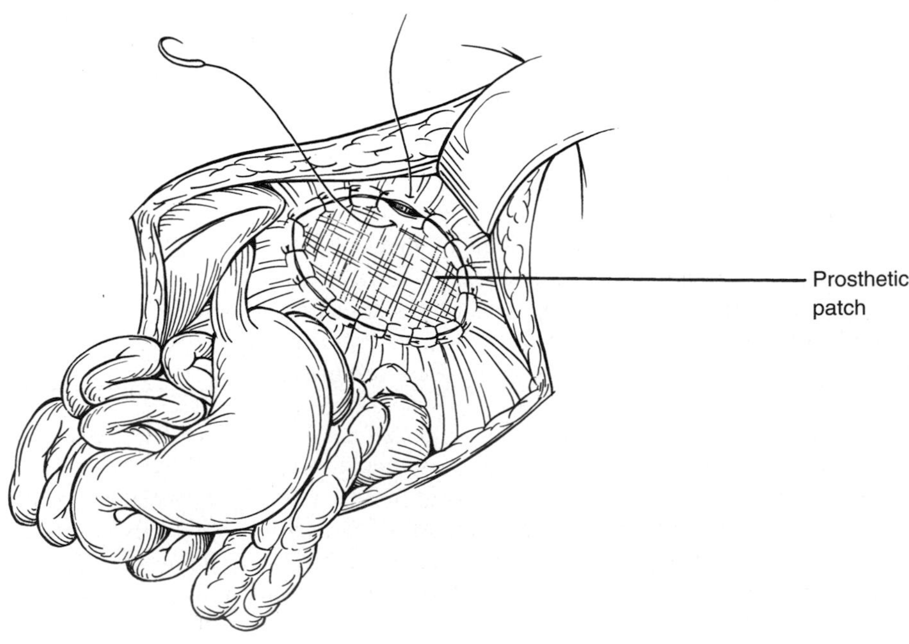

FIGURE 58-6. Patch repair of a large defect (not agenesis). The patch has been sewn to the edges of the defect.

materials. The size of the defect can make repair difficult in some patients. Agenesis of the diaphragm requires total reconstruction with a prosthesis. This may prove technically challenging, especially at the medial aspect of the diaphragm with repair around the esophageal and aortic hiatus, because these may not exist and will require creation. Patients with diaphragm agenesis are also usually more at risk physiologically than others and may require repair on ECMO.

The best time to repair the defect once a patient is on ECMO support is unknown. Some authors have recommended repair within 24 hours to avoid an operation in an edematous patient and to make clinical decision making easier after the repair is accomplished. Others have suggested delaying operation until the patient can be weaned from ECMO support. There is a risk of significant bleeding with repair on ECMO, due to the fact that the patient is systemically heparinized. Early reports of repair on ECMO demonstrated very high mortality in patients who developed significant hemorrhagic complications (77). The use of epsilon aminocaproic acid, started before operation and maintained for a period of time thereafter, has resulted in a marked decrease in the incidence of this complication (78).

Several authors have shown a high risk of recurrent hernia when large anatomic defects are repaired (79). Because much chest wall growth occurs postnatally, fixing a rigid prosthetic patch to the ribs must eventually result in separating the patch either from the chest wall or medially from the mediastinal contents. Although some recurrences occur early, others may not present for several years. It is unrealistic to expect a permanent and definitive repair in the neonatal period for infants with extremely large defects. It is best to view these as staged operations with the goal of the first procedure to close the defect as well as possible, leaving recurrent hernias to be repaired later at a time of physiologic stability. Although use of muscle tissue flaps, such as the latissimus dorsi, should be avoided in the acute phase due to the risk of bleeding, these have been reported to be a useful alternative later as they provide an autogenous, growing tissue replacement (80). Indeed, preemptive but elective resection of the patch with tissue reconstruction may be an approach to consider.

Repairing a diaphragmatic defect will often worsen pulmonary compliance by reducing elasticity of the chest wall and increasing intraabdominal pressure. Although delay in the time of repair allows one to select the moment for this, it is an unavoidable consequence of surgical closure. In some patients, the abdomen cannot be closed without significant tension. In this circumstance, the abdominal compartment can be decompressed using a temporary patch or silo. This is reduced and removed subsequently.

Use of tube thoracostomy for pleural drainage with CDH is controversial. Some authors recommend it routinely, whereas others avoid it. Many large centers do not use pleural drainage in most circumstances. There is generally no need to perform a separate Ladd's procedure for the malrotation, which most of these patients have because the CDH repair itself will cause adhesions to form and the longer operation and risk for bleeding is best avoided in most patients (76).

Chylothorax is a known complication after repair of CDH. Presumably, there is injury to the thoracic duct during repair, but it is possible that there is an abnormality in the chyle drainage. Although not well described in the literature, some infants with CDH will develop late bowel obstruction and wound hernias. Reoperative surgery is not uncommon, especially in the infants with large defects.

Long-term Follow-up

With improving survival in infants with CDH, the need for long-term follow-up has become apparent. Even those infants who undergo primary repair of the defect may have some late problems, and those with large defects will often have multiple problems for some time after hospital discharge. The optimal approach is to follow these infants in a multidisciplinary clinic where many issues can be addressed at the same time. Some of the CDH-associated problems that can occur include developmental delay; hearing loss; gastrointestinal problems, including gastroesophageal reflux, scoliosis and chest wall deformity; and recurrent herniation.

For some time, it has been known that CDH infants requiring ECMO support have significant subsequent neurological developmental delay, even when compared with other ECMO-treated infants (81,82). It is unclear why this occurs, but one contributing factor may be the fact that the ECMO-treated infants are a physiologically unstable subset of patients by the time ECMO is offered. As with other high-risk infant populations, parental socioeconomic status and education can profoundly affect the long-term outcome. It appears that these patients may also have a higher incidence of hearing abnormalities if ECMO is required early in the course of their illness (83).

Dilation of the esophagus acutely and foregut dysmotility subsequently has been reported in CDH patients by several authors, and this can be a cause of significant morbidity in some patients (84). Although initially believed to occur only in ECMO patients, this appears to be more widespread in CDH patients. Gastroesophageal reflux is a common finding in these infants and has been reported in more than 50% of patients in some series (85). Management of gastroesophageal reflux should focus on a conservative initial approach if at all possible. Surgical treatment should be approached cautiously as the cumulative effect of CDH repair and early fundoplication is substantial. A full 360-degree fundoplication should probably be avoided due to the underlying esophageal dysmotility that may be present, although meaningful data are absent and practices vary at this point. Besides gastroesophageal reflux, these infants can have other nutritional and eating-related problems. In a series of patients followed for up to 10 years, a high incidence of nutritional problems was reported; including gastroesophageal reflux, failure to thrive, and severe oral aversion (86). Long-term tube feedings may be required in some patients, although many of those who do require this type of feeding can be eventually transitioned to full oral feedings if they are not severely impaired. Even with attention to nutritional needs, there is a higher incidence of growth failure in CDH patients than in the general population.

As mentioned previously, hernia recurrence has been reported in CDH survivors with increasing frequency and appears to be quite prevalent in infants who require a synthetic patch to close the defect. As noted, the optimal material to repair large defects remains unknown because this type of repair requires fixation to the ribs and will clearly recur as the patch is a fixed size and the chest is growing (87). There are no reports of long-term follow-up in these patients after repair of a recurrent hernia.

As more infants with large diaphragmatic defects and significant degrees of pulmonary hypoplasia survive, it is apparent that some will develop abnormalities in chest wall and spine growth. Scoliosis and pectus excavatum deformities may be related to the tension on the repair or to the type of material used to patch large defects (88). Because there are no large cohorts of survivors with large defects who have reached late adolescence, it is unclear how many of these patients will develop such problems.

There is some controversy about the long-term pulmonary function in survivors with CDH. Some older reports suggest that there is no significant functional problem in these patients; however, survivors reported in earlier studies were probably less ill than patients who are surviving today. Muratore and colleagues describe a significant number of CDH-associated problems, including ventilation perfusion mismatch, chronic lung disease, and prolonged mechanical ventilation (89). Patients treated with ECMO and those requiring a patch to fix the defect had a higher incidence of long-term pulmonary problems. Some infants are discharged on home oxygen, and there is a high incidence of obstructive airway disease. Some series also highlight the postdischarge mortality risk (88). Surviving CDH infants with a patch repair, chronic lung disease, nutritional deficits, and other problems are clearly at high risk. It is not uncommon for these patients to be rehospitalized for pneumonia or other problems.

Although most surviving infants with CDH appear to have good outcomes on follow-up, a concerning number have significant long-term issues. These patients are best managed in a multidisciplinary clinic. Follow-up for these patients will be necessary throughout childhood, and some patients will need lifelong follow-up. Interestingly, despite the need for long-term follow-up in some patients, treatment of CDH remains a very cost-effective strategy (90).

MORGAGNI DIAPHRAGMATIC HERNIAS

This diaphragmatic hernia results from a defect in the anterior retrosternal muscle at one, or occasionally both, of the minor apertures where the superior epigastric arteries traverse the diaphragm. The location is parasternal rather than midline. It is a rare defect, representing 2% or less of all congenital diaphragmatic hernias. Patients are generally asymptomatic, and discovery typically results from diagnostic imaging undertaken for unrelated reasons. Air-filled viscera in the mediastinum on plain chest radiograph is the single most common scenario. Given the lack of symptoms, these patients are generally older than those with Bochdalek hernias. The hernia most often contains liver, but transverse colon, stomach, and small intestine are all possible. Incarcerated hollow viscera usually account for any related symptoms. Operative repair is straightforward and involves a transabdominal approach, reduction of involved viscera, and simple suture closure of the diaphragm to the posterior sheath of the rectus abdominis muscle. This may be done either via laparotomy or laparoscopically.

REFERENCES

1. Langham MR, Kays DW, Ledbetter DJ, et al. Congential diaphragmatic hernia: epidemiology and outcome. *Clin Perinatol* 1996;23:671–688.
2. Metkus AP, Essermn L, Sola A, et al. Cost per anomaly: what does a diaphragmatic hernia cost? *J Pediatr Surg* 1995;30:226–230.
3. The Congenital Diaphragmatic Hernia Study Group. Estimating disease severity of congenital diaphragmatic hernia in the first 5 minutes of life. *J Pediatr Surg* 2001;36:141–145.
4. Irish MS, Holm BA, Glick PL. Congenital diaphragmatic hernia: a historical review. *Clin Perinatol* 1996;23:625–654.
5. Hedblom CA. Diaphragmatic hernia: a study of three hundred and seventy-eight cases in which operation was performed. *JAMA* 1925;85:547–553.
6. Gross RE. Congenital hernia of the diaphragm. *Am J Dis Child* 1946;71:579–592.
7. Greer JJ, Cote D, Allan DW, et al. Structure of the primordial diaphragm and defects associated with nitrofen-induced CDH. *J Appl Physiol* 2000;89:2123–2129.
8. Babiuk RP, Zhang W, Clugston R, et al. Embryological origins and development of the rat diaphragm. *J Comp Neurol* 2003;455:477–487.
9. Iritani I. Experimental study of embryogenesis of congenital diaphragmatic hernia. *Anat Embryol* 1984;169:133–139.
10. Chinoy MR. Pulmonary hypoplasia and congenital diaphragmatic hernia: advances in the pathogenetics and regulation of lung development. *J Surg Res* 2002;106:209–223.
11. Tsang TM, Tam PK, Dudley NE, et al. Diaphragmatic agenesis as a distinct clinical entity. *J Pediatr Surg* 1994;29:1439–1441.
12. Cohen HS, Rychik J, Bush DM, et al. Influence of congenital heart disease on survival in children with congenital diaphragmatic hernia. *J Pediatr* 2002;141:26–30.
13. Garne E, Haeusler M, Barisic I, et al. Congenital diaphragmatic hernia: evaluation of prenatal diagnosis in 20 European regions. *Ultrasound Obstet Gynecol* 2002;19:320–333.
14. Hubbard AM, Crombleholme TM, Adzick NS, et al. Prenatal MRI evaluation of congenital diaphragmatic hernia. *Am J Perinatol* 1999;16:307–313.
15. The Congenital Diaphragmatic Hernia Study Group. Bilateral congenital diaphragmatic hernia. *J Pediatr Surg* 2003;38:522–524.

16. Elhalaby EA, Abo Sikeena MH. Delayed presentation of congenital diaphragmatic hernia. *Pediatr Surg Int* 2002;18:480–485.
17. Sbragia L, Paek BW, Filly RA, et al. Congenital diaphragmatic hernia without herniation of the liver: does the lung-to-head ratio predict survival? *J Ultrasound Med* 2000;19:845–850.
18. Fuke S, Kanzaki T, Mu J, et al. Antenatal prediction of pulmonary hypoplasia by acceleration time/ejection time ratio of fetal pulmonary arteries by Doppler blood flow velocimetry. *Am J Obstet Gynecol* 2003;188:228–233.
19. Wilcox DT, Glick PL, Karamanoukian HL, et al. Contributions by individual lungs to the surfactant status in congenital diaphragmatic hernia. *Pediatr Res* 1997;41:686–691.
20. Mysore MR, Margraf LR, Jaramillo MA, et al. Surfactant protein A is decreased in a rat model of congenital diaphragmatic hernia. *Am J Respir Crit Care Med* 1998;157:654–657.
21. Suen HC, Bloch KD, Donahoe PK. Antenatal glucocorticoid corrects pulmonary immaturity in experimentally induced congenital diaphragmatic hernia in rats. *Pediatr Res* 1994;35:523–529.
22. Ijsselstijn H, Pacheco BA, Albert A, et al. Prenatal hormones alter antioxidant enzymes and lung histology in rats with congenital diaphragmatic hernia. *Am J Physiol* 1997;272:L1059–1065.
23. Oue T, Shima H, Taira Y, et al. Administration of antenatal glucocorticoids upregulates peptide growth factor gene expression in nitrofen-induced congenital diaphragmatic hernia in rats. *J Pediatr Surg* 2000;35:109–112.
24. VanTuyl M, Hosgor M, Tibboel D. Tracheal ligation and corticosteroids in congenital diaphragmatic hernia: for better or worse? *Pediatr Res* 2001;50:441–444.
25. Ford WD, Kirby CP, Wilkinson CS, et al. Antenatal betamethasone and favourable outcomes in fetuses with 'poor prognosis' diaphragmatic hernia. *Pediatr Surg Int* 2002;18:244–246.
26. Losty PD, Pacheco BA, Manganaro TF, et al. Prenatal hormonal therapy improves pulmonary morphology in rats with congenital diaphragmatic hernia. *J Surg Res* 1996;65:42–52.
27. Harrison MR, Adzick NS, Longaker MT, et al. Successful repair in utero of a fetal diaphragmatic hernia after removal of herniated viscera from the left thorax. *N Engl J Med* 1990;322:1582–1584.
28. Harrison MR, Adzick NS, Flake AW, et al. Correction of congenital diaphragmatic hernia in utero: VI. Hardlearned lesions. *J Pediatr Surg* 1993;28:1411–1418.
29. Wilson JM, Fauza DO, Dennis P, et al. Antenatal diagnosis of isolated congenital diaphragmatic hernia is not an indicator of outcome. *J Pediatr Surg* 1994;29:815–819.
30. Sydorak RM, Harrison MR. Congenital diaphragmatic hernia: advances in prenatal therapy. *World J Surg* 2003;27:68–76.
31. Wilson JM, DiFiore JW, Peters CA. Experimental fetal tracheal ligation prevents the pulmonary hypoplasia associated with fetal nephrectomy: possible application for congenital diaphragmatic hernia. *J Pediatr Surg* 1993;28:1433–1439.
32. Hedrick MH, Estes JM, Sullivan KM, et al. Plug the lung until it grows (PLUG): a new method to treat congenital diaphragmatic hernia in utero. *J Pediatr Surg* 1994;29:612–617.
33. Chiba T, Albanese CT, Farmer DL, et al. Balloon tracheal occlusion for congenital diaphragmatic hernia: experimental studies. *J Pediatr Surg* 2000;35:1566–1570.
34. Tsuno K, Prato P, Kolobow T. Acute lung injury from mechanical ventilation at moderately high airway pressures. *J Appl Physiol* 1990;69:956–961.
35. Boix-Ochoa J, Peguero G, Seijo G, et al. Acid–base balance and blood gases in prognosis and therapy of congenital diaphragmatic hernia. *J Pediatr Surg* 1974;9:49–57.
36. Drummond WH, Gregory GA, Heymann MA, et al. The independent effects of hyperventilation, tolazoline, and dopamine on infants with persistent pulmonary hypertension. *J Pediatr* 1981;98:603–611.
37. Wung JT, Sahni R, Moffitt ST, et al. Congenital diaphragmatic hernia: survival treated with very delayed surgery, spontaneous respiration and no chest tube. *J Pediatr Surg* 1995;30:406–409.
38. Kays DW, Langham MR, Ledbetter DJ, et al. Detrimental effects of standard medical therapy in congenital diaphragmatic hernia. *Ann Surg* 1999;230:340–351.
39. Wilson JM, Lund DP, Lillehei CW. Congenital diaphragmatic hernia—a tale of two cities: the Boston experience. *J Pediatr Surg* 1997;32:401–405.
40. Boloker J, Bateman DA, Wung JT, et al. Congenital diaphragmatic hernia in 120 infants treated consecutively with permissive hypercapnea/spontaneous respiration/elective repair. *J Pediatr Surg* 2002;37:357–366.
41. Paranka MS, Clark RH, Yoder BA, et al. Predictors of failure of high-frequency oscillatory ventilation in term infants with severe respiratory failure. *Pediatrics* 1995;95:400–404.
42. Somaschini M, Locatelli G, Salvoni L, et al. Impact of new treatments for respiratory failure on outcome of infants with congenital diaphragmatic hernia. *Eur J Pediatr* 1999;158:780–784.
43. Cacciari A, Ruggeri G, Mordenti M, et al. High-frequency oscillatory ventilation versus conventional mechanical ventilation in congenital diaphragmatic hernia. *Eur J Pediatr Surg* 2001;11:3–7.
44. Bohn D. Congenital diaphragmatic hernia. *Am J Respir Crit Care Med* 2002;166:911–915.
45. Coppola CP, Gosche JR. Oxygen-induced vasodilation is blunted in pulmonary arterioles from fetal rats with nitrofen-induced congenital diaphragmatic hernia. *J Pediatr Surg* 2001;36:593–597.
46. Okazaki T, Sharma HS, McCune SK, et al. Pulmonary vascular balance in congenital diaphragmatic hernia: enhanced endothelin-1 gene expression as a possible cause of pulmonary vasoconstriction. *J Pediatr Surg* 1998;33:81–84.
47. Clark RH, Kueser TJ, Walker MW, et al. Low-dose nitric oxide therapy for persistent pulmonary hypertension of the newborn. Clinical Inhaled Nitric Oxide Research Group. *N Engl J Med* 2000;342:469–474.
48. Finer NN, Barrington KJ. Nitric oxide for respiratory failure in infants born at or near term. *Cochrane Database Syst Rev* 2001;(4):CD000399.
49. Okuyama H, Kubota A, Oue T, et al. Inhaled nitric oxide with early surgery improves the outcome of antenatally diagnosed congenital diaphragmatic hernia. *J Pediatr Surg* 2002;37:1188–1190.
50. Dillon PW, Cilley RE, Hudome SM, et al. Nitric oxide reversal of recurrent pulmonary hypertension and respiratory failure in an infant with CDH after successful ECMO therapy. *J Pediatr Surg* 1995;30:743–744.
51. Glick PL, Stannard VA, Leach CL, et al. Pathophysiology of congenital diaphragmatic hernia II: the fetal lamb CDH model is surfactant deficient. *J Pediatr Surg* 1992;27:382–387.
52. Thèbaud B, Barlier-Mur A-M, Chailley-Heu B, et al. Restoring effects of vitamin A on surfactant synthesis in nitrofen-induced congenital diaphragmatic hernia in rats. *Am J Respir Crit Care Med* 2001;164:1083–1089.
53. Guarino N, Oue T, Shima H, et al. Antenatal dexamethasone enhances surfactant protein synthesis in the hypoplastic lung of nitrofen-induced diaphragmatic hernia in rats. *J Pediatr Surg* 2000;35:1468–1473.
54. Lotze A, Knight GR, Anderson KD, et al. Surfactant (beractant) therapy for infants with congenital diaphragmatic hernia on ECMO: evidence of persistent surfactant deficiency. *J Pediatr Surg* 1994;29:407–412.
55. Moya FR, Thomas VL, Romaguera J, et al. Fetal lung maturation in congenital diaphragmatic hernia. *Am J Obstet Gynecol* 1995;173:1401–1405.
56. Glick PL, Leach CL, Besner GE, et al. Pathophysiology of congenital diaphragmatic hernia III: exogenous surfactant therapy for the high-risk neonate with CDH. *J Pediatr Surg* 1992;27:866–869.
57. Bae CW, Jang CK, Chung SJ, et al. Exogenous pulmonary surfactant replacement therapy in a neonate with pulmonary hypoplasia accompanying congenital diaphragmatic hernia—a case report. *J Korean Med Sci* 1996;11:265–270.
58. Janssen DJ, Tibboel D, Carnielli VP, et al. Surfactant phosphatidylcholine pool size in human neonates with congenital diaphragmatic hernia requiring ECMO. *J Pediatr* 2003;142:247–252.
59. Cogo PE, Zimmermann LJ, Rosso F, et al. Surfactant synthesis and kinetics in infants with congenital diaphragmatic hernia. *Am J Respir Crit Care Med* 2002;166:154–158.
60. Finer NN, Tierney A, Etches PC, et al. Congenital diaphragmatic hernia: developing a protocolized approach. *J Pediatr Surg* 1998;33:1331–1337.
61. Anderson JM, the Congenital Diaphragmatic Hernia Study Group. *Is surfactant use associated with worse outcomes in term infants with CDH?* Presented at the 19th annual CNMC ECMO Symposium, February 2003, Keystone, CO.

62. Colby CE, the Congenital Diaphragmatic Hernia Study Group. *Does surfactant replacement therapy on ECMO benefit the neonate with congenital diaphragmatic hernia?* Presented at the 19th annual CNMC ECMO Symposium, February 2003, Keystone, CO.
63. Lally KP. Extracorporeal membrane oxygenation in patients with congenital diaphragmatic hernia. *Semin Pediatr Surg* 1996;5:249–255.
64. Lally KP, the CEJ Study Group. *The use of ECMO for stabilization of infants with congenital diaphragmatic hernia—a report of the CDH Study Group*. Presented at the 18th–20th annual meeting of the Surgical Section of the American Academy of Pediatrics, October 2002, Boston, MA.
65. Dimmitt RA, Moss RL, Rhine WD, et al. Venoarterial versus venovenous extracorporeal membrane oxygenation in congenital diaphragmatic hernia: the Extracorporeal Life Support Organization Registry, 1990–1999. *J Pediatr Surg* 2001;36:1199–1204.
66. Reickert CA, Hirschl RB, Atkinson JB, et al. Congenital diaphragmatic hernia survival and use of extracorporeal life support at selected level III nurseries with multimodality support. *Surgery* 1998;123:305–310.
67. Stevens TP, Chess PR, McConnochie KM, et al. Survival in early- and late-term infants with congenital diaphragmatic hernia treated with extracorporeal membrane oxygenation. *Pediatrics* 2002;110:590–596.
68. DiFiore JW, Fauza DO, Slavin R, et al. Experimental fetal tracheal ligation and congenital diaphragmatic hernia: a pulmonary vascular morphometric analysis. *J Pediatr Surg* 1995;30:917–923.
69. Kay S, Laberge J-M, Flageole H, et al. Use of antenatal steroids to counteract the negative effects of tracheal occlusion in the fetal lamb model. *Pediatr Res* 2001;50:495–501.
70. Luks FI, Wild YK, Piasecki GJ, et al. Short-term tracheal occlusion corrects pulmonary vascular anomalies in the fetal lamb with diaphragmatic hernia. *Surgery* 2000;128:266–272.
71. Kitano Y, Kanai M, Davies P, et al. Lung growth induced by prenatal tracheal occlusion and its modifying factors: a study in the rat model of congenital diaphragmatic hernia. *J Pediatr Surg* 2001;36:251–259.
72. Nobuhara KK, Fauza DO, DiFiore JW, et al. Continuous intrapulmonary distension with perfluorocarbon accelerates neonatal (but not adult) lung growth. *J Pediatr Surg* 1998;33:292–298.
73. Walker GM, Kasem KF, O'Toole SJ, et al. Early perfluorodecalin lung distension in infants with congenital diaphragmatic hernia. *J Pediatr Surg* 2003;38:17–20.
74. Hirschl RB, Philip WF, Glick L, et al. A prospective, randomized pilot trial of perfluorocarbon-induced lung growth in newborns with congenital diaphragmatic hernia. *J Pediatr Surg* 2003;38:283–289.
75. Moyer V, Moya F, Tibboel R, et al. Late versus early surgical correction for congenital diaphragmatic hernia in newborn infants. *Cochrane Database Syst Rev* 2002;(3):CD001695.
76. Clark RH, Hardin WD Jr, Hirschl RB, et al. Current surgical management of congenital diaphragmatic hernia: a report from the Congenital Diaphragmatic Hernia Study Group. *J Pediatr Surg* 1998;33:1004–1009.
77. Lally KP, Paranka MS, Roden J, et al. Congenital diaphragmatic hernia. Stabilization and repair on ECMO. *Ann Surg* 1992;216:1048–1052.
78. Wilson JM, Bower LK, Lund DP. Evolution of the technique of congenital diaphragmatic hernia repair on ECMO. *J Pediatr Surg* 1994;29:1109–1112.
79. Moss RL, Chen CM, Harrison MR. Prosthetic patch durability in congenital diaphragmatic hernia: a long-term follow-up study. *J Pediatr Surg* 2001;36:152–154.
80. Sydorak RM, Hoffman W, Lee H, et al. Reversed latissimus dorsi muscle flap for repair of recurrent congenital diaphragmatic hernia. *J Pediatr Surg* 2003;38:296–300.
81. McGahren ED, Mallik K, Rodgers B. Neurological outcome is diminished in survivors of congenital diaphragmatic hernia requiring extracorporeal membrane oxygenation. *J Pediatr Surg* 1997;32:1216–1220.
82. Stolar CJH, Crisafi MA, Driscoll YT. Neurocognitive outcome for neonates treated with extracorporeal membrane oxygenation: are infants with congenital diaphragmatic hernia different? *J Pediatr Surg* 1995;30:366–372.
83. Rasheed A, Tindall S, Cueny DL, et al. Neurodevelopmental outcome after congenital diaphragmatic hernia: Extracorporeal membrane oxygenation before and after surgery. *J Pediatr Surg* 2001;36:539–544.
84. Stolar CJ, Levy JP, Dillon PW, et al. Anatomic and functional abnormalities of the esophagus in infants surviving congenital diaphragmatic hernia. *Am J Surg* 1990;159:204–207.
85. Fasching G, Huber, Uray E, et al. Gastroesophageal reflux and diaphragmatic motility after repair of congenital diaphragmatic hernia. *Eur J Pediatr Surg* 2000;10:360–364.
86. Muratore CS, Utter S, Jaksic T, et al. Nutritional morbidity in survivors of congenital diaphragmatic hernia. *J Pediatr Surg* 2001;36:1171–1176.
87. Lally KP, Cheu HW, Vazquez WD. Prosthetic diaphragm reconstruction in the growing animal. *J Pediatr Surg* 1993;28:45–47.
88. Jaillard SM, Pierrat V, Dubois A, et al. Outcome at 2 years of infants with congenital diaphragmatic hernia: a population-based study. *Ann Thorac Surg* 2003;75:250–256.
89. Muratore CS, Kharasch V, Lund DP, et al. Pulmonary morbidity in 100 survivors of congenital diaphragmatic hernia monitored in a multidisciplinary clinic. *J Pediatr Surg* 2001;30:133–140.
90. Poley MJ, Stolk EA, Tibboel D, et al. The cost-effectiveness of treatment for congenital diaphragmatic hernia. *J Pediatr Surg* 2002;37:1245–1252.

Chapter 59

Subglottic Airway

Richard G. Azizkhan

Many different airway disorders can cause airway obstruction and respiratory distress in children, and determining a precise diagnosis requires an understanding of each disorder. Due to distinctive anatomic features of the pediatric airway, symptoms of respiratory distress may rapidly progress and become life threatening. It is thus incumbent for physicians to quickly determine the problem and manage it appropriately.

Management strategy generally depends on the degree of respiratory insufficiency and information obtained from a thorough case history. Less severe respiratory insufficiency often manifests in subtle symptoms, such as irritability, restlessness, tachycardia, and feeding difficulties. Cyanosis, severe suprasternal and intercostal retractions, tachypnea, and lethargy indicate more severe respiratory compromise. Stridor, a harsh respiratory sound produced by turbulent airflow, is the most important physical sign in cases of upper airway obstruction. It can be present either in the inspiratory or expiratory phase of the respiration, or in both (1,2). Its characteristics, as well as its relationship to the respiratory cycle, may help in establishing a definitive diagnosis and in setting priorities for diagnostic evaluation (2). Reviewing the history of the child's symptoms may provide valuable clues to underlying etiology. Close attention should be paid to circumstances that may have triggered the onset of respiratory compromise, to the duration of symptoms, and to their progression over time. Questioning parents about a history of dysphagia or feeding problems, the nature of their child's cry, and the possibility of foreign-body aspiration can also yield important information. In addition, any previous history of endotracheal intubation, trauma, or cardiopulmonary abnormalities should be carefully reviewed.

In any patient with airway compromise, control of the airway is imperative and is the primary clinical concern. Once airway and ventilatory control has been obtained, a thorough evaluation should be initiated to delineate the structural lesions or functional abnormalities of the subglottic airway. This chapter focuses on these disorders, as well as the diagnostic and therapeutic techniques that are crucial to their successful management. To set the stage for this discussion, an overview of the embryogenesis and relevant anatomy of the pediatric airway is presented.

Richard G. Azizkhan: Cincinnati Children's Hospital Medical Center, University of Cincinnati School of Medicine, Cincinnati, Ohio 45229.

TRACHEOBRONCHIAL EMBRYOLOGY

The laryngotracheal groove arises from the ventral surface of the foregut during the third and fourth weeks of gestation (3). Cells lining the celomic cavity also divide during this time, becoming a proliferating primitive mesenchyme and eventually pulmonary muscle, cartilage, and connective tissue. During the fifth week of gestation, caudal progression of the embryonic trachea is followed by bifurcation and the appearance of lung buds. During the sixth week, the lobar bronchi lengthen and abut the esophagus. Asymmetric buds (the left bud being shorter and more nearly horizontal than the right) rapidly divide into lobar bronchi and tertiary bronchi by the seventh week. At this stage, pseudostratified epithelium lines the larger airways. Differentiation and branching of the epithelial bronchial tree depends on the presence of the mediastinal mesenchyme (3,4). The formation of new smaller bronchi continues through the sixteenth week. Bronchial subdivisions continue until the seventeenth order is established between the sixth and seventh month. At that time, alveolar differentiation occurs at the site of the distal terminal bronchi and continues until well after birth.

The initial vascular supply of the differentiating bronchial buds develops from the splanchnic plexus that originates from the dorsal aorta and drains into the plexus of cardinal veins. The bronchial arterial blood supply develops from gradual interconnection with the sixth aortic arch, and the bronchial vasculature is left as a remnant of the embryonic vascular system. Tracheal bifurcation is initially high in the cervical region, but descends to the level of the first thoracic vertebra by 8 weeks of gestation and to the fourth thoracic vertebra at birth. Cartilage appears in the trachea in approximately 10 weeks and in the segmental bronchi at 16 weeks (4). After this time, fetal lung development primarily consists of the successive generation of terminal airways and alveoli.

Congenital anomalies of the respiratory system are relatively uncommon and can occur along the entire tracheobronchopulmonary axis. Associated extrapulmonary anomalies are frequently present and may be part of a syndrome or association. Approximately 45% of children with congenital airway obstruction have associated congenital anomalies (1,2,5), some of which have a significant impact on prognosis. Although the cause of such anomalies is usually unknown, they are believed to result from causal mechanisms that differ in time, mode of action, and the embryonic region affected. As such, they are failures of normal growth and differentiation of different parts of the embryonic respiratory system. More specifically, defective mesodermal development in early embryogenesis may be responsible for the VACTERL[1] association. Primary abnormalities of the developing lung bud itself may lead to a variety of abnormalities, including congenital lobar emphysema, bronchogenic cysts, sequestrations, and cystic adenomatoid malformations, which are discussed elsewhere. Gestational teratogens may have selected effects on specific organ development. Experimental evidence suggests that vitamin A may play an important role in the development of the airway and lungs. In animal embryos, its deficiency causes a keratizing metaplasia of the tracheobronchial tree and pulmonary agenesis (6). Retinoic acid appears to be important for embryonic cell differentiation in many organ systems and has been studied intensely (3). Investigators have described a relationship between the maternal use of valproic acid and both tracheomalacia and laryngeal hypoplasia in offspring (7). Also, a constellation of abnormalities, including severe congenital tracheal stenosis, has been reported in infants of diabetic mothers (8).

PEDIATRIC AIRWAY ANATOMY

Several anatomic features of the airway in infants differ from those of older children or adults (5,9) and are important to keep in mind because of their impact on symptom progression, diagnosis, and disease management. The caliber of the airway is small and can be readily obstructed by secretions or mucosal swelling. The larynx is more cephalad and anterior, making visualization more difficult, especially for the inexperienced clinician. The cricoid, which is the only completely circumferential laryngeal cartilage, is the narrowest portion of the child's upper airway. Last, the length of the trachea is very short (approximately 4 to 5 cm), thus increasing the risk of unplanned extubation or right mainstem intubation during flexion or extension of the infant's head and neck.

Because of this unique subglottic anatomy, care must be taken to minimize trauma to this region during endotracheal intubation and airway procedures. Tightly fitting endotracheal tubes may cause mucosal or submucosal injury, thus resulting in stenosis at the level of the cricoid cartilage. A 50% reduction in cross-sectional area results for every millimeter of airway edema or narrowing of the lumen of an infant's airway. The correct fit of the child's uncuffed endotracheal tube can be estimated as follows (10):

$$4 + (\text{years of age}/4) = \text{tube size (mm)}$$

When positioning the endotracheal tube, there must be an air leak at less than 18 to 25 cm of water pressure to ensure an appropriate fit (10).

PATHOPHYSIOLOGY

Mapping the respiratory tract into three distinct regions helps identify possible pathologic correlates of stridor (10). The first area comprises a supraglottic and supralaryngeal region, which includes the pharynx; the second is an extrathoracic tracheal region, which includes the glottis and the subglottis; and the third is made up of an intrathoracic tracheal region, which includes primary and secondary bronchi. In certain regions, stridor occurs more frequently during inspiration, whereas in other regions, it occurs more frequently during expiration. These patterns of stridor are of utmost importance in that they indicate possible etiologies that warrant further investigation or signal imminent emergency. In the first region, stridor generally occurs during inspiration. A patient showing this pattern should undergo careful investigation for upper airway lesions (e.g., choanal atresia), expanding lesions in the tongue (e.g., a dermoid cyst or an internal thyroglossal duct cyst), or lack of structural airway support from mandibular hypoplasia, as seen in Pierre-Robin sequence or from macroglossia, as seen in Beckwith-Wiedeman syndrome. In the second region, stridor is heard during both inspiration and expiration, and is referred to as biphasic. When this pattern is heard, the glottic and subglottic lumina have reached a critically small size and tremendous effort is required to move air through a pinpoint opening. Biphasic stridor often signals impending respiratory collapse and is thus a medical emergency likely to require intubation or tracheotomy. In the intrathoracic bronchial region, the relative positive pressures of expiratory forces within the chest wall narrow the bronchial lumen in

[1] VACTERL = V, vertebral anomalies; A, anal anomalies; C, cardiac defects; T, tracheoesophageal fistula; E, esophageal atresia; R, renal anomalies; L, limb anomalies.

normal children. As air moves during expiration, the Venturi principle adds a constricting force. In the presence of a bronchial foreign body or a lesion, these forces act jointly to close the airway lumen. The expiratory phase sound can be heard as either stridor or wheezing.

AIRWAY ENDOSCOPY

Airway endoscopy, also referred to as laryngotracheobronchoscopy, is the instrument-aided visual examination of the airway. It can reveal airway structure and dynamics as well as airway contents, and also provide access to foreign bodies, secretions, and washings from the lower airways. As such, it has increasingly been used in infants and children for both diagnostic and therapeutic purposes (11–13). For a child with signs of respiratory distress, chest wall retractions, severe stridor, or tripod posture with drooling, airway endoscopy is urgent and imperative (10). Early endoscopic intervention in the setting of worsening stridor may avoid more extreme measures such as endotracheal intubation or a tracheotomy. Both of these procedures may interfere with establishing an accurate diagnosis. In cases where some degree of airway obstruction coexists with feeding difficulties and insufficient weight gain, airway endoscopy is warranted to determine the underlying cause. These circumstances are more likely to be found in chronic conditions such as laryngomalacia and bronchotracheomalacia. When diagnostic imaging techniques suggest an abnormality such as a vascular ring, endoscopy may be required to confirm the diagnosis. Because a significant percentage of children with stridor have more than one airway lesion, the entire upper and lower airway should be examined unless there are contraindications such as critical tracheal stenosis (11).

For airway endoscopy to be carried out safely and effectively, cooperation and collaboration between the surgeon and the anesthesiologist are absolutely essential, and an overall strategy must be discussed and agreed upon. Optimally, the attending pulmonologist should be included in the operative team, particularly when the patient has a history of pulmonary dysfunction. Also, essential resources should be available in the event of the need for urgent airway access by cannula or a tracheotomy.

RIGID AND FLEXIBLE BRONCHOSCOPY

Although rigid and flexible bronchoscopy offer different advantages and disadvantages, they are best viewed as complementary techniques to assess airway anatomy and function. They are often used concurrently, and of utmost importance, they both require gentle technique. They also both require an appreciation of the unique anatomy of infants and children, and the potential risks involved in attempting to visualize airway structures.

Rigid Bronchoscopy

Rigid bronchoscopy requires the administration of a general anesthetic to prevent pain and potentially dangerous movement that might cause tracheal or laryngeal damage. Because the rigid bronchoscope must be passed through the mouth, proper placement requires some degree of neck hyperextension, thus presenting a significant risk to children with certain physical disabilities such as Down syndrome and Arnold Chiari malformation. This bronchoscope does, however, offer superior visualization and greater suction capabilities. In addition, it allows for the use of a greater variety of instruments in the airways. The removal of foreign bodies is usually performed more safely using rigid bronchoscopy, although flexible bronchoscopy does have a role in the diagnosis of possible foreign-body aspiration (14). Rigid bronchoscopy can be useful in the diagnosis and treatment of massive hemoptysis, in dilatation of tracheal or bronchial stenosis, and in airway stent placement (10). It is also usually advantageous to use a rigid bronchoscope in the evaluation of children with suspected laryngoesophageal clefts, bilateral vocal cord paralysis, or H-type tracheoesophageal fistula. Confirming the importance of rigid bronchoscopy in the diagnostic process, a large-scale, long-term study conducted by Wiseman and colleagues found that it contributed to the final diagnosis in approximately 88% of patients. Further, there was no mortality and a morbidity rate of only 3.5% (15).

Rigid (open-tube) bronchoscopes range from approximately 2.5 to 8.5 mm in diameter to 20 to 50 cm in length. Due to their size, they can function as an endotracheal tube, allowing patients to ventilate. The airways distal to the tip of the bronchoscope are illuminated either with a prism inserted partially into the lumen or by a glass rod telescopic lens (Fig. 59-1). The optical characteristics of the rigid bronchoscope, when used with the glass rod telescope, are excellent and unequaled by any other bronchoscopic device (Fig. 59-2). When the telescope is not used, visualization through the bronchoscope is more difficult. This open-tube endoscopic configuration is often necessary to manipulate instruments (11).

The large lumen of the rigid bronchoscope allows for easy passage of instruments such as forceps, suction catheters, snares, and retrieval baskets into the airways. Because the glass rod telescope takes up a large part of the lumen, special instruments have been designed for use with this device. These include the optical forceps, which operate in conjunction with the telescope, and the ultrathin forceps, which can be passed alongside the telescope. Other endoscopic equipment, such as suction catheters, balloon-tipped catheters, and laser fibers, can also be passed through or around the bronchoscope (11).

Because glass rod telescopes significantly reduce the functional lumen of the rigid endoscope and increase airway resistance, ventilation is not necessarily assured.

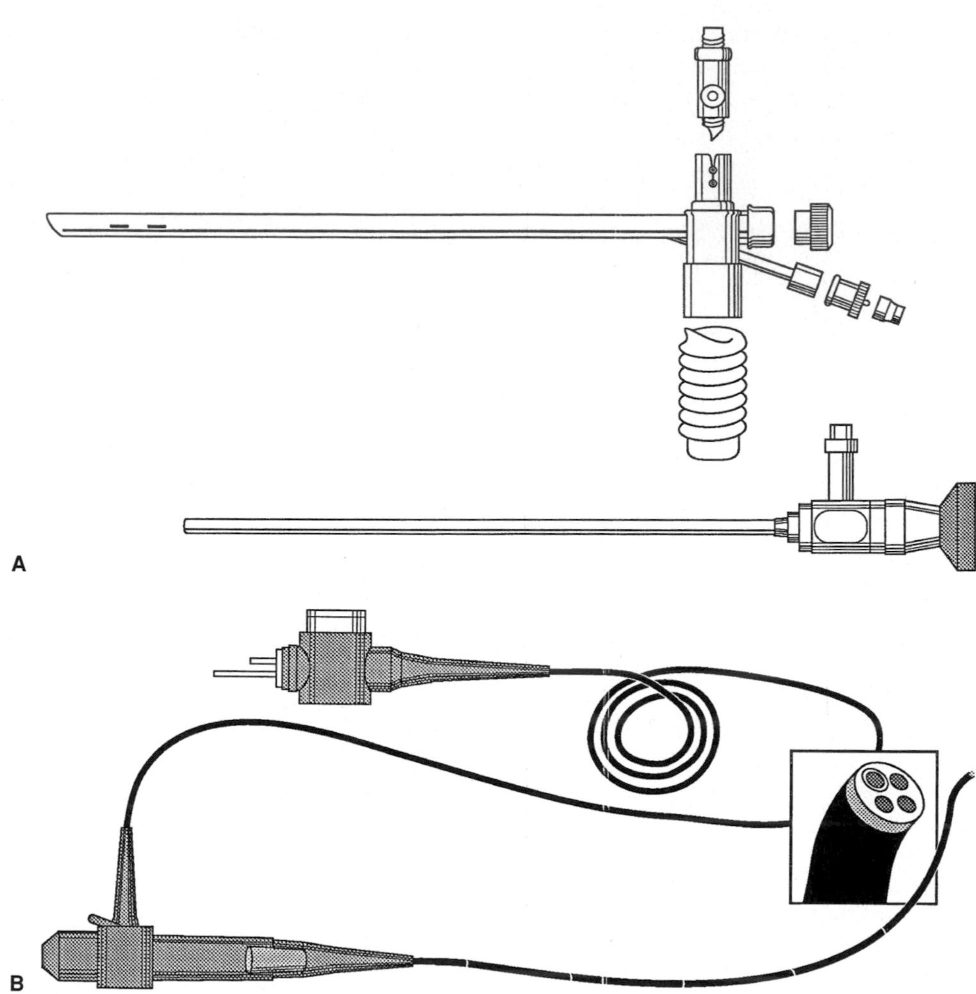

FIGURE 59-1. **(A)** A Storz pediatric ventilating bronchoscope *(top)* and a Hopkins rod lens telescope *(bottom)*. **(B)** Flexible pediatric bronchoscope.

This is particularly significant in infants because the most commonly used bronchoscope has an internal diameter of 3.5 mm and a corresponding telescope with a diameter of 2.5 mm. Therefore, it is essential that the patient's hemoglobin-oxygen saturation and ventilation be carefully monitored throughout the procedure. It is also important to evaluate airway dynamics, which may be altered by sedation or anesthesia, and to examine the airway with the patient spontaneously breathing. This is done because dynamic airway collapse can easily be missed during positive-pressure ventilation. The bronchoscope itself can also alter dynamics, either by stenting the airway or

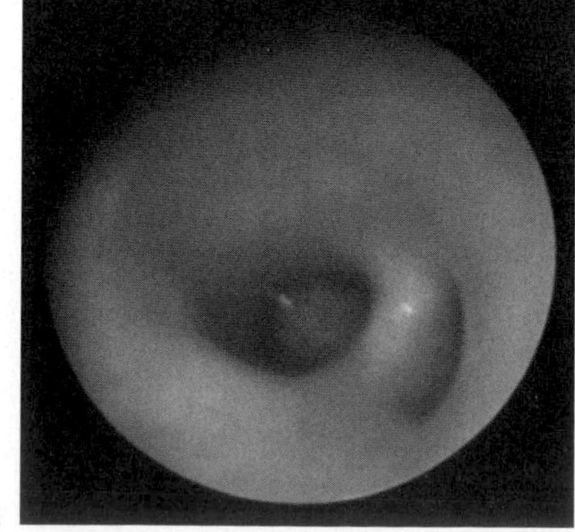

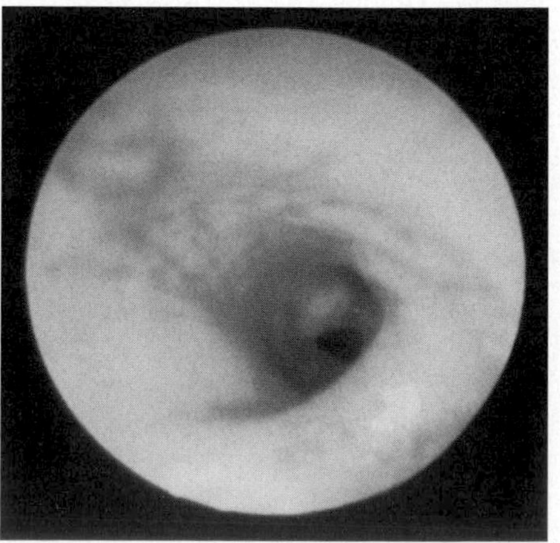

FIGURE 59-2. **(A)** The bronchus intermedius of a 600-g premature neonate who required prolonged ventilatory support and failed extubation is seen through a rigid bronchoscope. The right upper lobe orifice is seen at the 3 o'clock position and an obstructing granuloma is present in the bronchus intermedius itself. **(B)** After forceps extraction of the obstructing lesion, the airway was patent. The patient was rapidly weaned from the ventilator and successfully extubated.

by changing airway resistance and resultant pressure relationships (11).

Flexible Bronchoscopy

Although flexible fiberoptic bronchoscopy can be performed using a topical anesthetic and intravenous sedation, it is often performed under general anesthesia in infants and young children. The scope can be inserted either orally or nasally and can be passed through endotracheal or tracheostomy tubes of appropriate size. Flexible bronchoscopy has also been successfully performed through a laryngeal mask. Whereas the patient undergoing rigid bronchoscopy can use the endoscope for breathing, the patient undergoing flexible bronchoscopy must breathe around the instrument. This endoscopic approach is advantageous in maintaining difficult airways due to poor or limited neck mobility and cervicofacial trauma. Also important, flexible bronchoscopes are able to penetrate further into the bronchial tree with greater peripheral range. They can thus more easily detect distal foreign bodies that would not be seen with a rigid scope (11–13,16).

New pediatric flexible bronchoscopes have an outer diameter ranging from 2.8 to 3.7 mm and a 1.2 mm suction channel. They are distinguished by the ability to flex the distal end to as much as 180 degrees (Fig. 59-1B). These bronchoscopes can be used in infants weighing as little as 500 g, and most term infants can breathe around them spontaneously for short periods. The image produced by a flexible bronchoscope is composed of several thousand points of light, each representing the color and light intensity transmitted by a single glass fiber. Although the resolution of this image is lower than that with the glass rod telescope, the perceived image quality is quite good. This can be attributed to the fact that the surgeon's eye rapidly compensates for the lower resolution (11).

The standard flexible bronchoscope is diagnostically useful in the assessment of atelectasis, and can be used to obtain selected lobar or segmental bronchial washings for cytologic and microbiologic evaluation. Occasionally, lavage with mucolytic agents may be necessary, and rarely, a rigid bronchoscope with forceps extraction must be used in patients who have discrete mucous plugs (11). If the atelectasis is due to an impacted foreign body or a tissue mass, rigid bronchoscopy is needed.

The development of lasers that can be transmitted through fiberoptic light cables has led to the increasing use of laser bronchoscopy in the treatment of some intraluminal sublglottic airway lesions (17). Argon, neodymium-yttrium aluminum garnet (Nd:YAG), and potassium titanyl phosphate (KTP) are the three most common lasers used with this method of delivery, and all these laser systems can be deployed through either rigid or flexible endoscopes (Fig. 59-3). The use of small (300 to 600 μm) quartz fiberoptic laser cables allows clinicians to treat even distal bronchial lesions in small premature infants. The KTP and Argon lasers are most safely and effectively used in the noncontact mode, creating lesions 0.5 mm in diameter. These small spot sizes provide a significant advantage over the Nd:YAG laser, which requires a contact probe and direct contact with the tissues. The thermal effect (i.e., depth of penetration and spot size) of the Nd:YAG laser is more difficult to control and thus not as safe in children (18). Although both the Argon and KTP lasers are particularly useful for removing tracheal or endobronchial granulomas after repair of tracheal stenosis, the KTP laser is currently believed to be the most precise and effective in vaporizing lesions, while causing less destruction to overlying mucosa.

Ultrathin flexible bronchoscopes (1.8 to 2.2 mm in diameter) offer a number of advantages for examination of the lower airway of infants and small children. They

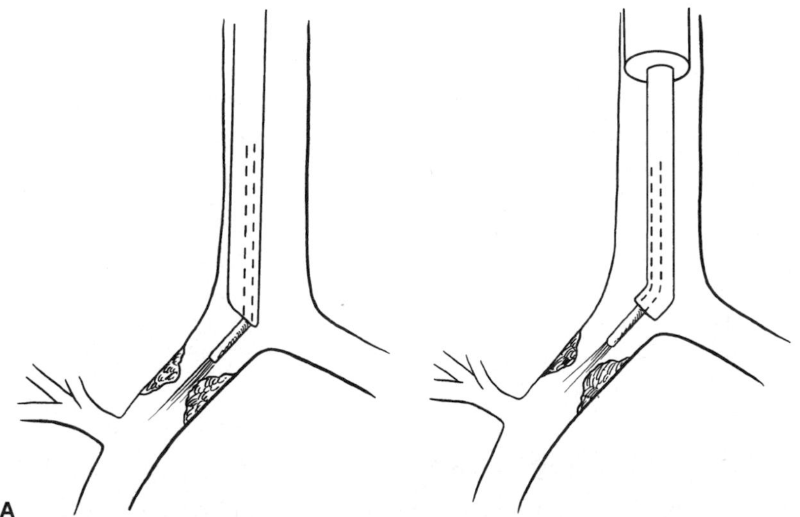

FIGURE 59-3. **(A)** A quartz fiberoptic laser cable is passed through the suction channel of a flexible bronchoscope and is positioned parallel to the bronchial wall and nearly perpendicular to the lesion. **(B)** The laser is fired with the laser cable tip positioned less than 1 mm from the target tissue. The obstructing lesion is outlined by the shaded areas.

are particularly useful in the critical care setting, where bedside endoscopy can be performed through small endotracheal tubes while maintaining effective ventilation. They are also extremely useful in evaluating the position of endotracheal tubes, examining the dynamics of the posterior wall of the trachea in relation to tracheostomy tubes, and for retrograde laryngoscopy in infants with tracheostomies. Flexible bronchoscopes can be used to direct placement of balloon catheters for bronchial dilatation, in positioning airway stents and fiberoptic laser fibers, and in examining the peripheral airway. A drawback of the ultrathin scope is that it is not equipped with a suction channel. Blood or secretions can thus easily obscure visualization.

Endoscopic techniques can also be useful during extubation in selected patients. When extubation has been unsuccessful, direct examination of the airway may define the problem (Fig. 59-2). The lower airways are initially examined through the endotracheal tube. The nasopharnyx and larynx are then examined with a flexible bronchoscope that has been passed through an appropriately sized clean endotracheal tube. The indwelling endotracheal tube is withdrawn after the tip of the bronchoscope is positioned just above the glottis. The bronchoscope is withdrawn if the anatomy and function appear favorable after several minutes of observation. If the child has evidence of obstruction or severe respiratory dysfunction, the bronchoscope is advanced into the trachea, and the fresh endotracheal tube is subsequently passed. Because subglottic edema that is significant enough to prevent successful extubation may not become apparent for 5 to 10 minutes after extubation, the airway should be examined in an unhurried manner (11).

Complications of Airway Endoscopy

Although airway endoscopy is a commonly used procedure, it is one that requires skill and experience to perform safely and effectively. The patient must be properly prepared and monitored before, during, and after the procedure. The endoscopist must be able to recognize and deal with any complications that may arise. The most commonly observed complications are due to direct or indirect tissue trauma. These complications include mucosal trauma, hemoptysis or epistaxis, pneumothorax, subglottic edema, tracheal or bronchial perforation, and trauma to the vocal cords. They occur more commonly with rigid bronchoscopy both because of the rigid physical characteristics of the instruments used and because of the types of procedures performed with this approach. Illustrating the latter, mucosal tears or bronchial perforation can occur during foreign-body extraction.

Physiologic complications include hypoxia, hypercarbia, laryngospasm, bronchospasm, and bradycardia or other cardiac arrhythmias. Hypoxia and hypercarbia may occur because a flexible instrument obstructs the airway for a significant period of time or because prolonged manipulation of an instrument through the open channel of a rigid endoscope interrupts positive-pressure ventilation. Cardiac arrhythmias and laryngospasm can result from direct vagal stimulation, often a consequence of insufficient topical anesthesia (11). Inadequate sedation or topical anesthesia can result in mechanical trauma from coughing. If the patient's stomach is not empty, endoscopy may induce regurgitation or gastroesophageal reflux and may cause aspiration. In addition, passage of a bronchoscope and the associated sedation or anesthesia alter the ability to breathe, placing patients at risk for other complications. Careful monitoring during any endoscopic airway examination is thus essential.

THE SURGICALLY CREATED AIRWAY

The surgeon treating infants and children with tracheobronchial abnormalities must be competent in performing different techniques of establishing a secure airway and with managing the postoperative care that each technique requires. Essential techniques include cricothyroidotomy, tracheotomy (temporary airway), and tracheostomy (long-term airway). The treatment selected is based on the surgeon's determination of whether securing the airway is emergent or elective and permanent versus temporary.

Cricothyroidotomy

Rarely, when establishing an airway is critical due to an acute airway obstruction episode and orotracheal intubation is not possible, the treatment of choice is a cricothyroidotomy. Immediate percutaneous tracheal access can be obtained with a needle cricothyroidotomy. A 14-gauge intravenous cannula is inserted through the cricothyroid membrane, and high-flow plastic tubing with 100% oxygen is connected to this cannula. Because this technique is a temporizing maneuver, a more secure surgical or orotracheal airway should be obtained as soon as possible. Another option is surgical cricothyroidotomy, which is also an excellent method of rapidly securing a difficult airway in an emergency. Subsequent to this procedure, a larger and more stable endotracheal tube can be inserted through the cricothyroid membrane. Because this approach is, however, known to cause irrevocable injury to the cricoid cartilage and subglottic region when performed in infants and small children, its use should be restricted to older children and teenagers. Conversion to a formal tracheostomy is recommended within a few days in cases likely to require prolonged airway support.

Tracheotomy and Tracheostomy

Whereas airway obstructions secondary to infection were the most common indication for emergency tracheotomy

TABLE 59-1 Indications for Tracheotomy in Infants and Children.

Bilateral choanal atresia
Severe micrognathia (e.g., Pierre Robin sequence)
Oropharyngeal tumors (e.g., lymphangioma, teratoma, hemangiopericytoma)
Cervical masses obstructing the larynx or trachea
Anomalies of the larynx (e.g., atresia, webs, laryngomalacia)
Bilateral vocal cord paralysis
Subglottic obstruction (e.g., stenosis, hemangioma)
Central apnea
Chronic respiratory failure and support
Chronic aspiration risk (e.g., severe oropharyngeal dysmotility, prolonged coma)
Acute obstruction from infection (e.g., epiglottitis)
Significant craniofacial trauma
Laryngeal trauma (e.g., fractured larynx)
Inability to achieve oral airway during resuscitation

in the past, this procedure is now commonly performed in infants and children with a wide range of congenital and acquired structural or functional airway abnormalities. Table 59-1 tracheostomy is also often required as an adjunct to airway reconstruction.

Knowledge of posttracheostomy complications has enabled surgeons to make modifications in tracheostomy technique. Important principles of this technique now include the preservation of tracheal tissue by not excising a window or flap and by not performing the procedure on an infant without a secured airway (19). In preparation for the procedure, the infant or child should be anesthetized in the operating room via endotracheal intubation or through a ventilating rigid bronchoscope. A small roll is placed under the child's shoulders and the neck is prepared with a surgical antiseptic solution. A transverse cervical skin incision is made 1 to 2 cm above the sternal notch, depending on the size of the child. The cervical fascia is then incised vertically and the thyroid isthmus retracted. Traction sutures made of Prolene are placed on both sides of the trachea, and a vertical tracheotomy is performed through the third and fourth tracheal rings. The surgeon and the anesthesiologist jointly coordinate the slow withdrawal of the endotracheal tube and placement of tracheostomy tube. The traction sutures are taped to the neck for use in guiding the replacement of this tube in the event of dislodgment or unexpected airway obstruction.

Meticulous care of the tracheostomy is necessary to avoid complications. Physicians and nurses responsible for this care must be adept in rapidly responding to possible urgent needs of a patient and be ready to perform one or more of the following life-saving steps:

- Suctioning the airway
- Establishing ventilation by bag-masking the child until the airway can be secured by an experienced clinician
- Reintubating the child through the glottis, if feasible
- Replacing the tracheostomy using a small suction tube to cannulate the trachea through the stoma
- Sliding the tracheostomy tube over the catheter

Attempting to blindly reinsert the tracheostomy tube at the bedside can have disastrous consequences if the tube enters the anterior mediastinum or perforates the posterior trachea. Until the first tracheostomy tube change, an intubation set, an appropriate endotracheal tube, and suction catheters that fit through the tracheostomy must be readily available.

Complications can occur early (less than 30 days) or late. The early complication rate ranges from 10% to 15%, with accidental decannulation, tracheal obstruction, bleeding, pneumothorax, and pneumomediastinum occurring most frequently. Late complications include formation of granulation tissue, tracheal obstructions, tube occlusion, and tracheoinnominate fistula (19).

Home Care

After receiving detailed and thorough hospital-based training in tracheostomy care and replacement, as well as emergency procedures, parents or other home care providers assume most of the routine care. Visiting nurses and respiratory therapists provide continued instruction, ongoing evaluation, and comprehensive support. Some children also benefit from home apnea monitors.

Decannulation

Prior to considering removal of the tracheostomy tube, flexible laryngotracheobronchoscopy is performed to examine the proximal and distal airways for intraluminal or extrinsic obstructing lesions or conditions that could preclude or complicate decannulation. Recognizing and treating serious pathologic lesions such as peristomal tracheal collapse or obstructing granulomas, is essential for safe, complication-free decannulation. Most children tolerate decannulation well; however, approximately 10% of infants with tracheostomies that have been in place for more than 1 year have significant cricoid collapse or severe peristomal tracheomalacia (20).

Sequential tracheal tube downsizing and operative stomal closure are commonly performed decannulation techniques. In uncomplicated cases, the tracheostomy tube is gradually downsized over several days to weeks. When a sufficiently small tube is in place, it is capped. If the child is able to tolerate this procedure, decannulation can be performed and an occlusive Vaseline gauze bandage applied to the stoma site. The stoma usually closes spontaneously over several days. If a persistent fistula occurs, operative primary closure can be performed (21).

An alternative one-stage operative procedure can be used to close the tracheocutaneous fistula and alleviate the cricoid collapse (20). With the child under orotracheal general anesthesia, the tracheostomy stoma is excised in a horizontal ellipse down to the tracheal wall, and scarred peristomal skin and subcutaneous tissue is removed. A small portion (1 mm) of the tracheal opening is circumferentially excised, along with any peristomal tracheal granulation tissue. The tracheal opening is then closed transversely with interrupted absorbable 4-0 or 5-0 monofilament sutures. The anterior cricoid suspension is performed by the extraluminal placement of three to four absorbable 3-0 monofilament sutures from the adherent tissue overlying the anterior trachea and cricoid ring through the musculofascial insertions of the cervical strap muscles adjacent to the sternum. Once tied, these sutures significantly elevate the anterior cricoid and peristomal trachea by pulling the airway ventrally and inferiorly. The strap muscles cover the tracheal suture line, and the skin and soft tissue are closed in a transverse fashion. Most patients can be extubated in the immediate perioperative period.

AIRWAY FOREIGN BODIES

Airway obstruction due to aspirated foreign bodies is common and potentially fatal, and is the fourth leading cause of accidental deaths (8%) in the under 5 age group in the United States (22). Approximately 15% of pediatric aspirations occur without an adult witness. Although foreign-body aspiration can occur at any age, approximately 90% of patients are younger than age 4 and two-thirds of patients are boys (23). Because children at this age do not have molars, they are unable to adequately chew on small, smooth, round, or hard food items. Hence nuts, particularly peanuts, account for more than one-half of all aspirated objects. Pieces of hard carrot, seeds, popcorn, and an array of toys and other small objects also put children at high risk. Aspirated foreign bodies may lie anywhere from the larynx to the lungs. The bronchi are the most common site, with the right main bronchi being the more common because its less angular orientation allows objects to enter it more easily. Foreign bodies may be mobile within the airway, thus causing varying degrees of obstruction.

The signs and symptoms of aspiration are variable, and may be subtle and nonspecific. Approximately 75% of the patients, however, have at least one element of the classic clinical triad of wheezing, coughing, and diminished or absent breath sounds (11). Although the sudden onset of coughing may be the only identifiable event, fever, sputum production, hemoptysis, and vomiting are also seen. Due to physiologic adaptation by sensory receptors in the respiratory tract, some patients may be asymptomatic by the time they present at a medical facility, thus making the diagnosis easy to miss unless a high index of suspicion is maintained. Characteristic physical findings include the unilateral presence of decreased breath sounds because of decreased ventilation of the affected lung and/or the partial occlusion of a main or lobar bronchus.

Radiographic Imaging

When case history and physical examination indicate possible foreign-body aspiration, inspiration and expiration chest films should be obtained. Because approximately 10% of aspirated foreign bodies are radiopaque, the signs of these films are usually the secondary results of airway obstruction rather than actual visualization of the foreign body. Thus, in most patients, indirect findings secondary to unilateral obstruction of the airway are required to make the diagnosis. Unilateral emphysema with air trapping secondary to a high-grade partial occlusion of the main bronchus is the classic radiographic finding (Fig. 59-4A). In patients with this finding, air may enter the affected lobe or lung on inspiration. On expiration, air trapping and focal alveolar overinflation results. Chest fluoroscopy and decubitus views of the chest may also demonstrate air trapping. In some patients, total occlusion of a bronchus may produce atelectasis or pneumonic infiltrates rather than emphysema (Fig. 59-4B). It is, however, important to appreciate that when a foreign object is lodged in the larynx or the trachea, the chest radiograph and physical examination may be unremarkable (24). Moreover, migration of foreign bodies may cause changing physical and radiographic findings.

Endoscopic Foreign-body Retrieval

If a foreign body is suspected, the presence of normal physical findings and normal chest radiographs does not obviate the need for endoscopic evaluation (11). If evidence for the presence of a foreign body in the lungs is uncertain, or if the sudden onset of wheezing or pneumonia has not responded to treatment, it may be beneficial to use a flexible bronchoscope for the diagnostic airway examination, switching to a rigid bronchoscope if foreign-body removal is required (25,26). Although some clinicians have more recently advocated the selected use of the flexible bronchoscope for foreign-body retrieval as well (27), rigid bronchoscopy remains the unequivocal procedure of choice for the removal of foreign bodies in infants and children (25,26). This should be performed only by an experienced pediatric endoscopist and an anesthesiologist experienced in the care of the pediatric airway, and excellent communication must be maintained between them throughout the procedure.

If a foreign body has been lodged in the airway for more than 24 hours, a parenteral antibiotic (ampicillin or penicillin) is usually administered. Modern pediatric ventilating bronchoscopes used with a Hopkins rod lens and appropriate extraction devices, including alligator, peanut, and fine foreign-body forceps, Fogarty catheters,

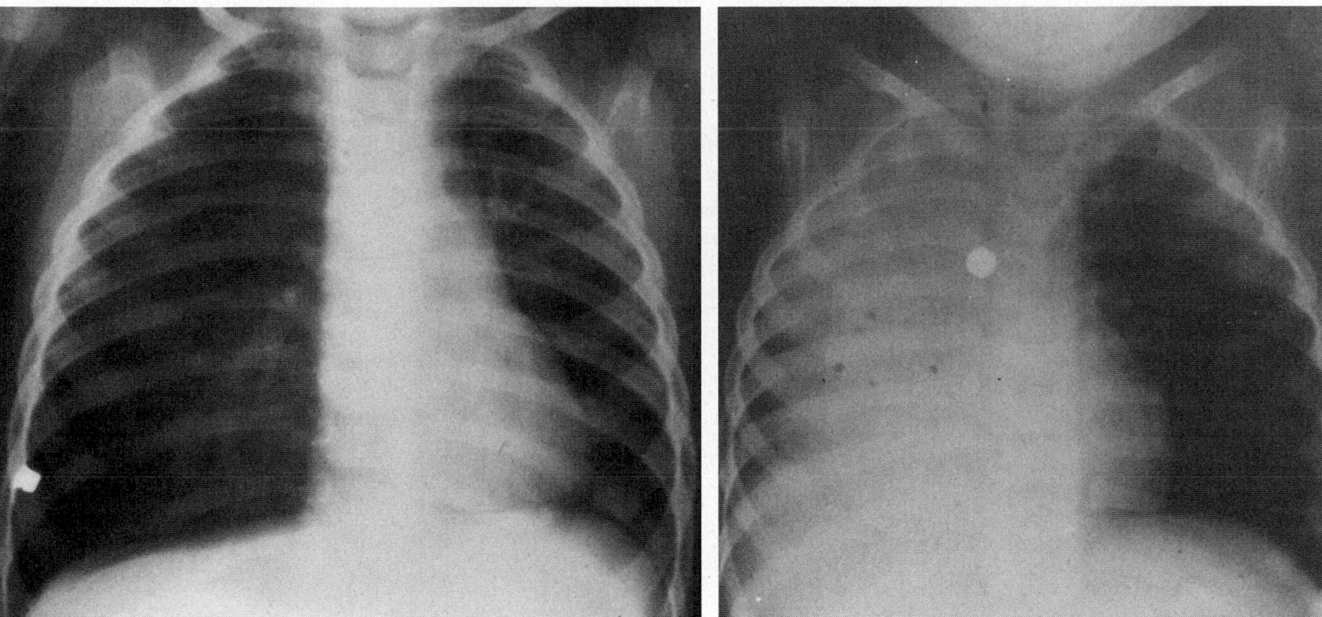

FIGURE 59-4. **(A)** Radiographic appearance of unilateral emphysema and air trapping secondary to a partial occlusion of the right main bronchus from a foreign-body aspiration. Mediastinal shift toward the contralateral hemithorax is common. **(B)** Total occlusion of the right main bronchus by a radiopaque foreign body has produced atelectasis and mediastinal shift toward the affected right side.

Dormia baskets, and other endoscopic equipment, are essential for successfully retrieving a variety of foreign bodies. Preendoscopic knowledge of the shape, size, and composition of the aspirated foreign body (i.e., toy fragments, screws, spherical objects) is extremely helpful in planning for extraction. It is also useful to practice grasping a similar or identical object *ex vivo* to ensure the instrumentation and technique are appropriate for successful extraction. Direct laryngoscopy is performed using a small laryngoscope with a straight blade. Instillation of a small amount of 1% lidocaine around the vocal cords and in the subglottis diminishes vagal reflexes during the procedure. Careful visualization of the subglottic and tracheal area is performed first. As the bronchoscope is advanced toward the carina, the foreign body is usually visualized in one of the mainstem bronchi. Prior to foreign-body extraction, the contralateral main bronchus is visualized to ensure the area is normal and free of additional foreign bodies. The type and shape of the foreign body determine which extraction instrument is most appropriate for removal. Flat foreign objects with an edge are easily extracted by forceps, whereas spherical foreign bodies such as peanuts, marbles, and round seeds may require a Fogarty catheter, peanut forceps, or a Dormia basket. The use of optical telescopic forceps has improved the visualization and removal of certain foreign bodies (Fig. 59-5) (11).

Once a foreign body has been grasped, the endoscopist generally manipulates the foreign body to the tip of the bronchoscope. The bronchoscope forceps and foreign body are then removed as a single unit. The surgeon carefully watches the extraction procedure to ensure the foreign body does not fall back into the airway. Occasionally, the foreign body is dislodged as it comes through the vocal cords and may lodge in back of the pharynx or in the piriform sinuses. Direct laryngoscopy with the use of McGill forceps is usually successful in removing the foreign body from these areas.

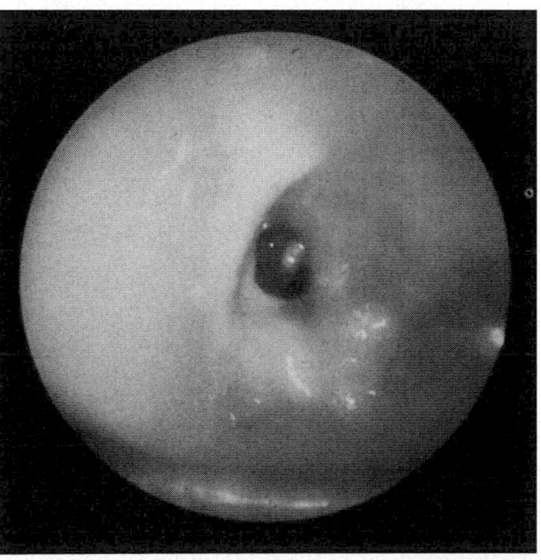

FIGURE 59-5. Metallic foreign body lodged in the bronchus intermedius as seen through a rigid bronchoscope using a Hopkins lens system.

In selected cases, the complementary use of the flexible bronchoscope can be very helpful. Foreign bodies occasionally migrate to a more distal segmental bronchus, beyond the reach of a rigid bronchoscope. The flexible bronchoscope can be passed through the ventilating bronchoscope to guide the passage of a 2F or 3F Fogarty catheter or a Dormia basket (11). In older children, examination of airways distal to the range of the rigid bronchoscope may reveal small foreign bodies not otherwise seen. Flexible instrumentation has also proved useful when follow-up examinations of patients who have had a foreign body removed earlier are necessary.

At the completion of the procedure, a repeat endoscopy is performed to rule out the presence of other foreign bodies or retained fragments, and bacterial cultures are obtained from the affected bronchus. In patients who have had vegetable material impacted in a main bronchus, an area of inflamed mucosa with granulation tissue is often present. This tissue usually contracts and heals once the foreign body has been extracted. Fulguration is generally not needed. Purulent secretions obstructing a main bronchus following extraction of a foreign body should be carefully suctioned and sent for appropriate microbiologic cultures.

Following endoscopic removal of foreign bodies, most infants and children experience hoarseness from edema of the vocal cords and the subglottic region, which typically resolves in 24 to 48 hours. Patients are usually placed on humidified oxygen and are closely monitored. They must remain well hydrated and occasionally require racemic epinephrine and bronchodilators. Chest physiotherapy and postural drainage may also be helpful in clearing purulent secretions from affected lobes. Following bronchoscopy, a chest radiograph is obtained. If symptoms persist after 1 week of intensive physiotherapy and antibiotics, another bronchoscopy may be required. Abnormalities seen on radiographs occasionally persist and are an indication for repeat endoscopy.

Operative Retrieval

Rarely, a foreign body may need to be extracted by a thoracotomy and bronchotomy, or even a lobectomy. When it is too large to be brought through the vocal cords, a tracheotomy should be performed over the bronchoscope and the foreign body removed in that fashion. Decannulation can be accomplished within 48 hours if the airway is otherwise normal. A foreign body that has been impacted for weeks is typically surrounded by dense inflammation and granulation tissue. In some patients, bronchiectasis and abscess formation may have occurred. Occasionally, a history of hemoptysis has been present. Such a history should alert the surgeon to the possibility of massive hemorrhage during foreign-body removal. These patients sometimes require segmental lung resection or lobectomy.

TRACHEAL ANOMALIES

Congenital Tracheal Stenosis (Complete Tracheal Rings)

Stenosis of the trachea is a rare condition in which either the trachea alone or both the trachea and bronchi are narrowed. The seriousness of this anomaly depends on the degree and extent of the narrowing. Although the etiologies of most congenital airway obstructions are unknown, one theory is that they are caused by interference with tracheobronchial organogenesis by teratogens, embryonic vascular accidents, or genetic or other environmental stresses at a critical stage of airway development (3). The different forms of tracheal stenosis, especially funnel-like stenosis or generalized tracheal hypoplasia, represent failure of normal growth and development. In more than 50% of infants with tracheal stenosis, a segmental stenosis is found. In such patients, the cartilaginous rings are abnormal in shape and form complete rings (28). The clinical manifestations of congenital tracheal stenosis vary from life-threatening respiratory distress at birth to subtle symptoms of airway compromise in older children. The most significant symptoms are pathologic airway sounds, including expiratory and inspiratory stridor, cough, and alterations of cry. Other signs and symptoms include atypical and persistent wheezing and rhonchi, respiratory distress, and sudden death. A wide spectrum of associated anomalies is seen, the most common of which are esophageal, cardiac, skeletal, and genitourinary anomalies.

In some patients, placing an endotracheal tube into the airway may exacerbate respiratory distress by causing acute swelling and inflammation. Partially obstructing congenital lesions of the trachea or distal airway may also become life threatening after the onset of a respiratory infection. In an infant or child with an abnormal trachea, the cross-sectional area of the airway can be decreased by one-third to one-half of its normal diameter with as little as 1 mm of edema. This accounts for the rapid progression of symptoms in some children who have acute inflammatory conditions superimposed on preexisting tracheal narrowing.

Diagnostic Evaluation

Expeditious diagnostic evaluation to define aberrant and normal tracheobronchial anatomy is required following the onset of airway symptoms. Although careful radiologic studies can provide significant clues as to the location of the obstruction, the precise location and extent of tracheal narrowing is now best achieved by endoscopic techniques (11,29).

Anteroposterior and lateral high-contrast radiographs (high kV) and fluoroscopy can provide a reasonably accurate assessment of the child's airway (Fig. 59-6). Computed

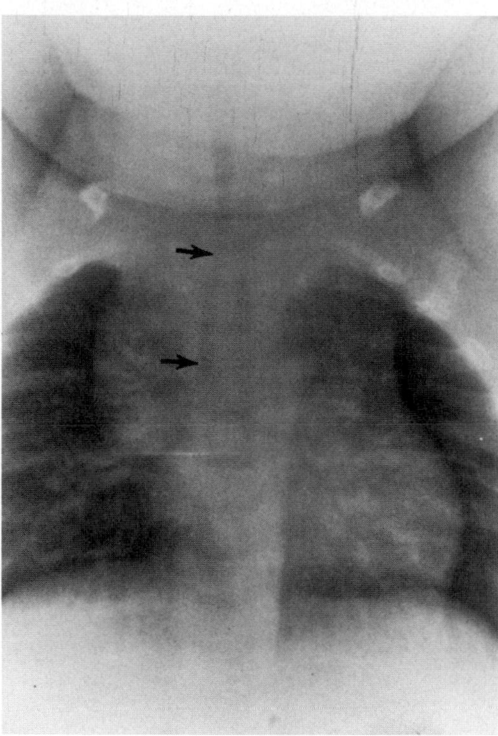

FIGURE 59-6. Chest radiograph demonstrating cervical and mediastinal tracheal stenosis in 4-month-old *(arrows)*.

tomography (CT) scans provide a rapid and more precise method of measuring the extent and length of airway narrowing or displacement. Visualization of the anatomic relationship between the airways and surrounding structures (e.g., the great vessels) can be enhanced with intravascular contrast. Three-dimensional image reconstruction is also possible with newer computer software and is helpful in planning surgical reconstruction. Magnetic resonance imaging (MRI) has the intrinsic advantage of not using ionizing radiation and is also useful in some patients. Unfortunately, however, the images take longer to obtain and are thus more prone to artifacts related to patient motion.

Bronchography is generally avoided because of the associated risk of sudden airway obstruction. The barium esophagogram is a useful preliminary study to look for evidence of esophageal and airway compression caused by a vascular lesion. Echocardiography and angiography may be indicated for suspected vascular ring or pulmonary artery sling abnormalities. Fifty percent of children with congenital tracheal stenosis have associated aortic and pulmonary artery vascular abnormalities, which must be identified prior to tracheal reconstruction. In older children, pulmonary function studies include inspiratory-expiratory flow volume curves to provide information regarding tracheal air movement. Most patients with these lesions are, however, too young for this to be helpful.

Operative Management

Tracheal Resection

The management of tracheal stenosis must be individualized, and depends on the extent of the pathologic process, the site of the lesion, and the age of the patient (Fig. 59-7). Several repair techniques have been used with varying success (30–33). Segmental tracheal resection with end-to-end anastomosis is considered the treatment of choice for short-segment tracheal stenosis secondary to complete tracheal rings (30). Segmental resection beyond five rings is generally possible only with bilateral release of the pulmonary hila through the pericardium.

Although laryngeal release is used in adults undergoing extensive tracheal resection to decrease anastomotic tension, this approach is avoided in children due to the high incidence of dysphasia and aspiration.

Several surgical principles govern the technical aspects of tracheal reconstruction. The trachea can be readily exposed from the cricoid to the carina through a sternotomy incision. Preserving the lateral blood vessels to the trachea is critical, and circumferential dissection is therefore limited to approximately 1 to 2 cm proximal and distal to the stenosis. To avoid recurrent laryngeal nerve injury, posterior and lateral dissections should be adjacent to the tracheal wall. The trachea should be divided as close as possible to the stenosis, leaving good cartilaginous rings both proximally and distally for the anastomosis. Insufficient excision of the stenosis leads to a prompt recurrence. Ventilation can be maintained through a separate anesthesia circuit or through translaryngeal jet cannulas placed through the endotracheal tube and past the area of resection into each main bronchus (33). Once the anastomosis is complete, the jet cannulas or distal circuit can be removed and the translaryngeal endotracheal tube can be advanced across the anastomotic site for postoperative ventilation management. Using this approach avoids tracheostomy. Alternative resection techniques for stenosis exceeding 50% of the length of the trachea are described as follows.

Patch Tracheoplasty

Anterior patch tracheoplasty usually involves incising the length of the tracheal stricture by interpositioning a supporting tissue, such as cartilage graft, dura, or pericardium, to enlarge the tracheal lumen (31,32). Although posterior incision of the tracheal rings has also been attempted with sutured interposition of the anterior wall of the esophagus to fill the gap, only one of three patients known to have had this procedure has survived long term (29).

The first successful reconstruction of subtotal tracheal stenosis with complete tracheal rings using patch tracheoplasty was reported in a 12-month-old infant in 1982 (32). Since that time, other patients have undergone

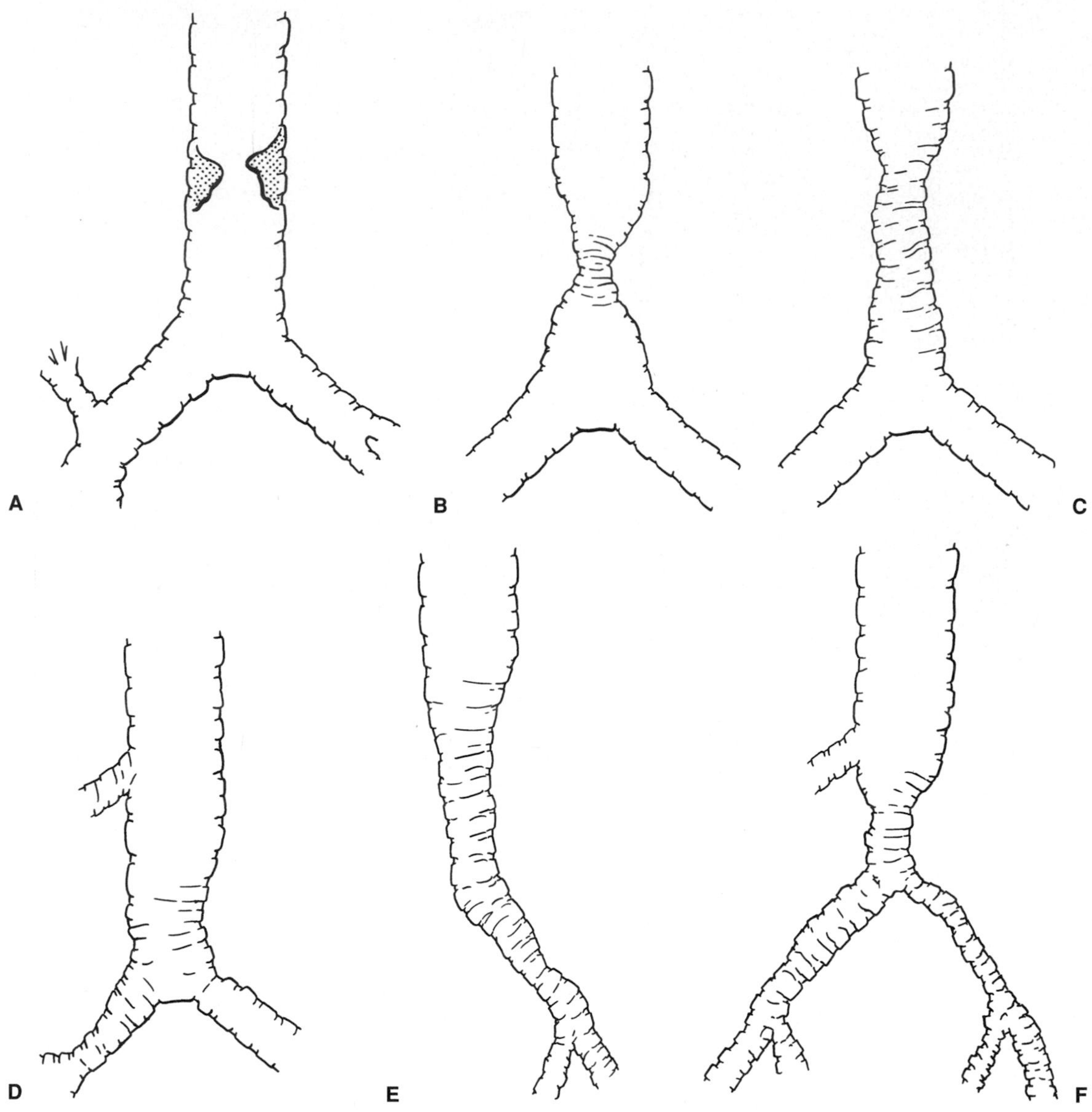

FIGURE 59-7. Variety of anatomic abnormalities of the trachea are seen in children with complete tracheal rings. Some of the possibilities are illustrated.

successful reconstruction with either cartilage or pericardial graft techniques (Fig. 59-8). Intraoperative airway control has been successfully managed with conventional and high-frequency jet ventilation or cardiopulmonary bypass (31,33). In some patients, postoperative symptoms of airway collapse have been minimized by suspending a cartilage graft from the innominate artery. The cartilage graft can be sealed with a vascularized pedicle of pericardium. An additional technique includes a partial tracheal resection, posterior end-to-end anastomosis, and anterior patching of the stenotic trachea with the opened resected trachea, a free tracheal autograft (34,35).

Slide Tracheoplasty

Developed more recently (35,36), slide tracheoplasty is currently the procedure of choice at our institution for long segments of tracheal involvement. The procedure uses only autologous tracheal tissue and is performed by transecting the trachea into two equal segments. The anterior wall of the lower half of the trachea and the posterior wall of the upper trachea are incised. These segments are then slid over each other and anastomosed with 5-0 monofilament and absorbable sutures (Fig. 59-9). The postoperative airway has four times the cross-sectional area and one-half the length of its previous dimension. The survival rate is greater than 80% and complications have been

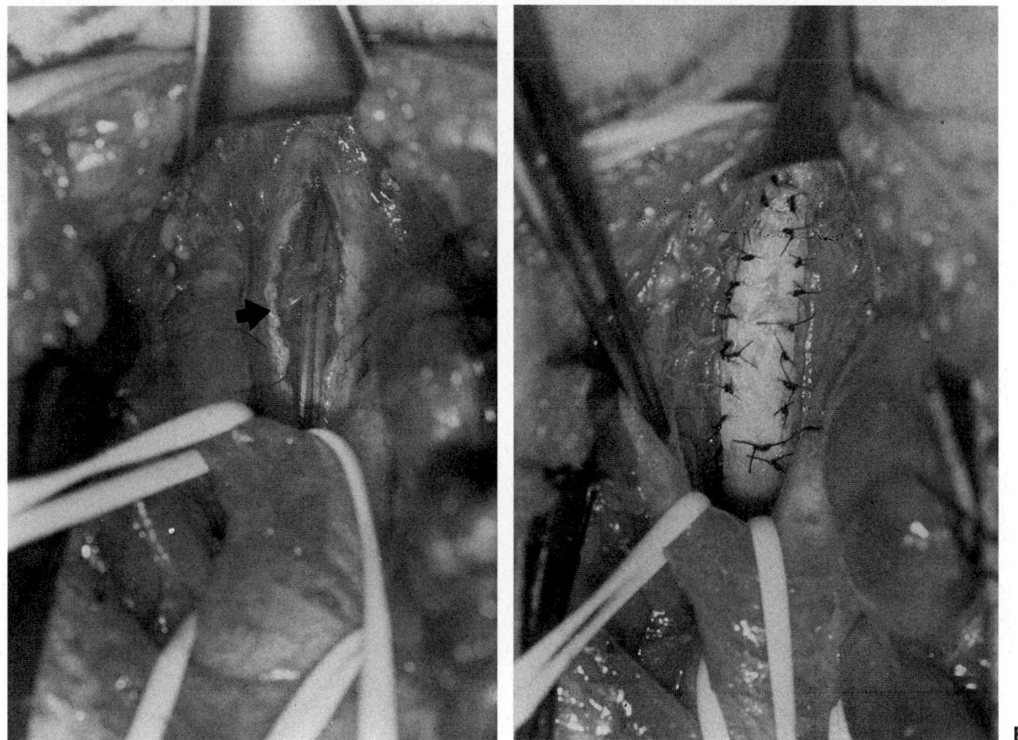

FIGURE 59-8. **(A)** Operative view of the opened trachea in an infant with tracheal stenosis from complete tracheal rings. Note the endotracheal tube with two jet ventilation cannulas that have been positioned into each main bronchus. **(B)** A patch tracheoplasty with autogenous cartilage graft was sutured in place.

considerably less than generally seen with patch tracheoplasty (36). Moreover, early results for continued tracheal growth are encouraging.

Balloon Dilatation

Balloon dilatation as a definitive treatment of long-segment tracheal stenosis remains a controversial and unproven technique, with only a limited number of published case reports and variable results (37). In a relatively recent case report (38), investigators used intraluminal balloon dilatation coupled with an expandable metallic stent in five infants. Although four of the five survived, the long-term effects are unknown.

Complications and Postoperative Management

Following reconstructive tracheal surgery, infants require endotracheal intubation for several days to 2 weeks. Although airway edema can cause obstruction in the perioperative period, the endotracheal tube acts as a stent, keeping the airway open and facilitating repair and healing of the reconstructed trachea. Nasotracheal intubation is used preferentially because the endotracheal tube can be stabilized in position more securely. To minimize the risk of damage to the newly reconstructed airway, unnecessary movements of the endotracheal tube or unplanned extubation must be avoided. For patients who have undergone extensive resection, a molded prosthetic brace to maintain head and neck flexion is recommended. Patients require continuous monitoring, careful pulmonary toilet, and endoscopic removal of any obstructing granulation tissue. Flexible fiberoptic endoscopy may be required through the endotracheal tube prior to extubation, and granulation tissue at the suture line may need to be endoscopically ablated using a KTP or Argon laser (28).

The selective and judicious use of steroids is primarily supported by anecdotal experiences. Although the use of systemic steroids or intralesional steroid injections to prevent local inflammation and edema remains controversial, a short course of high-dose steroids can significantly reduce postoperative edema of the airway and glottis. Also, in some patients, steroid administration dramatically improves abundant granulation tissue and associated inflammation within the airway.

Recurrent tracheal stenosis following tracheoplasty has been successfully treated with balloon dilatation (39).

Future Directions

Tracheal transplants using glutaraldehyde-treated homographs are now in the initial stages of clinical investigation

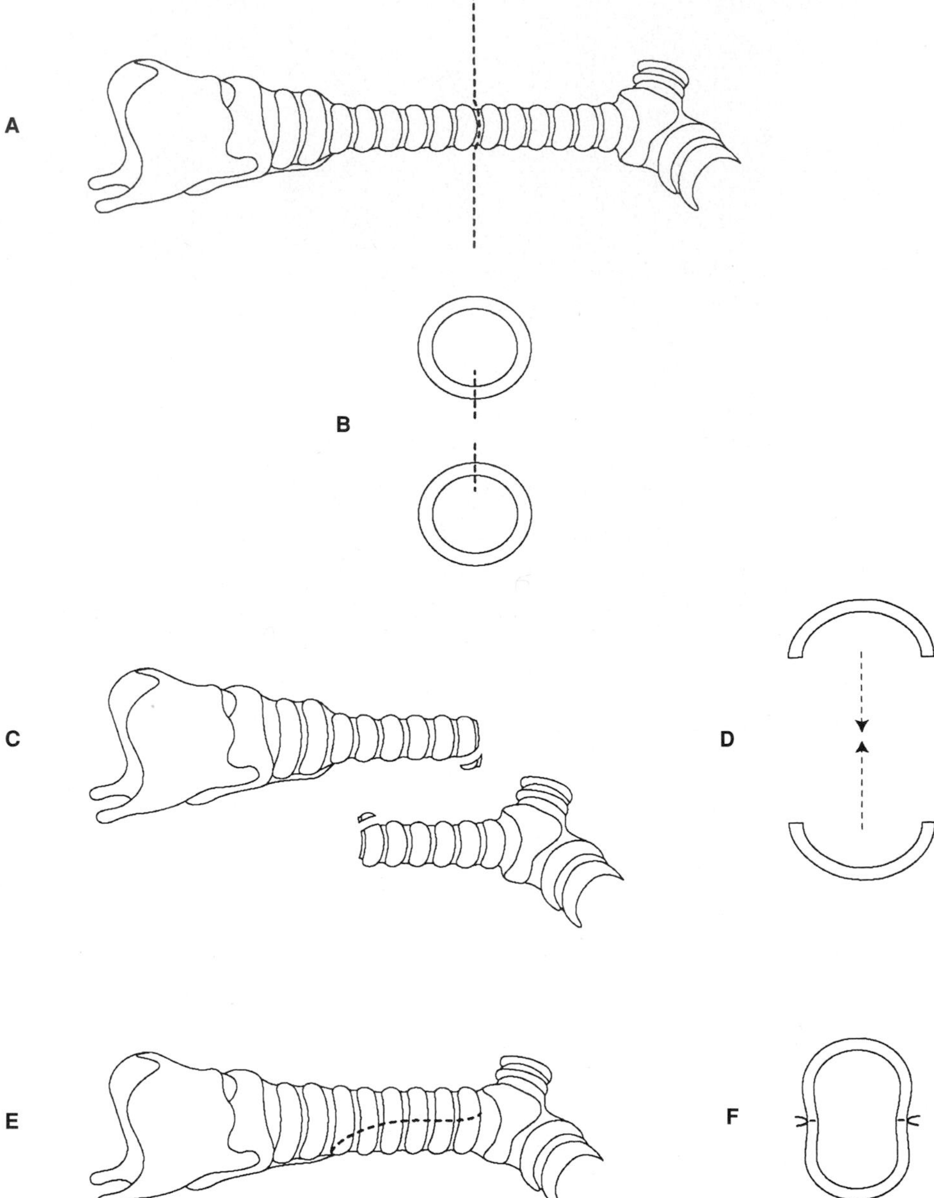

FIGURE 59-9. Schematic depicting salient features of a slide tracheoplasty in a child with lengthy tracheal stenosis. **(A)** The stenotic trachea is divided at the midpoint of the segment of complete rings. Each end of the transected trachea is mobilized by dissection, anterior and posterior. Care is taken during this dissection to preserve the lateral vascular attachments to the trachea. **(B)** The posterior wall of the proximal segment of rings is then incised until normal trachea is reached. The anterior wall of the distal segment is incised until normal rings or the carina are encountered. **(C)** Cartilage is trimmed off corners of the proximal and distal segments. **(D)** The proximal and distal tracheal segments are slid over each other. **(E)** The anastomosis is performed with a running 5.0 or 6.0 double-armed polydioxanone (PDS) suture, with a single knot securing the repair distally, well away from the innominate artery. Prior to final closure of the anastomosis, the patient is reintubated with an age-appropriate endotracheal tube, and the tip of the tube positioned under direct visualization. The anastomosis is then leak tested and further sealed with fibrin glue. The proximal and distal extent of the anastomosis is marked with small hemoclips to help identify the extent of the anastomosis on postoperative radiographs. **(F)** The airway cross-sectional area is doubled following the procedure in this illustration.

at several medical centers across the United States. In the future, biotracheal prostheses created through tissue engineering may be used to replace an absent trachea or missing portions of the airway (40).

Tracheal Diverticulum and Tracheal Bronchus

Anomalies of tracheal budding are relatively common. They occur during the third and fourth gestational weeks, when the trachea bifurcates and differentiates. Tracheal diverticula resemble a bronchus, but typically originate from the trachea and end blindly or communicate with a rudimentary lung. Tracheal bronchi most commonly affect the right upper lobe bronchus and may connect to an isolated intrathoracic lung segment or to the apical segment of an upper lobe. Most patients with tracheal diverticula or bronchi are asymptomatic and may not require treatment. In contrast, patients who are symptomatic generally experience symptoms such as pneumonia and respiratory distress in the neonatal period. In addition, they have an associated stenosis of the bronchus or other lung anomaly. Resection in these patients is usually curative. Clinicians must also be aware of a variety of other associated congenital anomalies, including dextrocardia, Down syndrome, and multiple fused ribs (41).

Tracheomalacia and Bronchomalacia

Airway malacia denotes a softening or weakening of the trachea or bronchi. Both tracheomalacia and bronchomalacia are conditions in which the structural integrity of the trachea or bronchi is diminished, and the cartilaginous rings of the airway do not have sufficient rigidity to prevent airway collapse during expiration. Malacia may occur in localized segments or diffusely throughout the airway. Although a number of etiologic explanations have been purported, one embryonic explanation is that extrinsic pressure or compression of the embryonic cartilaginous rings may cause gradual and progressive erosion of the structural elements of the airway. For example, vascular rings circumferentially entrap the trachea, preventing normal growth. In patients with vascular rings, constant pulsatile impingement may hinder normal structural development of the tracheal wall, resulting in segmental tracheomalacia. Tracheomalacia may also be idiopathic or associated with a number of conditions, including esophageal atresia or tracheoesophageal fistula, aberrant innominate artery, mediastinal masses, prolonged intubation for interstitial lung disease, or bronchopulmonary dysplasia. Children with bronchopulmonary dysplasia or chronic indwelling cuffed endotracheal or tracheostomy tubes are at particular risk for developing combined severe tracheal and bronchial malacia.

Diagnostic Evaluation

Although anteroposterior and lateral chest radiographs can show airway compression, cinefluoroscopy better demonstrates the dynamics of airway movement with tracheal expansion and collapse during inspiration and expiration. Esophageal contrast agents enhance the visualization of swallowing and define whether esophageal distention compresses the airway. Bronchoscopy, with the patient breathing spontaneously, is the best method of demonstrating dynamic distortion and compression of the trachea (Fig. 59-10) (11,19). In segmental tracheomalacia, the rigid bronchoscope can easily be passed through the region of compression. Vascular anomalies such as a vascular ring can be seen as a characteristic, pulsating compression through the tracheal wall.

Management Approaches

Most children are generally minimally symptomatic, presenting only with chronic cough or expiratory stridor on exertion, and thus do not require surgical intervention. Symptoms gradually improve and most often resolve by age 3 (42). Some children, however, experience a worsening of symptoms, including respiratory distress, severe stridor, and life-threatening events. When this occurs, more intensive medical and/or surgical intervention is required. Diffuse tracheobronchomalacia is successfully managed with prolonged positive-pressure respiratory support.

Trachael Supension (Aortopexy)

Surgery is clearly indicated when life-threatening airway obstruction and reflex apnea occur in infants with tracheomalacia. Vascular rings require division of the constricting vessels, with retraction and suspension of the vessels to ensure the tracheal lumen is no longer compressed. Infants with an aberrant innominate artery or tracheomalacia associated with esophageal atresia are treated by suturing the aortic arch and origin of the innominate artery to the underside of the sternum to suspend the anterior tracheal wall and to relieve the collapse. Although a sternal approach is effective, many prefer to approach this procedure extrapleurally through the left third interspace. The lobes of the thymus are first separated or partially

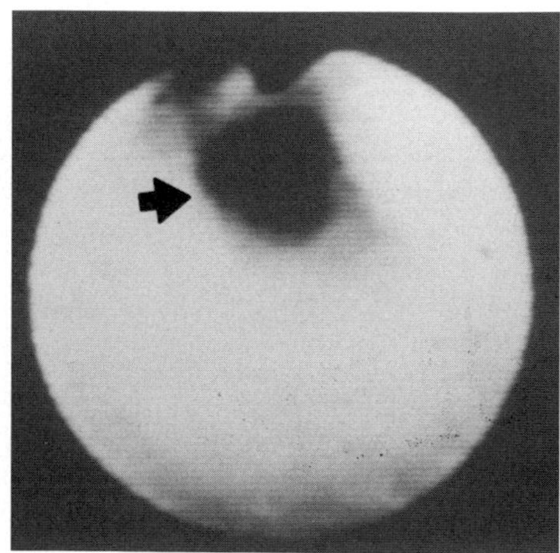
A

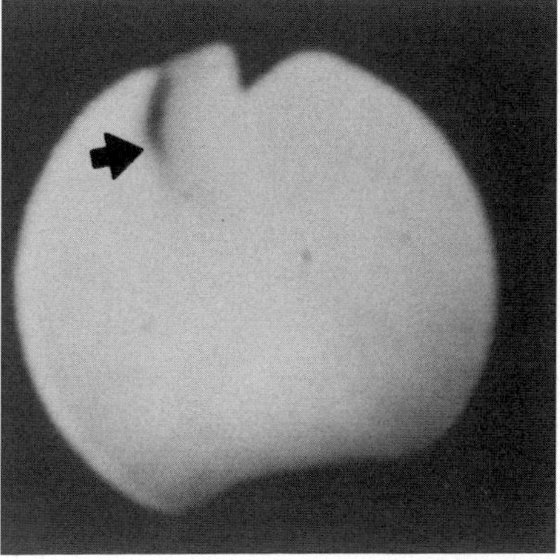
B

FIGURE 59-10. **(A)** Endoscopic view of the left main bronchus on inspiration in a child with severe tracheobronchial malacia *(arrow)*. **(B)** The same view during expiration demonstrating the collapsed airway *(arrow)*.

removed. To distribute the tension equally along the wall of the great vessels, a patch made of polytetrafluoroethylene or Dacron is first sutured to the origin of the innominate artery and the arch of the aorta with fine 5-0 nonabsorbable sutures. Additional 2-0 nonabsorbable sutures are placed from the graft through the sternum and tied on the ventral surface. Dissection between the trachea and the aorta must be avoided to prevent disrupting the connective tissue linking these two structures. Intraoperative tracheobronchoscopy is necessary to verify that the tracheal collapse has been alleviated once the suspension has been performed. Results have been excellent in more than 90% of children. Some surgeons are now performing tracheal suspension procedures using a thoracoscopic approach, and are achieving comparable results.

Endobronchial Stents

Airway stenting offers another treatment option for small children with severely problematic tracheomalacia or bronchomalacia that is unresponsive to nonoperative therapy or not suitable for surgical treatment. In addition, it is sometimes used as a complementary treatment after tracheal resection and reanastomosis or tracheoplasty have been performed. A wide variety of stents have been experimentally studied and are currently used clinically. Surgeons must be familiar with the advantages and limitations of each and be able to match the proper stent to the clinical situation at hand (43).

Because self-expanding metallic stents are large and difficult to place in the pediatric population and also put constant tension on the tracheal wall, balloon-expandable stents are preferable for relieving the airway in select cases of severe pediatric tracheomalacia and bronchomalacia in which conventional therapy has failed. These stents have the advantages of small size, accurate placement, and precise luminal diameter (42,44). Moreover, in the setting of refractory tracheomalacia or bronchomalacia, balloon-expandable stents can allow for growth and can help to avoid mechanical ventilation or tracheostomy (43). Removal of these stents is, however, not a simple procedure and not without concomitant risk. They sometimes become so incorporated into the airway wall that attempts at removal may cause tracheal tearing or major hemorrhage. Surgeons must thus be prepared to use whatever measures possible to relieve life-threatening airway compromise that might occur during stent removal (44). Because published series to date have been small and the results variable, long-term outcomes with balloon-expandable stents are difficult to assess. The primary complication associated with these stents has been granulation tissue formation over the stent. This tissue has been shown to grow numerous bacteria, including *Streptococcus viridans*, *Pseudomonas aeruginosa*, nonhemolytic streptococci, and *Staphylococcus aureus* (45). Stent technology continues to evolve, and investigations aimed at decreasing the complications associated with the currently available metallic stents are ongoing. In the future, alternative stent materials such as absorbable polytef-coated or temperature-sensitive stents may offer significant advantages.

OTHER BRONCHOPULMONARY FOREGUT ANOMALIES

Esophageal Bronchus

Bronchial connection between the esophagus and the airway is an extremely rare anomaly that is found twice as often in women as in men (46). This malformation is believed to develop from a supernumerary lung bud arising from the esophagus. Most often, a lower lobe is aerated by this ectopic bronchus, but occasionally an entire main bronchus and lung may be involved. In addition, the pulmonary vasculature may be abnormal, with the arterial supply coming off the aorta and the venous drainage going into either the systemic or pulmonary veins. These anatomic features may cloud the distinction between this anomaly and extralobar sequestration. As with other tracheoesophageal malformations, associated anomalies are common. These include cardiac, genitourinary, vertebral, and diaphragmatic defects (47).

Symptoms of recurrent pulmonary infection due to inadequate bronchial drainage usually occur early in childhood; however, associated malformations can overshadow the pulmonary manifestations of this anomaly. In rare cases, the abnormality is not discovered until adolescence or adulthood. Because of the spectrum of anatomic defects, radiographic findings of an esophageal bronchus are somewhat inconsistent. If an entire lung is involved, changes in the pulmonary parenchyma are usually identified in early infancy (48). If involvement is restricted only to isolated segments or lobes, radiographs may appear nearly normal for months or years. Collapse, consolidation, cavitation, and cyst formation within the pulmonary parenchyma are some of the typical presenting radiographic patterns. Although aggressive pulmonary toilet and antimicrobial therapy may improve the radiographic appearance, return to normal is unusual. The diagnosis is best confirmed by carefully performed contrast studies of the esophagus; however, false-negative results occasionally occur. Excision of the abnormal lung and closure of the bronchoesophageal fistula is the treatment of choice and is usually well tolerated. Prognosis depends on early diagnosis and treatment, as well as on the severity of associated anomalies.

Tracheobronchial-biliary Fistula

Congenital tracheobronchial-biliary fistulae are extremely rare, and may arise from the distal trachea or either mainstem bronchus. Virtually all children with this anomaly have significant respiratory problems in early infancy, but the cardinal symptom is bile-stained sputum. This indicates the need for bronchoscopy or bronchography in order to establish a definitive diagnosis. Surgical division of the fistulous tract is the only effective therapy for this condition (49,50).

Other bronchopulmonary foregut anomalies are discussed elsewhere in this text (see Chapter 61).

INTRALUMINAL LESIONS

Hemangiomas

Intraluminal hemangiomas are congenital vascular malformations causing inspiratory stridor and significant airway obstruction due to their critical anatomic location. Although vascular malformations can be seen anywhere within the tracheobronchial tree, the subglottic location is most common. The degree of obstruction varies and can be exacerbated by certain positions or crying, both of which increase venous pressure and lead to vascular engorgement. Most patients present in the first 6 months of life. More than one-half of these patients also have cutaneous hemangiomas, which provide a useful clue to the diagnosis. Female infants are twice as likely to be affected as males.

The diagnosis of subglottic hemangioma (SGH) is based on medical history and characteristic endoscopic findings. Lesions are typically asymmetric and may be covered by a normal smooth mucosa. Biopsy of vascular lesions is discouraged because of the risk of significant hemorrhage (11). Although spontaneous involution occurs after a proliferative growth phase, a SGH may seriously compromise the child's airway before this takes place. Most patients thus require definitive treatment. Many treatment modalities are used and often combined, depending on both the severity of airway compromise and surgeons' preferences. A number of treatment modalities have reduced the need for tracheotomy. These include intralesional or systemic corticosteroids, laser ablation, sclerosing agents, embolization, surgical procedures, interferon α-2a, and cryotherapy. The relative merits and drawbacks of each approach have been widely reported and remain controversial. Although the CO_2 laser has been widely used, a number of studies have reported that serial procedures result in a 20% incidence of posttreatment scarring and subglottic stenosis (51–53). Because the light of the KTP laser is preferentially absorbed by hemoglobin, it is currently believed by some clinicians to be more effective in vaporizing the SGH, with less destruction to overlying mucosa and normal adjacent tissue (54–55).

Tracheal Webs

Tracheal webs or stenoses that are not associated with gross deformity of the underlying cartilage may be amenable to laser treatment. Lesions in the proximal trachea can be treated with the CO_2, Argon, or KTP lasers (18,56). In contrast to the Argon and KTP lasers, however, the CO_2 laser cannot be used through small fiberoptic cables. This greatly restricts its use in the lower airways, especially in infants. Lesions in the distal trachea and bronchi of infants and small children are thus more safely and effectively treated with the Argon or KTP laser (57). Children with a stenosis longer than 1 to 2 cm or in whom the airway cartilage is either deficient or structurally abnormal may not be good candidates for laser treatment alone. Segmental tracheal resection or a cartilage interposition graft may also be necessary in these situations (29,31,32).

Bronchial Atresia

Localized bronchial atresia is a rare anomaly in which the atretic bronchus obstructs the flow of secretions and air from the distal lung to the main tracheobronchial tree. This condition may simulate lobar emphysema or a mediastinal mass. At birth the obstructed lung retains fluid, but eventually the affected lobe or segment becomes hyperaerated as air enters through the pores of Kohn (58). Patients accumulate secretions distal to the atresia, and a mucocele forms (59). Emphysema of the segment may cause compression of the normal lung tissue and may be associated with wheezing and stridor. Plain chest radiographs often demonstrate a hilar mass with radiating solid channels surrounded by hyperaerated lung. A CT chest scan may reveal a cystic central mucocele and can help differentiate bronchial atresia from a bronchogenic cyst or lobar emphysema. Children with bronchial atresia are at risk for serious pulmonary infection when entrapped secretions become infected. Although they may be asymptomatic for long intervals, resection is indicated (60).

Bronchial Stenosis

Acquired bronchial stenosis is a major cause of morbidity and mortality in infants who require prolonged intubation and respiratory support. Repeated endobronchial injury from suction catheters is a common, although preventable cause of this problem, which occurs in approximately 1% of chronically intubated infants (57,61). The Argon and KTP lasers are particularly useful for removing tracheal or endobronchial granulomas. Treatment with endoscopic-guided forceps resection, electroresection, and dilatation have had variable results.

REFERENCES

1. Holinger LD. Etiology of stridor in the neonate, infant and child. *Ann Otol Rhinol Laryngol* 1980;89:397–400.
2. Ryckman F, Rodgers BM. Obstructive airway disease in infants and children. *Surg Clin North Am* 1985;65:1663–1687.
3. Tibboel D, Kluth D. Embryology of congenital lesions of the tracheobronchial tree. In: Lobe TE, ed. *Tracheal reconstruction in infancy.* Philadelphia: WB Saunders, 1991:1–13.
4. Skandalakis JE, Gray SW, Symbas P. The trachea and the lungs. In: Skandalakis JE, Gray SW, eds. *Embryology for surgeons,* 2nd ed. Baltimore: Williams & Wilkins, 1994:414–450.
5. Holinger PH. Clinical aspects of congenital anomalies of the larynx, trachea, bronchi, and esophagus. *J Laryngol Otol* 1961;75:1–44.
6. Chytil F. Vitamin A and lung development. *Pediatr Pulmonol* 1985; S115–117.
7. Huot C, Gauthier M, Lebel M, et al. Congenital malformations associated with the maternal use of valproic acid. *Can J Neurol Sci* 1987;14:290–293.
8. Tack E, Perlman J. Tracheal stenosis. Lethal malformation in two infants of diabetic mothers. *Am J Dis Child* 1987;141:77–78.
9. Backofen JE, Rogers MC.Upper airway disease. In: Rogers MC, ed. *Textbook of pediatric intensive care.* Baltimore: Williams & Wilkins, 1987:171–197.
10. Bagwell CE, Elliot GR, Shapiro JH. Airway endoscopy and pathology. In: Ziegler MM, Azizkhan RG, Weber TR, eds. *Operative pediatric surgery.* New York: McGraw-Hill, 2003:295–305.
11. Wood RE, Azizkhan RG. Bronchoscopy and endobronchial procedures. In: Holcomb GW, ed. *Pediatric endoscopic surgery.* Norwalk, CT: Appleton & Lange, 1993:135–145.
12. Wood RE. Clinical applications of ultrathin flexible bronchoscopes. *Pediatr Pulmonol* 1985;1:244–248.
13. Wood RE, Azizkhan RG, Lacey SR, et al. Surgical applications of ultrathin flexible bronchoscopes in infants. *Ann Otol Rhinol Laryngol* 1991;100:116–119.
14. Wood RE, Gauderer MW. Flexible fiberoptic bronchoscopy in the management of tracheobronchial foreign bodies in children: the value of a combined approach with open tube bronchoscopy. *J Pediatr Surg* 1984;19:693–698.
15. Wiseman NE, Sanchez I, Powell RE. Rigid bronchoscopy in the pediatric age group: diagnostic effectiveness. *J Pediatr Surg* 1992;27:1294–1297.
16. Wood RE. Spelunking in the pediatric airways: exploration with a flexible bronchoscope. *Pediatr Clin North Am* 1984;31: 785–799.
17. Rimell FL. Pediatric laser bronchsocopy. *Int Anesthesiol Clin* 1997;35: 107–113.
18. Azizkhan RG. Lasers in pediatric surgery. *Surg Clin North Am* 1992; 72:1315–1333.
19. Johnson DG. Lesions of the larynx and trachea—tracheostomy. In: Welch KJ, Randolph JG, Ravitch MM, et al., eds. *Pediatric surgery,* 4th ed. Chicago: Year Book Medical, 1986:622–630.
20. Azizkhan RG, Lacey SR, Wood RE. Anterior cricoid suspension and tracheal stoma closure for children with cricoid collapse and peristomal tracheomalacia following tracheostomy. *J Pediatr Surg* 1993;28:169–171.
21. Pearl RH. Tracheotomy and laryngotracheal separation. In: Ziegler MM, Azizkhan RG, Weber TR, eds. *Operative pediatric surgery.* New York: Mc Graw-Hill, 2003:307–312.
22. Wagner MH. Foreign body aspiration. In: Loughlin GM, Eigen H, eds. *Respiratory disease in children: diagnosis and management.* Baltimore: Williams & Wilkins, 1994:343.
23. Blazer S, Naveh Y, Friedman A. Foreign body in the airway. *Am J Dis Child* 1980;134:68–71.
24. Johnson DG. Bronchoscopy. In: Welch KJ, Randolph JG, Ravitch MM, et al., eds. *Pediatric surgery,* 4th ed. Chicago: Year Book Medical, 1986:619–622.
25. Martinot A, Closset M, Marquette CH, et al. Indications for flexible versus rigid bronchoscopy in children with suspected foreign body aspiration. *Respir Crit Care Med* 1997;155: 1696–1699.
26. Godfrey S, Avital A, Maayan C, et al. Yield from flexible bronchoscopy in children. *Pediatr Pulmonol* 1997;23:261–269.
27. Swanson KL, Prakash UB, Midthun DE, et al. Flexible bronchoscopic management of airway foreign bodies in children. *Chest* 2002;121:1695–1700.
28. Lobe TE, Hayden CK, Nicholas D, et al. Successful management of congenital tracheal stenosis in infancy. *J Pediatr Surg* 1987;22:1137–1142.
29. Lobe TE. Operative technique and considerations for the reconstruction of congenital stenoses of the trachea in infants. In: Lobe TE, ed. *Tracheal reconstruction in infancy.* Philadelphia: WB Saunders, 1991:79–101.
30. Grillo HC, Zannini P. Management of obstructing tracheal disease in children. *J Pediatr Surg* 1984;19:414–416.
31. Idriss FS, DeLeon SY, Ilbawi MN, et al. Tracheoplasty with pericardial patch for extensive tracheal stenosis in infants and children. *J Thorac Cardiovasc Surg* 1984;88:527–536.
32. Kimura K, Mukohara N, Tsugawa C, et al. Tracheoplasty for congenital stenosis of the entire trachea. *J Pediatr Surg* 1982;17:869–871.
33. Schur MS, Maccioli GA, Azizkhan RG, et al. High frequency jet ventilation in the management of congenital tracheal stenosis. *Anesthesiology* 1988;68:952–955.
34. Backer CL, Mavroudis C, Dunham ME, et al. Repair of congenital tracheal stenosis with a free tracheal autograft. *J Thorac Cardiovasc Surg* 1998;115:869–874.
35. Grillo HC. Slide tracheoplasty for long-segment congenital tracheal stenosis. *Ann Thorac Surg* 1994;58:613–621.
36. Rutter MJ, Manning P, Azizkhan RG, et al. Slide tracheoplasty for the management of complete tracheal rings. *J Pediatr Surg* 2003;38:928–934.
37. Bagwell CE, Talbert JL, Tepas JJ III. Balloon dilatation of long-segment tracheal stenoses. *J Pediatr Surg* 1991;26:153–159.
38. Maeda K, Yasufuku M, Yamamoto T. A new approach to the treatment of congenital tracheal stenosis: balloon tracheoplasty and expandable metallic stenting. *J Pediatr Surg* 2001;36:1646–1649.
39. Philippart AI, Long JA, Greenholz SK. Balloon dilatation of postoperative tracheal stenosis. *J Pediatr Surg* 1988;23:1178–1179.
40. Vacanti CA, Paige KT, Kim WS, et al. Experimental tracheal replacement using tissue-engineered cartilage. *J Pediatr Surg* 1994;29:201–204.
41. McLaughlin FJ, Streider DJ, Harris GB, et al. Tracheal bronchus: associations with respiratory morbidity in childhood. *J Pediatr* 1985;106:751–755.
42. Furman RH, Backer CL, Dunham ME, et al. The use of balloon-expandable metallic stents in the treatment of pediatric tracheomalacia and bronchomalacia. *Arch Otolaryngol Head Neck Surg* 1999;125:203–207.
43. Jacobs JP, Quintessenza JA, Botero LM, et al. The role of airway stents in the management of pediatric tracheal, carinal, and bronchial disease. *Eur J Cardiothorac Surg* 2000;18:505–512.
44. Filler RM, Forte V, Chait P. Tracheobronchial stenting for the treatment of airway obstruction. *J Pediatr Surg* 1998;33:304–311.
45. Matt BH, Myer CM, Harrison CJ, et al. Tracheal granulation tissue. A study of bacteriology. *Arch Otolaryngol Head Neck Surg* 1991;117:538–541.
46. John S, Gopinath N, McPhall C. Congenital esophagobronchial fistula. *Br J Surg* 1965;52:941–943.
47. Toyama W. Esophageal atresia and tracheoesophageal fistula in association with bronchial and pulmonary abnormalities. *J Pediatr Surg* 1972;7:302–307.
48. Hanna EA. Broncho-esophageal fistula with total sequestration of the right lung. *Ann Surg* 1964;159:599–603.
49. Kalayoglu M, Olcay I. Congenital bronchobiliary fistula associated with esophageal atresia and tracheoesophageal fistula. *J Pediatr Surg* 1976;11:463–464.
50. Sane SM, Sieber WK, Girdany BR. Congenital bronchobiliary fistula. *Surgery* 1971;69:599–608.
51. Sie K, McGill T, Healy GB. Subglottic hemangioma: ten years' experience with the carbon dioxide laser. *Ann Otol Rhinol Laryngol* 1994;103:167–172.
52. Benjamin B, Carter P. Congenital laryngeal hemangioma. *Ann Otol Rhinol Laryngol* 1983;92:448–455.
53. Cotton RT, Tewfik TL. Laryngeal stenosis following carbon dioxide laser in subglottic hemangioma. *Ann Otol Rhinol Laryngol* 1985;104:494–497.

54. Madgy D, Ahsan SF, Kest D, et al. The application of the potassium-titanyl-phosphate (KTP) laser in the management of subglottic hemangioma. *Arch Otolaryngol Head Neck Surg* 2001;127:47–50.
55. Kacker A, April M, Ward RF. Use of potassium titanyl phosphate (KTP) laser in management of subglottic hemangiomas. *Int J Pediatr Otorhinolaryngol* 2001;59:15–21.
56. Bagwell CE. CO_2 laser excision of pediatric airway lesions. *J Pediatr Surg* 1990;25:1152–1156.
57. Azizkhan RG, Lacey SR, Wood RE. Acquired symptomatic bronchial stenosis in infants: successful management utilizing an argon laser. *J Pediatr Surg* 1990;25:19–24.
58. Schuster SR, Harris G, Williams A, et al. Bronchial atresia: a recognizable entity in the pediatric age group. *J Pediatr Surg* 1978;13:682–689.
59. Oh KS, Dorst JP, White JJ. Syndrome of bronchial atresia or stenosis with mucocele and focal hyperinflation of the lung. *Johns Hopkins Med J* 1976;138:48–53.
60. Haller JA, Tepas JJ, White JJ, et al. The natural history of bronchial atresia: serial observations of a case from birth to operative correction. *J Thorac Cardiovasc Surg* 1980;79:868–872.
61. Greenholz SK, Hall RJ, Lilly JR, et al. Surgical implications of bronchopulmonary dysplasia. *J Pediatr Surg* 1987;22:1132–1136.

Chapter 60

Mediastinum and Pleura

Bradley M. Rodgers and Eugene D. McGahren, III

THORACIC EMBRYOLOGY

Most of the important embryologic events in the development of the thorax are completed by the eighth or ninth week of gestation. The thoracic cavity fully separates from the abdominal cavity by closure of the pleuroperitoneal folds of the diaphragm during the eighth week of gestation (1). Failure of complete closure results in congenital diaphragmatic hernia. Diaphragmatic muscularization occurs principally by the ingrowth of muscle from the lateral chest wall. Arrest of this process may produce anomalies such as congenital eventration of the diaphragm. The paired pleural cavities begin to form by the invagination of the lung buds into the paired pericardioperitoneal canals, connecting the primitive pericardial and peritoneal cavities. The pleural cavities are isolated by the development of the pleuropericardial and pleuroperitoneal membranes, a process completed by the sixth week of gestation (2) (Fig. 60-1). During the sixth week of development, the lateral thoracic wall begins to form by extensions of the lateral vertebral processes, which form the ribs. During this same interval, the sternum forms anteriorly as a pair of bands of condensed mesenchyme. By the seventh week, these sternal bands begin to fuse cranially, displacing the heart caudally. Fusion of the sternum and its junction with the developing ribs is complete by the ninth week of gestation (3). Abnormalities of development at this stage may result in sternal clefts and complex abnormalities of chest wall development, such as Poland syndrome.

During the third week of gestation, the laryngotracheal groove forms at the cranial end of the foregut, giving rise to the primitive trachea. At the same time, proliferation of mesenchyme of the foregut mesentery leads to the development of the cartilage, muscle, and connective tissue of the lungs. By the fourth week of gestation, the elongating trachea has bifurcated into right and left mainstem bronchi, and by the sixteenth week, segmental bronchi have begun to form (4). Abnormalities of this segmentation may lead to forms of pulmonary agenesis or tracheal branching abnormalities, such as bronchogenic cysts. The close timing of parallel embryologic events occurring in the trachea and the esophagus during this interval often leads to complementary abnormalities in these two structures, such as tracheoesophageal fistula.

The pulmonary arteries begin as a capillary network extending caudally from the aortic sac. By the sixth week of gestation, there are bilateral sixth aortic arches carrying blood to the developing pulmonary mesenchyme. By the seventh week the right arch has involuted, leaving the left sixth arch, which is the primordium of the main pulmonary artery. Abnormalities occurring during this interval may lead to defects of pulmonary vascular development, such as pulmonary sequestration. The details of bronchopulmonary development are outlined in greater detail in Chapter 61.

Between the sixth and eighth weeks of gestation, the jugular lymphatic sacs are connected with the cisterna chyli through bilateral systems of thoracic lymphatic channels, which are interconnected by numerous branches (5). The inferior portion of the right channel and the superior portion of the left, together with a diagonal channel at the level of the fourth thoracic vertebra, persist to form the definitive thoracic duct by the ninth week of gestation. Abnormalities of this process explain the high incidence of anatomic variation of the thoracic duct system. The thymus arises from the third pharyngeal pouch in the fifth week of gestation. Between the seventh and eighth week, the thymus elongates caudally until, by the end of the eighth week, the left and right primordia have fused at the level of the aortic arch (6). By the end of the ninth week, the mesenchyme of the thymus begins to be populated with lymphoid cells, probably of systemic origin.

Bradley M. Rodgers and Eugene D. McGahren, III: Department of Surgery, University of Virginia Health System, Charlottesville, Virginia 22906.

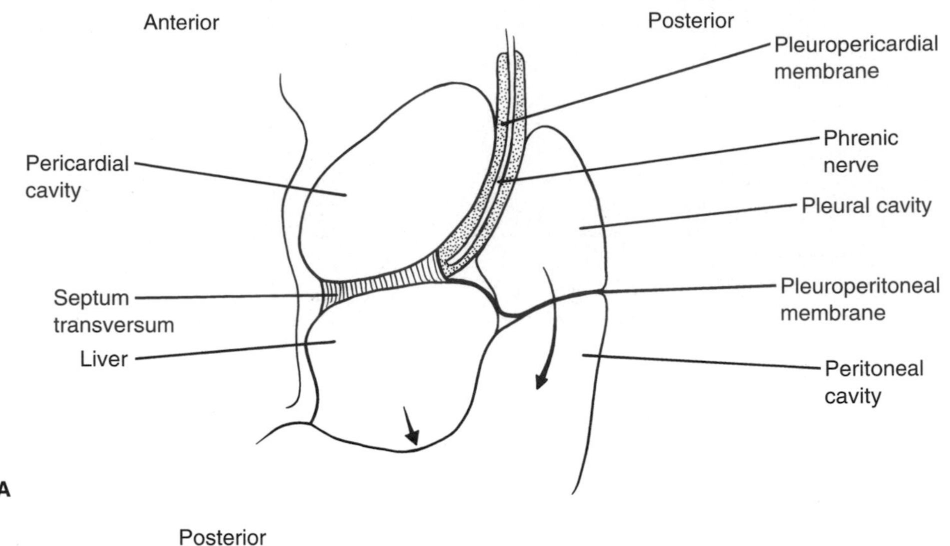

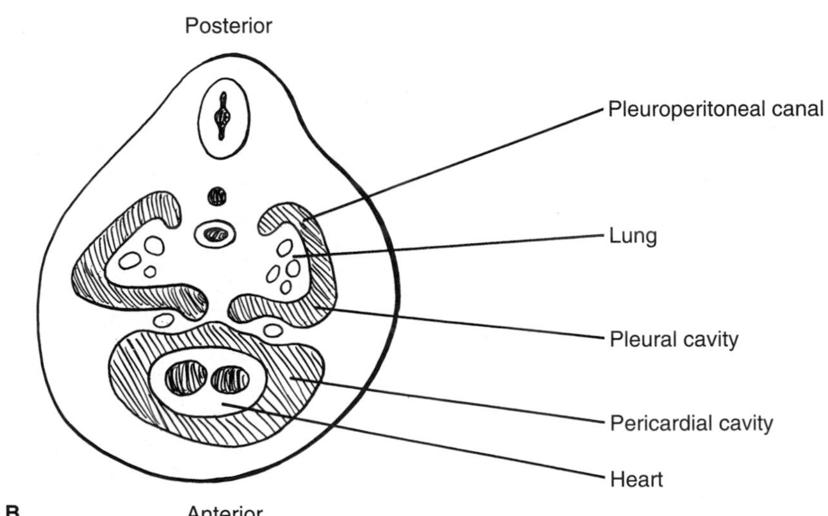

FIGURE 60-1. Formation of the pleural cavities. The pleura are separated from the pericardial cavity by the formation of the pleuropericardial membrane. The phrenic nerve descends through this membrane to meet the septum transversum, a major component of the diaphragm. The final step in isolation of the pleural cavities is completion of the pleuroperitoneal membrane with obliteration of the pleuroperitoneal canal. The lung buds project laterally into the pleural cavities, forming the separate visceral and parietal pleuras. (Adapted from O'Rahilly R, Müller F. *Human embryology and teratology*. New York: Wiley Liss, 1992;172.)

POSTNATAL THORACIC DEVELOPMENT

Structurally, the chest and mediastinum are almost fully developed at the time of birth; however, a few changes take place later. The first and most dramatic change is the shift from fetal to adult circulation. During the infant's first breaths, the pulmonary vascular resistance falls dramatically. This allows the pulmonary vasculature to accept the entire cardiac output, thereby facilitating closure of various fetal shunts, particularly the foramen ovale and the ductus arteriosus. The ductus functionally closes shortly after birth through contraction of its muscular wall; however, its anatomic closure is accomplished over 1 to 3 months by proliferation of the intimal layer (7,8).

The lungs continue their development after birth in a more subtle manner. Initially, in the postnatal period, the number of immature alveoli increases, and these alveoli are able to generate new immature alveoli, which subsequently enlarge into mature alveoli. Consequently, the area of the air–blood interface continues to increase as the alveoli and capillaries multiply. These changes continue through at least the eighth postnatal year. Only about 50 million, or one-sixth of the adult number of alveoli, are present at birth (9). The structural integrity of the airway improves after birth as the flexible cartilage of the infant's larynx and trachea becomes more rigid.

ANATOMY

Fully developed, the mediastinum and the pleural spaces represent a collection of complex organs interacting in a constant and literally fluid manner. The mediastinum represents the central portion of the thoracic cavity. Its boundaries are the sternum anteriorly, the vertebral column posteriorly, and the medial parietal pleural surfaces of the right and left lungs laterally. The mediastinum contains four compartments: the superior, anterior, middle, and posterior (Fig. 60-2). The superior mediastinum lies in the thoracic space cephalad to a plane joining the fourth

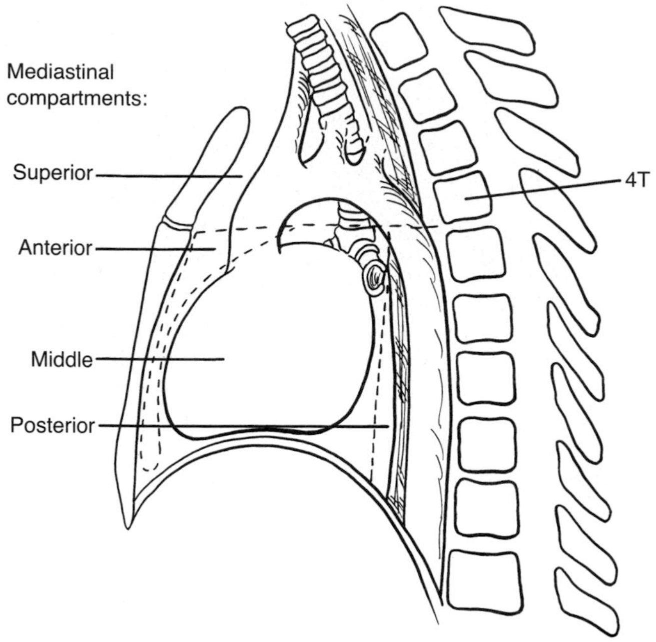

FIGURE 60-2. Anatomic division of the mediastinum into superior, anterior, middle, and posterior compartments.

thoracic vertebra and the sternomanubrial junction. The anterior mediastinum is bounded superiorly by the superior mediastinum, inferiorly by the diaphragm, anteriorly by the sternum, and posteriorly by the pericardium. The middle mediastinum is bounded by the anterior and posterior limits of the pericardium. The posterior mediastinum is bounded superiorly by the superior mediastinum, inferiorly by the diaphragm, anteriorly by the pericardium, and posteriorly by the vertebral column.

The right and left pleural spaces are separate entities that extend from the lateral aspects of the mediastinum as they envelope each lung. The parietal pleura lines the thoracic wall, whereas the visceral pleura adheres intimately to the pulmonary surface. A thin layer of mesothelial cells separates the two surfaces (10). In some areas, the parietal pleura may fold onto itself until the lung intercedes during inspiration. These areas are found inferiorly along the edges of the diaphragm, in the costodiaphragmatic sinus, and in a small cleft behind the sternum known as the costomediastinal sinus (10). The blood supply of the parietal pleura is derived from the intercostal, internal mammary, superior phrenic, and anterior mediastinal arteries. Corresponding veins drain the parietal pleura into the systemic veins. The visceral pleura is supplied by bronchial and pulmonary artery radicals; however, venous drainage is only to the pulmonary circulation (10). The parietal pleura receives sensory innervation from the intercostal and phrenic nerves. This results in relatively precise sensory localization. The visceral pleura receives vagal and sympathetic innervation and has far less precise sensory localization (10).

A dynamic relationship between the systemic and pulmonary vasculature and the lymphatic circulation maintains a relatively constant amount of pleural fluid, which is evenly distributed within the pleural space (11,12). Most pleural fluid is formed from the systemic circulation and travels along pressure gradients in the pleural space until it is primarily resorbed by parietal pleural lymphatics. Elevation of systemic venous pressure or lymphatic pressure results in excessive accumulation of pleural fluid either by increased production (venous congestion) or decreased absorption (lymphatic congestion). Normally, therefore, there is little interchange between pleural and pulmonary fluids. Pulmonary edema can disturb this balance by presenting a greater amount of fluid to the visceral pleura from the pulmonary parenchyma itself (13).

PHYSIOLOGY

The anatomy of the pleural space plays a significant role in respiratory physiology. During quiet respiration, the intrapleural pressure is −8 to −9 mm Hg during inspiration and −3 to −6 mm Hg during expiration. A positive gradient exists between the intrabronchial pressure and intrapleural pressure throughout the respiratory cycle, thus holding the pleural surfaces together (10). During inspiration, the lung is expanded by the negative pressure generated by the movement of the diaphragm and thoracic wall. In normal breathing, the diaphragmatic excursion is only about 2 cm. If the diaphragm is paralyzed, as seen in eventration of the diaphragm, it moves paradoxically upward during inspiration in response to the fall in intrathoracic pressure, interfering with ventilation of the ipsilateral lung (Fig. 60-3). The major accessory muscles of inspiration include the scalene and sternocleidomastoid muscles. These are usually quiescent during normal breathing, but may be quite active during exercise or respiratory insufficiency (14). Expiration is usually a passive event, but may become active during exercise and hyperventilation. The abdominal wall muscles are the most important muscles in active expiration, but are aided by intercostal muscles (14).

Various factors influence the efficiency of ventilation. First, the chest wall is quite elastic. There is an ongoing tension between the lung, which naturally tends to recoil inward, and the thoracic wall, which tends to recoil outward. This tension helps to keep the lung expanded. At rest, the upper lung is relatively more expanded than the lower lung because the intrathoracic pressure is less negative at the base than at the apex due to gravity. During inspiration, however, the lower lung expands more, relative to the upper lung, demonstrating a greater compliance (15). Gravity is not the lone determinant of this vertical gradient. The shapes of the intrathoracic organs, the chest wall orientation, and the tendency of the structures to resist displacement or deformation contribute to this gradient

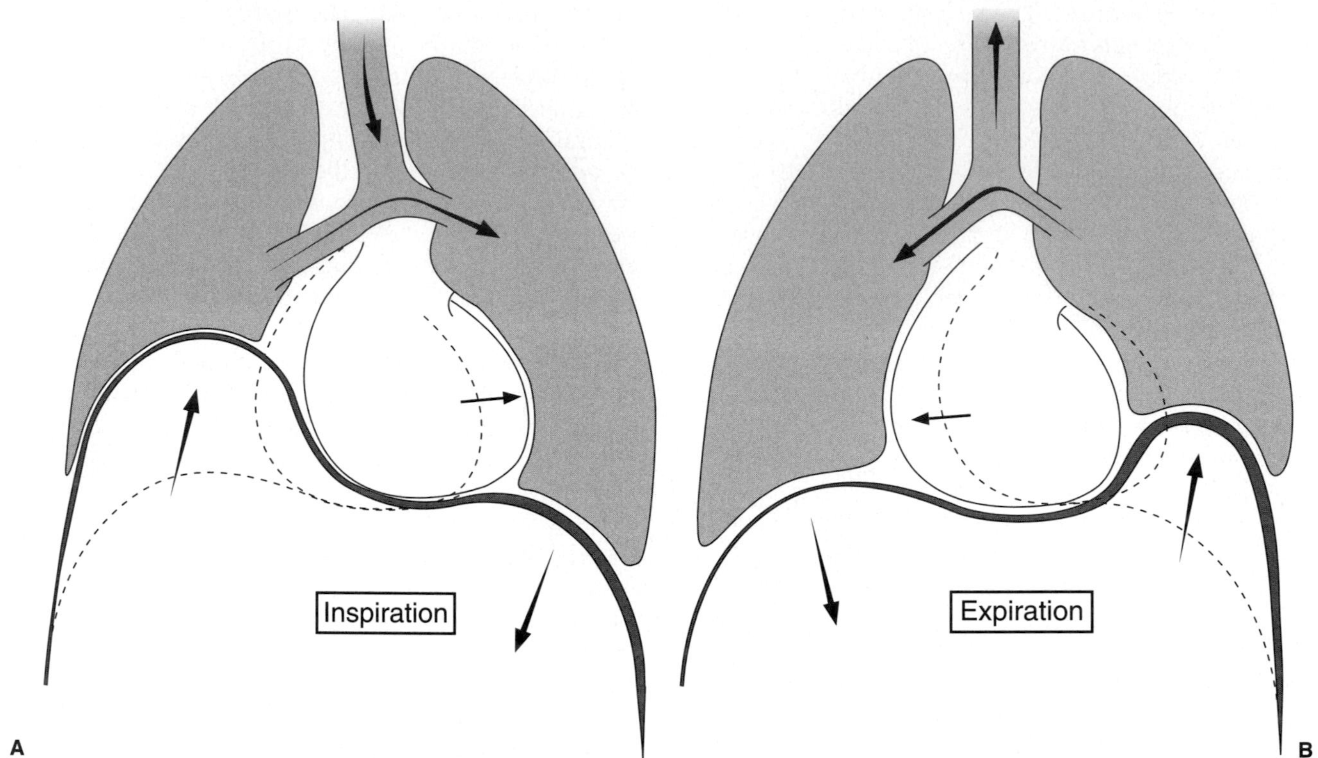

FIGURE 60-3. Pathophysiologic changes with paralysis of the right hemidiaphragm. **(A)** During inspiration, the normal left hemidiaphragm descends, increasing intraabdominal pressure. This elevates the right hemidiaphragm and shifts the mediastinal structures to the left. Gas in the right lung is forced into the left lung, increasing dead space ventilation. **(B)** During expiration, the normal left diaphragm elevates, reducing intraabdominal pressure and allowing the right diaphragm to descend. The mediastinal structures move back toward the right side. Gas in the left lung is forced into the right lung. The movement of air from one lung to the other during the respiratory cycle is dead space ventilation, termed *Pendelluft*. (Adapted from Rodgers BM, McGahren ED. Congenital eventration of the diaphragm. In: *Modern problems in pediatrics*, vol. 24. Basel: S Karger, 1989:121.)

(16,17). In fact, the two lungs can function almost as separate structures with different mechanical properties (16). The position of the patient may also affect the distribution of ventilation within the lung. For example, experimental studies have shown an improvement in oxygenation in animals placed in the prone versus the supine position because small airway patency is better maintained in the prone position (18).

The previous section describes the respiratory status of the child and the adult, but there are special considerations in the infant. Anatomic and physiologic dynamics are not fully developed in the neonate. The overly compliant chest wall is easily distorted during respiratory efforts. This is especially true during sleep because intercostal muscle activity is reduced, resulting in decreased lung dynamic compliance. Neonatal lung tissue is more viscous, peripheral airways offer more resistance, and mismatches of ventilation and perfusion are more marked than in the older child and adult. The upper airway is quite pliable and can close at pressures of 4 mm Hg. Neck extension can enhance airway patency, whereas flexion can hinder it. In addition, the functional residual capacity (FRC) in the neonate comprises a relatively higher proportion of lung capacity due to a decreased expiratory phase. This helps in the absorption of intrapulmonary fluid and the maintenance of a more uniform airway expansion, but leaves the infant vulnerable to atelectasis (19).

OPERATIVE PRINCIPLES

Anesthetic considerations are extremely important for infants and children undergoing thoracic surgery. The normal cardiopulmonary physiology in these young patients may compromise their ability to respond to the changes induced by general anesthesia. Infants and children have a relatively small FRC compared with tidal volume. In newborns, the FRC actually overlaps the closing volume of the lung (20). Thus, newborns are especially prone to alveolar collapse during open chest anesthesia. The use of positive end-expiratory pressure (PEEP) may prevent atelectasis and eliminate clinically significant hypoxia. The infant's myocardium is relatively less sensitive to the positive inotropic effects of isoproterenol and dopamine, and relatively more sensitive to the negative inotropic effects of propranolol (21). The infant's myocardium is also less compliant than that of the older child. Because of this difference in physiology, the cardiac output in infants is augmented principally by increasing heart rate, at a relatively fixed stroke volume. As the heart rate increases, however, there is less time for ventricular filling. A point is reached at which the infant can no longer increase cardiac output by this means and shock ensues. Shock may develop rapidly in infants, and is often heralded only by a progressive increase in heart rate, rather than a gradual decline in blood pressure. If the response to inotropic support is inadequate, vigorous volume resuscitation is necessary to support the peripheral circulation.

Pulmonary physiology in the lateral decubitus position has been thoroughly studied in adult patients, but poorly evaluated in children. Gravity increases the pulmonary blood flow to the dependent lung, as compared with the nondependent lung. Conversely, ventilation is superior in the nondependent lung because of elevation of the dependent diaphragm and gravitational shifts of the mediastinum (22) (Fig. 60-4). These changes in ventilation may be even more significant in small children because the mediastinum is more mobile and the abdominal organs are relatively larger. An anesthetized, paralyzed child in the lateral decubitus position, therefore, may experience significant ventilation–perfusion mismatch. The reduction of regional ventilation in the child's dependent lung may precipitate alveolar collapse and systemic hypoxia. This ventilation–perfusion mismatch may be further exacerbated by one-lung ventilation techniques, such as those used for many thoracoscopic procedures. In this instance, all the blood flow to the nondependent and nonventilated lung becomes shunt flow, creating an obligatory right-to-left shunt. Increasing the F_{IO_2} and respiratory rate may be enough to compensate for this shunt fraction and allow the procedure to be completed, but some infants and children become significantly hypoxic under these conditions and cannot tolerate one-lung ventilation in this position. The use of positive-pressure ventilation with PEEP prevents alveolar collapse and maximizes ventilation of the dependent lung.

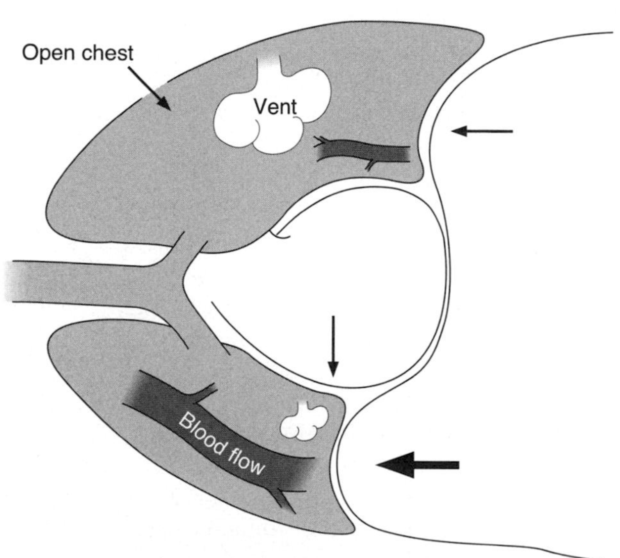

FIGURE 60-4. Pathophysiologic changes in the pleura and mediastinum in the lateral decubitus position during anesthesia with an open chest. Ventilation in the nondependent lung is superior to that in the dependent lung because of elevation of the dependent diaphragm and gravitational shifts of the mediastinum. Perfusion, however, is superior in the dependent lung because of gravitational forces. Both ventilation and perfusion in the nondependent, operated lung may be further impaired by compression during surgery.

Maintaining the fluid and glucose balance in children undergoing thoracic surgery is critical. Fluid overload in neonates may open a previously closed ductus arteriosus, creating a significant shunt. Likewise, excessive administration of crystalloid during an operative procedure may precipitate interstitial pulmonary edema, further aggravating the potential for systemic hypoxia. Infants undergoing thoracic surgery should generally receive no more than 75% of their calculated maintenance fluid volume in the first 24 to 48 hours postoperatively, unless there are ongoing fluid losses. Reductions in fluid intake are usually accompanied by reductions in glucose intake. Thus, careful glucose monitoring is important during this interval.

Intraoperative and perioperative monitoring of cardiac and respiratory function is essential in infants and children because their clinical condition may change rapidly. In the past, the size of these patients often made sophisticated monitoring of cardiopulmonary function difficult or impossible, but modern equipment has largely overcome these difficulties. As a minimum, all children undergoing thoracic surgery should have continuous monitoring of heart rate, blood pressure, electrocardiogram, oxygen saturation, and temperature. Blood pressure monitoring is facilitated by Doppler equipment, such as the Dinamap. This instrument can repeatedly measure systolic, diastolic, and mean blood pressure at preset time intervals in patients of all sizes. Automated blood pressure readings correlate closely with intraarterial readings, if appropriate size cuffs are used (23).

Oxygen saturation can be continuously measured with transcutaneous sensors. This equipment can be used on patients of all ages, and the readings are not adversely affected by the percentage of fetal hemoglobin in the circulation. Because of the shape of the oxyhemoglobin dissociation curve, oxygen saturation provides a better method for detecting levels of hypoxia than for detecting hyperoxia. This is not of practical importance, except in small premature infants in whom persistent excessive oxygenation can affect the retinal circulation. When oxygen saturations

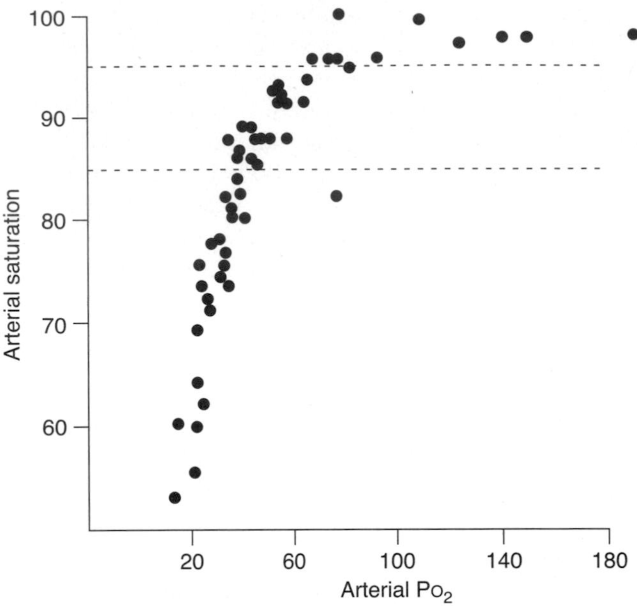

FIGURE 60-5. Measured relationship between Pao_2 (in mm Hg) and percent of transcutaneous oxygen saturation in human neonates. An oxygen dissociation curve for this patient population is generated. Maintaining saturation levels between 85% and 95% avoids Pao_2 levels higher than 100 or less than 50 mm Hg. Arterial saturation levels higher than 95% are associated with unacceptable levels of Pao_2 for premature human infants.

are maintained at or below 95%, the Pao_2 is not likely to exceed 100 mm Hg (24) (Fig. 60-5). Maintaining saturation levels between 85% and 95% assures a safe range of partial pressure of oxygen for premature infants. The ability to continuously monitor oxygen saturation has provided a sensitive method for detecting mechanical anesthetic complications, such as mainstem intubation or obstruction of the endotracheal tube. Using these devices in the postoperative period has greatly reduced the need for arterial blood gas sampling. Two oxygen saturation sensors can be used to detect right-to-left shunting through the ductus arteriosus. One sensor is placed proximal (right arm) and one is placed distal (legs) to the ductus arteriosus. A difference of greater than 5% saturation between the two sensors indicates significant shunting. Advances in technology have created accurate and practical end-tidal CO_2 monitors. These devices are connected to the endotracheal tube and sample expired gas concentrations. They provide an accurate correlation with arterial Pco_2, except in infants who weigh less than 4 kg. In these small patients, sampling errors of the small tidal volume may lead to inaccurate readings (25).

Catheters are available for measuring pulmonary capillary wedge pressure and performing calorimetric cardiac output in pediatric patients. In infants, these catheters (4F) may need to be inserted by cutdown techniques, but in older children they may be placed percutaneously. Percutaneous arterial catheters (22 gauge and 24 gauge) can be used in infants and children. Usually, these are placed in the radial artery, although the femoral artery may be used in small infants for short-term monitoring.

Certain relatively common thoracic surgical procedures in children require special anesthetic considerations. Airway endoscopy is frequently performed in children to evaluate the etiology of stridor or to remove airway foreign bodies. Most of these procedures are performed under general anesthesia, using a rigid ventilating bronchoscope. Insertion of this instrument in small children, even under general anesthesia, may precipitate laryngospasm. Applying topical anesthesia (lidocaine 4%) to the vocal cords before introducing the bronchoscope reduces the hazard of laryngospasm and eliminates much of the discomfort of the procedure. Positive-pressure ventilation through the bronchoscope is contraindicated in many of the bronchoscopic procedures performed in children. For example, positive pressure used in patients with airway foreign bodies may impact the foreign body onto the carina or into a distal bronchus. In addition, patients with pulmonary air trapping, such as children with lobar emphysema who are undergoing bronchoscopy for selective airway aspiration, may experience sudden respiratory collapse with positive-pressure ventilation because of the rapid expansion of the involved lobe or development of a pneumothorax. Rah et al. documented the inadequacies of ventilation with the smallest bronchoscopes (2.5 and 3 mm) when the rod lens telescope is in place (26). The lumen available for ventilation under these circumstances is very small, and exhalation of gas from the lung is impeded. When using these bronchoscopes, the surgeon is advised to remove the telescope intermittently, allowing periods of ventilation to avoid severe hypercarbia or pneumothorax.

Pain relief in children undergoing thoracic surgery is important to minimize respiratory complications. Intrapleural catheters inserted after the operation is completed provide excellent postoperative analgesia with intermittent or continuous infusion of bupivacaine (27,28). Regional anesthetic techniques, including local infiltration of the surgical wound and intercostal nerve blocks, may also help. Older children can be safely treated with patient-controlled analgesia pumps that allow intravenous infusion of measured doses of analgesics (29). Epidural catheters may be employed in some settings for perioperative analgesia (30).

The standard operative approach for most pediatric thoracic procedures has traditionally been the posterolateral thoracotomy. This incision divides a portion of the latissimus dorsi muscle and the serratus anterior muscle beneath it. For many years, a rib resection was advocated for the retropleural dissection used in correcting esophageal atresia with tracheoesophageal fistula.

Currently, however, an intercostal approach is preferred in an effort to avoid growth disturbances of the chest wall in these patients with considerable growth ahead of them. Chetcuti et al. reviewed a series of 302 patients who had survived esophageal atresia repair for four decades (31). Of patients who underwent a rib resection thoracotomy, 38% developed anterior chest wall asymmetry, scoliosis, or both. However, 25% of patients who underwent an intercostal thoracotomy without rib resection developed similar skeletal abnormalities. These deformities appeared to be progressive because their incidence increased with longer follow-up. Their incidence also increased significantly when more than one thoracotomy was necessary. The authors believed that the major factor that produced anterior chest wall asymmetry was partial denervation of the serratus anterior with subsequent atrophy of this muscle, rather than the rib resection itself. The development of scoliosis was more common in patients who had congenital vertebral anomalies, but was believed to be secondary to interference with intercostal muscle function in patients with normal spines. Jaureguizar et al. followed 89 patients after correction of esophageal atresia (32). Of these patients, 24% developed shoulder elevation on the side of the thoracotomy and 20% were found to have chest wall deformities, including asymmetric breast growth in female patients. Denervation of the serratus anterior muscle was also believed to be responsible for these abnormalities. Goodman et al. reported atrophy of both the serratus anterior and latissimus dorsi muscles in computed tomography (CT) studies of patients following a posterolateral thoracotomy (33). Because of these and similar studies, many pediatric surgeons advocate the of use muscle-sparing thoracotomy incisions (34–36). The incision for these thoracotomies extends posteriorly from the mid axillary line to avoid interference with breast development. The latissimus dorsi muscle can be mobilized and retracted either posteriorly or anteriorly, depending on the exposure required. With anterior retraction of the latissimus, the chest can be entered through the triangle of auscultation without dividing or mobilizing the serratus muscle. With posterior retraction, the inferior border of the serratus is mobilized and retracted anteriorly to allow entry through the fourth intercostal space (Fig. 60-6). These incisions lend themselves nicely to most intrathoracic procedures in infants and children. Although there are no long-term follow-up studies of chest wall development in children following these procedures, it is believed that avoiding division and denervation of these major muscles minimizes the chest wall and spinal deformities that occur following standard thoracotomy procedures. Ponn et al. evaluated 62 adult patients undergoing muscle-sparing thoracotomy 6 months after surgery. In these patients, forced vital capacity was significantly better preserved than in patients undergoing standard muscle-splitting thoracotomies (37).

THORACOSCOPY

The desire for a minimally invasive and minimally deforming thoracotomy has naturally led pediatric surgeons to explore thoracoscopy for many intrathoracic procedures. In thoracoscopy, the pleural cavity is accessed by instruments placed through trocars that are inserted through the intercostal space, without spreading the ribs. The intercostal muscles are not divided, and the muscles of the chest wall are left undisturbed. Initially proposed in 1976 as a technique for obtaining pulmonary biopsies in immunocompromised children, thoracoscopy has now been applied to a diverse range of thoracic disorders in children (38). With the development of sophisticated dissecting and retracting instruments, many therapeutic procedures can now be performed in the thoracic cavity with these instruments (Fig. 60-7). The success of thoracoscopy depends on the ability to establish a sufficient pneumothorax that allows visualization of the area of pathology. Patients with extensive pleural symphysis are thus not good candidates for thoracoscopic procedures. Careful preoperative imaging is essential for planning appropriate patient position and trocar location. Most thoracoscopy procedures are best performed in a full lateral decubitus position, although procedures involving lesions in the anterior or posterior mediastinum may be more easily accomplished by placing the patient in a 45-degree lateral position or an exaggerated lateral position, respectively.

Procedures involving retraction of the lung or extensive dissection within the mediastinum are best performed under general anesthesia, using either tracheal or selective mainstem ventilation. Selective mainstem intubation has the advantage of allowing complete collapse of the ipsilateral lung, thus avoiding the need for retraction. Positive-pressure ventilation in patients with tracheal ventilation may interfere with maintenance of an ipsilateral pneumothorax, reducing the visibility in the operated chest. Infusing carbon dioxide gas under low pressure (4 to 6 mm Hg) and low flow (100 mL per min) may alleviate this problem. Simple procedures, such as pleurodesis or pulmonary biopsy, can be performed under regional anesthesia, using an intercostal block with additional intravenous sedation as needed (39). After insertion of the initial trocar and telescope, the entire hemithorax is evaluated for areas of unsuspected pathology. Planning is then completed for insertion of the trocars for dissecting and retracting instruments. The lesion is then dissected entirely from its surrounding structures or biopsied. Hemostasis can be achieved either with the insulated electrocautery, metallic clips, endoscopic stapling, or ultrasonic dissecting shears. A chest tube is inserted through one of the trocar tracts, and the remaining tracts are closed in layers. In most patients, a small catheter is left through one of the trocar tracts for instillation of intrapleural analgesia.

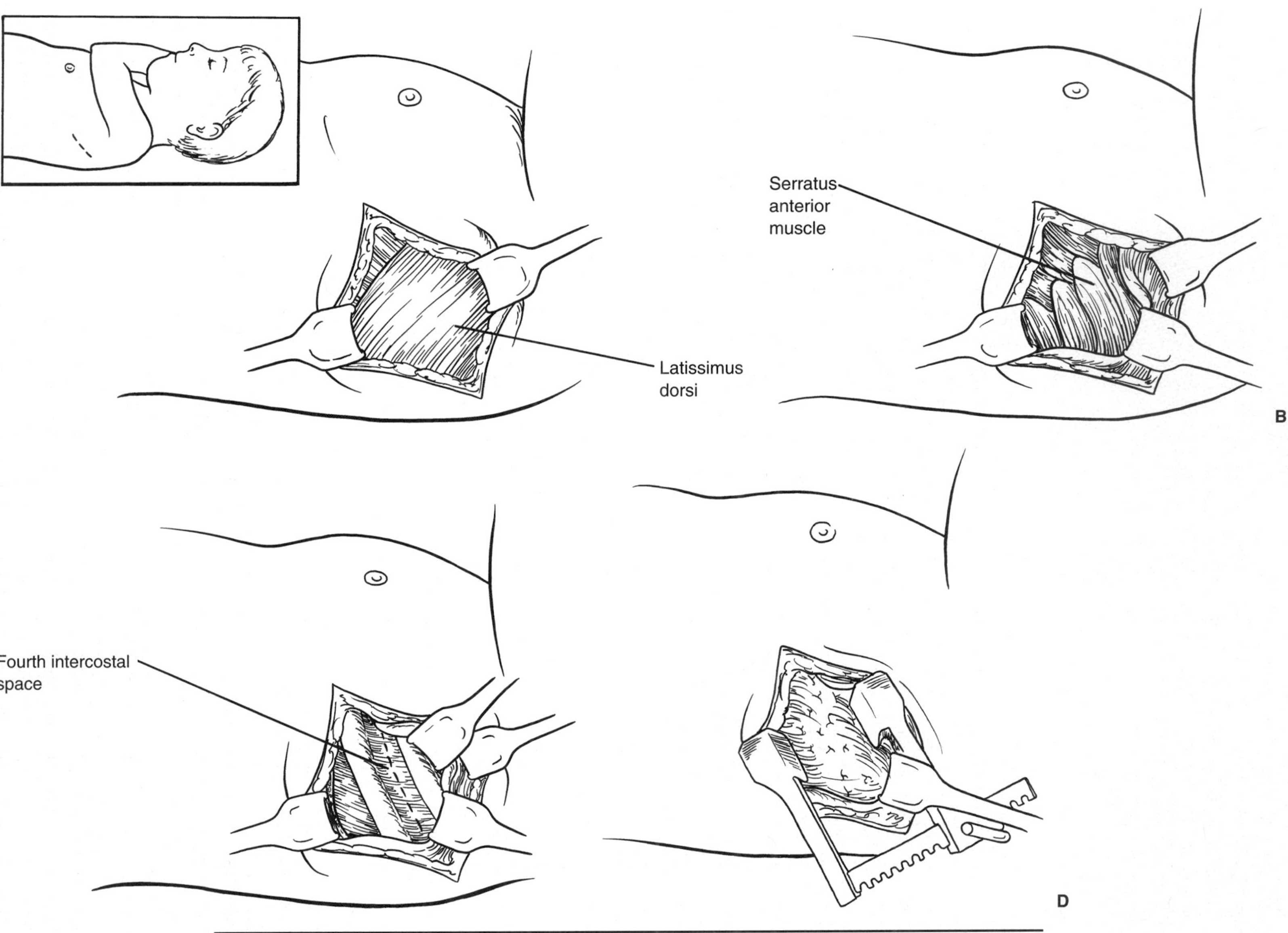

FIGURE 60-6. Muscle-sparing posterolateral thoracotomy incision. After mobilization of skin flaps superiorly and inferiorly **(A)**, the latissimus dorsi muscle is retracted posteriorly to expose the serratus anterior muscle **(B)**. **(C)** The serratus anterior muscle is mobilized superiorly to expose the intercostal space. Entry into the thorax may either be transpleural **(D)** or retropleural.

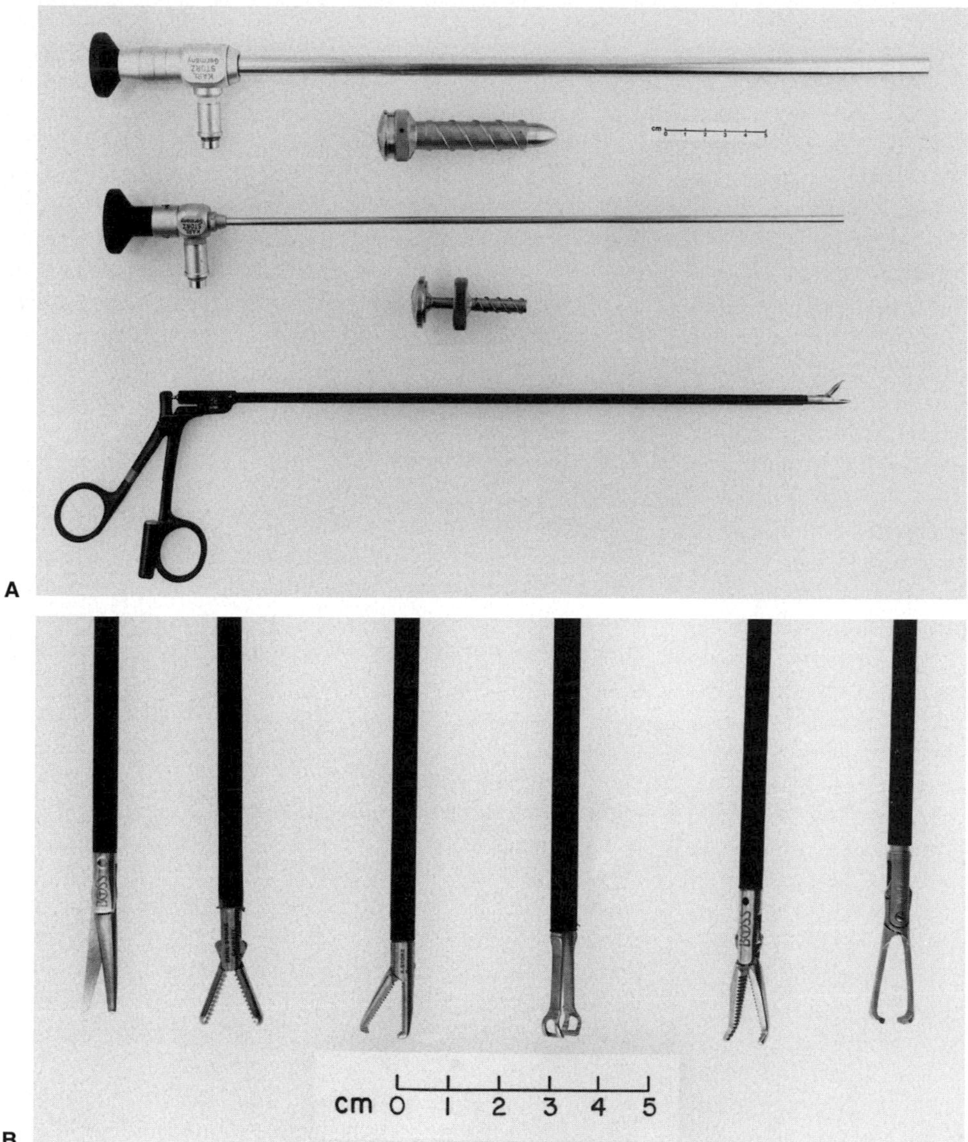

FIGURE 60-7. Examples of 10- and 5-mm thoracoscope telescopes and trocars. The trocars are straight, rigid sleeves through which telescopes and instruments can be passed. They contain no valves so an open pneumothorax can be maintained. The trocars are secured by twisting them into the intercostal space. (**A;** *top to bottom*) The 10- and 5-mm telescopes are forward viewing (0 degrees); the cup biopsy forceps are useful for simple biopsy. **(B)** The 5-mm instruments include (*left to right*) Metzenbaum scissors, nontoothed and toothed grasping forceps, Babcock clamp, right-angled dissector, and Alyce forceps. These instruments have insulated shafts so they can be used with the electrocautery.

Thoracoscopy has become widely accepted for use in pediatric patients for a variety of indications. Currently, one of the most frequent indications is for pleural debridement in children with fibrinopurulent empyema. This technique is easy to learn and has been virtually 100% successful in quickly clearing the pleural infection and facilitating discharge of these patients (40,41). Thoracoscopy is also commonly used for biopsy or excision of mediastinal lesions, for pulmonary biopsy in patients with diffuse or localized interstitial infiltrates, and for pleurodesis in treatment of spontaneous pneumothorax. Thoracoscopic biopsy or excision of mediastinal lesions has been successful in more than 95% of the children reported, and there have been no significant complications when using the technique for this purpose (42). Preoperative imaging is especially important for these patients to ensure they are appropriately positioned to allow access to the area of pathology. Cross-sectional scans are helpful to define the relationship of the lesion to vital structures in the vicinity. For simple biopsy of mediastinal lesions, two trocars are usually sufficient; one for the telescope and one for the biopsy forceps. Additional trocars may be necessary for retraction of the lung or if complete excision of the lesion is anticipated. Several authors have described complete excision of bronchogenic cysts and neurogenic tumors of the mediastinum in children using thoracoscopy (42–45). The cysts may be aspirated under direct vision and removed through one of the trocar tracts in an endosac. Mediastinal tumors should be placed in an Endosac and may be removed through a slightly expanded trocar tract. The use of thoracoscopy to biopsy mediastinal lymphadenopathy has proven particularly helpful in pediatric patients.

Patients with bulky lesions with some element of tracheal compression may be biopsied under regional anesthesia, thus reducing the anesthetic hazard of the procedure.

The use of thoracoscopy to provide accurate tissue diagnosis in children with diffuse or localized pulmonary infiltrates has been successful in nearly 100% of the patients reported (45). These biopsies may be rapidly obtained using the endoscopic stapling device to minimize postoperative air leaks or bleeding. This device must be passed through a 12-mm trocar and must be able to be passed at least 5 cm into the chest to fully open the anvil. It is therefore not applicable for use in very small patients, usually those younger than 3 or 4 years. More recently, the ultrasonic scalpel has been used for this purpose with success, and these instruments may be passed through a 5-mm trocar (46).

Most complications of thoracoscopy in children have occurred in patients undergoing lung biopsy who are immunocompromised and on mechanical ventilation (45). The problems in obtaining hemostasis and pneumostasis after these procedures have occasionally led to serious complications, including bleeding and bronchopleural fistulas. Many of these children should be biopsied by open techniques that provide better parenchymal control.

Thoracoscopic treatment of pneumothorax can be accomplished by various methods, including talc pleurodesis, mechanical pleural abrasion, and pleurectomy. Talc pleurodesis and pleurectomy have been successful in virtually 100% of the patients in whom they have been used (47). Mechanical pleural abrasion is successful in 90% to 95% of patients (48). Talc pleurodesis is simple to perform and can be completed under regional anesthesia, whereas pleurectomy and pleural abrasion cause more discomfort and require general anesthesia (39). With any of these techniques, blebs or cysts can be excised using either the endoscopic stapler or ultrasonic scalpel. Thoracoscopy can be used to treat chylothorax, either by occluding the thoracic duct with metallic clips or sutures or by spraying the mediastinum with fibrin glue (49).

As pediatric surgeons have become more comfortable with the technique of thoracoscopy and more sophisticated instruments have been developed, this technique is being applied to many more complicated intrathoracic procedures in children. Several authors have reported formal anatomic pulmonary lobectomy, even in very small children (50). Thoracoscopy is now frequently used for interruption of the ductus arteriosis in small infants and several authors have described using the technique for division of vascular rings (51,52). More recently, pediatric surgeons have begun to repair infants with esophageal atresia and tracheoesophageal fistula with thoracoscopic techniques with excellent results (53,54).

The introduction of robotic equipment for minimally invasive surgery has stimulated pediatric surgeons to explore its usefulness in pediatric thoracoscopy. This equipment, although somewhat complex to set up, has the important advantage of 6 or 7 degrees of movement of the endoscopic instruments, allowing for considerable flexibility while working in small spaces (55). Clinical reports have appeared of resection of mediastinal tumors with robotic equipment and patent ductus arteriosus, and vascular rings have been successfully divided in children as small as 2 to 3 kg (52,56,57). Repair of esophageal atresia has been simulated in experimental animals using robotic technology (58,59). It is anticipated that the use of this equipment will see wider application in pediatric surgical practice as the instruments are refined and scaled down for pediatric use.

PNEUMOTHORAX

A pneumothorax is an accumulation of air within the pleural space. It may occur spontaneously or as the result of trauma, surgery, or a therapeutic intervention. If the air accumulates under pressure, a tension pneumothorax ensues. A pneumothorax decreases pulmonary volume, compliance, and diffusing capacity. If the pneumothorax is greater than 50% of chest volume, hypoxia may result secondary to ventilation–perfusion mismatch. A normal lung can often compensate this for. Children with underlying chronic pulmonary disease may develop significant relatively smaller pneumothoraces secondary to diminished elastic recoil of their lungs, but the symptomatic consequences may be more significant because of their small margin of pulmonary reserve (60,61,62). Spontaneous pneumothorax may occur in children with no known underlying disease or may result from or, in fact, reveal an underlying condition, such as a congenital bleb, pneumonia with pneumatocele or abscess, tuberculosis, or cystic adenomatoid malformation. Traumatic pneumothorax may result from a tear in the pleura, esophagus, trachea, or bronchi. Iatrogenic causes include mechanical ventilation, thoracentesis or central venous catheter insertion, bronchoscopy, or cardiopulmonary resuscitation (60,63–65).

The most common presenting symptoms of pneumothorax are ipsilateral chest pain and dyspnea (60,64). Severe dyspnea should alert the surgeon to the presence of a tension pneumothorax. Physical examination may reveal diminished breath sounds on one side of the chest or a shift of the trachea from the suprasternal notch. A pneumothorax is usually detectable on a chest radiograph and is enhanced if the radiograph is taken at end expiration. It is common practice for the size of a pneumothorax to be described as a proportion of the chest field on an upright radiograph. The actual volume loss of the lung is greater than such a description because pulmonary volume is lost in three dimensions. The following formula is used to more accurately estimate this loss:

$$\frac{\text{diameter of lung}^3}{\text{diameter of hemithorax}^3} \times 100 = \%\ \text{pneumothorax}$$

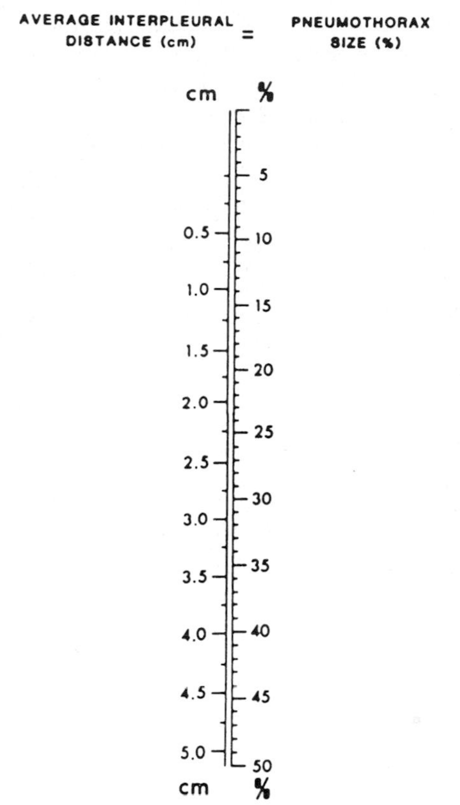

FIGURE 60-8. A nomogram for predicting the percentage of involvement with a pneumothorax in larger children and adolescents.

Other authors have developed a nomogram for this same purpose (Fig. 60-8) (66).

A number of factors determine the proper management of a pneumothorax. These include the initial size, symptomatology, ongoing expansion, presence of tension, and any contributing underlying condition. A spontaneous unilateral pneumothorax that is asymptomatic and less than 15% to 20% of the chest volume can usually be followed by observation alone (61,65). Pleural air reabsorbs at a rate of 1,25% per day, but this can be hastened by breathing supplemental oxygen (61,67). Classically, such a pneumothorax occurs in an ectomorphic, adolescent male. If there is no known underlying pathology, the chances are that such an episode represents the rupture of a subpleural bleb or cyst, the manifestation of a familial tendency, or perhaps even the presence of undetected tuberculosis (68). Pneumothorax recurs with a frequency of 50% after the first episode, 62% after the second, and 83% after the third (61,69).

Symptomatic or large pneumothoraces usually require intervention. Options for treatment of a small pneumothorax include thoracentesis, placement of a unidirectional (Heimlich-type) valve, or placement of a small pigtail catheter (70–72). However, if air is continuously aspirated or if the pneumothorax recurs, a standard chest tube should be inserted. A tension pneumothorax poses a surgical emergency and a chest tube should be placed immediately. If a chest tube is not immediately available or if the patient's condition deteriorates during preparation for placement, a large-bore (14-gauge) needle should be placed in the second intercostal space anteriorly to relieve the tension. If the pneumothorax recurs after tube thoracostomy, or if the air leak persists, further intervention is necessary. The choice of intervention is determined by the cause of the condition. In a posttraumatic pneumothorax, large or persistent air leaks may indicate damage to the airway or the esophagus. Appropriate diagnostic studies using esophagograms, bronchoscopy, esophagoscopy, thoracoscopy, or thoracotomy should be undertaken and direct repair of the injury, if present, performed. If the air leak is due to lung parenchymal injury, chest tube drainage is usually adequate. In a nontraumatic pneumothorax, the persistence of an air leak may accompany a chronic underlying condition, such as cystic fibrosis, bronchopulmonary dysplasia, lung cysts, or blebs. Treatment of these patients usually requires resection of the local pathology or pleurodesis.

Pleurodesis can be undertaken by instilling chemical agents into the pleural space through a chest tube, by thoracoscopy, or by thoracotomy. In the past, agents such as silver nitrate, quinacrine, iodized oil, and hypertonic glucose have been used, but currently, talc or tetracycline derivatives, such as doxycycline or fibrin sealant, are more commonly used (47,73–77). Talc is less painful and more uniformly successful than doxycycline. Treatment with talc has been shown to be particularly effective in treating pneumothoraces in children with cystic fibrosis (47). A more recent study in adults does suggest that talc may have systemic distribution and may rarely produce adult respiratory distress syndrome (78). Autologous blood patching may be useful in preventing pneumothorax after lung biopsy (79).

Traditionally, thoracotomy has been used for more aggressive interventions such as mechanical pleurodesis, pleurectomy, or resection of lung blebs or cysts. However, thoracoscopy has emerged as a preferred technique by many for all these interventions (80–83). It allows excellent visualization of the entire pleural space with a low surgical morbidity. It also allows use of a wider range of anesthetic techniques because older children can often undergo thoracoscopic pleurodesis under sedation with intercostal nerve block. The results of thoracoscopic pleurodesis for pneumothorax have been excellent, and complications of the technique are very uncommon (80,84).

CHYLOTHORAX

Chylothorax is an accumulation of lymphatic fluid in the pleural space. The main causes of chylothorax in children are idiopathic chylothorax of infancy, injury to lymphatic channels as a result of an operative procedure or trauma, malignancy, and innominate vein or superior vena cava thrombosis. Idiopathic chylothorax presents in infancy and is believed to be secondary to congenital defects of the thoracic lymphatics or to birth trauma. However, congenital pulmonary lymphangiectasia or lymphangiomatosis may be more frequent causes than appreciated. The most common etrology traumatic chylothorax is usually due to operative injury, often following cardiac surgical procedures. The incidence of chylothorax following thoracic surgery in children ranges from 0.25% to 0.9% (85). Traumatic injury to the thoracic duct has been reported secondary to either blunt or penetrating thoracic trauma. Chylothorax secondary to malignancy is seen in older children and is usually due to obstruction of the thoracic duct by lymphoma. The occurrence of chylothorax with thoracic duct obstruction by neuroblastoma has also been reported (86). If an older child presents with chylothorax but has no history of trauma or operation, an intrathoracic tumor should be suspected and investigated with chest CT or magnetic resonance imaging (MRI).

Chylothorax usually presents with significant respiratory insufficiency, although it may present as the incidental finding of a pleural effusion on an imaging study of the chest. Prenatal ultrasound may detect chylothorax in the fetus. The diagnosis of chylothorax is confirmed by evaluating the pleural fluid. Chyle is usually milky in color, but may be serosanguinous or straw colored in children who are receiving no enteral fats, such as those who have just undergone surgery. Chyle generally contains a total fat content of more than 400 mg per dL, triglycerides of more than 220 mg per dL, a protein content that is one-half that of plasma, and a specific gravity greater than 1.012. On Gram's stain of the fluid, more than 90% of the cells seen are lymphocytes, and Sudan red stain may demonstrate chylomicrons (87,88). Loss of significant volumes of chyle from the pleural space represents a considerable loss of protein and lymphocytes to these children. These losses must be monitored closely and replaced to avoid severe nutritional deficits.

Treatment of chylothorax has traditionally been nonoperative, with 70% to 80% of patients responding (87,89). The pleural space is drained by thoracentesis or tube thoracostomy to relieve symptoms and facilitate closure of the lymphatic leak. Feeding the patient a diet that principally contains medium-chain triglycerides can diminish lymphatic flow through the thoracic duct. These fats are absorbed directly into the portal venous system, unlike long-chain fatty acids, which are absorbed through the intestinal lymphatics. If chyle drainage persists, the patient can be placed on total parental nutrition, with no oral intake. If these measures fail to significantly reduce or eliminate lymphatic drainage in a 3- or 4-day interval, these patients should be started on intravenous octreotide in a progressively escalating dose. Several anecdotal reports have demonstrated efficacy of octreotide in these situations, presumably working by reducing splanchnic blood flow and chyle formation (90,91).

If nonoperative treatment fails to eliminate the lymphatic drainage, surgical therapy can be attempted to obliterate the thoracic duct or the area of leakage, or to create a pleurodesis. These objectives can be accomplished by either thoracotomy or thoracoscopy. Covering the area of leakage with fibrin glue has been effective in eliminating chylous drainage in some patients. Several reports have described the use of pleural-peritoneal shunts to treat refractory chylothorax (92,93). These shunts may be placed with the pumping chamber exteriorized to facilitate its compression (94). These shunts are easy to insert and have been effective in eliminating drainage in 85% to 95% of these patients (49,91,95).

The timing of surgical intervention has been a matter of some debate. An early report by Randolph and Gross recommended surgical intervention if the chylothorax did not respond to nonoperative treatment by 21 days (96). However, more recent reports recommend intervention as early as 5 to 7 days, particularly if less invasive procedures such as thoracoscopy or pleuroperitoneal shunts are to be used (49,95). This is especially true if the child has elevated right heart pressures or central venous thrombosis. Such children are unlikely to respond to nonoperative treatment (95). Ultimately, the results of treatment, either nonoperative or operative, are excellent.

EMPYEMA

Empyema refers to the accumulation of infected fluid in the pleural space. In children, this is usually the result of severe pneumonia (97). However, empyema may also result from infection of the retropharyngeal, mediastinal, or paravertebral spaces, thoracic trauma, or an immunocompromised state (97,98). In 1962, the American Thoracic Society described what are now the three classic stages of empyema (99). The first stage, or the exudative stage, is characterized by an accumulation of thin pleural fluid with few cells. The pleura and lung are mobile, and the fluid is amenable to drainage by thoracentesis. This stage may last only 24 to 72 hours. The second stage is the fibrinopurulent stage. Consolidation of infected pleural fluid results in an accumulation of fibrinous material, formation of loculations, and loss of lung mobility. This stage lasts 7 to 10 days. The third stage is the organizing stage. A pleural peel forms secondary to fibroblast proliferation and resorption of fibrin. The lung becomes entrapped, and capillary proliferation extends from the fibrinous peel into the visceral pleura itself. This usually occurs 2 to 4 weeks after the initial development of the empyema.

Before the widespread use of antibiotics, empyema was caused principally by infections of *Streptococcus pneumoniae*, *Streptococcus pyogenes*, *Staphylococcus aureus*, and

Haemophilus influenzae. The introduction of sulfapyridine and penicillin decreased the overall incidence of empyema, but *S. aureus* emerged as the primary offending pathogen. Since the mid-1980s, effective therapy for *S. aureus* has allowed the emergence of a variety of bacterial organisms, including anaerobic bacteria, as common causes of empyema in children (100):

More Common	*Less Common*
S. pneumoniae	Bacteroides species
S. aureus	Other streptococcal species
H. influenzae	*Pseudomonas aeruginosa*

Contemporary series report a preponderance of *H. influenza* and Streptococcal species in children (101–104). However, some series still report *S. aureus* as the most common pathogen (100,105–108). Interestingly, a number of these latter series are from developing countries (105–108). Children with empyema generally present with fever, cough, respiratory insufficiency, and chest pain (100,105,109). Physical signs may include dullness on chest percussion, tactile and vocal fremitus, decreased breath sounds, rales, and a pleural friction rub (100,109). A chest radiograph reveals a thickened pleura in addition to the primary pneumonic process and pleural fluid. Transthoracic ultrasound or chest CT scan are beneficial in assessing the degree of pleural thickening, fluid loculation, and lung consolidation (100,102,110). The diagnosis of empyema is confirmed by thoracentesis. The fluid is characteristically turbid and may be thick during the later stages of the infection. Laboratory analysis reveals a specific gravity greater than 1.016, protein greater than 3 g per dL, lactate dehydrogenase (LDH) greater than 200 U per L, pleural fluid protein/serum protein ratio greater than 0.5, pleural fluid LDH/serum LDH ratio greater than 0.6, and white blood cell count higher than 15,000 per mm^3. Fibrin clots may also be present (109). Once the diagnosis of empyema is made, appropriate antibiotics should be administered based on Gram's stain and culture of the pleural fluid or sputum. Frequently, however, antibiotics have already been started prior to drainage and the fluid is unrevealing. Complete drainage of the empyema should be accomplished either by thoracentesis or tube thoracostomy (111). Some children present with such advanced disease that the pleural involvement has passed the exudative stage. In these patients, thoracentesis or even tube drainage may not be adequate to obtain a clinical response. In general, the longer the prehospital or pretreatment illness has persisted, the more likely further interventions will be needed (112,113).

A suboptimal clinical response of the patient to antibiotics and drainage determines the need for additional intervention. Most patients are free of fever and residual pleural fluid within 3 to 5 days following institution of therapy. Persistence of fever or loculation of the pleural fluid requires the surgeon to consider further intervention (101,111–113). The nature and timing of this intervention has remained a subject of debate. The primary surgical objective must be to remove all the residual infected pleural fluid, to break up any loculations, and to free the lung to expand and fill the pleural space. The lung expansion allows better clearance of infection from the lung parenchyma itself. Many pediatric surgical series have discussed decortication for this objective. Properly used, the term *decortication* refers to the removal of a thick, fibrotic visceral peel that is restricting the underlying lung (114). In fact, the procedure actually described in most series is better termed *pleural debridement* because fluid and fibrinous peel from the visceral and parietal pleural surfaces are removed to extract truly infected material. This can be accomplished without the trauma and blood loss usually associated with true decortication procedures, and pleural debridement should be considered earlier in the course of the empyema. Although some more recent reports still advocate formal thoracotomy or minithoracotomy to accomplish this, (103,107,115) thoracoscopic debridement has clearly become a mainstream therapy (Fig. 60-9) (40,41,116–119). However, despite optimism that early thoracoscopic intervention may hasten recovery from empyema, no prospective studies have confirmed this. Pleural loculations in some patients can be lysed by instilling urokinase or streptokinase through existing chest tubes before resorting to surgical intervention (120,121).

In the event that a lung abscess develops, treatment may require pneumonostomy, wedge resection, or lobar resection (112,123). Radiographic findings often lag behind clinical response; therefore, they should not be used alone as indications for further intervention. With prompt and adequate treatment, the overall outcome for children with empyema is excellent. Pulmonary function after recovery is usually clinically normal, although some investigators have found mild restrictive or obstructive disease on follow-up spirometry (105,124).

MEDIASTINAL MASSES

The mediastinum is the most common location of intrathoracic masses in children. The large number of structures within the mediastinum creates a vast array of potential diagnoses. Dividing the mediastinum into arbitrary anatomic compartments has significantly helped to limit the differential diagnoses and to plan diagnostic studies. Although several schema have been proposed, this section discusses one that divides the mediastinum into four compartments: superior, anterior, middle, and posterior as delineated on the lateral chest radiograph (Fig. 60-2).

The superior mediastinal compartment contains the great vessels and most of the thymus gland. Tumors of the thymus, such as thymomas or germ-cell tumors, may

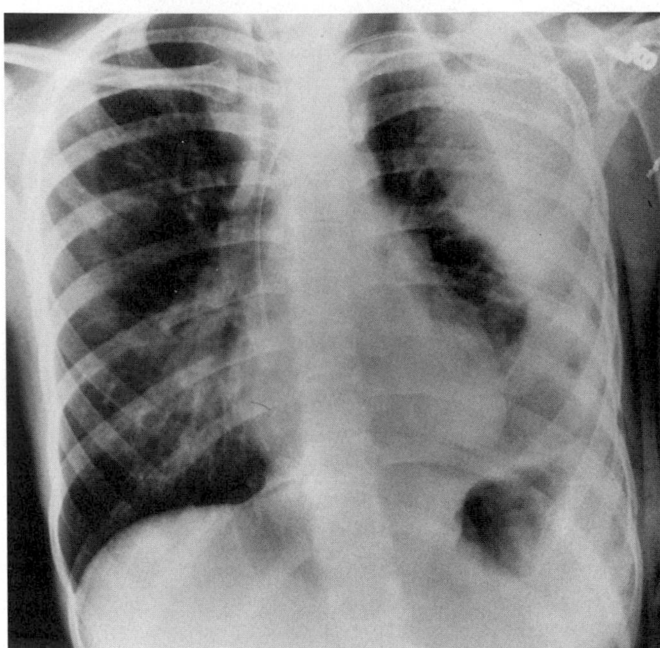

A

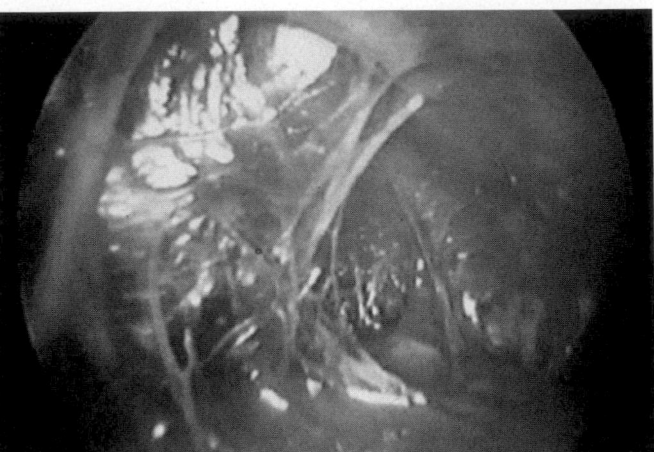

B

FIGURE 60-9. **(A)** Frontal chest radiograph of a 15-year-old boy who developed a posttraumatic empyema in the left hemithorax. A culture of chest tube drainage grew *Staphylococcus aureus*. **(B)** At the time of thoracoscopic pleural debridement, there were multiple thin pleural adhesions, which were completely lysed with blunt and sharp dissection. A single chest tube was left in place and removed 3 days later.

present in this compartment. Lymphangiomas are usually found in the superior mediastinum. The anterior mediastinum contains the lower portion of the thymus and scattered lymphatic tissue. In addition to thymic tumors, lymphomas may develop in this compartment. Bronchogenic cysts in the hilum occur within the middle mediastinum. The posterior mediastinum contains the esophagus, the descending aorta, and the sympathetic nerves and ganglia. The posterior compartment is the site of most neurogenic tumors, such as neuroblastomas and ganglioneuromas. Esophageal cysts also present within this compartment. Most mediastinal masses in children are found in the posterior compartment.

Most mediastinal masses in children are confined to a single compartment, although large masses may extend into adjacent compartments. Certain lesions, such as mediastinal lymphangiomas and hemangiomas, may primarily involve more than one compartment. Most mediastinal masses discovered in children younger than 6 years are benign, whereas masses diagnosed in older children are more likely to be malignant tumors. Almost one-half of the children with mediastinal masses are asymptomatic at the time of diagnosis (125). Those with symptoms may present either with respiratory symptoms or chest pain.

The principles of the diagnostic evaluation of a mediastinal mass in a child are to determine its primary location, define its morphology, and delineate its involvement of surrounding structures (126). Conventional chest radiographs are the primary radiologic examination and guide subsequent imaging. The presence and character of calcification noted on this study may help establish the diagnosis. Cross-sectional imaging is used to further define the location and extent of the mass. CT studies are most commonly used for lesions in the anterior and middle compartments. MRI may have significant advantages in evaluating lesions in the superior and posterior mediastinal compartments. In the superior mediastinum, the MRI can delineate the vascular structures and their relation to the lesion. In the posterior compartment, the MRI allows determination of intraspinal involvement of neurogenic tumors (127). The MRI in both areas has the distinct advantage of allowing multiplanar imaging (128). Transthoracic ultrasound may be helpful in differentiating between loculated pleural fluid and pleural masses, as well as in differentiating cystic from solid lesions in the anterior or posterior compartments (129).

GERM-CELL TUMORS

The mediastinum is the most common location for extragonadal germ-cell tumors, including teratomas, dysgerminomas, choriocarcinomas, endodermal sinus tumors, and dermoid cysts. Most of these lesions arise in the superior or anterior mediastinal compartments. These tumors are believed to arise from germ cells that have stopped migrating during embryogenesis and have persisted within the region of the thymus (130). Teratomas comprise 80% of primary germ-cell tumors found in the mediastinum.

The mediastinum is the second most common location for teratomas in children, next to the sacrococcygeal area. Mediastinal teratomas comprise approximately 10% to 20% of mediastinal tumors and approximately 10% of all teratomas (131,132). Most are located in the anterior or superior mediastinum, although they may occur within the pericardium or the posterior mediastinum (131–133). The rate of malignancy of these lesions varies from 10 to 25% (131–133). Males and females are equally affected. Characteristically, mediastinal teratomas are primarily, although not always entirely, cystic and are derived from more than one germinal layer. Ectodermal components predominate, and calcifications may be present (131–133).

Mediastinal teratomas may present in various ways. They may be detected on prenatal ultrasound, and be associated with fetal hydrops and polyhydramnios (134). The most common presenting symptom is respiratory insufficiency secondary to airway compression, compression of the pulmonary parenchyma, or intrapleural rupture of the teratoma (135,136). Interestingly, only a minority of mediastinal teratomas present with respiratory symptoms in the newborn period (137). Most of these tumors do not present until adolescence. Tissue within the teratoma may be functioning in a physiologic manner causing symptoms related to the particular hormone or enzyme secreted (138,139). Some teratomas may become infected, resulting in a febrile presentation (140). There have been reports of intrapericardial teratomas presenting with cardiac tamponade (141). Teratomas may also present as incidental findings on chest imaging studies (137). Once suspected, imaging of a mediastinal teratoma is best accomplished by CT or MRI. CT is particularly useful for evaluating these lesions because it allows for the identification of fat and calcifications (128). If a teratoma is intrapericardial or within the posterior mediastinum, angiography may be helpful to define the vascular anatomy. Laboratory evaluation should include measurement of serum alpha-fetoprotein, carcinoembryonic antigen, and human chorionic gonadotrophin to assist in patient follow-up if the lesion appears malignant.

Treatment of mediastinal teratomas is surgical excision either by thoracotomy or sternotomy. Usually, the lesions are well encapsulated with minimal vascularity, although pericardial and posterior mediastinal tumors may have significant vascular supply from the aorta. Malignant teratomas often envelop adjacent structures. The outcome for these malignant tumors is poor despite adjunctive chemotherapy and radiation therapy (131,132). Malignancy may be difficult to determine histologically at initial resection, and occasionally, patients present with malignant recurrence after removal of a teratoma initially believed to be benign (132); therefore, long-term follow-up is required for all children after removal of a mediastinal teratoma.

THYMOMA

Thymomas are the most common neoplasms of the anterior mediastinum in adults, but they are rare in children (142–145). Although thymomas are commonly associated with myasthenia gravis in adults, this association is extraordinarily rare in children (142). Immunodeficiency may sometimes be associated with thymoma (146). Thymomas represent neoplasms of epithelial or lymphocytic origin (144). Malignant potential is determined by the presence and extent of microscopic or macroscopic invasion beyond the capsule of the gland (143). Malignant thymomas are histologically similar to lymphoblastic lymphoma and must be differentiated from that disease (133,142). The treatment of these lesions is complete surgical excision. Radiation therapy and chemotherapy may be required for advanced stages of malignancy or partially resected or unresectable disease (144,147,148).

THYMIC CYSTS

Thymic cysts are uncommon lesions that may present as either mediastinal or neck masses in children (62,133,149,150). Mediastinal thymic cysts are generally asymptomatic and are found incidentally. If symptoms are present, they may include wheezing, cough, upper respiratory infection, and fever (151). Their origin has been a subject of debate, with some authors arguing that they are congenital in nature, whereas others suggest they are secondary to inflammation (149,150). Regardless, they are uniformly benign in children (150). Thymic cysts are lined by ciliated epithelium with components of lymphocytes, thymic tissue, cholesterol crystals, and Hassall corpuscles within the wall (150). When a thymic cyst is suspected, transthoracic ultrasound, CT scan, or fine-needle aspiration may help confirm the diagnosis, although preoperative diagnosis may sometimes be difficult (152). Thymic cysts rarely involve adjacent structures and are generally easily resected. Resection of a thymic cyst can be accomplished thoracoscopically (153,154).

BRONCHOGENIC CYSTS

Bronchogenic cysts are part of a spectrum of anomalies that arise from abnormalities of ventral foregut budding. Gerle proposed the term *bronchopulmonary-foregut malformations* to encompass the anomalies of bronchogenic cysts, pulmonary sequestrations, and abnormalities of tracheal budding (155). Most bronchogenic cysts are located in the middle mediastinum close to the trachea or mainstem bronchi. They may also be located more peripherally within the lung parenchyma itself (156). These are discussed in detail in Chapter 61. Mediastinal bronchogenic cysts are typically lined with ciliated columnar epithelium and contain thick mucous. The walls of the cysts are usually thin and may contain hyaline cartilage, scattered smooth muscle, mucous glands, and nerve fibers. The walls never contain the well-developed muscle layers and nerve plexuses characteristic of enteric cysts. Bronchogenic cysts rarely communicate with the airway, but they may densely adhere to it. The cysts may, however, communicate with the gastrointestinal tract, usually below the diaphragm (156). There may be associated vertebral anomalies (157). Bronchogenic cysts may cause symptoms ranging from stridor to frank respiratory distress. This is particularly true for cysts in infants and for cysts located near the carina (157). Bronchogenic cysts, however, are often discovered as incidental findings on chest radiographs. If the cyst itself is not always evident, associated findings of compression of the trachea, bronchi, or atelectasis may lead to the diagnosis. If a bronchogenic cyst is suspected, a contrast-enhanced CT scan of the chest should be obtained to confirm the diagnosis and to delineate the regional anatomy. MRI may be equally as helpful in this regard and avoids the risks of radiation (158,159).

Once detected, bronchogenic cysts should be excised. This has traditionally been accomplished by thoracotomy. However, these cysts can be completely excised using thoracoscopic techniques, and this is the preferred technique for centrally located lesions (42–44). Cysts that are asymptomatic at the time of diagnosis should still be removed because they are prone to causing airway obstruction and infection, and although rare, malignancies are reported with the passage of time (156,158,160,161). If the cyst cannot be completely excised, the epithelium should be fulgurated. These children must be monitored for recurrence (162).

LYMPHOMA

Lymphoma, both Hodgkin's and non-Hodgkin's, is the most common cause of anterior and middle mediastinal masses in children (163). Hodgkin's disease tends to have a predisposition to the cervical or mediastinal regions and may present as local or disseminated disease. Non-Hodgkin's lymphomas are assumed to be disseminated when first discovered (163). Most non-Hodgkin's tumors found in the mediastinum are of a lymphoblastic T-cell origin (126).

A mediastinal lymphoma may present as an incidental finding on a chest radiograph or by causing respiratory distress or superior vena cava syndrome (163,164). Non-Hodgkin's lymphomas grow quickly and tend to be more severe in their respiratory manifestations, with 50% to 70% having associated pleural effusions (163,165). A chest CT scan determines the size and location of the tumor and the degree of airway compression (166,167). Hodgkin's lymphoma may present with fever or systemic symptoms. The diagnosis of lymphoma is established by tissue biopsy. In some instances, a cervical or other lymph node can be biopsied, a chest effusion can be sampled, or a bone marrow aspirate can be obtained for diagnosis (168). However, when the mediastinal mass represents the only available tissue or when symptomatology does not allow delay in diagnosis, direct biopsy of the mediastinal mass is necessary (169,170). Fine-needle aspirates are unsuccessful in obtaining diagnostic material up to 50% of the time (171). Therefore, more aggressive procedures are usually needed. These include core-needle biopsies, thoracoscopic biopsy, or anterior thoracotomy (165,172). Local anesthesia can be used for needle aspirations or for biopsies requiring limited incisions. If general anesthesia is needed, it is best induced in a partial or total upright position with the patient breathing spontaneously. Airway collapse may ensue if muscle relaxants are used. In cases where complete anesthesia and relaxation are required, however, a rigid bronchoscope should be available to access and support the lower airway should difficulties arise (169). It is difficult to know ahead of time which patient will not tolerate anesthesia. Traditionally, it has been believed that the more significant the respiratory symptoms, the greater the risk of anesthesia. Shamberger et al. attempted to quantify this risk by measuring the cross-sectional area of the compressed trachea by CT. A tracheal cross-sectional area that is larger than 50% of expected suggests an uneventful anesthesia according to this study (167) (Fig. 60-10).

If respiratory symptoms truly prohibit manipulation of the patient, mediastinal radiation, perhaps supplemented by steroids, can rapidly shrink the tumor and relieve symptoms. However, this may also destroy any hope of obtaining reliable tissue to provide a precise diagnosis of the type of lymphoma (167,169,170,173). Therefore, the surgeon should try to obtain tissue before treatment if possible.

MEDIASTINAL LYMPH NODES

Mediastinal lymph nodes may become enlarged as part of several nonmalignant conditions. These include sarcoidosis, Castleman's disease, histoplasmosis, coccidiomycosis, tuberculosis, and rarely, bacterial and viral infections (174,175). Lymph node enlargement may result in respiratory symptomatology, dysphagia, or superior vena cava syndrome. A chest CT scan may be required to delineate the extent of mediastinal nodal pathology. Evaluation of these patients may ultimately require nodal biopsy if other diagnostic tests are inconclusive. Modalities commonly used for tissue sampling include needle biopsy, thoracoscopy, or thoracotomy.

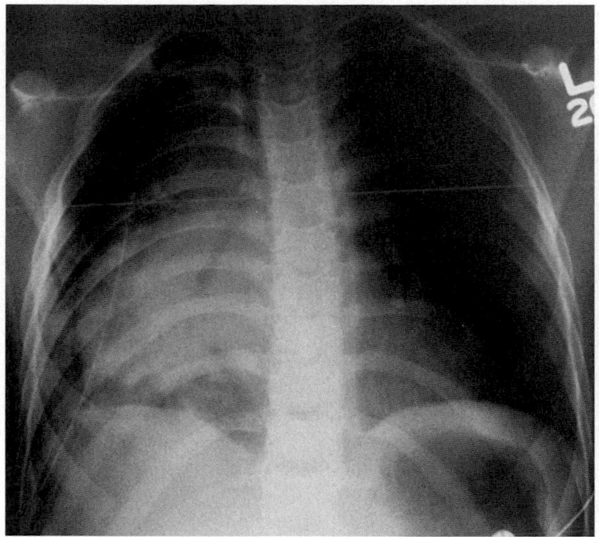
A

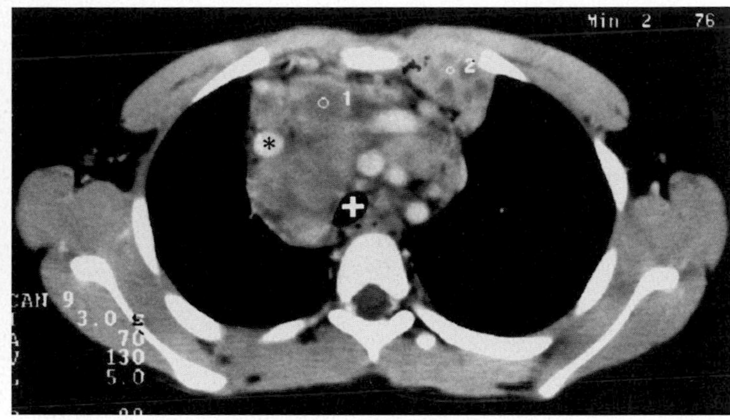

B

FIGURE 60-10. **(A)** Frontal chest radiograph of a 14-year-old girl with respiratory symptoms secondary to a large anterior mediastinal mass. **(B)** Chest computed tomography scan demonstrates a bulky mediastinal lesion displaying the trachea (*plus sign*) posteriorly and to the right, and compressing the tracheal lumen approximately 50%. The superior vena cava (*asterisk*) is displaced laterally. A percutaneous needle biopsy was nondiagnostic. Biopsy obtained by thoracosocpy under local anesthesia confirmed nodular sclerosing Hodgkin's disease.

PERICARDIAL CYSTS

Pericardial cysts result when the mesodermal lacunae fail to coalesce in the developing pericardium (149). These cysts are typically thin-walled, contain a flat mesothelial lining, and are generally found at the cardiophrenic angle in the middle mediastinum (62). These patients are usually asymptomatic, and the cysts present as incidental findings on chest images. Because of the benign and asymptomatic nature of these cysts, some authors believe that observation may be justified, although others make the case for surgical removal when they are found due to their potential for symptomatology (149,176). Even cardiac tamponade has been reported due to hemorrhage or effusion (177,178). The histology of pericardial cysts is uniformly benign (62,150). Ultrasound and CT scan usually confirm the diagnosis. Surgical excision is usually uncomplicated. Presently, some pericardial cysts may be removed by thoracoscopy (154,179,180).

LYMPHANGIOMA

Lymphangiomas are congenital lesions that contain abnormal proliferation of lymphatic and vascular tissue. They can be comprised principally of large lymphatic cysts, and thus bear the name *cystic hygroma*, or they can consist of denser tissue with more prominent vascular elements and be termed *lymphangiomas*. Lymphangiomatous tissue consists of vessels with a thin endothelial lining and some smooth muscle (181). There are several theories regarding the formation of lymphangiomas, but the most commonly accepted one suggests that lymphangiomas represent the failure in part of the embryonic lymph sacs to establish adequate drainage into the venous system (133,181).

Lymphangiomas occur with an incidence of approximately 1 in 6,000 births. Isolated mediastinal lymphangiomas represent only about 1% of these cases (182–185). Large cervical lymphangiomas, however, may extend into the mediastinum in 2% to 10% of cases (62,133,181). Isolated mediastinal lymphangiomas are usually found in the anterior mediastinum, although they can also be found in other compartments of the mediastinum (133). Cervical lymphangiomas often extend into the posterior mediastinum. Lymphangiomas of the neck and axilla usually present by 2 years of age and are readily apparent on physical examination; however, mediastinal lymphangiomas are often incidental findings on chest imaging or first come to the physician's attention with the onset of respiratory symptoms. Prenatal ultrasound may detect a mediastinal lymphangioma (184).

The presenting symptoms of mediastinal lymphangiomas are the result of their impingement on the airway, lungs, or other mediastinal structures. Infection or collections of chyle in the pleura or pericardium may occur. Hemorrhage into a lymphangioma with rapid enlargement and sudden onset of symptoms has been described (183,184,186–188). Mediastinal lymphangiomas appear as homogeneous masses on chest radiograph. Ultrasonography reveals their primarily cystic nature, sometimes containing debris. CT or MRI reveals the cystic nature of the lesion, as well as the extent of its involvement with other mediastinal structures. Calcifications are usually not present unless there is a significant vascular component (183,186).

There have been reports of spontaneous regression of lymphangiomas, but these are sporadic and not part of the natural course of this lesion. The optimal therapy of mediastinal lymphangiomas is total excision by thoracotomy or sternotomy, but it is widely agreed that vital structures should not be sacrificed during attempts at total excision (62,133,181,182). Because tissue must often be left behind and because some lesions are simply not resectable due to their extensive involvement of vital structures, alternative strategies for therapy have been advanced (182). Intralesional injection of bleomycin, OK-432, and fibrin sealant has been reported as primary therapy by some authors (189,190–193). Bleomycin, in particular, has been successful in shrinking some large lymphangiomas to resectable size (190). Injections of glucose, iodine, and tetracycline, or dexamethasone, have been used for sclerosis of residual tissue after resection with varying results (182,187). Irradiation of these lesions is discouraged (181).

The most common postoperative complication after resection of a lymphangioma is development of lymph accumulation. Repeated aspiration of the fluid often resolves this difficulty. Fibrin glue or chemical sclerosis with doxycycline may be helpful if aspiration fails (181). In some cases, resection of all or part of the residual tissue may be necessary. Lymphangiomas recur in at least 10% to 15% of cases if resection has not been complete; therefore, close long-term follow-up of these children is necessary.

NEUROFIBROMA

Mediastinal neurofibromas may occur as isolated tumors or may be manifestations of von Recklinghausen's disease. They often have a dumbbell shape and may extend from or along spinal nerve roots, intercostal nerves, the sympathetic chain, or the vagus nerve. Neurofibromas are often detected incidentally on chest radiographs. The presence of scoliosis, widened intervertebral foramina, or disruption of the costovertebral angle may suggest the diagnosis. A chest MRI scan can delineate the extent of the tumor and can detect any extension of the tumor into the spinal canal (194). Large tumors are known to undergo malignant change. Excision is recommended, although it may not be possible to completely resect portions extending deep within vertebral foramina or costovertebral junctions. Thoracic laminectomy may be required to completely excise some of these tumors. Occasionally, total excision may not be possible and subsequent attempts at resection may be required (194).

REFERENCES

1. Wells U. Development of the human diaphragm and pleural sacs. *Embryology* 1954;35:107.
2. Bremer JL. The diaphragm and diaphragmatic hernia. *Arch Pathol* 1943;36:539.
3. Chen JM. Studies of the morphogenesis of the mouse sternum. *J Anat* 1952;86:373.
4. Wells U, Boyden EA. The development of the bronchopulmonary segments in human embryos of horizons XIV to XIX. *Am J Anat* 1954;95:163.
5. Davis HK. A statistical study of the thoracic duct in man. *Am J Anat* 1915;17:211.
6. Weller GL. Development of the thyroid, parathyroid and thymus glands in man. *Embryology* 1933;24:93.
7. Adams FH, Lind J. Physiologic studies on the cardio-vascular status of the normal newborn infant (with special reference to the ductus arteriosus). *Am J Dis Child* 1957;93:13.
8. Joger VV, Wollerman OJ. An anatomical study of the closure of the ductus arteriosus. *Am J Pathol* 942;18:595.
9. Dunnill MS. Postnatal growth of the lung. *Thorax* 1962;17:329.
10. Davis RD, Oldham HN, Sabiston DC.The mediastinum. In: Sabiston DC, Spencer FC, eds. *Surgery of the chest,* 5th ed. Philadelphia: WB Saunders, 1990:444.
11. Agostoni E, D'Angelo E. Pleural liquid pressure. *J Appl Physiol* 1991;71:393.
12. Wang PM, Lai-Fook SJ. Upward flow of pleural liquid near lobar margins due to cardiogenic motion. *J Appl Physiol* 1992;73:2314.
13. Wiener-Kronish JP, Broaddus VC. Interrelationships of pleural and pulmonary interstitial liquid. *Annu Rev Physiol* 1993;55:209.
14. West JB.Mechanics of breathing. In: West JB, ed. *Respiratory physiology: the essentials,* 4th ed. Baltimore: Williams & Wilkins, 1990:87.
15. West JB.Ventilation. In: West JB, ed. *Respiratory physiology: the essentials,* 4th ed. Baltimore: Williams & Wilkins, 1990:11.
16. Hubmayr RD, Margulies SS. Effects of unilateral hyperinflation on the interpulmonary distribution of pleural pressure. *J Appl Physiol* 1992;73:1650.
17. Lai-Fook SJ, Rodarte JR. Pleural pressure distribution and its relationship to lung volume and interstitial pressure. *J Appl Physiol* 1991;70:967.
18. Mutoh T, Guest RI, Lamm WJE, et al. Prone position alters the effect of volume overload on regional pleural pressures and improves hypoxemia in pigs *in vivo. Am Rev Respir Dis* 1992;146:300.
19. Gross I. Respiratory diseases: developmental considerations. In: Oski FA, ed. *Principles and practice of pediatrics,* 1st ed. Philadelphia: JB Lippincott, 1990:329.
20. Smith CA, Nelson NM. *The physiology of the newborn infant.* Springfield, IL: Charles C Thomas, 1976:207.
21. Driscoll DJ. Use of inotropic and chronotropic agents in neonates. *Clin Perinatol* 1987;14:931.
22. Benumof JL. Physiology of the lateral decubitus position, the open chest, and one-lung ventilation. In: Kaplan JA, ed. *Thoracic anesthesia,* 2nd ed. New York: Churchill-Livingstone, 1991:193.
23. Darnall RA. Noninvasive blood pressure measurement in the neonate. *Clin Perinatol* 1985;12:31.
24. Solimano AJ, Smyth JA, Mann TK, et al. Pulse oximetry advantages in infants with bronchopulmonary dysplasia. *Pediatrics* 1986;78:844.
25. McEvedy BAB, McLeod ME, Kirpalani H, et al. End-tidal carbon dioxide measurements in critically ill neonates: a comparison of side-stream and mainstream capnometers. *Can J Anaesth* 1990;37:322.
26. Rah KH, Salzberg AM, Boyan CP, et al. Respiratory acidosis with small Storz-Hopkins bronchoscopes: occurrence and management. *Ann Thorac Surg* 1979;27:197.
27. McIlvaine WB, Chang JHT, Jones M. The effective use of intrapleural bupivacaine for analgesia after thoracic and subcostal incisions in children. *J Pediatr Surg* 1988;23:1184.
28. Tobias JD, Martin LD, Oakes L, et al. Postoperative analgesia following thoracotomy in children: intrapleural catheters. *J Pediatr Surg* 1993;28:1466.
29. Rodgers BM, Webb CJ, Stergois O, et al. Patient controlled analgesia in pediatric surgery. *J Pediatr Surg* 1987;23:259.

30. Rowney DA, Doyle E. Epidural and subarachnoid blockade in children. *Anesthesia* 1998;53:980.
31. Chetcuti P, Myers NA, Phelan PO, et al. Chest wall deformity in patients with repaired esophageal atresia. *J Pediatr Surg* 1989;24:244.
32. Jaureguizar E, Vazquez J, Murcia J, et al. Morbid musculoskeletal sequelae of thoracotomy for tracheoesophageal fistula. *J Pediatr Surg* 1985;20:511.
33. Goodman P, Balachandran S, Guinto FC. Postoperative atrophy of posterolateral chest wall musculature: CT demonstration. *J Comput Assist Tomogr* 1992;17:63.
34. Goh OW, Brereton RJ. Triangle of auscultation thoracotomy for esophageal atresia. *J Thorac Cardiovasc Surg* 1992;103:14.
35. Karwande SV, Rowles JR. Simplified muscle-sparing thoracotomy for patent ductus arteriosus ligation in neonates. *Ann Thorac Surg* 1992;54:164.
36. Rothenberg SS, Pokorny WI. Experience with a total muscle-sparing approach for thoracotomies in neonates, infants, and children. *J Pediatr Surg* 1992;27:1157.
37. Ponn RB, Ferneini A, D'Agostino RS, et al. Comparison of late pulmonary function after posterolateral and muscle-sparing thoracotomy. *Ann Thorac Surg* 1992;53:675.
38. Rodgers BM. The role of thoracoscopy in pediatric surgical practice. *Semin Pediatr Surg* 2003;12:62.
39. McGahren ED, Kern JA, Rodgers BM. Anesthetic techniques for pediatric thoracoscopy. *Ann Thorac Surg* 1995;60:927.
40. Kern JA, Rodgers BD. Thoracoscopy in the management of empyema in children. *J Pediatr Surg* 1993;28:1128.
41. Cohen G, Hjortdal V, Ricci M, et al. Primary thoracoscopic treatment of empyema in children. *J Thorac Cardiovasc Surg* 2003;125:79.
42. Kern JA, Daniel TM, Tribble CO, et al. Thoracoscopic diagnosis and treatment of mediastinal masses. *Ann Thorac Surg* 1993;56:92.
43. Dillon PW, Cilley RE, Krummel TM. Video-assisted thoracoscopic excision of intrathoracic masses in children: report of two cases. *Surg Laparosc Endosc* 1993;3:433.
44. Lobe TE. Pediatric thoracoscopy. *Semin Thorac Cardiovasc Surg* 1993;5:298.
45. Rodgers BM. Pediatric thoracoscopy: where have we come and what have we learned. *Ann Thorac Surg* 1993;56:704.
46. Tirabassi MV, Banever GT, Tashjiam DB, et al. Use of energy devices in thoracoscopy: quantitation of lung sealing capacity. *Pediatr Endosurg Innov Tech* 2003;7:104.
47. Tribble CG, Selden RF, Rodgers BM. Talc poudrage in the treatment of spontaneous pneumothoraces in patients with cystic fibrosis. *Ann Surg* 1986;204:677.
48. Urschel JD, Chan WKY. Technical report: thoracoscopic pleural abrasion for pneumothorax. *J Laparosc Surg* 1993;3:351.
49. Graham DD, McGahren ED, Tribble CG, et al. Use of video-assisted thoracic surgery in the treatment of chylothorax. *Ann Thorac Surg* 1994;57:1507.
50. Rothenberg SS. Experience with thoracoscopic lobectomy in infants and children. *J Pediatr Surg* 2003;38:102.
51. Laborde F, Hoirhomme P, Karam J, et al. A new video-assisted thoracoscopic surgical technique for interruption of patent ductus arteriosus in infants and children. *J Thorac Cardiovasc Surg* 1993;105:278.
52. LeBret E, Papadatos S, Folliguet J, et al. Interruption of patent ductus arteriosus in children: robotically assisted versus video-thoracoscopic surgery. *J Thorac Cardiovasc Surg* 2002;123:973.
53. Lobe TE, Rothenberg SS, Waldschmidt J, et al. Thoracoscopic repair of esophageal atresia in an infant: a surgical first. *Pediatr Endosurg Innov Tech* 1999;3:141.
54. Rothenberg SS. Thoracoscopic repair of tracheoesophageal fistula in newborns. *J Pediatr Surg* 2002;37:869.
55. Drasin T, Gracia C, Atkinson J. Pediatric applications of robotic surgery. *Pediatr Endosurg Innov Tech* 2003;7:377.
56. Mikaljevic T, Cannon JW, deNido PJ. Robotically assisted division of a vascular ring in children. *J Thorac Cardiov Surg* 2003;125:1163.
57. Morgan JA, Gensburg ME, Sonett JR, et al. Advanced thoracoscopic procedures are facilitated by computer-aided robotic technology. *Eur J Cardio-Thorac Surg* 2003;23:883.
58. Luebbe BN, Woo R, Wolf SA, et al. Robotically assisted minimally invasive surgery in a pediatric population: initial experience, technical considerations, and description of the daVinci surgical system. *Pediatr Endosurg Innov Tech* 2003;7:385.
59. Lorincz A, Langenburg S, Klein M. Robotics and the pediatric surgeon. *Curr Opin Pediatr* 2003;15:262.
60. DeMeester TR, Lafontaine E. The pleura. In: Sabiston DC, Spencer FC, eds. *Surgery of the chest,* 5th ed. Philadelphia: WB Saunders, 1990:444.
61. Kemp JS, Seilheimer DK. Diseases of the pleura. In: Oski FA, ed. *Principles and practice of pediatrics,* Ist ed. Philadelphia: JB Lippincott, 1990:1378.
62. Ravitch MM.Mediastinal cysts and tumors. II. In: Welch KJ, Randolph JG, Ravitch MM, et al., eds. *Pediatric surgery,* 4th ed. Chicago: Year Book Medical, 1986:602.
63. Benteur L, Canny G, Thorner P, et al. Spontaneous pneumothorax in cystic adenomatoid malformation. *Chest* 1991;99:1292.
64. Davis AM, Wensley DF, Phelan PD. Spontaneous pneumothorax in pediatric patients. *Respir Med* 1993;87:531.
65. Kemp JS, Seilheimer DK.Diseases of the pleura. In: Oski FA, ed. *Principles and practice of pediatrics,* Ist ed. Philadelphia: JB Lippincott, 1990:1378.
66. Rhea IT, DeLuca SA, Greene RE. Determining the size of pneumothorax in the upright patient. *Radiology* 1982;144:733.
67. Zierold D, Lee SL, Subramanian S, et al. Supplemental oxygen improves resolution of injury-induced pneumothorax. *J Pediatr Surg* 2000;35:998.
68. Kjaergaard H. Spontaneous pneumothorax in the apparently healthy. *Acta Med Scand Suppl* 1932;43:1.
69. Gaensler EA. Parietal pleurectomy for recurrent pneumothorax. *Surg Gynecol Obstet* 1956;102:293.
70. Vernejoux JM, Raherison C, Combe P, et al. Spontaneous pneumothorax: pragmatic management and long-term outcome. *Respir Med* 2001;95:857.
71. Gammie JS, Banks MC, Fuhrman CR, et al. The pigtail catheter for pleural drainage: a less invasive alternative to tube thoracostomy. *J Soc Laparoendosc Surg* 1999;3:57.
72. Noemi T, Hannukainen J, Aarnio P. Use of the Heimlich valve for treating pneumothorax. *Ann Chir Gynecol* 1999;88:36.
73. Austin EH, Flye MW. The treatment of recurrent malignant pleural effusion. *Ann Thorac Surg* 1979;28:190.
74. Spector ML, Stem RC. Pneumothorax in cystic fibrosis: a 26-year experience. *Ann Thorac Surg* 1989;47:204.
75. Stephenson LW. Treatment of pneumothorax with intrapleural tetracycline. *Chest* 1985;88:803.
76. Thorsrud GK. Pleural reaction to irritants. *Acta Chir Scand* 1965; 355:1.
77. Sarkar S, Hussain N, Herson V. Fibrin glue for persistent pneumothorax in neonates. *J Perinatol* 2003;23:82.
78. de Campos JR, Vargas FS, de Campos WE, et al. Thoracoscopy talc poudrage: a 15-year experience. *Chest* 2001;119:801.
79. Lang EK, Ghavami R, Schreiner VC, et al. Autologous blood clot seal to prevent pneumothorax at CT-guided lung biopsy. *Radiology* 2000;216:93.
80. Hazelrigg SR, Landreneau RJ, Mack M, et al. Thoracoscopic stapled resection for spontaneous pneumothorax. *J Thorac Cardiovasc Surg* 1993;105:389.
81. Stringel G, Amin NS, Dozor AJ. Video-assisted thoracoscopy in the management of recurrent spontaneous pneumothorax in the pediatric population. *J Soc Laparoendosc Surg* 1999;3:113.
82. Inderbitzi RGC, Furrer M, Striffeler H, et al. Thoracoscopic pleurectomy for treatment of complicated spontaneous pneumothorax. *J Thorac Cardiovasc Surg* 1993;105:84.
83. Cook CH, Melvin WS, Groner JI, et al. A cost-effective thoracoscopic treatment strategy for pediatric spontaneous pneumothorax. *Surg Endosc* 1999;13:1208.
84. Rodgers BM, McGahren ED. Endoscopy in children. *Chest Surg Clin North Am* 1993;3:405.
85. Allen EM, Van Heeckeren DW, Spector ML, et al. Management of nutritional and infectious complications of postoperative chylothorax in children. *J Pediatr Surg* 1991;26:1169.
86. Easa D, Balaraman V, Ash K, et al. Congenital chylothorax and mediastinal neuroblastoma. *J Pediatr Surg* 1991;26:96.
87. Bond SJ, Guzzetta PC, Snyder ML, et al. Management of pediatric postoperative chylothorax. *Ann Thorac Surg* 1993;56:469.

88. Telander RL, Moir CR. Acquired diseases of the lung and pleura. In: Ashcraft KW, Holder TM, eds. *Pediatric surgery,* 2nd ed. Philadelphia: WB Saunders, 1993:188.
89. Valentine VG, Raffin TA. The management of chylothorax. *Chest* 1992;102:586.
90. Au M, Weber TR, Fleming RE. Successful use of somatostatin in a case of neonatal chylothorax. *J Pediatr Surg* 2003;38:1106.
91. Tauber MT, Harris AG, Rochicciol P. Clinical use of the long acting somatostatin analogue octreotide in pediatrics. *Eur J Pediatr* 1994;153:304.
92. Murphy MC, Newman BM, Rodgers, BM. Pleuro-peritoneal shunts in the management of persistent chylothorax. *Ann Thorac Surg* 1989;48:195.
93. Engum SA, Rescorla FJ, West KW, et al. The use of pleuroperitoneal shunts in the management of persistent chylothorax in infants. *J Pediatr Surg* 1999;34:286.
94. Wolff AB, Silen ML, Kokoska ER, et al. Treatment of refractory chylothorax with externalized pleuroperitoneal shunts in children. *Ann Thorac Surg* 1999;65:1053.
95. Rheuban KS, Kron IL, Carpenter MA. Pleuroperitoneal shunts for refractory chylothorax after operation for congenital heart disease. *Ann Thorac Surg* 1992;53:85.
96. Randolph JG, Gross RE. Congenital chylothorax. *Arch Surg* 1957;74:405.
97. Fajardo E, Chang MG. Pleural empyema in children: a nationwide retrospective study. *South Med J* 1987;80:593.
98. Bartlett JC, Gorbach SL, Thadepalli HT, et al. Bacteriology of empyema. *Lancet* 1974;1:338.
99. American Thoracic Society. Management of nontuberculous empyema. *Am Rev Respir Dis* 1962;85:935.
100. Chonmaitree T, Powell KR. Parapneumonic pleural effusion and empyema in children. *Clin Pediatr* 1983;22:414.
101. Gustafson RA, Murray GF, Warden HE, et al. Role of lung decortication in symptomatic empyemas in children. *Ann Thorac Surg* 1990;49:940.
102. Hoff SJ, Neblett WW, Heller RM, et al. Postpneumonic empyema in childhood: selecting appropriate therapy. *J Pediatr Surg* 1989;24:659.
103. Gofrit ON, Englehard D, Abu-Dalu K. Post-pneumonic empyema in children: a continued surgical challenge. *Eur J Pediatr Surg* 1999;9:4.
104. Huang FL, Chen PY, Ma JS, et al. Clinical experience of managing empyema thoracis in children. *J Microbiol Immunol Infect* 2002;35:115.
105. Goeman A, Kipur N, Toppare M, et al. Conservative treatment of empyema in children. *Respiration* 1993;60:182.
106. Mangete ED, Kombo BB, Legg-Jack TE. Thoracic empyema: a study of 56 patients. *Arch Dis Child* 1993;69:587.
107. Sarihan H, Cay A, Aynaci M, et al. Empyema in children. *J Cardiovasc Surg* 1998;39:113.
108. Yilmaz E, Dogan Y, Aydinoglu AH, et al. Parapneumonic empyema in children: conservative approach. *Turk J Pediatr* 2002;44:134.
109. Lewis KT, Bukstein DA. Parapneumonic empyema in children: diagnosis and management. *Am Fam Physician* 1992;46:1443.
110. Ramnath RR, Heller RM, Ben-Ami T, et al. Implications of early sonographic evaluation of parapneumonic effusions in children with pneumonia. *Pediatrics* 1998;101:68.
111. Kosloske AM, Carwright KC. The controversial role of decortication in the management of pediatric empyema. *J Thorac Cardiovasc Surg* 1988;96:166.
112. Chan PW, Crawford O, Wallis C, et al. Treatment of pleural empyema. *J Pediatr Child Health* 2000;36:37.
113. Chan W, Keyser-Gauvin E, Davis GM, et al. Empyema thoracis in children: a 26-year review of the Montreal Children's Hospital experience. *J Pediatr Surg* 1997;32:870.
114. Hendren WH, Haggerty RL. Staphylococcal pneumonia in infancy and childhood. *JAMA* 1958;168:6.
115. Carey JA, Hamilton JR, Spencer DA, et al. Empyema thoracis: a role for open thoracotomy and decortication. *Arch Dis Child* 1998;79:510.
116. Kercher KW, Attori RJ, Hoover JD, et al. Thoracoscopic decortication as first-line therapy for pediatric parapneumonic empyema. A case series. *Chest* 2000;118:24.
117. Meier AH, Smith B, Raghavan A, et al. Rational treatment of empyema in children. *Arch Surg* 2000;135:907.
118. Chen LE, Langer JC, Dillon PA, et al. Management of late-stage parapneumonic empyema. *J Pediatr Surg* 2002;37:371.
119. Stovroff M, Teague G, Heiss KH, et al. Thoracoscopy in the management of pediatric empyema. *J Pediatr Surg* 1995;30:1211.
120. Cochran JB, Tecklenburg FW, Turner RB. Intrapleural instillation of fibrinolytic agents for treatment of pleural empyema. *Pediatr Crit Care Med* 2003;4:39.
121. Wells RG, Havens PL. Intrapleural fibrinolysis for parapneumonic effusion and empyema in children. *Radiology* 2003;228:370.
122. Kosloske AM, Ball WS, Butler C, et al. Drainage of pediatric lung abscess by cough, catheter, or complete resection. *J Pediatr Surg* 1986;21:596.
123. Lacey SR, Kosloske AM. Pneumonostomy in the management of pediatric lung abscess. *J Pediatr Surg* 1983;18:625.
124. Redding GJ, Walund L, Walund D, et al. Lung function in children following empyema. *Am J Dis Child* 1990;144:1337.
125. Azarow KS, Pearl RH, Zurcher R, et al. Primary mediastinal masses. *J Thorac Cardiovasc Surg* 1993;106:67.
126. Merten DL. Diagnostic imaging of mediastinal masses in children. *Am J Radiol* 1992;158:825.
127. Meza MP, Benson M, Siovis TL. Imaging of mediastinal masses in children. *Radiol Clin North Am* 1993;31:583.
128. Link KM, Samuels LJ, Reed LC, et al. Magnetic resonance imaging of the mediastinum. *J Thorac Imaging* 1993;8:34.
129. Rosenberg HK. The complementary roles of ultrasound and plain film radiography in differentiating pediatric chest abnormalities. *Radiographies* 1986;6:427.
130. Grosfeld JL, Billmire DF. Teratomas in infancy and childhood. *Curr Probl Cancer* 1985;IX:9.
131. Grosfeld JL, Skinner MA, Rescorla FJ, et al. Mediastinal tumors in children: experience with 196 cases. *Ann Surg Oncol* 1994;1:121.
132. Lakhoo K, Boyle M, Drake DP. Mediastinal teratomas: review of 15 pediatric cases. *J Pediatr Surg* 1993;28:1161.
133. Pokorny WJ. Mediastinal tumors. In: Ashcraft KW, Holder TM, eds. *Pediatric surgery,* 2nd ed. Philadelphia: WB Saunders, 1993:218.
134. Kuller JA, Laifer SA, Martin JG, et al. Unusual presentations of fetal teratoma. *J Perinatol* 1991;40:294.
135. Ashour M, Hawass NE, Adam KAR. Spontaneous intrapleural rupture of mediastinal teratoma. *Respir Med* 1993;87:69.
136. Mogilner JO, Fonseca J, Davies MRQ. Life-threatening respiratory distress caused by a mediastinal teratoma in a newborn. *J Pediatr Surg* 1992;27:1519.
137. Siebert J, Marvin L, Rose EF, et al. Mediastinal teratoma: a rare cause of severe respiratory distress in the newborn. *J Pediatr Surg* 1976;11:253.
138. Honicky RE, dePapp EW. Mediastinal teratoma with endocrine function. *Am J Dis Child* 1973;126:650.
139. Somrnerland BC, Cleland WP, Yong NK. Physiological activity in mediastinal teratoma. *Thorax* 1975;30:510.
140. Sidani AH, Oberson R, Deleze G, et al. Infected teratoma of lower posterior mediastinum in a six-year-old boy. *Pediatr Radiol* 1991;21:438.
141. Aldousany AW, Joyner JC, Price RA, et al. Diagnosis and treatment of intrapericardial teratoma. *Pediatr Cardiol* 1987;8:51.
142. Copper JD. Current therapy for thymoma. *Chest* 1993;103:3345.
143. Couture MM, Mountain CP. Thymoma. *Semin Surg Oncol* 1990;6:110.
144. Pokorny WJ.Thymomas. In: Oski FA, ed. *Principles and practice of pediatrics,* Ist ed. Philadelphia: JB Lippincott, 1990:1613.
145. Spigland N, Di Lorenzo M, Youssef S, et al. Malignant thymoma in children: a 20-year review. *J Pediatr Surg* 1990;25:1143.
146. Sicherer SH, Cabana MD, Perlman EJ, et al. Thymoma and cellular immune deficiency in an adolescent. *Pediatr Allergy Immnol* 1998;9:49.
147. Pollack A, Komaki R, Cox JD, et al. Thymoma: treatment and prognosis. *Intl Radiat Oncol Biosci Phys* 1992;23:1037.
148. Niches T, Harms D, Jurgens H, et al. Treatment of pediatric malignant thymoma: long-term remission in a 14-year-old boy with EBV-associated thymic carcinoma by aggressive, combined modality treatment. *Med Pediatr Oncol* 1996;26:419.

149. Rice TW. Benign neoplasms and cysts of the mediastinum. *Semin Thorac Cardiovasc Surg* 1992;4:25.
150. Wick MR. Mediastinal cysts and intrathoracic thyroid tumors. *Semin Diagn Pathol* 1990;7:285.
151. Hendrickson M, Azarow K, Eon S, et al. Congenital thymic cysts in children—mostly misdiagnosed. *J Pediatr Surg* 1998;33:821.
152. Taliesin I, You M, Bland JD, et al. Thymic cyst: is a correct preoperative diagnosis possible? Report of a case and review of the literature. *Eur J Pediatr* 2001;160:620.
153. Hazelrigg SR, Landreneau RI, Mack MJ, et al. Thoracoscopic resection of mediastinal cysts. *Ann Thorac Surg* 1993;56:659.
154. McGahren EM. Author's unpublished experience. 2003.
155. Gerle RD, Jaretzki A, Ashley CA, et al. Congenital bronchopulmonary-foregut malformation: pulmonary sequestration communicating with the gastrointestinal tract. *N Engl J Med* 1968;278:1413.
156. St. Georges R, Deslauriers J, Duranceau A, et al. Clinical spectrum of bronchogenic cysts of the mediastinum and lung in the adult. *Ann Thorac Surg* 1991;52:6.
157. Lazar RH, Younis BT, Bassila MN. Bronchogenic cysts: a cause of stridor in the neonate. *Am J Otolaryngol* 1991;12:117.
158. Suen GC, Mathisen DJ, Grillo HC, et al. Surgical management and radiological characteristics of bronchogenic cysts. *Ann Thorac Surg* 1993;55:476.
159. McAdams HP, Kirejczyk WM, Rosado-de-Christenson ML, et al. Bronchogenic cyst: imaging features with clinical and histopathological correlation. *Radiology* 2000;217:441.
160. Olsen JB, Clemmensen O, Andersen K. Adenocarcinoma arising in a foregut cyst of the mediastinum. *Ann Thorac Surg* 1991;51:497.
161. de Perrot M, Pache JC, Spiliopoulos A. Carcinoma arising in congenital lung cysts. *Thor Cardiovasc Surg* 2001;49:184.
162. Read CA, Moront M, Carangelo R. Recurrent bronchogenic cyst: an argument for complete surgical excision. *Arch Surg* 1991;126:1306.
163. Mauch PM, Kalish LA, Kaden M, et al. Patterns of presentation of Hodgkin disease: implication for etiology and pathogenesis. *Cancer* 1993;71:2062.
164. Ingram L, Rivera GK, Shapiro DN. Superior vena cava syndrome associated with childhood malignancy: analysis of 24 cases. *Med Pediatr Oncol* 1990;18:476.
165. Shorter NA, Fiston HC. Lymphomas. In: Ashcraft KW, Holder TM, eds. *Pediatric surgery,* 2nd ed. Philadelphia: WB Saunders, 1993;863.
166. Azizkhan RG, Dudgeon DL, Buck JR, et al. Life-threatening airway obstruction as a complication to the management of mediastinal masses in children. *J Pediatr Surg* 1985;20:816.
167. Shamberger RC, Holyman RS, Griscom NT, et al. CT quantitation of tracheal cross-section area as a guide to the surgical and anesthetic management of children with anterior mediastinal masses. *J Pediatr Surg* 1991;26:138.
168. Kurtyberg J, Graham ML. Non-Hodgkin's lymphoma. Biological classification and implication for therapy. *Pediatr Clin North Am* 1991;38:443.
169. Ferrari LR, Bedford RF. General anesthesia prior to treatment of anterior mediastinal masses in pediatric cancer patients. *Anesthesiology* 1990;72:991.
170. Halpern S, Chatten J, Meadows AT, et al. Anterior mediastinal masses: anesthesia hazards and other problems. *J Pediatr* 1983;102: 407.
171. King MR, Telander RL, Smithson WA, et al. Primary mediastinal tumors in children. *J Pediatr Surg* 1992;17:512.
172. Carr TF, Lockwood L, Stevens RF, et al. Childhood B cell lymphomas arising in the mediastinum. *J Clin Pathol* 1993;46:513.
173. Loeffler JS, Leopold KA, Recht A, et al. Emergency prebiopsy radiation for mediastinal masses: impact on subsequent pathologic diagnosis and outcome. *J Clin Oncol* 1986;4:716.
174. Lemonine G, Montupet P. Mediastinal tumors in infancy and childhood. In: Fallis JC, Filler RM, Lemoina G, eds. *Pediatric thoracic surgery.* New York: Elsevier, 1991:258.
175. Sills RH. The spleen and lymph nodes. In: Oski FA, ed. *Principles and practice of pediatrics.* Philadelphia: JB Lippincott, 1990: 1540.
176. Noyes BC, Weber T, Vogler C. Pericardial cysts in children: surgical or conservative approach? *J Pediatr Surg* 2003;38:1263.
177. Shiraishi I, Ymagishi M, Kawakita A, et al. Acute cardiac tamponade caused by massive hemorrhage from pericardial cyst. *Circulation* 2000;101:E196.
178. Bava GL, Magliani L, Bertoli D, et al. Complicated pericardial cyst: atypical anatomy and clinical course. *Clin Cardiol* 1998;21: 862.
179. Szinicz G, Taqxer F, Riedlinger J, et al. Thoracoscopic resection of a pericardial cyst. *Thorac Card Surg* 1992;40:190.
180. Eto A, Arima T, Nagashima A. Pericardial cyst in a child treated with video-assisted thoracoscopic surgery. *Eur J Pediatr* 2000;159: 889.
181. Glasson MJ, Taylor SF. Cervical cervico-mediastinal and intrathoracic lymphangioma. *Prog Pediatr Surg* 1991;27:62.
182. Hancock JF, St-Vil D, Luka FL, et al. Complications of lymphangiomas in children. *J Pediatr Surg* 1992;27:220.
183. Kostopoulos GK, Fessatidis JT, Hevas AL, et al. Mediastinal cystic hygroma: report of a case with review of the literature. *Eur J Cardiothorac Surg* 1993;7:166.
184. Zalel Y, Shalev E, Ben-Ami M, et al. Ultrasonic diagnosis of mediastinal cystic hygroma. *Prenat Diagn* 1992;12:541.
185. Wright CC, Cohen DM, Vegunta RK, et al. Intrathoracic cystic hygroma: a report of three cases. *J Pediatr Surg* 1996;31:1430.
186. Gupta AK, Bery M, Raghav B, et al. Mediastinal and skeletal lymphangiomas in a child. *Pediatr Radiol* 1991;21:129.
187. Pokorny WJ. Congenital malformations of the lymphatic system In: Oski FA, ed. *Principles and practice of pediatrics,* 1st ed. Philadelphia: JB Lippincott, 1990:1612.
188. Agartan C, Olguner M, Akgur FM, et al. A case of mediastinal hygroma whose only symptom was hoarseness. *J Pediatr Surg* 1998;33:642.
189. Ogita S, Tsuto T, Deguchi E, et al. OK-432 therapy for unresectable lymphangiomas in children. *J Pediatr Surg* 1991;26:263.
190. Okada A, Kubota A, Fukuzawa M, et al. Injection of bleomycin as a primary therapy of cystic lymphangioma. *J Pediatr Surg* 1992;27: 440.
191. Ogita S, Tsuto T, Nakamura K, et al. OK-432 therapy for lymphangioma in children: why and how does it work? *J Pediatr Surg* 1996;31:477.
192. Orford J, Barker A, Thonell S, et al. Bleomycin therapy for cystic hygroma. *J Pediatr Surg* 1995;30:1282.
193. Castanon M, Margarit J, Carrasco R, et al. Long-term follow-up of nineteen cystic lymphangiomas treated with fibrin sealant. *J Pediatr Surg* 1999;34:1276.
194. Lee CW, Shulman K, Morecki R, et al. Malignant degeneration of thoracic neurofibroma. *NY State J Med* 1975;75:347.

Chapter 61

Lung

Heidi J. Pinkerton and Keith T. Oldham

Infants and children manifest an extraordinary diversity of congenital and acquired abnormalities of the lung. Although none is truly common, all the surgical conditions presented in this chapter are important because physiologic lung dysfunction is a potential consequence. Because impaired respiratory gas exchange can be life threatening, it is of fundamental importance that those who care for infants and children are familiar with these lesions. A full understanding of respiratory physiology requires consideration of the chest wall, diaphragm, and airways, in addition to the lungs. This book considers each component separately for reasons of organizational and educational expediency. The reader is referred to other chapters for these specific related discussions, and also to Chapter 11, which considers respiratory physiology in detail.

EMBRYOLOGY AND ANATOMY

Lung Development

By the end of the third week of gestation, the laryngotracheal groove is discernible in the ventral aspect of the proximal foregut in human embryos. This groove develops into a tracheal diverticulum, a primordium that elongates caudally and lies ventral and parallel to the dorsal foregut, the primitive esophagus. By the middle of week 6, the trachea has undergone symmetric distal division into the left and right mainstem bronchi. Mesenchymal proliferation follows in the adjacent mediastinum and is necessary for normal lung organogenesis. This mesoderm is ultimately the source of cartilage, smooth muscle, and connective tissue to the developing lungs. Progressive bronchial branching follows, and by the seventh gestational week, three to five orders of bronchi are present. Tracheal and esophageal separation are normally complete at this time (1). All major bronchial beds are present by 8 to 9 weeks' gestation, when closure of the pleural peritoneal canal completes formation of the diaphragm. By this time, segmental and lobar lung development is complete. After about 16 weeks' gestation, the primary events in fetal lung development are related to the successive formation of terminal airways and alveoli—the critical sites for respiratory gas exchange. This process is of profound importance in understanding the physiologic consequences of mass lesions in the fetal thorax (2) (see Chapters 11 and 58). With regard to understanding the specific physiologic response to pulmonary surgery in infants, several points bear reiteration. Alveoli undergo highly significant maturation and development during the third trimester and during early postnatal life. Both the number and size of alveoli increase during this time. Most of this process is completed by 2 to 4 years of age, although it continues until about age 8 (2–4). Because of this age-related potential for compensatory lung growth, the tolerance of pulmonary resection in infants and children is generally good.

Heidi J. Pinkerton: Division of Pediatric Surgery, Children's Hospital of Wisconsin, Milwaukee, Wisconsin 53226.

Keith T. Oldham: Division of Pediatric Surgery, Medical College of Wisconsin, Children's Hospital of Wisconsin, Milwaukee, Wisconsin 53226.

Normal Anatomy

Key anatomic relations of the pulmonary hilar to adjacent structures are summarized in Fig. 61-1. The right lung is normally larger than the left, with an upper, middle, and lower lobe each supplied by its respective bronchus. The left lung is formed by upper and lower lobes similarly situated, and the lingula is analogous to the right middle lobe. The tracheal bifurcation is at the fourth or fifth vertebral body by the time of birth. The right mainstem bronchus is normally larger, more vertical, and about one-half the length of the left. These anatomic features account for the preferential drainage of endobronchial material or foreign bodies into the right lung, particularly the right lower lobe.

The circulation on which respiratory gas exchange depends is derived from the pulmonary artery and its branches. The circulation that provides nutritive support

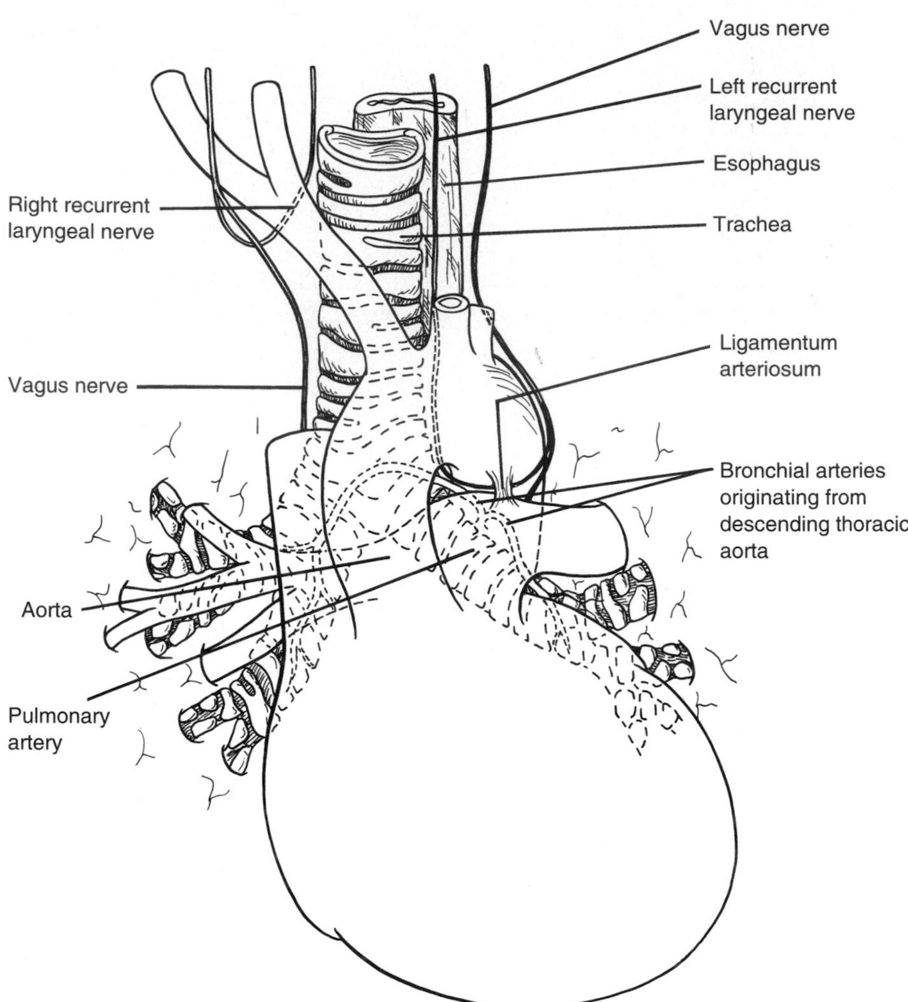

FIGURE 61-1. Key anatomic relations of the structures of the pulmonary hilum.

for the lung parenchyma and the bronchi, however, is systemic. The main left bronchus and its dependent airways are supplied by two bronchial arteries that arise from the anterior surface of the descending thoracic aorta. On the right, a single bronchial artery is usually present and is derived from either the third right intercostal artery or the more superior of the two left bronchial arteries. Intramural collateral flow from the trachea to the bronchi is derived from the inferior thyroid arteries, which are supplied by the thyrocervical trunks of the subclavian arteries. Venous bronchial drainage is into the azygous and hemiazygous systems. Generally, both arteries and veins follow the segmental and lobar architecture of the bronchi.

In large airways at the microscopic level, respiratory epithelium is ciliated, pseudostratified columnar epithelium. Smooth muscle demarcates the basal extent of the mucosa. Mucus-producing glands are apparent in the submucosa. Parasympathetic ganglion cells are abundant, and cartilage is present. Cartilage is an essential structural element for maintaining expiratory patency of the major conducting airways. Proceeding distally in the tracheobronchial tree, luminal size diminishes, and certain features are lost. In particular, as the bronchus becomes a bronchiole, cartilage is lost, the glands disappear, and the epithelium becomes simple, columnar, and ciliated. Smooth muscle and elastic tissues remain. More distally, these elements drop out of the terminal bronchiole as the need to conduct large volumes of air diminishes. Eventually, at the level of the respiratory bronchiole and the alveoli, where gas exchange occurs, capillaries and epithelial cells are juxtaposed intimately. Most oxygen and carbon dioxide diffusion actually occurs across a membrane composed only of thin cytoplasmic extensions of the type I epithelial cell and the capillary endothelial cell, bound by a common basement membrane. This is only nanometers in thickness.

Parenchymal lung lesions in infants and children are divided in the following discussion into those that are congenital and those that are acquired. Anomalies that result from disordered organogenesis during foregut development are reviewed in detail as follows (5–7). Certain conditions, such as cystic fibrosis (CF) and bullous disease, may have both congenital and acquired features, and these individual aspects are also reviewed in the following sections.

CONGENITAL DISORDERS

Congenital Lobar Emphysema

Congenital lobar emphysema, or congenital lobar overinflation, refers to the abnormal postnatal collection of air within a lobe of the lung that is otherwise anatomically normal. This condition is characterized by expiratory air-trapping within the affected lobe, resulting in lobar parenchymal distention. Compression of adjacent normal lung and mediastinal structures is expected, and physiologic impairment of gas exchange is common. The process is classically the result of developmental deficiency of the cartilage that supports the bronchus to the involved lobe, resulting in focal bronchial collapse and obstruction to expiratory air flow. This specific defect, however, is demonstrable in only one-third to two-thirds of surgically resected emphysematous lobes (8). The remainder of these infants and children have a variety of partially obstructing bronchial lesions. Some are endobronchial in origin and potentially reversible (e.g., viscid secretions, mucous plugs, or granulation tissue). Some are the result of extrinsic compression of the bronchus with partial obstruction. Causes include mediastinal lymphadenopathy; adjacent vascular structures, such as an aberrant or enlarged pulmonary artery or ductus arteriosus; mediastinal cysts or tumors that are bronchogenic in origin; or other congenital or acquired mediastinal lesions with an intimate hilar relation. For these reasons, preresection bronchoscopic evaluation is recommended with the expectation that reversible bronchial obstruction be corrected before sacrificing a lung lobe that is otherwise normal.

In addition, developmental abnormalities of the alveoli or the terminal airways may be associated with the clinical findings of congenital lobar emphysema. Of note in this regard is the finding of *polyalveolar morphology,* a descriptive histologic term that refers to a substantial and abnormal increase in the number of alveoli present. In this circumstance, postnatal air-trapping occurs within these many alveoli.

Congenital lobar emphysema is a rare lesion, with a 2:1 or 3:1 male predominance. It is most common in the white population. Unilobar involvement is the rule, with affected sites distributed in the following manner: left upper lobe, 40% to 50%; right middle lobe, 30% to 40%; right upper lobe, 20%; lower lobes, 1%; and multiple sites the remainder (7,8) (Fig. 61-2). Congenital lobar emphysema is associated with congenital heart disease or abnormalities of the great vessels in about 15% of infants (9–11). Indeed, extrinsic bronchial compression from vascular structures appears to be a common etiologic problem in this circumstance. For this reason, screening echocardiography is appropriate in all infants with congenital lobar emphysema.

Affected infants usually do not have symptoms at birth. With the onset of extrauterine life and spontaneous respiration, air-trapping and progressive lobar distention develop. Initial clinical symptoms are generally tachypnea and dyspnea, followed by cyanosis if oxygenation is sufficiently impaired. A cough or wheezing may also be present, but this is of little specificity. About one-half of affected infants develop symptoms in the first few days of life; the remainder develop symptoms within the first 6 months. Older infants and children may have few or no symptoms. Infants may have rapidly progressive respiratory failure, with up to 10% to 15% of patients requiring emergency thoracotomy. Generally, the clinical progression is slower, and some patients remain without symptoms.

The clinical presentation may be one of progressive respiratory distress; therefore, an affected infant may become increasingly agitated, anxious, and tachypneic. These normal responses to hypoxemia exacerbate the air-trapping phenomenon as the peak inspiratory and expiratory pressures escalate. In particular, focal bronchial collapse occurs with excessive expiratory effort; as this develops, the lobar emphysema worsens, and further compromise in gas exchange results. Likewise, positive-pressure ventilation can induce acute lobar distention with potentially catastrophic respiratory decompensation or mediastinal displacement. The physiologic derangements may be indistinguishable from those of tension pneumothorax. This is an important consideration during endoscopic evaluation of the endobronchial tree. Particularly in infants with preoperative symptoms, the surgeon must be prepared to decompress the thorax by emergent thoracotomy and then to proceed with definitive lobectomy.

Congenital lobar emphysema is typically found in term infants, but acquired emphysematous disease in preterm infants is common. The cause of this latter problem is multifactorial, including barotrauma from positive-pressure ventilation, oxygen toxicity, and lung immaturity. It is often seen in conjunction with, and as a complication of, bronchopulmonary dysplasia. Unlike congenital lobar emphysema, multiple areas of focal hyperinflation and interstitial emphysema are often present. Unilobar right lower lobe involvement is also common, probably as a consequence of endotracheal tube positioning, which selectively ventilates the right mainstem bronchus. These characteristics help differentiate congenital and acquired disease.

Physical findings of congenital lobar emphysema may include an asymmetric thorax, a shift in the apical cardiac impulse to the contralateral side, and focal hyperresonance and diminished breath sounds over the affected lobe. None of these findings, however, has the necessary sensitivity and specificity to demonstrate the precise nature of the problem.

The diagnosis is best established by plain chest radiograph (Fig. 61-2). Typical findings include lobar hyperinflation, contralateral shift of the mediastinum and trachea, compression or even lobar atelectasis of adjacent lung, and flattening of the ipsilateral hemidiaphragm. If these

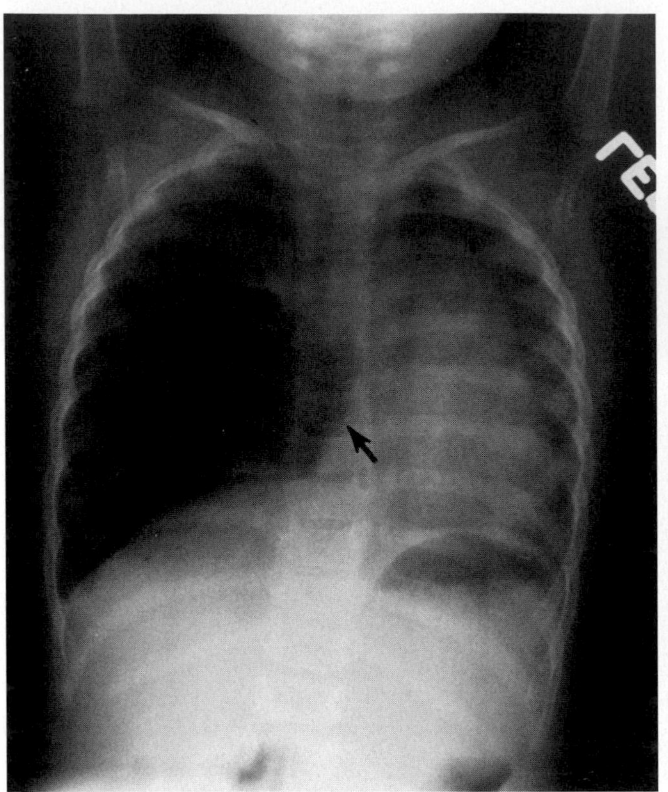

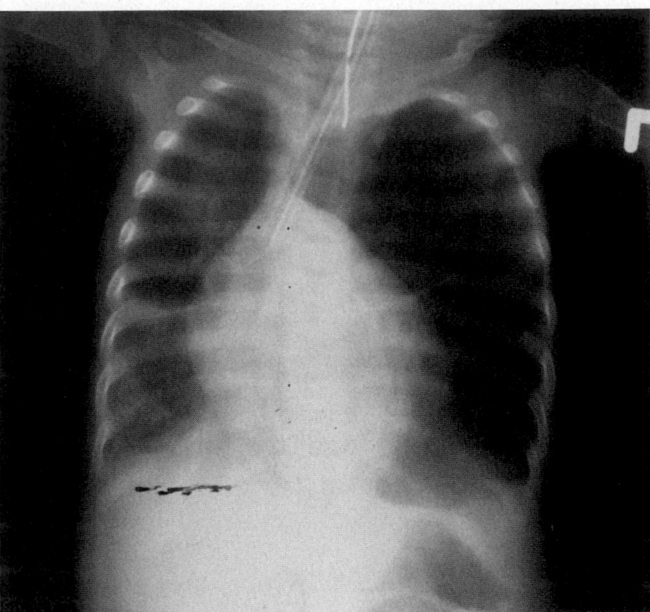

FIGURE 61-2. Congenital lobar emphysema involving the right middle lobe. **(A)** Herniation of the affected lobe across the midline has occurred (*arrow*), with compression of the adjacent right upper and right lower lobes. Mediastinal shift into the contralateral thorax is also apparent. **(B)** Similar abnormalities in a 4-month-old girl with involvement of the left upper lobe, the most common site of congenital lobar emphysema.

findings are all present, there is no need for additional imaging studies. Differentiating this presentation from tension pneumothorax is essential. The latter is characterized by collapse of the entire affected lung into the hilum. In contrast, although lobar emphysema can be dramatic in its radiographic appearance, adjacent compressed lung can almost always be discerned, most often the lower lobe at the base of the thorax. In addition, the occasional congenital cystic adenomatoid malformation (CCAM) with a single large cystic component can be mistaken for lobar emphysema. Because lobar emphysema rarely involves the lower lobes, this is an important differentiating feature. Nonetheless, the surgical management of these latter two lesions is similar so preoperative differentiation is less important than for tension pneumothorax, for which the treatment is different. As with most mass lesions in the chest, computed tomography (CT) and magnetic resonance (MR) imaging provide excellent anatomic information for infants with congenital lobar emphysema. These procedures are most helpful in elective situations when the diagnosis is in doubt. In addition, ventilation–perfusion scans have been employed to evaluate infants with lobar emphysema, particularly when the areas of involvement are multiple or the disease acquired (12). In this setting, specific areas of nonfunctional lung can be identified and resected if they appear to compromise adjacent normal lung.

Because the natural history of congenital lobar emphysema is often progressive and includes potentially life-threatening respiratory insufficiency, prompt surgical lobectomy is the treatment of choice for infants and young children. Because the underlying lesion is structural, medical treatment can be considered only a supportive adjunct in patients with symptoms. In patients without symptoms, particularly older children, this approach may be tempered reasonably because the likelihood of sudden decompensation in this circumstance is low. The rationale for routine endoscopic evaluation of the affected bronchus has been noted. The purpose is to identify and eliminate reversible endobronchial obstructions from secretions, mucous plugging, or granulation tissue. Clearly reversible endobronchial problems should be corrected without parenchymal lung resection.

Extrinsic bronchial compression is associated generally with a focal cartilaginous defect of the affected bronchus that is not adequately relieved by simple decompression.

Although congenital lobar emphysema results from a specific anatomic defect, reconstructive procedures, such as bronchoplasty or segmental bronchial resection and anastomosis, are generally inappropriate. The diminutive size of the infant bronchus and the possibility of nonfocal cartilaginous tracheobronchial defects present important technical obstacles to successful local reconstructive procedures. In addition, there is little reason to select this approach because the clinical results of lobectomy are generally excellent for this lesion (9–11,13).

Acquired emphysema is often seen in preterm infants with a multitude of other problems. Treatment is generally medical and supportive, with the natural history being one of slow resolution over a number of months. In the acute phase, selective ventilation of nonemphysematous areas of lung or the use of alternative strategies such as high-frequency oscillatory or jet ventilation can minimize the peak airway pressure, which is directly correlated to the formation of emphysema. These approaches can also help infants with congenital lobar emphysema if prolonged transport is necessary or there is delay in reaching the operating suite. Lobectomy may be beneficial in occasional selected patients with severe regional emphysematous disease; however, late death may result from associated bronchopulmonary dysplasia in these patients.

As noted, infants and children have an excellent response to lobectomy for congenital lobar emphysema (9–11,13). Even in those who are critically ill and require emergency thoracotomy, the physiologic response is a predictably prompt and dramatic return to normal after resection of the affected lobe. Mortality for this specific lesion is rare in a modern pediatric surgical environment. The general risks of thoracotomy and lung resection include morbidity related to anesthesia, empyema, pneumothorax, infection, bleeding, and bronchopleural fistula. These are not different than for any other neonatal thoracotomy and lobectomy, and are presented in detail in the section that deals with outcomes after lung resection. The cumulative incidence of these types of complications is about 5% to 10% in most modern pediatric surgical practices, although it has been as high as 20% to 40% in recent decades (7,9–11). Long-term pulmonary function is also predictably excellent after lobar resection, and this is discussed separately later. For infants with coexisting congenital heart disease, acquired pulmonary emphysema, or additional medical problems, the outcome is generally dictated by these other conditions.

In follow-up studies by Frenckner and Freyschuss, (14) actual lung volumes—residual volume, vital capacity, total lung capacity, and forced expiratory volume in 1 second (FEV_1)—in patients who had undergone neonatal lobectomy for congenital lobar emphysema were 90% of predicted values, and no long-term functional impairment was reported. Infants who had undergone neonatal lobectomy for congenital lobar emphysema were evaluated as adults by McBride and colleagues in 1980 (13). Ipsilateral and contralateral lung volumes were found to be equal, despite the previous lobectomy. This appeared to be the result of compensatory tissue growth, not simply distention of residual lung parenchyma. In this latter study, perfusion was found to be equally distributed between the operated and nonoperated lungs. These patients demonstrated diminished expiratory flow rates compared with expected values (FEV_1, 72% of predicted; maximal midexpiratory flow, 45% of predicted). These findings appear to result from disproportional growth between the conducting and the terminal airways during infancy. This concept does not diminish the excellent clinical prognosis for these infants, and is presented in detail at the end of this chapter.

Congenital Cystic Adenomatoid Malformation

Congenital cystic adenomatoid malformation (CCAM) is a term applied to a spectrum of lobar hamartomatous abnormalities of the lung. The pathologic definition requires an increase in terminal respiratory structures, usually bronchioles, in a glandular or adenomatoid pattern that is normally seen during organogenesis. It is suggested that developmental control of the lobar lung bud and the surrounding mediastinal mesenchyme is lost between 16 and 20 weeks' gestation, giving rise to a lesion that is composed of multiple interconnected cysts that are disorganized and variably sized. Involvement is generally unilobar, and communication with the tracheobronchial tree is usually present. Three types of CCAM lesions were described by Stocker and colleagues (15) in 1977 and are illustrated in Fig. 61-3. Subsequently, others used the terms *cystic, intermediate,* and *solid* to categorize the different lesions observed with this malformation. More recently, Adzick and colleagues (16) defined these lesions as either macrocystic (greater than 5-mm cyst diameter) or microcystic (solid or less than 5-mm cyst diameter), by use of prenatal ultrasound examination to differentiate between the two. Because the natural history is dependent on morphologic type, the distinctions have more than semantic import. Clinical treatment and outcomes are presented later.

Both before and after parturition, the important physiologic consequences of CCAM result from mediastinal or normal lung compression by the mass lesion. Lesions of great size, particularly those that are microcystic or solid in composition, are potentially associated with in utero mediastinal displacement, hydrops fetalis, and fetal death. As many as one-third of all newborns with CCAM have evidence of fetal hydrops at delivery. It is now routine to establish the diagnosis of CCAM by prenatal ultrasound. The data for the fetus diagnosed with CCAM are more limited and controversial, but as many as 40% of fetuses with CCAM lesions will progress to hydrops and fetal demise, whereas 15% will spontaneously regress (17). Adzick and

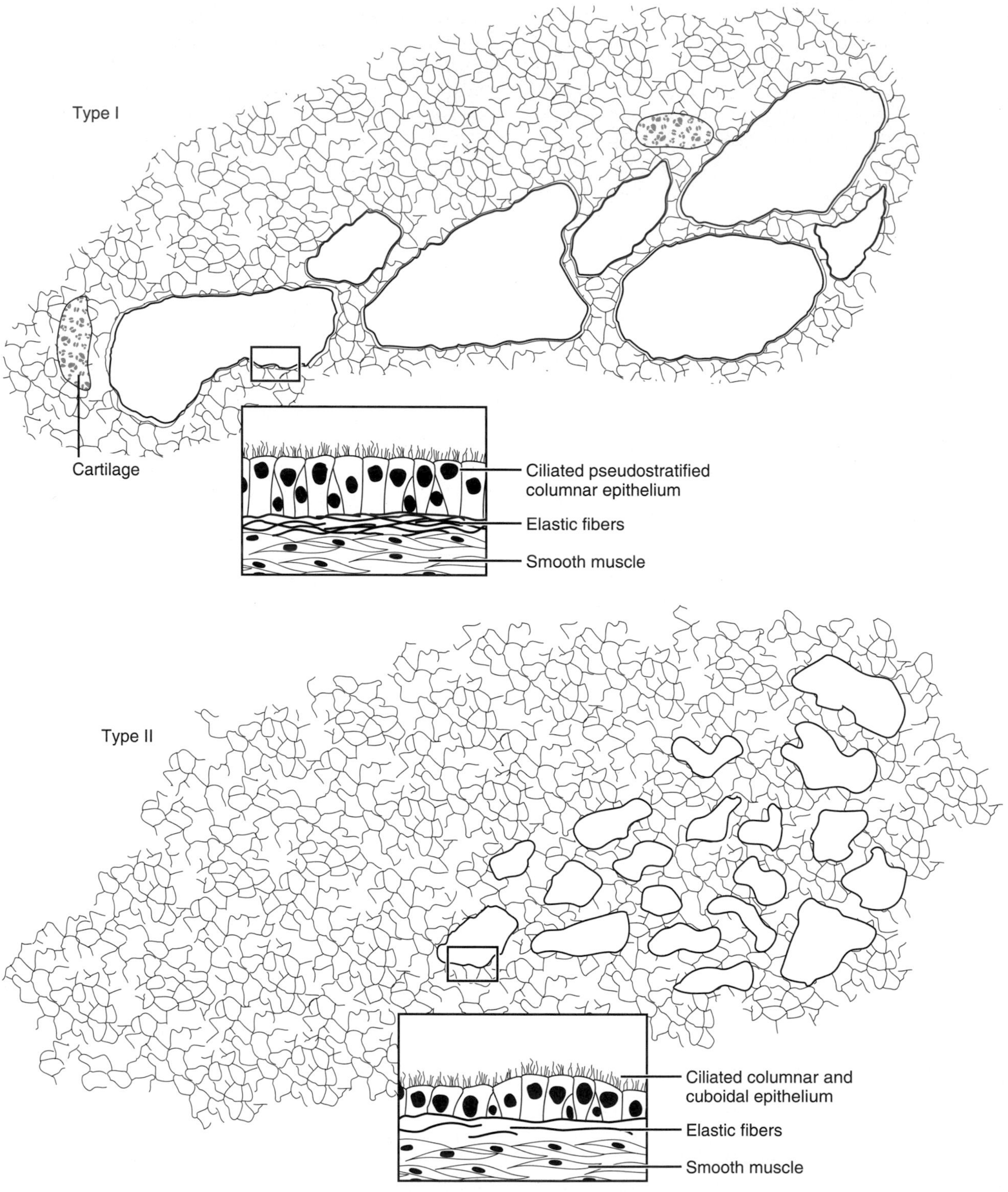

FIGURE 61-3. Congenital cystic adenomatoid malformation (CCAM) types. Type I lesions are composed of irregular cysts larger than 2 cm in diameter, elastic tissue is regularly present, and cartilage is present in 10% of lesions. The epithelium is ciliated, pseudostratified columnar epithelium. Relatively normal alveolar structures are adjacent to, or interspersed with, these cysts. Type II lesions have more and smaller cysts, less than 1 cm in diameter. The epithelium is ciliated cuboidal or columnar; there is less elastic tissue and no cartilage. The lesions blend into relatively normal lung parenchyma with large alveolus-like structures. Type III lesions occupy the entire affected lobe, and despite the CCAM nomenclature, there are no cystic spaces. Rather, masses of cuboidal epithelium line alveolus-like structures where no gas exchange can occur. (From Stocker JT, Madewell JE, Drake RM. Congenital cystic adenomatoid malformation of the lung. *Hum Pathol* 1977;8:155, with permission. (*continued*)

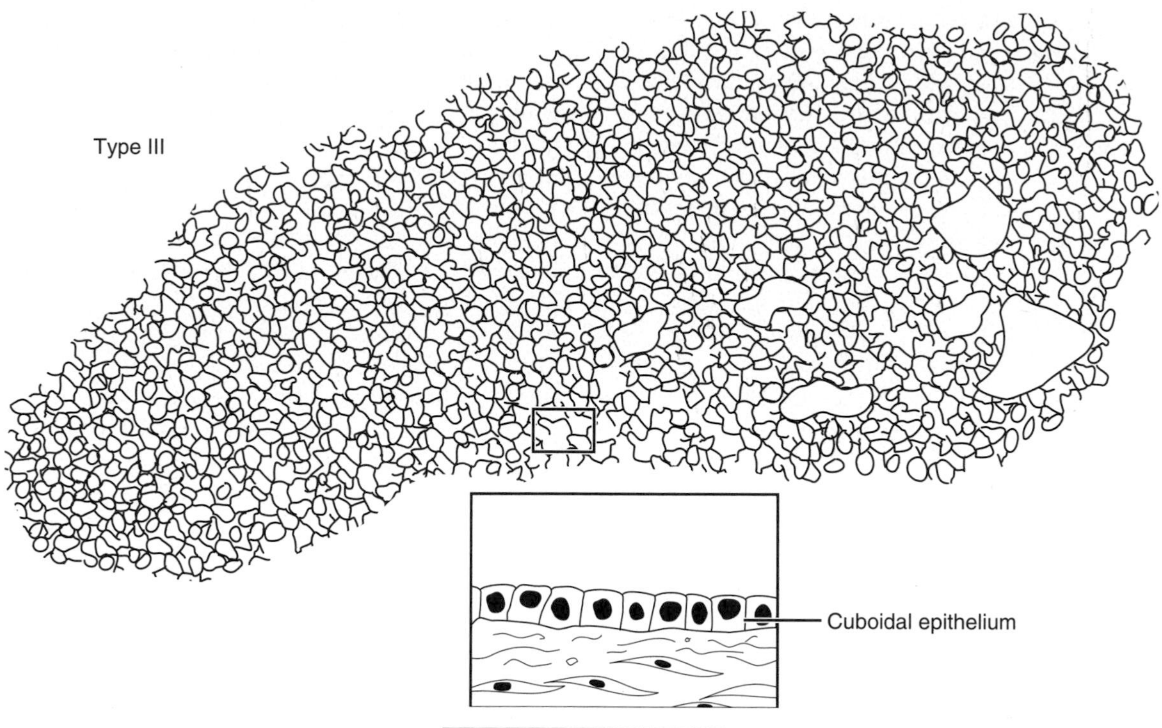

FIGURE 61-3. *(Continued)*

colleagues (18) suggested that the appearance of anasarca or hydrops in fetuses with microcystic CCAM is an indication of impending fetal demise; they have reported neonatal survival after fetal lobectomy in a small number of highly selected patients (19). Macrocystic lesions appear less threatening in utero, and although some have been managed with prenatal thoracoamniotic shunting or aspiration, most of these infants can be successfully treated after delivery at term. In addition, it appears that a substantial number of macrocystic lesions, perhaps one-third, diminish in size during fetal development (20,21). This is an important area of active investigation. Appropriate selection of patients for prenatal therapy depends on accurate information defining the natural history of CCAM.

Postpartum physiologic problems related to CCAM generally result from either pulmonary hypoplasia in newborns or inadequate tracheobronchial drainage with secondary infection in older infants and children. The former problem appears related to in utero compression and developmental arrest of the ipsilateral lung by the CCAM mass. In addition, some degree of contralateral pulmonary hypoplasia resulting from the shifted mediastinum is common. Pulmonary parenchymal hypoplasia and persistent pulmonary hypertension can result in acute respiratory failure in newborns. Severely affected infants with CCAM may have all the ventilatory instability of infants with congenital diaphragmatic hernias. This includes the potential need for conventional mechanical ventilation, high-frequency or jet ventilation, or extracorporeal life support. These issues are discussed in detail in Chapters 11 and 58. Although the spectrum of physiologic derangement includes both acute life-threatening respiratory failure and progressive newborn respiratory insufficiency, only about 30% of live-born infants with CCAM present in these ways. Many present with infectious pulmonary problems related to the persistent communication of the CCAM with the tracheobronchial tree. The abnormal lung parenchyma is exposed to environmental organisms, but lacks normal clearance mechanisms. This leads to a variety of infectious problems, such as recurrent pneumonia or lung abscess, or to more subtle chronic problems, such as failure to thrive. In contemporary practice, prenatal diagnosis yields a number of asymptomatic infants referred for treatment. In general, these infants should undergo elective lobectomy.

CCAM lesions are uncommon, representing about 30% to 40% of developmental lung bud anomalies in most reports. There is a slight male predominance and no apparent racial or geographic predilection. CCAM lesions are equally distributed between the left and right lobes, with bilateral disease being rare. Unilobar involvement is most common, with any lobe at risk, although there appears to be slight predilection for the lower lobes in most reports. Fortunately, multilobar disease when it occurs tends to be unilateral so surgical resection can be achieved by pneumonectomy, if necessary. A maternal history of polyhydramnios is common, and preterm delivery occurs in as many as one-half of these infants. Therefore, the many problems of preterm delivery may be superimposed.

Depending on the institutional environment, one-half or more of these lesions are detected and referred based on prenatal ultrasonography findings. As outlined earlier, about one-third of newborns with CCAM develop symptoms of tachypnea, dyspnea, cyanosis, or overt respiratory insufficiency in the first month of life. The remainder present with the consequences of pulmonary infection—one-half of these within the first year of life and the remainder at periods up to and including adulthood. Later presentations include recurrent or persistent pneumonia, lung abscess, pneumothorax, reactive airway disease, and failure to thrive, but not usually progressive respiratory insufficiency in older patients. Associated anomalies, including congenital heart disease, pectus excavatum, renal agenesis, skeletal anomalies, jejunal atresia, and others, have been reported, but the incidence is variable and may be no more than for the normal population (6,7).

The issues related to prenatal diagnosis have been discussed. The postnatal evaluation of infants with nonspecific respiratory symptoms is best begun with a plain chest radiograph. In infants with CCAM, however, the radiographic findings are variable. Images obtained shortly after birth may show retained fetal lung fluid within the lesion, and if it is a microcystic or solid lesion, this may not change with time. Macrocystic lesions tend to become aerated with ventilation, and the chest radiograph then has an area of air-filled cysts within the thorax. In infants, this appearance must be distinguished from congenital diaphragmatic hernia, particularly when the left side is involved. Although plain films alone are generally adequate, passage of a nasogastric tube into the stomach or an upper or lower gastrointestinal tract contrast study showing intrathoracic intestine may be helpful in distinguishing the two. Because the surgical approach is generally different for these two lesions, prospective distinction is important. Mediastinal displacement, compression of adjacent normal lung, and flattening of the intact ipsilateral diaphragm are also typical plain chest radiograph findings for CCAM. In older children with infectious complications, the findings are often less clear, and either CT with intravenous contrast or MR evaluation is necessary to provide definitive anatomic detail of the lesion (Fig. 61-4). Angiography has little or no role in the diagnosis of CCAM and other thoracic mass lesions in the modern environment because it has demonstrable risks and the information derived is available by less invasive means.

The principal goal of treatment for CCAM is to resect the area of abnormal lung promptly. Some carefully selected fetuses may benefit from prenatal intervention; however, concerns remain about the natural history of the lesions, appropriate patient selection, and the risk of preterm labor. Experience with this approach is limited and is

A

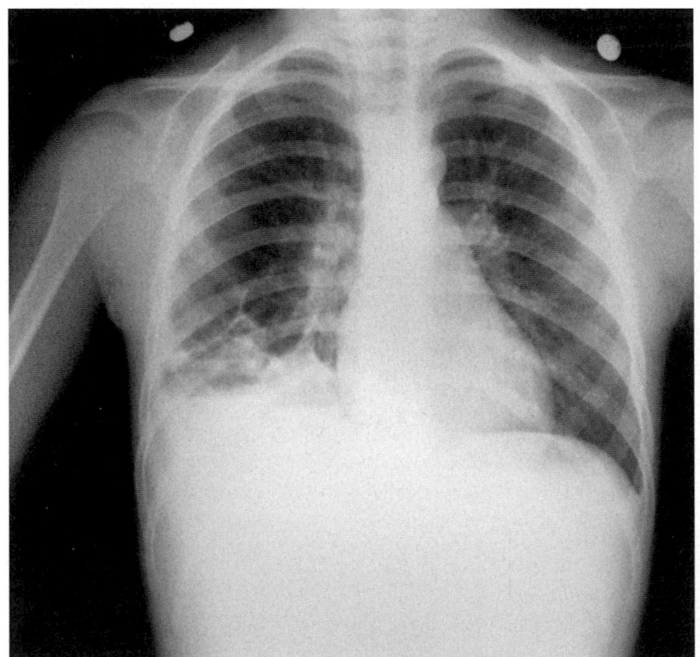

B

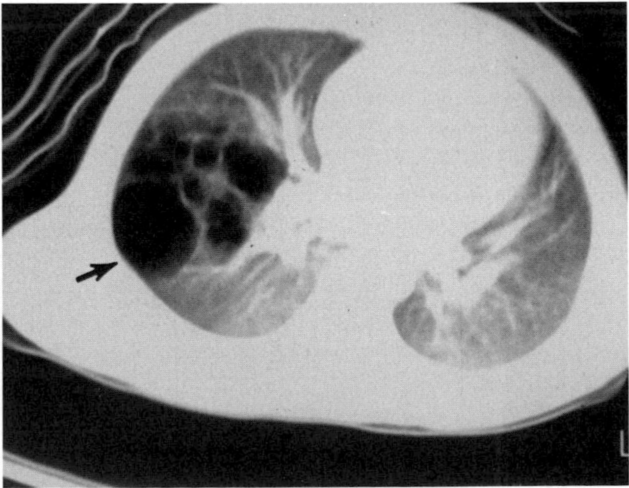

FIGURE 61-4. **(A)** Plain chest radiograph of a 9-year-old child who presented with fever, pleuritic chest pain, and cough. The lesion is an infected cystic adenomatoid malformation of the right lower lobe. **(B)** The lesion in **A** is shown on chest computed tomography scan after treatment with antibiotics and before surgical resection of the right lower lobe (From Coran AG, Oldham KT. The pediatric thorax. In: Greenfield LJ, Mulholland MW, Oldham KT, et al. *Surgery: scientific principles and practice.* Philadelphia: JB Lippincott, 1993:813, with permission.)

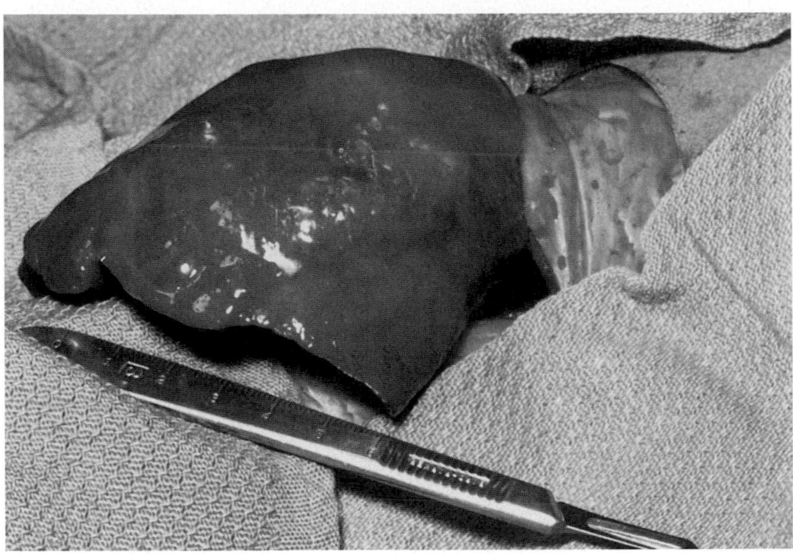

FIGURE 61-5. Right lower lobe cystic adenomatoid malformation that led to acute respiratory distress in a neonate. The size of the lobe after delivery from the thorax is much larger than the volume of the infant thoracic cavity. Delivery of such a space-occupying mass lesion from the thorax can lead to profound and immediate physiologic relief.

insufficient to be definitive. Generally, an in utero diagnosis and macrocystic disease are indications for sequential observation and delivery in a tertiary care environment where prompt thoracotomy and state-of-the-art critical care support are available. For the infant, treatment most often requires a thoracotomy with lobectomy. This can be life saving in critically ill newborns with mediastinal shift and normal lung compression from a ventilated and expanding CCAM. Fig. 61-5 demonstrates the relative size of a right lower lobe CCAM deliberately delivered from the thorax of an infant in extremis. The normal adjacent lung was allowed to ventilate, providing immediate physiologic relief before lobar resection. Because of the long-term risk of infectious complications, surgical resection is considered standard in older patients and in patients without symptoms. It is appropriate in the setting of an acute infectious process to treat a child preoperatively with systemic antibiotics to reduce acute inflammation. Long-term medical management, however, is not appropriate. Approximately 8% of primary lung malignant tumors and 4% of benign tumors are associated with cystic malformation of the lung, including CCAMs (22). To date, at least 24 reports of malignancy occurring within these and other congenital cystic lung lesions add further rationale for surgical resection (22–25). Pulmonary blastoma and rhabdomyosarcoma are the most common of these malignancies.

Pneumonectomy is required in as many as 15% to 20% of affected patients to achieve complete resection of a complex or multilobar CCAM (6,7,10). For the limited and well-demarcated CCAM, segmental resection has been reported, but data suggest that operative morbidity may be greater with this approach, and there is little or no apparent long-term benefit.

Outcome after surgical resection of CCAM is generally good. Adzick and colleagues (18) reported survival in four of six selected fetuses with microcystic CCAM after in utero thoracotomy and lobectomy between 24 and 32 weeks' gestation. For infants who are found at birth to have CCAM, the survival probability with resection is between 80% and 100% in most reports (6,7,10). When it occurs, death is usually the result of respiratory failure in newborns. In older children with infectious presentations, death is rare. The potential complications of neonatal lobectomy for CCAM are not different than for other similar lesions. Although many complications are possible, the overall incidence is less than 10%, and most can be readily managed. Most children have excellent long-term pulmonary function after lobectomy for CCAM. The experience after pneumonectomy is more limited and perhaps less optimistic given the larger extent of the resected lung (see discussion of outcomes after lung resection at the end of this chapter).

Pulmonary Sequestration

Pulmonary sequestration is a form of bronchopulmonary-foregut malformation that gives rise to a mass of lung tissue that is not normally related to the functional lung. In particular, the sequestration can reside outside the lung and be invested with its own visceral pleura (extralobar sequestration), or it can be located within the visceral pleura of the normal lung (intralobar sequestration) (26). The incidence of the two forms is roughly equal. In either case, a sequestration does not communicate with the tracheobronchial tree through a normal bronchus, and the blood supply is derived from one or more anomalous systemic arteries, most often rising from the descending thoracic aorta. In extralobar sequestrations, the arterial blood supply is derived from an infradiaphragmatic source in up to 20% of patients, and venous drainage is typically through the azygous vein. Typically, intralobar sequestrations have venous drainage through the appropriate pulmonary vein. Because of the foregut derivation, occasional communication with the esophagus or stomach is found. An extralobar sequestration may be located within the diaphragm or even in a subdiaphragmatic position.

Many anatomic variations occur with regard to location, the relation to the normal lung, and the systemic arterial blood supply. Conflicting theories of embryogenesis have been offered by way of explanation, distinguishing between disordered budding of the normal tracheobronchial tree and accessory budding from the primitive foregut. The developmental events remain unknown, but the spectrum of bronchopulmonary-foregut malformations is broad. The surgeon who treats these lesions simply must be prepared for variations in the blood supply and relations to the lungs and esophagus. The most important technical concern here is the need to identify the arterial blood supply. Infradiaphragmatic arteries to a pulmonary sequestration are typically elastic and found within the inferior pulmonary ligament. These require precise surgical control to avoid retraction below the diaphragm and occult intraoperative hemorrhage. Communication between the esophagus or stomach and a pulmonary sequestration occurs in about 10% of patients and must be specifically sought, either intraoperatively or possibly preoperatively, by contrast study of the gastrointestinal tract.

Prenatal diagnosis by maternal ultrasound screening is a common mode of discovery of pulmonary sequestrations, particularly for extralobar lesions (27). Typically, a posterior mediastinal or infradiaphragmatic solid mass is observed. The anomalous arterial blood supply may be demonstrable with Doppler ultrasound techniques. Some of these fetuses are vulnerable to the same in utero risks seen with CCAM and congenital diaphragmatic hernia. A large intrathoracic mass lesion can lead to mediastinal compression, hydrops fetalis, and fetal demise. Although relatively uncommon, this is an important possibility to consider in the perinatal care of these fetuses and mothers.

Pulmonary sequestrations are uncommon lesions, but represent about 20% to 40% of the congenital lung bud anomalies in most reports (6,7,10). The male predominance is as high as 3:1 in some reports, particularly for extralobar sequestration. No racial or geographic influence on incidence is known. Newborns have a broad spectrum of presentations, and the lesions can be discovered as asymptomatic posterior mediastinal or abdominal masses. Physiologic derangements include respiratory distress, pneumonia, feeding intolerance, hemorrhage, and congestive heart failure (26). The latter problem results from substantial arteriovenous shunting that can occur within the sequestered lobe, leading to high-output cardiac failure.

Most extralobar sequestrations are diagnosed within the first months or years of life. About 10% to 15% of infants with congenital diaphragmatic hernias have one or more extralobar sequestrations, and this association accounts for their frequent discovery (26). Other congenital anomalies are present in up to 40% of infants and children with extralobar sequestrations, unlike infants with intralobar sequestrations who are otherwise generally normal. Among the defects reported with extralobar sequestrations are ipsilateral diaphragmatic defects, chest wall and vertebral deformities, hindgut duplications, congenital heart disease, and a variety of others (6,7,10).

Intralobar pulmonary sequestrations generally present with infectious sequelae related to inadequate tracheobronchial drainage, either from the lesion or from the adjacent atelectatic lung. Recurrent or persistent pneumonia, lung abscess, and hemoptysis are among the more common presentations. Because these symptoms require temporal evolution, intralobar sequestration has usually presented in childhood or adult life, but not infancy. In published reports, one-half of patients with intralobar sequestrations present after the second decade of life. This pattern of presentation may be changing as prenatal discovery of these lesions by maternal ultrasound has become common (28–30).

The imaging evaluation of pulmonary sequestration is relatively straightforward. Prenatal ultrasound discovery is routine and has been mentioned. For newborns with respiratory symptoms, a plain chest radiograph is the standard initial investigation. Ninety percent of extralobar sequestrations appear as posterior mediastinal mass lesions in the left hemithorax. Most commonly, they appear as triangular retrocardiac density on the anteroposterior view (Fig. 61-6). On lateral view, they are posterior to the left

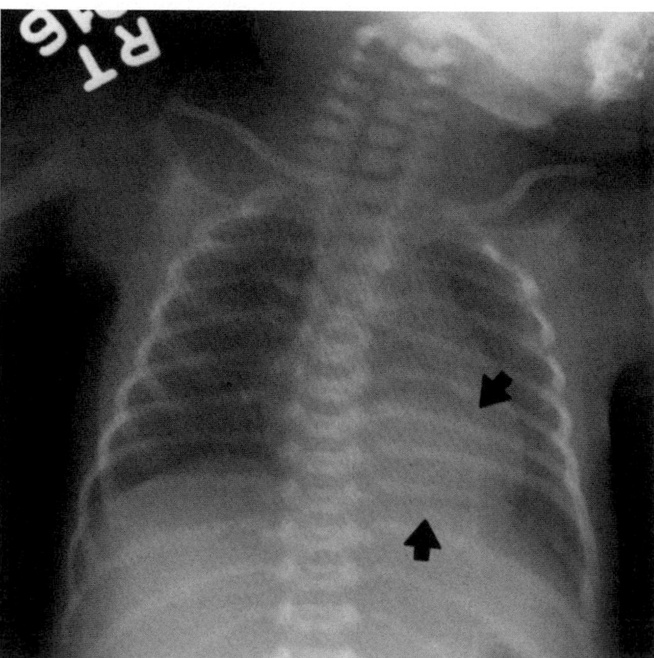

FIGURE 61-6. Chest radiograph of an extralobar pulmonary sequestration (*arrows*) in the left lower thorax. The contour of the retrocardiac left hemidiaphragm has been obliterated. This was a newborn with no symptoms whose lesion was first noticed on prenatal maternal ultrasound.

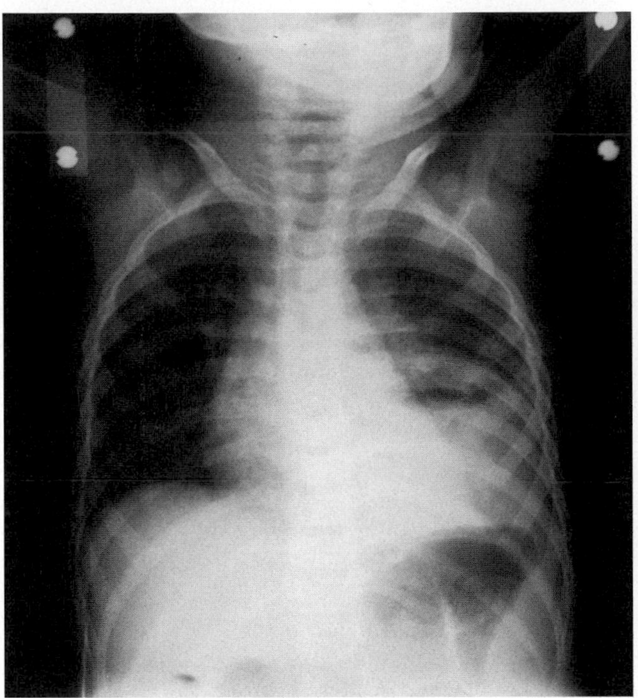

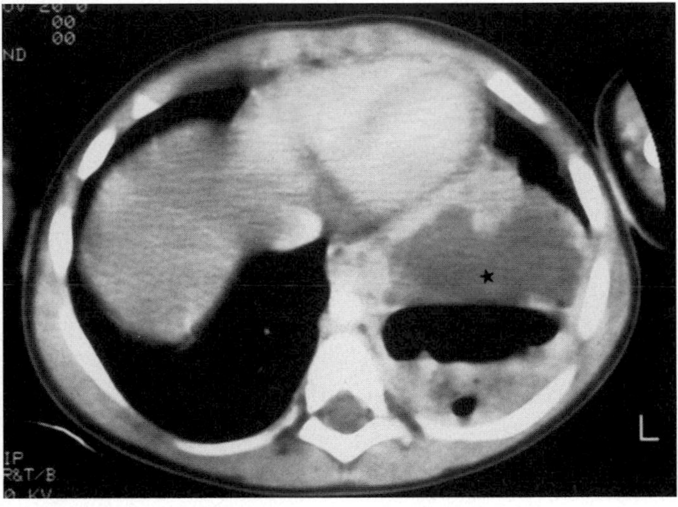

FIGURE 61-7. **(A)** Plain chest radiograph of a child with fever and cough who has an infected intralobar sequestration of the left lower lobe. **(B)** Computed tomography scan of the same lesion (*asterisk*).

lower lobe at or near the level of the diaphragm. Although many anatomic variations are possible, this appearance is nearly diagnostic on plain radiograph.

Sixty percent of intralobar sequestrations occur on the left, typically involving the posterior and basal segments of the left lower lobe (6,7,10) (Fig. 61-7). The appearance is generally that of lobar pneumonia and atelectasis. Air–fluid levels may be present if an abnormal communication with the tracheobronchial tree is patent. The intralobar mass, however, may be obscured and the plain films nondiagnostic. Although any lobe can be involved with a sequestration, upper lobe involvement is present in only 10% to 15% of cases, and bilateral sequestrations are rare.

Particularly for intralobar sequestrations, additional imaging is required to establish the diagnosis. Ultrasound, contrast-enhanced CT (see Fig. 61-7B), and MR imaging (Fig. 61-8) all provide excellent anatomic detail, including identification of the systemic vascular blood supply (31). Ultrasound has the potential advantage of Doppler blood flow assessment to identify the arterial supply. Particularly when prenatal ultrasound is the discovery tool, this provides gratifying, correlative data. Angiography, although emphasized in the past, is not required for either diagnosis or operative planning given the modern capabilities of less invasive imaging techniques.

Generally, resection is recommended for both intralobar and extralobar pulmonary sequestrations. Although extralobar sequestrations may be incidental autopsy

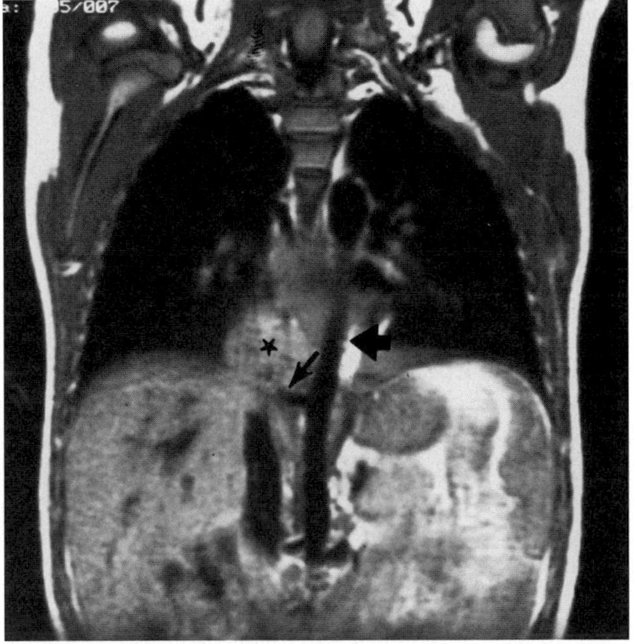

FIGURE 61-8. Magnetic resonance image of a right lower lobe extralobar pulmonary sequestration (*asterisk*), with the descending aorta visualized (*thick arrow*) and clear demonstration of the systemic arterial blood supply to the sequestration (*thin arrow*). (Courtesy of George Bissett, MD, Duke University Medical Center, Durham, NC.)

findings in the elderly, diagnostic uncertainty about the nature of a posterior mediastinal mass, as well as low but real risks of hemorrhage, infection, and malignancy over a lifetime, must be weighed against the risks of a relatively straightforward surgical resection. Certainly, any symptomatic extralobar pulmonary sequestration requires resection. Simple excision is generally straightforward. By definition, the lesion can be resected without the need to disturb the normal lung. The needs to establish vascular control and rule out foregut communication have been noted.

Patients with intralobar sequestrations are more likely to present with infection or hemorrhage; therefore, preoperative treatment with systemic antibiotics may be necessary. In the absence of this problem, prompt lobar resection is indicated. The principle for surgical management of an intralobar sequestration is to remove the affected area. In the face of acute or chronic inflammation, this generally requires a formal lobectomy. Although limited segmental resection is feasible in the absence of infection and when the surrounding lung parenchyma is normal, it is practical in only about 25% of patients. Most series report a predominance of lobectomies for intralobar sequestration (9,10). As with extralobar sequestrations, attention must be directed to the systemic arterial blood supply because all the technical issues are similar for intralobar and extralobar lesions. Although standard practice has been thoracotomy and appropriate resection, limited experience with thoracoscopic resection of extralobar sequestrations has been successful, and this approach appears to be appropriate in selected patients.

As with other pulmonary resections in a modern pediatric surgical environment, the survival rate approaches 100% for pulmonary sequestration in the absence of other medical problems. Likewise, the complications and postoperative morbidity are generally minimal. In particular, extralobar resections do not involve removal of normal lung parenchyma, so these children can be expected to have normal pulmonary function and excellent functional outcomes. Reports of intraoperative exsanguination from the loss of control of the systemic arterial blood supply have received considerable attention in the literature historically. This is an important but straightforward technical concern that does not diminish the expectation for an excellent outcome today.

Bronchogenic Cysts and Lung Cysts

A developmental cyst arising from the trachea or a bronchus is referred to as a *bronchogenic cyst.* These account for about 20% to 30% of congenital bronchopulmonary-foregut cystic malformations (9,10). Potential locations include the cervical or thoracic trachea, the hilar bronchi, or the more distal intraparenchymal bronchi. It has been reported that about 70% of thoracic bronchogenic cysts are located within the lung parenchyma, and the remainder are in the mediastinum, but this distribution varies considerably among different reports (5–7,10). Ectopic bronchogenic cysts, including those in paravertebral, paraesophageal, pericardial, subcarinal, and subcutaneous locations, have been reported.

Bronchogenic cysts are typically unilocular mucus-filled lesions arising from the posterior membranous portion of the airway. They do not usually communicate with the functional tracheobronchial tree. Many anatomic variations, however, have been described. By definition, the cyst has structural elements of the airway, including cartilage, smooth muscle, mucous glands, and respiratory epithelium. Likewise, these lesions have a normal bronchial arterial blood supply. The character of the epithelium depends on the site of origin; ciliated columnar, cuboidal, and squamous epithelium are all found within the tracheobronchial tree, and therefore, within these cysts (Fig. 61-9).

This section also considers cystic lung lesions that result from abnormal development of the more distal airways, alveoli, or pleural or lymphatic tissue. Even collectively, these true lung cysts are rare congenital lesions. They constitute a heterogeneous group of lung parenchymal cystic lesions with histologic features representative of their sites of origin. The spectrum is varied and can overlap with cysts that are bronchogenic in origin. Differentiation of the tissue of origin for simple lung cysts is principally of pathologic interest because the presentations are similar, and clinical management is generally straightforward with a good outcome. One important exception is when the developmental abnormality is lymphatic in origin. The result then may be pulmonary lymphangiectasis. This is typically characterized by diffuse bilateral pulmonary cystic disease, and the outcome is often lethal because resection is not feasible.

The discussion of bronchogenic and other lung cysts is consolidated because of the overlap in their clinical presentations and the similarity in their embryologic origins. As with other congenital cystic lung lesions, physiologic injury from bronchogenic and lung cysts generally results from either compression of adjacent hollow viscera, such as the airway or esophagus (Fig. 61-10), or inadequate drainage of secretions with secondary infection. Malignancies have also been reported within these lesions, and rhabdomyosarcoma, bronchogenic carcinoma, and adenocarcinoma have been described (22–25,32). In newborns with cysts adjacent to the trachea or proximal airways, respiratory distress or air-trapping with lobar emphysema are important and potentially life-threatening problems. More distal lesions may be asymptomatic or may present with evidence of infection. The latter usually occur in older children because time is necessary for the development of infection. Clinical presentations range from no symptoms to life-threatening respiratory distress, although the latter is rare. Infection and nonspecific respiratory symptoms,

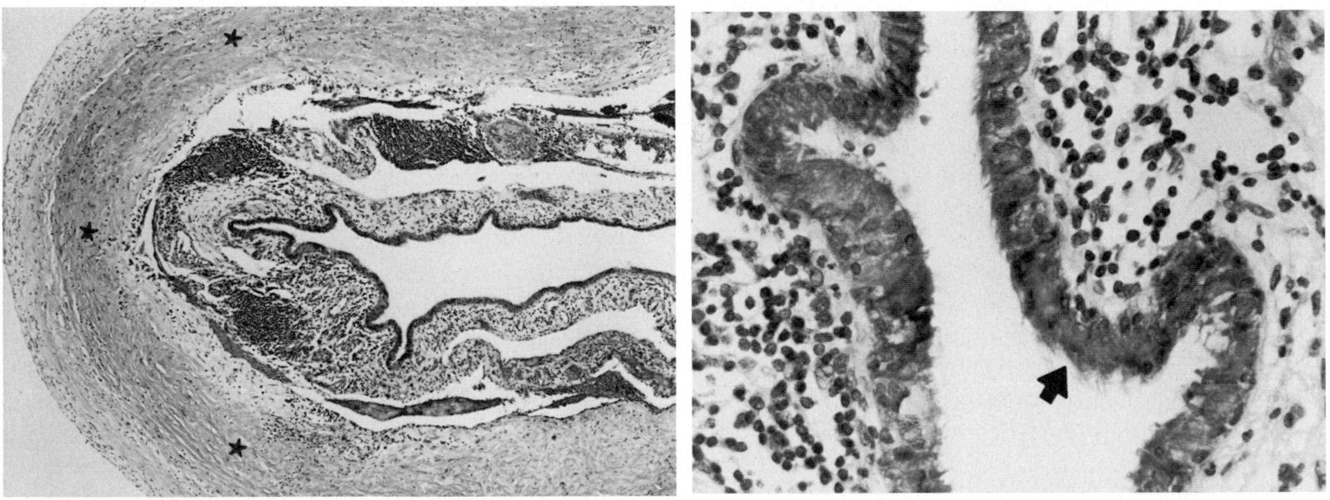

FIGURE 61-9. Bronchogenic cyst. The wall of this bronchogenic cyst consists of dense fibrous tissue (*asterisks*). Cartilage and seromucinous glands were also present (not shown). (Masson trichrome, ×52.) (Courtesy of Kay Washington, MD, Duke University Medical Center, Durham, NC.)

such as cough, dyspnea, tachypnea, wheezing, or chest pain, are typical. The usual chest radiographic appearance of a bronchogenic cyst is that of a smooth, roughly spherical, paratracheal, or hilar solid mass without calcification. Displacement of the adjacent airway and distal air-trapping are relatively frequent, even in patients without symptoms. Air–fluid levels suggest communication with the tracheobronchial tree or foregut, and this is a particularly likely finding in the presence of acute infection.

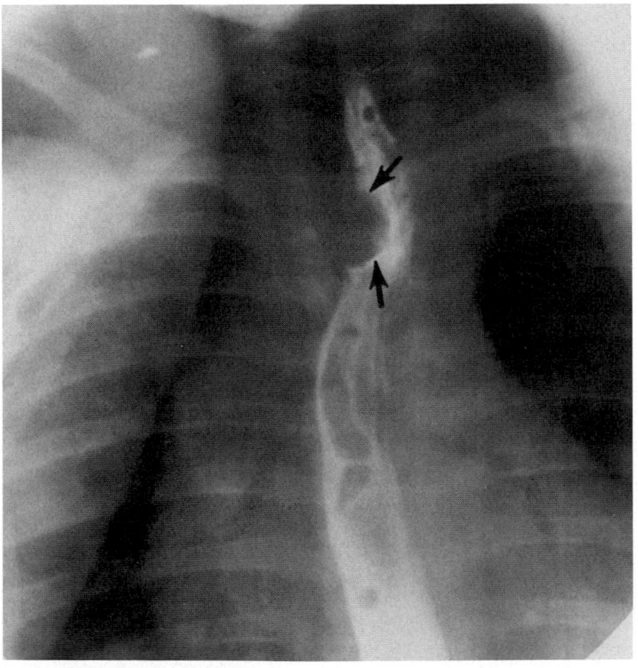

FIGURE 61-10. Esophogram demonstrating extrinsic compression (*arrows*) from a foregut-derived cystic lesion that caused symptomatic tracheal obstruction in an infant. At time of excision, this lesion had both esophageal and tracheal elements, consistent with a shared embryologic origin. Simple excision relieved the symptoms.

True lung cysts can occur anywhere. They are typically single, unilocular lesions. These can be large or small and difficult to distinguish from a lung abscess or macrocytic CCAM on chest radiograph. Discovery of a bronchogenic or true lung cyst after slow or incomplete radiographic resolution of acute pneumonia has also been well described. As with other thoracic mass lesions, CT and MR imaging provide both diagnostic accuracy and excellent definition of the anatomic relations of these lesions. In the patient with dysphagia and a paraesophageal bronchogenic cyst, a contrast esophagogram may demonstrate extrinsic compression at the site of the lesion. Likewise, endoscopic examination of the tracheobronchial tree or esophagus may show extrinsic compression.

Resection of the cystic abnormality is standard treatment for virtually all bronchogenic and lung cysts, even if asymptomatic. The risk of infection appears to be high, although no prospective data exist. Generally, simple local resection is easily accomplished and definitive. Occasionally, however, limited parenchymal lung resection or even lobectomy may be required. Preoperative treatment of pneumonia is helpful in diminishing perioperative morbidity and in minimizing the magnitude of parenchymal resection. Preservation of adjacent normal parenchyma is an important operative principle. Wedge resection, segmentectomy, and lobectomy have all been reported for individual circumstances. As with many other thoracic lesions, thoracoscopic resection of bronchogenic and lung cysts is feasible for selected patients. It is essential to establish precise anatomic relations preoperatively if a thoracoscopic approach is planned because bronchogenic cysts are often beneath the mediastinal pleura, and therefore, require pleural incision and mediastinal exploration to localize the lesion. Mediastinal exploration is important for infants with lobar emphysema because an occult bronchogenic cyst may be responsible, and relief is occasionally possible without lobar lung resection.

The long-term outcome for infants and children with bronchogenic and true lung cysts is excellent because they generally do not require sacrifice of significant normal lung parenchyma. Likewise, perioperative morbidity is low and mortality rare, particularly for mediastinal lesions without tracheobronchial communication. If lung resection is required, outcome is not different than for patients with other lung lesions, such as lobar emphysema or CCAM, and these outcomes are presented later in detail.

Pulmonary Agenesis, Aplasia, and Hypoplasia

Pulmonary Agenesis

Pulmonary agenesis refers to the unilateral or bilateral absence of the entire lung and bronchial tree. Bilateral pulmonary agenesis is rare enough to be reportable and is inconsistent with survival. Unilateral pulmonary agenesis is rare, with several hundred cases reported in the world literature, and is considered briefly (7). Involvement of the right and left sides is roughly equal, and no gender-related propensity is apparent. The pathogenesis is unknown, although it is presumed that agenesis represents a failure of bronchial budding from the trachea during early organogenesis. Associated anomalies are present in more than one-half of patients (33). Congenital abnormalities of the heart and the great vessels; esophageal abnormalities, including tracheoesophageal fistula; skeletal anomalies; genitourinary malformations; imperforate anus; cleft palate; asplenia; and many others have been reported (7,33,34). For unknown reasons, these anomalies are more commonly associated with right-sided agenesis; hence, left-sided involvement carries a considerably better long-term prognosis. Children with pulmonary agenesis present in one of three categories: (1) patients without symptoms for whom the finding is incidental, (2) patients with specific respiratory symptoms, or (3) patients with associated problems who come to medical attention. Among the latter, infants with congenital heart disease or tracheoesophageal fistula are notable and can present difficult joint management issues (Fig. 61-11). Respiratory symptoms may include an entire spectrum of nonspecific complaints. Dyspnea, tachypnea, cyanosis, exercise intolerance, wheezing, cough, and failure to thrive are among these. Recurrent pneumonia and bronchitis are the most common clinical problems. The physiologic basis for this vulnerability to

A

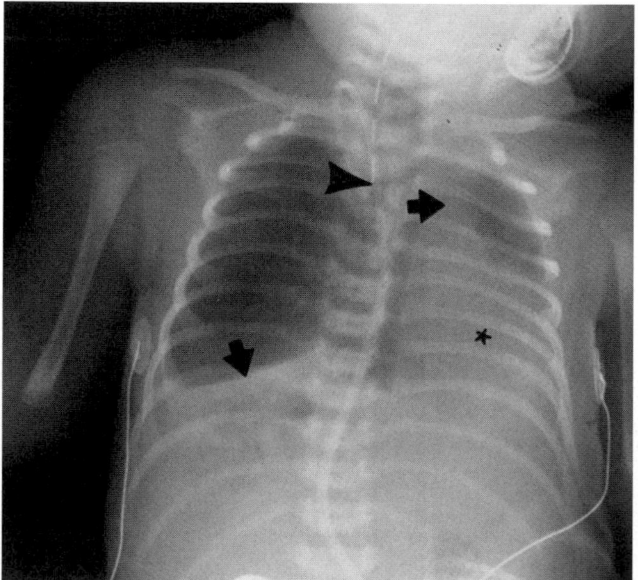

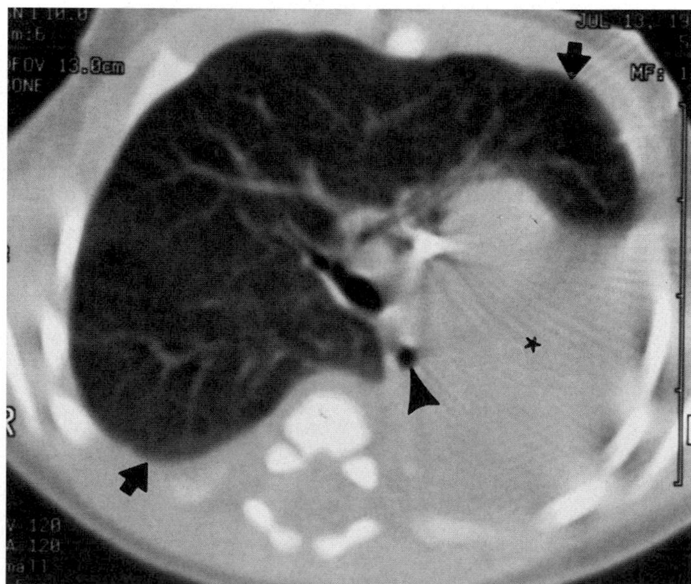

B

FIGURE 61-11. **(A)** Chest radiograph illustrating unilateral left pulmonary agenesis. The right lung is overinflated, and the ipsilateral diaphragm is flattened (*thick arrows*). The mediastinum is shifted to the left (*asterisk*). This diagnosis was confirmed endoscopically through the absence of a left mainstem bronchus. A confounding issue here is the presence of esophageal atresia with a distal tracheal esophageal fistula. On this radiograph, the nasoesophageal tube is positioned at the distal end of the proximal esophageal pouch (*arrowhead*). **(B)** Computed tomography scan of the chest for this lesion. The normal right lung is overinflated (*arrow*), with shift of the heart into the left hemithorax (*asterisk*). The distal esophageal fistula is also visible here (*arrowhead*).

pulmonary infection is unclear, although it has been suggested that the sole remaining bronchus is functionally abnormal and thus unable to clear secretions effectively. Regardless, infection in the single lung must always be considered a life-threatening problem, and aggressive nonoperative management is indicated.

The diagnosis of unilateral pulmonary agenesis is rarely obtained by history and physical examination alone. In older children, asymmetry of the chest or scoliosis may be present, although these are not often apparent in infants. Because the ipsilateral hemithorax is occupied by herniated contralateral lung and the heart, absent or diminished breath sounds and shifted heart sounds are predictable physical findings.

A plain chest radiograph is abnormal, but generally not definitive. The diagnosis is most simply confirmed by bronchoscopy. A normal trachea and contralateral mainstem bronchus with complete absence of the ipsilateral bronchus is diagnostic. CT, ultrasound, and MR imaging may also be helpful, although none of these is routinely required. Fig. 61-11 illustrates both plain chest radiographic and CT findings in an infant with unilateral pulmonary agenesis. In children with congenital heart disease, angiography or echocardiography shows complete absence of the ipsilateral pulmonary artery, and this too is pathognomonic. Contrast bronchography has been abandoned for this diagnosis because it has substantial risks to the single normal lung and is essentially unnecessary with modern imaging and endoscopic techniques.

Standard treatment for unilateral pulmonary agenesis consists of nonoperative respiratory support, particularly aggressive antibiotic treatment for recurrent infections. Lung transplantation has not been reported for this indication. The major surgical issues relate to the management of associated anomalies. The principles are to limit operative interventions to those that are physiologically essential and to time anesthesia for occasions when maximal lung function can be anticipated. Intrathoracic procedures that involve compression of the single lung, such as tracheoesophageal fistula repair, are potentially hazardous, although they can be accomplished by a coordinated and experienced surgical team without cardiopulmonary bypass.

Historically, about one-half to one-third of children with unilateral pulmonary agenesis failed to survive beyond the first 5 years of life (7). Most of this mortality is related to perinatal death, problems of associated anomalies, or recurrent pulmonary infections. In more recent years, the prognosis for these patients appears to be improving.

Pulmonary Aplasia and Hypoplasia

Pulmonary aplasia results from the interrupted development of the normal bronchial tree with either absence of, or reduction in, the number of normal alveoli. Pulmonary hypoplasia refers to the reduction in size of an entire lung and its individual components. Although these lesions generally arise for different reasons, the former as a primary defect in organogenesis and the latter secondary to extrinsic compression from an intrathoracic mass lesion, they are physiologically similar and are therefore presented jointly here. Although primary pulmonary hypoplasia does occur spontaneously, this problem is more often the result of lesions such as congenital diaphragmatic hernia or CCAM, which limit alveolar development in utero. These children present with newborn pulmonary hypertension, persistent fetal circulation, and respiratory failure.

Several forms of congenital thoracic dystrophy produce acute or chronic asphyxiation related to pulmonary hypoplasia. All are rare, but Jejune thoracic dystrophy is the least rare. The physiologic problem, pulmonary hypoplasia, results from in utero restriction of lung development by an abnormal chest wall. Most affected infants have many other problems and do not survive. The only circumstance in which surgical intervention appears rational is in potentially nonlethal forms of the disease. In this circumstance, procedures designed to enlarge the thorax have been attempted. Median sternotomy and several individualized forms of thoracoplasty have been described. Insufficient data are available for meaningful clinical analysis of these approaches.

ACQUIRED LUNG DISEASE

Infectious and inflammatory conditions of the lung share certain physiologic and morphologic features. It has become apparent that many of the humoral and cellular events that regulate acute lung injury are components of the endogenous inflammatory response. Although this response is an essential component of the normal host defense system, extraordinary stimuli that result in exuberant systemic activation generate a variety of end-organ injuries. The lungs appear to be uniquely vulnerable, and the interaction between host phagocytic cells and the pulmonary microvascular endothelial cell is fundamental. Whether the initial stimulus is barotrauma, oxygen toxicity, pneumonia, acid aspiration, sepsis, thermal injury, or some other proinflammatory stimulus, the inflammatory response is similar. This response regulates the progression of both adult and pediatric acquired lung disease (Fig. 61-12) (35). Depending on the clinical course of the underlying disease, chronic lung injury and fibrosis can result. In neonates, *bronchopulmonary dysplasia* is the most important example of this process.

Lung Abscess

Generally, a lung abscess develops when at least one of two fundamental problems exist: (1) a primary failure of host defenses is present, or (2) repeated aspiration of

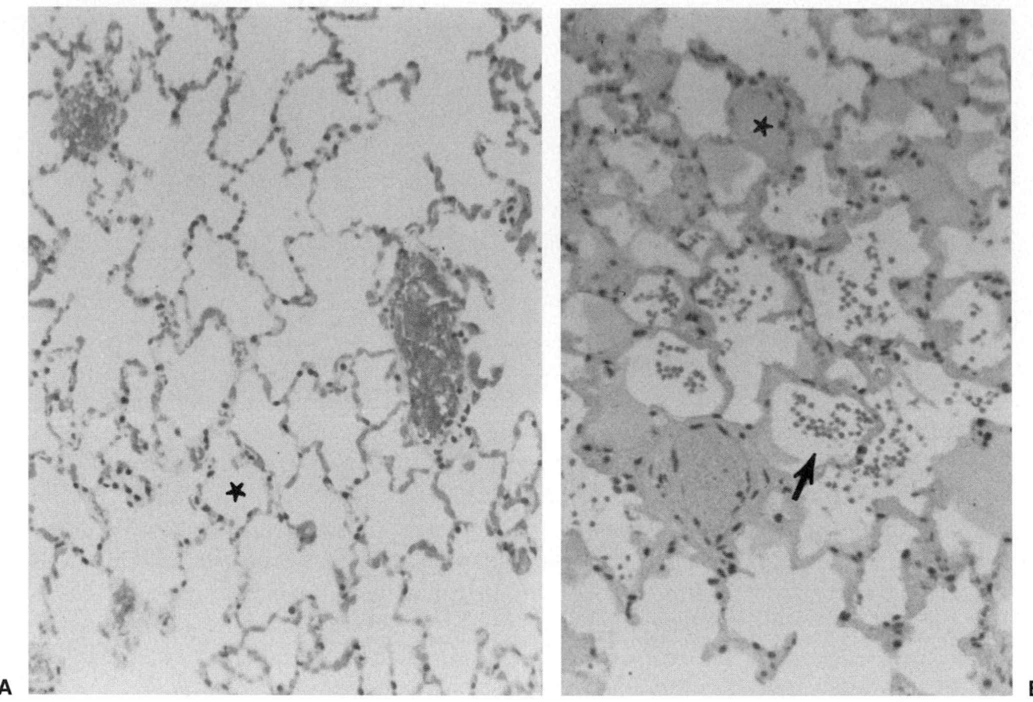

FIGURE 61-12. Photomicrographs of lung after experimental microvascular injury. **(A)** Normal lung histology with normal alveoli (*asterisk*). **(B)** Neutrophil infiltration, alveolar edema (*asterisk*), intraalveolar hemorrhage (*arrow*), and acute lung injury. (From Turnage RH, Guice KS, Oldham KT. Pulmonary microvascular injury following intestinal reperfusion. *New Horizons* 1994;2:463, with permission.

oral or intestinal bacteria into the tracheobronchial tree occurs. Some of the relevant deficiencies are provided in Table 61-1. As elsewhere, the abscess results from tissue necrosis related to pyogenic, toxin-producing bacterial organisms and to phagocytic cells that generate cytotoxic oxidants and proteases. Both cellular lung elements and the extracellular lung matrix are destroyed; tissue necrosis and cavitation within the lung parenchyma follow. The involved area is surrounded by atelectasis and pneumonia. A chronic lung abscess develops with varying degrees of circumferential fibrosis and may involve substantial destruction of parenchyma, usually in a lobar distribution. Typically, the abscess cavity communicates with the normal tracheobronchial tree, and this relation has important diagnostic and treatment implications.

Lung abscesses that form without underlying structural abnormalities are now uncommon in infants and children, although they are still potentially serious. Cowles et al. from Michigan found that 71% of children with lung abscesses had an accompanying anatomic or physiologic comorbidity, and more than 90% had been treated for prior pneumonia (36). In the modern medical environment, infants and children at particular risk are those who are immunocompromised.

Although aspiration is a common event in infants and children, lung abscesses do not ordinarily follow. Certain groups of children, however, appear to be at particular

TABLE 61-1 Deficiencies That Can Contribute to the Development of Lung Abscesses in Children.

Inadequate mechanical clearance mechanisms
Structural abnormalities
Retained endobronchial foreign body
Tracheostomy
Underlying cystic disease of the lung
Cystic fibrosis
α_1-Antitrypsin deficiency
Any cause of partial bronchial obstruction
Ineffective cough (neurologically impaired patients)
Immotile cilia (Kartagener syndrome)
Inadequate cellular host defenses
Transplantation, oncology, or other patients who are iatrogenically immunosuppressed by chemotherapy or antirejection regimens
Severe combined immunodeficiency syndrome
Chronic granulomatous disease
Other hereditary granulocyte deficiencies
Inadequate humoral host deficiencies
Hereditary complement deficiencies
Agammaglobulinemia
Immunoglobulin A deficiency
Iatrogenic manipulation of humoral defenses (monoclonal antibodies, receptor antagonists, and other strategies to alter the humoral component of the inflammatory response are currently in preclinical trials)

risk. Among these are children with cerebral palsy or other causes of neurologic dysfunction who may be unable to protect the airway adequately. Repetitive, incompletely cleared aspiration events result. Institutionalized children with periodontal and dental disease and patients who have been treated with antibiotics for some other reason may also be at high risk, presumably because of the presence of a larger than normal proximal reservoir of potentially pathogenic bacteria.

Lung abscesses are typically polymicrobial, with both anaerobic and aerobic bacteria. Since the 1970s, when anaerobic cultures became routine, oral anaerobic organisms have predominated in epidemiologic reviews of causative organisms. *Bacteroides* sp, group B β-hemolytic streptococci, *Streptococcus pneumoniae, Escherichia coli, Pseudomonas* sp, *Proteus* sp, and *Aerobacter aerogenes* are all important and relatively frequent pathogens in this setting (37,38). This is in contrast to *Staphylococcus aureus* and *Klebsiella pneumoniae,* which were the most common and important causes of lung abscesses in Western countries in the 1980s. It remains important, however, to recognize that the latter organisms are both associated with substantial parenchymal lung destruction and are still important pathogens. Both require long-term and aggressive antibiotic treatment.

Secondary and even primary pulmonary infection with a variety of fungal and other organisms may also lead to the development of a lung abscess. *Aspergillus, Actinomyces,* and *Nocardia* spp are among these pathogenic organisms. Cavitary tuberculosis was once an important risk factor for the development of secondary pyogenic lung abscesses in adults. Given the worldwide resurgence of tuberculosis, including among children in the United States, it may be worthwhile to recall this experience in coming years.

The clinical presentation of a patient with a lung abscess commonly includes systemic complaints, such as fever, chills, night sweats, anorexia, and weight loss. Nonspecific respiratory symptoms, such as coughing and wheezing, are also frequent. More specific and alarming symptoms, such as a productive cough, fetid sputum, or hemoptysis, are later events associated with suppurative disease and cavitation. These latter findings in particular should lead to a prompt laboratory and imaging evaluation because the physical examination generally yields only nonspecific signs of pulmonary consolidation. The most important examination is generally a plain chest radiograph. A single cavity in a dependent location with an air–fluid level is classic (Fig. 61-13). Predictably, lung abscesses occur in areas of the lung that are dependent. Two-thirds are found in the right lung; the superior segment of the lower lobe and the posterior segment of the upper lobe are most common (37,38). An ambulatory patient is more likely to have involvement of basal segments of the lower lobes because these are dependent on the upright position. Areas of surrounding consolidation, pneumonia, and a thick fibrous wall are all typical, but variable in appearance. It may be impossible to differentiate a lung abscess from an infected cystic lung lesion on radiographs obtained at a single point in time. Generally, sequential films demonstrate resolution of pneumonia or an abscess, whereas congenital cystic lesions remain and become conspicuous. A pneumatocele may develop after treatment of necrotizing pneumonia or a lung abscess and may have a residual cystic appearance; however, these air-filled cavities typically do not have air–fluid levels. In addition, patients generally improve clinically or have no symptoms after treatment when the typical air-filled cavity becomes apparent. CT and MR imaging are both excellent techniques for evaluating intrathoracic mass lesions such as a lung abscess; however, their routine use is not required, and their expense can be substantial.

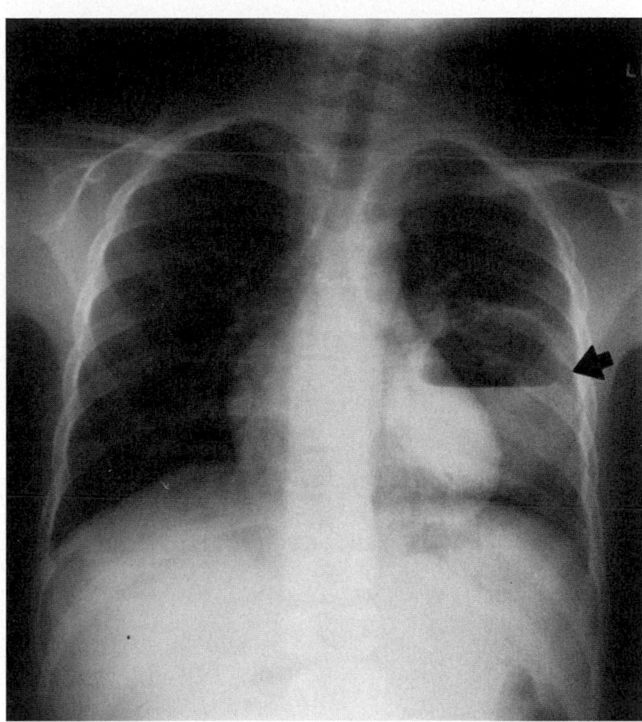

FIGURE 61-13. Plain chest radiograph showing the classic appearance of a thick-walled pulmonary parenchymal abscess with an obvious air–fluid level (*arrow*). (Courtesy of Don Frush, MD, Duke University Medical Center, Durham, NC.)

A lung abscess, like any other abscess, requires prompt drainage and treatment with appropriate antibiotics. Drainage may occur spontaneously into the tracheobronchial tree, and this is a time at which large amounts of purulent, malodorous sputum may be expectorated. Postural drainage and appropriate suctioning are simple yet fundamental aspects of care at this time. Infants, small children, and others who cannot eliminate sputum effectively may require more aggressive endoscopic or transpleural surgical drainage.

Endoscopic drainage of a lung abscess into the tracheobronchial tree can be achieved with a variety of needles, catheters, or other instruments passed through rigid or flexible instruments. If possible, this is preferred to other methods of surgical drainage. Intraoperative control of the airway is essential when endoscopic drainage of a lung abscess is performed because the decompression of purulent material into an adjacent bronchus or the contralateral lung may be life threatening if the abscess is sizable. The contralateral lung is best protected either by positioning the involved lung dependently or by selective intubation and balloon exclusion of the normal mainstem bronchus. A flexible endoscope has the advantage of better access to the peripheral airways, whereas a rigid bronchoscope allows the use of larger instruments and provides better visualization and control of the trachea and primary bronchi. The choice is best individualized. Most infants and children require general anesthesia for the initial endobronchial drainage procedure because of the absolute need for control of the airway. Fluoroscopy or ultrasound may provide valuable guidance in localizing the lesion intraoperatively, if necessary. Subsequent drainage or aspiration procedures may be needed, depending on the clinical response.

Transpleural diagnostic aspiration and both open and closed external drainage are all described and appropriate for selected patients. The risks of pleural contamination, empyema, and bronchopleural fistula, however, make these approaches desirable only in circumstances in which the abscess is peripheral in location and chronic enough that the visceral and parietal pleura are adherent. These approaches are best reserved for specific indications in complex abscesses after failure of initial drainage and antibiotics. Regardless of the drainage technique selected, the abscess contents require microbiologic evaluation to identify the organisms involved and to direct subsequent antibiotic therapy. Empiric initial therapy should cover anaerobic organisms, as well as gram-negative organisms and *S. aureus*. Clindamycin rather than penicillin G is recommended because increasing numbers of resistant oral anaerobes and resistant *S. aureus* organisms make penicillin therapy prone to failure. Antibiotic therapy is generally required for 6 to 12 weeks, although this depends on the patient's response and the rate at which the chest radiograph clears (37,38). Most patients with lung abscesses are successfully treated with drainage and antibiotics alone. Patients with underlying immunodeficiencies that can be corrected or modified should have this done. Modulation of immunosuppression drugs in transplant recipients, delay in chemotherapy for oncology patients, treatment with granulocyte colony-stimulating factor, and other similar approaches are appropriate when possible.

Operative management of a lung abscess is reserved for patients with specific related complications. Failure to control the initial infection or recurrent infection, massive or recurrent hemoptysis, bronchopleural fistula, and a persistent cavitary lesion are indications for operative resection of the affected lung. Immunosuppressed patients are at particular risk for these complications. Although a trial of medical therapy is appropriate in immunosuppressed patients, failure is much more probable, and prompt parenchymal resection is often required. The surgical principle that governs management of the complicated lung abscess is that resection of the involved parenchyma is required. This generally takes the form of a formal lobectomy; if done in the face of acute inflammation, this can be a formidable technical challenge. In this circumstance, the bronchial stump closure requires particular care to avoid an air leak and a bronchopleural fistula.

Pulmonary Surgery in Cystic Fibrosis

The molecular basis of CF has been defined progressively since the early 1990s. With regard to CF pulmonary disease, dysfunction of the adenosine triphosphate-dependent regulatory domain in the chloride channel of respiratory epithelial cell membranes results in the elaboration of abnormally viscid secretions that are chloride and water deficient (39,40). Bacterial clearance from the airways is impaired, and colonization by pathogenic organisms, particularly *Pseudomonas aeruginosa*, results. Chronic and recurrent respiratory infections follow, with a wide range of secondary pulmonary problems. All these complications are the result of chronic infection, inflammation, and lung parenchymal destruction. Today, most are adequately treated without surgical intervention.

Most affected patients are cared for in multidisciplinary centers with specific CF programs (63). Standard treatment for the pulmonary disease of CF includes many supportive measures, such as the use of mucolytic agents, physiotherapy, and aggressive antibiotic therapy, particularly aerosolized and systemic aminoglycosides. In addition, therapies such as DNAase (Pulmozyme) have shown sustained improvement in pulmonary function (41). This inhaled enzyme degrades neutrophil-derived DNA in respiratory secretions, making the mucus less viscid and therefore more easily cleared. Pharmacologic blockade of neutrophil elastase, a cytoplasmic protease, is also undergoing evaluation. The prospect for specific gene therapy, however, remains uncertain. The combined effect of these approaches is that the mean life expectancy for patients with CF is now about 28 years, with respiratory failure being the leading cause of death (42).

The pulmonary complications of CF that require surgical management are diminishing in frequency. It is not likely, however, that these will disappear in the near future because a substantial number of patients with chronic CF lung disease will exist for decades. Although none of these surgical problems is common, they are all potentially serious, and all physicians and surgeons who deal with CF patients must be familiar with them.

Bronchiectasis

Bronchiectasis refers to the structural and functional destruction of the bronchi by chronic or recurrent infection. Although many causes exist, CF is among the most common and important of these in childhood. Bronchiectasis results from recurrent pyogenic bacterial infection that injures and then destroys the cartilage, elastin, smooth muscle, and other structural elements of the airways, replacing them with collagen. Epithelial metaplasia also occurs, so ciliated respiratory epithelium is replaced by squamous epithelium. These structural changes in the conducting airways exacerbate the underlying problem with the clearance of secretions that characterizes CF. Therefore, successive pyogenic bronchial infections and additional injury occur.

Areas of bronchiectasis may be either localized or diffuse. Patients with CF have a systemic disease, and diffuse lung disease is always present. Bronchiectasis, however, tends to occur in specific lobar distributions; the lower lobes are more frequently involved (43). Symptoms of bronchiectasis in patients with CF are exceedingly difficult to differentiate from those of the underlying disease. Generally, the problem occurs in older children and adolescents because it requires a number of years for the bronchial destruction to occur. Diagnosis usually results from increasingly frequent bouts of infection and chronic cough, particularly with the expectoration of larger amounts of sputum, which may be fetid. Chest radiographs with persistent findings of focal pneumonia are also a harbinger of bronchiectasis. Plain radiographs are inadequate to evaluate the disease process in this circumstance. Historically, contrast bronchography was used to localize the disease and define its extent, but this is no longer necessary and has significant hazards. Likewise, bronchoscopy is of limited value because the distal airways must be evaluated and the pathology is often beyond the view of conventional instruments. Chest CT provides excellent definition of the areas of involvement, and MR imaging provides similar information (44). If surgical management is under consideration, ventilation–perfusion scans are also of substantial value because they identify areas of little or no gas exchange (6). Because correlation of anatomic disease with the site of physiologic dysfunction is possible, these data are potentially helpful in preoperative resectional planning. Pulmonary function studies are also helpful because these patients are generally old enough to cooperate, and the information obtained can help to anticipate tolerance for thoracotomy and lung resection.

The initial and often only treatment necessary for CF patients with bronchiectasis is nonoperative. Indications for resectional therapy for bronchiectasis, whether it results from CF or some other cause, all relate to specific complications of the process (45):

- Specific respiratory symptoms that progressively limit daily life, growth, or development, *and*
- Severe localized disease, *and*
- Evidence that parenchymal resection will not be physiologically limiting, *or*
- Recurrent or life-threatening hemorrhage

All are subjective and none are absolute. The number of children with CF who require resectional therapy for bronchiectasis has steadily diminished since the mid-1980s as their nonoperative care has improved. Decisions regarding the necessity for resection, the timing of resection, and the extent of resection require mature clinical judgment and substantial experience with CF patients.

The surgical principle that guides resectional therapy for bronchiectasis is to remove specific areas of severe involvement while preserving normal or less diseased areas of adjacent lung tissue. Generally, this means that segmental or lobar resection is performed. It is preferable to resect areas of disease that are known to be stable rather than those that are still evolving. It is essential to plan the resectional procedure preoperatively in detail by correlating areas of severe radiographic bronchiectatic change with zones of physiologic dysfunction on ventilation–perfusion scan. Patients with diffuse lung disease from CF are intolerant of the loss of functional lung parenchyma. Furthermore, the intraoperative assessment of the lung is generally unhelpful in CF patients because the parenchyma is all abnormal to some extent.

The most comprehensive study of outcomes for CF patients after surgical resection for bronchiectasis was published in 1979 (45). Despite improvements in medical care, this review remains relevant. After parenchymal lung resection for bronchiectasis, 61% of CF patients had substantially improved symptoms, 21% had some improvement, and 18% had no improvement or worsened. The authors reported no operative deaths in the last decade of the review. Similar experience has been repeated on a smaller scale at other institutions (46).

Hemoptysis is an important complication in CF patients with bronchiectasis. The chronic inflammatory and infectious destruction of the airways leads initially to exposure and then to erosion of the bronchial arteries. Pseudoaneurysm formation and hemorrhage can follow (Fig. 61-14). Most of these patients with hemoptysis have relatively minor bleeding that is self-limiting and that can be managed with the same general supportive approaches discussed earlier. For recurrent or refractory hemoptysis, angiographic localization and embolization of a bleeding site is the preferred method of management. For life-threatening bleeding, lobar resection is appropriate, with

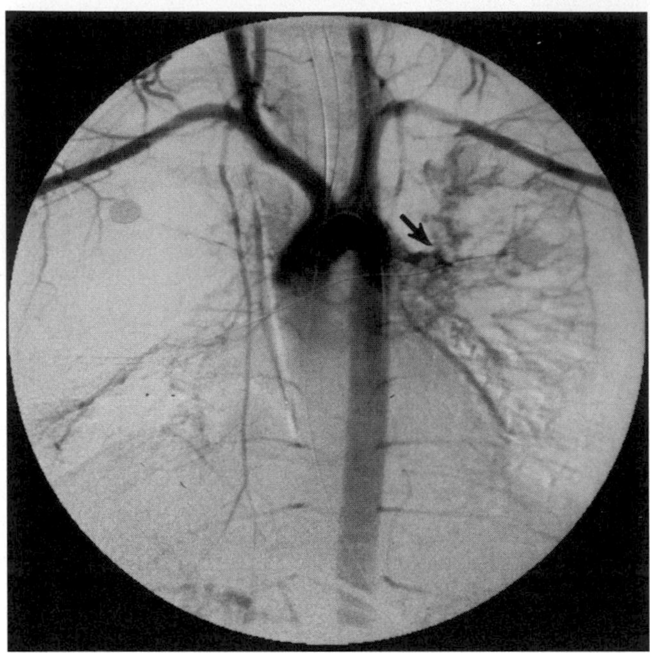

FIGURE 61-14. Angiogram in an adolescent with cystic fibrosis and refractory life-threatening pulmonary hemorrhage from the left upper lobe showing active bronchial arterial bleeding (*arrow*). Emergency left upper lobe resection was required because angiographic embolization was of only transient benefit.

two technical requirements: (1) before parenchymal resection, it is essential to localize the site of hemorrhage to at least the lobe that is bleeding; and (2) control of the airway must be achieved, preferably with selective intubation of the nonbleeding mainstem bronchus. In addition, balloon exclusion of the bleeding bronchus is desirable because the nonbleeding lung will be dependent intraoperatively, and therefore, will be at risk for obstruction from blood clot during the course of the thoracotomy and lung resection.

Pneumothorax

The subject of spontaneous pneumothorax is presented elsewhere in detail (see Chapter 60). With specific regard to patients who have CF, spontaneous pneumothorax occurs in 3% to 18% of patients, and is often a relatively late event in the course of the disease (46,47). Adolescents and young adults with advanced disease are at highest risk, and these patients also have significantly diminished physiologic tolerance. They may develop local infection with bleb formation and rupture, or alveolar rupture from localized air-trapping may occur. This diagnosis is rarely obscure in CF patients because the resulting chest pain and dyspnea are not well tolerated. The diagnosis is ordinarily confirmed by plain chest radiograph. As with any pneumothorax, the treatment objective is prompt evacuation of the air with approximation of the visceral and parietal pleura to seal the air leak. In patients with symptoms, conventional tube thoracostomy with sealed drainage to reexpand the lung is the safest and most effective therapy. Lesser maneuvers, such as needle aspiration, small catheter drainage, or oxygen therapy for transpleural air absorption, are of limited value in this population. In patients without symptoms, however, a therapeutic trial of these less morbid alternatives may be appropriate.

A major question in regard to surgical therapy in patients with spontaneous pneumothorax secondary to CF is whether pleurodesis should be done. The recurrence rate in these patients is about 50% in the absence of definitive treatment (45,48). Furthermore, the risks of pneumothorax may be substantial. For these reasons, it is appropriate to consider pleurodesis to CF patients at the time of an initial pneumothorax. Sclerosing agents placed into the pleural cavity through a chest tube can accomplish this, although the procedure is tedious and can be painful (48). In addition, if unsuccessful, subsequent entry into the pleural space may be hazardous. Open pleurodesis or pleurectomy through a limited thoracotomy is predictably successful and can be done without mortality, although the morbidity is substantial. Thoracoscopic pleurodesis using pleural abrasion or talc poudrage has emerged as the procedure of choice at present. This approach combines the advantages of excellent, direct visualization with a procedure that is highly successful, predictable, and has limited morbidity. In CF patients, it is important to consider that the major additional disadvantage to pleurodesis is the increased difficulty of lung transplantation. Given that lung replacement is feasible in these patients, this potential need must be weighed carefully because some consider pleurodesis a relative contraindication to lung replacement.

Therapeutic Bronchoscopy

Endobronchial toilet is effectively achieved routinely in patients with CF without the need for bronchoscopic suction or lavage. A 1982 trial demonstrated that, although the technique of endoscopic lavage and mucolytic agents is effective, the response is transient and short lived (49). Therefore, this approach has been abandoned for routine use, although it is periodically useful in selected patients with specific exacerbations of their disease. When it is done, cultures can be obtained to direct specific antibiotic therapy.

Lung Replacement

Lung replacement has become feasible as a treatment for the ultimate complication of CF, chronic and irreversible respiratory failure. The predominant approach has been bilateral (double) cadaveric lung transplant; however, living donor lung transplantation is sometimes an alternative (50). The Consensus Conference Statement of 1998 regarding lung transplantation in CF reports data from the International Lung Transplant Registry (through April 1996) and the CF Foundation National Patient Registry. These data indicate that 746 (14%) of the 5,208 lung transplants recorded worldwide were for patients with CF. The number of sites that perform lung transplants had increased to 62 as of 1995. The 3-year actuarial survival rate is 56% in patients with transplants after 1992, and 46% in patients who had operations before 1992. Five-year disease-specific survival rates are 48% (CF), 45% (chronic emphysema), and 38% (pulmonary fibrosis and primary pulmonary hypertension) among lung transplant recipients (51,52). A specific discussion of lung transplantation in children is presented in Chapter 49. Although definitive medical treatment for CF is likely in the future, many patients with chronic CF lung disease will require lung replacement for years to come.

Bullous Lung Disease

Bullae or blebs are saccular areas of subpleural air within the lung that are believed to result from an air leak from an adjacent alveolus. Generally, the term *bleb* refers to a smaller air collection and *bulla* to a larger one, although there are no specific numeric thresholds to distinguish between the use of the two terms. The important functional distinction is that the grossly apparent lesions (bullae) are associated with the loss of adjacent lung parenchyma, whereas this is not true of blebs. Blebs and bullae are not associated with normal alveoli or capillaries; hence, no gas exchange occurs within them, although they do communicate with the tracheobronchial tree (53).

Bullae and blebs are either congenital or acquired. Acquired lesions are usually a consequence of chronic infection related to a problem such as CF, α_1-antitrypsin deficiency, or another similar condition. Bullous emphysema is a common form of acquired chronic obstructive pulmonary disease in adults, but this is rarely seen in children. Congenital bullae and blebs apparently result from disordered development of alveoli and terminal airways during organogenesis. The discussion that follows deals principally with blebs and bullae rather than the underlying pulmonary diseases.

The clinical symptoms of blebs and bullae are generally the result of either spontaneous pneumothorax from rupture into the pleural space or exercise intolerance because of diminished lung volumes and inadequate respiratory reserve. The latter problem is generally associated with underlying diffuse lung disease. Plain chest radiographs and CT are usually adequate for definitive imaging. Apical disease is most common, and bilateral disease is frequent. α_1-Antitrypsin deficiency is unique in its propensity to form basal blebs (54).

The management of blebs and bullae is dependent on the degree of symptomatology and the underlying lung problem. Treatment of smaller lesions is usually limited to problems that result from air leak, specifically pneumothorax. Generally, tube thoracostomy is the appropriate treatment for the first spontaneous pneumothorax. Recurrent pneumothorax occurs in 20% to 50% of patients with congenital bullous disease, and this incidence increases significantly with each additional pneumothorax (55). It is therefore appropriate to consider definitive operative treatment after a first recurrent pneumothorax associated with congenital bullous disease.

The principles for operative management of lung bullae are to remove the area of involvement, to conserve all possible normal lung tissue, and to obtain a secure, airtight closure of the lung. The resections, therefore, generally are not segmental or lobar, but rather nonanatomic in nature (55,56). Resection of bullae with or without pleurodesis is highly effective. Closure of the bleb margin can present problems, but modern stapling devices confer more security and efficiency to this procedure than do traditional suture closure techniques. Therefore, stapled resections are considered routine for this problem. Resection of bullae can be done through either a thoracoscopic approach or an open thoracotomy, with limited morbidity and mortality (55–57). The thoracoscopic approach appears to be highly effective, rapid, and less morbid than open thoracotomy. Potential problems with air leak are best prevented by concurrent pleurodesis or pleurectomy.

The outcome after bleb resection is dependent on the amount of remaining lung and the extent of underlying disease. For congenital blebs with a large portion of the normal lung retained, the outcome is predictably excellent. For extensive local disease or for blebs acquired as a consequence of systemic disease, this is more problematic. Specifically, if preoperative evaluation shows that the bullae occupy more than one-third of the ipsilateral thorax, if ventilation–perfusion scan shows little or no function in the area of the bullae, and if pulmonary function studies indicate tolerance for thoracotomy and lung resection, the outcome is much more favorable (55).

Bronchiectasis

Bronchiectasis was discussed in some detail in the presentation of surgical problems associated with CF. The pathogenesis and treatment of the process are generally similar in patients without CF and are not repeated in detail here, although a number of other causes exist. Collectively, these conditions are relatively common, yet the complication of bronchiectasis is not. Those of particular importance in childhood are retained endobronchial foreign bodies, bronchial stenosis after a bout of pneumonia or acute bronchitis, endobronchial tumors, α_1-antitrypsin deficiency, Kartagener (immotile cilia) syndrome, structural lung lesions, chronic aspiration, and a variety of immunodeficiencies (6,58). In addition, congenital bronchiectasis can occur without an underlying cause. The fundamental lesion is one of chronic distal airway infection with loss of structural integrity of the conducting airways, inadequate clearance of secretions and bacteria, and sequential bouts of destructive inflammation and infection. Although many different bacterial and viral organisms can initiate the bronchiectatic process, specific pathogens of note include measles and pertussis, both of which have undergone a resurgence in the United States because of inadequate childhood immunization practices. Likewise, tuberculosis is an important and increasing cause of concern.

In previously healthy patients, the development of persistent respiratory symptoms and chronic, productive cough with fetid sputum or hemoptysis is highly suggestive of bronchiectasis. Unlike CF patients, these symptoms are easily identified in otherwise normal patients. The evaluation, treatment, and surgical principles are similar to those presented previously. Bronchoscopy is essential because clearly reversible lesions, such as endobronchial tumors or foreign bodies, must be corrected. Otherwise, the approach is to define the extent of disease and provide nonoperative treatment, principally in the form of antibiotics specific for oral bacterial pathogens. CT scanning is an excellent diagnostic technique (44) (Fig. 61-15). The underlying disease is treated, if possible. The spread of bronchiectasis to new areas of previously normal lung is unlikely with appropriate treatment, although progression at the site of previously injured lung occurs in about 25% of patients, even with appropriate treatment (6). Operative indications are related either to substantial disability or hemorrhage that is directly attributable to focal disease. Generally, segmental or lobar lung resection via thoracotomy is the procedure of choice. Conservation of uninvolved lung is a fundamental surgical principle, and in otherwise normal patients, this approach yields an excellent outcome. Using these principles, Wilson and Decker (59) reported that 75% of patients with focal bronchiectasis did not have symptoms or substantially improved postoperatively, while virtually none worsened. As expected, the prognosis in the presence of systemic or diffuse lung disease is substantially diminished.

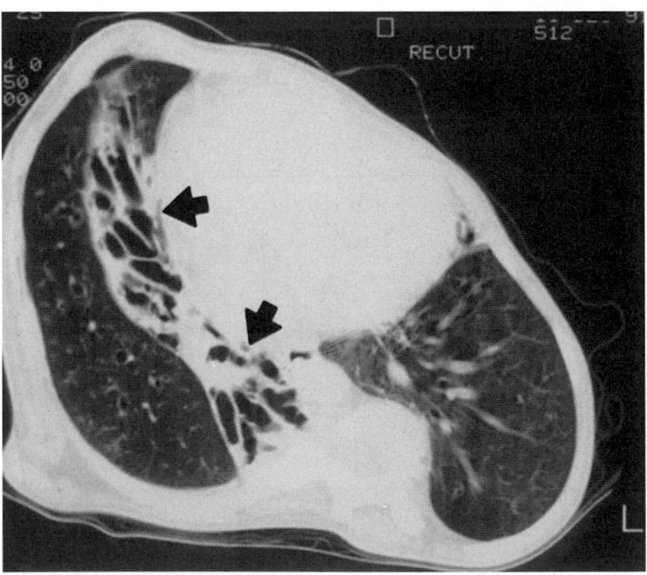

FIGURE 61-15. Computed tomography image of the chest showing severe bronchiectasis secondary to gastroesophageal reflux. This child had involvement of the right lower and the right middle lobes (*arrows*). Lesser involvement of the left lower lobe was also present. Substantial clinical improvement followed right middle and lower lobectomy.

Echinococcal Lung Disease

Echinococcus granulosus and *Echinococcus multilocularis* are parasites responsible for hydatid cystic lung disease in children. Echinococcal infection is endemic but rare among native populations of the Southwest United States, Northwestern Canada, and Alaska. The predominant vector in North America is the dog; in the Middle East, Australia, India, and the Mediterranean countries, exposure to sheep or cattle appears responsible for transmission to the human intermediate host. Humans become infected by eating food contaminated by the scoleces of these parasites. In adults, liver involvement is most common, followed by lung, brain, spleen, and other organs (60). In children, pulmonary echinococcus cysts are more common than liver cysts (61). The presentation of pulmonary disease includes patients without symptoms, as well as those with cough, dyspnea, fever, and chest pain. Those who do not have symptoms are believed to have been infected more recently because the hydatid cyst requires time to develop. Solitary lung cysts are often large, and air–fluid levels may be seen on chest radiograph. Calcification may also be present. The diagnosis can be confirmed with an accuracy of 80% or more with one or more of the following serologic tests: indirect hemagglutination, complement fixation, dot immunobinding, or enzyme-linked immunosorbent assay (60). Transpleural aspiration is also diagnostic, demonstrating *Echinococcus* sp hooklets and protoscoleces. Conventional therapy for pulmonary disease includes perioperative mebendazole treatment and prompt surgical resection of the thick-walled cyst, with care taken to avoid pleural contamination (55). The risks of anaphylaxis and local implantation of scolices appear low with lung disease, but most surgeons experienced with this disease attempt to prevent pleural spillage whether at the time of diagnosis or treatment. Antibiotic therapy alone is insufficient to eliminate the thick-walled cyst. Because of the risk of secondary bacterial infection, surgical resection of the cyst is recommended. Simple wedge resection is appropriate without scolecidal agents. Agents such as hypertonic saline or ethyl alcohol have been used in conjunction with resection, but the risk is substantial if drainage of these agents into the tracheobronchial tree occurs.

Opportunistic Lung Infections

The number of infants and children who have opportunistic pulmonary infections produced by mycobacterial, protozoan, viral, fungal, and bacterial pathogens is steadily growing because of progressive increases in the number of immunocompromised hosts. Transplant recipients, oncology patients, human immunodeficiency virus victims, and others offer a burgeoning at-risk population. Typically, at-risk patients develop diffuse interstitial pneumonitis with clinical symptoms that range from cough and fever to life-threatening respiratory distress (Fig. 61-16). Depending on the underlying disease, many receive empiric antibiotic therapy with trimethoprim-sulfamethoxazole or other agents to treat possible pathogens, such as *Pneumocystis carinii* (Fig. 61-17). A definitive tissue diagnosis becomes necessary for progressive or refractory disease. The most common surgical requirement for these immunosuppressed patients with interstitial lung disease is to provide tissue samples for histopathology and microbiologic analysis to direct specific therapy. Both transbronchial biopsy and percutaneous lung biopsy yield small tissue samples that may be helpful in differentiating among infectious, neoplastic, rejection-related, and inflammatory lung processes. Bronchoalveolar lavage may be helpful in identifying some pathogens in immunosuppressed children with pneumonia. Formal lung biopsy, however, whether by limited open thoracotomy or thoracoscopic means, is often preferred because of the larger specimen and its definitive nature. Although the surgical procedure is generally well tolerated, its combination with the underlying disease process yields substantial perioperative morbidity and mortality. In one review of open lung biopsies among childhood bone marrow transplant recipients with interstitial lung disease, the 30-day mortality rate was 45% and the overall mortality rate was 74% (62). A definitive diagnosis results from open lung biopsy in between 50% and 90% of immunosuppressed patients with interstitial lung disease, although the incidence of treatable disease is substantially lower (62,63).

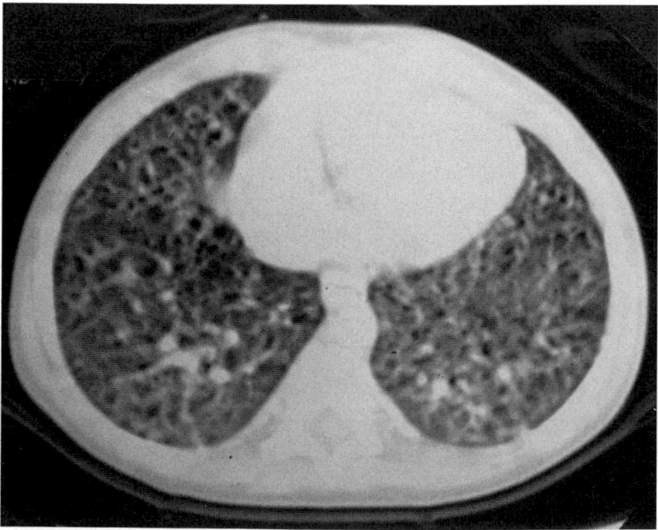

FIGURE 61-16. Child with acquired immunodeficiency syndrome and a bilateral interstitial pneumonitis. Appearance on chest computed tomography. Open lung biopsy is often necessary for definitive diagnosis in these circumstances. (Courtesy of Cindy Miller, MD, Duke University Medical Center, Durham, NC.)

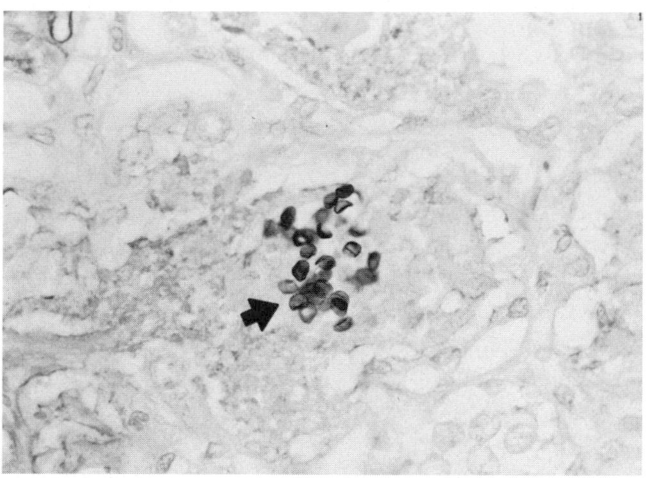

FIGURE 61-17. *Pneumocystis carinii* pneumonia. The 4- to 6-μm encysted form of *P. carinii* is round or helmet-shaped (*arrow*). These organisms are generally found within the intraalveolar transudative froth. (Methenamine silver, ×60.) (Courtesy of Kay Washington, MD, Duke University Medical Center, Durham, NC.)

From a technical standpoint, the thoracoscopic approach with use of a stapled wedge resection has rapidly gained acceptance in children with diffuse lung disease who are of sufficient size to use the commercially available stapling devices within the thorax (about 15 kg). Smaller children are also appropriate for thoracoscopic lung biopsy, although suture closure or coagulation of the lung may be needed. Conventional open biopsy remains an appropriate alternative, although the operative morbidity may be greater.

Pneumocystis Carinii

P. carinii is the most common protozoan lung infection that occurs in the immunocompromised host (62,63). It typically causes interstitial pneumonia, hypoxemia, fever, and tachypnea. Acute respiratory failure may follow. Bronchoalveolar lavage may be diagnostic, but the organisms are best demonstrated by methenamine silver staining of lung tissue, as shown in Fig. 61-17. Identification of these organisms is one of the diagnostic criteria for differentiating human immunodeficiency virus infection from clinical acquired immunodeficiency syndrome (see Chapter 13). Prophylaxis in high-risk patients or treatment for presumed or mild disease is initially with trimethoprim-sulfamethoxazole. If the disease is refractory or progressive, however, pentamidine isethionate is required (64). *Toxoplasma gondii* is a protozoan infection that can cause clinical pneumonitis indistinguishable from *P. carinii* except by pathologic evaluation. The distinction is important because the latter infection requires treatment with pyrimethamine sulfadiazine.

Fungi

Fungal infection, in particular, is an important and increasing source of pulmonary infection among immunocompromised children. Nosocomial infection with *Candida albicans* and other *Candida* species in critically ill hospitalized patients is quite common. Candidal pulmonary disease is often associated with sepsis and life-threatening systemic disease. Prophylaxis with oral antifungal agents is appropriate for high-risk patients to prevent pulmonary or systemic infection. Systemic amphotericin B is standard therapy for invasive or intracavitary candidal infection. Oral agents may be appropriate for airway colonization, but intravenous treatment with amphotericin B is necessary for candidal pneumonitis (64). Combination therapy with 5-fluorocytosine, ketoconazole, fluconazole, or other agents may also be useful, although no prospective studies address this question.

Fungi that are endemic pulmonary human pathogens in the United States include *Histoplasma capsulatum* in the Mississippi and Ohio River Valleys, *Blastomyces dermatitides* in the South and East, and *Coccidioides immitis* in California and the Southwest. Many people in these regions demonstrate serologic evidence of exposure, but few have clinical evidence of disease. Although any organ can be affected, lung involvement is most common, particularly for blastomycosis and coccidioidomycosis. Histoplasmosis may be associated with massive mediastinal lymphadenopathy. For all three of these organisms, a common clinical scenario is the discovery of a single lung nodule on a chest radiograph in an otherwise healthy patient who does not have symptoms. This may present a diagnostic dilemma that necessitates wedge resection for a definitive pathologic evaluation. In patients for whom the diagnosis is clear from the history and serology, this is not necessary. Typically, affected patients require no further treatment if they do not have symptoms.

Healthy individuals rarely develop fungal pneumonia or disseminated disease, but this is a particular risk in the immunosuppressed host. In at-risk patients, the diagnosis should be established and systemic antifungal treatment initiated. The appropriate diagnosis may be established if substantial elevations in acute complement fixation titers occur, but this is a time-consuming process because specimens obtained 4 to 6 weeks apart are required for comparison. Sputum, tracheobronchial aspirates, and lung tissue for culture are all useful as well. Amphotericin B remains the treatment of choice for fungal infection if the patient has systemic disease, has specific pulmonary symptoms, or is immunocompromised. Less serious disease can be treated with one of the azole class of antifungal agents, such as miconazole, ketoconazole, fluconazole, or itraconazole. Once the diagnosis is established, operation is indicated only for specific pulmonary complications, and these are rare.

Aspergillosis, mucormycosis, and other fungal infections are also seen in immunocompromised hosts. These are potentially life threatening when pulmonary infection is involved, and essentially all these infections require systemic amphotericin B treatment. Aspergillosis, in particular, is associated with cavitary tuberculosis and, in this setting, usually requires resection because it is difficult to eradicate the aspergilloma within the sequestered lung cavity. Mucormycosis is an aggressive and often lethal fungal infection resulting from the *Rhizopus* sp, which can occur anywhere. If a patient is to survive this invasive necrotizing infection, aggressive surgical debridement of involved tissue is necessary.

Mycobacteria

Childhood pulmonary infection from *Mycobacterium tuberculosis* and atypical mycobacterial forms is a substantial public health issue in the United States (65). The acquired immunodeficiency virus epidemic and concurrent resurgence of tuberculosis in the adult population appear to be important causes. The natural history of the disease does not appear fundamentally different in children than adults, but the emergence of atypical and antibiotic-resistant strains of mycobacteria is an increasingly important problem. Transmission is generally through a respiratory route, and the lung is the most common site of involvement. The initial treatment is always medical with multidrug antibiotic regimens, including combinations of isoniazid, rifampin, ethambutol, streptomycin, paraaminosalicylic acid, and pyrazinamide (64). Common atypical organisms include *M. avium*, *M. intracellulare*, and *M. kansasii*. These organisms all require treatment with rifampin and at least two additional agents, usually for 6 to 12 months or longer.

The goal of surgery in these patients is generally to obtain lung or lymph node tissue to establish the diagnosis or to deal with specific complications. Among these complications are bronchiectasis and cavitary disease with a secondary lung abscess, both of which are discussed previously. Other operative indications for pulmonary tuberculosis include recurrent or persistent hemorrhage, refractory nodular disease with resistant organisms, empyema with a restrictive component, irreversible lung destruction, and residual cavitary or caseous disease after 6 months of therapy. The surgical principle is to perform a minimal resection of the affected lung parenchyma, conserving lung that is normal or reversibly involved. The disease can be controlled or eradicated in most circumstances by appropriate concurrent antibiotic therapy, and the outcome is generally good (37).

Viral Infection

Herpes viruses, particularly the cytomegalovirus (CMV), are the most common pulmonary viral pathogens in immunosuppressed patients. Epstein-Barr virus, the herpes simplex viruses, and varicella-zoster virus are among this group. CMV infection in solid organ transplant recipients is especially common; evidence of infection is present in 30% or more of these patients. This is in part because of its transmission through the transplanted organ. In some series, CMV is the most common infectious pathogen among immunosuppressed children with diffuse alveolar and interstitial lung disease (62,63). Diagnosis by culture, polymerase chain reaction, or a rise in anti-CMV antibody titers is often too slow to be of clinical utility. The development of fluorescent anti-CMV monoclonal antibodies has allowed diagnosis to be established by direct staining of tissue or other specimens within 24 hours (64). In addition, specific antiviral therapy is available for CMV in the form of ganciclovir. Acyclovir is effective against other herpes viruses, and hyperimmune immunoglobulin G also appears to be beneficial in the treatment of clinical herpes infection.

LUNG TUMORS

Primary Lung Tumors

The definitive contemporary review of primary pulmonary neoplasms in children was by Hartman and Shochat in 1983 (66). They found that, of 230 primary tumors, 151 were malignant and 79 benign. Their findings are summarized in Table 61-2. Because this review represents the entire English language literature to that date, it is clear that the lesions are rare.

TABLE 61-2 Classification by Cell Type of 230 Primary Lung Tumors in Children.

Type of Tumor	*Patients*
Benign	79
Inflammatory pseudotumor	45
Hamartoma	15
Neurogenic tumor	9
Leiomyoma	6
Mucous gland adenoma	2
Myoblastoma	2
Malignant	151
Bronchial adenoma	65
Bronchogenic carcinoma	47
Pulmonary blastoma	14
Leiomyosarcoma	9
Rhabdomyosarcoma	6
Hemangiopericytoma	3
Lymphoma	3
Teratoma	2
Plasmacytoma	1
Myxosarcoma	1

(From Hartman GE, Shochat SJ. Primary pulmonary neoplasms of childhood: a review. *Ann Thorac Surg* 1983;36:108, with permission.)

Malignant Tumors

Bronchial Adenoma

The most common primary lung tumors in children are a heterogeneous group of low-grade adenocarcinomas incorrectly but irrevocably termed *bronchial adenomas*. These lesions have a variety of histologic features that have led to the use of several descriptive names: *carcinoid, mucoepidermoid carcinoma,* and *adenoid cystic carcinoma (cylindroma)*. In reality, all have the potential for metastatic spread, although this incidence is low, about 5% to 10% (66).

Endobronchial carcinoid tumors are the most common, generally representing 80% to 85% of this group. These lesions, like other carcinoid tumors, are derived from neural crest stem cells and retain their potential for serotonin and peptide hormone synthesis. Plasma serotonin and urine 5-hydroxyindoleacetic acid levels may be elevated in these patients, and they are therefore potentially useful tumor markers. The carcinoid syndrome has been reported in a single child with an endobronchial carcinoid tumor (67).

The clinical presentation is typically one of recurrent or persistent pneumonia because of partial or complete bronchial obstruction. Because of the critical anatomic location, the tumors generally become symptomatic while relatively small, although it appears that the rate of growth is slow. Radiographic imaging is generally nondiagnostic (Fig. 61-18). Bronchoscopic findings are, however, unique and compelling. The lesion is best described as a pink, friable mulberry. Although biopsy can be done, it is inadvisable for several reasons: (1) hemorrhage can be substantial or even life threatening, (2) the histopathology is difficult to evaluate with a small specimen and limited time, (3) the gross appearance is predictable from a diagnostic standpoint, and (4) obstructing bronchial adenomas require resection, the nature of which is generally dictated by anatomic rather than pathologic features.

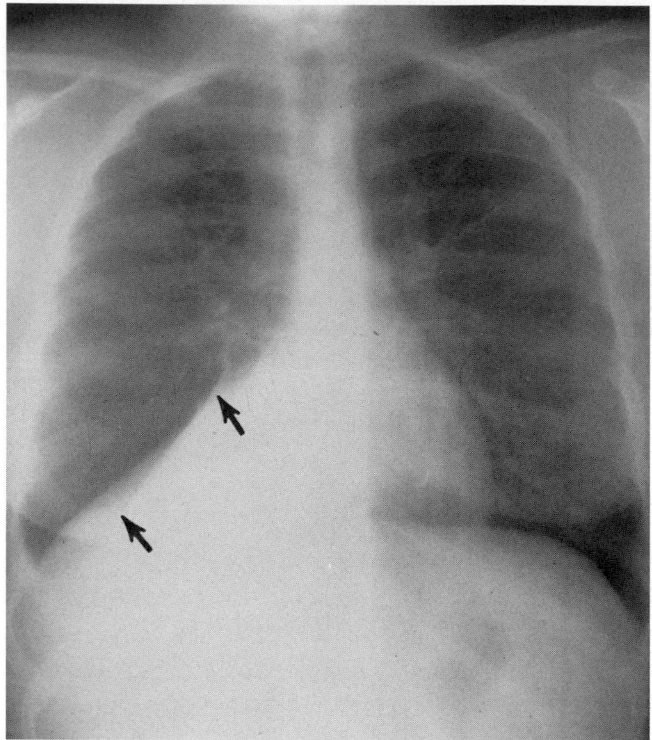

FIGURE 61-18. Chest radiograph of a 15-year-old girl with a 3-week history of refractory pneumonia. Right middle and right lower lobe collapse is obvious (*arrows*). At bronchoscopy, this patient was found to have a nearly completely obstructing carcinoid of the bronchus intermedius.

Careful endoscopic mapping under direct vision is essential to planning operative management. Endoscopy and video systems have evolved rapidly and offer substantial improvement in this aspect of care. Although endoscopic resection is reported, it is considered ill advised because of the risks of hemorrhage, bronchial stenosis, local recurrence, and the inability to examine regional lymph nodes. In older children and those with small tumors without lymphatic spread, successful segmental bronchial resection has been done. Most patients with endobronchial carcinoid tumors, however, require lobectomy or pneumonectomy, depending on the specific location of the tumor. Regional lymph node sampling, particularly in the presence of clinically suspicious nodes, is also appropriate. These carcinoid tumors are radiosensitive, and this may be an appropriate therapy for nonresectable disease, although available data are too limited for definitive guidelines. The 10-year survival rate in children after surgical resection for endobronchial carcinoid tumor is about 90% (66).

Endobronchial mucoepidermoid carcinomas represent 10% to 15% of bronchial adenomas. Their clinical features in childhood are similar to those of endobronchial carcinoid tumors, particularly with regard to presentation, diagnostic evaluation, and surgical treatment. The principal difference involves the histopathology. These lesions have both mucus-secreting and epidermoid cells. Only one child is reported to have had malignant spread of this lesion, and this tumor was characterized by a predominance of epidermoid cellular elements (66). The postoperative survival rate approaches 100%.

Adenoid cystic carcinoma (cylindroma) is the least common form of bronchial adenoma in childhood. The important distinction for this tumor is the observation that it is an indolent malignancy with a propensity for submucosal spread and late recurrence. Intraoperative frozen-section evaluation of the surgical margin of the bronchus is therefore appropriate when resecting a bronchial adenoma. These lesions are otherwise clinically indistinguishable from other forms of bronchial adenomas.

Bronchogenic Carcinoma

Primary bronchogenic carcinoma is rare in children; somewhat more than 50 cases have been reported in the world's literature. Only 10% of these were squamous cell carcinomas, and the remainder were adenocarcinomas or undifferentiated carcinomas. Although rare, persistent case reports suggest an important etiologic association with preexisting cystic bronchopulmonary-foregut abnormalities.

The unfortunate experience with this lesion is that patients often have hemoptysis, cough, dyspnea, chest pain, anemia, weight loss, or bone pain when diagnosed, and most have nonresectable or disseminated disease. The average survival in this circumstance is 7 months (66). For children with localized disease who undergo complete resection, a small Japanese experience suggests that about one-half have long-term survival (68).

Pulmonary Blastoma

Pulmonary blastoma is a rare tumor that is seen in both adults and children. About 25% of the patients are younger than 16 years of age at presentation, and 60% of these are younger than 4 years of age (66). The distinctive pathologic feature of pulmonary blastoma is that it is composed of cells that resemble fetal lung and that have metastatic potential. Most patients present with symptoms of cough, chest pain, hemoptysis, or frank hemorrhage, and the lesion is identified on plain chest radiograph. These are generally peripheral lesions, and lobar resection is the most common surgical procedure. Forty to 50% of patients have long-term survival with this approach. The roles of chemotherapy and irradiation have not been prospectively evaluated.

Other Malignant Neoplasms

The inventory of other rare primary lung malignancies are summarized in Table 61-2. Neurofibrosarcoma, fibrosarcoma, mesothelioma, and other lung malignancies have also been reported. The general clinical approach to these was detailed earlier. Radiographic imaging is best obtained for all primary lung neoplasms with either CT or MR imaging. The operative goal is to resect all gross disease and to conserve as much normal lung parenchyma as possible. The limited experience for each lesion precludes meaningful statistical analysis of adjuvant therapy, and treatment is generally individualized.

Benign Lung Tumors

Inflammatory Pseudotumor

Inflammatory pseudotumor is a rare lesion that presents as a solitary lung nodule in children. As the term suggests, it is not malignant, nor is it truly neoplastic. The histopathology typically shows a variety of inflammatory cells, including lymphocytes and fat-laden macrophages, as well as other lung parenchymal cell types. Descriptive pathologic names are abundant in the literature and reflect the fact that there is considerable variety in the appearance of the participant inflammatory cells (69). Among these names are *plasma cell granuloma, histiocytoma, xanthofibroma,* and *lung adenoma.* The pathogenesis of this unique local inflammatory process is unknown.

Inflammatory pseudotumor is the most common benign lung mass in infants and children. Seventy-five percent of the children are older than 5 years of age, 30% do not have symptoms when discovered, and 20% have a history of previous pulmonary infection (66). Other presentations include cough, fever, chest pain, hemoptysis, and airway obstruction. Pneumonia is diagnosed in about 10% of these children. Large inflammatory pseudotumors have resulted in esophageal obstruction and death from extrinsic compression of mediastinal structures.

The imaging approach is not different than for other mass lesions in the thorax. Plain chest radiographs are followed by either CT or MR imaging. The lesions appear as solid parenchymal nodules or larger masses that may be indistinguishable from neoplasms. Calcification can be dramatic (Fig. 61-19). The natural history of the process is generally one of either slow growth or spontaneous resolution. Metastatic spread has not been observed. If the diagnosis is clear, urgent surgical resection is not required because the lesion may resolve. In reality, the lesion is often indistinguishable from a primary malignancy with both preoperative imaging and intraoperative biopsy. Hence, surgical resection is often done for diagnosis, and this is appropriate. Formal lobectomy or local resection is required, depending on the level of diagnostic uncertainty and the anatomic relations involved.

Hamartomas

Hamartomatous lung nodules are seen commonly in adults, but are rarely discovered in children. They are considered congenital in origin, presumably because most are asymptomatic and therefore escape childhood detection.

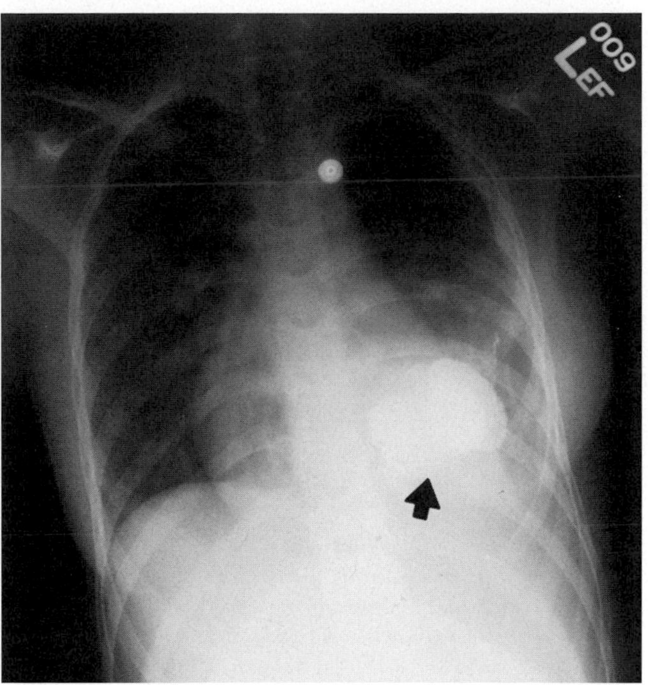

FIGURE 61-19. Radiograph illustrating a calcified pulmonary parenchymal lesion, which proved to be an inflammatory pseudotumor (*arrow*). This degree of calcification is unusual. The predominant histologic cell type involved was a plasma cell. (Courtesy of Don Frush, MD, Duke University Medical Center, Durham, NC.)

They may occur in either endobronchial or parenchymal lung sites and are characterized by the presence of cartilage, respiratory epithelium, and collagen (70). Endobronchial lesions cause clinical symptoms at a relatively small size. Lung parenchymal lesions in children may be large, however, and can produce symptoms of respiratory distress or mediastinal compression. Death in the neonatal period has been reported. Older children fare well after local resection. Most adults have small asymptomatic peripheral lesions readily excised by open or thoracoscopic wedge resection.

Other Benign Tumors

A number of primary benign lung tumors have been reported in children. Table 61-2 summarizes a number of these. The clinical approach detailed earlier is also applicable in these tumors because prospective differentiation between benign and malignant lesions is often not possible. When feasible, limited local resection of these tumors is performed. This is usually to establish the diagnosis because many of these patients do not have symptoms.

Mucous gland adenomas require particular mention. These benign endobronchial tumors are often included in the group of potentially malignant bronchial adenomas because their clinical presentation is virtually indistinguishable. These are truly benign entities, however, without known metastatic potential (66). This is important largely for prognostic purposes because their removal generally requires lobar resection, as detailed earlier in the discussion of endobronchial carcinoid tumors.

Metastatic Lung Tumors

The approach to children with metastatic lung tumors is considerably different than for adults with similar lesions because it is clear that patient survival is much more likely in the younger population. The most common causes of metastatic lung tumors in children are Wilms' tumor and osteogenic sarcoma (71). The approach to the child with metastatic (demonstrable in chest radiograph) Wilms' tumor in the lung involves standard initial surgical management, including radical nephrectomy and regional lymphadenectomy. In addition, the treatment includes systemic chemotherapy and bilateral lung irradiation. Surgical resection of lung metastatic lesions is generally performed for persistent or new metastases after the initial course of treatment is complete. About one-half of the children with pulmonary metastases from Wilms' tumor can be saved with this approach (71,72).

Adjuvant chemotherapy has reduced the incidence of metastatic lung lesions in patients with osteogenic sarcoma from about 80% to 30% during the past 10 to 15 years (71) (Fig. 61-20). National protocols in the United States include an aggressive surgical approach to pulmonary metastases after adequate chemotherapy and after appropriate resection of the primary tumor. With a combination of chemotherapy and sometimes multiple or bilateral pulmonary resections, about 40% of patients with metastatic lung disease from osteogenic sarcoma can be saved (71,73). The surgical principles are to perform limited wedge resections and conserve normal parenchyma because the lesions tend to be small, subpleural nodules, and may be numerous. It is common that operative exploration and bimanual palpation reveal lesions not discernible on preoperative imaging studies. This is a compelling argument for open thoracotomy rather than thoracoscopy in these particular patients, because with the closed approach, the surgeon surrenders the tactile input that is so important for detection of small metastases.

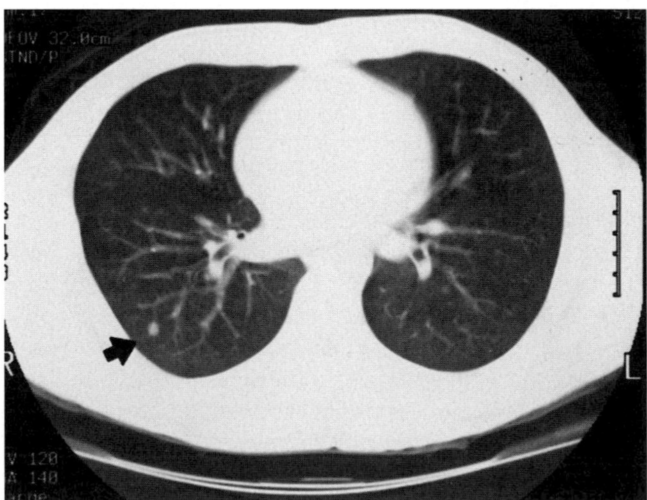

FIGURE 61-20. Computed tomography scan of the chest showing an obvious metastatic lung nodule in an adolescent with primary osteogenic sarcoma (*arrow*).

A host of other metastatic lung tumors have been treated surgically in children. The general principles are that the lesions must be stable, the primary disease controlled, the metastatic disease isolated to the lungs, and an aggressive effort endorsed by all participants. Generally, these patients first require adjuvant chemotherapy and receive irradiation for radiosensitive tumors. The surgical approach is to limit parenchymal resection to the metastatic sites and the immediately adjacent parenchyma, although lobectomy has been advocated to diminish the risk of recurrence and to resect larger metastatic deposits. These patients require individualized care, and the experience is too limited for meaningful statistical analysis.

PULMONARY RESECTION IN CHILDREN

Techniques

A detailed description of the technical aspects of lung resection and pulmonary surgery is beyond the scope of this text. Several noteworthy thoracic surgical atlases are available (55,56). There are few anatomic or technical differences between children and adults other than those related to overall size. Although technical precision is required for pulmonary surgery regardless of age or size, small infants in particular have little margin for error. One of the common lung resections, left lower lobectomy, is illustrated in Fig. 61-21. The principles of complete hilar dissection, meticulous vascular control, and bronchial stump closure are illustrated and apply to all lobar or whole lung resections. Bronchial stump closure is easily and reliably done in adults and older children with commercial surgical stapling devices. In infants and small children, this is undesirable because the size of the instrument may make its application insufficiently precise. When working with small airways, the difference between an acceptable and compromised residual bronchus can be exceedingly small. In addition, some staples may be too large for the secure closure of an infant bronchus. For these reasons, a carefully handsewn bronchial closure is preferable in infants and small children.

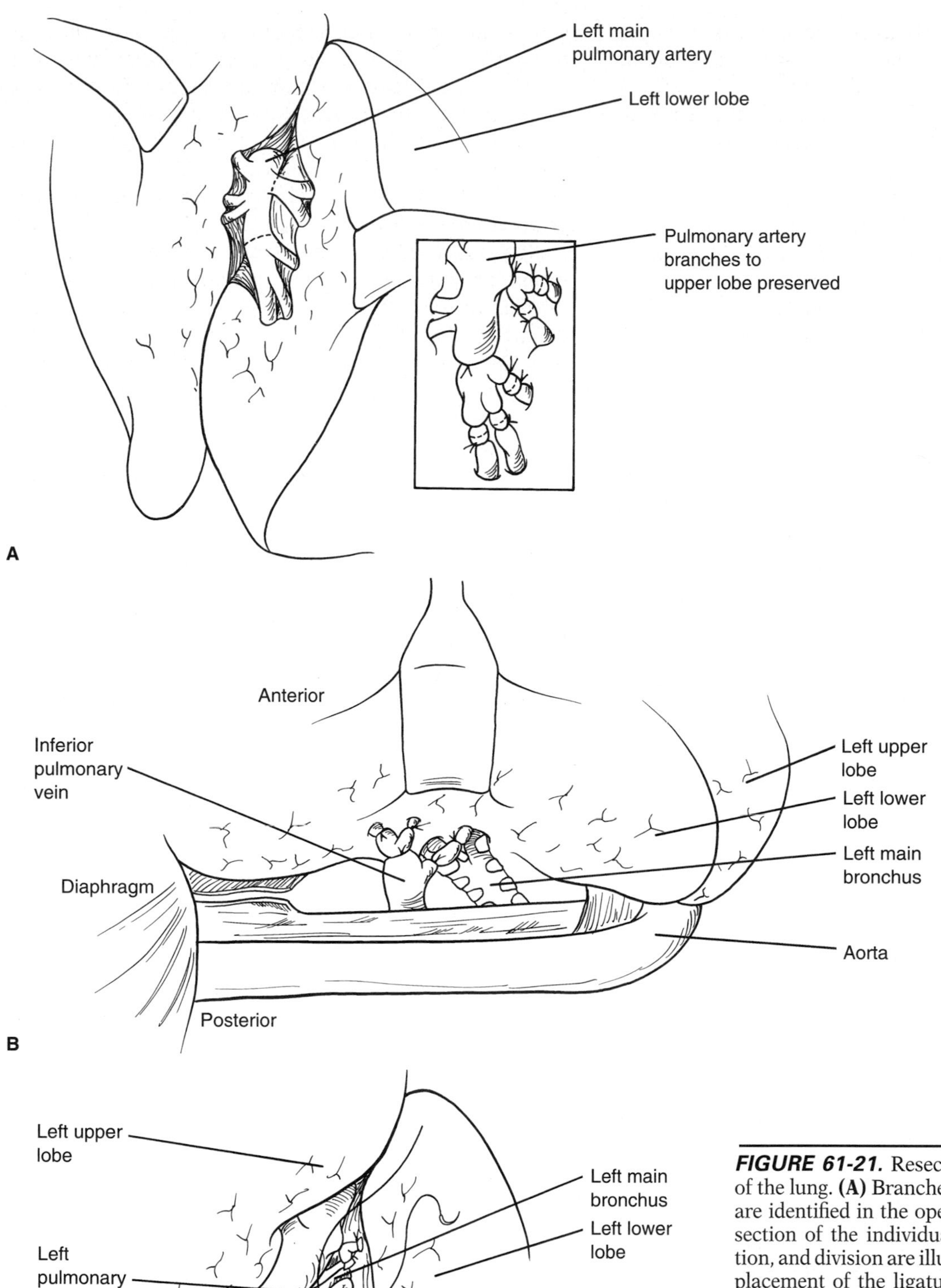

FIGURE 61-21. Resection of the left lower lobe of the lung. **(A)** Branches of the pulmonary artery are identified in the open fissure. Meticulous dissection of the individual arterial branches, ligation, and division are illustrated. (*Inset*) Peripheral placement of the ligatures is particularly important in small infants to avoid compromise of the arterial supply to the remaining upper lobe. Appropriate sites for arterial division are indicated. **(B)** The inferior pulmonary vein is controlled, ligated, and divided after the inferior pulmonary ligament is opened. **(C)** The left lower lobe bronchus is controlled and divided. Bronchial stump closure is best done with a handsewn closure in infants and small children. (Adapted from Nohl-Oser HC, Nissen R, Schreibe HN. *Surgery of the lung*. New York: Theime-Stratton, 1981.)

Wedge resections of peripheral lung lesions are common in pediatric thoracic surgery, and this is generally straightforward from a technical standpoint. Stapling devices can be used on lung parenchyma, even in small infants. These are more efficient and possibly more reliable than handsewn lung closures. Segmental lung resections are also sometimes appropriate, although a review of the literature suggests that the perioperative morbidity secondary to air leak and hemorrhage may be greater than for formal lobectomy (6). When appropriate, these more limited resections are individualized to follow the segmental anatomy of the lung. The principles of proximal and distal vascular control and bronchial closure are not different than for formal lobectomy.

Thoracoscopy in children has developed rapidly with the introduction of new instruments and particularly video camera systems. Its applications are expanding rapidly, and with prudent use, the technique offers the possibility of equivalent outcomes for a variety of selected intrathoracic procedures without the morbidity of a thoracotomy incision. It therefore has considerable appeal.

Outcomes After Lung Resection

In the absence of diffuse lung disease or pulmonary hypoplasia, pulmonary resection up to and including unilateral pneumonectomy is well tolerated by infants and children (13,14,74). Preservation of normal lung tissue is a fundamental surgical principle in pediatric thoracic surgery, although the surgeon must balance the need to definitively treat the underlying pathology. The age at which lung resection occurs is also relevant to outcome (13,14). It appears that adults have fixed lung volumes and pulmonary capacities, with little functional compensation after pulmonary resection. As detailed earlier, normal infants and children continue to undergo lung growth and alveolar development through much of the first decade of life. Their compensatory potential is inversely related to age during this time.

Although nonanatomic peripheral lung resections are common for diagnostic efforts, lobectomy is the most common resectional surgical procedure for primary lung pathology. McBride and colleagues performed a clinical follow-up and spirometry on 15 patients between 8 and 32 years of age who had undergone pulmonary resection for congenital lobar emphysema in early childhood (13). The volume of lung parenchymal tissue lost was estimated to be 8% to 45%. At follow-up, 11 of these children were without respiratory symptoms of any kind, 2 had reactive airway disease, and 2 had mild dyspnea on exertion. Height, weight, and chest radiographs were all within normal range. Lung volumes (total lung capacity and vital capacity) were within the range considered normal, although the mean value for each was slightly lower than expected (93% and 94%, respectively). The volume compensation was believed to be the result of unilateral increase in the volume of remaining lung on the ipsilateral side. Pulmonary artery blood flow after lobectomy was equal and normally distributed, suggesting compensatory growth of the vascular bed as well. At the cellular level, others have shown compensatory increases in the DNA, protein, collagen content, and weight of residual lung parenchyma after pulmonary resection (75).

McBride and colleagues (13) showed decreased expiratory flow rates and airway conductance after childhood lobectomy. This is consistent with a degree of persistent airway obstruction. Together, these findings suggest mild disproportion between the compensatory growth of airways and that of the alveoli. This is consistent with the observation that structural and functional maturation of the conducting airways occurs before similar maturation of the terminal airways and alveoli. Despite these findings, children generally have good or excellent functional results after lobectomy (14,74).

Childhood pneumonectomy is followed by contralateral lung overinflation and age-dependent compensatory growth, as outlined earlier. The affected hemithorax is occupied by a shift of the mediastinum, elevation of the hemidiaphragm, and serous fluid accumulation, which eventually evolves into a fibrothorax. The mediastinal shift in a newborn or infant may be dramatic, whether it occurs rapidly or over a period of time. Diminished venous return to the heart and compression of the trachea or residual mainstem bronchus by the aorta can be life threatening. This postpneumonectomy syndrome has been treated with a variety of tracheal and vascular reconstructive and suspension procedures and by the placement of an intrathoracic balloon prosthesis. This risk appears to diminish with age.

Spirometry shows predictable decrease of lung volumes after pneumonectomy, as well as higher than normal pulmonary arterial pressures, particularly with exercise. Significantly, however, even with this degree of parenchymal resection, functional outcomes are good or excellent in most children (76). Little or no restriction in lifestyle is to be expected in children who undergo major pulmonary resection in the absence of other lung disease. However, scoliosis and chest wall deformities are relatively frequent late complications after thoracic surgery in infants and young children.

REFERENCES

1. Gray SW, Skandalakis JE. The trachea and lungs. In: *Embryology for surgeons: the embryological basis for the treatment of congenital defects*. Philadelphia: WB Saunders, 1972:293.
2. DiFiore JW, Wilson JM. Lung development. *Semin Pediatr Surg* 1994; 3:221.
3. Thurlbeck WM. Postnatal growth and development of the lung. *Am Rev Respir Dis* 1975;111:803.
4. Davies GM, Reid L. Growth of the alveoli and pulmonary arteries in childhood. *Thorax* 1970;25:669.

5. Haller JA Jr, Golladay ES, Pickard LR, et al. Surgical management of lung bud anomalies: lobar emphysema, bronchogenic cyst, cystic adenomatoid malformation, and intralobar pulmonary sequestration. *Ann Thorac Surg* 1979;28:33.
6. Ryckman FC, Rosenkrantz JG. Thoracic surgical problems in infancy and childhood. *Surg Clin North Am* 1985;65:1423.
7. DeLorimer AA. Congenital malformations and neonatal problems of the respiratory tract. In: Welch KJ, Randolph JG, Ravitch MM, et al., eds. *Pediatric surgery*, 4th ed. Chicago: Year Book Medical 1986: 631.
8. Murray GF. Congenital lobar emphysema. *Surg Gynecol Obstet* 1967;124:611.
9. Buntain WL, Isaacs H Jr, Payne VC Jr, et al. Lobar emphysema, cystic adenomatoid malformation, pulmonary sequestration, and bronchogenic cyst in infancy and childhood: a clinical group. *J Pediatr Surg* 1974;9:85.
10. Wesley JR, Heidelberger KP, DiPietro MA, et al. Diagnosis and management of congenital cystic disease of the lung in children. *J Pediatr Surg* 1986;21:202.
11. Jones JC, Almond CH, Snyder HM, et al. Lobar emphysema and congenital heart disease in infancy. *J Thorac Cardiovasc Surg* 1965;49:1.
12. Markowitz RI, Mercurio MR, Vahjen GA, et al. Congenital lobar emphysema. *Clin Pediatr* 1989;28:19.
13. McBride JT, Wohl MEB, Strieder DL, et al. Lung growth and airway function after lobectomy in infancy for congenital lobar emphysema. *J Clin Invest* 1980;66:962.
14. Frenckner B, Freyschuss U. Pulmonary function after lobectomy for congenital lobar emphysema and congenital cystic adenomatoid malformation: a follow-up study. *Scand J Thorac Cardiovasc Surg* 1982;16:293.
15. Stocker JT, Madewell JE, Drake RM. Congenital cystic adenomatoid malformation of the lung. *Hum Pathol* 1977;8:155.
16. Adzick NS, Harrison MR, Glick PL, et al. Fetal cystic adenomatoid malformation: prenatal diagnosis and natural history. *J Pediatr Surg* 1985;20:483.
17. Cromblcholme TM, Coleman B, Hedrick H, et al. Cystic adenomatoid malformation volume ratio predicts outcome in prenatally diagnosed cystic adenomatoid malformation of the lung. *J Pediatr Surg* 2002;37:331.
18. Adzick NS, Harrison MR, Flake AW, et al. Fetal surgery for cystic adenomatoid malformation of the lung. *J Pediatr Surg* 1993;28:806.
19. Adzick NS, Harrison MR, Crombleholme TM, et al. Fetal lung lesions: management and outcome. *Am J Obstet Gynecol* 1998;179:884–889.
20. Budorick NE, Pretorius DH, Leopold GR, et al. Spontaneous improvement of intrathoracic masses diagnosed in utero. *J Ultrasound Med* 1992;11:653.
21. Revillon Y, Jan D, Plattner V, et al. Congenital cystic adenomatoid malformation of the lung: prenatal management and prognosis. *J Pediatr Surg* 1993;28:1009.
22. Hancock BJ, Di Lorenzo M, Youssef S, et al. Childhood primary pulmonary neoplasms. *J Pediatr Surg* 1993;28:1133.
23. Ozcan C, Celik A, Ural Z, et al. Primary pulmonary rhabdomyosarcoma arising within cystic adenomatoid malformation: a case report and review of the literature. *J Pediatr Surg* 2001;36:1062.
24. Granata C, Gambini C, Balducci T, et al. Bronchioloalveolar carcinoma arising in congenital cystic adenomatoid malformation in a child: a case report and review on malignancies originating in congenital cystic adenomatoid malformation. *Pediatr Pulmonol* 1998; 25:62.
25. Domizio P, Liesner RJ, Dicks-Mireaux C, et al. Malignant mesenchymoma associated with a congenital lung cyst in a child: case report and review of the literature. *Pediatr Pathol* 1990;10:785.
26. Landing BH. Congenital malformations and genetic disorders of the respiratory tract (larynx, trachea, bronchi and lungs). *Am Rev Respir Dis* 1979;120:151.
27. Dolkart LA, Reimers FT, Helmuth WV, et al. Antenatal diagnosis of pulmonary sequestration: a review. *Obstet Gynecol Surv* 1992; 47:515.
28. Buntain WL, Woolley MM, Mahour GH, et al. Pulmonary sequestration in children: a 25-year experience. *Surgery* 1977;81:413.
29. Smith RA. Some controversial aspects of intralobar sequestration of the lung. *Surg Gynecol Obstet* 1962;114:57.
30. Samji FM, Sachs HJ, Perkins DG. Cystic disease of the lungs. *Surg Clin North Am* 1988;68:581.
31. Stein SM, Cox JL, Hernanz-Schulman M, et al. Pediatric chest disease: evaluation by computerized tomography, magnetic resonance imaging, and ultrasonography. *South Med J* 1992;85: 735.
32. Ashizawa K, Okimoto T, Shirafuji T, et al. Anterior mediastinal bronchogenic cyst: demonstration of complicating malignancy by CT and MRI. *Br J Radiol* 2001;74:959.
33. Osborne J, Masel J, McCredie J. A spectrum of skeletal anomalies associated with pulmonary agenesis: possible neural crest injuries. *Pediatr Radiol* 1989;19:425.
34. Hoffman MA, Superina R, Wesson DE. Unilateral pulmonary agenesis with esophageal atresia and distal tracheoesophageal fistula: report of two cases. *J Pediatr Surg* 1989;10:1084.
35. Turnage RH, Guice KS, Oldham KT. Pulmonary microvascular injury following intestinal reperfusion. *New Horizons* 1994;2:463.
36. Cowles RA, Lelli JL Jr, Takayasu J, et al. Lung resection in infants and children with pulmonary infections refractory to medical therapy. *J Pediatr Surg* 2002;37:643.
37. Kosloske A. Infections of the lungs, pleura, and mediastinum. In: Welch KJ, Randolph JG, Ravitch MM, et al., eds. *Pediatric surgery*, 4th ed. Chicago: Year Book Medical 1986:657.
38. Alexander JC, Wolfe WG. Lung abscess and empyema of the thorax. *Surg Clin North Am* 1980;60:835.
39. Riordan J, Rommens JM, Kerem BS, et al. Identification of the cystic fibrosis gene: cloning and characterization of complementary DNA. *Science* 1989;245:1066.
40. Widdicombe JH, Wine JJ. The basic defect in cystic fibrosis. *Trends Biochem Sci* 1991;16:474.
41. Orenstein DM, Winnie GB, Altman H. Cystic fibrosis: a 2002 update. *J Pediatr* 2002;140:156.
42. Rosenstein BJ, Zeitlin PL. Recent advances in cystic fibrosis. *Curr Opin Pediatr* 1991;3:392.
43. Sanderson JM, Kennedy MCS, Johnson MF, et al. Bronchiectasis. Results of surgical and conservative management: a review of 393 cases. *Thorax* 1974;29:407.
44. Herman M, Michalkova K, Kopriva F. High-resolution CT in the assessment of bronchiectasis in children. *Pediatr Radiol* 1993;23: 376.
45. Schuster SR, Schwartz MZ. Surgical management of the pulmonary complications of cystic fibrosis. In: Ravitch MM, Welch KJ, Benson CD, et al., eds. *Pediatric surgery*, 3rd ed. Chicago: Year Book, 1979.
46. Marmon L, Schidlow D, Palmer J, et al. Pulmonary resection for complications of cystic fibrosis. *J Pediatr Surg* 1983;18:811.
47. Flume PA. Pneumothorax in cystic fibrosis. *Chest* 2003;123:217.
48. Luck SR, Raffensperger JG, Sullivan HJ, et al. Management of pneumothorax in children with chronic pulmonary disease. *J Thorac Cardiovasc Surg* 1977;74:834.
49. Rothman BF, Stone RT, Walker LH, et al. Bronchoscopic lavage for cystic fibrosis patients: an adjunct to therapy. *Ann Otol Rhinol Laryngol* 1982;91:641.
50. Barr ML, Baker CJ, Schenkel FA, et al. Living donor lung transplantation: selection, technique, and outcome. *Transplant Proc* 2001; 33:3527.
51. Yankaskas JR, Mallory GB Jr, the Consensus Committee. Lung transplantation in cystic fibrosis (Consensus Conference Statement). *Chest* 1998;113:217.
52. St. Louis International Lung Transplant Registry. *September 1994 report*. Barnes Hospital, Washington University, St, Louis Mo.
53. Miller WS. A study of the human pleura pulmonalis: its relation to the blebs and bullae of emphysema. *AJR* 1926;15:399.
54. Fitzgerald MX, Keelan PJ, Cugell DW, et al. Long-term results of surgery for bullous emphysema. *J Thorac Cardiovasc Surg* 1974;68:566.
55. Nohl-Oser HC, Nissen R, Schreiber HW. *Surgery of the lung*. New York: Theime-Stratton, 1981.
56. Ravitch MM, Steichen FM. *Atlas of general thoracic surgery*. Philadelphia: WB Saunders, 1988.
57. Nathanson LK, Shimi SM, Wood RA, et al. Videothoracoscopic ligation of bulla and pleurectomy for spontaneous pneumothorax. *Ann Thorac Surg* 1991;52:316.

58. Eliasson R, Mossberg B, Camner P, et al. The immotile-cilia syndrome. *N Engl J Med* 1977;297:1.
59. Wilson JF, Decker AM. The surgical management of bronchiectasis. *Ann Surg* 1982;195:354.
60. Lucy MR. Hepatic infection. In: Greenfield LJ, Mulholland MW, Oldham KT, et al., eds. *Surgery: scientific principles and practice*. Philadelphia: JB Lippincott, 1993:867.
61. Topcu S, Kurul IC, Tastepe I, et al. Surgical treatment of pulmonary hydatid cysts in children. *J Thorac Cardiovasc Surg* 2000;120:1097.
62. Snyder CL, Ramsay NK, McGlave PB, et al. Diagnostic open-lung biopsy after bone marrow transplantation. *J Pediatr Surg* 1990;25:871.
63. Bonfils-Roberts EA, Nickodem A, Nealon TF Jr. Retrospective analysis of the efficacy of open lung biopsy in acquired immunodeficiency syndrome. *Ann Thorac Surg* 1990;49:115.
64. Dunn DL. Infection. In: Greenfield LJ, Mulholland MW, Oldham KT, et al., eds. *Surgery: scientific principles and practice,* 2nd ed. Philadelphia: JB Lippincott, 1996.
65. Menzies D, Fanning A, Yuan L, et al. Current concepts: tuberculosis among health care workers. *N Engl J Med* 1995;332:92.
66. Hartman GE, Shochat SJ. Primary pulmonary neoplasms of childhood: a review. *Ann Thorac Surg* 1983;36:108.
67. Lack EE, Harris GB, Eraklis AJ, et al. Primary bronchial tumors in childhood. *Cancer* 1983;51:492.
68. Niitu Y, Kubota H, Hasegawa S, et al. Lung cancer (squamous cell carcinoma) in adolescence. *Am J Dis Child* 1974;127:108.
69. Cohen MC, Kaschula RO. Primary pulmonary tumors in childhood: a review of 31 years' experience and the literature. *Pediatr Pulmonol* 1992;14:222.
70. Fudge TL, Ochsner JL, Mills NL. Clinical spectrum of pulmonary hamartomas. *Ann Thorac Surg* 1980;30:36.
71. Filler RM. Tumors of the lung. In: Welch KJ, Randolph JG, Ravitch MM, et al., eds. *Pediatric surgery,* 4th ed. Chicago: Year Book Medical 1986:673.
72. Simone JV, Cassady JR, Filler RM. Cancers of childhood. In: DeVita VT Jr, Hellman S, Rosenberg SA, eds. *Cancer: principles and practice of oncology*. Philadelphia: JB Lippincott, 1982:1254.
73. Schaller RT Jr, Haas J, Schaller J, et al. Improved survival in children with osteosarcoma following resection of pulmonary metastases. *J Pediatr Surg* 1975;10:545.
74. Giammona ST, Mandelbaum I, Battersby JS, et al. The late cardiopulmonary effects of childhood pneumonectomy. *Pediatrics* 1966; 37:79.
75. Cowan MJ, Crystal RG. Lung growth after unilateral pneumonectomy: quantitation of collagen synthesis and content. *Am Rev Respir Dis* 1975;3:267.
76. Szots I, Toth T. Long-term results of the surgical treatment for pulmonary malformations and disorders. *Prog Pediatr Surg* 1977;10:277.

Chapter 62

Congenital Heart Disease

Stuart Berger and James S. Tweddell

Five to 8 out of 1,000 live born infants are diagnosed with a congenital cardiovascular defect (1–3) making congenital heart disease the most common birth defect. Cardiovascular abnormalities continue to be the leading cause of premature mortality from congenital abnormalities. The spectrum of cardiovascular involvement is quite variable and may include defects with minimal physiologic impact, such as a small ventricular septal defect, or more complex lesions, such as tetralogy of Fallot, which requires surgical intervention with a lifelong risk of sequelae.

Using data from the Pediatric Health Information System, an administrative database maintained by 32 major pediatric hospitals in the United States, the mean hospital charge for a patient undergoing surgical intervention for congenital heart disease is $88,042 per patient from 1997 to 2000 (4). The American Heart Association estimates that 40,000 children are born with congenital heart disease each year (5). In addition, there are 1,000,000 Americans with congenital heart disease alive today. If we assume that 25% of patients with congenital heart disease require hospital intervention for their congenital heart defect during the first year of life, and that 5% of the remaining patients with congenital heart disease older than 1 year will require a procedure each year, then the hospital charges for the diagnosis of congenital heart disease will be more than $5 billion per year. It should be noted that this figure underestimates the economic impact of congenital heart disease because it does not take into account all physician charges, outpatient medication costs, home health care costs, or days of school and work lost by patients and family members. It is clear that the cost and impact of congenital heart disease for the individual, the family, and society is large.

Stuart Berger and James S. Tweddell: Medical College of Wisconsin, Children's Hospital of Wisconsin, Milwaukee, Wisconsin 53226.

ETIOLOGY OF CONGENITAL HEART DISEASE

As much as 6% of congenital heart disease is associated with genetic factors, whereas 2% are known to be related to environmental causes. Well-known examples of environmental causes of congenital heart disease include rubella virus, which is associated with patent ductus arteriosus and branch pulmonary artery stenosis, and thalidomide, which is associated with tetralogy of Fallot and atrial septal defects. Additional environmental causes of congenital heart disease were identified by the Baltimore-Washington Infant Study (BWIS), a regional epidemiologic study of congenital heart disease (3,6,7). The BWIS took on the difficult task of identifying congenital heart disease among live births in a contiguous region of Maryland and northern Virginia from 1981 to 1986. Epidemiologic techniques were used to link congenital heart defects with environmental and genetic factors. Environmental factors apparently associated with congenital heart disease included paternal exposure to cold temperature and maternal exposure to solvents and hair dyes. In addition, the risks were increased with maternal exposure to diazepam, corticosteroids, phenothiazine, and gastrointestinal drugs. Paternal exposure to cocaine was also implicated. Other associations included an apparent link between maternal diabetes and tetralogy of Fallot, truncus arteriosus, and double-outlet right ventricle. Table 62-1 lists the reported associations of environmental influences and congenital heart disease.

Heritable syndromes, chromosomal abnormalities, and increasingly, specific gene defects have been linked to congenital cardiac abnormalities (8). Table 62-2 lists the syndromes and associated congenital cardiac defects, along with specific gene associations and/or chromosomal abnormalities where they are known. Mutation of the gene FBN1 that codes for fibrillin, a component of the aortic wall, results in Marfan syndrome (9). This disorder demonstrates autosomal dominant expression, and all

TABLE 62-1 Associations of Environmental Influences and Congenital Heart Disease.

Environmental Exposure	*Specific Form of Congenital Heart Disease*
Paternal exposure to cold	Nonspecific
Maternal exposure to solvents and hair dyes	Nonspecific
Maternal exposure to lithium	Ebstein's anomaly, tricuspid atresia, ASD
Maternal exposure to valproate	Coarctation, HLHS, asortic stenosis, interrupted aortic arch, ASD, pulmonary atresia with IVS, VSD
Maternal exposure to corticosteroids	Nonspecific
Maternal exposure to phenothiazine	Nonspecific
Maternal exposure to phenylketonuria (PKU) (especially if uncontrolled)	Tetralogy of Fallot
Maternal insulin-dependent diabetes (especially if uncontrolled)	VSD, TGA, tetralogy of Fallot, coarctation of the aorta
Maternal lupus	Congenital complete heart block
Maternal alcohol use	VSD, ASD
Maternal exposure to retinoic acid	Conotruncal defects
Maternal exposure to rubella	PDA, peripheral pulmonary artery stenosis, septal defects
Maternal exposure to hydantoin	Pulmonary stenosis, aortic stenosis, coarctation of the aorta, PDA
Maternal exposure to trimethadione	Tetralogy of Fallot, TGA, HLHS
Maternal exposure to thalidomide	Tetralogy of Fallot, septal defects, truncus arteriosus
Maternal HIV	Myocarditis
Maternal toxoplasmosis infection	Myocarditis
Maternal exposure to trichloethylene, trichloroethane, or dichloroethylene	Nonspecific
Environment of jewelry making, lead soldering, ionizing radiation, or paint stripping	Nonspecific

ASD, atrial septal defect; HLHS, hypoplastic left heart syndrome; IVS, intact ventricular septum; VSD, ventricular septal defect; TGA, transposition of the great arteries; PDA, patent ductus arteriosus.

heterozygotes express the trait to some degree. In addition to Marfan syndrome, trisomy 18 is associated with congenital heart disease in 100% of cases (10). In trisomy 18, however, the specific form of congenital heart disease is variable. Although ventricular septal defects predominate, other forms of congenital heart disease can occur. In other well-defined genetic syndromes, the association with congenital heart disease is less constant. For example, only 50% of children with Down syndrome (trisomy 21) have a congenital cardiac abnormality. The variable expression of congenital heart disease with a definite chromosomal abnormality is also demonstrated among patients with 22q11 deletion, where about one-half the affected individuals will have a conotruncal defect, an abnormality of the outflow of the heart and great vessels (11). Examples of specific gene mutations resulting in congenital heart disease include the gene NKX2-5, on chromosome 5, that results in atrial septal defects and conduction abnormalities (12). Holt-Oram syndrome, characterized by limb abnormalities and defects of the atrial septum, is caused by a mutation in the TBX5 gene located on chromosome 12 (13). The association of limb malformations and cardiac defects, "heart-hand syndromes," with a single gene defect suggests that the same gene may be responsible for several developmental processes. The more recent identification of several ion channel gene defects (HERG, SCN5A, KVLQT1, and MinK) associated with long QT syndrome have confirmed the genetic basis of this group of arrhythmias, which are known to be familial (14). The identification of genes fundamental for development of left–right asymmetry in animal models, such as nodal and Lefty2, defects of which are associated with cardiac abnormalities similar to heterotaxy syndromes in humans, suggests the role of homologous genes in congenital heart disease in humans (15). Genes responsible for cardiac development are being increasingly identified and mapped. Corresponding mutations that result in heart defects are being identified. Researchers will undoubtedly begin to identify additional gene mutations that result in isolated congenital heart defects. Although presently the cause of 85% of congenital heart disease is unknown, it is likely due to a combination

TABLE 62-2 Syndromes and Associated Congenital Cardiac Defects Along with Specific Gene: Associations and Chromosome Locations.

Syndrome	*Associated Congenital Heart Defects*	*Associated Gene Defect*	*Chromosome Location*	*Biochemical Screening*
Allagille syndrome	Branch pulmonary stenosis, pulmonary valve stenosis, PAPVC, TOF			
Barth syndrome	DCM, noncompaction of left ventricular			
Cardio-facio-cutaneous syndrome	ASD, PS			
Cat-eye syndrome	TAPVC, HLHS	Not identified	Isodicentric 22	
CHARGE (acronym)	Wide variety			
Down syndrome (trisomy 21)	AVSD, VSD, ASD, aberrant subclavian artery, ECD			
Duchenne muscular dystrophy	DCM, MVP, conduction abnormalities			Yes
Edwards syndrome (trisomy 18)	Various, VSD, PDA, BAV, bicuspid pulmonary valve			
Ehlers-Danlos syndrome	Arterial rupture, MVP, ASD			Yes
Ellis-Van-Creveld syndrome	ASD, single atrium	Not identified	4p13 (ASD)	
Familial dilated cardiomyopathy	Progressive cardiac dilation and dysfunction			
Friederichs ataxia	DCM, conduction abnormalities			
Goldenhars syndrome	TOF, ASD, VSD			
Hypertrophic cardiomyopathy	Cardiac hypertrophy, syncope, SCD			
Heterotaxy syndrome (multiple types)	Complex malformations			
Holt-Oram syndrome	ASD, VSD, conduction defects	TBX5 (ASD)	12q24.1	
Homocystinuria	Vascular thrombosis, aortic dilatation			Yes
Hurler syndrome	DCM, valve stenoses, valve insufficiency			
Jacobsen syndrome	ASD, VSD	a. BARX2 b. Not identified	a. 11q25 b. 11q23.3–24	
Jervell-Lange-Nielsen syndrome	Long QT syndrome, syncope, SCD			
LEOPARD syndrome (acronym)	PS, prolonged PR interval, DCM			
Marfan syndrome	Aortic dilatation, AI, MVP, aortic aneurysm	Defect(s) in the fibrillin gene(s) (FBN1)		
Myotonic dystrophy	Conduction defects, DCM, MVP			
Noonan syndrome	PVS, HOCM, ASD			
Osteogenesis imperfecta (multiple types)	MVP, aortic regurgitation, aortic dilatation			
Patau syndrome (trisomy 18)	Various (80%), VSD, ASD, PDA			
Pompe's disease (acid maltase deficiency)	Glycogen storage disease of the heart			Yes
Rubinstein-Taybi syndrome	HLHS	CBP	16p13.3	
Treacher Collins syndrome	VSD, PDA, ASD			
Tuberous sclerosis	Cardiac tumors, rhabdomyoma			
Turner syndrome	CoA, BAV, AS, HLHS, ASD, VSD			
VACTERL syndrome (acronym)	Wide variety			
VCFS (acronym); also known as 22q11, DiGeorge, or Shprintzen syndrome	Conotruncal abnormalities: IAA, truncus, TOF, right aortic arch, aberrant subclavian artery, VSD			
Williams syndrome	SVAS, supravalvar PS, AS, PS	Defect(s) in the elastin gene(s)?	7q11.23?	

PAPVC, partial anomalous pulmonary venous connection; TOF, tetralogy of Fallot; DCM, dilated cardiomyopathy; ASD, atrial septal defect; TAPVC, total anomalous pulmonary venous connection; HLHS, hypoplastic left heart syndrome; AVSD, atrioventricular septal defect; VSD, ventricular septal defect; ECD, endocardial cushion defect; MVP, mitral valve piolapse; PDA, patent ductus arteriosus; BAV, B. cuspid aortic valve; SCD, sudden cardiac death; QT, cardiac output; PR, PR; PVS, pulmonary valve stenosis; HOCM, hypertrophic destructive cardiomyopathy; CoA, coarctation of the aorta; IAA, interrupted aortic arch; SVAS, supravalvar aortic stenosis; AS, aortic stenosis.

or interaction between environmental causes and genetic susceptibility.

CARDIAC DEVELOPMENT

Congenital heart disease is by definition present at birth and is due to abnormalities of development. Most forms of congenital heart disease appear to be the result of arrested development, and therefore an understanding of basic cardiac development is essential to understanding congenital heart disease and its treatment. The vascular system of the human embryo begins to form when the developing embryo is no longer able to sustain nutritional requirements by diffusion alone; this occurs during the third gestational week (16). Two endocardial heart tubes develop at 18 to 20 days of gestation at the cephalad end of the embryo fusing into a single heart tube at 22 days of development. From caudad to cephalad, the heart tube is divided into segments: (1) sinus venosus, (2) primitive atria, (3) ventricle, and (4) bulbus cordis. These four segments will respectively develop into (1) the right atrium and coronary sinus, (2) the left atrium (3) the left ventricle, and (4) the right ventricle and outflow tracts of both ventricles. Differential growth of heart tube compared with the remaining embryo cause it to bulge ventrally (anteriorly) into the surrounding pericardial sac, and differential growth of the heart tube itself results in a rightward looping of the developing heart. By 28 days of development, the bulboventricular loop has formed and septation of the atrium has begun. The division of the ventricles and atrioventricular (AV) valves is initiated by the growth of the interventricular septum from the floor of the common ventricle at the bulboventricular sulcus (Fig. 62-1), and by the endocardial cushions that originate at the junction of the primitive atrium and left ventricle. Initially, this common AV orifice provides access only to the left ventricle; blood can only enter the primitive right ventricle (derivative of the bulbus cordis) through the bulboventricular foramen. With ongoing growth, the AV canal enlarges to the right (Fig. 62-1b). This provides direct access of the right side of the common AV valve, destined to become the tricuspid valve, to the bulbus cordis, which is destined to become the right ventricle. The endocardial cushion separates the common AV valve into the tricuspid and mitral valves. The valves themselves form from tissue at the AV junction, and the subvalvar apparatus forms from muscular cords that form from the endocardial surface and eventually develop into the chordae tendineae and papillary muscles (Fig. 62-2). Ventricular septation is completed by the seventh week. Separation of the outflow into pulmonary and systemic circuits is initiated during the fifth week of gestation by swellings on the right and left sides of the conus, and by right superior and left inferior swellings on the truncus arteriosus (Figs. 62-1b and c). Fusion of these opposing swellings results in the formation of the aorticopulmonary septum dividing the truncus into an aortic and pulmonary channel. The swellings within the conus separate the right and left ventricular outflow tracts and terminate proximally to complete ventricular septation. Formation of the heart is completed by 49 days of gestation. Congenital heart disease is nearly always the result of arrest of a portion of cardiac development. Common problems include defects of septation, such as atrial septal defects, ventricular septal defects, and AV septal defects, which result from failure of any of the components of the developing atrial and ventricular septa; conotruncal truncal abnormalities that result from failure of the outflow and proximal great vessels to complete septation and achieve proper alignment; and finally, lesions involving underdevelopment of the inflow or outflow of either ventricle that will result in a spectrum of hypoplastic lesions of either the left or right heart.

FETAL CIRCULATION

The demands of a permanent terrestrial existence required the development of a dual circulatory system: a low-pressure system for pumping desaturated blood through a low-resistance pulmonary circuit and a high-pressure system for pumping the oxygenated blood to the tissues. Although cardiac development is completed during the seventh week of development and results in two circulatory systems within one heart, the developing human is still more than 7 months away from breathing air. A functional single ventricle or Piscean circulatory system is maintained by the fetal circulatory pattern, which allows both the right and left sides of the heart to contribute to systemic work prior to delivery (16). Figure 62-3 is a drawing of the fetal circulation. In the fetus, gas exchange takes place in the placenta. Blood returning from the placenta via the single umbilical vein enters the fetus through the umbilicus and then empties into the inferior vena cava (IVC) via the ductus venosus. The IVC blood, with the umbilical vein contribution and therefore slightly higher oxygen saturation than blood from the superior vena cava (SVC), enters the right atrium and is preferentially shunted to the left atrium through the foramen ovale. The left ventricle now pumps this more oxygen-rich blood to the cerebral circulation. The right ventricle also performs systemic work by pumping blood to the descending aorta via the ductus arteriosus. The umbilical arteries arising from the iliac arteries now return to the placenta for gas and nutrient exchange.

Profound changes in the circulation occur following delivery, set in motion by the expansion of the lungs with the initial breaths of the newborn. The drop in pulmonary vascular resistance (PVR) that occurs with expansion of the lungs results in an increase in pulmonary blood flow and an elevation in the left atrial pressure. The increased oxygen tension in the blood normally results in involution of the ductus arteriosus. The elevated left atrial pressure

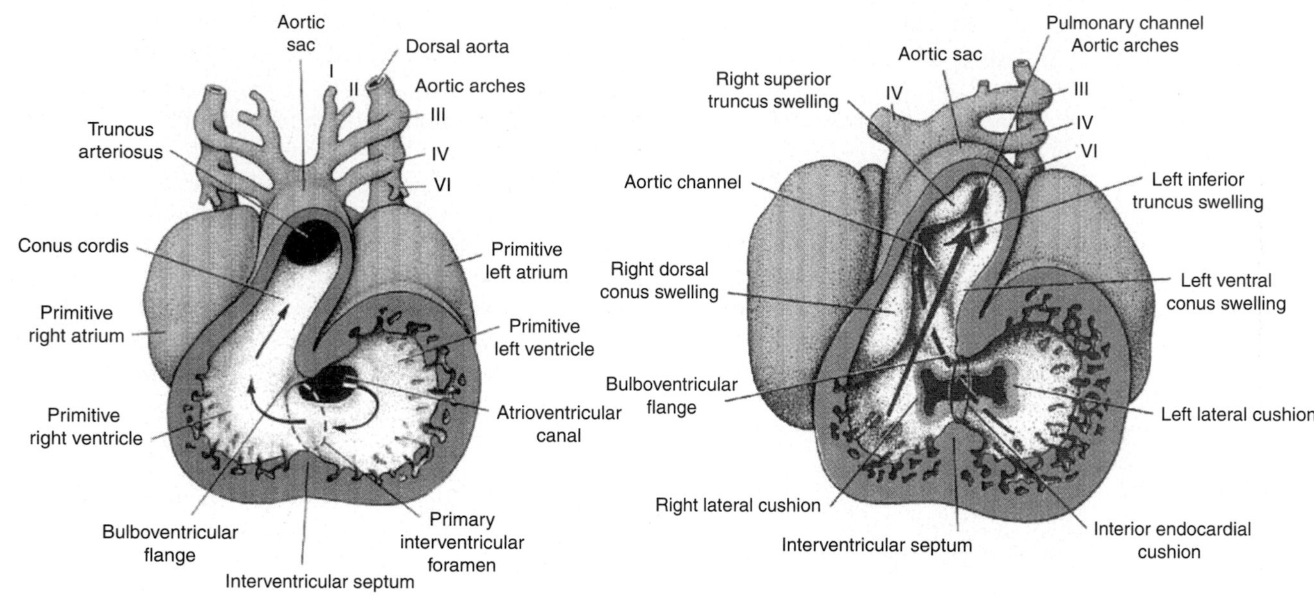

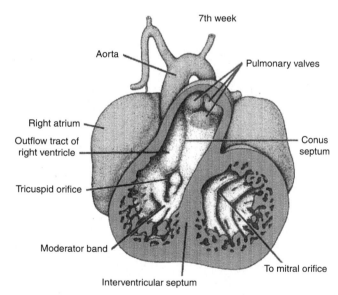

FIGURE 62-1. Cardiac development from formation of the bulboventricular loop to the completely formed heart takes place from 30 to 49 days and is depicted here. (**A**) 30 days. The right and left ventricles are becoming evident on either side of the interventricular foramen, and septation of the ventricles has been initiated. At this point, the atrioventricular canal, the opening from the atria to the ventricular loop, communicates with the primitive left ventricle only. (**B**) 35 days. Differential growth results in a shifting of the atrioventricular canal so blood enters both the primitive right and left ventricle. The endocardial cushions are evident and will participate in septation of the ventricles, along with separation of the atrioventricular valve into the tricuspid and mitral valves. Septation of the outflow tract is initiated by swellings on the right and left sides of the conus and right superior and left inferior swellings on the truncus arteriosus. (**C**) 49 days. Separation of the ventricles and atrioventricular valves is completed, the conus and truncus have completed septation, the left ventricle ejects to the aorta, and the right ventricle ejects to the pulmonary artery. Congenital heart disease is nearly always the result of arrest of a portion of cardiac development. Defects of septation, such as atrial septal defects, ventricular septal defects, and atrioventricular septal defects, are caused by failure of any of the components of the developing atrial and ventricular septa; conotruncal truncal abnormalities result from failure of the outflow and proximal great vessels to complete septation and achieve proper alignment; and finally, lesions involving underdevelopment of the inflow or outflow of either ventricle will result in a spectrum of hypoplastic lesions of either the left or right heart.

pushes septum primum against the edges of septum secundum, closing the foramen ovale. The result is separation of the pulmonary and systemic circulations. Abnormal cardiac development is frequently compatible with in utero existence because the fetal circulation allows one side of the heart to compensate for abnormal development of the contralateral side. Following delivery, significant malformations become evident. Most neonates, even those with congenital heart disease, have the ability to shunt blood across the foramen ovale, and ductal patency can be maintained with prostaglandin E_1 (PGE_1). Newborns with inadequate development of the right ventricular outflow tract, pulmonary valve, and main pulmonary artery, such as occurs with tetralogy of Fallot, can be managed by maintaining ductal patency. The patent ductus allows blood to shunt from the aorta to the pulmonary circuit and provides enough pulmonary blood flow to avoid lethal cyanosis. Similarly, the patient with severe coarctation and

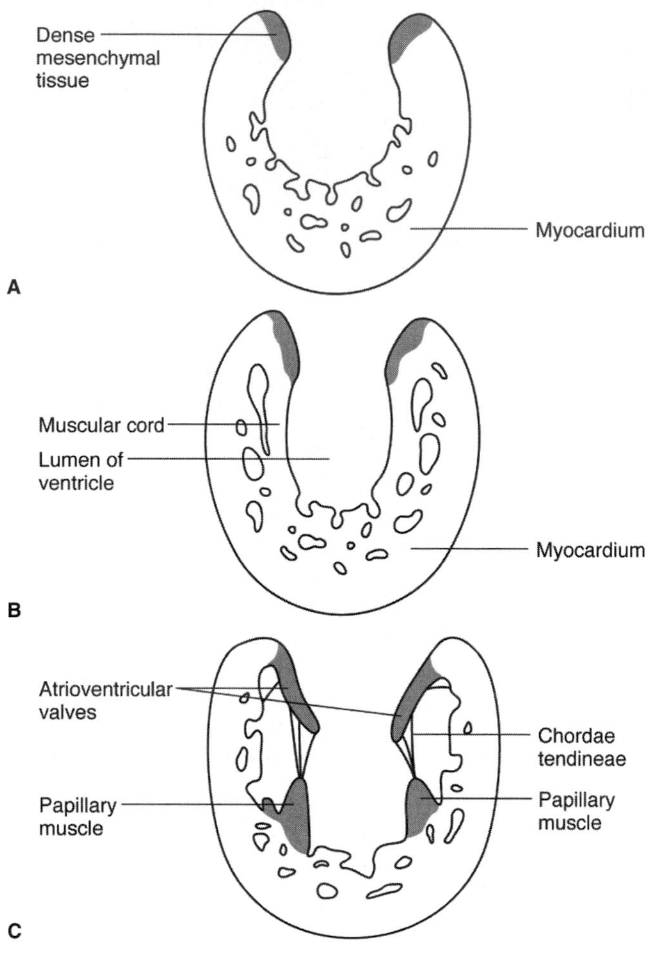

FIGURE 62-2. Formation of the valves is depicted.

arch hypoplasia is at risk for development of shock because of the obstruction of blood flow to the descending aorta. The use of PG-E_1 maintains patency of the ductus arteriosus, allowing the right side of the heart to continue to provide flow to the descending thoracic aorta, preventing critical tissue ischemia, and relieving congestive heart failure from increased resistance to left-sided output. In this way, ductal patency can be manipulated in order to resuscitate neonates with a variety of cardiac lesions with either systemic obstruction or inadequate pulmonary blood flow. Emergent procedures are avoided, and patients are allowed to recover before intervention is undertaken. Figure 62-4 is a drawing of ductal-dependent pulmonary blood flow (Fig. 62-4a) and ductal-dependent systemic blood flow (Fig. 62-4b).

PRESENTATION AND DIAGNOSIS

Cardiovascular disease in the neonatal and pediatric age groups can present with congestive heart failure, cyanosis, or both and may progress to shock (defined as critically low levels of oxygen delivery to the tissues), resulting in anaerobic metabolism. Neonates with cyanotic congenital heart disease may have ductal-dependent pulmonary blood flow and may develop life-threatening hypoxemia when the normal spontaneous closure of the ductus arteriosus occurs. Neonates with left heart obstructive lesions depend on the patency of the ductus arteriosus for perfusion of the proximal and distal aorta. When spontaneous ductal closure occurs, this group of neonates will develop low cardiac output as a result of left heart obstruction. Therefore, the presenting symptoms in this group include poor perfusion, diminished peripheral pulses, decreased urine output, acidosis, and all signs and symptoms associated with shock.

The signs and symptoms of congestive heart failure during infancy include tachypnea, tachycardia, poor feeding, slow growth, cardiomegaly, and hepatomegaly. In infants with left-to-right shunt lesions, it is common for heart failure to present within the first few weeks of life rather than immediately after birth. In the presence of a shunting defect, PVR can remain elevated for the first several weeks of life. The eventual decrease in PVR results in increased left-to-right shunting with the corresponding development of congestive heart failure. Infants and children with congenital heart disease may be first identified by the presence of a characteristic heart murmur. Although some serious congenital heart defects presenting in the neonatal period or early infancy do not have specific murmurs, less life-threatening congenital cardiac defects such as pulmonary stenosis, aortic stenosis, and restrictive ventricular septal defects often present with loud murmurs in patients who are asymptomatic.

The physical examination continues to be the mainstay of diagnosis for congenital heart disease, and a systematic approach to the physical examination increases the likelihood that a correct diagnosis will be made and that important findings will not be missed. Initial observation for obvious characteristic facial features of a specific syndrome should be done with care. In addition, one should get a general impression of the color and level of comfort of the neonate or infant so a rapid assessment of stability can be made. Respiratory distress can be ruled out by simple observation. The precordium should be palpated. Cardiac hyperactivity, often present in neonates and infants with serious cardiac abnormalities, can be easily determined. Pulses should be palpated in all four extremities. Decreased pulses in all four extremities suggest low cardiac output and shock. Strong upper-extremity pulses, but weak or absent lower-extremity pulses, suggest coarctation of the aorta. Bounding pulses suggest aortic runoff into the pulmonary vascular bed, the result of either a patent ductus arteriosus or arteriovenous malformation. It is important to routinely measure blood pressure in all four extremities in order to quantify any differences.

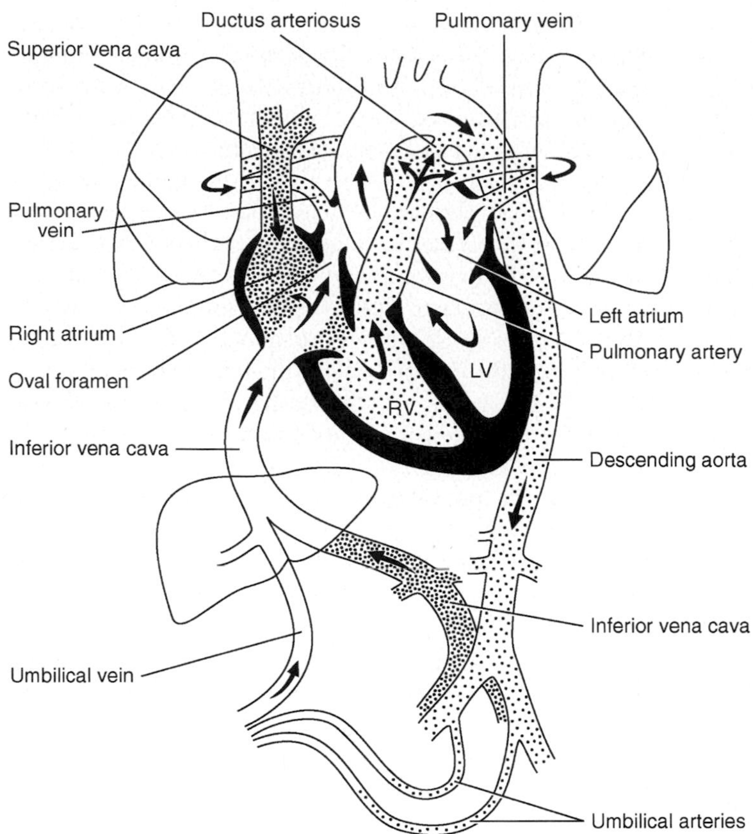

FIGURE 62-3. Fetal circulation. The circulation of the fetus following formation of the heart is depicted. The grayscale indicates the degree of desaturation of the blood. The darker shaded areas indicate more desaturated blood, whereas the white areas indicate more fully saturated blood. Umbilical venous return, the most saturated blood enters the inferior vena cava and is preferentially shunted across the patent foramen ovale to the left side of the heart to supply the cerebral circulation. Less fully saturated blood is pumped by the right ventricle through the ductus arteriosus to the descending thoracic aorta. Return to the placenta for gas exchange is via the umbilical arteries, which arise from the iliac arteries.

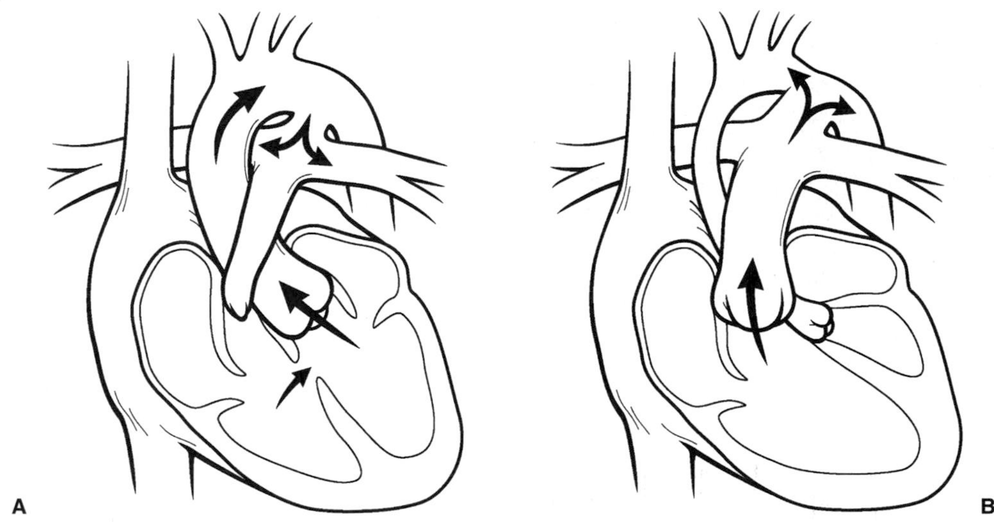

FIGURE 62-4. A patent ductus arteriosus can compensate for underdevelopment of either the right or left side of the heart. (**A**) Depicts ductal-dependent pulmonary blood flow in a case of pulmonary atresia and ventricular septal defect. Blood is shunted from the aorta to the pulmonary arteries to provide pulmonary blood flow. (**B**) Demonstrates ductal-dependent systemic flow in a patient with hypoplastic left heart syndrome. In this case, the single right ventricle ejects blood through the pulmonary root and systemic flow is supported by flow through the ductus arteriosus into the aorta. Flow to the head and coronary arteries is maintained via retrograde flow from the ductus.

Abdominal palpation will allow one to determine the position of the liver and whether it is enlarged. In syndromes of left–right isomerism (heterotaxy), it is possible for the liver and stomach to be reversed within the abdomen. In addition, it is not unusual to encounter hepatomegaly in patients with heart failure. One should inspect the nail beds for cyanosis and for clubbing. Cyanosis can be detected visually only if at least 5 g of unsaturated hemoglobin per 100 mL of blood is present in the capillary bed. Thus, anemia may mask important cyanosis. Routine measurement of pulse oximetry is therefore important in all neonates, infants, and children who are evaluated for congenital heart disease.

Auscultation often yields information with regard to the anatomic diagnosis, as well as the specific hemodynamic aspects of a specific lesion. Auscultation should also be undertaken in a systematic fashion. One should routinely listen to the precordium over the apex of the heart, left lower sternal border, left upper sternal border, and right upper sternal border. At each area, one should note the first heart sound, systole, the second heart sound, and diastole. These areas typically represent events associated with the mitral valve, tricuspid valve, pulmonary valve, and aortic valve, respectively. In addition, locations between the previously mentioned sites should be auscultated, as should the back and midaxillary areas of the chest. For example, the presence of a ventricular septal defect is often manifested by a harsh, holosystolic murmur at the left lower sternal border.

Two-dimensional echocardiography with Doppler and color flow Doppler mapping has revolutionized the noninvasive diagnostic capabilities for determining spatial anatomy and function of the heart in pediatric cardiology (17,18). This modality, developed since the mid-1980s, has become an effective, accurate, and safe technique for the elucidation of anatomic and hemodynamic details of all congenital cardiac abnormalities. The two-dimensional study provides tomographic images of the heart. Images are obtained via directing of the ultrasound transducer beam along standard cross-sectional planes through the heart. Based on these standard views, an accurate diagnosis can be made of the most complex of congenital heart defects along with the detailed relationships of the intracardiac anatomy and function of the heart.

In addition, Doppler ultrasound has aided in the evaluation of the hemodynamic severity of a particular cardiac defect by evaluating the blood flow pattern within the heart and peripheral vessels. Doppler echocardiography will detect normal and abnormal blood flow patterns, and can quantify the severity of a blood flow disturbance. The principle of Doppler is based on the fact that the frequency of a transmitted sound is altered when the source of the sound is moving. Doppler echocardiography provides information about the velocity and direction of blood flow, making possible calculation of pressure gradients across areas of stenosis. The simplified Bernoulli equation: $P_1 - P_2 = 4V_2^2$ ($P_1 - P_2$ = pressure gradient across the valve or defect in mm Hg; V_2 = peak velocity across the valve or defect as measured by Doppler echocardiography in meters per second) can be used to estimate the pressure gradient across a stenotic valve, or a septal defect.

Diagnostic cardiac catheterization provides important anatomic and physiologic data. Vascular anatomy can be defined by cardiac catheterization and corresponding hemodynamic data obtained, such as pressure and flow data that are necessary to make determinations of vascular resistance. Indications for diagnostic cardiac catheterization include incomplete or inconclusive noninvasive anatomic diagnoses. Cardiac catheterization is uniquely suited for the determination of pulmonary artery architecture and pulmonary vascular resistance. The impact of pulmonary vasodilators on pulmonary vascular resistance is ideally determined in the catheterization laboratory. Before the development of echocardiography, cardiac catheterization was the mainstay of physiologic and anatomic assessment of congenital heart disease (19) and, although the role of cardiac catheterization has diminished as a purely diagnostic tool, the catheterization laboratory is now more and more the venue for intervention. Increasingly, the catheterization laboratory is the site for treatment of patients with patent ductus arteriosus, atrial and ventricular septal defects, and branch pulmonary artery stenosis.

Developing diagnostic modalities include cardiac ultrafast computed tomography (CT) and magnetic resonance imaging (MRI) currently available as an adjunct to echocardiography and cardiac catheterization. These newer imaging techniques provide excellent noninvasive images of the pulmonary arteries and pulmonary veins, anomalies of the systemic veins, and anomalies of the aortic arch. CT and MRI may be useful in the postoperative evaluation of patients and in cases where precise flow and pressure data are not necessary.

TREATMENT OF CONGENITAL HEART DISEASE

Treatment of congenital heart disease is primarily focused on (1) relief of congestive heart failure, defined as excessively high filling pressures, and frequently the result of excessive pulmonary blood flow due to defects in either the atrial or ventricular septum, or (2) the treatment of cyanosis due to either right-to-left shunt or failure of development of an in-series pulmonary and systemic circulation.

The modern era of care for patients with congenital heart disease began when Dr. Robert Gross successfully ligated the patent ductus arteriosus of a 7-year-old girl in August 1938 (20). This was followed by the successful repair of coarctation of the aorta by Clarence Crafoord in Sweden in 1944 and subsequently by Dr. Gross in the

United States (21). Gross had shown that surgery on the great vessels around the heart was possible. Helen Taussig, a pediatric cardiologist, made the observation that patients with tetralogy of Fallot and a patent ductus arteriosus had improved survival and functional status compared with patients with tetralogy of Fallot and no patent ductus. She conjectured that for patients with cyanotic heart disease the addition of a ductus arteriosus would result in relief of cyanosis. Dr. Taussig found a receptive ear to her theories in Alfred Blalock. In 1944, Dr. Blalock performed the first systemic to pulmonary artery shunt in a patient with tetralogy of Fallot (22). This procedure was based on the largely unheralded work of his laboratory assistant Vivien Thomas. The Blalock-Taussig shunt was the first example of a novel anatomic solution to a physiologic problem. In 1952, Muller and Dammann reported pulmonary artery banding for the palliation of patients with congestive heart failure due to excessive pulmonary blood flow (23). In the 14 years between 1938 and 1952, fundamental steps had been taken in the therapy of congenital heart disease. Pathologic anatomy had been both corrected (ligation of a patent ductus arteriosus) and palliated. Patients with inadequate pulmonary blood flow could be managed by creation of a Blalock-Taussig shunt and patients with congestive heart failure (acyanotic congenital heart disease) could be managed with a pulmonary artery band. The development of these palliative procedures lead to the first classification of congenital heart disease into cyanotic and acyanotic lesions. This classification directed the initial palliative procedure. Blue babies were shunted; babies with heart failure underwent pulmonary artery banding.

Despite the simplicity and utility of this classification system, there were cyanotic patients in whom pulmonary blood flow was not limited and could at times even be excessive. These included patients with forms of transposition in whom desaturated systemic venous blood was pumped back to the body with little added oxygen, and fully saturated pulmonary venous blood was pumped back to the pulmonary circuit. The inefficiencies of this system are obvious. Early efforts directed at patients with transposition included efforts to improve mixing, as well as efforts to redirect blood to improve systemic oxygen saturations. Initial efforts included the Blalock-Hanlon atrial septectomy, a closed procedure in which an atrial septal defect was created by excising the interatrial septum in front of the right-sided pulmonary veins (24). This procedure would provide crucial mixing with relief of cyanosis in critically ill neonates. The Baffes procedure was an attempt at partial physiologic correction of transposition that predated cardiopulmonary bypass. The IVC was transected and anastomosed to the left atrium and the right-sided pulmonary veins were implanted into the right atrium (25). Now desaturated systemic venous blood returned to the left side of the heart and was pumped through the malpositioned great vessels to the pulmonary circuit. This provided significant relief of cyanosis and offered the first opportunity for prolonged survival in patients with transposition. Transposition of the great arteries also inspired the birth of interventional cardiology. In 1966, William Rashkind enlarged an atrial septal defect in an infant with transposition in the catheterization laboratory by passing a balloon catheter across the interatrial septum, inflating the balloon and drawing the catheter back across the interatrial septum, creating a tear in the septum (26). The balloon atrial septostomy is generally identified as the first interventional cardiac catheterization technique.

DEVELOPMENT OF OPEN HEART SURGERY

Tolerance to ischemia or decreased cardiac output is enhanced by hypothermia. In September 1952, F.J. Lewis, MD, at the University of Minnesota closed an atrial septal defect under direct vision using moderate surface-induced hypothermia with inflow occlusion (27). This technique was used early in the history of treatment of congenital heart disease and H. Swan used this strategy on hundreds of patients with defects in the atrial septum (28). It is noteworthy that these patients generally had very large defects with significant symptoms in order to be considered for this therapy. The atrial well technique developed by Dr. Gross was something of a hybrid technique in which the surgeon would create a funnel attached to the atrial appendage (29). By making the height of the well such that it was taller than the central venous pressure, the surgeon could operate through the well in the right atrium. Although complete visualization of the defect was not possible, sections of the atrial septum could be drawn up into the well to allow for direct visualization. Given the limitations of the era with less than optimal intraoperative and postoperative monitoring, including an inability to directly measure blood pressure, arterial blood gases, cardiac output, rhythm, and a lack of inotropic agents and antiarrhythmic agents, the results were excellent and many patients operated on with these techniques are alive today without residual lesions.

The real impact on congenital heart disease awaited the development of open heart techniques in which the cardiac output to the body could be maintained and allow surgeons to work within the heart. Following a long series of animal studies in which the circulation of one animal was supported by another, C. Walton Lillehei at the University of Minnesota embarked on a series of operations using an adult human as the source of oxygenated blood to perfuse a child (30). Using femoral access for both patients, arterial blood was pumped, with the help of a separate blood pump to control flow, from the adult patient to the child and venous blood was returned from the child to the adult. These cross-circulation operations allowed the surgeon to open the heart with enough time to perform complex corrections. For the first time, ventricular septal defects could be closed and patients with more complex heart problems, such as tetralogy of Fallot, could undergo complete repair. Despite a lack of sophisticated diagnostic techniques and postoperative support ability, the patients generally did well and many are alive today (31). Following decades of laboratory work inspired by his experience as an intern watching a postpartum woman die of pulmonary embolism, John Gibbon performed the first open heart procedure using a heart-lung machine on May 6, 1953 (32). During that procedure Dr. Gibbon closed an atrial septal defect in a teenage girl. Although Dr. Gibbon's operative career as a heart surgeon was short, the heart-lung machine he developed was adopted by other surgeons. In particular, Dr. John Kirklin at the Mayo Clinic began an historic series of open heart operations demonstrating the feasibility of open cardiac correction.

CURRENT CONDUCT OF CARDIOPULMONARY BYPASS

With few exceptions, open heart procedures are performed today using an open cardiopulmonary bypass circuit (33). Blood is drained from the patient using gravity or a low vacuum, into a calibrated reservoir. From there, blood is withdrawn by a pump and driven through a hollow-fiber oxygenator and returned to the arterial circuit of the patient. A combination of filters removes particulate matter, thereby minimizing systemic embolization. Two to three additional active suction pumps, usually roller pumps, are used to remove shed blood and actively drain specific parts of the heart such as the left ventricle. Modern cardiopulmonary bypass circuits are equipped with additional safety equipment to prevent injury. In addition to filters, they include bubble detectors and pressure monitors to prevent rupture of the bypass line and injury to the blood elements. A hemoconcentrator can be added to the circuit to remove excess water. Cardiopulmonary bypass is routinely combined with hypothermia, which is achieved with a countercurrent heat exchanger. Hypothermia is used to protect the patient from diminished oxygen delivery that may occur as a result of altered flow associated with cardiopulmonary bypass. Hypothermia will also increase the safe duration of circulatory arrest should bypass need to be interrupted. For simple procedures such as closure of an atrial septal or ventricular defect, mild hypothermia to 32°C may be employed. For more complex procedures such as an arterial switch for transposition of the great vessels, a temperature of 22°C may be used to provide additional protection and allow safe periods of diminished flow. Some procedures such as reconstruction of the aortic arch are routinely performed using cardiopulmonary bypass but also a period of deep hypothermic circulatory arrest (DHCA). Patients are placed on bypass and then cooled to a core temperature of 18°C. After reaching this temperature, circulation is halted, the blood is drained from the patient, and although the duration of safe circulatory arrest is not known, a period up to 45 to 60 minutes is generally accepted in contemporary practice. More recent studies suggest persistent behavioral and neurodevelopment abnormalities in patients subjected to prolonged circulatory arrest (34). Strategies to limit the duration and possibly the impact of DHCA include the use of regional cerebral perfusion in which circulation is maintained to the brain via one of the carotid arteries during the period of circulatory arrest or the use of intermittent circulatory arrest in which circulation is reestablished for a period of 5 to 10 minutes between periods of arrest of 20 minutes duration.

Most open heart procedures require a period of myocardial arrest to complete the repair. Cardioplegia is used to achieve myocardial arrest. Cardioplegia is a physiologic crystalloid solution or blood to which potassium is added to a concentration of 20 meq. This is introduced to the myocardium either via the coronary arteries or through the aortic root after cross-clamping. The result is diastolic cardiac arrest, allowing the surgeon to operate in a bloodless field. Cardioplegia has seen its own evolution, and various additives, delivery systems, and temperature strategies have been developed allowing prolonged periods of arrest with good recovery of systolic function.

TREATMENT OF SPECIFIC CONGENITAL HEART DEFECTS

Defects of Septation

Any communication between the atria constitutes an *atrial septal defect* (ASD). Figure 62-5 depicts the types of ASDs based on the location within the atrial septum. Shunting at the atrial level is dependent on the size of the defect and the relative compliances of the two ventricles. The right ventricle is far more compliant than the left ventricle and results in left-to-right shunting across the ASD with resultant right atrial and right ventricular volume overload. On physical exam, evidence of a volume-loaded right ventricle includes a peristernal heave and increased flow across a normal pulmonary valve, resulting in a pulmonary flow murmur. A diastolic murmur at the right lower sternal border suggests a relatively large shunt across the atrial septum and is caused by increased flow across a normal tricuspid valve. A fixed and widely split second heart sound is typical of patients with an ASD and right ventricular volume overload. The latter is present because of the increased flow across the pulmonary valve, minimizing the flow differential between the aortic and pulmonary valves that normally occurs during the respiratory cycle.

Most patients with an ASD are asymptomatic. Some patients with a large ASD can present with failure to thrive

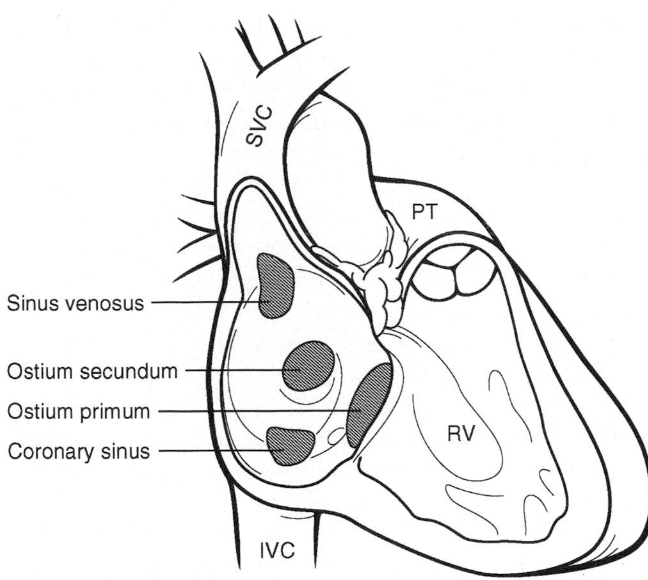

FIGURE 62-5. Diagram of the types of atrial septal defects (ASDs) and their location within the atrial septum. The most common type of ASD is the secundum defect located within the central portion of the atrial septum. The second most common type of atrial septal defect is the primum defect, a variant of an endocardial cushion defect. Primum ASDs are positioned directly above the atrioventricular valves. The sinus venosus type of ASD occurs third most often. The sinus venosus defect is located at the junction of the superior vena cava (SVC) and right atrium, and is frequently associated with anomalous drainage of the right-sided pulmonary veins. The coronary sinus type of ASD is the least common type of ASD and occurs in the inferior portion of the interatrial septum. PT, pulmonary trunk; RV, right ventricle; IVC, inferior vena cava.

and exercise intolerance. ASDs are easily diagnosed with echocardiography. Figure 62-5 shows the types of ASDs and their locations within the atrial septum. A primum ASD is actually a form of endocardial cushion defect and is associated with other features of endocardial cushion failure such as a cleft in the mitral valve (Fig. 62-5). Closure of ASD is recommended for those patients who have right heart dilatation on echocardiography.

As mentioned previously, the majority of the patients in this group will have no symptoms or only mild symptoms. Intervention is recommended to prevent future progression of right heart dilatation, pulmonary hypertension, and arrhythmias. The more recent development of catheter-based therapy for ASD has changed management of this defect. Secundum ASDs can be closed with one of several devices with excellent results on intermediate follow-up (35). Advantages of device closure include avoidance of cardiopulmonary bypass and a decreased likelihood of transfusion. Device closure has also been applied effectively to small atrial septal defects/patent foramen ovale associated with cryptogenic stroke (36). The currently available devices require a rim of tissue for positioning. Thus far, device closure has not been applied routinely to defects of the primum or sinus venosus type, where either a rim of tissue is absent or the defect is proximate to an atrioventricular valve. Catheter device closure of ASDs is generally reserved for children larger than 10 kg. Surgical intervention for ASDs will be necessary for primum defects in which the atrioventricular valves are adjacent to the defect, as well as sinus venosus defects or secundum with anatomy not suited to device closure.

As discussed previously in the section on fetal circulation, the ductus arteriosus is a normal intrauterine structure that allows right ventricular contribution to the systemic circulation. The ductus arteriosus is derived from the sixth aortic arch and connects the distal main pulmonary artery with the descending aorta. Elevation of arterial po_2 coincident with the first breaths triggers contraction of the muscular wall of the ductus arteriosus and normally results in closure during the first day of life. Between 0.02% and 0.006% of live births are complicated by a *patent ductus arteriosus* (PDA). Presence of a PDA is associated with neonatal respiratory distress, perinatal asphyxia, and prematurity. Thirty percent of neonates weighing less than 1,500 g will have a PDA. The mechanism of persistent PDA is believed to be arterial hypoxemia, as well as an incompletely developed ductal closure system in the premature newborn (37). Pulmonary arteriolar muscle, which can limit excessive pulmonary blood flow, is underdeveloped in the premature neonate and, as a result, a patent ductus can result in severe congestive heart failure. In neonates, initial management consists of indomethacin, a potent inhibitor of prostaglandin synthesis, which results in constriction of the ductus, the reverse effect of using PGE_1 to maintain ductal patency. Surgical ligation of the patent ductus in the neonate is reserved for those symptomatic patients who are unresponsive to indomethacin. In infants and older children, the presence of a large PDA can result in left-sided volume overload with excessive pulmonary blood flow, resulting in congestive heart failure and the eventual development of pulmonary vasculopathy. Patients with a small PDA are at risk of developing endocarditis. The risk of intervention, specifically occlusion of the PDA, is lower than the lifelong risk of developing endocarditis. Therefore, the presence of a patent ductus is indication for closure. As catheter-based therapies have shown their safety and effectiveness, few patients outside the neonatal intensive care unit are submitted for surgical closure (38,39).

Ventricular septal defects (VSD) are the most common congenital heart malformations and occur in 25% of patients with congenital heart disease. The perimembranous region, adjacent to the tricuspid annulus and below the aortic valve, is the most common location of a VSD. Other sites include the supracristal region below the pulmonary and aortic valves, the inlet septum, and the muscular septum (Fig. 62-6). VSDs result in left-to-right shunting from the left ventricle through the defect into the right ventricle

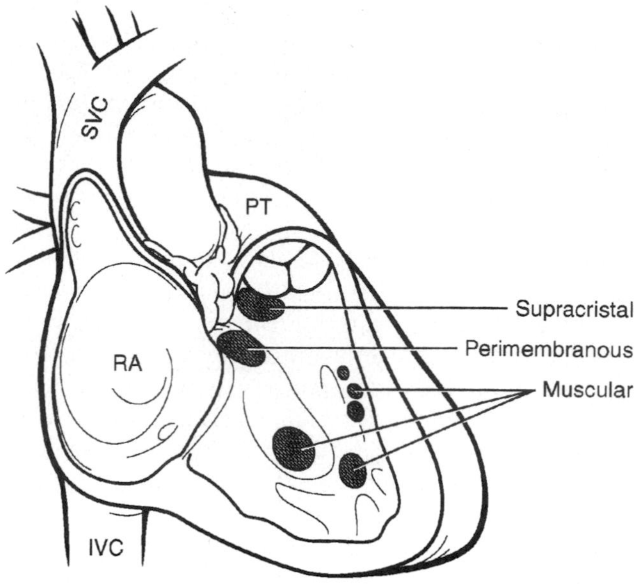

FIGURE 62-6. Typical location of ventricular septal defects is shown. Ventricular septal defects occur most commonly in the perimembranous region, the junction between the inflow and outflow septum. They can also occur in the supracristal region below the pulmonary valve, as well as within the muscular septum.

and pulmonary artery. The size of the shunt and therefore the severity of symptoms are due to both the size of the defect and the pulmonary vascular resistance. When a defect is larger than the aortic annulus, it is said to be nonrestrictive and flow is only limited by the pulmonary vascular resistance. Because the normal systemic vascular resistance is about six times greater than the PVR, large defects result in enormous shunts with elevation of pulmonary artery pressure to match the systemic arterial pressure. As the defects become smaller than the aortic annulus, the defect itself provides some restriction to flow and with still smaller defects the flow may become trivial. Provided they are not associated with malalignment of the outflow tract (such as occurs with conotruncal malformations), even large perimembranous VSDs as well as isolated muscular VSDs can close spontaneously. Fifty percent of muscular defects and 25% of perimembranous defects may close spontaneously in the first year of life (40). For this reason, unless profoundly symptomatic, infants with a VSD are usually managed with medical therapy directed at congestive heart failure while observing for spontaneous closure. This therapy includes the use of digoxin, diuretics, and afterload-reducing agents such as captopril or enalapril. Infants with symptoms of pulmonary overcirculation and/or pulmonary hypertension require surgical intervention during infancy. Therefore, a VSD that continues to produce a significant shunt should be surgically repaired if it has not spontaneously closed in infancy. Prolonged exposure of the pulmonary vasculature to excessive pulmonary flow and high pressure results in remodeling of the microcirculation, resulting in elevation of PVR. Although this remains reversible for some time, permanent elevation of PVR can occur. Irreversible elevation of PVR can render a patient inoperable.

Echocardiography has generally supplanted cardiac catheterization for the routine diagnosis of VSDs. Two-dimensional Doppler echocardiography can identify the precise location of the VSD and provide crucial physiologic data, such as the right ventricular pressure. As a result, cardiac catheterization plays a decreasing role in determining the need for VSD closure. However, in patients who present late with a large VSD, prolonged overcirulation can result in elevation of the PVR as discussed previously. As PVR reaches a critically elevated level, greater than 8 Wood units, VSD closure will result in acute right heart failure resulting in decreased cardiac output and increased risk of early mortality (41). Patients with suspected elevation of PVR should undergo cardiac catheterization with the calculation of the PVR. If the PVR is found to be increased, the patient should be acutely tested with pulmonary vasodilators, such as inhaled nitric oxide, in the catheterization laboratory to determine if the PVR can be reduced to a safe level to permit VSD closure. Irreversible elevation in PVR in association with a VSD is rarely encountered in patients less than 1 year of age.

Surgical closure of VSDs is the mainstay of treatment and is accomplished using cardiopulmonary bypass and mild hypothermia (Fig. 62-6). More recently, catheter-based techniques have been employed to close muscular VSDs. For defects in the perimembranous region, the proximity of the aortic valve and conduction system have limited the use of catheter-based devices, but recently modified devices have been used successfully to close perimembranous defects (42). This technique may be widely available in the future.

The endocardial cushions complete the septation of the inlet portion of the two ventricles, the atria and the separation of the common atrioventricular valve into separate tricuspid and mitral components. Failure of the endocardial cushions to complete this process results in an *atrioventricular septal defect* (AV). The combination of the significant left-to-right shunt from large VSDs and ASDs, as well as valvular insufficiency from the abnormal atrioventricular valve, can lead to substantial heart failure and failure to thrive in early infancy. Repair is performed using cardiopulmonary bypass and mild hypothermia. The ventricular and atrial septum are reconstructed with patch material, usually woven polyester or pericardium, which also accomplishes division and reconstruction of the common AV valve into tricuspid and mitral components (Fig. 62-7). Because of the risk of development of fixed elevation of pulmonary vascular resistance, elective repair of AV canal should be performed prior to 4 months of age. Results with early repair of complete endocardial cushion

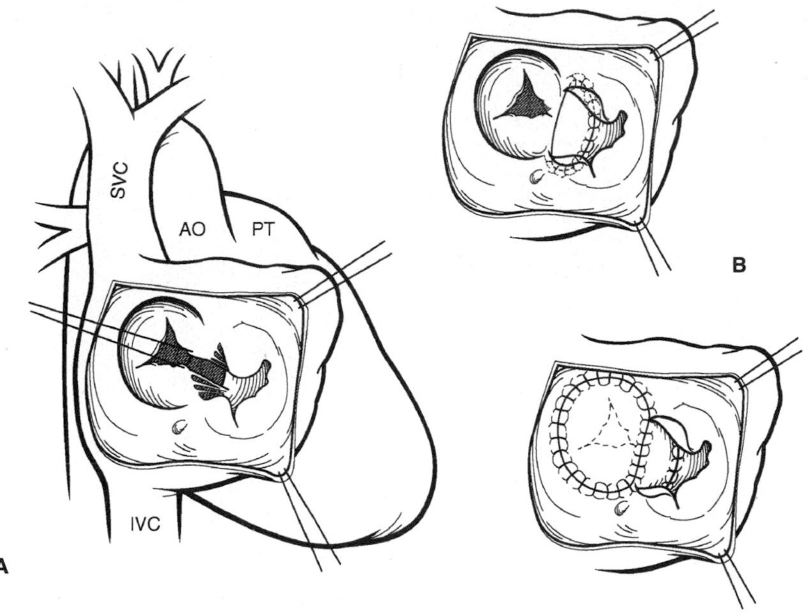

FIGURE 62-7. (**A**) A typical atrioventricular (AV) septal defect, also known as an endocardial cushion defect or atrioventricular canal, is shown. There is a common AV valve with an associated inlet ventricular septal defect and large atrial septal defect. (**B**) A patch is placed to close the ventricular septal defect and separates the left and right AV valves into mitral and tricuspid valves. (**C**) The atrial septal defect component is closed with a second patch. SVC, superior vena cava; AO, aorta; PT, pulmonary trunk; IVC, inferior vena cava.

defects are excellent. Early mortality is rare in cases uncomplicated by any comorbidity. Late reintervention occasionally is necessary for left-sided AV valve insufficiency (43).

Single Ventricles

Many forms of congenital heart disease are unsuitable for two-ventricle repair, but no single classification system exits (44). Isolated hypoplasia or atresia of the outlet portion of either ventricle does not rule out a two-ventricle repair. *Single ventricle* palliation is required for atresia or significant hypoplasia of either atrioventricular valve, severely unbalanced atrioventricular canal, or significant hypoplasia of either ventricle. A Fontan procedure is the treatment goal for patients with single ventricle anatomy. The Fontan operation and related procedures are also known as right heart bypass procedures (45,46). Initially, right heart bypass procedures were applied to patients with right heart obstructive lesions, most commonly tricuspid atresia. These procedures bypass the obstructed right ventricle, connecting the systemic venous return [superior (SVC) and inferior vena cava (IVC)] with the pulmonary arteries, and provide adequate pulmonary blood flow and cardiac output with minimal elevation of the systemic venous pressure. The Fontan procedure separates the systemic and pulmonary venous returns, relieves cyanosis, and decreases the volume load of the single ventricle (47). The Fontan procedure, therefore, achieves as closely as possible, a normal circulatory pattern for patients with single ventricle anatomy (SVA).

A standardized, staged approach to the management of patients with SVA ensures better preparation for the Fontan procedure and long-term outcome. Effective neonatal or early infant palliation is the first and most critical stage. During the neonatal or early infant period, the goal is complete relief of systemic obstruction and appropriate limitation of pulmonary blood flow to achieve a balanced circulation. Subsequent stages include a bidirectional superior cavopulmonary anastomosis, which is an anastomosis of the SVC to the confluent pulmonary arteries (Fig. 62-8). Later, connecting the IVC return to the pulmonary arteries completes the Fontan procedure (Fig. 62-9).

Following the completion Fontan procedure, central venous pressure is the force that drives pulmonary blood flow. Systemic output is derived from the pulmonary venous return. In this circuit, individual pressure gradients combine to elevate central venous pressure. Severe elevation of the gradient between the systemic veins and the pulmonary atrium results in intolerable elevation of central venous pressure and restrictive ventricular preload, resulting in reduced cardiac output. Risk factors for failure of the Fontan physiology include poor ventricular function with elevated end-diastolic pressure, insufficiency of the atrioventricular valve, elevated PVR, pulmonary artery distortion, and stenosis of the systemic venous to pulmonary artery connections. The goal of the staged approach to patients with single ventricle anatomy is to minimize the risk factors for subsequent Fontan palliation. The type of initial palliative intervention that may be necessary depends on the relative balance or imbalance of flow between the systemic and pulmonary circulations.

Many patients with single ventricle anatomy need palliative intervention shortly after birth. Whether palliative intervention is necessary and which palliative intervention

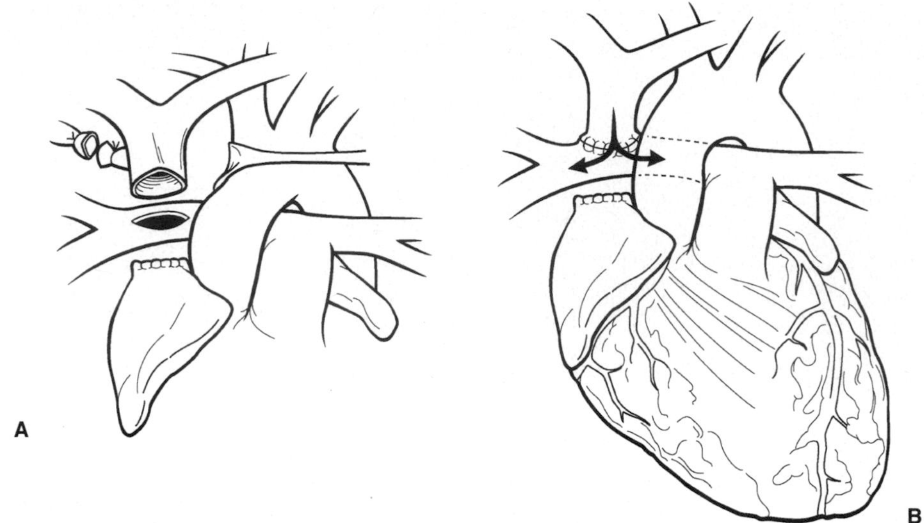

FIGURE 62-8. (**A**) Bidirectional Glenn shunt is created by dividing the superior vena cava and anastomosing this to the confluent pulmonary arteries. Desaturated venous blood is routed directly to the pulmonary circuit for gas exchange. (**B**) The bidirectional Glenn shunt relieves the single ventricle of the work excess volume load required to provide pulmonary blood flow through either a Blalock-Taussig shunt or through a stenotic pulmonary valve. In addition to relief of excess volume load, the bidirectional Glenn shunt further increases the efficiency of the circulation because more completely desaturated blood is routed to the pulmonary bed using venous pressure rather than actively pumping an arteriovenous admixture as occurs with either a Blalock-Taussig shunt or stenotic pulmonary valve.

is required depends on the specific anatomic details of the single ventricle anatomy. For example, the patient with a single ventricle and unobstructed flow to both the aorta and pulmonary artery will typically have pulmonary overcirculation. A pulmonary artery band will be appropriate to improve the symptoms of congestive heart failure and will also ensure a low distal pulmonary artery pressure. In contrast, the single ventricle patient with restrictive or ductal-dependant pulmonary blood flow (tricuspid atresia with normally related great arteries and a restrictive VSD or single ventricle with severe pulmonary stenosis) will likely require a systemic to pulmonary artery shunt so adequate pulmonary blood flow can occur in the absence of a ductus arteriosus (Fig. 62-10). In either of these two scenarios, this early palliation is necessary because the neonatal circulation, with its normal elevation in pulmonary artery pressure and PVR, will not allow a bidirectional shunt.

Finally, and most common, is the group of single ventricle patients with obstruction to systemic outflow. These patients can present in extremis when the ductus closes. The presenting symptoms include severe low cardiac output

FIGURE 62-9. A completion Fontan is depicted. (**A**) Shows a cutaway view of a patient with hypoplastic left heart syndrome who has undergone previous Norwood palliation and then subsequent bidirectional Glenn shunt. (**B**) A baffle, usually constructed of Gore-Tex, is used to route the inferior vena cava blood to the pulmonary artery confluence. A fenestration is commonly used, a small hole in the baffle. This allows some left-to-right shunting with a decrease in the central venous pressure and maintenance of cardiac output, albeit at the expense of mild desaturation.

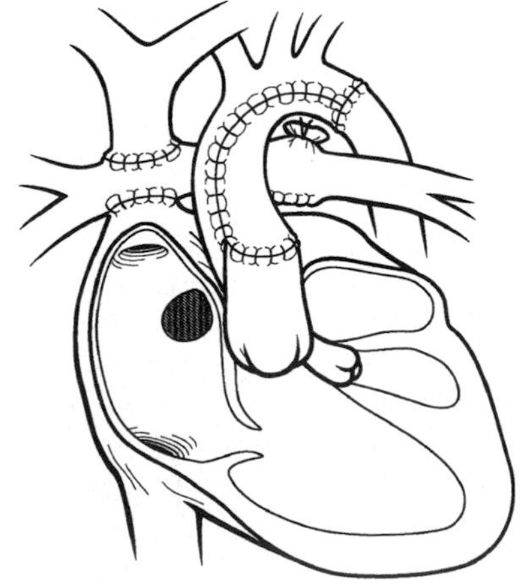

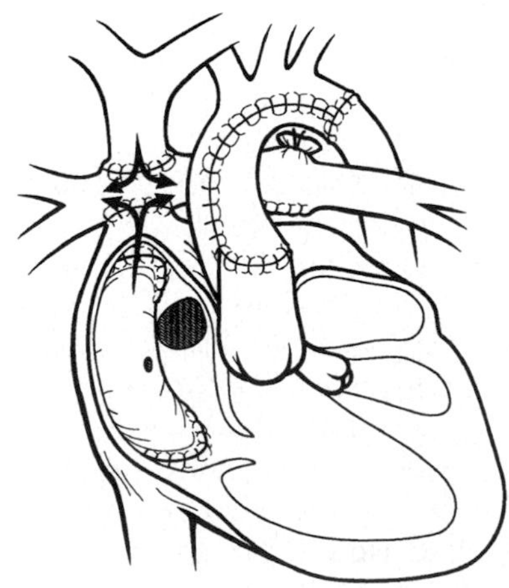

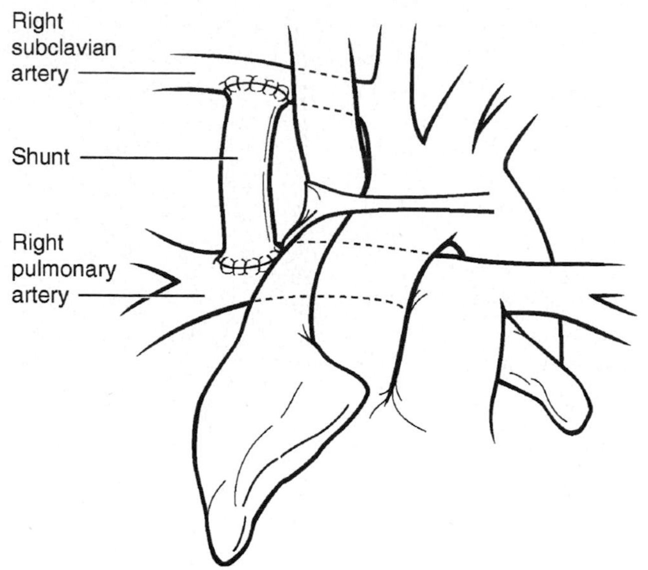

FIGURE 62-10. A modified Blalock-Taussig shunt is constructed using a synthetic graft between the right subclavian artery and the right pulmonary artery for provision of additional pulmonary blood flow in patients with excessive cyanosis.

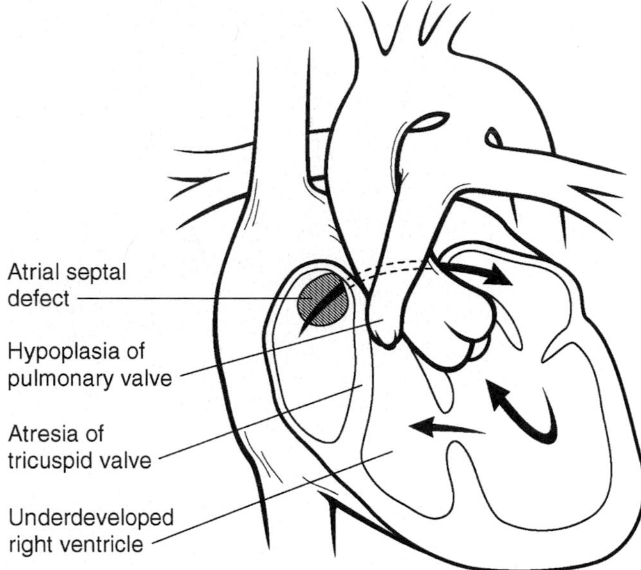

FIGURE 62-11. This diagram depicts the typical features of tricuspid atresia. The tricuspid valve does not develop. Systemic venous blood is shunted across the atrial septum through the nearly always-present atrial septal defect. Pulmonary blood flow is provided either through a stenotic pulmonary valve or by maintaining ductal patency with prostaglandin.

and pulmonary overcirculation. This group of patients requires complex reconstructive surgery, such as either a Damus-Kaye-Stansel or Norwood procedure. This approach is discussed in greater detail later in this chapter.

The durability of the Fontan circulation is unknown and survival beyond early adulthood is speculative. Despite optimal neonatal management and staged progression to a Fontan, some patients will develop well-recognized sequelae of the Fontan circulation, including protein-losing enteropathy, thrombosis in the Fontan circuit, atrial tachyarrhythmias, and cardiomyopathy. Heart transplantation has been offered to this group of patients with some success.

Right Heart Hypoplasia

As mentioned previously, *tricuspid atresia* is a single ventricle lesion characterized by absence of the tricuspid valve between the right atrium and the right ventricle (48). Also typically present is an ASD, a hypoplastic right ventricle, and a VSD. The VSD is usually perimembranous, and if the VSD is severely restrictive, pulmonary blood flow is markedly diminished and requires the maintenance of ductal patency. Therefore, depending on the size of the VSD, the pulmonary blood flow may be decreased, normal, or increased. Typical features of tricuspid atresia are demonstrated in Fig. 62-11. Infants with tricuspid atresia will follow the single ventricle pathway with aims toward a bidirectional cavopulmonary shunt followed by a Fontan operation. However, intervention in neonatal/infant period may be necessary prior to the cavopulmonary shunt, depending on the specific anatomy and clinical manifestations. For example, the neonate with tricuspid atresia and a small VSD may need a systemic-to-pulmonary artery shunt to provide for adequate pulmonary blood flow. An infant with tricuspid atresia and a large VSD may need a pulmonary artery band to treat symptoms of pulmonary overcirculation and to protect the pulmonary vasculature.

Following initial normal early cardiac development, the fetus with *pulmonary atresia and intact ventricular septum* fails to develop antegrade flow from the right ventricle to the pulmonary artery or alternatively develops atresia following early normal formation of a right ventricular to pulmonary artery connection (49). A principle of cardiac development is demonstrated by this lesion in that blood flow through cardiac structures promotes growth. With the development of pulmonary atresia with an intact ventricular septum, tricuspid inflow is severely limited. Therefore, growth of the tricuspid valve is impaired with resultant right ventricular hypoplasia. The size of the branch pulmonary arteries in this group of patients is usually favorable, but pulmonary blood flow is ductal dependent (50). The principal features of pulmonary atresia with intact septum are depicted in Fig. 62-12. There is a spectrum of right ventricular and tricuspid valve hypoplasia in this population group, and decisions regarding treatment focus on whether the right ventricle is adequate to sustain the work of the pulmonary circulation or whether the patient will be better served moving along the single ventricle palliative tract.

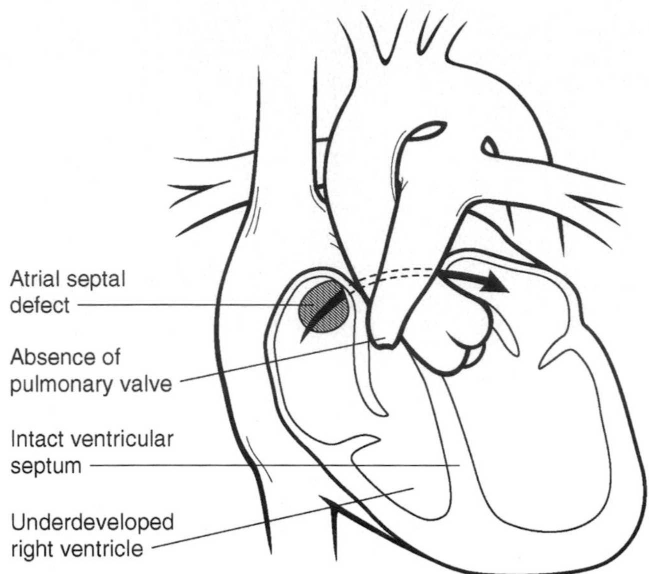

FIGURE 62-12. Pulmonary atresia with intact ventricular septum. Typical features of pulmonary atresia with intact ventricular septum are indicated here. It is believed that pulmonary atresia with intact septum is due primarily to absence of antigrade flow from the right ventricle. This results in hypoplasia of the right ventricular pumping chamber, as well as tricuspid valve hypoplasia. An atrial septal defect allows for right-to-left shunting maintenance of systemic blood flow. Ductal patency is maintained to provide pulmonary blood flow.

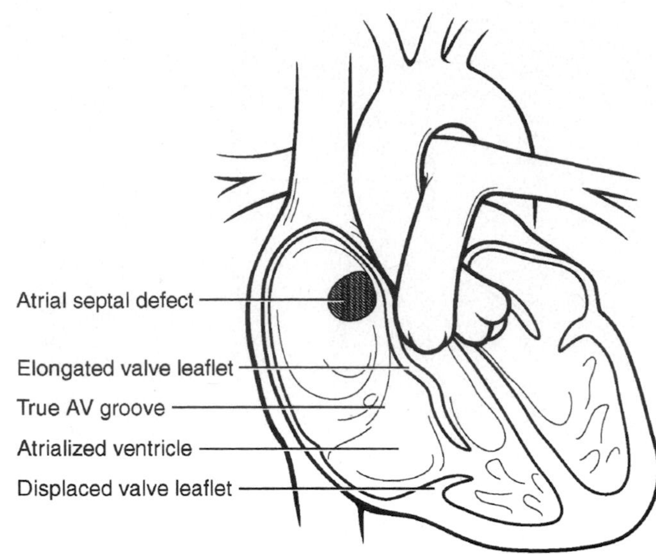

FIGURE 62-13. Displacement of the septal and posterior leaflets of the tricuspid valve associated with poorly functioning right ventricle and significant tricuspid insufficiency characterizes Epstein's anomaly. There is a broad spectrum of severity; some patients may be minimally impacted, whereas others may be symptomatic in the newborn period with evidence of right-sided failure and severe cyanosis. Cyanosis is due to inadequate antigrade flow from the dilated poorly contractile right ventricle combined with the right-to-left shunting across the atrial septal defect. AV, atrioventricular.

For those patients with a tricuspid valve that is not smaller than two standard deviations from normal and a right ventricle that is not severely hypoplastic, an intervention to open the pulmonary valve and right ventricular outflow tract, either surgical or transcatheter, may ultimately result in adequate pulmonary blood flow. Potential for growth of an initially hypoplastic right ventricle has been demonstrated and establishment of antegrade blood flow may promote growth of the tricuspid valve and right ventricle so two-ventricle repair might be possible. For patients with a severely hypoplastic tricuspid valve, less than two standard deviations below normal size, the likelihood of eventual two ventricle circulation is low. In addition, these patients can have abnormal connections between the right ventricular cavity and coronary arteries, usually the left anterior descending coronary artery. These connections are called coronary sinusoids and can be associated with proximal coronary artery stenosis. When coronary sinusoids are associated with proximal coronary stenosis, relief of right ventricular outflow tract obstruction in these patients will result in coronary steal and myocardial ischemia. Cardiac transplantation is recommended for this group because of the risk of sudden cardiac death as a result of coronary insufficiency.

Ebstein's anomaly is characterized by displacement of the septal and posterior leaflets of the tricuspid valve into the right ventricle resulting in tricuspid insufficiency. In addition, cephalad to the displaced tricuspid valve, is a portion of thinned right ventricle (atrialized right ventricle) that behaves like an aneurysm (Fig. 62-13). Ebstein's anomaly can be quite variable in its presentation as well as its severity (51). The clinical symptoms and physiology varies and depends on the degree of anatomic deformity of the tricuspid valve, along with the associated cardiac defects. With very mild displacement of the tricuspid valve and little or no tricuspid valve insufficiency, symptoms may be minimal or absent. In severe cases, cyanosis may be present due to right-to-left shunting across an ASD. In the neonatal period when PVR is elevated, shock may be present as the dysplastic right heart cannot maintain antegrade flow. As the PVR drops, the right ventricular function and tricuspid valve competence improve, and the infant may become less cyanotic. Twenty to 30% of patients with Ebstein's anomaly also have an accessory conduction pathway (Wolf-Parkinson-White syndrome) and may have associated supraventricular tachycardia.

Treatment must be individualized because the hemodynamic and physiologic abnormality is variable and depends on the associated anatomic abnormalities. In addition, the physiology can change with time. As stated previously, neonates with cyanosis may improve as the PVR decreases and may not need immediate intervention. If severe pulmonary stenosis or atresia is present, initial stabilization with PGE_1 may be necessary with a subsequent pulmonary valvotomy and systemic-to-pulmonary artery shunt. If symptoms of congestive heart failure secondary to severe tricuspid valve insufficiency are present, therapy with inotropic agents and diuretics may be necessary.

Surgical intervention is indicated for patients with Ebstein's anomaly who have severe tricuspid insufficiency and congestive heart failure, or who have persistence of cyanosis. Surgical repair includes tricuspid valvuloplasty, plication of the atrialized ventricle, closure of any ASD, and occasionally ablation of accessory conduction pathways. Surgery can be performed with good results. Some patients will require tricuspid valve replacement. Although a higher risk group, there is increasing success applying the techniques of tricuspid valve repair to the symptomatic neonate with Ebstein's anomaly (52).

Left Heart Hypoplasia

Coarctation of the aorta is a congenital narrowing of the aorta typically in the area of insertion of the ductus arteriosus at the junction of the distal aortic arch and proximal descending aorta. This narrowing results in a pressure gradient and proximal (upper extremity) hypertension and increased left ventricular developed pressure. Figure 62-14 shows the common forms of coarctation of the aorta: the juvenile or discrete form (Fig. 62-14a), which presents later in childhood, and the infantile form (Fig. 62-14b) associated with proximal arch hypoplasia that commonly presents during the newborn period. Neonates with severe coarctation of the aorta will present with shock and congestive heart failure and will require stabilization, including prostaglandins (53). Prostaglandins maintain ductal patency, allowing the right ventricle to support descending aortic blood flow. This allows for stabilization of the newborn followed by a complete evaluation of the extent of the defect. It is typical for these patients to have other lesions of the left side of the heart, such as distal arch hypoplasia, bicuspid aortic valve with or without aortic stenosis, and abnormalities of the mitral valve or subaortic region. Intervention is necessary for the relief of the obstruction. Surgical repair of coarctation is performed through a left thoracotomy and must also relieve any associated arch obstruction. A simple end-to-end anastomosis for relief of the discrete form of coarctation is shown in Fig. 62-14A. Figure 62-14B shows repair of coarctation of the aorta via using the extended end-to-end technique, which can be necessary to relieve proximal arch hypoplasia commonly present in newborns with coarctation. Recurrence of narrowing at the coarctation repair occurs in 10% of patients undergoing repair during infancy. Catheter intervention techniques are useful for recurrent narrowing at the site of previous surgical repair, but are rarely used as primary therapy in infants and children. The presence of coarctation is an indication for repair. Long-term proximal hypertension results in left ventricular hypertrophy, accelerated development of coronary artery disease, and an increased risk of cerebral aneurysms. Satisfactory repair in infancy is associated with a low risk of lifelong hypertension. In contrast, patients who undergo repair of coarctation beyond 12 months of age have an increased risk of chronic hypertension (54).

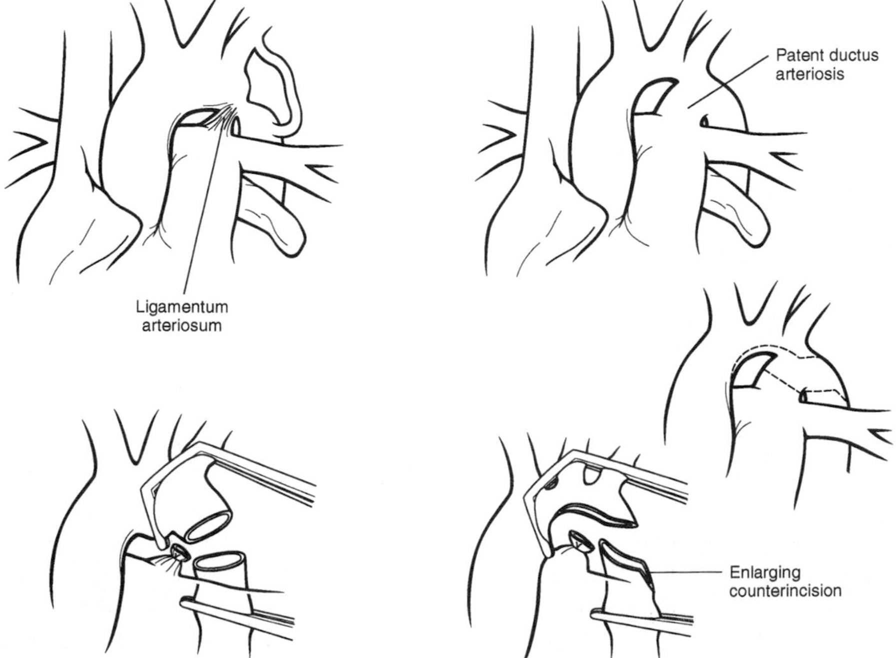

FIGURE 62-14. Coarctation of the aorta. (**A**) Coarctation of the aorta can present during childhood as depicted. Generally, this is a discrete coarctation, and commonly, there are large collateral vessels around the area of narrowing. Repair is accomplished by resection of the coarctation and end-to-end anastomosis. (**B**) The typical features of coarctation presenting during the neonatal period are depicted. Arch hypoplasia is nearly always present. Repair requires relief of distal arch hypoplasia using an extended end-to-end anastomosis.

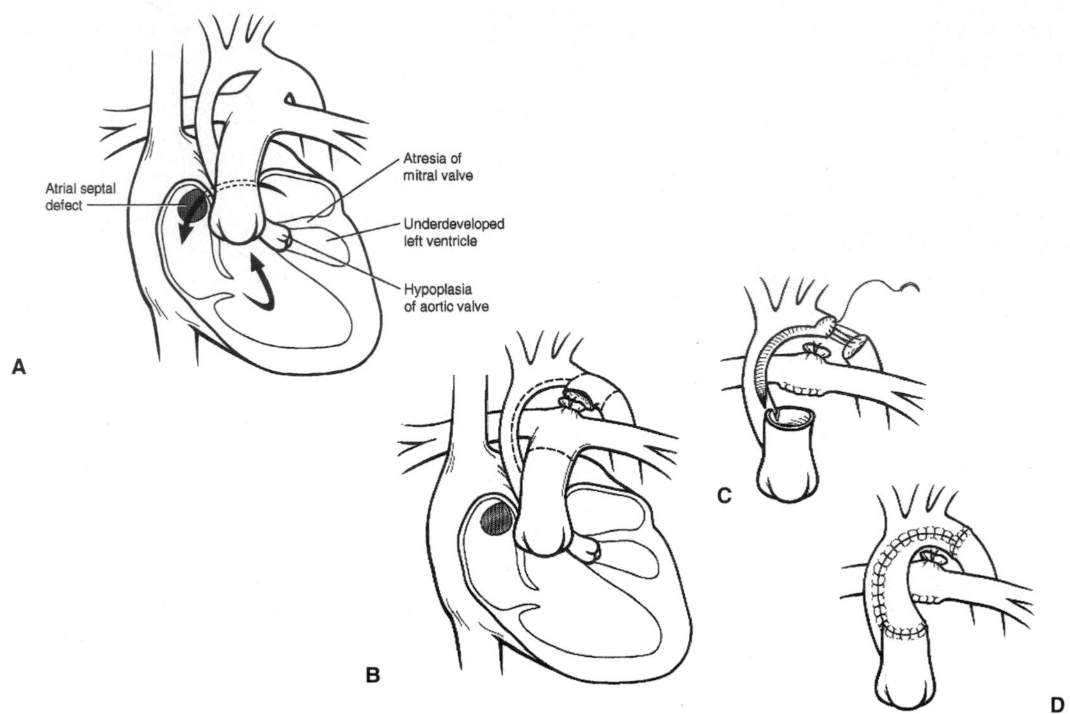

FIGURE 62-15. Hypoplastic left heart syndrome and the Norwood procedure. (**A**) Depicts the typical features of hypoplastic left heart syndrome, including complete underdevelopment of the left ventricle. An atrial septal defect is necessary to allow pulmonary venous return to enter the systemic circulation. Ductal patency is necessary to provide systemic output. (**B**) Surgery is performed using cardiopulmonary bypass and deep hypothermia. (**C**) The pulmonary outflow from the right ventricle is used to provide blood flow to the systemic circuit. (**D**) A connection is established between the ascending aorta, the pulmonary root, and the descending thoracic aorta, which is typically augmented with an additional patch of homograft as shown. In this way, permanent output from the right ventricle to the systemic circuit is constructed. A source of pulmonary blood flow, a Blalock-Taussig shunt is constructed during the final phase of the operation (not shown).

Hypoplastic left heart syndrome (HLHS) represents a continuum of congenital cardiac anomalies characterized by underdevelopment or atresia of aortic valve, mitral valve, and left ventricle, combined with hypoplasia of the aortic arch and coarctation. The extreme form is represented by aortic and mitral atresia, in which all output from the neonatal heart is from the right ventricle (Fig. 62-15a). As a consequence, systemic output is ductal dependent and the proximal arch, brachiocephalic vessels, and coronaries are supplied retrograde from the ductus arteriosus. Patients may present with congestive heart failure, tachypnea, and poor feeding secondary to excessive pulmonary blood flow. If the ductus arteriosus begins to close, the patients will have evidence of shock and low output in addition to congestive heart failure. Immediate measures to stabilize these patients include the use of prostaglandins to maintain ductal patency. If worsening congestive heart failure develops, neonates with HLHS are commonly intubated and PVR is intentionally elevated through medical gas manipulation in order to improve systemic output. These measures include hypoventilation or the addition of CO_2 to the circuit or the use of subatmospheric oxygen. These measures can restore systemic output with resultant resolution of acidosis and renal failure, thereby making the patient a candidate for surgical intervention.

The Norwood operation is the first-stage palliative approach for infants with HLHS (55) (Fig. 62-15). The Norwood procedure provides for a permanent unobstructed connection between the right ventricle and the systemic arteries. Pulmonary blood flow is provided either by a systemic to pulmonary artery shunt or a right ventricular to pulmonary artery shunt. In addition, a large ASD is created to prevent development of pulmonary venous obstruction. Subsequent surgical therapy is along a single ventricle pathway toward eventual Fontan anatomy. Current modifications in the surgical and postoperative approach have allowed experienced centers to achieve survival after the Norwood palliation in the 75% to 90% range (56,57).

The pulmonary venous plexus normally establishes connection with the left atrium at around 30 to 32 days of gestation. Following development of this connection, the pulmonary veins lose their connections with the systemic veins. If this process is interrupted, the pulmonary veins will continue to drain to the systemic veins returning eventually to the right atrium rather than the left atrium. This spectrum of anomalies is referred to as total anomalous pulmonary venous connection (58). In each patient, the details of the pulmonary venous return must be elucidated and typically can be diagnosed by echocardiography. There is potential for obstruction to pulmonary venous drainage at various sites, depending on the particular anatomic subgroup. These obstructive sites could include the atrial septum or the levocardinal vein as it crosses between the left mainstem bronchus and pulmonary artery. Anomalous pulmonary veins that drain below the diaphragm are uniformally obstructed to some degree as they course to the ligamentum venosum within the hepatic venous circulation. If obstruction to pulmonary venous drainage is present, the presenting symptoms include respiratory distress, hypoxemia, and a chest radiograph that shows a pulmonary venous obstructive pattern. Immediate surgical intervention is required in patients in this group. Patients without obstruction can undergo repair electively during the neonatal period or in early infancy.

Conotruncal Abnormalities

Conotruncal abnormalities involve maldevelopment of the outflow portion of the heart and proximal great vessels. This broad spectrum of lesions is unified by the frequent association with a deletion of the chromosome 22, specifically a 22q11 deletion. Conotruncal abnormalities include (1) tetralogy of Fallot in which there is anterior deviation of the outlet portion of the septum resulting in a large VSD, aortic override, and compensatory attenuation of the right ventricular outflow tract and pulmonary valve; (2) truncus arteriosus, which results from the failure of aorticopulmonary septation associated with a subarterial VSD; and (3) interrupted aortic arch with VSD in which there is posterior deviation of the outlet septum (opposite to tetralogy of Fallot) with hypoplasia of the left ventricular outflow tract and aortic valve. It is possible that a common genetic defect on the 22 chromosome results in aberrant formation of the outflow septum and aorticopulmonary septation that results in this spectrum of abnormalities. These defects are sometimes associated with DiGeorge syndrome also linked to abnormalities of the twenty-second chromosome. Features of DiGeorge syndrome include characteristic facies, athymia, hypocalcemia, and mental retardation. Although only rarely associated with 22q11 deletion, complete transposition of the great vessels, which results from failure of the aorticopulmonary septum to spiral as septation is completed, is also considered a conotruncal lesion.

Tetralogy of Fallot results from anterior deviation and underdevelopment of the outlet (infundibular) septum, resulting in a large perimembranous VSD, right ventricular outflow tract obstruction, and an aortic root that sits over the VSD with the secondary development of right ventricular hypertrophy, the classic tetrad of this lesion (Fig. 62-16). The severity may range from mild right ventricular outflow tract obstruction with physiology similar to an isolated VSD to complete absence of connection between the right ventricle and pulmonary arteries or pulmonary atresia. Tetralogy of Fallot was one of the first complex congenital heart lesions to be approached surgically. Prior to the development of open heart surgery, only palliation in the form of a systemic to pulmonary artery shunt was available for patients with tetralogy of Fallot. Following the development of cross-circulation and cardiopulmonary bypass, complete repair was performed with excellent early and late outcomes. Because of the difficulties of using early cardiopulmonary bypass equipment on infants, symptomatic infants and small children underwent initial palliation with a systemic to pulmonary artery shunt followed by complete repair when they were large enough to safely withstand cardiopulmonary bypass. Today palliative shunts are used rarely and then only in the newborn period. Results of complete repair of tetralogy of Fallot are excellent despite a decades long trend toward earlier surgery and the avoidance of initial palliation (59–62). Early complete repair also minimizes the occurrence

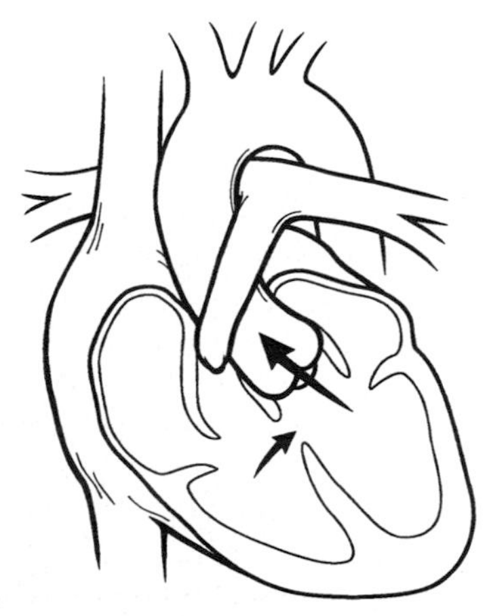

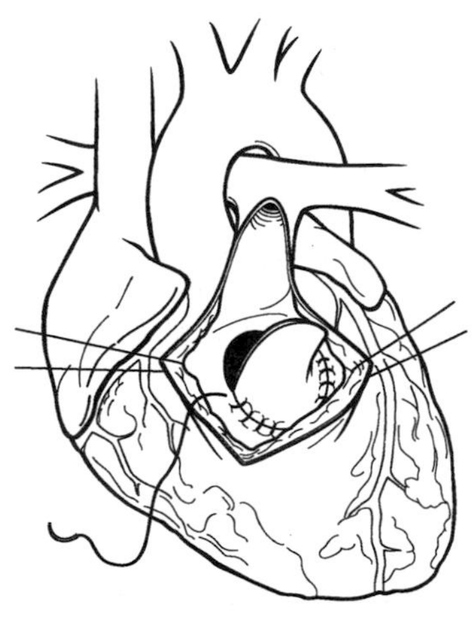

FIGURE 62-16. (**A**) The typical anatomic features of tetralogy of Fallot. There is underdevelopment of the right ventricular (RV) outflow tract and pulmonary valve. A ventricular septal defect is present, and commonly, there is shunting of desaturated blood from the right ventricle to the left ventricle. Repair involves relief of RV outflow tract obstruction, combined with closure of the ventricular septal defect. (**B**) Depicts an incision across the RV outflow tract into the main pulmonary artery; the ventricular septal defect is then closed through this exposure. A second patch is used to augment the RV outflow tract and proximal main pulmonary artery.

of hypercyanotic spells, which in and of itself may be associated with morbidity and mortality. Repair requires closure of the VSD and enlargement of the outflow tract between the right ventricle and the pulmonary artery. In the patients that have required a transannular patch (patch across the pulmonary valve annulus), severe pulmonary insufficiency is sometimes associated with the development of right ventricular dysfunction and ventricular arrhythmias originating from the right ventricular outflow tract. Some of these patients benefit from ablation of the origin of ventricular arrhythmias and/or placement of a valved conduit between the right ventricle and the pulmonary arteries.

The long-term outlook for patients with tetralogy of Fallot is promising. A more recent review of the outcomes of patients operated on during the period of cross-circulation, 1954 to 1955, showed that the majority did not require any additional cardiac intervention and are alive and well in NYHA heart failure class I or II.

Double-outlet right ventricle includes a variety of defects that have a VSD and origin of the majority of both great arteries from the right ventricle (63). The aorta and pulmonary arteries may be normally related, completely transposed, or intermediate. The VSD may be committed to (beneath) one or the other great vessels (subaortic or subpulmonary), committed to both (doubly committed), or remote from either great vessel (uncommitted). The detail of this variability determines the hemodynamics and the presenting symptoms of the specific patient, as well as the ultimate surgical repair. Therefore, it is possible that the patient with double-outlet right ventricle could have physiology similar to the patient with a large VSD, tetralogy of Fallot, or transposition of the great arteries. Despite the complexity of some of these defects, complete repair can be accomplished. This always entails closure of the VSD. In some instances, repair may also include an arterial switch or simultaneous repair of aortic coarctation. The specific repair depends on a careful analysis of the relationship of the VSD to the aorta, as well as the position and relationship of the great arteries to each other.

As the name implies, *truncus arteriosus* is the persistence of the truncal artery without division into a separate pulmonary artery and aorta. The pulmonary arteries arise directly off the truncal artery; the different types of truncus are classified on the basis of where the pulmonary artery arises from the truncal artery (Fig. 62-17). As PVR drops, excessive pulmonary blood flow occurs at the expense of systemic blood flow. The hemodynamics may rapidly deteriorate with resultant congestive heart failure and the development of compromised systemic output. Current practice and experience suggests that complete repair of this defect in the neonatal period is the preferred approach, and repair is planned as soon as the diagnosis is made (64). The pulmonary artery is detached from the truncal artery, the VSD is closed and continuity between the right ventricle and the pulmonary artery is established using a valved conduit, usually a homograft. Associated defects include abnormalities of the truncal valve most commonly truncal valve insufficiency. Figure 62-17 shows the repair of truncus arteriosus. A subset of patients with truncus arteriosus can also present with interrupted aortic arch. Among early survivors, long-term survival has been good and the majority of patients are in NYHA class I and II. A summary of results of 165 patients who survived truncus repair since 1975 has shown excellent survival and functional status (65).

Interrupted aortic arch is associated with posterior deviation of the infundibular septum (opposite to the anterior deviation associated with tetralogy of Fallot). As a result, there is a large perimembranous VSD and hypoplasia of the left ventricular outflow tract and aortic valve (Fig. 62-18). Patients can present with either (1) congestive heart failure due to pulmonary overcirculation as a consequence of the large VSD, or (2) shock/low output as a result of impending ductal closure. Therefore, prostaglandins are necessary to maintain ductal patency and perfusion of the lower body. Repair of both the interrupted aortic arch and VSD is performed as a single-stage procedure through a median sternotomy. Repair of the aortic arch is generally performed during deep hypothermia with or without continued perfusion to the cerebral circulation (66).

Transposition of the great arteries (TGA) is characterized by an abnormal connection between the ventricles and the great vessels such that the aorta arises from the right ventricle and the pulmonary artery arises from the left ventricle. Survival, even for a short period of time, is dependent on either a patent foramen ovale or a VSD to allow for mixing of pulmonary and systemic venous return so there is adequate systemic oxygen delivery. The majority of neonates with TGA have no extracardiac congenital defects. With the exception of the malpositioned great vessels and a VSD in 25% of patients with transposition, the heart itself is well formed with balanced ventricles and well-developed, competent atrioventricular valves. For neonates with TGA and excessive cyanosis, enlargement of the ASD via a balloon atrial septostomy will result in improved mixing, less cyanosis, and hemodynamic stabilization.

The arterial switch procedure, in which the great arteries (including the coronary arteries) are transferred to their appropriate ventricular connections, is the treatment of choice (Fig. 62-19). It is recommended that this procedure be performed within the first 2 weeks of life, before the PVR drops. Once the PVR decreases, there is a concomitant decrease in left ventricular systolic pressure; the left ventricle becomes deconditioned, and therefore, cannot pump against systemic afterload. Early results of the arterial switch are excellent with mortality in the 2% range (67). There is a small incidence of late death (3%) in the first 5 years following surgery presumably due to coronary

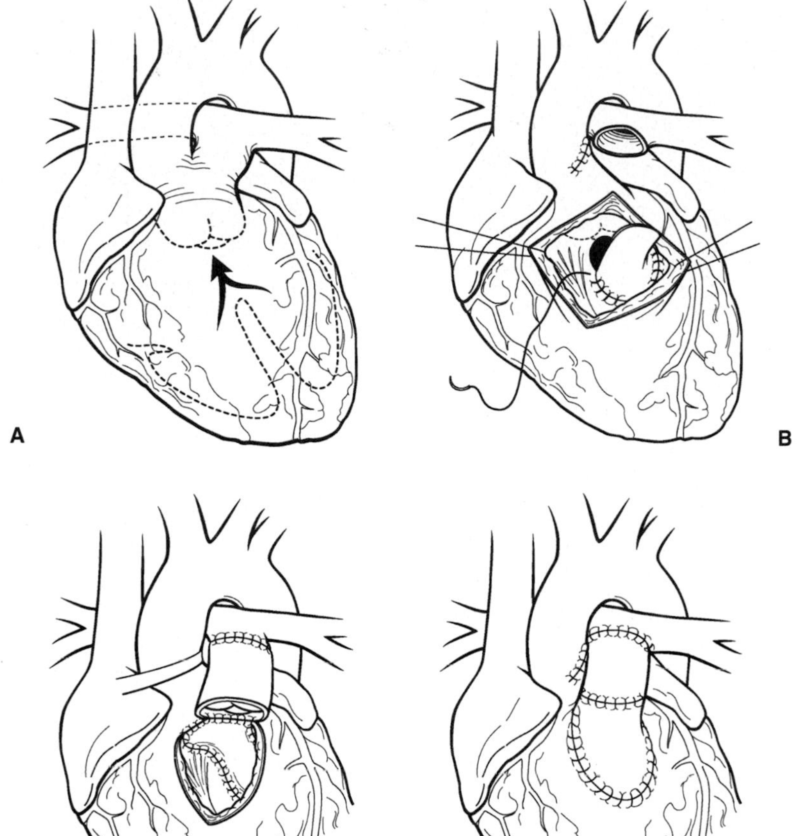

FIGURE 62-17. Truncus arteriosus. (**A**) Typical anatomic findings in truncus arteriosus. There is a common arterial trunk arising above a ventricular septal defect. Arterial venous ad mixture is pumped through the common atrioventricular (AV) valves, and patients may present with cyanosis, congestive heart failure, or both. (**B**) The initial steps of repair involve detaching the pulmonary arteries from the truncal artery. A ventriculotomy is then performed and the ventricular septal defect closed routing the left ventricular blood through the truncal artery to the aorta. (**C, D**) An RV to PA conduit is then used to establish RV to PA continuity.

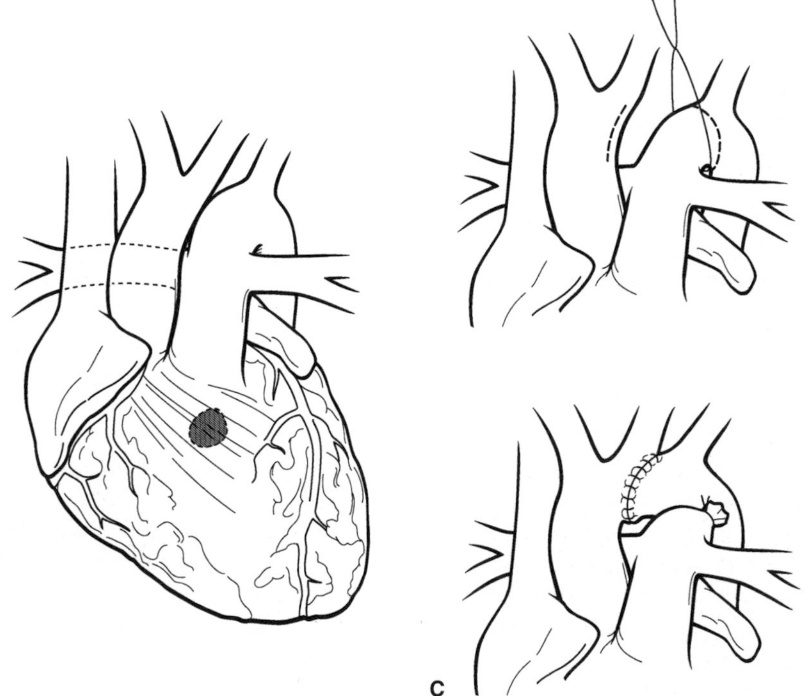

FIGURE 62-18. (**A**) Typical features of interrupted aortic arch. In this case, the left ventricle connects to an aorta, which terminates in the innominate artery and left common carotid artery. A ventricular septal defect shunts from the left side to the right side, and systemic output to the lower half of the body is maintained via the patent ductus arteriosus. Repair involves the use of bypass and deep hypothermia; the ventricular septal defect is closed (not shown). (**B**) The ductus arteriosus ligated. (**C**) The aortic arch is reconstructed.

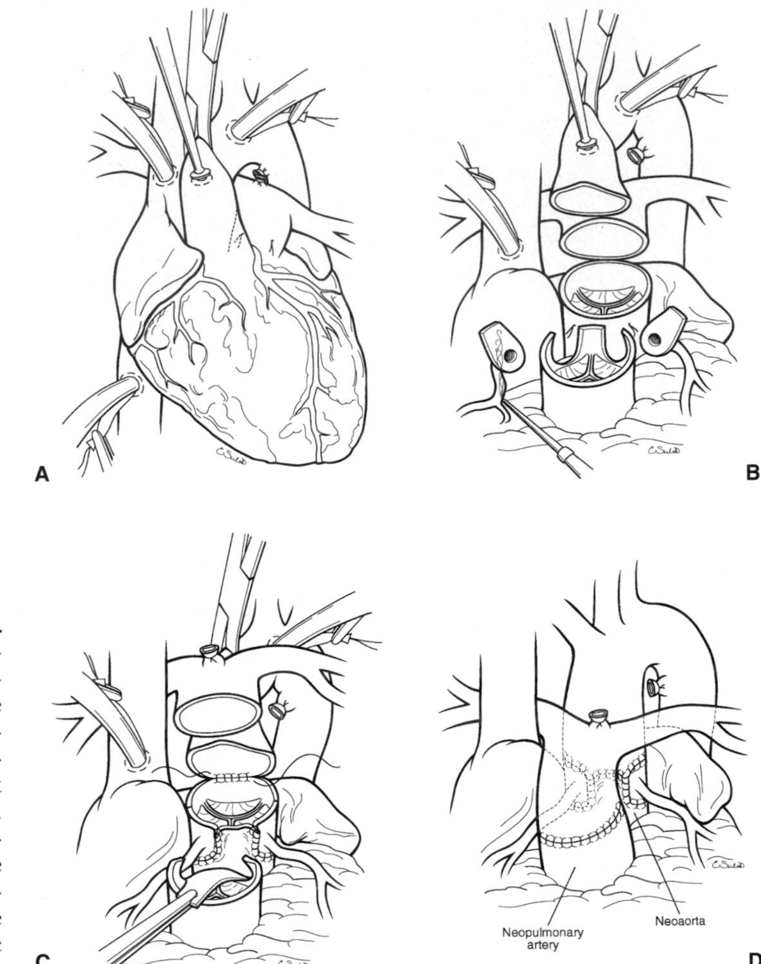

FIGURE 62-19. The arterial switch procedure for transposition of the great vessels. (**A**) Typical anatomic findings of transposition. The aorta arises anteriorly from the right ventricle, and the pulmonary artery arises posteriorly from the left ventricle. (**B**) After establishing cardiopulmonary bypass and cardioplegic arrest, the great vessels are transected; coronary ostial buttons are excised. (**C**) The coronary ostial buttons are then rotated posteriorly and implanted in the posterior great vessel. (**D**) The pulmonary artery confluence is brought in front of the ascending aorta (the LeCompte) maneuver and finally the pulmonary artery reconstructed in front of the neoaortic root.

insufficiency (68). There is also a tenfold increase in the likelihood of developing aortic insufficiency, compared with the general population, at 15 years of follow-up (69).

OUTCOMES AND CHALLENGES

Outcomes for children with congenital heart disease have improved significantly in a relatively short period of time. As described previously, severe abnormalities including those such as hypoplastic left heart syndrome, have until more recently been associated with a very high mortality, but currently have an expected survival in the 80% to 90% range after stage 1 palliation. As the population of patients with repaired congenital heart disease increases, attention has turned from simple survival to assessment of growth, development, and quality of life. Learning disabilities are being increasingly identified in survivors after repair of congenital heart disease. Neurodevelopmental sequelae are likely due to a combination of, or interaction between, neurologic abnormalities coexistent with the heart defect, sequelae of neurologic injury occurring before successful surgical intervention, and the adverse neurologic impact of surgery and cardiopulmonary bypass. Patients who have undergone repair of even simple congenital heart defects require lifelong follow-up and are at risk for late sequelae. For example, patients who have undergone repair of tetralogy of Fallot remain at risk for right ventricular dysfunction and life-threatening arrhythmias. Even patients with repaired VSDs require lifelong surveillance to identify potential conduction system abnormalities. Occlusion of a PDA and possibly closure of an ASD represent the only "curative" procedures we can offer to patients with congenital heart defects. Even the optimistic view that patients with secundum ASDs are cured has more recently been brought into question. A retrospective study of patients undergoing surgical intervention for ASD was found to have lower IQ compared with patients undergoing interventional catheterization device closure of the same type of defect. Despite the risk of developmental delay and the ongoing risk for the need for reintervention, quality-of-life studies among patients with repaired congenital heart disease suggest that they generally lead happy and productive lives (70–72).

The increasing population and age of survivors of congenital heart disease has spawned the development of a new specialty, adult congenital heart disease, to manage ongoing medical issues, such as the identification and treatment of residual or recurrent cardiac lesions, as well as issues complicated by the presence of repaired congenital heart disease such as pregnancy. Ongoing issues for survivors of congenital heart disease include access to health insurance without exclusion for preexisting conditions, as well as life insurance for a population whose long-term outlook is unknown. It is anticipated that the needs of adults with congenital heart disease will grow and coordination of care of these patients will be critical.

REFERENCES

1. Fyler DC. Report of the New England regional infant cardiac program. *Pediatrics* 1980;65(suppl):375–461.
2. Ferencz C, Rubin JD, Loffredo CA, et al. *Epidemiology of congenital heart disease: the Baltimore-Washington Infant Study 1981–1989.* Mount Kisco, NY: Futura, 1993.
3. Magee CA, Loffredo CA, Correa-Villansenor A, et al. Environmental factors in occupations, home and hobbies. In: Ferencz C, Rubin JD, Loffredo CA, et al. (eds.), *Epidemiology of congenital heart disease: the Baltimore-Washington Infant Study 1981–1989.* Mount Kisco, NY: Futura, 1993.
4. Pediatric Health Information System (PHIS). 2002. Child Health Corporation of America (CHCA).
5. Moller JH, Allen HD, Clark EB, et al. Report of the task force on children and youth. *Circulation* 1992;88:2479–2486.
6. Ferencz C, Rubin JD, Loffredo CA, et al. Maternal medical anthropometric characteristics. In: Ferencz C, Rubin JD, Loffredo CA, et al. (eds.), *Epidemiology of congenital heart disease: the Baltimore-Washington Infant Study 1981–1989.* Mount Kisco, NY: Futura, 1993.
7. Clark EB. Epidemiology of congenital cardiovascular malformations. In: Moss, Adams (eds.), *Heart disease in infants, children and adolescents,* 5th ed. Baltimore: Williams & Wilkins, 1995.
8. Burn J, Goodship J. *Principles and practice of medical genetics,* 3rd ed. New York: Churchill Livingstone, 1996.
9. Robinson PN, Booms P. The molecular pathogenesis of the Marfan syndrome. *Cell Mol Life Sci* 2001 Oct;58(11):1698–1707.
10. Bruyere HJ Jr, Kargas SA, Levy JM. The causes and underlying developmental mechanisms of congenital cardiovascular malformations: a critical review. *Am J Med Genet Suppl* 1987;3:411–431.
11. Payne RM, Johnson MC, Grant JW, et al. Toward a molecular understanding of congenital heart disease. *Circulation* 1995 Jan 15;91(2):494–504.
12. Schott, J-J, Benson D, Woodrow B, et al. Congenital heart disease caused by mutations in the transcription factor NKX2-5. *Science* 1998;281:108–111.
13. Li QY, Newbury-Ecob RA, Terrett JA, et al. Holt-Oram syndrome is caused by mutations in TBX5, a member of the Brachyury (T) gene family. *Nat Genet* 1997;Jan;15(1):21–29.
14. Moss AJ. Long QT syndrome. *JAMA* 2003;289:2041–2044.
15. Hamada H, Meno C, Watanabe D, et al. Establishment of vertebrate left–right asymmetry. *Nat Rev Genet* 2002;3:103–113.
16. Sadler TW. *Langman's medical embryology,* 9th ed. Philadelphia: Lippincott Williams & Wilkins, 2003:223–274.
17. Snider RR, Serwer GA. *Echocardiography in pediatric heart disease.* Chicago: Year Book Medical Publishers, 1990.
18. Silverman NH. *Pediatric echocardiography.* Baltimore: Williams & Wilkins, 1993.
19. Bargeron LM, Elliot LP, Bream PR, et al. Axial cineangiography in congenital heart disease. I: concept, technical and anatomic considerations. *Circulation* 1977;56:1075–1083.
20. Gross RE, Hubbard JP. Surgical ligation of a patent ductus arteriosus: report of first successful case. *JAMA* 1939;112:729–731.
21. Crafoord C, Nylin G. Congenital coarctation of the aorta and its surgical management. *J Thorac Surg* 1945;14:347–361.
22. Blalock A, Taussig HB. The surgical treatment of malformations of the heart in which there is pulmonary stenosis or pulmonary atresia. *JAMA* 1945;128:189.
23. Muller WH Jr, Dammann JF Jr. The treatment of certain congenital malformations of the heart by creation of pulmonary stenosis to reduce pulmonary hypertension and excessive pulmonary blood flow: a preliminary report. *Surg Gyenocol Obstet* 1952;95:213.
24. Blalock A, Hanlon CR. Surgical treatment of complete transposition of the aorta and pulmonary artery. *Surg Gynecol Obstet* 1950;90:1.
25. Baffes TG. A new method for surgical correction of transposition of the aorta and pulmonary artery. *Surg Gynecol Obstet* 1956;102:227.
26. Rashkind WJ, Miller WW. Creation of an atrial septal defect without thoracotomy: a palliative approach to complete transposition of the great vessels. *JAMA* 1966;196:991.
27. Lewis FJ, Taufic M. Closure of atrial septal defects with the aid of hypothermia: experimental accomplishments and the report of one successful case. *Surgery* 1953;33:52–59.
28. Swan H, Zeavin I, Blount SG Jr, et al. Surgery by direct vision in the open heart during hypothermia. *JAMA* 1953;153:1081–1085.
29. Gross RE, Pomeranz AA, Watkins E Jr, et al. Surgical closure of defects of the interauricular septum by the atrial well. *N Engl J Med* 1952;257:455–460.
30. Warden HE, Cohen M, Read RC, et al. Controlled cross circulation for open intracardiac surgery. *J Thorac Surg* 1954;28:331–343.
31. Lillehei CW, Varco RL, Cohen M, et al. The first open-heart repairs of ventricular septal defect, atrioventricular connumis, and tetralogy of Fallot using extracorporeal circulation by cross circulation: a 30-year follow-up. *Ann Thorac Surg* 1986;41:4–21.
32. Gibbon JH Jr. Application of a mechanical heart and lung apparatus to cardiac surgery. *Minn Med* 1954;37:171–185.
33. Myer JE. Cardiopulmonary bypass. In: Chang AC, Hanley FL, Wernovsky G, et al., eds. Pediatric intensive care. Baltimore: Williams & Wilkins, 1998:189–200.
34. David C, Bellinger D, Wypij K, et al. Developmental and neurological status of children at 4 years of age after heart surgery with hypothermic circulatory arrest or low-flow cardiopulmonary bypass. *Circulation* 1999;100:526–532.
35. Kim JJ, Hijazi ZM. Clinical outcomes and costs of Amplatzer transcatheter closure as compared with surgical closure of secundum atrial septal defects. *Med Sci Monit* 2002;8(12):787–791.
36. Onorato E, Melzi G, Casilli F, et al. Patent foramen ovale with paradoxical embolus: mid-term results of transcatheter closure in 256 patients. *J Interv Cardiol* 2003;16(1):43–50.
37. Pham JT, Carlos MA. Current treatment strategies of symptomatic patent ductus arteriosus. *J Pediatr Health Care* 2002;16:306–310.
38. Lloyd TR, Fedderly R, Mendelsohn AM, et al. Transcatheter occlusion of patent ductus arteriosus with Gianturco coils. *Circulation* 1993;88(4 Pt 1):1412–1420.
39. Shim D, Fedderly RT, Beekman RH, et al. Follow-up coil occlusion of patent ductus arteriosus. *J Am Coll Cardiol* 1996;28(1):207–211.
40. Lin MH, Wang NK, Hung KL, et al. Spontaneous closure of ventricular septal defects in the first year of life. *J Formos Med Assoc* 2001;100(8):539–542.
41. Clarkson PM, Frye RL, DuShane JW, et al. Prognosis for patients with ventricular septal defect and severe pulmonary vascular obstructive disease. *Circulation* 1968;38:129.
42. Hijazi ZM, Hakim F, Haweleh AA, et al. Catheter closure of perimembranous ventricular septal defects using the new Amplatzer membranous VSD occluder: initial clinical experience. *Catheter Cardiovasc Interv* 2002;56(4):508–515.
43. Tweddell JS, Litwin SB, Berger S, et al. Twenty-year experience with repair of complete atrioventricular septal defects. *Ann Thorac Surg* 1996;62:419–424.
44. Hagler DJ, Edwards WD. Univentricular atrioventricular connection. In: Moss, Adams, eds. *Heart disease in infants, children and adolescents,* 5th ed. Baltimore: Williams & Wilkins, 1995.
45. Fontan F, Baudet E. Surgical repair of tricuspid atresia. *Thorax* 1971;26(3):240–249.
46. Glenn WW, Gardner TH Jr, Talner NS, et al. Rational approach to the surgical management of tricuspid atresia. *Circulation* 1968; 37(4 Suppl II):62–67.

47. Tweddell JS, Litwin SB, Thomas JP, et al. Recent advances in the surgical management of the single ventricle patient. *Pediatr Clin North Am* 1999;46(2):465–480.
48. Sade RM, Fyfe DA. Tricuspid atresia: current concepts in diagnosis and treatment. *Pediatr Clin North Am* 1990 Feb;37(1):151–169.
49. Kutsche LM, Van Mierop LH. Pulmonary atresia with and without ventricular septal defect: a different etiology and pathogenesis for the atresia in the 2 types? *Am J Cardiol* 1983 Mar 15;51(6):932–935.
50. Freedom RM. Pulmonary atresia and intact ventricular septum. In: Moss, Adams, *Heart disease in infants, children and adolescents,* 5th ed. Baltimore: Williams & Wilkins, 1995.
51. Epstein ML. Congenital stenosis and insufficiency of the tricuspid valve. In: Moss, Adams, eds. *Heart disease in infants, children and adolescents.* 5th ed. Baltimore: Williams & Wilkins, 1995.
52. Knott-Craig CJ, Overholt ED, Ward KE, et al. Repair of Ebstein's anomaly in the symptomatic neonate: an evolution of technique with 7-year follow-up. *Ann Thorac Surg* 2002 Jun;73(6):1786–1792.
53. Beekman RH. Coarctation of the aorta. In: Moss, Adams, eds. *Heart disease in infants, children and adolescents,* 5th ed. Baltimore: Williams & Wilkins, 1995.
54. Celermajer DS, Greaves K. Survivors of coarctation repair: fixed but not cured. *Heart* 2002;88:113–114.
55. Norwood WI, Lang P, Hansen D. Physiologic repair of aortic atresia–hypoplastic left heart syndrome. *N Engl J Med* 1983;308:23.
56. Tweddell JS, Hoffman GM, Mussatto KM, et al. Improved survival of patients undergoing palliation of hypoplastic left heart syndrome: lessons learned from 115 consecutive patients. *Circulation* 2002;106(12 Suppl I):82–89.
57. Tweddell JS, Hoffman GM, Fedderly RT, et al. Patients at risk for low systemic oxygen delivery after the Norwood procedure. *Ann Thorac Surg* 2000;69(6):1893–1899.
58. Krabill KA, Lucas RV. Abnormal pulmonary venous connections. In: Moss, Adams, eds. *Heart disease in infants, children and adolescents,* 5th ed. Baltimore: Williams & Wilkins, 1995.
59. Kirklin JW, Blackstone EH, Pacifico AD, et al. Routine primary repair vs. two-stage repair of tetralogy of Fallot. *Circulation* 1979;60:373–386.
60. Kirklin JW, Blackstone EH, Jonas RA, et al. Morphologic and surgical determinants of outcome events after repair of tetralogy of Fallot and pulmonary stenosis: a two institution study. *J Thorac Cardiovasc Surg* 1992;103:706.
61. Vobecky SJ, Williams WG, Trusler GA, et al. Survival analysis of infants under age 18 months presenting with tetralogy of Fallot. *Ann Thorac Surg* 1993;56:944.
62. Uva MS, Lacour-Gayet F, Komiya T, et al. Surgery for tetralogy of Fallot at less than six months of age. *J Thorac Cardiovasc Surg* 1994;107:1291.
63. Ungerleider RM. Double outlet right ventricle. In: Sabiston DC Jr, ed. *Surgery of the chest*. Philadelphia: Hanley & Belfus, 1989:91.
64. Mavroudis C, Backer CL. Truncus arteriosus. In: Mavroudis C, Backer CL, eds. *Pediatric cardiac surgery.* St. Louis, MO: Mosby, 1994:237.
65. Rajasinghe HA, McElhinney DB, Reddy VM, et al. Long-term follow-up of truncus arteriosus repaired in infancy: a twenty-year experience. *J Thorac Cardiovasc Surg* 1997:113(5);869–878; discussion 878–879.
66. Menahem S, Rahayoe AU, Brawn WJ, et al. Interrupted aortic arch in infancy: a 10-year experience. *Pediatr Cardiol* 1992;13:214–221.
67. Lupinetti FM, Bove EL, Minich LL, et al. Intermediate-term survival and functional results after arterial repair for transposition of the great arteries. *J Thorac Cardiovasc Surg* 1992;103:421.
68. Wernovsky G, Mayer JE Jr, Jonas RA, et al. Factors influencing early and late outcome of the arterial switch operation for transposition of the great arteries. *J Thorac Cardiovasc Surg* 1995 Feb;109(2):289–301.
69. Losay J, Touchot A, Serraf A, et al. Late outcome after arterial switch operation for transposition of the great arteries. *Circulation* 2001 Sep 18;104(12 Suppl 1):1121–1126.
70. Mussatto KA, Frisbee SJ, Sachdeva RC, et al. (2002). Subjects with surgically treated complex congenital heart disease report health related quality of life equal to healthy peers. *J Am Coll Cardiol* 2002; 39(5 supp. A):413A.
71. Williams DL, Gelijns AC, Moskowitz AJ, et al. Hypoplastic left heart syndrome: valuing the survival. *J Thorac Cardiovasc Surg* 2000 Apr;119(4 Pt 1):720–731.
72. Dunbar-Masterson C, Wypij D, Bellinger DC. General health status of children with D-transposition of the great arteries after the arterial switch operation. *Circulation* 2001 Sep 18;104(12 Suppl 1):1138–1142.

Chapter 63

Pericardium and Great Vessels

Walter Pegoli, Jr.

PERICARDIUM

Embryology

The pericardial sac begins to take shape early in the fourth week of gestation. Clefts in the embryonic mesoderm develop and ultimately separate the somatic and splanchnic components. These individual clefts coalescence and form a single cavity. The central region of this cavity becomes the pericardial space, and the lateral aspects eventually form the pleural cavities. The floor of the pericardial cavity contains a layer of splanchnopleure that develops into the cardiogenic plate. This plate ultimately forms the myocardium and the visceral pericardium.

Early in gestation, the pericardial cavity is large, and the pleural cavities are relatively small. With development of the fetal lungs, the size of the pleural cavities increases rapidly. Abnormalities in the formation of the pleuropericardial membrane result in pericardial defects. These defects are attributable to abnormal organogenesis during the fifth week of gestation. Most abnormalities are located on the left side.

Anatomy

The pericardium surrounds the heart and is lined by simple squamous epithelium or mesothelium. It has both visceral and parietal layers. The visceral pericardium is intimately associated with the heart; the parietal pericardium forms the sac. The two components of the pericardium are contiguous at the sites where great vessels enter and exit the heart. The area between the visceral and parietal pericardia is the pericardial space. The pericardial space is filled with a small volume of serous fluid that acts as a lubricant.

The anterior pericardium separates the heart from the sternum. The posterior pericardium is adjacent to the esophagus and thoracic aorta. Superiorly, the pericardium separates the heart from the thymus. The inferior pericardium is contiguous with the central tendon and anterior aspect of the diaphragm. Laterally, the pericardium and the parietal pleura are in intimate contact.

The blood supply to the pericardium is derived from branches of the internal thoracic arteries and the descending thoracic aorta. The venous drainage is through the azygous system. The sympathetic trunks and the phrenic and vagus nerves innervate the pericardium. Lymph drains through the thoracic duct and the right lymphatic duct. The absorptive capacity of the pericardium is limited. Therefore, situations that increase fluid formation, such as inflammatory states, can lead to pericardial effusions.

Physiology

The pericardium performs several important functions. It fixes the heart anatomically within the thorax, it minimizes the friction between the heart and surrounding structures during the cardiac cycle, it prevents mechanical distortion of the great vessels, and it helps prevent spread of infection from contiguous sites. Because collagen is the major structural component, the pericardium has a limited ability to distend acutely. When the contents of the pericardial sac exceed a particular volume, a point of pericardial nonextensibility is reached, and the pericardium limits cardiac filling and therefore cardiac output. This is the physiologic basis for tamponade. Clinical evidence for tamponade includes the Beck triad: (1) elevated central venous pressure (distended neck veins); (2) a small, quiet heart (diminished QRS-complex amplitude); and (3) systemic hypotension. A paradoxical pulse may be demonstrated on physical examination. Experiments in dogs have shown that hydrostatic distending pressures of 3 to 8 mm Hg can produce a noncompliant pericardium and result in tamponade (1). In children, the most frequent condition that produces a pericardial effusion that exceeds pericardial reserve volume is a viral infection. Chronic pericardial effusions of considerably greater size can be tolerated without physiologic decompensation because the pericardium is

Walter Pegoli, Jr.: Pediatric Surgery, University of Rochester School of Medicine and Dentistry, Rochester, New York 14642.

capable of modest distention without hydrostatic pressure increases under these conditions.

Anatomic Defects

Anatomic defects in the pericardium are uncommon and usually occur on the left side. These defects communicate with the ipsilateral pleural space. If the defect is large, segments of the heart or the entire heart can be located within the pleural space. More often, a small portion of the heart is herniated into the pleural space, most commonly the auricular appendage. The phrenic nerve usually courses along the anterior margin of these smaller defects.

Pericardial defects are often associated with cardiac anomalies; the most common are the tetralogy of Fallot, patent ductus arteriosus (PDA), mitral valve prolapse, and mitral stenosis. Bronchogenic cysts and enteric cysts are also associated with these defects. The Cantrell pentalogy is present when pericardial defects are associated with diaphragmatic defects, abdominal wall defects, lower sternal defects, and intracardiac abnormalities.

Most patients with pericardial defects do not have symptoms. Chest pain, shortness of breath, dizziness, and hemoptysis can occur with cardiac displacement, however, and sudden death with cardiac herniation and strangulation has been described.

On physical examination, patients exhibit a systolic murmur, accompanied by a shift of the point of maximal cardiac impulse to the side of the defect. Electrocardiographic findings can include right-axis deviation, incomplete right bundle branch block, or right ventricular hypertrophy. On plain chest radiograph, there is elongation of the left heart border. Echocardiography is routinely done, but is relatively nonspecific. The finding of a left atrial aneurysm should raise the possibility of a partial pericardial defect. The diagnosis of a pericardial defect is most reliably established with computed tomography (CT) or magnetic resonance (MR) imaging.

Patients with large or complete pericardial defects have little or no potential for herniation and strangulation, and are not considered for surgical intervention. Patients with partial defects are at risk for cardiac herniation and sudden death. These patients should undergo surgical reconstruction by enlarging the defect, resecting the pericardium, or patching the defect with prosthetic material or local tissue transfer.

Pericardial Cysts and Diverticula

Diverticula or cystic sequestrations of the pericardium typically occur at the cardiophrenic angle. Like the pericardium itself, they are lined by simple squamous epithelium and filled with serous fluid.

Pericardial cysts and diverticula have a male predominance and are twice as likely to occur on the right side. Ninety percent are unilocular; the remainder are multilocular. Although most patients with these findings do not have symptoms, precordial or substernal chest pain, dyspnea, and chronic nonproductive cough have been noted. Complications of pericardial cysts are rare. As with any benign cystic lesion, infection, rupture, and compression of adjacent structures from local enlargement can occur. Malignancy is rare. These cysts are not known to regress spontaneously.

On plain chest radiograph, the typical pericardial cyst appears as a smooth, rounded mass in the region of the cardiophrenic angle. The differential diagnosis includes foramen of Morgagni hernia, mediastinal cystic hygroma, and mediastinal teratoma. As for most thoracic structural anomalies, contrast-enhanced CT is a sensitive diagnostic tool. The lesion is seen as a thin-walled oval or tubular structure filled with fluid. It typically displaces rather than infiltrates surrounding structures.

Surgical excision is advised for these lesions. Resection is both diagnostic and prophylactic. When symptomatic, cysts should certainly be removed. The blood supply is limited so the cyst can be excised without difficulty. Diverticula require ligation and removal. This is technically straightforward and either a conventional transthoracic or a thoracoscopic approach can be used (2). Aspiration has been performed in high-risk patients, using either fluoroscopic or ultrasonographic guidance; however, recurrence is an important concern with this approach. In one 3-year follow-up of a small group of patients who underwent aspiration, no recurrences were reported (3).

Infections

The classic clinical triad for acute pericarditis includes chest pain, pericardial friction rub, and electrocardiographic abnormalities. The most common causes of acute pericarditis in children are viral infection, bacterial infection, uremia, and trauma. Precordial pain is characteristic of the acute condition. The onset usually coincides with fever, but can follow a shaking chill. The pain is usually intensified by respiration, coughing, swallowing, or lying the supine position. In some patients, the pain is diminished by the assumption of an upright position.

Specific Forms of Viral Pericarditis

Acute viral pericarditis can follow infection with the coxsackievirus B, echovirus 8, mumps, Ebstein-Barr virus, influenza, poliomyelitis, or varicella virus. Patients with infectious mononucleosis can present with acute pericarditis and cardiac tamponade followed by progressive pericardial restriction. Viral pericarditis evokes significant inflammation. The inflammatory process can be serous, serofibrinous, fibrinous, suppurative, hemorrhagic, or some combination of these. Viral pericarditis is usually of the fibrinous or serofibrinous variety; suppurative pericarditis is often the result of bacterial infection. With resolution of the acute process, the fibrin either undergoes fibrinolysis or becomes organized to obliterate the pericardial space. The latter outcome is more frequent after severe infections.

Patients with viral pericarditis usually have an antecedent history of an upper respiratory tract infection. Seventy percent of patients have temperatures as high as 39°C. Pleuritic chest pain, a pericardial friction rub, cough, and a pericardial effusion are common. The pericardial fluid typically is clear and serous, resolving spontaneously in most cases.

A specific virus rarely can be retrieved from pericardial fluid, stool, or blood. The diagnosis is commonly established by demonstrating a fourfold increase in serial neutralizing antibody titers in serum. The electrocardiogram may demonstrate sequential ST-T-segment and T-wave changes. Sinus tachycardia is often present (4). Atrial and ventricular arrhythmias result from inflammation of the underlying myocardium. In otherwise healthy children, the differential diagnosis should include blunt chest trauma, systemic lupus erythematosus, rheumatic pericarditis, and bacterial endocarditis.

Patients with viral pericarditis have no symptoms for about 1 to 2 weeks. Those with coxsackievirus or echovirus infections are at particular risk for myocarditis with cardiac insufficiency and cardiomegaly. The cardiac dysfunction can resolve completely or result in persistent physiologic dysfunction that can take the form of chronic ventricular failure or even sudden death. Patients with coxsackievirus infections are at risk for the development of coronary artery aneurysms and therefore require vigorous and regular follow-up.

The basic treatment for patients with acute viral pericarditis is bed rest and analgesics. Specific antiviral agents are not available for the responsible pathogens. During the acute phase, patients should be observed for evidence of cardiac tamponade, myocarditis, and heart failure. Patients with significant pain are treated with a 3- to 7-day course of systemic steroids. In patients with mild symptoms, aspirin or indomethacin are adequate. This therapy generally results in the rapid resolution of symptoms within 12 to 24 hours.

Bacterial Pericarditis

Children who present with bacterial pericarditis commonly have a history of acute pharyngitis, pneumonia, meningitis, otitis media, anemia, impetigo, or purulent arthritis. The most common organism is *Staphylococcus aureus,* followed in frequency by *Haemophilus influenzae* type B, *Neisseria meningitidis,* other gram-negative organisms, *Streptoccocus pneumoniae,* and β-hemolytic streptococcal organisms.

Bacterial pericarditis presents as an acute illness with high fever, shaking chills, dyspnea, night sweats, and cough. Chest pain is an uncommon symptom. Patients can manifest tachycardia, a pericardial friction rub, pulsus paradoxicus, and in severe cases, systemic hypotension. The white blood cell count usually exceeds 17,000 cells per μL, with a shift toward immature forms on the differential count.

A plain chest radiograph may show findings that correlate with the cause. In particular, pulmonary parenchymal disease, pneumonia, pleural effusion, or mediastinal widening may be evident radiographically. Nonspecific ST-T-wave changes are present on electrocardiogram. The leukocyte count of the pericardial fluid is usually greater than 50,000 cells per μL, consisting mostly of polymorphonuclear leukocytes; the glucose level is usually less than 35 mg per dL; and the protein content is more than 3 g per dL (5).

Antibiotic therapy alone is inadequate treatment for acute bacterial pericarditis. Mortality rates are reduced by surgical drainage combined with appropriate antibiotic treatment. The initial antibiotic coverage should include an agent effective against *S. aureus* and an aminoglycoside. Patients with a penicillin allergy should receive systemic vancomycin. Either closed or open drainage should be instituted as outlined later, and early pericardiectomy should be considered to prevent the development of constrictive pericarditis.

Surgical Intervention

Pericardiocentesis

Aspiration of pericardial fluid can be a life-saving maneuver in patients with cardiac tamponade, regardless of the cause. In addition, it is an indispensable adjunct to the diagnosis and treatment of idiopathic pericardial effusions. The most common approach is a subxiphoid route. The procedure is optimally done with full cardiac monitoring. A long needle is attached to a syringe and electrocardiograph lead. The needle is usually inserted to the left of the xiphoid and directed to the ipsilateral shoulder posteriorly at a 45-degree angle. The needle is slowly advanced until fluid is retrieved or until electrocardiographic changes occur (Fig. 63-1). An adjunct to this procedure is to use this needle as a guide for placing a catheter into the pericardial space. This can be done by threading a catheter through the needle, or by placing a wire through the needle and using the wire to direct a larger catheter. This latter technique is especially valuable in patients who had recurrent effusions requiring repeated pericardiocentesis.

The potential risks of pericardiocentesis include pneumothorax, myocardial or coronary artery injury, and arrhythmias. The use of sonographic guidance techniques has lessened the incidence of these potentially life-threatening complications.

Pericardiostomy

Open drainage of the pericardium is most commonly required in cases of malignant effusions or acute pyogenic pericarditis. The former is rare in children. For the latter,

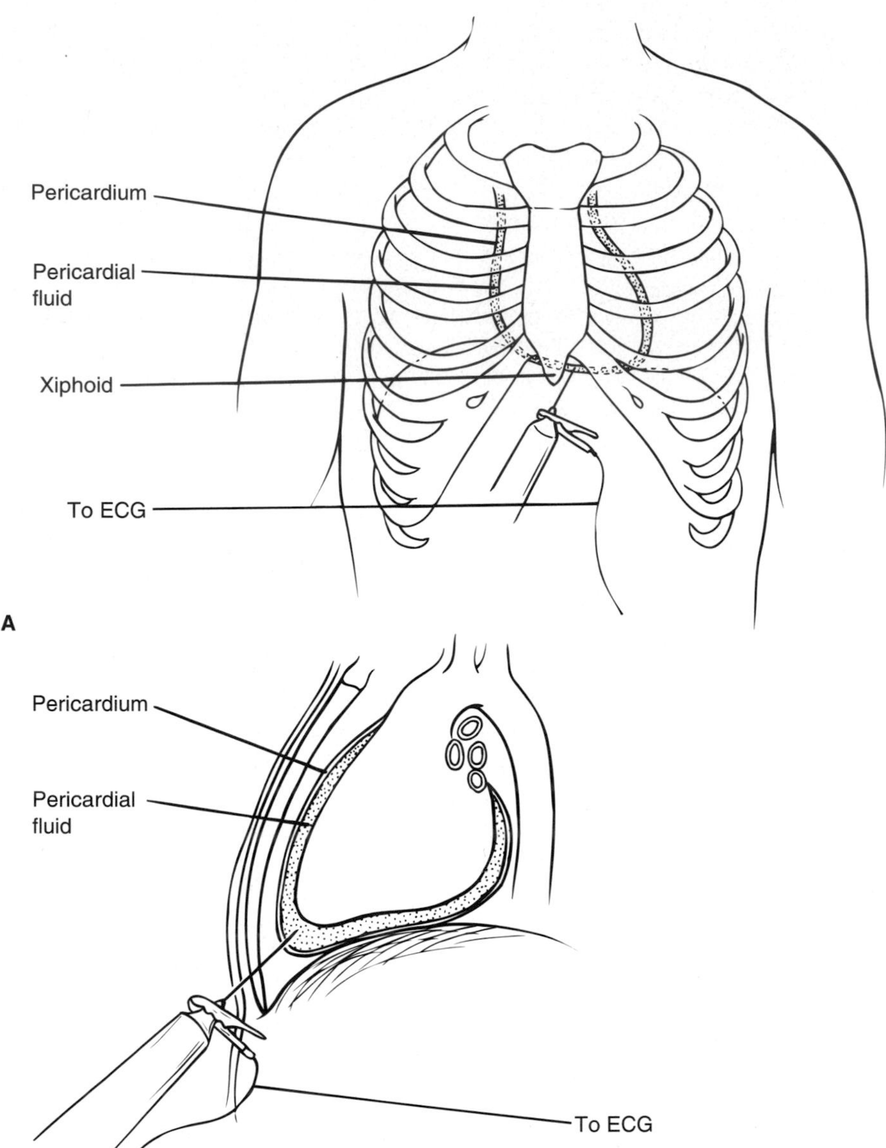

FIGURE 63-1. Technique of pericardiocentesis. Needle is inserted to the left of the xiphoid and directed toward the ipsilateral shoulder, posteriorly at a 45-degree angle. The electrocardiographic lead is attached to the needle. ECG, electrocardiogram. (Adapted from Ebert PA, Najafi H. The pericardium. In: Sabiston DC Jr, Spencer FC, eds. *Gibbons' surgery of the chest*, 5th ed. Philadelphia: WB Saunders, 1990:1234.)

this procedure may be necessary if the effusion is fibrinous or fibrinopurulent and has multiple loculations. Classically, this procedure was done through an open subxiphoid approach that allowed dependent drainage while avoiding contamination of the pleural space.

Pericardiostomy can be performed using thoracoscopic techniques (6). The patient is positioned supine at 45 degrees to allow the lung to fall posteriorly after pneumothorax has been achieved. Access ports are placed in the seventh intercostal space, midaxillary line; fourth intercostal space, midclavicular line; and sixth intercostal space, anterior axillary line (Fig. 63-2). The thoracoscope is inserted through the port in the seventh intercostal space. Dissection using monopolar current is avoided because it can fibrillate the heart and result in cardiac arrest if used in proximity to the myocardium. The laser or bipolar cautery is recommended for hemostasis. Segments of the lateral pericardium can be excised under direct vision. During dissection, it is important to identify the vagus and phrenic nerves on the pericardial surface. An advantage of the thoracoscopic approach is complete visualization of the pericardium. Three-dimensional video imaging technology and the use of the harmonic scalpel improve efficiency and precision (7). The ability to identify both the phrenic and vagus nerves, improved cosmesis, and less postoperative discomfort are additional benefits. The major disadvantage is that drainage is into the pleural cavity. When this is an undesirable clinical outcome, such as with bacterial pericarditis, an alternative route is indicated.

Pericardiectomy

Open resection of the pericardium is performed for patients with constrictive pericarditis. The procedure can be

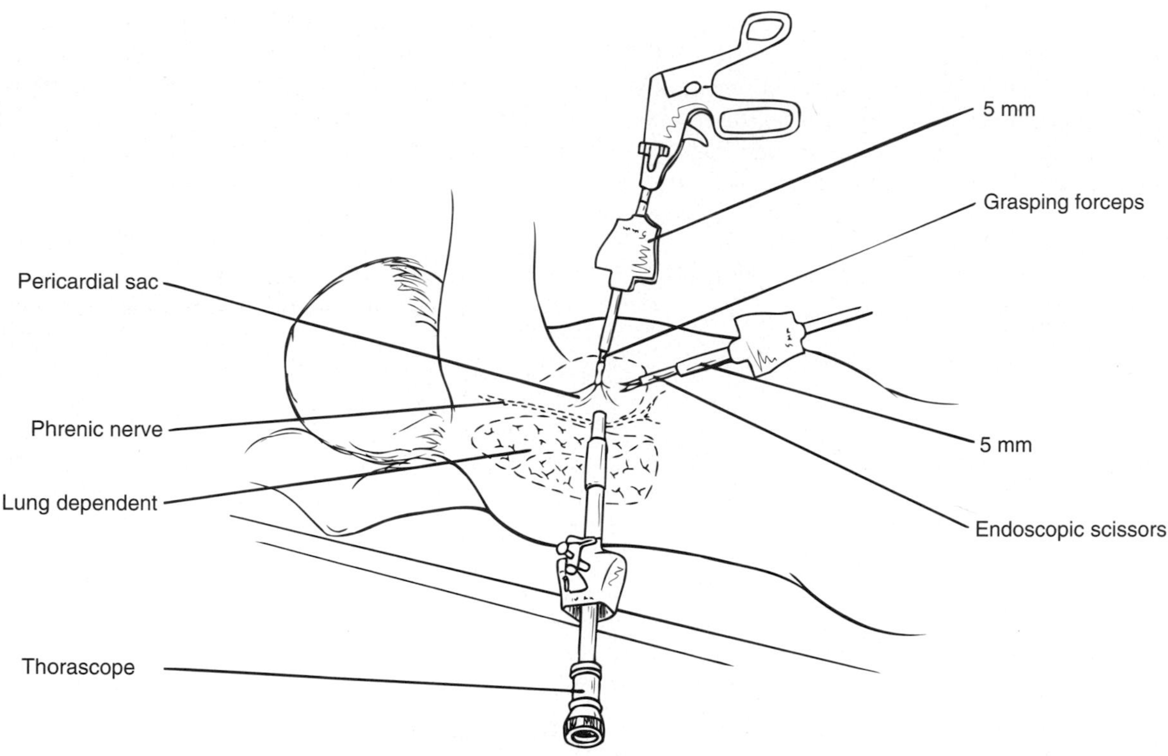

FIGURE 63-2. Thoracoscopic pericardiostomy using three-puncture technique. The course of the phrenic nerve can been seen along anterolateral surface of the pericardium. (Adapted from Lobe TE, Schropp KP. Pericardiectomy. In: *Pediatric laparoscopy and thoracoscopy*. Philadelphia: WB Saunders, 1994:239.)

performed through either a median sternotomy or an anterolateral thoracotomy. Cardiopulmonary bypass may be an advantage in that the heart can be manipulated to a greater degree. In addition, the posterior, lateral, and diaphragmatic aspects of the pericardium can be resected, which is difficult via conventional thoracotomies. The major risks in the use of cardiopulmonary bypass are systemic heparinization and concomitant bleeding. The principal alternative approach is the anterolateral thoracotomy, usually through the left fifth intercostal space. The advantage is that cardiopulmonary bypass is not required, and the risk of bleeding is therefore diminished.

GREAT VESSELS

Embryology

The earliest embryonic blood vessels develop from yolk sac mesoderm. These take the form of arborizing cords of angioblasts. The heart forms ventral to the foregut. Paired aortic arches pass laterally from the ventral heart, around the gut, and eventually unite to form the dorsal aorta. During the fifth week of development, a series of paired vessels that supply the six branchial clefts form, segments of which develop into the aortic arch and its major branches. Nearly all important anomalies of the aorta and its branches can be explained by the abnormal growth and involution of one or more portions of the primitive arch system. The six pairs of arches are not all present simultaneously. The first and second arches develop initially, and most segments undergo involution. The remnants of the first branchial arch form part of the mandibular artery. Remnants from the second arch form the hyoid artery and arteries of the inner ear. A large portion of the third arch remains and eventually forms part of the common carotid artery and the internal carotid artery. The right fourth arch forms the proximal portion of the right subclavian artery, and the distal segment is derived from a portion of the right dorsal aorta. A remnant of the left fourth arch forms the segment of the aorta between the origin of the left common carotid artery and the left subclavian artery. The fifth aortic arch pairs are transient and regress early. The right sixth arch forms the proximal right pulmonary artery; the proximal left sixth arch develops into the proximal left pulmonary artery, and the distal portion remains as the ductus arteriosus.

In the embryo, the heart and great vessels begin as cervical structures that later migrate caudally. On rare occasions, the aortic arch fails in this migration and remains in the cervical position, forming a *cervical aortic arch*. This structure is an anatomic curiosity and typically produces no symptoms, but this possibility should be considered in the evaluation of a pulsatile neck mass.

Critical events in the embryologic development of the great vessels occur during the eighth week of gestation. A double aortic arch results if the left and right fourth arches both persist. If the left fourth arch regresses and the right fourth arch persists, a right aortic arch results. Abnormal segmental regression of the left fourth arch results in abnormalities in the aorta that range from coarctation to complete interruption of the aortic arch.

Anatomy

The ascending aorta originates at the heart and travels through the pericardium, where it emerges to become the aortic arch. The superior vena cava lies to the right, and the pulmonary artery crosses posterior to the ascending arch. The aortic arch passes anterior to the trachea, giving rise to the brachiocephalic trunk or innominate artery, the first of three great arteries originating from the aortic arch. The brachiocephalic artery divides promptly into the right common carotid artery and the right subclavian artery. The second great branch of the aortic arch is the left common carotid artery, which runs almost vertically cephalad between the left pleural sac and the trachea to the base of the neck. The third and most distal artery arising from the aortic arch is the left subclavian artery, which passes along the cephalad aspect of the left pleural sac. As it gives rise to its three great branches, the anterior aspect of the arch of the aorta is covered by the left brachiocephalic vein. The aorta normally passes to the left of the trachea. The left phrenic nerve and the vagus nerve cross the anterior aspect of the aorta. On the right, at the level where the vagus nerve lies directly anterior to the subclavian artery, the nerve gives rise to the right recurrent laryngeal nerve, which passes posterior and then cephalad, thereby encircling the right subclavian artery. At about the level of the origin of the left subclavian artery, the aortic arch is joined on its inferior border by the ligamentum arteriosum extending from the left pulmonary artery. The vagus nerve on the left side courses anterior to the arch of the aorta in the vicinity of the ligamentum arteriosum and gives off the left recurrent laryngeal nerve, which passes around the arch in intimate contact with the junction of the aorta and ligamentum arteriosum (Fig. 63-3).

Anomalies of the Aortic Arch

During the past several decades, surgical correction of the major anomalies of the aortic arch has become routine.

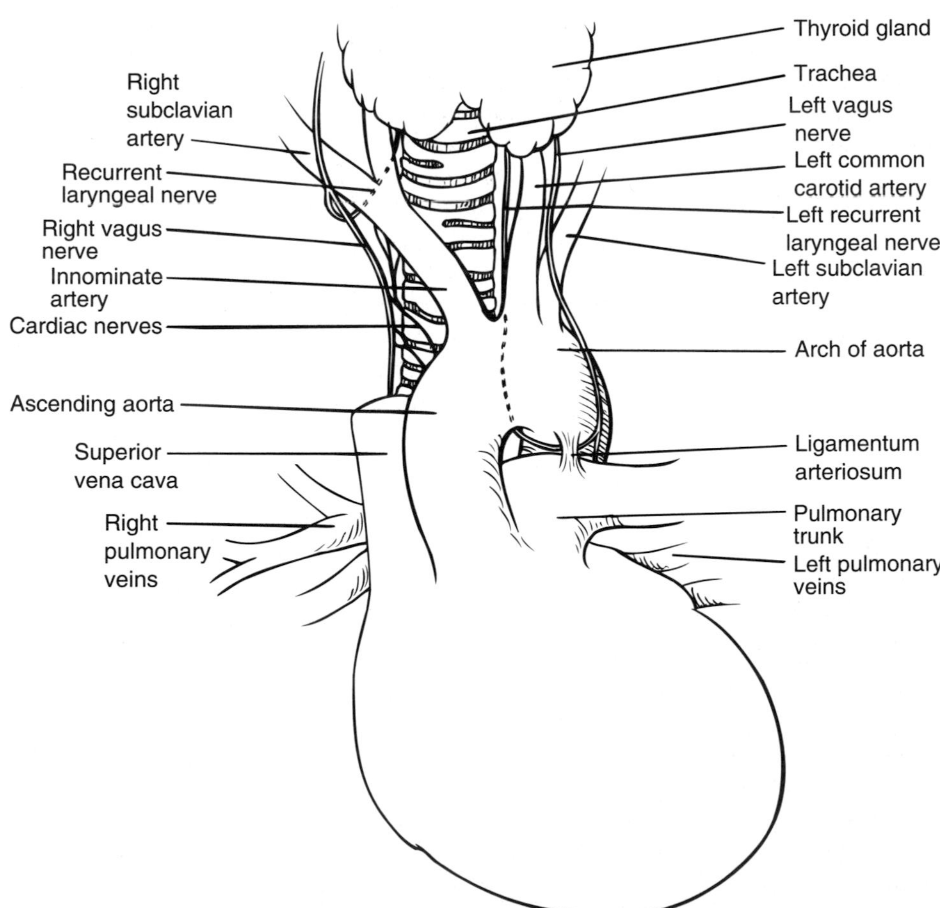

FIGURE 63-3. Anterior view of normal aortic arch anatomy and its relation to the aerodigestive tract and major nerves.

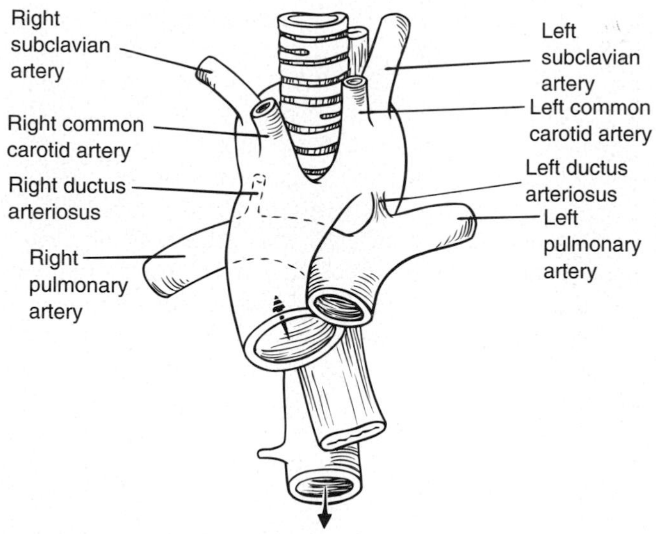

FIGURE 63-4. Schematic illustration of double aortic arch encircling esophagus and trachea.

Although some malformations are asymptomatic, patients with potentially life-threatening obstruction of the trachea or esophagus can be offered a predictably curative surgical procedure in most instances (8,9).

Double Aortic Arch

The most common type of symptomatic aortic arch abnormality is the double aortic arch. It is derived embryologically from persistence of the paired aortic arches and presents anatomically as a bifurcation of the ascending aorta. The right and left arches encircle the trachea and esophagus, and then join posteriorly to form the descending aorta (Fig. 63-4). In its most usual form, each common carotid artery and subclavian artery arises independently from its respective arch. The ligamentum arteriosum can be found on either or both arches. Usually the right (posterior) arch is larger than the left (anterior) arch, although the arches can be equal in size or asymmetric with a dominant anterior arch.

Seventy-five percent of patients with these anatomic variations have symptoms. Physiologically limiting tracheal compression leads to inspiratory stridor, dyspnea, and wheezing. The presentation is generally during infancy, and the urgency can be great. Because of concurrent esophageal obstruction and the risk of aspiration, symptoms are often exacerbated by feeding; dysphagia may be the presenting symptom. About 20% of these infants have associated cardiac anomalies, with ventricular septal defects and tetralogy of Fallot being most common.

On plain chest radiograph, a vascular shadow to the right of the trachea and esophagus is noted (Fig. 63-5). If a vascular anomaly is suspected, the next step in the evaluation is a barium esophagogram (Fig. 63-6). On anteroposterior view, there is bilateral compression of the esophagus. Lateral projections show anterior and posterior indentation as the arch crosses the midline. Historically, angiography was routine for evaluation of these patients. Today, MR imaging and contrast-enhanced CT have replaced angiography for the definitive evaluation of vascular rings (Fig. 63-7). MR imaging depicts vascular and tracheobronchial anatomy with a high degree of spatial resolution without the need for intravascular contrast agents (10). However, definitive intraoperative delineation of arch anatomy optimizes surgical success (11).

Treatment for a symptomatic double aortic arch is surgical. The aim of surgery is to relieve tracheal and esophageal compression and their attendant symptoms by dividing the constricting vascular ring while preserving distal perfusion. As with all vascular rings, exposure is achieved through a left posterolateral thoracotomy incision through the third or fourth intercostal space. All major vascular structures are dissected and definitively identified. The nondominant arch is then divided; this usually means that the anterior arch is divided and oversewn at its junction with the descending aorta distal to the left common carotid and subclavian arteries. When the right (posterior) arch is dominant or equal in size, it is preferentially divided near the origin of the descending aorta. It is prudent to ensure radial and carotid pulses are preserved during temporary vascular clamp occlusion at the planned site of arch interruption before surgical division for this and other vascular ring corrections, regardless of the anatomic configuration. It is also essential to divide any residual fibrous tissue meticulously around the trachea and esophagus after the vascular ring is divided. During this portion of the procedure, great care must be taken to avoid injury to the recurrent laryngeal nerve. Intraoperative monitoring of electromyograms to identify location and route of the recurrent laryngeal nerve has been shown to decrease the risk of injury (12). If a diverticulum of Kommerell is present at the origin of the aortic portion of the ligamentum arteriosum, it should be sewn to the prevertebral fascia to prevent the possibility of future recurrence. If persistent tracheal compression by the anterior arch remains after the vascular ring has been divided, sutures can be placed through the undersurface of the sternum and tied to suspend and open the trachea and esophagus.

Right Aortic Arch

Three abnormalities of clinical significance are related to a persistent right aortic arch. The most common is an independent right aortic arch that is a mirror image of the normal left arch. This abnormality is associated with situs inversus. The second variation is a right aortic arch associated with a right thoracic descending aorta. This type is not associated with situs inversus, but may be associated with a double superior vena cava and a retroesophageal left subclavian artery. The third type is a right-sided aortic

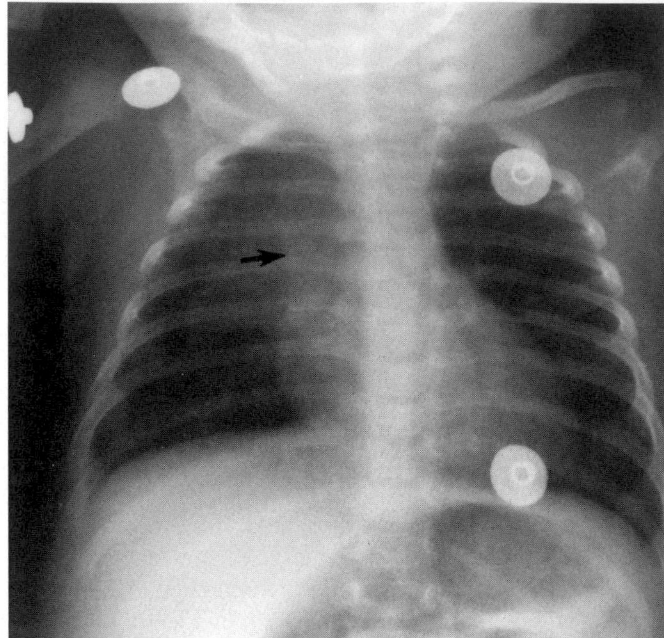

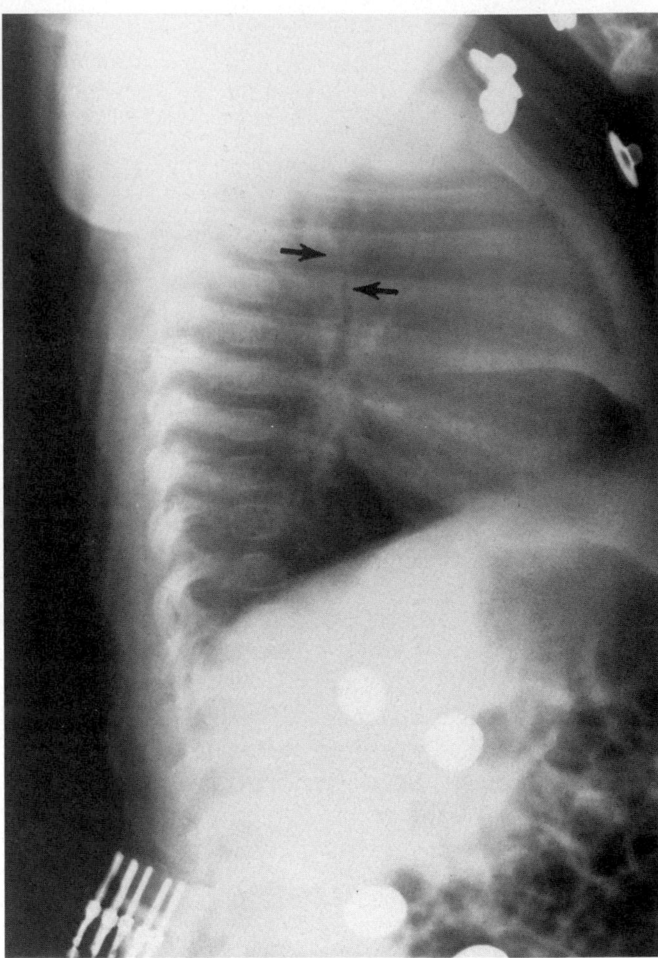

FIGURE 63-5. Anteroposterior (**A**) and lateral (**B**) chest radiographs of a 6-week-old child with stridor and dysphagia. The anteroposterior view shows a right aortic knob (*arrow*), and the lateral view exhibits narrowing of the tracheal air column (*arrows*). The findings are consistent with a vascular ring.

arch that courses behind the esophagus into a normal left descending thoracic aorta. Compression of the trachea and esophagus by a vascular ring mechanism can occur if a right aortic arch is associated with a left ligamentum arteriosum. The ring is formed by the aorta and the pulmonary artery to the right and anterior; the left ligamentum arteriosum completes the ring around the trachea and esophagus (Fig. 63-8). These anomalies occur in less than 1% of the population. The most common associated defect is congenital heart disease. Tetralogy of Fallot, double-outlet right ventricle, pulmonary atresia, and ventricular septal defect have been described (13,14).

Patients who have isolated right aortic arches without structural cardiac anomalies usually have neither symptoms nor evidence of esophageal or tracheal obstruction. Patients with restrictive vascular rings exhibit progressive respiratory symptoms. Stridor and wheezing can be absent in the infant, but these symptoms develop over time because normal growth of the aorta results in symptomatic tracheal compression. These children generally present within the first several years of life, but not in the neonatal period. Evaluation of these lesions is the same as that described for a double aortic arch. A plain chest radiograph commonly identifies a right aortic arch. Thereafter, echocardiography and MR imaging further elucidate the anatomy (15).

Patients with symptoms require surgical division of this vascular ring. The approach is through a left posterior lateral thoracotomy. It is important to identify the arch and its branches, as well as the ligamentum arteriosum. The ligamentum is then doubly ligated and divided, taking care not to injure the recurrent laryngeal nerve. It is occasionally necessary to divide the left subclavian artery at its origin to achieve adequate release of the entrapped esophagus and trachea.

Anomalous Right Subclavian Artery

In about 0.5% of the population, the right subclavian artery originates as the terminal branch from a normal left aortic arch and passes posterior to the esophagus and trachea, but anterior to the vertebral column. This results from the embryologic persistence of a portion of the distal right fourth aortic arch. This anomaly is associated with the classic presentation of interference with swallowing (*dysphagia lusoria*), described by Bayford in 1787 (8). Because

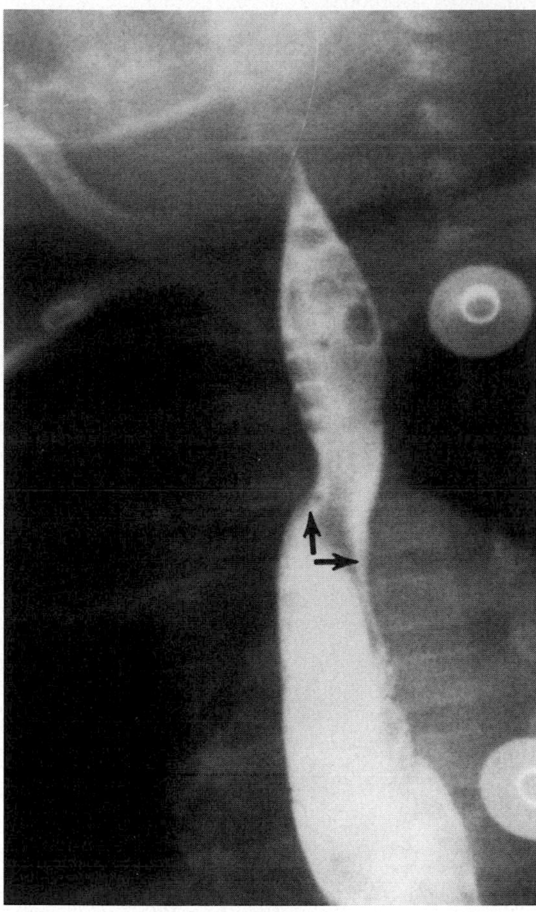

FIGURE 63-6. Barium esophagogram of the patient in Fig. 63-9. There is anterior and posterior indentation of the esophagus at the sites of encirclement by the left and right aortic arches. This is consistent with compression by a vascular ring, in this case, a double aortic arch.

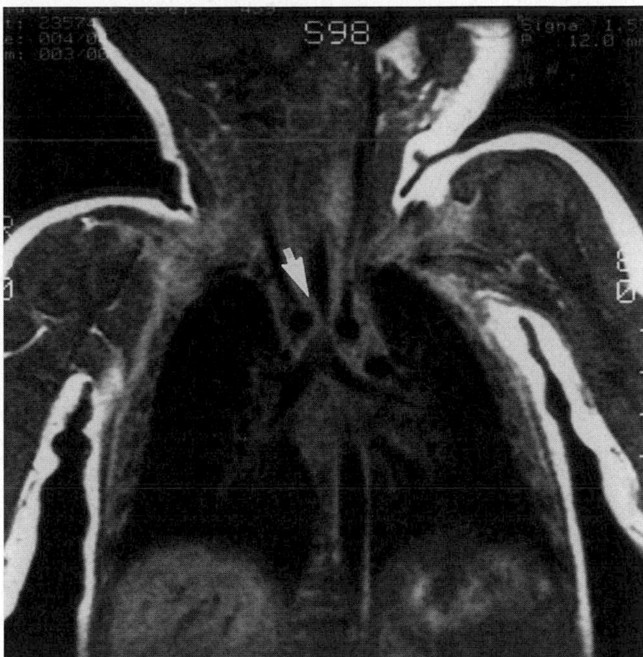

FIGURE 63-7. Magnetic resonance image of double aortic arch. Note the symmetry of cephalic vessels and compression of the trachea (*arrow*).

this form of vascular ring is incomplete, however, most of these patients do not have symptoms. Plain chest radiographs usually are nondiagnostic. If the index of suspicion is high, barium esophagogram shows a shallow oblique posterior indentation slanting upward from left to right, which is caused by the impression of the right subclavian artery. Evaluation and treatment are undertaken as outlined earlier for other vascular rings. Patients with symptoms should undergo surgical correction. The aortic arch and the aberrant right subclavian artery are identified. On occasion, the anomalous subclavian artery arises from a bulbous diverticulum that is a remnant of the right distal fourth arch. The classic treatment for this anomaly is ligation and division of the right subclavian artery at its anomalous origin. During this segment of the dissection, it is important to identify the recurrent laryngeal nerve that normally encircles the portion of the subclavian artery derived from the right fourth arch. As described earlier, the ligamentum arteriosum is also divided.

Pulmonary Artery Sling

The pulmonary artery sling is not truly related to aortic arch abnormalities, but it is in this clinical context that the lesion is generally encountered. The distal trachea, right mainstem bronchus, or both are compressed by an aberrant left pulmonary artery. This is an important diagnosis to establish prospectively. Although it can be approached via left thoracotomy as with other forms of vascular rings, some surgeons prefer a median sternotomy with the option of cardiopulmonary bypass. The principles of management previously articulated apply here as well, although division of the left pulmonary artery and release of the vascular ring must be followed by repositioning of the pulmonary artery anterior to the trachea and surgical reconstruction. In addition, segmental resection of the trachea or right mainstem bronchus may be necessary to relieve intrinsic tracheobronchial stenosis. Endoscopic assessment of the airway is essential for this purpose.

Treatment Results

The prognosis for patients with symptomatic vascular rings who undergo surgical release is excellent. Relief of esophageal and tracheal compression is predictable and immediate. Modern imaging and surgical techniques make unexpected findings and intraoperative complications unusual. Coexisting conditions, however, particularly congenital heart disease, impose important attendant morbidity. Tracheomalacia can follow the surgical release

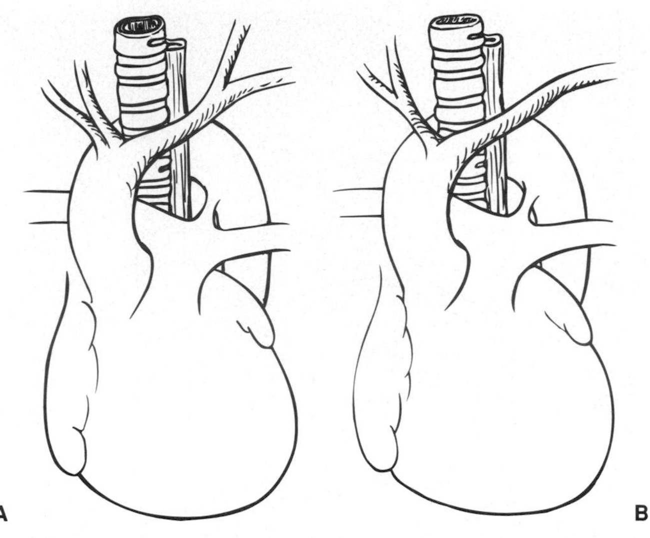

FIGURE 63-8. Anomalies of the aortic arch and its branches. (**A**) Right aortic arch with left ligamentum arteriosum, left descending aorta, and left innominate artery. (**B**) Right aortic arch with left ligamentum arteriosum, left descending aorta, and left subclavian and carotid arteries. (Adapted from Haryle HRS. The development and anomalies of the aortic arch and its branches. *Br J Surg*1959;46:561.)

of a vascular ring, and this is one specific indication for aortopexy. These issues are discussed elsewhere in this text.

Coarctation of the Aorta

Coarctation of the aorta is a constriction of the lumen that results in obstruction to blood flow. The lesion is either focal or elongated, and the site is categorized as *preductal,* proximal to the ductus arteriosus, or *postductal,* distal to this landmark (Fig. 63-9). Postductal coarctation is the most common type, and typically the ductus arteriosus involutes normally. In patients with preductal coarctation, the ductus arteriosus is usually patent.

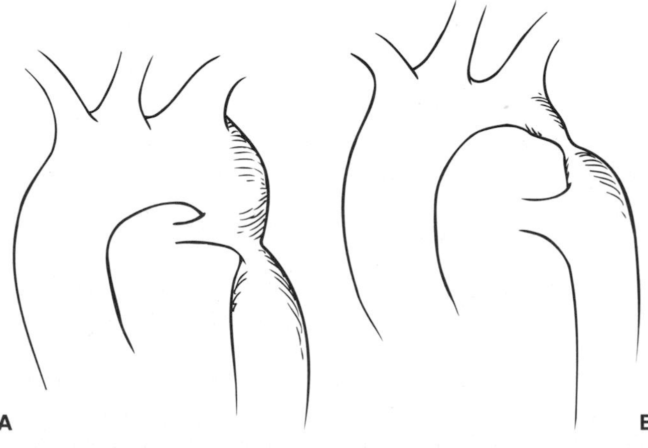

FIGURE 63-9. Schematic representations of coarctation of the aorta. (**A**) Postductal. (**B**) Preductal.

When coarctation of the aorta is classified as a type of congenital cardiac lesion, it is the third most common type of congenital heart disease in infants, ranking behind ventricular septal defect and PDA in frequency. This lesion accounts for about 10% of cases of congenital heart disease. Ninety percent of patients with aortic coarctation have associated intracardiac anomalies; the most common are ventricular septal defects, aortic and mitral valve abnormalities, and PDA (16). Twenty percent of infants admitted to the hospital with congestive heart failure have coarctation of the aorta. There is 3:1 male predominance, and the autopsy incidence is about 1 in 4,000. Coarctation is also relatively common in a number of noncardiac conditions, such as Turner syndrome and congenital lobar emphysema.

The cause of the lesion is unknown. It has been suggested that there may be an abnormally large extension of the ductus arteriosus into the wall of the adjacent aorta. If so, it is feasible that this tissue contracts and undergoes fibrosis during the transition to extrauterine life, and that this process leads to coarctation. There is histologic evidence to support this concept. In patients with aortic coarctation, the media is abnormally prominent, and there is evidence of intimal hyperplasia. Another theory is that the coarctation results from a transient reduction in aortic blood flow during the neonatal period. Compensatory increases in flow through the ductus may produce a jet effect, leading to aortic intimal injury opposite the ductus and generating fibrosis, narrowing, and classic coarctation (17).

The symptoms in patients with coarctation depend on the site. Patients with preductal coarctation often present during the neonatal period or infancy with failure to thrive and congestive heart failure. The latter problem may be exacerbated by associated intracardiac defects. Patients with postductal coarctation have much more diverse symptoms that depend on the degree of obstruction to blood flow. In infants, the nonspecific findings of failure to thrive, poor feeding, and irritability can result from minor narrowing. In contrast, high-grade obstructions to distal flow can present as an acute emergency with all the end-organ consequences of inadequate regional perfusion, oliguria, lactic acidosis, and multisystem organ failure.

On physical examination, a harsh systolic murmur over the back or left lateral chest is classic. A blood pressure gradient between the upper and lower extremities in a child is highly suspicious. Proximal hypertension is expected, with lower-extremity hypotension. Likewise, bounding upper-extremity pulses with diminished femoral and lower-extremity pulses raises the possibility of coarctation. Aortic coarctation should always be considered in the evaluation of an infant or child with hypertension. As in older patients, evidence of collateral flow through the intercostal and internal thoracic arteries is often present. This finding is supported by notching of the inferior rib margins by enlarged intercostal arteries on plain chest radiograph.

The diagnosis can be confirmed using a number of different modalities. Duplex Doppler echocardiography gives excellent and noninvasive resolution of the lesion and provides additional information about associated intracardiac anomalies. With advanced technology, this evaluation can also yield physiologic information by estimating the pressure gradient across the lesion. Angiography, however, remains the gold standard for diagnosis and may provide an avenue for therapy. It provides definitive information concerning the anatomy and associated cardiac anomalies and precise measurement of the pressure gradient across the obstruction.

Balloon angioplasty was first reported in 1982 by Singer et al. (18). The technique was initially used as rescue for recurrent coarctation, but has gained acceptance as an initial treatment modality. Proper patient selection is of utmost importance for favorable outcome. Children with hypoplasia of the transverse aortic arch are poor candidates for balloon angioplasty and should undergo surgical repair (19). Beneficial results from balloon angioplasty have been reported in approximately 80% of patients. Rates of restenosis and aneurysm formation are less than 10% (20).

Placement of an endovascular stent at the time of balloon angioplasty has been shown to improve overall long-term outcome in adults. Translation to the younger pediatric population has been tempered by concerns surrounding subsequent growth. However, results for primary balloon dilation and stent implantation in selected patients older than 15 years of age have been favorable (21).

The surgical management of coarctation of the aorta began in the 1940s. The procedure described by Gross consisted of resection of the area of aortic narrowing with a primary end-to-end aortic anastomosis. This concept was elegant and simple. Although its implementation was initially complex, it is now routine. Through a posterolateral thoracotomy, the aortic arch, descending aorta, and great vessels are identified. The aorta and the ligamentum arteriosum are then controlled (Fig. 63-10). The ligamentum is then divided and the area of aortic coarctation resected. If the lesion is elongated, proximal and distal aortic mobility can be enhanced by ligating and dividing adjacent intercostal vessels. A primary end-to-end anastomosis is then performed using interrupted monofilament suture. The outcome is excellent in this circumstance. In one series, a 92% success rate was reported at 5-year follow-up with this technique (22). Advantages include the resection of all abnormal aortic tissue and restoration of normal aortic anatomy without prosthetic material.

In patients for whom a primary anastomosis is not possible because of inadequate aortic arch length, an interposition graft is used. In 1961, Schuster and Gross reported the use of aortic homografts in 70 patients. Although there were no deaths noted and complication rate was minimal, (23) subsequent experience with these and other similar patients suggests important long-term risks related to degenerative changes and aneurysm formation. Others subsequently described the use of Dacron, polytetrafluoroethylene, and other prosthetic grafts in patients with complex lesions, with recurrent coarctation after primary repair, and with aneurysmal changes after homograft placement.

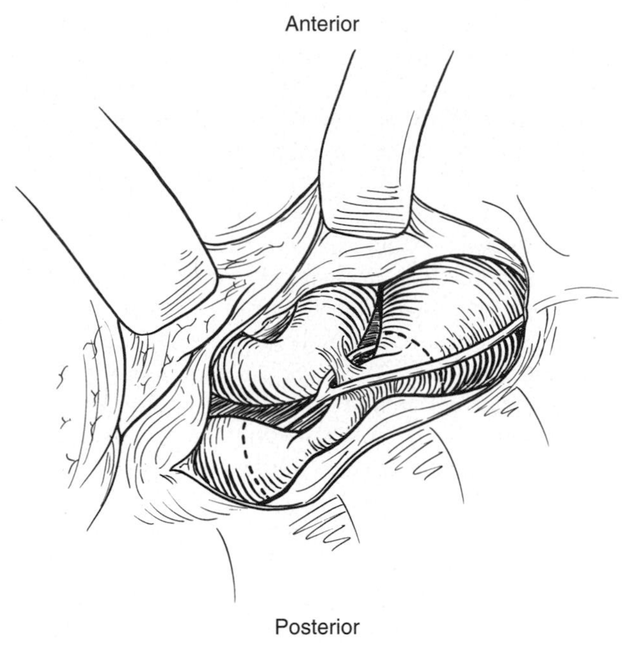

FIGURE 63-10. Illustration of the operative view of preductal coarctation as seen through a left thoracotomy. Dotted lines depict sites of aortic transection. Note courses of vagus and recurrent laryngeal nerves with regard to the aorta and the ligamentum arteriosum.

During the past 15 years, a technique has been developed to avoid the potential problems of prosthetic conduits and the real problems of aortic anastomosis under tension—the subclavian patch aortoplasty. In this procedure, the origin of the left subclavian artery is dissected to its first branch, and the vertebral artery is ligated to prevent subclavian steal. The subclavian artery is then ligated and divided just proximal to its first branch. The aorta is incised longitudinally through the area of coarctation into the subclavian artery. The resultant subclavian flap is then rotated downward and sutured into place with a series of fine interrupted monofilament sutures, providing autologous arterial tissue for reconstruction. Advantages include the use of autologous tissue, a limited dissection, and a relatively short operative time. Because spinal cord ischemia injury is a risk in all operations on the thoracic aorta, this latter advantage is potentially significant.

Campbell and associates (24) performed this technique in 53 infants, with a mortality rate of 4%. Concerns remain, however, about long-term growth and development of the left upper extremity because decreased limb lengths and mass in children after flap aortoplasty have been described (25).

Regardless of technique, postoperative complications after coarctation repair are relatively infrequent, but potentially serious. These consist of hemorrhage, hemothorax, recurrent laryngeal nerve paralysis, infection, thrombosis, late stenosis, and spinal cord injury. A complication particular to coarctation repair is postoperative paradoxical hypertension. This problem occurs in 7% to 28% of patients and initially presents within the first 24 hours after surgery as an elevation in systolic blood pressure (26). This is generally amenable to pharmacologic control in an intensive care or other hospital setting and lasts a few days. Subsequently, longer-lasting diastolic hypertension can develop. This is believed to be due to aberrant activation of the sympathetic nervous system. The late phase can be prolonged, and there is evidence that it is renin dependent (27).

Patients with postcoarctation hypertension can develop splanchnic vasoconstriction and mesenteric ischemia. Abdominal pain, ileus, and lactic acidosis can lead to presentation as an acute abdominal crisis. Histologic examination of mesenteric blood vessels shows necrotizing mesenteric arteritis (28). The most successful treatment of postcoarctectomy syndrome is that of prevention by aggressive medical intervention when hypertension becomes evident. Sodium nitroprusside, propanolol, and reserpine are among the most useful agents.

The least common but most disabling complication after coarctation repair is paraplegia, which occurs in 0.7% to 1.5% of patients (26). In an attempt to avoid this complication, some have monitored distal aortic pressure during cross-clamping to ascertain the efficacy of collateral circulation, with the concept that if the distal aortic perfusion pressure falls to less than 50 mm Hg, bypass perfusion should be instituted. An alternative approach is to monitor electromyographic-evoked potential in the lower extremities because these are reliably maintained at perfusion pressures greater than 60 mm Hg (29). In this instance, shunting is instituted to maintain distal aortic pressures of more than 60 mm Hg during surgical repair.

The overall mortality rate using classic surgical techniques is about 10%. Comparable results are described using either a subclavian flap or a primary anastomotic technique. Stenosis at the coarctation site can occur and is believed to be due to either failure of anastomotic growth or an inadequate aortic resection. These patients present with similar signs and symptoms as de novo patients. If hypertension cannot be controlled readily by medical management, angiography with gradient determination should be undertaken and reoperation considered. Reoperation is made difficult by scarring at the previous operative site, and as with all reoperations, morbidity and mortality rates are higher (30).

Patent Ductus Arteriosus

The ductus arteriosus is indispensable to the maintenance of fetal circulation. It is a conduit that shunts most of the right ventricular outflow from the pulmonary artery and developing lung into the descending thoracic aorta and systemic circulation (Fig. 63-11). Normally, this vessel closes within days of birth and is obliterated during the first year of life. It is then referred to as the *ligamentum arteriosum.* Failure of closure should be considered an anomalous condition and is associated with significant morbidity and mortality. PDA is the most common type of extracardiac shunt.

The ductus arteriosus is derived from the dorsal aspect of the left sixth aortic arch, and forms a circuit between the pulmonary artery and the descending thoracic aorta just distal to the origin of the left subclavian artery. Structurally, the normal ductus arteriosus is 5 to 7 mm in diameter and 7 to 10 mm in length. It has a conical shape, with a smaller pulmonary orifice. Ductal closure occurs as a natural part of the transition from fetal to adult circulation. Closure occurs in two phases. The first phase is functional, and the second is anatomic. In utero, ductal patency is maintained by low oxygen tension and autocrine regulation of endogenous prostaglandin synthesis (31). Functional closure occurs when the vascular smooth muscle in the wall of the ductus constricts and the intimal cushions become opposed. The functional closure usually occurs within the first day of life in normal full-term infants. Anatomic closure marked by fibrosis occurs much later. Cristie (32) reported that 88% of infants had an anatomically closed ductus arteriosus after 60 days of extrauterine life, and this rate was 99% at 1 year of age.

Patency of the ductus arteriosus is clinically significant in about 1 in 5,000 live full-term births, but is much more common in premature infants. A direct relation exists between gestational age and the incidence of PDA. Histologic analysis of the ductus arteriosus in operated infants has shown altered architecture of the medial smooth muscle cells, as well as an abnormality of the intimal endothelial cushions (33). The defect is often associated with other congenital abnormalities. Among these, cardiac malformations are common, and certain conditions, such as pulmonary hypertension, are predictable. Infants with severe pulmonary hypertension, such as that with congenital diaphragmatic hernia and pulmonary hypoplasia, often depend on a PDA to sustain cardiac function. For reasons that are unknown, PDA is twice as frequent in girls as in boys.

The natural history of a PDA is well documented. Untreated, ductal patency in the infant has significant

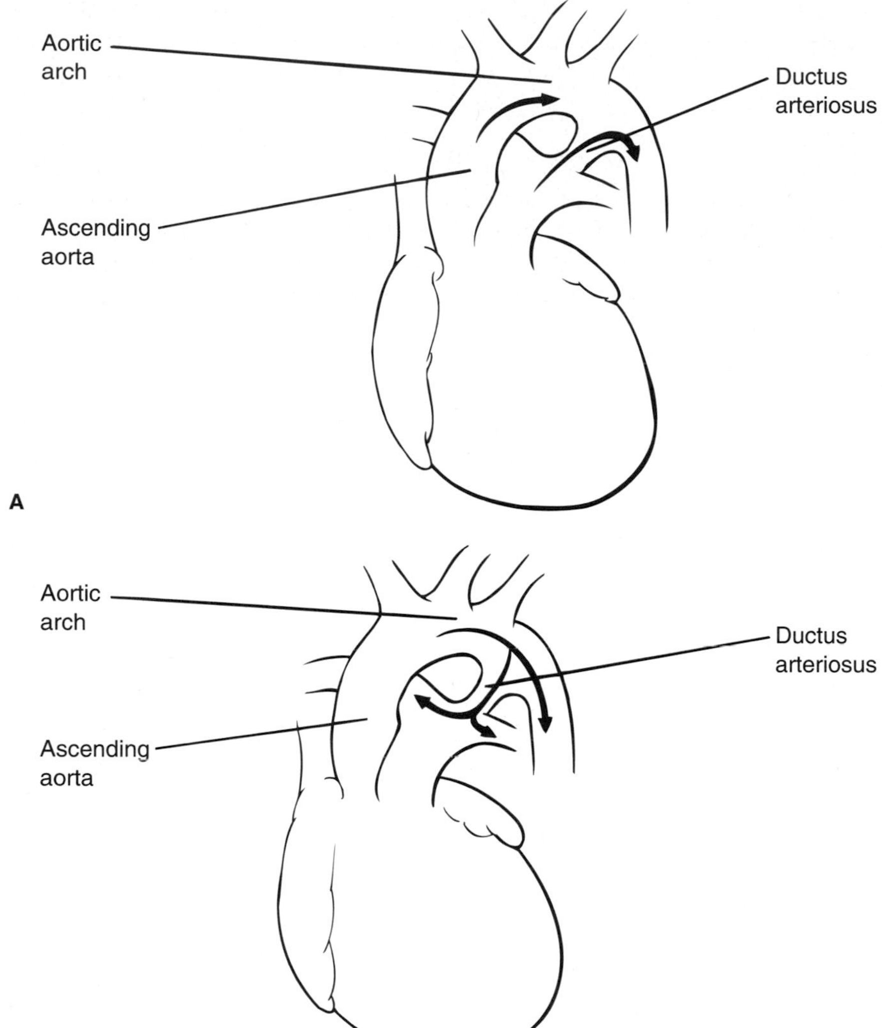

FIGURE 63-11. Drawing of circulatory patterns through the ductus arteriosus before (**A**) and after (**B**) birth.

morbidity and a mortality rate as high as 30% (16). The usual cause of death in untreated patients is congestive heart failure. In patients more than 1 year old, bacterial endocarditis is a common cause of morbidity. Aneurysmal dilation of the ductus arteriosus, left-to-right shunting, and pulmonary hypertension can occur in patients who survive to adulthood (34).

In preterm infants with respiratory distress syndrome, the incidence of PDA is as high as 80%. Symptoms in these patients include intolerance of feeding and high-output cardiac failure. Bounding peripheral pulses, tachypnea, and tachycardia are characteristic. The physical examination typically reveals a classic "machinery" murmur over the left upper sternal border. Doppler ultrasonography has shown a marked reduction in splanchnic blood flow in patients with PDA, and an important clinical correlation with neonatal necrotizing enterocolitis exists (35).

The diagnosis of PDA can be made using several modalities. Chest radiography can show cardiomegaly and pulmonary congestion. Doppler echocardiography is routinely used for screening. It is highly accurate, noninvasive, and portable. Shunt flow can be quantitated with Doppler echocardiography, and the diagnosis of associated cardiac anomalies often can be made. Doppler is often sufficient to make management decisions, but cardiac catheterization can be used as an adjunct to elucidate complex intracardiac anomalies.

As noted earlier, certain circumstances require that ductal patency be maintained to preserve cardiac function and aortic blood flow. This is most successfully accomplished pharmacologically using prostaglandin E_1 or E_2 (36) (see Chapter 62).

In most normal infants, persistent ductal patency leads to significant morbidity and mortality. Generally, the presence of prolonged or symptomatic ductus arteriosus patency is an indication for closure. Since 1939, the traditional therapy for PDA has been surgical ligation (37); however, nonoperative management has been successful in selected term infants. Indomethacin, by means of inhibition of prostaglandin synthesis, is effective in closing a PDA in most preterm infants (38). Its use, however, has been associated with necrotizing enterocolitis, bowel perforation, reduced renal function, and delayed closure. Indomethacin is contraindicated in infants with renal impairment, sepsis, coagulopathy, intracranial hemorrhage, liver failure, or a physiologically urgent need for closure.

More recently, successful transcatheter PDA embolization has been reported in highly selected patient populations. Closure rates of up to 92% using prosthetic sponges or metal coils have been achieved (39). Adolescents with small to moderate size lesions (less than 3.5 mm) have the best outcomes (40).

For infants who are inappropriate for or nonresponsive to pharmacologic treatment, and who are not candidates for transcatheter embolization, surgical PDA ligation is indicated. Video-assisted thoracoscopic surgery (VATS) has assumed an expanded role in the management of the PDA. VATS-assisted PDA ligation has been accomplished safely and effectively. Burk et al. reported excellent results in low-birth-weight infants (less than 1,000 g). Operative mortality was zero, and four patients required conversion to open thoracotomy (41). Advanced laparoscopic skills and optimal patient selection are required to ensure a favorable outcome.

Patients who are not candidates for minimally invasive PDA ligation should undergo open ligation. The procedure is done through a left posterior lateral thoracotomy using

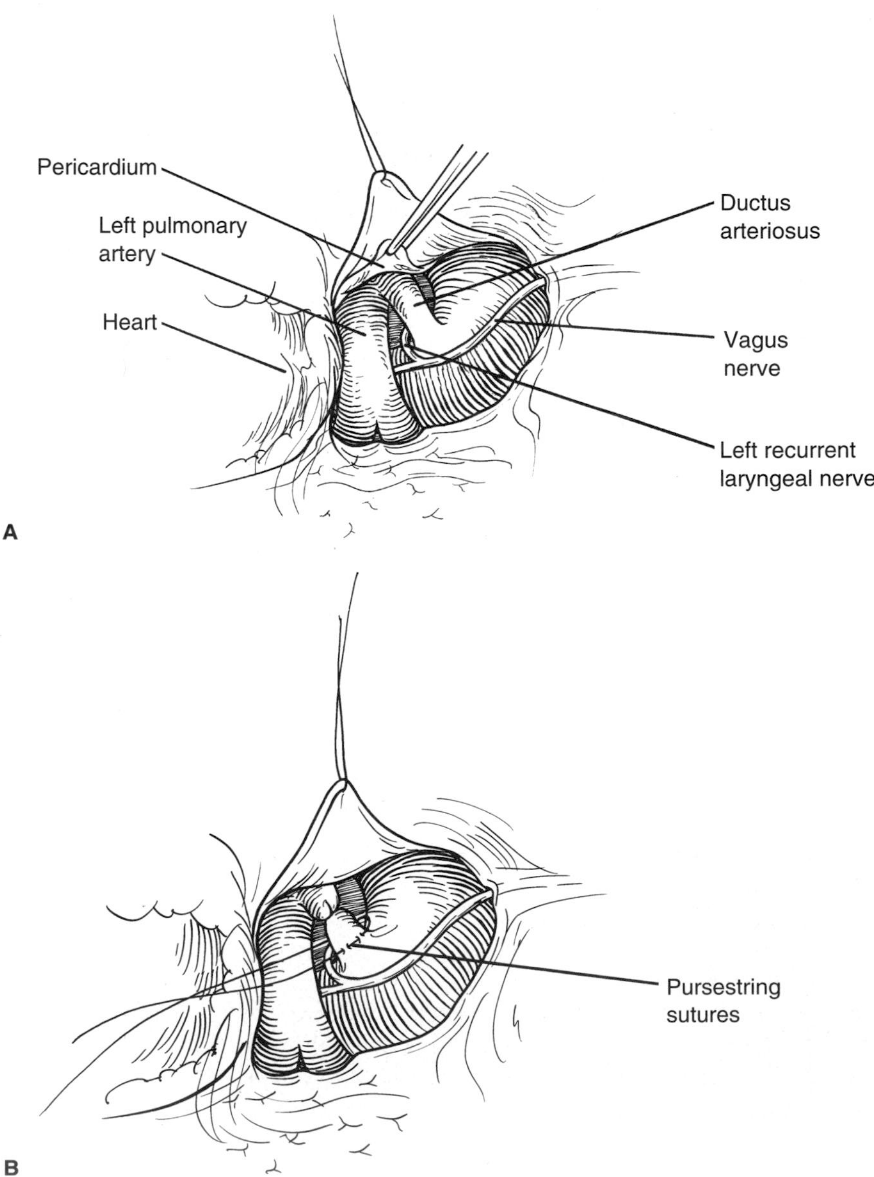

FIGURE 63-12. Operative view of ligation of ductus arteriosus. (**A**) Normal anatomy depicted through left posterolateral thoracotomy. (**B**) Suture ligation using large multifilament nonabsorbable sutures. Several alternative techniques for closure are also commonly used.

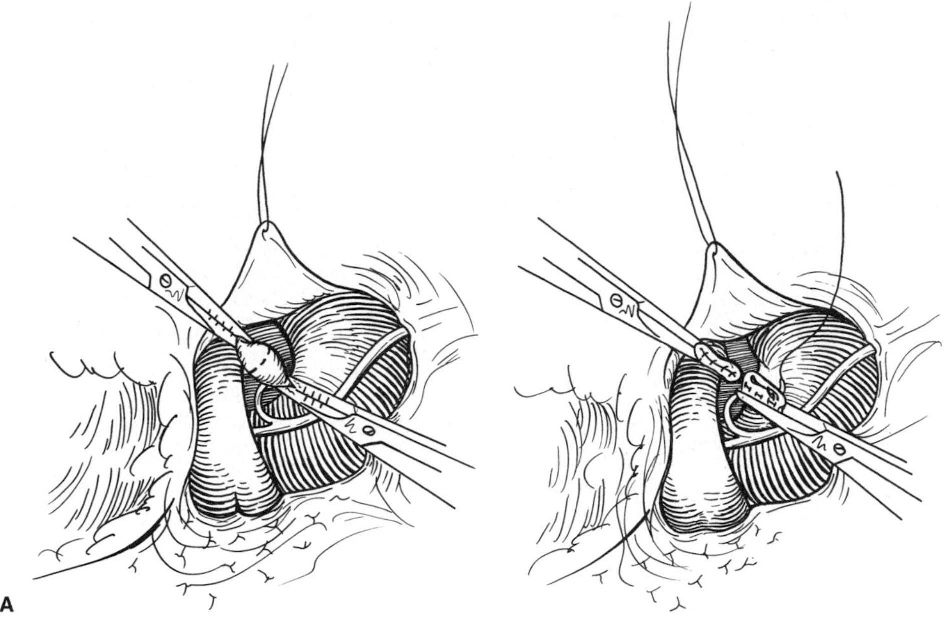

FIGURE 63-13. The ductus arteriosus can be divided, particularly in older infants and children. The ductus is viewed here through a left posterolateral thoracotomy. (**A**) Proximal and distal control is obtained by vascular clamps. (**B**) Double-suture ligation of both proximal and distal ends before division.

either a transpleural or an extrapleural approach. The pulmonary artery, aorta, ductus arteriosus, and left recurrent laryngeal nerve require identification. This is often facilitated by identifying the origin of the left subclavian artery, which is easily found; the ductus arteriosus is close by on the inferior medial aspect of the aorta at this point. Proximal and distal control of the ductus is obtained, taking care not to injure the recurrent laryngeal nerve. In certain instances, the ductus can be as large or larger than the descending thoracic aorta. Care must be taken to differentiate the ductus and the left pulmonary artery. The ductus is then either simply ligated or ligated and divided. The ductus can be ligated with large multifilament nonabsorbable sutures or surgical clips (Fig. 63-12). It can be divided between vascular clamps and oversewn with monofilament nonabsorbable sutures (Fig. 63-13), although this is potentially hazardous in preterm infants. Postoperative complications are minimal, but include hemorrhage, infection, pneumothorax, pneumonia, hemothorax, and injury to the recurrent laryngeal nerve. Outcome is determined by other medical conditions. In patients undergoing simple ligation, there have been occasional reports of recanalization requiring reoperation with division and oversewing of the proximal and distal ends of the ductus (42).

In infants with asymptomatic PDA, treatment is not recommended unless signs of cardiovascular compromise become evident. Initially, fluid restriction and diuretic therapy are all that is required. If these modalities fail, then indomethacin is used. Given intravenously, indomethacin results in a permanent PDA closure rate of 70% to 90% (43). Infants in whom indomethacin therapy fails should undergo surgical PDA closure. The results of surgical closure are excellent. In infants, the mortality rate is less than 1%. In older children with evidence of pulmonary hypertension and right ventricular dysfunction, the mortality rate is substantially greater.

REFERENCES

1. Freeman G, LeWinter MM. Pericardial adaptations during cardiac dilatation in dogs. *Circ Res* 1984;54:294.
2. Umemori Y, Kotani K, Makihara S. Video assisted thoroscopical surgery for pericardial cyst: report of two cases. *Jap J Thorac Surg* 2001;54–1125.
3. Klatte EC, Yune HY. Diagnosis and treatment of pericardial cysts. *Radiology* 1972;104:541.
4. Surawicz B, Lassiter KC. Electrocardiogram in pericarditis. *Am J Cardiol* 1970;26:471.
5. Rubin RH, Moellering RC Jr. Clinical, microbiologic, and therapeutic aspects of purulent pericarditis. *Am J Med* 1975;59:68.
6. Geissbuhler K, Leiser A, Fuhrar J, et al. Video assisted thorascopic pericardial fenestration for loculated or recurrent effusions. *Eur J Cardio-Thorac Surg* 1998;14:403.
7. Luison F, Boyd WD. Three dimensional video-assisted thorascopic pericardectomy. *Ann Thorac Surg* 2000;70:2137.
8. McNally PR, Rak KM. Dysphagia lusoria caused by persistent right aortic arch with aberrant left subclavian artery and diverticulum of Kommerell. *Dig Dis Sci* 1992;37:144.
9. Gross RE. Surgical relief for tracheal obstruction from a vascular ring. *N Engl J Med* 1945;233:586.
10. Brockmeirer K, Demirakca S, Metzner R, et al. Double aortic arch. *Circulation* 2000;102:93.
11. Woods R, Sharp R, Holcomb G. Vascular anomalies and tracheoesophageal compression: a single institutions 25-year experience. *Ann Thorac Surg* 2001;72:434.
12. Odegard K, Kirse D, Delvido, et al. Intraoperative recurrent laryngeal nerve monitoring during video-assisted thoroscopic surgery for patent ductus arteriosis. *J Cardiothorac Vasc Anesth.* 2000;14:562.
13. Moës CA.Vascular rings and anomalies of the aortic arch. In: Keith JD, Rowe RD, Vlad D, eds. *Heart diseases in infancy and childhood,* 3rd ed. New York: Macmillan, 1978:869.
14. Paris M. Retrecissement considerable de laorte paetorale observe a la Hotel Dieu de Paris. *J Chir Desault* 1791;2:107.

15. Zachary C, Myers J, Eggli K. Vascular ring due to right aortic arch with mirror image branching and left ligamentum arteriosis: complete perioperative diagnosis by magnetic resonance imaging. *Pediatr Cardiol* 2001;22:71.
16. Gaynor JW, Sabiston DC.Patent ductus arteriosus, coarctation of the aorta, aortopulmonary window, and anomalies of the aortic arch. In: Sabiston DC, Spenser FC, eds. *Surgery of the chest*. Philadelphia: WB Saunders, 1990.
17. Nugent EW, Plauth WH Jr, Edwards JE, et al.The pathology, abnormal physiology, clinical recognition, and medical and surgical treatment of congenital heart disease. In: Hurstt JW, ed. *The heart,* 7th ed. New York: McGraw Hill, 1990.
18. Singer MI, Rowan M, Dorsey TJ, Transabdominal aortic balloon angioplasty for coarctation of the aorta in the newborn. *Am Heart J* 1982;103:131.
19. Ovaert C, McCrindle BW, Nykanau D, et al. Balloon angioplasty of native coarctation: clinical outcomes and predictors of success. *J Am Coll Cardiol* 2000;35:988.
20. Kaine SF, Smith ED, Mott AR, et al. Qualitative echocardiographic analysis of the aortic arch predicts outcome of balloon angioplasty of the native coartation of the aorta. *Circulation* 1996;94:1056.
21. Hornung, TS, Benson LN, McLaughlin PR. Interventions for aortic coarctation. *Cardiol Rev* 2002;10:139.
22. Cobanoglu A, Teply JF, Gronkemeier GL, et al. Coarctation of the aorta in patients younger than three months: a critique of the subclavian flap operation. *J Thorac Cardiovasc Surg* 1985;89:121.
23. Schuster SR, Gross RE. Surgery for coarctation of the aorta: a review of 500 cases. *J Thorac Cardiovasc Surg* 1962;43:54.
24. Campbell DB, Waldhausen JA, Pierce WS, et al. Should elective repair of coarctation of the aorta be done in infancy? *J Thorac Cardiovasc Surg* 1984;88:979.
25. Todd DJ, Dangerfield DH, Hamilton DI, et al. Late effects of the left upper limb of subclavian flap aortoplasty. *J Thorac Cardiovasc Surg* 1983;85:678.
26. Lerberg DB, Hardesty RL. Coarctation of the aorta in infants and children: 25 years of experience. *Ann Thorac Surg* 1982;33:159.
27. Leandro J, Balfe JW, Smallhorn JF, et al. Coarctation of the aorta and hypertension. *Child Nephrol Urol* 1992;12:124.
28. Kawanchi M, Tada Y, Asano K, et al. Angiographic demonstration of mesenteric arterial changes in post coarctation syndrome. *Surgery* 1985;98:602.
29. Hughes RK, Reemsta K. Correction of coarctation of the aorta: manometric determination of safety during test occlusion. *J Thorac Cardiovasc Surg* 1971;62:31.
30. Footer ED. Re-operation for aortic coarctation. *Ann Thorac Surg* 1984;38:81.
31. Barst RJ, Garsony WM. The pharmacologic treatment of patent ductus arteriosus. *Drugs* 1989;38:249.22.
32. Cristie A. Normal closing time of the foramen ovale and the ductus arteriosus: anatomic and statistical study. *Am J Dis Child* 1930;40:323.
33. Slaup J, van Monsteron JC, Poelmann RE, et al. Formation of intimal cushions in the ductus arteriosus as a model for vascular intimal thickening: an immunohistochemical study of changes in extracellular matrix components. *Atherosclerosis* 1992;93:25.
34. Colermyer DS, Shoker GF, Hughes CF, et al. Persistent ductus arteriosus in adults: a review of surgical experience with 25 patients. *Med J Aust* 1991;155:233.
35. Wong SN, Lor NS, Hui PW. Abnormal neural and splanchnic arterial Doppler pattern in premature babies with symptomatic patent ductus arteriosus. *J Ultrasound Med* 1990;9:125.
36. Buck ML. Prostaglandin E1 treatment of congenital heart disease: use prior to neonatal transport. *Drug Intell Clin Pharm* 1991;25: 408.
37. Gross RE, Hubbard JP. Surgical ligation of a patent ductus arteriosus: reports of first successful case. *JAMA* 1939;112:729.
38. Bhatt V, Nahata MC. Pharmacologic management of patent ductus arteriosus. *Clin Pharmacol* 1989;8:17.
39. Hoskinig MCK, Benson LN, Musewe N, et al. Transcatheter occlusion of the persistently patent ductus arteriosus: forty month follow-up and prevalence of residual shunting. *Circulation* 1991;84:2313.
40. Laohaprasitipooru D, Nana A, Durongpisitwik et al. Transcatheter coil occlusion of small patent ductus arteriosis: experience at Siriraj Hospital. *J Med Assoc Thailand* 2002;85:5630.
41. Burke RP, Jacobs JP, Cheng W, et al. Video-assisted thoroscopic surgery for patent ductus arteriosis in low birth weight neonates and infants. *Pediatrics* 1999;104:227.
42. Ghani SA, Hashima R. Surgical management of patent ductus arteriosus: a review of 413 cases. *J R Coll Surg Edinb* 1989;34:33.
43. Hammerman C, Aramburo MJ. Prolonged indomethacin therapy for the prevention of recurrences of patient ductus arteriosus. *J Pediatr* 1990;117:771.

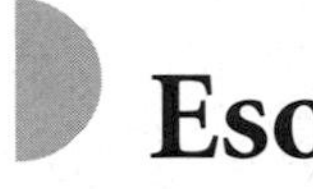

Esophagus

Patrick A. Dillon

EMBRYOLOGY

Although the normal esophagus can be identified as a distinct structure by the fourth week of embryogenesis, the development of the esophagus has remained controversial. The development of the esophagus is intimately related to the embryology of the trachea, and the separation of these two foregut structures is complete before the fifth week of gestation. The separation usually proceeds in a caudad to cephalad direction. During subsequent development, the esophagus increases in length more rapidly than the fetus as a whole and reaches its final length (8 to 10 cm at birth) by 7 weeks (1). A more recent theory supports the idea of the respiratory epithelium developing from the ventral foregut and creating a stalk (Fig. 64-1) of tissue that will form the trachea. Experimental studies support aspects of both theories (2,3). Ciliated columnar epithelium appears in the esophagus at approximately 10 weeks' gestation and stratified squamous epithelium replaces it at around 20 to 25 weeks, a process that begins in the midesophagus and proceeds both caudad and cephalad. The muscular fibers of the esophagus appear to develop at different rates. Circular muscle is present at 8 weeks, whereas longitudinal muscle becomes apparent by approximately 13 weeks' gestation in the human embryo. In fetuses, the thickness of the muscularis externa increases linearly from 8 weeks to term (40 weeks), then growth slows postnatally (4,5). Neurons can be recognized concomitantly with circular muscle at 8 weeks, with peak density occurring by 16 to 20 weeks. Subsequently, there is rapid decline in the number of neurons during the second trimester, and this is reduced further toward adult levels during infancy. The numbers of ganglion cells and nerve fibers in the myenteric plexus are also maximal at 16 to 20 weeks. However, their density decreases with increasing gestational age, and by 30 weeks, it becomes constant despite further esophageal growth (4,5). Relationships between neuropeptides, neuronal function, and the ontogeny of esophageal motor activity have yet to be characterized (5).

Maturation of esophageal motility appears to progress in an orderly fashion postnatally. However, the relevance of certain developmental events in utero is not known. For example, we do not know whether the functional status of preterm infants [reduced lower esophageal sphincter pressure, simultaneous contractions and noncoordinated peristalsis, and frequent transient lower esophageal sphincter (LES) relaxations] represents merely delayed development or confers some specific adaptive advantage to the third-trimester human fetus. Fetal swallowing can be detected as early as 11 weeks' gestation, with sucking movements beginning as early as 18 and 20 weeks (6). The swallowing of amniotic fluid begins very slowly with a few milliliters per day and increases to 450 mL per day in the third trimester (7). In animals, fetal swallowing defects have been correlated with failure of growth of the gastrointestinal (GI) tract, as well as ultrastructural abnormalities (8). Careful studies of human fetuses are not available.

ANATOMY

The arterial blood supply to the esophagus is generally considered with regard to the cervical, thoracic, and abdominal segments of the esophagus.

The arterial blood supply to the pharyngoesophageal junction and the cervical esophagus is derived from branches of the inferior thyroid artery. In addition, the junctional area of the esophagus is supplied by small arterial branches of the subclavian, common carotid, vertebral, superior thyroid, and costocervical trunk vessels (9). The thoracic esophagus is supplied from branches of the aorta, the bronchial arteries, and the right intercostal arteries. Bronchial artery branches enter the esophagus at the level of the carina and proceed inferiorly along the ventral aspect of the esophagus. Accessory esophageal branches are also present directly from the aorta, the internal

Patrick A. Dillon: Washington University School of Medicine, St. Louis Children's Hospital, St. Louis, Missouri 63110.

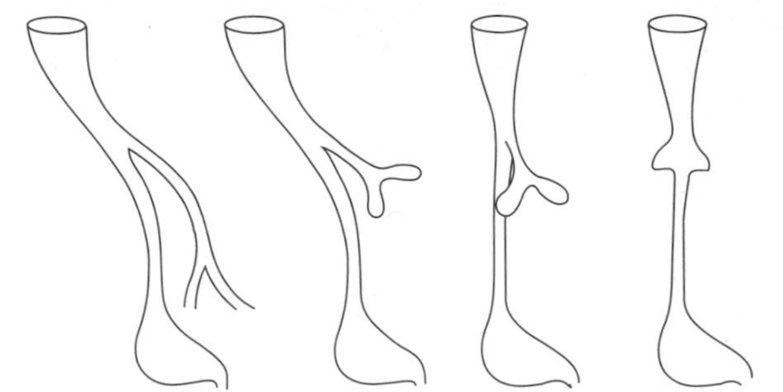

FIGURE 64-1. The description of the tracheobronchial tree developing as a stalk off the foregut.

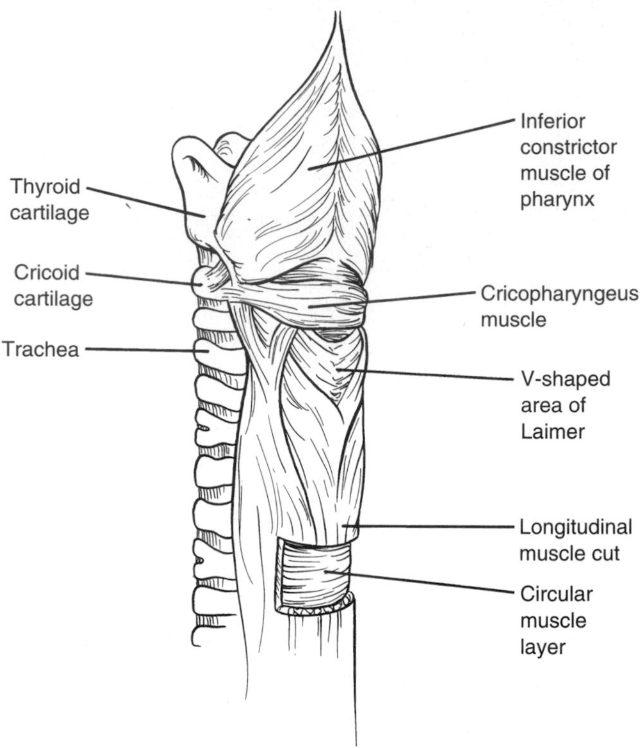

FIGURE 64-2. The muscular wall of the pharynx and esophagus. The longitudinal muscle fibers decussate superiorly to produce an area of weakness, the area of Laimer. This represents the location of most instrumental esophageal perforations. (Adapted from Netter FH. *Ciba collection of medical illustrations*, vol. 3, part I, sec. II, plate 3. I. Upper digestive tract. West Caldwell, NJ: Ciba Pharmaceutical Co., 1983.)

mammary, common carotid, and superior intercostal arteries (10). Esophageal branches of the aorta supply the esophagus immediately below the level of the carina. These vessels have ascending and descending branches that form anastomoses with the inferior thyroid and left gastric arterial branches (10). The left gastric artery provides esophageal blood supply to the abdominal segment of the esophagus in most individuals. Rarely, esophageal arteries will arise from an accessory left hepatic artery. In fewer than one-half of individuals, the esophagus receives arterial blood via the left inferior phrenic artery, and rarely from the right inferior phrenic artery (9). A well-developed subepithelial network of capillaries is present in the esophageal mucosa and submucosa (11,12). Venous drainage from the esophagus includes intrinsic, extrinsic, and longitudinal vessels. The intrinsic system includes subepithelial and submucosal veins that join gastric veins, and perforating veins that join with the extrinsic system of veins. The extrinsic veins include larger longitudinal vessels that run on the outer surface of the esophagus and are close to the vagus nerves. These vessels connect the left gastric vein to the azygous or hemiazygous veins either directly or indirectly or via the posterior bronchial veins. Extrinsic veins include the cervical drainage into the inferior thyroid, vertebral, and deep cervical veins. Esophageal veins at the level of the cardia join the phrenic and abdominal esophageal veins to drain primarily into the left gastric vein, as well as the gastroepiploic and splenic veins (13). This may be a point of importance when dealing with a patient with portal hypertension.

Oblique muscular fibers that fuse with pharyngeal constrictor muscles and transverse fibers that encircle the esophagus compose the cricopharyngeal (CP) muscle. The CP muscle is a unique striated muscle in that contraction occurs while at rest. During swallowing, belching, and vomiting, relaxation of the muscle occurs and the upper esophagus opens (14). The CP muscle is located at the pharyngoesophageal junction, attaches to the cricoid cartilage, and forms a C-shaped muscular band with innervation by the pharyngeal plexus of the vagus nerve and the recurrent laryngeal nerve (Fig. 64-2). The recurrent laryngeal nerve projects to the anterior motor units located in the anterior segments of the horizontal part of the muscle, whereas the pharyngeal plexus projects to the posterior motor units of the muscle (15). The main function of the CP muscle is to control luminal flow between the pharynx and esophagus. The CP sphincter muscle is tonically contracted at rest and relaxes during swallowing. The major component of the upper esophageal sphincter (UES) is the CP muscle, although the inferior pharyngeal constrictor and striated muscles of the proximal esophagus also contribute (16). The CP muscle posteriorly is where the longitudinal muscles diverge to attach to the cricoid cartilage. This area is vulnerable to perforation during esophagoscopy. Videofluoroscopy and manometry studies have been the source of data used to link the CP muscle to the UES in deglutition (17).

The LES area corresponds to the position of the CP muscle in the cervical esophagus, although there is no specific muscle to correspond at the LES. There is a sphincter equivalent at the level of the gastroesophageal (GE) junction. The primary role of the LES is to prevent gastroesophageal reflux (GER). The LES relaxes as a primary esophageal wave moves through the esophagus toward the

GE junction. The LES is also responsive to intraabdominal pressure, gastrin, secretin, narcotics, benzodiazepines, theophylline, and its derivatives, caffeine, chocolate, and alcohol.

ESOPHAGOSCOPY

Pediatric esophagoscopy was first used for the removal of foreign bodies. Presently, it is used to evaluate symptoms of dysphagia and GER, to evaluate and dilate congenital or acquired esophageal strictures, to evaluate the esophagus after trauma, for sclerotherapy for bleeding esophageal varices, and to carry out gastrostomy tube or button placement. Before esophagoscopy, an evaluation of the child should be undertaken that is appropriate for the condition being addressed. The radiologic evaluation of most esophageal disorders begins with a frontal and lateral chest radiograph, a contrast esophagogram, or a chest computed tomography (CT) imaging study. The definitive diagnosis, however, of many of the disorders in childhood depends on direct observation by esophagoscopy.

Both flexible and rigid esophagoscopes are available that are suitable for use in children. The advantage of the flexible esophagoscope is that it may be used with topical anesthesia and sedation for routine diagnostic endoscopy in children. The disadvantages of this instrument are that the biopsy and foreign-body instruments that pass through the operating channel are relatively small, and therapeutic esophagoscopy can be impractical.

Rigid esophagoscopes are available in sizes suitable for use in any infant or child (Fig. 64-3). These instruments employ the same Hopkins rod-lens telescope used for rigid bronchoscopy and provide superior visualization compared with flexible instruments. Foreign-body and biopsy instruments may be passed through a separate channel of the esophagoscope, or larger instruments may be coupled to the telescope and passed directly through the lumen of the scope. In addition to the availability of a broader range of sizes of endoscopes, the rigid esophagoscope allows passage of larger instruments, thus facilitating therapeutic esophagoscopy.

Diagnostic esophagoscopy with the flexible gastroscope may be performed under topical anesthesia with intravenous sedation. Pretreatment with atropine is used to reduce oral secretions and block reflex bradycardia. These children should be observed with cardiac and oxygen saturation monitors during the procedure. The child is placed in the left lateral position with the neck slightly extended. A plastic mouth guard may be used in older children, but is not needed for infants without teeth. The esophagoscope is passed gently over the tongue, and a slight deflection is placed in the tip as the patient is induced to swallow. With gentle pressure, the scope is pushed through the CP sphincter into the upper esophagus. It is then passed through the length of the esophagus, keeping the lumen under direct

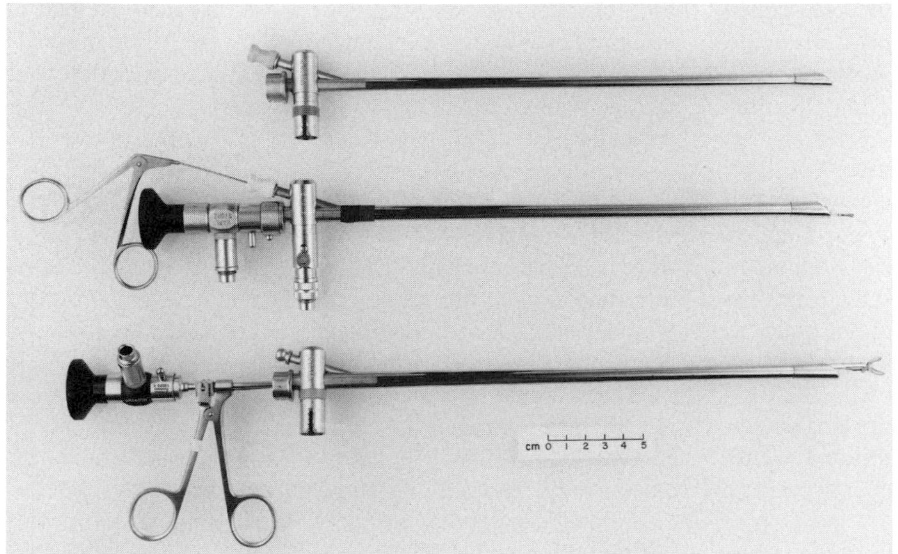

A

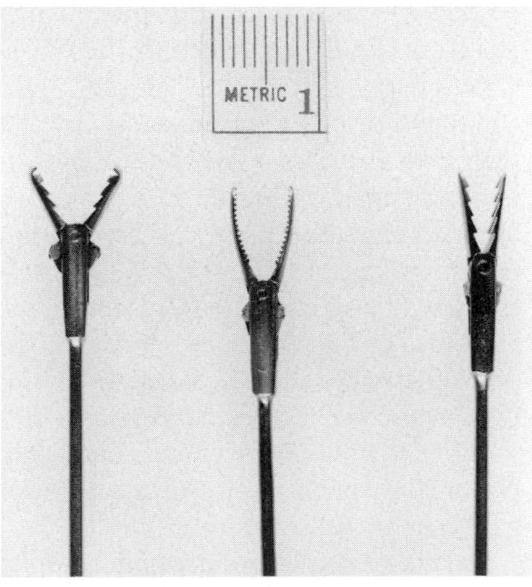

B

FIGURE 64-3. Rigid pediatric esophagoscopes. **(A)** The 3-mm, 30-cm rigid esophagoscope (*top*) is suitable for use in infants. The 5-mm (*center*) and 6-mm (*bottom*), 30-cm esophagoscopes can be used in older children. Each esophagoscope accepts the Hopkins rod lens telescope. Foreign-body and biopsy instruments can be passed directly through the lumen of the esophagoscope (*bottom*) or through the offset instrument channel (*center*). **(B)** Specialized foreign-body forceps used through these esophagoscopes include grasping forceps (*left and right*) and peanut forceps (*center*).

vision. The GE junction may be visualized from below by passing the instrument into the stomach and retroflexing. Care must be taken not to insufflate excessive air because many smaller children experience respiratory distress with gastric distension. The region of the CP sphincter is more carefully examined as the esophagoscope is withdrawn.

The technique of rigid esophagoscopy is more difficult to learn and has a higher incidence of complications in inexperienced hands. Rigid esophagoscopy is performed under general anesthesia in children. Because of the flexibility of the larynx and upper airway, these children should be intubated for airway control before insertion of the esophagoscope. The patient is placed supine, and a soft roll is placed under the shoulders to extend the cervical spine. The appropriate-size esophagoscope is passed gently along the right border of the tongue into the right piriform sinus under direct vision. The scope is then moved medially to visualize the right arytenoid cartilage and the posterior wall of the larynx. The tip of the scope is gently insinuated behind the posterior laryngeal wall and directed anteriorly to expose the CP sphincter. Under general anesthesia, this sphincter is usually relaxed and open, and the esophagoscope can be passed under direct vision into the upper esophagus. If the sphincter is in spasm, a small filiform dilator or a nasogastric tube can be passed through the esophagoscope into the upper esophagus and used as a guide. The esophagoscope is supported and manipulated by the surgeon's left hand, which also protects the child's teeth. The endoscope is passed through the body of the esophagus under direct vision. To pass the esophagoscope through the GE junction, the head must be hyperextended and the instrument passed to the left, anteriorly. It should be possible to visualize the entire length of the esophagus from the CP sphincter to the GE junction with this equipment.

Complications of esophagoscopy are more common than with bronchoscopy. The complications of passage of either the rigid or flexible scopes are usually encountered at the level of the CP muscle. Perforation of the cricopharyngeus occurs in about 0.03% of patients with flexible esophagoscopy, but mucosal lacerations are not unusual. Perforation of the piriform sinus or the posterolateral aspect of the CP sphincter is more common with the rigid esophagoscope and occurs in about 0.1% of patients. Perforation of the body of the esophagus is rare and occurs principally when biopsy specimens are taken or in patients with esophageal stricture.

Iatrogenic perforation of the esophagus is the most common cause of perforation encountered in children. The diagnosis is suspected with the development of a spiking fever or pain and crepitation in the cervical region after esophagoscopy. The diagnosis is confirmed by demonstration of mediastinal or cervical emphysema on plain radiograms and extravasation of contrast on esophagogram. Most iatrogenic perforations are small and well contained. These may be treated with intravenous antibiotics, with the child receiving nothing by mouth. Larger perforations and those communicating with a pleural space need open drainage and attempts at closure. Pleural flaps or intercostal muscle flaps may be used to secure the esophageal closure.

FOREIGN-BODY INGESTION

The accidental ingestion of aerodigestive foreign bodies by children occurs frequently and, although is usually associated with minimal morbidity, can occasionally result in significant morbidity and even mortality (18). More than one-half of the children are less than 4 years old. In most cases, the episode is either witnessed by an adult or the child tells of the ingestion. Young children tend to sample their environment by placing things in their mouth. For this reason, all manner of objects may be swallowed. The majority of them are not excessively large in proportion to the esophagus and are not sharp edged. They can be swallowed and not become impacted in the esophagus. If the object enters the stomach, there is good likelihood that it will pass through the remainder of the GI tract. An exception is the child with a congential or acquired intestinal stricture, such as a child after an episode of necrotizing enterocolitis. Coins continue to be the most common objects swallowed. Of note, there is increasing incidence of small button-type batteries being ingested (19). These batteries can leak chemicals, which can cause esophageal scarring or perforation. Approximately 20% of ingested foreign bodies become lodged in the esophagus and will require removal (20). The inability of the esophagus to propel the object into the stomach may be due to the size of the object, its configuration, or the degree or lack of esophageal peristalsis.

Dysphagia, excessive salivation, neck pain, and occasional choking are the symptoms commonly seen in these children. Approximately 10% may be asymptomatic (21). This is a high enough incidence that if there is a clinical suspicion of ingestion, radiologic evaluation should be carried out. Patients at increased risk for foreign-body obstruction are those who have undergone repair of an esophageal atresia or tracheoesophageal fistula, who are neurologically impaired, or who are psychiatric patients. The diagnosis is usually made at the initial evaluation, but a delay in recognition is not unusual and is directly related to the incidence and severity of complications in removal of the foreign body (22).

The most common sites of foreign-body impaction are at points of relative narrowing in the neck at the level of the CP muscle, in the thorax at the level of the aortic arch and left mainstem bronchus, and at the GE junction. Another point of obstruction can be at an anastomotic stricture. Objects lodged at the level of the CP muscle can cause neck pain. A foreign body in the upper third of the thoracic esophagus can produce respiratory symptoms because of its position in the esophagus directly contiguous with the membranous trachea. Pain may be produced throughout the length of the esophagus due to mucosal irritation or erosion and perforation. This process is usually acute; however, occasionally an object may be chronically impacted and cause obstruction due to its presence as an inflammatory mass (23). Foreign bodies lodged in the upper and middle third of the esophagus should be removed because it is unlikely they will spontaneously pass. In contrast, the majority of coins in the distal esophagus will pass spontaneously (24). Allowing the patient to drink some liquids and a short period of waiting is reasonable in selected instances (25).

The incidence of esophageal perforation is low, approximately 1%. However, if the diagnosis of an esophageal foreign body is delayed, there is a greater risk of morbidity, including perforation and mediastinitis (26). All retained foreign bodies and those with sharp edges should be removed.

The removal of the foreign body can be done in several ways. The majority of cases are treated by endoscopic removal with a rigid esophagoscope under a general anesthetic to protect the airway. The rigid esophagoscope has ports large enough to pass the appropriate foreign-body graspers and telescopes. For smooth foreign objects, particularly in the upper half of the esophagus, balloon extraction performed with procedural sedation in the radiology suite or in the operation room is a reasonable option. Antegrade bougilnage and flexible endoscopy are appropriate in selected cases.

Patients with esophageal perforation may present with respiratory distress, including tachypnea, stridor, retractions, and supplemental oxygen requirement. The child may present in this manner initially, or this may be seen shortly after foreign-body extraction. Hematemesis or hemoptysis may signal a vascular erosion (26).

Treatment of the patient with an esophageal perforation includes removal of the foreign body, surgical drainage of the mediastinum, and repair or diversion of the perforation. In selected cases with a contained mediastinal perforation, endoscopic removal of the foreign body, intravenous antibiotics, and avoidance of oral intake may suffice.

CAUSTIC ESOPHAGEAL INJURY

Although federal legislation has greatly improved product labeling, packaging, and their contents, caustic ingestion in children continues to be a significant problem. Anderson et al. estimated approximately 17,000 ingestions in children (27). The vast majority of these cases are accidental and seen in children younger than 5 years old. These caustic substances are usually separated into acids and alkalis. Household and industrial acids include hydrochloric acid (toilet bowl and swimming pool cleaners), sulfuric acid (storage batteries), and phosphoric acid (metal cleaners).. Strong acids, usually with a pH less than 2, produce a coagulation necrosis, and penetrating injury may occur if a sufficient volume of acid is ingested. Ingested hydrofluoric acid, in contrast, results in a liquefaction necrosis of the esophagus and can cause death secondary to an imbalance in calcium metabolism from fluoride absorption. Most and the most severe caustic injuries are due to household cleaning alkalis (28). The volume and nature of the alkali will determine the depth and extent of injury to the esophagus. Alkalis produce a liquefaction necrosis often deep and transmural, and are frequently more severe when compared with acid ingestion. There may be associated vascular thrombosis, perforation, and contracture of the esophagus. Sodium hydroxide, commonly used as a drain cleaner, can be especially dangerous. It often comes in liquid form, is easily ingested and may cause injury to the surrounding organs, such as the larynx, trachea, aorta, colon, or pancreas (29). Although household bleach may be the most frequently ingested material, this rarely causes serious injury. Newer dishwashing agents are known to have a high pH and can be especially injurious to the esophagus (30).

The signs and symptoms seen in children with an ingestion injury include oropharyngeal pain, irritability, vomiting, drooling, and at times, respiratory distress. The mouth and the pharynx should be inspected for evidence of injury, although the absence of visible oral burns does not preclude esophageal or gastric involvement. Initial care is aimed at control of the airway, if necessary, administering intravenous fluids, and control of pain. Chest and abdominal radiographs are obtained to evaluate for mediastinal or intraperitoneal air. With the patient stabilized, endoscopic evaluation for esophageal injury beyond the cricopharyngeus should be carried out within the initial 24 hours following injury to avoid the time of maximum edema. This procedure is performed under general anesthesia and preferably uses the rigid esophagoscope, although a flexible endoscope can also be used. The esophagoscope should be passed only to the first area of injury beyond the cricopharyngeus to prevent iatrogenic injury. If respiratory symptoms are also present, laryngoscopy and bronchoscopy should also be performed. Endoscopic assessment of the injury can be graded (Table 64-1) according to the extent of mucosal injury and can be useful in planning future management. First-degree injuries of the esophagus usually result in mucosal erythema and edema, and no additional therapy is required. Second- and third-degree injuries are characterized by mucosal ulceration and the formation of pseudomembranous plaques. Second-degree injuries are noncircumferential, whereas third-degree injuries are circumferential and may involve mucosal sloughing and thrombosis of submucosal esophageal vessels (31).

Patients with second- and third-degree burns are generally treated with parenteral antibiotics. The use of corticosteroid for caustic ingestions of the esophagus remains

TABLE 64-1 Endoscopic Grading of Caustic Esophageal Injuries.

First degree	Mucosal hyperemia and edema
Second degree	Mucosal ulceration with vesicles and exudates, pseudomembrane formation
Third degree	Deep ulceration with charring and eschar formation, severe edema obliterating the lumen

(From Orringer MB. Tumors, injuries, and miscellaneous conditions of the esophagus. In: Greenfield LJ, ed. *Surgery: scientific principles and practice.* Philadelphia: Lippincott Williams & Wilkins, 2001:692–735, with permission.)

controversial (27,32–34). Many surgeons favor treatment for several weeks with prednisone 2.0 to 2.5 mg per kg per day and ampicillin 50 mg per kg per day to attempt to minimize an inflammatory response and subsequent stricture formation. However, there is no contemporary evidence-based study to support this protocol. Steroids may be more effective in the established stricture by allowing a significant increase in time between dilatations (30). Esophageal perforation or hemorrhage is an indication for emergency thoracotomy and esophagectomy. Twenty-five percent of patients will develop strictures and require dilation. Triamcinolone injection into the stricture may be helpful (35). Esophageal dilations have remained the mainstay of treatment for esophageal strictures. There has been some more recent use of esophageal stents to treat refractory strictures. The development of obstructing granulation tissue and stent migration has limited their effectiveness in the pediatric population. Despite these drawbacks, stents may provide limited relief and may reduce the overall frequency of esophageal dilatations (30,36). Determining when to abandon esophageal dilatation and proceed to esophageal replacement surgery can be difficult. Factors making esophageal replacement surgery more probable include a delay in the time of ingestion injury to the start dilatations (more than 1 month), the length of the stricture (more than 5 cm), and esophageal perforation during dilatation (36).

There is increased risk of the development of esophageal adenocarcinoma in these patients. Long-term follow-up and surveillance is necessary.

ESOPHAGEAL CYSTS

Esophageal cysts and duplications comprise approximately 10% of all GI tract duplications. Fallon et al. proposed two classes of esophageal cysts: intramural esophageal cysts and enteric cysts (37). Intramural esophageal cysts occur within the wall of the esophagus and are believed to represent defects of vacuolation of the primitive esophagus (38). During the fourth week of development, the esophageal mucosa proliferates to obliterate the esophageal lumen completely. At 6 weeks' gestation, vacuoles begin to form within this solid mass of epithelial cells, gradually coalescing to reestablish an esophageal lumen. Disruption of this process presumably leaves epithelial cells within the wall of the esophagus, which can lead to development of intramural esophageal cysts (39). These cysts are lined by columnar or pseudostratified columnar epithelium with cilia, which is consistent with the foregut epithelium of a 4- to 6-week embryo. These lesions have been referred to as true duplications of the esophagus and archenteric cysts, although the term *intramural esophageal cysts* seems most appropriate. The embryology of enteric cysts is more controversial, but most authors believe they are caused by abnormalities that occur during separation of the endoderm from the notochord. Persistence of neuroenteric canals or a split notochord syndrome is often used to explain the development of posterior mediastinal cysts when there are vertebral abnormalities or an extensive duplication (40). The notochord appears at the third week of gestation and simultaneously is believed to begin separation from the endoderm (Fig. 64-4). A gap in the notochord can occur during separation, and a diverticulum of the foregut can lead to a number of anomalies. Vertebral anomalies indicate spina bifida and hemivertebrae. In addition, a tract can form, and the gut may form short or long diverticula or fistulas along any portion of the GI tract (41). Esophageal duplications are usually identified in the thoracic esophagus, although cervical esophageal duplications have been reported (42). Two-thirds of enteric cysts in the esophagus are identified during childhood.

Enteric cysts may be incidentally identified by plain chest radiograph prior to the development of symptoms. However, the continued secretion of mucin by the lining of the cysts will result in expansion and growth that usually results in respiratory symptoms, dysphagia, or feeding intolerance (42). The presence of a vertebral anomaly makes the diagnosis of an enteric cyst likely. A complete evaluation of the cyst usually involves an esophagogram to rule out a common enteric lumen and a CT scan or magnetic resonance imaging (MRI) to establish the relationship of the cyst with the surrounding mediastinal structures. The MRI is particularly helpful in regard to identifying any intraspinal anomaly that may be present.

Esophageal cysts should be surgically excised (43,44). An intramural esophageal cyst may be enucleated by division of the esophageal musculature overlying the cyst and careful dissection of the cyst from the esophageal wall. Usually, this can be accomplished without violation of the esophageal lumen. An enteric cyst is totally separate from the true esophageal wall, but usually has a fibrous connection to the anterior vertebral body, which should be removed with the cyst. Often, this connection may pass cephalad out of the thorax to communicate with a lower cervical vertebra. Small esophageal cysts of either type are

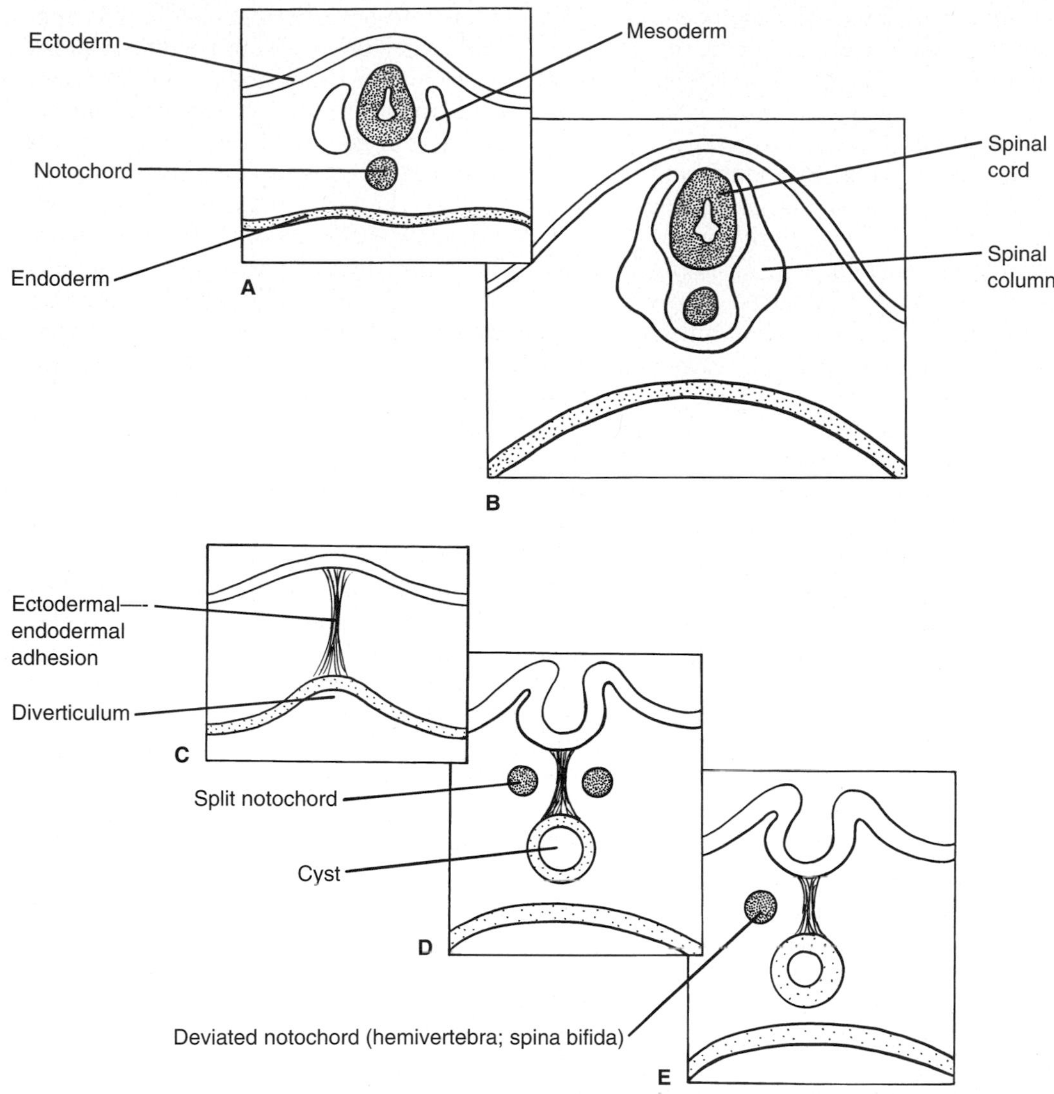

FIGURE 64-4. Development of the split notochord syndrome. **(A, B)** The normal process of enclosure of the spinal cord and notochord by the paraxial mesodermal cell mass to form the vertebral body. **(C** through **E)** In the cephalic end of the embryo, the ectoderm and endoderm are in close proximity. Adhesions between the two can interfere with the cephalad growth of the notochord. A split notochord can result in the development of spina bifida, and deviation of the notochord can result in hemivertebra formation. (Adapted from Beardmore HE, Wiglesworth FW. Vertebral anomalies and alimentary duplications. *Pediatr Clin North Am* 1958;5:457.)

potentially resectable by thoracoscopic techniques, thus avoiding some of the morbidity of a formal thoracotomy.

INFECTION/INFLAMMATION

Eosinophilic Esophagitis

The presence of intraepithelial eosinophils on esophageal biopsy is commonly associated with pediatric gastroesophageal reflux disease (GERD) (45). Eosinophilic esophagitis is a distinct disease entity in children (46). Careful review of the clinical presentation, endoscopic, and pathologic findings of these patients, as well as the response to treatment, is required to make the diagnosis. The majority of patients are male, and the symptoms may be multiple and overlap with reflux esophagitis. Although pain and vomiting are frequent occurrences, obstructive symptoms such as dysphagia and food impaction without evidence of esophageal stricture are present. Diarrhea, which may be a marker for the presence of eosinophilic GI involvement, and a positive allergy history are also noted in these patients (46,47). Moreover, the patients have often been diagnosed with GERD and have been unresponsive to adequate medical therapy.

In patients with eosinophilic esophagitis, a upper GI fluoroscopy and an esophageal pH probe study often show little evidence of GERD (46). Endoscopic evaluation should include esophagogastroduodenoscopy. Gross findings on endoscopy may include the presence of multiple esophageal rings throughout the length of the esophagus. These rings are concentric, spaced approximately 1 to 2 cm apart, and do not resolve with insufflation of the esophagus. Despite the presence of the rings, no definitive stricture is found (48). Biopsies obtained during the endoscopy should be from the proximal and distal esophagus, as well as from the antrum and duodenum. Although the presence of eosinophils on esophageal biopsy may reflect GERD, a number of studies have suggested that an increased number of eosinophils (more than 20 per high-powered field), preferential distribution of eosinophils to the squamous mucosa and superficial epithelium, and eosinophilic aggregates identifies an individual with eosinophilic esophagitis (46,47,49,50). Although documentation of eosinophilic infiltration is required to establish the diagnosis, the role of eosinophils in the pathophysiology remains unclear. The activation status of eosinophils and the release of potentially toxic granules is hypothesized to play a role in other inflammatory bowel conditions, although this has not been clearly established in patients with eosinophilic esophagitis (51).

The presence of severe eosinophilia and a lack of response to standard medical therapy should prompt a discussion of etiologies other than GERD. Once the diagnosis of eosinophilic esophagitis is suspected, a proper immunologic and food allergy workup should be completed prior to referral for surgical antireflux procedures (52). Treatment for eosinophilic esophagitis includes elimination of suspected food allergies, but may require an elemental amino acid-based diet (46,47). In addition, suspected patients have been treated with a course of steroids. Methylprednisolone (1.5 mg per kg) administered twice daily over a 4-week period has resulted in both a marked improvement in clinical symptoms, as well as improvement in the histologic appearance of the esophagus (50).

Barrett's Esophagus

Barrett's esophagus is a condition in which specialized columnar epithelium extends for more than 3 cm above the top of the top of the LES. Whereas islands of normal-appearing gastric epithelium are relatively common in the esophagus, Barrett's goblet epithelium is specialized in nature and contains cells that stain positive with Alcian blue at a pH of 2.4 (53). Barrett's epithilium is frequently associated with severe and unrelenting strictures of the esophagus, often in the proximal and middle thirds (54). Although Barrett's esophagus was at one time believed to be congential, most now agree that this disorder is acquired. GER is believed to be a major precursor to the development of Barrett's epithelium in children (55,56). In addition to GER, other predisposing conditions include esophageal atresia, lye ingestion, and mental retardation (57,58). The incidence of Barrret's epithelium appears to be exceptionally high in the esophagus just proximal to the cervical anastomosis in gastric tube reconstruction of the esophagus (59). Children with Barrett's esophagus usually present with symptoms of severe GER in the first year of life. Often, these patients have significant dysphagia secondary to esophagitis or esophageal stricture. Hematemesis and respiratory symptoms secondary to chronic aspiration are often seen. The diagnosis of Barrett's esophagus requires multiple biopsy specimens of the esophageal mucosa, obtained well proximal to the LES. Unlike adult patients, most children with Barrett's epithelium do not show any gross changes on endoscopic observation, and these specimens must be obtained in blind fashion (56). The diagnosis of Barrett's esophagus is made on observation of the specialized metaplastic epithelium characteristic of this disorder, although many pediatric series have described patients with Barrett's esophagus in whom only normal-appearing gastric mucosa was identified at biopsy (55). The true frequency of Barrett's esophagus in children is unknown.

Treatment of patients with Barrett's esophagus focuses on the elimination of GER and chronic esophagitis. Treatment with histamine-2-blocking agents, proton pump inhibitors, and antacids may eliminate the acid reflux, but does nothing for the alkaline reflux characteristic in these patients. Most authors believe that the alkaline reflux is primarily responsible for the development of esophagitis and perhaps dysplasia of the epithelium. For this reason, the surgical elimination of GER is universally recommended (54,56). Even with successful operation, however, Barrett's epithelium rarely completely regresses in children with this disorder (60,61).

Barrett's epithelium of the special columnar variety is a premalignant condition. Patients with Barrett's epithelium have a 30- to-125-fold increased incidence of adenocarcinoma of the esophagus (62,63). Hassall and colleagues reported the case of a 17-year-old boy with Barrett's esophagus and severe dysphagia who was found to have adenocarcinoma of the esophagus on esophagoscopy (63). They reviewed nine additional cases of adenocarcinoma developing in young patients with Barrett's epithelium reported in the literature. The prognosis of these patients is particularly poor, even after esophageal resection. Children with Barrett's esophagus require careful long-term follow-up with esophageal biopsies to detect the development of dysplasia within the epithelium. Younes and colleagues demonstrated accumulation of p53 protein, as well as intraepithelial adenocarcinoma, in patients with dysplastic Barrett's epithelium (64). This analysis may prove helpful in differentiating those patients who are likely to develop malignancy, thus allowing earlier treatment.

FUNCTIONAL ESOPHAGEAL DISORDERS

Achalasia

Functional esophageal disorders in the pediatric population remain rare, although the exact incidence is difficult to establish. The incidence of achalasia, a motor disorder affecting almost the entire esophagus, is believed to be four to six cases per million population per year, with only 5% of those cases attributed to patients 15 years of age or youngers (65). Problems with relaxation of the LES muscle may be related to nitric oxide (66). Achalasia may be associated with neuromuscular disorders such as glucocorticoid deficiency and familial dysautonomia. In older children, dysphagia, regurgitation of food, and weight loss are present. A chest radiograph may show mediastinal widening and an air–fluid level. An esophagogram shows dilation of the esophagus ending in a bird's beak narrowing at the GE junction. The diagnosis is confirmed by esophageal manometry. The LES is elevated (more than 40 mm Hg), and with swallowing, there is often incomplete or absent relaxation of the LES. In addition, peristaltic waves are lacking or incomplete in the body of the esophagus.

Treatment for children with achalasia involves a variety of modalities. This includes the use of pharmacologic agents, such as nifedipine and botulinum toxin, and endoscopic therapy, with the use of bougie and balloon dilatation of the esophagus. Although the experience in children with these treatments is limited, they appear to have less effectiveness when compared with adult series.

Endoscopic evaluation may differentiate esophageal achalasia from esophageal changes seen with GERD. The distal esophagus demonstrates a smooth narrowing, which allows easy passage of the endoscope. The mucosa is normal, and there is no lower esophageal stenosis or inflammatory changes seen with GERD (65). Preoperatively, these patients should be placed on a clear liquid 24 to 48 hours prior to surgery to decrease the potential of food obstructing the distal esophagus. In addition, prior to induction of anesthesia, the esophagus should be drained with a lavage tube to minimize the chance of aspiration (67).

Dilatation of the esophagus with bougie dilators and with pneumatic balloon dilatation have both been used in pediatric patients with achalasia. There is an ongoing debate concerning the efficacy of esophageal dilatation, although there appears to be more success associated with pneumatic balloon dilatation (68,69).

Surgical treatment consists of a Heller esophagomyotomy. This may be accomplished with an open operation, although reports describing both a laparoscopic and a thoracoscopic approach are increasing in frequency. A laparoscopic approach allows fundoplication to be performed easily. Performance of an antireflux operation at the time remains a point of debate; however, a review of more recent literature advocates at least a partial fundoplication to prevent postoperative reflux (67). A transthoracic approach, whether through a minimally invasive or open operation, provides access for a longer, more cephalad extension of the myotomy. If extended esophageal involvement is documented radiographically or with manometry, a transthoracic approach appears superior to the abdominal approach (65).

The technical aspects of the myotomy are vital to the success of the operation (Fig. 64-5). The myotomy extends

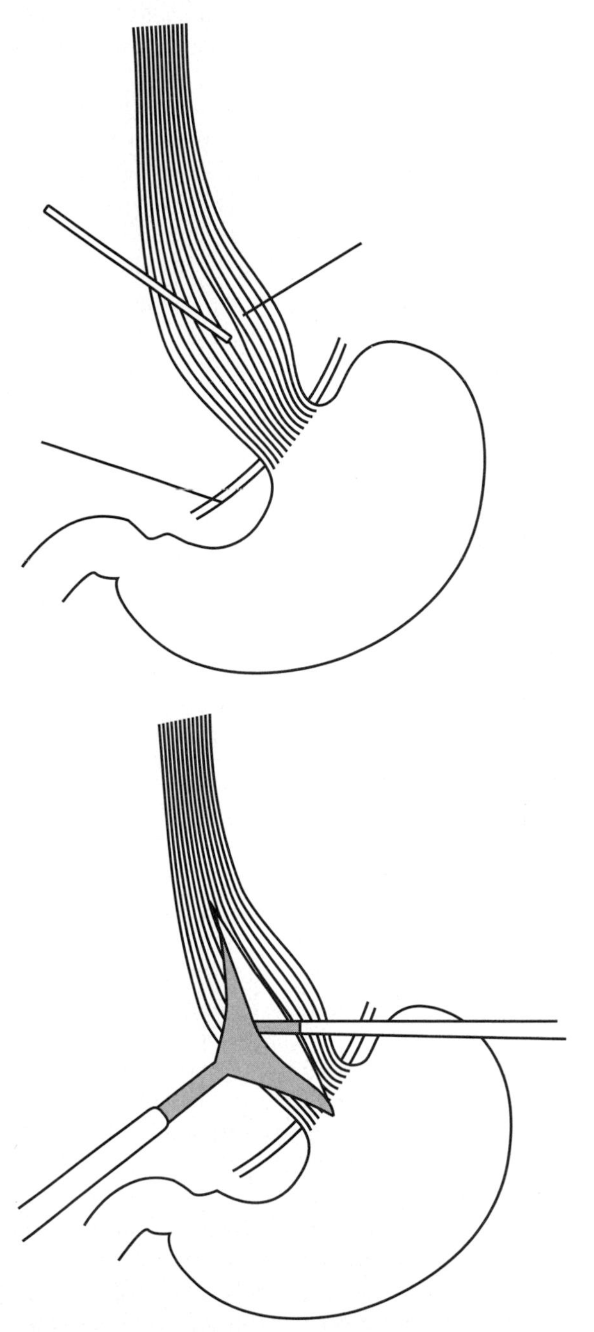

FIGURE 64-5. A Heller myotomy extending 2 to 3 cm across the gastroesophageal junction and well up onto the thoracic esophagus.

across the GE junction for approximately 2 to 3 cm to minimize the chance of postoperative recurrence. Appropriate downward retraction at the level of the GE junction allows exposure of the anterior esophagus and cephalad extension of the myotomy for a total myotomy distance of approximately 7 to 8 cm (70). Placement of an esophageal dilator or esophagoscope can facilitate the myotomy. Complications from the esophagomyotomy can occur, regardless of the surgical approach. Perforation of the esophagus along the site of myotomy can occur in any location, although the GE junction is particularly vulnerable and a fundoplication that is too constrictive may lead to continued dysphagia (71).

CP achalasia is a rare condition that will usually present much earlier when compared with esophageal achalasia. Chronic dysphagia may be present in patients with CP achalasia. Symptoms may include choking, excessive salivation, and nasal reflux when feeding. There are reports describing the use of botulinum toxin for the initial treatment of CP achalasia. Decreased spasm was documented with postinjection cineradiography and manometry, and allowed the ingestion of food without previous difficulties. Patients who benefited the most from botulinum toxin did not have associated dysmotility or prior surgery (72). Alternatively, in those patients with mild symptoms, initial bougienage of the narrowing may be of benefit with surgery reserved for those who do not respond to dilatation. In patients with severe symptoms and no associated abnormalities, CP achalasia is better treated with initial cricopharyngeus myotomy (14,73).

ESOPHAGEAL STENOSIS

Esophageal stenosis caused by an intrinsic congenital deformity is extremely uncommon in infants and children. The main forms of congenital esophageal stenosis (CES) consist of a membranous esophageal web or diaphragm, stricture caused by ectopic tracheobronchial remnants (TBRs), and congenital idiopathic fibromuscular hypertrophy (FMH) (74). A modification of this classification has been proposed, which includes patients with multiple stenoses, and is based on the type of stenosis and the association of the stenosis with other abnormalities of foregut separation (75). TBRs are usually located in the distal one-third of the esophagus, whereas membranous obstruction and FMH are more commonly noted in the middle one-third of the esophagus. Given that treatment options vary according to the etiology of the stricture, accurate diagnosis is essential for proper care. Symptoms are usually related to feeding intolerance and dysphagia, although a stenosis in the upper esophagus may have more respiratory symptoms. There is no evidence of extrinsic compression of the esophagus, and there is an absence of GERD. In addition, with regard to TBRs, there may be a history of esophageal atresia and tracheoesophageal fistula (76,77). Diagnosis of CES usually requires an esophagogram, pH probe study, and upper endoscopy to rule out esophagitis and GERD. More recently, endoscopic high-frequency ultrasound has been used to differentiate TBR from FMH and can also be used to identify other submucosal lesions (76,78,79). Despite these measures, the etiology of the CES can remain difficult, often resulting in attempts to dilate lesions that will require surgery (80).

Treatment of tracheobronchial remnants with esophageal dilatation is generally unsuccessful, and adequate treatment entails a segmental esophageal resection of the TBR with end-to-end anastomosis of the esophagus or rarely enucleation of the cartilaginous remnant. The TBR lesion is usually approached through a left thoracotomy, given the lower esophageal location of the lesion. Palpation of the cartilaginous lesion and intraoperative endoscopy can be helpful in identifying the exact location for resection (78). For patients with TBR resections that involve the gastroesophageal junction (GE), an antireflux procedure should be considered in order to prevent subsequent GERD.

FMH is classically located in the middle third of the esophagus and has a length of 1 to 4 cm, resulting in an hourglass shape to the esophagus on esophagogram studies (75). Although there is no consensus on the exact therapy for suspected FMH, esophageal dilatation appears to be successful in a number of series and should be the initial treatment of choice for this patient group (75,78,80). Pneumatic balloon dilatation and traditional bouginage can be used for dilatation with minimal risk of perforation of the esophagus. With balloon dilatation, the force is transmitted only to the stenotic segment of the esophagus, and correct placement of the balloon can be determined by direct endoscopic visualization (78). If dilations are required frequently and remain ineffective, consideration should be given to an alternative diagnosis and surgical intervention should be undertaken.

In patients with a membranous diaphragm as the cause of stenosis, balloon dilation is recommended. Endoscopic incision or partial resection of the diaphragm may be required prior to dilatation if the stenosis is severe. Balloon dilations and endoscopic incision of the membrane (as needed) are currently the treatments of choice (74,81).

ESOPHAGEAL VARICES

The development of esophageal varices is associated with portal hypertension and is often seen in conjunction with ascites and hypersplenism. The optimal treatment of esophageal varices continues to evolve with a number of therapeutic modalities available to the practicing physician. Endoscopic diagnosis and treatment is commonly used. In addition, pharmacologic methods are often used, and selective use of transjugular intrahepatic portosystemic shunting (TIPS) has been successful in selected cases. Shunt operations are presently used rarely, and liver transplantation is applicable for children with end-stage liver disease not related to presinusoidal portal hypertension. The optimal treatment is often based on the etiology of the portal hypertension.

The clinically significant portosystemic collaterals develop from the portal vein through the coronary vein and short gastric veins to the esophageal veins. The portal venous gradient must exceed 10 mm Hg for varices to develop, although a gradient at or above this level does not guarantee the development of varices (82). Variceal rupture can be precipitated by erosions caused by GER and sudden increases in portal pressure (82).

Initial treatment for bleeding esophageal varices includes the maintenance of an adequate airway and proper volume resuscitation. Placement of a nasogastric tube for decompression and correction of coagulopathy should also be accomplished.

TIPS provides decompression of the portal system by establishing a connection from the intrahepatic portal system to the hepatic vein. The technique is not useful in children with extrahepatic portal hypertension. There are a number of technical limitations related to the size of the involved vessels and the possible complications of capsular bleeding and portosystemic encephalopathy. In patients with biliary atresia, the associated periportal fibrosis and tortuous collateral development make TIPS especially challenging. Moreover, there is a higher incidence of stent restenosis and reintervention required for these patients (83).

The smaller size of the vessels involved and the liver itself result in a higher chance of technical problems. The most common associated complication is extrahepatic bleeding. The bleeding is often the result of puncture through the hepatic capsule with the needle (84).

TUMORS

Leiomyoma

Leiomyoma of the esophagus is rarely seen in children, but should be considered in the differential diagnosis of esophageal obstruction and mediastinal masses (85). Localized lesions are found in approximately 10% of cases, whereas the diffuse form predominates in 90% of cases. The entire esophagus may be involved in one-third of cases. Encroachment on the cardia or upper stomach occurs in 70% of patients. Major symptoms can include dysphagia, dyspnea, vomiting, retrosternal pain, and coughing. The initial diagnosis following contrast studies is most often achalasia. The diagnosis of leiomyoma is made only with subsequent endoscopy. Treatment consists of removal of the mass.

ESOPHAGEAL REPLACEMENT

The most common indication for esophageal replacement surgery include long-gap esophageal atresia corrosive injuries with stricture or dysfunction, GER with the development of refractory strictures, a variety of infections and inflammatory conditions, and rare esophageal conditions, such as tumors, congenital stenosis, trauma, achalasia, and postoperative complications. The conduits that can be used include colon, stomach, and small bowel. None is ideal, and none is as good as the native esophagus. When considering esophageal replacement surgery, several goals should be kept in mind:

1. The conduit should be short and straight, and should be able to drain by dependent drainage. None of the conduits have effective peristalsis.
2. If possible, one should preserve the CP muscle and the area of the LES.
3. An antireflux procedure may be necessary to decrease GER.
4. Because all options are complex, the simpler the better. Three major factors are considered: the choice of the visceral conduit, followed by determination of the location for the replacement, and finally, a decision as to whether to remove the native esophagus.

Esophageal atresia without fistula may require esophageal replacement after failed esophagoesophagostomy. In nearly all situations, an attempt is made to salvage the native esophagus; however, replacement surgery is required in some circumstances. The choice of esophageal replacement remains the subject of debate (Table 64-2). Established choices of replacement include the stomach, a gastric tube formation, either the left or right colon, and rarely, small bowel interposition. Depending on the replacement choice, the route of replacement may be through the chest, through the mediastinum, or retrosternally.

The left colon has been used most extensively as an alternative to the native esophagus. The left colon is believed to have a more favorable blood supply because the left colic artery lies favorably, and using the left colon, and does not require removal of the terminal ileum (86). There is experimental evidence that isoperistaltic colon segment responds to acid stimulation and promotes rapid clearing into the stomach. The colon may be brought through the chest retrosternally or through a left transthoracic approach. Postoperative function appears to be similar when comparing the retrosternal approach with the left thoracic approach (86). Anastomosis of the left colon to the remaining esophagus is generally performed through a left cervical incision. A gastrostomy is also performed (Fig. 64-6). Cervical anastomotic leak and stricture are the most common complications in most series. Over time, the colon replacement has been known to dilate and become

TABLE 64-2 Summary of Esophageal Replacement Literature.

Esophageal Replacement	No. of Studies	No. of Patients	Deaths n (%)	Leaks n (%)	Strictures n (%)
Colon interposition	26	918	63 (7)	267 (29)	174 (19)
Jejunal interposition	6	64	6 (9)	12 (18)	9 (14)
Gastric tube esophagoplasty	7	156	7 (4)	108 (69)	83 (53)
Gastric transposition	5	143	9 (6)	30 (21)	31 (22)

(From Hirschl RB, Yardeni D, Oldham K, et al. Gastric transposition for esophageal replacement in children: experience with 41 consecutive cases with special emphasis on esophageal atresia. *Ann Surg* 2002;236(4):531–539, with permission.)

redundant, often resulting in dysphagia and reflux-type symptoms. Placement of the isoperistaltic left colon segment in the posterior mediastinum may reduce the incidence of progressive dilatation over time and also prevent kinking of the replacement graft that can be seen when using the retrosternal approach.

Another option for esophageal replacement is to use the stomach. This can entail either a gastric transposition or the use of a gastric tube esophagoplasty—a reversed gastric tube. In a single large series, the most common diagnosis requiring gastric transposition was esophageal atresia, and the overall survival was good (87). An excellent description of the gastric transposition operation, with placement of the conduit in the posterior mediastinum, has been provided by Hirschl et al. (88) (Fig. 64-7). Patients undergo preoperative bowel preparation so the colon is available if the gastric conduit proves to be unacceptable. The abdomen, chest, neck, and left arm are prepped and easily accessible to the operative field. After a left subcostal incision, the stomach is carefully examined, and the gastrostomy is taken down and closed. The greater omentum is divided, while maintaining the gastroepiploic arcade. The left gastric artery is test-occluded with a Heifitz clamp and then divided and ligated. The right gastric artery is identified and preserved. An ample Kocher maneuver is required to mobilize the duodenum, and a pyloromyotomy or pyloroplasty is recommended. The esophageal hiatus is opened to allow passage of the stomach, and the initial dissection of the lower esophagus is performed bluntly; however, with proper retraction, an

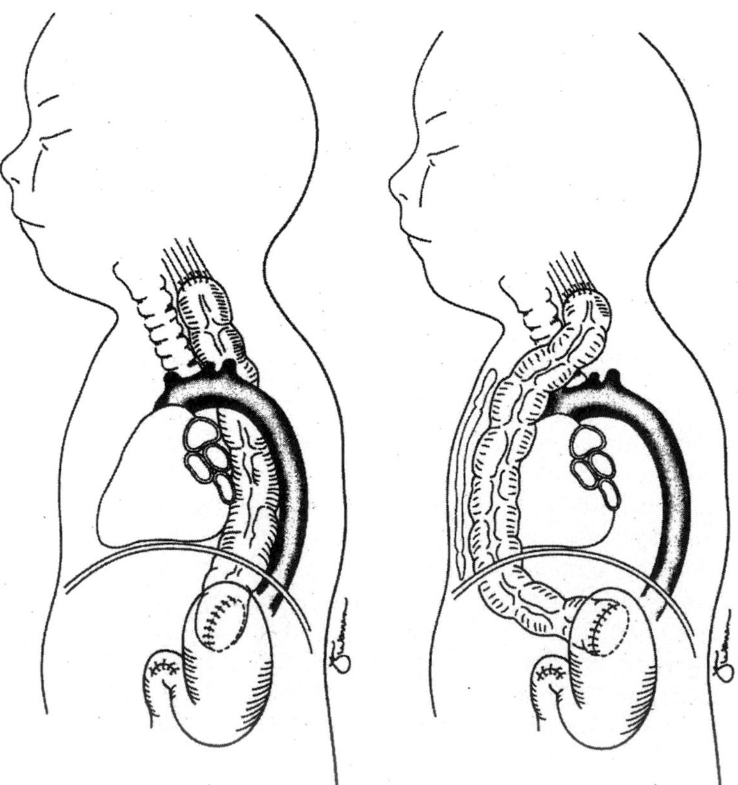

FIGURE 64-6. Colon interposition as an esophageal replacement via either a retrohilar (left) or retrosternal (right) approach.

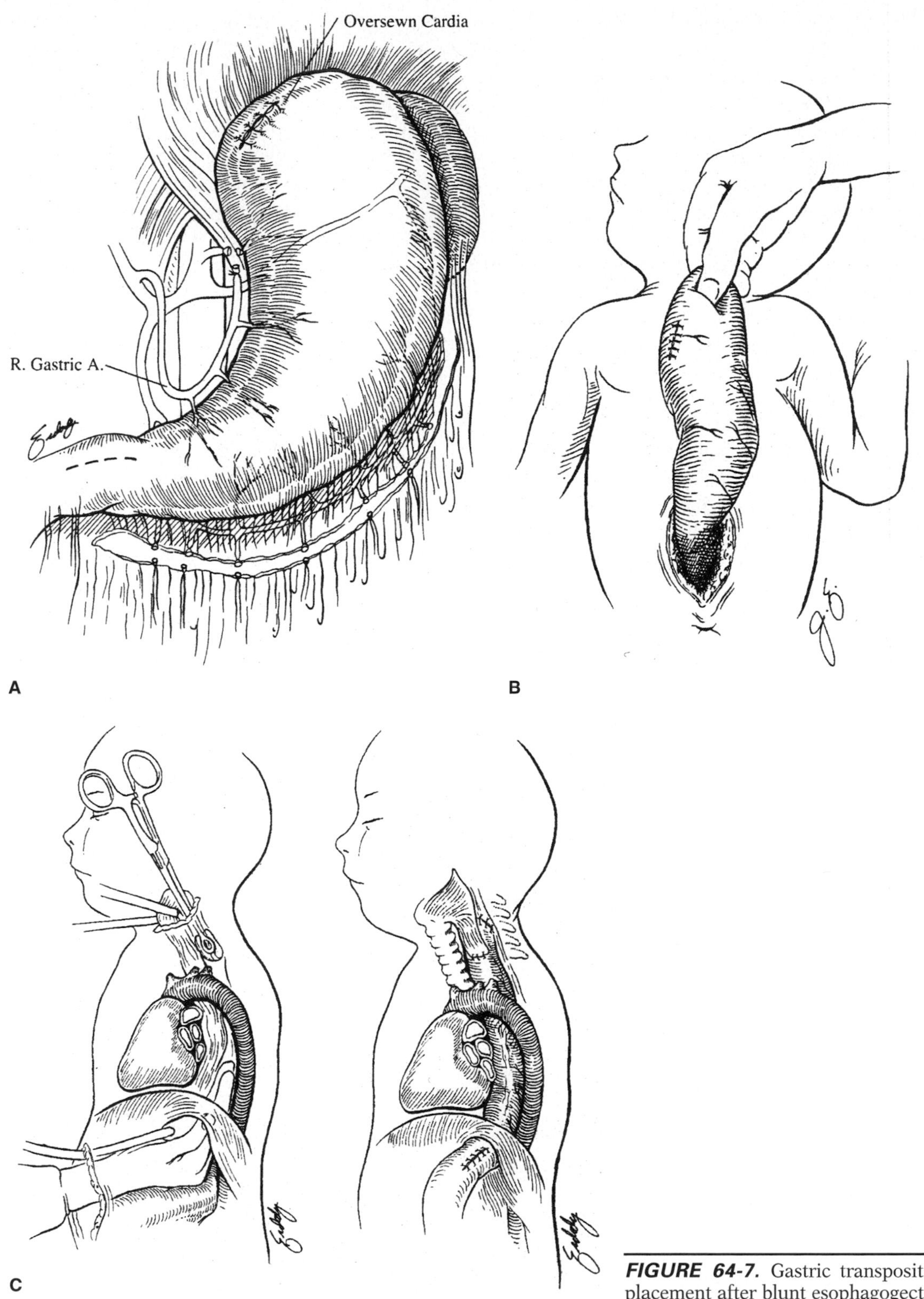

FIGURE 64-7. Gastric transposition for esophageal replacement after blunt esophagogectomy using cervical and abdominal incisions.

increased amount of the dissection can be performed under visualization. The left cervical incision provides access to the cervical esophagus. If an esophagostomy is present, this should be mobilized for a distance of 2 to 3 cm. Identification of the recurrent laryngeal nerve may be difficult. The cervical esophagus is encircled, and by primarily using blunt dissection, mobilization of the cervical, thoracic, and abdominal esophagus is completed. The cervical esophagus may then be divided and a 28 French chest tube is sutured to the distal cervical esophagus. The esophagus, along with the end of the chest tube, is then delivered into the abdomen. In patients with esophageal atresia, the mediastinum is bluntly dissected until a passage is formed from the cervical incision to the esophageal hiatus. The GE junction is divided with a stapling device and the staple line oversewn. The apex of the fundus is then sutured to the chest tube and passed through the hiatus and chest to the cervical incision. There should be minimal tension on the stomach as it passes to the cervical incision. The left triangular ligament of the liver may be mobilized to provide a shorter path to the neck if tension on the stomach is excessive. To prevent slippage of the esophagogastric anastomosis into the mediastinum, the esophagus is then sutured to the sternocleidomastoid and strap muscles. A single-layer anastomosis is performed between the apex of the fundus and the distal cervical esophagus, and a new gastrotomy is then created (Fig. 64-8). A drain is placed in the cervical incision, and the platysma and skin of the neck and the fascia and skin of the abdomen are closed. A contrast study of the conduit is obtained on the seventh postoperative day (88).

Previous esophageal and gastric procedures, which may result in a scarred posterior mediastinum and compromised gastric blood supply, have been relative contraindications for the posterior approach and the use of the gastric conduit. However, more recent studies have demonstrated that this approach may be performed safely and with acceptable complications (88,89). Moreover, placement of the gastric conduit in the posterior mediastinum may limit long-term distension, making it more tubular and preventing potential respiratory compromise (88). Anastomotic leaks and stricture formation are the most commonly encountered early postoperative complication and occur, respectively, in approximately 10% of patients. Treatment is generally conservative for these complications. However, significant feeding difficulties often arise postoperatively that may take several months to improve. This was particularly true in patients with pure esophageal atresia (90).

Delayed gastric emptying, feeding intolerance, and delayed gastric emptying are common postoperative complications. In addition, poor weight gain and feeding aversion may be present. Pulmonary function, although less than predicted for age, was better in those children who had a primary gastric transposition compared with those with complicated thoracic procedures before the gastric transposition. This finding may suggest that the underlying lung

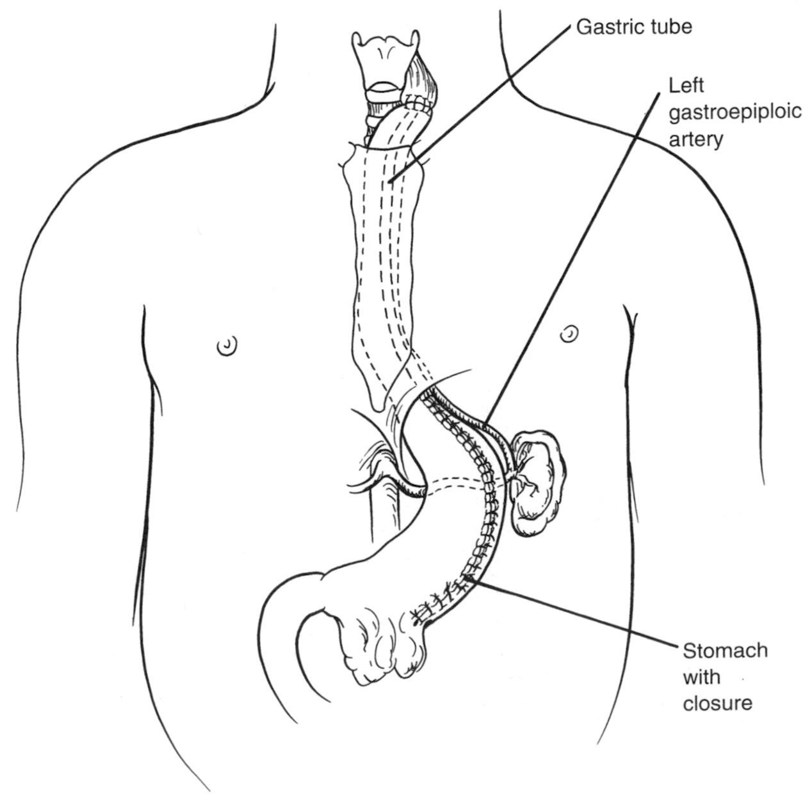

FIGURE 64-8. Reverse gastric tube esophageal substitute.

disease, rather than the stomach itself, might be the cause for the decrease in pulmonary function (88).

The above issues notwithstanding, there are concerns regarding gastric transposition in young children in regard to acid reflux and the volume of the postprandial stomach in the chest and its effect on ventilation. For these and other reasons, some pediatric surgeons favor the construction of a reversed gastric tube. In this procedure a gastric tube is constructed from the greater curvature of the stomach based on the left gastroepiploic artery. This is typically done with a series of firings of a GIA stapler with a 20 to 24 French chest tube along the greater curvature of the stomach as a stent. The tube can be brought up to the neck either by a restrosternal or a left thoracotomy approach. The anastomosis is done in the neck. A pyloroplasty is performed to allow for improved gastric emptying (Figure 64-8).

These three techniques tend to have comparable complication rates and long term results. The outcomes for the procedures are difficult to compare objectively due to their infrequency of use and the number of variations in the procedures. Both technical and functional complications are not uncommon, though mortality is unusual.

REFERENCES

1. Skandalakis JE, Ellis H. Embryologic and anatomic basis of esophageal surgery. *Surg Clin North Am* 2000;80(1):85.
2. Sanudo JR, Domenech-Mateu JM. The laryngeal primordium and epithelial lamina. A new interpretation. *J Anat* 1990;171:207–222.
3. Williams A, Quan Q, Beasley S. Three-dimensional imaging clarifies the process of tracheoesophageal separation in the rat. *J Pediatr Surg* 2003;38(2):173–177.
4. Hitchcock RJ, Pemble MJ, Bishop AE, et al. Quantitative study of the development and maturation of human oesophageal innervation. *J Anat* 1992;180(Pt.1):175–183.
5. Montgomery RK, Mulberg AE, Grand RJ. Development of the human gastrointestinal tract: twenty years of progress. *Gastroenterology* 1999;116(3):702–731.
6. Dumont RC, Rudolph CD. Development of gastrointestinal motility in the infant and child. *Gastroenterol Clin North Am* 1994;23(4):655–671.
7. Grand RJ, Watkins JB, Torti FM. Development of the human gastrointestinal tract. A review. *Gastroenterology* 1976;70(5 Pt.1):790–810.
8. Trahair JF, Harding R. Restitution of swallowing in the fetal sheep restores intestinal growth after midgestation esophageal obstruction. *J Pediatr Gastroenterol Nutr* 1995;20(2):156–161.
9. Swigart LL. The esophageal arteries. *Surg Gynecol Obstet* 1950;90: 234–243.
10. Geboes K, Geboes KP, Maleux G. Vascular anatomy of the gastrointestinal tract. *Best Pract Res Clin Gastroenterol* 2001;15(1):1–14.
11. Potter SE. Observations on the intrinsic blood supply of the esophagus. *Arch Surg* 1950;61:944–948.
12. Shapiro AL. The esophageal arteries: their configurational anatomy and variations in relation to surgery. *Ann Surg* 1950;131:171–185.
13. Butler H. The veins of the oesophagus. *Thorax* 1951;6:276–296.
14. Muraji T, Takamizawa S, Satoh S, et al. Congenital cricopharyngeal achalasia: diagnosis and surgical management. *J Pediatr Surg* 2002;37(5):e12.
15. Sasaki CT, Kim YH, Sims HS, et al. Motor innervation of the human cricopharyngeus muscle. *Ann Otol Rhinol Laryngol* 1999;108(12):1132–1139.
16. Goyal RK, Martin SB, Shapiro J, et al. The role of cricopharyngeus muscle in pharyngoesophageal disorders. *Dysphagia* 1993;8(3):252–258.
17. Ertekin C, Aydogdu I. Electromyography of human cricopharyngeal muscle of the upper esophageal sphincter. *Muscle Nerve* 2002;26(6): 729–739.
18. Lyons MF, Tsuchida AM. Foreign bodies of the gastrointestinal tract. *Med Clin North Am* 1993;77:1101.
19. Litovitz T, Schmitz BF. Ingestion of cylindrical and button batteries: an analysis of 2382 cases. *Pediatrics* 1992;89:747.
20. Nandi P, Ong GB. Foreign body in the esophagus: review of 2394 cases. *Br J Surg* 1978;65:5.
21. Paul RI, Christoffel K, Binns HJ, et al. Foreign body ingestions in children: risks of complications varies with the site of initial health care contact. *Pediatrics* 1993;91:121.
22. Reilly J, Thompson J, MacArthur C, et al. Pediatric aerodigestive foreign body injuries are complications related to timeliness of diagnosis. *Laryngoscope* 1997;107(1):17–20.
23. Burton DM, Stith JA. Extraluminal esophageal coin erosion in children: case report and review. *Int J Pediatr Otol* 1992;23:187.
24. Conners GP, Chamberlin JM, Ochsensalger DW. Symptoms and spontaneous passage of esophageal coins. *Arch Pediatr Adolesc Med* 1995;149:36.
25. Robbins MI, Shortsleeve MJ. Treatment of acute esophageal food impaction with glucagon, an effervescent agent and water. *AJR* 1994; 162:325.
26. Kerschner JE, Beste DJ, Conley SF, et al. Mediastinitis associated with foreign body erosion of the esophagus in children. *Int J Pediatr Otorhinolaryngol* 2001;59(2):89–97.
27. Anderson KD, Rouse TM, Randolph JG. A controlled trial of corticosteroids in children with corrosive injury of the esophagus. *N Engl J Med* 1990;323(10):637–640.
28. Scott JC, Jones B, Eisele DW, et al. Caustic ingestion of the upper aerodigestive tract. *Laryngoscope* 1992;102:1.
29. Hugh TB, Kelly MD. Corrosive ingestion and the surgeon. *J Am Coll Surg* 1999;189(5):508–522.
30. Broto J, Asensio M, Jorro CS, et al. Conservative treatment of caustic esophageal injuries in children: 20 years of experience. *Pediatr Surg Int* 1999;15(5–6):323–325.
31. Hugh TB, Kelly MD. Corrosive ingestion and the surgeon. *J Am Coll Surg* 1999;189(5):508–522.
32. Ulman I, Mutaf O. A critique of systemic steroids in the management of caustic esophageal burns in children. *Eur J Pediatr Surg* 1998;8(2):71–74.
33. Karnak I, Tanyel FC, Buyukpamukcu N, et al. Combined use of steroid, antibiotics and early bougienage against stricture formation following caustic esophageal burns. *J Cardiovasc Surg (Torino)* 1999;40(2):307–310.
34. Howell JM, Dalsey WC, Hartsell FW, et al. Steroids for the treatment of corrosive esophageal injury: a statistical analysis of past studies. *Am J Emerg Med* 1992;10(5):421–425.
35. Holder TM, Ashcraft KW, Leape L. The treatment of patients with esophageal strictures by local steroid injections. *J Pediatr Surg* 1969;4:646.
36. Panieri E, Rode H, Millar AJ, et al. Oesophageal replacement in the management of corrosive strictures: when is surgery indicated? *Pediatr Surg Int* 1998;13(5–6):336–340.
37. Fallon M, Gordon ARG, Landrum AC. Mediastinal cysts of foregut origin associated with vertebral abnormalities. *Br J Surg* 1954;41:520.
38. Carachi R, Azmy A. Foregut duplications. *Pediatr Surg Int* 2002;18 (5–6):371–374.
39. Kirwan WO, Walbaum PR, McCormack RJM. Cystic intrathoracic derivatives of the foregut and their complications. *Thorax* 1973;28:424.
40. Almog B, Leibovitch L, Achiron R. Split notochord syndrome—prenatal ultrasonographic diagnosis. *Prenat Diagn* 2001;21(13): 1159–1162.
41. Qi BQ, Beasley SW, Williams AK. Evidence of a common pathogenesis for foregut duplications and esophageal atresia with tracheoesophageal fistula. *Anat Rec* 2001;264(1):93–100.
42. McCullagh M, Bhuller AS, Pierro A, et al. Antenatal identification of a cervical oesophageal duplication. *Pediatr Surg Int* 2000;16(3):204–205.

43. Stringer MD, Spitz L, Abel R, et al. Management of alimentary tract duplication in children. *Br J Surg* 1995;82(1):74–78.
44. Holcomb GW III, Gheissari A, O'Neill JA Jr, et al. Surgical management of alimentary tract duplications. *Ann Surg* 1989;209(2):167–174.
45. Winter HS, Madara JL, Stafford RJ, et al. Intraepithelial eosinophils: a new diagnostic criterion for reflux esophagitis. *Gastroenterology* 1982;83(4):818–823.
46. Orenstein SR, Shalaby TM, Di Lorenzo C, et al. The spectrum of pediatric eosinophilic esophagitis beyond infancy: a clinical series of 30 children. *Am J Gastroenterol* 2000;95(6):1422–1430.
47. Walsh SV, Antonioli DA, Goldman H, et al. Allergic esophagitis in children: a clinicopathological entity. *Am J Surg Pathol* 1999;23(4): 390–396.
48. Siafakas CG, Ryan CK, Brown MR, et al. Multiple esophageal rings: an association with eosinophilic esophagitis: case report and review of the literature. *Am J Gastroenterol* 2000;95(6):1572–1575.
49. Ruchelli E, Wenner W, Voytek T, et al. Severity of esophageal eosinophilia predicts response to conventional gastroesophageal reflux therapy. *Pediatr Dev Pathol* 1999;2(1):15–18.
50. Liacouras CA, Wenner WJ, Brown K, et al. Primary eosinophilic esophagitis in children: successful treatment with oral corticosteroids. *J Pediatr Gastroenterol Nutr* 1998;26(4):380–385.
51. Justinich CJ, Ricci A Jr, Kalafus DA, et al. Activated eosinophils in esophagitis in children: a transmission electron microscopic study. *J Pediatr Gastroenterol Nutr* 1997;25(2):194–198.
52. Furuta GT. Eosinophilic esophagitis: an emerging clinicopathologic entity. *Curr Allergy Asthma Rep* 2002;2(1):67–72.
53. Hassall E. Barrett's esophagus: congential or acquired? *Am J Gastroenterol* 1993;88:819.
54. Hassall E, Weinstein WM, Ament ME. Barrett's esophagus in childhood. *Gastroenterology* 1985;89:1331.
55. Hassall E. Barrett's esophagus; new definitions and approaches in children. *J Pediatr Gastroenterol Nutr* 1993;16:345.
56. Otherson HB, Ocampo RJ, Parker EF, et al. Barrett's esophagus in children. *Ann Surg* 1993;217:676.
57. Snyder JD, Goldman H. Barrett's esophagus in children and young adults. Frequent association with mental retardation. *Dig Dis Sci* 1990;35(10):1185–1189.
58. Krug E, Bergmeijer JH, Dees J, et al. Gastroesophageal reflux and Barrett's esophagus in adults born with esophageal atresia. *Am J Gastroenterol* 1999;94(10):2825–2828.
59. Lindahl H, Rintala R, Sariola H, et al. Cervical Barrett's esophagus: a common complication of gastric tube reconstruction. *J Pediatr Surg* 1990;25:466.
60. Cheu HW, Grosfeld JL, Heifetz SA, et al. Persistence of Barrett's esophagus in children after antireflux surgery: influence on follow-up care. *J Pediatr Surg* 1992;27(2):260–264.
61. Cooper JE, Spitz L, Wilkins BM. Barrett's esophagus in children: a histologic and histochemical study of 11 cases. *J Pediatr Surg* 1987;22(3):191–196.
62. Shamberger RC, Eraklis AJ, Kozakewich HP, et al. Fate of the distal esophageal remnant following esophageal replacement. *J Pediatr Surg* 1988;23(12):1210–1214.
63. Hassall E, Demmick JE, Magee JF. Adenocarcinoma in childhood Barrett's esophagus: case documentation and the need for surveillance in children. *Am J Gastroenterol* 1993;88;281.
64. Younes M, Lebovitz RM, Lachago LV, et al. p53 Protein accumulation in Barrett metaplasia, dysplasia, and carcinoma: a followup study. *Gastroenterology* 1993;105:1637.
65. Karnak I, Senocak ME, Tanyel FC, et al. Achalasia in childhood: surgical treatment and outcome. *Eur J Pediatr Surg* 2001;11(4):223–229.
66. Murray J, Du C, Ledlow A, et al. Nitric oxide: mediator of nonadrenergic noncholinergic responses of opossum esophageal muscle. *Am J Physiol* 1991;6:G401.
67. Miller KA, Holcomb GW III. Laparoscopic adrenalectomy and esophagomyotomy. *Semin Pediatr Surg* 2002;11(4):237–244.
68. Babu R, Grier D, Cusick E, et al. Pneumatic dilatation for childhood achalasia. *Pediatr Surg Int* 2001;17(7):505–507.
69. Nakayama DK, Shorter NA, Boyle JT, et al. Pneumatic dilatation and operative treatment of achalasia in children. *J Pediatr Surg* 1987;22(7):619–622.
70. Esposito C, Cucchiara S, Borrelli O, et al. Laparoscopic esophagomyotomy for the treatment of achalasia in children. A preliminary report of eight cases. *Surg Endosc* 2000;14(2):110–113.
71. Esposito C, Mendoza-Sagaon M, Roblot-Maigret B, et al. Complications of laparoscopic treatment of esophageal achalasia in children. *J Pediatr Surg* 2000;35(5):680–683.
72. Blitzer A, Brin MF. Use of botulinum toxin for diagnosis and management of cricopharyngeal achalasia. *Otolaryngol Head Neck Surg* 1997;116(3):328–330.
73. Brooks A, Millar AJ, Rode H. The surgical management of cricopharyngeal achalasia in children. *Int J Pediatr Otorhinolaryngol* 2000;56(1):1–7.
74. Nihoul-Fékété C. Congenital esophageal stenosis: a review of 20 cases. *Pediatr Surg Int* 1987;2:86–92.
75. Ramesh JC, Ramanujam TM, Jayaram G. Congenital esophageal stenosis: report of three cases, literature review, and a proposed classification. *Pediatr Surg Int* 2001;17(2–3):188–192.
76. Usui N, Kamata S, Kawahara H, et al. Usefulness of endoscopic ultrasonography in the diagnosis of congenital esophageal stenosis. *J Pediatr Surg* 2002;37(12):1744–1746.
77. Yeung CK, Spitz L, Brereton RJ, et al. Congenital esophageal stenosis due to tracheobronchial remnants: a rare but important association with esophageal atresia. *J Pediatr Surg* 1992;27(7):852–855.
78. Takamizawa S, Tsugawa C, Mouri N, et al. Congenital esophageal stenosis: therapeutic strategy based on etiology. *J Pediatr Surg* 2002;37(2):197–201.
79. Das A, Sivak M, Chak A, et al. High-resolution endoscopic imaging of the GI tract: a comparative study of optical coherence tomography versus high-frequency catheter probe EUS. *Gastrointest Endosc* 2001;54(2):219–224.
80. Vasudevan SA, Kerendi F, Lee H, et al. Management of congenital esophageal stenosis. *J Pediatr Surg* 2002;37(7):1024–1026.
81. Grabowski ST, Andrews DA. Upper esophageal stenosis: two case reports. *J Pediatr Surg* 1996;31(10):1438–1439.
82. Karrer FM, Narkewicz MR. Esophageal varices: current management in children. *Semin Pediatr Surg* 1999;8(4):193–201.
83. Huppert PE, Goffette P, Astfalk W, et al. Transjugular intrahepatic portosystemic shunts in children with biliary atresia. *Cardiovasc Intervent Radiol* 2002;25(6):484–493.
84. Heyman MB, Laberge JM. Role of transjugular intrahepatic portosystemic shunt in the treatment of portal hypertension in pediatric patients. *J Pediatr Gastroenterol Nutr* 1999;29(3):240–249.
85. Lee H, Morgan K, Abramowsky C, et al. Leiomyoma at the site of esophageal atresia repair. *J Pediatr Surg* 2001;36(12):1832–1833.
86. Khan AR, Stiff G, Mohammed AR, et al. Esophageal replacement with colon in children. *Pediatr Surg Int* 1998;13(2–3):79–83.
87. Spitz L. Esophageal atresia: past, present, and future. *J Pediatr Surg* 1996;31(1):19–25.
88. Hirschl RB, Yardeni D, Oldham K, et al. Gastric transposition for esophageal replacement in children: experience with 41 consecutive cases with special emphasis on esophageal atresia. *Ann Surg* 2002;236(4):531–539.
89. Spitz L. Gastric transposition for esophageal substitution in children. *J Pediatr Surg* 1992;27(2):252–257.
90. Ruangtrakool R, Spitz L. Early complications of gastric transposition operation. *J Med Assoc Thai* 2000;83(4):352–357.

Chapter 65

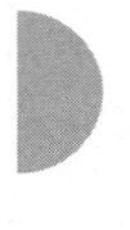

Esophageal Atresia and Tracheoesophageal Fistula

Spencer W. Beasley

Esophageal atresia is a congenital abnormality in which the midportion of the esophagus is absent. Its estimated live birth incidence is between 1 in 3,570 and 1 in 4,500. Most patients have an additional abnormal communication between the trachea and lower esophageal segment called a *distal tracheoesophageal fistula.* The remainder of the patients have either no fistula ("pure atresia") or a fistula between the trachea and upper esophageal segment (proximal tracheoesophageal fistula). There is a history of maternal polyhydramnios in about 35% of patients with a distal fistula, and in about 95% of patients with no distal fistula. Prematurity is also common. More than one-half the patients with esophageal atresia have other major congenital anomalies, of which congenital heart disease, urinary tract abnormalities, and gastrointestinal tract abnormalities are the most common. Esophageal atresia and tracheoesophageal fistula are correctable surgically, with generally good results. The diagnosis should be suspected in any newborn infant who appears to have excessive mucus or saliva at birth, with or without respiratory distress.

EMBRYOLOGY

Abnormal Development of the Esophagus

The esophagus develops from the primitive foregut immediately distal to the pharynx. It is likely that the insult that causes esophageal atresia occurs before 32 days' gestation. The morphologic changes that occur during the embryogenesis of esophageal atresia have been well described, but their interpretation and causes are poorly understood. This has led to a variety of theories being proposed (1), but many of them are now of historical interest only.

Esophageal atresia appears to result from aberrations of differential growth rate, cellular differentiation, and apoptosis. The exact timing and location of the apoptosis in the region of the tracheoesophageal septum seems to be critical for normal separation of the trachea and esophagus (2).

It appears that one or more (as yet unconfirmed) factors alter the rate and timing of cell proliferation and differentiation, and of apoptosis in the region of the esophagus and developing lung bud before 34 days' gestation. There is some evidence to suggest that the notochord may play a pivotal role (3), possibly through the sonic hedgehog-Gli signaling pathway. The *Shh* –/– and *Gli* –/– mutant mice develop esophageal atresia, implying that this signaling pathway is important during foregut development (4).

Spencer W. Beasley: Christchurch Hospital, Christchurch, New Zealand.

ANATOMIC AND PHYSIOLOGIC CONSIDERATIONS

Anatomic Variations

Esophageal atresia with distal tracheoesophageal fistula is by far the most common type of abnormality (Fig. 65.1). The length of the upper esophageal segment is variable, but usually reaches within 1 cm of the level of the arch of the azygos vein. The length of the upper esophagus can be estimated preoperatively by the length of tube that can be introduced through the mouth into the esophagus, or by air in the upper esophageal segment seen on plain radiography. At operation, the upper esophagus can be identified when the anesthetist introduces a stiff catheter into the esophagus. The lower esophageal segment commences from the posterior wall of the trachea, usually just proximal to the carina. The level of the tracheoesophageal fistula can be assessed by identifying the carinal air shadow, knowing that the distal esophagus extends at least that far superiorly into the mediastinum. Although the upper esophageal segment is relatively thick walled as a result of hypertrophy from obstruction in utero, the lower segment

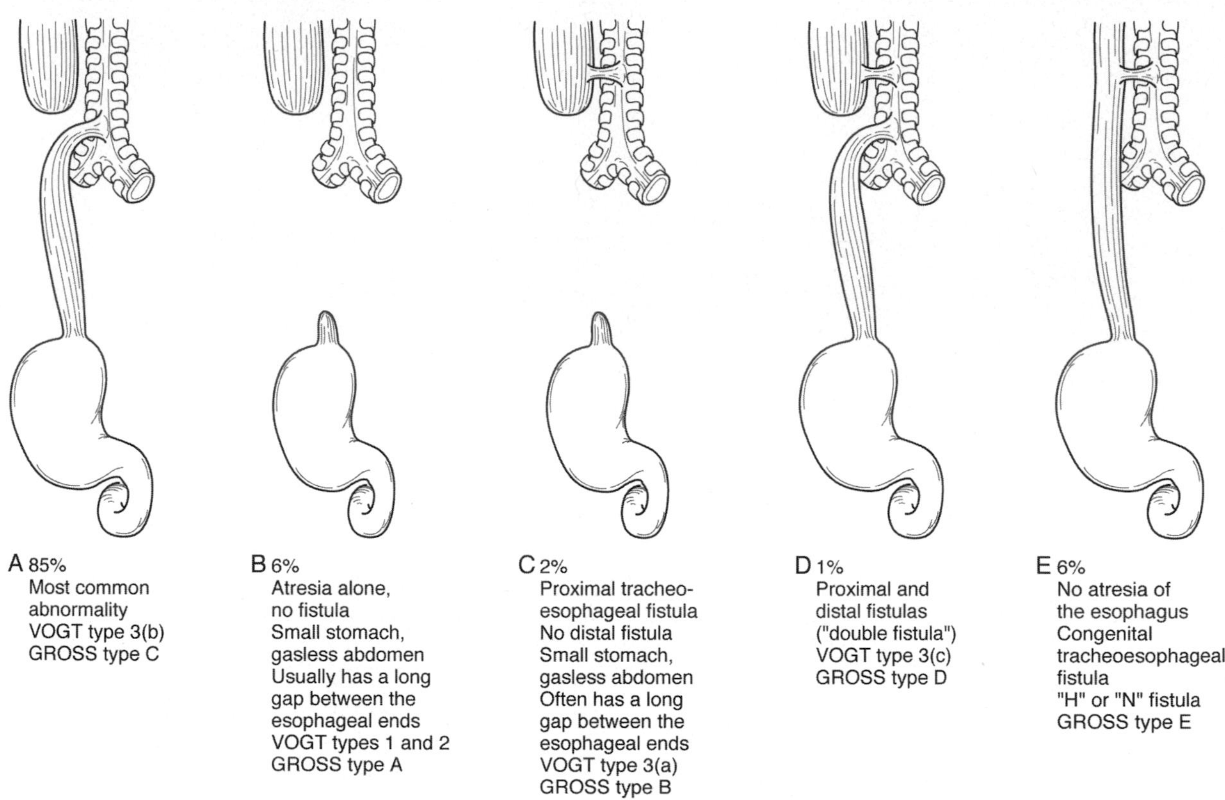

FIGURE 65-1. Types of esophageal atresia. **(A)** Esophageal atresia and distal tracheoesophageal fistula. **(B)** Esophageal atresia alone (no fistula). **(C)** Esophageal atresia with proximal distal fistula. **(D)** Esophageal atresia with double fistula. **(E)** "H" fistula—percentage reflects approximate incidence.

has a smaller caliber. At thoracotomy, however, the lower segment may be seen to expand with air during assisted ventilation. Vagal fibers coursing over its surface assist in its identification at operation.

The most important varieties of esophageal atresia and tracheoesophageal fistula are summarized in Fig. 65-1. Various systems of classification have been used, of which the Vogt (1929) and Gross (1953) systems have been the most popular, but do not accommodate all the variations observed (5). Confusion with other classifications and difficulties in their application to unusual variants have gradually led to their abandonment in favor of descriptive terms.

Surgical Approach

The approach employed for any thoracotomy in a neonate is determined by the need for good exposure, as well as the effect the incision will have on subsequent growth and function of the chest wall. An intercostal approach offers little morbidity and satisfactory exposure. Rib resection is no longer employed because of the deformity it may produce, and the posterior fibers of serratus anterior are either retracted anteriorly or divided low at their origin off the chest wall to preserve their innervation.

Many years ago, multiple thoracotomies were performed deliberately as part of staged repairs and in the management of major esophageal complications. It is now evident that multiple thoracotomies increase the likelihood and severity of anterior chest wall deformity, scoliosis, decreased total lung capacity, and decreased vital capacity. In part, this may be a consequence of the reasons for which multiple thoracotomies were performed, such as anastomotic dehiscence or empyema (6). Improvements in neonatal care and surgical technique have meant that staged procedures for repair of esophageal atresia are now performed rarely.

Some surgeons repair esophageal atresia using a thoracoscopic minimally invasive technique (7). To date, thoracoscopy has involved a transpleural approach, and provides a magnified view of the structures in situ. It is not anticipated that it will produce any long-term adverse effects on chest wall development.

Vascular Supply of the Esophagus and Its Influence of Esophageal Mobilization

The cervical portion of the esophagus is supplied by the inferior thyroid artery, which gives off esophageal branches. These branches run vertically downward to the level of the arch of the aorta, where, in the normal esophagus, they anastomose with esophageal branches that come directly from the aorta and bronchial arteries. The remainder of the thoracic esophagus, particularly that part inferior to the tracheal bifurcation, is supplied by segmental branches from the aorta, but these are of relatively small caliber. They form anastomoses with adjacent vessels, including branches from the intercostal arteries. The distal esophagus is supplied by the ascending branch of the left gastric artery, with some assistance from branches of the inferior phrenic artery. In esophageal atresia, the blood supply to the esophagus is believed to follow the same pattern.

The surgical significance of the vascular supply to the esophagus is that the cervical and abdominal portions are supplied by vessels that run along the esophagus, whereas the thoracic portion is supplied segmentally, and thus has the most tenuous connections. There is a risk that excessive mobilization of the thoracic esophagus may render it ischemic. In esophageal atresia with an extensive gap between the two esophageal segments (so-called "long-gap" esophageal atresia), an anastomosis may only be achievable after mobilization of both segments. Knowledge of the vascular anatomy enables the surgeons to be confident of the blood supply of the upper esophageal segment. Even when its mobilization is extensive and continues well up into the neck, there is little risk of it becoming ischemic. However, extensive mobilization of the lower esophageal segment may disrupt its segmental supply and devascularize it. This influences the approach to long-gap esophageal atresia: The lower segment is mobilized only as much as is required to achieve an end-to-end anastomosis without excessive tension.

Circular or spiral esophageal myotomies may further compromise the blood supply of the esophagus, which explains their high complication rate. They may also compromise the innervation of the esophagus, adversely affecting its motility. There are few situations where myotomies are indicated.

Innervation of the Esophagus

The esophagus is supplied by the autonomic nervous system. The sympathetic supply comes from preganglionic neurons in the thoracic and upper lumbar spinal cord. Postganglionic fibers enter the esophagus by way of visceral branches of the sympathetic trunks and greater splanchnic nerves.

Parasympathetic neurons located in the nuclei of the vagus have preganglionic fibers that pass with the vagus nerves. They synapse with short postganglionic neurons situated within the intramural myenteric and submucosal plexuses. These innervate the smooth muscle and secretory cells. An inherent abnormality of the parasympathetic supply in esophageal atresia and the vulnerability of vagal fibers during surgical dissection and mobilization of the esophagus may be responsible for the abnormalities of esophageal function seen in repaired esophageal atresia.

Esophageal Dysmotility

Esophageal motility is abnormal both before and after repair of esophageal atresia. Evidence of inherent congenital motor dysfunction has come from preoperative manometric studies (including studies in patients with H-type tracheoesophageal fistulae) and from observations in rats with Adriamycin-induced esophageal atresia (8). Postoperative manometric and radiologic studies after repair of esophageal atresia have shown that almost the entire length of the esophagus has abnormal motility, regardless of the extent of dissection or tension at the anastomosis.

The surgical procedure may further adversely affect esophageal motility if the fine vagal fibers are injured during mobilization of the esophagus. Esophageal function tends to improve gradually with age, but patients often need to drink with their meals, even into adulthood. Abnormal esophageal motility may contribute to tracheal aspiration. Poor esophageal clearance allows acidic gastric juice to remain in the lower esophagus for a longer period of time than is normal, which may explain the observation that children with esophageal atresia are more likely to suffer complications of gastroesophageal reflux, particularly esophageal stricture. Anastomotic stricture, esophagitis, recurrent tracheoesophageal fistula, and tracheal instability from tracheomalacia all contribute to disordered esophageal motility.

Gastroesophageal Reflux

Gastroesophageal reflux is common in infants with esophageal atresia. Esophageal dysmotility, poor esophageal clearance, and anastomotic narrowing make gastroesophageal reflux more significant and hazardous in infants with esophageal atresia than in normal infants. Esophageal dilatation alone is not effective as definitive treatment for an esophageal stricture secondary to gastroesophageal reflux because ongoing reflux causes the stricture to recur rapidly, often within weeks. Omeprazole may limit stricture formation and reduce esophagitis. It has even been observed to resolve strictures, often without the need for dilatation (9). Where treatment with omeprazole or other proton pump inhibitors fails, or a stricture redevelops despite dilatation, fundoplication (either laparoscopic or open) is required to control the reflux, at which time further esophageal dilatation (radial balloon dilatation under fluoroscopic control) may be performed. Most strictures resolve after the fundoplication, but dysphagia may persist for many months.

Tracheoesophageal Fistula

A distal tracheoesophageal fistula can compromise an infant in two ways. First, escape of air down the tracheoesophageal fistula into the stomach and beyond results in gaseous distension of the abdomen, causing elevation of the diaphragm (so-called "splinting" of the diaphragm) and

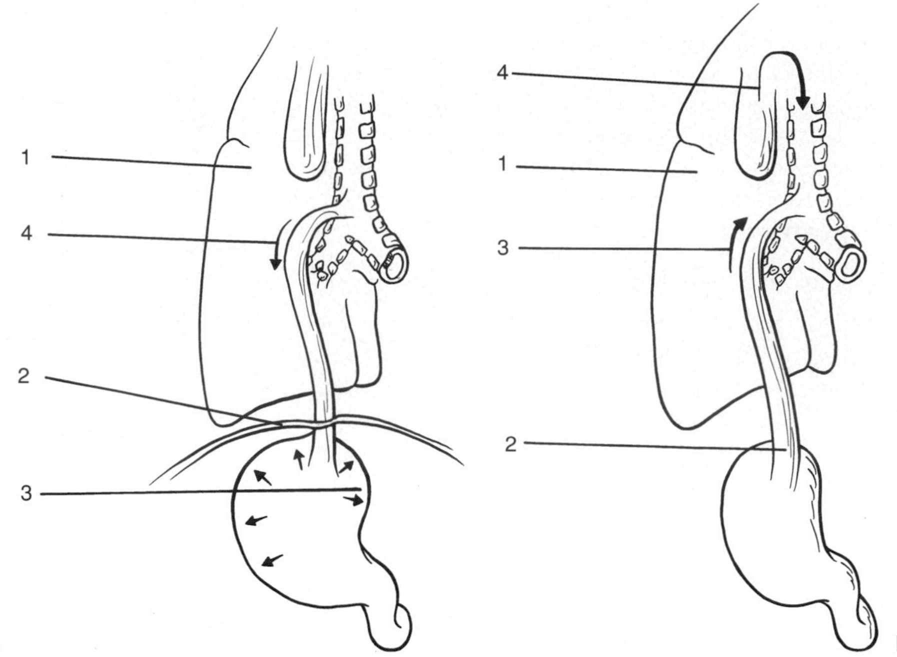

FIGURE 65-2. Physiologic effects of distal tracheoesophageal fistula **(A)** 1. Hyaline membrane disease may necessitate higher ventilator pressures, which encourage air to pass through the distal fistula. 2. A distended abdomen elevates and "splints" the diaphragm. 3. Gastric distension may result in gastric rupture and pneumoperitoneum. 4. Passage of air through a distal tracheoesophageal fistula diminishes the effective tidal volume. **(B)** 1. Aspiration of gastric juices leads to soiling of the lungs and pneumonia. 2. Gastroesophageal reflux. 3. Direction of gastric fluid proximally through distal fistula. 4. Overflow of secretions or inadvertent feeding may contribute to aspiration and contamination of the airway.

restriction of ventilation (Fig.65-2a). The neonate depends almost entirely on diaphragmatic movement for effective ventilation because the relatively transverse (rather than oblique) configuration of the neonatal ribs means that intrathoracic volume increases little with intercostal contraction. Clinically, the infant is observed to be in respiratory distress, with tachypnea and abdominal distension.

Second, in the presence of gastroesophageal reflux (which is common) in esophageal atresia, gastric juice may ascend the esophagus and enter the airway through the fistula (Fig. 65-2b). The frequency with which this mechanism causes contamination of the airway in esophageal atresia is unclear, but in isolated tracheoesophageal fistula (H-fistula), passage of food through the fistula accounts for the recurrent chest infections so often seen. Pneumonia also occurs from overflow of secretions from the blind upper esophageal segment into the airways and by inadvertent feeding before diagnosis. This is the reason infants diagnosed with esophageal atresia must have frequent and regular suctioning of their upper pouch, and must not be fed.

Tracheomalacia

Some degree of structural and functional weakness of the trachea is expected in all infants with esophageal atresia, but in some it may be severe enough to cause respiratory obstruction. There is a deficiency in the tracheal cartilage and an increase in the length of the transverse muscle of the posterior tracheal wall. The cartilage is unable to support the tracheal wall, which has a perimeter greater than normal. The section of the trachea most affected is at the level of the blind-ending proximal esophageal segment. The lower half of the trachea and, occasionally, the whole trachea may be involved. Aberrant vessels (e.g., vascular ring) may increase the severity of tracheomalacia of the adjacent trachea (10). When the abnormality is confined to the intrathoracic trachea, the signs are those of expiratory obstruction. Conditions that increase intrathoracic pressure, such as lower respiratory infection, exacerbate the degree of tracheal collapse. The usual signs of tracheomalacia are those of intermittent expiratory obstruction and normal inspiration. There may be feeding difficulties and vomiting. An esophageal stricture predisposes to inhalation of saliva and food. Distension of the proximal esophagus may compress the trachea and worsen the obstruction of tracheomalacia. In turn, the expiratory obstruction promotes gastroesophageal reflux by increasing intraabdominal pressure. Gastroesophageal reflux, therefore, may be both a cause and result of tracheomalacia.

The natural history of tracheomalacia is one of spontaneous improvement in time. When symptoms are mild, no active intervention is necessary, although the "seal bark" cough may persist into adult life. When tracheomalacia is more severe, careful attention must be paid to feeding. The infant should be offered small amounts of soft foods until late in the first year. Associated gastroesophageal reflux should be managed initially by positioning the head 30 degrees upright and by thickening the feeds. If respiratory symptoms persist, or an esophageal stricture develops, a loose fundoplication should be performed. Aortopexy (tracheopexy) is employed when these measures have failed and the child has recurrent cyanotic episodes due to expiratory obstruction. The rationale for aortopexy relies on the observation that there are fibrous connections between the posterior surface of the aorta and the anterior wall of the trachea. Drawing the ascending arch of the aorta anteriorly and suturing it to the body of the sternum holds the tracheal lumen open by tightening these fibrous connections.

Prematurity

The combination of hyaline membrane disease in premature infants and splinting of the diaphragm from preferential entry of air through the distal tracheoesophageal fistula may produce respiratory embarrassment severe enough to necessitate positive pressure ventilatory support. This may exacerbate the problem of air passing through the fistula, further compromising ventilation. For this reason, management should be directed at maintaining the lowest possible ventilatory pressure to achieve adequate oxygenation, followed by early surgical division of the tracheoesophageal fistula. Because hyaline membrane disease takes 24 to 48 hours to develop, there is time to divide the fistula before the respiratory distress becomes fully established and the complications of inadequate ventilation against an elevated diaphragm or ruptured stomach occur. The earlier practice of performing an emergency gastrostomy alone in infants with major escape of air through a distal tracheoesophageal fistula has been abandoned. This is because the massive air leak often continued after gastrostomy and made ventilation even more ineffective as the air continued to pass preferentially through the fistula.

Closure of the fistula improves the ease of ventilation because

- There is no further escape of air down the fistula.
- There is no diaphragmatic splinting interfering with ventilation.
- Soiling of the lungs with gastric secretions is prevented.

In most infants, esophageal continuity can be achieved at the time of thoracotomy to divide the fistula. If gastric perforation results in a tight pneumoperitoneum, the infant will become extremely difficult to ventilate and will deteriorate rapidly; in this situation, immediate insertion of a wide bore needle into the peritoneal cavity to decompress the abdomen will allow the infant to survive until the fistula is controlled.

DIAGNOSIS OF ESOPHAGEAL ATRESIA

Antenatal Diagnosis

Esophageal atresia may be suspected on antenatal ultrasonography when maternal polyhydramnios, a small stomach, a distended upper esophageal pouch, or abnormal swallowing is observed (11). Diagnostic suspicion is increased when abnormalities known to be associated with esophageal atresia are identified.

Clinical Diagnosis

Any excessively drooling infant should be assumed to have esophageal atresia until proven otherwise. The diagnosis is made when a stiff 10-gauge French catheter introduced through the mouth (Fig. 65-3a) becomes arrested at about 10 cm from the gums. Failure to pass the catheter into the stomach confirms the diagnosis of esophageal atresia. Fluid aspirated up the catheter (saliva) does not usually turn blue litmus pink, as would be expected with gastric aspirate. A tube of smaller caliber may curl up in the proximal pouch and give a misleading impression of esophageal continuity (Fig. 65-3b). A plain radiograph will confirm the tube has not reached the stomach. The tube should not be introduced through the nose because it may injure the nasal passages. Contrast studies, on the rare occasions that they are required, should be performed by an experienced pediatric radiologist, or after transfer to the tertiary institution, and with the use of a small amount (0.5 to 1 mL) of water-soluble contrast. Care must be taken to avoid aspiration.

Diagnosis of Anatomic Type

The choice of definitive treatment is dependent on the anatomic variant (Fig. 65-1). It is necessary to know whether there is a fistula between the trachea and one or other esophageal segment. It is also useful to have information about the distance between the esophageal ends when there is no distal fistula. A plain chest radiograph with a tube introduced through the mouth shows the blind upper esophageal segment ending in the upper mediastinum. The lateral view may display an open fistula and air in the lower esophagus. Visualization of the tracheal bifurcation shows the approximate level of the tracheoesophageal fistula. The role of routine bronchoscopy to identify the presence and level of a fistula is debated (12).

The Gasless Abdomen

Absence of gas in the abdomen suggests that the patient has either atresia without a fistula or atresia with a proximal fistula only (Fig. 65-1b or c). A carefully performed upper-pouch contrast study demonstrates the presence of a proximal fistula in about 20% of cases. Bronchoscopy will also identify a proximal tracheoesophageal fistula. If no upper-pouch fistula is found, it is reasonable to assume that the infant has esophageal atresia without fistula. The length of the lower esophagus can be demonstrated at the time of gastrostomy by passing a metal bougie through the opening in the stomach and through the gastroesophageal junction into the lower esophageal segment. Simultaneous insertion of a radioopaque catheter into the upper esophageal pouch by the anesthetist enables an estimation of the length of gap between the esophageal ends

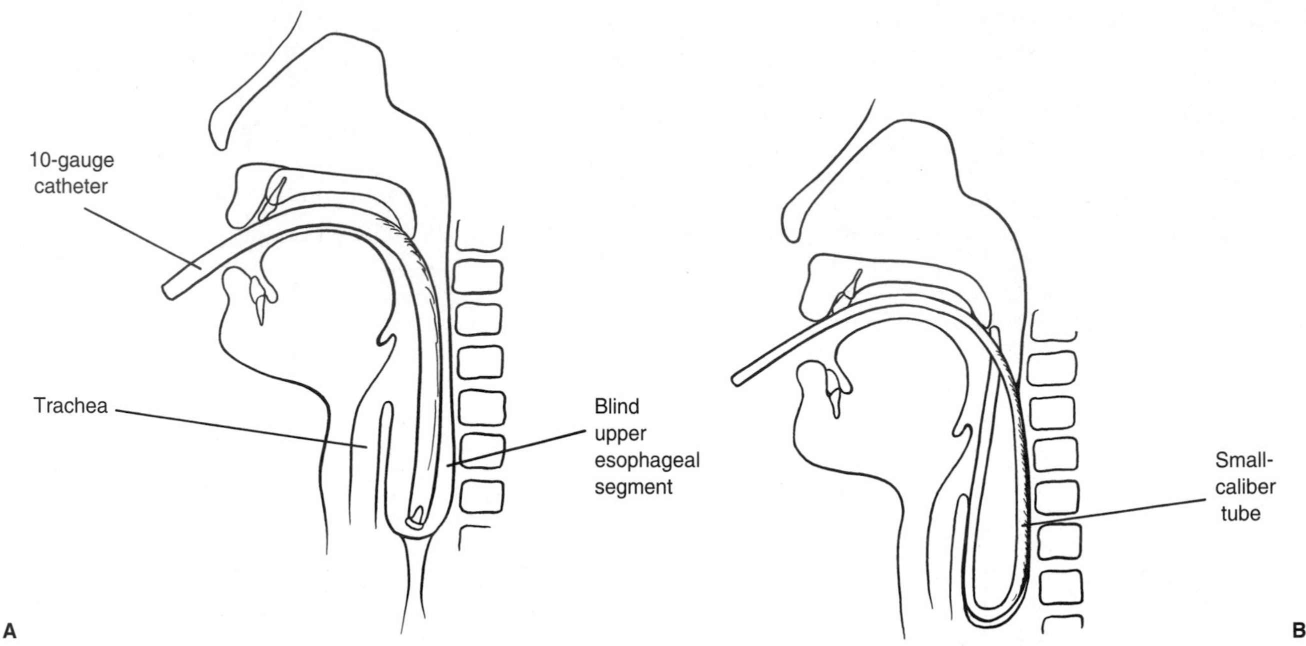

FIGURE 65-3. **(A)** Diagnosis of esophageal atresia is confirmed when a 10-gauge (French) catheter cannot be passed beyond 10 cm from the gums. **(B)** A smaller-caliber tube is not used because it may curl up in the upper esophageal segment, giving a false impression of esophageal continuity.

so a decision can be made as to whether it is possible to proceed to immediate definitive repair (esophageal anastomosis).

Distal Tracheoesophageal Fistula

If there is gas below the level of the diaphragm on plain radiographs of the abdomen, it can be safely assumed that there is a distal tracheoesophageal fistula. Only a small proportion of these patients have an upper-pouch fistula, and this becomes evident at the time of thoracotomy. Some surgeons, however, prefer to perform a preoperative upper contrast study or bronchoscopy routinely.

H-fistula

The presenting features of an infant with an isolated tracheoesophageal fistula are different because the esophagus is intact. These infants can swallow, but may choke and cough when eating. When air escapes through the fistula, they may present with abdominal distension. Recurrent aspiration from food may lead to repeated chest infections. The diagnosis is confirmed on a midesophageal contrast study or by endoscopy (12).

Associated Abnormalities

More than one-half of infants born with esophageal atresia have one or more associated congenital abnormalities (Table 65-1). Not all affect the management of the esophageal atresia, and not all require treatment with the same urgency (Table 65-2). Those that require treatment should be diagnosed early. The VATER (or VACTERL) association describes a commonly encountered spectrum of associated anomalies: vertebral, anorectal, tracheoesophageal, radial, and renal abnormalities, as well as congenital heart disease, duodenal atresia, and a number of other abnormalities. It is best to regard the VATER or VACTERL association as encompassing a spectrum of anomalies that frequently occur at the same time.

Trisomy 18 and 21 occur more commonly in patients with esophageal atresia than might be expected (in about 7% of patients) (13). When trisomy 18 is suspected clinically, the chromosomes should be analyzed immediately and the surgery postponed until the results are known;

TABLE 65-1 Incidence of Associated Anomalies in Esophageal Atresia.

Anomaly	*Frequency (%)*
Congenital heart disease	25
Urinary tract	22
Orthopaedic (mostly vertebral and radial)	15
Gastrointestinal (e.g., duodenal atresia, imperforate anus)	22
Chromosomal (usually trisomy 18 or 21)	7
Total with one or more associated anomalies	**58**

TABLE 65-2 Relevance of Associated Anomaly to Esophageal Atresia.

Anomalies	*Relevance*
▪ Meckel diverticulum ▪ Duplex kidney	Interesting, but not relevant in relation to management of esophagus
▪ Vertebral anomalies	Relevant because of frequency of association (treatment in later childhood may be required for scoliosis)
▪ Pelviureteric junction obstruction ▪ Vesicoureteric reflux	Demands treatment, but not urgently; esophageal atresia takes undisputed priority
▪ Duodenal atresia and anorectal anomaly	Demands treatment early, following closure of tracheoesophageal fistula; needs to be coordinated with treatment of esophageal atresia
▪ Congenital dislocation of the hip	Does not need to be coordinated with treatment of esophageal atresia
▪ Duct-dependent congenital heart disease	Prostaglandin E_1 infusion should be commenced preoperatively; occasionally, if infant remains unstable, the heart may take priority over complete repair of the esophageal atresia
▪ Trisomy 18 ▪ Bilateral renal agenesis	Incompatible with survival; definitive surgery not indicated.

this is because the prognosis is so poor in trisomy 18 that surgery is not justified. When there are features of Down syndrome, the possibility of associated duodenal atresia, congenital heart disease, and Hirschsprung disease must be considered.

The CHARGE association (*c*olobomata, *h*eart malformations, choanal *a*tresia, *r*etardation, *g*enital hypoplasia, *e*ar anomalies) is seen in about 2% of patients with esophageal atresia. Central nervous system abnormalities occur in more then 80% of these children, the most common of which is cerebral atrophy (14). Despite this, the outlook in these children is better than previously believed: They exhibit a broad spectrum of developmental outcomes, with some demonstrating normal abilities (15).

MANAGEMENT OF ESOPHAGEAL ATRESIA

Initial Management

Handling of the infant should be kept to a minimum because excessive disturbance may lead to crying, increases the infant's oxygen consumption, exposes the infant to cold stress, and may cause dramatic cardiovascular responses in an unstable newborn. Crying tends to fill the stomach with air; this increases the likelihood of regurgitation of gastric contents into the trachea and increases abdominal distension, which in turn impedes ventilation. Care must be taken to avoid excessive cooling in the delivery room and during subsequent stabilization and transport.

A number of infants with esophageal atresia have respiratory distress because of prematurity, other congenital abnormalities, aspiration pneumonia, or diaphragmatic splinting caused by excessive escape of air through the distal fistula into the stomach. If blood gas monitoring facilities are not available, the infant must be kept pink at all times; a short period of hypoxia is more dangerous than several hours of hyperoxia. Pulse oximetry for monitoring is considered standard.

Aspiration is prevented by maintaining a partly upright position and by repeated suction of the upper esophageal pouch. This keeps the proximal esophagus empty and reduces the likelihood of overflow of saliva into the lungs. The upper esophagus should be suctioned every 10 minutes, or more often if the child appears to have excessive mucus or air bubbles.

On no account should infants with esophageal atresia be fed. Any material swallowed is likely to end up in the lungs and cause aspiration pneumonia. Attending staff must be aware that the only thing to be introduced through the mouth should be the suction catheter.

Resuscitation by vigorous "bagging" may force air through the distal fistula and cause abdominal distension. The stomach may distend rapidly and cause elevation and splinting of the diaphragm, increasing respiratory difficulty.

Transfer to a major tertiary pediatric institution is best not delayed. The Neonatal Emergency Transport Service, or regional equivalent, should be notified early, and arrangements should be made to continue suctioning of the upper esophageal pouch before and during transport. In general, the infant should be position in a partly upright position with the head elevated to allow emptying of the proximal blind-ending pouch (13). This position minimizes regurgitation of gastric contents up the distal tracheoesophageal fistula, decreases the work of breathing, and improves oxygenation.

Management of Associated Abnormalities

Congenital Heart Disease

Antenatal ultrasonography often identifies congenital cardiac abnormalities. Irrespective of this, preoperative echocardiography should be performed routinely in all infants with esophageal atresia. An echocardiogram defines any significant congenital heart disease and determines the position of the aortic arch.

Infants with non–duct-dependent conditions should have early repair of the esophageal atresia while pulmonary vascular resistance is high, and the cardiac condition should be treated definitively later (16). Infants with severe right or left heart obstructive lesions, in whom either the pulmonary or systemic circulation is duct dependent, may deteriorate rapidly when the duct closes. Most of these patients present on the first day of life because of their heart disease; others deteriorate during repair of the esophageal atresia, or early in the postoperative period if the diagnosis was not made preoperatively. They should be supported hemodynamically with prostaglandin E_1 infusion (to keep the duct open), and the esophagus should be repaired when their clinical condition is stable. Any palliative or reparative cardiac surgery is performed subsequently.

A right aortic arch can be suspected on plain film of the chest or by preoperative echocardiography. When diagnosed preoperatively, the esophagus is best repaired through a left thoracotomy in this circumstance. If first recognized at the time of thoracotomy, it may still be possible to repair the esophagus from the right side; otherwise, the wound is closed, and a left thoracotomy performed.

Urinary Tract Abnormalities

Most urinary tract abnormalities are not life threatening, but are best detected early before irreversible damage to the kidneys has occurred. Reflux-associated nephropathy occurs in about 5% of patients with esophageal atresia. It is worthwhile to identify patients with bilateral renal agenesis or severely multicystic dysplastic kidneys before operation because repair of the esophageal atresia in these patients is probably inappropriate. When kidneys cannot be found on ultrasound examination, a nuclear renal scan confirms the absence of functioning renal tissue. Patients with both esophageal atresia and bilateral renal agenesis may not have features of Potter syndrome because there is no oligohydramnios. A renal sonogram should be performed before surgery, unless the infant has been observed to pass urine. A micturating cystourethrogram is requested if the renal ultrasound is abnormal, but can be delayed for some weeks after repair of the esophageal atresia. In the meantime, the infant is placed on prophylactic antibiotics.

Gastrointestinal Abnormalities

All children with esophageal atresia should have careful examination of the anorectal region. When an anorectal anomaly is identified, the esophageal atresia is repaired first, after which the anorectal anomaly is treated: Depending on the type of anorectal malformation, this may involve anoplasty, colostomy, or primary neonatal anorectoplasty. When esophageal atresia occurs with duodenal atresia and high imperforate anus, a thoracotomy is performed first to correct the esophageal atresia, followed by a duodenoduodenostomy and then colostomy, usually under the same anesthetic.

Chromosomal Aberrations

The two most common chromosomal aberrations are trisomy 18 and 21. It is important to recognize trisomy 18 early because its poor prognosis represents a contraindication to surgical repair of the esophageal atresia. The overall mortality rate of infants born with esophageal atresia and a major chromosomal abnormality is about 70% (13).

Orthopedic Abnormalities

Congenital vertebral anomalies (e.g., hemivertebrae) may produce progressive scoliosis, for which later surgical stabilization of the spine is required in about 15% of patients. Limb abnormalities include radial club hand, absent thumb, and isolated thumb abnormalities. Congenital dislocation of the hip and congenital talipes equinovarus also occur more frequently than might be expected.

Anterior chest wall deformity and secondary scoliosis were common when the rib was resected at thoracotomy, when staged procedures were employed, and when intrathoracic sepsis necessitating multiple thoracotomies was common. The current intercostal approach in esophageal atresia makes this late complication infrequent. In the absence of hemivertebrae, significant chest wall deformity or scoliosis is now rare.

Summary of Preoperative Investigations

A plain radiograph of the torso provides information on the lungs (evidence of aspiration), the vertebral column (hemivertebrae form part of the VATER association), and most important, the presence of gas in the bowel below the diaphragmly, which indicates the presence of a distal tracheoesophageal fistula. Conversely, absence of gas signifies that there is no distal tracheoesophageal fistula: Most of these infants have a wide gap between the esophageal ends and no fistula at all, whereas a few have a proximal tracheoesophageal fistula. This can be demonstrated by endoscopy or a careful midesophageal contrast study performed in a tertiary center. In some centers, bronchoscopy is performed routinely in all infants with esophageal atresia. Renal ultrasonography and echocardiography are routine preoperative investigations.

Operative Repair of Esophageal Atresia

Operation is performed after the preoperative evaluation (including renal ultrasonography and echocardiography) is complete. If the infant has evidence of respiratory compromise (i.e., pneumonitis or lobar collapse), especially if this involves the left lung, operation may be delayed 1 or 2 days to optimize the pulmonary status before repair.

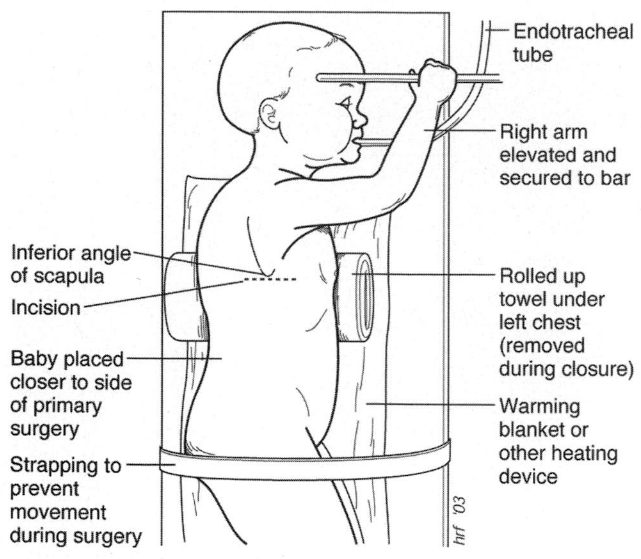

FIGURE 65-4. Positioning of the infant for repair of esophageal atresia by open thoracotomy.

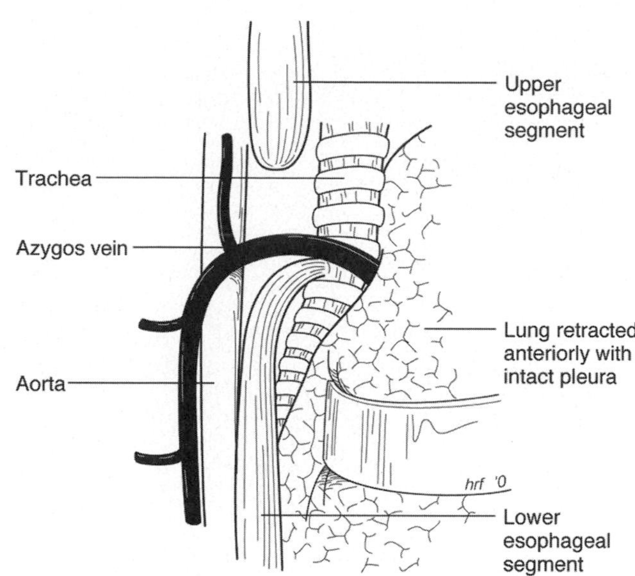

FIGURE 65-5. The anatomic relationships at thoracotomy prior to division of the azygos vein.

During this period, the upper pouch must be kept empty by regular suctioning, and the infant is given antibiotics.

In preparation for thoracotomy, the infant is placed with the right side uppermost and a towel folded underneath the left chest to give lateral flexion (Fig. 65-4). A transverse incision is centered on the inferior angle of the scapula. After division of fibers of the latissimus dorsi, the serratus anterior is retracted anteriorly and the chest entered by a fourth intercostal extrapleural approach. The extrapleural approach is favored because an empyema is less likely to develop following an anastomotic leak. Once the pleura has been swept off the chest wall, the structures of the posterior mediastinum can be identified (Fig. 65-5). The azygos vein is ligated and divided.

The connection of the distal esophagus to the trachea is identified. Absorbable transfixion sutures (e.g., interrupted 4/0 Vicryl®, PDS® or Monocryl®) close the fistula, which is then divided. Care is taken to avoid damage to the vagal fibers and blood supply to the distal esophageal segment.

The upper esophagus is mobilized enough to allow an end-to-end, one-layer, interrupted esophageal anastomosis between the upper pouch and the lower esophageal segment (Fig. 65-6): It can be extensively mobilized along its full length without risk of significant ischemia. On occasions where extensive mobilization of the proximal esophagus fails to provide adequate length, the lower esophagus also may be mobilized to prevent undue tension on the anastomosis. It is possible to mobilize the lower esophagus without complete disruption of its segmental vascular supply (17). Care should be taken to avoid excessive or rough handling of the esophagus. If an anastomosis cannot be preformed without excessive tension, despite extensive mobilization of the two esophageal segments, an esophageal myotomy (usually of the upper pouch) can be performed, but this causes significant damage to the nerve and blood supply distal to the myotomy and predisposes to diverticulum formation and strictures. Placement of a chest drain is not indicated unless there are concerns about the integrity of the anastomosis. An alternative to open thoracotomy is thoracoscopy using a transpleural approach (7). In other respects, the steps of the thoracoscopic procedure are similar to the open operation, although there is little information on the relative merits of the procedures.

Ventilation may be difficult in premature infants because of progressive hyaline membrane disease and air passing preferentially down the tracheoesophageal fistula into the stomach—the fistula acts as a low-pressure vent. Major morbidity can occur because of gastric distension and perforation, pneumoperitoneum, and elevation of the diaphragm, which worsens ventilation. Immediate needle decompression of the abdomen should be followed by urgent laparotomy to control the air leakage. The technique involves insertion of a Foley catheter through the gastric perforation into the lower esophagus (18). This occludes the distal tracheoesophageal fistula and allows thoracotomy to proceed, at which time the distal tracheoesophageal fistula is divided.

Esophageal Atresia Without Fistula

This variant of esophageal atresia presents some specific problems that may be difficult to overcome. There is almost always a substantial gap between the esophageal ends when there is no distal tracheoesophageal fistula.

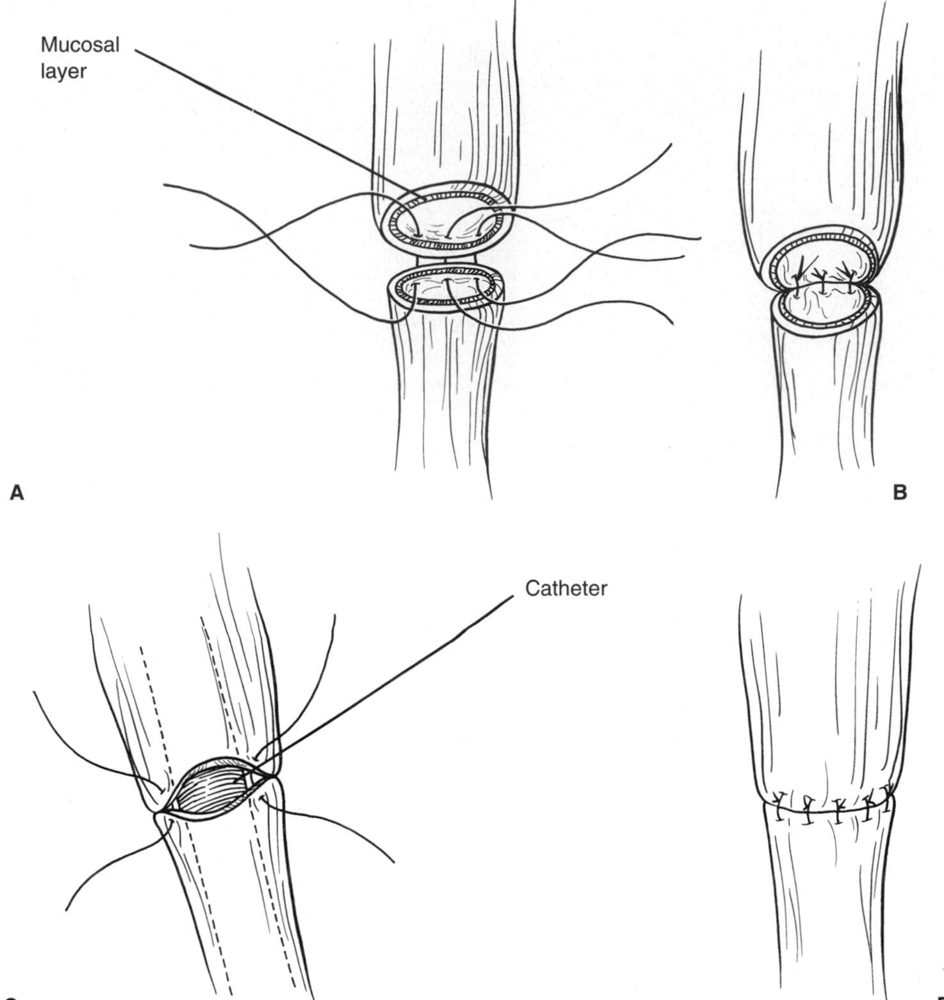

FIGURE 65-6. The esophageal anastomosis. **(A)** Three or four interrupted all-layered sutures are inserted in the far wall of the esophageal segments. It is important to ensure each suture includes mucosa because the mucosal layer tends to retract out of view. **(B)** The sutures are ligated with the knots tied on the mucosal side, drawing the esophageal ends together. **(C)** A catheter is introduced through the upper pouch into the lower esophageal segment. **(D)** The end-to-end all-layered interrupted 5/0 absorbable anastomosis is completed. On the near wall, the knots are tied on the outside.

(Fig. 65-7). Sometimes, the upper esophagus is short and there is virtually no lower esophageal segment above the level of the diaphragm.

The length of the upper esophageal segment can be demonstrated by the contrast study that is performed to exclude a proximal fistula, and can be confirmed at the time of gastrostomy by the passage of a radioopaque catheter through the mouth into the esophagus by the anesthetist. The lower esophageal segment is also evaluated at the time of gastrostomy by introducing a metal bougie through the stomach into the lower esophagus and observing its position using an image intensifier. On the basis of this information, a decision can be made as to whether immediate primary repair is feasible. Where it is not, because of the great distance between the esophageal ends, an attempt at primary anastomosis is delayed for up to 3 months during which time there may be further growth of the upper pouch. Anastomosis of the esophageal ends may be facilitated by the maneuvers outlined in Table 65-3. Even when the gap is extensive, it is usually possible to obtain esophageal continuity without resorting to esophageal replacement.

Isolated Tracheoesophageal Fistula (H-fistula)

Tracheoesophageal fistula without atresia presents an entirely different clinical spectrum from esophageal atresia. The esophagus is intact and patent, but there is an oblique fistula running downward from the trachea to the esophagus, usually at the level of T1 to T3; this is at a level somewhat higher than seen in most patients with esophageal atresia. Apart from gastroesophageal reflux, other congenital abnormalities are less common than in patients with esophageal atresia.

As most fistulas are in the root of the neck, at about the level of the second thoracic vertebra, a cervical approach provides the best surgical access. The recurrent laryngeal nerves, which lie in the grooves between the esophagus and the trachea, are closely related to the

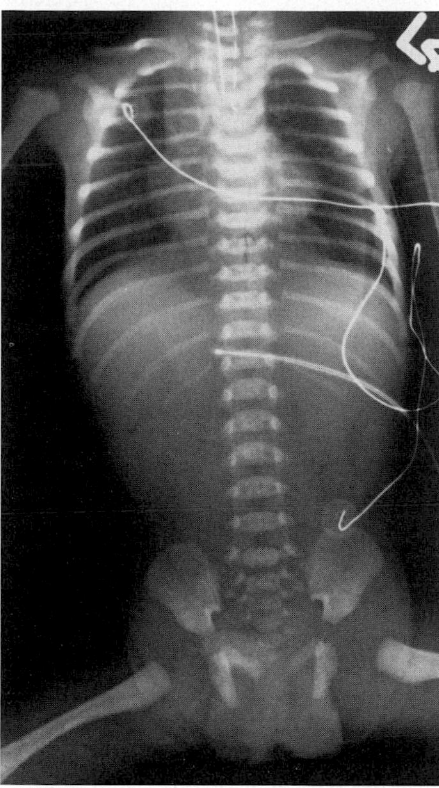

FIGURE 65-7. Radiologic diagnosis of an esophageal atresia without fistula; note the gasless abdomen.

TABLE 65-3 Maneuvers to Achieve Esophageal Anastomosis in Long-gap Esophageal Atresia.

Full mobilization of upper esophageal segment

- Can be extensive and taken proximally to the level of the cricopharyngeus
- Should always be done first
- Little risk of ischaemia

Dissection of lower esophageal segment

- Preserve segmental vessels where possible
- Dissection can be taken to (or through) esophageal hiatus

Myotomy (usually of upper pouch):

- Circular or spiral
- Causes significant damage to blood and nerve supply

Mobilization of stomach into chest:

- Through esophageal hiatus
- Division of lesser curve (19)
- Gastric transposition

If the previous measures fail, esophagostomy and gastrostomy may be required, with later esophageal replacement using one of the following options:

- Isoperistaltic gastric tube or reversed gastric tube
- Gastric transposition (20,21)
- Jejunal interposition
- Esophagocoloplasty

fistula and may be vulnerable to damage during operative dissection.

The obliquity of the fistula and the close apposition of the trachea and esophagus mean that the fistula is occluded for much of the time. Pressure changes and the upward movement of the esophagus during swallowing may open the fistula, allowing air from the trachea to enter the esophagus, or esophageal contents to enter the trachea. The symptoms produced by an H-fistula result from this "two-way traffic" through the fistula. Typical symptoms of a congenital tracheoesophageal fistula include choking and cyanotic attacks with feeding, aspiration pneumonia, and abdominal distension with air. A few patients appear to have excessive secretions; this is presumably related to irritation of the respiratory tract from the passage of saliva and milk through the fistula. Unfortunately, choking with or without cyanotic episodes may be attributed to other causes, leading to delay in diagnosing the fistula. The clinical picture may be further confused if the patient has minimal or intermittent symptoms. When a fistula is suspected on clinical grounds, it can be demonstrated by radiology or bronchoscopy. Swallowed contrast is viewed on continuous fluoroscopy and recorded on video to see whether it enters the fistula. If the initial barium swallow is negative or when contrast appears in the trachea but the route is obscure, the examination should be repeated with contrast introduced through a midesophageal catheter (12).

The fistula should be divided surgically. This may be delayed in some patients with severe pneumonia, who may first require resuscitation and several days of antibiotic treatment. Initial bronchoscopic cannulation of the fistula to assist in its identification at surgery may be helpful, but is not always easy to achieve.

The fistula is usually best approached through a right-sided supraclavicular incision 1 to 1.5 cm above the clavicle; this minimizes the likelihood of injury to the thoracic duct. Dissection may be facilitated by division of the sternomastoid muscle. The strap muscles are retracted medially, and the dissection is continued medial to the carotid sheath. The fistula should be divided, rather than ligated, to reduce the likelihood of recurrence. Placement of a muscle flap between the divided ends of the fistula may also decrease the recurrence rate. A contrast esophagogram is usually obtained 1 week after repair. This assesses the presence of an anastomotic leak, any stricture, and the amount of gastroesophageal reflux. Drainage of the wound is not normally necessary, and gastrostomy is not used. At completion of the operation, the anesthetist inspects the vocal cords for movement.

COMPLICATIONS OF REPAIR OF ESOPHAGEAL ATRESIA

A variety of complications can occur after repair of esophageal atresia. These complications are listed in Table 65-4 and described in the following sections in more detail.

Anastomotic Leak

Anastomotic leakage can vary enormously in significance, from a minor radiologic leak in an otherwise well infant to complete anastomotic disruption with mediastinitis, empyema, pneumothorax, and septicemia. Factors that contribute to anastomotic leakage include insecure or incorrectly placed sutures, excessive tension at the anastomosis, ischemia of the esophageal ends, and sepsis. The extent of the esophageal dissection undertaken is the balance between that required to gain adequate length to avoid excessive tension at the anastomosis, and that resulting in potential injury to the blood supply of both esophageal ends causing them to become ischemic, which may occur when the esophagus is mobilized extensively or when esophageal myotomy is performed. An interrupted one-layer, end-to-end esophageal anastomosis using absorbable sutures appears to have the lowest rate of leakage, stricture, and recurrent fistula.

Most leaks are successfully managed nonoperatively. Total parenteral nutrition enables oral feeding to be ceased. Antibiotics are commenced, and the leak usually closes spontaneously. A long-standing leak may require gastrostomy to allow continuation of enteral feeding. Cervical esophagostomy is necessary only rarely, when supportive therapy has been unsuccessful and when ongoing major sepsis has proved difficult to control.

TABLE 65-4 Esophageal Complications After Repair of Esophageal Atresia.

Incidental leaks with no clinical symptoms
■ Observe on postoperative contrast study
■ No specific treatment
Minor leakage
■ Saliva in chest drain (if used), but infant clinically well
■ Cease oral feeds, antibiotics
■ Will close spontaneously
Major leak
■ Mediastinitis or abscess
■ Pneumothorax or empyema
■ Radiologically confirmed major esophageal disruption
■ Cease oral feeds, antibiotics, may require further surgery
Recurrent tracheoesophageal fistula
■ Close surgically
■ Transpleural thoracotomy when infant well
■ Endoscopic ablation (?)
Anastomotic stricture
■ Check for gastroesophageal reflux
■ Can be due to technical errors suturing anastomosis
Motility problems; delayed esophageal clearance
■ Tends to improve with age
■ Adjust diet, drink with meals
Esophageal pseudodiverticulum after leakage or circular myotomy
■ Occurs after anastomotic leakage or circular myotomy
Shelf at site of anastomosis (secondary to eccentric anastomosis)
■ Technical error
Gastroesophageal reflux
■ Potent cause of esophageal stricture at anastomosis
■ Initial treatment with proton pump inhibitor
■ Fundoplication if conservative treatment fails and stricture develops
■ Long-term malignancy risk

Anastomotic Stricture

Anastomotic stricture is the most common reason for further surgery after repair of esophageal atresia. Factors that predispose to stricture formation include rough handling of the esophagus at the time of repair, ischemia of the esophageal ends, excessive tension of the esophageal anastomosis, the choice of suture material (e.g., silk), anastomotic leak or dehiscence, the use of a two-layer anastomosis, and gastroesophageal reflux. Gastroesophageal reflux is the most common cause of late stricture development.

Infants with a stricture develop feeding difficulties and dysphagia. The first symptom may be that the infant appears to eat slowly with excessive regurgitation, with or without cyanotic episodes. Older children present with foreign-body impaction of food in the esophagus, most commonly between 1 and 5 years of age. The diagnosis of a stricture is confirmed by barium swallow or on esophagoscopy.

In refluxing infants with mild narrowing of the esophagus, proton pump inhibitor therapy is commenced, although one or two dilatations (e.g., radial balloon dilatation under fluoroscopic control) may also be required. An antireflux operation involving open or laparoscopic fundoplication may be necessary for severe gastroesophageal reflux, where symptoms or a stricture persist despite pharmacologic therapy.

Recurrent Tracheoesophageal Fistula

A recurrent tracheoesophageal fistula is a relatively rare but severe and potentially dangerous complication. Failure to close the fistula adequately at the time of initial thoracotomy, as well as an anastomotic leak with local infection and abscess formation, may contribute to the development of a recurrent fistula.

Coughing, gagging, choking, cyanosis, apnea, and recurrent chest infections are symptoms suggestive of a recurrent tracheoesophageal fistula. The typical presentation is that of the infant who coughs and splutters with each feed. The diagnosis can be confirmed by performing cineradiographic tube esophagography with the patient prone. A nasogastric tube is introduced into the esophagus, and the esophagus is filled with contrast while the tube is gradually withdrawn. Bronchoscopy is an alternative diagnostic method. Spontaneous closure of a recurrent fistula is unlikely. When the child is in optimal respiratory and general condition (usually after a period of intravenous nutrition), thoracotomy is performed through the original incision. The fistula is divided using a transpleural approach. Various other techniques to close a recurrent fistula by endoscopic ablation have been attempted, with mixed results.

Gastroesophageal Reflux

Radiographically demonstrable reflux can be seen in most infants after tracheoesophageal fistula repair. If there has been mobilization of the distal esophageal segment, the angle of His may be altered. The degree of functional consequence of the reflux is variable. The combination of reflux and poor esophageal motility means that acid can bathe the esophagus for protracted periods of time and can cause esophagitis. Dysphagia can be marked when an esophagitis stricture forms at the anastomosis or in the distal esophagus. About 25% of infants with repaired esophageal atresia subsequently require an antireflux operation, although use of proton pump inhibition may be reducing this number. There are now several reports of esophageal malignancy in adults following repair of esophageal atresia: reflux causing esophagitis and a Barrett's esophagus may be predisposing factors in the development of malignant degeneration of the esophagus.

OUTCOME

A steady decline in mortality rates has been seen in patients with esophageal atresia. In the past, most deaths resulted from respiratory failure, inadequate resuscitation, and complications of prematurity. The other major cause of mortality related to the complications of the surgical repair of the esophageal atresia itself, particularly sepsis after dehiscence of the esophageal anastomosis and prolonged poor nutrition. Currently, a major cause of mortality is from associated major congenital abnormalities. It is now rare that infants die from prematurity or esophageal complications; consequently, the previously used Waterston classification has little relevance today in predicting outcome.

Most adults with esophageal atresia can lead a comparatively normal life, although most will drink water with their meals, suggesting that they have some degree of ongoing esophageal dysmotility.

It is possible that long-term survival in repaired esophageal atresia patients may be limited by the effects of gastroesophageal reflux and poor esophageal clearance. There is some concern that dysplastic changes in the lower esophageal mucosa may predispose to esophageal carcinoma. There have been several reports of esophageal malignancy in relatively young adults after repair of esophageal atresia, as well as malignant degeneration in the retained bowel segment after esophageal replacement. The exact risk of late malignancy is not yet clear, although ongoing gastroesophageal reflux in those patients may be more significant than previously realized, and there may be a role for regular surveillance in some patients.

REFERENCES

1. Beasley SW. Embryology. In: Beasley SW, Myers NA, Auldist AW, eds. *Osophageal atresia.* London: Chapman & Hall Medical, 1991:31.
2. Williams AK, Qi BQ, Beasley SW. Temporo-spatial aberrations of apoptosis in the rat embryo developing esophageal atresia. *J Pediatr Surg* 2000;35(11):1617–1620.
3. Vleesch Dubois VN, Qi BQ, Beasley SW. Abnormal branching and regression of the notochord and its relationship to foregut abnormalities. *Eur J Pediatr Surg* 2002;12(2):83–89.
4. Arsic D, Qi BQ, Beasley SW. Hedgehog in the human: a possible explanation for the VATER association. *J Paediatr Child Health* 2002;38(2):117–121.
5. Kluth D. Atlas of esophageal atresia. *J Pediatr Surg* 1976;11:901–919.
6. Chetcuti P, Myers NA, Phelan PD, et al. Chest wall deformity in patients with repaired esophageal atresia. *J Pediatr Surg* 1989;23:244–247.
7. Bax KM, Van Der Zee DC. Feasibility of thoracoscopic repair of oesophageal atresia with distal fistula. *J Pediatr Surg* 2002:37(2);192–196.
8. Qi BQ, Merei J, Farmer P, et al. The vagus and recurrent laryngeal nerves in the rodent experimental model of esophageal atresia. *J Pediatr Surg* 1997;32(11):1580–1586.
9. Hassall E, Israel D, Shepherd R, et al. Omeprazole for treatment of chronic erosive oesophagitis in children: a multicenter study of efficacy, safety, tolerability and dose requirements. *J Pediatr* 2000; 137:800–807.
10. Beasley SW, Qi BQ. Understanding tracheomalacia [Annotation]. *J Paediatr Child Health* 1998;34:209–210.
11. Shulman A, Mazkereth R, Zalel Y, et al. Prenatal identification of oesophageal atresia: the role of ultrasonography for evaluation of functional anatomy. *Prenat Diagn* 2002;22(8):669–674.
12. Pigna A, Gentili A, Landuzzi V, et al. Bronchoscopy in newborns with oesophageal atresia. *Pediatr Medi Chir* 2002;24(4):297–301.
13. Beasley SW, Allen M, Myers NA. The effect of Down syndrome and other chromosomal abnormalities on survival and management in oesophageal atresia. *Pediatr Surg Int* 1997;12(8):550–551.
14. Tellier AL, Cormier-Daire V, Abadie V, et al. CHARGE syndrome: report of 47 cases and review. *Am J Med Genetics* 1998;76:402–409.
15. Harvey AS, Leaper PM, Banker A. CHARGE association: clinical manifestations and developmental outcome. *Am J Med Genetics* 1991; 39:48–55.

16. Mee RBB, Beasley SW, Myers NA, et al. Influence of congenital heart disease on the management of oesophageal atresia. *Pediatr Surg Int* 1992;7(2):90–93.
17. Farkash U, Lazar L, Erez I, et al. The distal pouch in oesophageal atresia—to dissect or not to dissect, that is the question. *Eur J Pediatr Surg* 2002:12(1)19–23.
18. Maoate T, Myers NA, Beasley SW. Gastric perforation in infants with oesophageal atresia and distal tracheo-oesophageal fistula. *Pediatr Surg Int* 1999;15(1):24–27.
19. Scharli AF. Esophageal reconstruction in very long atresia by elongation of the lesser curvature. *Pediatr Surg Int* 1992;7:101–107.
20. Spitz L. Gastric replacement of the oesophagus. In: Spitz LV, Nixon HH, eds. *Rob and Smith's operative surgery, paediatric surgery,* 4th ed. London: Butterworths, 1998:142–145.
21. Hirschl RB, Yardeni D, Oldham K, et al. Gastric transposition for oesophageal replacement in children: experience with 41 consecutive cases with special emphasis on oesophageal atresia. *Ann Surg* 2002;236(4):531–539.

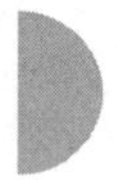

Gastroesophageal Reflux

Robert P. Foglia

Gastroesophageal reflux (GER) is a major cause of morbidity in children. In many children's hospitals, related operations are one of the most common intraabdominal procedures performed. Its incidence is difficult to quantitate because the definition and evaluation vary among institutions. GER is a relatively newly described disease entity. Research in the 1960s generally ascribed GER to the presence of a partial thoracic stomach and identified a hiatal hernia as a prominent component of the pathophysiology. The 1960s and 1970s saw progressive improvement in diagnostic studies used to assess GER. The first large report of surgically treated infants with GER opened the modern era of evaluation and treatment of this entity in the pediatric population in 1974 (1).

ANATOMY AND PHYSIOLOGY

The anatomy and physiology of GER can be considered in terms of the dynamic events occurring in three distinct areas: the esophagus, the gastroesophageal (GE) junction, and the stomach (Fig. 66-1). The esophagus functions as a conduit to transport material from the pharynx to the stomach. The initial propulsion of food into the esophagus is under skeletal muscle control. After the bolus begins to descend in the esophagus, propulsion is due to smooth muscle function from the pharynx and the cricopharyngeus. In the normal circumstance, a coordinated primary esophageal stripping wave moves the food through the esophagus. A secondary esophageal wave serves to clear any residual material not moved distally by the primary wave, or any gastric contents that reflux into the esophagus. The propulsion of a bolus of food down the length of the esophagus can be considered as a pump function which allows the bolus to move from a negative pressure area (the thorax, with an average intrathoracic pressure of –6 torr to the stomach with an intraperitoneal pressure of +6 torr).

Robert P. Foglia: Department of Surgery, Washington University School of Medicine, St. Louis Children's Hospital, St. Louis, Missouri 63110.

Normally, there is an intraabdominal segment of the distal esophagus below the diaphragm. Although there is not a true anatomic sphincter present, the lower esophageal segment at the level of the diaphragm functions as a physiologic sphincter. Factors contributing to the GE junction function include the length of the intraabdominal esophagus, the configuration of the muscle fibers at the GE junction, the relative difference in the diameters of the intraabdominal portion of the esophagus and the fundus of the stomach, and the presence of a high-pressure zone at the GE junction. Typically, this sphincterlike area remains closed until a peristaltic wave transfers a bolus of food to the GE junction, at which time the sphincter relaxes. After the peristaltic wave passes and the foodbolus traverse the area, the sphincter again closes (2). It appears that lower esophageal sphincter pressure (LESP) and relaxation at the GE junction are controlled by several mechanisms, both neural and hormonal.

The lower esophageal sphincter (LES) is regulated by the adrenergic anatomic nervous system. However, LESP is decreased with alpha blockers or beta-adrenergic stimulation. In addition, both excitatory and inhibitory impulses are conducted by the vagus nerves to the esophagus and the GE junction. Hormones such as gastrin and motilin increase LESP as do peptides such as bombesin, beta enkephalin, and substance P. In contrast, LESP is lowered by secretin, cholecystokinin, glucagon, somatostatin, and estrogen. Likewise, mediators such as vasoactive intestinal peptide, neuropeptide Y, and gastric inhibitory peptide all decrease LESP. Pharmacologic agents that increase LESP include antacids, metoclopramide, cholinergics, domperidone, and prostaglandin F. Other agents such as barbiturates, narcotics, benzodiazepines, theophylline, calcium channel blockers, caffeine, alcohol, and prostaglandin E all lower LESP.

The stomach acts a reservoir, and the competency of the GE junction prevents pathologic reflux. If there is an obstruction to gastric emptying, either from a true mechanical problem or a physiologic abnormality, the contents

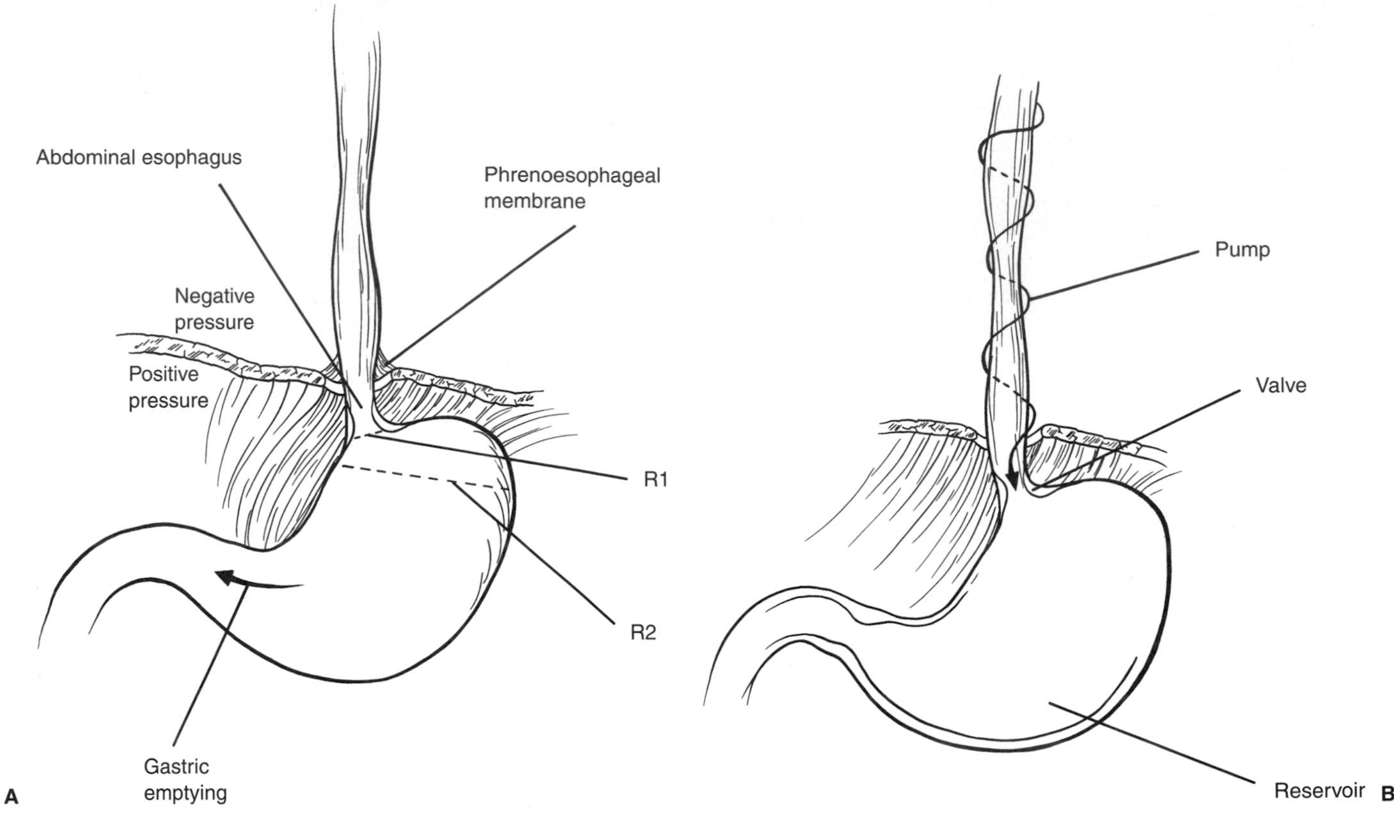

FIGURE 66-1. (**A**) Anatomic and physiologic factors that influence gastroesophageal competency. (**B**) Schematic representation of the interaction of the esophagus, gastroesophageal junction, and stomach. R1 and R2 designation illustrate the diameters of the distal esophagus and fundus, respectively.

remain in the stomach for a protracted period, and intragastric pressure increases within the stomach in an attempt to more forcefully empty the gastric contents into the duodenum. However, this contraction and its force is not directed solely toward the gastric outlet. If there is concomitant dysfunction at the GE junction, acid reflux can occur.

PATHOPHYSIOLOGY

Initially, pathologic GER was believed to result from a hiatal hernia and this was described as a "partial thoracic stomach". In adult screening tests, about one-half of people 50 years of age have a radiographically demonstrable hiatal hernia. Most of these individuals do not have significant symptoms of GER. In children with pH probe-proven pathologic GER, the incidence of a hiatal hernia is 3% to 6%.

GER may be of marked significance or of little or no functional consequence. If a patient has brief episodes of acid reflux into the lower esophagus, but has no clinical symptoms, this is considered physiologic. An understanding of the elements that allow for a greater degree and amount of GER helps to explain both the process and the strategies that can be used to correct the reflux (Fig. 66-1). The normal position of an intraabdominal segment of esophagus allows for the development of a high-pressure zone. The acute angle (angle of His) between the intraabdominal portion of the esophagus and the cephalad end of the greater curvature of the stomach allows for a marked difference in the diameter of the intraabdominal portion of the esophagus and the superior portion of the stomach. The law of LaPlace states that the tension in two areas that are in continuity is inversely related to their radii. Thus, if the diameter (or radius) of the stomach at the level of the fundus (R2) is five times longer than the diameter (or radius) of the intraabdominal portion of the esophagus (R1, Fig. 66-1), then the pressure is five times greater in the esophagus than in the stomach, and this tends to prevent reflux. If the angle of His is not present, the relation of the distal esophagus and the proximal stomach becomes more like the shape of a funnel. The difference in the esophageal and gastric diameters is smaller, and the pressure differential between the two areas is less, affording greater potential for reflux. This problem is seen in patients with hiatal hernias, in whom a portion of the stomach is above the diaphragm and the angle of His may be absent.

In the evaluation of a patient with suspected GER, it is important to identify whether the child is receiving any medication that might adversely alter LESP. A classic situation is a premature infant who is receiving theophylline as treatment for apnea and bradycardia. The medication is given to increase the respiratory drive; however, the apnea and bradycardia might result from silent reflux, and the theophylline may actually exacerbate GER. Conversely, metoclopramide both increases LESP and acts as a prokinetic agent. These and other drugs or stimulation of other hormones can modulate GER.

As noted previously, the esophagus can be considered to be a type of pump that moves liquids and solids into the stomach. In the semiupright or upright position, esophageal motility and gravity transport food down the esophagus into the stomach and clear the esophagus of refluxed material (Fig. 66-1B). The LES and the GE junction function as a physiologic valve and depend on an intraabdominal length of esophagus and a high-pressure zone. The LES opens in response to an esophageal peristaltic wave and then closes afterward. In the pathologic circumstance, LESP decreases in the absence of a peristaltic wave and the GE junction opens. This allows gastric contents to reflux into the esophagus. The GE junction is highly influenced by medications and inflammation. A mechanically inadequate lower esophageal sphincter can result from inadequate sphincter pressure, inadequate intraabdominal esophageal length, or decreased abdominal pressure (3). The final component of this mechanical model is the stomach, which functions as a reservoir. Gastric abnormalities that can result in GER include increased gastric pressure caused by decreased or delayed gastric emptying, and increased acid secretions. Likewise, gastric dilation and retching can alter the anatomy in the area of the cardia and fundus, and afford greater likelihood of reflux. Note that, as the stomach fills and becomes distended, the upper portion of the stomach distends, and this may decrease the overall length of the high-pressure zone at the GE junction. In addition, reflux of duodenal contents into the stomach and subsequent duodenogastric reflux may affect the distal esophagus and the GE junction and cause more pathology than acid reflux alone. In summary, the antireflux barrier at the GE junction is a function of three components: (1) an adequate LESP, (2) adequate length of the LES, and (3) appropriate portion of intraabdominal esophagus subjected to positive abdominal pressure.

In some patients, GER is a component of a foregut motility disorder and can be associated with dyscoordinate esophageal peristalsis and motility, as well as delayed gastric emptying. GER can be quantitated by the number of times that acid is noted in the esophagus on a pH probe study. Fifteen to 20 brief episodes of incompetency of the GE junction occur normally daily (referred to as *eructation* or *burping*). If there is prompt esophageal clearance, this is not of functional significance. The combination of acid reflux and poor esophageal motility causes the esophagus to be bathed in acid for a protracted period. This inflammation serves to decrease LESP, and this leads to a vicious cycle of potentiating GER. Patients with associated tracheoesophageal fistulas often have dyscoordinate esophageal peristalsis; thus, they are at high risk for the development of pathologic acid reflux. These children can develop an anastomotic stricture due to technical problems with the anastomosis, such as tension and a marginal blood supply, combined with the subsequent effect of acid at the anastomosis. They also are at risk for esophagitis and stricture formation in the distal esophagus.

Strategies to correct GER should address abnormalities of the esophageal motility, ineffective LESP due to anatomic or pharmacologic causes, and gastric anomalies, especially delayed gastric emptying.

Reflux

With regard to the esophagus, the functional consequences of GER are the result of the refluxed material from the stomach. Previously, if was believed that the acidic pH of the gastric contents caused irritation of the esophageal mucosa leading to inflammation and pain, and manifested by esophagitis. Over a period of time, there could be associated bleeding and stricture formation. It is now known that acid reflux alone causes only mild esophageal mucosal damage. However, if the esophagus is exposed to both acid and pepsin, there will be a significant mucosal injury (4). Similarly, refluxed duodenal contents alone do not cause a significant esophageal injury, whereas duodenal contents and gastric contents combined cause a marked esophageal mucosal injury (5). The interplay of refluxed gastric and duodenal contents can have a mild or profound effect in regard to esophageal injury. For example, duodenal reflux can blunt peptic esophagitis in a patient in whom the acid inactivates trypsin, and the bile salts modulate pepsin. Conversely, if a patient refluxes duodenal contents into the stomach with a limited degree of acidity present, the net result would be the reflux of an alkaline bolus of duodenal and gastric contents into the esophagus. Thus, trypsin's activity would be optimized, resulting in a greater degree of esophageal injury. One can see that hypothetically lowering the gastric pH might be beneficial in treating GER alone, but that it could be detrimental in the child with concomitant GER and duodenal reflux.

PRESENTATION

GER is defined by a lack of competency of the GE junction, allowing gastric contents to ascent into the esophagus. Virtually all humans have this occur regularly; the clinical objective is to differentiate those individuals with pathologic GER who are at risk for complications related to this event. Presentation of pathologic GER vary, and not all children with reflux have emesis. Clinically significant GER can be categorized in three broad patterns of presentation. The first is characterized by overt emesis. The other two presentations are referred to as *silent reflux* because emesis is absent. The second involves reflux to the level of the epiglottis, with gastric contents spilling into the tracheobronchial tree and causing acid aspiration with respiratory symptoms. The third type of reflux involves the esophagus alone.

Infants normally have some degree of emesis, ranging from a wet burp to regurgitation of a significant amount, if not all, of a recent feeding. Children with pathologic GER, however, often regurgitate large volumes more frequently. The differential diagnosis of children with emesis should take into account the character of the emesis. Bilious emesis in young children is considered to be caused by obstruction until proved otherwise. The emesis with GER is nonbilious and typically occurs during a feeding or shortly after a feeding. Often, the parent finds the crib sheet or pillow stained by the vomited material. In the child who is several weeks of age, the major differential diagnosis is pyloric stenosis. If the GER is severe, weight loss and failure to thrive can occur. Parents may describe the number of times the child's clothes must be changed each day. In older children, the repeated emesis can lead to social problems and poor self-esteem. The presence of emesis makes the diagnosis of reflux easy to identify; however, the lack of emesis does not rule out GER.

Aspiration of gastric contents into the tracheobronchial tree can cause apnea, pneumonia, bronchitis, and asthma (6). Gastric contents can be a potent trigger for apnea and bradycardia from reflex laryngospasm. A decrease in esophageal pH can be associated with the simultaneous development of respiratory symptoms. These respiratory symptoms can be as mild as coughing or as critical as apnea, which can be a mechanism for sudden infant death syndrome (7). In infants and children with recurrent episodes of pneumonia believed to be aspiration related, the association with GER may be relatively straightforward. Conversely, a number of patients with reflux may have asthma or bronchitis for many years, and this may be the primary or even sole symptom of the GER. Although the concept of reflux causing pulmonary symptoms from aspiration has been well known, there and now data which show that exposure of the distal esophagus to acid is associated with reflex bronchoconstriction (8).

Symptoms related solely to acid bathing the esophagus include poor feeding, dysphagia, and Sandifer syndrome. In the older child, there may be a complaint of heartburn. Findings may include esophagitis, esophageal ulceration, stricture formation, melena, bleeding, anemia, and Barrett's esophagus. A symptom constellation may be relatively acute or chronic in regard to its presentation.

ASSOCIATED ANOMALIES

Children with esophageal atresia are likely to have reflux for several reasons. Because of the discontinuity of the esophagus, there is a lack of the normal innervation into the area of the LES. In addition, at the time of repair of esophageal atresia, there may be a need to mobilize the distal esophageal segment to achieve sufficient length to carry out an anastomosis without tension. This can change the configuration of the angle of His, thereby disrupting one anatomic antireflux mechanism. Extensive mobilization of the distal esophagus can actually pull part of the stomach up through the diaphragm, decreasing or eliminating the intraabdominal portion of the esophagus and creating a hiatal hernia. This may be true in the typical tracheoesophageal fistula repair with the distal esophageal segment attached to the trachea, and is of even more concern in children with pure esophageal atresia and a long gap between the two esophageal segments. If GER is present, its sequelae may be more severe in these patients because of esophageal dysmotility and ineffective acid clearance from the distal esophagus. In this event, the gastric acid contents remain in contact with the esophagus longer, causing further inflammation of the distal esophagus.

After repair of a diaphragmatic hernia, patients are more likely to have pathologic GER, with an incidence as high as 35% (9,10). Closure of the diaphragmatic defect can place tension on the esophageal crura, pulling the left crus laterally and altering the anatomy of the GE junction. Hiatal hernia is uncommon in children with GER, but when present, this confers a high likelihood that the reflux will not respond to medical therapy. Finally, there is a high incidence of GER in neurologically impaired patients. It is unclear whether this is due to a central mechanism or whether chronic retching in some of these children causes reflux.

DIAGNOSIS

The evaluation of the infant or child with suspected pathologic GER begins with a detailed history and physical examination. In the infant, pyloric stenosis and GER can be confused. The pattern of emesis, both in terms of frequency and severity, often allows for differentiation. Emesis with GER is typically nonbilious. Bilious emesis should be considered in the young child to be due to malrotation until proved otherwise (11). The patient may have a history of recurrent upper respiratory infections, bronchitis, pneumonitis, pneumonia, or asthma. Any of these can be indicative of GER. Poor feeding can be due to repetitive bouts of reflux and subsequent esophagitis or esophageal stricture formation.

Physical examination can reveal obvious emesis, a cough related to GER, pneumonia, or Sandifer syndrome. In the latter circumstance, the infant repetitively turns his or her head to one side to improve peristalsis in the esophagus. This can be confused with torticollis. It is associated with neck extension and arching of the back, presumably the consequences of esophagitis induced pain. In some patients, a period of hospitalization may ascertain whether there is a significant feeding problem. Specific questions about the amount of food the infant is taking can help define failure to thrive and potential causes of emesis. A period of observation also allows for identification of the frequency and severity of GER, as well as assessment of the effect of treatment strategies.

The diagnostic tests available to evaluate the patient with suspected GER include an esophagogram, esophageal pH probe measurement, scintigraphy, esophageal manometry, esophagoscopy, and biopsy. Each test has advantages and disadvantages, and is not performed in every patient.

Esophagogram

The esophagogram is the most commonly used diagnostic test in the evaluation of GER. It is an good as a screening test, is arguably the easiest test to perform, and provides information about the anatomy of the esophagus, stomach, and duodenum, as well as their respective function. Fluoroscopy can identify the presence of GER and whether the refluxed material remains in the esophagus alone or results in aspiration of acid into the tracheobronchial tree. Abnormalities of the esophagus, such as esophagitis, ulceration, stricture, and dilation, are identified (Figs. 66-2 and 66-3). The presence of normal peristalsis in the esophagus and stomach can be evaluated. The presence of a hiatal hernia, the position of the GE junction, the configuration of the stomach, and the angle of His can also be evaluated. In addition, a number of abnormalities that cause a delay in gastric emptying, such as pyloric stenosis, malrotation, or a duodenal web, can be identified. The esophagogram is reviewed with spot films and cinefluoroscopy. The latter gives a representation of the dynamic process of swallowing and GER. Another point of evaluation in this study is the rapidity of esophageal clearance of refluxed gastric contents. In the esophagus with poor peristalsis, refluxed contrast may remain for a lengthy period of time. In the patient who has had repair of esophageal atresia, the esophagogram can identify abnormal esophageal motility, an anastomotic stricture, a more distal stricture, and GER. The overall sensitivity of the esophagogram in the evaluation of GER is about 85% (12). A major limitation is the short interval used to evaluate the subject. If reflux is noted during the deglutition of barium, or if it is noted when the stomach is filled with contrast, a positive diagnosis is made. The absence of reflux during the relatively short evaluation, however, does not rule out its presence.

The esophagogram is also valuable in patients who have a clinical history of reflux and who have had an antireflux procedure. In these patients, the study allows for an evaluation of the GER and determination of whether a

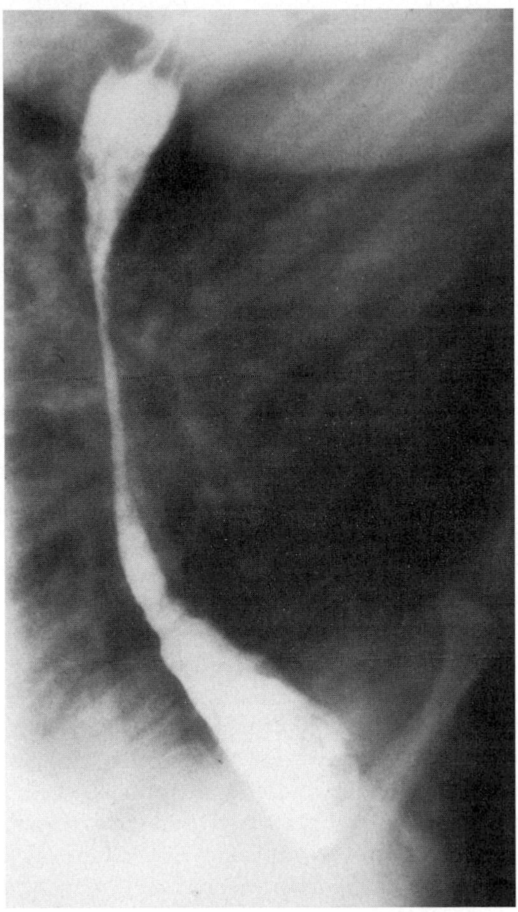

FIGURE 66-2. Esophagogram showing a long narrow esophageal stricture secondary to gastroesophageal reflux.

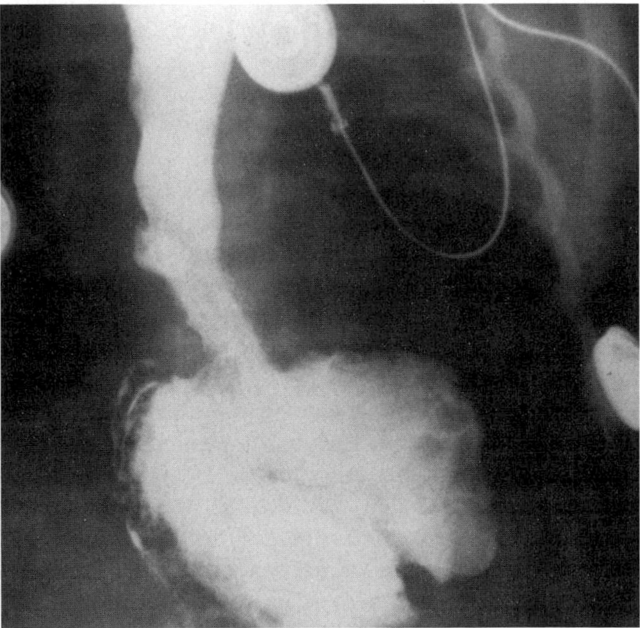

FIGURE 66-3. Esophagogram showing a large esophageal ulcer induced by pathologic acid gastroesophageal reflux.

fundoplication is still intact, its position, any difficulty with esophageal peristalsis delivering contrast through the area of the fundoplication, and any delay in gastric emptying. Contrast can be given by mouth or if need be via a gastroesophageal button in neurologically impaired patients.

Esophageal pH Monitoring

Since the early 1980s, the prolonged monitoring of esophageal pH has become the standard for evaluation of GER (11,13). The test consists of placing a 2F catheter through the nose with probes both in the proximal thoracic and the distal esophagus. Continuous pH monitoring is performed during the following 24 hours. The study measures the presence of acid in the distal esophagus, the number of reflux episodes, and typically reports the length of time acid is present for each episode, the total amount of time that acid is present in the esophagus, and the longest continuous periods of time that acid is present in the esophagus. Evaluation is carried out while the child is awake, asleep, supine, sitting, or upright. It is important to feed the child during the study. Fasting status throughout the study may give a false-negative result because the stomach is not filled. The two most important measurements are the total percent of time that the pH is less than 5 and the total number of episodes of GER lasting longer than 5 minutes. Associated problems, such as cough, choking, cyanosis, oxygen desaturation, or apnea, should be recorded. Because the esophageal pH monitoring test is performed for a number of hours, it is a much more representative study for the presence of pathologic GER than an esophagogram. Shortening the length of the study can cause difficulties in interpretation. For example, 12-hour monitoring does not identify up to 20% of patients with pathologic reflux (14).

The data are recorded by computerized telemetry in a nearly physiologic setting and can be combined with an apnea study.

The major advantages of the pH probe study are that it has a 98% specificity for the identification of GER and that it is carried out under normal physiologic conditions (no sedation or anesthesia), over an extended length of time, and with the child carrying out normal activities. Corroborative information regarding esophageal motility and acid clearance can be obtained by analysis of the time it takes for esophageal pH to return to normal after feeding. A disadvantage of the study is that most food buffers the gastric pH to a level near that of the esophageal pH. A false-negative evaluation of GER may be assumed during the postprandial period. To avoid this problem, feeding times should be recorded. Feeding with a highly acidic liquid, such as apple juice, can be done if necessary to clarify this. A similar limitation is its inability to identify intrinsic alkaline reflux (i.e., duodenogastric reflux).

Radionuclide Scan

Scintigraphy for GER involves the ingestion of a radionuclide-labeled liquid or semisolid material; alternatively, the material is administered through a tube in the stomach. Semisolids are now used more frequently than liquids alone. The patient is subsequently placed under a gamma counter, and for 90 minutes, the amount of the nuclide leaving the stomach is measured. This study serves two major purposes: (1) It identifies the presence of GER and the aspiration of gastric contents into the tracheobronchial tree by the presence of the nuclide in the lungs, and (2) it provides physiologic information regarding the efficacy of gastric emptying. The norm is that one-half of the meal passes out of the stomach into the small intestine within 1 hour of its ingestion.

Advantages of the radionuclide study include the quantitative measurement of gastric emptying, which can be used for subsequent comparison. The study is more accurate than an upper gastrointestinal series in identifying a delay in gastric emptying. Although a point of controversy, many consider it an important test in the identification of a foregut motility disorder.

Disadvantages of the radionuclide study include low-dose radiation exposure, the necessity for the patient to remain under the gamma counter for a lengthy period, and the potential difficulty obtaining an accurate assessment of gastric emptying if the patient has significant pathologic GER and loses a portion of the nuclide label with emesis.

Esophageal Manometry

Measurement of the intraluminal pressures in the esophagus and at the GE junction gives useful physiologic information about GER and esophageal motility. Manometry provides information regarding LES function, pressure, and length. Normal LESP is considered to be 15 mm Hg or more. When properly performed, the manometic evaluation has a sensitivity for detecting pathologic GER of about 70%. Esophageal manometry is more useful and has better-developed normal standards in adults than in children. It is generally considered the most difficult of the studies available to assess GER, and, in children, is used infrequently.

Endoscopy and Biopsy

Esophagoscopy allows visualization of the distal esophagus, the GE junction, and the stomach, and affords the opportunity to obtain biopsy specimens. A biopsy can help to identify the presence and degree of esophagitis. The degree of inflammatory change may not correlate with histologic change, particularly when comparing acid reflux with duodenal reflux. Multiple biopsies should be performed to obtain representative samples. An important related finding is that of Barrett's esophagus (see Chapter 64). Esophagoscopy can also provide a baseline for following the patient postoperatively, especially if a distal esophageal stricture is present. Bronchoscopy can be helpful in patients with pulmonary symptoms and suspected GER. The bronchoscopy can allow for aspiration of material from the bronchial segments with analysis for the presence of lipid-laden macrophages, which correlate with GER and aspiration (15,16). In addition, endoscopy can also visualize the vocal cords. If inflammation of the cords is noted, this may be another sequela of GER.

MEDICAL TREATMENT

Management of the infant or child with GER should take into account whether there is an anatomic cause for the reflux and the severity of the reflux. Concomitant anatomic anomalies may contribute to severe reflux, which is difficult to obviate without operative intervention. Patients who have undergone esophageal atresia or diaphragmatic hernia repair, and those with a hiatal hernia may be refractory to nonoperative management. Patients with these associated anatomic problems, however, make up only a small number of all patients with GER. In patients with pathologic reflux, the goal of treatment is to decrease the amount of reflux and to relieve symptoms. Overall, nonoperative treatment of GER is successful in the majority of children, with this success rate 80% or more in young children. The patients most likely to respond well are those with mild to moderate reflux. Children with moderate to severe reflux are less likely to do well without surgical intervention. Other factors that influence the prognosis of GER are patient age, the presence of a significant neurologic deficit, and whether the GER is part of a foregut motility disorder.

Infants without complications related to their GER are likely to do well with medical treatment. There appears to be physiologic maturation of the LES during the first 4 to 6 months of age. As infants begin to sit up and stand, gravity also helps minimize the reflux. Also, this time usually corresponds with the beginning of solid feedings. These factors work together to decrease the amount of GER in most infants. In contrast, children with poor or dysfunctional esophageal peristalsis, GER, and significant delay in gastric emptying components of foregut motility disorders are likely to have synergism of these factors, limiting the probability of a good response to medical treatment.

GER in neurologically impaired patients can be particularly difficult to treat. The reflux in many of these patients may be potentiated by hypertonicity, which raises intraabdominal and intragastric pressures. In addition, many of these patients have behavioral retching. This is difficult to stop and often contributes to reflux. GER to the level of the epiglottis is a particular problem in neurologically impaired children who cannot protect the airway and thus are at higher risk for aspiration-related problems.

Symptomatic GER in patients older than 6 to 8 years of age is usually not associated with the spontaneous improvement seen in infants and younger children. These children are already upright and eating solid food. It is likely that reflux has been present, if not obvious, for a number of years in these children. Therefore, it is reasonable to have an increased concern regarding reflux complications in these children. This would include stricture formation, Barrett's esophagus, and chronic pulmonary disease.

The major medical components of GER treatment, especially in young children, include upright positioning, frequent and low-volume feedings, thickened feedings, and pharmacologic treatment with antacids and prokinetic agents. Placing the child in an upright position exploits gravity and promotes better clearance from the esophagus. The infant seat has been advocated for many years for this purpose. Young children tend to slide downward in this device, however, and it is not always effective in achieving a semiupright position for any length of time. Since the early to mid-1990s, the use of the prone position with the head upright 30 degrees has proven to be a significant improvement in the therapy of GER (17). This position should be kept for at least 60 minutes after feedings. The major disadvantage of this technique is that it can be difficult to maintain for an older, more mobile infant. A second important consideration is the frequency and character of the feedings. More frequent, smaller-volume feedings distend the stomach less. Thickening the milk or formula with rice cereal and similar substances also decreases the amount of GER. The combination of frequent, smaller, and thickened feedings is a mainstay in the management of these children.

LESP is decreased by inflammation, as seen with peptic esophagitis. Medications that reduce gastric acid production have become mainstays in the medical treatment of GER. An array of pharmacologic agents can have a salutary effect. H_2-antagonists, such as ranitidine, and proton pump inhibitors, such as omeprazole, have demonstrated efficacy (18,19). Their mechanism of action is likely from antiinflammatory effects on the distal esophagus via decreased gastric acidity. This causes an increase in LESP and thus ameliorates GER. Prokinetic agents, such as metoclopramide and cisapride (Propulsid), improve peristalsis and gastric emptying. Cisapride not only aids in gastric emptying, but also improves esophageal peristalsis and helps clear gastric contents from the distal esophagus. Unfortunately, it is no longer approved for use in the United States. In addition to improving peristalsis, metoclopramide increases LESP.

In patients with mild reflux, strategies to decrease acid production and to improve motility are effective. In patients with more severe GER, the response to nonoperative treatment is usually not as satisfying. Because long-term pharmacologic treatment can pose additional problems, there comes a point when other options, such as surgery, should be considered. Relevant pharmacologic agents have associated side effects, including extrapyramidal reactions, sedation, and diarrhea (20). A fundamental consideration with the use of pharmacologic agents is whether they are modifying the symptoms of pathologic reflux or actually decreasing the reflux itself. A management strategy that deals with the causes of reflux and thereby prevents the event is appealing.

SURGICAL CORRECTION

Gastroesophageal reflux should be corrected surgically if the symptoms cannot be controlled medically or if an anatomic abnormality is contributing significantly. In addition, if a patient has significant GER and cannot protect the airway (e.g., a neurologically impaired patient), then operative intervention is indicated.

Indications for operative intervention in the treatment of GER include the following:

- Unremitting emesis
- Failure to grow adequately
- Recurrent pneumonitis
- Apnea
- Refractory reactive airway disease
- Esophagitis
- Esophageal stricture
- Hiatal hernia

The child with multiple episodes of emesis each day often fails to thrive because of a lack of appropriate nutrition. Parents and physicians are hard pressed to miss the bouts of emesis, the need to have clothes changed, and the associated lack of appropriate weight gain. The decision to perform an operative procedure to correct GER is straightforward in the patient with recurrent emesis who has not improved with medical management. Many patients have silent reflux and may have primarily respiratory symptoms. If, despite medical therapy, the child is having repetitive bouts of pneumonitis, aspiration pneumonia, or apneic spells, it is clear that nonoperative management is not achieving the desired result. Other patients may have evidence of long-standing lung disease manifested by chronic bronchitis or asthmalike symptoms (21). Personal experience with a group of pediatric lung transplant recipients indicates that GER is not uncommon in this setting. Acid reflux with aspiration into the tracheobronchial tree can cause life-threatening pulmonary infection in this immunocompromised group. Pulmonary symptoms due to GER that are unresponsive to medical therapy are well treated by an antireflux operation (21).

Operation is also indicated for chronic esophagitis. Reflux in these patients can lead to a cycle of acute and chronic inflammation, fibrosis, and stricture formation. The inflammation can progress to the point of chronic bleeding and can cause iron-deficiency anemia. Patients may develop hematemesis or melena. Chronic esophagitis is associated with the development of Barrett's esophagus (see Chapter 64).

In the older child who can verbalize, the complaint of persistent lower chest discomfort or persistent dysphagia is an indication for operation. In the younger child, there may be a significant aversion to food. This poor appetite may improve markedly after the reflux is obviated.

The principles for surgical treatment of GER include the establishment of an intraabdominal portion of the esophagus and the development of a LES that resists the passage of gastric contents from the stomach to the esophagus. The mechanical model of the esophagus, GE junction, and stomach (Fig. 66-1) allows for an understanding of the goals of operation. The surgeon creates an antireflux valve around a segment of the intraabdominal esophagus by bringing a portion of the fundus of the stomach around the esophagus. The fundoplication may be a circumferential (360° Nissen) wrap or partial (270° Toupet or modified Thal). Both techniques have good functional results and each has enthusiastic proponents. An important tenet is that the 360-degree fundoplication should never be tight or snug, but floppy. The goal is not to have the fundoplication impinge on or constrict the esophagus during the resting state. Before operation, if intragastric pressure increases, gastric contents can easily pass from the stomach into the esophagus because no effective antireflux mechanism is in place. After an antireflux procedure, an increase in intragastric pressure temporarily causes the portion of the stomach positioned around the intraabdominal esophagus to act as a pinchcock valve (Fig. 66-4). As soon as intragastric pressure decreases, the enfolded stomach around the esophagus collapses and does not impinge on the esophagus. The floppy characteristic of the fundoplication is integral to the repair. It should not function as an impediment to passage of food from the esophagus to the stomach. If there is esophageal dysmotility and the fundoplication is tight, liquids or solids may not be able to pass from the esophagus into the stomach. Likewise, material refluxed into the esophagus may not be able to clear easily. This problem is particularly significant in patients with previous esophageal atresia repair because they have predictably poor peristalsis. In these cases, nothing should be done to create a further impediment to the prograde passage of material from esophagus to stomach. These patients appear to do better with a partial fundoplication such as a Toupet.

The pump function of the esophagus depends on peristalsis. The valve mechanism is created by the fundoplication around the intraabdominal portion of the esophagus.

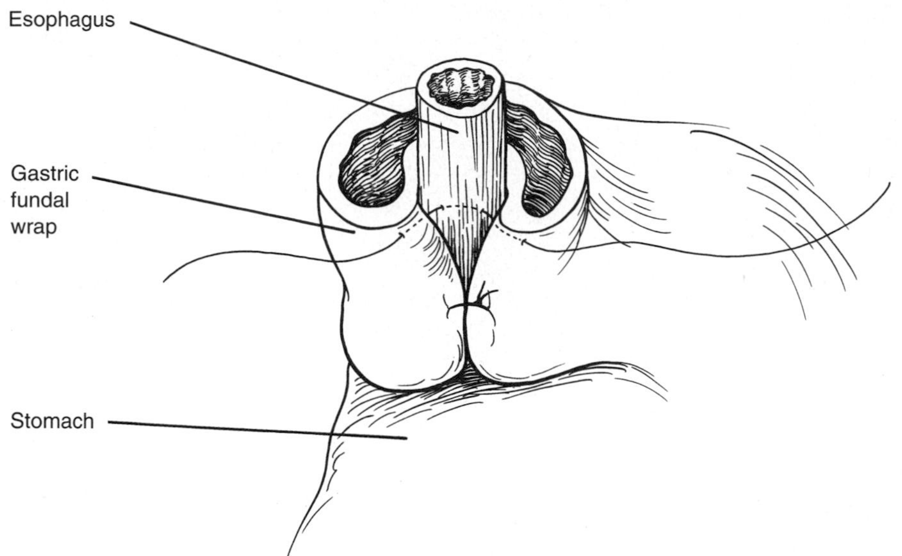

FIGURE 66-4. Formation of an antireflux valve around the intraabdominal esophagus. As intragastric pressure increases, it presses inward on the esophagus. As intragastric pressure returns to normal, there is no impingement on the esophagus.

The third component of a successful repair relates to the function of the stomach itself. Malrotation, pylorospasm, and idiopathic causes of delayed gastric emptying all create an increase in the reservoir capacity of the stomach. Dilation causes an increase in gastric pressure, which can lead to retching. In addition, gastric distension or dilation can shorten the length of the intraabdominal esophagus. This may contribute to the development of GER. In this case, the fundoplication prevents egress of material retrograde into the esophagus. Retching can disrupt or displace the fundoplication into the mediastinum. Correction of GER by an antireflux procedure in the presence of continued poor gastric emptying can be associated with a subsequent disruption of the fundoplication or a "slipped" fundoplication, where the fundoplication has migrated into the mediastinum. If the stomach cannot empty well, gastric contractility increases. This is not directed solely at the pylorus, but the gastric peristaltic wave can be directed toward the gastric fundus. This can cause the disruption of the fundoplication. If there is objective evidence of delayed gastric emptying, the fundoplication should be combined with a gastric emptying procedure.

Operative Technique

Pediatric surgeons generally prefer an abdominal approach for operation. The Nissen fundoplication is the most commonly performed procedure, but many recommend a partial anterior (modified Thal) or a partial posterior (Toupet) antireflux procedure. Each of these procedures includes the principles of creating an intraabdominal segment of esophagus, creating a high-pressure zone in this portion of the esophagus, and preserving the angle of His. The procedure can be performed with equally good results via either an open technique or laparoscopically. Long-term outcome data using the laparoscopic approach are not yet available.

In a Nissen fundoplication, the intraabdominal esophagus is circumferentially encircled. If a hiatal hernia is present, the stomach is reduced from the chest, and mobilization is carried out so the distal esophagus is below the diaphragm. The esophageal hiatus is assessed. If it is patulous posterior to the esophagus, several nonabsorbable sutures are used to reapproximate the crura (Fig. 66-5A). This decreases the likelihood of a displacement of the fundoplication, cranially through the hiatus. The posterior part of the fundus is then brought posterior and to the right side of the esophagus. The anesthesiologist passes a bougie through the mouth, down the esophagus, and into the stomach. The largest bougie that easily passes through the esophagus should be used. The fundoplication is then carried out over the bougie, wrapping the esophagus within the fundus creating a loose or floppy fundoplication. A series of interrupted nonabsorbable sutures are placed in the fundus to the left of the esophagus, superficially through the anterior wall of the esophagus, and then to the portion of the fundus brought to the right of the esophagus. When these sutures are tied, a 360-degree fundoplication results (Fig. 66-5B). The most superior suture of the fundoplication is used to secure it to the esophagus just ventral to the esophageal hiatus. This also helps prevent movement of the fundoplication. Several nonabsorbable sutures are used to secure the fundus to the left of the fundoplication to the diaphragm. This tends to reform a normal angle of His. The bougie is then removed. In children younger than 2 years of age, in neurologically impaired children, and in those requiring tube feedings, a gastrostomy tube is placed. The gastrostomy tube or button is used for feeding purposes in the latter case. In young or neurologically impaired children, it is used to prevent

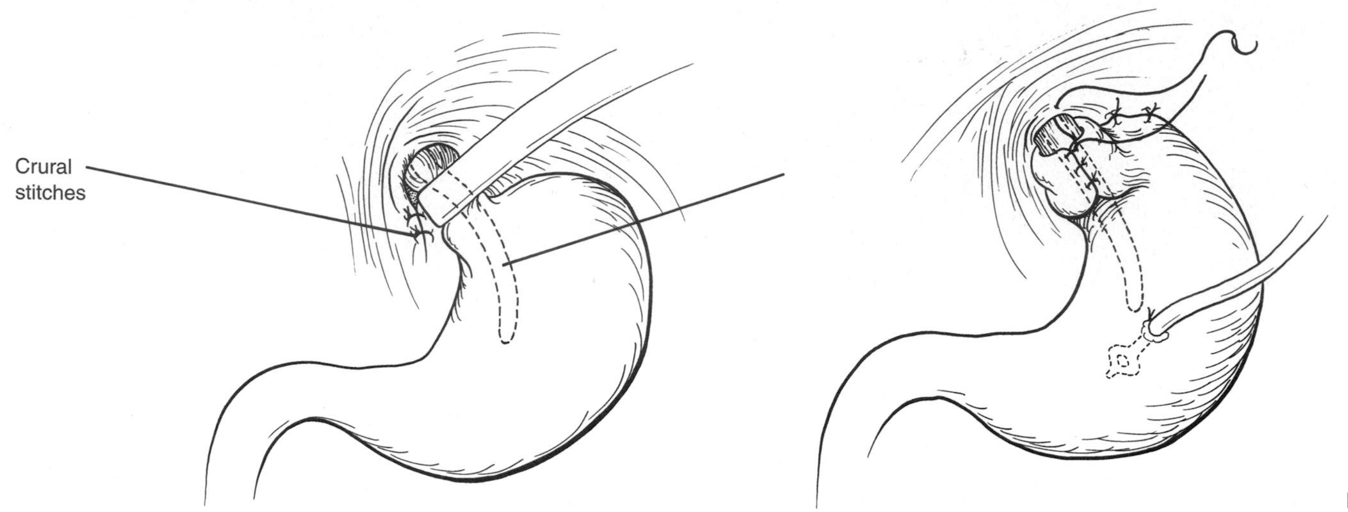

FIGURE 66-5. Creation of a 360-degree Nissen fundoplication. (**A**) The esophageal hiatus is closed. (**B**) The completed fundic wrap is secured to the diaphragm, and a gastrostomy tube is placed.

a gas bloat syndrome. In patients with a significant delay in gastric emptying, a gastric emptying procedure is often carried out. This can consist either of a pyloroplasty, pyloromyotomy, or antroplasty (22). In these patients where there has been an operative intervention at both the upper and lower portions of the stomach, a gastrostomy tube is placed for at least a temporary period of time.

Some surgeons contend that the 360-degree wrap significantly inhibits the child's ability to clear material from the esophagus. Gas bloat syndrome is seen in about 3% of these patients (23). A postoperative patient with a small bowel obstruction who cannot vomit can develop massive gastric dilation. Because of these problems, some surgeons favor a fundoplication in which the fundus is not brought circumferentially around the entire esophagus. This partial fundoplication is also believed to be of benefit in children after a repair of a tracheoesophageal fistula. The partial fundoplication may diminish the risk of distal esophageal obstruction in these patients with impaired esophageal peristalsis. In patients with a short esophagus, as can be seen in some children with long-standing GER, an appropriate segment of intraabdominal esophagus cannot be achieved. The Collis-Nissen procedure nicely lengthens the intraabdominal esophageal segment needed.

A number of complications can be related to the technical aspects of the operative repair. These include problems with the esophageal hiatus. If this is widely patent, appropriate reapproximation of the crura needs to be performed to prevent migration of a portion of the fundoplication above the diaphragm. If an insufficient portion of the abdominal esophagus is mobilized, the fundoplication and therefore the functional LES may be inadequate. Another problem in the patient with insufficient intraabdominal esophagus mobilized is the inadvertent wrapping of the stomach rather than the lower esophagus. If the fundoplication is too tight around the esophagus, it may impede passage of food into the stomach. Care must be taken to bring the fundus loosely around the esophagus. The fundus can also be twisted as it is brought posterior to the esophagus, which causes malfunction of the wrap. Other technical considerations include avoidance of vagal nerve injury. This can be a particular problem in the patient with a previously failed fundoplication. Placing the gastrostomy tube in the antrum of the stomach and directing it toward the pylorus can lead to partial gastric outlet obstruction, due to a balloon of the gastrostomy button.

Results

Many centers report 80% to 90% good to excellent results with an antireflux operation for the infant or child with GER who has not responded satisfactorily to medical therapy. These results include both the Nissen fundoplication and various partial fundoplications, either anterior or posterior (23–26). The treatment of GER in patients without associated anomalies has a more than 90% success rate. Children with symptoms of failure to thrive often show a significant compensatory weight gain, pulmonary symptoms improve, and esophagitis and strictures can be substantially resolved. Further, the use of multiple medications to treat GER can often be stopped.

Operative intervention often results in improvement in the overall health of children with congenital heart disease who have failure to thrive and GER. Almost all pediatric reports have a high incidence of associated anomalies in patients with GER. The outcomes in these patients are more disparate.

In a combined study from two institutions, Fonkalsrud reviewed 1,200 consecutive patients who underwent fundoplication for GER (6). Similar to other reports, many (39%) patients were neurologically impaired. At the time of these initial operations, 871 patients underwent a fundoplication alone, whereas 286 children underwent both fundoplication and a gastric emptying procedure. A significant neurologic abnormality was present in 25% of the children who had fundoplication alone; in contrast, 75% of patients who had a gastric emptying procedure added to the fundoplication were neurologically impaired. The most common symptoms in the children operated on were repeated emesis (75%), feeding disorders in neurologically impaired children (39%), failure to thrive (32%), and respiratory problems, including repeated pneumonia (29%), asthma, or reactive airway disease (10%). Esophageal pH probe studies identified GER in 99% of the patients, and barium esophagogram with slight abdominal pressure applied showed GER in 86% of 1,147 patients studied. A hiatal hernia was present in only 6% of the children. Manometry was used in a small number of children, and LESP was less than 15 mm Hg in 61% of patients studied. Endoscopy and biopsy showed histologic evidence of esophagitis in 65% of the patients thus evaluated.

This study showed relief of emesis in essentially 100% of patients, and weight gain in almost all patients as well. There was cessation or marked improvement of pulmonary symptoms in 91% of the children. Operation is generally considered to result in improvement in more than 90% of patients who have significant esophagitis or stricture.

The results of antireflux procedures for the treatment of GER in neurologically impaired children vary. Indications for surgical intervention include the common problems related to GER and the concomitant need for gastrostomy button placement to aid in feeding. Controversy exists regarding whether an antireflux procedure should be performed routinely at the time of gastrostomy tube placement in these children, whether evaluation for GER should be carried out, or whether the gastrostomy placement should be performed alone.

Central nervous system disorders, both congenital and acquired, are associated with GER (27). Because gastrostomy placement can result in a decrease in LESP, which can add to the likelihood of reflux, we believe it is appropriate to evaluate the neurologically impaired child for GER before gastrostomy tube placement. If GER is identified, further evaluation to identify the presence of delayed gastric emptying is done. If the patient has evidence of reflux, an antireflux procedure is performed concurrent with the gastrostomy tube placement. If the child also has delayed gastric emptying, a gastric emptying procedure is added to the gastrostomy tube placement and antireflux procedure.

Complications

The incidence of death after fundoplication in most large series is approximately 1% to 2%. It is largely skewed to patients who have major associated problems and is usually not related directly to the operation. A variety of complications can be seen after an antireflux procedure. These include

- Pulmonary dysfunction
- Wound infection
- Gas bloat syndrome
- Herniation of fundoplication
- Intestinal obstruction
- Dysphagia
- Gastrostomy tube problems

Atelectasis or pneumonia is seen in 3% to 5% of patients, and wound infection is seen in about 1% to 2% of patients. The gas bloat syndrome is seen in about 3% of patients after a Nissen fundoplication. It is usually transient in nature, lasting several weeks, and avoided by forming a floppy wrap. It can be dealt with effectively by venting through a gastrostomy tube or button.

Since the mid-1990s, increasing evidence has shown a strong association between pathologic GER and delayed gastric emptying. The failure of a fundoplication, either with disruption or slippage of the fundoplication into the mediastinum, is often related to delayed gastric emptying. The incidence of delayed gastric emptying in patients with pH-proven GER has been reported to be 22% (28). This association is more common in neurologically impaired children.

Recurrent GER recurs in about 10% of all patients and in about 25% of neurologically impaired children after fundoplication (29). In children with clinical evidence of emesis or regurgitation after fundoplication, evaluation should include an upper gastrointestinal study to assess for GER and to evaluate the presence and position of the fundoplication. If GER is present, a gastric emptying study should be done to ensure that delayed gastric emptying is not a contributing factor. This may be a major issue if the patient cannot empty the stomach in a prograde manner and therefore retches. If this is the case, reconstruction of the fundoplication should be done concomitant with a gastric emptying procedure. The addition of the gastric emptying procedure decreases the failure rate of the fundoplication and is very infrequently associated with dumping problems or alkaline reflux (30). Some believe that because of the possibility of injury to the vagal nerve trunks at the time of the reconstruction of the fundoplication, a gastric emptying procedure should be performed even without obvious evidence of delayed gastric emptying in the reoperative setting (6).

Dysphagia is seen infrequently in patients after fundoplication. It is associated with esophagitis, stricture

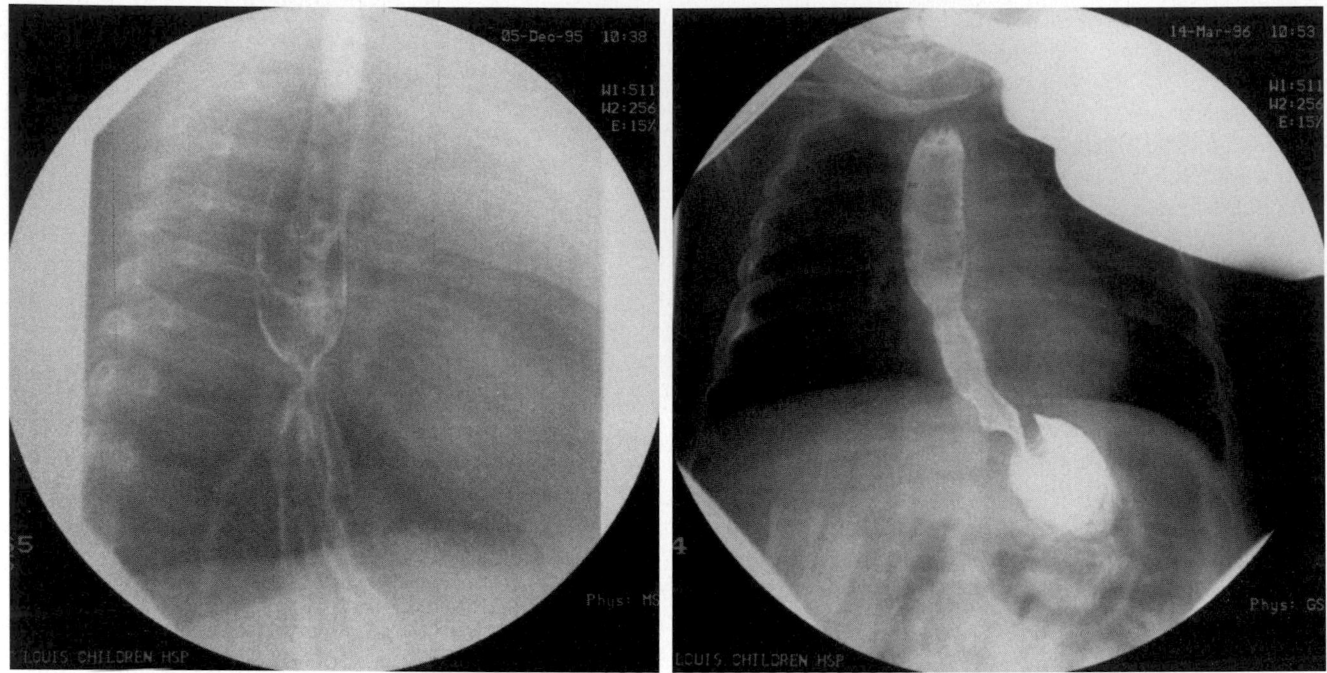

FIGURE 66-6. (**A**) Esophagogram showing a tight esophageal stricture in a child after repair of a pure esophageal atresia. This patient had severe gastroesophageal reflux. (**B**) In the same patient 2 months after a Nissen fundoplication and two esophageal dilations, there is resolution of the stricture. In addition, the fundal wrap around the intraabdominal esophagus can be seen.

formation, a tight fundoplication, and poor esophageal peristalsis. Typically, esophagitis resolves in patients promptly after successful fundoplication. A stricture, however, may take some time and several esophageal dilations before appreciable improvement is noted (Fig. 66-6). Dysphagia can be caused by a snug fundoplication. This is best avoided by performing the wrap over an appropriate-size bougie so the fundal wrap does not collapse or constrict the esophagus. Dysphagia is almost nonexistent in patients who have had a partial fundoplication. Attention to the laxity of the circumferential fundoplication is especially important in patients with poor or discoordinate esophageal motility. In these children, the passage of a bolus of semisolid or solid food through the esophagus may be largely dependent on gravity. Any esophageal obstruction due to the fundic impingement on the esophagus can cause obstruction and dysphagia.

Intestinal obstruction develops in 1% to 10% of patients after fundoplication. The likelihood of its occurrence appears to be lessened if additional intraabdominal procedures are limited, if handling of the small intestine is kept to a minimum, and if the dissection involves only the stomach and adjacent structures.

Potential gastrostomy site problems include excoriation at the exit site on the skin and obstruction of the gastric outlet or proximal small intestine. These are primarily related to the gastrostomy tube not being well secured. If the balloon or bulbous end of the catheter is not pulled up against the anterior gastric wall, gastric juice can leak out along the gastrostomy tract and cause skin irritation. If the tube is not anchored well, a balloon can migrate to the pylorus and cause obstruction, or it can pass into the duodenum and become a source of obstruction there. One of the common causes of emesis in a child with a gastrostomy tube in place is malposition of the tube. The development of the gastrostomy button has largely resolved these problems.

REFERENCES

1. Randolph JG, Lilly JR, Anderson KD. Surgical treatment of gastroesophageal reflux in infants. *Ann Surg* 1974;180:479.
2. Skinner DB. Pathophysiology of gastroesophageal reflux. *Ann Surg* 1985;202:546.
3. DeMeester TR, Wang CI, Wernly JA, et al. Technique, indications and clinical use of 24 hour esophageal pH monitoring. *J Thorac Cardiovasc Surg* 1980;79:665.
4. Lillemoe KD, Johnson LF, Harmon JW. Role of the components of gastroduodenal contents in experimental acid esophagitis. *Surgery* 1982;92:276–284.
5. Kauer WKH, Peters JH, DeMeester TR. Mixed reflux of gastric juice is more harmful to the esophagus than gastric juice alone: the need for surgical therapy reemphasized. *Ann Surg* 1995;222:525–533.
6. Berquist WE, Rachelefsky GS, Kadden M, et al. Gastroesophageal reflux, associated recurrent pneumonia and chronic asthma in children. *Pediatrics* 1981;68:29.
7. Jolley SG, Halpern LM, Tunell WP, et al. The risk of sudden infant death from gastroesophageal reflux. *J Pediatr Surg* 1991;26:691.

8. ElSerag HB, Sonnenberg A. Comorbid occurrence of laryngeal or pulmonary disease with esophagitis in United States military veterans. *Gastroenterology* 1997;113:755–760.
9. Stolar CJH, Levy JP, Dillon PW, et al. Anatomic and functional abnormalities in the esophagus in infants surviving congenital diaphragmatic hernia. *Am J Surg* 1990;159:204.
10. Koot VC, Bergmeijer JH, Bos AP, et al. Incidence and management of gastroesophageal reflux after repair of congenital diaphragmatic hernia. *J Pediatr Surg* 1993;28:48.
11. Jolley SG, Johnson DG, Herbst JJ, et al. An assessment of gastroesophageal reflux in children by extended pH monitoring of the distal esophagus. *Surgery* 1978;84:16.
12. Fonkalsrud EW, Ellis DG, Shaw A, et al. A combined hospital experience with fundoplication and gastric emptying procedure for gastroesophageal reflux in children. *J Am Coll Surg* 1995;180:449.
13. De Meester TR, Dunnington GL. Esophageal anatomy and physiology. In: Greenfield LJ, Mulholland MW, Oldham KT, et al., eds. *Surgery: scientific principles and practice.* Philadelphia: JB Lippincott, 1993.
14. Friesen CA, Holder TM, Ashcraft KW, et al. Abbreviated esophageal pH monitoring as an indication for fundoplication in children. *J Pediatr Surg* 1992;27:776.
15. Nussbaum E, Maji JC, Mathis R, et al. Association of lipid-laden alveolar macrophages and gastroesophageal reflux in children. *J Pediatr* 1987;110:190.
16. Collins KA, Geisinger KR, Wagner PH, et al. The cytologic evaluation of lipid laden alveolar macrophages as an indicator of aspiration pneumonia in young children. *Arch Pathol Lab Med* 1995;119:229.
17. Meyers WF, Herbst JJ. Effectiveness of positioning therapy for gastroesophageal reflux. *Pediatrics* 1982;79:768.
18. Gunasekcran TS, Hassall E. Efficacy and safety of omeprazole for severe gastroesophageal reflux in children. *J Pediatr* 1993;123:148.
19. Hassall E. Wrap session: is the Nissen slipping? Can medical treatment replace surgery for severe gastroesophageal reflux in children? *Am J Gastroenterol* 1995;90:1212.
20. Harrington RA, Hamilton CW, Brogden RN, et al. Metoclopramide: an updated review of its pharmacologic properties and clinical use. *Drugs* 1983;25:451.
21. Foglia RP, Fonkalsrud EW, Ament ME, et al. Gastroesophageal fundoplication for the management of chronic pulmonary disease in children. *Am J Surg* 1980;140:72.
22. Fonkalsrud EW, Ament ME, Vargas J. Gastric antroplasty for the treatment of delayed gastric emptying and gastroesophageal reflux in children. *Am J Surg* 1992;164:327.
23. Ashcraft KW.Gastroesophageal reflux. In: Ashcraft KW, Holder TM, eds. *Pediatric surgery,* 2nd ed. Philadelphia: WB Saunders, 1993.
24. Bliss D, Hirschl R, Oldham K, et al. Efficacy of anterior gastric fundoplication in the treatment of gastroesophageal reflux in infants and children. *J Pediatr Surg* 1994;29:1071.
25. Bensoussan AL, Yazbeck S, Carcellar-Blanchard L. Results and complications of Toupet partial posterior wrap: 10 years experience. *J Pediatr Surg* 1994;29:1215.
26. Randolph JG. Experience with the Nissen fundoplication for correction of gastroesophageal reflux in infants. *Ann Surg* 1983;198:579.
27. Halpern LM, Jolley SG, Johnson DG. Gastroesophageal reflux: a significant association with central nervous system disease in children. *J Pediatr Surg* 1991;26:171.
28. Fonkalsrud EW, Foglia RP. Operative treatment for the gastroesophageal reflux syndrome in children. *J Pediatr Surg* 1989;24:525.
29. Martinez DA, Ginn-Pease ME, Caniano DA. Sequelae of antireflux surgery in profoundly disabled children. *J Pediatr Surg* 1992;27:267.
30. Buchmiller TL, Curr M, Fonkalsrud EW. Assessment of alkaline reflux in children after Nissen fundoplication and pyloroplasty. *J Am Coll Surg* 1994;178:1.

PART C

Abdomen and Abdominal Wall Defects

Chapter 67

Clinical Principles of Abdominal Surgery

George W. Holcomb, III and Daniel J. Ostlie

PERITONEUM

The peritoneal cavity is divided into two separate cavities connected by the epiploic foramen. This opening connects the lesser sac behind the stomach and liver with the greater peritoneal cavity. Anatomically, the general peritoneal sac is divided into several spaces, owing to the fixed visceral attachments to the retroperitoneum. The right and left subphrenic spaces are common locations for abscess formation. The left and right subhepatic spaces are located between the liver and transverse mesocolon, and are separated by the epiploic foramen. The right subhepatic space is a common site for inflammatory processes arising from the biliary system, the head of the pancreas, and the duodenum. Located to the right of the small bowel mesentery, the right infracolic space has direct communication with the right subhepatic space. Viscera included in this space are the appendix, cecum, and right female adnexa. Because of its location, inflammatory processes from the right infracolic region may spread to the lesser sac. Similarly, the left infracolic space is located left of the obliquely oriented small bowel mesentery and contains the sigmoid colon and left female adnexa. The remaining spaces include the pelvis and lateral paracolic gutters. Inflammatory processes tend to remain localized to these spaces if host-defense mechanisms are effective.

George W. Holcomb, III and Daniel J. Ostlie: Children's Mercy Hospital, University of Missouri at Kansas City School of Medicine, Kansas City, Missouri 64108.

The peritoneum is the serous membrane that encloses the abdominal cavity and is reflected onto its associated viscera. This monolayer lining consists of mesothelial cells in a continuous layer resting on a basement membrane constructed from a collagen lattice. The apical surfaces of the mesothelial cells are lined with microvilli so the entire surface area of the peritoneum is approximately equal to that of the skin.

A complex circulation system present within the peritoneum provides a small volume of fluid for lubricating purposes that promotes mobility between visceral organs. Excess fluid accumulates in the subdiaphragmatic spaces and is actively pumped into the thoracic duct with diaphragmatic contraction. Although clearance of excess peritoneal fluid is effective, this process may also promote entry of bacteria into the systemic circulation, causing bacteremia. An additional fluid transfer mechanism is the lymphatic system. The diaphragmatic and peritoneal lymphatics are large and do not have valves or occlusive junctions. With certain diseases and during peritoneal dialysis, these lymphatics play an important part in transport of fluids. In addition to clearance through the previously mentioned transport mechanisms, the peritoneum contains resident macrophages, mast cells, basophils, and eosinophils, which respond to inflammation and infection.

In response to injury, peritoneal healing differs from skin. The entire peritonea defect becomes endothelialized simultaneously, not from the borders, as occurs with epidermalization of skin wounds (1,2). Moreover, the granulation and contraction that occurs around the edges of skin wounds does not occur during peritoneal healing. Reepithelialization of the parietal peritoneum occurs within 5 to 6 days of injury with complete repair by 8 days. Healing of the visceral peritoneum does not differ significantly from that of the parietal peritoneum, but it may occur 1 to 2 days earlier. Several studies have confirmed that reepithelialization from peritoneal injury appears to occur faster in immature versus mature rats.

Innervation

The parietal peritoneum is derived from the somatopleural mesoderm, whereas the splanchnopleural mesoderm gives rise to the visceral peritoneum. Because of this different derivation, the parietal peritoneum shares its neurovascular and lymphatic connections with the musculoskeletal abdominal wall, and the visceral peritoneum shares its connections with its associated visceral organs. For this reason, perception of painful stimuli is markedly different between the visceral and parietal peritoneum.

Visceral pain is perceived through neuronal pathways from the lower thoracic and lumbar splanchnic nerves and from the parasympathetic pathways of the vagus and sacral plexus. As such, visceral pain is usually dull and aching, and may be poorly localized. A steady, vague pain usually occurs after inflammation of the visceral peritoneum, whereas severe, intermittent, colicky pain results from hollow visceral obstruction. Moreover, nausea, vomiting, and sweating commonly occur with visceral inflammation.

Generalized discomfort in the epigastric, periumbilical, and hypogastric regions, respectively, may correspond with foregut, midgut, and hindgut inflammation. Inflammatory processes in the stomach, pancreas, duodenum, and biliary system may initially be manifested with vague epigastric discomfort. Similarly, small bowel and right and transverse colon inflammation is sensed as periumbilical discomfort, whereas left colon, sigmoid, and rectal pain is perceived as lower abdominal pain.

Because neuronal innervation to the parietal peritoneum is derived from the somatic nerves supplying the adjacent abdominal wall structures and skin, inflammatory stimulation is usually more localized, intense, and constant than with visceral pain. Stimulation of the parietal peritoneum is usually responsible for localization of the disease process. An example of the difference between recognition of visceral and parietal stimuli is found with appendicitis. Early appendiceal distention may be manifested by a periumbilical dull or cramping discomfort. With inflammation of the overlying parietal peritoneum, localization of the pain to the right lower quadrant typically develops, leading to the diagnosis of appendicitis.

Adhesions

Peritoneal adhesions occur as a by-product of laparotomy and inflammation. A number of pharmacologic agents, including corticosteroids, nonsteroidal antiinflammatory agents, and dextran have been used to decrease postoperative adhesions. Although corticosteroids have not been found to be useful, some benefit is suggested for ibuprofen and dextran (3,4). Barrier agents, such as polytetrafluoroethylene and oxidized regenerated cellulose, have been used in gynecologic studies (5–7). With intact hemostasis, these agents have been observed to be effective in localized peritoneal injury. Instillation of crystalloid solution has also been tried in an effort to decrease postoperative adhesions, but this isolated agent has not been effective (4,8).

Controversy exists as to whether peritoneal closure to cover areas denuded by previous dissection is beneficial. Animal studies demonstrate enhanced adhesion formation to suture lines when the peritoneum is closed over denuded tissue (9). Experimental evidence indicates that areas stripped of peritoneum heal satisfactorily. Moreover, suturing of the peritoneum may actually increase the formation of adhesions (10,11). It has been postulated that one way to reduce postoperative adhesions is through the use of laparoscopic surgery. In a prospective multicenter trial, second-look laparoscopy and adhesiolysis were performed (12). Of the areas where laparoscopic adhesiolysis had been previously performed, 67% contained adhesions at second-look laparoscopy. De novo adhesion formation, however, was substantially reduced by the laparoscopic surgery—new adhesions were noted in only 16% of the patients. Reduced adhesions were also found by Garrard and colleagues (13) in an experimental study comparing laparotomy with laparoscopy. Therefore, it appears that laparoscopic surgical techniques may reduce de novo adhesion formation, although reformation of old adhesions that have been lysed continues to be a major problem.

ACUTE ABDOMINAL CONDITIONS

Acute abdominal diseases in infants, children, and adolescents are often different from those conditions found in adults. Congenital abnormalities are usually the cause for abdominal symptoms in infants and young children. As the child grows older, diseases and symptoms common to adults become more prevalent.

The approach to the patient depends largely on the patient's age. Historical data may be lacking in infants and children too young to verbalize their complaints specifically. Often, young parents are not as perceptive as grandparents in detailing an accurate history of the young child's symptoms. Moreover, children may be placed in day-care centers, and a detailed history may actually be unknown to the parents.

Physical examination is key to determining the cause of a child's illness. The young child may be frightened and apprehensive, thus precluding an accurate examination. It may be helpful to examine an infant or young child in the parent's lap where they feel secure and comfortable, allowing a more accurate evaluation. In addition, abdominal palpation may be easier to perform and more information may be gained with the use of a stethoscope rather than the physician's hand. Often, children relax their abdominal muscles if they believe the physician is merely trying to listen to abdominal sounds rather than attempting to elicit tenderness. It is usually best to examine the region of suspected abdominal pathology last to get a more accurate interpretation of the abdominal examination. When examining the location of symptoms first, the child may become apprehensive and sense that the remainder of the examination will also be painful. When examining young children and adolescents, another helpful maneuver is to distract the child from the examination through talking. Questions about school, play, siblings, family, and so forth may distract the child from the palpation and permit a more accurate evaluation.

The rectal and pelvic examination in infants and children may not be as helpful as in adults. Rectal examination is not necessary in every case of abdominal discomfort. When indicated, however, it may be useful in eliciting a cause for the symptoms. Similarly, rarely do prepubescent girls need a pelvic examination. Rectal examination may serve the same purpose by documenting the presence of a cervix, uterus, or pelvic abscess and other masses. External genitalia examination, however, is an important component to evaluation of the child with abdominal symptoms because vaginal atresia, imperforate hymen, or foreign bodies can cause abdominal symptoms.

Laboratory data can be useful in children with abdominal symptoms. Hematocrit, leukocyte count, and urinalysis are helpful in most children with relevant complaints. Other, more specific tests, such as serum amylase, sedimentation rate, liver function tests, and clotting tests, are reserved for investigation of suspected organ cause. Sometimes, radiographic tests are the most helpful in evaluating abdominal symptoms in infants and children. These may be especially advantageous in infants who present with abdominal distention, nausea, and vomiting. In general, supine and upright radiographs should be performed when plain films are requested. In infants, a left decubitus radiograph serves the same purpose as an upright and may demonstrate evidence of pneumoperitoneum and obstruction. A prone cross-table lateral radiograph is helpful in documenting the presence or absence of air in the rectum. The absence of rectal gas may be useful in diagnosing conditions, such as small bowel obstruction, intestinal atresia, and meconium ileus. Chest radiographs may also be helpful because pneumonia can cause upper abdominal discomfort, particularly with pleurisy. When evaluating a child with fever and abdominal complaints, it is important to realize that pneumonia may not be apparent if the child is dehydrated, but will be evident on subsequent chest radiographs after rehydration (Fig. 67-1). Ultrasound examination can also be useful in evaluating

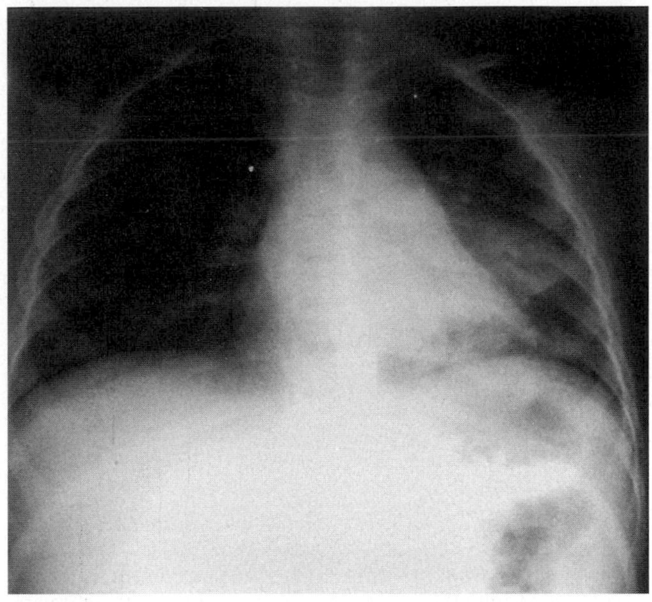

FIGURE 67-1. This chest radiograph was taken in a $2^1/_2$-year-old girl who presented with generalized abdominal pain. A chest radiograph taken the previous day was normal. In this radiograph, there is evidence of left lower lobe pneumonia accounting for the child's symptoms. She was treated with oral antibiotics and recovered uneventfully.

abdominal symptoms. Most pediatric radiologists are adept at imaging both solid and hollow intestinal viscera and frequently can determine the cause of a child's complaints. It is important, however, to provide the ultrasonographer with as much information as possible relating to the history and examination so the study is directed toward the suspected organ. Computed tomography (CT) examination may also be employed in cases in which plain radiographs and sonographic studies have failed to determine the diagnosis. Moreover, CT and even magnetic resonance imaging may be required when a neoplasm is suspected. Specific abdominal conditions are addressed in individual chapters.

SURGICAL TECHNIQUES

Diagnostic Laparoscopy

Although Stephen Gans (14) described laparoscopy for several pediatric uses in the 1970s, few pediatric surgeons incorporated this into their practices prior to the late 1980s. Most laparoscopic procedures in adults were performed by gynecologists. After the sentinel report of laparoscopic cholecystectomy by Reddick and Olsen in 1989 (15), a revolution in endoscopic surgery began. Now, almost every open procedure in an adult has an endoscopic counterpart. Application of this endoscopic approach was less rapid in children, however, primarily because the apparent advantages, such as decreased hospitalization, reduced discomfort, improved cosmesis, and a faster return to work, were

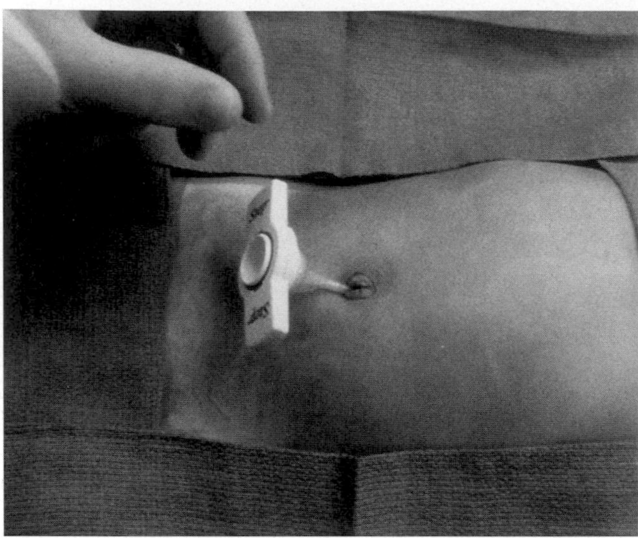

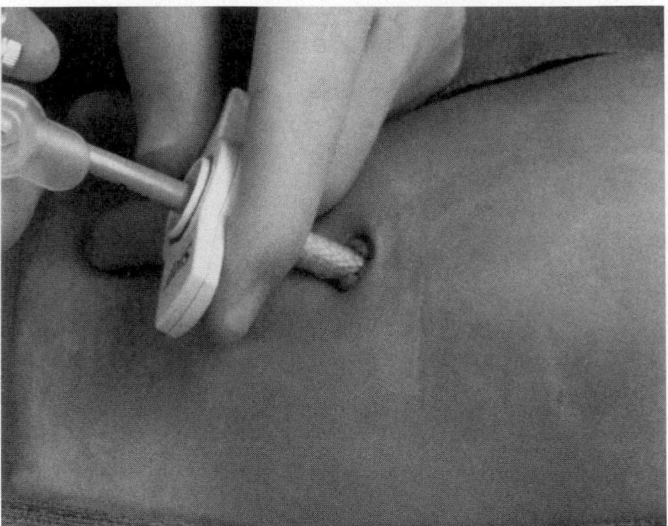

FIGURE 67-2. When introducing the initial umbilical cannula for laparoscopy, we prefer a direct umbilical cutdown technique with insertion of the expandable Step sheath (*on the left*), followed by introduction of the cannula with a blunt trocar through the sheath (*on the right*). In this way, injuries from the use of the Veress needle technique are minimized in infants and small children.

not believed to be as important to children by many pediatric surgeons. Moreover, small incisions are routinely employed for a variety of pediatric surgical procedures, and use of several small incisions for endoscopic surgery was not obviously beneficial. However, during the late 1990s and subsequent, the use of laparoscopy and thoracoscopy by pediatric surgeons has increased dramatically and these endoscopic approaches are now considered routine rather than revolutionary.

Although the principles of laparoscopic surgery for children are similar to those in adults, several unique differences require special attention. Because of the smaller abdominal cavity in children, especially infants, it is important to separate the cannulas as widely as possible to provide adequate working space. Placement of the ports too closely hinders the operation. As an example, for cholecystectomy in adults, the epigastric cannula is usually positioned in the midline of the epigastrium, and the right lower port is often placed just below or just above the level of the umbilicus. In a young child, however, the epigastric incision should be situated more to the patient's left, and the right lower port may be placed in the inguinal crease to allow sufficient separation.

Infants and young children have pliable abdominal walls. Therefore, when introducing cannulas with sharp trocars, it is critical to advance the trocar cautiously as it penetrates the peritoneum in order to prevent injury to the underlying viscera and intestine. Once the sharp stylet has penetrated the peritoneum, it is prudent to direct it anteriorly above the underlying intestine, viscera, and major vessels as the trocar and cannula are inserted deeper into the abdominal cavity. In addition, use of the Veress needle in children and, in particular, infants, is discouraged for creation of pneumoperitoneum. A much safer technique is an umbilical cutdown with insertion of the umbilical cannula into the peritoneal cavity under direct vision. This cutdown technique should prevent serious injury related to a blind puncture of the peritoneal cavity with the Veress needle.

Because of the previous concerns with the pliable abdominal wall in infants and young children, many pediatric surgeons prefer using the Step™ technique (US Surgical, Norwalk, CT). When introducing the initial umbilical cannula, we prefer to insert the expandable sheath (without the Veress needle) into the abdominal cavity followed by the cannula with the blunt trocar (Fig. 67-2). If an accessory cannula is used, then the Veress needle and expandable sheath are inserted into the abdominal cavity under telescopic visualization. The Veress needle is removed, and the cannula with blunt trocar is inserted through the expandable sheath. In this way, a sharp stylet is not used and potential injury to underlying viscera is minimized. Currently, these cannula sheaths are available as disposable units or reusable instruments. With the reusable instrument, the disposable portion is the cap, sheath, and Veress needle, but the blunt stylet and shaft of the cannula are reusable. Despite the resuable nature, there is added cost to using the disposable portion of these cannulas. Because of this added cost, several years ago, we began to insert the instruments directly through the abdominal wall without the use of a cannula, when possible. Between November 1999 and March 2003, we used minimal access stab incisions, rather than cannulas, for patients undergoing foregut, biliary, adrenal, splenic, colonic, and genitourinary operations. A single cannula was used for telescope access and, in select cases, a second cannula was needed for unique instruments, such as endoscopic staplers or ultrasonic shears. The abdominal wall stab incisions were used in the remaining patients (Fig. 67-3). During this time

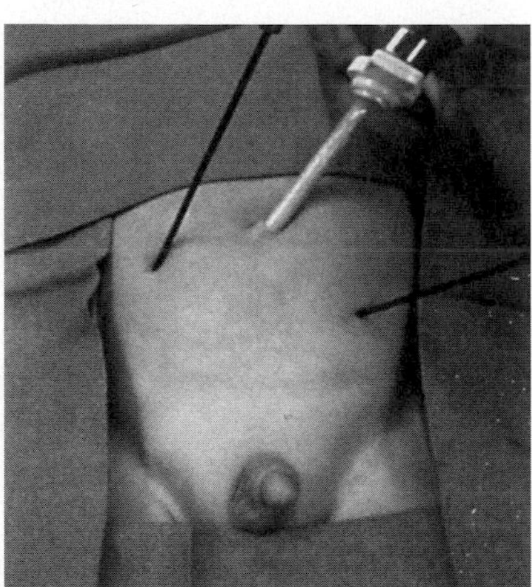

FIGURE 67-3. This photograph depicts the use of stab incisions with introduction of the instruments through the abdominal wall without the use of accessory cannulas. There is an umbilical cannula through which the telescope is introduced and insufflation is achieved. This infant is undergoing laparoscopic ligation of the right testicular vessels as the first stage of a planned two-stage management for an intraabdominal testis. [From Ostlie DJ, Holcomb GW III. The use of stab incisions for instrument access in laparoscopic operations. *J Pediatr Surg (in press),* with permission.]

period, 511 minimal access procedures were performed and pneumoperitoneum was maintained in all cases. In 308 of these cases, a single cannula was used and a second cannula was placed in 203 patients. In total, 1,337 reusable cannula systems (Veress needle, expandable sheath and cap) were saved using this minimal access technique. At a charge to the patient of $140 per cannula system, overall cost savings were $187,180 (16).

Another special concern in children is excessive abdominal insufflation. In a research model, Liem and associates (17) demonstrated a direct correlation between insufflation pressure using CO_2 and hypercapnea. In addition, there was marked acidemia, hypoxia, and increased exhaled CO_2 with higher insufflation pressures. The authors recommended using insufflation pressures of less than 15 mm Hg. Many pediatric surgeons, however, continue to use 15 mm Hg as the maximum inflating pressure without apparent adverse clinical sequelae.

Absolute contraindications to laparoscopy include abdominal wall sepsis at the cannula site, an uncorrectable bleeding disorder and the inability to create a pneumoperitoneum. A common scenario arises when an infant with severe lung disease, such as respiratory distress syndrome and/or an oxygen requirement, requires a fundoplication. Depending on the patient's condition, it may not be possible to establish a pneumoperitoneum without compromising oxygenation or ventilation. Whether a laparoscopic operation is possible depends on the individual patient's condition. A preoperative discussion with the anesthesiologist is beneficial before scheduling the laparoscopic operation.

Diagnostic Laparoscopy

Laparoscopy can be employed for diagnostic purposes or for performance of a definitive operation. Diagnostic laparoscopy can be valuable in infants and children. Indications for diagnostic laparoscopy include evaluation of a nonpalpable testis, determination of the presence or absence of a contralateral patent processus vaginalis (CPPV) in a child with a known unilateral inguinal hernia, evaluation for chronic abdominal pain, diagnostic assessment for the presence of appendicitis, evaluation of traumatic injury, and in children with cancer.

A thorough preoperative conference is arranged with the parents and child, if age appropriate, at which time the procedure, risks, and benefits are discussed. General endotracheal anesthesia is usually preferred, but mask anesthesia is possible for short cases (18). An orogastric tube is inserted for gastric decompression, and the bladder is emptied using a Credé maneuver. The bladder is generally not catheterized, especially in young boys, to avoid iatrogenic urethral injury.

The abdomen is prepped and draped widely. As previously mentioned, an umbilical cutdown is performed for initial access to the abdominal cavity. The expandable sheath is introduced into the abdominal cavity followed by insertion of the cannula with a blunt trocar through the sheath. Use of the Veress needle for initial insufflation is discouraged, owing to the risk of injury to the abdominal viscera and vasculature. In general, a 5-mm cannula and telescope are used for most diagnostic procedures. The incision is well hidden in the umbilicus, and the visualization is better than with a 3-mm telescope. Moreover, the 5-mm umbilical fascial defect is easier to close than the smaller 3-mm opening. When operative laparoscopy is required, additional ports can be inserted as needed. Insufflation pressures up to 15 mm Hg have not caused significant adverse clinical sequelae in the authors' experience with more than 1,000 laparoscopic operations.

Evaluation for a Nonpalpable Testis

The use of laparoscopy in boys with nonpalpable testes has a number of advantages and few disadvantages. Some surgeons who do not favor this approach argue that a complete examination of the inguinal region and abdominal cavity can be performed through an inguinal approach and that it is rarely necessary to resort to a two-stage procedure for orchiopexy (19). Proponents of the laparoscopic approach emphasize two valid points. First, some intraabdominal testes are not identified at the time of inguinal exploration and are missed even by experienced surgeons (20,21). Second, a laparoscopic approach allows the surgeon to defer the second-stage Fowler-Stephens orchiopexy, when indicated, preventing disruption of the vasal collateral vessels that might occur with extensive dissection using an initial inguinal incision. With a two-stage approach for the abdominal testis (initial laparoscopy with

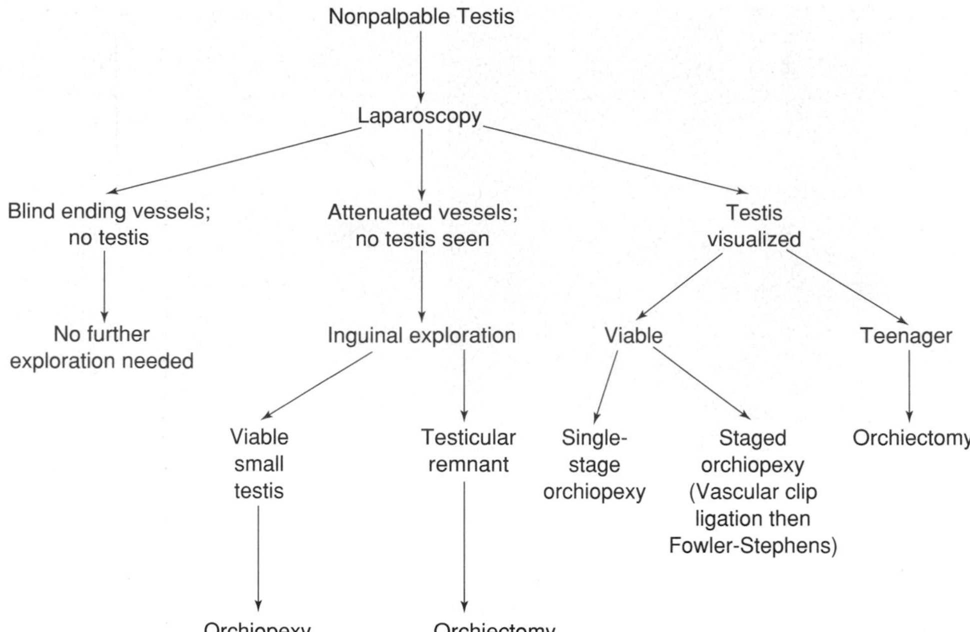

FIGURE 67-4. Algorithm depicting the operative management of patients with nonpalpable testes undergoing initial diagnostic laparoscopy. The next operative step depends on the findings at diagnostic laparoscopy.

vascular ligation followed later by Fowler-Stephens orchiopexy), the success rate should be greater than a one-stage approach, although the reported data are at present insufficient (22,23).

Under general anesthesia before laparoscopy, a final examination is performed to ensure the testicle is not palpable. When the testis is located in the inguinal canal or scrotum with the patient under anesthesia, then laparoscopy is not necessary. When the testis is not palpated, however, laparoscopy is performed, and the findings help the surgeon determine whether vessel ligation, orchiectomy, or an inguinal exploration is indicated (Fig. 67-4).

At diagnostic laparoscopy for the nonpalpable testis, several findings may be apparent. If a testis is found intraabdominally and the vascular leash appears short, then initial endoscopic vessel ligation can be performed. Great care should be taken to ensure the ureter is not injured. Six to 9 months later, the patient returns for a Fowler-Stephens orchiopexy, with the testicle then being nourished by collateral vessels surrounding the vas deferens. At the initial diagnostic laparoscopy, if there is no evidence of a testis, but a normal vascular pedicle and vas deferens are seen entering a closed internal ring, then inguinal exploration is indicated. Although the vas deferens and testicular vessels are likely to lead the surgeon to an atrophic testicular remnant, Turek and colleagues (24) found 6% of such specimens to have seminiferous tubules with germal elements. They recommended excision of these testicular remnants because of increased malignant potential. On occasion, however, a small, but viable, testis is found, and orchiopexy is possible. If the testis is identified to be high in the inguinal canal, but not truly intraabdominal (so-called peeping testis), then a one-stage orchiopexy may be possible. At laparoscopy, if the testicular vessels are noted to end blindly and do not enter the internal ring, then inguinal exploration is not indicated. Finally, in teenagers with intraabdominal testes or in younger children with atrophic intraabdominal testes, orchiectomy can be performed laparoscopically or through a separate inguinal incision.

Laparoscopy for Contralateral Patent Processus Vaginalis (CPPV)

A controversial subject among pediatric surgeons continues to be whether to perform a contralateral exploration under the same anesthesia in an infant or child with a known unilateral inguinal hernia. Advocates of routine bilateral exploration note that between 40% and 60% of children have a CPPV, and bilateral exploration prevents the need for a repeat operation with hernia repair in the future. A second anesthesia and the cost of a second procedure are avoided using this approach (25,26). Proponents for repair of the unilateral hernia alone argue that only 10% to 30% of children undergoing unilateral hernia repair return with a symptomatic contralateral hernia; therefore, in most children, an unnecessary contralateral operation would be avoided (27,28). Moreover, there is a small risk of injury to the testicle and vas deferens during inguinal exploration, which would also be avoided. One report of 313 children undergoing inguinal herniorrhaphy documented segments of vas deferens in five specimens (1.6%) (25). In another review, 160 infants with unilateral or bilateral repair were followed for up to 20 years and were discovered to have a 2% incidence of testicular atrophy (27).

With the increased use of diagnostic laparoscopy, a study was undertaken to ascertain whether laparoscopy would be beneficial in the evaluation of a CPPV in a child with a known unilateral inguinal hernia (29). After

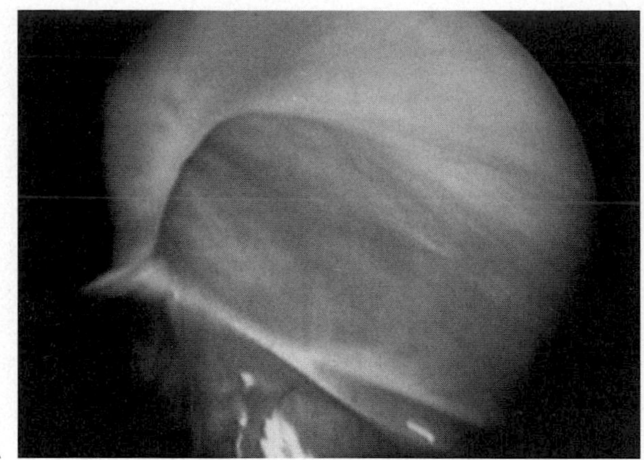

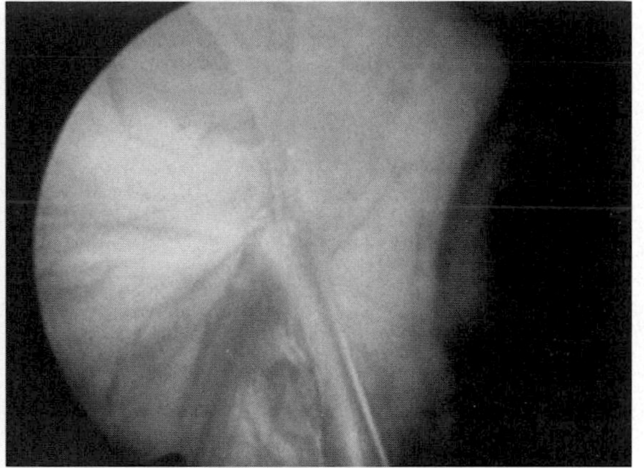

FIGURE 67-5. Diagnostic laparoscopy through the umbilicus is performed in a 6-month-old patient with a known right inguinal hernia **(A)**. There is no evidence of a left patent processus vaginalis **(B)**, and unnecessary left inguinal exploration is avoided.

induction of general endotracheal anesthesia, the patient was examined and the surgeon asked to document if a CPPV was present on clinical examination under anesthesia (EUA). Diagnostic peritoneoscopy was then performed. Pneumoperitoneum was created to a pressure of 15 mm Hg, and the inguinal canal and scrotum were inspected to see if insufflation alone would be sufficient for the diagnosis of CPPV. Diagnostic peritoneoscopy was then performed (Fig. 67-5). These patients (1,432 of them) younger than 10 years of age were evaluated and laparoscopy was possible in 94.9% of them. In 548 patients (38%), a CPPV was identified. At EUA, it was predicted that 427 of these 1,359 patients would have a CPPV. The presence of a CPPV was confirmed in 188 (44%). Also, it was believed that 932 would not have a CPPV on EUA, but a CPPV was seen in 361 (39%). Thus, it is concluded that physical examination, even under anesthesia, is a poor prediction of a CPPV. In addition, a bulge was seen or crepitus palpated on the contralateral side with creation of the pneumoperitoneum in less than 10% of patients found to have a CPPV on laparoscopy. Therefore, laparoscopy should be considered the gold standard for evaluating for a CPPV (30). However, in no way does laparoscopy select who will have a symptomatic CPPV in the future.

Other Indications

Evaluation for chronic abdominal pain is another valid indication for diagnostic laparoscopy in children. Despite multiple radiographic studies, laboratory tests, and physical examinations, an open laparotomy may be necessary in selected circumstances when abdominal pain persists or recurs. Laparoscopy has been very helpful in this circumstance (31). Telander reported an incidence of positive findings in 60% of 40 cases using laparoscopy for evaluation of chronic abdominal pain (Telander W.H., 1999 personal communication). Moreover, 30% of these 40 patients had an abnormal appendix on pathologic examination.

Diagnostic laparoscopy may also be useful in children with suspected appendicitis. In addition, this technique can be used to direct the best location for an open incision when the surgeon, for any reason, is not comfortable with continuation of the laparoscopic approach.

In addition to the previously mentioned indications, diagnostic laparoscopy may also be useful in other selected circumstances. Infants with ambiguous genitalia are good candidates for diagnostic laparoscopy for determination of their internal anatomy (32). It can be used in the evaluation of traumatic injuries in children in whom the radiographic and other noninvasive evaluations are equivocal. This is especially applicable to penetrating trauma in which the surgeon does not believe that the traumatic event, whether a low-velocity gunshot or stab injury, penetrated the abdominal cavity. Moreover, it does allow the surgeon to evaluate for internal injuries if the peritoneum was violated. Finally, diagnostic laparoscopy can be used in selected circumstances in children with cancer, especially when the radiographic evaluations are not diagnostic. It can be useful for determining resectability of a large lesion, such as a hepatoblastoma or neuroblastoma, followed by open exploration and resection, if appropriate. Second-look laparoscopy can be useful following adjuvant therapy in certain circumstances (Fig. 67-6). In a review several years ago from the Children's Cancer Group, 24 children were documented to have undergone laparoscopy as part of their surgical management (33). Indications include evaluation for possible metastatic tumor or recurrent disease, consideration of a new mass for suspected cancer, and evaluation of hepatoblastoma for resectability.

Procedural Laparoscopy

Cholecystectomy

Laparoscopic cholecystectomy is now considered the standard approach for removal of the gallbladder in children requiring cholecystectomy (34,35). There are

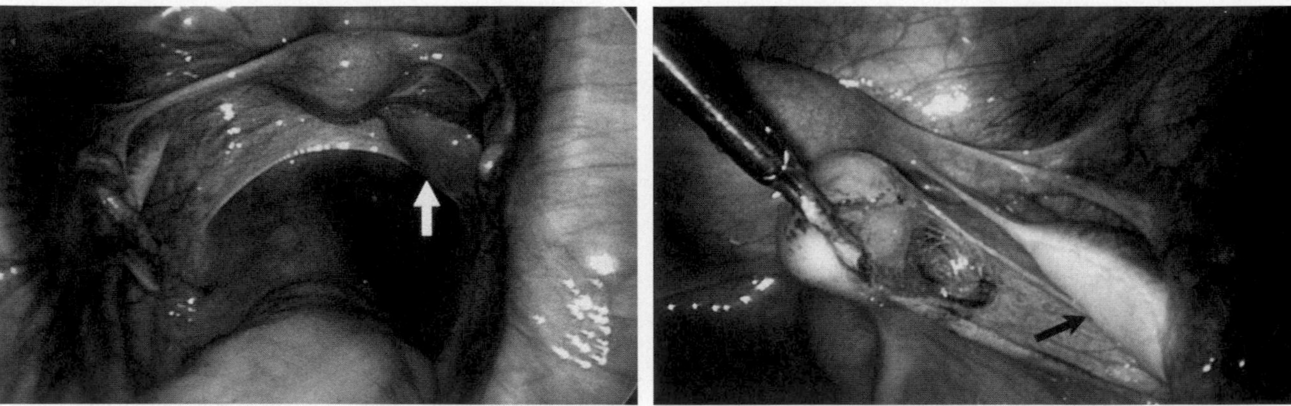

FIGURE 67-6. Second-look laparoscopy can be useful followed adjuvant therapy in certain circumstances. In this teenage patient who previously had undergone laparotomy and resection of a large germ-cell tumor, second-look laparoscopy was performed to see if there was evidence of residual disease. In the photograph on the left, residual disease is seen along the right pelvic side wall (*white arrow*). On the right, the tumor is being removed from the peritoneum. The right ovary is well visualized in this frame (*black arrow*).

multiple advantages of the laparoscopic route, including an abbreviated hospital stay, reduced postoperative pain, and improved cosmesis (36). The data supporting a faster return to activity in children are retrospective and imperfect; however, there is a clear benefit to the family with regard to hospital stay. The cost–benefit relationship with regard to loss of parental work days is evident.

Indications for laparoscopic cholecystectomy are essentially unchanged from those for open cholecystectomy. Previously, prior abdominal surgery and obesity, as well as young age, were considered contraindications to laparoscopic cholecystectomy. Currently, these are not contraindications, and laparoscopic cholecystectomy is the preferred operation in all children who require removal of the gallbladder.

The technique used in children uses four access sites. The operating telescope is placed through a 10-mm cannula placed into the abdomen through a vertical incision in the umbilicus. The primary reason a 10-mm cannula is used is that a relatively large incision is required for removal of the gallbladder. Moreover, a 10-mm cannula allows the use of a 10-mm camera, which optimizes the visual field. There are three remaining instrument insertion sites in the upper abdomen. In the epigastric region, a 5-mm cannula is placed near the lower edge of the liver margin and, ideally, passes through the membranous portion of the falciform ligament. A retracting nonlocking grasping instrument is placed in the right upper midabdomen through a stab incision. The final instrument is inserted through the right lower abdominal wall at a distance sufficient to allow grasping of the dome of the gallbladder with retraction in a cephalad manner. This instrument is often a toothed instrument with a locking mechanism.

The technique for cholecystectomy is similar to the technique used in adult laparoscopic cholecystectomy and has been reported elsewhere (15,34,36,37). The dome of the gallbladder is grasped with the right lower quadrant locking instrument and reflected in a cephalad fashion. With the surgeon's left-hand instrument, the infundibulum of the gallbladder is retracted inferior and lateral. This maneuver is of critical importance as the cystic duct is retracted in an inferior and lateral direction away from the common duct. The dissection is carried out with the right hand of the surgeon through the epigastric port. Either a Maryland dissector or a spatula-tipped instrument attached to electrocautery can be used for the dissection of the infundibulum. The peritoneum overlying the infundibulum and distal cystic duct is cauterized. This peritoneum and underlying fat are dissected toward the common duct. The cystic duct is then circumferentially dissected, and the cystic duct-gallbladder junction identified. This technique should reduce the possibility of injury to the common duct as a result of too proximal dissection on the cystic duct. If a cholangiogram is indicated (hyperbilirubinemia, evidence of common duct dilation on ultrasound, previous history of gallstone pancreatitis, or unclear anatomy), it is performed at this point.

After completion of the cholangiogram, if indicated, the proximal cystic duct is doubly clipped. In all but rare occasions, 5-mm clips are sufficient to ligate the cystic duct. If indeed the cystic duct is of such size that the 5-mm clip is not adequate, the epigastric port can be converted to a 10-mm cannula, and two 10-mm clips can be placed proximally. The cystic duct is subsequently transsected. Dissection is continued along the infundibulum, and the cystic artery is identified. In a similar fashion, the artery is circumferentially dissected and two clips are placed on the proximal aspect of the cystic artery. A single clip is placed distally, and the artery is transsected. The gallbladder is subsequently removed in a retrograde fashion. The gallbladder bed is inspected meticulously and any bleeding is controlled with electrocautery prior to removal of the gallbladder from its superior peritoneal attachments. The 10-mm camera is removed from the umbilical site, and a 5-mm telescope is placed through the epigastric cannula. The gallbladder can either be removed intact or placed into an endoscopic retrieval bag and removed intact through the umbilical incision. In our practice, all children are admitted to the hospital for an overnight stay. The diet is begun with clear liquids initially and advanced to a regular diet as tolerated. Pain control is initially managed with intravenous narcotics and transitioned to oral narcotics once the children are tolerating a diet. Rarely, a child may require hospitalization for 2 days because of ongoing discomfort not controllable with oral narcotics.

Appendectomy

The use of laparoscopy for the management of acute and perforated appendicitis has not gained universal acceptance within the pediatric surgical population. From a historical standpoint, in 1980, Leape and Ramenofsky used diagnostic laparoscopy to identify noninflamed appendices to reduce the number of appendectomies performed in patients without acute appendicitis (38). It has become evident in the last decade that laparoscopic appendectomy is as effective as open appendectomy in the presence of acute appendicitis (39–41), and in some hands, it is effective in the face of uncomplicated perforated appendicitis. There are two techniques that may be employed for laparoscopic appendectomy. The authors prefer the endoscopic stapler technique. We use a 12-mm cannula placed through a vertical incision in the umbilicus. Following insufflation, we position a 5-mm cannula in the left lower abdomen, and use either a 5-mm or 3-mm instrument through a stab incision in the left lateral suprapubic position. A 5-mm 45-degree operating telescope is placed through the umbilical cannula, and the cecum and terminal ileum are identified as landmarks for locating the appendix. The appendix is dissected using blunt and electrocautery dissection with nonlocking atraumatic graspers placed through the two operating sites. Occasionally, this dissection can be difficult, especially if an inflamed retrocecal appendix is encountered. Care should be taken to avoid injury to the ureter and iliac vessels when this is the case. After dissection of the appendix, its tip is retracted inferomedially. This allows the surgeon to use the retroperitoneal attachments for countertraction during the creation of a window in the mesoappendix. This is usually performed near the base of the appendix with care taken not to injure the cecum. After the window in the mesoappendix has been created, the mesoappendix is stapled and divided using an endoscopic stapler with a vascular load. The base of the appendix is then inspected and, in a similar fashion, an endoscopic stapler with a gastrointestinal staple load is placed across the base of the appendix with care not to encroach upon the cecum or the ileocecal valve.

The patient population chosen for laparoscopic appendectomy is based on individual surgeon preference. We proceed with laparoscopic appendectomy in all patients, except those with complicated appendicitis of more than 7 days' duration. In these patients, we employ percutaneous drainage, intravenous antibiotics, and internal laparoscopic appendectomy 6 weeks later. The risk of intraabdominal abscess after laparoscopic appendectomy in children with perforated appendicitis has not been shown to be higher than after open appendectomy (42). Moreover, the laparoscopic approach in a patient with a well-defined abscess is also controversial. Laparoscopy does allow irrigation and debridement within the generalized peritoneal cavity with suction evacuation of the infected material under direct visualization. However, reduced hospitalization has not been shown to be a benefit of the laparoscopic approach in children with complicated appendicitis, as most require prolonged hospitalization for antibiotics and recovery of intestinal ileus (43).

Laparoscopic Pyloromyotomy

The laparoscopic approach for pyloric stenosis is gaining acceptance within the pediatric surgical community (44,45). Its primary benefit lies in improved cosmesis in relation to the open technique. Our technique uses a single 5-mm umbilical cannula. The insufflating pressure in these neonates is usually reduced to approximately 10 to 12 mm Hg, and accordingly, the flow rate is decreased. A nonlocking, grasping forceps is placed through a stab incision in the lateral right upper abdominal wall at a site just above the lower edge of the right lobe of the liver. Placing the instrument in this position allows for cephalad retraction of the liver using the shaft of the instrument. An arthroscopy knife is placed through a stab incision in the left upper abdominal wall (Fig. 67-7). Using the grasping instrument, the proximal duodenum is secured while the arthroscopy knife is used to incise the serosa of the pyloric channel from just proximal to the duodenal pyloric junction to well onto the antrum. This incision should be approximately 2 cm in length. The pyloric musculature is subsequently divided using a pyloric spreader. The stomach is insufflated with air to ensure mucosal perforation has not occurred. The air is suctioned from the stomach, and omentum is placed over the pyloromyotomy site.

The stab incisions are not closed with suture, but use a steristrip for skin approximation. The baby's diet is advanced beginning 2 hours postoperatively, and the patients are usually discharged within 24 hours. Narcotics are not routinely used.

Fundoplication

The laparoscopic approach to fundoplication is becoming the preferred technique for many pediatric surgeons.

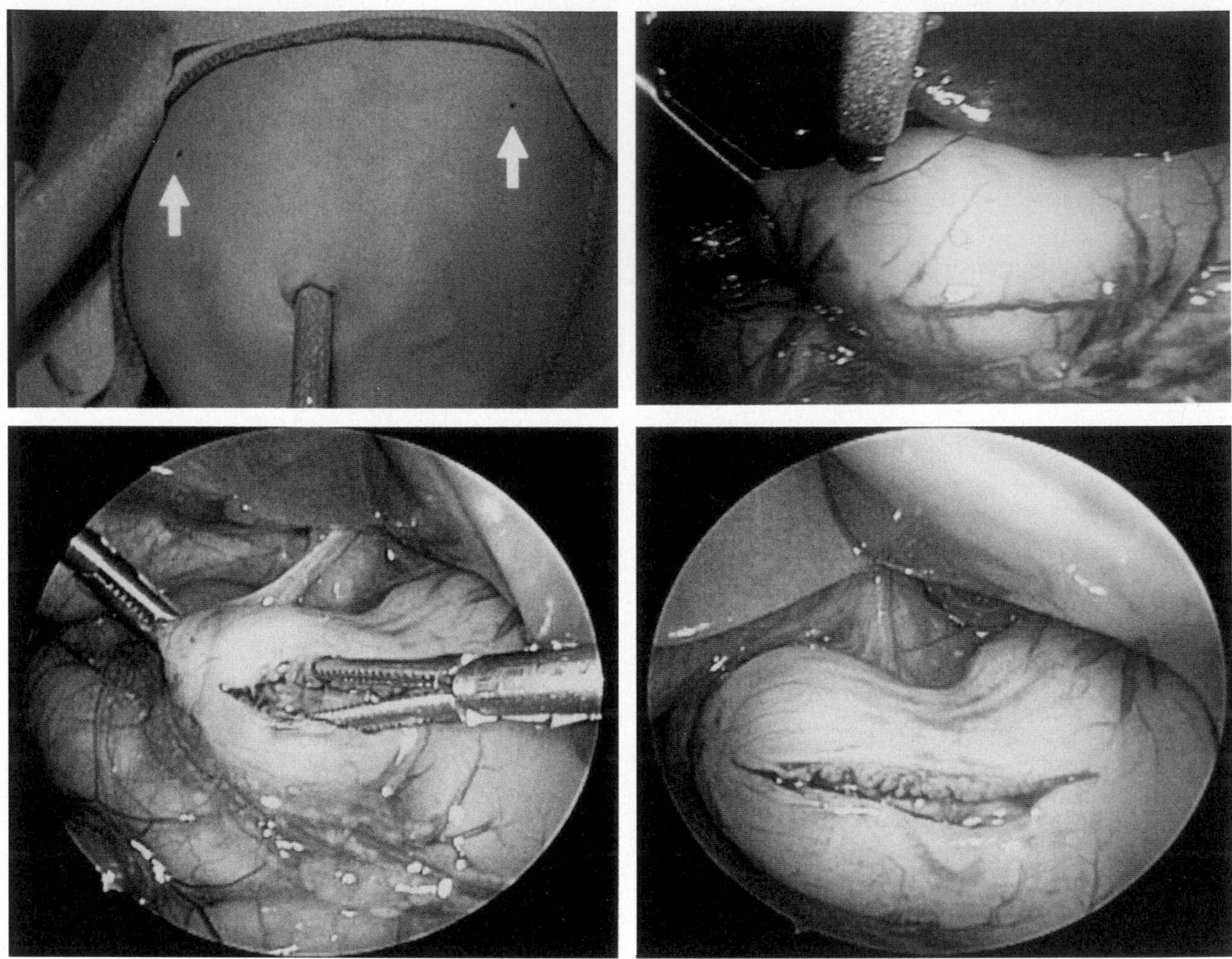

FIGURE 67-7. In an infant undergoing laparoscopic pyloromyotomy, a 5-mm cannula is inserted through an incision in the umbilical fascia. The sites of the stab incisions in the left and right upper quadrants are shown (*white arrows; upper left photograph*). Using an arthroscopy knife, an incision is made in the seromuscular portion of the hypertrophied pylorus (*upper right*). The knife is removed and a pyloric spreader is introduced through this same incision and the hypertrophied muscle bluntly divided (*lower left*). The pyloromyotomy incision is usually approximately 2 cm in length (*lower right*).

Numerous authors have reported excellent results with the laparoscopic technique (46–48). A key to any laparoscopic procedure is that the basic principles of the operation should not change from the open approach. For laparoscopic Nissen fundoplication, we use five incisions. A single 5-mm cannula is placed through the umbilicus. Four stab incisions are positioned in the epigastric region two through the left upper and two through the right upper abdominal wall. If a gastrostomy tube is to be placed, the left upper stab incision is positioned so the gastrostomy may be placed through this stab incision. The actual technique of fundoplication does not differ from the open approach. The short gastric vessels are divided for approximately one-half the length of the greater curve. The phrenoesophageal ligament is divided, and an adequate length of intraabdominal esophagus is mobilized to perform a circumferential Nissen fundoplication. We attempt to mobilize 2 to 3 cm of esophagus into the abdomen, thereby creating an adequate length for the lower esophageal sphincter mechanism. The crura are reapproximated using silk sutures. We routinely secure the esophagus to the diaphragmatic hiatus at the 12, 3, and 9 o'clock positions using a single interrupted silk suture at each position in an attempt to prevent transmigration of the fundoplication through the esophageal hiatus, the most common complication. A standard 360-degree Nissen fundoplication is created and secured using silk sutures. We attempt to create a 2-cm long fundoplication as this has been shown to provide an adequate lower esophageal sphincter mechanism without causing dysphagia (49). Other techniques, such as the Thal anterior fundoplication or the Toupet posterior fundoplication, can also be performed laparoscopically.

As noted, many children undergoing fundoplication require gastrostomy. This can be performed laparoscopically or by the use of percutaneous techniques. Moreover, pyloromyotomy or pyloroplasty may be performed laparoscopically, if indicated.

Splenectomy

The removal of the spleen for childhood disease processes, such as idiopathic thrombocytopenia purpura and hereditary spherocytosis, can be accomplished using the laparoscopic approach, and this is done routinely in some institutions. Rescorla and his colleagues reported the safety of laparoscopic splenectomy with decreased postoperative length of hospitalization and diminished analgesic requirements (50). We begin with a 15-mm cannula, which is inserted following incision of the umbilical skin and fascia. A 5-mm incision is placed in the lower epigastric midline and two 3-mm stab incisions are created in the upper epigastric midline. Although we orientate the access sites in the midline, placement in the left subcostal region can also be used if desired. The 5-mm telescope is introduced through the 5-mm cannula and the primary working port is the umbilical cannula. Three-millimeter instruments are placed through the upper epigastric stab incisions for retraction. The ultrasonic scalpel is used to perform most of the dissection, which begins with division of the short gastric vessels along the length of the spleen. The lienocolic ligament is opened and divided along the inferior border of the spleen. The spleen is then reflected anteriorly, and the lienorenal ligament is identified and divided. The lateral diaphragmatic attachments are then divided and the vascular pedicle isolated. There are two alternatives for management of the vascular pedicle. First, a 35-mm endoscopic stapler with a vascular load may be placed across the pedicle in its entirety, with care taken not to include any portion of the pancreas or stomach. The stapler is fired, thereby transecting the pedicle and the remaining attachments. Alternatively, the vasculature can be dissected independently and controlled using endoscopic clips. If any diaphragmatic attachments remain, they are divided, thereby completing the splenectomy. The spleen is then placed into an endoscopic bag, which is exteriorized through the umbilical fascial defect. The spleen is morcellated manually and the splenic fragments are removed in a piecemeal fashion.

Adrenalectomy

Laparoscopic adrenalectomy has been shown to be safe and effective in the removal of adrenal tumors, including pheochromocytomas, in adults and children (51–53). We position the patient in a lateral position and use two cannulas and two stab incisions. On the right side, the right triangular ligament of the liver is incised and the liver retracted to the patient's left. On the left side, the spleen is mobilized and retracted cephalad and to the patient's right. The colon is mobilized from its retroperitoneal position using electrocautery and the ultrasonic scalpel. The kidney is identified, and the dissection is carried anteriorly and superiorly over the kidney to identify the adrenal gland. If a left adrenalectomy is being performed, the venous drainage is identified entering the left renal vein. A single or multiple arteries are usually identified arising from the aorta; however, these can sometimes be quite small and can usually be divided using the ultrasonic scalpel. The remainder of the dissection is straightforward, and the organ is placed into an endoscopic bag. Conversely, if a right adrenal gland is being removed, the key venous drainage is to the vena cava. The gland is mobilized and the vein is ligated as the last step using endoscopic clips. Again, the organ is removed via an endoscopic bag through the largest incision. For larger lesions, the gland can be morcellated. Also, the largest incision can be enlarged to extract the whole specimen.

Achalasia

As with fundoplication, the laparoscopic approach to patients with achalasia has been shown to be safe and effective with improved outcomes in regard to length of hospitalization, postoperative pain, and cosmesis (54,55). The access sites are similar to a laparoscopic fundoplication. The initial dissection is identical, including division of the short gastric vessels and mobilization of the esophagus after division of the phrenoesophageal ligament. The esophagomyotomy is performed using either the ultrasonic scalpel or hook cautery. Extreme care should be taken to clearly identify the musculature of the esophagus and the submucosa. We carry the myotomy approximately 5 to 7 cm superiorly onto the esophagus and 2 to 3 cm distally into the stomach. Following the myotomy, we perform an anterior fundoplication to help prevent the need for a subsequent operation for reflux.

Anorectal Pull-through Procedures

The management of patients with Hirschsprung's disease has changed since the mid-1990s. Some authors now advocate a transanal pullthrough procedure for Hirschsprung's disease (56). We prefer the traditional pull-through technique, which entails intraabdominal dissection that is performed laparoscopically with perineal dissection. The technique was originally described by Georgeson (57,58). A 5-mm cannula is initially introduced in the right subhepatic region using a cutdown approach. Following insufflation, the telescope is inserted through this port. A 5-mm cannula is placed in the right abdominal wall through which the ultrasonic scalpel is introduced. After insufflation, the colon and rectum are identified. The rectosigmoid colon is mobilized from its rectoperitoneal attachments using either electrocautery or ultrasonic scalpel. An adequate length of proximal colon is mobilized on its mesentery to allow for the pull-through to be accomplished without significant tension. The rectal dissection is then carried out using electrocautery distally to a point where the perineal dissection can be accomplished, thereby connecting the two dissecting fields. The perineal dissection is performed in a standard fashion, and the rectum and colon are exteriorized through the perineum. Biopsies are then performed at the apparent transition zone and proximal. It is imperative that histologic examination for ganglion cells is accurate to ensure a proper level of the pull-through. A diverting stoma is not employed when using this primary technique.

Other Indications

A number of additional laparoscopic procedures have been reported with increasing frequency in children. These include laparoscopic surgery for Crohn's disease, ulcerative colitis, and duodenal atresia (59–61). In addition, laparoscopic assistance for insertion or removal of ventricular-peritoneal shunts, gonadectomy for intersex anomalies, ovarian cystectomy, and testicular vein ligation in the presence of varicoceles have been established (32,62). In patients with Crohn's disease, laparoscopic surgery is particularly beneficial in identifying the diseased segment and minimizing the abdominal incision. The diseased segment can usually be exteriorized through an enlarged cannula site with a standard intestinal anastomosis performed extracorporally. An alternative is to perform a stapled anastomosis in a side-to-side fashion within the abdomen. For patients with ulcerative colitis, a two-stage approach has been used to perform the total abdominal colectomy with ileal J pouch formation and ileoanal anastomosis with a diverting ileostomy (63). The mesentery of the colon can either be controlled using multiple endoscopic vascular staplers, or the colon can be exteriorized with standard mesenteric division using suture ligatures. The J pouch is usually created extracorporally with a stapled or hand sewn anastomosis. It is then returned to the abdominal cavity and, after standard perineal dissection, the ileal pouch is brought down to the anus and sewn into place. A diverting ileostomy can be exteriorized through one of the cannula sites. The advantages of the laparoscopic approaches to Crohn's disease and ulcerative colitis include earlier discharge from the hospital after the initial procedure, improved cosmesis, and possible reduced operative times.

With dedicated institutional and programmatic commitment, many operations formerly requiring open abdominal access can now be performed successfully using contemporary laparoscopic techniques (Table 67-1).

TABLE 67-1 The Laparoscopic Experience at Children's Mercy Hospital (Kansas City): November 1999–December 2002.

Diagnostic laparoscopy for contralateral processus vaginalis	743
Fundoplication	268
Appendectomy	254
Gastrostomy	146
Pyloromyotomy	108
Cholecystectomy (without cholangiogram)	59
Cholecystectomy (with cholangiogram)	23
Ovarian procedures	24
Splenectomy	23
Nephrectomy	18
Pull-through procedures	20
Adrenalectomy	9
Esophagomyotomy	7
Total	1,702

Complications

Most complications associated with laparoscopy occur following introduction of the Veress needle or sharp trocars. Routinely, use of a Veress needle is to be avoided in pediatric patients unless it is used for the placement of subsequent ports after the operating telescope has been inserted using a cutdown technique. In this setting, the Veress needle is directly observed as it enters the abdomen to ensure there is no injury to the intestine or intraabdominal vessels. Other complications include inadvertent cautery injury to the intestine during the dissection or coagulation because the electrical current may arc outside the visual field, thereby injuring the adjacent intestinal wall. With careful and constant attention to the use of cautery, however, this should rarely occur. Moreover, the use of bipolar instruments may help prevent this complication. Two other complications are bleeding and infection. One reason to use the laparoscopic approach with small incisions is to reduce the incidence of postoperative wound infections. Excessive bleeding may develop, particularly with procedures such as splenectomy, adrenalectomy, or nephrectomy. However, in most instances, the bleeding can be controlled laparoscopically, especially in the hands of an experienced surgeon. Conversion to an open procedure, however, should be performed without hesitation if bleeding becomes excessive during any endoscopic operation.

Robotics

Over the last several years, there has been further advancement in minimally invasive surgery with the development of robotic surgical assistants (Aesop, Computer Motion, Santa Barbara, CA) and surgical systems (Zeus, Computer Motion, Santa Barbara, CA, and daVinci, Intuitive Surgical, Culver City, CA). These devices should be considered further evolution of minimally invasive surgery and have developed as a result of the demands to perform a number of complex operations using a minimally invasive approach.

Aesop (Automated Endoscopic System for Optimal Positioning) began development in 1991 as a robotic telescopic assistant to surgeons performing minimally invasive operations. In 1994, Aesop 1000 was the first U.S. Food and Drug Administration-approved robotic surgical assistant. It could be controlled by ancillary surgical staff or by a surgeon using a foot pedal. Subsequently, a rudimentary voice control recognition panel was developed to give the surgeon control over the assisted maneuvers, but there remained an element of difficulty in relaying the surgeon's commands to the telescopic visual field. Currently, new technical developments have increased maneuverability compared with the earlier models, and this device is easily controlled through the surgeon's voice using advanced speech recognition technology. In addition, integrated operating room networking systems that allow the surgeon to control robotic devices, capture pictures, operate a videocassette recorder, and perform other tasks are commercially available. Reported experiences with robotic telescopic assistance have primarily been limited to adult and animal studies for a variety of operations in general, urology, gynecology, cardiac, and vascular surgery (64–66).

Robotic arms are advantageous for certain procedures, but not helpful for others. Advantages include a consistent and steady visual field throughout the operation, which is especially important when operating on infants and small children. Moreover, there is no sudden movement or loss of the visual field due to human fatigue. In an infant, there is not enough space available for more than two people (surgeon and assistant) around a small patient, and this can be invaluable (Fig. 67-8). In addition, we have found there is much better utilization of the operating room personnel because there was dissatisfaction on the part of the personnel asked to hold the camera prior to use of the robotic arm. With a robotic arm in a teaching environment, the teaching surgeon often has a free hand if he or she is not manipulating the camera and can help the operating surgeon as needed. The robotic arm is advantageous for common operations that are performed similarly each time, the operation is centered in one anatomic area, and there is little movement of the telescope/camera. Moreover, an ideal case would be one with a duration of longer than 1 hour. Using these criteria, laparoscopic fundoplication, laparoscopic cholecystectomy, laparoscopic esophagomyotomy, and laparoscopic adrenalectomy are good uses. It is not routinely used for operations such as laparoscopic pyloromyotomy or laparoscopic appendectomy, which are of short duration, nor is the robotic arm especially useful for laparoscopic splenectomy because the camera and telescope are manipulated many times during the operation to ensure a safe procedure.

The use of robotic surgical systems remains in its infancy, especially in the pediatric surgical arena (67,68). In adults, there are reports of the use of these systems for almost every operation for which laparoscopy is currently being used. The list of these operations ranges from laparoscopic fundoplication to laparoscopic-assisted radical prostectomy (69–72). Moreover, there is an evolving experience in adult cardiac surgery with mitral valve repair also using these systems (73,74). The concept for these robotic devices is not to replace surgeons, but rather to enhance the surgeon's ability and improve what the surgeon is already able to accomplish. At this time, further investigation is required to determine the appropriate utilization of these surgical systems in the clinical arena. It will likely be several years before pediatric surgeons fully understand the advantages of these robotic systems in the pediatric patients.

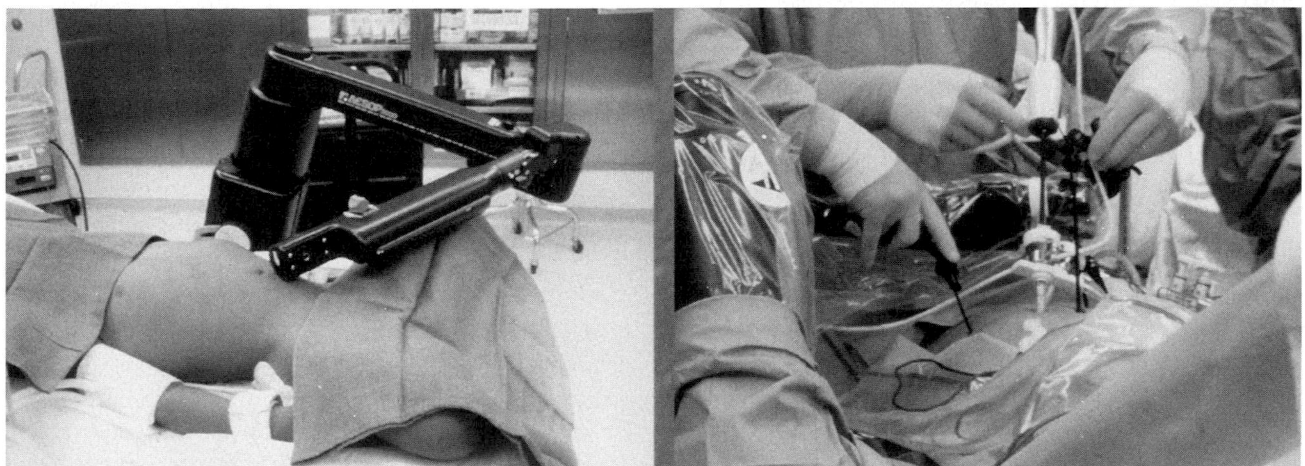

FIGURE 67-8. A robotic telescopic holder has been invaluable for certain laparoscopic procedures in children. On the left, the robot has been attached to the left side rail of the operating table and placed in a full downward tilt and a –1-degree angulation in a young child undergoing a laparoscopic fundoplication. On the right, the surgeon and assistant are seen working over the robotic arm during performance of a laparoscopic fundoplication.

Incisions

The location of the abdominal incision for entry into the peritoneal cavity should be individualized according to the proposed operation. Other factors include the experience and training of the surgeon, the size and age of the patient, and the possibility of previous abdominal operations. In general, a laparotomy is performed through a transverse incision in the newborn, as compared with a midline incision used in adolescents. In newborns, the transverse incisions are usually either supraumbilical or infraumbilical and are located on the right side of the abdomen because of diseases specific to newborns. A supraumbilical transverse incision is usually preferred for correction of malrotation, repair of duodenal stenosis or atresia, and biliary exploration. Some pediatric surgeons also prefer the supraumbilical approach for necrotizing enterocolitis (NEC). A right infraumbilical transverse incision may be used for exploration for NEC and for exploration for intussusception, distal intestinal atresia, or obstruction and meconium ileus.

For some neonatal conditions, stomas are required as a temporary measure if the infant is critically ill, is too small for primary anastomosis, or has NEC. Although location of the stoma is an individual decision, some surgeons prefer placement through the lateral or medial aspect of the incision. Because the abdominal cavity is usually explored through a transverse right lower quadrant incision for most diseases requiring a stoma, the stoma may be exteriorized either medially or laterally through that incision. A side-by-side double-barreled enterostomy is the preferred technique because, at subsequent closure, a formal laparotomy is not required. Also, access to the distal bowel is preferred in some circumstances for radiographic evaluation of obstruction or distal strictures. An alternative technique, however, is a single functioning stoma with closure of the distal end, which is positioned just beneath the peritoneum.

Stomas

Stomas are frequently required in pediatric surgery. Most are temporary, although in selected cases, a permanent ostomy is necessary.

Gastrostomy

An open or laparoscopic gastrostomy is often performed in infants and children for nutritional supplementation either in conjunction with fundoplication or as an isolated procedure. The most common site for placement is along the greater curvature of the stomach, with exteriorization of the tube or button in the left upper abdominal quadrant. If a lesser curvature gastrostomy site is selected, exteriorization may be preferable in the right upper abdominal quadrant. Regardless of site selection, it is important to position the stoma away from the costal margin because the stoma tends to rise superiorly as the child grows, which can cause complications later. A Janeway gastrostomy may also be employed, although it has the disadvantage of possible leakage of gastric contents, with resulting skin irritation and breakdown. It is entirely satisfactory, however, if leakage does not occur.

Enterostomy

In infants too small for primary anastomosis or in those with large discrepancies between proximal and distal intestines, a temporary enterostomy is often required. Several different techniques are available for creation of an enterostomy in infants and children. In 1957, Bishop and Koop (75) described an end-to-side Roux-en-Y anastomosis between proximal and distal ileum for intestinal obstruction due to meconium ileus. The distal ileum is brought out as a single ileostomy stoma. The advantage of this technique is that a small catheter may be inserted through the ileostomy into the distal bowel with instillation of liquefying solutions for passage of the remaining tenacious meconium. Moreover, ileostomy closure can often be accomplished by oversewing the cutaneous stoma, leaving the patent functional end-to-side anastomosis intact. A disadvantage of this technique is the creation of an intraabdominal anastomosis usually between bowel of widely disparate size, which may leak causing peritonitis. Santulli and Blanc (76) described a reverse of the Bishop-Koop stoma for management of this problem. Using this technique, the proximal dilated intestine is exteriorized as a single stoma, and the narrow distal intestine is anastomosed end-to-side just below the peritoneum. Irrigation can also be accomplished using this single stoma, but a formal ileostomy closure is usually required.

Another stomal technique is exteriorization of the two limbs of intestine side by side, either through the laparotomy incision or through a separate incision. The advantage of this technique is the absence of an intraabdominal anastomosis. Formal closure is usually required, however, although it is often a procedure confined to the area of the stoma without general abdominal exploration and an accompanying ileus. This is the preferred technique in very small or very sick infants.

A loop ileostomy is often used for intestinal diversion in children after colectomy and mucosal proctectomy with ileoanal anastomosis for ulcerative colitis. The intent of diversion is prevention of leakage of the ileoanal anastomosis with resulting pelvic sepsis. This stoma is usually closed within 2 months after the original procedure.

A final technique for ileostomy is end-ileostomy with closure of the distal segment. This is certainly acceptable in cases in which access to the distal bowel is not required. In patients with NEC, however, when radiographic examination of the distal ileum is desired before stomal closure, it is usually preferable to exteriorize the two limbs of bowel side by side. With this technique, a prograde study for stricture evaluation is possible through the mucous fistula.

Colostomy

In contrast to adults, in whom an end-colostomy is used almost exclusively, three techniques for colostomy can be employed in infants and children. Although a primary pull-through can be performed in many patients with Hirschsprung's disease at the time of diagnosis, some patients still may be best managed by a colostomy. A loop colostomy brought through the incision works well, as does an end-colostomy with closure of the distal colon. A divided colostomy is another technique. Because the anus is patent in infants with Hirschsprung's disease, spillover from the functioning ostomy to the distal limb is not a significant concern. Whether the laparoscopic or traditional posterior sagittal approach is used for correction of high anorectal atresia, most, if not all, babies undergo initial diversion with a colostomy. In cases of high anorectal atresia, however, it is important to separate the proximal and distal fecal streams, and a divided colostomy is preferred. It is important to allow urine to drain from the distal orifice because of the bladder fistula; this tends to prevent hyperchloremic acidosis. The functioning stoma is usually brought out through the lateral aspect of a left lower quadrant incision and the distal stoma exteriorized through the medial aspect of the incision. Regardless of the type of colostomy, it is important to secure the anterior and posterior fascial layers to the bowel to prevent herniation of small intestine with resulting obstruction. Use of silk sutures for fascial attachment is also preferred because visualization of the sutures at subsequent takedown makes fascial dissection easier and helps prevent entry into the colon.

Appendicovesicostomy

Appendicovesicostomy is a stoma unique to pediatric practice. The appendix is used as a catheterizable conduit after bladder augmentation (77). It can be positioned either in the lower abdominal quadrant or in the perineum to provide easy access for bladder catheterization. Because of this potential use, incidental appendectomy should not be performed in patients who may need bladder augmentation at a later date, such as children with spina bifida.

The umbilicus merits special emphasis as a site for placement of intestinal stomas. Fitzgerald et al. (78) recommended the use of the umbilicus for temporary ostomies in infants and children, and reported their experience in 47 patients. Advantages include its convenience for placement of appliances and cosmesis after closure.

Complications

Complications from stomas are not infrequent, but can be minimized with careful attention to technique (79). Mild complications include skin irritation from contact with intestinal contents. This usually occurs because the care provider is not able to place a tight seal with the appliance around the stoma. The likely reason is that the stoma is flush with the skin and not elevated for easy placement of the appliance. Another reason is that the stoma may be positioned in a place that does not lend itself well to placement of an appliance. For instance, if a colostomy is placed too low in the left or right lower quadrant areas, the appliance may not sit well and may leak because of the contour of the underlying pelvis and hip elevations.

Other complications include stomal prolapse, which is usually confined to the distal colon with a loop or divided colostomy. Small bowel obstruction may develop either around the stoma or from herniation of small bowel loops if the fascial approximation to the colon is not properly sutured. As previously mentioned, it is important to secure the colon to the anterior and posterior layers of the fascia with a number of interrupted silk sutures to prevent this complication. In infants with an ileostomy for NEC, it is often not necessary to secure the ileum to the fascia because the dense inflammatory reaction within the abdominal cavity does not allow the small intestine sufficient mobility for herniation. The inflammatory response also helps the ileostomy to attach to the fascial stoma. An important concept to remember is that rarely is a stoma too elevated above the skin in an infant, but a stoma that is flush with the skin is usually difficult to manage.

SPECIFIC SURGICAL PROBLEMS

Small Bowel Obstruction

Congenital lesions causing small intestinal obstruction usually present in the neonatal period. Examples include intestinal malrotation and other anomalies of rotation, small intestinal atresia, meconium ileus, intestinal aganglionosis, and intestinal duplication anomalies. Acquired causes of small intestinal obstruction include inguinal hernia, intussusception, inflammatory strictures from NEC, appendiceal abscess or Crohn's disease, and neoplastic disorders. Lymphoma is the most frequent malignant neoplasm that causes obstruction of the small intestine, and polyps are the most common benign tumor in children. Detailed discussions of these lesions are presented elsewhere.

Small intestinal obstruction may also occur after laparotomy, usually from adhesions. An incidence of 2.2% was reported by Festen (80) in 1,476 laparotomies. Seventy percent of the obstructions in this series were due to a single adhesion. Adhesive bowel obstruction appears infrequently after a laparoscopic operation. The authors have performed more than 1,000 laparoscopic procedures and have not had a single patient return with symptoms suggestive of adhesive intestinal obstruction. However, any child who has had a previous abdominal surgery is at risk for adhesive small bowel obstruction. Early symptoms include crampy abdominal pain, anorexia, nausea, and vomiting. Lethargy and reduced activity also often occur, but are usually later signs. Bowel sounds may be hyperactive initially and high pitched. Occasionally, borborygmi are present. As intestinal distention increases, the intermittent peristaltic discomfort disappears and is replaced by constant pain from peritoneal irritation and intestinal distention. Pain is greater with a lower intestinal obstruction because of increased abdominal wall and intestinal distention. In fact, with a proximal small bowel obstruction, abdominal distention may not be apparent because vomiting may empty the obstructed intestinal loops. Indications of intestinal ischemia and necrosis include fever, a rapid pulse, leukocytosis, and peritonitis.

Evaluation initially should include supine and upright abdominal films for evaluation of air–fluid levels and free intestinal air. A prone cross-table lateral film is useful in infants to determine if air is present in the rectum. Rectal gas is usually indicative of partial rather than complete obstruction unless the film has been taken so soon after the onset of complete obstruction that the air has not been evacuated. Initial treatment is directed toward rehydration and electrolyte correction. A nasogastric tube should be placed for decompression and antibiotics administered. Operative intervention should be reserved for a complete bowel obstruction or failure of nonoperative management by 24 hours. In general, if the original incision was made transversely in one of the abdominal quadrants, then the midline approach is preferable because intestinal loops may have adhered to the old scar, making access to the peritoneal cavity difficult and hazardous.

Akgür and colleagues (81) reviewed 230 adhesive small bowel obstructions in 181 children. Immediate operation was performed for 81 children who presented with fever, leukocytosis, abdominal tenderness, or complete obstruction. Of the remaining 149, 110 were successfully managed conservatively; however, 39 of these subsequently required surgical intervention. The recurrence rate after surgical management was 18.75% and for nonoperative treatment was 36.47% ($P < .01$). Using a conservative approach in selected patients, 40% were spared operation without any adverse consequences.

Postoperative intussusception is a problem unique to pediatric patients (82). The diagnosis is often delayed owing to the protean manifestations of the disorder (distention, nausea, and vomiting) that, when encountered shortly after an abdominal operation, usually result in a low index of suspicion because these symptoms are confused with the routine occurrence of postoperative ileus. Most patients with postoperative intussusception develop symptoms within 1 to 2 weeks after operation (83). This is in contrast to adhesive obstruction, in which most patients present 2 weeks or more after surgery. Therefore, a high index of suspicion is required for an early diagnosis in the postoperative period, particularly if nasogastric suction has been instituted. In that situation, abdominal distention and cramping pain are minimized, but the real clue is a marked increase in the volume of gastric drainage. Surgical exploration is required in all cases of postoperative intussusception (Fig. 67-9).

Ascites

Although many causes for the development of ascites are known, only a few conditions account for most childhood cases. Ascites can develop as a result of congenital cardiovascular disease and cardiac failure; hepatorenal

A

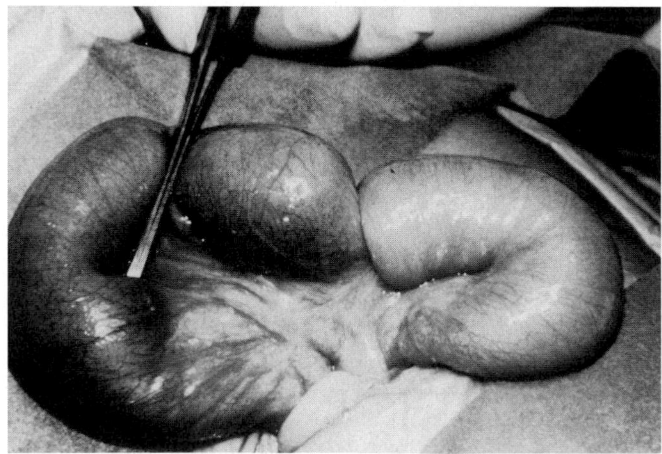

B

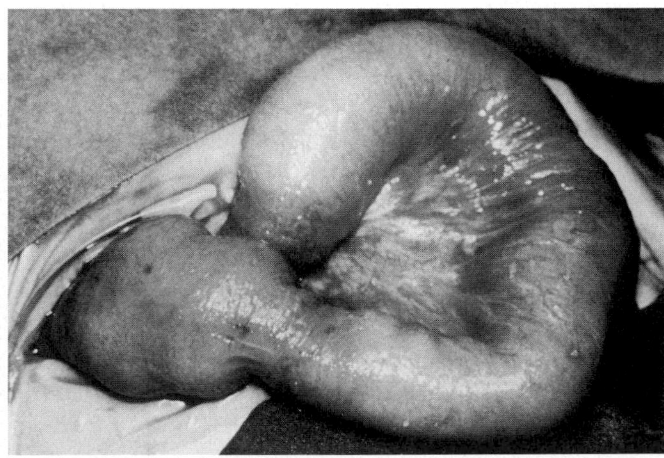

FIGURE 67-9. Postoperative jejunojejunal intussusception (*top*) found at laparotomy is manually reduced (*bottom*). There is no lead point for the postoperative small bowel intussusception. (From Holcomb GW III, Ross AJ III, O'Neill JA Jr. Postoperative intussusception: increasing frequency or increasing awareness? *South Med J* 1991;84:1334, with permission.

syndrome; lymphatic and urinary obstruction; prenatal bowel perforation with meconium peritonitis; and pancreatic, biliary, and ovarian conditions. In some instances, the development of ascites is expected, such as in infants with biliary atresia with failed surgical portoenterostomy. In other cases, the reason is unclear, and paracentesis is important for diagnosis and relief of tension. After paracentesis, the cause is usually apparent. A large mesenteric or omental cyst may be mistaken for ascites.

Ascitic chylous fluid may be clear in newborns, but is usually cloudy and turbid after feedings have been initiated. There is an increase in the total fat and triglyceride content and a decrease in protein. Leukocytosis usually occurs with lymphocyte predominance. In a review of 59 children with chylous ascites, Vasko and Tapper (84) found congenital malformation in 39%, no apparent etiology in 31%, inflammation in 15%, and neoplasm in 3%. Most infants and children respond to nonoperative therapy directed toward reducing the fat and elevating the protein content in diets. Medium-chain triglycerides are often employed for this purpose. Total parenteral nutrition may be preferable. If identifiable causes are present, such as abdominal cyst, trauma, or malrotation, those conditions should be corrected. Exploration is reserved for failure of nonoperative therapy for 4 to 6 weeks. Preoperative feedings of cream with a lipophilic dye may help identify the site of the leak at operation. On occasion, a peritoneal venous shunt is required when repeated attempts at nonoperative and operative therapy have failed.

Ascites may also develop secondary to spontaneous or traumatic biliary tract perforation (85,86). In one review of 50 cases of biliary ascites in infancy, laparotomy was required in all cases, and biliary tract drainage was performed in 45 patients. Thirty-six patients survived local drainage alone without repair of the biliary perforation. With traumatic injuries in older children, drainage, possible cholecystectomy, and ductal repair are sometimes indicated. Biliary ascites may also occur after failed therapy for biliary atresia, blunt liver injury, neonatal hepatitis, or cytomegalovirus. Paracentesis reveals biliary fluid with a bilirubin content usually greater than 400 mg per mL.

Pancreatic ascites in children is usually related to traumatic injury. Most cases are related to the development of a pancreatic pseudocyst. The major reason for delayed or incorrect preoperative diagnosis of pancreatic ascites appears to be the failure to analyze the acidic fluid for amylase (87). Pancreatic ascites usually resolves after pseudocyst drainage. Persistent ascites requires surgical correction.

Ovarian ascites may occur after birth, rarely develops in older children, and may be related to large cysts in neonates. In adolescent girls, ascites may accompany ovarian tumors, such as thecoma, and may be a part of Meigs syndrome.

Urinary ascites usually results from mechanical obstruction of the urinary tract. Causes reported include posterior urethral valves, urethrocele, urethral atresia, neurogenic bladder, and bladder neck obstruction (88,89). Bladder perforations have also been reported as the cause for ascites (90). The infant usually develops abdominal distention, sometimes with extensive ascites. An elevated serum creatinine and urea may result from peritoneal absorption of urine. Urinary function, however, may be relatively normal. A voiding cystourethrogram and intravenous urography can detect urinary leakage in most cases.

REFERENCES

1. Rodgers KE, DiZerega GS. Modulation of peritoneal re-epithelialization by postsurgical macrophages. *J Surg Res* 1992;53:542.
2. DiZerega GS. The peritoneum and its response to surgical injury. *Prog Clin Biol Res* 1990;358:1.
3. Nishimura K, Nakamura RM, DiZerega GS. Ibuprofen inhibition of postsurgical adhesion formation: a time and dose response biochemical evaluation in rabbits. *J Surg Res* 1984;36:115.
4. Adhesion Study Group. Reduction of postoperative pelvic adhesions with intraperitoneal 32% dextran 70: a prospective, randomized clinical trial. *Fertil Steril* 1983;40:612.
5. Interceed (TC7) Adhesion Barrier Study Group. Prevention of postsurgical adhesions by INTERCEED (TC7), an absorbable adhesion barrier: a prospective, randomized multicenter clinical study. *Fertil Steril* 1989;51:933.
6. Interceed (TC7) Adhesion Barrier Study Group II. Pelvic sidewall adhesion reformation: microsurgery alone or with Interceed absorbable adhesion barrier. *Surg Gynecol Obstet* 1993;177:135.
7. Surgical Membrane Study Group. Prophylaxis of pelvic sidewall adhesions with Gore-Tex surgical membrane: a multicenter clinical investigation. *Fertil Steril* 1991;57:921.
8. Jansen RPS. Failure of intraperitoneal adjuncts to improve the outcome of pelvic operation in young women. *Am J Obstet Gynecol* 1985;153:363.
9. DiZerega GS, Rodgers KE. *The peritoneum*. New York: Springer-Verlag, 1992.
10. Thomas JW, Rhoades JE. Adhesions resulting from removal of serosa from an area of bowel: failure of "oversewing" to lower incidence in the rat and the guinea pig. *Arch Surg* 1950;61:565.
11. Trimpe HD, Bacon HE. Clinical and experimental study of denuded surfaces in extensive surgery of the colon and rectum. *Am J Surg* 1952;34:596.
12. Operative Laparoscopy Study Group. Postoperative adhesion development after operative laparoscopy: evaluation at early second look procedures. *Fertil Steril* 1991;55:700.
13. Garrard LC, Nanney L, Richards WO. *Adhesion formation is reduced after laparoscopic surgery* [Abstract]. SAGES 1994, Complications of Laparoscopy and Flexible Endoscopy. Nashville, TN, April 16–19, 1994.
14. Gans SL. Historical development of pediatric endoscopic surgery. In: Holcomb GW III, ed. *Pediatric endoscopic surgery*. Norwalk, CT: Appleton & Lange, 1993:1.
15. Reddick EJ, Olsen DO. Laparoscopic laser cholecystectomy. *Surg Endosc* 1989;3:131.
16. Ostlie DJ, Holcomb GW III. The use of stab incisions for instrument access in laparoscopic operations. *J Pediatr Surg* 2003;38:1837.
17. Liem TK, Applebaum H, Herzberger B. Hemodynamic and ventilatory effects of abdominal CO_2 insufflation at various pressures in the young swine. *J Pediatr Surg* 1994;29:966.
18. Tobias JD, Holcomb GW III, Brock JW III, et al. General anesthesia by mask with spontaneous ventilation during brief laparoscopic inspection of the peritoneum in children. *J Laparoendosc Surg* 1996;6:175.

19. Duckett JW. Pediatric laparoscopy: prudence please. [Editorial]. *J Urol* 1994;151:742.
20. Elder JS. Laparoscopy for the non-palpable testis. *Semin Pediatr Surg* 1993;2:168.
21. Bloom DA, Ritchey ML, Manzoni G. Laparoscopy for the nonpalpable testis. In: Holcomb GW III, ed. *Pediatric endoscopic surgery*. Norwalk, CT: Appleton & Lange, 1993:41.
22. Elder JS. Two-stage Fowler-Stephens orchiopexy in the management of intra-abdominal testes. *J Urol* 1992;148:1239.
23. Holcomb GW III, Brock JW III, Neblett WW III, et al. Laparoscopy for the nonpalpable testis. *Am J Surg* 1994;60:143.
24. Turek PJ, Ewalt DH, Snyder HM, et al. The absent cryptorchid testis: surgical findings and their implications for diagnosis and etiology. *J Urol* 1994;151:718.
25. Sparkman RS. Bilateral exploration in inguinal hernia in juvenile patients. *Surgery* 1962;51:393.
26. Kiesewetter WB, Oh KS. Unilateral inguinal hernias in children: what about the opposite side? *Arch Surg* 1980;115:1443.
27. McGregor DB, Halverson K, McVay CB. The unilateral pediatric inguinal hernia: should the contralateral side be explored? *J Pediatr Surg* 1980;15:313.
28. Surana R, Puri P. Is contralateral exploration necessary in infants with unilateral inguinal hernia? *J Pediatr Surg* 1993;28:1026.
29. Holcomb GW III, Morgan WM III, Brock JW III. Laparoscopic evaluation for an a contralateral patent processus vaginalis II. *J Pediatr Surg* 1996;31:1170.
30. Ostlie DJ, Spilde TL, Morgan JW III, et al.Laparoscopic evaluation for contralateral processus vaginalis with unilateral inguinal hernia. Submitted for publication.
31. Schier F, Waldschmidt J. Laparoscopy in children with ill-defined abdominal pain. *Surg Endosc* 1994;8:97.
32. Powell DM, Newman KD. Laparoscopy for intersex abnormalities. In: Holcomb GW III, ed. *Pediatric endoscopic surgery*. Norwalk, CT: Appleton & Lange, 1993.
33. Holcomb GW III, Tomita SS, Haase GM, et al. Minimally invasive surgery in children with cancer. *Cancer* 1995;76:121.
34. Holcomb GW III. Laparoscopic cholecystectomy. In: Holcomb GW III, ed. *Pediatric endoscopic surgery*. Norwalk, CT: Appleton & Lange, 1993:29.
35. Davidoff AM, Branum GD, Chong WK, et al. The technique of laparoscopic cholecystectomy in children. *Ann Surg* 1992;215:186.
36. Holcomb GW III, Sharp KW, Neblett WW III, et al. Laparoscopic cholecystectomy in infants and children: modifications and cost analysis. *J Pediatr Surg* 1994;29:900.
37. Holcomb GW III. Laparoscopic cholecystectomy. *Semin Pediatr Surg* 1993;2:159.
38. Leape LL, Ramenofsky ML. Laparoscopy for questionable appendicitis: can it reduce the negative appendectomy rate? *Ann Surg* 1980; 191:410.
39. Holcomb GW III. Laparoscopic appendectomy in children. *Laparosc Surg* 1993;1:145.
40. Valla JS, Limonne B, Valla V, et al. Laparoscopic appendectomy in children: report of 465 cases. *Surg Laparosc Endosc* 1991;1:166.
41. Naffis D. Laparoscopic appendectomy in children. *Semin Pediatr Surg* 1993;2:174.
42. McKinlay R, Neeleman S, Klein R, et al. Intraabdominal abscess following open and laparoscopic appendectomy in the pediatric population. *Surg Endosc* 2003;17:730.
43. Lintula H, Kokki H, Vanamo K, et al. Laparoscopy in children with complicated appendicitis. *J Pediatr Surg* 2002;37:1317.
44. Downey EC Jr. Laparoscopic pyloromyotomy. *Semin Pediatr Surg* 1998;7:220.
45. Campbell BT, McLean K, Barnart DC, et al. A comparison of laparoscopic and open pyloromyotomy at a teaching hospital. *J Pediatr Surg* 2002;37:1068.
46. Georgeson KE. Results of laparoscopic antireflux procedures in neurologically normal infants and children. *Semin Laparosc Surg* 2002;9:172.
47. Rothenberg SS. Laparoscopic Nissen procedure in children. *Semin Laparosc Surg* 2002;9:146.
48. Ostlie DJ, Miller KA, Woods RK, et al. Single cannula technique and robotic telescopic assistance in infants and children requiring laparoscopic Nissen fundoplication. *J Pediatr Surg* 2003;38:111.
49. Ostlie DJ, Miller KA, Holcomb GW III. Effective Nissen fundoplication length and bougie diameter size in young children undergoing laparoscopic Nissen fundoplication. *J Pediatr Surg* 2002;37:1664.
50. Rescorla FJ, Engum SA, West KW, et al. Laparoscopic splenectomy has become the gold standard in children. *Am J Surg* 2002;68: 297.
51. Matsuda T, Murota T, Oguchi N, et al. Laparoscopic adrenalectomy for pheochromocytoma: a literature review. *Biomed Pharmacother* 2002;1:132s.
52. Miller KA, Albanese C, Harrison M, et al. Experience with laparoscopic adrenalectomy in pediatric patients. *J Pediatr Surg* 2002; 37:979.
53. Stanford A, Upperman J, Nguyen N, et al. Surgical management of open versus laparoscopic adrenalectomy: outcome analysis. *J Pediatr Surg* 2002;37(7):1027–1029.
54. Patti MG, Albanese C, Holcomb GW III, et al. Laparoscopic Heller myotomy and Dor fundoplication for esophageal achalasia in children. *J Pediatr Surg* 2001;36:1248.
55. Rothenberg SS, Partrick DA, Bealer J, et al. Evaluation of minimally invasive approaches to achalasia in children. *J Pediatr Surg* 2001; 36:808.
56. Langer JC, Durrant AC, de la Torre LM, et al. One-stage transanal Soave pullthrough for Hirschsprung's disease: a multicenter experience with 141 children. *Ann Surg* (in press).
57. Georgeson KE, Fuender MM, Hardin WD. Primary laparoscopic pullthrough for Hirscusprung's disease in infants and children. *J Pediatr Surg* 1995;30:1.
58. Georgeson KE. Laparoscopic-assisted pull-through for Hirschsprung's disease. *Semin Pediatr Surg* 2002;11:205.
59. Tabet J, Hong D, Kim CW, et al. Laparoscopic versus open bowel resection for Crohn's disease. *Can J Gastroenterol* 2001;4: 237.
60. Hamel CT, Hildebrandt U, Weiss EG, et al. Laparoscopic surgery for inflammatory bowel disease. *Surg Endosc* 2001;15:642.
61. Rothenberg SS. Laparoscopic duodenoduodenostomy for duodenal obstruction in infants and children. *J Pediatr Surg* 2002;37:1088.
62. Holcomb GW III. Wherein lies the future? *Semin Pediatr Surg* 1993;2: 195.
63. Georgeson KE. Laparoscopic-assisted total colectomy with pouch reconstruction. *Semin Pediatr Surg* 2002;11:233.
64. Merola S, Weber P, Wasielewski A, et al. Comparison of laparoscopic colectomy with and without the aid of a robotic camera holder. *Surg Laparosc Endosc Percutan Tech* 2002;12:46.
65. Kondraske GV, Hamilton EC, Scott DJ, et al. Surgeon workload and motion efficiency with robot and human laparoscopic camera control. *Surg Endosc* 2002;16:1523.
66. Allaf ME, Jackman SV, Schulam PG, et al. Laparoscopic visual field. Voice vs. foot pedal interface for control of the Aesop robot. *Surg Endosc* 1998;12:1415.
67. Hollands CM, Dixey LN. Robotic-assisted esophagoesophagostomy. *J Pediatr Surg* 2002;37:983.
68. Gutt CN, Markus B, Kim ZG, et al. Early experiences of robotic surgery in children. *Surg Endosc* 2002;16:1083.
69. Talamini M, Campbell K, Stanfield C. Robotic gastrointestinal surgery: early experience and system description. *J Laparoendosc Adv Surg Tech* 2002;12:225.
70. Weber PA, Merola S, Wasielewski, et al. Telerobotic-assisted laparoscopic right and sigmoid colectomies or benign disease. *Dis Colon Rectum* 2002;45:1689.
71. Menon M, Shrivstava A, Tewari A. Laparoscopic and robot assisted radical prostatectomy: establishment of a structured program and preliminary analysis of outcomes. *J Urol* 2002;168:945.
72. Horgan S, Vanuno D, Sileri P, et al. Robotic-assisted laparoscopic donor nephrectomy for kidney transplantation. *Transplantation* 2002;73:1474.
73. Nifong LW, Chu VF, Bailey BM, et al. Robotic mitral valve repair: experience with daVinci system. *Ann Thorac Surg* 2003;75:438.
74. Mohr FW, Falk V, Diegeler A, et al. Computer-enhanced "robotic" cardiac surgery: experience in 148 patients. *J Thorac Cardiovasc Surg* 2001;121:842.
75. Bishop HC, Koop CE. Management of meconium ileus: resection, Roux-en-Y anastomosis and ileostomy irrigation with pancreatic enzymes. *Ann Surg* 1957;145:410.

76. Santulli TV, Blanc WA. Congenital atresia of the intestine: pathogenesis and treatment. *Ann Surg* 1961;154:939.
77. Duckett JW, Lotfi AH. Appendicovesicostomy (and variations) in bladder reconstruction. *J Urol* 1993;149:567.
78. Fitzgerald PG, Lau GYP, Cameron GS. Use of the umbilical site for temporary ostomy: review of 47 cases. *J Pediatr Surg* 1989;24:973.
79. Festen C, Severijnen RS, vdStaak FH. Enterostomy complications in infants. *Acta Chir Scand* 1988;154:525.
80. Festen C. Postoperative small bowel obstruction in infants and children. *Ann Surg* 1982;196:580.
81. Akgür FM, Tanyel FC, Büyükpamukçu N, et al. Adhesive small bowel obstruction in children: the place and predictors of success for conservative treatment. *J Pediatr Surg* 1991;26:37.
82. Holcomb GW III, Ross AJ III, O'Neill JA Jr. Postoperative intussusception: increasing frequency or increasing awareness? *South Med J* 1991;84:1334.
83. Mollitt DL, Ballentine TV, Grosfeld JL. Postoperative intussusception in infancy and childhood: analysis of 119 cases. *Surgery* 1979;86:402.
84. Vasko JS, Tapper RI. Surgical significance of chylous ascites. *Arch Surg* 1967;95:355.
85. Prevot J, Rickham PP. Acute biliary peritonitis. *Prog Pediatr Surg* 1971;1:196.
86. Hansen RC, Wasnich RD, DeVries PA, et al. Bile ascites in infancy: diagnosis with ^{131}I-rose bengal. *Pediatrics* 1974;84:719.
87. Rubin SZ, Ein SH. The unusual presentation of pancreatitis in infancy. *J Pediatr Surg* 1979;14:146.
88. Mann CM, Leape LL, Holden TM, et al. Neonatal urinary ascites: a report of 2 cases of unusual etiology and a review of the literature. *J Urol* 1974;111:124.
89. Cywes S, Wynne J, Louw JH, et al. Urinary ascites in the newborn, with a report of two cases. *J Pediatr Surg* 1968;3:350.
90. Tank ES, Davis R, Hoit JF, et al. Mechanisms of trauma during breech delivery. *Obstet Gynecol* 1971;38:761.

Chapter 68

Hernias and Umbilicus

Frederick J. Rescorla

INGUINAL HERNIA

Embryology

Most inguinal hernias in infants and children are indirect inguinal hernias due to a patent processus vaginalis. The pertinent embryology of the inguinal region relates to the development and descent of the testes and their relation to the processus vaginalis.

The gonads develop near the kidney as a result of migration of primitive germ cells from the yolk sac to the genital ridge, which is completed by 6 weeks' gestation. Differentiation into testes or ovaries occurs by 7 or 8 weeks' gestation under hormonal influences. The gubernaculum forms from the caudal end of the mesonephros and is attached to the lower pole of the testes. The lower portion of the gubernaculum has several thin, cordlike structures that appear to guide the testes into the scrotum. These occasionally pass to ectopic locations (perineum *or* femoral region) outside the line of normal scrotal descent. Downward retroperitoneal migration of the gonads starts at about 3 months' gestation. The ovary reaches the pelvic brim at about 12 weeks' gestation and remains at this level. The remnant of the gubernaculum in girls forms the ovarian and uterine ligaments. The testes continue to descend, reaching the level of the internal ring by 7 months' gestation.

The peritoneum bulges into the inguinal canal as the processus vaginalis during the third month prior to testicular descent. The gubernaculum precedes the testes and begins to shorten as it approaches the bottom of the scrotal sac. The testes descends from the internal inguinal ring during the seventh month of gestation and passes through the inguinal canal in a few days, but takes about 4 weeks to migrate from the external ring to the lower scrotum. As the testis evaginates the abdominal wall, the layers of the spermatic cord are formed from the layers of the abdominal wall. The internal spermatic fascia forms from the transversalis fascia, the cremasteric fascia from the internal oblique and transversus abdominis muscle, and the external spermatic fascia from the fascia of the external oblique.

The processus vaginalis normally closes during the last few weeks of term gestation after the completion of testicular descent. It obliterates initially both at the level of the internal inguinal ring and just above the testes. The portion adjacent to the testes becomes the tunica vaginalis. In girls, the canal of Nuck corresponds to the processus vaginalis, opens into the labium majus, and usually obliterates earlier than the male processus vaginalis.

Failure of the processus vaginalis to close accounts for nearly all inguinoscrotal abnormalities seen in infancy and childhood. Although reason for failure of closure is unknown, it is more common in cases of testicular nondescent and prematurity. In addition, persistent patency is twice as common on the right side, which is probably related to later descent of the right testis.

Pathology

An indirect inguinal hernia occurs when intestinal contents enter the inguinal region through a patent processus vaginalis. Depending on the degree of patency of the distal processus, the hernia may be confined to the inguinal region or pass down into the scrotum (Fig. 68-1). A communicating hydrocele occurs when the opening is narrow, allowing fluid but not intestinal structures to pass into the inguinoscrotal region. A scrotal hydrocele occurs when the proximal portion of the processus vaginalis obliterates and the tunica vaginalis fills with fluid. A hydrocele can also occur along the cord because the processus may obliterate proximal and distal to an isolated cystic dilation. In little girls, the processus (canal of Nuck) may remain patent and may fill with fluid, or allow the ovary and fallopian tube to enter the inguinal region.

Frederick J. Rescorla: Indiana University School of Medicine, Indianapolis, JW Riley Hospital for Children, Indianapolis, Indiana 46202.

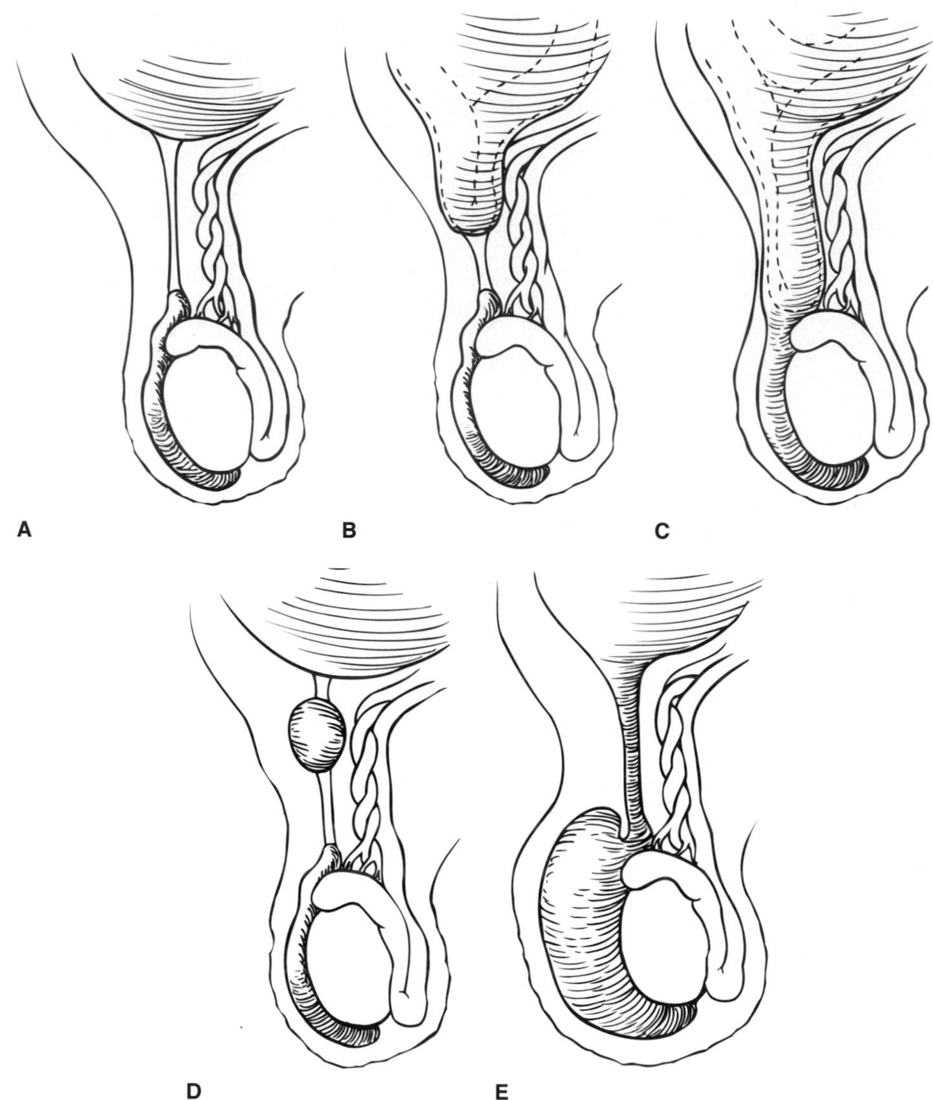

FIGURE 68-1. **(A)** Normal inguinoscrotal anatomy with an obliterated processus vaginalis. **(B)** Inguinal hernia. **(C)** Scrotal hernia. **(D)** Hydrocele of the cord. **(E)** Communicating hydrocele.

Clinical Presentation and Initial Management

Presenting Symptoms

A *hernia* is generally identified as a bulge in the area of the lower abdominal crease, with varying degrees of extension from the area of the internal inguinal ring down along the path of the cord structures to the hemiscrotum. The differential diagnosis includes a communicating hydrocele, which usually has a history of size fluctuation, transilluminates on examination, and is usually not reducible on physical examination. Other, less common abnormalities include torsion of the testes and inguinal lymphadenopathy. In addition, a retractile testis frequently is felt as a mass just below the external ring. In girls, an asymptomatic labial mass is frequently identified. If not repaired, this can lead to torsion and strangulation of the ovary and fallopian tube. In most patients, the hernia reduces either spontaneously or with gentle pressure by the parent or physician.

Conditions associated with an increased occurrence of inguinal hernias include prematurity, undescended testes, epispadias, bladder exstrophy, ambiguous genitalia, and a family history. Inguinal hernias are more common in children with increased intraabdominal pressure secondary to abdominal wall defects and in children in whom ventriculoperitoneal shunts or peritoneal dialysis is used.

At initial examination, an attempt should be made to reduce the hernia. This can be facilitated with one hand applying gentle pressure on the lowest aspect of the hernia and the other hand forming an inverted V at the level of the internal inguinal ring to force the hernia contents back through and not superficial to the external inguinal ring (Fig. 68-2). If reduction is not possible, the hernia is incarcerated.

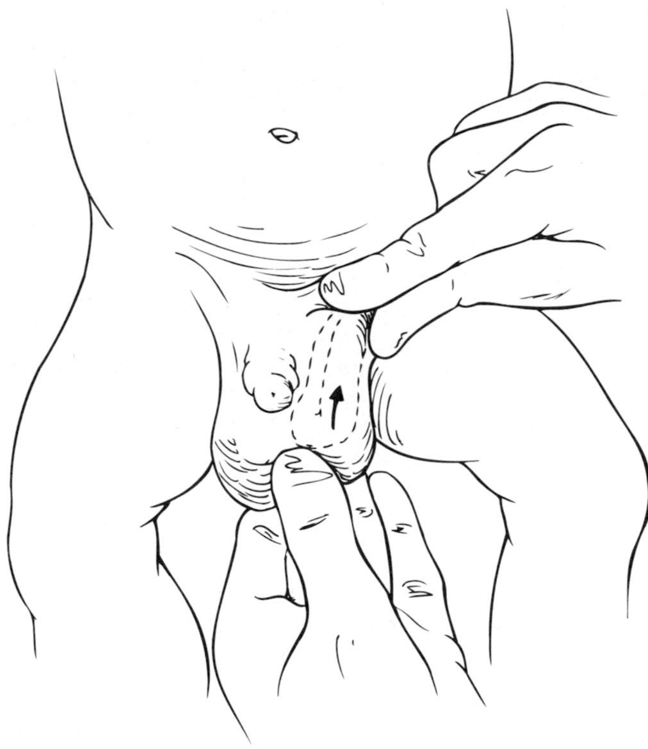

FIGURE 68-2. Manual reduction of an inguinal hernia. Two fingers form an inverted V to allow reduction through the external inguinal ring.

Incarceration

Incarceration represents the most common complication associated with inguinal hernias. Incarceration is reported in 6% to 18% of patients in several large series (1–3), and several researchers have reported rates of about 30% for infants less than 2 months of age (1,4). Contained structures can include small bowel, appendix, omentum, colon, or, rarely, Meckel diverticulum. In girls, the ovary, fallopian tube, or both are usually incarcerated. Rarely, the uterus is drawn into the sac along with the fallopian tube.

It is essential at the time of the initial evaluation to attempt reduction of an incarcerated hernia. The only exception to this is a long-standing incarceration with evidence of peritoneal irritation. Reduction can be attempted in the presence of uncomplicated clinical and radiographic bowel obstruction. An attempt by the surgeon with several minutes of gentle pressure is usually successful. If unsuccessful, sedation administered intramuscularly or intravenously may allow adequate relaxation to allow reduction.

Indications for Surgery

Due to the high rate of complications associated with inguinal hernias, repair is generally recommended shortly after the diagnosis is established. In an otherwise healthy child with an easily reducible hernia, outpatient surgery is scheduled within a few weeks at the convenience of the parents and surgeon. If reduction is moderately difficult, repair should be performed within a few days and the parents advised to return if incarceration occurs. If reduction is difficult or requires sedation, most surgeons admit the child for close observation and perform the procedure within the next 24 hours. The child with one episode of incarceration may have another and should be observed closely. An irreducible hernia requires immediate exploration.

In girls, hernias frequently appear as asymptomatic labial masses that can be difficult to reduce. The ovary is usually not strangulated, and the question arises as to the urgency of repair of an irreducible structure that is not compromised and that may have been incarcerated for days or weeks. The occurrence of strangulation of ovaries in this location is well documented so same day or next day repair is probably the most prudent.

Premature infants diagnosed with hernias while hospitalized in the neonatal units can be safely repaired before discharge. The neonatal staff can observe these patients, and as long as reduction is easy, repair can be delayed. Premature infants with inguinal hernias diagnosed after discharge may have surgery delayed to allow a general anesthetic on an outpatient basis if the hernia is easily reducible. Because the natural history of communicating and noncommunicating hydrocele can result in spontaneous closure and resolution, a period of observation until 1 year of age is generally warranted.

Contralateral Side

Few topics in pediatric surgery have drawn as much attention or generated more controversy than the management of the contralateral side in children presenting with a unilateral hernia. The only purpose of a contralateral exploration is to avoid the occurrence of a hernia on that side at a later date. The advantages of routine contralateral exploration are related to avoiding the issues associated with the development of a contralateral hernia, including parental anxiety, cost, anesthesia, and risk of contralateral incarceration. The disadvantages include potential injury to the vas deferens and testes, increased operative time, and the fact that in many infants it is an unnecessary procedure. The relevant issues in the debate revolve around the frequency of occurrence of contralateral hernias and the relation of this to age, gender, and side of the clinically apparent hernia. A more recent survey by Levitt et al. (5) found that 51% of surgeons routinely explore the contralateral side in prematures, 40% do so in boys younger than 2 years and 13% in boys ages 2 to 5 years. Routine contralateral exploration in girls younger than 5 years was performed by 39% of surgeons.

Rothenberg and Barnett (6) in 1955 reported that the contralateral processus vaginalis was patent in all the infants in their study who were younger than 1 year and in 65% of those older than 1 year. Kiesewetter and Parenzan (7) attempted to determine the role of contralateral exploration in children younger than 2 years. They performed contralateral exploration in 100 infants with clinical unilateral hernias and identified a contralateral patent processus vaginalis in 61% of cases. A second group of 237 infants underwent unilateral repair only, and 31% went on to have contralateral hernias. In view of these data, Kiesewetter and Parenzan recommended bilateral repairs for children younger than 2 years.

A similar study by Sparkman (8) in 1962, involving 918 infants and children, identified a contralateral patent processus vaginalis (CPPV) in 57%. A second group of 1,944 children underwent unilateral repair only, and 15.8% had subsequent contralateral hernias. In a review of 2,764 patients undergoing routine contralateral exploration, Rowe and colleagues (9) reported a decreasing patency rate with advancing age. Patent processus vaginalis was seen in 63% of infants younger than 2 months, gradually decreasing to an incidence of about 40% after 2 years of age.

Two more recent reports of unilateral repairs at all ages observed a somewhat lower incidence of contralateral hernias, but also focused on the side of recurrence. A 20-year follow-up study reported an overall contralateral hernia occurrence rate of 22%, with a 41% occurrence rate of a right hernia after an initial left hernia repair and a 14% occurrence rate of a left hernia after an initial right repair (10). In a review of 904 unilateral repairs, Given and Rubin (11) reported a contralateral occurrence rate of 6.8%, with subsequent occurrence of a right hernia in 9.6% of patients and left hernia in 5.4%. This study may be somewhat flawed in that the mean delay between hernia repairs was 26.8 months and the follow-up period of the study patients was only 9 to 32 months.

Several series of unilateral repairs have also reported low rates of development of contralateral hernias, although the accuracy of follow-up is questionable. The occurrence rates of a contralateral hernia were 5.8% in Kobe, Japan, (12) 3.7% in Jakarta, Indonesia, (13) and 2% in Karachi, Pakistan (14). These investigators found no significant prediction for occurrence based on the original side or gender.

In an attempt to focus on infants, Surana and Puri (15) reviewed infants between 1 week and 6 months of age (excluding premature infants who underwent bilateral exploration) undergoing unilateral repair. Ten percent of those with long-term follow-up (5 to 17 years) had contralateral hernias. Of those with initial right hernias, left hernias developed in 8.7%; of those with initial left hernias, right hernias developed in 16.6%. Only 1 of 12 girls had a contralateral hernia.

The case for premature infants is less clear, with several of the previously mentioned series including routine bilateral explorations for premature infants younger than 6 months. In a review of 222 very-low-birthweight (less than 1,500 g) neonates with hernias, 61% had bilateral presentation (16). Many researchers reporting on premature infants have observed bilateral rates exceeding 80%, but many consider a patent processus vaginalis equivalent to a hernia (4,17,18). Misra and associates, (19) in a follow-up study of 251 infants younger than 6 months who underwent unilateral repair, observed that contralateral hernias developed in 8%. Only 13% of the premature infants in this group experienced contralateral hernias. In general, these studies appear to draw into question the routine bilateral management of premature and young infants.

The issue of young girls with hernias is also controversial. In one study of 117 girls with hernias, the rates of significant contralateral sacs (more than 1 cm) was 60% for patients younger than 1 year, 28% for patients 1 to 7 years of age, and 33% for patients older than 7 years (20). Although these rates are similar to those for boys, the rate of contralateral hernia occurrence is unknown in girls compared with boys or with advancing age among girls. Several studies have reported a similar 2:1 ratio for right-sided and left-sided hernias, but a more even distribution of hernias in older girls than in older boys (20,21). In addition, if unilateral repairs are performed, the contralateral hernia rate is between 8% and 25% and appears unrelated to age or the original side of repair (20,21).

The basic question remains: How many infants and children have a CPPV, and what percentage of these have a subsequent hernia? The initial data by Rowe and colleagues (9) of contralateral patency rates of 63% in infants younger than 2 months decreasing to 40% after 2 years of age appear secure, with subsequent hernias developing in about 25% to 50% of these patients, although this latter point is perhaps the area of most controversy. Another factor rarely discussed is the actual size of the CPPV and the relationship of this size to the risk of subsequent development of a hernia. Schier et al. (22), in a laparoscopic (three-port) approach, identified wide open CPPV in 26% of boys and 11% of girls presenting with initial right hernia and wide open CPPV in 30% of boys and 38% of girls presenting with left hernias. In all four groups, small (undefined size or depth) CPPV were noted in 15% to 20%. This later group of small CPPVs may be recorded as true CPPV in many open and laparoscopic series.

The pediatric surgeon is then left with three options: (1) never exploring the contralateral side, (2) exploring up to a certain age (e.g., premature infants, 6 months, 1 or 2 years), or (3) attempting to determine contralateral patency and thus avoid negative explorations. If the other side is to be explored, it may be more reasonable to operate on the clinically uninvolved right sides more often or to an older age than the uninvolved left sides owing to the 2:1 ratio for occurrences of contralateral right hernias compared with left hernias. If a reliable and safe method were available to determine patency, negative contralateral explorations could be eliminated; however, even with this approach, at least two contralateral repairs would be performed to prevent one clinical hernia. Many authors therefore recommend avoiding contralateral exploration (23). A relatively recent prospective study followed 656 infants, children, and adolescents with unilateral inguinal hernias after unilateral repair only, without consideration of age, gestational age, or gender (24). At a mean follow-up of 25.5 months, they noted development of metachronous contralateral hernias in 8.8 months at a median interval of 6 months (range 4 days to 7 years) with the rate of 12.4% in infants less than 6 months of age, 14.8% in premature infants, 10.6% in infants less than 2 years of age, and 27.6% in children with an incarcerated hernia.

Several methods have been used in an attempt to avoid negative contralateral explorations. The use of a Bakes dilator through the hernia sac to evaluate the contralateral side has been advocated (25), but has been difficult and unreliable in other reports (26). Herniography has also been used, but has disadvantages, including pain with injection, radiation, and time and cost of a radiologist. As a result, this technique has not been widely accepted. Pneumoperitoneum has also been used. In a series of 64 children, only 5 (8%) had CPPV, although one later developed a contralateral hernia (27). This technique was shown to be unreliable for determining patency of the processus vaginalis in a study using pneumoperitoneum followed by laparoscopy (28). The use of ultrasound to detect a CPPV was reported to have an accuracy of 91% in one early report (29). Chen et al. (30) more recently noted an accuracy of 97.9% using a measurement of 4 mm at the internal ring as the upper limit of normal.

The introduction of laparoscopy into pediatric surgery has allowed diagnostic visualization of the opposite side. Several reports have documented initial diagnostic laparoscopy in children presenting with unilateral hernias (28,31,32). The incidence of CPPV detected by this method ranges from 30% to 53%, again consistent with previous reports on intraoperative patency determinations. Of interest, several reports have noted that the incidence of patent processus vaginalis does not decrease with advancing age during the first 5 years of life (28,31). Another approach that is currently widely used is to evaluate the other side by passing a 30- or 70-degree oblique scope through the open hernia sac. A meta-analysis of 964 laparoscopic evaluations identified a sensitivity of 99.4% and specificity of 99.5% (33). In these reports, the average additional time was 6 minutes. This technique appears attractive in that it may avoid negative contralateral exploration in cases in which it would be routinely performed by the surgeon. It appears to have little advantage in older children who would normally undergo unilateral repair only. If performed in the latter setting, laparoscopy may actually lead to an increased rate of contralateral exploration, although it should reliably eliminate the occurrence of any subsequent indirect inguinal hernias.

From the preceding discussion, it is clear that this topic remains controversial. My preferred method in boys younger than 2 years old and girls younger than 5 or 6 years old who present with unilateral hernias is to examine the contralateral side by passing a 70-degree angled scope through the open hernia sac (Fig. 68-3). To minimize cost, this should be performed with nondisposable materials. The bladder is emptied with a Crede's maneuver before the procedure. A 5-mm reusable trocar is passed under

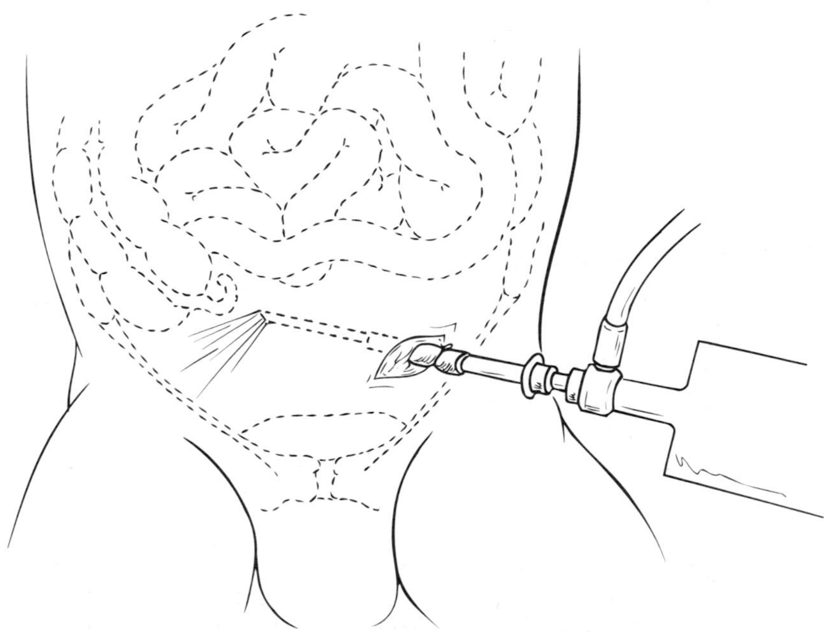

FIGURE 68-3. Nonpuncture laparoscopy. A 70-degree oblique, 4-mm diameter telescope through a 5-mm nondisposable cannula is used to visualize the contralateral internal inguinal ring.

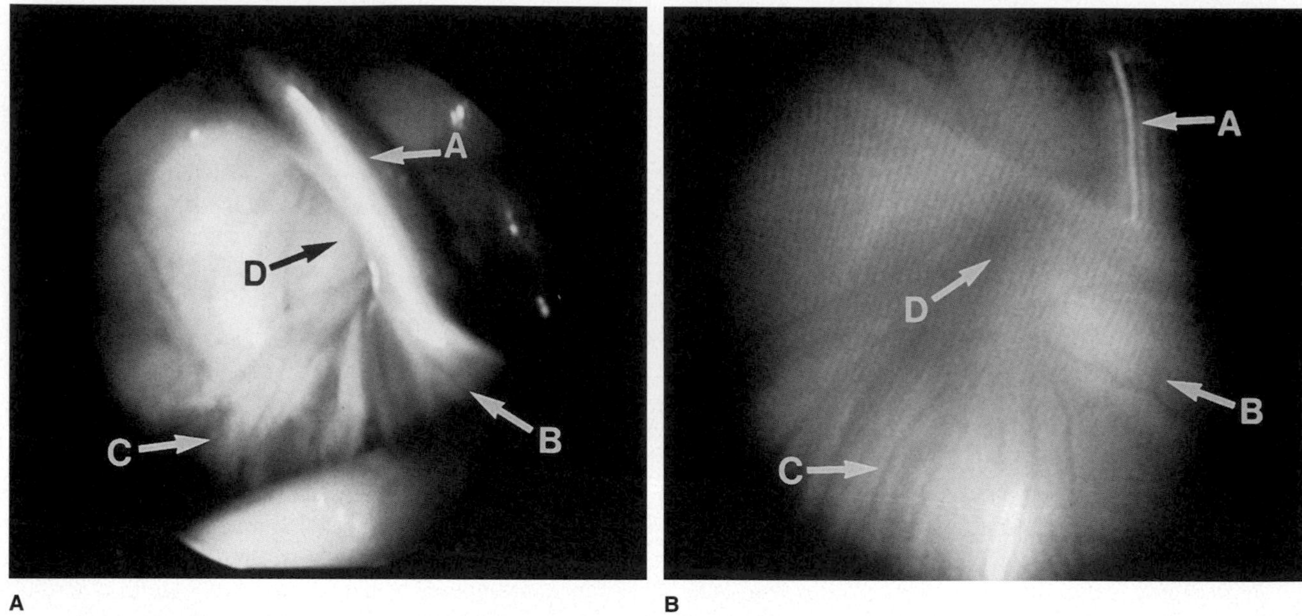

FIGURE 68-4. Photographs of left internal inguinal ring showing **(A)** lateral umbilical fold, **(B)** vas deferens, **(C)** testicular vessels, and **(D)** patent processus vaginalis.

direct vision through the open hernia sac into the peritoneal cavity. A silk tie is passed around the sac and trocar above the level of the internal ring and secured to maintain the pneumoperitoneum. After low-pressure insufflation, the 70-degree angled telescope is passed through the trocar and the contralateral side examined (Fig. 68-4). If a CPPV is identified, contralateral exploration is performed. Because of the angle of approach, it is not always possible to determine the length of the patent processus vaginalis. In cases that are inconclusive due to inability to determine the depth of a small defect or to rule out a veil of peritoneum obscuring a patent processus, a probe may be passed through a 14-gauge angiocatheter to directly measure the length (34).

Operative Management

The operative procedure for repair of an indirect inguinal hernia involves high ligation of the hernia sac at the level of the internal ring. A transverse incision is placed in the lowest inguinal crease. Scarpa fascia is incised and the external oblique fascia identified. Dissection is continued laterally just above the external oblique to the inguinal ligament, which is then followed inferiorly to expose the external inguinal ring. The external oblique fascia is opened in the direction of its fibers, taking care to avoid injury to the ilioinguinal nerve. Some surgeons prefer to perform the repair in young infants without opening the external oblique (Mitchell-Banks technique) (35). The rationale for this modification is based on the proximity of the external and internal inguinal rings in neonates. The cremaster muscle fibers are gently dissected in a direction perpendicular to the axis of the cord structures. This exposes the hernia sac on the anteromedial surface of the cord. The sac is gently elevated, and the spermatic vessels and vas deferens are separated from the sac. When the sac is free, it is divided between clamps. The proximal sac is gently elevated and the cord structures dissected free to the level of the internal ring where the sac is ligated. The distal sac is examined and, if short, may be left in place. If the sac extends into the scrotum, the anterior aspect can be excised. Levitt et al. (5) found that 78% of pediatric surgeons leave the distal sac alone, other than to drain fluid. If a hydrocele is present, it should also be excised, taking care to avoid injury to the testes and epididymis. In addition, the testes should not be separated from the scrotal attachments. If the testis is undescended or retractile and will not remain in the scrotum, an orchiopexy is performed. The external oblique is then closed. Local anesthetic can be placed in the area of the ilioinguinal nerve and in the subcutaneous tissue to provide postoperative pain relief. The remaining layers are closed, and a collodion topical dressing is placed over the wound in infants. A standard dressing is used for older children.

This procedure is adequate for nearly all indirect inguinal hernias. Occasionally, particularly in neonates with large hernias, the internal ring appears excessively dilated. In these cases, the internal ring can be closed along its medial aspect, below the cord structures. Another approach in the neonate with a difficult hernia is to use a technique of direct closure of the hernia sac through the open sac at the level of the internal ring (36). The suture includes

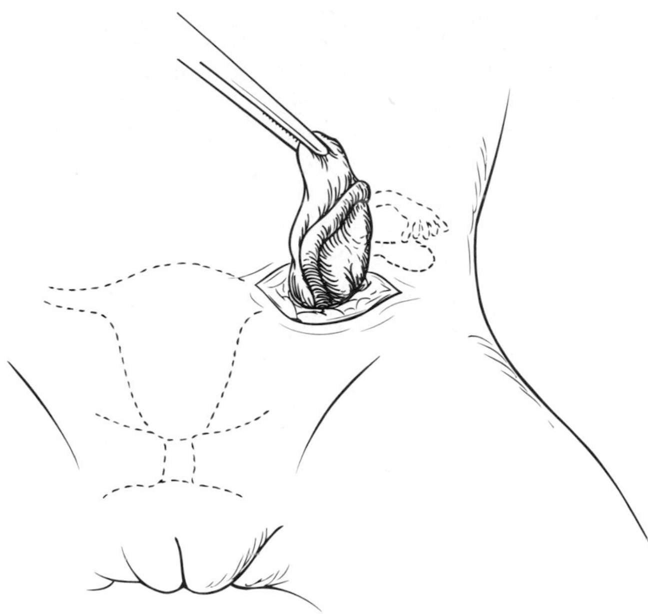

FIGURE 68-5. Sliding hernia in a girl with the fallopian tube in the wall of the sac.

peritoneum and, where available, muscle surrounding the internal ring taking care to avoid injury to the vas deferens and cord vessels.

In girls, the initial exposure is identical. The hernia sac and round ligament are dissected free, and the distal attachments are divided. The sac is then mobilized to the level of the internal ring. The fallopian tube is frequently within the wall of the hernia sac as a sliding hernia (Fig. 68-5). This can occasionally be identified by looking through the sac to ensure the ligature is placed distal to the fallopian tube. I prefer to open the sac, gently pull on the round ligament until the fallopian tube is identified, and if a slider is not present, simply ligate the sac. The internal ring is closed, and the remainder of the closure is identical to that in boys. A survey of pediatric surgeons noted that 41% of surgeons tighten the internal ring in girls (5). If a slider of the fallopian tube is present, the sac can be ligated distal to the fallopian tube, divided, and invaginated into the peritoneal cavity, with closure of the internal ring. Another method, described by Goldstein and Potts (21), involves incising the sac along the borders of the fallopian tube to the level of the internal ring. A pursestring suture is then placed in the remainder of the sac at the level of the internal ring. The tube with the attached portion of the sac is then placed into the peritoneal cavity, the suture is tied, and the internal ring is closed.

Laparoscopic Herniorrhaphy

Although several laparoscopic techniques using various prosthetic materials have been widely used since the early 1990s in adults, the experience in children has been more limited. In 1997, El-Gohary (37) reported the use of an endoscopic loop around the base of the inverted hernia sac as definitive management in girls.

This was not used in boys because the cord structure would be within the loop (38). In 1998, Schier presented a technique of an intracorporeal laparoscopic "Z" suture closure of the hernia sac in girls. He later, however, adapted this technique to boys (39). He placed sutures to close the internal ring lateral to the vas deferens and vessels, leaving these structures unimpaired, and he had one recurrence among 202 internal inguinal ring closures. A subsequent series from the same institution of 403 hernias in 279 children with mean follow-up of 22.8 months noted a 2.7% recurrence rate and a 1.7% postoperative hydrocele rate (40). Montupet and Esposito (41) performed intracorporeal pursestring suture closure of the hernia sac in 45 boys, although they had two recurrences (4.4%) that were repaired laparoscopically. A subsequent multicenter series of 933 laparoscopic repairs noted a recurrence rate of 3.4% (follow-up time ranged from 2 months to 7 years) well above the open recurrence rate (42).

Laparoscopic extraperitoneal closure has been reported by several groups (43,44). Prasad and associates (45) more recently described a needleoscopic herniorrhaphy in which a curved awl was used to place an extraperitoneal suture around the hernia sac at the level of the internal ring. The knot is tied extracorporeally and rests in the subcutaneous tissue. This technique uses three to four stab incisions, and according to the authors, allows excellent visualization of the vas and vessels, which are excluded from the repairs. The authors do not recommend this technique if a hydrocele is present. One laparoscopic technique more recently reported succeeded in closing a direct defect by patching it with the vesical ligament as an autologous patch (46). Although this technique closed the defect, it remains difficult to determine if such a closure will be adequate over time.

Incarceration

An irreducible hernia requires immediate exploration. Occasionally, the hernia reduces on induction of anesthesia. Nonviable bowel is unlikely to reduce spontaneously, and the patient in this setting can undergo a standard exploration. The sac should be opened, and if cloudy or bloody fluid or foul odor is encountered, the previously entrapped bowel should be identified. This can usually be accomplished through the open sac, but may require a lateral extension of the internal ring or a separate abdominal incision to allow visualization.

If the bowel remains entrapped, the sac is opened and the bowel inspected. Clearly viable bowel is returned to the abdominal cavity. This may require gentle retraction at the level of the internal ring or actual lateral extension of the internal ring. If the entrapped bowel is ischemic or discolored, it should be delivered further into the wound so clearly viable bowel is identified. This may also require enlargement of the internal ring. The bowel is then covered with a warm, saline-soaked laparotomy pack for several minutes. The bowel is examined for signs of viability, such as color, antimesenteric pulsations, and peristalsis. If viability is questionable or if it is clearly necrotic, a resection with an end-to-end anastomosis is performed. A standard hernia repair is performed after return of the bowel to the abdominal cavity. Separation of the sac from the cord structures is frequently difficult in these cases, and care should be taken to avoid injury to the vas deferens and gonadal vessels, as well as to ensure complete ligation of the sac at the level of the internal ring. Some researchers have advocated a transperitoneal approach with closure of the internal ring in infants with irreducible hernias to avoid this difficult dissection (47).

A discolored or blue testis may be seen at the time of exploration in irreducible cases or in situations of recent reduction of an incarcerated hernia. If the testis is clearly necrotic, it may be removed, but if questionable, it should be left in place. Several infants with blue testes observed intraoperatively have had normal-size testes on follow-up examination (48).

Direct Inguinal Hernia

Although rare in children, an initially observed direct inguinal hernia should be repaired with a standard direct hernia repair. The conjoined tendon can be secured to the inguinal ligament in a Bassini repair. If there is concern about a possible femoral hernia, the surgeon can proceed with a Cooper ligament (McVay) repair. Many direct hernias present as recurrent hernias and may represent direct hernias missed at the original procedure or a direct occurrence due to disruption of the floor at the initial procedure (49,50). A Cooper ligament repair is preferred in this setting.

Femoral Hernia

Femoral hernias are unusual in childhood. They present as masses lateral to the pubic tubercle and below the inguinal ligament. They are also reported in some series after an initial inguinal exploration, which may be due to an original missed femoral hernia or iatrogenic disruption of the femoral canal (51). Repair can be accomplished by three methods. A standard inguinal approach with a Cooper ligament (McVay) repair is the most common repair. A low infrainguinal approach involves ligation of the sac and approximation of the inguinal ligament to the Cooper ligament. A suprainguinal (transperitoneal or extraperitoneal) approach is occasionally useful in incarcerated cases to allow easier intestinal repair, although incarcerated femoral hernias are extremely rare in childhood.

Complications

Complications after inguinal hernia repair are unusual. The data on complications are inherently deficient because patients with complications may not seek follow-up at the original institutions. Some complications are related to technical factors (recurrence, iatrogenic cryptorchidism), whereas others are related to the underlying process, such as bowel ischemia, gonadal infarction, and testicular atrophy related to an incarcerated hernia. Wound infection occurs in less than 1% of all reported series and is disproportionately represented in cases that progress to irreducible hernias.

Recurrent Hernia

The occurrence rate of recurrent inguinal hernias after uncomplicated open inguinal hernia repairs is generally reported at 0.5% to 1%, (3,52,53) with rates as high as 2% for premature infants (17,19). The rate of recurrence after repair of an incarcerated hernia has been reported at 3% to 6% (3,54). The true incidence, however, is probably unknown owing to problems of accurate long-term follow-up. Recurrence generally occurs in 50% of the patients within 1 year of the original repair; this rate is more than 75% by 2 years (50,52).

Recurrent hernias have a number of causes. Indirect recurrences can result from failure to identify the sac at the original procedure, failure to ligate the sac at the level of the internal ring, or a tear in the sac in which a strip of peritoneum remains along the cord structures. Direct recurrences are the result of damage to the floor at the original procedure or a missed direct hernia at the original exploration. Wright, (52) in a review of 13 recurrent hernias from an original group of 1,600 hernia repairs, observed that 5 were indirect, 7 direct, and 1 both direct and indirect. In a review of 71 recurrent hernias, Grosfeld and colleagues (50) reported that 51 were indirect and 20 direct. In this series, 15 of the patients had increased abdominal pressure (ventriculoperitoneal shunts, ascites), which may predispose to recurrence.

Technical ways to avoid a recurrence were discussed earlier. Management of recurrent hernias can usually be accomplished through an inguinal approach. An indirect sac is managed with high ligation at the level of the internal inguinal ring. If the internal ring is large, it may be partially closed medial to the cord structures. If a direct hernia is present, the posterior wall of the inguinal canal should be repaired, bringing the transversalis fascia to the inguinal ligament or Cooper ligament (McVay repair). The preferred method is the Cooper ligament repair. Some researchers advocate a transperitoneal approach if an immediate recurrent hernia develops. This allows easier visualization of the hernia sac, enabling the surgeon to avoid injury to the cord structures (47).

Iatrogenic Cryptorchidism

Iatrogenic cryptorchidism can occasionally result after hernia repair, although it is a preventable problem (55,56). If an undescended testis is observed preoperatively, an orchiopexy should be performed at the time of hernia repair. In addition, at the conclusion of a routine herniorrhaphy, the testis should be placed in an intrascrotal position. The presence of a retractile testis associated with a hernia may predispose to this, owing to disruption of the cremasteric fibers. If the testis will not remain in a scrotal position, an orchiopexy should be performed at the time of hernia repair.

Incarceration

Intestinal complications requiring bowel resection are relatively unusual, occurring exclusively with incarcerated hernias. Intestinal resections have been reported in about 1.4% to 1.8% of the total group of incarcerated hernias and in 4% to 7% of the irreducible cases (1,3).

The reported incidence of testicular infarction and subsequent atrophy with incarceration ranges from 4% to 12% (1,54), with higher rates among the irreducible cases. This presumably occurs from compression of the gonadal vessels by the irreducible hernia, although some atrophic testes develop as a result of damage incurred during repair of a difficult incarcerated hernia. In their series of 351 incarcerated hernias, Rowe and Clatworthy (1) reported that 8 of 68 irreducible cases (12%) were associated with vascular compromise of the testes. Others have also observed an increased rate of gonadal atrophy with irreducible cases (57). Many of these testes are atrophic on follow-up, although there have been several cases of blue testes that are normal in size at long-term follow-up (48). Young infants are at higher risk, with testicular infarction rates of 30% to 33% reported in infants younger than 2 or 3 months (48,57). These problems underscore the need for prompt reduction of incarcerated hernias and avoidance of repeat episodes of incarceration.

Preoperative and Postoperative Care

The anesthetic management of neonates with inguinal hernias is also controversial. The main issues involve the risk of apnea relative to (1) the postconceptional age (PCA) for premature and term infants, and (2) the risk of apnea based on the type of anesthetic (general vs. spinal or epidural).

One of the initial studies by Steward (58) reported that 18% of preterm infants developed apnea after general anesthesia for herniorrhaphy, compared with zero episodes in term infants. Of those who developed apnea, all were 8 weeks old or younger, and therefore, based on inclusion criteria, less than 47 weeks' PCA. Liu and colleagues (59) documented a 40% incidence of postoperative apnea in preterm infants with a PCA of less than 44 weeks. Gregory and Steward (60) subsequently recommended 18 hours of postoperative monitoring for preterm infants less than 44 weeks' PCA. Welborn and colleagues (61) confirmed these recommendations in another study, in which periodic breathing occurred in premature infants with a PCA of less than 44 weeks. Kurth and colleagues, (62) however, in 1987 reported a 37% incidence of apnea in 47 preterm infants less than 60 weeks' PCA, and therefore, extended the recommendation to 60 weeks. Unfortunately, several infants in this study had more extensive procedures. Apnea was seen in three healthy outpatients with PCAs of 43, 52, and 54 weeks, although only the 43-week-old infant had apnea past the recovery room period (12 hours).

More recent studies have questioned the need for extended monitoring of these neonates. In 1991, Melone and colleagues (63) presented a series of 124 premature infants (average gestational age, 32.7 weeks; average PCA, 45.3 weeks) who underwent herniorrhaphy with general anesthesia. They reported one early apneic episode and one episode identified on a home monitor in a child with a prior history of apnea. One patient required ventilatory support in the recovery room and another for 24 hours. They concluded that these patients could be managed safely as outpatients, although this conclusion was later criticized by Peutrell and Hughes (64). Naylor and colleagues (65) stratified a group of term and premature infants by gestational age as well as risk factors defined as history of apnea and bradycardia, anemia (hemoglobin less than 10 g per dL), chronic respiratory disease, or need for theophylline. They reported a 34.5% incidence of postoperative apnea and bradycardia for those younger than 40 weeks' PCA. The incidence was much lower for those 40 weeks' PCA or older, and all these could be identified by their preoperative risk factors. In addition, no episodes of postoperative apnea and bradycardia occurred in term infants. The researchers therefore recommended outpatient management at 40 weeks' PCA or older in the absence of risk factors.

Although these two studies favor outpatient management of premature infants, they must be balanced against some of the earlier reports. In addition, a 1993 report by Gollin and colleagues (66) on hospitalized premature infants who underwent herniorrhaphy before discharge reported a high rate of complications (23% had apnea or bradycardia). Although these neonates were hospitalized, they had a mean PCA of 38.9 weeks (range, 33 to 47 weeks), and if at home, some may have been candidates for outpatient management at other medical centers. The researchers reported that a history of respiratory distress syndrome or bronchopulmonary dysplasia, history of patent ductus arteriosus, and low absolute weight were independent risk factors for postoperative complications.

The management of term infants is also somewhat unclear. Several studies have failed to demonstrate any apnea in term infants (61,65), but there have been several case reports of postoperative apnea in term infants (PCA, 41.5 to 44.5 weeks) (67–69). Two of the episodes occurred within 1 hour of anesthetic administration, but one episode involving a 44.5-week PCA child occurred 6 hours after the end of anesthesia (68).

Several other groups have reported on the use of spinal anesthesia to decrease the risk of apnea in high-risk infants. In a study of 84 high-risk infants (mean PCA, 41.5 weeks; range, 27 to 60 weeks) who underwent inguinal hernia repair under spinal anesthesia, Veverka and colleagues (70) observed no occurrences of postoperative apnea. Sartorelli and colleagues (71) reported on 140 high-risk infants (PCA, 44.8 ± 7.8 weeks), with only one case of apnea occurring in a child who received a supplemental dose of midazolam. Webster and colleagues, (72) in a report on spinal anesthesia in 44 premature infants (PCA, 40.54 ± 2.18), observed 5 with postoperative apnea (4.5 to 29 hours after surgery), although all 5 infants had received supplemental mask inhalation anesthesia. In these series and others reviewed, a small percentage of patients required supplementation with intravenous or inhalation agents, thus increasing the risk of apnea. The use of caudal epidural catheters in awake expremature babies is another technique with advantages of longer action and postoperative pain relief (73). In addition, many centers use a caudal epidural to supplement the general anesthesia.

Anesthetic management at a given institution is primarily determined in conjunction with an anesthesiologist. An unsupplemented spinal anesthetic is preferable, but these have limited duration. If supplemental agents are required, patients may be at risk for postanesthetic apnea. In a comparative review of these techniques, Gallagher (74) recommended 12-hour postoperative apnea monitoring for all preterm infants with PCAs of less than 44 to 46 weeks. His practice was to monitor all preterm infants with PCAs of less than 60 weeks. On review of the literature, he recommended monitoring all term infants with PCAs of less than 44 weeks and all premature infants with PCAs of less than 51 to 54 weeks for at least 12 to 18 hours.

DISORDERS OF THE UMBILICUS

Embryology and Pathology

Disorders of the umbilical region are due either to persistence of structures, which usually obliterate before birth, or failure of closure of the umbilical ring. The umbilicus in early gestation is formed as the result of a fusion of the body stalk containing the umbilical vessels and allantois with the extracoelomic yolk stalk containing the vitelline (omphalomesenteric) duct and vessels.

The vitelline or omphalomesenteric duct normally obliterates at 7 or 8 weeks' gestation. Failure of obliteration results in persistence of remnants, which can lead to a wide variety of disorders depending on the stage of arrest. Persistence of the omphalomesenteric duct most frequently leads to a Meckel diverticulum with no connection to the umbilicus; however, the omphalomesenteric duct can occasionally have a vessel extending to the umbilicus (Fig. 68-6A). In addition, the omphalomesenteric duct may remain attached to the umbilicus as an umbilical fistula (Fig. 68-6B). Other disorders include an umbilical polyp (Fig. 68-6C) and a sinus or an enteric cyst located below the umbilicus.

Urachal anomalies occur when the allantois fails to involute into the usual cordlike urachus. Early in development, the allantois and cloaca are in communication. As the bladder forms from the ventral portion of the cloaca, it descends toward the pelvis with the urachus, the apical connection of the bladder to the umbilicus. The urachus is located between the peritoneum and transversalis fascia in the space of Retzius, and this investment usually limits extension of urachal disorders. The urachus normally becomes a fibrous cord at 4 or 5 months' gestation and is identified as the median umbilical ligament. Failure of this process may result in several anatomic abnormalities. A patent urachus (Fig. 68-7A) represents a total lack of involution. A urachal sinus (Fig. 68-7B) occurs when the cephalad portion of the urachus remains open, and a urachal cyst (Fig. 68-7C) occurs when the central portion fails to involute. An alternating sinus can drain into the umbilicus and bladder. A vesicourachal diverticulum represents a remnant at the top of the bladder, but this does not affect the umbilicus. Various theories have attempted to explain urachal abnormalities. Although an association with obstruction of the lower urinary tract has been reported, this is unusual.

The fetal midgut normally returns to the abdominal cavity by 10 to 12 weeks' gestation, and the abdominal wall proceeds to close. The umbilicus closes as mesoderm migrates in to form the abdominal wall. Failure of this closure can lead to an omphalocele, hernia of the umbilical cord, or an umbilical hernia. The first two present at delivery as abdominal wall defects and are discussed in other chapters. The umbilical ring continues to close until birth as the linea alba narrows and the rectus muscles approach the midline. The round ligament and a thickening of the transversalis fascia (umbilical fascia) also protect this area. The round ligament usually crosses the ring to insert on the inferior margin, but it can instead attach to the superior ring. In addition, the umbilical fascia can be absent or incompletely cover the umbilical ring, predisposing to defects.

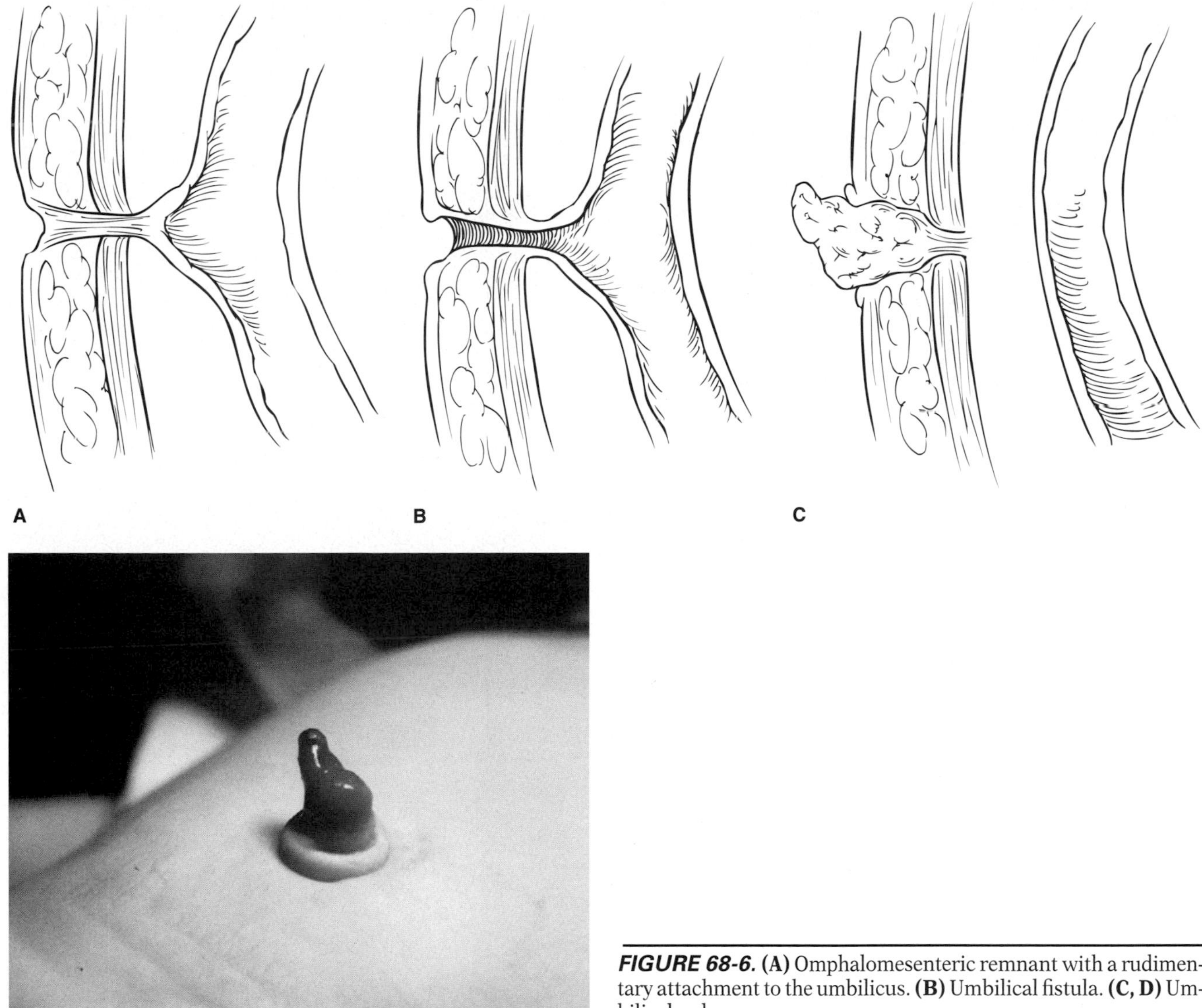

FIGURE 68-6. **(A)** Omphalomesenteric remnant with a rudimentary attachment to the umbilicus. **(B)** Umbilical fistula. **(C, D)** Umbilical polyp.

Urachal Abnormalities

Clinical Presentation and Diagnosis

The patent urachus accounts for about one-half of anomalies and generally presents in the newborn period with urine draining from the umbilicus. The umbilical cord in these infants is often enlarged and edematous. The diagnosis can be confirmed by catheterization of the tract. A lateral voiding cystourethrogram demonstrates the opening, and intravesical methylene blue confirms the diagnosis.

Urachal cysts account for about 30% of cases that occur primarily in the lower third of the urachus. They are usually asymptomatic, and only one-third of cases are identified in infancy or childhood (75). Most present in older children and adults as urachal abscesses. These patients have a tender infraumbilical mass that may drain into the umbilicus or bladder. Intraperitoneal rupture has also been reported (76), but some patients have only umbilical erythema (77). A urachal sinus (15% of cases) usually presents with intermittent periumbilical pain and tenderness. This can usually be diagnosed either by probing the tract or with a lateral contrast injection study of the sinus. A vesicourachal diverticulum is a remnant at the top of the bladder and accounts for about 5% of urachal abnormalities.

The location of the urachus allows excellent evaluation by ultrasound or computed tomography. Routine ultrasound, however, demonstrates a small elliptical, hypoechoic structure above the bladder in up to 62% of children given the test, and these should not be mistaken for pathologic processes (78). Rich and colleagues (79) recommended an intravenous pyelogram to evaluate for concomitant urinary anomalies, although others have

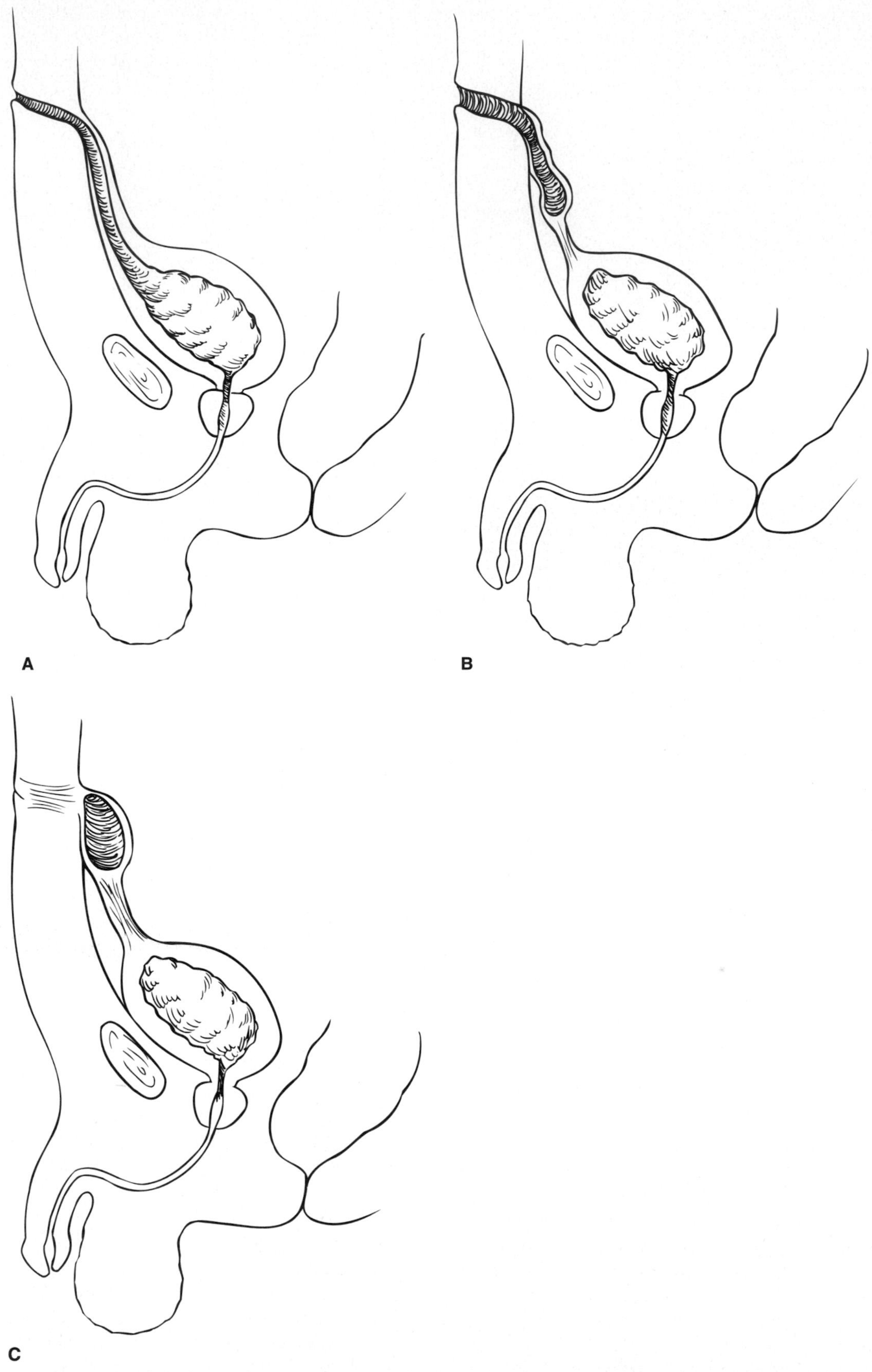

FIGURE 68-7. Urachal abnormalities. **(A)** Urachal fistula. **(B)** Urachal sinus. **(C)** Urachal cyst.

suggested that a voiding cystourethrogram may be more useful to aid in identification of a urachal cyst and to allow evaluation of vesicoureteral reflux (75). An ultrasound of the urachal region, kidney, and bladder and a voiding cystourethrogram are usually adequate.

Treatment

If lower urinary tract obstruction is identified, it should be managed before the urachal anomaly. The standard of treatment for urachal anomalies consists of complete excision of the urachus, generally with a cuff of bladder. The rationale for excision of a cuff of bladder is based on the risk of malignancy, and so long as the distal margin of the mucosa of a urachal sinus or cyst is excised, excision of a portion of bladder is not necessary (76,77).

The management of an infected urachal cyst may occasionally merit initial incision and drainage or percutaneous drainage with antibiotic therapy followed by delayed excision. Resection of the urachus can be achieved through a transverse or vertical incision. In addition, laparoscopic excision of an infected urachal cyst has been reported (80).

Umbilical Hernia

Incidence and Natural History

Umbilical hernia is one of the more common pediatric surgical problems. The factors of interest center on the incidence based on age and race, as well as on spontaneous closure rates. Several older observational studies provide most of the available data. The actual incidence is unknown, but in one large infant clinic (consisting of only 1% black infants), umbilical hernia was identified in 18.5% of infants younger than 6 months (81). The incidence of umbilical hernia has been observed to be higher in black children. In a large comparative study, Evans (82) reported an incidence of 24.7% among black infants and 3% among white infants. The cause for the racial difference is unknown, but the most likely factors are related to differences in the incidence of umbilical fascia defects.

The incidence of umbilical hernias decreases with advancing age in all races. In a study evaluating a large black population, Crump (83) reported an incidence of umbilical hernias of 41.6% in those younger than 1 year, declining to 15.9% at 4 years, 9.3% at 5 years, and 0% between 8 and 16 years of age. Crump also reported a higher incidence among premature infants. Walker (84) performed a 6-year follow-up study of 314 black infants younger than 3 months. He observed that 96% of initial fascial defects of less than 0.5 cm closed spontaneously, but no defects greater than 1.5 cm closed during the 6-year observation period. Spontaneous closure of defects greater than 1.5 cm in internal diameter has been reported, although at a lower rate than smaller defects (85).

The increased incidence of umbilical hernias in premature children was mentioned already. In one follow-up study (86), 75% of very-low-birthweight infants (501 to 1,500 g) had hernias at 3 months of age, with resolution occurring during the next 12 months to a 0% incidence at 12 months.

Clinical Presentation and Management

Most infants present with asymptomatic umbilical hernias. Incarceration and strangulation remain the only absolute indicators for surgical repair, and both of these are rare, occurring not at all in several large series (81,84), and as scattered occurrences in other reports (85,87,88). Haller and colleagues (88) reported incarceration in 6 children and 102 adults during a 15-year period, and recommended childhood repair to prevent adult incarceration. Others have observed that adult umbilical hernias generally do not result from unrepaired childhood hernias.

It appears that the low rate of incarceration and strangulation does not support a policy of early repair. Although some have recommended repair of large defects (more than 1.5 cm in diameter) at 1 to 2 years of age, spontaneous closure does occur in some of these defects (89). Based on a review of the available data on closure rates, umbilical hernias that persist at 5 years of age should be repaired.

Surgical Management

Operative repair is accomplished through an infraumbilical curvilinear incision. The fascia inferior to the hernia sac is identified and the sac encircled at the level of the fascia. The fascial closure can be open or closed. In the former, the sac is excised and the fascia closed. In the closed technique, the sac is sharply detached from the umbilicus and inverted, and the fascia is closed over the sac. The dermis underlying the center of the umbilicus is secured to the fascia to restore the normal umbilical contour.

Some children with very large proboscis-like hernias can present the surgeon the problem of redundant skin with a large circumference. Techniques describe to handle this problem include use of a pursestring (90) or flap closure (91–93). Billmire (93) described a caudal-based umbilicoplasty technique with excision of the top "half moon" wedge of skin. The inferior flap is then tubularized to form the neoumbilicus with a resultant vertical scar to close the skin above the umbilicus. This report also reported normal umbilical diameters (5-year-old boy, 1.1 cm; girl, 1.2 cm).

OMPHALOMESENTERIC DUCT ANOMALIES

An umbilical fistula (Fig. 68-6B) usually presents with intestinal contents draining from the umbilicus after cord separation and needs no other formal diagnostic studies. An umbilical polyp (Figs. 68-6C and 68-6D) can appear similar to a granuloma, but does not respond to silver nitrate. It can contain small bowel or gastric mucosa. An enteric cyst can be asymptomatic or can present as an umbilical mass as the cyst fills with fluid.

Excision of these structures can usually be achieved with an intraumbilical incision. If the opening in the fascia is inadequate, a vertical extension allows adequate exposure. Complete excision is performed, and if a connection to the ileum is present, it is delivered into the wound and closed in a transverse fashion.

Umbilical Granuloma

An umbilical granuloma typically appears after cord separation as a mass of pink granulation tissue at the base of the umbilicus. Successful treatment consists of one or more applications of silver nitrate. If the lesion persists after several treatments, it should be excised because it may actually represent an umbilical polyp.

Periumbilical Necrotizing Fasciitis

Necrotizing fasciitis is a rare soft-tissue infection that occurs in neonates. These cases usually start as omphalitis, which itself is rare with routine umbilical care. In the largest reported series, seven of eight patients died (94). Most cases present with progressive erythema, abdominal wall induration, and discoloration of the umbilicus. One successful case report (95) emphasized the need for debridement and wide excision, as well as excision of the umbilical vessels and urachal remnant to a point where they appear normal. A temporary Silastic patch is usually necessary for closure of the abdominal wall.

REFERENCES

1. Rowe MI, Clatworthy HW. Incarcerated and strangulated hernias in children. *Arch Surg* 1970;101:136.
2. DeBoer A. Inguinal hernia in infants and children. *Arch Surg* 1957;75:920.
3. Farrow GA, Thompson S. Incarcerated inguinal hernia in infants and children: a five year review at the Hospital for Sick Children, Toronto, 1955–1959 inclusive. *Can J Surg* 1963;6:63.
4. Rescorla FJ, Grosfeld JL. Inguinal hernia repair in the perinatal period and early infancy: clinical considerations. *J Pediatr Surg* 1984;19:832.
5. Levitt MA, Ferraraccio D, Arbesman MC, et al. Variability of inguinal hernia surgical technique: a survey of North American pediatric surgeons. *J Pediatr Surg* 2002:37:745.
6. Rothenberg RE, Barnett T. Bilateral herniotomy in infants and children. *Surgery* 1955;37:947.
7. Kiesewetter WB, Parenzan L. When should hernia in the infant be treated bilaterally? *JAMA* 1959;171:127.
8. Sparkman RS. Bilateral exploration in inguinal hernia in juvenile patients. *Surgery* 1962;51:393.
9. Rowe MI, Copelson LW, Clatworthy HW. The patent processus vaginalis and the inguinal hernia. *J Pediatr Surg* 1969;4:102.
10. McGregor DB, Halverson K, McVay CB. The unilateral pediatric inguinal hernia: should the contralateral side be explored? *J Pediatr Surg* 1980;15:313.
11. Given JP, Rubin SZ. Occurrence of contralateral inguinal hernia following unilateral repair in a pediatric hospital. *J Pediatr Surg* 1989;24:963.
12. Muraji T, Noda T, Higashimoto Y, et al. Contralateral incidence after repair of unilateral inguinal hernia in infants and children. *Pediatr Surg Int* 1993;8:455.
13. Wardhani H, Arianto A, Halimun EM. Inguinal hernia in children in Indonesia. *Pediatr Surg Int* 1993;8:464.
14. Hasan N. Management of inguinal hernia of childhood as practiced in Karachi, Pakistan. *Pediatr Surg Int* 1993;8:462.
15. Surana R, Puri P. Is contralateral exploration necessary in infants with unilateral inguinal hernia? *J Pediatr Surg* 1993;28:1026.
16. Rajput A, Gauderer MWL, Hack M. Inguinal hernias in very low birth weight infants: incidence and timing of repair. *J Pediatr Surg* 1992;27:1322.
17. Krieger NR, Shochat SJ, McGowan V, et al. Early hernia repair in the premature infant: long-term follow-up. *J Pediatr Surg* 1994;29:978.
18. Moss RL, Hatch EI. Inguinal hernia repair in early infancy. *Am J Surg* 1991;161:596.
19. Misra D, Hewitt G, Potts SR, et al. Inguinal herniotomy in young infants, with emphasis on premature neonates. *J Pediatr Surg* 1994;29:1496.
20. Wright JE. Inguinal hernia in girls: desirability and dangers of bilateral exploration. *Aust Paediatr J* 1982;18:55.
21. Goldstein IR, Potts WJ. Inguinal hernia in female infant and children. *Ann Surg* 1957;148:819.
22. Schier F, Danzer E, Bondartschuk M. Incidence of contralateral patent processus vaginalis in children with inguinal hernia. *J Pediatr Surg* 2001;36:1661.
23. Burd RS, Heffington SH, Teague JL. The optimal approach for management of metachronous hernias in children: a decision analysis. *J Pediatr Surg* 2001;36:1190.
24. Tackett LD, Breuer CK, Luks FI, et al. Incidence of contralateral inguinal hernia: a prospective analysis. *J Pediatr Surg* 1999;34:684.
25. Kramer SG, Davis SE. Transperitoneal detection of occult inguinal hernia. *Milit Med* 1967;132:512.
26. Kiesewetter WB, Oh KS. Unilateral inguinal hernias in children. *Arch Surg* 1980;115:1443.
27. Harrison CB, Kaplan GW, Scherz HC, et al. Diagnostic pneumoperitoneum for the detection of the clinically occult contralateral hernia in children. *J Urol* 1990;144:510.
28. Holcomb GW III, Brock JW III, Morgan WM III. Laparoscopic evaluation for contralateral patent processus vaginalis. *J Pediatr Surg* 1994;29:970.
29. Erez I, Kovalivker M, Schneider N, et al. Elective sonographic evaluation of inguinal hernia in children: an effective alternative to routine contralateral exploration. *Pediatr Surg Int* 1993;8:415.
30. Chen KC, Chu CC, Chou TY, et al. Ultrasonography for inguinal hernias in boys. *J Pediatr Surg* 1998;33:1784.
31. Wolf SA, Hopkins JW. Laparoscopic incidence of contralateral patent processus vaginalis in boys with clinical unilateral inguinal hernias. *J Pediatr Surg* 1994;29:1118.
32. Chu CC, Chou CY, Hsu TM, et al. Intraoperative laparoscopy in unilateral hernia repair to detect a contralateral patent processus vaginalis. *Pediatr Surg Int* 1993;8:385.
33. Miltenburg DM, Nuchtern JG, Jaksic T, et al. Laparoscopic evaluation of the pediatric inguinal hernia—a meta-analysis. *J Pediatr Surg* 1998;33:874.
34. Geiger JD. Selective laparoscopic probing for a contralateral patent processus vaginalis reduces the need for contralateral exploration in inconclusive cases. *J Pediatr Surg* 2000;35:1151.
35. Kurlan MZ, Wels PB, Piedad OH. Inguinal herniorrhaphy by the Mitchell Banks technique. *J Pediatr Surg* 1972;7:427.
36. Applebaum H, Bautista N, Cymerman J. Alternative method for repair of the difficult infant hernia. *J Pediatr Surg* 2000;35:331.
37. El-Gohary MA. Laparoscopic ligation of inguinal hernia in girls. *Pediatr Endosurg Innov Tech* 1997;1:185.
38. Schier F. Laparoscopic herniorrhaphy in girls. *J Pediatr Surg* 1998;33:1495.

39. Schier F. Laparoscopic surgery of inguinal hernias in children—initial experience. *J Pediatr Surg* 2000;35:1331.
40. Gorsler CM, Schier F. Laparoscopic herniorrhaphy in children. *Surg Endosc* 2003;17:571.
41. Montupet P, Esposito C. Laparoscopic treatment of congenital inguinal hernia in children. *J Pediatr Surg* 1999;34:420.
42. Schier F, Montupet P, Esposito C. Laparoscopic inguinal herniorrhaphy in children: a three-center experience with 933 repairs. *J Pediatr Surg* 2002;37:395.
43. Lee Y, Liang J. Experience with 450 cases of micro-laparoscopic herniotomy in infants and children. *Pediatr Endosurg Innov Tech* 2002;6:25.
44. Endo M, Ukiyama E. Laparoscopic closure of patent processus vaginalis in girl with inguinal hernia using specially devised suture needle. *Pediatr Endosurg Innov Tech* 2001;5:187.
45. Prasad R, Lovvorn H III, Wadie GM, et al. Early experience with needleoscopic inguinal herniorrhaphy in children. *J Pediatr Surg* 2003:38;1055.
46. Lima M, Ruggeri G, Domini M, et al. Laparoscopic treatment of bilateral direct inguinal hernia by using the vesical ligament as an autologous patch. *Pediatr Endosurg Innov Tech* 2002;6:277.
47. Misra D, Hewitt G, Potts SR, et al. Transperitoneal closure of the internal ring in incarcerated infantile inguinal hernias. *J Pediatr Surg* 1995;30:95.
48. Slowman JG, Mylius RE. Testicular infarction in infancy: its association with irreducible inguinal hernia. *Med J Aust* 1958; 1:242.
49. Wright JE. Direct inguinal hernia in infancy and childhood. *Pediatr Surg Int* 1994;9:161.
50. Grosfeld JL, Minnick K, Shedd F, et al. Inguinal hernia in children: factors affecting recurrence in 62 cases. *J Pediatr Surg* 1991;26:283.
51. Wright JE. Femoral hernia in childhood. *Pediatr Surg Int* 1994;9:167.
52. Wright JE. Recurrent inguinal hernia in infancy and childhood. *Pediatr Surg Int* 1994;9:164.
53. Zhang JZ, Li XZ. Inguinal hernia in infants and children in China. *Pediatr Surg Int* 1993;8:458.
54. Clatworthy HW, Thompson AG. Incarcerated and strangulated inguinal hernia in infants: a preventable risk. *JAMA* 1954;154:123.
55. Puri P, Guiney EJ, O'Donnel B. Inguinal hernia in infants: the fate of the testis following incarceration. *J Pediatr Surg* 1984;19:44.
56. Kaplan GW. Iatrogenic cryptorchidism resulting from hernia repair. *Surg Gynecol Obstet* 1976;142:671.
57. Fasching G, Hollwarth ME. Risk of testicular lesions following incarcerated inguinal hernia in infants. *Pediatr Surg Int* 1989;4: 265.
58. Steward DJ. Preterm infants are more prone to complications following minor surgery than are term infants. *Anesthesiology* 1982;56:304.
59. Liu LMP, Cote CJ, Goudsouzian NG, et al. Life threatening apnea in infants recovering from anesthesia. *Anesthesiology* 1983;59:506.
60. Gregory GA, Steward DJ. Life threatening perioperative apnea in the ex-"premie." *Anesthesiology* 1983;59:495.
61. Welborn LG, Ramirez N, Oh TH, et al. Postanesthetic apnea and periodic breathing in infants. *Anesthesiology* 1986;65:658.
62. Kurth CD, Spitzer AR, Broennle AM, et al. Postoperative apnea in preterm infants. *Anesthesiology* 1987;66:483.
63. Melone JH, Schwartz MZ, Tyson KRT, et al. Outpatient inguinal herniorrhaphy in premature infants: is it safe? *J Pediatr Surg* 1992;27:203.
64. Peutrell JM, Hughes DG. To the editor. *J Pediatr Surg* 1992;27:1487.
65. Naylor B, Radhakrishnan J, McLaughlin D. Postoperative apnea in infants. *J Pediatr Surg* 1992;27:955.
66. Gollin G, Bell C, Dubose R, et al. Predictors of postoperative respiratory complications in premature infants after inguinal herniorrhaphy. *J Pediatr Surg* 1993;28:244.
67. Tetzlaff JE, Annand DW, Pudimat MA, et al. Postoperative apnea in a full-term infant. *Anesthesiology* 1988;69:426.
68. Karayan J, LaCoste L, Fusciardi J. Postoperative apnea in a full-term infant. *Anesthesiology* 1991;75:375.
69. Cote CJ, Kelly DH. Postoperative apnea in a full-term infant with a demonstrable respiratory pattern abnormality. *Anesthesiology* 1990;72:559.
70. Veverka TJ, Henry DN, Milroy MJ, et al. Spinal anesthesia reduces the hazard of apnea in high-risk infants. *Am Surg* 1991;57: 531.
71. Sartorelli KH, Abajian JC, Kreutz JM, et al. Improved outcome utilizing spinal anesthesia in high-risk infants. *J Pediatr Surg* 1992;27:1022.
72. Webster AC, McKishnie JD, Kenyon CF, et al. Spinal anaesthesia for inguinal hernia repair in high-risk neonates. *Can J Anaesth* 1991;38:281.
73. Peutrell JM, Hughes DG. Epidural anaesthesia through caudal catheters for inguinal herniotomies in awake expremature babies. *Anaesthesia* 1993;47:128.
74. Gallagher TM. Regional anaesthesia for surgical treatment of inguinal hernia in preterm babies. *Arch Dis Child* 1993;69:623.
75. MacNeily AE, Koleilat N, Kiruluta HG, et al. Urachal abscesses: protean manifestations, their recognition and management. *Urology* 1992;40:530.
76. Iuchtman M, Rahav S, Zer M, et al. Management of urachal anomalies in children and adults. *Urology* 1993;42:426.
77. Newman BM, Karp MP, Jewett TC, et al. Advances in the management of infected urachal cysts. *J Pediatr Surg* 1986;21:1051.
78. Cacciarelli AA, Kass EJ, Yang SS. Urachal remnants: sonographic demonstration in children. *Radiology* 1990;174:473.
79. Rich RH, Hardy BE, Filler RM. Surgery for anomalies of the urachus. *J Pediatr Surg* 1983;18:370.
80. Siegel JF, Winfield HN, Valderrama E, et al. Laparoscopic excision of urachal cyst. *J Urol* 1994;151:1631.
81. Woods GE. Some observations on umbilical hernia in infants. *Arch Dis Child* 1953;28:450.
82. Evans A. The comparative incidence of umbilical hernias in colored and white infants. *J Natl Med Assoc* 1941;33:158.
83. Crump EP. Umbilical hernia. I. Occurrence of the infantile type in Negro infants and children. *J Pediatr* 1952;40:214.
84. Walker SH. The natural history of umbilical hernia: a six-year follow-up of 314 Negro children with this defect. *Clin Pediatr* 1967;6:29.
85. Sibley WL, Lynn HE, Harris LE. A 25-year study of infantile umbilical hernia. *Surgery* 1964;55:462.
86. Vohr BR, Rosenfeld AG, Oh W. Umbilical hernia in low birth weight infants (less than 1500 grams). *J Pediatr* 1977;90:807.
87. Lassaletta L, Fonkalsrud EW, Tovar JA, et al. The management of umbilical hernias in infancy and childhood. *J Pediatr Surg* 1975;10:405.
88. Haller JA Jr, Morgan WW, Stumbaugh S, et al. Repair of umbilical hernias in childhood to prevent adult incarceration. *Am Surg* 1971;37:246.
89. Neblett WW III, Holcomb GW III.Umbilical and other abdominal wall hernias. In: Ashcraft KW, Holder TM, eds. *Pediatric surgery*, 2nd ed. Philadelphia: WB Saunders, 1993:557.
90. Cone JB, Golladay ES. Purse-string skin closure of umbilical hernia repair. *J Pediatr Surg* 1983;18:297.
91. Reyna TM, Hollis HW, Smith SB. Surgical management of proboscoid hernia. *J Pediatr Surg* 1987;22:911.
92. Blanchard H, St-Vil D, Carceller A, et al. Repair of the huge umbilical hernia in black children. *J Pediatr Surg* 2000;35:696.
93. Billmire DF. A technique for the repair of giant umbilical hernia in children. *J Am Coll Surg* 2002;194:677.
94. Lally KP, Atkinson JB, Woolley MM, et al. Necrotizing fasciitis: a serious sequela of omphalitis in the newborn. *Ann Surg* 1984;199:101.
95. Kosloske AM, Bartow SA. Débridement of periumbilical necrotizing fasciitis: importance of excision of the umbilical vessels and urachal remnant. *J Pediatr Surg* 1991;26:808.

Chapter 69

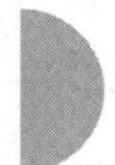

Abdominal Wall Defects

Robert K. Minkes

Management challenges of infants with abdominal wall defects begin in the prenatal period and can extend many years into the child's life. The use of prenatal ultrasound and maternal alpha-fetoprotein has led to an increasing number of abdominal wall defects diagnosed before birth. This provides the opportunity to influence neonatal outcome through changes in the management of the pregnancy or delivery, and by prenatal education and counseling of the family (1). Survival of infants with gastroschisis and isolated omphalocele has improved markedly; however, many challenges remain. Our understanding of the normal and abnormal development of the abdominal wall continues to improve and the prenatal and postnatal management of infants with these defects is evolving. Prior to the late 1960s, survival for infants with gastroschisis was rare. Three major advances led to a marked improvement in survival in these babies: parenteral nutrition, the ability to use a silo when primary closure was not possible, and advances in perinatal care in the neonatal intensive care unit (NICU). This chapter reviews the relevant embryology, anatomy, etiology, and management of common abdominal wall defects.

EMBRYOLOGY

The embryology of the anterior abdominal wall and umbilicus is well described (2,3). The details on the molecular and genetic level are less clear. From a descriptive standpoint, the embryo is seen to grow, curl, and fold in on itself. This process represents several integrated events that are specific regarding time and location. Cellular differentiation, proliferation, migration, and deposition of cells occur at different times and rates with respect to the developing embryo and are likely stimulated and regulated by specific growth factors. Several events coincide with the formation of the abdominal wall, and it is not surprising that other anomalies are associated with abdominal wall defects.

The embryo begins as a flat structure within the umbilical ring and is comprised of the epiblast (ectoderm), destined to become neuroectoderm or surface epithelium, and the hypoblast (endoderm), which becomes the inner epithelium of the gut-derived organs. Formation of the third germ layer (mesoblast) occurs with the change in the embryo's shape. The processes involved to form the mesoblast cell layer include apoptosis of the epithelial basement membrane, phagocytosis of the dead cells and migration of the ectoderm cells from the epithelial layer to the mesodermal layer. Defects in these processes may lead to body stalk abnormalities. As the neuroectoderm and underlying mesoderm proliferate, the embryonic disc is seen to grow and the embryo folds ventrally. During this time, the thoracic and abdominal cavities become distinct from the extraembryonic coelom. The folding of the embryo occurs along two perpendicular axes and involves folding from four directions—the cranial, the caudal, and two lateral aspects of the embryo. The cranial fold contains the embryonic derivatives that will develop into the thoracic and epigastric walls. The hindgut, bladder, and hypogastric wall are derived from the caudal fold. The lateral folds are involved in midgut and lateral abdominal wall development. The ectoderm is continuous with the amnion, and as the embryo elongates, it curls and wraps around, eventually putting the ectoderm-amnion border on the ventral body wall where it forms the umbilical ring around a diminishing yolk sac. The umbilical ring contains the allantois, umbilical vessels, extraembryonic coelom, the vitelline duct, and the associated vitelline vessels.

Following the completion of folding in the fourth week of gestation, the next embryologic event significant in the development of abdominal wall defects is the rapid growth of the midgut from the sixth to the tenth week. During this stage, the midgut elongates at a rate greater than the growth of the abdominal cavity and the bowel herniates

Robert K. Minkes: Section of Pediatric Surgery and Department of Surgery, Louisiana University School of Medicine, Pediatric Surgery, Department of Surgery, Children's Hospital of New Orleans, New Orleans, Louisiana 70118.

through the umbilical ring into the extraembryonic coelomic space in the umbilical cord. In normal development, the midgut rotates and returns into the abdominal cavity from the tenth to the twelfth week. Without proper abdominal wall development, the viscera remain herniated in the umbilical cord. By the end of the twelfth week the extraembryonic space is obliterated and the intestine return to the abdominal cavity. Similarly, the allantois, vitelline duct, and accompanying vessels are obliterated, leaving one umbilical vein and two umbilical arteries covered by amnion. Defects in these processes result in defects of the abdominal wall.

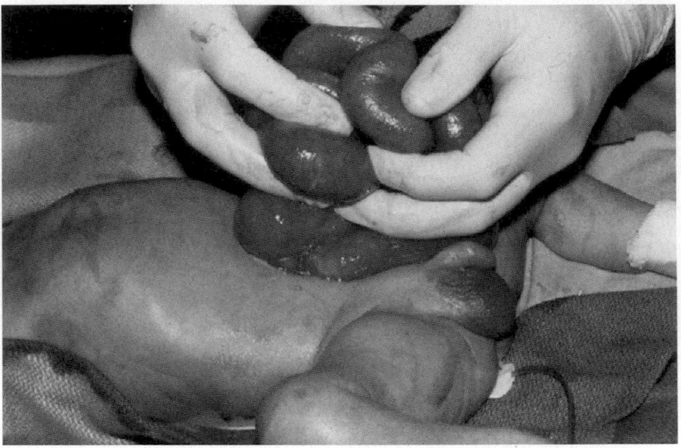

FIGURE 69-1. Gastroschisis demonstrating thickening of eviscerated bowel and lack of normal markings and folds.

PATHOGENESIS OF ABDOMINAL WALL DEFECTS

The pathogenesis of abdominal wall defects is not completely understood and the etiology likely differs depending on the timing of the embryologic abnormality. In general, the earlier the embryologic defect, the more complex the structural anomaly (Table 69-1). Abdominal wall defects may result from failure of mesoderm ingrowth and decreased apoptosis, failure of the umbilical ring to develop, failure of the amnion to approximate with the yolk sac and body stalk, abnormal neuronal differentiation, or nerve ingrowth, and may be under the influence of maternal or environmental factors.

Body stalk anomalies are produced when the embryologic defect occurs in the fourth to sixth week of gestation. Head, spine, and extremity anomalies are observed in addition to the defect of the abdominal wall. Gastroschisis results when the defect occurs in the sixth or seventh week. During normal development, the paired umbilical veins supply the abdominal wall until the omphalomesenteric arteries branch from the aorta and replace them. In the seventh week, the right umbilical vein and the left umbilical artery atrophy. The left umbilical vein and the right omphalomesenteric artery remain to supply the anterior abdominal wall. Gastroschisis (Fig. 69-1) is believed to result from vascular compromise of the right abdominal wall. Ischemia of the right paraumbilical abdominal wall could result from premature atrophy or persistence of the right umbilical vein that may interfere with development of aortic collaterals (4) or a vascular accident of the right omphalomesenteric artery. Ischemia of the right omphalomesenteric artery can produce intestinal atresia, a finding associated with gastroschisis (5). Despite clear differences in the origin of the various abdominal wall defects, there are a small number of fetuses in whom gastroschisis results from prenatal rupture of an omphalocele (6).

Embryologic anomalies during the seventh and eight weeks can affect multiple areas of the developing abdominal wall and usually involve the cranial or caudal folds

TABLE 69-1 Embryology of Abdominal Wall Defects.

Gestational Age	*Defect*	*Anomaly*
4–6 weeks	Failure of anterior abdominal wall development	Body stalk defect Short or absent umbilical cord, other anomalies
6–7 weeks	Defective mesenchymal development or vascular accident leading to paraumbilical ischemia	Gastroschisis (usually a right paraumbilical defect)
7–8 weeks	Defective fusion of myotomes in midline of the cranial fold Failed formation of septum transversum and fibrous pericardium	Pentalogy of Cantrell: thoracoabdominal ectopia cordis or cardiac defect, omphalocele, sternal defect, diaphragmatic defect, pericardial defect
	Defective fusion of myotomes in midline of the caudal fold Abnormal development of cloacal membrane, urorectal septum	Bladder or cloacal extrophy Imperforate anus Lower neural tube defect
7–12 weeks	Failure of fusion of the myotomes in the midline Failure of closure at the umbilical ring	Omphalocele

producing a predictable pattern of defects. During this time, the abdominal wall is completed by the fusion of mesodermal myotomes in the midline. The diaphragm and fibrous pericardium are also formed during this time. In addition, the urorectal septum and anterior wall of the bladder and overlying abdominal wall are formed. Defective fusion of the mesodermal myotomes in the upper midline is associated with lack of formation of the septum transversum and failure of the fibrous pericardium to form. The resulting defect termed the *pentalogy of Cantrell* (Fig. 69-2) is associated with thoracoabdominal ectopia cordis and other cardiac defects, omphalocele, cleft sternum, and diaphragmatic and pericardial defects. The urorectal septum arises between the allantois and hindgut at this time, and separates the cloaca into the urogenital sinus and the anorectal canal. Failure of these structures to form results in cloacal exstrophy: extrophy of the bladder, imperforate anus, omphalocele, and lower neural tube defects. Bladder exstrophy results from failure of the cloacal membrane to develop and defective fusion of the mesodermal myotomes in the lower midline.

The most widely accepted mechanism of omphalocele (Fig. 69-3) formation is the improper migration and fusion of the lateral embryonic folds resulting in failure of closure at the umbilical ring. This results in persistent herniation of the midgut. The herniated abdominal viscera are contained within an opaque omphalocele sac. The sac is composed of peritoneum internally, amnion externally, and may contain Wharton's jelly. The umbilical cord inserts into the sac, and the umbilical vessels radiate onto the wall of the sac. The fascial defect associated with an omphalocele can vary greatly in size. The smallest omphaloceles are sometimes referred to as congenital hernias of the umbilical cord and have a small fascial defect and minimal abdominal contents herniating into the small sac. The larger omphaloceles are more challenging to manage and may have a fascial defect up to 12 cm in diameter and involve almost the entire anterior abdominal wall. Stomach, small bowel, and large bowel often make up the contents of the sac. The liver is found herniating into the sac approximately one-half the time (7). Giant omphaloceles can include the entire gastrointestinal tract, liver, spleen, bladder, and gonads. Because the abdominal viscera develop outside the peritoneal cavity, there is no impetus for the peritoneal cavity to grow and increase in capacity. The small, underdeveloped peritoneal cavity presents a challenge in the management of infants with a giant omphalocele and gastroschisis. Gross' observation that the abdominal contents had lost its right of domicile to the peritoneal cavity is apropos to these abdominal wall defects.

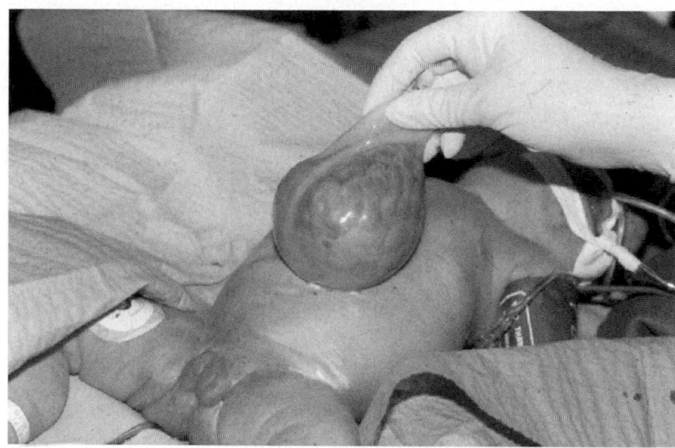

FIGURE 69-3. Appearance of omphalocele. Note umbilical cord originating from omphalocele sac.

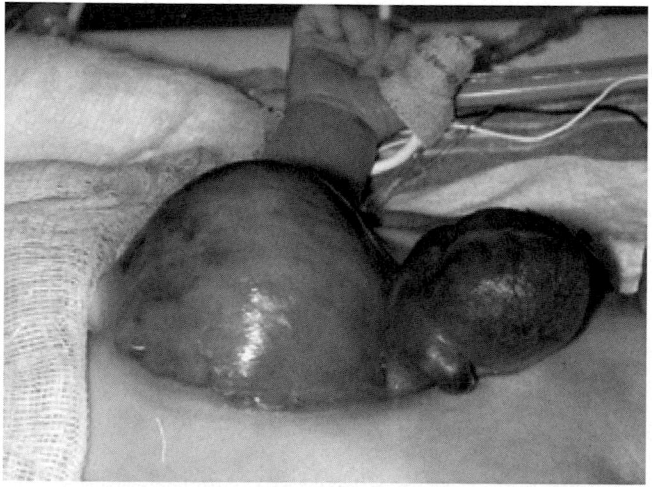

FIGURE 69-2. Pentalogy of Cantrell. Note omphalocele and ectopia cordis.

ETIOLOGY

The precipitating cause leading to abdominal wall defects is unclear, but may involve genetic predisposition, environmental, or maternal factors. Socioeconomic factors, reproductive immaturity, medications, illnesses, and nutritional status may contribute. It is postulated that these factors produce placental insufficiency and may also be responsible for the small for gestational age or prematurity that is common among infants with abdominal wall defects. Gastroschisis is associated with an average maternal age younger then 20 years. Folic acid deficiency, hypoxia, and salicylates have been shown to produce abdominal wall defects in laboratory animals, and a more recent population-based study demonstrated periconceptional multivitamin use was associated with a 60% reduction in the risk for nonsyndromic omphalocele (8,9). Several studies suggest that maternal ingestion of certain medications or drugs, especially those producing vasoconstriction early in pregnancy increases the risk of gastroschisis. Medications that are commonly used for colds, coughs, and pain early in pregnancy may increase both the risk of gastroschisis and small intestine atresia. Among the medications implicated are aspirin, acetaminophen, ibuprofen, pseudoephedrine, and phenylpropanolamine (10–13). Caution must be used when attributing ingestion of medication as causative because it may have been an underlying illness or a combination of the illness and medication that ultimately produces the defect. There are data to suggest that the risk of abdominal wall defects is increased in conjunction with cigarette smoking (10–14). Marijuana, cocaine, alcohol, and other agents have also been implicated (12,15–19).

GENETICS

Familial cases of both omphalocele and gastroschisis have been reported (20). Omphalocele is associated with trisomy 13, 14, 15, 18, and 21 (12) and other genetic syndromes. New syndromes that include omphalocele have more recently been described (21,22). The reports of gastroschisis coinciding with other anomalies such as Hirschsprung's disease and oromandibular limb hypogenesis suggest that these are sporadic events (23,24). The association of gastroschisis and specific genetic conditions in humans is less well defined. However, gastroschisis can be induced in laboratory animals by both chemicals and radiation (12). In addition, certain strains of mice, such as the HLG inbred mouse, show an increased prevalence of gastroschisis and are more susceptible to radiation injury (25,26). Gastroschisis is also seen in p53-deficient mice exposed to radiation (27). Methods for genome analysis allow for identification of genes that may be responsible for multifactorial or polygenic diseases. A mutation in the bone morphogenic protein gene 1 produces gastroschisis in mice; however, a more recent study found no mutation of this gene in 11 patients with gastroschisis (28). The use of transgenic and knockout animals has begun to shed some light on the complex nature of these defects.

INCIDENCE

The prevalence of congenital abdominal wall defects is 4 to 5 per 10,000 live births. Prenatal ultrasound data indicate an incidence of 1 in 2,500 fetuses. Historically, the incidence of omphalocele has been reported to be 1 in 4,000 births and gastroschisis 1 in 6,000 to 10,000 births. Both gastroschisis and omphalocele occur in males and females equally. More recent reports have indicated that the birth prevalence of gastroschisis is on the increase worldwide, whereas the prevalence of newborns with omphalocele in most regions has not changed or decreased slightly during the same time periods (29). Even where increases in the prevalence of omphalocele have been seen, they are less dramatic than the increases seen for gastroschisis. The reason for the increase is not well defined (29–32).

PATHOPHYSIOLOGY

Table 69-2 lists the salient differences of these two types of abdominal wall defects. The physiologic impact of an omphalocele is related to its size and, more important, to associated anomalies that can occur in approximately 60% of neonates with an omphalocele. Structural malformations are more common in infants with omphalocele than in those with gastroschisis (33–36). These included cardiac, renal, limb, and facial anomalies, as well as genetic syndromes such as Beckwith-Wiedemann and pentalogy of Cantrell (37,38). Chromosomal anomalies are more commonly associated with omphalocele, especially small omphaloceles that do not contain liver (39,40). Babies with large or giant omphaloceles have an increased association with respiratory difficulties, including pulmonary hypoplasia and other pulmonary anomalies. The cause of the pulmonary hypoplasia is unknown. These infants have small narrow thoracic cavities and minimal pulmonary reserve. Mortality is high in these infants and reduction and repair in some babies may not be possible. Normal gastrointestinal (GI) motility and function is usual when the omphalocele sac is intact. Serositis is seen with ruptured omphaloceles. Lack of intestinal fixation is present in almost all these infants, and delayed complications may occur due to rotation.

In contrast to omphalocele, gastroschisis has a low incidence of associated anomalies. Intestinal atresia is seen in approximately 10% of infants with gastroschisis, and undescended testis may be present in up 30% of boys (41–43). It is not clear if this represents a common vascular etiology or the result of vascular compromise secondary to constriction of eviscerated bowel at the abdominal wall (44). Gastroschisis can result in severe abnormalities of fetal bowel function and prognosis of these infants is determined by the condition of the exteriorized bowel (7,45). Bowel damage results in morbidity through direct

TABLE 69-2 Abdominal Wall Defects.

	Gastroschisis	*Omphalocele*
Defect	Open	Membrane covered
Defect size	2–5 cm	2–15 cm
Umbilical cord	Left of the defect	Center of the membrane
Bowel	Serositis, edematous	Normal
Alimentation	Delayed	Normal
Associated anomalies	10%	60%

interference with intestinal function and by leading to intrauterine growth retardation, amniotic fluid abnormalities, and preterm labor (46,47). The etiology of intestinal damage remains unclear. Animal models have been used to test several etiologic theories, including (1) damage is due to contact between the bowel and the amniotic fluid, and (2) damage is due to constriction of the bowel at the abdominal wall defect and may be partially dependent on exposure to meconium (48). In the chick embryo, bowel exposed to allantoic content but not amniotic fluid alone became thickened, edematous, and covered with a fibrous peel, suggesting that bowel damage is likely caused by urine in the amniotic fluid (49). This theory is supported by studies demonstrating that amnioallantoic fluid exchange can prevent damage in these models (50). Similarly, amniotic fluid-induced intestinal damage has been demonstrated in rabbit and sheep models. Mucosal absorption, decreased enzymatic function, altered gene expression, increased collagen production, and decreased smooth muscle function has been demonstrated in response to amniotic fluid exposure (51–55). Other studies have shown that the inflammatory peel is a result of amniotic fluid exposure and that bowel wall thickening and dilation is due to constriction at the abdominal wall defect. Moreover, the mechanism of constriction-induced bowel damage has been shown to result from mechanical obstruction and not ischemia (56,57). Bowel damage increases in severity with time of exposure to amniotic fluid, and both histologic and contractility changes are most severe toward the end of gestation (52,58).

Analysis of human intestinal tissue is only available when damage is severe enough to require resection. Histologic studies of intestinal samples have found the fibrinous peel to be a feature that begins at 30 weeks' gestation. The peel consists of type I collagen and fibrin, and it dissolves postnatally after repair with the involved bowel now in the peritoneal cavity and exposed to peritoneal fluid. The fascinating problem is that there is not a clear reason why the exposure of the serosa of the bowel to amniotic fluid should cause a motility disorder that can be severe in some babies (59,60). No enteric systemic abnormalities were observed that could account for hypomotility (59). Villous atrophy was identified as the structural basis for the clinical problem of altered nutrient uptake in the newborn.

PRENATAL DIAGNOSIS

Imaging

The diagnosis of gastroschisis or omphalocele can be made after 14 weeks' gestation when the fetal midgut has normally returned to the abdominal cavity. If an abdominal wall defect is seen on screening maternal ultrasound, a subsequent examination should be performed to search for associated anomalies. Ultrasonographic features demonstrating a major abdominal wall defect, severe kyphoscoliosis, limb abnormalities, neural tube defects, and a malformed, short umbilical cord with a single artery suggest a more complex body stalk anomaly (61). The ultrasound examination includes biparietal skull diameter and femur length to determine the extent of growth retardation. The size of the defect should be determined, as should the diameter of the bowel and abdomen. Attempts should be made to identify associated malformations. These include central nervous system, cardiac, craniofacial, and renal anomalies. These initial findings are then followed throughout pregnancy. Results of regional surveys show that ultrasound is accurate in the diagnosis of associated anomalies in greater than 70% of cases. Although ultrasound is useful, it is not perfect and anomalies may not be seen until after birth.

Serial ultrasound examinations concentrate on the appearance of eviscerated bowel in gastroschisis and the degree of growth retardation. The presence of bowel dilation and the development of bowel thickening or a fibrotic peel should be documented. The development of bowel dilation and thickening late in gestation may suggest an atresia or other form of mechanical obstruction. The thickening may also result from exposure of the gut to amniotic fluid. Progressive bowel dilation or thickening seen on ultrasound suggests ongoing bowel damage. Delivery may be induced once lung maturity is confirmed by amniocentesis.

Magnetic resonance imaging (MRI) has shown promise for diagnosing and defining the extent of many pediatric surgical conditions prenatally. There are several reports showing the possibility of MRI for abdominal wall defects (62–66). For selected cases, MRI may be useful for diagnosing the extent and content of abdominal wall defects, as well as the presence of associated anomalies.

Fetal Markers

An elevated maternal alpha-fetoprotein (AFP) is an indication for a fetal ultrasound to determine the presence of an abdominal wall defect. Elevated AFP in the serum suggests either a neural tube or ventral defect. Ninety percent of cases of omphalocele and 100% of gastroschisis cases are associated with elevated AFP. Amniotic acetylcholinesterase is elevated in neural tube defects and gastroschisis, but not in omphaloceles.

Prenatal Management

An amniocentesis for karyotype is performed on all fetuses with omphalocele and may be indicated for gastroschisis. Some centers routinely karyotype all children with gastroschisis, whereas other centers reserve it for when other anomalies are found in conjunction with the gastroschisis. A multidisciplinary approach is needed to aid in the decision-making process when lethal anomalies have been identified. Counseling must begin once the diagnosis of an abdominal wall defect has been established.

Prenatal Counseling

Prenatal diagnosis gives expectant mothers and families the time to learn more about their child with an abdominal wall defect and come to terms with their child's condition. In addition, it has been demonstrated that prenatal counseling by a multidisciplinary team has a positive effect on maternal anxiety (67). A mother whose fetus has been diagnosed with an abdominal wall defect should have the opportunity to meet a neonatologist and a pediatric surgeon in order to better understand the implications of their child's condition. Table 69-3 lists important issues to be addressed during the prenatal consultation. It is imperative to stress that, although certain fundamentals are applied to infants with abdominal wall defects, each infant is different and care will be individualized based on the child's needs. The families should be introduced to all participants in the fetal management team, including the perinatal center where the child will be born, the NICU, neonatologists, pediatric surgical staff, and clinical nurse specialists. Providing reading material or references to parents and a means by which they can contact the surgical or NICU team should be done. A tour of the NICU helps parents become more comfortable with the staff, high technology, and stressful environment they will be a part of following the birth of their child. Based on the diagnosis of gastroschisis or omphalocele, the specifics about that defect, pathophysiology, expected fetal course, and potential complications are introduced. The associated conditions of growth retardation, respiratory distress, and the possibility of potential preterm labor and delivery should be discussed, and arrangements for follow-up and delivery at an appropriate perinatal center should be suggested. Delivery at or near a perinatal center is associated with the need for less postoperative ventilatory support and a trend toward earlier feeding and discharge.

There is still debate regarding timing and mode of delivery, especially for infants with gastroschisis. Improving or preventing damage to the eviscerated intestine is believed to improve outcome. Potential sources of bowel injury include ongoing prenatal exposure to amniotic fluid, decreased perfusion or visceral compression from uterine contractions during delivery and postnatally from increased abdominal distention secondary to ingestion of air, exposure to pathogens and heat and fluid loss and obstruction of the mesenteric vessels at the level of the fascial defect, particularly in a gastroschisis with a small defect. In theory, intervention to prevent these insults could improve outcome. Nevertheless, no randomized, prospective trials have been performed showing a clear benefit to early delivery, avoidance of labor and vaginal delivery by performing elective cesarean section or prenatal transfer to a tertiary center. Thus far, no studies have clearly demonstrated an advantage of routine cesarean delivery for gastroschisis (1,68). Some authors have suggested that elective delivery by cesarean section prevents ongoing damage and improves outcome; however, it is likely that the benefit is a result of the timing rather than the mode or location of delivery (69–72). Because most of the bowel damage is in infants with gastroschisis is believed to occur late in pregnancy, early delivery has been proposed for those infants who had bowel dilation in utero. Unfortunately, there is no convincing evidence that preterm delivery actually improves outcome (73). It is also clear that the risks of prematurity must always be weighed against the potential advantages of preterm delivery for these infants (1,74). Furthermore, there is some evidence that intestinal damage may occur postnatally because both repair of the defect in the delivery room (75) and routine early application of a spring-loaded silo have been associated with improved outcome (76). As long as there are no signs of fetal distress or bowel injury, delivery can be planned between 37 and 40 weeks' gestation.

There is less controversy regarding mode of delivery when it comes to omphalocele. Fetuses with small omphaloceles can be delivered vaginally with minimal risk. In infants with giant omphalocele, cesarean section may be necessary to prevent dystocia. Although many obstetricians prefer to deliver infants with omphalocele by cesarean section to prevent injury to the sac (77,78), this approach is not supported by the literature (68).

TABLE 69-3 Prenatal Counseling.

Description and cause of abdominal wall defects
Size of the defect and how that may influence management
What organs are involved in the abdominal wall defect
Other anomalies the infant may have
Timing of delivery
Management following birth, including resuscitation and the possible need for intubation
Neonatal intensive care unit
Treatment goals
Surgical options
Anticipated fetal course
Treatment options and timeline of treatment
Potential complications
Prognosis and quality-of-life issues

Management

Common principles of newborn resuscitation and preoperative management apply to infants with abdominal wall defects. Initial assessment and care is provided in the delivery room and continues as the child is transported. All infants with abdominal wall defects should be transported to a facility with a NICU and pediatric surgery capabilities. Intubation is performed based on the infants' respiratory status and not on the presence of an abdominal wall defect. The goal of surgical treatment for both omphalocele and gastroschisis is complete closure of the muscle, fascia, and skin. Arterial catheters may be needed for ventilator management and blood drawing, and central venous access is often required to give total parenteral nutrition (TPN).

Gastroschisis

Immediate care focuses on protecting the eviscerated bowel, preventing hypothermia, and providing appropriate fluid resuscitation. Inappropriate or careless coverage and positioning of the eviscerated bowel may cause vascular compromise and bowel ischemia. The viscera are initially wrapped in saline-moistened gauze and stabilized so the intestine does not kink at the fascial level. The infant can be placed in a bowel bag up to the torso or wrapped in clear thermoplastic wrap such as plastic kitchen wrap. The infant should be transported in a lateral position with bowel contents supported. This position affords less chance for the extraperitoneal intestine to have its blood supply compromised. Gastric decompression is essential, and an orogastric or nasogastric tube should be placed on suction immediately after birth. Babies in respiratory distress may respond to gastric decompression; however, intubation should be performed if indicated. Venous access is secured and preferably should be in an upper extremity.

Once in the NICU, the patient is completely evaluated and resuscitated. Infants with gastroschisis may need up to two times the usual maintenance fluid requirements in the first 24 hours of life. In addition, gastric output should be replaced. Appropriate fluid resuscitation is needed to ensure adequate urine output and acid–base balance. An initial normal saline bolus of 20 mL per kg followed by 5% to 10% dextrose one-fourth normal saline at one and one-half times the maintenance fluid rate is initiated. The neonate is monitored for adequate urine output, and a bladder catheter may be needed. Antibiotics should be started. The baby should be placed under a radiant heater to prevent heat loss. The child is evaluated for growth retardation and any other anomalies. The pediatric surgeon inspects the bowel and assesses for midgut volvulus, segmental bowel ischemia, intestinal perforation, or atresia. The degree of serositis and inflammatory peel should be documented. When the inflammatory peel is thick, an atresia may not be seen. No attempt should be made to remove the reactive peel.

The optimal management of abdominal wall defects continues to be sought. In the case of gastroschisis, in at least one-half of the cases, there is a large enough volume of extraperitoneal viscera and lack of abdominal domain, that one cannot achieve a primary abdominal wall closure. Prior to 1970, the mortality rate in gastroschisis approached 90%. Inability to achieve some type of coverage led to the development of peritonitis, and to the child's demise. In circumstances in which the fascia could not cover the viscera, Gross' technique of broad skin flap mobilization and closure with skin allowed for coverage of the viscera. Months to years later the often massive abdominal wall hernia was then repaired. In the decade beginning in 1967, several developments and techniques occurred that had a major effect on improving the survival of infants with large abdominal wall defects. The advent of the silo offered the pediatric surgeon the ability to temporarily cover the exposed viscera and to gradually reduce the viscera into the peritoneal cavity over a series of days. Dudrick's development of TPN meant that with intravenous access alone an anabolic state could be achieved. The third element was the development of improved NICUs and particularly ventilators specifically designed for neonates. These three factors were associated with a quantum improvement in gastroschisis survival. A number of other improvements since the mid-1970s have resulted in a survival rate in excess of 90% for infants born with this anomaly at the present time.

Definitive Closure

There is no question that if the extraperitoneal viscera can be placed in the peritoneal cavity without difficulty and without undue intraabdominal pressure, then a one-stage closure is preferable. Most centers perform definitive closure in the operating room under general anesthesia. In the emergent setting, the bowel is inspected as described previously. The eviscerated contents may include stomach, small and large intestine, bladder, ovaries, fallopian tubes, or testes. An inspection for an intestinal atresia is performed. An atresia may not be apparent if the bowel is inflamed and matted together. No attempts should be made to separate the matted bowel. The peritoneal cavity is manually stretched and reduction of the abdominal contents is attempted. Care must be taken while handling the edematous bowel. Once the bowel is reduced, attempts are made to close the fascia primarily. The fascial defect may be closed in a vertical or transverse fashion, and the umbilicus may be preserved (Fig. 69-4). The skin is closed over the defect. If the umbilicus is resected, a neoumbilicus can be created.

Staged Closure

In more than one-half the cases, a primary closure cannot be performed and alternatives must be selected. Options include skin coverage without closing the fascia, the use of a synthetic or biologic patch to close the defect if

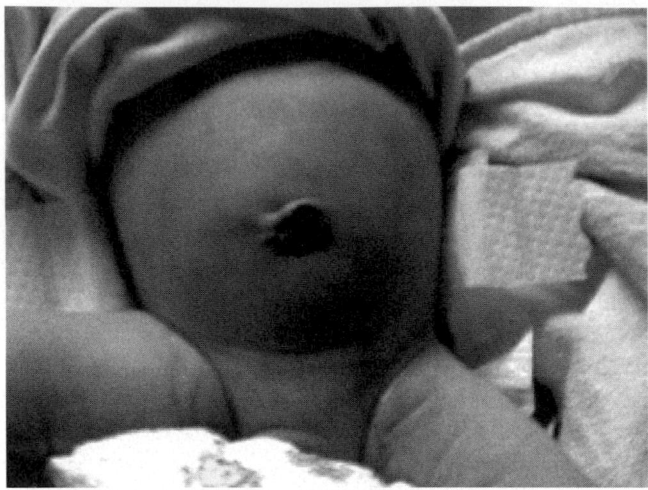

FIGURE 69-4. Appearance of gastroschisis closure with preservation of umbilicus.

reduction is complete but closure of the fascia is unsafe, or the use of an abdominal wall silo (76,79–82). When a silo is used, management typically consists of bringing the infant to the operating room and under a general anesthetic suturing Dacron reinforced Silastic sheeting to the medial aspect of the rectus fascia on either side. The two sheets are then sutured closed superiorly, inferiorly and across the top (Fig. 69-5A). Often an arterial catheter and Broviac catheter are also placed. These patients usually remain on ventilator support over the next week as the viscera in the silo is gradually reduced into the peritoneal cavity. This reduction takes place at the bedside (Fig. 69-5B). When the silo is fully reduced of viscera, the child is brought back to the operating room, the silo removed, and the fascia and skin closed. This usually requires continued ventilator support for several days afterwards.

Spring-loaded Silo

Recent development of spring-loaded silos has changed the management of many of these patients. There are several commercially available types of preformed silos. These silos have a ring opening larger than the gastroschisis defect. Thus, when the eviscerated intestine and other contents are placed in the silo, the ring can be placed below the fascia (Fig. 69-6A). The silo can be placed in the delivery room, at the bedside, or in the operating room. Routine sedation or intubation is not needed. However, if the infant is intubated for respiratory distress, sedation and paralysis may aid in the subsequent reduction of the eviscerated contents. After venous access and oro- or nasogastric decompression are established, the eviscerated contents are elevated and the abdomen is prepped and draped sterilely. The intestine is inspected for atresia, ischemia, or perforation. The stomach, bladder, and testes or ovaries can usually be manually reduced into the peritoneal cavity. A finger should be passed circumferentially around the fascia to ensure the abdominal wall is free. Adhesions to the bowel can be disrupted manually, divided sharply, or cauterized. The fascial defect can also be enlarged, if needed. If there is a concern regarding adhesions to the fascial rim or if the defect needs to be enlarged, the child should be sedated or anesthetized. The eviscerated bowel is placed within the transparent silo bag, and the ring is placed in the abdomen and allowed to expand below the fascia opening (Fig. 69-6B). The abdominal wall is palpated to ensure proper expansion of the ring. An initial reduction can be performed; however, this is usually kept to a minimum. The base of the sac can be covered with an antibiotic impregnated gauze. The sac is then suspended and permits gravity to begin the reduction. The silo is reduced each day until a definitive closure can be performed (Fig. 69-6C and 69-6D). The transparent silo allows frequent inspection

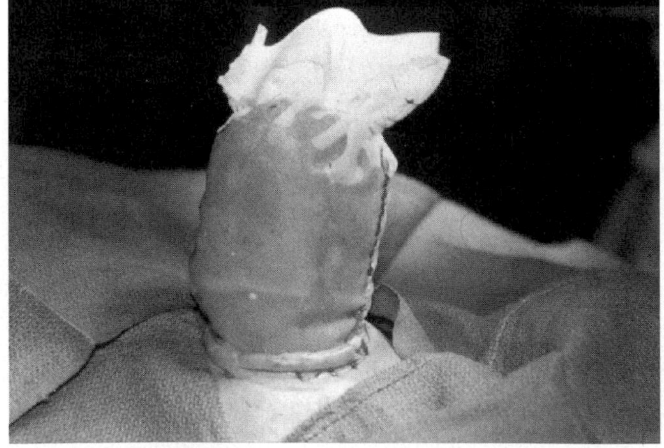
A

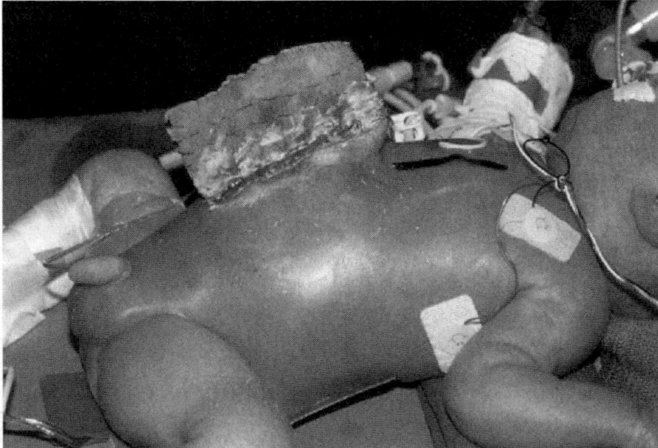
B

FIGURE 69-5. Management of gastroschisis. **(A)** Use of silo if primary closure is not possible. **(B)** Staged ligation of silo with reduction of viscera into the abdominal cavity.

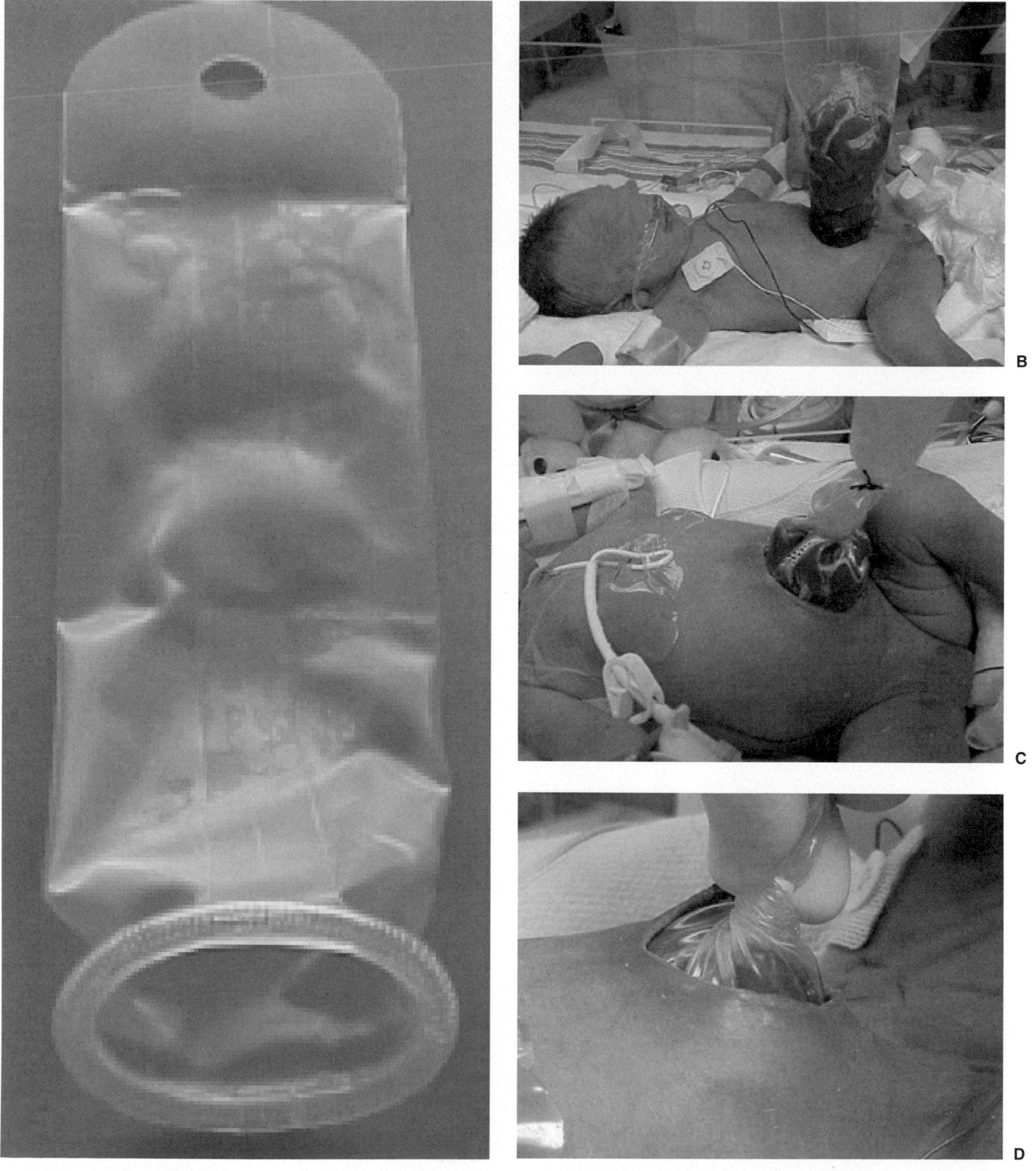

FIGURE 69-6. **(A)** Preformed transparent Silastic silo. **(B)** The intestine has been placed into the sac and the ring placed within the abdominal cavity. **(C)** Gradual reduction of the silo. Note central line for total parenteral nutrition. **(D)** Final reduction.

of the bowel. Umbilical tapes are used to reduce the sac and may be easily removed if the bowel becomes dusky.

Complications

Problems that can be seen in both primary and staged repairs include decreased venous return and an abdominal compartment syndrome. The major direct consequence of too tight a closure is an abnormally elevated intraabdominal pressure. This can cause renal failure, necrotizing enterocolitis, bowel perforation, and worsening respiratory failure. Elevation of abdominal pressure results in decreased venous return, decreased cardiac output, increased pulmonary compliance, decreased ventilation, and decreased splanchnic perfusion. Several methods to determine whether the closure is too tight exist. The findings of increased respiratory rate, decreased lower extremity perfusion, and low urine output may be appreciated. Monitoring central venous pressure, intragastric pressure, urinary bladder pressure, end-tidal carbon dioxide, ventilator pressure, and gastric tonometry have been used as means to assess intraabdominal pressure and predict safe closure. An intraabdominal pressure of less than 20 mm Hg as measured by intragastric or urinary catheters or an elevation in central venous pressure of less than 4 mm Hg is associated with successful closure (83–86). An elevation of end-tidal carbon dioxide greater than 50 mm Hg (87) or an elevation of peak airway pressure greater than 25 cm H_2O is associated with problems with the primary closure. Prompt reduction in intraabdominal pressure is mandatory. This may mean silo placement if a primary repair was performed, or allowing some of the viscera to come back into the silo if a silo was placed. If the silo was removed for a second-stage closure, this wound may need to be reopened and Silastic sheet placed across the fascia.

Advantages of a Preformed, Transparent Silo

There appears to be several advantages with this type of silo. The placement of the silo is simple and can be done in the NICU or even in the delivery room under controlled, sterile conditions. General anesthesia or sedation is not routinely required. The transparent nature of the bag permits continuous inspection of the bowel. In addition, the umbilical tapes can be removed if the bowel becomes ischemic, systemic perfusion becomes compromised, or ventilation becomes difficult following reduction. The use of a preformed silo and elective closure decreases manipulation of the intestine and eliminates forceful reduction, appearing to obviate the need for intraoperative measures of intragastric, bladder, or central venous pressures as advocates by some surgeons. Arterial catheters for monitoring are rarely needed because these children typically are not intubated. In addition, a peripherally placed intravenous central catheter (PICC) can be placed at the bedside, avoiding the need for a surgical line in many instances. More recent reports have demonstrated that the routine use of a preformed silo is associated with decreased trauma to the fascia and decreased operative time when compared with Silastic silo formation, improved fascial closure rates, lower ventilatory pressures, fewer days on the ventilator, and fewer complications when compared with initial primary closure (76,79,81, 88–91). Potential problems associated with the use of a preformed silo include silo dislodgement and a widening of the defect, which can make fascial closure more difficult.

Management of Intestinal Atresia and Bowel Ischemia

Intestinal atresia is noted in approximately 8% to 10% of infants with gastroschisis. In some cases, it is obvious due to a very small fascial defect or if there is an obvious mesenteric defect. In other cases, it may be hard to identify due to the degree of serositis and bowel wall thickening. A significant size discrepancy between contiguous segments of bowel can often make one quite suspicious of this diagnosis. Atresia can involve the small and large bowel and may be multiple. Management is individualized. A proximal atresia is often treated by nasogastric drainage, closure of the abdominal wall defect, and repair of the atresia after the serositis has resolved. This usually takes 6 to 8 weeks for the serositis to resolve. A distal atresia is more difficult to keep decompressed. Formation of a stoma at the point of atresia often allows decompression of the intestine, primary abdominal wall closure, and possibly the initiation of enteral feedings in several weeks. Stoma takedown and repair of the atresia is performed 6 to 8 weeks later.

A subset of children with gastroschisis have impaired intestinal peristalsis. However, one normally expects coordinated peristalsis to occur by several weeks after abdominal wall closure. If this is not seen, the possibility of an associated intestinal atresia should be entertained. A contrast enema is the diagnostic procedure of choice.

On occasion, bowel ischemia is noted in patients with gastroschisis. This is particularly true with a narrow silo in place and in other cases of a forced abdominal closure. If the bowel is ischemic, reducing the intraabdominal pressure is of significant benefit. In some cases, particularly those where there is a narrow silo at the base, widening of the fascial defect is efficacious. If there is obvious intestinal necrosis, treatment requires resection and stoma formation.

Management of Undescended Testis

Undescended testis is occasionally found in males with gastroschisis. The testis may be intraabdominal or prolapsed through the fascial defect. The majority of testes will descend normally when replaced into the peritoneal cavity. Those that do not descend can be safely treated with an orchiopexy at a later time (41,42).

Omphalocele

Specific considerations for omphalocele relate to a close examination for the integrity of the sac and a search for associated anomalies. Typically, initial evaluation of these infants include evaluation for a cardiac murmur, evidence of cyanosis, a chest X-ray, cardiac echo, and renal ultrasound. Consideration of associated anomalies has priority over surgical repair unless there is disruption of the sac and evisceration. Pulmonary hypoplasia or other factors may be significant and preclude immediate surgical closure of large and giant omphaloceles. In those circumstances, the omphalocele is treated with a topical bacteriocidal agent to induce formation of an eschar and eventual epithelialization. Escharotic agents should be chosen carefully because several used in the past were associated with systemic absorption and significant toxicity. Current agents used include silver sulfadiazine cream, povidone-iodine solution, and triiodomethane-petroleum gauze. Iodinated agents may produce thyroid suppression (92–94).

Small and medium-size defects can usually be closed primarily. Pressure monitoring, using the principles described for gastroschisis, may be needed to prevent large increases in intraabdominal pressure and subsequent cardiopulmonary compromise. Patients are intubated and paralyzed for the procedure. Ventilation and paralysis may be used postoperatively. In general, attempts are made to remove the sac. With larger defects, the sac may be adherent to the liver and preclude removal. Care must be taken not to injure the liver. If the sac is removed, the umbilical vessels should be identified and ligated individually. When primary closure is possible, skin flaps are elevated from the fascia. Interrupted sutures are placed in the fascia and sequentially tied, and the skin is closed. A neoumbilicus can be created.

The surgical management of infants with large and giant omphaloceles poses a greater challenge. Treatment options include short-term silo reduction, which may take up to 2 weeks, followed by fascial closure or closure with prosthetic material, long-term silo reduction over 2 to 6 weeks followed by closure, or a staged reduction closing skin flaps over the amnion, followed by delayed closure of the ventral hernia at 6 to 12 months of age (Fig. 69-7). External compression techniques prior to repair may facilitate delayed closure (95–97).

Figure 69-8 demonstrates the coverage and repair for a giant omphalocele. A Dacron reinforced Silastic membrane sheet, GoreTex or Alloderm, is attached to the fascial edges and closed in the midline. Aggressive mobilization of the fascia is not performed and the amniotic membrane may be left in situ. Tightening the midportion of the silo progressively reduces the abdominal contents. Several techniques and materials have been described for silo reduction. The most common are the use of stapling devices or suture techniques. The base of the silo must be inspected for disruption from the fascia.

Postoperative Management and Complications

The initial postoperative management centers on the need for respiratory support, nutritional support, and wound care. TPN is needed for most infants, and a PICC or central line is placed. Paralysis and heavy sedation may be used to aid in ventilatory support and prevent increases in intraabdominal pressure. Prolonged paralysis may cause generalized edema and produce deleterious effects. It is common to see abdominal wall erythema postoperatively, and antibiotics are continued until the erythema resolves. The wound and abdominal wall must be inspected frequently for evidence of cellulitis or fasciitis. Gastric decompression is maintained in the postoperative period.

Poor intestinal motility and absorption are common in infants with gastroschisis. Signs of bowel function, as evidenced by a decrease in the volume and clearing of the gastric aspirate and bowel movements, suggest that enteral feeds can be initiated. A more recent report has suggested that early enteral feeds are associated with improved outcome (98). A major source of morbidity and mortality in these infants is related to the use of TPN. Central line infections are not uncommon, especially when TPN is needed long term. TPN-associated cholestasis causes jaundice, cirrhosis, and may lead to liver failure, which may be fatal. Liver transplantation may be an option for these infants.

The duration of postoperative mechanical ventilation varies. Most infants with gastroschisis can be weaned and extubated within the first few days postoperatively. Infants with large or giant omphaloceles, especially those with associated pulmonary hypoplasia require long-term ventilation.

Failure to achieve abdominal closure in infants with constructed silos within 2 weeks is associated with increased risk of infectious and mechanical complications (95,96,99–101).

Postoperative Necrotizing Enterocolitis, Intestinal Perforation, and Obstruction

The incidence of necrotizing enterocolitis following repair for gastroschisis has been reported to be as high as 18.5%,

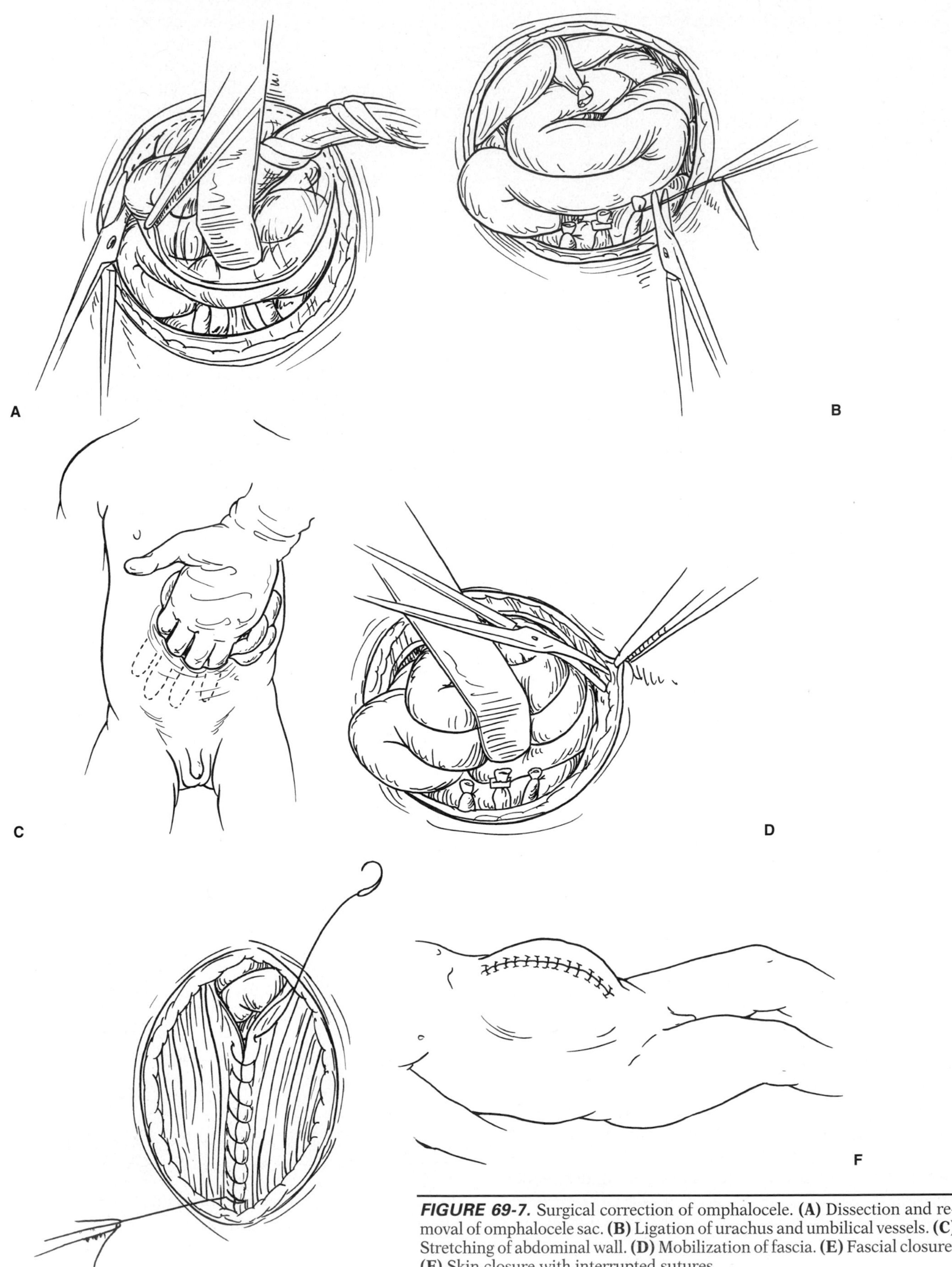

FIGURE 69-7. Surgical correction of omphalocele. **(A)** Dissection and removal of omphalocele sac. **(B)** Ligation of urachus and umbilical vessels. **(C)** Stretching of abdominal wall. **(D)** Mobilization of fascia. **(E)** Fascial closure. **(F)** Skin closure with interrupted sutures.

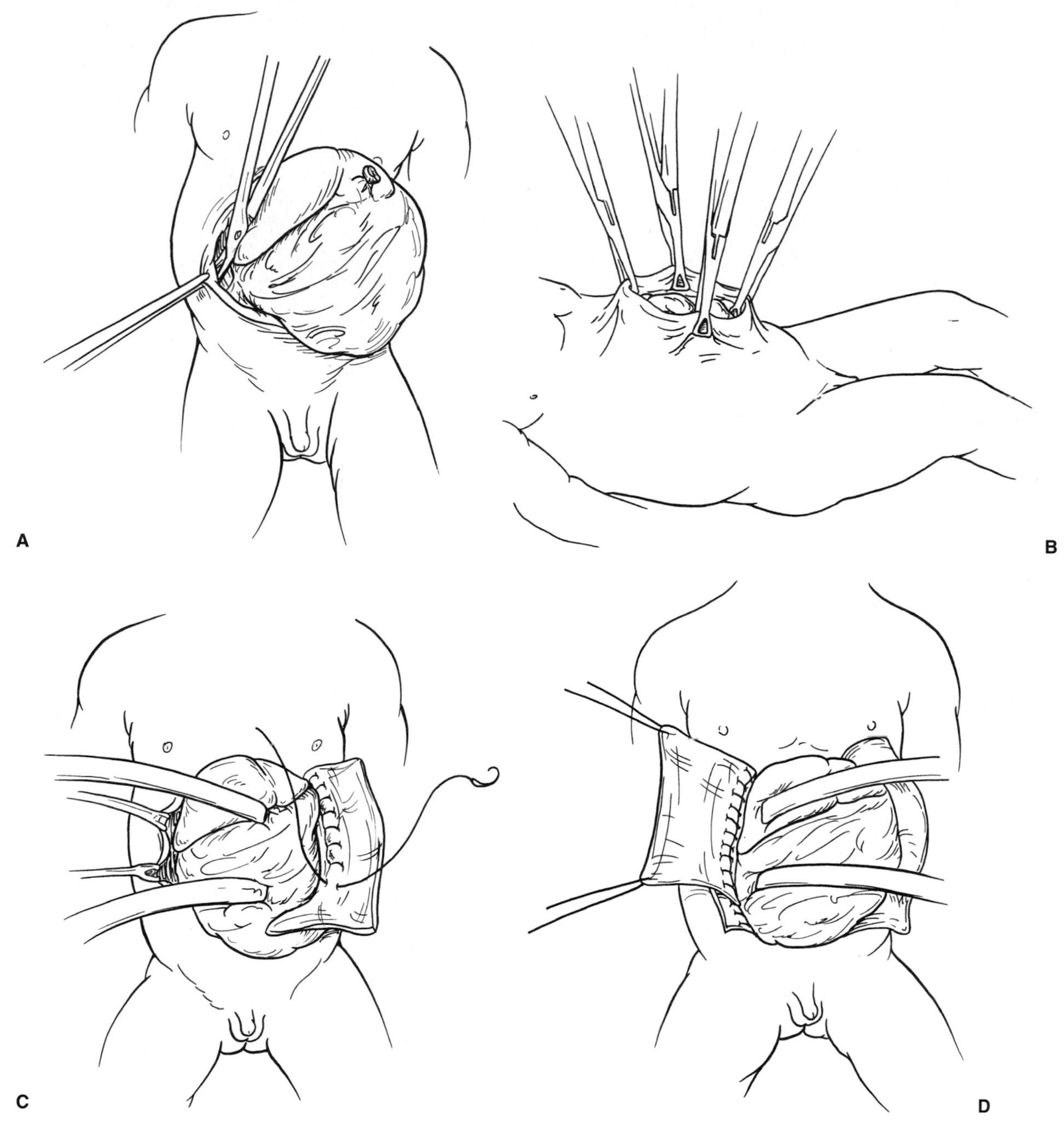

FIGURE 69-8. Surgical management of large (giant) omphalocele. **(A)** Dissection and removal of omphalocele sac. **(B)** Stretching and extension of abdominal wall. **(C)** Application of Goretex patch to left abdominal wall. **(D)** Application of patch to right abdominal wall. *(continued)*

and typically occurs several weeks after closure. Delayed enteral feedings, TPN-associated cholestasis, and other intestinal anomalies such as atresia are associated with the development of necrotizing enterocolitis. The form of necrotizing enterocolitis in these infants appears to be more benign, and operative intervention is unusual in the acute setting. Early intestinal perforations are also well described and are believed to be associated with aggressive reduction to achieve primary closure.

Small bowel obstructions resulting from adhesions, strictures, stenotic anastomoses, or complications from malrotation may be observed. Unless there is bowel compromise, the symptoms may be subtle, and diagnosis is often not easily distinguishable from the feeding intolerance that is usually observed in these infants. The use of water-soluble contrast studies may facilitate the diagnosis. However, multiple studies may be needed before the diagnosis is confirmed. Progressive bowel dilation or failure to

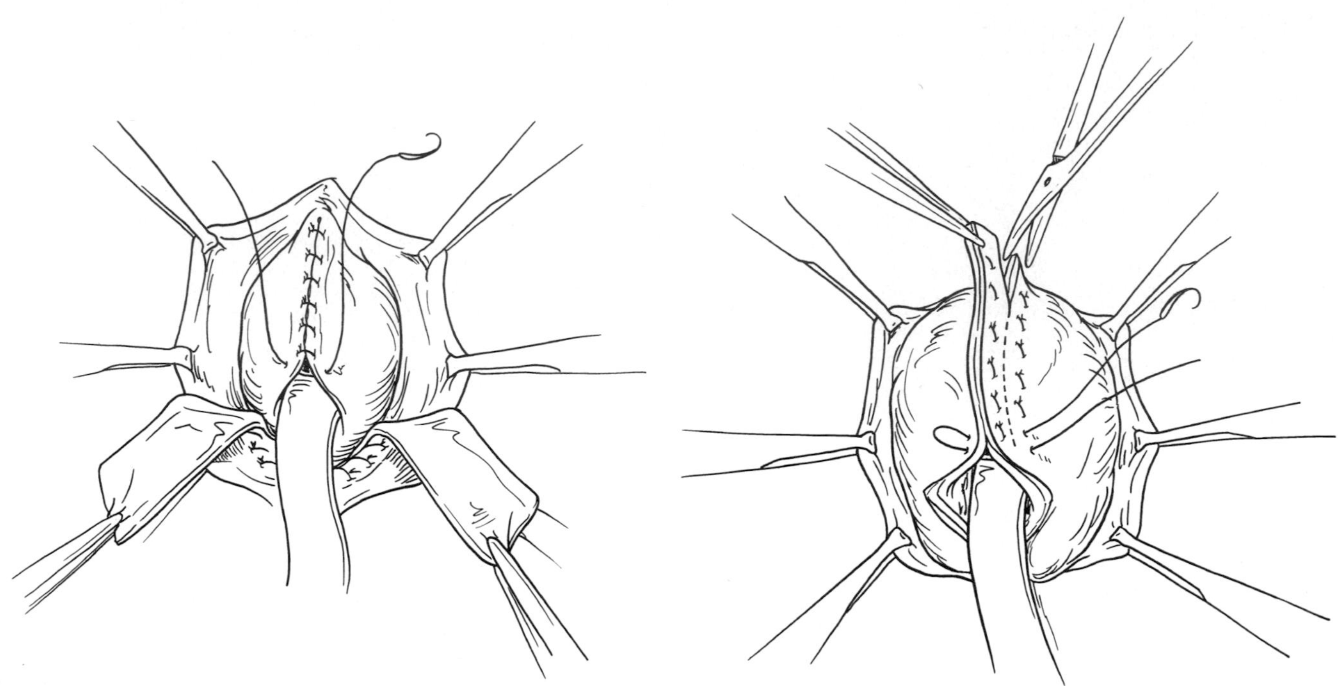

FIGURE 69-8. *Continued* **(E)** Approximation and creation of GorTex silo. **(F)** Secondary shortening of silo and staged closure of abdominal wall.

advance feeds after several weeks may suggest the presence of a mechanical obstruction. Infants with gastroschisis can develop severe malabsorption or short-gut syndrome and require small bowel transplantation for survival (102).

Outcome

The prognosis for infants undergoing surgical repair of abdominal wall defects is good in contemporary practices. Outcome following repair of abdominal wall defects not associated with other anomalies is excellent. However, concerns of short-gut syndrome, respiratory compromise, and developmental delay require continued attention. There are clearly high- and low-risk groups for both gastroschisis and omphalocele (103). The outcome of patients with omphalocele largely depends on the severity of associated anomalies. The mortality for patients with omphalocele is increased significantly when associated with chromosomal syndromes or a cardiac defect (104). Similarly, giant omphaloceles and those associated with pulmonary hypoplasia have a worse outcome.

A more recent report separated gastroschisis patients into risk groups based on the presence of intestinal defects (103). The high-risk or complex group included infants with intestinal atresia, perforation, necrotic segments, or volvulus, whereas the low-risk or simple group had no intestinal anomalies. The high-risk, complex group had increased morbidity and mortality characterized by longer periods of mechanical ventilation; longer ileus; and time to tolerate full feeds, longer length of stay, and an increased complication and mortality rate. Ventral hernias are common following repair of abdominal wall defects, and surgery may be needed for gastroesophageal reflux disease.

There have been recent reports summarizing the long-term outcome of survivors following surgery for abdominal wall defects. Although there have been reports suggesting that survivors may have congnitive or growth problems, the majority of children with isolated abdominal wall defects attend mainstream schools and have normal mental development (105,106). Although most adults report satisfactory health, some report poor stamina and inadequacy at sports (107,108). A study of 28 patients demonstrated that 7 patients were sedentary and 21 participated in recreational sports (109). A more recent study evaluating the cardiopulmonary performance of children and adolescents born with large abdominal wall defects demonstrated normal cardiopulmonary function, except for a decrease in exercise tolerance and maximal oxygen consumption (110). There were no differences noted in cardiorespiratory function as expressed by heart rate, blood pressure, and forced vital capacity, and the authors concluded that the decreased exercise tolerance was related to a lack of physical activity. The reason for sports abstinence in these patients was reported to be parental or physician's advice. The authors concluded that there should be no limitations to regular social and sports participation. Education of parents and primary physicians is imperative in this regard (110). A more recent survey of 75 adult survivors in Finland demonstrate the most frequent cause of morbidity to be related to the abdominal scar, gastrointestinal disorders, and low self-esteem; however, these rarely caused serious problems (111). There were no differences in quality-of-life assessment and educational level from the general population.

REFERENCES

1. Langer JC. Abdominal wall defects. *World J Surg* 2003;27:117–124.
2. Vermeij-Keers C, Hartwig NG, van der Werff JF. Embryonic development of the ventral body wall and its congenital malformations. *Semin Pediatr Surg* 1996;5:82–89.
3. Robinson JN, Abuhamad AZ. Abdominal wall and umbilical cord anomalies. *Clin Perinatol* 2000;27:947–978, ix.
4. deVries PA. The pathogenesis of gastroschisis and omphalocele. *J Pediatr Surg* 1980;15:245–251.
5. Hoyme HE, Jones MC, Jones KL. Gastroschisis: abdominal wall disruption secondary to early gestational interruption of the omphalomesenteric artery. *Semin Perinatol* 1983;7:294–298.
6. Glick PL, Harrison MR, Adzick NS, et al. The missing link in the pathogenesis of gastroschisis. *J Pediatr Surg* 1985;20:406–409.
7. Stringel G, Filler RM. Prognostic factors in omphalocele and gastroschisis. *J Pediatr Surg* 1979;14:515–519.
8. Nagao T, Saitoh Y, Yoshimura S. Possible mechanism of congenital malformations induced by exposure of mouse preimplantation embryos to mitomycin C. *Teratology* 2000;61:248–261.
9. Botto LD, Mulinarc J, Erickson JD. Occurrence of omphalocele in relation to maternal multivitamin use: a population-based study. *Pediatrics* 2002;109:904–908.
10. Torfs CP, Katz EA, Bateson TF, et al. Maternal medications and environmental exposures as risk factors for gastroschisis. *Teratology* 1996;54:84–92.
11. Werler MM, Mitchell AA, Shapiro S. First trimester maternal medication use in relation to gastroschisis. *Teratology* 1992;45:361–367.
12. Drongowski RA, Smith RK Jr, Coran AG, et al. Contribution of demographic and environmental factors to the etiology of gastroschisis: a hypothesis. *Fetal Diagn Ther* 1991;6:14–27.
13. Martinez-Frias ML, Rodriguez-Pinilla E, Prieto L. Prenatal exposure to salicylates and gastroschisis: a case-control study. *Teratology* 1997;56:241–243.
14. Werler MM, Sheehan JE, Mitchell AA. Association of vasoconstrictive exposures with risks of gastroschisis and small intestinal atresia. *Epidemiology* 2003;14:349–354.
15. Chun K, Andrews HG, White JJ. Gastroschisis in successive siblings: further evidence of an acquired etiology. *J Pediatr Surg* 1993;28:838–839.
16. Torfs CP, Velie EM, Oechsli FW, et al. A population-based study of gastroschisis: demographic, pregnancy, and lifestyle risk factors. *Teratology* 1994;50:44–53.
17. Wakefield MR, Steinbecker KM, Krambeck AE, et al. Primary surgical repair of combined gastroschisis and bladder exstrophy. *J Pediatr Surg* 2002;37:1634–1636.
18. Martin ML, Khoury MJ, Cordero JF, et al. Trends in rates of multiple vascular disruption defects, Atlanta, 1968–1989: is there evidence of a cocaine teratogenic epidemic? *Teratology* 1992;45:647–653.
19. Viscarello RR, Ferguson DD, Nores J, et al. Limb-body wall complex associated with cocaine abuse: further evidence of cocaine's teratogenicity. *Obstet Gynecol* 1992;80:523–526.
20. DiLiberti JH. Familial omphalocele: analysis of risk factors and case report. *Am J Med Genet* 1982;13:263–268.
21. Viot G, Pannier E, Faivre L, et al. A new case of exomphalos, short limbs, and macrogonadism syndrome. *J Med Genet* 2001;38:E8.
22. Keppler-Noreuil KM. OEIS complex (omphalocele-exstrophy-imperforate anus-spinal defects): a review of 14 cases. *Am J Med Genet* 2001;99:271–279.
23. Hipolito R, Haight M, Dubois J, et al. Gastroschisis and Hirschsprung's disease: a rare combination. *J Pediatr Surg* 2001;36:638–640.
24. Kilic N, Kiristioglu I, Balkan E, et al. Oromandibular limb hypogenesis and gastroschisis. *J Pediatr Surg* 2001;36:E15.
25. Hillebrandt S, Matern S, Lammert F. Mouse models for genetic dissection of polygenic gastrointestinal diseases. *Eur J Clin Invest* 2003;33:155–60.
26. Hillebrandt S, Streffer C, Muller WU. Genetic analysis of the cause of gastroschisis in the HLG mouse strain. *Mutat Res* 1996;372:43–51.
27. Baatout S, Jacquet P, Michaux A, et al. Developmental abnormalities induced by X-irradiation in p53 deficient mice. *In Vivo* 2002;16:215–221.
28. Komuro H, Mori M, Hayashi Y, et al. Mutational analysis of the BMP-1 gene in patients with gastroschisis. *J Pediatr Surg* 2001;36:885–887.
29. Di Tanna GL, Rosano A, Mastroiacovo P. Prevalence of gastroschisis at birth: retrospective study. *BMJ* 2002;325:1389–1390.
30. Laughon M, Meyer R, Bose C, et al. Rising birth prevalence of gastroschisis. *J Perinatol* 2003;23:291–293.
31. Baerg J, Kaban G, Tonita J, et al. Gastroschisis: a sixteen-year review. *J Pediatr Surg* 2003;38:771–774.
32. McDonnell R, Delany V, Dack P, et al. Changing trend in congenital abdominal wall defects in eastern region of Ireland. *Ir Med J* 2002;95:236, 238.
33. Moore TC. Gastroschisis and omphalocele: clinical differences. *Surgery* 1977;82:561–568.
34. Venugopal S, Zachary RB, Spitz L. Exomphalos and gastroschisis: a 10-year review. *Br J Surg* 1976;63:523–525.
35. Lindham S. Omphalocele and gastroschisis in Sweden 1965–1976. *Acta Paediatr Scand* 1981;70:55–60.
36. Chen CP, Liu FF, Jan SW, et al. Prenatal diagnosis and perinatal aspects of abdominal wall defects. *Am J Perinatol* 1996;13:355–361.
37. Greenwood RD, Rosenthal A, Nadas AS. Cardiovascular malformations associated with omphalocele. *J Pediatr* 1974;85:818–8121.
38. Nicolaides KH, Snijders RJ, Cheng HH, et al. Fetal gastro-intestinal and abdominal wall defects: associated malformations and chromosomal abnormalities. *Fetal Diagn Ther* 1992;7:102–115.
39. Nyberg DA, Fitzsimmons J, Mack LA, et al. Chromosomal abnormalities in fetuses with omphalocele. Significance of omphalocele contents. *J Ultrasound Med* 1989;8:299–308.
40. Benacerraf BR, Saltzman DH, Estroff JA, et al. Abnormal karyotype of fetuses with omphalocele: prediction based on omphalocele contents. *Obstet Gynecol* 1990;75:317–319.
41. Lawson A, de La Hunt MN. Gastroschisis and undescended testis. *J Pediatr Surg* 2001;36:366–367.
42. Chowdhary SK, Lander AD, Buick RG, et al. The primary management of testicular maldescent in gastroschisis. *Pediatr Surg Int* 2001;17:359–360.
43. Levard G, Laberge JM. The fate of undescended testes in patients with gastroschisis. *Eur J Pediatr Surg* 1997;7:163–165.
44. Hoyme HE, Higginbottom MC, Jones KL. The vascular pathogenesis of gastroschisis: intrauterine interruption of the omphalomesenteric artery. *J Pediatr* 1981;98:228–231.
45. Luck SR, Sherman JO, Raffensperger JG, et al. Gastroschisis in 106 consecutive newborn infants. *Surgery* 1985;98:677–683.
46. Adair CD, Rosnes J, Frye AH, et al. The role of antepartum surveillance in the management of gastroschisis. *Int J Gynaecol Obstet* 1996;52:141–144.
47. Luton D, De Lagausie P, Guibourdenche J, et al. Prognostic factors of prenatally diagnosed gastroschisis. *Fetal Diagn Ther* 1997;12:7–14.
48. Correia-Pinto J, Tavares ML, Baptista MJ, et al. Meconium dependence of bowel damage in gastroschisis. *J Pediatr Surg* 2002;37:31–35.
49. Kluck P, Tibboel D, van der Kamp AW, et al. The effect of fetal urine on the development of the bowel in gastroschisis. *J Pediatr Surg* 1983;18:47–50.
50. Aktug T, Erdag G, Kargi A, et al. Amnio-allantoic fluid exchange for the prevention of intestinal damage in gastroschisis: an experimental study on chick embryos. *J Pediatr Surg* 1995;30:384–387.

51. Shaw K, Buchmiller TL, Curr M, et al. Impairment of nutrient uptake in a rabbit model of gastroschisis. *J Pediatr Surg* 1994;29:376–378.
52. Langer JC, Bell JG, Castillo RO, et al. Etiology of intestinal damage in gastroschisis, II. Timing and reversibility of histological changes, mucosal function, and contractility. *J Pediatr Surg* 1990;25:1122–1126.
53. Srinathan SK, Langer JC, Wang JL, et al. Enterocytic gene expression is altered in experimental gastroschisis. *J Surg Res* 1997;68:1–6.
54. Srinathan SK, Langer JC, Botney MD, et al. Submucosal collagen in experimental gastroschisis. *J Surg Res* 1996;65:25–30.
55. Langer JC, Longaker MT, Crombleholme TM, et al. Etiology of intestinal damage in gastroschisis. I: effects of amniotic fluid exposure and bowel constriction in a fetal lamb model. *J Pediatr Surg* 1989;24:992–997.
56. Srinathan SK, Langer JC, Blennerhassett MG, et al. Etiology of intestinal damage in gastroschisis. III: morphometric analysis of the smooth muscle and submucosa. *J Pediatr Surg* 1995;30:379–383.
57. Langer JC. Fetal abdominal wall defects. *Semin Pediatr Surg* 1993;2:121–128.
58. Haller JA Jr, Kehrer BH, Shaker IJ, et al. Studies of the pathophysiology of gastroschisis in fetal sheep. *J Pediatr Surg* 1974;9:627–632.
59. Tibboel D, Kluck P, van der Kamp AW, et al. The development of the characteristic anomalies found in gastroschisis—experimental and clinical data. *Z Kinderchir* 1985;40:355–360.
60. Amoury RA, Beatty EC, Wood WG, et al. Histology of the intestine in human gastroschisis—relationship to intestinal malfunction: dissolution of the "peel" and its ultrastructural characteristics. *J Pediatr Surg* 1988;23:950–956.
61. Smrcek JM, Germer U, Krokowski M, et al. Prenatal ultrasound diagnosis and management of body stalk anomaly: analysis of nine singleton and two multiple pregnancies. *Ultrasound Obstet Gynecol* 2003;21:322–328.
62. Song A, McLeary MS. MR imaging of pentalogy of Cantrell variant with an intact diaphragm and pericardium. *Pediatr Radiol* 2000;30:638–639.
63. Dell'Acqua A, Mengozzi E, Rizzo F, et al. Ultrafast MR imaging of the foetus: a study of 25 non-central nervous system anomalies. *Radiol Med (Torino)* 2002;104:75–86.
64. Saguintaah M, Couture A, Veyrac C, et al. MRI of the fetal gastrointestinal tract. *Pediatr Radiol* 2002;32:395–404.
65. Verswijvel G, Gyselaers W, Grieten M, et al. Omphalocele: prenatal MR findings. *Jbr-Btr* 2002;85:200–202.
66. Hormann M, Pumberger W, Scharitzer M, et al. [MR imaging in congenital complicated anterior body wall defects]. *Rofo Fortschr Geb Rontgenstr Neuen Bildgeb Verfahr* 2003;175:536–539.
67. Aite L, Trucchi A, Nahom A, et al. Multidisciplinary management of fetal surgical anomalies: the impact on maternal anxiety. *Eur J Pediatr Surg* 2002;12:90–94.
68. Carpenter MW, Curci MR, Dibbins AW, et al. Perinatal management of ventral wall defects. *Obstet Gynecol* 1984;64:646–651.
69. Lenke RR, Hatch EI Jr. Fetal gastroschisis: a preliminary report advocating the use of cesarean section. *Obstet Gynecol* 1986;67:395–398.
70. Fitzsimmons J, Nyberg DA, Cyr DR, et al. Perinatal management of gastroschisis. *Obstet Gynecol* 1988;71:910–913.
71. Moore TC, Collins DL, Catanzarite V, et al. Pre-term and particularly pre-labor cesarean section to avoid complications of gastroschisis. *Pediatr Surg Int* 1999;15:97–104.
72. Sakala EP, Erhard LN, White JJ. Elective cesarean section improves outcomes of neonates with gastroschisis. *Am J Obstet Gynecol* 1993;169:1050–1053.
73. Huang J, Kurkchubasche AG, Carr SR, et al. Benefits of term delivery in infants with antenatally diagnosed gastroschisis. *Obstet Gynecol* 2002;100:695–699.
74. Langer JC, Khanna J, Caco C, et al. Prenatal diagnosis of gastroschisis: development of objective sonographic criteria for predicting outcome. *Obstet Gynecol* 1993;81:53–56.
75. Coughlin JP, Drucker DE, Jewell MR, et al. Delivery room repair of gastroschisis. *Surgery* 1993;114:822–826; discussion 826–827.
76. Minkes RK, Langer JC, Mazziotti MV, et al. Routine insertion of a silastic spring-loaded silo for infants with gastroschisis. *J Pediatr Surg* 2000;35:843–846.
77. Cameron GM, McQuown DS, Modanlou HD, et al. Intrauterine diagnosis of an omphalocele by diagnostic ultrasonography. *Am J Obstet Gynecol* 1978;131:821–822.
78. Hasan S, Hermansen MC. The prenatal diagnosis of ventral abdominal wall defects. *Am J Obstet Gynecol* 1986;155:842–845.
79. Fischer JD, Chun K, Moores DC, et al. Gastroschisis: a simple technique for staged silo closure. *J Pediatr Surg* 1995;30:1169–1171.
80. Bianchi A, Dickson AP, Alizai NK. Elective delayed midgut reduction-No anesthesia for gastroschisis: Selection and conversion criteria. *J Pediatr Surg* 2002;37:1334–1336.
81. Jona JZ. The 'gentle touch' technique in the treatment of gastroschisis. *J Pediatr Surg* 2003;38:1036–1038.
82. Bianchi A, Dickson AP. Elective delayed reduction and no anesthesia: 'minimal intervention management' for gastrochisis. *J Pediatr Surg* 1998;33:1338–1340.
83. Yaster M, Scherer TL, Stone MM, et al. Prediction of successful primary closure of congenital abdominal wall defects using intraoperative measurements. *J Pediatr Surg* 1989;24:1217–1220.
84. Wesley JR, Drongowski R, Coran AG. Intragastric pressure measurement: a guide for reduction and closure of the silastic chimney in omphalocele and gastroschisis. *J Pediatr Surg* 1981;16:264–270.
85. Lacey SR, Carris LA, Beyer AJ III, et al. Bladder pressure monitoring significantly enhances care of infants with abdominal wall defects: a prospective clinical study. *J Pediatr Surg* 1993;28:1370–1374; discussion 1374–1375.
86. Rizzo A, Davis PC, Hamm CR, et al. Intraoperative vesical pressure measurements as a guide in the closure of abdominal wall defects. *Am J Surg* 1996;62:192–196.
87. Puffinbarger NK, Taylor DV, Tuggle DW, et al. End-tidal carbon dioxide for monitoring primary closure of gastroschisis. *J Pediatr Surg* 1996;31:280–282.
88. Schlatter M, Norris K, Uitvlugt N, et al. Improved outcomes in the treatment of gastroschisis using a preformed silo and delayed repair approach. *J Pediatr Surg* 2003;38:459–464.
89. Schlatter M. Preformed silos in the management of gastroschisis: new progress with an old idea. *Curr Opin Pediatr* 2003;15:239–242.
90. Kidd JN, Levy MS, Wagner CW. Staged reduction of gastroschisis: a simple method. *Pediatr Surg Int* 2001;17:242–244.
91. Kidd JN Jr, Jackson RJ, Smith SD, et al. Evolution of staged versus primary closure of gastroschisis. *Ann Surg* 2003;237:759–764; discussion 764–765.
92. Hatch EI Jr, Baxter R. Surgical options in the management of large omphaloceles. *Am J Surg* 1987;153:449–452.
93. Adam AS, Corbally MT, Fitzgerald RJ. Evaluation of conservative therapy for exomphalos. *Surg Gynecol Obstet* 1991;172:394–396.
94. Nuchtern JG, Baxter R, Hatch EI Jr. Nonoperative initial management versus silon chimney for treatment of giant omphalocele. *J Pediatr Surg* 1995;30:771–776.
95. Yazbeck S. The giant omphalocele: a new approach for a rapid and complete closure. *J Pediatr Surg* 1986;21:715–717.
96. DeLuca FG, Gilchrist BF, Paquette E, et al. External compression as initial management of giant omphaloceles. *J Pediatr Surg* 1996;31:965–967.
97. Sander S, Elicevik M, Unal M. Elastic bandaging facilitates primary closure of large ventral hernias due to giant omphaloceles. *Pediatr Surg Int* 2001;17:664–667.
98. Singh SJ, Fraser A, Leditschke JF, et al. Gastroschisis: determinants of neonatal outcome. *Pediatr Surg Int* 2003;19:260–265.
99. Ein SH, Rubin SZ. Gastroschisis: primary closure or Silon pouch. *J Pediatr Surg* 1980;15:549–552.
100. Swartz KR, Harrison MW, Campbell JR, et al. Ventral hernia in the treatment of omphalocele and gastroschisis. *Ann Surg* 1985;201:347–350.
101. Schwartz MZ, Tyson KR, Milliorn K, et al. Staged reduction using a Silastic sac is the treatment of choice for large congenital abdominal wall defects. *J Pediatr Surg* 1983;18:713–719.

102. Nishida S, Levi D, Kato T, et al. Ninety-five cases of intestinal transplantation at the University of Miami. *J Gastrointest Surg* 2002;6:233–239.
103. Molik KA, Gingalewski CA, West KW, et al. Gastroschisis: a plea for risk categorization. *J Pediatr Surg* 2001;36:51–55.
104. Hughes MD, Nyberg DA, Mack LA, et al. Fetal omphalocele: prenatal US detection of concurrent anomalies and other predictors of outcome. *Radiology* 1989;173:371–376.
105. Boyd PA, Bhattacharjee A, Gould S, et al. Outcome of prenatally diagnosed anterior abdominal wall defects. *Arch Dis Child Fetal Neonatal Ed* 1998;78:F209–F213.
106. Lunzer H, Menardi G, Brezinka C. Long-term follow-up of children with prenatally diagnosed omphalocele and gastroschisis. *J Matern Fetal Med* 2001;10:385–392.
107. Tunell WP, Puffinbarger NK, Tuggle DW, et al. Abdominal wall defects in infants. Survival and implications for adult life. *Ann Surg* 1995;221:525–528; discussion 528–530.
108. Davies BW, Stringer MD. The survivors of gastroschisis. *Arch Dis Child* 1997;77:158–160.
109. Clausner A, Lukowitz A, Rump K, et al. Treatment of congenital abdominal wall defects. A 25 year review of 132 patients. *Pediatr Surg Int* 1996;11:76–81.
110. Zaccara A, Iacobelli BD, Calzolari A, et al. Cardiopulmonary perfomances in young children and adolescents born with large abdominal wall defects. *J Pediatr Surg* 2003;38:478–481.
111. Koivusalo A, Lindahl H, Rintala RJ. Morbidity and quality of life in adult patients with a congenital abdominal wall defect: a questionnaire survey. *J Pediatr Surg* 2002;37:1594–1601.

Bladder/Cloacal Exstrophy, and Prune Belly Syndrome

John P. Gearhart and Dominic Frimberger

BLADDER EXSTROPHY

Incidence

The incidence of bladder exstrophy has been estimated between 1 in 10,000 and 1 in 50,000 live births (1,2). However, data from the International Clearinghouse for Birth Defects monitoring system estimated the incidence to be 3.3 per 100,000 live births (3). A 5:1 to 6:1 ratio of male-to-female rate exists (1).

Embryology

Mesodermal ingrowth between the ectoderm and endodermal layers of the bilaminar cloacal membrane results in formation of the lower abdominal musculature and pelvic bones. After mesenchymal ingrowth occurs, downward growth of the rectal septum divides the cloaca into a bladder anteriorly and a rectum posteriorly. The genital tubercles migrate medially and fuse in the midline cephalad to the dorsal membrane before it perforates. The cloacal membrane is subject to premature rupture, depending on the extent of the infraumbilical defect. The stage of development when the membrane rupture occurs determines whether bladder exstrophy, cloacal exstrophy, or epispadias results (4).

The most likely theory of embryonic development in exstrophy describes the basic defect as an abnormal lower overdevelopment of the cloacal membrane, preventing medial migration of the mesenchymal tissue, and therefore, proper abdominal wall development (5). The timing of the rupture of this cloacal defect determines the severity of the disorder. The highest incidence with 60% is central perforations resulting in classic exstrophy, where 30% have exstrophy variants and 10% cloacal exstrophy.

Other theories have been offered concerning the cause of the exstrophy-epispadias complex. These include (1) abnormal development of the genital hillocks, with fusion in the midline below rather than above the cloacal membrane; (2) abnormal caudal insertion of the body stalk, with failure of the interposition of the mesenchymal tissue in the midline so translocation of the cloaca into the depths of the abdominal cavity does not occur; or (3) a cloacal membrane that remains in a superficial infraumbilical position, and remains in an unstable embryonic state with a strong tendency to disintegrate (4,6,7).

Predisposing Factors

Some evidence exists for genetic predisposition of exstrophy and epispadias. The risk for recurrence of bladder exstrophy and epispadias in any given family is 1 in 275 births (8). The likelihood of an exstrophic parent producing a child with exstrophy is about 1 in 70, or 500 times the risk of the general population. More recent data have shown a sevenfold increase in exstrophy and cloacal exstrophy associated with the use of assisted reproductive technology such as introcystoplasmic sperm injection (9).

Prenatal Diagnosis

Exstrophy of the bladder is rarely diagnosed by prenatal ultrasound. The main criteria for the prenatal diagnosis of exstrophy includes absence of bladder filling; lower abdominal mass, which becomes more protuberant as the pregnancy proceeds; a low-set umbilicus; normal scrotum; separation of the pubic rami; and difficulties determining the sex of the baby. In addition to these data, bladder exstrophy should always be suspected on the basis of nonvisualization of the bladder and a low-set umbilicus.

John P. Gearhart: Department of Urology, Johns Hopkins Children's Center, Baltimore, Maryland 21287.

Dominic Frimberger: Department of Urology, Johns Hopkins University School of Medicine, Baltimore, Maryland 21287.

Anatomic Malformations and Histologic Differences in the Exstrophy Complex

The diagnosis is made at birth. The bladder plate characteristically protrudes just beneath the umbilical cord with divergent rectus muscles on either side leading to separated pubic bones (Fig. 70-1). This separation is caused by outward rotation of the innominate bones, eversion of the pubic rami, and a 30% shortage of bone in the pubic ramus. In boys, there is a short phallus due to 50% deficiency of corporal length (10) with a dorsourethral plate, splayed glans, and dorsal chordee. The scrotum is generally normally developed, although the testes are often located in the distal inguinal canal. In girls, the mons, clitoris, and labia are separated, and the vaginal orifice is displaced anteriorly (Fig. 70-2).

Bilateral inguinal hernias are common due to a lack of obliquity of the inguinal canal combined with large internal/external rings. Inguinal hernia is reported in 82% of males and 11% of females (11).

Three-dimensional computed tomography (CT) demonstrates the anterior segment of the levator ani to be shorter and the posterior segment of the levator ani longer in exstrophy patients compared with normal controls. In addition, the transverse diameter of the levator hiatus is two times larger and the length 1.3 times greater, respectively.

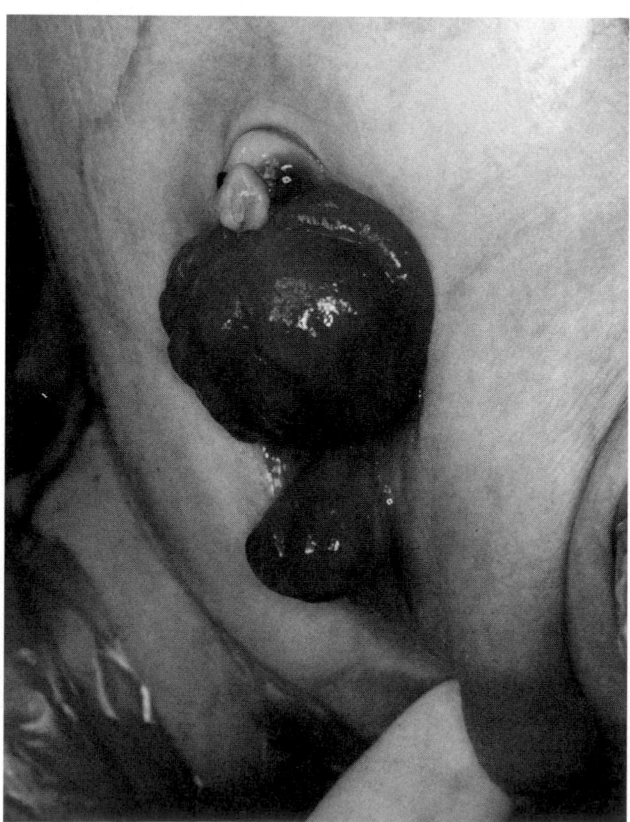

FIGURE 70-1. Male classic bladder exstrophy.

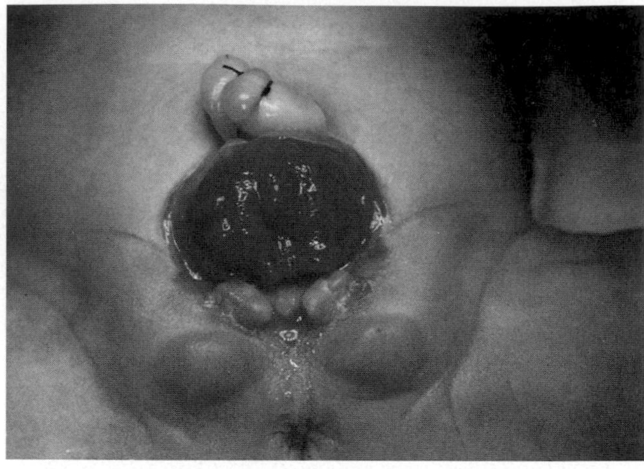

FIGURE 70-2. Female classic bladder exstrophy.

These anatomic findings cause a more anterior/superior rotation of the pelvic floor in exstrophy patients vs. normal controls. Although the levator muscle group in normal controls is evenly distributed anteriorly and posteriorly to the rectum, there is an uneven 70% to 30% posterior to anterior distribution in the exstrophic pelvis. Subsequently, the anus is anteriorly placed and sometimes patulous as part of the posterior extent of the myofascial defect (12,13). These musculoskeletal malformations explain the increased rate of rectal prolapse especially in the female exstrophy population (1).

The collagen/smooth muscle ratio was found to be 0.833 ± 0.46 instead of the 0.33 ± 0.11 ratio in normal control children, but the ratio normalized after successful closure (14). Although there is a decrease in the neural innervation of the bladder exstrophy muscle at the time of birth, the bladder musculature contains a normal compliment of muscarinic receptors for contractile stimulation staining (15). Using neuropeptides, evidence of abnormal innervation was not found in the classic bladder extrophy, but was found in the cloacal exstrophy children. Bladder specimens from newborns with classic bladder exstrophy were stained antibodies to the S 100 protein. Although the large nerve fibers were preserved, there was a significant reduction in myelinated and smaller nerve fibers (15). Using electron microscopy, significant differences in the ultrastructural nature of the intracellular organelles appear even more severe after failed initial bladder closure. Although these ultrastructural abnormalities are also seen if the bladder fails to grow, the group that obtained an adequate capacity after initial closure for bladder neck repair had only minimal changes of the bladder smooth muscle cells (16).

CT scans of patients with bladder exstrophy have shown that the posterior and anterior pelvic segments are externally rotated by a mean of 12 and 18 degrees on each side, respectively, with significant acetabular retroversion of the anterior pelvic segment. No difference was found either in the length of the posterior segment or in the width of the sacrum (17).

Assessment and Management in the Neonatal Period

It is essential that the newborn with exstrophy be seen by a pediatric genitourinary surgeon with a special interest and experience in this problem because the impact of a major birth defect is significantly worsened by inappropriate initial management.

The bladder mucosa is easily injured and inflamed; therefore, the umbilical cord should be ligated with a strong silk suture, rather than clamped to avoid mucosal abrasion. The bladder is best protected with a clear plastic wrap and should not be covered with moistened or petroleum-coated gauze. Each time the diaper is changed, the bladder surface is irrigated with sterile saline and the plastic wrap replaced.

General pediatric and cardiopulmonary assessment should be completed with an eye toward the likelihood of major surgery in the first 48 hours of life. An ultrasound of the kidneys is performed to rule out hydronephrosis and a radionucleotide scan added if abnormalities are seen.

The parents have to be reassured that children with classic bladder exstrophy are in general healthy, robust infants with the prospect of a very normal life (1). Effective reconstruction to allow urinary storage, drainage, and control can be expected with an acceptable cosmetic appearance. The support of psychologists, nurses, and parents of other children with exstrophy is invaluable and is available at a large medical center with an interest in this problem. There are also multiple international support groups, the most prominent being the Association for the Bladder Exstrophy Community.

Role and Technique of Osteotomy

Closure of the pelvic ring is important to the eventual attainment of urinary continence and appropriate cosmesis of the abdominal wall. If the operation can be carried out within the first 72 hours of life, the pelvic ring can sometimes be closed effectively without the need for osteotomy (1). When the pubic diastasis is greater than 4 cm or in the condition of a failed prior closure, osteotomy is essential to the closure of the pelvic ring and should be performed at the same time as the bladder closure (18).

The most widespread pelvic osteotomy used in the world today is the transverse innominate and vertical iliac osteotomy performed from an anterior approach dividing the innominate bone above the acetabulum (17,18) (Fig. 70-3). An incision is made at the junction of the trunk and the legs, both sides of the innominate bone are exposed simultaneously, and horizontal osteotomies are performed

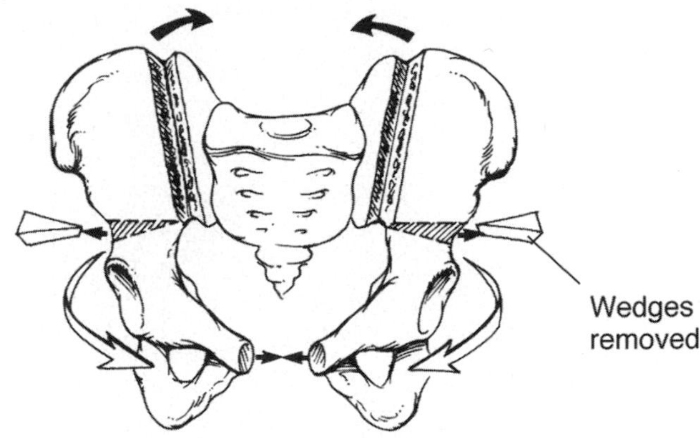

FIGURE 70-3. Transverse innominate and vertical iliac osteotomy. (From Frimberger D, Gearhart JP. Bladder exstrophy and epispadias. In: Graham SD Jr, Keane TE, Glenn JF, eds. *Glenn's urologic surgery*, 6th ed. Philadelphia: Lippincott Williams & Wilkins, 2004, with permission.)

using a Gigli saw. The osteotomy extends from 5 mm above the anterior inferior iliac spine to the most cranial part of the sciatic notch. Bilateral iliac osteotomies are performed at the same time using an osteotome and leaving the posterior table intact, giving the pelvis a better contour and mobility. The infant is already in supine position and prepared so the bladder closure can begin immediately. Pins for the external fixating device are inserted after bladder, but before the wound closure. This approach provides improved symphyseal approximation, making the midline closure easier and decreasing the likelihood of dehiscence. Postoperatively, the external fixator is left in place for 4 to 6 weeks, whereas Buck's traction is maintained with the legs supported only on a pillow. Newborns undergoing exstrophy closure without osteotomy are maintained in modified Bryant's traction for 4 weeks. The hips are kept at 90 degrees flexion with the knees straight.

Bladder and Posterior Urethra Closure in the Modern Repair

A strip of mucosa 2 cm wide extending from the distal trigone to below the verumontanum and out onto the penis in boys and to the vaginal orifice in girls outlines the prostatic and posterior urethral construction (Fig. 70-4). The male urethral groove is usually of adequate length to allow for primary closure. This is necessary, especially when the prostate is up near the base of the glans. The groove can be elongated by using paraexstrophy skin flaps (19). When these flaps are needed, great care should be exercised to follow plastic surgical principles of rotational skin flaps. An incision is made outlining the bladder mucosa and the prostatic plate. The urethral groove is transected distal to the verumontanum. In the staged approach, it is no longer necessary to free the corpora extensively or dissect

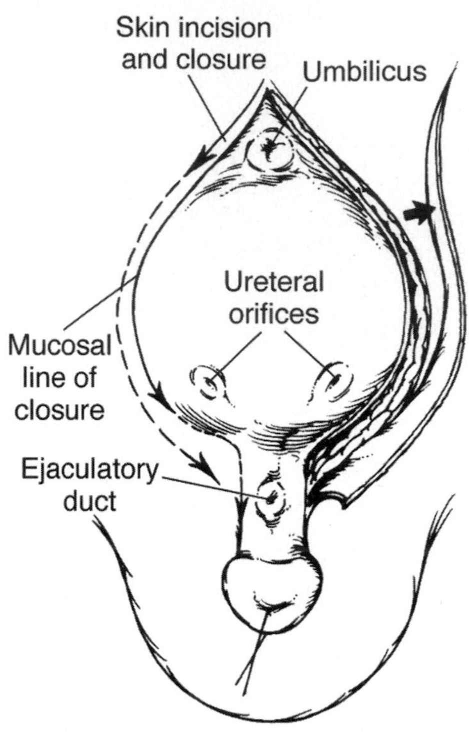

FIGURE 70-4. Male classic bladder exstrophy. Outline and initial incision. (From Frimberger D, Gearhart JP. Bladder exstrophy and epispadias. In: Graham SD Jr, Keane TE, Glenn JF, eds. *Glenn's urologic surgery*, 6th ed. Philadelphia: Lippincott Williams & Wilkins, 2004, with permission.)

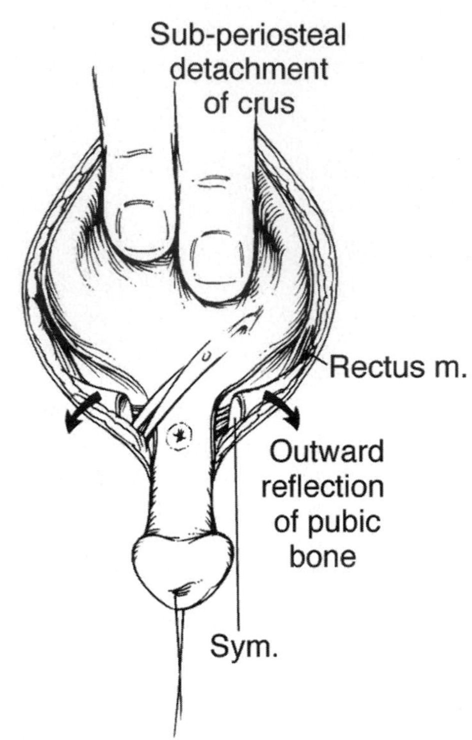

FIGURE 70-5. Radical bilateral dissection of the urogenital diaphragm fibers to detach the vesicourethral unit from the pubic bone. (From Frimberger D, Gearhart JP. Bladder exstrophy and epispadias. In: Graham SD Jr, Keane TE, Glenn JF, eds. *Glenn's urologic surgery*, 6th ed. Philadelphia: Lippincott Williams & Wilkins, 2004, with permission.)

them completely in the midline because of the preference for later epispadias repair, as described in the modified Cantwell-Ransley approach. The urethra in the female patient does not require lengthening at the time of initial bladder closure, but can still be very short. By cutting the hymenal ring at 3 o'clock and 9 o'clock, an additional 0.5 cm or so of urethral length can be obtained.

The umbilical area is dissected free and discarded. The bladder muscle is freed from the rectus sheath on each side. The peritoneum is exposed above the bladder, and a careful extraperitoneal dissection reveals the retropubic space on each side. The peritoneum is taken down from the dome of the bladder to allow the bladder to be sunken deep into the pelvis at the time of closure. Dissection is carried distally along the border between the bladder and the rectus down to the level of the urogenital diaphragm fibers. These fibers are incised sharply, and the diaphragm is detached subperiostally from the pubis bilaterally. This dissection must be carried onto the inferior ramus, and taken laterally and caudally down to the level of the levator hiatus to allow the bladder neck and posterior urethra the mobility to fall deeply within the pelvic ring (Fig. 70-5). A double-pronged skin hook can be inserted into the pelvic bone and pulled laterally to accentuate the urogenital diaphragm fibers. If this maneuver is not performed adequately, the vesicourethral unit will be brought anteriorly with pelvic closure in an unsatisfactory position for later reconstruction. The mucosa and muscle of the bladder are closed in the midline (Fig. 70-6). The urethra is closed proximally and out onto the penis so it can easily accommodate a 12 to 14 sound. This allows enough resistance to stimulate bladder growth and prevent bladder prolapse, but not too much to cause upper tract changes. The posterior urethra and bladder neck are buttressed to a second layer of local tissue, if possible. The bladder is drained by a suprapubic Malecot catheter for 4 weeks. The urethra is not stented. Ureteral stents provide urinary drainage for the first 3 weeks after surgery to avoid ureteral obstruction and hydronephrosis. The pelvis is closed by placing pressure on both greater trochanters, where horizontal mattress sutures using no. 2 nylon are placed in the pubis with the knot directed away from the urethra. A second stitch is placed caudal to the insertion of the rectus fascia, if possible, for added support. A simple umbilicoplasty is performed with a V-shaped flap, and the drainage tubes are brought out through this site.

In females, the mons and external genitalia are reconstructed at the time of initial exstrophy closure. The bifid clitoris is denuded medially and brought together in the

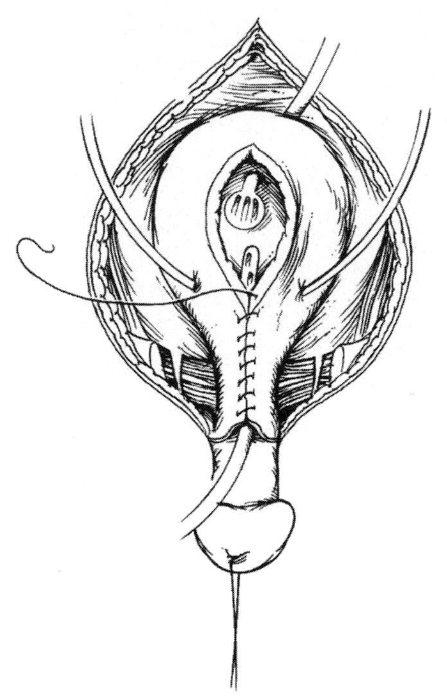

FIGURE 70-6. Bladder and proximal urethral closure. Placement of ureteral stents and suprapubic tube. The urethral stent used intraoperatively is removed at the end of the procedure. (From Frimberger D, Gearhart JP. Bladder exstrophy and epispadias. In: Graham SD Jr, Keane TE, Glenn JF, eds. *Glenn's urologic surgery*, 6th ed. Philadelphia: Lippincott Williams & Wilkins, 2004, with permission.)

midline, along with labia minora reconstruction, creating a fourchette.

Postoperative Care After Initial Closure

Broad-spectrum antibiotics are administered before and during the procedure to convert a contaminated area into a clean surgical wound. These antibiotics are continued postoperatively and then converted to low-dose prophylactic antibiotics. The factors in achieving successful primary closure have been well documented. Urethral catheters, abdominal distension, infection, and poor nutrition appear to be associated with bladder prolapse and dehiscence (20). In addition, a review of a large series of failed exstrophy patients referred to Johns Hopkins stressed the importance of osteotomy, avoidance of urethral tubes, use of postoperative antibiotics, pelvic immobilization, ureteral stenting catheters, and maintaining patient comfort, as well as decreasing the amount of postoperative movement (21). The modern application of continuous caudal catheter anesthesia has been a great asset to the anesthesia techniques in these patients. After placing the catheter in a subcutaneous tunnel, it can be left in place for up to 2 weeks postoperatively and provides excellent continuous pain control.

Four weeks after closure, the residual urine is estimated by clamping the suprapubic tube and a urine culture is obtained before the child leaves the hospital. An ultrasound is performed to assess the status of the upper tracts and repeated regularly. The bladder outlet and urethra are calibrated with a sound or catheter and, if adequate and residual urines are low, the suprapubic tube is removed. Because primary closure creates a complete epispadias with incontinence, it is unusual to have much of a continent interval after the operation. Consequently, urethral calibration and cystoscopy, as well as renal ultrasound, should not only be performed for urinary retention, but also for prolonged continent periods. If uncontrollable hydronephrosis develops, revision of the bladder outlet must be considered. Rarely, a child requires urinary diversion because of upper tract deterioration, but if necessary it is usually performed using a nonrefluxing colon conduit to preserve renal function.

Epispadias Repair

Repair of the epispadias adds to the outlet resistance of the urinary stream and can subsequently contribute significantly to the development of a larger bladder capacity (22). Epispadias repair is carried out between 6 months and 1 year of age. To stimulate penile skin growth, preoperative testosterone is given intramuscularly. Regardless of the time of epispadias repair, the five goals include (1) achievement of potential penile length, (2) correction of dorsal chordee, (3) reconstruction of the penile urethra, (4) reconstruction of the glans penis, and (5) adequate skin coverage.

Penile lengthening has been described as a key component in initial bladder exstrophy closure and is best done at the time of initial exstrophy closure. Techniques for achieving penile length vary, but all have in common release of corporal tissue from the inferior pubic ramus, preservation of the neurovascular bundles, and achievement of maximal urethral length.

A penile disassembly technique where the urethral plate is totally taken from the corporal bodies, rolled into a tube, and then brought to the tip of the penis has been described. Initial reports of a small series of this technique have been favorable (23). However, in some patients, when the urethral plate is totally dissected from the glans it will not reach the tip of the penis and either a graft has to be used or the patient is made into a hypospadias condition, which will need to be repaired later (24,25). Considering the description of a 50% shortage in penile length between exstrophy patients and controls, it is the author's opinion that any minimum of extra length obtained is not worth sacrificing the urethral plate and creating a hypospadias condition (10). The techniques of epispadias repair are described elsewhere in this text.

Bladder Neck Reconstruction

Timing is crucial to the success of bladder neck reconstruction. An adequate bladder capacity is an absolute prerequisite for success (26). The patient must have the desire to be dry and old enough to cooperate with toilet training. Under anesthesia, the bladder capacity is measured yearly after the child reaches 3 years of age. If the capacity is 85 mL or greater, bladder neck reconstruction can be considered. If the bladder does not achieve an adequate capacity after epispadias repair, injecting a bulking agent around the bladder neck, or ultimately, augmentation cystoplasty can be performed. Nearly all these children exhibit vesicoureteral reflux and antireflux procedure is required at the time of bladder neck repair (1).

Modified Young-Dees-Leadbetter Bladder Neck Reconstruction

The bladder is opened using a lower transverse incision. This is extended vertically in the midline, and the cervical closure of this incision narrows the area of the bladder neck at the end of the procedure. Reimplantation of ureters can be done in a transtrigonal or cephalotrigonal fashion.

Bladder neck reconstruction is begun by outlining a posterior mucosal strip 15 to 18 mm wide by 3 cm in length, which extends from the midtrigone to the prostate and posterior urethra. A transverse, full thickness muscular incision is not performed because there is a significant risk of denervation and ischemia for the bladder neck. The bladder muscle lateral to the strip is denuded of mucosa. Multiple small incisions in the free edges of these triangles of muscle allow the reconstruction to assume a more cephalad position (Fig. 70-7). A mucosal strip is formed into a tube using interrupted sutures of 4-0 polyglycolic acid. Denuded mucosal flaps are overlapped, and sutures are placed with 3-0 polydioxanone sutures to reinforce the neobladder neck (Fig. 70-8). Reconstruction is performed over an 8F urethral catheter, which is removed at the end of the procedure. It is essential that the bladder neck be dissected completely free from the surrounding structures. This allows suspension of the bladder neck to the anterior fascia. Often, it is advantageous to split the symphyseal bar to enhance visualization. The bar is simply closed at the end of the procedure with heavy sutures of polydioxanone. Mobility should be restricted in the postoperative period to allow healing.

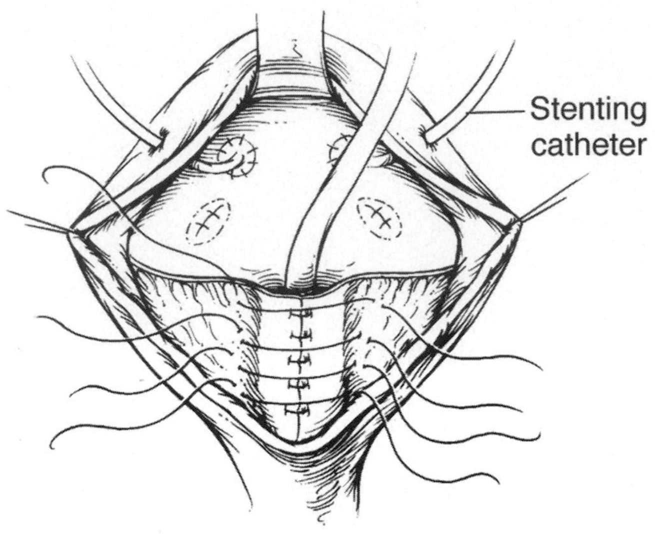

FIGURE 70-8. Mucosal strip is formed into a tube over an 8F catheter, which is removed at the end of the operation. Overlapping of the denuded mucosal flaps to reinforce the bladder neck. (From Frimberger D, Gearhart JP. Bladder exstrophy and epispadias. In: Graham SD Jr, Keane TE, Glenn JF, eds. *Glenn's urologic surgery*, 6th ed. Philadelphia: Lippincott Williams & Wilkins, 2004, with permission.)

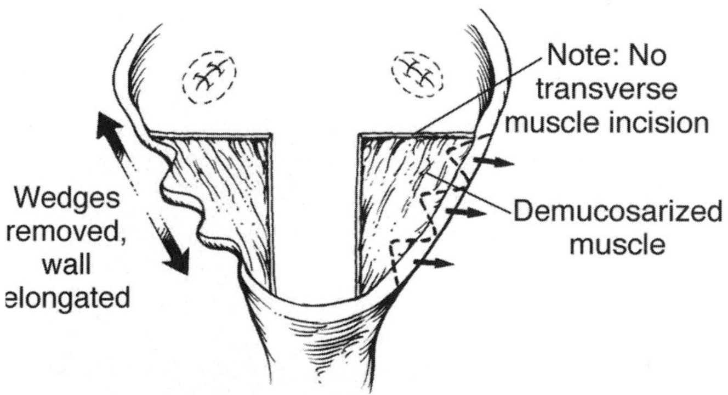

FIGURE 70-7. Modified Young-Dees-Leadbetter bladder neck reconstruction. Bladder muscle lateral to the mucosal strip for the bladder neck is denuded, and small incisions are made in the free edges. (From Frimberger D, Gearhart JP. Bladder exstrophy and epispadias. In: Graham SD Jr, Keane TE, Glenn JF, eds. *Glenn's urologic surgery*, 6th ed. Philadelphia: Lippincott Williams & Wilkins, 2004, with permission.)

Postoperative Management After Continence and Reflux Procedures

The patients are kept on broad-spectrum antibiotics and intravenous (IV) fluids until taking food by mouth well. The ureteral stents are removed after 2 to 3 weeks. At 3 weeks, the suprapubic tube is clamped intermittently to initiate a voiding trial. Initially, the tube should not be clamped for more than 1 hour. Once the child is emptying the bladder satisfactorily, the suprapubic tube is removed. Frequent bladder and renal ultrasounds are obtained in the first few months after bladder neck reconstruction to ensure adequate emptying and to observe the status of the upper tracts. If voiding does not occur after clamping the suprapubic tube, a Foley catheter is placed under anesthesia. Sometimes cystoscopy and placement of a catheter over a guide wire is necessary to negotiate the urethral channel. The catheter is then left in place for 5 days, at which point another voiding trial is attempted. Children failing repeated voiding trials are typically placed on intermittent catheterization. In some cases, these patients may have adequate storage capacity, but are unable to initiate bladder contractions sufficient for voiding. In other patients, bladder capacity may not increase necessitating bladder augmentation. If hydronephrosis is observed, the cause is likely ureterovesical junction obstruction or high voiding pressures. Urodynamics and a Lasix scan will aid in determining the correct diagnosis.

Suppressive antibiotics are continued until complete bladder emptying is achieved. In some patients, recurrent infections will become a problem. After exclusion of high postvoid residuals, long-term antibiotic suppression is recommended. The bladder should be carefully monitored to ensure progress over time as the bladder function improves. Postoperative irritations may result in an extremely small bladder capacity at first. Patients are not familiar with the sensation of bladder filling or the need for detrusor contraction. Several months for adjustment are often required before a reasonable dry interval can be developed.

Combined Bladder Exstrophy and Epispadias Repair

Newborn exstrophy closure can be combined with epispadias repair. However, this approach requires good phallic length, a deep urethral groove, and an adequate amount of penile skin (24,25,27). This technique should only be attempted by an experienced exstrophy surgeon as the complications can be severe (28,29). One of the best applications of combined exstrophy and epispadias repair is in the patient undergoing delayed primary closure or reoperative exstrophy closure (29).

The combined closure of bladder exstrophy and epispadias repair is very similar to the beginning of the closure of bladder exstrophy and posterior urethra alone. Evaluation of the bladder template is performed by everting the bladder into the abdomen with a sterile gloved finger. This allows evaluation of the extent of the bladder plate, which may be larger than noted on visual inspection of the abdominal wall defect. The operative procedure begins and proceeds as with the standard closure of the bladder, posterior urethra, and abdominal wall with only a few differences. In reclosure, great care must be used to divide any remnants of the urogenital diaphragm fibers that were left behind after the failed initial closure. Once the urogenital diaphragm fibers have been incised, the entire vesicoureteral unit can be moved posteriorly into the pelvis. Placing the bladder neck and posterior urethra deep within the pelvic ring allows approximation of the levator and puborectalis sling, and provides an improved eventual continence rate.

After adequate dissection of the bladder and posterior urethra, attention is given to the dissection of the penis, corporal bodies, and urethral plate. This part of the procedure progresses much as in a standard epispadias repair and exstrophy closure with a few exceptions. The corporal bodies are not brought over the urethra until the pelvic bones are sewn together in the midline, thus rotating the corpora more medially and allowing less tension on the corpora in the midline. A small oblique drain is placed next to the bladder closure, and abdominal wall closure is completed. An 8F Firlit stent is used to stent the urethra for 2 weeks. The external fixating device is then attached to intrafragmentary pins and tightened. External fixation of the pelvis is maintained for 4 weeks in children undergoing primary closure and 6 to 8 weeks for those undergoing reclosure of the bladder. Follow-up is very much the same as in standard exstrophy closure with monitoring residual urine and upper tract imaging by ultrasonography before suprapubic tube removal. Although some patients have achieved long-term continence after the procedure, most ultimately require bladder neck reconstruction to become dry.

Overall Results After Bladder Exstrophy Repair

The overall outcome after bladder exstrophy repair has improved remarkably since the mid-1970s. The standard treatment of exstrophy in the United States has evolved from urinary diversion to functional reconstruction in almost all cases. Favorable overall long-term outcome depends on the success of all phases of surgical reconstruction. The importance of a successful initial closure cannot be overemphasized and should be performed in centers with a large experience. Failure of the initial closure markedly decreases the attainment of successful continence and, in most cases, ultimately required bladder augmentation (30). Continence is correctly defined as being dry for more than 3 hours. Socially continent patients achieve that goal during the day, but have bed-wetting incidences during nighttime. After modern repair, continence rates can be expected to be as high as 75% to 80% with preservation of renal function as documented in several large series (26,31–33). Appropriate patient selection, meticulous surgical technique and careful postoperative care are essential to obtaining consistent outcomes. The functional and cosmetic outcomes of the genital reconstruction are of high quality. Patients have a very low rate of urethrocutaneous fistula with a very acceptable cosmetic appearance (34). Most postpubertal patients were able to participate in satisfactory intercourse (35).

Not all patients are candidates for immediate postnatal reconstruction. In patients with bladder template size at birth not sufficient for closure, primary closure should be delayed to permit growth of the bladder to a feasible size. In a series of 19 affected patients seen at our institution, primary closure was delayed and performed at a mean age of 13 months (36). Nine of them became dry after bladder neck reconstruction and 4 patients are currently awaiting the procedure. Four others perform intermittent catheterization, 1 required a colonic conduit, and 1 underwent an ureterosigmoidostomy.

A one-stage closure in the newborn period without reimplanting the ureters, reconstructing the bladder neck, or performing osteotomies has been proposed (24). Initial results using the penile disassembly technique for epispadias repair left some children with a residual hypospadias, necessitating later repair. Moreover, 50% of children presented with urinary breakthrough infections, despite antibiotic prophylaxis, and subsequently required ureteral reimplantation. Bladder closure, ureteral reimplantation, epispadias repair, and bladder neck reconstruction in the newborn period can be accomplished, using the same technique even for older children without osteotomies (37). Combining newborn exstrophy closure with later bladder neck reconstruction and epispadias repair has also been described (38). A completely different approach is the creation of an ureterosigmoidostomy as an initial procedure after bladder and abdominal wall closure in one procedure (39). These procedures allowed children continence and, once nonrefluxing ureterocolonic anastomosis was performed, protected the upper tracts. Long-term complications of ureterosigmoidostomy include pyelonephritis, hypercalemic metabolic acidosis, ureteral obstruction, and the late development of colonic malignancy.

Although all these approaches have merit and supporters, the quality and size of the bladder template, appropriate patient selection, and experience of the surgeon and supporting staff will ultimately determine the outcome in a particular child.

CLOACAL EXSTROPHY

Incidence

Cloacal exstrophy, also known as vesicointestinal fissure, ileovesical fissure, or splanchnic exstrophy, is the most severe defect that can occur in the formation of the ventral abdominal wall. Fortunately, this entity is extremely rare, occurring in 1 in 200,000 to 400,000 live births (40). Formerly, the incidence between sexes was believed to be similar; however, current reports indicate a 2 : 1 male/female ratio (41). The mode of inheritance of this condition is unknown because offspring have never been produced from people with this disorder.

Embryology and Anatomy

Two main theories on the embryology of cloacal exstrophy have been proposed. The first proposed that the paired primordial of the genital tubercles are displaced caudally. This permits persistence of the more cephalad cloacal membrane. Thus, if there is incomplete urorectal septal division and disintegration of the unstable cloacal membrane, then both the exstrophied bladder and bowel would be on the ventral abdominal surface (42). The second theory suggests that the cloacal membrane is overly developed. This overdevelopment prevents migration of the mesenchymal layer between the inner endodermal and outer ectodermal layers. As previously mentioned, the unstable membrane ruptures, and if this occurs before fusion of the genital tubercles and before caudal movement of the urorectal septum, then the ventral abdominal defect arises (5).

A gridlike schema has been used to describe cloacal exstrophy and to better delineate its variants. In type I classic cloacal exstrophy, the hemibladders may be confluent cranial to the bowel patch, lateral to the bowel (most common), or confluent caudal to the bowel. Type IIA grids show variations of the bladder (covered bladder or hemibladder), type IIB grids show variations of distal exstrophied bowel segments (duplications), and type IIC grids depict the situation in which both bowel and bladder variations occur. The grid also describes the penis (hemi or united) and the clitoris and vaginal status (duplications). The authors modified the grid concept to describe the status of the hindgut remnant (Fig. 70-9).

Two more recent reports with appropriate intrauterine follow-up have found the presence of a cloacal membrane at 17 to 18 weeks, with rupture of the membrane up to 26 weeks of embryonic life (43,44). These findings are discordant with previous theories of the embryogenesis of cloacal exstrophy. More recently, there appears to be an increased incidence of cloacal exstrophy in patients who were the products of modern assisted reproductive technology (45).

Anatomically, there is exstrophy of the foreshortened hindgut or cecum, which displays its bulging mucosa between the two hemibladders. The orifices of the terminal ileum, the rudimentary hindgut, and a single or paired appendix are apparent on the surface of the everted cecum.

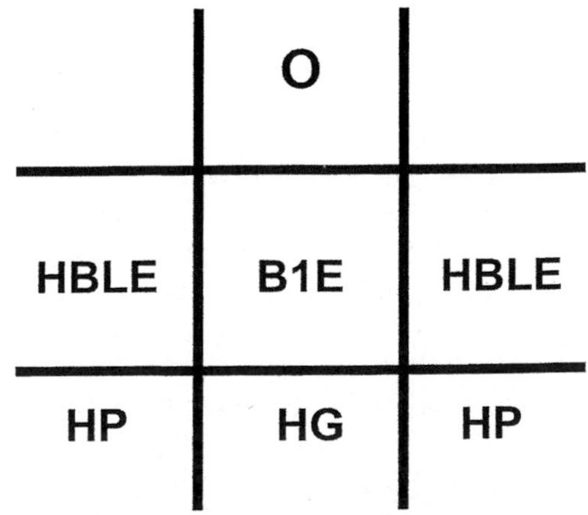

FIGURE 70-9. Modified coding grid used to describe classic cloacal exstrophy and variants. O, omphalocele; HBLE, hemibladder; B1E, everted bowel; HP, hemiphallus; HG, hindgut.

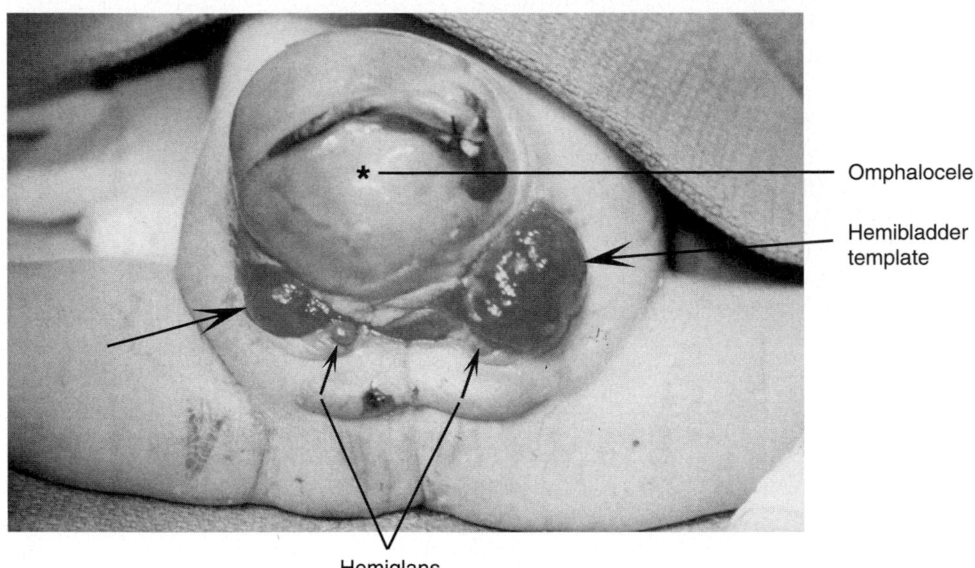

FIGURE 70-10. Male cloacal exstrophy.

The hindgut is blind ending, and the ileum is usually prolapsed. The anatomy of the bony pelvis in cloacal exstrophy was generally described in the past as a widened pubic symphysis with hips that are externally rotated and abducted (Fig. 70-10).

Markedly severe abnormalities of the bony pelvis can be associated with cloacal exstrophy. Using CT scans of the pelvis in controls and patients with cloacal exstrophy, the interpubic diastasis was found to have a mean of 0.5 cm in controls and 8 cm in cloacal exstrophy patients with extreme external rotation of the iliac wings. Overall, patients with cloacal exstrophy have extreme abnormalities of the pelvis, as well as asymmetry between the sides, sacroiliac joint malformations, and occasional hip malformations (46).

In cloacal exstrophy, the autonomic innervation to the bladder halves and corporal bodies arises from a pelvic plexus on the anterior surface of the sacrum. The phallus is usually separated into a right and left half with adjacent scrotum or labia. Occasionally, the penis is together in the midline, but the structure is usually diminutive and the corporal bodies small.

The nerves to the hemibladders travel along the midline on the posteroinferior surface of the pelvis and extend laterally to the hemibladders. The autonomic innervation of the phallic halves arises from the sacral pelvic plexus, travels in the midline, perforates the inferior portion of the pelvis floor, and courses medially to the hemibladder (47).

Associated Anomalies

Of the anomalies associated with cloacal exstrophy, those involving spinal dysraphism associated with myelomeningocele are the most devastating. The incidence of spina bifida in various series ranges from 29% to 75%, but of course figures include patients with meningoceles and lipomeningoceles (48). Evaluation of the full spinal cord with CT reveals an incidence of spinal cord vertebral anomalies approaching 100%. In two series, the level of the myelomeningocele was 72% lumbar, 14% sacral, and 14% thoracic (49–51). Magnetic resonance imaging (MRI) of the spinal cord should be part of the initial evaluation of newborns with cloacal exstrophy. Close consultation with a pediatric neurosurgeon must be established to determine the distinction between meningocele, myelomeningocele, and lipomeningocele, and to develop a plan of treatment priorities.

Several series have demonstrated the common occurrence of upper tract urinary anomalies in up to one-third of patients involving pelvic kidney and renal agenesis (11). Hydronephrosis and hydroureter were found in one-third of patients in series, but in only 1 of 22 patients in another series (13,14). Ectopia of the ureter draining into the vasa in boys and into the uterus, vagina, or fallopian tube in girls has also been reported.

Duplication of the vagina can occur in up to 65% of patients (2,52). Vaginal agenesis occurs in 25% to 43% and partial or complete duplication of the uterus in up to 95% of patients. An increased incidence of large ovarian cysts after menarche was noted in one group of cloacal exstrophy patients. All became symptomatic with long-term follow-up and required oophorectomy. In most series, the testes were undescended and found in the groin or abdomen in the majority of patients (2,53).

Vertebral anomalies have been reported in up to 80% of patients (11). Lower limb abnormalities are seen in 12% to 65% of patients (11). These include club foot, congenital hip dislocation, agenesis, and severe deformity of both the foot and leg.

Omphaloceles are reported in more than 85% of cases (11). Immediate closure is often required to prevent rupture of the omphalocele with its attendant problems. Omphalocele defects are usually closed primarily without using prosthetic materials. The use of a silicone silo has been reported when the omphalocele is extremely large. Other serious anomalies of the gastrointestinal tract have been described, including malrotation, bowel duplication, duodenal atresia, duodenal web, and Meckel's diverticulum (2). The short-gut syndrome has been variously reported in 25% to 50% of patients (11).

Life-threatening anomalies of the cardiovascular and pulmonary systems are extremely rare. Cyanotic heart disease and aortic duplication have been described, as has duplication of the vena cava (10). A bilobular lung and atretic upper lobe bronchus have been reported.

Prenatal Diagnosis

Prenatal diagnosis is important to allow referral to a major center for counseling and delivery. Major and minor criteria for the prenatal evaluation of cloacal exstrophy have been proposed (54). Major criteria included nonvisualization of the bladder, a large midline infraumbilical defect, omphalocele, myelomeningocele, and appearance of prolapsed bowel below the umbilical. The minor criteria included lower-extremity defects, renal anomalies, ascites, pubic separation, narrow thorax, hydronephrosis, and single umbilical artery.

Surgical Management

Surgical reconstruction of cloacal exstrophy was first described in 1900 (55). The omphalocele was corrected at birth, and the atretic colon was pulled through to the perineum; however, the neonate died at 5 days of age. In general, surgical reconstruction of cloacal exstrophy was considered futile, and untreated neonates usually died from prematurity, sepsis, short bowel syndrome, or renal and central nervous system deficits. When the importance of separating the genitourinary tract from the gastrointestinal tract became apparent, survival increased. Rickham reported on the first patient with cloacal exstrophy to survive surgical reconstruction. The omphalocele was repaired, the intestinal strip was separated from the hemibladders, and the blind-ending colon was pulled through to the perineum. The hemibladders were then reapproximated. An ileal conduit was constructed at age 18 months, and a cystectomy was subsequently performed. After early reconstructive efforts, the patient was left with two stomata: one to collect urine and the other to collect stool (56). Survival is no longer the major issue; instead, the achievement of a good quality of life is now the greatest challenge facing these patients (57).

Immediate Neonatal Assessment

The infant's condition at birth may be critical, and attempts to reconstruct and repair may be futile or morally or ethically unwise. Often, the severity of cloacal exstrophy is enhanced by the nature and severity of the associated anomalies. The more robust infant will survive, and reparative surgery is initiated at birth. A one-stage closure when the infant is in excellent condition and has favorable anatomy with minimal associated anomalies is preferred. However, many of these infants are premature, are small for gestational age, and have such severe associated anomalies that it is difficult for them to undergo an extensive one-stage procedure in the newborn period.

Surgical management and preoperative assessment should only be undertaken by a multidisciplinary team that includes surgeons who are familiar with the principles of exstrophy treatment, its options, and later reconstructive techniques. Also included in the team should be a neonatologist, a neurosurgeon, and an orthopedic surgeon familiar with the osteotomy techniques needed for a secure pelvic closure.

Surgical Options in the Neonatal Period

Gender Assignment

The need for gender reassignment is limited to the 46 XY patients with cloacal exstrophy. Male gender assignment is appropriate for infants with adequate bilateral or unilateral phallic structures. A most difficult reconstructive and ethical decision presents when a male newborn has minimal phallic structures available for repair. Although modern phallic surgical techniques allow better genital reconstruction, patients will be seen in whom these structures are inadequate for the male sex of rearing, and these represent the "ultimate challenge." In one study of eight genotypic boys with cloacal exstrophy, all had phallic inadequacy, and of four who have reached puberty, two are impotent, and three have required intense psychiatric counseling (58). Thus, sexual conversion still should be part of the treatment algorithm in all genotypic boys with the cloacal exstrophy syndrome. Any decision concerning gender reassignment must occur after consultation from multiple disciplines and parental input. More recent reports from two major centers are at odds concerning long-term outcomes of these gender-reassigned patients. Thus, research is certainly needed on gender development and quality of life.

Among the important decisions to be made during this period is whether to perform a one- or two-stage closure. A one-stage closure is preferred, if at all possible. During either a one- or two-stage procedure, the omphalocele is excised and the bowel is separated from the bladder halves. The lateral vesicointestinal fissure is closed in continuity, and a short colostomy is created from the end of the distal colon segment. The hemibladders then are reapproximated in the midline to create a single exstrophic bladder. If a one-stage procedure is selected, the entire bladder is closed completely after a bilateral anterior innominate osteotomy and vertical iliac osteotomy is performed. Also, an anterior approach allows placement of pins for external fixation and is preferred when severe lumbosacral dysraphism is present. With a large omphalocele defect, bladder closure and osteotomy may be delayed until respiratory and gastrointestinal stability is achieved (21).

Management of the Bowel in Cloacal Exstrophy

The management of the bowel in cloacal exstrophy must be closely integrated with the management of the urinary tract. The grid coding system for cloacal exstrophy has previously been mentioned and ensures a precise description of the bowel anomalies is undertaken, that variant patterns are identified, and that appropriate early decisions are made concerning the exstrophied bowel and hindgut.

The principles guiding the management of the bowel in cloacal exstrophy are to conserve all bowel segments, to minimize fluid and electrolyte loss, and to maximize nutritional potential of all these elements. Formerly, patients died from fluid and electrolyte loss with a short bowel and terminal ileostomy. Early total parenteral nutrition is used to help these infants grow so the short-gut syndrome becomes less of a problem as the patients get older (21). Careful preservation of the hindgut segment is important because this segment can enlarge considerably if it is used initially as a fecal colostomy, and it may help absorption and prevent fluid loss. Also, as the hindgut enlarges if used for a fecal colostomy, it later can be used as a bladder augmentation or vaginal replacement if nutritional circumstances allow (21).

Placement of the colostomy or ileostomy at a favorable location is of prime importance. It should be placed where it can easily be managed with an appliance. In the rare instance in which there is an adequate hindgut and no neurologic deficit, a colostomy can be created with a later posterior sagittal anorectoplasty to bring the colon to the perineum. A more recent series has reported some patients able to have continence of stool, mainly by enema washout through a perineal opening (59). These patients must have limited to no neurologic deficits, a good pelvic floor by MRI, along with adequate nerve response to stimulation and enough colonic length for solid stool before this approach is taken. Finally, every effort must be expended to save the appendiceal structures for later continent stoma construction, if needed.

Management of the Phallic Structures and Vagina

In boys with cloacal exstrophy, the penis is usually represented by two widely separated and small phallic structures. Because these structures are rudimentary and wide apart, attempts at reconstruction have been generally unsatisfactory. However, in the rare instance with adequate corporal tissue, epispadias repair can be performed at the time of initial closure, or later, depending on the situation.

If the female sex of rearing is chosen, the medial aspects of the bifid phallus are denuded of mucosa and brought together in the midline. This is usually done at the time of bladder closure and osteotomy. If there is a single phallic structure in the midline (20% of patients), the urethral plate is dissected and the corporal bodies dropped between them to the perineum for a urethral opening. The corpora and glans are then recessed for more appropriate female appearance and the labial folds are created from the scrotum by a posterior Y-V plasty. Correction of genital anomalies in girls is usually done at the time of bladder closure and osteotomy. The medial aspect of the hemiclitoris is denuded of mucosa, and the halves are brought together with 5-0 Vicryl for the subcutaneous layer and fine 6-0 Vicryl for the epithelial layer. Commonly, duplicate vaginas are far apart and on opposite sides of the pelvis. In the unusual case of the vaginas being close together, they should be joined in the midline and used for later reconstruction. The ostia of the vaginas may be difficult to find at the time of the initial closure, and the surgeon should be aware that they can enter the posterior wall of the bladder. It is acceptable to leave the vaginas in situ, but further surgery will be needed to bring one of these to the perineum.

In the genotypic male patient raised as a female, the vagina is usually created at the time of puberty. In the past, vaginas have been created by anatomic "scraps" such as portions of duplicated bowel, unneeded dilated ureter, or a few centimeters of the distal colonic segment. Therefore, it is probably better to wait until puberty and construct a vagina from intestine or from a free full-thickness skin graft. There is a paucity of literature on the construction of a neovagina in the cloacal exstrophy patient, but as more of these patients reach puberty, experience with this entity will increase, and long-term information will be available.

Reconstruction of the Lower Urinary Tract

Bladder Closure

The bladder closure is performed much as that of classic bladder exstrophy described earlier. Care must be taken when the bowel is separated from the bladder halves to avoid damage to the blood supply of the bowel mesentery and the autonomic vesical innervation, which becomes exposed at the medial aspect of the hemibladder. In girls, a double vagina may complicate closure of the urethra. If possible, the vaginas are joined and positioned posteriorly, and the tissue on the anteromedial aspect is tabularized to form a urethra. If this tissue is unavailable, then local tissues are used to form a urethral channel. As mentioned previously, in the genotypic male patient raised as a girl, the urethral plate is raised from the corpora, much as in the initial part of a Cantwell-Ransley repair, and then brought ventral to the corpora as a perineal urethra.

Drainage of the urinary tract is accomplished by ureteral stents and suprapubic catheter all exiting from the abdomen. No urethral stent or catheter is used. After bladder closure, free incontinent drainage of urine through the urethra is expected, but antibiotic suppression and close monitoring are necessary to avoid retention, infection, and reflux nephropathy.

Osteotomy should be performed in all patients with cloacal exstrophy, based on success with this procedure for classic bladder exstrophy. The goal is to achieve tension-free approximation of the widely separated pubic bones and of the anterior abdominal wall. Anterior osteotomy also provides large cancellous surfaces with good healing potential. Furthermore, in cases of extreme pubic diastasis, combined anterior innominate and posterior osteotomy may be done within the periosteum through the same skin incision for better correction. Immobilization is provided by an eternal fixator and modified Bryant traction or Buck traction for 4 to 6 weeks.

The importance of osteotomy at the time of cloacal exstrophy closure has been demonstrated. In one study of 22 patients with cloacal exstrophy, of 9 who underwent closure without osteotomy, 89% had significant complications (dehiscence, vesicocutaneous fistula, prolapse), whereas there were complications in only 2 of 12 who had osteotomy at the time of initial cloacal exstrophy closure (14). A novel approach to osteotomy in cloacal exstrophy patients with failed prior closures or extreme diastasis has been reported. In this approach, osteotomy is performed, along with external fixator placement followed by soft-tissue and pelvic ring closure 2 to 3 weeks later, after the pelvis has been gradually reduced by fixator approximation (60).

Management of Urinary Incontinence

Incontinence of urine is managed by diapering only during the early years. Intermittent catheterization is likely to be needed for emptying after any procedure to enhance outlet resistance. This may be due in part to spinal defects, which can cause a neurologic deficit in bladder function, or to a small bladder capacity, which may require augmentation. In both instances, bladder detrusor activity is usually impaired. The role of bladder outlet repair in cloacal exstrophy is minimal. More recent data clearly show a very marked different in continence results between cloacal exstrophy and classic exstrophy, which is mainly due to coexisting neurologic abnormalities (22). Surgery to produce a continent reservoir should be delayed until the child is old enough to participate in self-care. The choice between a catheterizable urethra and an abdominal stoma depends on the adequacy of the urethra and bladder outlet, the intellect and dexterity of the child, and the child's orthopedic status as regards the spine, hip joints, braces, and ambulation.

Occasionally, hindgut is available for bladder enhancement, but ileum has traditionally been used. To avoid further loss of absorptive surface by preserving both hindgut and ileum, gastrocystoplasty has been used with good success (61). Regardless of which bowel segment is chosen, bladder augmentation should be delayed until bowel function is mature and until nutrition and acidosis are no longer a problem.

Some patients with a minimal neurologic lesion have a functioning bladder and can void through a reconstructed bladder outlet. Innovative methods may be needed, however, to construct a continent outlet in patients without substantial native urethral tissues. These techniques include use of the vagina to form a urethra, with reimplantation of the vagina into the bladder for continence, or an ileal nipple (62).

Using a variety of continence procedures and augmentation, more than one-half of patients can achieve significant urinary continence (57).

A scoring system has been developed to analyze both bladder and bowel continence. In the absence of multiple cases, owing to the rarity of this condition, use of this scoring system may allow a collective experience to be analyzed and thus optimization of future management of this complex disorder (15).

Long-term Psychological and Psychosexual Issues

With improved survival and reconstructive surgery, long-term adjustment issues have become paramount. One report on six children who had undergone gender reassignment documented that all had developmental difficulties. None had undergone replacement with exogenous female hormones and most expressed typical male behavior. Two had spontaneous gender reassignment and assigned themselves back to the male sex of rearing. All had extensive family counseling at birth, as well as continued counseling through childhood for the parents and children (63). A series from the Great Ormond Street Hospital contrasts that with 46 XY cloacal exstrophy patients, all with feminine-typical core gender identity on long-term follow-up. The patients will have to be followed into adult life for appropriate decision making and information to be obtained. Also, in the same study, regardless of karyotype, the quality of life of those patients raised in the female sex of rearing was very good. All disliked their colostomy and the need to catheterize, but the quality of life was rated high (64).

CONCLUSION

The management of cloacal exstrophy has improved to provide more quality of life for these children. Complete reconstruction in the newborn period seems to be the best approach if the infant's condition allows. Neurologic and GI management takes precedence over urologic and genital repair. Improvements in neurologic evaluation have served to reduce life-threatening complications and the progression of neurologic deficits. Urinary continence is now possible in most children. Currently, information is insufficient to make an informative decision about optimal gender assignment in patients with XY chromosomes and cloacal exstrophy. Advances in tissue engineering and stem cell research will likely allow congruent rearing of all male patients with cloacal exstrophy. Further long-term research is mandatory to continue progress in the treatment of these interesting children.

PRUNE BELLY SYNDROME

Incidence

The prune belly syndrome is known by many other names, including Eagle-Barrett syndrome and, more commonly, the triad syndrome (65,66). This syndrome has three distinguishing features: (1) deficient abdominal wall musculature; (2) undescended, usually intraabdominal testes; and (3) urinary tract abnormalities. Strictly speaking, only boys can be affected by all these findings, but a triad of abdominal wall laxity, urinary tract dilation, and genital anomalies, most commonly vaginal atresia or bicornuate uterus, has been described in girls. The incidence of prune belly syndrome is estimated to be between 1 in 29,000 and 1 in 40,000 live births (67).

Embryogenesis

Theories proposing a disorder of embryogenesis postulate a lateral mesenchymal defect, affecting both the development of the abdominal wall musculature and the smooth muscle of the urinary tract (68). The association of omphalocele and gastroschisis with prune belly syndrome supports these theories. Another widely held belief considers transient severe bladder outlet obstruction as the inciting event, perhaps due to prostatic hypoplasia and subsequent collapse of the posterior urethra (69). Furthermore, theories have been advanced such as temporary prominence of the mullerian tubercle or valvular obstruction with spontaneous rupture before birth. This obstruction is believed to cause dilation of the urinary tract, urinary ascites, abdominal wall stretching, and maldevelopment, and cryptorchidism owing to obstruction of the inguinal canals by the bladder (70). An animal model of urethral and urachal obstruction in the first trimester fetal lamb appears to support this theory (71).

Contrary to those who advance transient posterior urethral obstruction as the cause of prune belly, one group has suggested the point of obstruction to be the junction of the penile and glandular urethra (72). This is supported by an increasing incidence of megalourethra in prune belly syndrome and by the timing of other embryologic events, such as prostatic development at week 11 and closure of the urachus at week 15. Last, some propose that the etiology of prune belly syndrome is a result of teratogenic stimuli to mesodermal precursors. Because all precursor layers of the genitourinary tract are in close proximity at 6 to 10 weeks' gestation, a teratogenic insult at this time could cause maldevelopment and dysplasia of both the lower and upper urinary tracts.

The genetic basis of prune belly syndrome is unclear. Several associations have been reported with prune belly syndrome, and a multifactorial inheritance or a teratogenic mechanism might best explain the range of associations. Prune belly syndrome has been associated with trisomy 13, 18, and 21; interstitial deletion of the long arm of chromosome 1; 8q interstitial deletion; 45XO phenotype; Beckwith-Wiedeman syndrome; exposure to teratogens; and paucity of interlobular bile ducts. It will take careful study of greater numbers of patients to allow any scientific genetic counseling. Parents should be made aware that prune belly syndrome has occurred in siblings, although the relative risk of this occurrence is unknown.

Anatomic Malformations

Prune belly syndrome represents a spectrum of involvement. Patients can be divided into three categories. Category I patients have oligohydramnios, pulmonary hypoplasia, possible urethral obstruction, a patent urachus, and will frequently die in the neonatal period. Category III patients have mild or incomplete abdominal wall involvement and a near-normal urinary tract. Most patients, however, fall into category II, with abdominal wall and urinary tract abnormalities, but no immediate threat to survival.

The abdominal wall in the affected patient has a characteristic appearance at birth and presents lax, wrinkled, thin, and redundant with prominent bulges at the flanks. The liver edge and intestinal peristalsis are often clearly visible. Although electromyograph (EMG) studies have shown that the lower medial abdominal musculature is most severely affected, it can be patchy and asymmetric in its distribution (73). The enlarged upper urinary tract and the distended bladder are usually palpable. The umbilicus is displaced upward because the upper abdominal muscles are often relatively spared. Because of the absence of the lower rectus abdominus, the arms are used to assist when sitting up from a supine position.

The complete urinary tract is usually involved. The kidneys are often dysmorphic, with large calyces, long infundibuli, and dilated pelves. In addition, pathologic changes consistent with segmental or total dysplasia are frequently seen (74). The ureters are tortuous and markedly dilated, usually more distally pronounced. Fluoroscopic examination of the ureters demonstrates diminished or absent peristalsis, especially in the lower two-thirds of the lower ureter, whereas the upper ureters are usually less dilated and more apt to demonstrate effective peristalsis (75).

A high-resolution color image video analysis system morphometrically quantified the smooth muscle and collagen content of various abnormal ureters types. Collagen content of the lower ureters from prune belly patients demonstrated significantly elevated collagen levels, especially in those demonstrating reflux (62%) (76). It is proposed that this increase in collagen associated with reflux is due either to repetitive stretching stimulating collagen production, or a primary ureteral bud abnormality leading to reflux and increased collagen. These impressive megaureters are rarely truly obstructed, and the radiographic appearance correlates poorly with renal function. Ureteropelvic junction obstruction, horseshoe kidney, and renal hypoplasia are other upper tract anomalies reported (74).

The bladder is characteristically large with thickened walls, but trabeculation is generally absent. There is commonly a pseudodiverticulum at the dome, which is conceptually an urachal extension, and occasionally the urachus is patent (74). An autopsy study of fetuses with posterior urethral valves and prune belly syndrome found that patients with prune belly bladders can be divided into two groups. The first group of patients has increased muscle mass and connective tissue, as well as bladder outlet obstruction similar to patients with posterior urethral valves. In addition, the ureteral orifices are laterally placed on a large trigone often causing vesicoureteral reflux. The second group demonstrated no histologic evidence of bladder thickening or outlet obstruction (77).

The posterior urethra is dilated with the bulbous configuration beginning proximally at a wide, open bladder neck and ending with an abrupt narrowing at the membranous urethra, which can be confused with posterior urethral valves. Valves are usually not demonstrated in children with the syndrome, although they have been documented in severe cases with oligohydramnios and neonatal death. The histology of the dilated posterior urethra is consistent with a deficiency in the development of the prostate (74). The bladder neck is wide and not hypertrophied, as is often the case in valves. The verumontanum is usually not apparent radiographically or cystoscopically, but present on pathologic examination (78). The sexual ducts can demonstrate a spectrum of abnormalities, including narrowing of the junction between the rete testis and efferent ducts, straightening of the epididymis, segmental atresia of the vas deferens, and either an absent or hypoplastic tortous seminal vesicle.

The anterior urethra is usually normal, although a narrow, underdeveloped urethra or a megalourethra may be found. Urethral atresia is usually associated with fatal pulmonary hyperplasia, but may be compatible with survival in the presence of a patent urachus. Megalourethra comes in two forms: The fusiform deformity involves absence or hypoplasia of all the penile bodies, and the scaphoid megalourethra is due to an isolated defect in the spongiosum. The fusiform megalourethra is generally found in severe cases and often associated with neonatal death. The scaphoid megalourethra was associated with azotemia or death in more than one-half of patients (79). Megalourethra may be associated with significant urethral obstruction, and improvement of the upper urinary tracts has been seen after megalourethra repair. Hypospadias is rarely associated with the prune belly syndrome, but has been reported.

One of the defining features of the prune belly syndrome is bilateral cryptorchidism. The testes may be located anywhere along the normal course of descent, but are most commonly found in the abdomen. The fertility potential of these testicles is a matter of controversy. The histologic examination of testes at the time of orchidopexy has been described as consistent with Sertoli-cell-only syndrome, but in other cases found to be similar to age-matched controls (80). Spermatogonia in reduced numbers are present (81). However, there also appears to be a significant risk for testicular malignancy in these cryptorchid testes. One study demonstrated an atypical appearance of the germ cells in early orchidopexy biopsy specimens, suggesting intratubular neoplasia (82).

Associated Abnormalities

One of the potentially devastating associations with prune belly syndrome is the tendency for respiratory difficulties. Respiratory compromise either due to pulmonary hypoplasia or pneumothorax (74) may be seen in the severely affected neonate. The pulmonary hypoplasia is almost certainly related to the occurrence of oligohydramnios rather than to compression by the distended abdomen (83). In addition, the lack of abdominal muscles to assist in coughing predisposes these children to respiratory infection and postoperative atelectasis (83). Gastrointestinal abnormalities such as intestinal malrotation, small bowel atresia, large bowel atresia, megacolon (not due to aganglionosis), and imperforate anus are found frequently (84). Chronic constipation, probably due to lack of abdominal musculature, can be a feature of the syndrome. Fecal impaction, volvulus, and splenic torsion have been described, and a high index of suspicion must be maintained in cases of intestinal obstruction or abdominal pain (85).

Cardiovascular abnormalities are present in more than 10% of patients. These include patent ductus arteriosus, atrial septal defect, ventricular septal defect, and bicuspid aortic valve (86).

Orthopedic anomalies occur in most patients, the most common being clubfoot, but also including congenital dislocation of the hip and atresia or agenesis of the lower limb, perhaps due to iliac artery compression by the distended bladder (87). Pectus deformities and scoliosis are also more common in prune belly syndrome than in the general population (88). Dimpling at the knee is a common finding, even in children who have no other orthopedic deformities (74).

Diagnosis

Prune belly syndrome is frequently diagnosed on prenatal ultrasound examination. The findings are similar to those of posterior urethral valves, with an enlarged bladder, bilateral hydronephrosis, and in some cases, oligohydramnios (89). One case has been documented in which an apparent transient bladder outlet obstruction was associated with the prune belly phenotype. Other aspects of the syndrome, such as undescended testicles and megalourethra, have been detected prenatally.

The diagnosis of prune belly syndrome is usually easily made on initial examination of the newborn. Initial radiologic evaluation should consist of renal and bladder ultrasound examination. The urinary tract dilation that is evident in most cases is not necessarily obstructive in nature, but is always consistent with significant urinary stasis. Despite the appearance of the urinary tract, the renal function is often within the normal range for age. Serial creatinine values should be obtained in the neonate, and further evaluation and surgical treatment for obstruction is necessary if the values are rising.

A voiding cystourethrogram often reveals the entire urinary collecting system owing to bilateral vesicoureteral reflux, but this test may be inadvisable initially, owing to the high risk of urinary tract infection. Diuretic renal scintigraphy and intravenous pyelography may be inaccurate owing to pooling in the large renal pelves and ureters. Alternatively, a Whitaker pressure perfusion test may be helpful to determine obstruction.

Treatment

Two schools of thought have emerged on the treatment of the urinary tract in prune belly syndrome (90,91). Some children do well with no surgical treatment for reflux or gross dilation of the urinary tract. An initial conservative stance is reasonable, keeping in mind that there are indications for aggressive surgical management. The impetus for an aggressive reconstructive approach is the assumption that pooling of urine and reflux lead to progressive renal damage, or that the appearance of the urinary tract is due to obstruction. With improvements in renal imaging and better antibiotics, the observational approach has become more widespread. Conservative therapy, consistcing of prophylactic antibiotics and monitoring of urine cultures and serial renal function studies, is properly undertaken when the urinary tract has a balanced nature. However, even a balanced urinary tract can decompensate over time, and serial monitoring is of the utmost importance.

Temporary urinary diversion is usually preferable to major reconstruction in the neonate because of the unpredictability of the pulmonary reserve (74). Vesicostomy addresses the issues of poor bladder emptying and vesicoureteral reflux, and is occasionally indicated for recurring infections or a rising creatinine. Upper urinary tract diversion is rarely necessary because true ureterovesical junction obstruction is rare. When needed, pyelostomy is the procedure of choice because it spares the upper ureter, which is needed for later reconstruction of the urinary tract (91). The lower ureter can also be brought to the skin as an end-cutaneous ureterostomy because this portion of ureter is generally discarded.

Surgery of the dilated ureters is performed for obstruction at the ureteropelvic or ureterovesical junction, or for reflux with recurrent infection. The stasis of urine in the dilated ureters predisposes to urinary infection, and any surgery to correct reflux or obstruction should address this redundancy. Generally, the lower more dilated and tortuous ureters are discarded. The more normal upper ureter is tapered as necessary and then reimplanted into the bladder in a nonrefluxing fashion. Preservation of the vascular adventitia of the ureter is extremely important, especially if correction of ureteropelvic junction obstruction is carried out during the operation.

The function of the urinary bladder in prune belly syndrome can change over time. These bladders may empty poorly, and double voiding, Crede maneuver, or intermittent catheterization have to be employed as necessary to reduce postvoid residuals. Urethrotomy is occasionally performed to improve bladder emptying, but prior urodynamic evidence of obstruction should be obtained because it is unclear how often urethrotomy is actually necessary and effective (92). The function of the urinary bladder can change and potentially decompensate with aging. Onset of recurrent urinary infections, worsening renal function, urinary incontinence, or frequency should prompt reevaluation of bladder function. It seems obvious that the function of the bladder should improve by removing the often found large dome diverticulum, but there is no urodynamic evidence that reduction cystoplasty actually aids the emptying ability (93).

The one clear indication for surgical intervention is orchidopexy for the bilaterally undescended testes (94). It is unknown whether early orchidopexy results in improved spermatogenesis, but the ease of orchidopexy decreases after the patient is 1 or 2 years of age. Options for orchidopexy include a conventional transabdominal approach maintaining the integrity of the spermatic vessels with high success rates when undertaken early in life. The other procedure used frequently is the Fowler-Stephens long-looped vas orchidopexy (95), with division of the spermatic vessels. This has been associated with a 20% to 30% atrophy rate in the hands of experienced surgeons. The two-stage Fowler-Stephens approach, involving ligation of the spermatic vessels followed by orchidopexy, may enhance success rates. Microvascular orchidopexy has been performed with reasonable success on boys with prune belly syndrome (96). These alternatives to conventional transabdominal orchidopexy may be necessary in children who present for orchidopexy after 1 year of age.

Surgical repair of the abdominal wall defect has been attempted for both cosmetic and functional indications. The psychological implications of the unusual abdominal appearance in these boys have been stressed. Voiding can improve after abdominoplasty, although this does not represent a primary indication for surgery (97). There are two major alternatives to the reconstruction of the abdominal wall. The first involves vertical plication and overlapping to reduce abdominal girth and to bring the more normally formed lateral muscles toward the midline. This can be done with excision of the midline abdominal wall and preservation of the umbilicus or by overlapping the deficient anterior abdominal fascial layers with or without umbilical preservation. The abdominoplasty popularized by Randolph et al. (97) involves a transverse excision of the lower abdominal wall, under the assumption that the upper abdominal musculature is more normally developed and can be brought down to the lower fascia. This can be performed with the adjunct of electromyographic data to optimize the removal of nonmuscular abdominal wall.

Other techniques involve overlapping the fascia to strengthen the abdominal wall and eliminate redundancy (98). Reconstruction of the abdominal wall offers not only cosmetic and psychological benefits, but also improves voiding parameters and decreases postvoid residual.

Long-term Results

The long-term outlook depends in large part on the neonatal course and presentation. Renal function tends to remain normal in children with a balanced or reconstructed urinary tract who start life with reasonable renal function. In severe cases with dysplastic kidneys, there is often early death due to pulmonary or renal failure. Those children who fall somewhere in between often go on to require dialysis or transplantation. The prognosis of renal transplantation is not adversely affected by the diagnosis of prune belly or by the need for intermittent catheterization. Most patients require preoperative bilateral native nephrectomy.

The prognosis for sexual function and fertility is mixed. Although there is no documented fertility in men with prune belly syndrome, other aspects of sexual function can be expected to be normal. Boys have several causes of impaired fertility. The first is bilaterally undescended testicles, which until recently, were not brought to a scrotal position until later in life. Whether the spermatogenic potential of these testicles is normal is a matter for debate because semen analysis in adults who ejaculate is generally acellular. This question may be answered more definitively as children who have undergone neonatal orchidopexies mature. The other cause of infertility is the hypoplastic nature of the prostate and most do not ejaculate at all. Although prenatal diagnosis and testing are decreasing the incidence of prune belly syndrome, infants continue to be born with this malady. Modern reconstructive surgery will continue to play a role in the ultimate goal to protect renal function in this interesting group of patients.

REFERENCES

1. Gearhart JP. The bladder exstrophy-epispadias-cloacal exstrophy complex. In: Gearhart JP, Rink RC, Mouriquand PDE, eds. *Pediatric urology.* Philadelphia: WB Saunders, 2001:511–546.
2. Clementson C, Kockum C, Hansson E, et al. Bladder exstrophy in Sweden: a long term follow-up study. *Eur J Pediatr Surg* 1996;6:208.
3. Lancaster PAL. Epidemiology of bladder exstrophy: a communication from the International Clearinghouse for Birth Defects monitoring system. *Teratology* 1987;36:221.
4. Ambrose SS, O'Brian DP. Surgical embryology of the exstrophy-epispadias complex. *Surg Clin North Am* 1974;54:1379.
5. Marshall VF, Muecke C. Congenital abnormalties of the bladder. In: *Handbuch der urologie.* New York: Springer-Verlag, 1968:165.
6. Mildenberger H, Lkuth D, Dziuba M. Embryology of bladder exstrophy. *J Pediatr Surg* 1988;23:116.
7. Johnson JH, Kogan SJ. The exstrophic anomalies and their surgical reconstruction. *Curr Prob Surg* August 1974;1–39.
8. Shapiro E, Lepor H, Jeffs RD. The inheritance of classic bladder exstrophy. *J Urol* 1984;132:308.
9. Woodhouse CR. Prospects for fertility in patients born with genitourinary anomalies. *J Urol* 2001;165:2354–2360.
10. Silver RI, Partin AW, Epstein JI, et al. Penile length in adulthood after bladder exstrophy reconstruction. *J Urol* 1997;158:999–1003.
11. Connolly JA, Peppas DS, Jeffs RD, et al. Prevalence and repair of inguinal hernias in children with bladder exstrophy. *J Urol* 1995; 154.
12. Stec AA, Pannu HK, Tadros YE, et al. Pelvic floor anatomy in classic bladder exstrophy using 3-dimensional computerized tomography: initial insights. *J Urol* 2001;166:1444.
13. Stec AA, Pannu HK, Tadros YE, et al. Evaluation of the bony pelvis in classic bladder exstrophy by using 3D-CT: further insights. *Urology* 2001;58:1030.
14. Lee BR, Pearlman EJ, Partin AW, et al. Evaluation of smooth-muscle and collagen subtypes in normal newborns and those born with bladder exstrophy. *J Urol* 1996;156:2034–2036.
15. Mathews RI, Wills M, Pearlman E, et al. Neural innervation of the newborn exstrophy bladder: an immunohistological study. *J Urol* 1999;162:506–508.
16. Frimberger D, Lakshmanan Y, Gearhart JP. Continent urinary diversions in the exstrophy complex: why do they fail? *J Urol* 2003 Oct;170(4 Pt 1):1338–1342.
17. Sponseller PD, Bisson LJ, Gearhart JP, et al. The anatomy of the pelvis in the exstrophy complex. *J Bone Joint Surg Am* 1995;77:177–189.
18. Gearhart JP, Forsher DC, Jeffs RD, et al. A combined vertical and horizontal pelvic osteotomy for primary and secondary repair of bladder exstrophy. *J Urol* 1996;155:689–693.
19. Duckett JW. Use of paraexstrophy skin pedicle grafts for correction of exstrophy and epispadias repair. *Birth Defects* 1977;13:171.
20. Husmann DA, McLorie GA, Churchill BM. Closure of the exstrophic bladder: an evaluation of the factors leading to its success and its importance on urinary continence. *J Urol* 1989;142:522–524.
21. Gearhart JP, Ben-Chaim J, Scortino C, et al. The multiple reoperative bladder exstrophy closure: what affects potential to the bladder. *Urology* 1996;47:240–243.

22. Gearhart JP, Jeffs RD. Bladder exstrophy: increase in capacity following epispadias repair. *J Urol* 1989;142:525–526.
23. Zaontz MR, Steckler RE, Shortliffe LMD, et al. Multicenter experience with the Mitchel technique for epispadias repair. *J Urol* 1998;160:172.
24. Grady R, Mitchell ME. Complete repair of bladder exstrophy. *J Urol* 1999;162:1415–1420.
25. Gearhart JP. Complete repair of bladder exstrophy in the newborn: complications and management. *J Urol* 2001;165:2431–2433.
26. Chan YD, Jeffs RD, Gearhart JP. Determinants of continence in the bladder exstrophy population: predictors of success? *Urology* 2001;57:774–777.
27. Gearhart JP, Mathews R, Taylor S, et al. Combined bladder closure and epispadias repair in the management of bladder exstrophy. *J Urol* 1998;160:1182–1185.
28. Lattimer JK, Smith MJ. Exstrophy closure: a followup on 70 cases. *Trans Am Assoc Genitourin Surg* 1965;57:102–105.
29. Gearhart JP, Jeffs RD. Management of the failed exstrophy closure. *J Urol* 1991;146:610–612.
30. Meldrum KK, Gearhart JP. *Methods of pelvic immobilization following bladder exstrophy closure: associated complications and impact on surgical success.* Presented at the 2nd International Symposium on Exstrophy and Epispadias, Baltimore, October 2002.
31. Perlmutter AD, Weinstein MD, Rademan C. Vesical neck reconstruction in patients with the bladder exstrophy complex. *J Urol* 1991;146:613–615.
32. Mollard P, Mouriquand PE, Buttin X. Urinary continence after reconstruction of classic bladder exstrophy (73 cases). *Br J Urol* 1994;73:298–302.
33. McMahon DR, Kane MP, Husmann DA, et al. Vesical neck reconstruction in patients with the exstrophy-epispadias-complex. *J Urol* 1996;155:1411–1413.
34. Surer I, Baker LA, Jeffs RD, et al. The modified Cantwell-Ransley technique repair in exstrophy and epispadias. *J Urol* 2000;164:1040.
35. Ben-Chaim J, Jeffs RD, Reiner WG, et al. The outcome of patients with classic bladder exstrophy in adult life. *J Urol* 1996;155:1251.
36. Dodson JL, Surer I, Baker LA, et al. The newborn exstrophy bladder inadequate for primary closure: evaluation, management and outcome. *J Urol* 2001;165:1656–1659.
37. Schrott KM. Komplette einzeitige aufbauplastik der blasenekstrophie. In: Schreiter F, ed. *Plastisch-rekonstruktive chirurgie in der urologie.* Stuttgart-New York: Georg Thieme-Verlag, 1999:430–438.
38. Baka-Jakubiak M. Combined bladder neck, urethral and penile reconstruction in boys with exstrophy-epispadias complex. *BJU Int* 2000;86:513–518.
39. Stein R, Fisch M, Black P, et al. Strategies for reconstruction of unsuccessful or unsatisfactory primary treatment of patients with bladder exstrophy or incontinent episapdias. *J Urol* 1999;161:1934–1941.
40. Hurwitz RS, Manzoni GA, Ransley PG, et al. Cloacal exstrophy: a report of 34 cases. *J Urol* 1987;138:1060.
41. Woodhouse CRJ. Sexual function in boys with exstrophy, myelomeningocele and micropenis. *Urol* 1998;52:3.
42. Patten BM, Barry A. The genesis of exstrophy of the bladder and epispadias. *Am J Anat* 1952;90:35.
43. Langer JC, Brennan B, Lappaliainen RF, et al. Cloacal exstrophy: prenatal diagnosis before rupture of the cloacal membrane. *J Pediatr Surg* 1992;27:1352–1355.
44. Bruch SW, Adzick NS, Goldstein RB, et al. Challenging the embryogenesis of cloacal exstrophy. *J Pediatr Surg* 1996;31:768–770.
45. Surer I, Ferrer FA, Baker LA, et al. Continent diversion and the exstrophy-epispadias complex. *J Urol* 2003;169:1102–1105.
46. Sponseller PD, Bisson LJ, Gearhart JP, et al. The anatomy of the pelvis in the exstrophy complex. *J Bone Joint Surg Am* 1995;77:177–189.
47. Schlegel PN, Gearhart JP. Neuroanatomy of an infant with cloacal exstrophy: a detailed microdissection with histology. *J Urol* 1989;141:583.
48. Diamond DA. Management of cloacal exstrophy. *Dial Pediatr Urol* 1990;13:2.
49. McLaughlin KP, Rink RC, Kalsbeck JE, et al. Cloacal exstrophy: the neurological implications. *J Urol* 1995;154:782–784.
50. Howell C, Caldamone A, Snyder H, et al. Optimal management of cloacal exstrophy. *J Pediatr Surg* 1983;18:365–369.
51. Ben-Chaim J, Sponseller PD, Jeffs RD, et al. Application of osteotomy in cloacal exstrophy patients. *J Urol* 1995;154:865–867.
52. Tank ES, Lindenauer SM. Principles of management of exstrophy of the cloaca. *Am J Surg* 1970;119:95–98. Geiger JD, Corn AG. The association of large ovarian cysts with cloacal exstrophy. *J Pediatr Surg* 1998;33:1719–1727.
53. Ricketts RR, Woodard JR, Zwiren GT, et al. Modern treatment of cloacal exstrophy. *J Pediatr Surg* 1991;26:444–450.
54. Austin P, Holmes YL, Gearhart JP, et al. Prenatal diagnosis of cloacal exstrophy. *J Urol* 1998;160:1179. Hamada H, Takno K, Shiina A, et al. New ultrasound criteria for the prenatal diagnosis of cloacal exstrophy: elephant trunk-like image. *J Urol* 1999;162:2123–2124.
55. Steinbuchel W. Ueber nabelschnurbruch und blasenbauchspalte mit kloakenbildung von seiten des duenndarms. *Arch Gynaekol* 1900;60:456.
56. Rickham PP, Stauffer UG. Exstrophy of the bladder progress of management during the last 25 years. *Prog Pediatr Surg* 1984;17:169–188.
57. Mathews RI, Jeffs RD, Reiner WG, et al. Cloacal exstrophy—improving the quality of life. The Johns Hopkins experience. *J Urol* 1998;160:2452–2456.
58. Husmann DA, Vanderstein Dr, McLorie GH, et al. Urinary incontinence after staged bladder reconstruction for cloacal exstrophy. The affect of co-existing neurological abnormalities on urinary continence. *J Urol* 1999;162:1598–1602.
59. Hendren WH. Cloaca, the most severe degree of imperforate anus: experience with 195 cases. *Ann Surg* 1998;228:331–346.
60. Silver RI, Sponseller PD, Gearhart JP. Staged closure of the pelvis in cloacal exstrophy: first description of a new approach. *J Urol* 1999;161:263–266.
61. Adams MC, Mitchell ME, Rink RC. Gastrocystoplasty: an alternative solution to the problem of urological reconstruction in the severely compromised patient. *J Urol* 1988;140:1152.
62. Hendren WH. Ileal nipple for continence in cloacal exstrophy. *J Urol* 1992;148:372.
63. Reiner WG. Psychosocial concerns in bladder and cloacal exstrophy. *Dial Pediatr Urol* 1999;22:8.
64. Shober JM, Carmichael PA, Hines M, et al. The ultimate challenge of cloacal exstrophy. *J Urol* 2002;167:300–304.
65. Eagle JF, Barret GS. Congenital deficiency of abdominal musculature with associated genitourinary anomalies: a syndrome: reports of nine cases. *Pediatrics* 1950;6:721.
66. Greskovich FJ, Nyberg LN Jr. The prune-belly syndrome: a review of its etiology, defects, treatment and prognosis. *J Urol* 1988;140:707.
67. Garlinger P, Ott J. Prune-belly syndrome—possible genetic implications. *Birth Defects* 1974;10:173.
68. Manzoni GA, Ransley PG, Hurwitz RS. Cloacal exstrophy and cloacal exstrophy variants: a proposed system of classification. *J Urol* 1987;138:1065–1068.
69. Stumme EG. Ueber die symetrischen kongenitalen bauchmuskeldefekte und ueber die kombination derselben mit anderen bildungsanomalien des rumpfes. *Mii Grenzgebiete Med Cir* 1903;11:548.
70. Pagon RA, Smith DA, Shepard TH. Urethral obstruction malformation complex: a cause of abdominal muscle deficiency and the "prune belly". *J Pediatr* 1979;94:900–906.
71. Docimo SG, Luetic T, Crone RK, et al. Pulmonary development in the fetal lamp with severe bladder outlet obstruction and oligohydramnios: a morphometric study. *J Urol* 1989;142:657.
72. Beasley SW, Bettenay F, Hudson JM. The anterior urethra provides clues to the etiology of the prune belly syndrome. *Pediatr Surg Int* 1988;3:169–172.
73. Smith AS, Woodard JR. Prune-belly syndrome. In: Gearhart JP, Rink RC, Mouriquand PDE, eds. *Pediatric urology.* Philadelphia: WB Saunders, 2001:577–592.
74. Rogers LW, Ostrow PT. The prune-belly syndrome: report of 20 cases and description of a lethal variant. *J Pediatr* 1973;83:786.
75. Williams DI, Burkholder GV. The prune belly syndrome. *J Urol* 1967;98:244.
76. Gearhart JP, Lee BR, Partin AW, et al. Quantitative histological evaluation of the dilated ureter of childhood II: ectopia, posterior urethral valves and the prune-belly syndrome. *J Urol* 1995;153:172–176.
77. Workman SJ, Kogan BA. Fetal bladder histology in posterior urethral valves and the prune-belly syndrome. *J Urol* 1990;144:337–339.

78. Stephens FD, Gupta D. Pathogenesis of the prune-belly syndrome. *J Urol* 1994;152:2328–2331.
79. Appel RA, Kaplan RW, Brock WA, et al. Megalourethra. *J Urol* 1986;135:747.
80. Nunn IN, Stephens FD. The triad syndrome: a composite anomaly of the abdominal wall, urinary system and testes. *J Urol* 1961;86: 782.
81. Orvis BR, Bottels K, Kogan BA. Testicular histology in fetuses with prune-belly syndrome and posterior urethral valves. *J Urol* 1988; 139:335.
82. Massad CA, Cohen MB, Kogan BA, et al. Morphology and histochemistry of the infant testis in prune-belly syndrome. *J Urol* 1991; 146:1598.
83. Alford BA, Peoples WM, Resnick JS, et al. Pulmonary complication associated with the prune-belly syndrome. *Pediatr Radiol* 1978; 129:401.
84. Wright JR, Barth RF, Neff JC, et al. Gastrointestinal malformations associated with the prune-belly syndrome. *Pediatr Pathol* 1986;5: 421.
85. Heydenrych J, DuToit PE. Torsion of the spleen and associated prune-belly syndrome—case report and review of the literature. *S Afr Med J* 1978;53:637.
86. Adebonojo FO. Dysplasia of the abdominal musculature with multiple congenital anomalies: prune-belly or triad syndrome. *J Natl Med Assoc* 1973;65:327.
87. Green NE, Lowery ER, Thomas R. Orthopedic aspects of prune-belly syndrome. *J Pediatr Orthop* 1993;13:496.
88. Loder RT, Guiboux JP, Bloom DA, et al. Musculoskeletal aspects of prune-belly syndrome. *Am J Dis Child* 1992;146:1224.
89. Bovicelli L, Rizzo N, Orsini LF, et al. Prenatal diagnosis of the prune-belly syndrome. *Clin Genet* 1980;18:79.
90. Woodard JR, Smith EA.Prune-belly syndrome. In: Walsh PC, Retik AB, Vaughn ED Jr, et al. eds. *Campbell's urology,* 7th ed. Philadelphia: WB Saunders, 1980:9.
91. Woodhouse CRJ, Kellett MJ, Williams DI. Minimal surgical interference in prune-belly syndrome. *Br J Urol* 1979;51:475–480.
92. Snyder HM, Marrison NW, Whitfield HN, et al. Urodynamics in the prune-belly syndrome. *Br J Urol* 1976;48:663.
93. Bukowski TP, Perlmutter AD. Reduction cystoplasty in the prune-belly syndrome. A long term follow-up. *J Urol* 1994;152:2113–2116.
94. Woodard JR, Parrott TS. Orchidopexy in prune-belly syndrome. *Br J Urol* 1978;50:348.
95. Fowler R Jr, Stephens FD.The role of testicular vascular anatomy in the salvage of high undescended testes. In: Stephens FD, ed. *Congenital malformations of the rectum, anus, and genitourinary tract.* Baltimore: Williams & Wilkins, 1963.
96. Wacksman J, Dinner M, Staffon RA. Technique of testicular autotransplantation using a microvascular anastomosis. *Surg Gynecol Obstet* 1980;150:399.
97. Randolph J, Cavatt C, Eng G. Surgical correction and rehabilitation for children with the "prune-belly" syndrome. *Ann Surg* 1981;6:757.
98. Monfort G, Guys JM, Bocciardi A, et al. A novel technique for reconstruction of the abdominal wall in the prune-belly syndrome. *J Urol* 1991;146:639.

PART D

Intestine

Chapter 71

Gastrointestinal Bleeding

Michael G. Caty and B. Robert Gibson

Gastrointestinal (GI) hemorrhage is an alarming situation for both parent and surgeon. Fortunately, GI bleeding in most children is due to benign causes and is usually self-limited (Table 71-1). Nevertheless, an aggressive diagnostic approach to the child with significant bleeding is warranted. A diagnostic approach based on the frequency of age-related causes of bleeding usually results in the establishment of a cause for the bleeding.

INITIAL APPROACH AND RESUSCITATION

The initial steps in the evaluation of the child with GI bleeding are to identify the source as upper or lower, assess the magnitude of the bleeding, and initiate resuscitation of the child.

Upper GI hemorrhage is defined as bleeding that originates proximal to the ligament of Treitz. This is manifested by either hematemesis, melena, or occult blood loss. Lower GI hemorrhage may present with hematochezia, melena, or occult blood loss. Elements of the patient's history that suggest an upper GI source include preexisting liver disease, recent surgical stress or injury, or a family history of ulcer disease. A recent diarrheal illness, history of weight loss with abdominal pain, or family history of polyps or colon resections may suggest a lower source of GI bleeding. Following examination of the nasopharynx to exclude a non-GI source of bleeding, the initial diagnostic maneuver is to place a nasogastric tube. The absence of blood in the presence of aspirated bile rules out an upper GI source with reasonable certainty. If blood is detected, the nasogastric tube allows lavage of the stomach to assess the rate of bleeding. It also removes blood that would impair endoscopic evaluation.

To direct the diagnostic evaluation and guide the resuscitation, an estimate of the rate of bleeding must be made. An initial impression can be formed from observation of the volume of blood from the nasogastric tube or amount of melenic stool. The most important information comes from the physiologic status of the infant or child. Children tolerate blood loss of less than 10% of blood volume (8 mL per kg) extremely well and may demonstrate only minimal elevation of the pulse rate. Increasing heart rate and the presence of orthostatic hypotension suggest a 10% to 20% loss. The findings of hypotension and poor capillary refill are associated with blood loss in excess of 30% of blood volume. Patients with greater than 10% blood loss should be monitored in an intensive care unit.

The resuscitation of the child with GI hemorrhage is directed by the magnitude of the bleeding. A history is obtained, and the location and magnitude of the bleeding is estimated. A history of medications that affect the coagulation system is elicited. A complete blood count, platelet count, liver function tests, and coagulation studies are obtained. The resuscitation itself is as one would conduct for a patient with hemorrhage from any site.

After the initial resuscitation, the management plan shifts to that of diagnosis and treatment. The following section presents a discussion of organ-specific sources of GI bleeding followed by an age-related approach to the diagnostic evaluation of children with upper and lower GI hemorrhage.

SOURCES OF UPPER GASTROINTESTINAL BLEEDING

Esophagitis

Esophagitis is responsible for 15% to 19% of upper GI hemorrhage found in childhood (1). In infancy, esophagitis

Michael G. Caty: Division of Pediatric Surgery, State University of New York at Buffalo, Women and Children's Hospital of Buffalo, Buffalo, New York 14222.

B. Robert Gibson: Department of Surgery, State University of New York at Buffalo, Erie County Medical Center, Buffalo, New York 14215.

TABLE 71-1 Common Causes of Gastrointestinal Hemorrhage in Children.

Upper GI tract
Newborn
Gastritis
Esophagitis
Swallowed maternal blood
Infant
Gastritis
Esophagitis
Peptic ulcer disease
Preschool age
Gastritis
Esophagitis
Peptic ulcer disease
Esophageal varices
School age and adolescent
Gastritis
Esophagitis
Esophageal varices
Peptic ulcer disease
Vascular malformation
Lower GI tract
Newborn
Necrotizing enterocolitis
Malrotation with midgut volvulus
Anal fissure
Vascular malformation
Hirschsprung's disease with enterocolitis
Infant
Anal fissure
Allergic proctocolities
Vascular malformation
Intussusception
Meckel's diverticulum
Lymphonodular hyperplasia
Intestinal duplication
Preschool age
Colonic polyps
Lymphonodular hyperplasia
Meckel's diverticulum
Intestinal duplication
Hemolytic uremic syndrome
Henoch-Schönlein purpura
Infectious colitis
School age and adolescent
Inflammatory bowel disease
Infectious colitis
Colonic polyps

often results from gastroesophageal reflux (GER). Although biopsy evidence of esophagitis is present in 61% to 83% of infants with GER, clinically apparent bleeding is unusual (2). Esophagitis usually causes occult blood loss and anemia. Acute bleeding from esophagitis is treated with nasogastric decompression, histamine-2 (H_2) antagonists, proton pump inhibitors, or oral antacids, and positional therapy. If nonoperative therapy is successful, reflux is documented, and medical management is instituted. If medical management does not control reflux, an antireflux operation is performed. Severity of esophagitis has not been shown to correlate with the need for antireflux surgery (3).

Esophageal Varices

Variceal hemorrhage is an important cause of 7% to 10% of upper GI hemorrhage in children and adolescents (4). Most children with portal hypertension and variceal hemorrhage present before 5 years of age. Portal hypertension in children results from both extrahepatic and intrahepatic causes. Among the known causes of extrahepatic portal hypertension are neonatal omphalitis, umbilical vein catheterization, and portal vein hypoplasia associated with Klippel-Trenaunay syndrome. Intrahepatic portal hypertension most commonly results from cirrhosis secondary to biliary atresia. Nonoperative management includes endoscopic variceal ligation or injection, placement of a Sengkstaken-Blakemore tube, and use of intravenous octreotide or vasopressin (5). Operative management includes portosystemic shunts, variceal ligation, esophageal division, and esophageal devascularization.

Stress Ulceration and Gastritis

Gastritis is responsible for 13% to 22% of pediatric upper GI hemorrhage and may be defined as primary or secondary. Primary gastritis in children is most often due to *Helicobacter pylori* infection. This rarely results in symptomatic gastritis (6). Its importance lies in its relation to peptic ulcer disease in children. Secondary gastritis resulting in GI hemorrhage can occur secondary to mechanical injury to the gastric mucosa as occurs with long-term nasogastric suction, or due to stress ulceration of the stomach. Premature infants and children sustaining trauma, burns, or serious medical illnesses are at risk for developing stress ulcers. Stress ulceration has been found to be responsible for approximately 10% of GI hemorrhage in pediatric intensive care patients (7). The pathophysiology of stress ulceration of the stomach is not fully defined. Important concepts include loss of mucosal barrier function, alterations in gastric microcirculation, back diffusion of hydrogen ion, and duodenogastric bile reflux. Neonates and children present with either "coffee ground" emesis or frank hematemesis. Children with significant ongoing bleeding should undergo prompt diagnostic endoscopy. Initial nonoperative management includes transfusion, correction of any coagulopathy, and the use of antacids, H_2-antagonists, proton pump inhibitors, or sucralfate. If correctable causes of stress exist, such as burn wound infection or intraabdominal abscess, they should be treated concurrently. If initial management does not succeed, operative exploration should be performed, although this is uncommon in contemporary pediatric surgical practice.

Preoperative endoscopy can identify bleeding sites in the stomach in most patients. The presence or absence of associated duodenal bleeding from either duodenitis or peptic ulcer disease should be established prospectively. In the absence of duodenal bleeding, the initial operative maneuver should be a gastrotomy and the walls of the stomach inspected. The least ablative surgery should be performed. If possible, superficial erosions should be oversewn. Focal ulcers, Dieulafoy lesions, or isolated areas of bleeding can be resected locally or with a standard partial gastrectomy, but this is rarely necessary. Problems arise in patients with life-threatening hemorrhage from multiple sites on the gastric wall. Gastric devascularization has been used successfully to treat this condition (8). If this fails to stop the bleeding, total gastrectomy is an option. It is difficult to identify the appropriate application of vagotomy in these situations, but it may be recommended in children with associated duodenal ulcer disease.

Having discussed the operative management of the child with stress gastritis, it is important to emphasize the importance of prophylaxis. Stressed children should have aggressive attempts to raise their gastric pH to above 4.5 with either H_2-antagonists, proton pump inhibitors, or antacids. This is usually sufficient therapy.

Peptic Ulcer Disease

Peptic ulcer disease can afflict children in all age groups. The capacity of the stomach to produce acid is present in the premature and full-term newborn infant (9). About one-half of children with acute ulcers present with GI hemorrhage. Gastric and duodenal ulcer disease is responsible for 18% and 11% of upper GI hemorrhage, respectively. Fortunately, this bleeding is usually not life threatening. Endoscopy should accurately localize the ulcer. Endoscopic techniques, such as heater probe coagulation or bipolar cautery, may be used to arrest the bleeding focus. If this fails, operation is necessary. Standard therapy includes exposure of the ulcer and three-point suture ligation of the ulcer bed. Ligation of the gastroduodenal artery may be beneficial. Vagotomy and a drainage procedure do not appear necessary for acute bleeding ulcers in children. After successful medical or surgical management, children are placed on an H_2-antagonist for 3 to 6 months. The Zollinger-Ellison syndrome should be considered in any child with multiple ulcers or recurrent ulcers. Serum gastrin levels are obtained to rule out this syndrome.

SOURCES OF LOWER GASTROINTESTINAL BLEEDING

Meckel's Diverticulum

Lower GI hemorrhage is a common complication of a Meckel's diverticulum. Most children affected are younger than 5 years of age (10). In 95% of cases, bleeding results from ulceration of adjacent ileal mucosa by heterotopic acid secreting gastric or pancreatic mucosa contained in the diverticulum. Bleeding is usually painless. The diagnostic test of choice is a technetium-99m pertechnetate scan (Fig. 71-1). Uptake of the isotope by the heterotopic mucosa allows identification of the bleeding source. The technetium scan is 85% sensitive and 95% specific for a Meckel's diverticulum presenting with hemorrhage. Diagnostic yield of the scan can be increased by

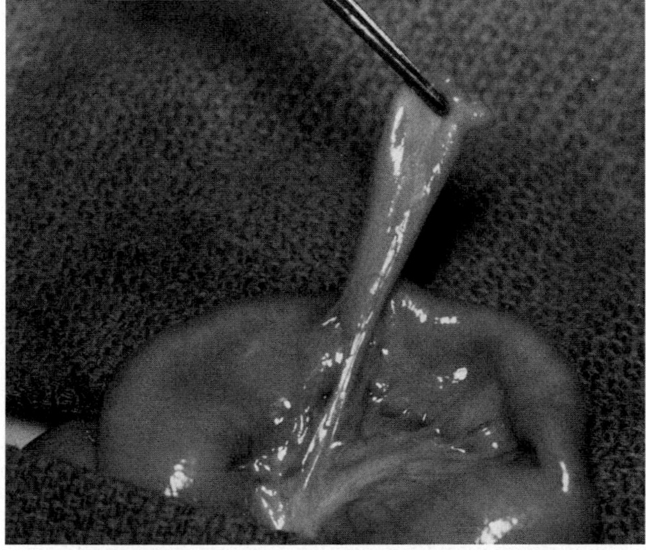
A

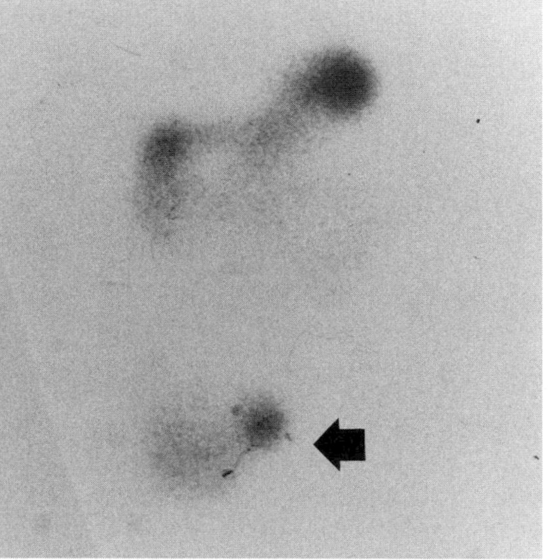
B

FIGURE 71-1. **(A)** Meckel's diverticulum. **(B)** Technetium scan positive for bleeding Meckel's diverticulum (*arrow*).

pharmacologic intervention with H_2-blockers to inhibit isotope excretion from ectopic gastric mucosa. In addition, pentagastrin stimulates isotope uptake by the ectopic mucosa and glucagon decreases peristalsis, thereby increasing isotope retention time within the diverticula (11). Nonbleeding Meckel's diverticuli can also be diagnosed by visceral angiography (12).

After the child is stabilized, the diverticulum is excised surgically. Care is taken to assess the adjacent ileum for the presence of an ulcer that may need to be resected with the diverticulum. Many Meckel's diverticuli are amenable to laparoscopic excision.

Intestinal Polyps

Juvenile Polyps

Juvenile polyps have an estimated prevalence of 1% to 2% in the general population. The most common presentation for a juvenile polyp is painless rectal bleeding, which occurs in 92% of these patients (13). Bleeding from juvenile polyps usually occurs in preschool-age children. These polyps, also known as *hamartomatous* or *retention polyps*, are benign, with less than 5% of polyps showing signs of dysplasia (14). Bleeding originates from the friable surface of the polyps. The cause of these polyps is unknown. The presence of interstitial eosinophils raises the possibility of an allergic reaction of the colonic mucosa. Recent application of pancolonoscopy has revealed that greater than 55% of polyps are found in the rectosigmoid colon, 15% in the descending colon, 15% in the transverse colon, and 15% in the right colon. Colonoscopy has refuted the assumption that juvenile polyps are usually solitary because multiple polyps are found in greater than 50% of patients presenting with a lower GI hemorrhage (15). This finding has taken on new significance, as the presence of three to five polyps is consistent with the premalignant condition juvenile polyposis coli (JPC) (16). Curative treatment by colonoscopic polypectomy or transanal excision is achieved in 97% of cases.

Juvenile Polyposis Coli

JPC is an autosomal dominant disorder that typically presents with rectal bleeding associated with abdominal pain and diarrhea. At the time of presentation, colonic polyps may number from 10 to 200 and may be located throughout the colon. Although rare, the stomach and small bowel may also be involved. JPC is distinguished from other disorders by polyp number and the presence of a family history of colon cancer. Those with greater than three juvenile polyps on colonoscopy have a 50% lifetime risk of developing colon cancer (17). Patients should be managed with upper endoscopy and complete colonoscopy every 2 years, with random biopsy of mucosa and polyps. If symptoms persist or a dysplastic polyp is found, prophylactic colectomy may be considered. Given the lifelong risk of cancer, and the necessity of invasive screening, prophylactic colectomy may be considered after adolescence. Because JPC is an inherited disorder, first-degree relatives must also be screened for the disease with complete colonoscopy after 12 years of age (14).

Familial Adenomatous Polyposis

Familial adenomatous polyposis (FAP) is found in 1:5,000 to 17,000 patients and is inherited in an autosomal dominant pattern. Patients with FAP present with 100 to 1,000 adenomatous polyps located throughout the colon, carrying a 100% lifetime risk of colonic neoplasia. Variants of FAP such as Gardner and Turcot syndrome are associated with extraintestinal tumors and have the same lifetime risk of colonic neoplasia. Once FAP or a variant is diagnosed, prophylactic colectomy is considered the treatment of choice (18). Because the disease is inherited in an autosomal dominant pattern, genetic screening is recommended for first-degree relatives. Nonoperative therapy may include cyclooxygenase-2 inhibitors, which have been found to reduce the number of polyps by 28% (19). However, there is yet no evidence that this reduction in polyp number translates into a decreased risk of malignancy. For those with positive genetic screening, annual screening sigmoidoscopy should be performed until the presence of polyposis is noted, total colectomy should then be performed after adolescence (17).

Peutz-Jeghers Syndrome

Peutz-Jeghers syndrome is a rare autosomal dominant disorder that frequently presents with intussusception, abdominal pain, and bleeding. Symptoms arise from hamartomatous polyps, which can be located throughout the GI tract: 78% of affected individuals with polyps located in the small bowel, 42% in the colon, 38% in the stomach, and 28% in the duodenum (18). Those diagnosed with Peutz-Jeghers syndrome are at increased risk of developing intestinal and extraintestinal malignancy, such as ovarian or testicular cancer. Less than 5% of polyps are associated with neoplastic change and management consists of polypectomy with upper and lower endoscopy every 2 years starting at age 10. First-degree relatives should also be screened for polyps with complete colonoscopy every 3 years, starting in adolescence.

Hamartoma Tumor Syndromes

Hamartoma tumor syndromes are also known as phosphatase and tensin homologue hamartoma tumor syndromes (PTEN). These hamartoma tumor syndromes are a rare cause of hamartomatous polyps in children and are inherited in an autosomal dominant pattern. Diagnosis of a particular subtype of PTEN syndrome is dependent on a constellation of other findings. Cowden syndrome is associated with goiter and increased risk of thyroid cancer and breast cancer. Gastrointestinal polyps are found in as many as 40% of patients with Cowden syndrome. Bannayan-Riley-Ruvacaba syndrome (BRRS) is associated with pigmented macules on the penis, macrocephaly, multiple lipomas, and intestinal hamartomas. Diagnosis of BRRS may be facilitated by finding ganglia within biopsied polyps. Neither Cowden's or BRRS is known to be associated with increased risk of GI malignancy. Hereditary nonpolyposis colorectal cancer syndrome (HNPCC) is a rare cause of polyps in children, but has been associated with cancer in patients as young as 6 years of age. This PTEN syndrome is associated with malignancy in multiple extraenteric sites: uterus, ovaries, stomach, small bowel, genitourinary tract, pancreas, biliary tract, skin, and the larynx. In those diagnosed with HNPCC, screening colonoscopy should be performed before age 20. Genetic screening should also be performed in first-degree relatives of any patient diagnosed with a PTEN syndrome due to the autonomic dominant inheritance pattern.

Lymphoid Polyps

Lymphoid polyps result from lymphonodular hyperplasia of the colon. They are benign lesions that cause bleeding in infants and preschool-age children. This entity is believed to be due to an immunologic response to intraluminal antigens because food allergy coexists with 75% of endoscopically proven cases (20). Diagnosis can be made with either sigmoidoscopy or air contrast enema. Endoscopy reveals multiple small friable nodules scattered throughout the colon. Air contrast enema shows raised nodules with a characteristic central umbilication. These lesions resolve spontaneously without treatment.

Anorectal Lesions

Anal fissures are a common cause of rectal bleeding in infants. Infants present with bright red blood on the outside of the stool or with blood in the diaper. Physical examination reveals a small tear at the anal verge. The fissure is often posterior. Fissures result from a superficial tear of the squamous lining of the anal canal during the passage of a firm stool. Bowel movements cause significant discomfort to the infant. Reluctance to defecate results in worsening constipation and increased pain with bowel movements. Treatment consists of breaking this cycle by softening the stool and using warm Sitz baths. It is unusual for breast-fed infants to have anal fissures. Anal fissures may also be a presentation of child abuse. This should be suspected in patients with multiple fissures, perianal condylomata, or other indications of perineal trauma.

Other, less common lesions of the anorectum may cause lower GI bleeding. Anorectal varices result from portal hypertension in children and are rarely symptomatic. Treatment includes sclerotherapy, banding, embolization, and portosystemic shunting.

The solitary rectal ulcer syndrome may also cause bleeding in children. Ulceration is believed to be due to either ischemia or degeneration of a rectal polyp. Treatment is conservative and consists of observation and laxative administration (21).

Heterotopic gastric mucosa in the colon or rectum can also cause bleeding. Lesions are identified by either endoscopy or technetium scan. Treatment consists of local excision.

Intestinal Vascular Malformations

Vascular malformations of the intestine are rare lesions that can involve any part of the alimentary tract. Approximately 25% present in infancy (22). Hemorrhage is the presenting symptom in 71%. Vascular malformations may also present as intussusception, obstruction, congestive heart failure, or portal hypertension (23). Hemorrhage may be slow and chronic, or massive. Lesions may be associated with the Blue-Rubber-Bleb nevus syndrome, Klippel-Trenaunay syndrome, or Rendu-Osler-Weber syndrome. Hemorrhage from the Blue-Rubber-Bleb nevus syndrome is typically occult and chronic (24). Endoscopy can identify vascular malformations in the colon and stomach. Endoscopy may not identify lesions during massive hemorrhage or in atypical locations such a Dieulafoy's lesion in the small bowel. Radionuclide scanning, selective angiography, or both are useful in this instance. Preoperative localization allows directed resections of prepared bowel. Endoscopic laser ablation has been described as an excellent method of palliation of anorectal lesions (25).

Miscellaneous Causes of Lower Gastrointestinal Bleeding

Malrotation with midgut volvulus may cause lower GI hemorrhage. This results from mucosal injury secondary to ischemia of the volvulized bowel. This diagnosis must be considered in the newborn with bilious emesis or abdominal distention. An upper GI series identifies the location of the ligament of Treitz and establishes the diagnosis. Such a child should be immediately explored and a Ladd's procedure performed with resection to nonviable bowel.

The premature infant who has rectal bleeding is evaluated for necrotizing enterocolitis (NEC). Bleeding indicates mucosal ischemia. Findings supportive of the diagnosis of NEC include pneumatosis intestinalis or pneumoperitoneum on abdominal radiograph, abdominal wall erythema, and thrombocytopenia. Initial management includes nasogastric decompression, administration of broad-spectrum antibiotics, and fluid resuscitation. Operation is reserved for patients with pneumoperitoneum or clinical deterioration. Although the stomach is rarely involved in NEC, heme-positive nasogastric aspirates may alert the clinician to the diagnosis in the at-risk newborn. Hemorrhage is rarely significant in magnitude to warrant surgical exploration.

Intestinal duplications can occur in any part of the intestine along its length from mouth to anus, and can be multiple in as many as 5% to 15% of cases (11). Among the complications, they may cause is bleeding. Because 50% of duplications are located in the ileum, bleeding complications usually result in lower GI hemorrhage. Duplications cause bleeding by one of three mechanisms: (1) the presence of heterotopic gastric mucosa in a duplication can result in local acid ulceration, (2) necrosis and bleeding of the bowel wall can result from local ischemia, and (3) a duplication can serve as an intussusceptum. Approximately 25% of duplications contain ectopic gastric mucosa. These duplications can be diagnosed with a technetium scan with 98% sensitivity. Detection of an abdominal mass in a patient with lower GI hemorrhage should raise the suspicion of a duplication. Surgical excision of the duplication is curative.

Intussusception occurs in infants and young children. Rectal bleeding occurs frequently and is described as "currant jelly." This bleeding is rarely hemodynamically significant; its importance relates to helping recognize the diagnosis of intussusception in the infant with crampy abdominal pain.

Invasive bacteria, such as *Salmonella, Shigella,* and *Campylobacter* sp and *Escherichia coli*, can cause colitis presenting with hematochezia. A history of vomiting and diarrhea suggests this cause. Stool cultures and the presence of fecal leukocytes confirm it.

Viral infection from cytomegalovirus can cause life-threatening lower GI hemorrhage. Affected children usually have acquired immunodeficiency syndrome. Multiple, deep mucosal ulcerations of the colon and small intestine are the source of the bleeding. Bleeding can be localized by arteriography or colonoscopy. This entity is often fatal.

Allergic proctocolitis is a common cause of hematochezia in young infants. It results from an allergic response to exposure to cow milk, soy milk, or breast milk. Diagnosis is made on clinical grounds after serious illnesses, such as infectious diarrhea and Hirschsprung's disease, have been ruled out. The implicated formula is stopped, and an alternative formula used. Reinstitution of the previous formula should result in a similar symptom complex. Most cow milk and soy milk allergies resolve by 2 years of age. In cases of chronic lower GI hemorrhage of unknown etiology, a trial of cow's milk exclusion should be made.

Lower GI bleeding may also result from acquired bleeding disorders. The hemolytic uremic syndrome is characterized by fever, hemolytic anemia, and renal dysfunction. Lower GI hemorrhage can result from microvascular thrombosis and mucosal ischemia. Henoch-Schönlein purpura causes a diffuse vasculitis that often involves the intestine. In 25% of cases, bloody stools result from diffuse mucosal hemorrhage. Intussusception associated with Henoch-Schönlein purpura can also cause GI hemorrhage.

AGE-RELATED APPROACH TO THE DIAGNOSIS OF GASTROINTESTINAL BLEEDING IN CHILDREN

The age at which a child with GI bleeding presents defines the differential diagnosis and guides the diagnostic approach. For the sake of simplicity, newborns and infants are considered together, as are preschool-age children, school-age children, and adolescents. Algorithms outlining these approaches are presented in the next section.

Upper Gastrointestinal Bleeding in Newborns and Infants

Newborns and infants with upper GI hemorrhage present with hematemesis or heme-positive nasogastric aspirates (Fig. 71-2). A hospitalized newborn or infant usually has stress gastritis or ulcer disease as a cause of the bleeding. Following nasopharyngeal examination, a nasogastric tube is passed and the stomach lavaged. If the blood clears with irrigation, the nasogastric tube is placed on suction, and the patient is observed. In stressed newborns and infants, intravenous cimetidine or ranitidine is administered, and a blood type and screen is sent for analysis. Failure to clear continued bleeding warrants upper endoscopy for diagnosis. Endoscopy may not be possible in extremely premature infants, but in rare instances, an ultrathin bronchoscope may be used for diagnostic esophagogastroduodenoscopy. If this is unsuccessful and the hemorrhage refractory, laparotomy serves as the diagnostic procedure. Patients with bleeding that fills the stomach and prevents endoscopic diagnosis, as well as patients that are unstable, should also undergo laparotomy. At laparotomy, the stomach and duodenum are inspected. The absence of pathology in the stomach or duodenum warrants examination of the esophagus and gastroesophageal junction for esophagitis or a Mallory-Weiss tear. The full-term infant with hematemesis on the first day of life should be suspected of having swallowed maternal blood. This can be confirmed with the Apt test. This is performed by adding sodium hydroxide to the observed blood. Fetal blood remains pink, whereas adult blood turns brown (26). Approximately 1% of healthy newborns have symptoms of upper GI hemorrhage. Endoscopic examination in these patients reveals esophagitis in 45%, gastric erosions in 40%, gastric ulcers in 33%, gastric petechiae in 10%, and duodenal ulcers in 2% (27). All newborns with bleeding must be

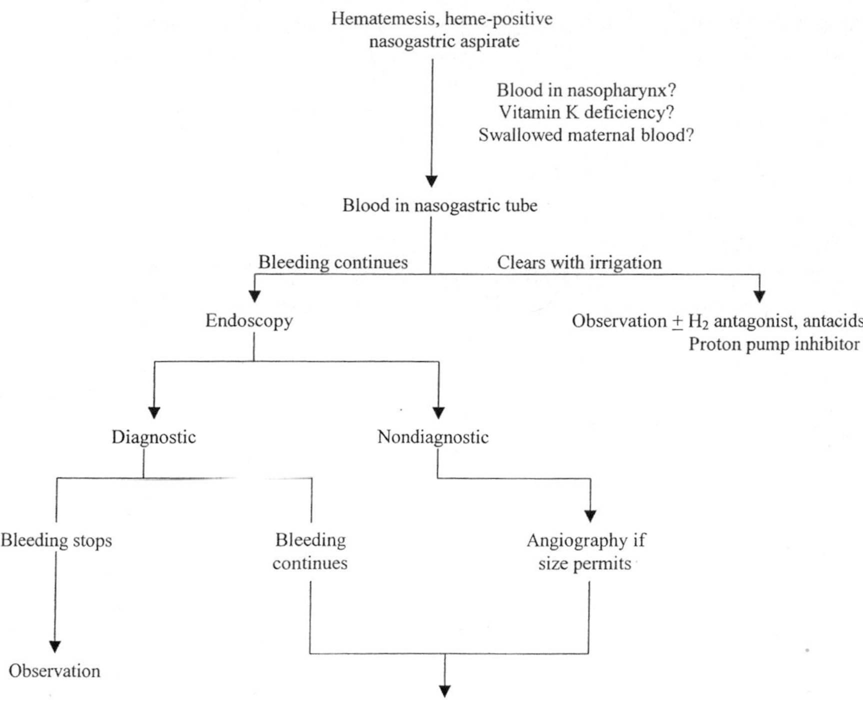

FIGURE 71-2. Diagnostic approach to upper gastrointestinal hemorrhage in infants and children.

considered to have vitamin K deficiency, and 1 mg of vitamin K should be administered intramuscularly. If no underlying coagulopathy exists, nearly all newborns ccase symptomatic bleeding in 48 hours. If symptoms persist past 48 hours, endoscopy should be performed.

Upper Gastrointestinal Bleeding in Children and Adolescents

Children and adolescents with upper GI hemorrhage may present with hematemesis or heme-positive nasogastric aspirates. Older children may also develop massive rectal bleeding or melena as a manifestation of upper GI hemorrhage (Fig. 71-3). The history and physical examination contribute important clues to the cause of the bleeding in this age group. The presence of von Willebrand disease and hemophilia should be sought. A history of placement of an umbilical vein catheter, omphalitis, or biliary atresia suggests esophageal varices as a cause. A family history of ulcer disease should be sought. Following nasopharyngeal exam, a nasogastric tube is placed, confirming the location of the bleeding and estimating its magnitude. Prompt

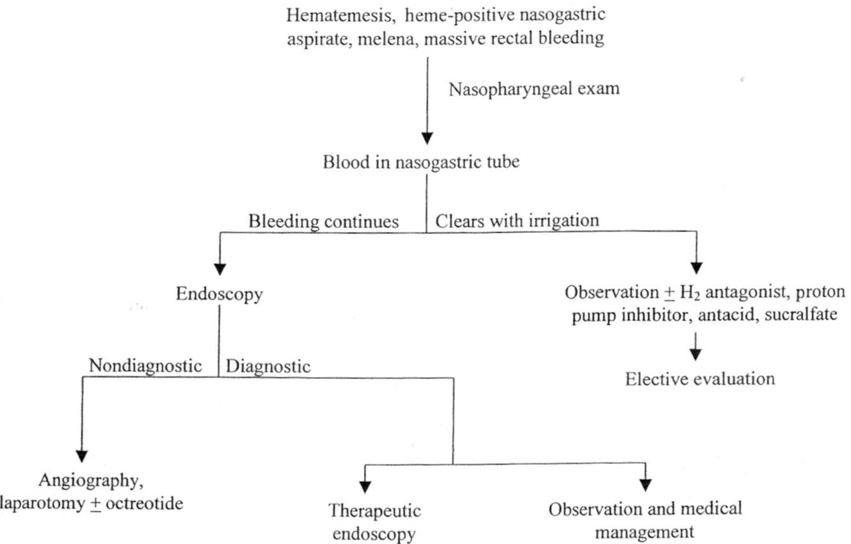

FIGURE 71-3. Diagnostic approach to upper gastrointestinal hemorrhage in children and adolescents.

clearing of the blood merits observation and elective evaluation with endoscopy or an upper GI series. Continued bleeding warrants immediate endoscopy, which can determine the cause of upper GI hemorrhage in 90% of cases (28). In these age groups, therapeutic endoscopy should be performed at the initial examination. Endoscopic findings associated with hematemesis in school-age children include prolapse gastropathy 26%, gastritis 22%, esophagitis 19%, duodenal ulcer 11%, and esophageal varices 7% (1). Endoscopy should include injection or banding of varices and heater probe or cautery treatment of bleeding ulcers. Laparotomy, with or without intravenous octreotide therapy, should be reserved for patients with ongoing bleeding despite therapeutic endoscopy, life-threatening hemorrhage at presentation, or recurrent bleeding (5).

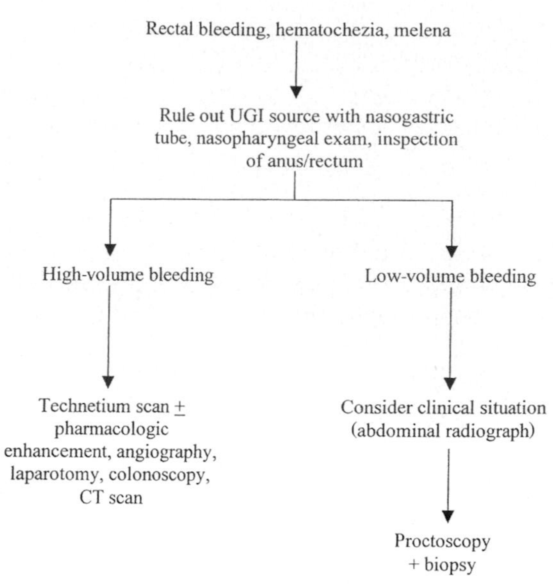

FIGURE 71-4. Diagnostic approach to lower gastrointestinal hemorrhage in infants and children. UGI; upper gastrointestinal; CT, computed tomography.

Lower Gastrointestinal Bleeding in Newborns and Infants

The newborn infant with rectal bleeding should have an upper GI source ruled out by passage of a nasogastric tube. The clinical situation in which the bleeding occurs suggests the diagnosis (Fig. 71-4). The premature infant must be suspected of having NEC. The newborn or infant with bilious emesis must have malrotation ruled out. Intussusception is considered in the older infant with associated crampy abdominal pain. Inspection of the anal area confirms the diagnosis of an anal fissure. Anal fissure and allergic colitis are the most common cause of lower GI hemorrhage in infants younger than 12 months of age. Abdominal radiographs help to evaluate for Hirschsprung's disease, malrotation, NEC, and intussusception. The infant with significant hematochezia should undergo a technetium scan. If this scan is negative, it should be repeated with pharmacologic enhancement. If the scan is again negative, a computed tomographic scan can be performed to evaluate for a duplication. Alternatively, in the presence of significant bleeding, an angiogram can be performed to evaluate for a duplication, vascular malformation, or Meckel's diverticulum not detected by nuclear medicine scan. Patients believed to have allergic proctocolitis by history can have this diagnosis confirmed by proctoscopy and biopsy with Wright's stain for eosinophils.

Lower Gastrointestinal Bleeding in Children and Adolescents

The evaluation of the child or adolescent with rectal bleeding begins with a thorough history and physical examination (Fig. 71-5). The presence of associated symptoms, such as diarrhea and vomiting, should be ascertained. A family history of inflammatory bowel disease or familial polyposis should be sought. Stool should be inspected

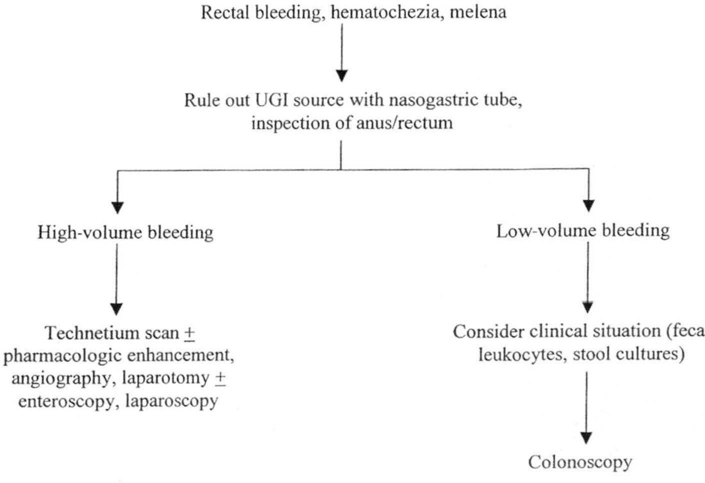

FIGURE 71-5. Diagnostic approach to lower gastrointestinal hemorrhage in children and adolescents. UGI, upper gastrointestinal.

for fecal leukocytes and cultures sent when infection is suspected. Patients with significant bleeding should undergo a technetium scan. If this does not prove diagnostic, colonoscopy is 80% sensitive, and should be performed to evaluate for polyps, infectious colitis, and inflammatory bowel disease (28). If inflammatory bowel disease is restricted to the small bowel, an upper GI series with small bowel follow-through may be necessary to make the diagnosis. Colonoscopy may not be effective with massive bleeding, and angiography or laparoscopy may be necessary. Angiography can potentially identify bleeding from vascular malformations, Meckel's diverticuli, and intestinal duplications. Laparoscopic examination establishes the diagnosis in 76% of patients in this age range with lower GI bleeding, and the port site may be enlarged to deliver pathologic bowel for resection and reanastomosis (29).

REFERENCES

1. Bishop PR, Nowicki MJ, Parker PH. Vomiting-induced hematemesis in children: Mallory-Weiss tear or prolapse gastropathy? *J Pediatr Gastroenterol Nutr* 2000;30:436.
2. Shub MD, Ulshen MH, Hargrove CB, et al. Esophagitis: a frequent consequence of gastroesophageal reflux in infancy. *J Pediatr* 1985;12:881.
3. Black DD, Haggitt RC, Orenstein SR, et al. Esophagitis in infants: morphometric histological diagnosis and correlation with measures of gastroesophageal reflux. *Gastroenterology* 1990;98:1408.
4. Fox VL. Gastrointestinal bleeding in infancy and childhood. *Gastroenterol Clin North Am* 2000;29:37.
5. Siafakas C, Fox VL, Nurko S. Use of octreotide for the treatment of severe gastrointestinal bleeding in children. *J Pediatr Gastroenterol Nutr* 1998;26:356.
6. Drumm B. *Helicobacter pylori* in the pediatric patient. *Gastroenterol Clin North Am* 1993;22:169.
7. Chaibou M, Tucci M, Dugas MA, et al. Clinically significant upper gastrointestinal bleeding acquired in a pediatric intensive care unit: a prospective study. *Pediatrics* 1998;102:933.
8. Udassin R, Nissan S, Lernau OZ, et al. Gastric devascularization—an emergency treatment for hemorrhagic gastritis in the neonate. *J Pediatr Surg* 1983;18:579.
9. Brownlee KG, Kelly EJ. When is the fetus first capable of gastric acid, intrinsic factor and gastrin secretion? *Biol Neonate* 1993;63:153.
10. St-Vil D, Brandt ML, Panic S, et al. Meckel's diverticulum in children: a 20-year review. *J Pediatr Surg* 1991;25:1289.
11. Brown RL, Azizkhan RG. Gastrointestinal bleeding in infants and children: Meckel's diverticulum and intestinal duplication. *Semin Pediatr Surg* 1999;8:202.
12. Routh WD, Lawdahl RB, Lund E, et al. Meckel's diverticula: angiographic diagnosis in patients with non-acute hemorrhage and negative scintigraphy. *Pediatr Radiol* 1990;20:152.
13. Pillai RB, Tolia V. Colonic polyps in children: frequently multiple and recurrent. *Clin Pediatr* 1998;37:253.
14. Hyer W. Polyposis syndromes: pediatric implications. *Gastroenterol Clin North Am* 2001;11:659.
15. Lehmann CU, Elitsur V. Juvenile polyps and their distribution in pediatric patients with gastrointestinal bleeding. *W Va Med J* 1996;92:133.
16. Sandeep KG, Fitzgerald JF, Croffie JM, et al. Experience with juvenile polyps in North American children: the need for pancolonoscopy. *Am J Gastroenterol* 2001;96:1695.
17. Hyer W, Beveridge I, Domizio P, et al. Clinical management and genetics of gastrointestinal polyps in children. *J Pediatr Gastroenterol Nutr* 2000;31:469.
18. Erdman SH, Barnard JA. Gastrointestinal polyps and polyposis syndromes in children. *Curr Opin Pediatr* 2002;14:576.
19. Corredor J, Wambach J, Barnard J. Gastrointestinal polyps in children: advances in molecular genetics, diagnosis, and management. *J Pediatr* 2001;138:621.
20. Kokkonen J, Karttunen TJ. Lymphonodular hyperplasic on the mucosa of the lower gastrointestinal tract in children: an indication of enhanced immune response? *J Pediatr Gastroenterol Nutr* 2002;34:42.
21. De la Rubia L, Ruiz Villaespesa A, Cebrero M, et al. Solitary rectal ulcer syndrome in a child. *J Pediatr* 1992;122:533.
22. Irish MS, Caty MG, Azizkhan RG. Bleeding in children caused by gastrointestinal vascular lesions. *Semin Pediatr Surg* 1999;8:210.
23. Fishman SJ, Burrows PE, Leichtner AM, et al. Gastrointestinal manifestations of vascular anomalies in childhood: varied etiologies require multiple therapeutic modalities. *J Pediatr Surg* 1998;33:1163.
24. Ertem D, Acar Y, Kotiloglu E, et al. Blue rubber bleb nevus syndrome. *Pediatrics* 2001;107:418.
25. Azizkhan RG. Life-threatening hematochezia from a rectosigmoid vascular malformation in Klippel-Trenaunay syndrome: long term palliation using an argon laser. *J Pediatr Surg* 1991;26:1125.
26. Apt L, Downey WS. "Melena" neonatorum: the swallowed blood syndrome. *J Pediatr* 1955;46:6.
27. Lazzaroni M, Petrillo M, Tornaghi R, et al. Upper GI bleeding in healthy full-term infants: a case-control study. *Am J Gastroenterol* 2002;97:89.
28. Arain Z, Rossi TM. Gastrointestinal bleeding in children: an overview of conditions requiring nonoperative management. *Semin Pediatr Surg* 1999;8:172.
29. Lee KH, Yeung CK, Tam YH, et al. Laparoscopy for definitive diagnosis and treatment of gastrointestinal bleeding of obscure origin in children. *J Pediatr Surg* 2000;35:1291.

Chapter 72

Stomach and Duodenum

David K. Magnuson and Marshall Z. Schwartz

Congenital anomalies and acquired abnormalities of the stomach and duodenum are common problems in children. The proper management of these abnormalities, many unique to infants and children, requires an understanding of the anatomy and physiology of the proximal gastrointestinal (GI) tract. The stomach is a complex organ with two distinct physiologic functions: a secretory function effected by the cells of the epithelial lining, and a storage, mixing, and propulsive function effected by the three muscular layers of the gastric wall. These functions are regulated by a complex variety of stimulatory and inhibitory feedback mechanisms that employ neurocrine, endocrine, and paracrine components. The duodenum produces a large number of peptides, many with unknown physiologic roles, and contains the structures that convey bile and pancreatic secretions to the intestinal lumen for mixing with the gastric effluent. Although anatomically, histologically, and functionally distinct, the stomach and duodenum are often considered together because of their proximity and their many interrelated physiologic properties and pathophysiologic responses to disease and stress. This chapter reviews the developmental anatomy of the stomach and duodenum, examines the physiology and pathophysiology of gastric secretory and motor activity, and discusses the treatment of both congenital and acquired gastroduodenal abnormalities in children.

ANATOMY AND PHYSIOLOGY

Developmental Gross Anatomy

The primordial digestive tube forms from the lateral and craniocaudad folding of the embryo during gestational weeks 3 and 4. During this process, the germinal endodermal layer forms the interior of the tube and is surrounded by splanchnic mesoderm. Differentiation of endodermal precursors into surface and glandular epithelium, and of mesodermal precursors into smooth muscle and peritoneal attachments, occurs over the next 6 to 8 weeks. Development of the specialized neuroendocrine cell population of the stomach occurs at about the same time.

Grossly, the stomach begins as a dilation of the foregut, which occurs at about 5 weeks' gestation. Both the stomach and duodenum are suspended between the posterior and anterior body walls by a dorsal and ventral mesentery. During gestational weeks 6 to 10, the stomach undergoes rotation in two planes. A 90-degree rotation occurs around the longitudinal axis in the clockwise direction when viewed from a craniocaudad perspective, and a lessor rotation around the anteroposterior axis occurs in a clockwise fashion when viewed from the front. Differential growth of the ventral wall of the stomach occurs concurrently. These processes result in the following developmental relations: the greater curvature of the stomach migrates inferiorly and to the left of midline, the gastroesophageal junction is placed superior and to the left, the pylorus moves inferiorly and to the right of midline, the dorsal mesogastrium becomes the gastrosplenic ligament and greater omentum and forms the anatomic boundary of the lessor sac, and the ventral mesogastrium becomes the gastrohepatic ligament. Rotation of the vagal trunks results in the left vagus innervating the anterior gastric wall and liver, and the right vagus innervating the posterior gastric wall, small intestine, and retroperitoneum.

The shape of the stomach and the various epithelial cell types that constitute its mucosal lining create several histologically and functionally distinct zones: the cardia, which surrounds the gastroesophageal junction; the fundus, which projects cephalad from the gastroesophageal junction; the corpus, or body, which represents the largest portion of the gastric reservoir; and the antrum, which describes that portion of the stomach immediately preceding the pylorus (Fig. 72-1). The outer longitudinal and

David K. Magnuson: Department of Surgery, Case Western Reserve University, Rainbow Babies and Children's Hospital, Cleveland, Ohio 44106.

Marshall Z. Schwartz: Thomas Jefferson University, Philadelphia, Pennsylvania 19107.

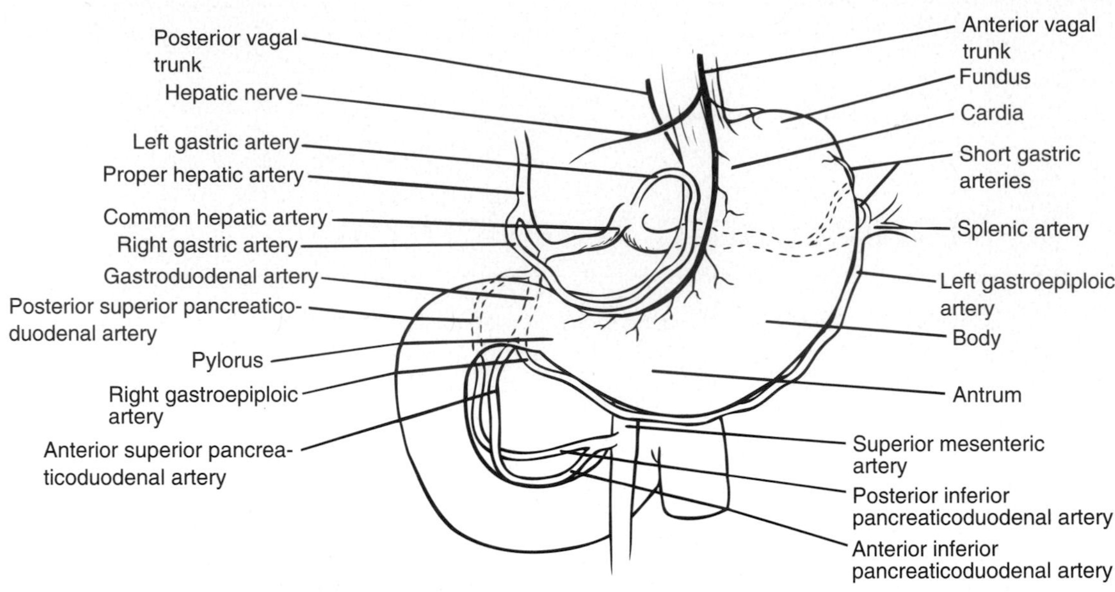

FIGURE 72-1. Gross anatomy of the stomach and duodenum.

intermediate circular muscle layers (which are concentrated on the greater and lesser curvatures) and the inner oblique layer (concentrated over the anterior and posterior surfaces) compose the three muscular layers of the gastric wall. The gastric wall in the neonate is extremely thin initially, but grows rapidly in the postnatal period in response to the propulsive work associated with enteral feeding.

The gastric blood supply is redundant and derived principally from branches of the celiac axis. The left gastric artery supplies the cardia and proximal lesser curvature; the splenic artery gives off short gastric arteries to the fundus and the left gastroepiploic artery to the proximal greater curvature; the common hepatic artery gives off both the gastroduodenal artery, from which derives the right gastroepiploic artery to the distal greater curvature, and the right gastric artery to the pylorus and distal lesser curvature. Venous return is to the portal vein through the splenic, left gastric (coronary), and superior mesenteric veins.

The duodenum occupies a section of the primitive digestive tube that spans the transition from foregut to midgut. The foregut is proximal to the liver bud and subserved by branches of the celiac trunk, whereas the midgut is distal to the liver bud and subserved by the superior mesenteric artery. The duodenum also undergoes a rotational process. The proximal duodenum is drawn superiorly and to the right during anteroposterior rotation of the stomach, whereas the distal duodenum is drawn leftward by the counterclockwise rotation of the midgut as it returns to the abdomen from the umbilical stalk. The net result of these movements is the C-loop configuration of the normal duodenum. Superimposed on these rotational events is a shortening of the dorsal mesoduodenum, which fixes the duodenum in a retroperitoneal location.

During the sixth to tenth weeks of gestation, the proximal duodenum (along with the esophagus and rectum) undergoes a process of rapid epithelial proliferation that obliterates the hollow lumen, converting the duodenum into a solid, cordlike structure. Vacuoles appear in this homogenous epithelial interior after 8 weeks' gestation, and gradual recanalization occurs as these vacuoles coalesce into larger cavities. The distal duodenum is believed not to pass through a solid phase.

The duodenum is divided into four portions corresponding to the curvatures of the C loop. A consistent landmark is the ampulla of Vater, which is located medially in the second portion and represents the confluence of the common bile and pancreatic ducts and their entry into the duodenum. The duodenal blood supply is derived from the celiac axis through superior pancreaticoduodenal branches of the gastroduodenal artery, and the superior mesenteric artery through inferior pancreaticoduodenal branches. Venous drainage is through corresponding branches to the portal vein.

During this same period, the pancreas develops from separate dorsal and ventral anlagen. The ventral anlage arises to the right of midline, and as the intestinal tract undergoes rotation, this structure also rotates posterior to the duodenum and fuses with the dorsal anlage to the left of the duodenal C loop. The two separate ductal systems fuse, forming the main pancreatic duct of Wirsung and a minor accessory duct of Santorini. Abnormalities of pancreatic migration and fusion result in ductal anomalies (pancreas divisum) and parenchymal anomalies (annular pancreas). The frequent coexistence of annular pancreas with congenital duodenal obstruction suggests that the anatomic development of these structures is closely interrelated.

Developmental Neuroanatomy

The stomach is richly innervated by all three components of the autonomic nervous system—sympathetic, parasympathetic, and enteric—although functionally the latter two predominate. Sympathetic fibers in which the postganglionic neurotransmitter is primarily norepinephrine are generally inhibitory to GI function, whereas parasympathetic pathways mediated by acetylcholine are generally stimulatory. In contrast, the enteric nervous system (ENS) is characterized by a wider variety of neurotransmitters, including dopamine, somatostatin, vasoactive intestinal peptide (VIP), gastrin-releasing peptide, ghrelin, and cholecystokinin (CCK), and a wider variety of effector and regulatory functions. Many of the peptides used by the ENS as neurocrine mediators are also elaborated by enteroendocrine cells as endocrine and paracrine mediators.

The sympathetic and parasympathetic innervation of the stomach is well defined. Sympathetic innervation originates from cell bodies within the thoracic spinal cord and extends through presynaptic fibers in the greater splanchnic nerve to postsynaptic neurons in the celiac ganglion, whose axonal fibers follow blood vessels into the gastroduodenal wall. This arrangement correlates well with the principal sympathetic function of vasomotor control. Sympathetic innervation of the muscular layers is sparse and is concentrated chiefly in the pyloric sphincter. Parasympathetic presynaptic nerves originate in the brainstem and follow the vagus nerves to the stomach. Interestingly, efferent impulses constitute only about 20% of the total neural traffic in the vagus nerves. The entire gastric wall is richly innervated by terminal vagal fibers branching off the left (anterior) and right (posterior) vagal trunks as they give off their hepatic and celiac divisions, respectively. These presynaptic fibers synapse with intramural ganglia and also integrate at this level with ENS ganglion cells. Parasympathetic innervation mediates predominantly prosecretory and prokinetic functions.

The ENS is the largest and most complex compartment of the autonomic nervous system and comprises more than 10^8 resident neurons within the walls of the GI tract. It is distinguished from the sympathetic and parasympathetic systems by its anatomic separation from the central nervous system (CNS). It has long been recognized that the ENS functions more or less independently, but receives modulatory input from the central autonomic system, mostly by way of the vagus (parasympathetic) nerves. When one considers that the efferent fibers of the vagal trunks at the esophageal hiatus number only about 2,000, it is clear that most of the ENS neurons receive stimulatory and inhibitory inputs from other ENS neurons (1). Thus, the inherent myoelectric activity of GI smooth muscle is under both intrinsic (ENS) and extrinsic (CNS) control.

ENS precursors differentiate from neuroblasts located in the vagal area of the neural crest and migrate with the vagus nerves to the developing stomach and GI tract (2). Once incorporated into the gastric wall, these ENS neurons further differentiate, proliferate, and establish connections to each other, to other autonomic pathways, and to developing gastric secretory and muscle cells. Although the migrating precursors transiently express immunoreactivity for catecholamines, once established within the gastric wall, they no longer express catecholamines. ENS plexuses are found within virtually every histologic layer of the stomach, integrating with ganglia found in the mucosa, the intermyenteric plane, and the subserosa.

Developmental Histology of the Gastric and Duodenal Epithelium

The gastric epithelium is an aggregation of diverse cell populations that are distributed in a regionally specialized manner and that account for the various secretory functions of the stomach. Seen from the luminal surface, the gastric mucosa is a monotonous sheet of mucus-secreting columnar epithelial cells riddled with tiny openings referred to as *gastric pits*. At the base of these pits are the gastric glands, which are specialized tubular invaginations of the mucosa that contain the effector and regulator cells of gastric secretion. Gastric glands are composed of different cell populations in various regions of the stomach, allowing the stomach to be compartmentalized by histologic and functional characteristics.

The cells that occupy the surface zone throughout the entire stomach secrete mucus, which provides a protective barrier between luminal acid and the gastric wall. These surface mucous cells are simple columnar epithelium with projecting microvilli. Immediately subjacent to the villi are mucous granules, which fuse with the apical cell membrane and deliver mucus by exocytosis. An extensive and active Golgi apparatus and rough endoplasmic reticulum are seen in the cytoplasm. These cells continuously recycle every 72 hours. Mucous neck cells are found deeper in the neck of the gland and have a similar morphology and function. They appear to renew every 7 days.

Parietal cells are perhaps the most functionally unique cells found in the gastric epithelium. They produce both hydrochloric acid (HCl) and intrinsic factor (IF) and are under a complicated system of regulatory controls. In the resting state, these cells contain unusual intracellular smooth membranes termed *tubulovesicles*. When stimulated, these structures are replaced by extensive intracellular canaliculi that communicate directly with the glandular lumen at the apical interface and that contain numerous microvilli. These microvilli appear to be the site of greatest concentration of the H^+-K^+-ATPase (proton pump) that drives HCl secretion against a large concentration gradient. Consistent with such an energy-intensive process, these cells contain large mitochondria in a concentration exceeded only by the myocardium. Parietal cells are found throughout the isthmus and neck regions of the glands, predominately in the gastric fundus and body and less often in the proximal antrum. They can be identified in gastric glands as early as gestational week 10.

Chief cells are found exclusively at the base of the gastric glands. They synthesize, store, and secrete pepsinogen, which is hydrolyzed to the active proteolytic enzyme pepsin in the acid environment of the gastric lumen. Pepsinogen is stored in apical zymogen granules in preparation for release by exocytosis. These cells are found principally in the gastric fundus and body, and first appear in the twelfth week of gestation.

Enteroendocrine cells are present throughout the stomach, duodenum, and distal intestine (Fig. 72-2). These cells have in common the ability to internalize certain precursor molecules and produce biologically active amines and peptides by intracellular decarboxylation. They are therefore referred to as *amine precursor uptake and decarboxylation* cells. Enteroendocrine cells also interact with ENS fibers within the gastric and duodenal walls. Together, the enteroendocrine cells and ENS fibers produce a variety of signaling molecules that integrate and regulate the complex events underlying acid secretion, motility, digestion, and metabolic response (Table 72-1).

Many distinct types of enteroendocrine and neurocrine cells are found in the gastric mucosa. The most common and well-characterized are the G cells, which produce gastrin, and the D cells, which produce somatostatin and amylin. Others produce such diverse amines and peptides as serotonin, histamine, dopamine, vasoactive intestinal peptide (VIP), glucagon, gastrin releasing peptide (GRP), motilin, and ghrelin. Because these substances function in endocrine and paracrine regulation, the cells that produce them tend to have high concentrations of secretory granules at their basolateral (i.e., abluminal) membranes. Microvilli on their apical (luminal) membranes contain the chemoreceptors and pH receptors necessary to sense environmental changes and function in feedback inhibition. Another enteroendocrine cell, the enterochromaffin-like (ECL) cell, produces histamine, perhaps the primary stimulus for acid secretion. Enteroendocrine cells are ubiquitous both within the gastric glands and within the duodenal wall. The most common types, the G and D cells, predominate in the gastric antrum.

Enteroendocrine cells are among the first to populate the gastric glands, emerging at 8 to 9 weeks' gestation. They derive from stem cells located within the base of the gastric gland. Certain cells, referred to as *A cells,* appear to produce glucagon and are only present in fetal and neonatal glands. Such observations, along with the recognition that many GI hormones have trophic effects, have led to the hypothesis that some enteroendocrine cells may participate

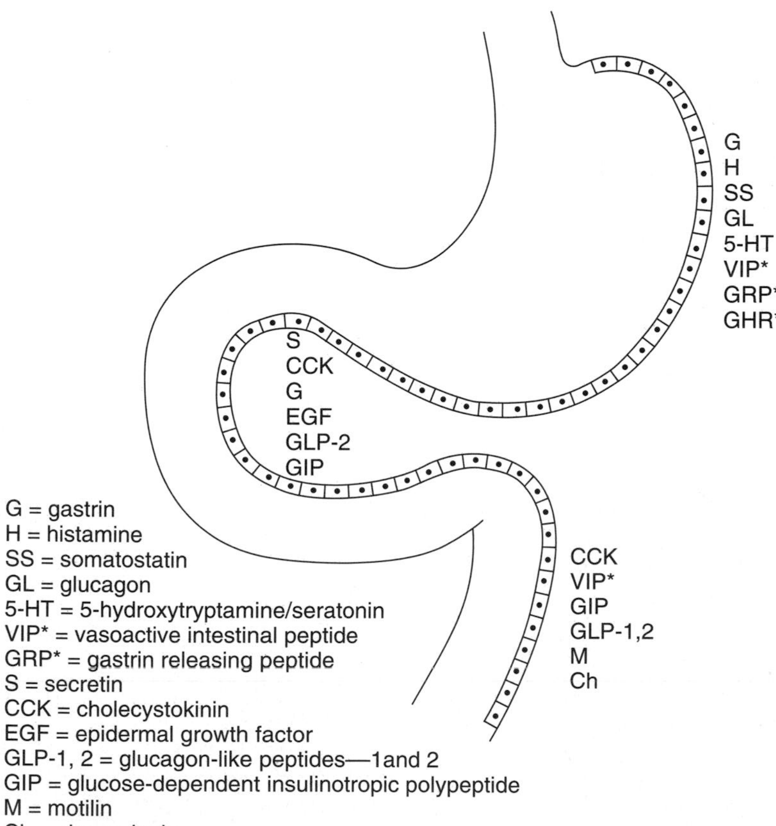

FIGURE 72-2. Distribution of selected enteroendocrine and neurocrine (*asterisk*) cells and their products in the proximal gastrointestinal tract.

TABLE 72-1 Important Intercellular Signaling Molecules in the Stomach and Duodenum.

Mediator	*Location*	*Cell Type*[a]	*Primary Physiologic Effects*
Gastrin family			
Gastrin	Fetal duodenum, postnatal stomach	G	Stimulates enterochromaffin-like (ECL) cell histamine release and potentiates parietal cell stimulation; trophic effects on mucosal growth
Cholecystokinin	Duodenum	I	Stimulates gallbladder contraction and exocrine pancreatic secretion in response to fatty acids and amino acids
	Stomach	ENS	Possible role in ECL cell inhibition
Secretin family			
Secretin	Duodenum	S	Stimulates bicarbonate production in pancreas, liver, and duodenal mucosa
Vasoactive intestinal peptide	Stomach, duodenum	ENS	Stimulation of G-cell gastrin secretion in peptide response to low-level gastric distention
Glucagon family			
Glucagon	Fetal stomach	A	Undefined; possible role in mucosal development
Glucagon-like peptide 1	Duodenum	L	Potentiates glucose-mediated insulin release, stimulates pancreatic beta-cell proliferation, inhibits gastric acid secretion and motility
Glucagon-like peptide 2	Duodenum	L	Stimulates proliferation and inhibits apoptosis of gut epithelium, inhibits gastric acid secretion and motility
Gastric inhibitory peptide	Duodenum	K	Mediates insulin response to enteral sugars; (glucose-dependent inhibits gastric secretory and motor activity insulinotropic polypeptide, GIP)
Others			
Somatotstatin	Ubiquitous	D	Generally inhibitory to enteroendocrine cells and gastric acid secretion
	Amylin stomach	D	Inhibits gastric acid secretion and motility
Histamine	Stomach	ECL	Final mediator of parietal cell acid secretion
Serotonin (5-HT)	Stomach, duodenum	EC	Mediates central nervous system and duodenal effects on stomach
Gastrin-releasing peptide	Stomach	ENS	Stimulates G-cell gastrin secretion in response to aromatic amino acids
Ghrelin	Stomach	ENS	Stimulates growth hormone release, increases gastric acid secretion and motility, increases food intake and decreases energy expenditure

[a]ENS, enteric nervous system; ECL, enterochromaffin-like; EC, .

in the growth and differentiation of the fetal stomach GI tract. Finally, a large number of undifferentiated cells can be seen interspersed with other cell types in the gastric glands. Their role is postulated to be the regeneration of all nonenteroendocrine components of the epithelium after injury. Enteroendocrine regeneration appears to result from type-specific precursors.

Based on the cell types previously described, it is possible to segregate the stomach into three histologically and functionally distinct regions characterized by the presence of one of three specific gland types: cardiac, oxyntic, or pyloric. Cardiac glands are devoid of parietal and chief cells, and occupy a 1- to 2-cm ring around the gastroesophageal junction. Oxyntic glands are the most prevalent; they occupy the fundus and most of the body. These glands contain all the cell types listed earlier, and are especially rich in parietal and chief cells. Pyloric glands, found in the distal 10% of the stomach, have few parietal and no chief cells, but are well endowed with enteroendocrine cells, especially G and D cells.

The duodenal mucosa is also richly populated with enteroendocrine cells. These cells are stimulated by nutritional substrates delivered from the stomach, and they secrete mediators that regulate a variety of digestive processes. Secretin is produced by duodenal S cells in response to luminal acid, stimulating bicarbonate secretion from the pancreas, liver, and duodenal Brunner glands and mucosal cells. CCK is produced by duodenal I cells in response to certain fatty acids and amino acids; it stimulates gallbladder contraction and pancreatic exocrine secretion. Secretin and CCK have also been proposed to have trophic effects on the fetal intestinal tract and pancreas, respectively. Glucagon-like peptides 1 and 2, previously termed *enteroglucagons*, are produced by L cells in the duodenal and distal gastrointestinal mucosa, and govern such diverse events as insulin secretion and gastric motility (3). A partial list of these cells and their putative functions is found in Table 72-1.

Physiology of Gastric Motor Function

The coordinated muscular activity of the stomach and duodenum, like that of the rest of the GI tract, is the net result of many complex interactions between mural smooth muscle cells and the ENS. The stomach is divided into two distinct functional zones based on marked differences in motor activity. The proximal stomach, including the fundus and proximal third of the body, exhibits the properties of receptive relaxation and accommodation, and serves as a reservoir in which the ingested meal is stored. The ability to distend without a concomitant increase in intraluminal pressure is important during bolus feeding. In addition, the proximal stomach generates slow, sustained, tonic contractions that elevate mean intragastric pressure above duodenal pressure and provide a constant pressure gradient that controls the passage of liquids through the stomach. These properties are under significant CNS modulation by nonadrenergic, noncholinergic vagal fibers. Therefore, vagotomy significantly impairs these functions and causes rapid emptying of liquids. The remainder of the stomach distal to the first third of the body is functionally and physiologically distinct from the proximal stomach. Motor activity in the distal stomach is characterized by spontaneous myocyte membrane depolarizations that result in phasic, directional contractions. These contractions account for the ability of the distal stomach to mix and grind solid food and to empty mixed food particles into the duodenum in a controlled fashion.

A basic property of smooth muscle cells in the distal stomach and duodenum (but not the proximal stomach) is a spontaneous slow depolarization of their membrane potential from a resting level of about −70 mV toward zero. Because myocytes are physiologically linked through gap junctions, the slow wave depolarizations of one cell are communicated to adjacent and more distant cells through serial connections. This leads to a spreading wave of depolarization in which cells with the most frequent spontaneous membrane depolarizations entrain those with lower frequencies. In the stomach, the cell population with the highest rate of spontaneous depolarization, referred to as the *gastric pacemaker*, is located along the greater curvature at the proximal boundary of the distal zone. Depolarizations spread aborally through the body, antrum, and pylorus without being propagated into the proximal zone. The rhythmic activity of the gastric pacemaker is about 3 to 4 cycles per minute (in the duodenum, which can be considered to be a small intestine pacemaker, slow waves are generated at a rate of about 10 to 12 cycles per minute).

Slow wave depolarizations are electrical events. They are coupled to mechanical contractions only when the depolarizations exceed a threshold potential, at which time a rapid depolarization to 0 mV occurs (termed an *action potential*) and triggers smooth muscle contraction by a rapid increase in intracellular calcium. When an action potential of sufficient magnitude is generated, a series of rapid action potentials follows before repolarization can occur (termed a *spikeburst*); this results in a sustained muscular contraction sufficient to elevate intragastric pressure. The underlying organization of slow wave depolarization dispersion ensures contractions are organized in a propulsive or peristaltic fashion. The frequency, direction, and magnitude of muscular contraction is under intrinsic and extrinsic neurocrine controls that alter resting membrane potentials, threshold potentials, and action potentials as a means of regulating the translation of slow wave depolarizations into mechanical contractions.

During the fasting state, gastric myoelectric activity follows a repetitive pattern with a period of about 90 to 120 minutes, called the *interdigestive migrating motor* (myoelectric) *complex* (MMC). The MMC can be divided into four phases. Phase I is mechanically silent, without the generation of action potentials or muscular contractions. In phase II, random, low-amplitude contractions occur. Phase III is characterized by regular, intense muscular contractions resulting from the conversion of every slow wave depolarization into an action potential with spikebursts. This phase empties the gastric lumen of all indigestible materials and is responsible for imparting the term *housekeeper* to describe the MMC. A short phase IV is marked by a gradual return to phase I quiescence.

The fed state occurs when the interdigestive MMC is interrupted by the arrival of ingested food in the stomach. The regular pattern of MMC activity is replaced with forceful, nonpropagated contractions in the distal stomach, coupled with coordinated contractions of the pyloric sphincter, that serve to churn and grind food into small particles. Distal gastric motor activity appears to be controlled by multiple factors: Vagal cholinergic activity, gastrin, GRP, CCK, neurotensin, motilin, and ghrelin stimulate contractions, whereas adrenergic and noncholinergic vagal activity, somatostatin, secretin, VIP, GLP 1 and 2, and GIP inhibit them.

When the average particle size approximates 1 mm in diameter, chyme is allowed to empty into the duodenum. The particulate composition and osmolality of chyme affects the rate of emptying: Carbohydrates empty faster than proteins, which empty faster than fats. Isocaloric amounts of nutrients, however, empty in about equal times. Intraduodenal acid, carbohydrate, and fat stimulate intramural, cholinergic ENS feedback loops that result in pyloric contraction, slowing gastric emptying. This complex set of interactive factors ensures the rate of gastric emptying is adjusted to provide an isocaloric flow of nutrients into the duodenum over time.

Physiology of Gastric Secretion

Production and secretion of HCl by gastric parietal cells is governed by a complex, highly redundant network of stimulatory and feedback controls that involve neurocrine, endocrine, and paracrine pathways. Establishing a dominant or final common pathway has been difficult because the parietal cell and other regulatory cells have been shown to possess cell surface receptors for a wide variety of molecular secretagogues. The parietal cell receives input from cholinergic and noncholinergic nerve terminals of the autonomic nervous systems (sympathetic, parasympathetic, and enteric), from hormones delivered through the microvasculature from distant sources (e.g., gastrin from antral G cells), and from peptide and amine messengers secreted into the local interstitial environment (e.g., histamine from fundic ECL cells). Each cell elaborating these regulatory substances is, in turn, subject to regulatory inputs equally complex.

Functions of acid include initiating and facilitating the hydrolysis of peptide bonds during protein digestion by denaturing ingested proteins and exposing specific amino acid sequences to pepsin, an endopeptidase that requires an acidic environment for activation. Because patients with chronic achlorhydria do not often suffer from malabsorption, the importance of acid-peptic digestion may not be critical. Nevertheless, when acid secretion is normal, it plays an integral role in initiating the digestive process.

An additional function of gastric acid is to create a barrier to the entrance of bacteria into the GI tract. Gastric acidity not only protects the upper aerodigestive tract from potentially pathogenic bacteria found in the lower GI tract, but also insulates the various populations of indigenous bacteria inhabiting the lower tract from constant challenges by new strains of ingested microorganisms. Chronic neutralization of gastric acidity results in bacterial overgrowth, which can lead to nosocomial respiratory tract infections, digestive abnormalities, and possibly generation of carcinogenic nitrosamines.

Gastric secretory function evolves early in development. By 10 weeks' gestation, parietal and enteroendocrine cells have begun to differentiate, and by 12 to 13 weeks, gastrin, HCl, pepsin, and IF can all be detected. Mucus and bicarbonate secretion commences later, at about the sixteenth week of gestation. Further prenatal growth and development is probably under enteroendocrine control. In the newborn, the gastric luminal pH is neutral, owing to swallowed amniotic fluid. Within the first several hours of life, however, acid secretion is sufficient to reduce the pH to 3.5. Further secretion lowers the pH to 1.0 to 3.0 by 48 hours, with little distinction between basal and stimulated outputs. Thereafter, acidity declines until the third week, when HCl secretion begins to increase again. By the age of 3 to 4 years, acid secretion approximates adult levels. Premature infants have a prolonged period of alkalinity, often extending for several days. As expected, the smallest premature infants display the most prolonged delay in acid secretion.

Control of Acid Secretion

Parietal cells in the fundus and corpus display surface membrane receptors for a variety of substances that stimulate or inhibit production and secretion of HCl. Stimulatory substances and their receptors include histamine (H_2 receptor), acetylcholine (M3 receptor), and gastrin (gastrin receptor); inhibitory substances include somatostatin (somatostatin receptor), epidermal growth factor (EGF) receptor, prostaglandin E (PGE) series prostaglandins (EP_3 receptor), and possibly adrenergic neurotransmitters (β-adrenergic receptors). Although the heterogeneity of receptors suggests that receptor-mediated acid secretion can be effected through a number of pathways, the observation that competitive inhibition of H_2 receptors can abolish acid output in response to all secretagogues strongly supports a central role for histamine as the final common pathway for most acid secretion under physiologic conditions. Gastrin alone is a relatively weak activator of isolated parietal cells in culture (4). The primary function of both acetylcholine and gastrin at the parietal cell membrane is probably to potentiate the effect of histamine because synergistic responses in acid secretion are seen with combinations of histamine and either gastrin or acetylcholine (5).

Although the source of gastric histamine was originally presumed to be the mast cell, gastrin has no demonstrable effect on mast cell histamine secretion. It is now widely accepted that the cell responsible for histamine-mediated parietal cell activation is the ECL cell (6). These enteroendocrine cells are intimately associated with the much larger parietal cells and possess numerous vacuoles containing histamine, which is released by exocytosis. Cell surface receptors for gastrin and acetylcholine have been purified from ECL membrane preparations, suggesting that the ECL cell directly integrates these inputs and releases histamine in a paracrine fashion (Fig. 72-3).

The major inhibitory regulator of ECL cell function is somatostatin, which causes receptor-mediated suppression of histamine release in response to the secretagogues mentioned earlier. Somatostatin-secreting D cells also exert a tonic inhibitory effect on acid secretion by directly suppressing parietal cell function. The principal stimulators of D-cell activity are hydrogen ion, resulting in a negative feedback loop, and noncholinergic neurons,

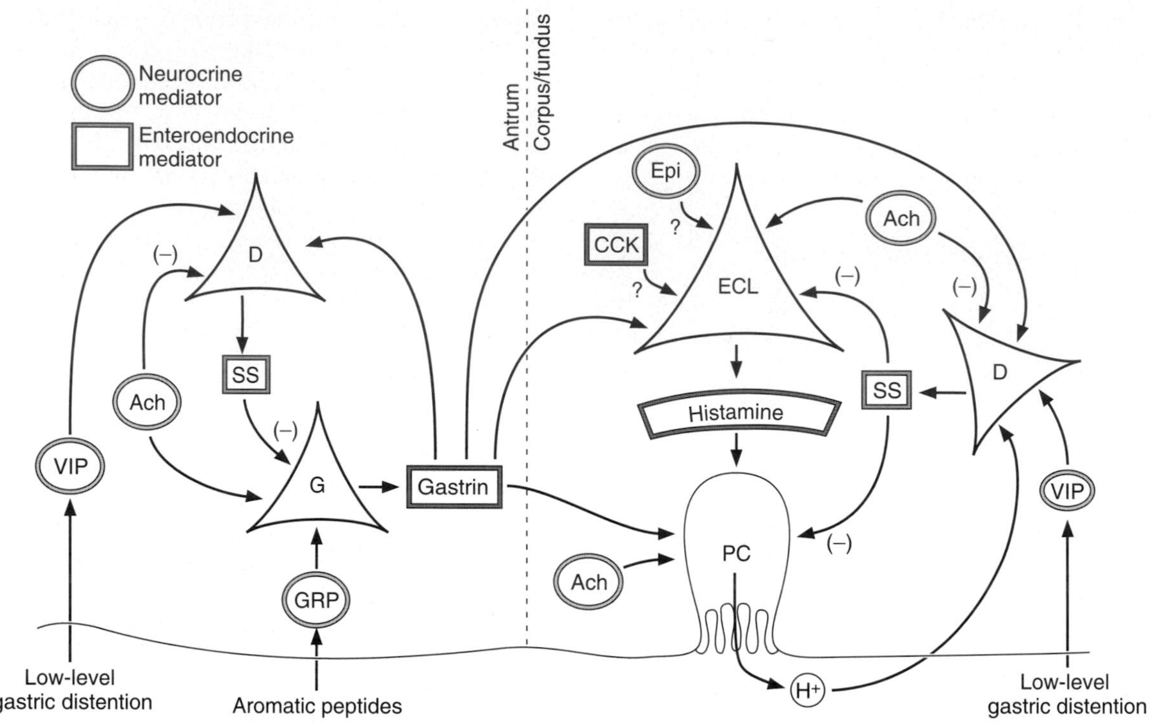

FIGURE 72-3. Regulation of gastric acid secretion by neurocrine, endocrine, and paracrine agents. Ach, acetylcholine; CCK, cholecystokinin; ECL, enterochromaffin-like cell; Epi, epinephrine; GRP, gastrin-releasing peptide; PC, parietal cell; VIP, vasoactive intestinal peptide; SS, somatostatin.

releasing VIP in response to low-grade distention. Other stimulators of fundic somatostatin release include gastrin and epinephrine, but their roles have not been clarified. Acetylcholine exerts a negative effect on somatostatin secretion, potentiating cholinergic enhancement of acid secretion by ECL and parietal cell stimulation.

The dominant pathway of parietal cell activation is paracrine stimulation of parietal cells by ECL cell-secreted histamine. The more proximal mechanisms that transduce physiologic stimuli into ECL cell histamine release involve the production of gastrin by antral G cells and the transmission of impulses through gastric effector neurons of the enteric autonomic system directly to the ECL cells. G cells are responsive to two stimulatory neurocrine agents: acetylcholine from cholinergic neurons, and GRP from noncholinergic neurons. Vagal cholinergic activity governs gastrin release from both cephalic-phase (CNS) stimulation and high-level gastric distention (i.e., after ingesting a meal). GRP appears to mediate gastric-phase activation of G cells by luminal protein fragments, particularly aromatic amino acids (7). On stimulation by either acetylcholine or GRP, antral G cells secrete gastrin into adjacent capillaries. This neurocrine stimulation accounts for the entire gastrin response to central and local factors.

Gastrin is actually a heterogeneous collection of at least three peptides: big gastrin (34 amino acids), little gastrin (17), and minigastrin (14). Big gastrin predominates physiologically because it has the longest half-life. Actions of gastrin include the direct stimulation of ECL cells and potentiation of the parietal cell response to histamine. Proposed physiologic effects of gastrin are trophic effects on oxyntic gland mucosa, secretion of IF and pepsin, and augmentation of lower esophageal sphincter (LES) pressure, intestinal motility, and pancreatic exocrine secretion.

G cells are under constant, ambient inhibitory influences exerted by somatostatin secreted from adjacent D cells. Histologically, D cells are linked to G cells through cell membrane processes that abut directly on the G-cell plasma membrane. Somatostatin, released into the interface, binds to receptors on the G cells that downregulate gastrin secretion. Somatostatin secretion is stimulated by gastrin, resulting in a negative feedback loop. In addition to gastrin, somatostatin secretion is elicited by VIP released from noncholinergic neurons in response to low-level gastric distention (i.e., after partial emptying of a meal) (8). This constitutive inhibition by somatostatin must be blocked for maximal stimulation of gastrin secretion to occur. Acetylcholine inhibits somatostatin secretion, potentiating its direct stimulation of gastrin secretion.

Mechanism of Acid Secretion

Activating agents bind with high affinity to parietal membrane receptors that are linked to second messenger systems, resulting in either the generation of cyclic adenosine monophosphate (cAMP) or an increase in the intracellular calcium concentration ($[Ca]_i$). The H_2 receptor appears to be a typical seven-membrane segment, G-protein–coupled receptor that activates adenylate cyclase on the cytoplasmic surface of the plasma membrane, resulting in the hydrolysis of adenosine triphosphate (ATP) and generation of cAMP. cAMP then triggers the phosphorylation and activation of various cytoplasmic protein kinases (9). The critical component in this linkage is the stimulatory guanosine triphosphate-binding protein (G_s) that translates external receptor occupation to internal adenylate cyclase activation. Both acetylcholine and gastrin receptors result in increased $[Ca]_i$, presumably owing to phospholipase C-dependent inositol turnover and protein kinase C activation, increased surface membrane Ca^{2+} conductance, or both. Receptors for inhibitory substances (somatostatin, PGE, opioids, EGF) are linked to an inhibitory G protein (G_i) that suppresses adenylate cyclase activity.

When the appropriate stimulatory signals converge on the parietal cell basolateral membrane, a number of distinct morphologic changes occur that coincide with acid secretion from the apical end of the cell. Cytoplasmic tubulovesicles, which have been shown to contain the quiescent proton pump, coalesce into a larger membrane system termed the *secretory canaliculus,* which communicates with the gastric gland lumen at the apical cell surface. At the same time, the K^+-Cl^- channel, which provides exchangeable K^+ ions to the extracellular portion of the proton pump, is also inserted into the membrane of the secretory canaliculus. These changes occur within minutes of activation and persist throughout the entire period of increased acid secretion.

Although the sequence of events after the activation of cAMP is undefined, these events eventually result in the activation of the proton pump—an H^+-K^+-ATPase that effects an electroneutral exchange of H^+ for K^+ at the luminal surface of the secretory canaliculus. Omeprazole, a substituted benzimidizole, is a weak base that becomes protonated and trapped within the low-pH canaliculus. There, it undergoes conversion to a sulfenamide, which reacts with the exposed portions of the catalytic subunit of the H^+-K^+-ATPase pump, forming stable disulfide bonds and preventing the conformational change that allows for ion transport.

Other Gastric Secretory Products

Pepsinogen

Pepsin refers to a family of digestive enzymes synthesized and secreted by the chief and mucous neck cells of the gastric glands. The pepsinogen family can be divided into two groups: A (or I), and C (or II). Pepsinogen A has a molecular weight of about 43 kd and is secreted by the proximal stomach; pepsinogen C is of similar size and is secreted by the entire gastric mucosal surface as well as by the duodenum, prostate, and seminal vesicles. The enzymes are actually synthesized and stored in zymogen granules as prepepsinogens, which undergo intracellular conversion to their zymogen forms, pepsinogens, by cleavage of an N-terminal sequence before secretion through exocytosis. In addition to pepsinogen A and C, two other acid proteinases are secreted by the gastric mucosa: cathepsin D and E. Their physiologic importance is not well defined.

After secretion as an inactive zymogen, an N-terminal sequence is cleaved by acid-mediated hydrolysis, converting pepsinogen to active pepsin. Thereafter, pepsin autocatalyzes its own conversion from pepsinogen. Pepsin is an acid proteinase that has an abundance of aspartate residues at the catalytic site (hence, an aspartic proteinase). At pH below 5, pepsin is progressively more efficient at cleaving internal peptide bonds between aromatic amino acids, thus generating protein fragments with exposed aromatic residues known to stimulate gastrin secretion maximally by GRP-dependent neurocrine stimulation. Pepsinogens can be detected in the fetal stomach by 8 weeks' gestation, but peptic activity is absent until about 16 weeks.

Stimulation of pepsinogen secretion is primarily governed by cholinergic and β-adrenergic inputs. Paracrine and endocrine stimulation also occurs through histamine, CCK, secretin, and VIP. Gastrin does not elicit pepsinogen secretion. Inhibitory regulation is mediated by somatostatin and PGE.

Lipase

Gastric lipase activity is demonstrable at birth. Its optimal pH for activity (5.5) is higher than that of pepsin, but is still slightly acidic. Intragastric lipolysis liberates long-chain fatty acids, which stimulate duodenal CCK secretion, and medium-chain fatty acids, which are directly absorbed through the gastric epithelium.

Intrinsic Factor

Intrinsic factor is a 60-kd mucoprotein that is secreted from parietal cells in the fundus and body. Regulatory controls for IF closely parallel those for acid secretion, suggesting a physiologic coupling of IF and acid secretion. In the infant and young child, however, this coupling is dissociated, allowing a constant, basal secretion of IF, which exceeds that of acid (10).

In the stomach, IF competes with a second ligand, R protein, for binding to vitamin B_{12} cobalamins. Although vitamin B_{12} preferentially binds R protein in the stomach, pancreatic enzymes in the intestine degrade R protein, allowing IF to bind available vitamin B_{12}. The IF-B_{12} complex is then absorbed in the terminal ileum.

Mucus

Mucus is a complex gel consisting of mucin, desquamated epithelial cells, salts, and water. In the stomach, bicarbonate is also secreted and trapped in this gel and is an important protective component of gastric mucus. Mucin, consisting of proteins, glycoproteins, and mucopolysaccharides, is secreted by surface epithelial cells and mucous neck cells in a manner that appears coupled to acid secretion—synthesis and secretion are stimulated by acetylcholine, histamine, and gastrin (11). The mucus layer is about 180-μm deep and displays a thin layer of hydrophobic phospholipids on its luminal surface.

The physiologic function and importance of mucus is controversial. Previously, the mucus–bicarbonate barrier was considered important in maintaining a pH-neutral environment overlying the surface epithelium by preventing back-diffusion of HCl and pepsin, and by preventing the dissipation of epithelial-secreted bicarbonate. Indeed, a pH gradient of nearly 5 logs exists between the gastric lumen and the epithelial surface. Disruption of the mucus layer by mucolytic agents, however, does not render the underlying epithelium more susceptible to acid-mediated injury, but it does exacerbate epithelial disruption by other injurious agents. It may be reasonable to conclude that the physiologic role of gastric mucus is not in preventing injury, but in protecting the already injured epithelial surface during the regenerative phase. Other functions of mucus include lubricating the gastric surface to minimize mechanical trauma during mixing, and trapping ingested microbes until they can be processed and phagocytized by immunocompetent cells.

Mucosal Defense Mechanisms

Mucosal defense is a critical ongoing function for an organ whose luminal surface is regularly exposed to a highly acidic environment, a wide range of osmolarities, and activated proteolytic enzymes. The components of mucosal defense, their relative importance, and the precise mechanisms by which they confer protection to the gastric epithelium are, however, poorly understood. Certain mechanisms have been proposed to constitute a hierarchical system of mucosal defense. Those that are best described include (1) mucus and bicarbonate secretion, (2) epithelial resistance and restitution, (3) mucosal blood flow, and (4) subepithelial activity of immunoinflammatory cells.

CONGENITAL ABNORMALITIES OF THE STOMACH AND DUODENUM

Abnormal Gastric Fixation and Gastric Volvulus

Congenital deficiencies of mesenteric fixation of the stomach to the surrounding structures predispose to gastric volvulus and can take two distinct forms. Normally, the stomach is suspended in a peritoneal leaflet that is tethered in four quadrants by the gastrohepatic, gastrophrenic, and gastrosplenic ligaments and the retroperitoneal fixation of the duodenum. The gastrocolic ligament (greater omentum) may also provide stabilization. Absence or laxity of the gastrohepatic and gastrosplenic ligaments allows the stomach to rotate around its longitudinal axis, producing an *organoaxial volvulus* (Fig. 72-4). Similar abnormalities

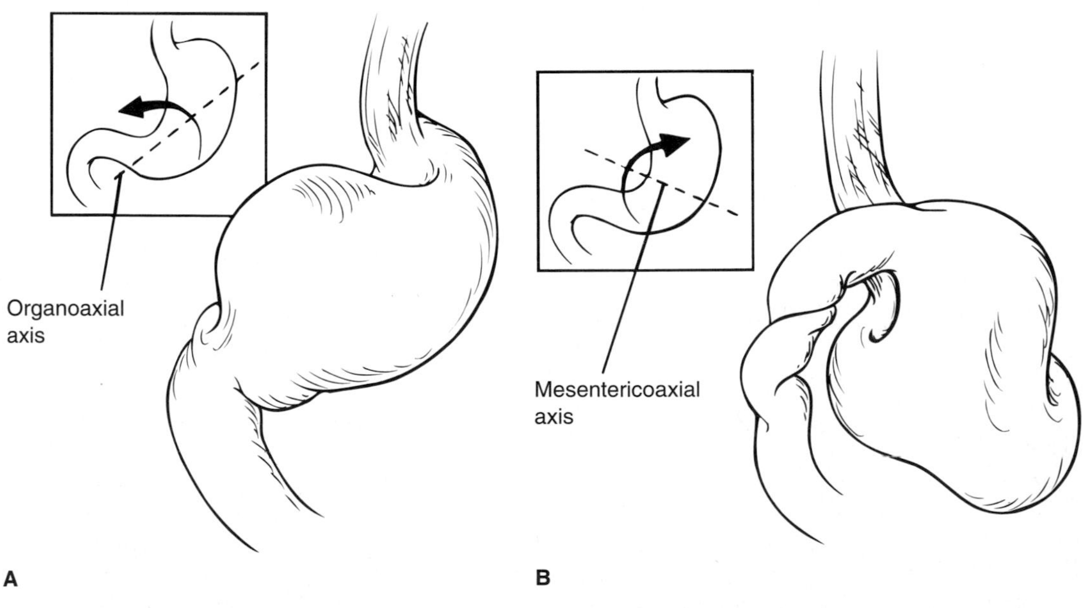

FIGURE 72-4. Two variants of gastric volvulus. **(A):** Organoaxial axis, **(B):** Mesentericoaxial axis.

of the gastrophrenic ligament and duodenal attachments allow rotation around the stomach's transverse axis, referred to as a *mesentericoaxial volvulus*. Organoaxial volvulus is the more common of the two types in infants and children.

A strong association has been found between gastric volvulus and several other developmental anomalies. These include malrotation, asplenia, and congenital abnormalities of the diaphragm (e.g., hiatal hernia, posterolateral "Bochdalek" hernia, eventration) (12). Because these entities all result in abnormalities of the stabilizing peritoneal attachments listed earlier, a causative role is assumed. Gastric volvulus may also be associated with conditions resulting in the stretching and laxity of the peritoneal attachments caused by gastric distension (e.g., aerophagia, prior hypertrophic pyloric stenosis).

Although gastric volvulus can occur as either an acute or chronic problem, the acute form is more common in children. The classic presentation of sudden catastrophic epigastric pain, intractable retching without emesis, and inability to advance a nasogastric tube into the stomach is rarely encountered in the actual clinical setting. Children may experience emesis, which can be bilious or nonbilious, and may not have abdominal distention. Intermittent gastric volvulus may be considered in the workup of infants presenting with apparent life-threatening episodes (13). Any combination of symptoms suggesting a partial or complete proximal mechanical obstruction may be present. Profound physiologic decompensation, hemodynamic instability, or unrelenting metabolic acidosis suggest strangulation, ischemic necrosis, and possibly perforation. Obviously, such a presentation mandates emergent surgical intervention concurrent with ongoing resuscitation. Older children may present with chronic, intermittent volvulus exhibited by postprandial pain, early satiety, and belching.

Radiologic assessment can reveal several characteristic findings. On plain abdominal radiographs, massive gastric dilation can usually be seen, often with a distinct incisura pointing toward the right upper quadrant. The spleen and small intestine may be displaced inferiorly. If a contrast study has been attempted, the contrast column may be confined to the esophagus, with a long, gradual tapering at the bottom. Occasionally, a paraesophageal hiatal hernia is detected (Fig. 72-5).

Chronic idiopathic volvulus may be medically managed in selected cases (14). Operative treatment of acute gastric volvulus includes gastric decompression by nasogastric suction or needle aspiration and reduction of the volvulus. Perforations are closed primarily or, depending on their location, around a Malecot tube; more extensive necrosis requires resection. Coexisting anomalies, such as malrotation and diaphragmatic defects, should be corrected. Recurrent volvulus is prevented by performing an anterior gastropexy. Historically, a Stamm-type gastrostomy has often been employed to increase the stability of the gastropexy, although there are no data that suggest this is

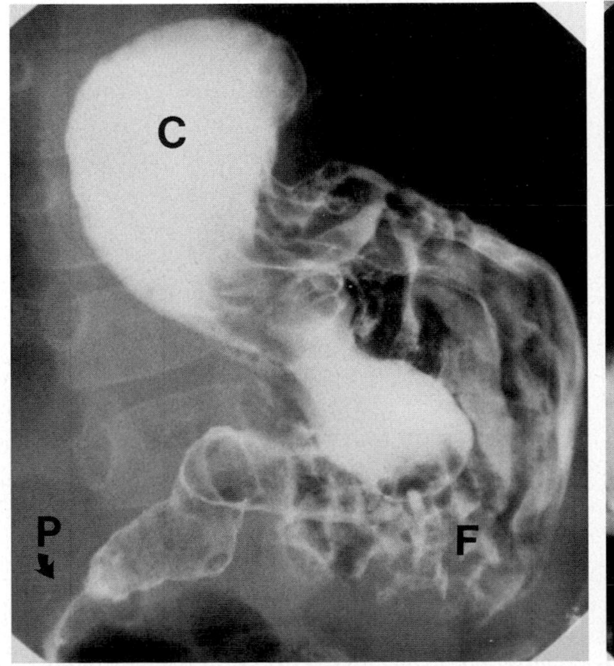

A

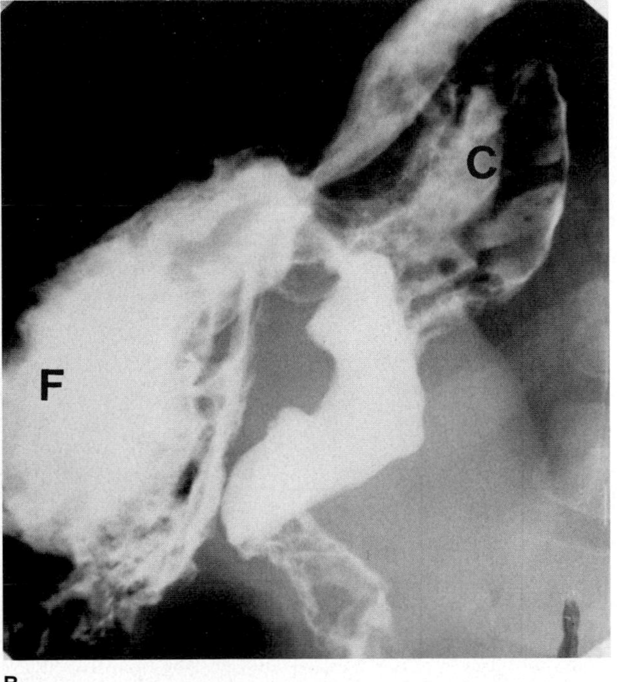

B

FIGURE 72-5. Organoaxial gastric volvulus defined by upper gastrointestinal tract contrast study. **(A):** Anteroposterior projection shows a caudad rotation of the upper corpus and fundus (F), a cephalad rotation of the antrum and lower corpus (C), and a nondisplaced pylorus (P). **(B):** Lateral projection.

mandatory. Both laparoscopic and open approaches are effective. Recurrence is rare.

Microgastria

Congenital microgastria is a rare anomaly in which the stomach retains a tubular morphology, fails to develop its normal rotation and fixation, and attains a much smaller volume than normal. Follow-up involving one long-term survivor has documented that the gastric volume remains small indefinitely (15). Other abnormalities of the abdomen frequently accompany this condition, including megaesophagus, gastroesophageal reflux (GER), intrinsic duodenal obstruction, malrotation, biliary anomalies, situs inversus, asplenia, and skeletal defects.

Microgastria presents with vomiting and failure to thrive in the infant, often associated with persistent diarrhea. Vomiting may be due to gastric insufficiency, GER, or duodenal obstruction. Diarrhea is presumed to be due to rapid gastric transit and dumping. The diagnosis is established by contrast upper GI tract study, which reveals a small stomach with a transverse lie and frequently a large, patulous esophagus (Fig. 72-6). Particular attention should be given to the anatomy of the duodenum and ligament of Treitz.

The initial management of microgastria is usually by continuous drip feeding. This approach has been variably successful in providing adequate fluids and calories. In most cases, parenteral nutrition is necessary. When continuous feedings can be maintained for several weeks, the stomach may undergo significant enlargement, allowing for a gradual transition to bolus and ad lib feeds. Antireflux precautions, including small frequent meals, may be required indefinitely. If this strategy is unsuccessful, fundoplication may be necessary, and may require a more limited procedure (e.g., Thal or Dor gastropexy). Although case reports of successful management by gastrojejunostomy exist, the favored approach involves construction of a Roux-en-Y jejunal reservoir—the Hunt-Lawrence pouch (16).

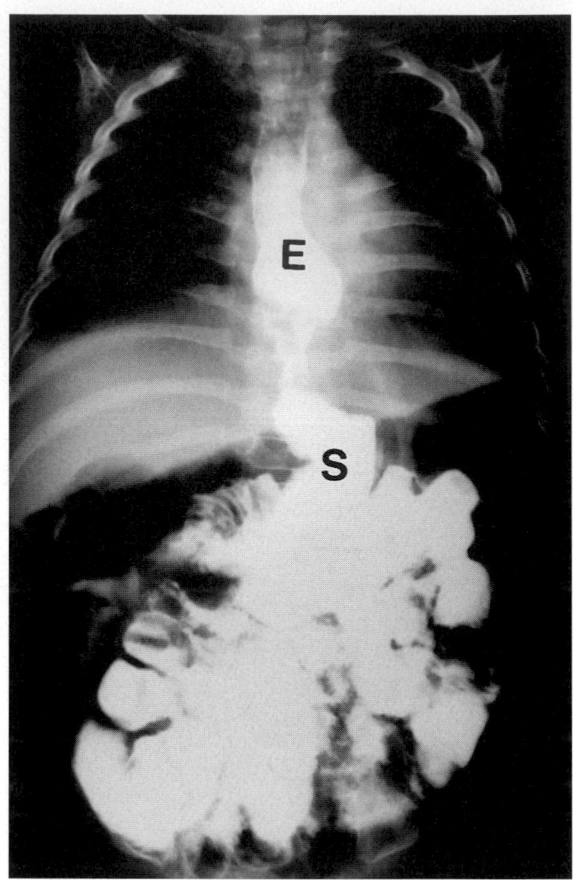

FIGURE 72-6. Characteristic upper gastrointestinal tract contrast study findings in congenital microgastria, including a small, tubular stomach (S) and free reflux into a patulous esophagus (E).

Congenital Gastric Outlet Obstruction

Congenital causes of partial or complete gastric outlet obstruction are much less common than acquired causes in children. The obstruction may involve either the antrum or pylorus and may take the form of a segmental defect (gap), which is sometimes bridged by a fibrous cord, or a membrane (web), which can have one or more apertures through which gastric contents pass. Histologically, such membranes consist of mucosa and submucosa without a muscularis. Prepyloric membranes can become redundant after exposure to antegrade propulsive pressures, creating a "windsock" web that can prolapse through the pyloric channel. This can be the source of considerable confusion and lead to strategic errors in surgical management. Pyloric webs account for two-thirds of these obstructions, pyloric atresia accounts for about one-fourth, and most of the remainder are antral webs and atresias. Another rare cause for the obstruction is the presence of ectopic pancreatic tissue within the submucosa of the pyloric channel, bulging into the lumen and producing a partial obstruction.

The etiology of antral and pyloric atresia is not understood. Unlike jejunoileal atresias, infarction and resorption from an in utero vascular accident is unlikely, owing to the stomach's redundant blood supply and extensive peritoneal fixation. As the stomach does not undergo a solid embryonic phase like the duodenum, failure of recanalization cannot account for these anomalies. Instead, some form of foregut segmentation mechanism is proposed but unproved. A genetic cause has been identified for some cases of pyloric atresia that occur in association with epidermolysis bullosa lethalis (Herlitz syndrome), which is inherited in an autosomal recessive manner. A hemidesmosome defect has been identified in the gastric mucosal epithelium in this syndrome, and genetic studies have documented a variety of mutations in the genes coding for cell surface integrins.

Clinical manifestations depend primarily on the degree of obstruction. Complete membranes or atresias present in the first few days of life as acute gastric outlet obstruction with nonbilious projectile vomiting. There is often a history of maternal polyhydramnios. Gastric distention leading to respiratory compromise can occur, and frank gastric perforation has been reported as early as 12 hours of life. Incomplete gastric outlet obstruction due to perforated membranes or heterotopic pancreatic tissue can present early in the neonatal period or later in childhood. Epigastric pain, vomiting, and weight loss can all occur in the child. Older patients may present with an incomplete prepyloric web, but whether such a web is congenital or acquired from peptic ulcer disease and mucosal inflammation is debatable.

Radiologic evaluation characteristically reveals a large gastric air bubble, either without any gas distal to the obstruction (Fig. 72-7), or with a nondistended distal small intestine in cases with a fenestrated membrane. Because neonatal gastric hypotonia can reproduce these radiographic findings, upper GI tract contrast studies are mandatory. These studies either show nonfilling of the duodenum or delineate the membrane when viewed laterally (Fig. 72-8). Ectopic pancreatic tissue can cause an eccentric protrusion into the pyloric channel. The typical string sign and bulging muscle of hypertrophic pyloric stenosis (HPS) is absent. In situations in which a contrast study is equivocal, flexible endoscopy may be helpful.

Preoperative resuscitation and preparation of the infant with antral or pyloric obstruction is similar to that for HPS, but intermittent gastric decompression is necessary in infants with complete gastric outlet obstruction. A chloride-responsive contraction alkalosis is often seen, and requires specific measures to restore fluid volume and correct chloride and potassium deficits. Prolonged vomiting in the neonate can also lead to profound hypoglycemia, which must be anticipated and corrected.

Anatomic obstructions that require surgical correction must be distinguished from nonoperative causes, such as neonatal gastroparesis. Surgical management is dictated by anatomy. In general, webs can be excised through a longitudinal incision that bisects them, followed by transverse closure to avoid stenosis. Complete atresias with anatomic disconnection can usually be corrected by primary anastomosis, such as gastroduodenostomy. Gastrojejunostomy

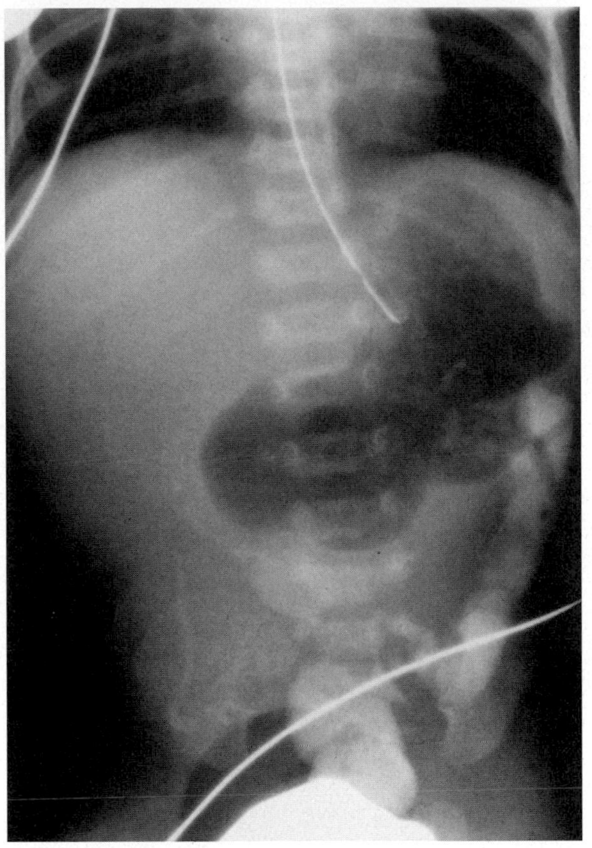

FIGURE 72-7. Plain radiograph of isolated gastric distention in pyloric atresia.

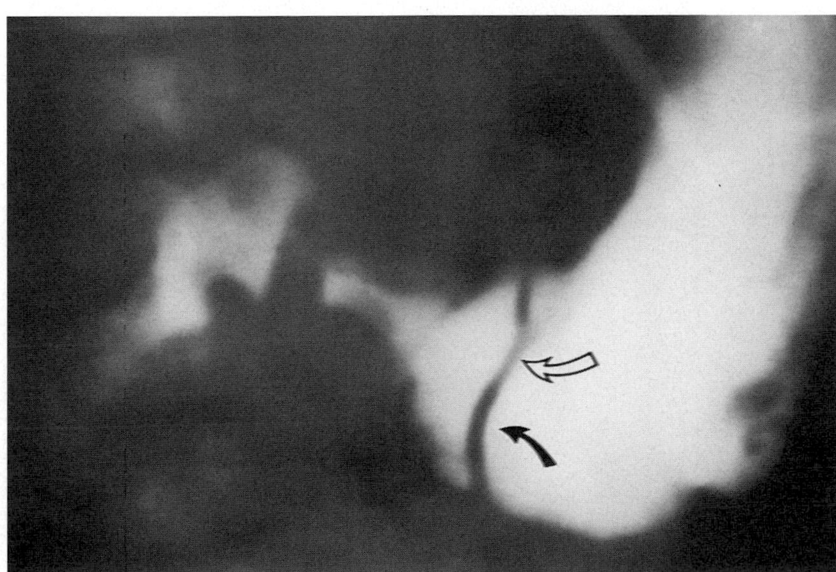

FIGURE 72-8. Upper gastrointestinal tract contrast study showing an antral web (*closed arrow*) with a central aperture (*open arrow*).

is poorly tolerated in the neonate and should be avoided whenever possible. Recognition of windsock deformities and distal atresias by passage of a balloon catheter proximally and distally can be helpful in defining the exact anatomy and in detecting additional distal obstructions. Ectopic pancreatic tissue in the pylorus requires excision of the mass and reconstruction of the pylorus.

Duplications

The stomach and duodenum are the least common regions of the GI tract in which duplications occur. For most congenital lesions of the stomach and duodenum included in this category, the term *duplication* may be a misnomer. The actual embryologic cause of these lesions is unknown, but the designation of enterogenous cyst or congenital diverticulum may be more accurate. Nevertheless, it is important to recognize that gastric and duodenal duplications are occasionally associated with other GI duplications or with vertebral anomalies. Communications with or attachments to an abnormal vertebral column suggest they may be caused by aberrant splitting of the primitive notochord during early embryonic development.

Classically, four pathologic criteria are considered necessary to establish the diagnosis of gastric duplication: (1) contiguity with the stomach, (2) an outer smooth muscle layer, (3) a shared blood supply with the stomach, and (4) a gastric epithelial lining (which may also contain pancreatic tissue). Most gastric duplications are cystic, do not communicate with the gastric lumen, and are located along the greater curvature of the stomach. When a luminal communication is present, it may be due to peptic ulceration of the common wall between the two structures. Tubular duplications are less common, frequently communicate with the gastric lumen, and are also most commonly found on the greater curvature (Fig. 72-9). Extragastric cystic structures lined by gastric epithelium and exhibiting a muscular wall, however, are usually referred to as gastric duplications, regardless of their proximity to the stomach.

In the neonatal period, duplications often present with symptoms and signs of proximal GI obstruction. Vomiting is common and can be bilious or nonbilious, depending on the location of the extrinsic compression relative to the ampulla of Vater. Case reports of gastric duplications, both adjacent to the stomach and in the retroperitoneum, have described connections to the pancreatic ductal system and have resulted in chronic pancreatitis and pseudocyst formation. Connections to the biliary system and to extrapulmonary sequestrations have also been reported. Duodenal duplications most commonly occur in the first or second portion, usually on the posterior surface, and may be lined with gastric mucosa. These may also cause pancreatitis by compression of the pancreatic duct within the duodenal wall. Gastroduodenal hemorrhage or perforation secondary to peptic ulceration are the usual emergency indications for surgery. Upper and lower GI hemorrhage secondary to ulcer penetration from a noncommunicating duplication cyst into an adherent loop of intestine or colon have been reported.

Gastroduodenal duplications are being detected by antenatal ultrasound with increasing frequency and should be considered along with choledochal cysts and omental cysts in the differential diagnosis of a fetal right upper quadrant cystic mass (17). Postnatally, an upper GI tract contrast study may demonstrate an extrinsic compression of the stomach or duodenum, but ultrasound and computed tomography can definitively reveal the mass itself. Technetium-99m scans may identify duplications distant from the stomach if they contain ectopic gastric mucosa but are not specific for duplications per se.

Resection of the entire duplication, either by enucleation or limited gastric resection, is the treatment of choice. Successful laparoscopic resection has been

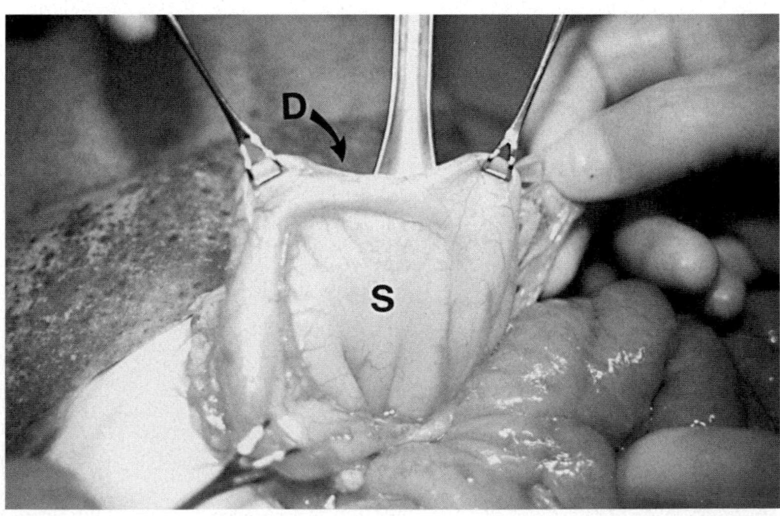

FIGURE 72-9. Tubular gastroduodenal duplication (D) adjacent to the greater curvature of the stomach (S).

reported and may be advisable for smaller, uncomplicated lesions. Extensive duplications, however, require removal of the entire mucosal cyst lining to avoid potential malignant degeneration. Adenocarcinoma arising from the gastric epithelium has been described in later life (18). Partial excision of the duplication with stripping of the residual mucosa is acceptable for lesions around the pylorus and duodenum for which en bloc resection of the contiguous gastroduodenal wall would necessitate sacrificing important structures (e.g., the common bile duct). Internal drainage into the adjacent duodenum or a Roux-en-Y jejunal limb is reserved for the rare circumstance in which resection or mucosal stripping is not feasible. Partial resection of a contiguous aberrant pancreatic lobe or internal drainage of an associated pseudocyst may also be required. Marsupialization should be avoided.

Congenital Duodenal Obstruction

Congenital duodenal obstruction is a relatively common abnormality in the newborn period and may be complete or partial, intrinsic or extrinsic. Intrinsic atresias or stenoses are relatively common; a population-based study documented that duodenal atresias and stenoses have an incidence of about 1 in 7,000 live births and account for 49% of all small intestinal atresias (19). Extrinsic obstruction has many causes, including malrotation with Ladd bands, preduodenal portal vein, gastroduodenal duplications, cysts or pseudocysts of the pancreas and biliary tree, and annular pancreas. Annular pancreas is almost invariably associated with an intrinsic cause of duodenal obstruction.

Intrinsic duodenal obstructions and annular pancreas are developmental abnormalities that occur during early

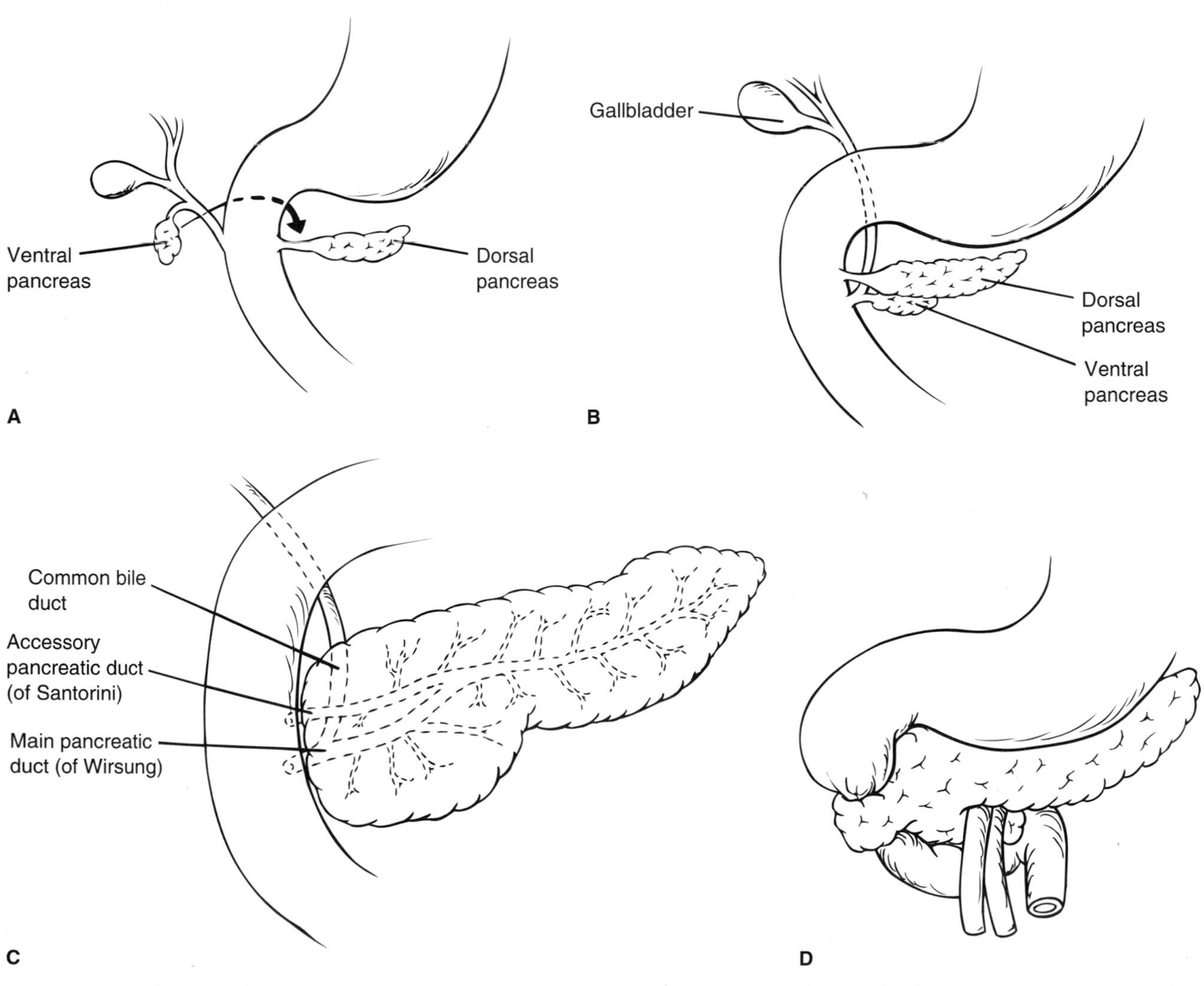

FIGURE 72-10. Proposed cause of annular pancreas. **(A** to **C)** Normal process of migration of the ventral pancreas and bile duct behind the duodenum. The ventral pancreatic duct fuses with the dorsal duct, producing the major pancreatic duct (of Wirsung) and the major papilla. **(D)** Persistent annulus of pancreatic parenchyma results from failure of ventral pancreatic migration.

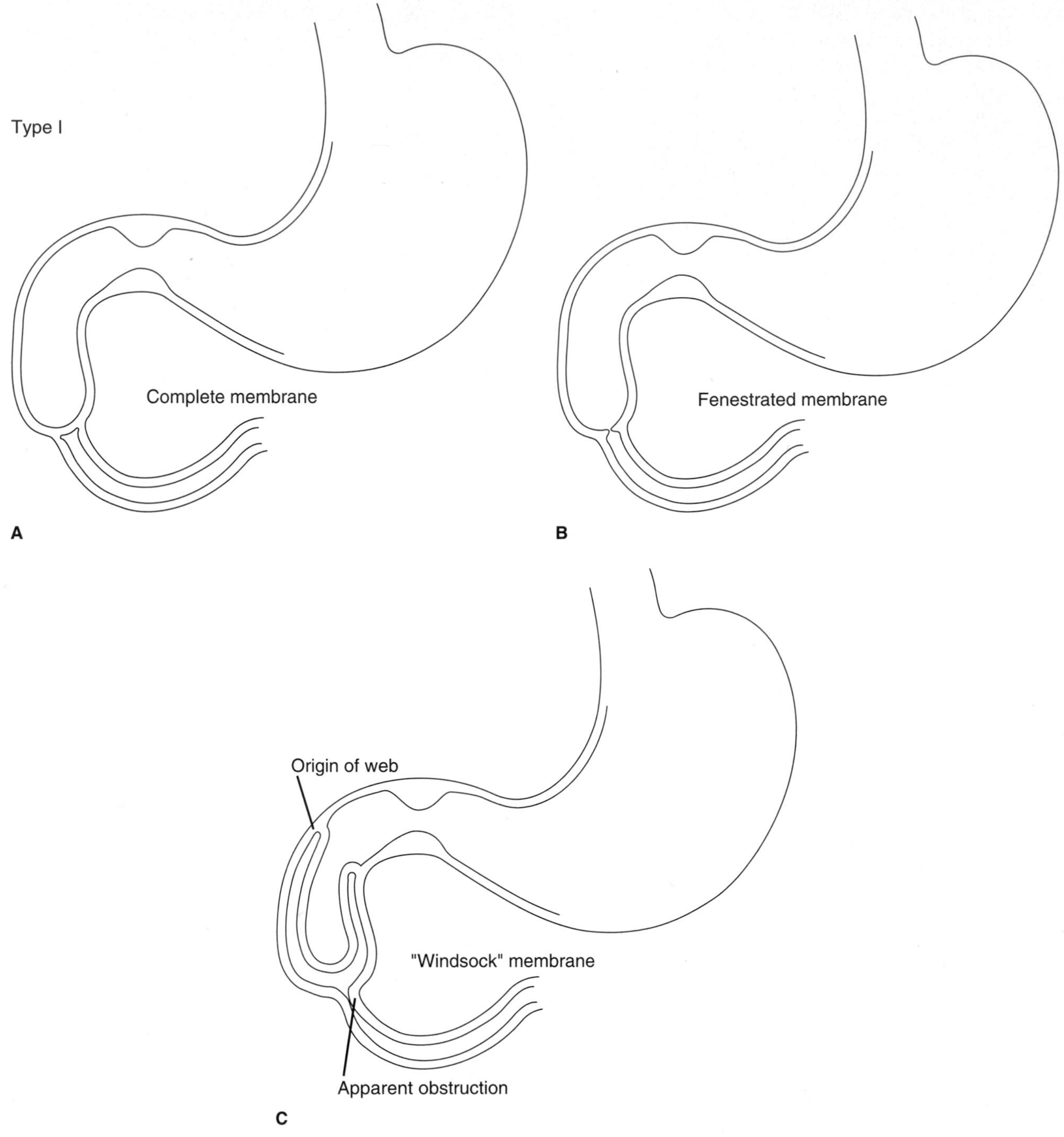

FIGURE 72-11. Variants of congenital duodenal obstruction. Type I refers to a luminal membrane, which can be **(A)** simple, **(B)** fenestrated, or **(C)** elongated (windsock). Types II and III describe atresias with complete mural discontinuity **(D)** with or **(E)** without a connecting fibrous cord, respectively.

development of the foregut. Duodenal atresia and stenosis are believed to result from a failure of the recanalization process that follows epithelial proliferation and obliteration of the developing duodenal lumen during the first trimester. Annular pancreas was originally suggested by Lecco (20) to occur when the ventral bud fails to rotate behind the duodenum, leaving pancreatic tissue fully encircling the second portion of the duodenum. This results in a nondistensible ring of pancreatic parenchyma and a functional stenosis (Fig. 72-10). Immunohistochemical studies of the annular tissue have identified pancreatic polypeptide-rich islets, known to predominate in the ventral anlage, and lend credence to this hypothesis (21). Annular pancreas frequently coexists with intrinsic

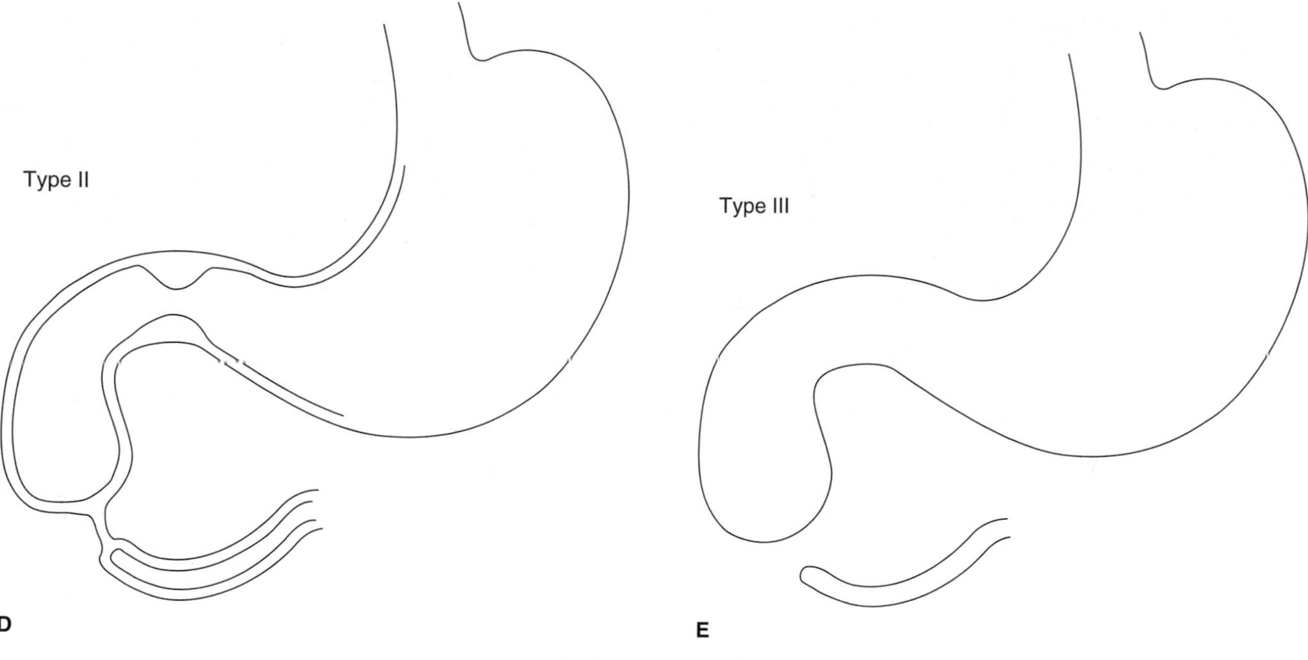

FIGURE 72-11. *(Continued)*

duodenal anomalies and anomalies of the pancreaticobiliary ductal system, suggesting closely linked mechanisms of pancreatic, duodenal, and biliary development during this stage.

Atresias of the duodenum have three basic morphologic appearances (Fig. 72-11). Type I atresias are characterized by luminal webs or membranes, which include mucosal and submucosal layers. Endoluminal membranes usually span the duodenal lumen at the level where the dilated proximal duodenum changes to a smaller, distal segment. Of particular interest are membranes that take on a windsock morphology, in which the endoluminal membrane extends distally for a variable distance from its origin. An external transition zone then occurs at the leading edge of the windsock; a significant portion of the dilated duodenum may therefore be distal to the point of obstruction. Type II atresias have dilated proximal and diminutive distal segments connected by a fibrous cord. Type III atresias are characterized by a complete discontinuity or gap between the segments. Congenital intrinsic stenoses are caused by luminal membranes identical to type I atresias, but contain a crescentic defect or central fenestration of variable size. Large openings can provide a conduit of sufficient size to postpone symptoms until later in life.

The relation between the point of obstruction and the ampulla of Vater is important. Most series document a predominance of postampullary obstructions, approaching 80% in some studies (22). A European report described a preampullary predominance (23). Obstructions caused by a membrane are frequently associated with anomalies of the common bile duct. Instead of opening into the medial wall of the duodenum, the common bile duct may terminate within the membrane itself.

Congenital duodenal obstruction is commonly associated with other serious congenital anomalies, which account for most of the morbidity and mortality in these patients. Various reports put the incidence of associated conditions between 50% and 80%. Congenital heart disease and trisomy 21 (Down syndrome) are the most common associated conditions, each occurring in about 30% of cases (24). Not infrequently, all three conditions coexist in the same patient (25). In patients with trisomy 21 who underwent prenatal ultrasonography, about 4% were found to have prenatal evidence of duodenal atresia (26). Other associated anomalies include intestinal malrotation (20%), esophageal atresia or imperforate anus (10% to 20%), heterotaxia, and gallbladder agenesis. The outcome for patients with duodenal atresia depends more on the severity and correctability of these associated anomalies than on the surgical management of the obstruction.

The diagnosis of duodenal atresia is often suggested by prenatal ultrasound (Fig. 72-12). A maternal history of polyhydramnios is common in congenital duodenal obstruction, approaching 75% in one series (27). Prenatal sonographic evaluation of the fetus in these instances can detect two fluid-filled structures consistent with a double-bubble reliably at 22 to 23 weeks' gestation, with the earliest detection having been reported at 18 weeks (28). About 15% to 20% of patients with duodenal atresia have the diagnosis suggested by prenatal ultrasonography. The relatively late availability of a sonographic diagnosis results frequently in an ethical dilemma for prospective parents

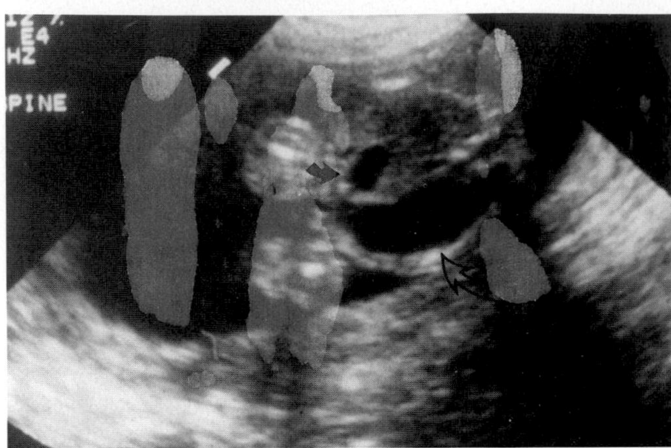

FIGURE 72-12. Prenatal ultrasound of a fetus with duodenal atresia showing the dilated duodenum (*closed arrow*) and stomach (*open arrow*).

who may consider elective termination of pregnancy based on the association of duodenal atresia with Down syndrome. Reliable data regarding the rate of false-positive examinations for duodenal obstruction in the fetus are unavailable.

The clinical presentation of the infant with congenital duodenal obstruction depends on the presence or absence of a membranous aperture, its size, and the location of the obstruction relative to the ampulla. The classic presentation of a complete postampullary obstruction includes bilious vomiting within 24 hours of birth in an otherwise stable infant with a nondistended abdomen. Plain radiographs of the abdomen typically show the classic double-bubble sign—two distinct gas collections or air–fluid levels in the upper abdomen resulting from the markedly dilated stomach and proximal duodenal bulb (Fig. 72-13). If the infant's stomach has been decompressed by vomiting or previous nasogastric aspiration, 40 to 60 mL of air may be injected carefully through the nasogastric tube and the double-bubble reproduced. Air makes an excellent contrast agent, obviating an upper GI tract contrast study in routine cases. The distal intestinal tract may be gasless or may reveal a small amount of intraluminal air, owing to a membranous aperture, a microperforation of an otherwise complete web (29), or a bile duct with openings on both sides of the obstructing diaphragm (30).

The importance of differentiating intrinsic duodenal obstruction from intestinal malrotation with a midgut volvulus in the infant who presents with bilious vomiting cannot be overstated. A clue may be derived from the appearance of the duodenum on the plain radiograph. In the classic double-bubble sign, the duodenum appears distended and round, owing to chronic intrauterine obstruction. When a distended stomach is associated with a normal caliber duodenum, the diagnosis of malrotation with duodenal obstruction secondary to Ladd's bands or volvulus must be entertained. In an unstable patient, echocardiography and upper GI tract contrast study may be required to distinguish between hemodynamic compromise caused by volvulus or cardiac anomalies because therapy obviously differs for congenital heart disease and midgut volvulus. Even when the diagnosis of duodenal atresia

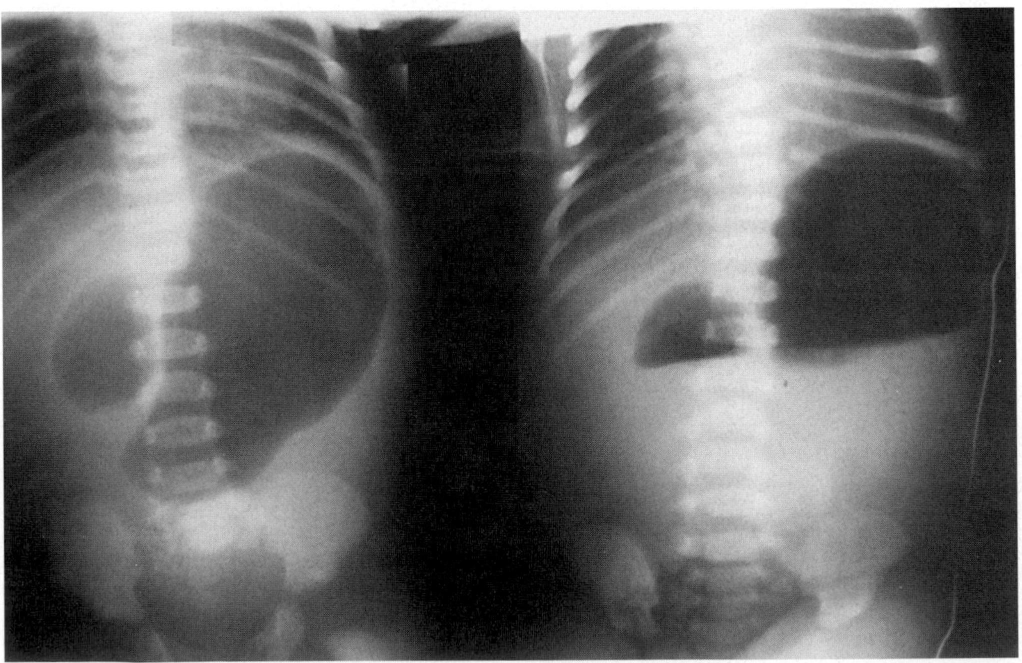

FIGURE 72-13. Supine and upright air contrast radiographs displaying the classic appearance of a double bubble in duodenal atresia.

is established in the stable patient, cardiac anatomy and function should be evaluated before surgical correction.

Preoperative preparation includes nasogastric decompression, fluid and electrolyte replacement, and a thorough evaluation for associated anomalies. If malrotation is ruled out, surgical correction of duodenal atresia can be temporarily postponed, and more urgent conditions evaluated and treated. Prophylactic perioperative antibiotics, usually ampicillin and gentamicin, are begun preoperatively.

Surgical management of intrinsic duodenal obstruction is performed through a transverse right upper quadrant incision. The ligament of Treitz is identified to exclude concomitant intestinal malrotation. It may be necessary to mobilize the hepatic flexure of the colon to expose the duodenum. True atresia with mural discontinuity and annular pancreas is easily recognized. More often, mural continuity is maintained, and the presence of an intraluminal membrane is inferred. When a windsock diaphragm is present, however, the transitional region may not coincide with the location of the obstruction.

The most widely accepted surgical management of both true atresia and annular pancreas involves constructing an anastomosis between the dilated proximal duodenum and the diminutive distal duodenum. The long side-to-side duodenoduodenostomy is an effective procedure, but has been associated with a high incidence of anastomotic dysfunction and prolonged obstruction. The duodenojejunostomy, commonly employed in the past, is also associated with greater morbidity and is now reserved for special circumstances, such as the presence of a long gap between proximal and distal duodenal segments or a large ventral pancreatic remnant that prevents apposition of the duodenal segments. Gastrojejunostomy is an unacceptable alternative, given the high incidence of marginal ulceration and bleeding.

The diamond duodenoduodenostomy, as described by Kimura and colleagues (31), has yielded consistently good results and remains the procedure of choice. Limited mobilization of the duodenum distal to the atresia may be necessary to facilitate apposition of the segments. A transverse incision is made in the anterior wall of the distalmost portion of the dilated proximal duodenal pouch, and an incision of similar length is made in a longitudinal orientation on the antimesenteric border of the distal duodenum. The anastomosis is fashioned in such a way as to approximate the ends of one incision to the midpoints of the other incision. The tension resulting from this orientation tends to hold the anastomosis open in a self-stenting manner (Fig. 72-14).

One of the most problematic issues following repair of duodenal atresia by any method is delayed transit, usually associated with a persistently dilated and dyskinetic proximal duodenum. In Kimura's series of patients managed with the diamond-type duodenoduodenostomy, two-thirds were followed up with contrast studies and displayed no

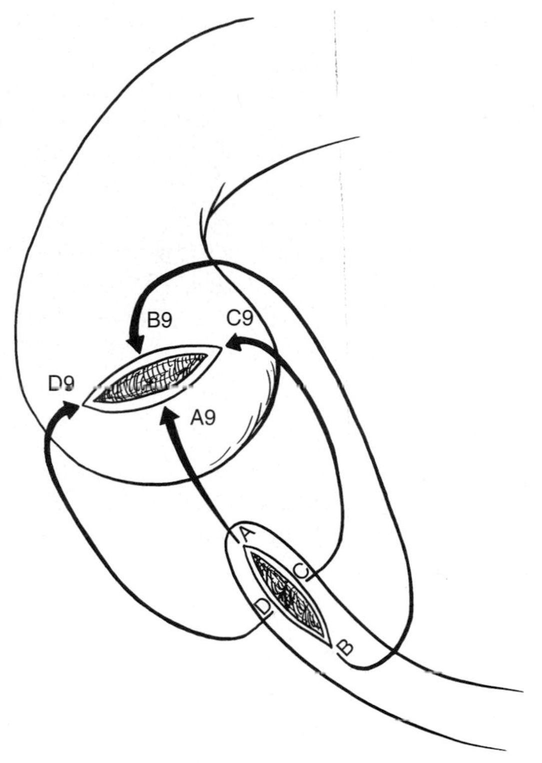

FIGURE 72-14. Technique of diamond duodenoduodenostomy as described by Kimura and colleagues. (Adapted from Kimura K, Mukohara N, Nashijima E, et al. Diamond-shaped anastomosis for duodenal atresia: an experience with 44 patients over 15 years. *J Pediatr Surg* 1990;25:977.)

significant anastomotic dysfunction or residual megaduodenum. In contrast, a contemporary series of standard side-to-side anastomoses reported a 30% incidence of radiographic abnormalities related to anastomotic dysfunction, including megaduodenum with delayed transit (27). An additional 17% displayed GER, which may have been due, in part, to a relative impairment in gastric emptying. Even with the diamond anastomosis, however, a persistent megaduodenum with symptomatic partial obstruction and stasis can occur. This complication may be managed either by tapering duodenoplasty or lateral seromuscular resetion (32).

The surgical management of an intrinsic duodenal web begins with a longitudinal incision centered over the web origin. The site of origin, however, may not be easily identified. Palpation of the duodenal wall may reveal a thickened circumferential ridge. When this is not detected, a catheter can be advanced by the anesthesiologist and guided into the duodenum by the surgeon. When the advancing catheter encounters the web, further advancement produces an indentation on the wall of the duodenum. This may be at or proximal to the actual transition zone. Once the site of attachment has been determined, stay sutures are placed in the antimesenteric wall and the duodenum opened longitudinally for a short distance (less than 1 cm) in both directions.

Because of the high incidence of bile duct anomalies, a thorough search for the ampulla and accessory ductal ostia is important. If these are separate from the membrane, a portion of the web on the antimesenteric aspect of the lumen can be excised. If anomalous bile ducts involve the web itself, the uninvolved portion of the web can be incised from the antimesenteric border to the center. In either case, the longitudinal incision is closed transversely, widening the lumen at that point. An additional option is a diamond anastomosis, bypassing the web to avoid injury to the common bile duct.

A feeding gastrostomy should not be necessary for postoperative management of an uncomplicated duodenal repair. Gastroduodenal function usually returns within 5 to 7 days, but may be delayed. Regardless, enteral feeding can be initiated when appropriate with small boluses and progressively advanced in volume as tolerated. Results of surgery are generally good. As mentioned earlier, complications related to surgery are directly related to the underlying pathology and choice of operation. Survival rates of 95% are commonly reported in those for whom surgery is deemed appropriate, and virtually all the mortality in these series was due to associated conditions.

ACQUIRED ABNORMALITIES OF THE STOMACH AND DUODENUM

Hypertrophic Pyloric Stenosis

HPS is an acquired condition in which the circumferential muscle layer of the pyloric sphincter becomes thickened, resulting in narrowing and elongation of the pyloric channel. This produces a high-grade gastric outlet obstruction with compensatory dilation, hypertrophy, and hyperperistalsis of the stomach. The thickening of the smooth muscle layer results from muscular hypertrophy as opposed to hyperplasia.

The first accurate clinicopathologic description of HPS in an infant is credited to Hirschsprung in the late nineteenth century, who considered it to be a congenital disease. At that time, surgical management consisted of gastrojejunostomy, which resulted in a mortality rate of 60%. Extramucosal pyloroplasty proved unsatisfactory, owing in large part to excessive hemorrhage that occurred when sutures tore through the edematous muscle that had been closed. In 1911, Ramstedt omitted this unnecessary muscle closure and thus defined pyloromyotomy—recognized as the definitive procedure ever since.

The incidence of HPS ranges between 0.1% and 1% in the general population and appears to be rising. Studies conducted in the mid-1960s reported rates of 1 in 300 to 1 in 900. More recent population-based studies from the United Kingdom have documented a rise in incidence from 0.1% to 0.2% up to 0.8% during the past several decades. A large population-based study conducted by the Mayo Clinic documented an overall incidence of 0.26% from 1950 to 1984 in Olmsted County, Minnesota, but reported that the rate approached 0.5% by the end of the study period (33). A longitudinal study employing ultrasonographic evaluation of 1,400 randomly selected term neonates documented that all 9 infants (0.65%) in whom HPS later developed had normal pyloric dimensions at birth (34). There is a significant male predominance of about 4 : 1, although the long-held belief that HPS primarily afflicts first-born males has not been confirmed. The incidence in whites exceeds that in blacks by severalfold; the incidence in Asian infants is low. The transmission of HPS appears to involve multifactorial threshold inheritance or the effects of multiple interacting loci (35). Transmission from mothers is more common than from fathers: HPS develops in 19% of boys and 7% of girls whose mothers had HPS as infants and in 5% of boys and 2.5% of girls whose fathers were previously affected (36).

The cause of HPS remains unknown. One hypothesis is that dyscoordination between gastric peristalsis and pyloric relaxation results in simultaneous gastric and pyloric contraction and work hypertrophy of the pyloric muscle (37). This initiates a cycle of escalating pyloric obstruction and gastric hyperperistalsis. Although functional disturbances in gastric emptying in the first weeks of life have not been proven to occur in neonates in whom HPS later develops, a report of in utero gastric dilation in a neonate who later developed HPS suggests a possible role for prenatal gastric emptying dysfunction (38). More recently, an association between maternal and infant exposure to erythromycin and development of HPS has been identified, and a causal link postulated (39,40). Erythromycin stimulates phase III MMC activity and may expose the immature pylorus to markedly elevated gastric pressures.

The underlying pathophysiology of pyloric dysfunction in HPS has not been defined. Observations of decreased ganglion cell density in the pyloric region have not been consistently reproduced, nor does such an observation explain the curative role of pyloromyotomy. Attempts to establish a causative link between the hypergastrinemia and hyperacidity seen in these patients and HPS have also been unsuccessful. In fact, gastrin-mediated acid secretion is an expected consequence of any gastric outlet obstruction that produces gastric distention. Elevated levels of certain prostaglandins (e.g., PGE_2 and PGF_2-α) have been described in these patients and have been proposed to cause pyloric constriction with the eventual development of HPS. Gastric outlet obstruction due to pylorospasm has been reported in neonates receiving PGE infusions. Pyloric dysfunction in these infants, however, does not lead to muscular hypertrophy (41).

Perhaps a more promising hypothesis for the pathophysiology of HPS is a primary abnormality of the ENS. Investigations have focused on finding evidence of altered neural control of muscular contraction. Studies have documented both decreased and disordered innervation of the circumferential muscle layer in specimens of pyloric muscle taken at the time of pyloromyotomy (42–44). Furthermore, the muscle layer in HPS appears to be nearly devoid of neurotrophins—peptides that govern differentiation and survival of ENS neurons (45). Circumstantial evidence exists to suggest that such neural immaturity is transient, accounting for the fact that HPS does not recur after temporary myotomy (46).

Immunohistochemical identification of a variety of neuropeptides, such as GRP, VIP, somatostatin, and substance P, has revealed a marked reduction in these neuropeptides in patients with HPS as compared with normal controls (47,48). VIP, in particular, demonstrates significant activity in mediating pyloric smooth muscle relaxation. Another observation has implicated a local deficiency of nitric oxide, a ubiquitous paracrine and neurocrine mediator of smooth muscle relaxation, as a causative factor in the development of HPS. Nitric oxide synthase (NOS), which can be identified in significant concentrations in the pyloric circular and longitudinal muscle layers and the myenteric plexus in normal controls, has been shown to be selectively absent in the circular muscle layer in patients with HPS (49). This has also been documented for NOS mRNA (50). Another study has reported axonal degeneration in both the myenteric plexus and the intramuscular nerves in patients with HPS (51).

The typical clinical presentation is a term male infant between 3 and 6 weeks of age who has progressive, nonbilious, projectile vomiting. Many infants are initially believed to have a food allergy or GER until the vomiting consistently follows every feeding and is forceful. Many infants with HPS are significantly dehydrated at the time of presentation, although inanition is fortunately no longer a common finding. Serum chemistries reflect a hypochloremic, hypokalemic contraction metabolic alkalosis, which may be associated with paradoxical aciduria when severe. Significant hypoglycemia can also be present and may precipitate seizures. Unconjugated hyperbilirubinemia is common and correlates with a decrease in hepatic glucuronyltransferase activity. The jaundice is transient and resolves as soon as the gastric outlet obstruction is corrected, making it attractive to speculate that the hepatic defect is secondary to abnormal enteroendocrine feedback between the stomach and the hepatocyte.

The hallmark of the diagnosis is the finding of a small, mobile, ovoid mass referred to as an *olive* (because of its size and shape) in the epigastrium. The process of detecting the olive may be quite difficult. Two or three fingertips are gently placed in the upper abdomen and gently advanced into the deeper tissues below the liver edge. They are then slowly swept inferiorly toward the umbilicus. The olive can be felt to roll under the fingertips during this sweeping motion—no other structure gives this sensation. A positive examination is very accurate, with a selectivity value of more than 97% (52). The art of detecting the olive lies in performing the examination under conditions conducive to deep abdominal palpation in a quiet, cooperative infant. Sometimes considerable time—15 to 20 minutes—may be required to obtain conditions that are conducive for palpation of the hypertrophied pylorus. Prior nasogastric suctioning to empty the stomach followed by removal of the tube allows the surgeon to examine the abdomen while the baby is sucking on a small amount of sugar water. This often permits a more thorough palpation of the pyloric region. If the pylorus is unequivocally felt, the diagnosis is established, and no further diagnostic maneuvers are necessary.

If the pylorus is not detected and the clinical presentation is sufficiently suggestive to warrant further evaluation, radiologic evaluation can be definitive. Real-time ultrasonography has supplanted barium upper GI tract study as the procedure of choice. Teele and Smith (53) observed the hypertrophied pylorus to have a characteristic appearance on B-mode ultrasound, and subsequently it has been shown that measurement of pyloric dimensions accurately establishes the diagnosis of HPS. Parameters measured include overall diameter, single wall thickness, and pyloric channel length, with the latter two being the most commonly used (Fig. 72-15). Measurements found to have greater than 90% positive predictive value include diameter 17 mm or more, muscular wall thickness 4 mm or greater, and channel length 17 mm or greater. In infants 30 days of age or younger, it has been suggested that diagnostic criteria for wall thickness be reduced to 3 mm (54). When parameters are equivocal (e.g., wall thickness 2 to 3 mm, channel length 12 to 16 mm), especially in younger infants, calculation of the pyloric volume has been reported to have greater diagnostic accuracy than the individual measurements alone (55). Finally, upper GI tract study can be diagnostic in cases in which ultrasound is equivocal by demonstrating an elongated and narrowed pyloric channel, with the characteristic shoulders of the hypertrophied pylorus bulging into the gastric lumen (Fig. 72-16).

Although an accurate diagnosis based on physical examination should be possible in most cases, and should be attempted in all, it is evident that an increasing reliance on ultrasonography will continue to erode the skills of examiners. A review comparing diagnostic accuracy between two eras in a single pediatric institution found that the sensitivity of physical examination declined by one-half during a period of increasing reliance on ultrasound (56). It is likely that ultrasound, a noninvasive, highly accurate, and relatively inexpensive technology, will continue to experience great popularity among primary care providers who first evaluate these infants.

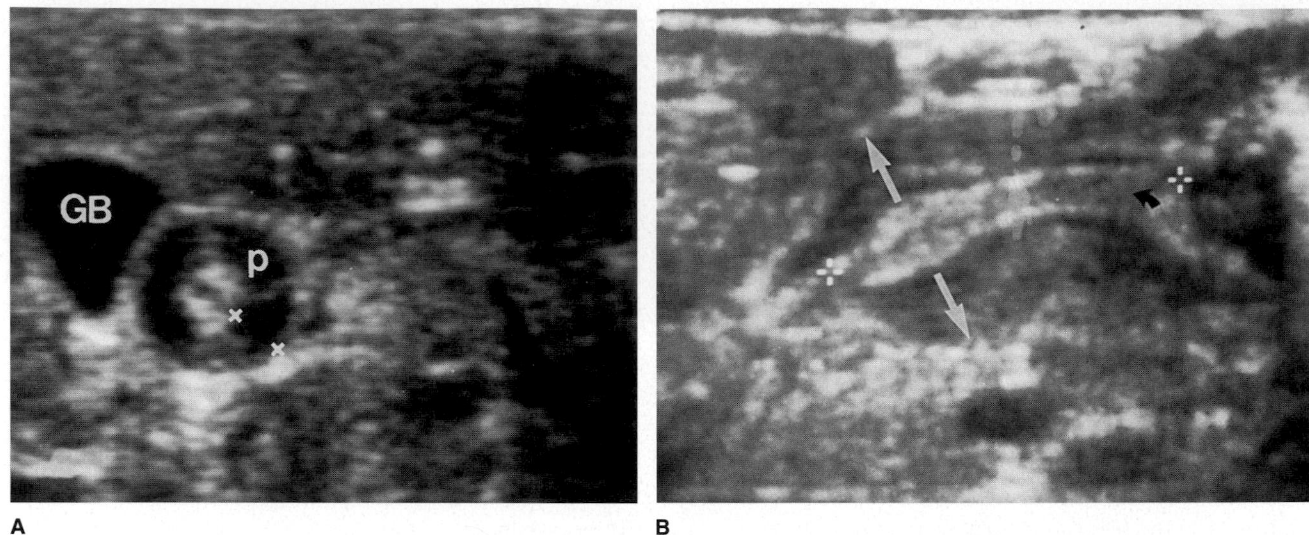

FIGURE 72-15. Two-dimensional ultrasonographic findings in hypertrophic pyloric stenosis. **(A)** Transverse view showing cross section of hypertrophied pylorus (P) and adjacent gallbladder (GB). The thickness of the echolucent circumferential muscle layer is measured by the distance between the cursors. **(B)** Longitudinal view showing echolucent muscle walls in profile (*white arrows*). They are separated by two echogenic lines that represent the submucosa and an echolucent core that represents the pyloric channel lumen (*black arrow*). The channel length between the cursors is increased in hypertrophic pyloric stenosis.

Preoperative preparation is critical once the diagnosis is made. HPS is not a surgical emergency, so careful correction of fluid and electrolyte losses should be accomplished before operative intervention. The infant who presents early in the course of the disease with no clinical dehydration, normal serum electrolytes and glucose, and a normal urine output can be operated on at the earliest convenience. Many patients, however, present with dehydration, hypoglycemia, or a contraction alkalosis of sufficient severity to require preoperative resuscitation for 24 to 48 hours. Infants with severe intravascular fluid deficits causing hypoperfusion should first be resuscitated with isotonic lactated Ringer solution in boluses of 10 to 20 mL per kg until hemodynamic stability is restored. Most preexisting deficits can be replaced with 5% dextrose in 0.45% NaCl, which is administered intravenously at one and one-half times the maintenance rate. Because total body potassium and chloride deficits are considerable in these

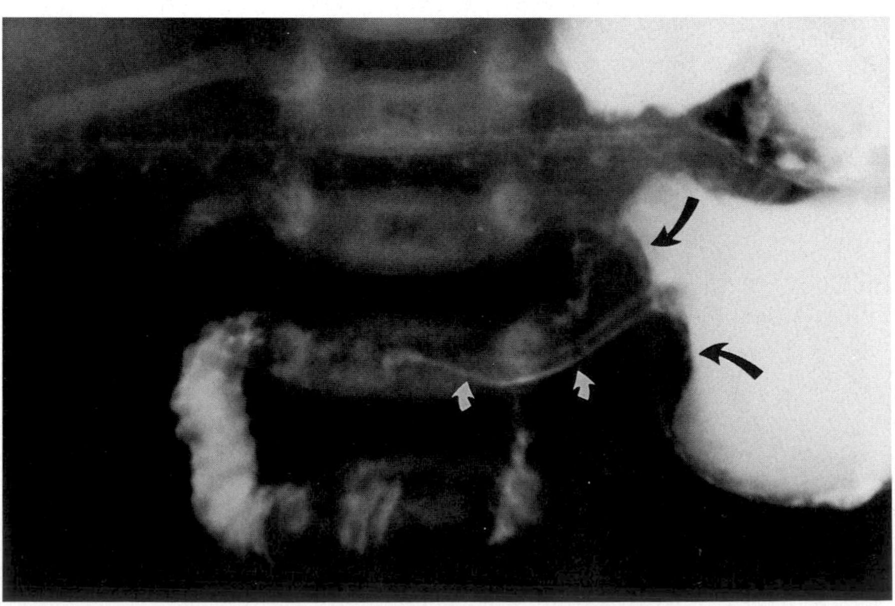

FIGURE 72-16. Upper gastrointestinal tract contrast study findings in hypertrophic pyloric stenosis, displaying the "string sign" of a stenotic channel lumen (*white arrows*) and the bulging "shoulders" of the hypertrophic pyloric muscle (*black arrows*).

patients, maintenance fluid is supplemented with potassium chloride (KCl) at a concentration of 20 to 40 mEq per L. The serum potassium level underestimates the potassium deficit because alkalosis shifts extracellular potassium ions into the intracellular compartment. The presence of paradoxical aciduria indicates a significant total-body potassium deficit. Once volume status and urine output have normalized, serum chloride and potassium have normalized, and serum bicarbonate is normalizing, surgery can be safely conducted.

The treatment of HPS is pyloromyotomy. Historically, the operation is performed through a transverse right upper quadrant incision over the rectus muscle at or above the liver edge. The pylorus may be identified by delivering the greater curvature of the stomach through the wound and using it as a lever to externalize the pylorus. The pylorus usually has a pale white appearance and a rubbery texture. A superficial incision is made through the serosa on the anterior surface from the distal antrum to a point just proximal to the duodenum. The duodenal end is usually easily identified by the color change from the pale to pink, and is further delimited by a prominent pyloric vein. The duodenal mucosa may prolapse over the bulging distal shoulder of the pylorus, causing the duodenal lumen to be entered if the myotomy is deepened too aggressively. The myotomy is deepened bluntly to the submucosa, and the overlying muscle fibers are gently spread and mobilized to allow the submucosa and mucosa to bulge out to the level of the serosa (Fig. 72-17). Care must be taken to avoid tearing the underlying mucosa, particularly at the duodenal end. Deliberate attention to mucosal integrity is important because the morbidity associated with a recognized injury is minimal, whereas that associated with delayed recognition is not. When the hypertrophied muscle has been adequately mobilized and the two halves of the pylorus can be moved back and forth independently, the pyloromyotomy is complete. Venous congestion caused by delivering the pylorus through a relatively small incision under moderate traction can result in venous bleeding from the submucosa and the cut surface of the muscle. This bleeding ceases when the pylorus is returned to the abdomen, and electrocautery is unnecessary. The wound is closed in layers as usual.

Since the mid-1990s, the minimally invasive approach to pyloromyotomy has gained widespread popularity. Most surgeons employ an umbilical port for placement of the laparoscope, and two tiny unported instrument sites in the upper abdomen. Conceptually, the operation is identical to the open procedure. After a steep learning curve, operative time is no longer and the complication rate no greater than for open pyloromyotomy. The time to full feedings and discharge may be slightly shorter when the operation is done laparoscopically, and cosmesis is better (57,58). Both approaches to pyloromyotomy are accepted, and the choice of one or the other depends on individual factors and operator preference.

If the mucosa of the underlying pyloric channel or duodenum is violated, the management of the perforation should be individualized. If the lumen is entered early in the conduct of the pyloromyotomy, the mucosa is closed with fine absorbable sutures as attempts to continue muscle spreading only enlarge the rent. The muscle is closed over the mucosal repair, and a second myotomy is performed by rotating the pylorus 180 degrees. If, however, the tear occurs at a point when the myotomy is essentially complete, the tear can be closed with fine absorbable sutures and covered with a portion of the gastrocolic omentum, obviating a second myotomy. In this situation, some surgeons prefer to decompress the stomach for 1 or 2 days until GI function fully returns. Others contend that the

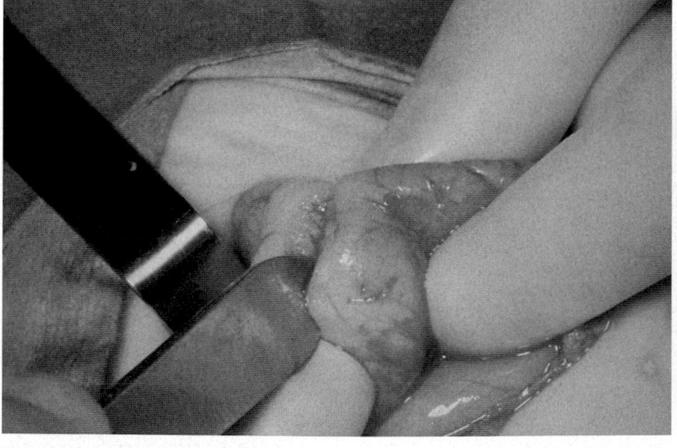

A

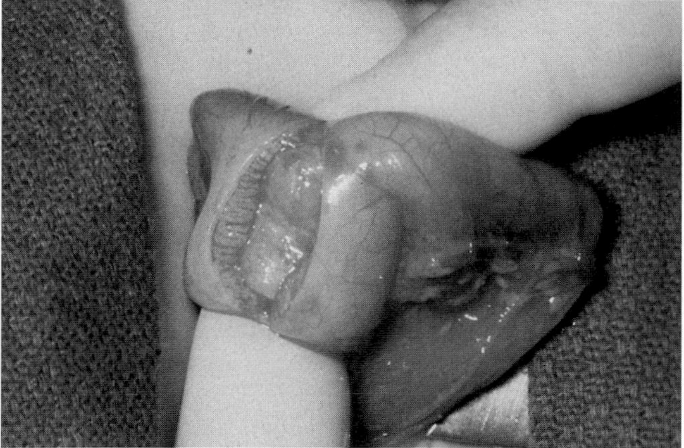

B

FIGURE 72-17. Operative technique of pyloromyotomy. **(A)** The pyloric muscle is split longitudinally with the blunt end of a scalpel handle. **(B)** Completed myotomy allows the submucosal layer to bulge out to the level of the serosa.

nasogastric tube represents a risk of reperforation and simply withhold feeding for several days. Contrast studies are not necessary before feeding unless clinically indicated for other reasons.

The postoperative management of an uncomplicated pyloromyotomy is straightforward. A feeding regimen is begun 4 to 8 hours after operation with a small volume of sugar water, advancing volume and osmolarity every 2 to 3 hours until the infant is taking formula or breast milk ad libitum. It is common for occasional emesis to occur after pyloromyotomy; this should not delay the progression of the feeding schedule in most cases. In general, most infants so managed are able to be discharged within 24 to 48 hours of surgery.

Persistent postoperative vomiting beyond 48 hours is uncommon. In this circumstance, the possibilities of an incomplete myotomy or unrecognized perforation should be considered. Radiologic studies are of little value in evaluating the completeness of the myotomy because the fluoroscopic and sonographic appearance of the hypertrophied pylorus before and after myotomy are similar. A contrast study should be obtained to exclude a mucosal leak, which may produce a fluid collection that compresses the gastric outlet. In the absence of a leak or complete obstruction, an interval of at least 2 weeks is allowed to pass before the presumptive diagnosis of incomplete myotomy prompts reexploration.

Most children treated for HPS can expect excellent short- and long-term outcomes. With appropriate resuscitation, expert anesthesia, and a standard surgical approach, mortality has been virtually eliminated. The reported rates of duodenal perforation range from 3% to 30% (depending on whether the procedures were performed by pediatric surgeons), although rates higher than 10% are unusual. Wound infection and dehiscence, significant problems in previous eras, are relatively uncommon today. Postoperative ultrasound studies have documented a return to normal muscle thickness within 4 weeks, associated with healing of the pyloric muscle and return of function. A study addressing gastric emptying and abdominal symptoms after pyloromyotomy found no differences between treatment and control groups several decades after surgery (59).

Acid-peptic Disease

The most common clinical disorders implicating the stomach and duodenum in human disease involve acid-peptic injury to the mucosa, resulting in inflammation, superficial erosions, and ulcerations. Hence, the physiologic and pharmacologic regulation of acid secretion have become important areas of investigation. Despite significant progress in the understanding of the physiology of acid secretion, the many causes of acid-peptic disease (APD) still lack complete explanation.

Although the incidence of APD in adults is gradually declining, it appears to be increasing in children. This is in part due to the increased use of endoscopy in evaluating children with abdominal symptoms, but there are indications that the prevalence of the disease in children is also increasing. Increased usage of ulcerogenic drugs (e.g., nonsteroidal antiinflammatory agents) and an increase in the numbers of children subjected to and surviving physiologically stressful events (e.g., trauma, burns, cancer chemotherapy, bone marrow transplantation) may contribute to this increased incidence.

It is commonly accepted that most ulcers follow a progression from mucosal inflammation to superficial erosions to deeper ulcerations. Superficial erosions are defined as discrete, punctate defects in the mucosa that extend only into the submucosa. An ulcer must extend at least through the submucosa and muscularis mucosa into the muscularis propria. Ulcers are usually accompanied by significant inflammation and edema, as well as by thickened rugal folds that radiate away from the lesion. Both erosions and ulcers can disrupt underlying blood vessels and cause hemorrhage. True ulcers can extend through the entire wall, leading to hemorrhage from major adjacent arteries (e.g., the gastroduodenal artery), free perforation, or retroperitoneal penetration (e.g., into the head of the pancreas).

The process of peptic ulceration requires an imbalance between the aggressive forces of HCl and activated pepsin, and the protective mechanisms that defend the gastroduodenal mucosa from chemical and autodigestive injury. Any one of a large number of abnormalities in this homeostatic balance can lead to progressive mucosal injury. Although maximal and basal acid outputs are often increased in children with APD, a significant degree of overlap exists between the APD patients and normal controls. Furthermore, the level of acid output correlates poorly with duration and severity of symptoms (although it correlates somewhat better with prognosis and need for surgical intervention). It is therefore difficult to ascribe a causal relation between hyperacidity and clinical disease. Simple acid hypersecretion is probably the principal cause of APD in only a small minority of patients.

Gastroduodenal ulcers in children can be defined as either primary or secondary. Primary ulcers are the result of an intrinsic ulcer diathesis and are not associated either with contributing extrinsic factors or with other acute medical illnesses. They are usually located in the duodenum, but concurrent pyloric channel ulcerations can also occur. Primary gastric ulcers in children are rare. These ulcers are chronic and usually present with long-standing complaints of abdominal symptoms. Acute primary ulcers are probably present for a considerable time before causing symptoms.

Although most patients with primary APD do not have any definable underlying condition, a small number of patients have a known cause for acid hypersecretion.

The most well characterized of these conditions is the Zollinger-Ellison syndrome (ZES), caused by a secreting gastrinoma. Other conditions associated with primary APD include G-cell hyperplasia, G-cell hyperfunction, and systemic mastocytosis.

Much attention has focused on a possible infectious etiology for primary APD. *Helicobacter pylori*, is a fastidious, spiral-shaped gram-negative rod that inhabits the microaerobic mucus layer and invades the gastric wall with great frequency, causing localized inflammation. *H. pylori* has been recovered from antral biopsy specimens in virtually all adults and children with chronic active gastritis or duodenal ulcers. The organism is occasionally recovered from the duodenum as well, but only from areas of gastric metaplasia. Most or all children with *H. pylori*-associated antral gastritis do not have symptoms, and their gross endoscopic findings are frequently normal. Those with endoscopic abnormalities display a characteristic antral nodularity, but no inflammation. Histopathologic examination of biopsy material in all patients, however, uniformly reveals chronic inflammatory changes with mononuclear cell infiltrates.

The high correlation between *H. pylori*-associated chronic gastritis and primary duodenal ulcer suggests a causative link between the two conditions. The virulence factors influencing the ability of *H. pylori* to invade and colonize the antral mucosa involve urease production, flagellar-mediated motility, and specific membrane-associated adhesins that allow the microorganism to attach to gastric cells. Bacterial urease degrades urea to bicarbonate and ammonia, which is toxic to gastric epithelial cells. More virulent strains also express a vacuolating cytotoxin. The pathophysiologic mechanisms that translate antral colonization into duodenal ulceration are unknown, but probably involve gastrin hypersecretion by the chronically inflamed antral mucosa. Basal, peak, and 24-hour integrated gastrin levels are increased in patients with *H. pylori* gastritis and duodenal ulcer; elevations in basal or stimulated acid outputs, however, have not been consistently observed (60). Although the causal link has not been firmly established, the prevention of recurrence of primary APD in children appears to require the pharmacologic eradication of *H. pylori* (61). This usually requires a multidrug regimen that may include amoxicillin, metronidazole, and bismuth.

Secondary ulcers occur in association with other unrelated disorders or extrinsic factors that are considered to be pathophysiologically linked to ulcer formation. This association may be through either acid hypersecretion or compromise of mucosal defense mechanisms. These include physiologically stressful events (hence, the term *stress ulcer*), such as neonatal hypoxia, sepsis, trauma, head injury (Cushing ulcer), and severe burns (Curling ulcer). Drug-related ulcers in children most commonly occur with the use of aspirin and other nonsteroidal antiinflammatory drugs. These compounds decrease mucosal blood flow by inhibiting prostaglandin synthesis; inhibit other defense mechanisms, such as bicarbonate and mucus secretion; and induce other cytotoxic inflammatory mediators. Secondary APD is more common in most pediatric series than is primary disease and involves the stomach as often as the duodenum. In addition, the incidence of complications (e.g., hemorrhage and perforation) and death are much higher in secondary APD than in primary APD (62).

As in adults, the treatment of choice for most children with primary APD is medical management. Strategies to control the adverse effects of gastric acid include acid neutralization (antacids), stimulus inhibition (H_2 blockers, such as ranitidine), inhibition of acid production (proton pump blockade, such as omeprazole), and mucosal protection (binding resins, such as sucralfate). Sucralfate functions not only by providing a protective physiochemical barrier, but also by enhancing mucosal microvascular flow and by the protective binding of basic fibroblast growth factor, a prime regulator of angiogenesis and ulcer healing (63).

The treatment of secondary APD involves all these approaches and also includes PGE replacement (e.g., misoprostol, a PGE_1 analogue) to restore mucosal perfusion in patients receiving nonsteroidal antiinflammatory drugs. Obviously, the single most important component of stress ulcer management is to remove the precipitating event. This, of course, is not often possible, accounting for the high degree of treatment failure and complications in this group.

Because of the high morbidity associated with stress ulceration, treatment has focused on prevention in high-risk patients. Maintenance of an intragastric pH higher than 4 clearly reduces the incidence of APD-associated hemorrhage. Although this can be accomplished with equal efficacy using antacids or H_2 blockers, H_2 blockade is usually more practical. Evidence also suggests that the incidence of bleeding can be further reduced by administering the H_2 blocker by continuous infusion, reducing the number of episodes of breakthrough hyperacidity. Intravenous proton pump inhibitors (pantoprazole) are now available, and may be more effective than histamine blockade. Frequent monitoring of gastric pH to assess the adequacy of acid suppression is important.

Attention has also focused on the beneficial antimicrobial effects of gastric acidity, suggesting that the stomach's acid environment may reduce the incidence of gastric colonization and subsequent nosocomial infections in critically ill ventilated patients. In adults, sucralfate has been shown to prevent stress ulcer-related complications as effectively as H_2 blockade. A concomitant decrease in the incidence of nosocomial pneumonia has not been seen, however (64). The efficacy of sucralfate compared with H_2 blockers for prophylaxis against nosocomial infections has not been adequately studied in children.

The absolute indications for surgery in children are the same as in adults: perforation, persistent hemorrhage, obstruction, and intractability. A relative indication is recurrence—the risks of surgery and its side effects must be weighed against a lifelong dependency on medication. Primary APD in children has an extremely high recurrence rate, exceeding 50% in many series. In the past, such high recurrence rates constituted an indication for definitive surgery in a significant number of patients, approaching 40% in a retrospective series (65). Today, with a wide variety of effective pharmacologic approaches and an expectation that *H. pylori* eradication will lead to a higher cure rate, definitive surgery for primary APD is less commonly performed. Intractability or rapid recurrence off medication should prompt a thorough workup for gastrinoma.

The number of children requiring surgery for APD has declined dramatically since the introduction of effective antisecretory agents (66). When surgery is performed for APD in children, it is usually performed for hemorrhage or perforation resulting from secondary ulcers. Nearly 50% of children with endoscopically proven secondary APD ultimately require emergent surgical intervention for either hemorrhage or perforation. Historically, hemorrhage and perforation have been relatively equivalent in their frequencies as indications for emergency surgery in children.

The indications for surgical intervention in children with hemorrhage from APD are subjective. Persistent or repeated bleeding in the face of failed medical and endoscopic therapy are noncontroversial indications. Other recommendations include hemorrhage of sufficient magnitude to require transfusion of one-half the calculated blood volume in 8 hours, or one total blood volume in 24 hours (some consider one-half the blood volume in 24 hours to be an indication). A visible vessel at the ulcer base, identified during endoscopic examination, is associated with a high risk of rebleeding and is commonly considered another indication for surgical therapy. Perforation, marked by pneumoperitoneum and peritonitis, is an absolute indication for surgery. Recommendations in the adult literature regarding nonoperative management of contained perforations in stable patients of advanced age are difficult to translate to children, and experience with such management is anecdotal.

The choice of operation depends on several factors: the indication for surgery, the chronicity of disease, the anticipated need for surgical control of future ulcer diathesis, the stability and preoperative condition of the patient, and the child's age. Most data regarding the efficacy and risks of surgery for APD have been from studies in adults. The application of conclusions and recommendations from these studies to infants, children, and adolescents must be individualized.

For most adolescent and adult patients, the curative options available to the surgeon include truncal vagotomy and drainage (usually by pyloroplasty; VP), truncal vagotomy and antrectomy (VA), or proximal gastric vagotomy (PGV). Mortality, morbidity, and recurrence rates for these procedures performed electively in adults have been well established. All three have minimal mortality rates. Both VP and VA have significant long-term side effects associated with GI denervation and impaired gastric emptying that approach 15% for both procedures. The rate of recurrence for VA (about 2%) is, however, considerably lower than for VP (10% to 15%). Although PGV has a rate of recurrence similar to VP, the virtual absence of side effects, greater acceptance by patients as scored by the Visik grading scale, and availability of effective new drugs to control recurrence makes PGV the procedure of choice whenever possible (67).

In the rare child with primary APD refractory to medical therapy, or in whom multiple recurrences have occurred after cessation of medications, PGV is the recommended procedure after eliminating ZES as a potential cause. A modification of this procedure, which includes a posterior truncal vagotomy and an anterior PGV (lesser curve seromyotomy), has been reported to be as effective and free of side effects as PGV, while having the additional advantages of preserving the blood supply to the lesser curve and lending itself to laparoscopic techniques (68). Experience with either of these procedures in children is limited.

More commonly, surgical intervention is necessitated by hemorrhage or perforation occurring in the setting of stress- or steroid-related secondary duodenal ulcers. Support can be found both for limited intervention to control the complication and for combining control of the complication with definitive antiulcer surgery. Simple oversewing of the bleeding ulcer followed by pharmacologic suppression of acid secretion is the preferred treatment in infants and young children. Because most older patients who present with uncontrolled hemorrhage do so despite maximal attempts at prophylaxis, antisecretory therapy, and endoscopic control, it is prudent to advocate definitive ulcer surgery in most of these patients. The risk of recurrent bleeding in patients who have failed medical control, and the consequences of repeated life-threatening hemorrhage, argue against limited surgery simply to ligate the involved vessel. VP provides both a simple approach to expose the duodenal ulcer for vessel ligation and relatively effective antisecretory therapy. Although VA is considered to be superior to VP for bleeding duodenal ulcers in stable, healthy adults, there is little enthusiasm for (or experience with) VA in children. In the well-resuscitated stable patient, consideration should be given to ligation of the duodenal ulcer through a pylorus-sparing duodenotomy, followed by anatomic duodenal closure and either formal or modified PGV. This approach has gained favor in adults, but is unstudied in children.

For children with perforated duodenal ulcers, most pediatric surgeons support simple closure of the perforation with an omental buttress (Graham patch), relying on aggressive postoperative medical therapy, including continuously infused histamine blockers or omeprazole, to facilitate ulcer healing. Avoidance of a suture line and hiatal dissection in the face of peritonitis are believed to be reasonable tenets. In adults, historical evidence documenting high rates of recurrence and eventual surgery has led to an acceptance of combining PGV with closure of the perforation as a definitive procedure in this setting. The rationale for and results of this approach in children are not defined.

As noted earlier, patients with a particularly aggressive ulcer diathesis should be evaluated for ZES before deciding on the surgical approach. ZES is a condition of severe ulcer diathesis caused by a gastrin-secreting neoplasm. Gastrin levels are markedly and continuously elevated and do not show any evidence of physiologic regulation. Parietal cell hypersecretion and peptic ulceration are severe, and the incidence of multifocal disease, recurrence, and ulcer-related complications is high. Diagnosis relies on the demonstration of elevated gastrin levels, both at baseline and after stimulation with secretin. The primary tumor, or gastrinoma, is usually found in the duodenal wall, the pancreas (as a non-β islet cell tumor), or in the adjacent retroperitoneum. In the familial form of the disease, associated with multiple endocrine neoplasia syndrome type I, there is a high incidence of multicentricity, with multiple tumor nodules dispersed diffusely throughout the pancreas. In the sporadic form, fewer tumors (one to three) are usually observed. Noninvasive imaging has been disappointing in localizing the primary tumor, but computed tomography is recommended to evaluate the liver for metastatic deposits. Angiography and intraoperative ultrasonography may offer improvements in definitive localization. Although total gastrectomy was formerly required to control the effects of hypergastrinemia, management with aggressive H_2 blockade and proton pump inhibitors has largely controlled the severe ulcer diathesis. Surgical management involves extirpation of the gastrinoma, if possible, by tumor enucleation or distal pancreatic resection in the sporadic form. Even though only one-half of the patients who undergo tumor excision are rendered biochemically free of disease, surgical resection of the primary gastrinoma appears to reduce the incidence of eventual metastasis (69). In patients with multiple endocrine neoplasia syndrome type I, curative surgery is unlikely given the diffuse nature of the disease. Medical management with antisecretory agents and somatostatin analogues has been successful in achieving long-term survival, in part owing to the indolent nature of the disease. Long-term prognosis in the face of metastatic disease is poor.

Gastric Dysmotility

Rarely, infants younger than 1 year of age present with persistent nonbilious vomiting and are presumed to have GER. Evaluation for GER by manometric and pH probe studies documents normal LES function. An upper GI tract contrast study reveals a funnel-shaped, atonic antrum with delayed gastric emptying and reflux of contrast. The pylorus is normal. These patients have antral dysmotility, a primary motility disorder of unknown etiology. Usually, the condition is transient and responds to conservative measures, such as altering the feeding regimen. In one series, nearly 40% of patients underwent pyloroplasty with good results (70). Alternatively, pyloromyotomy can be used and has proved to be effective.

Neonatal Gastric Perforation

The causes of gastric perforation in neonates can be categorized as traumatic, ischemic, or spontaneous. Traumatic perforations are generally caused by pneumatic gastric distention from bag-mask ventilation or positive-pressure ventilation in an infant with a tracheoesophageal fistula, or by puncture of the stomach during gastric intubation. Usually, these appear as short lacerations or discrete puncture wounds.

Ischemic perforations occur in the setting of severe physiologic stress, such as extreme prematurity or birth asphyxia, and sometimes accompany necrotizing enterocolitis involving the distal GI tract. The pathophysiology of these lesions is unknown but is presumed to be associated with locoregional redistribution of blood flow resulting in impaired mucosal defense and even infarction of a small area of the gastric wall. It is possible that some of these lesions represent perforated stress ulcers. The perforations are often accompanied by a surrounding zone of necrosis and devitalized tissue.

Occasionally, a healthy neonate presents with a spontaneous gastric perforation of unknown cause. Some of these infants are premature or small for gestational age, but otherwise are stable. Therefore, a plausible explanation for the perforation is lacking. One hypothesis suggests that a congenital abnormality of the muscularis causes a focal weakness prone to rupture (71). The most common location is high on the greater curvature near the gastroesophageal junction.

The most constant diagnostic feature of gastric perforation in the neonate is massive pneumoperitoneum, unless the perforation is posterior and contained within the lesser sac. Exploration requires mobilization to evaluate the gastroesophageal junction and lesser sac to locate perforations that do not occur on the anterior aspect of the stomach. Surgical management is individualized to either simple debridement and closure or closure around a temporary gastrostomy tube. Extensive gastric resections have not been necessary. Perforations of the greater curvature of the stomach at the gastroesophageal junction, which usually resemble ruptures or lacerations, can be difficult to repair because of their location. We prefer to debride the edges and perform a two-layer closure. Outcomes depend on the cause of the perforation and associated disease, such as respiratory failure and complex congenital malformations. Although mortality rates have historically ranged from 25% to 60% (72,73), current mortality rates should be significantly lower for most types of neonatal gastric perforations.

Foreign Bodies and Bezoars

Foreign bodies within the stomach and duodenum constitute an unusual indication for surgical intervention in the current era. Coins are the most commonly ingested objects and usually lodge in the esophagus. Those that reach the stomach are passed through the GI tract without incident 80% to 90% of the time; most of the remainder are endoscopically retrievable, and a small number (about 1%) require surgical removal (74). Round objects greater than 2 cm in diameter and linear objects longer than 3 cm in the infant or toddler, or longer than 5 cm in the older child, are unlikely to pass spontaneously. Objects that are sharp at one end are usually passed through with the blunt end in front. Objects that are sharp at both ends are more likely to cause penetration of the bowel wall and have been observed to migrate into the chest, liver, and retroperitoneum. For these reasons, endoscopic removal of gastroduodenal foreign bodies is recommended at the outset for high-risk objects and for those of large size. Others can be managed expectantly with serial abdominal films to follow movement and examination of the stools to detect passage. Objects remaining in the stomach after 4 weeks should be retrieved. If endoscopic removal is unsuccessful, open gastrotomy is indicated.

Disk-shaped batteries used in cameras and other electronic devices represent a special problem. Complications from battery ingestion include pressure necrosis, low-voltage electrical burn, corrosive alkaline injury, and rarely, mercury toxicity. Although impaction in the esophagus mandates immediate removal, passage into the stomach usually results in spontaneous transit. Some surgeons favor immediate retrieval of all batteries to minimize the risk of mucosal injury. If immediate removal is judged unnecessary, endoscopic or surgical retrieval should be performed if the battery remains in the gastric lumen longer than 48 hours or if abdominal symptoms develop.

Bezoars represent aggregations of multiple foreign bodies ingested over time. The most common type in children is the trichobezoar, which is composed of hair (ingested due to an emotional disorder) and other indigestible fibers from carpets, blankets, toys, and so forth. Less common types include phytobezoars (derived from vegetable matter) and lactobezoars (derived from precipitates of milk and usually occurring in premature infants). Bezoars commonly form a cast of the stomach with a tail that extends a variable distance through the pylorus.

The most common symptoms associated with bezoars relate to gastric outlet obstruction, with abdominal distention, early satiety, pain, and vomiting being common. Less common manifestations include anemia and hypoproteinemia from chronic gastritis, as well as jaundice, pancreatitis, and steatorrhea from pancreaticobiliary obstruction. Plain radiographs often display a frothy appearance in the gastric lumen. An upper GI tract contrast series and endoscopy are diagnostic.

Treatment depends on the type of bezoar and the associated symptoms. Trichobezoars virtually always require surgical removal. Phytobezoars can often be fragmented endoscopically or partially digested with papain, acetylcysteine, or cellulase. Lactobezoars usually respond to nasogastric decompression with intravenous rehydration and parenteral nutrition (75).

ENTERAL ACCESS FOR NUTRITION

Surgically placed gastrostomy tubes for enteral access have revolutionized the long-term care of many children with neurologic deficits, GI anomalies, complex congenital heart disease, and inanition due to cancer and chemotherapy. The effectiveness of aggressive nutritional intervention in these patients is undisputed, and permanent access to the gastric lumen has simplified the care rendered by nurses, nutritionists, and parents. Gastrostomies, however, are not without considerable complications. Furthermore, although they may be beneficial for feeding, caution must be exercised when they are used for decompression because they may be less reliable than standard nasogastric tubes used for this purpose. For patients who may require permanent gastric decompression, such as the spastic, neurologically impaired child, they offer a distinct advantage over nasogastric placement.

The two open surgical techniques employed for gastrostomy are the Stamm and Janeway procedures. The Stamm gastrostomy is most common and involves placing a mushroom-tipped catheter into the gastric lumen through a double pursestring suture, which inverts the tract (Fig. 72-18). The gastrostomy site is then fixed to the anterior abdominal wall, through which the tube exits, to minimize the risk of leakage. In 2 or 3 weeks, the anterior surface of the stomach fuses with the parietal peritoneum of the abdominal wall, and a secure gastrocutaneous fistula develops through which the feeding tube passes. It is necessary to keep the tube inserted to maintain the tract. Removal of the tube usually results in closure of the fistula within 24 hours. Its reversibility is one of the principal advantages of this procedure.

The Janeway gastrostomy entails creating a gastric tube from the anterior wall or the greater curvature, and bringing the tube through the rectus sheath to be matured as a permanent stoma. Although the stoma is designed to be

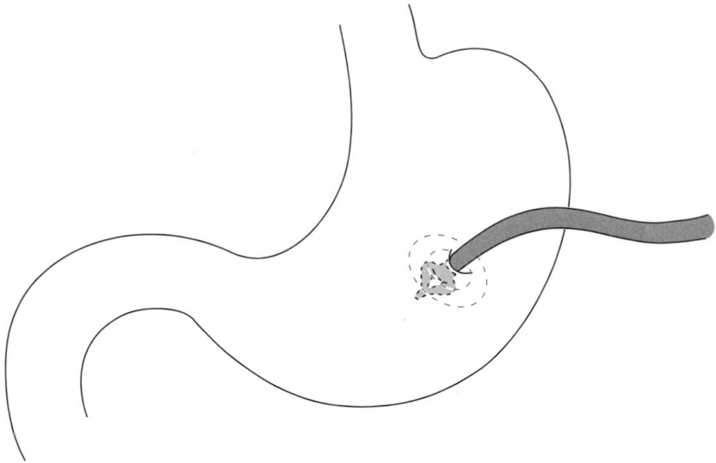

FIGURE 72-18. Technique of Stamm gastrostomy.

continent, problems with difficult catheterization and with incontinence plague this procedure in common practice. Furthermore, it is reversible only with a second procedure. Its present use is limited to unusual cases.

The risks and complications associated with gastrostomy tubes are numerous and are usually associated with the medical comorbidity in this patient population. Reported complications include exacerbation of GER with aspiration, tract infections with abdominal wall cellulitis, intraperitoneal leakage, external leakage with cutaneous excoriation, accidental dislodgement and removal of the tube, inadvertent advancement of the tube causing gastric outlet obstruction, internal herniation around the gastrostomy, gastric volvulus, and duodenal perforation. Many of these complications are avoided by immobilization of the tube at the skin level. The reported incidence of significant complications has been between 2% and 10% in most series.

The incidence of GER in these patients merits special attention. The apparent increased incidence of GER after gastrostomy in neurologically impaired children has led many to hypothesize that gastrostomy worsens subclinical GER or produces GER in some previously unaffected patients (76), apparently by distorting the angle of His and causing incompetence of the LES (77,78). These observations have led to a recommendation that an antireflux procedure be routinely added to a feeding gastrostomy in these patients (79). Newer data have supported the selective use of antireflux procedures only in those patients documented to have GER preoperatively (80). It seems reasonable to evaluate all neurologically impaired children referred for enteral access for GER by upper GI tract study, radionuclide scan, and pH monitoring, and to perform concomitant fundoplication only in those displaying GER before operation. In patients who do not require fundoplication initially, consideration should be given to positioning the gastrostomy on the lesser curvature in an effort to preserve LES function and reduce postgastrostomy GER (81,82).

In 1980, a percutaneous, endoscopically assisted technique of gastrostomy placement (PEG) was introduced to reduce the need for general anesthesia and to reduce the ileus and discomfort associated with the open procedure (83). Since its introduction, PEG has become the predominant method of providing enteral access in patients who do not require laparotomy for other reasons. Its safety and efficacy have been well documented (84). Modifications include the development of a "push" technique that obviates transoral passage of the gastrostomy device and may reduce the number of catheter-related infections (85), as well as nonendoscopic techniques that rely on fluoroscopic guidance (86). Recognition of GER in many of these patients has generated enthusiasm for percutaneous placement of dual-lumen tubes comprising a gastric decompression port and a transpyloric jejunal feeding port (PEJ). Studies in adults, however, have failed to document a significant difference between PEG and PEJ with respect to reflux episodes and aspiration pneumonia (87).

Another development in enteral access has been the low-profile tube with a one-way valve—the gastrostomy "button." Several designs are commercially available, and all are relatively effective in preventing tube movement and dislodgement—two problems that lead to many of the complications listed earlier. Acceptance by patients and parents is high because of the practical and cosmetic advantages associated with the lack of an external tube. In the past, a standard gastrostomy was established either by percutaneous or open technique, and the catheter was exchanged for a button about 6 weeks later when the tract was sufficiently secure to tolerate manipulation. This procedure can be done without general anesthesia in most cases. Experience with primary surgical button placement is increasing, and it does not appear to be associated with an increase in the complication rate. Primary placement of low-profile gastrostomy "buttons" using endoscopic or laparoscopic guidance is rapidly gaining popularity. These techniques require stabilizing the stomach to the anterior abdominal wall with bolstered full-thickness sutures or toggled fasteners prior to tract dilation and button placement. These techniques have now made it possible to avoid staged procedures for most patients requiring enteral access.

REFERENCES

1. Furness JB, Costa M. Types of nerves in the enteric nervous system. *Neuroscience* 1980;5:1.
2. Newgreen D, Young HM. Enteric nervous system: development and developmental disturbances—part 1. *Pediatr Dev Pathol* 2002 May–Jun;5(3):224.
3. Drucker DJ. Gut adaptation and the glucagon-like peptides. *Gut* 2002 Mar;50(3):428.
4. Prinz C, Kajimura M, Scott D, et al. Acid secretion and the H,K ATPase of the stomach. *Yale J Biol Med* 1992;65:577.
5. Wolfe MM, Soll AH. The physiology of gastric acid secretion. *N Engl J Med* 1988;319:1707.
6. Hakanson R, Boettcher F, Ekblad E, et al. Histamine in endocrine cells in the stomach. *Histochemistry* 1986;86:5.
7. Schubert ML, Coy DH, Makhlouf GM. Peptone stimulates gastrin secretion from the stomach by activating bombesin/GRP and cholinergic neurons. *Am J Physiol* 1992;262:G685.
8. Schubert ML, Hightower J. Release of gastric somatostatin during distension is mediated by gastric VIP neurons: a mechanical reflex for inhibition of gastrin. *Gastroenterology* 1989;96:A455.
9. Gantz I, Schaeffer M, DelValle J, et al. Molecular cloning of a gene encoding the histamine H_2-receptor. *Proc Natl Acad Sci U S A* 1991;88:429.
10. Agunod M, Yamaguchi N, Lopez R, et al. Correlative study of hydrochloric acid, pepsin, and intrinsic factor secretion in newborns and infants. *Am J Digest Dis* 1969;14:400.
11. Shimamoto C, Takao Y, Asada S, et al. Regulation of human and rat gastric mucin synthesis: assessment by histochemical and biochemical methods. *Gastroenterology* 1991;100:A159.
12. McIntyre RC Jr, Bensard DD, Karrer FM, et al. The pediatric diaphragm in acute gastric volvulus. *J Am Coll Surg* 1994 Mar;178(3):234.
13. Okada K, Miyako M, Honma S, et al. Discharge diagnoses in infants with apparent life-threatening event. *Pediatr Int* 2003 Oct;45(5):560.
14. Canazza L, Bianchini E, Cerri M, et al. Chronic idiopathic gastric volvulus in children. *Pediatr Med Chir* 2002 Jul–Aug;24(4):302.
15. Blank E, Chisholm AJ. Congenital microgastria: a case with a 26-year followup. *Pediatrics* 1973;51:1037.
16. Velasco AL, Holcomb GW III, Templeton JM Jr, et al. Management of congenital microgastria. *J Pediatr Surg* 1990;25:192.
17. Borgnon J, Durand C, Gourlaouen D, et al. Antenatal detection of a communicating duodenal duplication. *Eur J Pediatr Surg* 2003 Apr;13(2):130.
18. Coit DG, Mies C. Adenocarcinoma arising within a gastric duplication cyst. *J Surg Oncol* 1992;50:274.
19. Cragan JD, Martin ML, Moore CA, et al. Descriptive epidemiology of small intestinal atresia in Atlanta, Georgia. *Teratology* 1993;48:441.
20. Lecco TM. Zur morphologie des pankreas annulare. *Sitzungsb Akad Wissensch Cl* 1910;119:391.
21. Suda K. Immunohistochemical and gross dissection studies of annular pancreas. *Acta Pathol Jpn* 1990;40:505.
22. Fonkelsrud EW, de Lorimier AA, Hays DM. Congenital atresia and stenosis of the duodenum: a review compiled from the members of the Surgical Section of the American Academy of Pediatrics. *Pediatrics* 1969;43:79.
23. Schier F, Schier C, Waldschmidt J, et al. Duodenal atresia: experiences with 145 patients. *Zentralbl Chir* 1990;115:135.
24. Grosfeld JL, Rescorla FJ. Duodenal atresia and stenosis: reassessment of treatment and outcome based on antenatal diagnosis, pathologic variance, and long-term follow-up. *World J Surg* 1993;17:301.
25. Fogel M, Copel JA, Cullen MT, et al. Congenital heart disease and fetal thoracoabdominal anomalies: associations in utero and the importance of cytogenetic analysis. *Am J Perinatol* 1991;8:411.
26. Nyberg DA, Resta RG, Luthy DA, et al. Prenatal sonographic findings of Down syndrome: review of 94 cases. *Obstet Gynecol* 1990;76:370.
27. Spigland N, Yazbeck S. Complications associated with surgical treatment of congenital intrinsic duodenal obstruction. *J Pediatr Surg* 1990;25:1127.
28. Stubbs TM, Horger EO. Sonographic detection of fetal duodenal atresia [Letter]. *Obstet Gynecol* 1989;73:146.
29. Bickler SW, Harrison MW, Blank E, et al. Microperforation of a duodenal diaphragm as a cause of paradoxical gas in congenital duodenal obstruction. *J Pediatr Surg* 1992;27:747.
30. Panuel M, Bourliere-Najean B, Delarue A, et al. Duodenal atresia with bifid termination of the common bile duct. *Arch Fr Pediatr* 1992;49:365.
31. Kimura K, Mukohara N, Nashijima E, et al. Diamond-shaped anastomosis for duodenal atresia: an experience with 44 patients over 15 years. *J Pediatr Surg* 1990;25:977.
32. Kimura K, Perdzynski W, Soper RT. Elliptical seromuscular resection for tapering the proximal dilated bowel in duodenal or jejunal atresia. *J Pediatr Surg* 1996 Oct;31(10):1405.
33. Jedd MB, Melton LJ III, Griffin MR, et al. Trends in infantile hypertrophic pyloric stenosis in Olmsted County, Minnesota, 1950–1984. *Paediatr Perinat Epidemiol* 1988;2:148.
34. Rollins MD, Shields MD, Quinn RJ, et al. Pyloric stenosis: congenital or acquired? *Arch Dis Child* 1989;64:138.
35. Mitchell LE, Risch N. The genetics of infantile hypertrophic pyloric stenosis. A reanalysis. *Am J Dis Child* 1993 Nov;147(11):1203.
36. Carter CO, Evans KA. Inheritance of congenital pyloric stenosis. *J Med Genet* 1969;6:233.
37. Kawahara H, Imura K, Yagi M, et al. Motor abnormality in the gastroduodenal junction in patients with infantile hypertrophic pyloric stenosis. *J Pediatr Surg* 2001 Nov;36(11):1641.
38. Katz S, Basel D, Branski D. Prenatal gastric dilatation and infantile hypertrophic pyloric stenosis. *J Pediatr Surg* 1988;23:1021.
39. Mahon BE, Rosenman MB, Kleiman MB. Maternal and infant use of erythromycin and other macrolide antibiotics as risk factors for infantile hypertrophic pyloric stenosis. *J Pediatr* 2001 Sept;139(3):380.
40. Sorensen HT, Skriver MV, Pedersen L, et al. Risk of infantile hypertrophic pyloric stenosis after maternal postnatal use of macrolides. *Scand J Infect Dis* 2003;35(2):104.
41. Mercado-Deane MG, Burton EM, Brawley AV, et al. Prostaglandin-induced foveolar hyperplasia simulating pyloric stenosis in an infant with cyanotic heart disease. *Pediatr Radiol* 1988;24:45.
42. Kobayashi H, O'Brian DS, Puri P. Immunochemical characterization of neural cell adhesion molecule (NCAM), nitric oxide synthase, and neurofilament protein expression in pyloric muscle of patients with pyloric stenosis. *J Pediatr Gastroenterol Nutr* 1995 Apr;20(3):319.
43. Langer JC, Berezin I, Daniel EE. Hypertrophic pyloric stenosis: ultrastructural abnormalities of enteric nerves and the interstitial cells of Cajal. *J Pediatr Surg* 1995 Nov;30(11):1535.
44. Kobayashi H, Miyahara K, Yamataka A, et al. Pyloric stenosis: new histopathologic perspective using confocal laser scanning. *J Pediatr Surg* 2001 Aug;36(8):1277.
45. Guarino N, Yoneda A, Shima H, et al. Selective neurotrophin deficiency in infantile hypertrophic pyloric stenosis. *J Pediatr Surg* 2001 Aug;36(8):1280.
46. Kobayashi H, Wester T, Puri P. Age-related changes in innervation in hypertrophic pyloric stenosis. *J Pediatr Surg* 1997 Dec;32(12):1704.
47. Wattchow DA, Cass DT, Furness JB, et al. Abnormalities of peptide-containing nerve fibers in infantile hypertrophic pyloric stenosis. *Gastroenterology* 1987;92:443.
48. Abel RM, Bishop AE, Dore CJ, et al. A quantitative study of the morphological and histochemical changes within the nerves and muscle in infantile hypertrophic pyloric stenosis. *J Pediatr Surg* 1998 May;33(5):682.
49. Vanderwinden JM, Mailleux P, Schiffmann SN, et al. Nitric oxide synthase activity in infantile hypertrophic pyloric stenosis. *N Engl J Med* 1992;327:511.

50. Kusafuka T, Puri P. Altered messenger RNA expression of the neuronal nitric oxide synthase gene in infantile hypertrophic pyloric stenosis. *Pediatr Surg Int* 1997;12(8):576.
51. Dieler R, Schroder JM. Myenteric plexus neuropathy in infantile hypertrophic pyloric stenosis. *Acta Neuropathol (Berl)* 1989;78:649.
52. Godbole P, Sprigg A, Dickson JA, et al. Ultrasound compared with clinical examination in infantile hypertrophic pyloric stenosis. *Arch Dis Child* 1996 Oct;75(4):335.
53. Teele RL, Smith EH. Ultrasound in the diagnosis of idiopathic hypertrophic pyloric stenosis. *N Engl J Med* 1977;296:1149.
54. Lamki N, Athey PA, Round ME, et al. Hypertrophic pyloric stenosis in the neonate: diagnostic criteria revisited. *Can Assoc Radiol J* 1993;44:21.
55. Westra SJ, de Groot CJ, Smits NJ, et al. Hypertrophic pyloric stenosis: use of the pyloric volume measurement in early US diagnosis. *Radiology* 1989;172:615.
56. Macdessi J, Oates RK. Clinical diagnosis of pyloric stenosis: a declining art. *Br Med J* 1993;306:553.
57. Greason KL, Thompson WR, Downey EC, et al. Laparoscopic pyloromyotomy for infantile hypertrophic pyloric stenosis: report of 11 cases. *J Pediatr Surg* 1995 Nov;30(11):1571.
58. Fujimoto T, Lane GJ, Segawa O, et al. Laparoscopic extramucosal pyloromyotomy versus open pyloromyotomy for infantile hypertrophic pyloric stenosis: which is better? *J Pediatr Surg* 1999 Feb;34(2):370.
59. Ludtke FE, Bertus M, Voth E, et al. Gastric emptying 16 to 26 years after treatment of infantile hypertrophic pyloric stenosis. *J Pediatr Surg* 1994;29:523.
60. Levi S, Beardshall K, Haddad G, et al. *Campylobacter pylori* and duodenal ulcers: the gastrin link. *Lancet* 1989;1:1167.
61. Yeung CK, Fu KH, Yuen KY, et al. *Helicobacter pylori* and associated duodenal ulcer. *Arch Dis Child* 1990;65:1212.
62. Kumar D, Spitz L. Peptic ulceration in children. *Surg Gynecol Obstet* 1984;159:63.
63. Folkman J, Szabo S, Stovroff M, et al. Duodenal ulcer: discovery of a new mechanism and development of angiogenic therapy that accelerates healing. *Ann Surg* 1991;214:414.
64. Maier RV, Mitchell D, Gentilello L. Optimal therapy for stress gastritis. *Ann Surg* 1994;220:353.
65. Drumm B, Rhoads JM, Tringer DA, et al. Peptic ulcer disease in children: etiology, clinical findings, and clinical course. *Pediatrics* 1988;82:410.
66. Azarow K, Kim P, Shandling B, et al. A 45-year experience with surgical treatment of peptic ulcer disease in children. *J Pediatr Surg* 1996 Jun;31(6):750.
67. Jordan PH, Thornby J. Twenty years after parietal cell vagotomy or selective vagotomy antrectomy for treatment of duodenal ulcer. *Ann Surg* 1994;220:283.
68. Taylor TV, Gunn AA, MacLeod DA, et al. Morbidity and mortality after anterior lesser curve seromyotomy with posterior truncal vagotomy for duodenal ulcer. *Br J Surg* 1985;72:950.
69. Fraker DL, Norton JA, Alexander JR, et al. Surgery in Zollinger-Ellison syndrome alters the natural history of gastrinoma. *Ann Surg* 1994;220:320.
70. Byrne WJ, Kangarloo H, Ament ME, et al. Antral dysmotility: an unrecognized cause of chronic vomiting during infancy. *Ann Surg* 1984;193:521.
71. Herbut PA. Congenital defect in the musculature of the stomach with rupture in a newborn. *Arb Pathol* 1943;36:91.
72. Rosser SB, Clark CH, Elechi EN. Spontaneous neonatal gastric perforation. *J Pediatr Surg* 1982;17:390.
73. Tan CE, Kiely EM, Agrawal M, et al. Neonatal gastrointestinal perforation. *J Pediatr Surg* 1989;24:888.
74. Schwartz GF, Polsky HS. Ingested foreign bodies of the gastrointestinal tract. *Am Surg* 1985;51:173.
75. Yoss BS. Human milk lactobezoars. *J Pediatr* 1984;105:819.
76. Mollitt DL, Golladay ES, Seibert JJ. Symptomatic gastroesophageal reflux following gastrostomy in neurologically impaired patients. *Pediatrics* 1985;75:1124.
77. Jolley SG, Tunnell WP, Hoelzer DJ, et al. Lower esophageal pressure changes with tube gastrostomy: a causative factor of gastroesophageal reflux in children? *J Pediatr Surg* 1986;21:624.
78. Papaila JG, Vane DW, Colville C, et al. The effect of various types of gastrostomy on the lower esophageal sphincter. *J Pediatr Surg* 1987;22:1198.
79. Jolley SG, Smith EI, Tunell WP. Protective antireflux operation with feeding gastrostomy: experience with children. *Ann Surg* 1985;201:736.
80. Wheatley MJ, Wesley JR, Tkach DM, et al. Long-term follow-up of brain-damaged children requiring feeding gastrostomy: should an antireflux procedure always be performed? *J Pediatr Surg* 1991;26:301.
81. Stringel G. Gastrostomy with antireflux properties. *J Pediatr Surg* 1990;25:1019.
82. Seekri IK, Rescorla FJ, Canal DF, et al. Lesser curvature gastrostomy reduces the incidence of postoperative gastroesophageal reflux. *J Pediatr Surg* 1991;26:982.
83. Gauderer ML, Ponsky JL, Izant RJ Jr. Gastrostomy without laparotomy: a percutaneous endoscopic technique. *J Pediatr Surg* 1980;15:872.
84. Marin OE, Glassman MS, Schoen BT, et al. Safety and efficacy of percutaneous endoscopic gastrostomy in children. *Am J Gastroenterol* 1994;89:357.
85. Crombleholme TM, Jacir NN. Simplified "push" technique for percutaneous endoscopic gastrostomy in children. *J Pediatr Surg* 1993;28:1393.
86. Malden ES, Hicks ME, Picus D, et al. Fluoroscopically guided percutaneous gastrostomy in children. *J Vasc Interven Radiol* 1992;3:673.
87. Kadakia SC, Sullivan HO, Starnes E. Percutaneous endoscopic gastrostomy or jejunostomy and the incidence of aspiration in 79 patients. *Am J Surg* 1992;164:114.

Chapter 73

Surgical Implications of Pediatric Obesity

Michael A. Helmrath, Thomas H. Inge, Mary L. Brandt, and Victor Garcia

Obesity is now considered the most common nutritional disorder of children and adolescents in the United States, with 15% of children and adolescents classified as overweight and almost 30% either overweight or at risk of being overweight (1,2). No longer a disease limited to adults, pediatric specialists are now confronted with a new set of diagnostic and therapeutic dilemmas in overweight and obese children and adolescents (2–6). Direct and indirect costs attributed to obesity in the United States have been estimated to approach \$75 to \$100 billion per year (7,8). Twenty-five percent to 83% of obese children become obese adults, suggesting that early intervention will be not only effective, but also essential. Numerous studies have shown that obesity in childhood is associated with increased morbidity and mortality, both in childhood and in adulthood (3,5,9–11). Being morbidly obese at age 20 is associated with a predicted 13-year reduction in life span for white males, and a 20-year reduction in life span for African American males (11). In a 55-year follow-up of school children in Boston, Must et al. demonstrated a twofold increase in death from all causes in boys who had been overweight [body mass index (BMI) > 75th percentile] in adolescence (9). The risk of dying from atherosclerotic disease was increased 2.3-fold, from cerebrovascular disease 13.2-fold, and from colon cancer 9.1-fold (9). This increased mortality risk was not seen in the girls followed in this study (9). However, the girls did have an eight times higher risk of difficulty with personal care and activities of daily living as adults, when compared with the lean control group and a 1.6 times increased risk of arthritis (9).

Michael A. Helmrath: Baylor College of Medicine, Texas Children's Hospital Care Center, Houston, Texas 77030.

Thomas H. Inge: Comprehensive Weight Management Center Division of Pediatric General and Thoracic Surgery, Cincinnati Children's Hospital Medical Center, Cincinnati, Ohio 45229.

Mary L. Brandt: Michael E. DeBakey Department of Surgery, Baylor College of Medicine, Houston, Texas 77030.

Victor Garcia: University of Cincinnati, Cincinnati, Ohio 45267.

Childhood obesity also affects physical and psychological growth and development, a consequence that cannot be quantified in a monetary sense, but is perhaps the most significant "cost" this disorder inflicts on these children (5,12,13). Obese children are more at risk for poor self-esteem, withdrawal from social interactions, depression, and anxiety (2). Obese adolescents are more likely to remain unmarried, have lower incomes, and live in poverty than their matched normal weight controls (14). They are less likely to be accepted into college than normal weight adolescents with comparable scholastic achievement (5). In a more recent study, the health-related quality of life experienced by obese children and adolescents was the same as that of children undergoing chemotherapy for cancer (15).

All children seen in a health care setting should have a height and weight obtained, with percentiles based on growth charts recorded. In addition, these two measurements allow easy calculation of the BMI, which is weight (kg) per height $(m)^2$. BMI changes with age; the 50th percentile for male BMI at 6, 12, and 18 years of age is 15.4 kg per m^2, 18 kg per m^2, and 22 kg per m^2, respectively. BMI values recorded on BMI growth charts [available on the Centers for Disease Control and Prevention (CDC) web site, www.cdc.gov] allow tracking of percentile changes over time to identify children at risk for obesity. One of the problems in interpreting the literature on obesity in children is the different ways obesity has been defined in the pediatric population. Growing children have been classified as normal (BMI < 85th percentile), at risk for overweight (BMI 85th to 95th percentile), or overweight (BMI > 95th percentile) (13). In adolescents, who have completed linear growth, it may be more appropriate to use adult criteria: A BMI of greater than 25 is considered overweight and a BMI greater than 30 obese. Obese adolescents can further be classified using the criteria defined by the National Institutes of Health (NIH): class 1 obesity (BMI 30–34.9), class 2 obesity (35–39.9), and class 3 or "morbid" obesity (BMI greater than 40). Finally, in the surgical literature, patients with a BMI greater than 50 have been termed "super obese." The patient's BMI and the medical issues associated with obesity should be discussed at every clinic visit with the child and family. In this way, appropriate interventions and/or referrals can be initiated (2,16). The medical and psychosocial rather than cosmetic implications of obesity should be discussed. It should be stressed that weight management efforts that result in a loss of 5% to 10% of body weight can result in a significant reduction of obesity-related health risks (17).

COMORBIDITIES OF OBESITY

Obesity can cause or contribute to the development of numerous comorbidities (Table 73-1). These comorbid conditions may be silent, and it is incumbent upon the pediatric surgeon to screen for these disorders prior to planning any elective surgery in obese children. In addition, the presence of one or more of these major comorbid states in a child mandates aggressive intervention to treat the underlying obesity.

Cardiac risk factors are common in obese children and include insulin resistance, hyperlipidemia, sleep apnea, and hypertension. Fifty percent of overweight adolescents have one risk factor for developing cardiovascular disease and 20% have two factors (3). Hyperlipidemia in obese children is most often manifested by elevated low-density lipoprotein-cholesterol, elevated triglycerides, and decreased high-density lipoprotein-cholesterol (12). Twenty percent to 30% of obese children between ages 5 and 11 have elevated systolic or diastolic blood pressure (5). Clinical hypertension is 9 to 10 times more common in obese children than in lean children (12,18). Significant, irreversible consequences of hypertension, such as hypertensive cardiac disease, can present in childhood. In one study, 38% of children with hypertension had left ventricular hypertrophy by echocardiography (18). More important, nearly 30% of obese adolescents have already developed the metabolic syndrome (syndrome X; the clustering of abdominal obesity, high fasting blood glucose, hypertension, and hyperlipidemia). This dangerous condition may have profound public health implications given the fact that up to 910,000 adolescents in the United States may be affected based on current population trends (19).

TABLE 73-1 Comorbidities of Obesity.

Major comorbidities

- Type 2 diabetes mellitus
- Sleep apnea (including obesity hypoventilation syndrome)
- Pseudotumor cerebri

Minor comorbidities

- Abnormal glucose metabolism
- Hyperlipidemia
- Hypertension
- Venous stasis disease
- Nonalcoholic fatty liver disease
- Skeletal disorders (Blount's disease, slipped capital femoral epiphysis)
- Polycystic ovary syndrome
- Psychosocial pathology (depression, withdrawal)
- Significant impairment in activities of daily living
- Gastroesophageal reflux
- Hidradenitis suppurativa
- Sleep disorders

Glucose metabolism and insulin sensitivity are altered by obesity (20). There has been a dramatic increase in the prevalence of type II diabetes in the pediatric population, and this is primarily the result of the increased prevalence of obesity (20,21). The ramifications of the obesity epidemic are major and worrisome. Current projections by the CDC include scenarios in which up to one-third of the children born today will develop type 2 diabetes mellitus during their lifetime, a percentage that rises to one-half for Hispanics and blacks (22). Because type 2 diabetes is often asymptomatic in the early stages, obese children undergoing surgery may benefit from a screening fasting blood glucose. Acanthosis nigrans, or increased thickness and pigmentation of skin in the intertriginous folds, is associated with hyperinsulinemia (12). The presence of acanthosis nigrans, most commonly diagnosed by examining the back of the neck, may indicate the need for formal glucose tolerance testing by a pediatric endocrinologist. The history of vaginal yeast infections in an obese adolescent should also prompt further workup for diabetes (20).

Sleep disorders are extremely common with childhood obesity. Up to 37% of obese children have an abnormal polysomnogram when studied (10,23). Most of these abnormalities are minor, with true sleep apnea occurring in only 7% of obese children (12). Symptoms of sleep apnea may include snoring, poor school performance, daytime sleepiness, enuresis, and hyperactivity (10). However, there is no clear correlation between symptoms and the severity of the sleep apnea, making this difficult to diagnose (12). Weight loss results in improvement of sleep apnea. In addition, many of these children demonstrate clinical improvement with tonsillectomy and/or adenoidectomy, suggesting that many of these patients would benefit from otorhinolaryngologic examination (23–25). Obesity hypoventilation syndrome, previously called Pickwickian syndrome, is an extreme version of sleep apnea and can result in hypoxia, hypercarbia, right ventricular hypertrophy or failure, and polycythemia (10).

Blount's disease (*tibia vara*) is defined as overgrowth of the medial aspect of the proximal tibial metaphysis, which occurs in response to and then accentuates "bowing" of the legs under the pressure of excess weight (12). Sixty-six percent to 80% of patients with Blount's disease are obese (5,12). Obesity in childhood may also result in slipped capital femoral epiphyses (12). Fifty to 70% of children with slipped capital femoral epiphyses are obese, and severe obesity complicates the orthopedic management of this deformity (5).

Polycystic ovarian syndrome, previously called Stein-Leventhal syndrome, is the most common endocrinopathy in women (26). It is a complex metabolic disease that may present in adolescents and is associated with obesity (12). This syndrome is manifested by oligomenorrhea or amenorrhea associated with obesity, insulin resistance, hirsutism, acne, and acanthosis nigricans (5). Ultrasound of the ovaries, particularly in adolescent girls, is often normal, with no evidence of pathologic ovarian cysts. Patients with suspected polycystic ovarian syndrome should be evaluated by a pediatric endocrinologist.

Nonalcoholic fatty liver disease (NAFLD) is one of the silent, but potentially dangerous comorbidities of obesity in childhood (27). NAFLD is a spectrum of disease ranging from fatty infiltration of the liver to steatohepatitis (termed NASH for nonalcoholic steatosis/hepatitis) to fibrosis and cirrhosis (28). Up to 40% of obese children have findings on ultrasound suggestive of fatty infiltration of the liver (10). Approximately 10% of obese children and 40% to 50% of severely obese children have abnormal liver function tests and this is frequently, but not always, associated with NAFLD (5,12,13). Serum liver enzyme levels can be used as a screening test, but the definitive diagnosis is made by liver biopsy. Liver biopsy should be considered in any obese child with abnormal liver function tests or ultrasound, or visible changes in the parenchyma of the liver. Up to 20% of adult patients with this disorder eventually develop cirrhosis, and this may progress to liver failure (27). NAFLD is almost universally associated with insulin resistance and, therefore, appropriate testing should be done in children with this diagnosis to screen for this disorder (28). Weight loss is the only known treatment for NAFLD (12,27).

Biliary disease is also common in obese children. Fifty percent of adolescent patients undergoing cholecystectomy for cholelithiasis are obese (13). Eight percent to 33% of all gallstones seen in childhood are related to obesity (5).

Pseudotumor cerebri is a rare disorder characterized by a gradual and idiopathic increase in intracranial pressure (12). The usual presentation is headaches, but patients may also experience dizziness, unsteadiness, or diplopia (10,12). Approximately 50% of children with pseudotumor cerebri are obese (12). There is no effective therapy other than weight loss. If untreated, this syndrome may result in visual impairment, need for optic nerve fenestration, or even blindness (12).

MEDICAL TREATMENT OF OBESITY

The mainstay of medical therapy for obesity is dietary and behavioral change (29–31). The abundance and variety of diet books and programs available in our society is reflective of how ineffective most of these strategies are for adults. It is not surprising that 90% to 95% of adult patients who lose weight with dietary changes alone regain the weight (29). One pound of fat (0.45 kg) is the equivalent of 3,500 kcal of energy. Thus, to lose 1 lb of excess weight, an overall change of 3,500 kcal must be made from the patient's baseline. As an example, a change of 500 kcal per day for a week will result in a loss of 1 lb of body weight. This can be accomplished by reducing daily intake by 500 kcal, increasing daily caloric expenditure (exercise) by 500 kcal, or a combination. Education concerning the relationship between food intake, caloric expenditure, and weight gain can result in effective weight control in some patients. However, most patients require more intensive diet control and behavioral modification for success, which is limited even in the most intensive programs. Physician-controlled diets, such as the protein-sparing modified diet or ketogenic diet, may have some utility in the treatment of severely obese adolescents, but the long-term effects and outcomes in the pediatric population are not known (31).

Pharmacologic interventions for weight control have been used with limited success in adult patients and are not recommended currently for routine use in children (32). Two drugs are in clinical trials but are not approved currently for use in children and adolescents: sibutramine, a serotonin-mediated appetite suppressant, and orlistat, which inhibits fat absorption (31). A more recent randomized controlled study of sibutramine in severely obese adolescents (mean BMI 37 kg per m^2) demonstrated an average 10% weight loss, with a side effect profile requiring dose reduction or medication cessation in 33 of 88 (37%) patients (33). Further clinical trials of these two drugs will be needed before treatment recommendations can be made.

SPECIAL PERIOPERATIVE CONSIDERATIONS IN OBESE CHILDREN

Obese children undergoing any surgical procedure have unique physiologic and anatomic issues that must be understood to provide optimal care. Obesity may be associated with restrictive pulmonary disease (from restriction of chest wall and diaphragm movement), as well as obstructive airway disease (from upper airway collapse or obstruction) (10). Airway management of the obese child poses specific challenges to the anesthesiologist because many of the normal anatomic landmarks are difficult to visualize and control of the airway may be problematic (25). Postoperatively, obese patients are at increased risk for atelectasis and incentive spirometry, and ambulation should be encouraged. If the patient has a history of sleep disorders or symptoms consistent with a sleep disorder, monitoring with pulse oximetry may be indicated after surgery (34). Meticulous positioning and padding of the morbidly obese patient undergoing a surgical procedure is critical to prevent pressure necrosis, rhabdomyolysis, and peripheral nerve damage (35). Obesity is a known risk factor for developing deep venous thrombosis (DVT) and pulmonary embolism (PE) after surgery in adults. All adults and adolescents undergoing bariatric surgery receive prophylaxis for DVT (low-molecular-weight heparin and intermittent sequential compression devices) because the risk of DVT is approximately 2.6% and the risk of PE is 0.95% following these procedures (13). More data are needed before definitive recommendations can be made, but obese adolescents undergoing other surgical procedures may also benefit from DVT prophylaxis. Antibiotic and other drug dosing are complicated by obesity due to the body composition and relatively high volume of distribution (13,36). In severely obese adolescents, standard dosing of cephalosporins may be inadequate (37). Aminoglycosides dosing may require the use of special formulas or help from a clinical pharmacologist (36).

SURGICAL TREATMENT OF OBESITY

Surgery has been a viable option for morbid obesity in adults in the United States for almost 50 years. Surgery for the treatment of obesity is called bariatric surgery (G. *baros*, weight + *iatria*, medical treatment) (38). Bariatric surgery has proven to be an effective method of decreasing morbidity and mortality in obese adults (13,39–41). The indications for bariatric surgery in adults were derived by an NIH consensus panel in 1991 (42). In general, adults with a BMI greater than 40 kg per m^2 with no comorbidities and greater than 35 kg per m^2 with comorbidities who have failed multiple attempts at medical management of their obesity are considered candidates for bariatric surgery. Adolescents represent a unique subset of patients and were not included as potential patients in this consensus development process. Because of the risks unique to the adolescent population, the current guidelines for bariatric procedures in adolescents are much more conservative than those for adults (6) (Table 73-2). Issues that are unique to adolescent patients include the possibility of adverse effects of bariatric surgery on growth and development, ethical concerns in obtaining assent from adolescent patients who are at a uniquely vulnerable point of psychological development, effect on future reproductive ability, and the outcome of future pregnancies (6,13). Inducing significant weight loss, such as with bariatric surgery, is not without consequences in the growing child. Even mild restrictions of calories in obese children have been associated with a decrease in linear growth (30). In addition, there is risk of decreasing intake of specific nutrients needed for growth and development, such as iron, calcium, zinc, folate, and vitamins A, B, C, and E (30). However, treatment of the obesity early in life theoretically could prevent or reverse many of the serious comorbidities of obesity, such as diabetes (41).

TABLE 73-2 Guidelines for Patient Selection for Bariatric Surgery in Adolescents.

- Failure to lose weight after at least 6 mo of organized attempts at weight loss
- Attainment or near attainment of physiologic maturity (Tanner stage IV or V)
- BMI $\geq$ 40 with major comorbidities or BMI $\geq$ 50 with minor comorbidities
- Commitment to medical and psychological evaluation before and after surgery
- Commitment to avoid pregnancy for 1 y after surgery
- Capability and willingness to adhere to postoperative nutritional guidelines
- Presence of supportive family environment
- Ability to provide informed assent (patient) and consent (family)

Preoperative Evaluation

Preoperative evaluation of adolescents being considered for bariatric surgery should be comprehensive and conducted in a multidisciplinary environment with the ability to provide specific expertise relational to children's and adolescent's needs. The evaluation should be planned to identify major medical comorbidities and behavioral problems. Preoperative evaluations should include fasting glucose and hemoglobin (Hb) A1C, liver function tests, lipid profile, complete blood count, thyroid function tests, pregnancy tests for females, and screening for micronutrient deficiencies. For patients with abnormal fasting glucose or HbA1C, an oral glucose tolerance test is obtained. For patients with symptoms of obstructive sleep apnea, a polysomnogram is suggested. Bone age assessment should be considered for younger patients to document the degree of skeletal maturity. In addition to a structured clinical interview with an adolescent psychologist, consideration should also be given to age-appropriate objective testing to assess personality traits, cognitive maturity, depression, eating behaviors, and weight-related quality of life, which may have a bearing on candidacy for bariatric surgery or on postoperative adherence to medical and nutritional regimens.

Surgical Procedures for Morbid Obesity

The ideal bariatric surgical procedure would be safe, effective (i.e., reverse medically significant comorbidities), and potentially reversible. Bariatric surgical procedures can be divided into two general categories: restrictive and malabsorptive. Purely restrictive procedures create a small, proximal gastric pouch that induces early satiety and decreased oral intake. The original restrictive procedures divided the intact stomach with staple lines (horizontal gastroplasty, vertical gastroplasty, and vertical banded gastroplasty). These gastroplasties resulted in weight loss, but there was

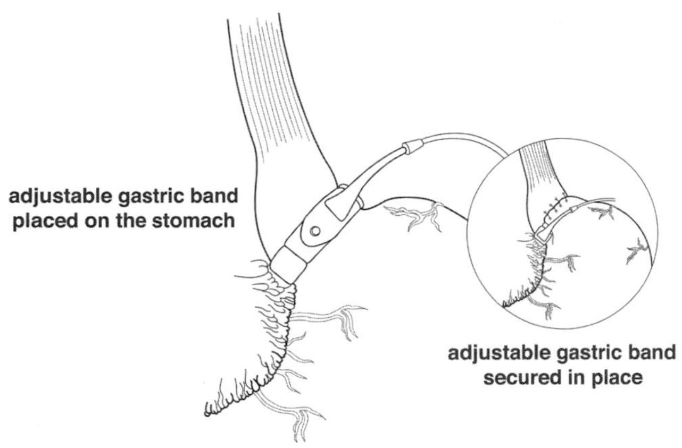

FIGURE 73-1. The adjustable gastric band is typically placed laparoscopically and is currently the only commonly performed purely restrictive procedure for morbid obesity performed in the United States.

frequent subsequent weight gain from overeating or dilitation of the gastric stoma. Currently, the adjustable gastric band is the only purely restrictive procedure commonly performed in the United States (Fig. 73-1). In this procedure, which is almost universally performed laparoscopically, an inflatable ring is placed around the proximal stomach, creating a small proximal gastric pouch. The ring is inflated and adjusted with injections into a subcutaneous port. The adjustable gastric band has the advantage of being relatively safe and reversible. Unfortunately, data concerning efficacy are conflicting. For that reason, the Roux-en-Y gastric bypass (Fig. 73-2) has become the "gold standard" procedure in bariatric surgery (40). In this procedure, which is most often performed laparoscopically, the stomach is divided in order to leave a small (30-cc) proximal gastric pouch. The small bowel is divided distal to the ligament of Treitz and a Roux limb of variable length (based on BMI) is then brought up in either an antecolic or retrocolic position and anastomosed to the proximal gastric pouch. The Roux-en-Y gastric bypass is relatively safe and is effective in reversing obesity-related comorbidities. It is, however, reversible only with great technical difficulty. Malabsorptive procedures bypass a portion of the small bowel to decrease absorption. The jejunoileal bypass was the original malabsorptive procedure. That particular procedure was abandoned, however, due to an unacceptably high rate of complications. The biliopancreatic bypass or diversion, with or without duodenal switch is currently the primary malabsorptive procedure being performed. This procedure essentially bypasses the jejunum with a distal enteroenterostomy, with or without moderate gastric reduction (40,43). Because of an increased risk of malabsorption of critical nutrients, malabsorptive procedures are rarely used in adolescent patients.

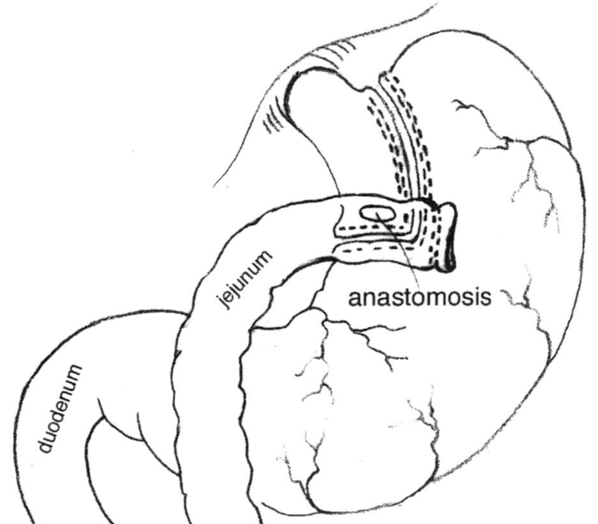

FIGURE 73-2. The Roux-en-Y gastric bypass combines both restrictive and malabsorptive features. The jejunal limb is of variable length. This is the most common procedure for control of morbid obesity in adolescents in the United States.

Postoperative Complications of Bariatric Procedures

All surgeons should be familiar with the unique postoperative problems encountered by patients undergoing bariatric procedures. Early complications occur in 1% to 5% of adult patients undergoing a Roux-en-Y gastric bypass, and include acute gastric distention, pulmonary embolism (1% to 2%), anastomotic leak (1% to 2%), and wound infection (1% to 5%) (13,44). Acute gastric distention may occur in the bypassed (distal) stomach. Patients present with hiccups, bloating, left shoulder pain, or frank shock (45). A plain radiograph of the abdomen is often diagnostic. However, because the distal bypassed stomach is no longer in continuity with the esophagus, air may not be visible in the dilated stomach on plain X-ray. In this case, ultrasound is diagnostic (45). If not treated, acute gastric distention can lead to gastric perforation. Acute gastric distention is treated by image-guided needle decompression, usually performed by an interventional radiologist. If the distention recurs, an image-guided percutaneous gastrostomy tube can be placed (45). The diagnosis of an anastomotic leak in the early postoperative period is notoriously difficult in patients who have undergone bariatric surgery (45). The abdomen may not be tender and the absence of peritoneal signs is the rule, not the exception. In addition, an upper gastrointestinal (UGI) series may be interpreted as normal in many patients, without evidence of leak. Patients who develop unexplained tachycardia, particularly in the presence of fever, shoulder pain, or pelvic pain, should undergo abdominal reexploration. Late complications of the Roux-en-Y gastric bypass include anastomotic stricture (up to 10%), marginal ulcer (up to 10%), and small bowel obstruction (up to 3%) (13,43). Dumping syndrome has been reported after Roux-en-Y gastric bypass, although this is not common (44). Anastomotic strictures can usually be treated by balloon dilitation, but may require surgical revision (46). Marginal ulcers may result from an unrecognized leak or tension (ischemia) at the gastrojejunostomy (45). *Helicobacter pylori* may also play a causal role (45). These ulcers usually respond to medical therapy with proton pump inhibitors (45). Small bowel obstruction can be adhesive or from an internal hernia. Internal hernias can occur at the jejunojejunostomy mesentery, the transverse mesocolon (if the Roux limb is retrocolic), or behind the Roux limb (Petersen hernia) (45). Internal hernias are difficult to diagnose. Patients with these hernias often present with recurrent periumbilical abdominal pain as their only symptom. Plain films and UGI contrast series may be normal. Computed tomography scan may be diagnostic, but may also be normal. The presence of persistent periumbilical pain, even in the face of normal imaging studies, mandates exploration (45). In many cases, the diagnosis is made at the time of surgical exploration. Up to 38% of adults undergoing bariatric surgery develop postoperative cholelithiasis, although this risk has been substantially reduced by routine use of ursodeoxycholic acid postoperatively (47).

Nutritional Complications after Bariatric Surgery

Protein calorie malnutrition is a potential complication of the reduced intake enforced by bariatric surgery. Patients must be encouraged to eat protein first, and limit carbohydrate intake to avoid protein deficit. Micronutrient deficiencies occur relatively commonly following bariatric procedures. Because the stomach, duodenum, and proximal small bowel are bypassed, there is an increased risk of folate, B1 (thiamine), B12, iron, and calcium deficiency following gastric bypass (48,49). B12 and iron deficiency occur in 30% of patients after Roux-en-Y gastric bypass, but can easily be prevented and/or treated in most patients (44). Iron-deficiency anemia is common in menstruating women, but can usually be avoided by appropriate use of iron supplements. Thiamine stores can be depleted in as little as 4 to 6 weeks (50). Patients with postprandial vomiting after bariatric surgery are at risk for developing beriberi, or thiamine deficiency, with cardiac and neurologic sequelae (49). Early symptoms of thiamine deficiency include numbness in the extremities and ataxia. Nystagmus, ophthalmoplegia, and loss of position sense may be present on physical examination (50). If left untreated, the patient may develop irreversible (Wernicke-Korsikoff) encephalopathy. If thiamine deficiency is suspected, glucose should never be given prior to thiamine repletion because this can cause progression to encephalopathy (50). Nutritional complications can be avoided by adherence to the five basic "rules" given to patients after bariatric surgery: (1) eat protein first, (2) drink at least 64 oz of water or sugar-free liquids daily, (3) no snacking between meals, (4) exercise at least 30 minutes per day, and (5) always remember vitamins and minerals.

Postoperative Management of the Bariatric Surgery Patient

The postoperative management of patients who have undergone bariatric surgery is intensive and lifelong. Bariatric procedures work primarily by restricting the amount of food that can be ingested or absorbed, although it is likely that there are also changes in the hormonal signals responsible for hunger and satiety. The ultimate success of all bariatric procedures depends on the patient's ability to adhere to a markedly changed diet (51). Given the propensity of adolescents to rebel against strict regimens, this raises an additional concern about performing bariatric surgery in this age group. Decreased intake and absorption of vitamins, essential fatty acids, and other specific nutrients has the potential to result in significant deficiencies, the long-term results of which are not completely understood and thus are of legitimate concern. This is particularly relevant given the fact that a majority (approximately 80%) of adolescents seeking bariatric surgery are females who are or soon will be considering planning families of their own. Pregnancies can be safely supported after bariatric surgery, but reliable contraception should be used for at least the first 2 years following the operation due to the increased risk to the fetus posed by the period of rapid weight loss and extreme hypocaloric intake.

Gastric bypass essentially results in surgically enforced very low-calorie, low-carbohydrate dietary intake. Attention to an adequate (0.5 g per kg) daily protein intake is important to preserve lean body mass, particularly during the period of most rapid weight loss. Postoperative vitamin and mineral supplementation is critical and typically consists of two pediatric chewable multivitamins, in addition to a calcium supplement (1,200 to 1,500 mg of calcium citrate per day) (48). Calcium carbonate (e.g., Tums) is not favored because absorption is decreased in the absence of gastric acid (48). Calcium supplementation is particularly important in the growing adolescent to decrease the risk of osteoporosis and bone fractures in later life (52,53). Almost one-half of the adult bone mass is accrued during adolescence (53). Serum calcium levels may be normal, even in the face of severe osteopenia, underscoring the need for routine supplementation. Many surgeons recommend additional supplementation of B-complex vitamins beyond what is contained in most multivitamin preparations to augment thiamine supplementation. All menstruating women should have supplemental iron (ferrous fumarate) included in their postoperative regimen.

TABLE 73-3 Bariatric Surgery in Adolescents: Published Results.[a]

Number of Patients	*Procedure*	*Results*	*Complications*	*Ref.*
19	Open vertical banded gastric bypass	80% Low of excess body weight	2 Revisions for gastrogastic fistula	(70)
11 (age 11–17)	Laparoscopic gastric band	Mean BMI decreased from 46.6 to 32.1 at mean follow-up of 23 mo, improvement of all comorbidities	None	(61)
12 (average age 15.9)	Laparoscopic Roux-en-Y gastric bypass ($n = 8$) Lap-band ($n = 4$)	"Satisfactory"	Not published	(13)
4 (age 17–19)	Laparoscopic Roux-en-Y gastric bypass	87% Decrease in excess body weight	None	(66)
33 (age 12.4–17.9)	Horizontal gastroplasy ($n = 1$) Vertical banded gastroplasty ($n = 2$) 15 Open gastric bypass 2 Laparoscopic gastric bypass distal gastric bypass ($n = 3$) Long limb gastric bypass ($n = 10$)	5 pt with weight regained at 5 yr 28 pt: 77% excess body weight loss No "impaired physical or sexual maturation"	2 Revisions for insufficient weight loss 6 incisional hernia 1 SBO 2 deaths, 2 and 6 years postop (not believed to be related to procedure)	(67)
10 (age 15–17)	Open Roux-en-Y gastric bypass	59% of Excess weight lost in 9 pt Weight gain of 14 kg at 144 mo in 1 pt 3 Patients with uncomplicated pregnancies	No perioperative complications Incisional hernia at 18 mo (1 pt) Protein calorie malnutrition at 12 mo (1 pt) Sympomatic cholelithiasis at 36 mo (2 pt) SBO at 153 mo (1 pt) Iron-deficiency anemia (5 pt) Transient folic acid deficiency (3 pt) Vitamin D deficiency (2 pt) 2 Late deaths: 3.5 yr (unknown cause) and 15 mo (protein malnutrition and seizures)	(47)
14	Vertical banded gastroplasty	79% with >25% loss of excess weight	Not published	(69)
22	Vertical banded gastroplasty ($n = 3$) Open Roux-en-Y gastric bypass ($n = 14$) Biliopancreatic diversion ($n = 4$)	59% excess weight loss in pt without sleep apnea, 45% in pt with sleep apnea	No perioperative complications Vitamin deficiency ($n = 2$, BPD) Protein malnutrition ($n = 3$, BPD) Cholelithiasis ($n = 1$) Nephrolithiasis ($n = 1$) Incisional hernia ($n = 1$)	(68)
34 (age 11–19)	Open Roux-en-Y gastric bypass ($n = 30$) Vertical banded gastroplasty ($n = 4$)	66% excess body weight lost at 6 yr	No perioperative complications 5 pt required revision for inadequate weight loss	(51)
16	Jejunoileal bypass	Average total weight loss 48 kg	Diarrhea	(63)
23 pt (11 additional pt with Prader-Willi syndrome excluded) average age 17	Open gastric bypass (gastrogastostomy or gastoenterostomy) ($n = 16$) Gastroplasty ($n = 7$)	Decrease from 238% IBW to 171% IBW at 3 yr and 187% IBW at 5 yr	1 Death POD 3 1 Death 36 mo postop Wound infection (5 pt) Subphrenic abscess (1 pt) Wound dehiscence (2 pt) Early anastomotic stricture (1 pt) Atalectasis (3 pt) Pneumonia (2 pt) 4 Revisions for failure to lose weight 3 Incisional hernias	(62)
4	Jejunoileal bypass	Average 32% total weight loss	Diarrhea	(64)

[a]BMI, body mass index; SBO, Small bowel obstruction; BPD, Bilopancreatic diversion; IBW, Ideal body weight; POD, Post operative day.

Iron-deficiency anemia due to menstrual bleeding can also be minimized with oral contraception. When there is any question of compliance with supplement intake, it is reassuring to document adequacy of intake by measuring specific micronutrient levels (e.g., folate, iron, vitamins A, B_1, B_6, B_{12}), although this is not necessary for most patients. Prothrombin time can be used as an inexpensive indicator of vitamin K adequacy. Nonsteroidal antiinflammatory medications should be avoided to reduce the risk of intestinal ulceration and bleeding. Ursodiol and ranitidine are prescribed for 6 months postoperatively to decrease the risk of cholelithiasis and marginal ulcer.

Outcome following surgery for morbid obesity has been extensively reported in retrospective adult cohorts (39–41,43,44). Unfortunately, few studies have been appropriately controlled with a matched comparison group of patients that did not undergo operation. The Roux-en-Y gastric bypass, which is considered the "gold standard" for bariatric surgery, results in 84% to 90% of patients achieving a loss of more than 50% of their excess weight with marked improvement of comorbidities (13,44,47). Most patients lose 20 to 30 lb in the first month, with 5 to 10 lb per month in subsequent months (13). This weight loss plateaus after 12 to 18 months for most patients (13). If the patient is compliant with the strict postoperative diet, a weight loss of 80% of excess body weight is expected at 1 year (13). There is some recidivism noted 3 to 5 years after surgery, with 20% to 30% of patients regaining most, if not all, the weight lost after surgery (54,55). Surgical mortality for the Roux-en-Y gastric bypass is 0.5% to 1% (13,44). Most patients undergoing laparoscopic Roux-en-Y gastric bypass have a hospital stay of 1 to 2 days and a rapid return to normal activities (13).

The adjustable gastric band offers an enticing alternative to the gastric bypass, particularly for adolescent patients, because it is reversible and has a lower morbidity and the mortality rate is 0.1% (43). However, American series have shown disappointing short- and long-term efficacy for this technique with 15% to 38% excess weight loss reported (56,57). Complications of the adjustable gastric band include erosion of the band through the stomach, slippage of the band proximally or distally, gastric mucosal intussusception through the band, pouch dilitation, esophagitis, and malfunction of the balloon or port (43,56). Complications leading to reoperation have been reported in up to 41% of patients (43,56,57). It should be noted that in Europe, Israel, and Australia the adjustable gastric band has been used with greater success, perhaps due to protocols with more intense postoperative monitoring and adjustments. In Europe, Israel, and Australia, reported weight loss after placement of the adjustable gastric band is 51% to 68% of excess body weight with complications occurring in 5% to 13% of patients (56,58–60). As more experience is accrued in the United States and more data obtained, the adjustable gastric band may become an important option in the treatment of adolescent morbid obesity. More experimental procedures, including intragastric balloon and gastric pacing, have been proposed in the literature but, due to lack of data, poor outcomes, or risk of complications, are not recommended currently for the treatment of obesity in children or adolescents (32).

Bariatric surgery outcomes have been reported in adolescents in 13 published series (13,47,51,61–70) (Table 73-3). Other publications include small numbers of adolescents as part of a larger adult series, making separate evaluation of these patients difficult. Excluding adolescent series prior to 1985, when procedures now abandoned were in use, there have been 159 adolescent patients who have undergone bariatric procedures reported in the literature, 162 had open procedures, and 27 had laparoscopic procedures. The short and intermediate outcome data for these patients are very similar to that reported in the adult literature. The long-term results of bariatric surgery on growth and development, however, are not known. For that reason, it is strongly recommended that these procedures be done only in centers with expertise in the unique problems of pediatric and adolescent patients, multidisciplinary support, surgeons who are adequately trained, and the capability of participating in multicenter prospective studies (6). Unlike adult trials, which may be able to concentrate on the short- and intermediate-term success of bariatric surgery, long-term outcome studies will be essential in determining the accurate risk-to-benefit ratio of these procedures in the pediatric and adolescent population.

REFERENCES

1. Hedley AA, Ogden CL, Johnson CL, et al. Prevalence and trends in overweight among US children and adolescents, 1999–2000. *JAMA* 2002;288(14):1728–1732.
2. Deckelbaum RJ, Williams CL. Childhood obesity: the health issue. *Obes Res* 2001;9(Suppl 4):239S–243S.
3. Freedman DS, et al. Relationship of childhood obesity to coronary heart disease risk factors in adulthood: the Bogalusa Heart Study. *Pediatrics* 2001;108(3):712–718.
4. Whitaker RC, et al. Predicting obesity in young adulthood from childhood and parental obesity. *N Engl J Med* 1997;337(13):869–873.
5. Must A, Strauss RS. Risks and consequences of childhood and adolescent obesity. *Int J Obes Relat Metab Disord* 1999;23 (Suppl. 2):S2–11.
6. Inge T, et al. Bariatric surgery for adolescents: concerns and recommendations. *Pediatrics (in press)*.
7. *Obes Res*. 2004.
8. Finkelstein EA, Fiebelkorn IC, Wang G. State-level estimates of annual medical expenditures attributable to obesity. *Obes Res* 2004;12(1):18–24.
9. Must A, et al. Long-term morbidity and mortality of overweight adolescents. A follow-up of the Harvard Growth Study of 1922 to 1935. *N Engl J Med* 1992;327(19):1350–1355.
10. Styne DM. Childhood and adolescent obesity. Prevalence and significance. *Pediatr Clin North Am* 2001;48(4):823–854, vii.
11. Fontaine KR, et al. Years of life lost due to obesity. *JAMA* 2003;289(2):187–193.
12. Dietz WH. Health consequences of obesity in youth: childhood predictors of adult disease. *Pediatrics* 1998;101(3 Pt 2):518–525.
13. Garcia VF, Langford L, Inge TH. Application of laparoscopy for bariatric surgery in adolescents. *Curr Opin Pediatr* 2003;15(3):248–255.

14. Gortmaker SL, et al. Social and economic consequences of overweight in adolescence and young adulthood. *N Engl J Med* 1993;329(14):1008–1012.
15. Schwimmer JB, Burwinkle TM, Varni JW. Health-related quality of life of severely obese children and adolescents. *JAMA* 2003;289(14):1813–1819.
16. Greger N, Edwin CM. Obesity: a pediatric epidemic. *Pediatr Ann* 2001;30(11):694–700.
17. Finer N. Obesity. *Clin Med* 2003;3(1):23–27.
18. Sorof J, Daniels S. Obesity hypertension in children: a problem of epidemic proportions. *Hypertension* 2002;40(4):441–447.
19. Cook S, et al. Prevalence of a metabolic syndrome phenotype in adolescents: findings from the third National Health and Nutrition Examination Survey, 1988–1994. *Arch Pediatr Adolesc Med* 2003; 157(8):821–827.
20. Steinberger J, Daniels SR. Obesity, insulin resistance, diabetes, and cardiovascular risk in children: an American Heart Association scientific statement from the Atherosclerosis, Hypertension, and Obesity in the Young Committee (Council on Cardiovascular Disease in the Young) and the Diabetes Committee (Council on Nutrition, Physical Activity, and Metabolism). *Circulation* 2003;107(10):1448–1453.
21. Pinhas-Hamiel O, et al. Increased incidence of non-insulin-dependent diabetes mellitus among adolescents. *J Pediatr* 1996;128 (5 Pt. 1):608–615.
22. Narayan KM, et al. Lifetime risk for diabetes mellitus in the United States. *JAMA* 2003;290(14):1884–1890.
23. Wing YK, et al. A controlled study of sleep related disordered breathing in obese children. *Arch Dis Child* 2003;88(12):1043–1047.
24. Spector A, et al. Adenotonsillectomy in the morbidly obese child. *Int J Pediatr Otorhinolaryngol* 2003;67(4):359–364.
25. Ray RM, Senders CW. Airway management in the obese child. *Pediatr Clin North Am* 2001;48(4):1055–1063.
26. Silfen ME, et al. Early endocrine, metabolic, and sonographic characteristics of polycystic ovary syndrome (PCOS): comparison between nonobese and obese adolescents. *J Clin Endocrinol Metab* 2003;88(10):4682–4688.
27. Roberts EA. Nonalcoholic steatohepatitis in children. *Curr Gastroenterol Rep* 2003;5(3):253–259.
28. Schwimmer JB, et al. Obesity, insulin resistance, and other clinicopathological correlates of pediatric nonalcoholic fatty liver disease. *J Pediatr* 2003;143(4):500–505.
29. Rosenbaum M, Leibel RL, Hirsch J. Obesity. *N Engl J Med* 1997; 337(6):396–407.
30. Ikeda JP, Mitchell RA. Dietary approaches to the treatment of the overweight pediatric patient. *Pediatr Clin North Am* 2001;48(4):955–968, ix.
31. Copperman N, Jacobson MS. Medical nutrition therapy of overweight adolescents. *Adolesc Med* 2003;14(1):11–21.
32. Yanovski JA. Intensive therapies for pediatric obesity. *Pediatr Clin North Am* 2001;48(4):1041–1053.
33. Berkowitz RI, et al. Behavior therapy and sibutramine for the treatment of adolescent obesity: a randomized controlled trial. *JAMA* 2003;289(14):1805–1812.
34. Shikora S. Pre-, intra-, and postoperative care of the bariatric patient. In: *Essentials of bariatric surgery.* Boston: American Society of Bariatric Surgery, 2003.
35. Torres-Villalobos G, et al. Pressure-induced rhabdomyolysis after bariatric surgery. *Obes Surg* 2003;13(2):297–301.
36. Cheymol G. Effects of obesity on pharmacokinetics implications for drug therapy. *Clin Pharmacokinet* 2000;39(3):215–231.
37. Forse RA, et al. Antibiotic prophylaxis for surgery in morbidly obese patients. *Surgery* 1989;106(4):750–756; discussion 756–757.
38. *Stedman's medical dictionary.* Baltimore: Lippincott Willams & Wilkins; 2000.
39. Sugerman HJ, et al. Diabetes and hypertension in severe obesity and effects of gastric bypass-induced weight loss. *Ann Surg* 2003;237(6):751–756; discussion 757–758.
40. Livingston EH. Obesity and its surgical management. *Am J Surg* 2002;184(2):103–113.
41. Schauer PR, et al. Effect of laparoscopic Roux-en-Y gastric bypass on type 2 diabetes mellitus. *Ann Surg* 2003;238(4):467–484; discussion 84–85.
42. NIH conference. Gastrointestinal surgery for severe obesity. Consensus Development Conference Panel. *Ann Intern Med* 1991;115 (12):956–961.
43. Fisher BL, Schauer P. Medical and surgical options in the treatment of severe obesity. *Am J Surg* 2002;184(6B):9S–16S.
44. Brolin RE. Bariatric surgery and long-term control of morbid obesity. *JAMA* 2002;288(22):2793–2796.
45. Sugerman H. Postoperative complications after bariatric surgery. In: *Essentials of bariatric surgery.* Boston: American Society of Bariatric Surgery, 2003.
46. Ahmad J, et al. Endoscopic balloon dilation of gastroenteric anastomotic stricture after laparoscopic gastric bypass. *Endoscopy* 2003;35(9):725–728.
47. Strauss RS, Bradley LJ, Brolin RE. Gastric bypass surgery in adolescents with morbid obesity. *J Pediatr* 2001;138(4):499–504.
48. Elliot K. Nutritional considerations after bariatric surgery. *Crit Care Nurs Q* 2003;26(2):133–138.
49. Gollobin C, Marcus WY. Bariatric beriberi. *Obes Surg* 2002;12(3): 309–311.
50. Brolin R. Postoperative follow up and nutritional management. In: *Essentials of bariatric surgery.* Boston: American Society of Bariatric Surgery, 2003.
51. Rand CS, Macgregor AM. Adolescents having obesity surgery: a 6-year follow-up. *South Med J* 1994;87(12):1208–1213.
52. Lytle LA, Kubik MY. Nutritional issues for adolescents. *Best Pract Res Clin Endocrinol Metab* 2003;17(2):177–189.
53. Rourke KM, et al. Effect of weight change on bone mass in female adolescents. *J Am Diet Assoc* 2003;103(3):369–372.
54. Hsu LK, et al. Nonsurgical factors that influence the outcome of bariatric surgery: a review. *Psychosom Med* 1998;60(3):338–346.
55. Deitel M. Avoidance of weight regain after gastric bypass. *Obes Surg* 2001;11(4):474.
56. DeMaria EJ. Laparoscopic adjustable silicone gastric banding. *Surg Clin North Am* 2001;81(5):1129–1144, vii.
57. Doherty C, Maher JW, Heitshusen DS. Long-term data indicate a progressive loss in efficacy of adjustable silicone gastric banding for the surgical treatment of morbid obesity. *Surgery* 2002;132(4):724–727; discussion 727–728.
58. Fielding GA, Rhodes M, Nathanson LK. Laparoscopic gastric banding for morbid obesity. Surgical outcome in 335 cases. *Surg Endosc* 1999;13(6):550–554.
59. Szold A, Abu-Abeid S. Laparoscopic adjustable silicone gastric banding for morbid obesity: results and complications in 715 patients. *Surg Endosc* 2002;16(2):230–233.
60. O'Brien PE, et al. Prospective study of a laparoscopically placed, adjustable gastric band in the treatment of morbid obesity. *Br J Surg* 1999;86(1):113–118.
61. Abu-Abeid S, et al. Bariatric surgery in adolescence. *J Pediatr Surg* 2003;38(9):1379–1382.
62. Anderson AE, Soper RT, Scott DH. Gastric bypass for morbid obesity in children and adolescents. *J Pediatr Surg* 1980;15(6):876–881.
63. Organ CH Jr, Kessler E, Lane M. Long-term results of jejunoileal bypass in the young. *Am Surg* 1984;50(11):589–593.
64. Randolph JG, Weintraub WH, Rigg A. Jejunoileal bypass for morbid obesity in adolescents. *J Pediatr Surg* 1974;9(3):341–345.
65. Soper RT, et al. Gastric bypass for morbid obesity in children and adolescents. *J Pediatr Surg* 1975;10(1):51–58.
66. Stanford A, et al. Laparoscopic Roux-en-Y gastric bypass in morbidly obese adolescents. *J Pediatr Surg* 2003;38(3):430–433.
67. Sugerman HJ, et al. Bariatric surgery for severely obese adolescents. *J Gastrointest Surg* 2003;7(1):102–107; discussion 107–108.
68. Breaux CW. Obesity surgery in children. *Obes Surg* 1995;5(3):279–284.
69. Greenstein RJ, Rabner JG. Is adolescent gastric-restrictive antiobesity surgery warranted? *Obes Surg* 1995;5(2):138–144.
70. Capella JF, Capella RF. Bariatric surgery in adolescence. Is this the best age to operate? *Obes Surg* 2003;13(6):826–832.

Small Intestine

Martin H. Ulshen and William R. Treem

The small intestine is the major digestive and absorptive portion of the gastrointestinal tract. Any pathologic process that disrupts the normal function of the small intestine profoundly affects the normal growth and metabolism of the child. Pediatric surgeons are involved in the care of patients with chronic conditions of the small intestine that preclude normal enteral nutrition. These include conditions resulting in short bowel syndrome and protracted diarrhea in infancy; motility disorders causing pseudoobstruction and bacterial overgrowth; acquired inflammatory immune-mediated conditions, such as Crohn's disease and graft versus host disease; and acquired conditions believed to be triggered by viral or bacterial infections, such as Henoch-Schönlein purpura and hemolytic uremic syndrome. Parenteral nutrition has provided a means of supporting these patients, while treating their underlying disease and waiting for growth, development, and regeneration of the damaged small intestine. This chapter briefly reviews the ontogeny of small intestine development, the basic gross and microscopic anatomy, the physiology of nutrient digestion and absorption, and normal small intestinal motility. The second portion of the chapter highlights some of the disease processes that disrupt normal function in these areas and lead to the potential need for surgical intervention to provide parenteral or selective enteral nutrition.

DEVELOPMENTAL ANATOMY

The gut lengthens rapidly between 6 and 12 weeks' gestation. During this time, the small intestine transiently herniates into the umbilical cord. On reentry into the abdominal cavity, the intestine rotates counterclockwise 270 degrees around an axis formed by the superior mesenteric artery. Further positioning of the small intestine continues until 20 weeks' gestation, when the gastrointestinal tract achieves its final anatomic position. The small intestine continues to lengthen throughout gestation and measures 200 to 300 cm at birth in a full-term neonate (1). Between 26 and 38 weeks' gestation, the overall length of the gastrointestinal tract doubles. The small intestine does not achieve its maximum length of 600 to 800 cm until at least 4 years of age. These changes in overall length, the doubling of the intestinal diameter, and the development of the plicae circulares, villi, and microvilli combine to enlarge the absorptive surface area of the small intestine from about 950 cm^2 at birth to 7,500 cm^2 in the adult (2).

The circular muscles of the small intestine appear at 6 weeks' gestation, and the longitudinal muscles at 8 weeks' gestation. Neuroblasts appear at 7 weeks' gestation, and differentiation into the myenteric and submucosal plexuses occurs at 9 and 13 weeks' gestation, respectively. Peristalsis first occurs shortly thereafter, but jejunal contractions remain disorganized in the premature infant before 30 weeks' gestation (3). When radiographic contrast material is injected into the gastrointestinal tract of a fetus in utero before 30 weeks' gestation, there is little movement of the marker out of the stomach (4). With the appearance of the migrating motor complexes (MMCs) at 32 to 34 weeks' gestation, duodenal and jejunal contractions become more coordinated, but are still immature. Despite the greater frequency of MMCs in premature infants, transit time through the small intestine can be as long as 9 hours, or twice as long as that in term infants, because of the twofold shorter propagation rate of the MMCs. By 38 weeks' postconception, the MMCs are fully present, and fasting motor activity is mature (5). Feedings increase the number of duodenal contractions in infants as young as 25 weeks' postconception; in very premature infants, there is often the coexistence of an active fed pattern with an immature fasting pattern and no MMCs (6). The administration of corticosteroids accelerates maturation of neonatal small intestinal motility, whereas ischemia and central nervous system disease slow maturation.

Martin H. Ulshen and William R. Treem: Division of Pediatric Gastroenterology and Nutrition, Duke University Medical Center, Durham, North Carolina 27710.

Villi appear in the duodenum at 8 weeks' gestation and proliferate aborally, reaching the terminal ileum by 11 weeks' gestation. The crypt compartment of the small intestine, which is the site of enterocyte proliferation, appears in the duodenum by 10 weeks' gestation. The villi acquire their tall, fingerlike shape in the proximal intestine by 14 weeks' gestation, but remain shorter in the distal small intestine, resulting in a fourfold greater absorptive surface area in the jejunum than in the ileum. Microvilli also appear at 8 weeks' gestation, and by 14 weeks' gestation, enterocytes are morphologically mature and display a well-organized brush border. The entire process of enterocyte migration from crypt to villus in the newborn infant is slower than that in adults and requires at least 6 days for epithelial renewal.

ONTOGENY OF DIGESTION AND ABSORPTION

Carbohydrates

The proportion of carbohydrate ingested as starch increases progressively during the first year of life. Starch digestion is dependent on pancreatic α-amylase activity in the duodenal fluid, which is reduced during the first 6 months of life. Below this age, salivary amylase may be important in starch digestion. In addition, α-amylase activity is higher in human milk than in the duodenal contents of infants younger than 3 months of age. By 1 year of age, the capacity for starch digestion is comparable to that of an adult.

Despite the mature appearance of the intestinal epithelium by the end of the second trimester, its brush-border membrane is functionally immature. The disaccharidases lactase and sucrase-isomaltase can be detected by 8 weeks' gestation, but lactase activity remains low until 36 weeks' gestation (7). Peak lactase activity is found in the full-term newborn and during early postnatal life. Within the first few years of life, lactase activity decreases to adult levels (one-tenth that at birth). In contrast, sucrase-isomaltase activity rises throughout gestation so 70% of adult levels is achieved at 34 weeks' gestation and adult levels are reached at birth. Glucoamylase (maltase) has been detected at 13 weeks' gestation, and the presence of this α-glucosidase together with sucrase-isomaltase allows the premature infant to digest glucose polymers more readily than lactose. These enzymes are also important in the final steps of starch digestion. Despite the apparent lactase deficiency, term infants tolerate lactose-containing formulas and human milk owing to the process of carbohydrate salvage through fermentation to short-chain fatty acids by colonic bacteria. Infant formulas designed for preterm infants often contain lower lactose and higher glucose polymer concentrations.

The rate of glucose transport is low in the first trimester and increases as the number of sodium-coupled transport sites increases first in the jejunum and then in the ileum. The maximal glucose transport rate in the jejunum of infants is 20% to 25% that of adults and increases throughout the first year of life (8).

Proteins

Most protein hydrolysis occurs in the proximal gut and is dependent on the presence of enterokinase, pancreatic proteases, and brush-border and cytosolic peptidases. Enterokinase initiates the process of protein digestion by the activation of trypsinogen. Enterokinase activity is detected in the duodenum at 24 weeks' gestation and increases during the latter part of gestation to 10% of eventual adult levels, which are finally achieved by about 4 years of age. Despite the relative deficiency of enterokinase, the presence of the pancreatic proteases (trypsin, chymotrypsin, and carboxypeptidase B) permits efficient digestion of protein to peptides. Most of the activities of both the brush-border and cytosolic peptidases are present at 8 weeks' gestation and soon reach levels similar to those found in adults.

Fats

The efficiency of long-chain triglyceride absorption ranges from 70% to 90% in term infants and from 40% to 90% in premature infants. Medium-chain triglycerides are digested and absorbed more efficiently than are long-chain triglycerides because they do not require bile salts for esterification or solubilization in mixed micelles. Medium-chain triglycerides are taken up directly in the portal vein. The multiple factors that contribute to the immaturity of bile acid metabolism and the enterohepatic circulation of bile acids in the newborn are collectively termed *physiologic cholestasis* (9,10) (Fig. 74-1). These factors include decreased rates of bile acid synthesis, the lack of an active transporter of bile salts in the ileum, and the resultant smaller pool size (11). Although taurine-conjugated bile acids are passively absorbed by the fetal gut, active ileal transport does not begin until after birth. Together, these factors contribute to the relative paucity of bile salts appearing in the infant duodenum; these may not reach the critical micellar concentration necessary for long-chain fat absorption, especially in premature infants. Hormones such as glucocorticoids and thyroxine, growth factors such as epidermal growth factor, and dietary factors including long-chain fatty acids are all believed to regulate and enhance the development of bile acid metabolism and the enterohepatic circulation in the fetus and premature infant (12).

NORMAL ANATOMY AND PHYSIOLOGY

Gross Anatomy

Although a distinct demarcation between jejunum and ileum is not apparent, structural differences are present

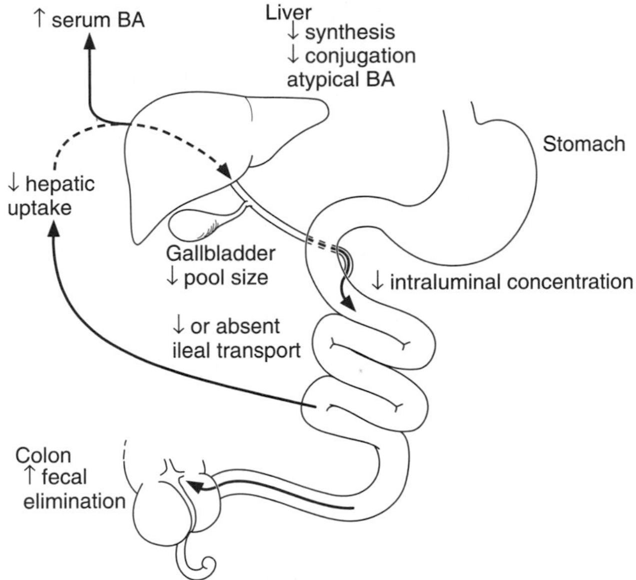

FIGURE 74-1. Manifestations of immature bile acid (BA) transport and metabolism in early life. Most facets of the enterohepatic circulation are defective, allowing spillover of bile acids into the systemic circulation (physiologic cholestasis) and loss through fecal elimination.

that reflect the functional compartmentalization of the small intestine. The thickness of the small bowel wall, the overall luminal diameter, and the prominence of the circular submucosal folds (plicae circulares) are all greatest in the proximal jejunum and decrease with progression through the ileum. Absorptive surface area, as a consequence, is much greater in the jejunum than in the ileum. The direct stimulatory effect of nutrients on the growth of the absorptive mucosa is believed to be responsible for the normal proximal to distal absorptive gradient; proximal jejunal villi are taller and have greater absorptive capacity because of abundant exposure to nutrients, most of which are depleted by the time intestinal chyme reaches the distal small intestine. The ileum of animals undergoing jejunectomy experiences marked hyperplasia when exposed to enteral nutrients. Similarly, when a segment of ileum is transplanted proximally and exposed to the jejunal nutrient environment, that segment becomes hyperplastic and takes on the morphologic and functional absorptive characteristics of proximal intestine (13). Conversely, a jejunal segment transposed to the ileal environment undergoes opposite changes and decreases its mucosal mass.

The mucosa is the innermost layer of the small intestine and is composed of three distinct layers: the muscularis mucosa, lamina propria, and surface epithelial cell lining (Fig. 74-2). As noted, the most striking feature of the small intestinal mucosa is the formation of villi, which are about 1.5 mm tall in the jejunum and progressively shorter through the ileum. Surrounding the base of each villus are several pitlike crypts, called the *crypts of Lieberkühn,* which average one-third to one-fourth the height of the villi and are the site of epithelial cell proliferation.

Cells that populate the epithelial layer differ depending on whether they overlay the villi, crypts, or lymphoid aggregates of Peyer patches. The most abundant cells in the crypt epithelium are undifferentiated columnar epithelial cells, with fewer goblet cells, enteroendocrine cells, and Paneth cells. These stem cells are responsible for cell renewal and can differentiate into all other cellular components. In addition, the crypt epithelial cells regulate water and ion secretion. Epithelial cells differentiate and develop mature digestive and absorptive function as they migrate from proximal crypt to villus tip. Structurally distinct M cells that are found in the epithelium overlaying Peyer patches appear to be important in antigen processing and presentation to immunocompetent gut lymphocytes.

The small intestine is in a perpetual state of turnover, with intense mitotic activity in the crypts, uniform migration of all cell types (with the exception of Paneth cells) luminally up the side of the villus, and eventual extrusion at the villus tip. As cells make this journey, they acquire the special structure and intracellular elements needed for their mature function, including the development of specific digestive and absorptive functions. Epithelial cell migration and maturation occur about every 3 to 5 days; the entire mucosal lining is replaced in 1 week.

Cellular Anatomy

Enterocytes are tall columnar epithelial cells that are responsible for absorption. These cells rest tightly on their basal laminae and are attached at the apical pole to adjacent enterocytes by tight junctions. In the jejunum, however, these tight junctions are actually permeable, and back diffusion of fluid and electrolytes into the lumen allows the luminal contents to remain isotonic even as the bulk of nutrients are absorbed. Conversely, in the ileum, the tight junctions are less permeable; there is less back diffusion resulting in increased concentration of luminal contents.

The luminal surface of the enterocyte has numerous membrane extensions, termed *microvilli,* which are about 1 mm tall. The microvilli (collectively known as the *brush border)* are in direct contact with the luminal contents and contain the membrane-bound digestive enzymes, transport proteins, and other elements necessary for nutrient absorption. The brush border can be damaged by multiple small bowel pathogens such as rotavirus or *Giardia* sp, leading to transient reduction in digestive enzyme function. Interposed between and lying on top of the microvilli is a glycoprotein coat called the *glycocalyx* or the "fuzzy coat." Glycoproteins that make up this layer are resistant to removal by enzymatic activity (14). Fluid and electrolyte trafficking between cells is controlled by the junctional complexes between adjacent cells and the basolateral membrane. This portion of the cell membrane lacks the disaccharidases and peptidases present on the

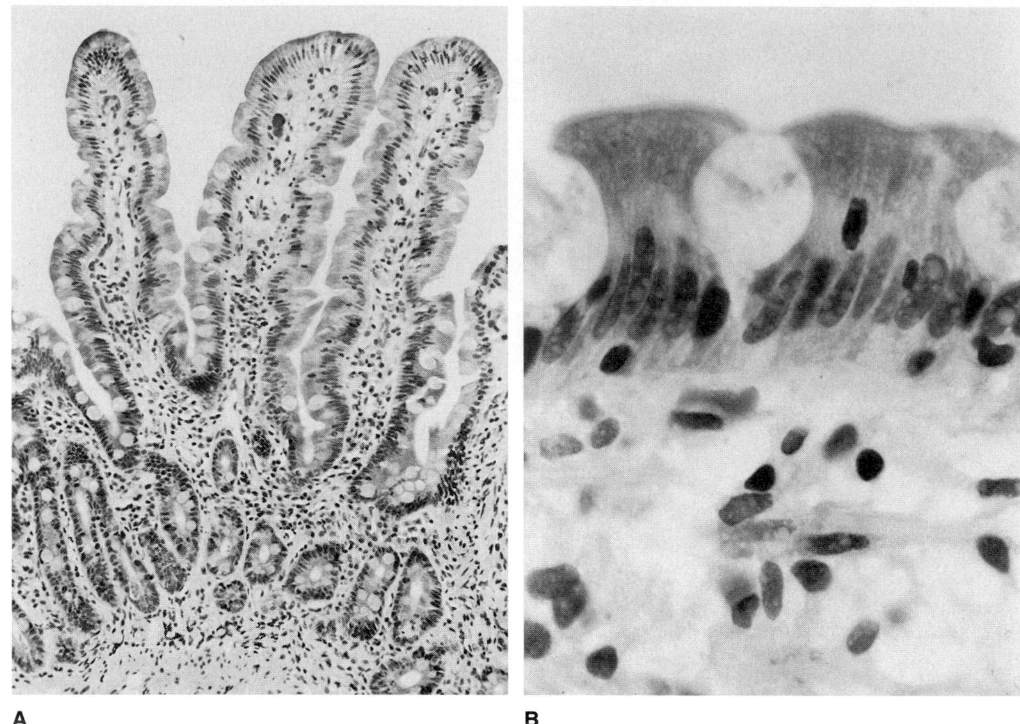

FIGURE 74-2. **(A)** Light photomicrograph of the normal mucosa of the human jejunum. The villi are tall, thin, and most prominently developed within the jejunum. In the ileum, the villi are broader and shorter, goblet cells are more prominent, and the lamina propria contains more lymph follicles and lymphoid cells. (Hematoxylin-eosin stain, ×100.) (Courtesy of M. Gottfried, MD.) **(B)** High-powered view of brush border showing columnar epithelium with interspersed goblet cells. Deep to the epithelial layer of the mucosa is the lamina propria, a thin layer of connective tissue filled with arterioles, capillaries, veins, lacteals, small nerve fibrils, and numerous additional cellular elements. At the luminal surface of the epithelial cell is the brush border or microvillus membrane, shown here by the lucent band running along the apical enterocytes.

apical membrane, but is rich in Na^+-K^+-ATPase, glycosyl transferase, and adenyl cyclase, all of which are involved in the major energy-dependent mechanisms that control solute and, thereby, fluid transport.

Small Intestinal Motility

The two functions of small intestinal motor activity are to mix and propel ingested food, promoting effective digestion and absorption of luminal contents, and to sweep the small intestine clear of undigestible food particles, bacteria, and desquamated cells during periods of fasting. Coordinated peristalsis, consisting of contractions and relaxations, is regulated by the intrinsic activity of the smooth muscle together with the modulating actions of the autonomic nervous system and gastrointestinal hormones. The human enteric nervous system (ENS) consists of cell bodies and processes of the neural plexuses within the gut wall. It contains more than 10^8 neurons, which is roughly equivalent to the number of neurons in the spinal cord. Complexity of this neural control network has led to its being called the "little brain in the gut" (15).

During fasting, small intestinal motility is organized into a recurrent pattern of sequential periods, which together make up the MMCs. The MMCs have been called the "intestinal housekeeper" because they clear the small intestine of bacteria and undigestible food residue. Absence of MMCs in patients with pseudoobstruction is associated with bacterial overgrowth(16). MMCs consist of three phases. Phase 1 is a period of quiescence characterized by slow transit and maximal absorption of nutrients. It is followed by phase 2, a period of random, intermittent contractions similar to the normal postprandial pattern, designed for mixing rather than propulsion. Phase 3 is a brief period of high-amplitude contractions occurring at maximal frequency. Phase 3 can start anywhere from the lower esophageal sphincter to the distal jejunum, and propagates at a rate of 5 to 15 cm per minute toward the ileum. Phase 3 is also associated with an increase in intestinal secretions, which may aid in clearing the small intestine of bacteria and residue (17). As one complex reaches the terminal ileum, another starts in the proximal intestine. A complete MMC occurs every 90 to 300 minutes in adults and every 40 to 100 minutes in infants.

Ingestion of a nutrient meal disrupts the cyclic pattern of the migrating motor complexes (MMC), leading to a prolonged period of irregular activity similar to phase 2 during fasting. The fed pattern, however, has even fewer propagating contractions than phase 2 of the MMC and results in slow transit and more time for intraluminal digestion and absorption of nutrients in the proximal small intestine (18). The duration of the fed pattern correlates with the time of gastric emptying and is influenced by the characteristics of nutrients ingested. Fat meals are slower to empty the stomach and inhibit the MMC longer than isocaloric amounts of sucrose, which in turn inhibit the MMC longer than protein. Hormonal influences also play a role. Intravenous infusions of secretin, insulin, glucagon, cholecystokinin, or gastrin disrupt the MMC and induce a fed motility pattern, even in the absence of luminal nutrients. Neural control is also important because vagotomy inhibits the fed pattern, suggesting that vagal activity has a role in suppressing the fasting pattern (19). Local perfusion of anticholinergic compounds disrupts the MMC for a considerable distance proximal and distal to the perfusion site.

The ENS is comprised of the myenteric plexus (Auerbach plexus), situated between the longitudinal and circular muscle layers, and the submucosal plexus (Meissner plexus), located in the submucosa. The two plexuses contain networks of neurons, communicate through connecting nerve axons, and generate stereotypic patterns of electrical activity that regulate motility, secretion, and blood flow. These intrinsic patterns are essential, as illustrated by numerous animal models of extrinsically denervated intestinal segments that retain peristalsis and cycled MMCs. When the small intestine is divided into small segments by multiple transections and reanastomoses, each segment generates its own MMC, which cycles independently from other segments (20). Stimulation of motilin receptors by erythromycin, which ordinarily induces MMCs in adults, fails to induce similar motility changes in preterm infants who lack a mature ENS necessary for normal intestinal cyclic motor activity (21).

In the presence of a mature ENS, extrinsic neurogenic, chemical, and hormonal control is important in regulating small bowel motility. The small intestine is supplied by parasympathetic nerves from the vagus and by sympathetic nerves from the thoracolumbar spinal cord. Blocking the parasympathetic input by vagotomy or the administration of atropine reduces the duration of phase 2 of the MMC, and initiating an MMC by injections of motilin into the stomach requires an intact vagus (22). In contrast, extrinsic sympathetic nerves are important inhibitory efferents to the small intestine and mediate the disappearance of MMCs, as seen in patients who develop a postoperative ileus (23). Chemical excitatory substances that stimulate small bowel contraction include acetylcholine, tachykinins, and substance P. Likely candidates for postsynaptic inhibitors of contraction include vasoactive intestinal polypeptide (VIP), calcitonin gene-related peptide, nitric oxide, high doses of somatostatin, and β-endorphin. The peptide hormone motilin appears to stimulate MMCs that originate in the stomach, but MMCs that begin below the pylorus do not correlate with plasma motilin variation. Eating a meal produces an increase in the serum concentration of motilin (24).

Physiology of Water and Electrolyte Absorption

Osmotic differences of as little as 1.6 mOsm per L across the apical enterocyte membrane and of only an additional 0.7 mOsm per L across the basolateral membrane are believed to account for the transfer of water from the luminal space to the capillary space in the small intestine (25). Solute entry into the enterocyte to maintain this small osmotic gradient is achieved primarily by active transport processes. The apical (luminal) membrane of the enterocyte contains numerous active transporters of solutes, including glucose and amino acids, which transfer sodium in an obligatory process. The basolateral membrane contains an active transporter for sodium in the form of the Na^+-K^+-ATPase pump. Together, these processes maintain a small gradient of relative hypotonicity in the lumen, intermediate tonicity in the cell, and mild hypertonicity within the lateral intracellular space. Increasing hydrostatic pressure in this space helps push water across the freely permeable basal lamina and interstitial space into the capillaries of the lamina propria.

Ion transport across the small intestinal epithelium occurs by passive diffusion down a chemical concentration gradient or because of electrical potential differences, by solvent drag from the passive flow of solutes secondary to water flow, or by active transport carrier-mediated processes that are energy dependent and move ions against either an electrical or a chemical concentration gradient. In all segments of the small intestine, the final determinant of the driving force for all active ion transport is the Na^+-K^+-ATPase pump located along the basolateral membrane. This pump actively transports sodium out of the cell at the basolateral membrane in exchange for potassium. Absorption of sodium and other ions is regulated by the intestinal epithelium covering the villi, and secretion of chloride is predominantly handled by the crypt cells.

Chloride secretion occurs in intestinal crypt cells because of two mechanisms. Chloride is carried into the cell by a cotransporter located in the basolateral membrane, which results in the electroneutral transport of one sodium, one potassium, and two chloride molecules. Chloride carried across the basolateral membrane is then secreted from the cell through chloride-selective channels located in the apical membrane of crypt cells (26). These chloride-selective channels are generally closed, but they can be opened by activating cyclic adenosine monophosphate (cAMP), cyclic guanosine monophosphate (cGMP), or protein kinase C, or by calcium. cAMP is stimulated by cholera toxin, VIP, and prostaglandins (27). cGMP stimulation can result from *Escherichia coli* enterotoxin and calcium. As chloride is secreted across the apical membrane, sodium is lost through the paracellular pathway in response to the outwardly directed electrochemical gradient created by the chloride secretion.

Physiology of Nutrient Digestion and Absorption

Carbohydrates

Starches and oligosaccharides are the major form of carbohydrate in the human diet, but must undergo digestion to monosaccharides before they can be absorbed. Table 74-1 summarizes the extraintestinal and brush-border enzymes that participate in carbohydrate digestion to monosaccharides. A small amount of dietary disaccharide, and as much as 10% to 20% of starch, are not normally absorbed in the small intestine and pass into the colon to be fermented by colonic bacteria to short-chain fatty acids reabsorbed in the colon. This colonic reclamation of carbohydrate prevents loss of energy and the osmotic diarrhea that would result from carbohydrate malabsorption. It is also probably important in limiting diarrhea in patients with lactose intolerance, sucrase-isomaltase deficiency, and short bowel syndrome.

The most important enzyme in the digestion of starch is α-amylase, which acts on the interior α_{1-4} bonds of starch. Salivary amylase makes a minor contribution to overall starch digestion, except perhaps in neonates, because it is inactivated at gastric pH. Human milk, in contrast to cow milk, is rich in α-amylase activity (28). Pancreatic amylase activity is low in the first months of life, but in older children with normal pancreatic function, it is present in excess of normal requirements for starch hydrolysis. Therefore, starch digestion is essentially complete when intestinal contents reach the distal duodenum (29). Exposure of the duodenum to nutrient is the major stimulus for pancreatic amylase secretion. This effect is likely mediated through both the cholinergic nervous system and gut hormones because administration of a cholecystokinin receptor antagonist reduces meal-stimulated pancreatic enzyme secretion by 60%, and atropine causes nearly complete suppression of pancreatic enzyme secretion (30). Secretin, the major stimulant of pancreatic bicarbonate and fluid secretion, also promotes α-amylase secretion, but has less effect on lipase and little effect on pancreatic protease release.

Fats

Figure 74-3 provides an overview of the major steps of lipid digestion and absorption. Despite the complexity of the process, absorption from the lumen into the enterocyte and then to the lamina propria requires only about 12 minutes, and beyond infancy, more than 95% of intraluminal fat is normally absorbed. Triglycerides, which comprise about 90% of dietary fat intake, are emulsified into tiny particles and stabilized by other dietary components, such as phospholipids and polysaccharides or endogenous bile salts. Bile salts are important in solubilization and in the promotion of pancreatic lipase activity, but 75% of dietary triglyceride can be absorbed without bile salts. Cholesterol and fat-soluble vitamin absorption are affected more severely by bile acid deficiency than is triglyceride absorption.

TABLE 74-1 Extraintestinal and Brush-border Enzymes of Carbohydrate Digestion.

Enzyme	*Substrate*	*Products*
Amylase (human milk, saliva, pancreas)	Starch (amylose, amylopectin)	Maltose, maltotriose, oligosaccharide with terminal 1–6 linkage (α-limit dextrins)
Lactase	Lactose	Glucose, galactose
Sucrase	Sucrose, maltose, maltotriose, α-limit dextrins with terminal α_{1-4} links	Glucose, fructose, maltooligosaccharide with α_{1-6} linkage
Glucomylase	Maltose, maltotriose, maltooligosaccharide (glucose polymers with maximal affinity for chains of 6–10 residues)	Glucose, maltooligosaccharide with terminal α_{1-6} linkage
Isomaltase (α-dextrinase)	Maltose, isomaltose, α-limit dextrins (maltooligosaccharide with terminal α_{1-6} links)	Glucose, maltooligosaccharide
Trehalase	Trehalose (found principally in mushrooms)	Glucose

Adapted from Treem WR. Congenital sucrase-isomaltase deficiency. *J Pediatr Gastroenterol Nutr 1995; 21:1–14.*

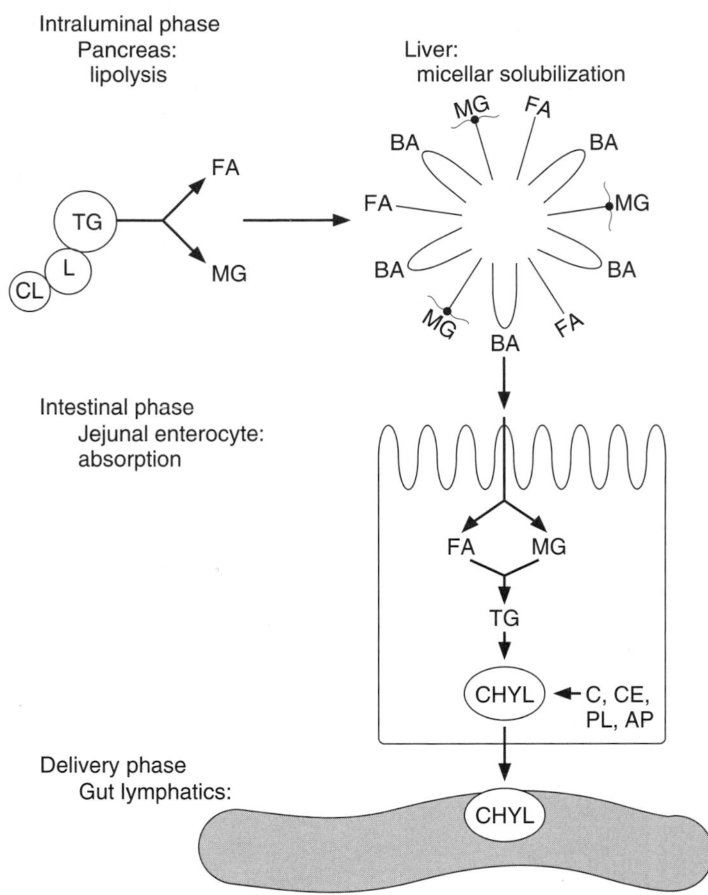

FIGURE 74-3. Overview of the major steps of lipid digestion and absorption. (1) Lipase (L) and colipase (CL) bind to the triglyceride (TG) droplet. (2) Intraluminal lipolysis of TG to fatty acids (FA) and monoglycerides (MG). (3) Formation into micelles with bile acids (BA). (4) Absorption of the FA and MG into the enterocyte. (5) Reesterification into TG and formation of chylomicrons (CHYL) made up of cholesterol (C), cholesterol ester (CE), phospholipid (PL), and apoproteins (AP). (6) Secretion of CHYL into intercellular spaces and gut lymphatics in lamina propria.

Multiple lipases have a role in the hydrolysis of the ester bonds of triglycerides and phospholipids, but pancreatic lipase, in conjunction with its cofactor colipase, is responsible for the major proportion of triglyceride hydrolysis. Lingual and gastric lipases initiate hydrolysis in the stomach and can be of great importance in the neonatal period when pancreatic lipase is deficient. Gastric lipase hydrolyzes medium-chain triglycerides five to eight times faster than long-chain triglycerides. In neonates, medium-chain triglycerides disappear more rapidly from the stomach after a meal than do long-chain triglycerides because neonates appear to absorb medium-chain triglycerides directly from the stomach (31). This factor, in addition to the necessity for bile salts for long-chain triglyceride solubilization, may explain the relative advantage of medium-chain triglyceride-containing formulas for premature neonates. Fat digestion in breastfed infants also benefits from a separate lipase found in human milk (32). This enzyme is resistant to stomach acid and is activated by bile salts in the duodenum.

In the presence of bile salts and phospholipid in the proximal intestinal lumen, colipase binds pancreatic lipase to the triglyceride emulsion for hydrolysis of fatty acids off the glycerol backbone. Colipase is initially synthesized as procolipase and subsequently activated by trypsin. The functions of colipase are to attach to the ester bond of the triglyceride and to bring lipase close to this bond, facilitating hydrolysis. In patients with steatorrhea secondary to pancreatic insufficiency, fecal fat loss correlates better with colipase secretion than with lipase secretion (33). As little as 2% of normal lipase secretion can be compatible with normal fat digestion if colipase secretion is adequate. Phospholipase A_2 is a calcium-dependent bile salt-activated lipase secreted by the pancreas. It is the major enzyme in the digestion of intestinal phopholipids, both from the diet and contained in bile.

As a solute passes from the bulk phase within the lumen toward the enterocyte, it first passes through the unstirred water layer, adjacent to the microvillus membrane. The layer acts as a diffusion barrier and is the rate-limiting step for the absorption of fats in the small intestine (34). The products of fat digestion are free fatty acids, monoglycerides, phosphatidylcholine (phospholipid), free cholesterol, and free sterols (vitamins), which are solubilized in bile acid micelles. Most absorption of the contents of these mixed micelles occurs in the proximal small intestine at the villus tips and is complete by the midjejunum. Dissociation of micelles into an absorbable form is promoted by the acid pH of the microenvironment at the surface of the microvillus membrane (35). A change in luminal pH can affect the pH of the microenvironment, and therefore, can affect lipid absorption. Once the products of lipolysis reach the enterocyte membrane, they rapidly diffuse by passive transport into the cell.

A small proportion of the bile acids that previously formed the micelle are absorbed by passive diffusion in the jejunum. The bulk are reabsorbed in a conjugated form by active transport in the terminal ileum. Deconjugation of intraluminal bile acids by small bowel bacterial overgrowth and loss of active transport of bile salts by ileal disease or resection can compromise the enterohepatic circulation of bile acids and adversely affect fat absorption. In addition, jejunal hyperacidity, which occurs in cystic fibrosis and other forms of pancreatic insufficiency, can cause precipitation of bile acids, further compromising fat absorption.

Once inside the enterocyte, the products of lipolysis are bound to fatty acid-binding protein and transported to the smooth endoplasmic reticulum for reassembly into triglycerides, phophatidylcholine, and cholesterol. Chylomicrons, made up of phospholipid and apoprotein surface coats and inner triglyceride, cholesterol esters, and free cholesterol, are synthesized inside the enterocyte and subsequently released across the basolateral membrane. They enter lacteals within the lamina propria and subsequently reach gut lymphatic vessels.

Proteins

Protein digestion begins in the stomach, where gastric acid denatures dietary protein and promotes pepsin digestion of protein into large polypeptides. Pancreatic proteases, secreted into the small intestine, then act to further split large polypeptides into oligopeptides of six or fewer amino acid residues. Pancreatic proteases are initially secreted in an inactive form. Conversion of the inactive pancreatic trypsinogen into trypsin is catalyzed by the brush-border enzyme enterokinase, which is localized to the proximal small intestine. Trypsin then activates the other pancreatic proteases, including chymotrypsin and elastase. Animals with ligation of the pancreatic duct can still absorb nearly 40% of a protein meal, and patients with severe pancreatic insufficiency can still absorb a portion of ingested protein (36). This ability is due to the presence of three neutral endopeptidases expressed in the mature region of the villus, which can also hydrolyze intact large peptides (37). Although dietary protein can be identified in the proximal ileal contents, digestion and absorption are nearly completed by the time the intestinal contents arrive at the terminal ileum. Less than 1 g of protein, oligopeptides, and free amino acids normally pass into the colon each day.

A large proportion of the protein undergoing gastrointestinal digestion had been endogenously produced. In adults, this includes about 20 to 30 g of glycoproteins and mucins secreted by the gastrointestinal tract and accessory organs of digestion. In addition, in adults about 1 lb of intestinal epithelial cells is shed each day, providing an additional 30 g of protein for digestion. More than one-half of the dietary protein intake is used initially by the small intestine, primarily to produce glycoproteins for secretion and also for production of mucosal cell proteins and for energy needs (38). About one-half the dietary protein intake ultimately enters the systemic circulation as amino acids; one-third of this comes from recycled intestinal secretions. The major energy source of the intestine is oxidation of the amino acids glutamate, glutamine, and aspartate, as well as glucose (39). As a result, systemic requirements for these amino acids must be met by synthesis within the body rather than intestinal absorption.

CHRONIC SMALL INTESTINAL DISEASES

This section describes some clinical syndromes and specific disease entities that are often characterized by diffuse involvement of the small intestine and that present with chronic vomiting, diarrhea, failure to thrive, or gastrointestinal bleeding. The pediatric surgeon is frequently involved in the treatment of patients with these problems because of the acute need for surgical intervention, the need for chronic enteral or parenteral nutrition, or consideration of special procedures to relieve strictures of the small intestine, lengthen the intestine, or restore more normal small bowel motility. This discussion concentrates on the recognition of the clinical symptoms and complications that characterize these syndromes and the diagnostic tests available to evaluate them. Treatment of these complicated patients is often a collaborative effort among the pediatric surgeon, pediatric gastroenterologist, and other pediatric subspecialists. Studies that are useful for anatomic evaluation of the small bowel include upper gastrointestinal radiographic series with small bowel follow-through and endoscopic small bowel biopsy. Functional studies of the small bowel include stool fat evaluation for malabsorption (72-hour collection is most reliable), stool pH and reducing substance for carbohydrate malabsorption, fecal α-1-antitrypsin for protein-losing enteropathy, fecal elastase to rule out pancreatic insufficiency, serum folate, fat-soluble vitamins, albumin and vitamin B_{12} levels, and small bowel biopsy for disaccharidase assay. Carbohydrate hydrogen breath tests are useful in identifying carbohydrate malabsorption and small bowel bacterial overgrowth.

Short Bowel Syndrome

Compromise of the normal anatomic and physiologic mechanisms that facilitate small bowel function is perhaps best illustrated by the complex problems encountered in children with short bowel syndrome. Abnormalities in small bowel motility, digestion, and absorption characterize these patients and contribute to significant morbidity, and even mortality, in some patients. Two major developments have dramatically altered the prognosis for even the most severely affected infants and children with short bowel syndrome. For more than 30 years, parenteral nutrition has been an indispensable part of the acute and chronic management of short bowel syndrome. More recently, limited success with small intestine transplantation has offered hope to those without sufficient intestinal adaptation to support enteral feedings (40).

Short bowel syndrome is defined as malabsorption, fluid and electrolyte loss, and malnutrition after massive resection of the small intestine. Wilmore defined short bowel syndrome as less than 75 cm of residual small intestine, or less than 40% of the normal length of the small intestine in a full-term neonate (41). Resection of more than 75% of the small intestine with preservation of the ileocecal valve invariably produces initial intractable malabsorption and diarrhea. As much as one-half of the small intestine can be lost, however, without significant long-term problems in sustaining normal nutrition, provided the duodenum, distal ileum, and ileocecal valve are spared.

In contrast, distal ileal resections that include the ileocecal valve can cause severe diarrhea, even though only 25% of the small intestine has been resected. This is most likely due to several important functions peculiar to the ileum. First, the ileum is capable of undergoing much more dramatic compensatory hyperplasia in response to jejunal resection than is the jejunum in response to ileal resection. Second, resection of the ileum has more profound effects on the volume and tonicity of intestinal contents reaching the colon because it is only in the ileum that decreased permeability of the intracellular tight junctions allows for increased concentrations of luminal contents. Also, only the ileum and right colon can absorb sodium chloride against a steep concentration gradient. Third, resection of the ileum also causes diarrhea and even steatorrhea if the resection is massive enough, secondary to the malabsorption of bile salts. Finally, loss of the ileocecal valve is one of the major permissive factors in the development of bacterial overgrowth in the small intestine.

Nutrients in the lumen of the small intestine are essential for the maintenance of mucosal mass. Not only starvation, but also the provision of adequate protein and calories exclusively by total parenteral nutrition, results in mucosal atrophy in humans and experimental animals. Numerous studies in animals have demonstrated that, even in the presence of resection of the small intestine (the most potent trigger of small intestinal mucosal hyperplasia), no adaptation occurs unless luminal nutrients are provided. These findings suggest that after intestinal resection, parenteral nutrition should be supplemented with enteral nutrients as soon as possible to stimulate small intestine adaptation. Early enteral feeding of infants with short bowel has been associated with development of a mild, noninfectious colitis that does not usually require discontinuing feedings. In animal models, complex nutrients stimulate greater mucosal growth than more elemental nutrients (e.g., long-chain vs. medium-chain triglycerides). The use of glutamine supplementation and/or administration of growth hormone, insulinlike growth factor (IGF)-1, epidermal growth factor, or enteroglucagons has been studied to promote adaptive growth and recovery of function of the small bowel mucosa, but remains controversial (42–44).

Table 74-2 summarizes the causes of short bowel syndrome in infants (41,45–51). The most common causes include necrotizing enterocolitis, volvulus, jejunoileal atresia, and gastroschisis. Short bowel syndrome has been reported in 7% to 38% of infants who survive surgical therapy for necrotizing enterocolitis (40). Midgut volvulus and diffuse small bowel Crohn's disease predominate in older children. Less frequent causes of short bowel syndrome include trauma to the gastrointestinal tract and total colonic aganglionosis with proximal extension into the small intestine.

Specific clinical consequences of massive resection of the small intestine include the following:

- Nutrient malabsorption
  - Steatorrhea
  - Fat-soluble vitamins
  - Starch, disaccharides
  - Iron, folate, vitamin B_{12}, zinc
- Electrolyte loss
- Hypocalcemia, hypomagnesemia
- Bile acid malabsorption
- Bacterial overgrowth
- Gastric acid hypersecretion
- D-Lactic acidosis
- Hyperoxaluria (renal stones)
- Cholelithiasis
- Total parenteral nutrition-induced hepatotoxicity
- Central venous catheter-related infections

Small intestinal adaptation to short bowel correlates with the length of residual bowel (51,52). Recovery takes twice as long in infants with less than 40 cm versus those with 40 to 80 cm of residual small bowel (52). Furthermore, the time to adaptive recovery from short bowel is inversely correlated with the length of residual ileum. In many studies, the absence of ileocecal valve prolongs the time to complete intestinal adaptation. In general, necrotizing enterocolitis and gastroschisis are associated with greater symptoms of short bowel and slower resolution than other etiologies (e.g., congenital atresia or volvulus). Patients

TABLE 74-2 Causes of Short Bowel Syndrome in Infants.

Cause	Wilmore, 1972[41]	Bohane et al., 1979[46]	Cooper et al., 1984[47]	Dorney et al., 1985[48]	Grosfeld et al., 1986[49]	Caniano et al., 1989[50]	Goulet et al., 1991[51]
Volvulus	30	2	6	6	5	1	22
Atresia	14	6	3	3	13	5	36
Gastochisis	5	3	2	1	5	5	10
Necrotizing enterocolitis	0	4	5	2	24	2	11
Other[a]	1	0	0	1	7	1	8
Total	**50**	**15**	**16**	**13**	**54**	**14**	**87**

[a]Meconium peritonitis, extensive intestinal angioma, complicated intussusception, congenital short bowel syndrome.
From Treem WR. Short bowel syndrome. In: Wyllie R, Hyans J, eds. *Pediatric gastrointestinal disease: pathophysiology, diagnosis, management.* Philadelphia: WB Saunders, 1993:574, with permission.

who have undergone partial or total colectomy in addition to extensive resection of the small intestine are more prone to experience severe dehydration, hypokalemia, hypomagnesemia, and hyponatremia (53). The large potential reserve capacity of the intact healthy adult colon has been demonstrated by the absorption of 6 L of water and 800 mEq of sodium, slowly perfused into the cecum of normal healthy adult volunteers (54). The colon also salvages malabsorbed carbohydrate by bacterial fermentation to short-chain fatty acids, which are absorbed and used as fuel by colonic epithelial cells or exported to the liver for energy-yielding metabolic processes.

An infant with short bowel syndrome with ileostomy can experience chronic sodium depletion with secondary hypovolemia and may require 5 to 10 mEq of sodium per kilogram body weight per day to compensate for excessive sodium loss. Hypokalemia and/or acidosis can also occur in short bowel syndrome. Deficiencies of divalent cations, especially magnesium, are common and lead to symptoms of tetany, osteopenia, osteomalacia, and spontaneous fractures. Luminal absorption of both calcium and magnesium can be compromised by fat malabsorption. Zinc deficiency can occur in the setting of chronic diarrhea or fat malabsorption. Pancreatic secretions are rich in zinc, which may be lost and inadequately replaced because of decreased ability to absorb zinc in short bowel syndrome. Malabsorption of fat-soluble vitamins (vitamins A, D, E, and K) increases with steatorrhea. Iron and folate deficiency occur when proximal small intestine has been lost. Vitamin B_{12} malabsorption is almost invariably present when more than 100 cm of terminal ileum has been resected. However, deficiency may not become apparent until after 1 to 2 years of age, as a result of in utero transfer of vitamin B_{12} stores. Terminal ileal resection can result in bile acid malabsorption. With the colon in continuity, bile acid malabsorption can lead to diarrhea, which responds to treatment with cholestyramine.

In both adults and children, gastric acid hypersecretion occurs after massive resection of the small intestine. Its magnitude appears to be proportional to the length of intestine resected; gastric acid hypersecretion is more prevalent in patients with less than one-third of the small intestine remaining (55). Treatment with an H_2-receptor antagonist for 6 to 12 months after resection is advisable.

As many as 10% of infants and children with short bowel syndrome develop cholelithiasis, and the majority of these require cholecystectomy for acute cholecystitis, biliary colic, or both (48–51). Both chronic total parenteral nutrition and ileal resection appear to be important predisposing factors for cholelithiasis (56). Early institution of enteral nutrition to stimulate the elaboration of gut hormones, gallbladder motility, and bile flow, and the use of choleretic agents, such as ursodeoxycholic acid, may prevent bile stasis and the formation of biliary sludge and stones, as well as total parenteral nutrition hepatotoxicity. Renal stones can also occur, as a result of steatorrhea with secondary increase in oxalate absorption and recurrent dehydration.

Bacterial Overgrowth Syndrome

Bacterial overgrowth may occur in short bowel syndrome and in other small bowel disorders (stagnant loop, partial small bowel obstruction, pseudoobstruction, etc.). It exacerbates malabsorption of almost all nutrients secondary to its detrimental effects on bile acid conjugation, enterocyte microvillus membrane integrity, vitamin B_{12} absorption, small intestinal motility, and the normal turnover and regeneration of the small bowel mucosa and mucosal enzymes. Factors that promote bacterial overgrowth in patients with short bowel syndrome include absence of the ileocecal valve; presence of a partial small intestine obstruction from a tight anastomosis, an ischemic stricture, or an adhesion; presence of a dilated hypotonic intestinal segment with disordered motility; presence of an enteroenteral fistula secondary to an underlying inflammatory disease, such as Crohn's disease, or a surgical complication; and relative achlorhydria secondary to the prolonged use of H_2-receptor antagonists to prevent gastric acid hypersecretion. Treatment of bacterial overgrowth consists of periodic use of oral antibiotics, such as trimethaprim-sulfamethoxazole, metronidazole, ciprofloxacin, vancomycin, or gentamicin.

Patients with small bowel bacterial overgrowth can develop D-lactic acidosis, a syndrome of encephalopathy and metabolic acidosis brought on by liberalization of the diet to include more lactose and bacterial fermentation of the lactose to D-lactic acid. Effective treatment consists of correction of the acidosis, cessation of enteral carbohydrates, and reduction of the intestinal flora with oral antibiotics.

Protracted Diarrhea in Infancy

Another group of infants with severe chronic malabsorption are those with protracted diarrhea from a variety of causes. Protracted diarrhea is defined as greater than 20 mL per kg per day of stool output that begins any time after birth, persists for more than 2 weeks, and requires change not only in the composition, but also in the mode of delivery of nutrition. The most frequent causes of protracted diarrhea produce a combined osmotic and secretory diarrhea due to severe mucosal injury. These include congenital disorders of enterocyte proliferation and differentiation, disorders of immune regulation, severe intraluminal infections, congenital mucosal ion transport defects, tumors producing intestinal secretagogues, and bacterial overgrowth secondary to functional or mechanical obstruction (Table 74-3).

TABLE 74-3 Differential Diagnosis of Protracted Diarrhea in Infancy and Childhood.

Impaired intraluminal digestion
Cystic fibrosis
Short bowel syndrome
Crohn's disease (with marked small bowel resection)
Bacterial overgrowth
Shwachman syndrome
Congenital enterokinase deficiency
Biliary atresia (other cholestatic syndromes)
Impaired microvillus membrane function
Flat villous lesion
Celiac disease
Food allergy/eosinophilic gastroenteritis
Giardia sp, *Cryptosporidium* sp, other parasites[a]
IgA deficiency, severe combined immunodeficiency, common variable hypogammaglobulinemia, acquired immune deficiency syndrome
Graft versus host disease
Rotavirus (other viral infections), usually associated with immune deficiency
Microvillus inclusion disease
Normal villi
Congenital chloridorrhea
Primary bile acid malabsorption
Congenital sucrase-isomaltase deficiency
Congenital glucose-galactose malabsorption
Congenital lactase deficiency
Impaired chylomicron formation and delivery
Abetalipoproteinemia
Congenital lymphangiectasia
Extraintestinal causes (normal villi)
Neural crest tumors (neuroblastoma, ganglioneuroma)
Laxative abuse (Munchausen by proxy, anorexia nervosa)
Iatrogenic (e.g., excess sorbitol or fructose intake)

[a]Occurs mainly in immunocompromised hosts.

Diarrhea usually begins in the first few weeks of life and is often initially accompanied by vomiting, poor feeding, and failure to thrive. Dietary manipulation with multiple formula changes and the institution of oral rehydration solutions with dilute formulas is usually the first intervention and contributes to the spiral of malnutrition that further compromises gut regeneration. In some of these infants, a trial of a hydrolyzed casein formula containing glucose polymers as the carbohydrate source may ameliorate the diarrhea. The persistence of the diarrhea with concomitant fluid and electrolyte problems and protein calorie malnutrition dictates that central venous access be established for parenteral alimentation.

It is rare that viral gastroenteritis (rotavirus, adenovirus) or enteric bacterial infections cause protracted diarrhea in infancy, unless they are associated with immune deficiency or superimposed on previous mucosal injury caused by malnutrition, cow milk or soy protein allergy, or bacterial overgrowth. In patients with congenital or acquired immunodeficiency states, chronic diarrhea can be associated with opportunistic pathogens, including *Cryptosporidium* sp, *Giardia* sp, *Isospora belli, Microsporida* sp, cytomegalovirus, and *Mycobacterium avium-intracellulare.* Bacterial overgrowth, particularly with strains of *Escherichia coli* that adhere to the enterocyte brush border, can damage the microvillus membrane and cause patchy villus atrophy and depression of brush-border enzymes (57,58).

A primary immunodeficiency state or acquired immunodeficiency syndrome should be suspected in infants with chronic diarrhea who have persistent shedding of pathogens that usually cause a self-limited diarrhea. These include *Salmonella* sp, *Giardia* sp, adenovirus, and rotavirus. Other potential clues to an underlying immunodeficiency disease include chronic thrush and diarrhea with *Candida albicans;* recurrent otitis media, sinusitis, and bronchopulmonary infections; the presence of opportunistic pathogens in the stool; chronic skin rashes; and recurrent hematologic abnormalities, including hemolytic or aplastic anemia, neutropenia, or thrombocytopenia. In T-cell or combined cellular and humoral immunodeficiency diseases, chronic diarrhea is often a presenting or prominent syndrome. Even in patients with isolated B-cell deficiencies, including isolated IgA deficiency, flat, villus lesions have been described (59). Unlike patients with gluten-sensitive enteropathy (celiac disease) or cow milk protein allergy, the flat, villus lesion seen in patients with immunodeficiency syndromes usually does not respond to removal of any food protein from the diet. Children with chronic granulomatous disease of childhood can have gastrointestinal findings that mimic Crohn's disease.

Autoimmune enteropathy should be considered in an infant with intractable diarrhea in the first 6 months of life. Infants with this disorder are typically males with secretory diarrhea who have diffuse inflammatory flat, villus lesions of the small intestine, and features of autoimmune disease, including circulating enterocyte autoantibodies and concurrent extraintestinal disease (60–62). Extraintestinal disease can take the form of membranous glomerulonephritis, interstitial nephritis, thyroiditis, hemolytic anemia, autoimmune thrombocytopenia, neutropenia, diabetes mellitus type 1, and polyarteritis nodosa. Circulating antibodies against renal epithelial cells, anti-smooth muscle antibodies, antinuclear antibodies, and antithyroid microsomal antibodies have also been detected in selected cases. Treatment with a variety of immunosuppressive agents, including azathioprine, methylprednisolone, cyclosporine, tacrolimus, and infliximab, has been effective in some cases (63). In many cases, however, the response is short lived, and relapses are common once the medication has been discontinued.

In the presence of normal small intestinal villus architecture, potential causes of protracted diarrhea include congenital transport defects, secretory tumors, and laxative-induced diarrhea as a manifestation of Munchausen syndrome by proxy (64). Congenital chloridorrhea is a rare autosomal recessive disorder resulting from a selective defect in the Cl^-, HCO_3^- exchange transport system of the ileum and colon (65). Abdominal distention, severe secretory diarrhea, and high stool chloride content are present from birth. Electrolyte disturbances in untreated patients include hyponatremia, hypochloremia, and alkalosis. Protracted diarrhea in young children can also be an important clinical manifestation of neural crest tumors such as ganglioneuromas and neuroblastomas (66,67). Laxative abuse in infants and young children can be a clinical manifestation of child abuse or Munchausen syndrome, as noted. The clinical picture of surreptitious laxative ingestion includes abdominal pain, vomiting, muscle weakness, lassitude, hypokalemia, and nonspecific inflammation, melanosis, or both on rectal biopsy. Factitious diarrhea can be recognized by a stool osmolality less than 280 mOsm per kg (i.e., diluted with water). Protracted diarrhea can also be the result of unsuspected osmotic agents used as vehicles for the suspension of common medications such as Sorbitol.

Any infant who presents with diarrhea in the first week of life and/or any child who is admitted with severe diarrhea of greater than 2 weeks' duration associated with weight loss should be given nothing by mouth and started on continuous enteral drip of an elemental formula or, if enteral feedings are not tolerated, on intravenous nutrition. It is a mistake to delay nutritional repletion while the diagnostic evaluation is taking place because malnutrition is a potential complicating factor in the perpetuation of severe protracted diarrhea. If the diarrhea ceases within 24 to 48 hours after the child is given nothing by mouth, secretory diarrhea is not present, and an evaluation for a secretory tumor by assay of serum VIP levels or urine vanillymandelic acid is not indicated. Trials of formulas that do not contain cow milk or soy protein are warranted if there are no signs of intestinal obstruction or enterocolitis. Avoidance of lactose- or sucrose-containing formulas excludes the rare genetic abnormalities of congenital lactase deficiency and sucrase-isomaltase deficiency. The persistence of the diarrhea with the use of a formula that contains glucose polymers as its sole carbohydrate helps to identify patients who have acquired monosaccharide malabsorption. This usually is secondary to a severe diffuse small intestinal injury from viral gastroenteritis or other causes.

The diagnostic evaluation suggested by the differential diagnosis should include an assessment for infectious causes, immunodeficiencies, and secretory diarrhea. Small intestine and often colonic biopsies are extremely useful in the evaluation and treatment of infants and children with protracted diarrhea. Aside from the routine histologic assessment afforded by such biopsies, special stains can be performed that illuminate infectious organisms, such as cytomegalovirus, *Cryptosporidium* sp, and *Giardia* sp. Electron microscopy is invaluable in the identification of congenital microvillus atrophy, enteroadherent bacterial overgrowth, and certain viral pathogens. Measurement of intestinal disaccharidase activity can be helpful in determining the diagnosis of congenital or acquired problems of carbohydrate absorption and direct the choice of the proper carbohydrate composition of the formula.

Celiac Disease

Celiac disease (gluten-sensitive enteropathy) is a disorder in which permanent sensitivity to dietary gluten results in small bowel mucosal damage. Symptoms at presentation are variable and can include diarrhea, failure to thrive, abdominal distention, vomiting, irritability, or poor appetite. Rarely, children may present with iron-deficiency anemia alone. Presentation is most common between 6 months and 2 years of age, but can occur at any age.

The disorder develops only after chronic dietary exposure to the gliadin fraction of the protein gluten, found in wheat, rye, and barley (not oats, as previously believed). The immunologic response to gluten results in villus atrophy, crypt hyperplasia, and damage to the surface epithelium in the small bowel, greatest in proximal small bowel. A decrease in absorptive and digestive capacity leads to maldigestion and malabsorption. Pancreatic secretion is decreased as a result of lowered small bowel secretion of cholecystokinin and secretin.

Serum antibody tests, especially endomysial antibody and tissue transglutaminase antibody, have high sensitivity and specificity for celiac disease. The diagnosis is confirmed by findings on endoscopic small bowel biopsy, as described previously. The occurrence of celiac disease is increased in children with selective IgA deficiency, diabetes mellitus, chronic rheumatoid arthritis, and Down syndrome compared with unaffected children. Endomysial and tissue transglutaminase antibodies are IgA antibodies and, therefore, may not be identified in a child with celiac disease and selective IgA deficiency. A serum IgA level should always be measured when evaluating for celiac disease.

Treatment is strict gluten-free diet, which should be planned in collaboration with an experienced dietitian. Resolution of irritability and improved appetite are usually the first signs of response to diet, and resolution of other signs and symptoms follows. If correctly diagnosed, this is a disorder requiring lifelong treatment.

Chronic Intestinal Pseudoobstruction

Chronic intestinal pseudoobstruction is characterized by signs of intestinal blockage in the absence of an anatomic obstruction. The most common signs and symptoms are abdominal distention, failure to thrive, abdominal pain, vomiting, and constipation or diarrhea. The following discussion is limited to syndromes that affect the small intestine in childhood. Causes of chronic pseudoobstruction in children are summarized in Table 74-4. These include primary congenital forms and acquired causes related to an underlying chronic disease.

The occurrence of pseudoobstruction in infants with fetal alcohol syndrome and in those who were exposed to narcotics in utero suggests that substances that potentially alter neuronal migration or maturation might affect the development of the myenteric plexus and cause severe small intestine motility problems. Some premature infants with bronchopulmonary dysplasia or with a past history of necrotizing enterocolitis appear to develop severe gastrointestinal motility disturbances, presumably related to ischemia and chronic hypoxemia that causes myenteric plexus injury. In a few cases, chronic intestinal pseudoobstruction results from a familial inherited disease (68).

Many affected children develop symptoms in the first year of life. Of children presenting with symptoms at birth, about 40% have malrotation. Abdominal distention and vomiting are the most common features. Constipation, abdominal pain, and poor weight gain are also present in many patients. Urinary tract smooth muscle is affected in about one-fifth of all intestinal pseudoobstruction patients, including those who present at birth with the aptly named megacystis-microcolon intestinal hypoperistalsis syndrome (69). The radiographic signs are usually those of intestinal obstruction (dilated small intestine loops and air–fluid levels) and the presence of a microcolon because of obstruction at birth. Antroduodenal manometry is the confirmatory test for the diagnosis of small intestinal pseudoobstruction syndrome. Once true mechanical obstruction has been excluded and the diagnosis of intestinal pseudoobstruction has been made, antroduodenal manometry can help differentiate between neuropathic and myopathic pseudoobstruction, offer prognostic information, and suggest potential responses to pharmacologic intervention (70).

TABLE 74-4 Causes of Chronic Intestinal Pseudoobstruction in Children.

Primary
Familial, sporadic, visceral neuropathies
Aganglionosis affecting the small bowel
Familial, sporadic, visceral myopathies
Neuronal intestinal dysplasia with trisomy 21, neurofibromatosis, multiple endocrine neoplasia type IIb
Megalocystis—microcolon intestinal hypoperistalsis syndrome
Acquired or associated with systemic causes
Fetal alcohol syndrome
Infants of cocaine- or narcotic-abusing mothers
Drugs—anticholinergics, opiates, calcium-channel blockers, phenothiazines, tricyclic antidepressants, vincristine
Central nervous system or spinal cord injury
Muscular dystrophies (Duchenne, myotonic)
Scleroderma, other connective tissue disorders
Familial dysautonomia
Diabetes, hypothyroidism
Chagas disease (*Trypanosoma cruzi* infection)

Food Allergy

Symptoms of food allergy are common, occurring in as many as 6% of children during the first 3 years of life (71). Although allergic proctocolitis is the most frequent manifestation in infancy, small bowel involvement with protracted diarrhea, vomiting, malabsorption, and failure to thrive may occur. This presentation is associated with patchy villus atrophy on small bowel biopsy. With small bowel involvement, reaction to food challenge, as well as resolution of symptoms on removal of the offending food, may take several days to weeks.

In making the diagnosis of food allergy, other nonallergic mechanisms of food intolerance should be considered (e.g., lactose intolerance). Response to food challenge and elimination diet suggests the diagnosis. Skin tests or radioallergosorbent tests (RASTs) measure the presence of specific IgE. In children younger than 1 year of age, a positive skin test or RAST is likely to be meaningful, whereas a negative test does not rule out allergy. The reverse is true in children older than 1 year of age; a positive test for specific IgE does not mean that a specific food is the cause of symptoms, but only that it may be.

Treatment for food allergy is elimination diet. At least 30% of infants allergic to cow milk are also allergic to soy protein. Furthermore, some infants continue to demonstrate allergic manifestations when fed protein hydrolysate formula and require a crystalline amino acid formula (72).

Symptoms with food challenge resolve by 3 years of age in 85% of infants with food hypersensitivity. Resolution of symptoms from cow milk or soy protein hypersensitivity is common by 1 year of age. When milk is reintroduced, 1 tsp or less should be offered at first. For a child who has previously demonstrated a severe reaction to a food allergen, challenge should be performed only in a medical setting where anaphylaxis can be treated. In older children, symptoms caused by allergy to peanut, nuts, fish, or shellfish rarely resolve.

Hemolytic-Uremic Syndrome

Strictly speaking, the definition of hemolytic-uremic syndrome includes the triad of microangiopathic hemolytic anemia, thrombocytopenia, and acute renal failure. In the United States, it is most often associated with an enteric infection with the verotoxin-producing bacteria *E. coli* 0157:H7, and typically presents with a prodrome of bloody diarrhea before the onset of obvious hemolysis, thrombocytopenia, or oliguria and renal failure (73,74). The association with *E. coli* 0157:H7 is much less striking in other parts of the world. For example, in Argentina, only 2% of children with hemolytic-uremic syndrome are infected with *E. coli,* but 55% have evidence of an antecedent infection with *Shigella* sp (75). Epidemic outbreaks of hemolytic-uremic syndrome have been associated with the ingestion of raw or poorly cooked ground beef and unpasteurized milk.

Both the intestinal wall and renal injury appear to be caused by endothelial cell damage, intravascular platelet activation, and subsequent ischemic intestinal and renal disease. Endothelial damage may occur by a variety of proposed mechanisms, including direct bacterial cytotoxin-induced cytolysis, systemic endotoxin release, cell membrane lipid peroxidization, or immune complex-mediated injury. In addition to bloody diarrhea, crampy abdominal pain and vomiting may be part of the prodrome. At times, peritoneal signs are prominent, leading to consideration of an exploratory laparotomy. Usually, as the gastrointestinal symptoms subside, the other features of pallor, severe anemia, petechiae, easy bruising, thrombocytopenia, oliguria, edema, hypertension, electrolyte disturbances, and renal failure become evident.

Stool cultures for routine pathogens are usually negative. Many laboratories can culture for *E. coli* 0157:H7 if it is specifically requested. A careful examination of the blood smear may reveal early changes of microangiopathic hemolytic anemia and a disproportionately low platelet count in the setting of inflammatory enterocolitis. A flat plate of the abdomen often shows "thumbprinting," indicative of edema and mucosal hemorrhage in the intestinal wall. The endoscopic appearance of the colon is nonspecific, and the mucosa usually appears hyperemic, edematous, and friable (76). Perforations of the small intestine and colon are recognized complications of the ischemic bowel disease (although the latter can be caused by the insertion of a peritoneal dialysis catheter). Intussusception has also been reported, and intestinal strictures and fistulas are late complications.

Henoch-Schönlein Purpura

Henoch-Schönlein purpura is a vasculitis that primarily affects the postcapillary venules of the intestine, skin, kidneys, and joints. It commonly presents with a prodrome of abdominal pain, a purpuric rash, and then later manifestations of nephritis, arthritis, and edema. Occult gastrointestinal blood loss is common, but only about 3% of children have gross lower intestinal bleeding. Henoch-Schönlein purpura generally affects children younger than 7 years of age, and most cases occur in clusters in the winter and early spring (77). Almost all pediatric cases are preceded by a viral or bacterial illness, including cases associated with hepatitis A and B and parvovirus (78).

The central pathogenic mechanism appears to be the deposition of IgA immune complexes on postcapillary venules throughout the body, triggered by some unknown antigen (79). The alternate complement pathway is activated, resulting in the depletion of plasma C_3 and the deposition of C_3 in immune complexes. The rash has a predilection for the lower extremities and buttocks, and is described as *palpable purpura*. Abdominal pain and blood in the stool may appear as early as 1 month before the rash, leading to erroneous diagnoses of infectious colitis, intussusception, or inflammatory bowel disease. Joint pain and overt pauciarticular arthritis occur in more than one-half of affected patients, with the knees and ankles most commonly involved. Renal involvement with overt hematuria and proteinuria occurs in about 40% of patients. Less common manifestations include central nervous system vasculitis, leading to encephalopathic changes and even seizures (80); pancreatitis; orchitis; cholecystitis; hydrops of the gallbladder; and pulmonary hemorrhage. Intussusception may occur with edematous intestine acting as a lead point; rarely, the intestine perforates or becomes strictured secondary to the transmural ischemia. Both upper and lower gastrointestinal endoscopy reveal purpuric lesions of the stomach, small intestine, and colon that are similar to those seen in the skin. Punctate hemorrhages may also be seen. Biopsy of the skin or intestine shows vasculitis with selective IgA and C_3 deposition on the wall of small veins, a finding that differentiates Henoch-Schönlein purpura from other vasculitides.

REFERENCES

1. Siebert JR. Small-intestinal length in infants and children. *Am J Dis Child* 1980;134:593.
2. Klish WJ, Putnam TC. The short gut. *Am J Dis Child* 1981;35:1056.
3. Morriss FH Jr, Moore M, Weisbrodt NW, et al. Ontogenic development of gastrointestinal motility. IV. Duodenal contractions in preterm infants. *Pediatrics* 1986;78:1106.
4. McLain CR. Amniography studies of the gastrointestinal motility in human fetus. *Am J Obstet Gynecol* 1963;86:1079.
5. Bisset WM.Intestinal motor activity in the preterm infant. In: Milla PJ, Welburn P, eds. *Disorders of gastrointestinal motility in childhood.* Chichester, UK: Wiley, 1988:29.
6. Berseth CL. Neonatal small intestinal motility: motor responses to feeding in term and preterm infants. *J Pediatr* 1990;117:777.
7. Antonowicz I, Lebenthal E. Developmental pattern of small intestinal enterokinase and disaccharidase activities in the human fetus. *Gastroenterology* 1977;72:1299.
8. Younoszai MK. Jejunal absorption of hexose in infants and adults. *J Pediatr* 1986;85:446.
9. Watkins JB, Szczepanik P, Gould JB, et al. Bile salt metabolism in the human premature infant. *Gastroenterology* 1975;69:706.
10. Heubi JE, Balistreri WF, Suchy FJ. Bile salt metabolism in the first year of life. *J Lab Clin Med* 1982;100:127.
11. Lester R, Smallwood RA, Little JM, et al. Fetal bile salt metabolism: the intestinal absorption of bile salts. *J Clin Invest* 1977;59:1009.
12. Henning SJ. Postnatal development: coordination of feeding, digestion, and metabolism. *Am J Physiol* 1981;241:G199.
13. Mienge H, Robinson JWL. Functional and structural characteristics of the rat intestinal mucosa following ileojejunal transposition. *Acta Hepatogastroenterol* 1986;25:150.
14. Madara JL.Functional morphology of epithelium of the small intestine. In: Field M, ed. *Handbook of physiology, vol. 4, sec. 6: the gastrointestinal system.* New York: Oxford University Press, 1991:83.
15. Wood JD. Intrinsic neural control of intestinal motility. *Annu Rev Physiol* 1981;43:33.
16. Vantrappen G, Janssens J, Ghoos Y. The interdigestive motor complex of normal subjects and patients with bacterial over-growth of the small intestine. *J Clin Invest* 1977;59:1158.
17. Vantrappen GR, Peeters TL, Janssens J. The secretory component of the interdigestive migrating motor complex in man. *Scand J Gastroenterol* 1979;14:663.
18. Sarna SK, Soergel KH, Harig JM, et al. Spatial and temporal patterns of human jejunal contractions. *Am J Physiol* 1989;257:G423.
19. Thompson DG, Ritchie HD, Wingate DL. Patterns of small intestinal motility in duodenal ulcer patients before and after vagotomy. *Gut* 1982;23:517.
20. Sarna SK, Otterson MF. Small intestinal physiology and pathophysiology. *Gastroenterol Clin North Am* 1989;18:375.
21. Tomomasa T, Miyazki M, Igarashi T, et al. The effect of erythromycin on the gastroduodenal motility in human premature infants. *J Gastrointest Motil* 1991;3:205.
22. Hall KE, Greenberg GR, El-Sharkawy TY, et al. Relationship between porcine motilin-induced migrating motor complex-like activity, vagal integrity, and endogenous motilin release in dogs. *Gastroenterology* 1984;87:78.
23. Bueno L, Fioramonti J, Ruckebusch Y. Postoperative intestinal motility in dogs and sheep. *Dig Dis Sci* 1978;23:682.
24. Boivin M, Raymond MC, RiBerdy M, et al. Plasma motilin variation during the interdigestive and digestive states in man. *J Gastrointest Motil* 1990;2:240.
25. Sullivan SK, Field M. Ion transport across mammalial small intestine. In: Field M, ed. *Handbook of physiology, vol. 4, sec. 6: the gastrointestinal system.* New York: Oxford University Press, 1991:287.
26. Field M. Intestinal ion transport mechanisms. In: *Diarrheal diseases.* New York: Elsevier, 1991:3.
27. Dobbins JW, Laurenson JP, Forrest JN. Adenosine and adenosine analogues stimulate adenosine cyclic 3′,5′-monophosphate-dependent chloride secretion in the mammalial ileum. *J Clin Invest* 1984;74:929.
28. Jones JB, Mehta NR, Hamosh M. Alpha-amylase in preterm human milk. *J Pediatr Gastroenterol Nutr* 1982;1:43.
29. Fogel MR, Gray GM. Starch hydrolysis in man: an intraluminal process not requiring membrane digestion. *J Appl Physiol* 1973;35:263.
30. Adler G, Beglinder C. Hormones as regulators of pancreatic secretion in man. *Eur J Clin Invest* 1990;20:S27.
31. Hamosh M, Bitman J, Liao TH, et al. Gastric lipolysis and fat absorption in preterm infants: effect of medium-chain triglyceride- or long-chain triglyceride-containing formulas. *Pediatrics* 1989;83:86.
32. Bernback S, Blackberg L, Hernell O. The complete digestion of human milk triacylglycerol *in vitro* requires gastric lipase, pancreatic colipase-dependent lipase and bile salt-stimulated lipase. *J Clin Invest* 1990;85:1221.
33. Gaskin KJ, Durie PR, Lee L, et al. Colipase and lipase secretion in childhood-onset pancreatic insufficiency: delineation of patients with steatorrhea secondary to relative colipase deficiency. *Gastroenterology* 1984;86:1.
34. Proulx P, Aubry H, Brglez I, et al. Studies on the uptake of fatty acids by brush border membranes of the rabbit intestine. *Can J Biochem Cell Biol* 1984;63:249.
35. Shiau Y-F, Levine GM. pH dependence of micellar diffusion and dissociation. *Am J Physiol* 1980;239:G177.
36. Curtis KJ, Graines HD, Kim YS. Protein digestion and absorption in rats with pancreatic duct occlusion. *Gastroenterology* 1978;74:1271.
37. Guan D, Yoshioka M, Erickson RH, et al. Protein digestion in human and rat small intestine: role of new neutral endopeptidases. *Am J Physiol* 1988;255:G212.
38. Van der Schoor SR, Reeds PJ, Stoll B, et al. The high metabolic cost of a functional gut. *Gastroenterology* 2002;123:1931.
39. Wu G. Intestinal mucosal amino acid catabolism. *J Nutr* 1998;128:1249.
40. Vanderhoof JA, Antonsen DL, Kaufman SS, et al. Combined liver/intestinal versus isolated intestinal transplantation in children. *Gastroenterology* 1995;108:A221.
41. Wilmore DW. Factors correlating with a successful outcome following extensive intestinal resection in newborn infants. *J Pediatr* 1972;80:88.
42. Hwang TL, O'Dwyer ST, Smith RJ, et al. Preservation of small bowel mucosa using glutamine enriched parenteral nutrition. *Surg Forum* 1986;37:56.
43. Taylor B, Murphy GM, Dowling RH. Effect of food intake and the pituitary on intestinal structure and function after resection [Abstract]. *Gut* 1975;16:397.
44. Burne TA, Morrissey TB, Ziegler TR, et al. Growth hormone, glutamine, and fiber-enhanced adaptation of remnant bowel following massive intestinal resection. *Surg Forum* 1992;43:151.
45. Gillingham MB, Dahly EM, Murali SG, et al. IGF-I treatment facilitates transition from parenteral to enteral nutrition in rats with short bowel syndrome. *Am J Physiol* 2003;284:R363.
46. Bohane TD, Haka-Ikse K, Biggar WD, et al. A clinical study of young infants after small intestinal resection. *J Pediatr* 1979;94:552.
47. Cooper A, Floyd TF, Ross AJ, et al. Morbidity and mortality of short-bowel syndrome acquired in infancy: an update. *J Pediatr Surg* 1984;19:711.

48. Dorney SFA, Ament ME, Berquist WE, et al. Improved survival in very short small bowel of infancy with use of long-term parenteral nutrition. *J Pediatr* 1985;107:521.
49. Grosfeld JL, Rescorla FJ, West JW. Short bowel syndrome in infancy and childhood. *Am J Surg* 1986;151:41.
50. Caniano DA, Starr J, Ginn-Pease ME. Extensive short-bowel syndrome in neonates: outcome in the 1980's. *Surgery* 1989;105:119.
51. Goulet OJ, Revillon Y, Jan D, et al. Neonatal short bowel syndrome. *J Pediatr* 1991;119:18.
52. Sondheimer JM, Cadnapaphornchai M, Sontag M, et al. Predicting the duration of dependence on patenteral nutrition after neonatal intestinal resection. *J Pediatr* 1998;132:80.
53. Allard JP, Jeejeebhoy KN. Nutritional support and therapy in the short bowel syndrome. *Gastroenterol Clin* 1989;18:589.
54. Debongnie JC, Phillips SF. Capacity of the human colon to absorb fluid. *Gastroenterology* 1978;74:468.
55. Hyman PE, Everett SL, Haranda T. Gastric acid hypersecretion in short bowel syndrome in infants: association with extent of resection and enteral feeding. *J Pediatr Gastroenterol Nutr* 1986;5:191.
56. Roslyn JJ, Berquist WE, Pitt HA, et al. Increased risk of gallstones in children receiving total parenteral nutrition. *Pediatrics* 1983;71:784.
57. Sherman P, Drum B, Karmali M, et al. Adherence of bacteria to the intestine in sporadic cases of enteropathogenic *Escherichia coli*-associated diarrhea in infants and young children: a prospective study. *Gastroenterology* 1989;96:86.
58. Hill SM, Phillips AD, Walker-Smith JA. Enteropathogenic *Escherichia coli* and life-threatening chronic diarrhea. *Gut* 1991;32:154.
59. Anderson KE, Finlayson NDC, Deschner EE. Intractable malabsorption with flat jejunal mucosa and selective IgA deficiency. *Gastroenterology* 1974;67:709.
60. Walker-Smith JA, Unsworth DJ, Hutchins P, et al. Autoantibodies against gut epithelium in child with small intestinal enteropathy. *Lancet* 1982;1:566.
61. Colletti RB, Guillot AP, Rosen S, et al. Autoimmune enteropathy and nephropathy with circulating autoantibodies. *J Pediatr* 1991;118:853.
62. Hill SM, Milla PJ, Bottazzo GF, et al. Autoimmune enteropathy and colitis: is there a generalized autoimmune gut disorder? *Gut* 1991;32:36.
63. Seidman EG, Lacaille F, Russo P, et al. Successful treatment of autoimmune enteropathy with cyclosporine. *J Pediatr* 1990;117:929.
64. Ackerman NB, Strobel CT. Polle syndrome: chronic diarrhea in Munchausen's child. *Gastroenterology* 1981;81:1140.
65. Bieberdorf FA, Gorden P, Fordtran JS. Pathogenesis of congenital alkalosis with diarrhea. *J Clin Invest* 1985;51:1958.
66. Kaplan SJ, Holbrook CT, McDaniel HG, et al. Vasoactive intestinal peptide secreting tumors in childhood. *Am J Dis Child* 1980;134:21.
67. Mitchell CH, Sinatra FR, Crast FW, et al. Intractable watery diarrhea, ganglioneuroblastoma and vasoactive intestinal peptide. *J Pediatr* 1976;89:593.
68. Mayer EA, Schuffler MD, Rotter JI, et al. Familial visceral neuropathy with autosomal dominant transmission. *Gastroenterology* 1986;91:1528.
69. Vargas JH, Sachs P, Ament ME. Chronic intestinal pseudo-obstruction syndrome in pediatrics: results of a national survey of members of the North American Society of Pediatric Gastroenterology and Nutrition. *J Pediatr Gastroenterol Nutr* 1988;7:323.
70. Hyman PE, McDiarmid SV, Napolitano JA, et al. Antroduodenal motility in children with chronic intestinal pseudo-obstruction. *J Pediatr* 1988;112:889.
71. Sampson HA. Food allergy. *JAMA* 1997;278:1888.
72. Vanderhoof JA, Murray ND, Kaufman SS, et al. Intolerance to protein hydrolysate infant formulas: an underrecognized cause of gastrointestinal symptoms in infants. *J Pediatr* 1997;131:741.
73. Martin DL, MacDonald KL, White KE. The epidemiology and clinical aspects of the hemolytic-uremic syndrome in Minnesota. *N Engl J Med* 1991;323:1161.
74. Neill MA, Agosti J, Rosen H. Hemorrhagic colitis with *Escherichia coli* 0157:H7 preceding adult hemolytic uremic syndrome. *Arch Intern Med* 1985;145:2215.
75. Lopez EL, Diaz M, Grinstein S, et al. Hemolytic uremic syndrome and diarrhea in Argentine children: the role of Shiga-like toxins. *J Infect Dis* 1989;160:469.
76. Berman W Jr. The hemolytic uremic syndrome: initial clinical presentation mimicking ulcerative colitis. *J Pediatr* 1972;81:275.
77. Allen DM, Diamond LK, Howell DA. Anaphylactoid purpura in children (Schönlein-Henoch syndrome). *Am J Dis Child* 1960;99:833.
78. LeFrere J, Courouce A, Soulier J, et al. Henoch-Schönlein purpura and human parvovirus infection. *Pediatrics* 1986;78:183.
79. Stevenson JA, Leong LA, Cohen AH, et al. Henoch-Schönlein purpura: simultaneous demonstration of IgA deposits in involved skin, intestine, and kidney. *Arch Pathol Lab Med* 1982;106:192.
80. Belman A, Leicher C, Moshe S, et al. Neurologic manifestations of Schönlein-Henoch purpura: report of three cases and review of the literature. *Pediatrics* 1985;75:687.

Chapter 75

Short Bowel Syndrome

Richard A. Falcone, Jr. and Brad W. Warner

Short bowel syndrome (SBS) is a term that is loosely used to define the pathophysiologic disorders that result from the removal of a large portion of the small intestine. Although this problem most commonly results from an anatomic loss or deficiency of intestinal surface area; it may also occur in the context of normal intestinal mucosal surface area due to perturbed intestinal absorption, motility, or both. The clinical syndrome leads to malnutrition, weight loss, steatorrhea, and diarrhea as a consequence of the inability of the gastrointestinal tract to absorb nutrients.

The introduction of total parenteral nutrition (TPN) (1) has resulted in a remarkable improvement in survival for patients with SBS. Unfortunately, the most common cause of death associated with SBS is TPN-induced hepatic dysfunction. However, the survival for patients with less than or equal to 40 cm of residual small bowel is routine, and long-term survival of infants with as little as 20 to 30 cm of small bowel can be expected. More recently, an infant was reported who survived off TPN with only 11 cm of small bowel and without an ileocecal valve (2). Fortunately, the dismal outcomes reported by Haymond in 1935, including a 33% operative mortality and 20% 1-year survivals, are of historic interest only. More recent estimates suggest that at least 70% of patients with SBS leave the hospital and nearly all are alive at the end of 1 year (3). The goals of management in these patients are to reduce the duration of TPN use and to intervene to maximize intestinal nutrient absorption. Multiple nutritional, hormonal, and surgical therapies have evolved to manage patients with SBS in an attempt to improve quality of life and decrease the duration of TPN dependence.

Richard A. Falcone, Jr.: Division of Pediatric and Thoracic Surgery, Cincinnati Children's Hospital Medical Center, Department of Surgery, University of Cincinnati College of Medicine, Cincinnati, Ohio 45229.

Brad W. Warner: University of Cincinnati College of Medicine, Department of Pediatric Surgery, Cincinnati Children's Hospital Medical Center, Cincinnati, Ohio 45229.

ETIOLOGY

The specific causes of SBS in the pediatric population have changed over time. Previously, the most common causes were midgut volvulus and intestinal atresia; however, in more contemporary reports, the most common cause of SBS is neonatal necrotizing enterocolitis (NEC) (4–8). Other causes of SBS in children include loss of bowel from mesenteric vascular occlusion, such as may occur from invasive aortic monitoring devices, neonatal aortic thrombosis, or cardiogenic emboli. Reduced perfusion states secondary to cardiogenic, hypovolemic, or septic shock, as well as the use of vasoconstrictive inotropic agents, may result in ischemic or necrotic bowel. Meconium ileus or plugging may promote the development of a volvulus with necrosis. Volvulus with intestinal necrosis may follow adhesive bowel obstruction associated with prior abdominal surgery or an intraabdominal inflammatory process.

Functional disorders in which the anatomic bowel length is normal, but motility and absorption capacity are impaired, include long-segment aganglionosis and the syndrome of idiopathic intestinal pseudoobstruction. Gastroschisis can be associated with SBS due to a combination of foreshortening of intestinal length, as well as dysfunctional peristalsis of the thickened bowel loops. Crohn's disease may be associated with SBS because of multiple, extensive resections, bypassed absorptive mucosa due to fistulae, or impaired mucosal absorptive capacity.

Clinical Course

The normal small intestine length for a full-term infant is approximately 200 to 250 cm. In the fetus, the overall rate of growth of the gastrointestinal tract increases with age. The period of most rapid growth occurs during the third trimester. In fact, the small bowel can be expected to double in length between the second and third trimester. The rate of small intestinal lengthening due to growth alone is rapid during infancy with continued elongation until crown-heel length (CHL) reaches about 60 cm. Slower intestinal growth then occurs between a CHL of 60 to 100 cm, and there is little change above 100 to 140 cm (9). Therefore, after massive enterectomy, consideration should be given to the expected rate of bowel lengthening due to growth alone. Further, prognosis should be based not on absolute intestinal length, but on the percentage of normal for a given gestational age following resection. Survival and complete return of gastrointestinal function may be predicted when the postresection length of intestine exceeds 5% of normal for gestational age when the ileocecal valve remains, or greater than 10% of normal if the ileocecal valve has been lost (10).

The clinical course of patients with SBS involves several stages. There is an initial perioperative period of extreme fluid and electrolyte loss. This is followed by initial enteral feeding and a period of intestinal adaptation. Finally, a chronic or plateau stage is reached after 1 to 2 years if the adaptive intestinal response is inadequate. It is this final phase when the persistent problems of malabsorption, diarrhea, parenteral nutrition, and chronic nutritional deficiencies occur. The initial postoperative management is therefore directed toward fluid and electrolyte replacement. Large volumes of fluid may be lost from an ostomy, and replacement with a solution containing comparable electrolyte composition may be required to avoid fluid and electrolyte imbalance. The early postoperative care may be further complicated by the need for reoperation because of intraabdominal infections and/or fistulae. This early stage generally lasts about 1 to 2 weeks (11).

By removing specific portions of the small bowel, certain complications become more prevalent. Jejunectomy produces no permanent defect in the absorption of macronutrients and electrolytes because the ileum is capable of taking over these absorptive functions. Several of the intestinal hormones responsible for inhibiting gastric secretion are distributed mainly in the jejunum, and therefore, jejunectomy is more likely to result in gastric hypersecretion (11). In contrast, the ileum has a pronounced effect in slowing intestinal transit. Thus, ileal resection generally results in more rapid intestinal transit. The ileum is also an essential site for the absorption and recycling bile salts. As such, bile salt waste is associated with extensive ileal resection. Under these circumstances, the bile salt pool becomes depleted, leading to a high incidence of cholelithiasis and malabsorption of fat (11). It is for this reason that prophylactic cholecystectomy may be beneficial in the setting of SBS. The malabsorption of fat leads to deficiency of fat-soluble vitamins A, D, E, and K. In addition, vitamin B_{12} malabsorption after ileal resection may necessitate parenteral vitamin B_{12} on a monthly basis (12).

Patients with SBS are also at increased risk of developing hyperoxaluria, and this is associated with nephrolithiasis. Rarely, children with extensive small bowel resections may develop D-lactic acidosis. This occurs secondary to alterations in colonic pH and inhibition of the growth of Bacteroides species of bacteria. This leads to the increased growth of acid-resistant anaerobes capable of producing D-lactate.

The final stage following massive small bowel resection is the plateau phase, which occurs following maximal adaptation. This stage is generally reached within 1 to 2 years from the time of resection. It is during this final stage that decisions regarding additional surgical intervention are generally undertaken. Remedial surgical procedures may be indicated earlier in the face of the appearance of liver dysfunction or failure to advance enteral calories.

INTESTINAL ADAPTATION

Following massive small bowel resection (SBR), adaptive changes in the remaining intestine are detected as soon as 48 hours (13). This process probably continues for more than 1 year in humans. The adaptive response is mediated primarily by a mitogenic signal culminating in significantly taller villi, deeper crypts, and greater caliber and length of the intestine. In face of massive SBR, these morphologic alterations serve to expand the mucosal digestive and absorptive surface area (14). The key elements that control enterocyte proliferation and intestinal adaptation are incompletely understood. The magnitude of the adaptive response is directly related to the time interval following resection (13,15) and the amount of intestine removed. The degree of adaptation is greater after proximal SBR when compared with a distal resection of similar magnitude.

Studies by Loran et al. confirmed that the augmented villus height and crypt depth are the result of increased proliferation and accelerated cellular migration along the villus (16,17). Furthermore, similar villus cell densities, unaltered RNA/DNA ratios, and increased protein content suggest it is epithelial hyperplasia rather than hypertrophy that accounts for these changes (16,17). The increase in crypt epithelial cell proliferation occurs shortly after surgical resection.

Previously, it was believed that the increased cell proliferation during intestinal adaptation was balanced simply by the natural loss of senescent enterocytes from the villi into the intestinal lumen. However, more recent work has highlighted the importance of apoptosis or programmed cell death in the cellular homeostasis of the intestinal epithelium (18). Helmrath et al. reported significantly increased rates of crypt apoptosis in the remnant ileum of mice that had undergone SBR when compared with control mice (15).

Specific members of the bcl-2 gene family appear to be important in the regulation of resection-induced enterocyte apoptosis. Stern et al. reported a significant reduction in the antiapoptosis protein bcl-w coincident with an increase in the expression of the proapoptosis member of the bcl-2 family bax in the remnant intestine following SBR (19). Further, this group reported that the increase in postresection apoptosis was prevented in bax-null mice (20). Bax therefore appears to be a key regulator of postresection apoptosis.

In addition to various morphologic changes, the remnant intestine undergoes functional adaptation to counteract the acute loss of digestive and absorptive capacity after resection. Like the structural alterations, changes in enterocyte function are more prominent after a proximal intestinal resection. Because diarrhea is a common complication of massive intestinal resections, adaptive increases in sodium and water absorption are particularly important. Active Na^+/substrate transporters, Na^+/H^+ exchangers (NHE), and passive Na^+ channels facilitate sodium absorption and the subsequent passage of water and chloride (21). NHE activity, as well as mRNA and protein levels of the NHE-3 isoform, are increased in the residual intestine after resection (21). The Na^+/glucose cotransporter is the primary mechanism for sodium transport in the small bowel (22). Schulzke et al. found a 2.5-fold increase in glucose-dependent sodium absorption per centimeter of intestine following 70% SBR in rats (23).

Multiple mechanisms and mediators have been proposed to be required for the initiation and maintenance of the postresection adaptation response. There is strong evidence to implicate a role for luminal nutrients, gastrointestinal secretions, and humoral factors in the genesis of adaptation. Further, the nutritional status of the host, as well as neural, bacterial, and mechanical factors, have become more clear recently.

The important contributions of luminal nutrients to the adaptive response of the intestine is underscored by the observations that gut mucosal atrophy is associated with starvation and is reversed by refeeding. Further, under normal conditions, indicators of adaptation such as bowel wall thickness, villus height, and crypt depth are greatest in the proximal jejunum and decrease as one moves toward the terminal ileum. This aboral gradient coincides with the nutrient composition of the ingested luminal contents. Because absorption of luminal carbohydrate, fat, and protein is virtually completed in the jejunum, the ileal mucosa is not normally exposed to high concentrations of these nutrients. In fact, surgical transposition of a segment of the ileum into the more proximal intestinal stream results in structural and functional "jejunalization" of the transposed ileum (24).

The most compelling evidence that luminal nutrients play a significant physiologic role is the observation that postresection adaptive changes in animals receiving only parenteral nutrition are attenuated (25). However, it is likely that the effect of luminal nutrients is indirect, including hormones, various gastrointestinal secretions, intestinal peristalsis, and mucosal blood flow. An indirect effect of luminal nutrients is best demonstrated in experiments where enteral feeding of an animal results in reversal of mucosal atrophy within a Thiry-Vella loop, which is not in continuity with the remainder of the gastrointestinal tract (26).

Not only is the presence of luminal nutrition important for adaptation, but also the composition of the nutrients. More complex nutrients require more metabolic energy to absorb and digest. They appear to induce the greatest adaptive response, the so-called *functional workload hypothesis* (27). Enteral fats appear to be the most effective of the trophic macronutrients in inducing adaptation. More specifically, longer-chain and more unsaturated fats may provide an even greater stimulus for adaptation (28). Further, supplementation of the enteral diet with pectin (a source of short-chain fatty acids) has revealed an enhanced adaptation response.

Another important luminal nutrient to consider is glutamine, an enterocyte-specific fuel. Enteral supplementation with glutamine after intestinal resection in animal and human models has yielded conflicting results (29,30). It appears that glutamine contributes to the proliferative effects of several different endogenous growth factors such as epidermal growth factor (EGF) (31) and insulinlike growth factor-1.

Multiple experimental observations contribute to the notion that endogenous gastrointestinal secretions are important for adaptation. Similar to the previous arguments related to luminal nutrition, there is a declining aboral gradient in bowel thickness from the origin of the pancreaticobiliary secretions (ampulla of Vater) toward the ileum. Transposition of the ampulla to areas more distal in the gastrointestinal tract results in villus hyperplasia beyond the transposed ampulla. Bile alone has been demonstrated to stimulate intestinal RNA and DNA content when directly delivered to the mid-small bowel, but the effect seems to be more profound when combined with the pancreatic secretions. In other studies, pancreatic secretions seem to be more trophic to the intestinal mucosa when compared with bile.

Further evidence that pancreaticobiliary secretions are important for postresection adaptation is the observation that somatostatin, an agent that dramatically diminishes the output of endogenous gastrointestinal secretions, also inhibits the adaptation response. The inhibitory effect of somatostatin is reversible with growth factor administration *in vivo* (32). However, the results of an *in vitro* study suggest that somatostatin perturbs the proliferative effects of growth factor administration (33). Along these lines, it is unclear what component(s) of the pancreaticobiliary secretions may be trophic to the intestinal mucosa. Because many growth factors are concentrated within the pancreaticobiliary secretions, it is possible that these are the necessary constituents for mucosal stimulation.

Increased serum or tissue levels of multiple hormones, growth factors, and cytokines after massive SBR have been taken as support for the concept that these factors play a role in the pathogenesis of adaptation. Coupled with these observations, exogenous administration of many of these substances has been shown to enhance various components of the adaptation response. One of the more compelling experiments to substantiate the contribution of hormones to adaptation is the parabiosis model. In animals that share a common circulation, it has been shown that intestinal resection in one animal induces adaptive changes in the intestine of the unoperated animal (34). The most important circulating factor(s) is unknown, but this question is presently under intense investigation.

Although a multitude of hormones and growth factors have been proposed to mediate postresection adaptation, there is significant evidence to support the hypothesis that EGF and its intestinal receptor [epidermal growth factor receptor (EGFR)] are crucial (35). Similar to other known trophic substances, exogenous administration of EGF enhances adaptation. The optimal route (orogastric gavage), dose (50 μg per kg per day), and timing of EGF administration (immediately following intestinal resection, not prior to or after adaptation had already taken place) in a murine model of SBR have been detailed. Following a 50% proximal enterectomy, there is evidence for increased expression of mRNA and protein, as well as activation of the ileal EGFR. The direct effect of EGF on the intestine was proven by demonstrating that transgenic mice with targeted intestinal overexpression of EGF "superadapt" to massive small bowel resection. In these mice, EGF was overexpressed only in the remnant intestine, without affecting serum levels of EGF.

However, surgical removal of the major source of EGF in the mouse (bilateral submandibular gland resection) prior to SBR resulted in a significantly blunted adaptation response in the remnant ileum (36). Exogenous EGF rescued this impaired adaptation. Adaptation after intestinal resection is substantially impaired in a mutant strain of mice with defective EGFR signaling (37). Taken together, the evidence accumulated in the murine model for intestinal resection would strongly support the hypothesis that EGF and the intestinal EGFR are requisite for the normal adaptation response.

Glucagon-like peptide 2 (GLP-2) is another intestinotrophic peptide that has been shown to enhance intestinal adaptation (38). The glucagon-like peptides are synthesized in and released from enteroendocrine cells in the small and large intestine. In rat models of massive small bowel resection, GLP-2 has been shown to produce significant increases in segmental and mucosal wet weight. In addition, crypt-villus height and mucosal sucrase activity are enhanced postresection following the administration of GLP-2. GLP-2 appears to enhance adaptation by both increased cellular proliferation and decreased crypt epithelial cell apoptosis (39).

In a clinical study of short bowel patients, GLP-2 has been shown to provide modest improvement in intestinal absorption and nutritional status (40). Despite these limitations, the data supporting potential use of GLP-2 for the pharmacologic management of SBS is encouraging.

Growth hormone (GH) has also been investigated for its potential role in improving intestinal function in patients with SBS. There have been several studies demonstrating the beneficial effect of GH on nitrogen balance in patients receiving parenteral nutrition; however, these studies have not evaluated the effects of GH on intestinal absorption. It is possible that the effects of GH on protein catabolism and nitrogen excretion rather than on intestinal adaptation may account for these findings (41).

INTESTINAL BARRIER FUNCTION FOLLOWING MASSIVE INTESTINAL RESECTION

A major cause of morbidity and mortality in patients with SBS is sepsis. Because patients with SBS are typically receiving parenteral nutrition, the nidus for most episodes of infection is often attributed to the central venous catheter. However, in this group of patients, there is mounting evidence to suggest that the intestine itself may be an important source of pathogens. In contrast with the expected gram-positive bacteremia associated with central venous catheter sepsis, there is a high frequency of gram-negative bacteremia during septic episodes in patients with SBS. Further, the clinical incidence of liver injury and cholestasis may be reduced when measures are taken to reduce bacterial levels in the gut lumen (42).

Studies that have examined the role of postresection adaptation on intestinal permeability are conflicting and limited in number. Disparate experimental results likely reflect the different times the ileum was studied after resection and underscore the dynamic nature of intestinal adaptation. In one study, O'Brien et al. were unable to demonstrate significant alterations in intestinal epithelial permeability in mice at multiple time points following a 50% SBR (43). Despite the similar permeability to two markers of varied molecular weight, the SBR animals demonstrated greater translocation of bacteria to mesenteric lymph nodes and liver. These findings suggest that increased postresection bacterial translocation is likely not due to simple alterations in intestinal permeability.

The exact mechanism for increased bacterial translocation in patients with SBS is not well understood. Alverdy et al. demonstrated a dramatic decrease in the biliary production of secretory IgA, which reduces bacterial passage *in vitro*, in rats 2 weeks after the initiation of parenteral nutrition (44). Alterations in postresection immune function may therefore contribute to changes in the barrier function of the intestinal mucosa. Further research to characterize the complex pathophysiology of permeability and bacterial translocation during intestinal adaptation is ongoing.

MEDICAL AND NUTRITIONAL MANAGEMENT

The most important therapeutic objective in the management of the SBS is to maintain the patient's nutritional status and to support continued growth. TPN should begin early to prevent significant weight loss and to establish a positive nitrogen balance. It is essential to start enteral nutrition as soon as possible with the ultimate aim for the patient to eat as normal a diet as possible (4). The first decision that needs to be made is the type of feeding to use. In infants under 1 year of age, increased permeability to food antigens may occur resulting in the development of an allergic reaction to any protein in the formula. Hypoallergenic formulas therefore have theoretical advantage and include Nutramigen, Pregestimil (Mead Johnson Laboratories, Evansville, IN), and Alimentum (Ross Laboratories, Columbus, OH). To reduce the allergic risk even further in highly susceptible patients, an amino acid formula such as Neocate (SHS, Liverpool, England) can be used. Another advantage of these formulas is that a high percentage of their calories are in the form of fat, which appears to be better tolerated than carbohydrates in infants. Breast milk, when available, is probably the best source of nutrition for neonates. It is known that human milk can have a positive influence on cell proliferation and on the adaptive transformation of the residual intestine. The probable explanation for these benefits is the presence of a plethora of trophic growth factors that are yet to be completely characterized (2). Older children tolerate more complex and less costly enteral feedings. Rarely is protein absorption a problem in older children (45).

Gastrostomy tubes are important in the management of these patients as they allow access for continuous or bolus enteral feeding. Continuous feeding is preferred over bolus feeding in SBS patients because the total percentage of calories absorbed is greater due to continuous saturation of transporter proteins in the small intestine. The enteral infusion should be isotonic and advanced at an extremely slow rate. Ultimately, the volume of enteral feedings can be gradually increased as the volume of parenteral feedings is decreased, based on the patient's tolerance. Stool output increasing by more than 50% in a 24-hour period is usually a contraindication to advancing enteral feeding, suggesting either an intercurrent illness or osmotic diarrhea secondary to overloading of the glucose transporters in the small intestine. Stool losses greater than 40 to 50 mL per kg per day and that are strongly positive for reducing substances suggests that enteral feedings should not be advanced. These observations indicate that the rate of feeding has reached or exceeded the limit of the patient's absorptive capacity (5).

Once the SBS patient has been stabilized on a combination of parenteral and enteral nutrition, the TPN should be transitioned from an around-the-clock continuous infusion to a cyclic nighttime infusion. This infusion schedule is safe and permits fewer limitations in daytime activities for the patient and parent.

Feeding behavior is an important component in the management of these patients. Young infants should be encouraged to continue sucking and swallowing, and provision of small amounts of the continuous enteral infusion formulation as intermittent bottle feedings should be provided. It is difficult to completely withhold food from older children, and they should be allowed to experiment with foods that are both palatable and not associated with a large stool output.

Pharmacologic agents are used primarily to reduce gastric hypersecretion and to slow the rapid intestinal transit. Due to the increase in the volume of gastric secretions, acid production, and serum gastrin levels in patients with SBS, drugs aimed at decreasing gastric acid and secretions should be started early in the postoperative course. The histamine-2 (H_2) receptor antagonists are quite effective. In clinical trials of patients with SBS, cimetidine has been shown to improve nutrient absorption, decrease stool mass, and reduce levels of fecal Na^+ and K^+. These effects are likely due to the decreased acid and volume load presented to the duodenum because more alkaline duodenal contents favor micellar aggregation and fatty acid solubilization. Cimetidine has also been shown to have a positive influence on intestinal adaptation in animal models (46). Gastric hypersecretion has been noted to decrease after 6 to 12 months following small bowel resection, suggesting that treatment with H_2 blockers for only the first year may be sufficient.

In cases of refractory hypersecretion, proton pump blockers such as omeprazole may be useful. In 11 short bowel patients, omeprazole resulted in a significant reduction in gastrointestinal output in patients that had net secretory losses, but it did not uniformly prevent the need for parenteral supplementation of fluids and electrolytes. In two patients, omeprazole was effective only when administered parenterally (47).

Pharmacologic agents can also be used to slow intestinal transit, thus improving nutritional absorption and potentially allowing the patient to wean from parenteral nutrition. The mainstay of pharmacologic therapy to slow intestinal transit has been the use of opioid substances. Opioid agents most commonly used to treat diarrhea include codeine, diphenoxylate, and loperamide. Loperamide has been demonstrated to be more effective than diphenoxylate in the control of diarrhea in several clinical trials (48,49). Codeine, although quite effective for the control of diarrhea, has significant central nervous system side effects and a clear abuse potential.

Somatostatin and its long-acting analogue octreotide have been investigated in the management of severe refractory diarrhea in SBS. Octreotide inhibits essentially all exocrine and endocrine gastrointestinal and pancreatic secretions. In clinical trials of patients with SBS, the need for supplemental electrolytes and nutrition was decreased, secretory fluid and electrolyte losses were reduced, and quality of life improved (50). The use of octreotide in the pediatric population has been limited primarily because of concern regarding the effect of this agent on somatic growth. In addition, octreotide has also been shown to inhibit intestinal adaptation perhaps by decreasing the significant adaptive enhancing effects of exocrine gastrointestinal secretions (51). For these reasons, octreotide cannot be endorsed for routine use in the patient with SBS.

Cholestyramine may be beneficial in the management of diarrhea. It is effective only when the diarrhea is related to the cathartic effect of unabsorbed bile salts reaching the colon. It should be considered in patients with diarrhea who have had an ileal resection greater than 100 cm (52).

In addition to the myriad of fluid, electrolyte, and nutritional obstacles that the patient with SBS faces, several other complications must be anticipated. These include central venous catheter complications, TPN-induced liver disease, and intestinal bacterial overgrowth. TPN-induced liver disease is frequent in infants with SBS and, along with sepsis, is the leading cause of death in these patients. It appears to be a multifactorial process that is often reversible, but may lead to severe steatosis, cholestasis, and eventually cirrhosis. It occurs more frequently in children than adults and accounts for one-third of deaths of patients receiving long-term parenteral nutrition. TPN-induced liver disease remains one of the main indications for liver/small bowel transplant. Avoidance of parenteral overfeeding and provision of as many calories as possible via the enteral route may help to prevent this complication (52). Either cholecystokinin (CCK) or the bile salt ursodeoxycholic acidmay lead to improvement in liver function when administered to patients with SBS and TPN-induced liver disease. Avoiding central venous line sepsis and aggressively managing small bowel bacterial overgrowth may help to decrease the progression of cholestasis.

Detection of bacterial overgrowth requires a high degree of suspicion. Colonization of the small intestine leads to decreased luminal concentration of conjugated bile acids with resultant fat malabsorption. Secretory diarrhea then develops as a consequence of malabsorbed fatty acids, increased formation of short-chain fatty acids with increased osmotic load and gas, and impaired vitamin B_{12} absorption. In addition, bacterial overgrowth causes mucosal inflammation, exacerbating malabsorption of all nutrients. Patients without an ileocecal valve may be at increased risk for this complication due to the potential for reflux of bacteria from the colon. Colonization should be suspected when the patient's absorptive capacity and diarrhea acutely change and dilated bowel loops are present (52). Treatment is often empiric with antibiotics targeted at both gram-positive and gram-negative organisms. Typical regimens include combinations of cephalexin-metronidazole or monotherapy with metronidazole, trimethoprim-sulfamethoxazole, or oral gentamicin. Further studies are needed to confirm whether probiotics may play a role in prevention and treatment by inhibiting the growth of pathogenic bacteria (53).

SURGICAL OPTIONS

Prevention of SBS is the earliest and best approach to this problem. Timely surgical intervention in patients with NEC and/or volvulus and a conservative approach to intestinal resection are important principles. Once the patient is beyond the initial operation, the ultimate goal is to provide all calories via the enteral route and to discontinue parenteral nutrition. Patients often develop complications related to parenteral nutrition or reach a point where stool output and/or electrolyte losses limit the ability to advance enteral feeding. In addition, some patients may actually worsen and require increasing, rather than decreasing amounts of parenteral nutrition. Those that fall into these groups (complications of parenteral nutrition, failure to advance enteral nutrition, worsening tolerance of enteral feeding) are those in whom operative intervention should be considered.

The optimal timing of remedial operative intervention is important. If surgery is performed too early, it might be unnecessary, as the normal postresection adaptation or intestinal lengthening due to normal growth may prevent the need for long-term parenteral nutrition. If offered too late, the patient may suffer complications, as well as the added cost of prolonged parenteral nutritional support. A period of at least 1 year should be the minimum interval that intestinal adaptation should be allowed to improve the ability to tolerate enteral feeding. After this length of time, if a patient is still making progress with regard to tolerance of enteral feeding, operative intervention should be postponed. However, this approach may need to be reconsidered in the context of complications of parenteral nutrition.

The major goal of surgical intervention is to increase intestinal absorptive capacity. Most surgical procedures have been created to address the specific anatomic and physiologic abnormalities of the intestine in patients with SBS. These abnormalities include rapid intestinal transit, decreased mucosal surface area, ineffective peristalsis, and reduced intestinal length. The various surgical procedures may therefore be categorized based on the primary abnormality they address.

Determining the indications for each procedure requires a careful preoperative workup and a meticulous operative plan. As a first step, a thorough understanding of the patient's intestinal anatomy and function should be obtained. This is gleaned through plain abdominal radiographs and a contrast upper gastrointestinal series with small bowel follow-through. Information regarding areas of partial obstruction and efficiency of transit should be sought. Surgical procedures designed to slow intestinal transit are obviously not indicated in a patient with obvious delay in transit. Although not entirely accurate, small intestinal length and caliber may also be deduced from the upper gastrointestinal series. In patients with a proximal stoma, it is also prudent to obtain a contrast enema, which will provide information as to how much distal bowel is available for subsequent reanastomosis and identify areas of stricture.

INTESTINAL VALVES

The importance of the ileocecal valve (ICV) has been well appreciated by those caring for patients with SBS. In 1972, Wilmore documented that survival in infants with an ICV required a minimum bowel length of 15 cm. However, in those infants without an ICV, the minimum bowel length required for survival was significantly longer (40 cm). More recently, it has been reported that up to 89% of patients without an ICV and with less than 40 cm of small bowel will survive (54). In this same report, it was also noted that an absent ICV was associated with a significantly longer duration of TPN. Preservation of the ICV should therefore be a major goal during any operative intervention.

Based on the observed importance of the ICV, multiple techniques for the construction of similar valves have been described. The simplest techniques include the placement of sutures or an external Teflon collar around the circumference of the bowel (55). A more technically involved procedure involves everting a segment of bowel to create a small intussusceptum and thus retard transit (Fig. 75-1). The more variable and less well understood aspects of these procedures are the optimum length of bowel to be everted, as well as the direction of the intussusception. If too large a segment of bowel is intussuscepted, a functional bowel obstruction will result. Too short of a segment of intussuscepted bowel will not have any effect. In a canine model, the ideal length of bowel to be intussuscepted was found to be 4 cm. Overall survival, weight loss, intestinal transit time, and bacterial counts within the small bowel were more favorable in the group with the valve following an 80% enterectomy (56). The clinical experience with intestinal valves is mostly anecdotal and of varying success.

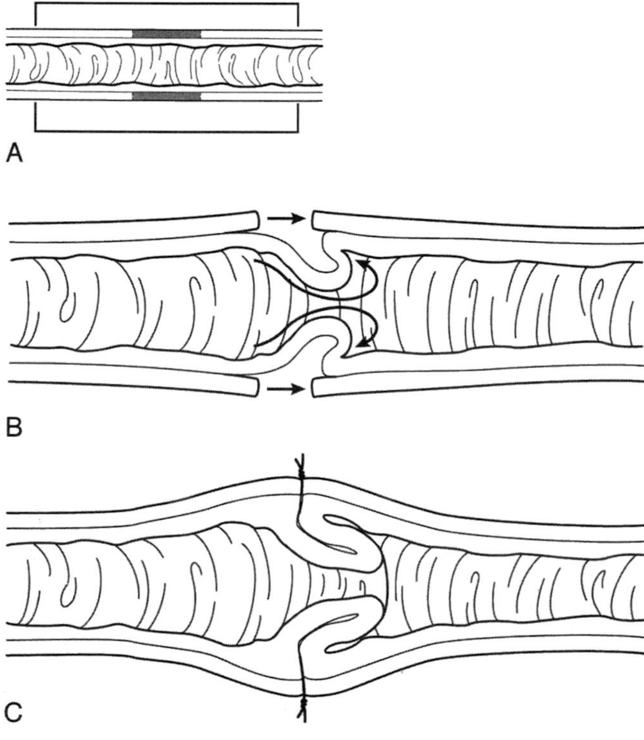

FIGURE 75-1. **(A)** Intestinal valve in which the outer seromuscular layer is circumferentially stripped, leaving the underlying mucosa intact. **(B)** The now redundant mucosa is intussuscepted to create a valve. **(C)** Finally, the serosa is reapproximated.

REVERSED INTESTINAL SEGMENTS

Some experience has developed with the use of reversed segments of intestine to slow peristalsis in patients with postvagotomy diarrhea or dumping syndrome. A "physiologic" valve is believed to be created by the interposition of a segment of bowel in which peristalsis is in the opposite direction. Using electromyography, Tanner et al. demonstrated a disruption of the intrinsic nerve plexus within the reversed segment and slowing of the distal myoelectrical activity (57). The radiographic appearance of reversed peristalsis, however, does not always correlate with intestinal function in terms of efficiency of absorption.

The exact length of bowel to be reversed is critical because a segment that is too short may be ineffective in slowing peristalsis, whereas too long a segment may create a functional bowel obstruction. Various lengths of reversed bowel probably contribute to the disparate results obtained in many experimental and clinical series. Although 10 cm seems to be the most common length used in adult patients, beneficial effects have been described in infants when as little as 3 cm has been reversed (58). From a technical standpoint, the reversed segment should be placed in the most distal aspect of the bowel to derive maximal benefit in terms of retarded transit and enhanced mucosal absorption. Reversed segments may have limited applicability in patients with extremely short bowel as the construction of the reversed segment may compromise an already tenuous small bowel mucosal mass.

Favorable results have been reported using reversed intestinal segments in more than 30 adult patients with

SBS (59). The long-term success of reversed segments is presently unclear. In children, the reversed segment may continue to grow, leading to possible bowel obstruction. In addition, the reversed segment may not function normally and thus effectively shorten the intestinal remnant, particularly if complications such as obstruction or ischemia occur. The use of a reversed segment has also been proposed to provide benefit over a short period while adaptation occurs (60). Most of the reports of reversed intestinal segments remain anecdotal and infrequent compared with some of the other surgical options. There may be a role for this procedure and for intestinal valves when the bowel caliber is normal and transit is rapid.

RECIRCULATING LOOPS

Theoretically, if a loop of intestine were created so enteral contents recirculate several times prior to proceeding distally, then the exposure time of the nutrients and mucosa would be prolonged. Further, overall intestinal transit would be slowed. Unfortunately, these theoretical advantages are seldom realized. Several experimental studies have failed to show any benefit of these procedures. Morbidity and mortality are generally increased in direct relationship to the complexity of the loop. Another interesting observation is that, although enteral contents can be demonstrated to recirculate radiographically, absorption is not improved.

Recirculating loops have been performed in a few patients with discouraging results. At the present time, the clinical utility of recirculating loops in the management of SBS is limited. Morbidity is prohibitive, while efficacy is unproven. Recirculating intestinal loops should probably not be performed in contemporary practice and are mentioned only for completeness.

COLON INTERPOSITION

The interposition of a segment of colon between two limbs of small bowel in patients with rapid intestinal transit has been studied experimentally and tried clinically, although the exact mechanism by which this procedure is effective is not well understood. The interposed colon segment is generally placed proximally and probably slows intestinal transit by virtue of its slow, segmental peristaltic contractions. It thereby slows the rate at which nutrients are delivered to the distal small intestine. The interposed colon has also been demonstrated to absorb nutrients, water, and electrolytes.

Colon interposition has been successful in both children and adults. In the largest series of children with SBS, isoperistaltic colon interposition allowed three of six patients to wean from parenteral nutrition completely. The other three patients died from complications secondary to parenteral nutrition. No reported morbidity or mortality was associated with the interposition procedure itself. However, the surviving patients were younger and had a greater length of small bowel at the time of interposition (61).

The ideal length of colon to use for the interposition is unknown. In the previously mentioned series, the length of colon ranged from 8 to 15 cm. Others have reported segments as long as 24 cm. The small number of patients reported precludes determination of the most appropriate length of colon to use in interposition. This appears to be a useful technique for increasing intestinal transit, with success in about 50%, while not compromising the viability of the small bowel. This procedure may be considered when the small bowel has a normal caliber in SBS patients who have an intact colon.

TAPERING ENTEROPLASTY

Dilated segments of intestine are a known cause of functional bowel obstruction. The mechanism appears to be ineffective peristalsis due to failure of bowel wall apposition during contraction. The dilated bowel has low contraction pressures, resulting in a back-and-forth motion of the enteric contents. This situation sets the stage for stasis, bacterial overgrowth with associated toxin production, and malabsorption. In patients with a short segment of affected bowel and a sufficient length of remaining intestine, resection of the dilated bowel may be optimal management. Unfortunately, in the patient with SBS, the majority of the bowel is dilated and the overall length is short. Resection is therefore not a viable option.

Tapering enteroplasty reduces the caliber of the bowel, while preserving intestinal length. This is accomplished by excising an antimesenteric portion of the bowel, leaving the mesenteric tube of bowel intact (Fig. 75-2). The tapered intestine has a significantly smaller caliber, and therefore, peristalsis becomes more effective (62).

A variation of this technique consists of antimesenteric plication of the bowel. Instead of resecting the antimesenteric portion of intestine, the bowel is folded into the lumen and plicated. This theoretically results in preservation of the mucosa for better absorption, while decreasing the overall caliber of the bowel (63). Unfortunately, the suture lines tend to break down with time and bowel dilation, and functional obstruction tends to recur.

In a more recent review of 11 children, ages 6 months to 9 years, with dilated intestinal segments and remnant lengths longer than 30 cm, all had associated bacterial overgrowth and malabsorption, and only 3 had a mechanical small bowel obstruction. Enteroplasty was performed

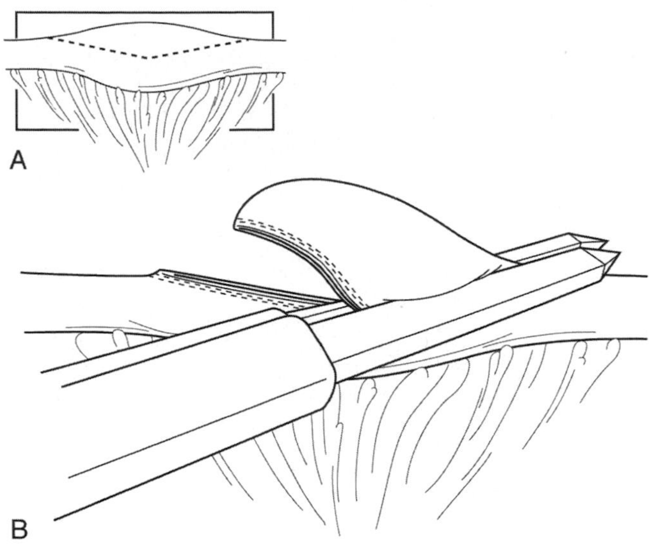

FIGURE 75-2. Tapering enteroplasty. **(A)** The antimesenteric portion of the dilated bowel is removed. **(B)** The remaining bowel is tabularized to create a segment that is smaller in caliber.

on the duodenum ($n = 3$), jejunum ($n = 3$), or ileum ($n = 5$), with the length of the tapered segment longer than 15 cm in 7 of the 11 patients. Nine of the 11 patients were weaned completely from parenteral nutrition, and the other 2 required decreased amounts of parenteral support. Two patients subsequently underwent intestinal lengthening because of recurrent malabsorption (64). Tapering has less morbidity than a lengthening procedure and is usually the procedure of choice as long as the patient has more than 40 cm of remaining small intestine.

INTESTINAL LENGTHENING PROCEDURES

An important procedure to actually increase the length of the intestine was first described by Bianchi in 1980 (65). This procedure, like other surgical options, appears to be most successful for patients who have undergone a period of normal bowel adaptation following initial bowel resection (66). This method takes advantage of the anatomic features of the mesenteric blood supply to the bowel. Just prior to reaching the edge of the bowel wall, the blood vessels within the mesentery bifurcate to supply one-half of the bowel circumference. This segmental blood supply pattern permits the bowel to be safely divided along a longitudinal axis into two tubes that measure one-half of the circumference of the original bowel. This is facilitated with a gastrointestinal anastomosis (GIA) stapling device, but can be accomplished by hand suturing. Once the bowel has been divided along its longitudinal axis, the two newly constructed tubes of bowel are sewn together in an isoperistaltic fashion. The overall result is a segment of bowel in which the length is doubled and overall circumference is halved (Fig. 75-3). Thus, this procedure not only lengthens the bowel to increase absorption, but also improves peristalsis by decreasing bowel caliber.

Dilated bowel is generally easier to lengthen because the GIA stapler may be used. In addition, the larger diameter of the newly divided bowel facilitates the performance of the subsequent anastomoses. Extensive intraperitoneal adhesions from prior surgery are often encountered in patients subjected to the lengthening procedure, and care must always be taken to avoid injury to the mesenteric blood supply. In addition, variability in blood supply to the bowel wall may be present, possibly contributing to technical failures (67).

In patients without the significant spontaneous dilation of the bowel that makes the Bianchi procedure technically feasible, a staged sequential lengthening procedure as described by Georgeson may be undertaken (68). This procedure involves the initial creation of a 4-cm nipple valve in the small intestine to induce proximal bowel dilation, followed in 3 to 9 months by a Bianchi lengthening procedure.

Thompson et al. reported a series of six patients who underwent the Bianchi procedure (69). One patient died of sepsis, four patients were weaned completely off parenteral nutrition, and the final patient had a decreased requirement for parenteral nutrition. More recently, Figueroa-Colon et al. reported a series of seven patients who underwent intestinal lengthening and showed that the tolerance of enteral calories increased significantly at 9 months. They also showed that all growth parameters were either maintained or improved and that the number of hospitalization days decreased during the second year following the lengthening procedure (70). Overall, at least 40 children have been treated using this technique, with 90% of patients having improved tolerance of enteral nutrition. In 17 of these patients, parenteral nutrition was discontinued altogether (69–71).

The Iowa procedure was described as a means of treating SBS in patients who are not candidates for the Bianchi procedure or who have limited mesentery associated with very short bowel. The procedure is a two-stage process. The first step is initial coaptation of the antimesenteric surface of the bowel to a host blood supply. This is performed by first making a longitudinal seromyotomy, which is extended along the antimesenteric border of the bowel, exposing the submucosa. Then the capsule of the anterior liver margin and the parietal peritoneum on the undersurface of the right abdominal wall muscles are removed to create a denuded tissue surface. The submucosa and the denuded tissue surface of the liver and abdominal wall muscles are coapted using two continuous sutures to form a hepatomyoenteropexy. Approximately 8 weeks later, the second step may be performed, which involves a

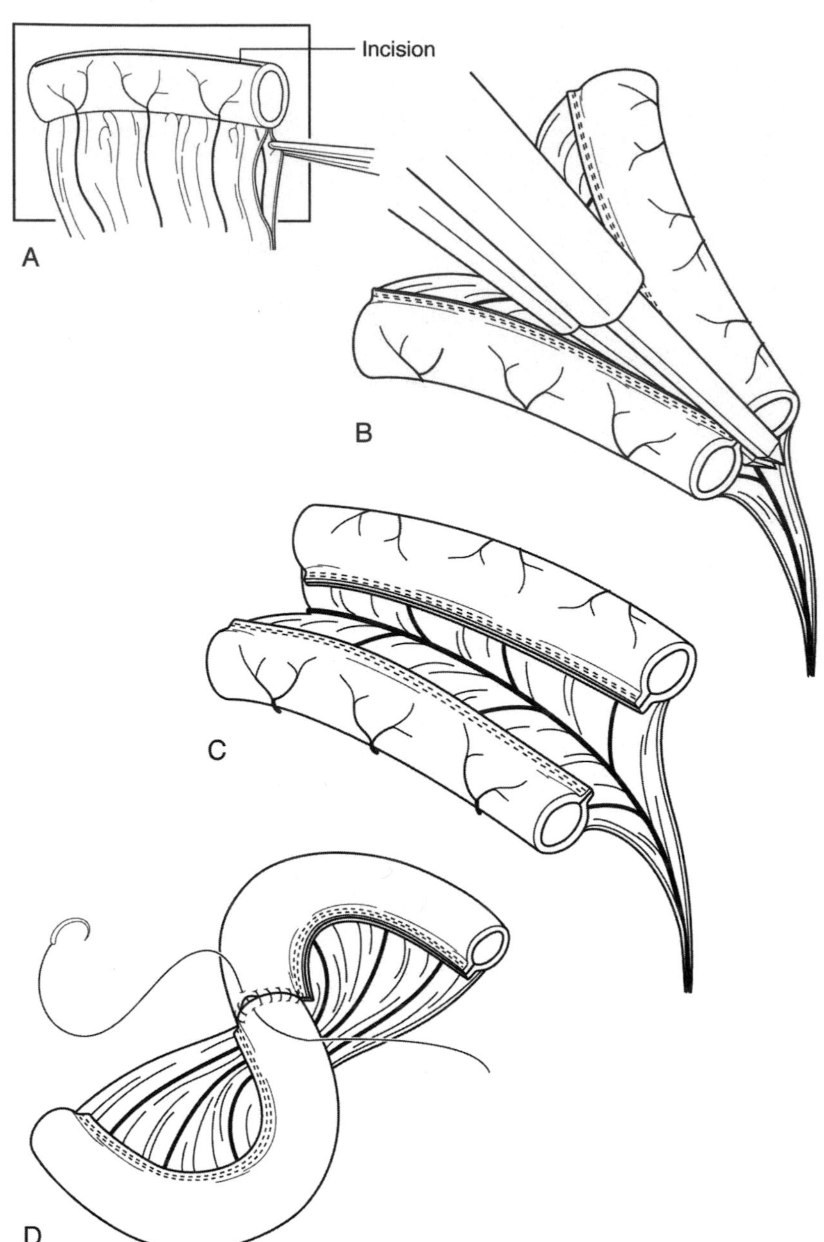

FIGURE 75-3. **(A)** Dissection between peritoneal leaves of the mesentery. **(B)** Bowel loop between jaws of gastrointestinal anastomosis stapler prior to division of the bowel. **(C)** Hemiloops resulting from stapling and division of the bowel. **(D)** Isoperistaltic anastamosis between hemiloops.

longitudinal split of the bowel to provide two bowel loops. These bowel loops may then be arranged in series by end-to-end anastamosis to double the bowel length. So far, there are only anecdotal reports of the use of this procedure (71). It appears to be specifically useful in children in whom the remaining bowel is limited to the duodenum, thus limiting the applicability of the Bianchi procedure. A similar procedure has also been proposed using the omentum as a source of neovascularization. In a preliminary study using dogs, it was demonstrated that the neovascularization improved both absorption and adaptation (72).

More recently, a novel bowel-lengthening operation termed *serial transverse enteroplasty procedure* (STEP) has been described (73). This procedure has been reported using a pig model in which dilated small bowel was lengthened by serial transverse applications of a GIA stapler, from opposite directions, to create a zigzag channel (Fig. 75-4). This procedure provided near doubling of bowel length. This procedure has been subsequently applied to one patient with SBS with a favorable outcome. Further studies are required, and careful clinical evaluation in relation to the traditional Bianchi lengthening technique is needed.

Tissue engineering of neomucosa represents an exciting new frontier and is presently in the early stages of investigation. These models use tubular microporous biodegradable polymers that are seeded with intestinal epithelial organoid units. The blood supply is derived from the mesentery. The neointestinal cysts are then anastamosed

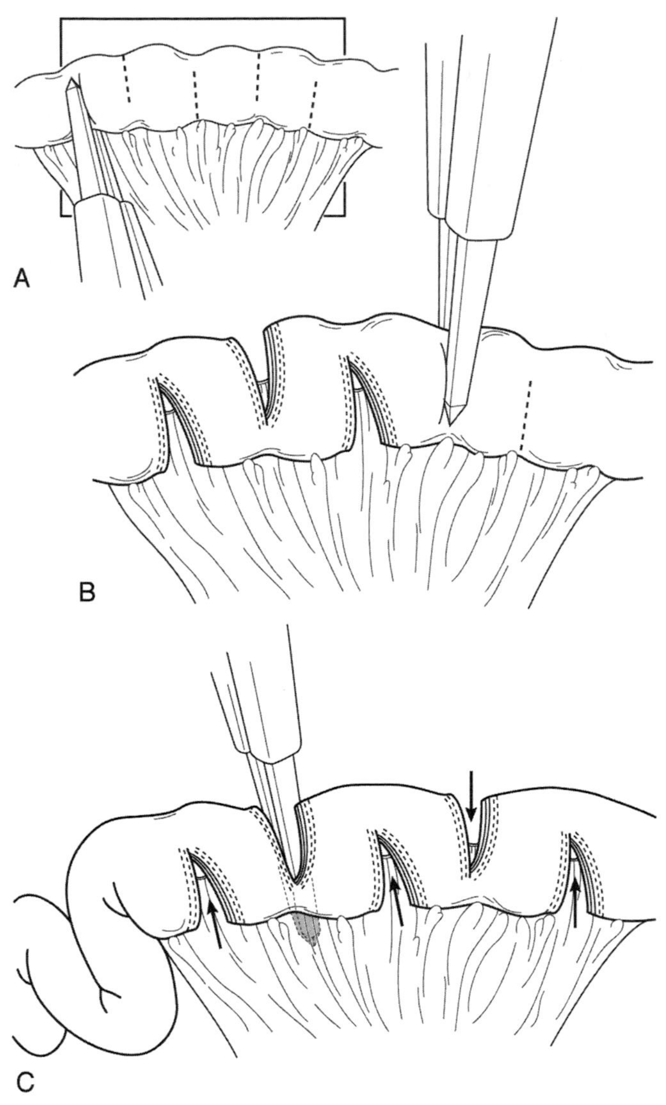

FIGURE 75-4. Schematic of the serial transverse enteroplasty procedure. **(A)** Segment of bowel is identified and staple points planned. **(B)** Gastrointestinal anastomosis stapler fired in 90- and 270-degree orientations. **(C)** Final appearance with bowel lengthened and tapered.

to the native intestine (74–76). The use of neointestine in humans has not yet been reported, but the field of tissue engineering may play a significant role in the future treatment of SBS.

INTESTINAL TRANSPLANTATION

Transplantation of the small bowel is an important final option for management of SBS and is covered elsewhere in this text. Intestinal transplantation is promising definitive therapy, but is associated with significant morbidity and mortality. Current reported results demonstrate 1-year patient and graft survival rates of 70% and 65%, respectively. At 3 years posttransplant, however, the patient and graft survival are reduced to 55% and 50%, respectively (77). The complex immunosuppression, as well as the myriad of infectious complications, continue to be a difficult hurdle in the management of these complex patients.

CONCLUSION

Overall, the care of the patient with SBS has advanced significantly in recent years, although it remains problematic. Although multiple surgical procedures have been devised to address the intestinal abnormalities that develop following massive SBR, they have not been tried in sufficient numbers of patients to permit valid outcome comparisons. The ultimate goal of all procedures should be to allow the patient to advance to enteral feeding so the complications of TPN are avoided and the patient may return to as normal a lifestyle as possible. Perhaps as important in the management of patients with SBS is an understanding of endogenous regulation of mucosal growth and the genetic regulation of postresection adaptation.

REFERENCES

1. Wilmore DW, Dudrick SJ. Growth and development of an infant receiving all nutrients exclusively by vein. *JAMA* 1968;203:860.
2. Iacono G, Carroccio A, Montalto G, et al. Extreme short bowel syndrome: a case for reviewing the guidelines for predicting survival. *J Pediatr Gastroenterol Nutr* 1993;16:216.
3. Wilmore DW, Robinson MK. Short bowel syndrome. *World J Surg* 2000;24:1486.
4. Warner BW, Ziegler MM. Management of the short bowel syndrome in the pediatric population. *Pediatr Clin North Am* 1993;60:1335.
5. Vanderhoof JA. Short bowel syndrome. *Clin Perinatol* 1996;23:377.
6. Caniano DA, Starr J, Ginn-Pease ME. Extensive short bowel syndrome in neonates: outcome in the 1980s. *Surgery* 1989;104:119.
7. Georgeson KE, Breaux CW. Outcome and intestinal adaptation in neonatal short bowel syndrome. *J Pediatr Surg* 1992;27:344.
8. Grosfeld JL, Rescorla FJ, West W. Short bowel syndrome in infancy and childhood: analysis of survival in 60 patients. *Am J Surg* 1986;151:41.
9. Skandalakis JE, Gray SW. *Embryology for surgeons,* 2nd ed. Baltimore: Williams & Wilkins, 1994.
10. Touloukian RJ, Walker-Smith GJ. Normal intestinal length in preterm infants. *J Pediatr Surg* 1983;18:720.
11. Shanbhogue LKR, Molenaar JC. Short bowel syndrome: metabolic and surgical management. *Br J Surg* 1994;81:486.
12. Vanderhoof JA, Langas AN, Pinch LW, et al. Short bowel syndrome. *J Pediatr Gastroenterol Nutr* 1992;14:359.
13. Hanson WR, Osborne JW, Sharp JG. Compensation by the residual intestine after intestinal resection in the rat. II. Influence of postoperative time interval. *Gastroenterology* 1977;72:701.
14. Williamson RC, Bauer FL, Ross JS, et al. Proximal enterectomy stimulates distal hyperplasia more than bypass or pancreaticobiliary diversion. *Gastroenterology* 1978;74:16.
15. Helmrath MA, Erwin CR, Shin CE, et al. Enterocyte apoptosis is increased following small bowel resection. *J Gastrointest Surg* 1998;2:44.
16. Williamson RC. Intestinal adaptation. Structural, functional and cytokinetic changes. *N Engl J Med* 1978;298:1393.
17. Williamson RC. Intestinal adaptation. Mechanisms of control. *N Engl J Med* 1978;298:1444.

18. Gavrieli Y, Sherman Y, Ben-Sasson SA. Identification of programmed cell death in situ via specific labeling of nuclear DNA fragmentation. *J Cell Biol* 1992;119:493.
19. Stern LE, Falcone RA, Huang F, et al. Epidermal growth factor alters the bax:bcl-w ratio following massive small bowel resection. *J Surg Res* 2000;91:38.
20. Stern LE, Huang F, Kemp CJ, et al. Bax is required for increased enterocyte apoptosis after massive small bowel resection. *Surgery* 2000;128:165.
21. Falcone RA, Shin CE, Stern LE, et al. Differential expression of ileal Na(+)/H(+) exchanger isoforms after enterectomy. *J Surg Res* 1999;86:192.
22. Hines OJ Bilchik Aj, Zinner MJ, et al. Adaptation of the Na^+/glucose cotransporter following intestinal resection. *J Surg Res* 1994;57:22.
23. Schulzke JD, Fromm M, Bentzel CJ, et al. Ion transport in the experimental short bowel syndrome of the rat. *Gastroenterology* 1992;102:497.
24. Altmann GG, Leblond CP. Factors influencing villus size in the small intestine of adult rats as revealed by transposition of intestinal segments. *Am J Anat* 1970;127:15.
25. Levine GM, Deren JJ, Yezdimir E. Small bowel resection. Oral intake is the stimulus for hyperplasia. *Am J Dig Dis* 1976;21:542.
26. Dworkin LD, Levine GM, Farber NJ, et al. Small intestinal mass of the rat is partially determined by indirect effects of intraluminal nutrition. *Gastroenterology* 1976;71:626.
27. Warner BW, Vanderhoof JA, Reyes JD. What's new in the management of short gut syndrome in children. *J Am Coll Surg* 2000;190:725.
28. Booth IW. Enteral nutrition as primary therapy in short bowel resection in rats. *Gastroenterology* 1994;35:S69.
29. Vanderhoof JA, Blackwood DJ, Mohammadpour H, et al. Effects of oral supplementation of glutamine on small intestinal resection and pectin feeding. *J Am Coll Nutr* 1992;11:223.
30. Scolapio JS, Camilleri M, Fleming CR, et al. Effect of growth hormone, glutamine, and diet on adaptation in short bowel syndrome: a randomized, controlled study. *Gastroenterology* 1997;113:1074.
31. Ko TC, Beauchamp RD, Townsend CM, et al. Glutamine is essential for epidermal growth factor stimulated intestinal cell proliferation. *Surgery* 1993;114:147.
32. Liu CD, Rongione AJ, Shin MS, et al. Epidermal growth factor improves intestinal adaptation during somatostatin administration *in vivo*. *J Surg Res* 1996;63:163.
33. Hodin RA, Saldinger P, Meng S. Small bowel adaptation: counterregulatory effects of epidermal growth factor and somatostatin on the program of early gene expression. *Surgery* 1995;118:206.
34. Williamson RC, Buchholtz TW, Malt RA. Humoral stimulation of cell proliferation in small bowel after transaction and resection in rats. *Gastroenterology* 1978;75:249.
35. Stern LE, Erwin CR, O'Brien DP, et al. Epidermal growth factor is critical for intestinal adaptation following small bowel resection. *Microsc Res Tech* 2000;51:138.
36. Helmrath MA, Shine CE, Fox JW, et al. Adaptation after small bowel resection is attenuated by sialoadenectomy: the role for endogenous epidermal growth factor. *Surgery* 1998;124:848.
37. Helmrath MA, Erwin CR, Warner BW. A defective EGF receptor in waved-2 mice attenuates intestinal adaptation. *J Surg Res* 1997;69:76.
38. Drucker DJ, Boushey RP, Wang F, et al. Biologic properties and therapeutic potential of glucagon-like peptide 2. *J Parenter Enteral Nutr* 1999;25:S98.
39. Drucker DJ. Gut adaptation and the glucagon-like peptides. *Gut* 2002;50:428.
40. Jeppesen PB, Hartmann B, Thulesen J, et al. Glucagon-like peptide 2 improves nutrient absorption and nutritional status in short bowel patients with no colon. *Gastroenterology* 2001;120:806.
41. Tavakkolizadeh A, Whang EE. Understanding and augmenting human intestinal adaptation: a call for more clinical research. *J Parenter Enteral Nutr* 2002;26:251.
42. O'Brien DP, Nelson LA, Kemp CJ, et al. Intestinal permeability and bacterial translocation are uncoupled after small bowel resection. *J Pediatr Surg* 2002;37:390.
43. O'Brien DP, Nelson LA, Stern LE, et al. Epithelial permeability is not increased in rats following small bowel resection. *J Surg Res* 2001;97:65.
44. Alverdy JC, Aoys E, Moss GS. Total parenteral nutrition promotes bacterial translocation from the gut. *Surgery* 1998;104:185.
45. Vanderhoof JA, Young RJ. Enteral nutrition in short bowel syndrome. *Semin Pediatr Surg* 2001;10:65.
46. Tomas-de la Vega JE, Banner BF, Haklin MF. Effect of cimetidine on intestinal adaptation following massive resection of the small intestine. *Surg Gynecol Obstet* 1983;156:41.
47. Nightingale JMD, Walker ER, Farthing MJG. Effect of omeprazole on intestinal output in the short bowel syndrome. *Aliment Pharmacol Ther* 1989;45:77.
48. Ericsson CD, Johnson PC. Safety and efficacy of loperamide. *Am J Med* 1990;88:10S.
49. O'Brien JD, Thompson DG, McIntyre A. Effect of codeine and loperamide on upper intestinal transit and absorption in normal subjects and patients with postvagotomy diarrhea. *Gut* 1988;29:312.
50. Nightingale JMD, Walker ER, Burnham WR. Octreotide (a somatostatin analogue) improves the quality of life in some patients with the short bowel syndrome. *Aliment Pharmacol Ther* 1989;3:367.
51. Bass BL, Fischer BA, Richardson C. Somatostatin analogue treatment inhibits post-resection adaptation of the small bowel in rats. *Am J Surg* 1991;161:107.
52. Thompson JS. Management of the short bowel syndrome. *Gastroenterol Clin North Am* 1994;23:403.
53. Hwang ST, Shulman RJ. Update on management and treatment of short gut. *Clin Perinatol* 2002;29:181.
54. Chaet MS, Farell MK, Ziegler MM, et al. Intensive nutritional support and remedial surgical intervention for extreme short bowel syndrome. *J Pediatr Gastroenterol Nutr* 1994;19:295.
55. Stahlgren LH, Roy RH, Umana G. A mechanical impediment to intestinal flow: physiological effects on intestinal absorption. *JAMA* 1964;187:41.
56. Ricotta J, Zuidema GD, Gadacz TR, et al. Construction of an ileocecal valve and its role in massive resection of the small intestine. *Surg Gynecol Obstet* 1981;152:310.
57. Tanner WA, O'Leary JF, Byrne PJ. The effect of reversed jejunal segments on the myoelectrical activity of the small bowel. *Br J Surg* 1978;65:567.
58. Warden MJ, Wesley JR. Small bowel reversal procedure for treatment of the "short gut" baby. *J Pediatr Surg* 1978;13:321.
59. Panis Y, Messing B, Rivet P, et al. Segmental reversal of the small bowel as an alternative to intestinal transplantation in patients with short bowel syndrome. *Ann Surg* 1997;225:401.
60. Shanbhogue LKR, Molenaar JC. Short bowel syndrome: metabolic and surgical management. *Br J Surg* 1994;81:486.
61. Glick PL, DeLorier AA, Adzick NS, et al. Colon interposition for the short bowel syndrome. *J Pediatr Surg* 1986;19:719.
62. Warner BW, Chaet MS. Nontransplant surgical options for management of the short bowel syndrome. *J Pediatr Gastroenterol Nutr* 1993;17:1.
63. DeLorimier AA, Harrison MR. Intestinal placation in the treatment of atresia. *J Pediatr Surg* 1983;18:734.
64. Thompson JS, Langnas AN, Pinch LW, et al. Surgical approach to short bowel syndrome. Experience in a population of 160 patients. *Ann Surg* 1995;222:600.
65. Bianchi A. Intestinal loop lengthening—a technique for increasing small intestinal length. *J Pediatr Surg* 1980;2:145.
66. Bianchi A. Autologous gastrointestinal reconstruction. *Semin Pediatr Surg* 1995;4:54.
67. Thompson JS, Vanderhoof JA, Antonson DL. Intestinal tapering and lengthening for short bowel syndrome. *J Pediatr Gastroenterol Nutr* 1985;4:495.
68. Vernon AH, Georgeson KE. Surgical options for short bowel syndrome. *Semin Pediatr Surg* 2001;10:91.
69. Thompson JS, Pinch LW, Murray N, et al. Experience with intestinal lengthening for the short bowel syndrome. *J Pediatr Surg* 1991;26:721.
70. Figueroa-Colon R, Harris PR, Birdsong E, et al. Impact of intestinal lengthening on the nutritional outcome for children with short bowel syndrome. *J Pediatr Surg* 1996;31:912.
71. Georgeson BK, Figueroa R, Vicente Y, et al. Sequential intestinal lengthening procedures for refractory short bowel syndrome. *J Pediatr Surg* 1994;2:316.
72. Williams JK, Carlson GW, Austin GE, et al. Short gut syndrome:

treatment by neovascularization of the small intestine. *Ann Plastic Surg* 1996;1:84.
73. Kim HBK, Fauza D, Garza J, et al. Serial transverse enteroplasty (STEP): a novel bowel lengthening procedure. *J Pediatr Surg* 2003;38:425.
74. Perez A, Grikscheit TC, Blumberg RS, et al. Tissue-engineered small intestine: ontogeny of the immune system. *Transplantation* 2002;74:619.
75. Choi RS, Riegler M, Pothoulakis C, et al. Studies of brush border enzymes, basement membrane components, and electrophysiology of tissue-engineered neointestine. *J Pediatr Surg* 1998;33:991.
76. Kaihara S, Kim SS, Kim BS, et al. Long-term follow up of tissue engineered intestine after anastomosis to the native small bowel. *Transplantation* 2000;69:1927.
77. Reyes J. Intestinal transplantation for children with short bowel syndrome. *Semin Pediatr Surg* 2001;10;99.

Chapter 76

Introduction to Neonatal Intestinal Obstruction

George B. Mychaliska

Through advancements in surgical technique, neonatal anesthesia, neonatal intensive care, and total parenteral nutrition, significant progress has been made in the management of neonates with intestinal obstruction. Despite improvements in care, neonatal intestinal obstruction continues to provide a diagnostic challenge for clinicians. In this chapter, we describe the common clinical manifestations of neonatal intestinal obstruction and outline a diagnostic algorithm.

A variety of lesions exist that cause intestinal obstruction in the neonatal period. The lesions can be separated into high anatomic obstructions, low anatomic obstructions, and functional obstructions. High anatomic obstructions are caused by lesions that interrupt bowel continuity proximal to the midportion of the jejunum. The high lesions include pyloric atresia, duodenal obstruction from atresia, stenosis, annular pancreas, preduodenal portal vein, malrotation with or without midgut volvulus, and proximal jejunal atresia or stenosis. Low anatomic obstructions are distal to the midportion of the jejunum. Low obstructive lesions include ileal atresia or stenosis, colonic atresia or stenosis, meconium ileus, Hirschsprung's disease, imperforate anus, small left colon syndrome, meconium plug syndrome, intussusception, and anorectal malformations. Functional obstructions may be caused by sepsis, electrolyte imbalance, necrotizing enterocolitis (NEC), and hypothyroidism. Table 76-1 lists the common causes of intestinal obstruction in the neonate.

Most clinical series have examined each obstructive lesion individually. However, studies by Reyes et al. (1) and Santulli (2) reviewed the broad topic of intestinal obstruction in the neonate. With advancements in surgical technique and medical management, outcomes in neonates with intestinal obstruction have dramatically improved. In 1954, Santulli reported a mortality rate of 44.8% (2), compared with the mortality rate of 2.8% in 1989 (1). These data are consistent with other more recent studies that looked at lesions responsible for neonatal bowel obstruction. In three series that reviewed intestinal atresia, the operative mortality for jejunoileal atresia was 0.8% and increased to 4% for duodenal atresia when associated with a cardiac anomaly (3). The long-term survival ranged from 86% to 93% (4–6).

PRENATAL DIAGNOSIS

Many of the anomalies that lead to intestinal obstruction in the neonate develop during fetal life. With the current technical capabilities of ultrasonography, many obstructive lesions can be accurately diagnosed during the prenatal period. Diagnosis in the prenatal setting facilitates the care of the pregnant mother and future patient. Prenatal diagnosis provides the opportunity for appropriate counseling and for planning the delivery in a tertiary care center with a pediatric surgeon and a neonatal intensive care unit. Timely resuscitation and appropriate surgical management can be optimized.

The accuracy of prenatal ultrasonography is dependent on the level of intestinal obstruction. Corteville et al. reviewed the ultrasonographic findings of 16,471 consecutive fetuses, 89 of which had a suspected bowel lesion (7). The study revealed a sensitivity of 100% and positive predictive value of 73% for the diagnosis of small bowel lesions. Large bowel lesions had a low sensitivity of 8% and positive predictive value of 18%. Therefore, prenatal ultrasound accurately predicts the presence of high lesions, but it is a poor test for detecting low lesions.

Specific ultrasound criteria is useful in defining obstructive lesions. Isolated gastric distention and polyhydramnios is usually seen in rare cases of pyloric atresia (8).

George B. Mychaliska: Division of Pediatric Surgery, Washington University School of Medicine, St. Louis Children's Hospital, St. Louis, Missouri 63110.

TABLE 76-1 Cause of Neonatal Intestinal Obstruction.

High Obstructive Lesions	Low Obstructive Lesions	Functional Obstruction
Pyloric atresia or pyloric stenosis (rare)	Ileal atresia or stenosis	Necrotizing enterocolitis
Duodenal obstruction: atresia, stenosis, annular pancreas, congenital peritoneal bands, preduodenal portal vein	Meconium ileus	Sepsis
Malrotation	Intussusception (rare)	Hypothyroidism
Malrotation with volvulus	Colonic atresia or stenosis (rare)	Electrolyte imbalance
Proximal jejunal atresia or stenosis	Small left colon syndrome	
	Meconium plug syndrome	
	Hirschsprung's disease	
	Anorectal malformation	

In duodenal atresia, a sonographic "double-bubble" is usually diagnostic, and polyhydramnios is present in one-half of the fetuses with duodenal atresia (9,10). Jejunoileal atresias are diagnosed by dilated fluid filled loops of bowel with increased peristalsis. Only 24% of cases of jejunal atresia are associated with maternal polyhydramnios. Distal atresias are less often associated with polyhydramnios (11). Midgut volvulus may also present with distended fluid-filled loops of bowel, increased mural thickness, and increased peristalsis (10). Intraabdominal calcifications and ascites should raise suspicion for meconium peritonitis from intestinal obstruction with perforation. However, calcifications and ascites can be produced by a variety of other causes (10). Low obstructive lesions, such as meconium ileus, colonic atresia, Hirschsprung's disease, and imperforate anus, are difficult to reliably identify by prenatal ultrasound.

POSTNATAL DIAGNOSIS

Although intestinal obstruction may be suggested in the prenatal period, the definitive diagnosis is made in the neonatal period. The diagnosis is based on the clinical presentation, physical examination, and imaging studies. Symptoms typically begin to manifest within the first 24 hours of life. The clinical presentation differs based on the level of intestinal obstruction. The severity of the obstruction determines the clinical manifestations in the neonate. Partial obstructions often initially produce minimal or no findings.

SYMPTOMS AND SIGNS

Vomiting is one of the earliest and most consistent signs of intestinal obstruction in neonates. The onset, character, and severity of the vomiting is dependent on the cause of obstruction. Bilious vomiting is characteristic of obstruction distal to the to the ampulla of Vater. Bilious emesis should be considered to be due to malrotation until proven otherwise. With proximal lesions, bilious vomiting has a sudden presentation and may be forceful in nature. The frequency of bilious emesis in neonates with duodenal obstruction ranges from 66% to 91% (3,4) and was 46% to 100% in neonates with intestinal malrotation (12–14) In approximately 15% of neonates with duodenal atresia, the obstruction is proximal to the ampulla of Vater, and emesis will be nonbilious. However, bilious vomiting may also be a clinical symptom present in low obstructive lesions, such as ileal atresia, intussusception, colonic atresia or stenosis, and Hirschsprung's disease. Bilious emesis is usually a late manifestation of imperforate anus. Nonbilious vomiting may also be encountered in the neonate with obstruction due to any type of lesion.

Failure to pass meconium is another sign of intestinal obstruction. Meconium should be passed within 24 hours of birth in 95% of full-term infants, and the remainder will usually pass meconium within 48 hours (15). Failure to pass meconium within the first 24 hours of life is a classic finding for meconium ileus, meconium plugging, anorectal malformations, and Hirschsprung's disease. Failed passage of meconium is also present in jejunoileal atresia, colonic atresia or stenosis, and intussusception. Neonates with proximal intestinal obstructions may pass meconium within the first 24 to 48 hours, but they will fail to have subsequent stools. With more proximal lesions, sufficient cells can be shed from the intestine distal to the point of obstruction to account for the meconium. Some patients with anorectal anomalies will pass meconium through abnormal anatomic structures, such as small perineal openings or fistulae, or in males with high anorectal lesions, through the urethra. Neonates with incomplete obstruction may pass meconium and subsequent stool.

Abnormal findings in the stool of a neonate may suggest threatened bowel. Passage of blood per rectum is an ominous sign that represents intestinal ischemia. This may be present in neonates with malrotation with midgut volvulus and necrotizing enterocolitis. Neonates with intussusception may pass blood-tinged mucus or stool that resembles red current jelly. Any finding that may be consistent with threatened bowel viability must be immediately diagnosed to allow for prompt definitive care.

Abdominal distention is a common sign of neonatal intestinal obstruction, and is a characteristic and frequent finding of low obstructive lesions of the neonate. The degree of distention caused by low obstructive lesions tends to be progressive and severe. In neonates with high obstructive lesions, abdominal distention is variably present. When present, the distention tends to be confined to the epigatrium. The remainder of the abdomen may have a scaphoid appearance due to the lack of air passing the point of obstruction into the distal areas of bowel. Frequent vomiting relieves gastric distention; therefore, abdominal distention is an unreliable finding in intestinal obstruction due to high lesions.

PHYSICAL EXAMINATION

Physical examination provides clues to aid in the diagnosis of the neonate with intestinal obstruction. The clinician should determine if the neonate has a distended or flat abdomen. The abdomen should be palpated to assess for tenderness and guarding. Peritoneal signs are often present in cases of volvulus, NEC, bowel perforation, and bowel ischemia. Abdominal wall erythema is also consistent with peritonitis. A palpable mass in the right upper quadrant and an empty right lower quadrant may be seen in intussusception. However, few patients with neonatal intussusception will present with an abdominal mass. Fixed masses may be present in neonates with advanced NEC.

Inspection of the anus and examination of the rectum should be performed. The perineum is inspected to determine the patency and location of the anus. If an anorectal anomaly is present, the surgeon should inspect for an anal stenosis, membrane, perineal fistula, or a vestibular fistula. Rectal examination should be performed. In neonates with Hirschsprung's disease the anal sphincter is often hypertonic and the rectum is usually empty. In anal stenosis, the anus will be tight. Meconium should be guaiac tested. Passage of meconium as a result of rectal examination should raise suspicion for Hirschsprung's disease. Explosive watery discharge should alert the clinician to the presence of enterocolitis.

RADIOGRAPHIC EXAMINATION

After a thorough history and physical examination, all neonates with suspected intestinal obstruction should have plain abdominal films. The plain radiographs should consist of an anteroposterior abdominal radiograph and a left-side down decubitus or cross-table lateral. A prone cross-table lateral view may also be helpful. Radiographic examination in the neonate is often challenging. It is usually difficult to differentiate large and small bowel on plain films in infants younger than 1 year old. Colonic gas may not be visible until meconium has passed, making early evaluation of the colon difficult. Small and large bowel are often difficult to distinguish due to the close apposition of loops of bowel and lack of haustral markings in the colon (16,17). In their review of 225 distended neonates, Carty and Brereton described three pitfalls that must be avoided in the radiologic evaluation of the neonate. First, films may have been taken before characteristic changes have had time to develop. Second, the presence of meconium in the colon does not automatically indicate patency of bowel. If an atresia forms during fetal life after the passage of meconium, then meconium will be present in the distal segment of bowel. Third, there may be multiple distinct abnormalities in the same patient (16). Characteristic findings on plain films, coupled with the history and physical examination, will place the neonate in the category of a high or low intestinal obstruction. High lesions are characterized by few dilated loops with a paucity of distal gas. In contrast, low lesions typically have multiple loops of dilated bowel, often with air–fluid levels.

HIGH INTESTINAL OBSTRUCTION

Plain films of patients with pyloric atresia reveal a distended stomach with no distal gas. Although pyloric stenosis in the newborn period also presents with a distended stomach bubble, there is usually distal air present. A limited upper gastrointestinal (UGI) study helps to delineate the anatomy. Patients with duodenal obstruction are diagnosed by plain abdominal films. Patients with duodenal obstruction will have a characteristic "double-bubble" sign. The "double-bubble" sign represents distended stomach and proximal duodenum with concomitant air–fluid levels. In duodenal atresia, no distal air will be present in the bowel. This is pathognomonic and no other imaging study is needed. A "double-bubble" with distal air suggests partial duodenal obstruction from duodenal stenosis, a web, an annular pancreas, a preduodenal portal vein, or extrinsic compression of the duodenum by malrotation with Ladd's bands. In the series by Reyes, all patients with duodenal obstruction were diagnosed with plain films (1). In some cases of duodenal stenosis or a duodenal web, an upper gastrointestinal contrast study may be helpful. For example, one may see a "windsock" deformity with a duodenal web.

Malrotation may present with a number of radiographic findings. Although there may be a paucity of bowel gas, plain films can be entirely normal. If there is complete obstruction of the duodenum, the "double-bubble" sign may be present, although there is usually distal air in the gastrointestinal tract. In the setting of volvulus, a "gasless" abdomen may be present. However, a nonspecific bowel gas pattern does not rule out volvulus. Bowel thickening and edema are other findings that may be appreciated on plain films. Abdominal plain films are nondiagnostic for malrotation with or without volvulus. A limited UGI contrast study is the "gold standard" to diagnose malrotation. The diagnosis of volvulus should be based on clinical grounds, and further diagnostic studies should not delay operative intervention in a sick neonate. Findings on UGI study consistent with malrotation include failure of the duodenojejunal junction to cross to the left of the spine, obstruction of the duodenum, and an abnormal right-sided jejunum. Volvulus will have a characteristic "corkscrew" appearance of the small bowel and the "bird's beak" sign representing the passage of contrast into the volvulized segment of bowel. Although a barium enema can be used to define the location of the cecum, malrotation cannot be excluded with a cecum in the right lower quadrant. The finding of the reversal of the relationship between the superior mesenteric artery and vein on ultrasound is neither sensitive nor specific and should not be used in the acute setting to diagnose malrotation (17).

Jejunal atresia is usually diagnosed with plain films. Plain films will display dilated loops of bowel to the site of the most proximal atresia. In more distal lesions, air–fluid levels are often present. No distal gas beyond the obstruction is identified. A UGI study is not necessary and, if performed may be problematic because there will be a considerable amount of contrast in the intestine with no means of egress.

In summary, a history, physical, and plain abdominal films are usually sufficient to diagnose most high intestinal obstructions. Occasionally, a UGI is helpful to delineate the anatomy. An urgent UGI is required in any neonate suspected of having malrotation.

LOW INTESTINAL OBSTRUCTION

The characteristic findings on plain films for a low intestinal obstruction are multiple dilated loops of bowel, often with air–fluid levels. Although plain films may be suggestive of a particular type of low intestinal obstruction, they are rarely diagnostic. All neonates with suspected low intestinal obstruction require a contrast enema.

Neonates with a distal small intestinal obstruction will have plain films showing multiple dilated loops of bowel. Air–fluid levels are usually present. The diagnosis of a small bowel atresia is confirmed by contrast enema. The contrast enema will show a microcolon, which is indicative of an unused colon. A microcolon may not be present if the atresia formed shortly before birth.

A neonate with meconium ileus will have plain films showing multiple distended loops of small bowel often without air–fluid level because of the thick, tenacious meconium. The classic radiologic finding for meconium ileus is Neuhauser's or Singleton's sign representing distended loops of small bowel with a "soap bubble" pattern of meconium in the right lower quadrant. However, this is not a consistent finding in patents with meconium ileus (16). The most common plain film finding is moderately severe distention of the small bowel with no obvious colonic gas. A contrast enema should be performed in patients with suspected meconium ileus for diagnostic and therapeutic purposes. Findings on contrast enema include a microcolon and multiple small filling defects representing meconium pellets present in the microcolon. Reflux into the inspissated meconium of the terminal ileum is essential for accurate diagnosis. Subsequent gastrograffin enemas may also provide a therapeutic benefit and avoid operative intervention. If contrast is not refluxed into the terminal ileum, it may be difficult to distinguish meconium ileus from a distal small intestinal obstruction such as an atresia.

Patients with complicated meconium ileus that results from in utero perforation have a different constellation of findings from simple meconium ileus. Plain films must be examined for the presence of calcifications, meconium, and free air. With the discovery of the previous findings, no other tests are warranted.

A variety of findings on plain films may indicate the diagnosis of intussusception. Early in the course of disease, the bowel gas pattern may be nonspecific. With progression of disease, dilated loops of small bowel and decreased air in the colon will be present. The absence of air-filled bowel loops in the right lower quadrant is suggestive of intussusception. A right upper quadrant density is highly diagnostic of intussusception. Diagnosis and initial treatment is performed by contrast enema if there is no evidence of peritonitis.

Obstructive lesions of the colon require a contrast enema for definitive diagnosis. Patients with meconium plug syndrome will have filling defects in the presence of a normal-appearing colon. Neonates with small left colon syndrome will reveal a normal-size rectum, but the left colon will have the appearance of a microcolon. This can be distinguished from Hirschsprung's disease based on the lack of dilatation in the proximal colon, and a smaller caliber left colon than the typical aganglionic segment in Hirschsprung's patients. Patients with colonic atresia will show a microcolon that terminates at the point of atresia on contrast enema.

In Hirschsprung's disease, plain films demonstrate findings consistent with a low intestinal obstruction and the rectum is usually small to normal if it can be visualized. Seventy percent of patients have involvement of the rectum or rectosigmoid alone. The aganglionic bowel is usually normal in caliber, whereas the normal ganglionic bowel proximal to the bowel with Hirschsprung's disease is dilated. Contrast enema is used to define the transition zone between the normal-size aganglionic bowel and the dilated proximal ganglionic bowel. The delineation of a transition zone is often difficult and only present in 65% of neonates. Retention of barium after 24 hours is present in 80% of neonates with Hirschsprung's disease, but it is less specific because it is present in 60% of patients without Hirschsprung's disease (17). A suction rectal biopsy should be performed in any patient suspected of having Hirschsprung's disease.

Anorectal malformations are diagnosed by physical examination. Radiological studies may be used to aid in the planning of corrective surgery and ruling out associated anomalies.

In summary, a history, physical examination and plain films are sufficient to diagnose a low intestinal obstruction. However, a contrast enema is required in all neonates to provide a definitive diagnosis of the type of low intestinal obstruction.

FUNCTIONAL INTESTINAL OBSTRUCTION

Plain radiographs are important in the diagnosis of neonates with functional obstructions. Once mechanical obstructions are ruled out, functional obstruction may be present in infants with NEC, sepsis, and congenital hypothyroidism. Plain films of neonates with NEC will have edema of the bowel wall, generalized bowel distention, pneumatosis intestinalis, and often portal venous gas. In the setting of intestinal perforation, pneumoperitoneum or intraperitoneal fluid may be present. Left lateral decubitus films aid in the recognition of pneumoperitoneum. In the correct clinical setting, the constellation of plain film findings listed previously eliminate the need for further studies. Clinical history, physical examination, laboratory data, and plain abdominal films are usually sufficient to diagnose functional intestinal obstruction.

After the definitive diagnosis is made in the neonate with intestinal obstruction, initial management consists of bowel decompression, fluid resuscitation, antibiotics, correction of metabolic abnormalities, and ventilatory support where needed. The patients should then undergo definitive management according to the lesion causing obstruction.

In summary, intestinal obstruction in the neonate can provide the surgeon with a diagnostic challenge. The lesions causing obstruction can be divided into high, low, or functional obstructive lesions. A diagnostic and therapeutic algorithm is presented in Fig. 76-1. High lesions may have a prenatal history of polyhydramnios and are easily recognizable by prenatal ultrasound. Low lesions

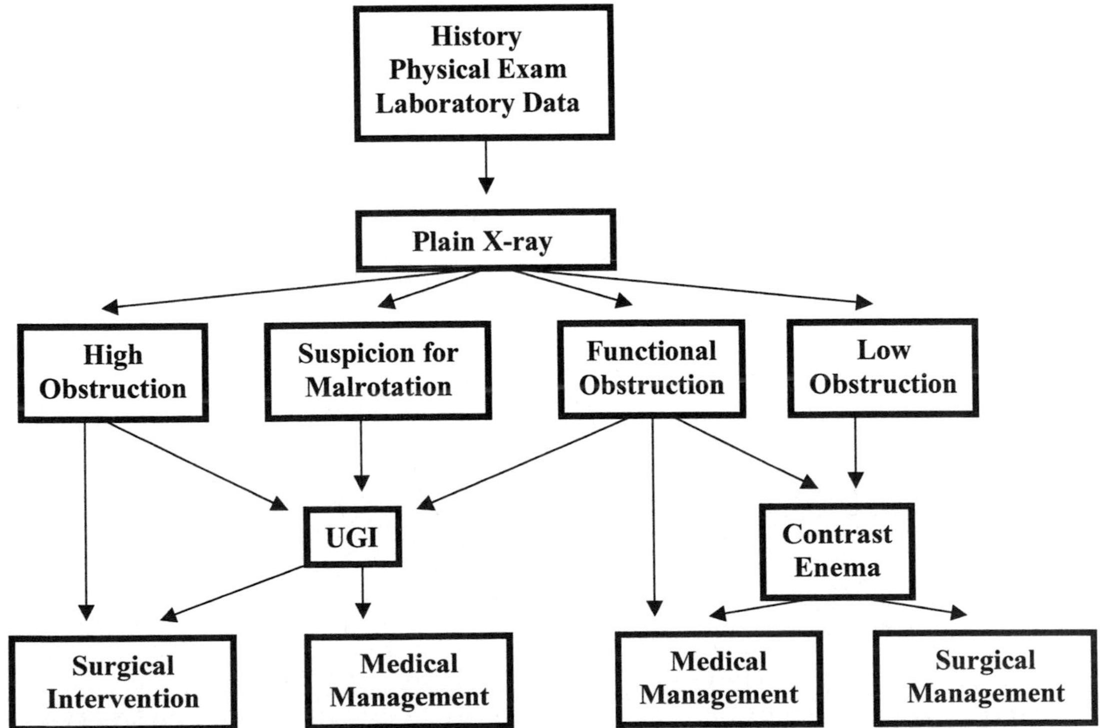

FIGURE 76-1. Algorithm for diagnosis and treatment of neonatal intestinal obstruction. After preliminary evaluation, the majority of infants can be categorized as having a high, low, or functional obstruction. Subsequent radiographic studies and treatment is dictated based on the lesion. All infants suspected of malrotation require an emergent upper gastrointestinal (UGI) unless peritonitis is present.

often do not have prenatal manifestations and are uncommonly detected by prenatal ultrasound. High obstructive lesions will present with bilious emesis as the most common sign at presentation. Bilious emesis occurs later with low lesions. High lesions often do not have a significant amount of abdominal distension. Low lesions will present with generalized abdominal distention and no or late passage of meconium after 24 hours. The integration of the data provided from the presenting symptoms and signs, physical examination, laboratory data, and radiological studies will guide the surgeon to the proper diagnosis and treatment of neonates with intestinal obstruction.

REFERENCES

1. Reyes HM, Meller JL, Loeff D. Neonatal intestinal obstruction. *Clin Perinatol* 1989;16(1):85–96.
2. Santulli TV. Intestinal obstruction in the newborn infant. *J Pediatr* 1954;44:317–337.
3. Dalla Vecchia LK, Grosfeld JL, West KW, et al. Intestinal atresia and stenosis: a 25-year experience with 277 cases. *Arch Surg* 1998;133(5): 490–496; discussion 496–497.
4. Bailey PV, Tracy TF Jr, Connors RH, et al. Congenital duodenal obstruction: a 32-year review. *J Pediatr Surg* 1993;28(1):92–95.
5. Hancock BJ, Wiseman NE. Congenital duodenal obstruction: the impact of an antenatal diagnosis. *J Pediatr Surg* 1989;24(10):1027–1031.
6. Harberg FJ, Pokorny WJ, Hahn H. Congenital duodenal obstruction. A review of 65 cases. *Am J Surg* 1979;138(6):825–828.
7. Corteville JE, Gray DL, Langer JC. Bowel abnormalities in the fetus—correlation of prenatal ultrasonographic findings with outcome. *Am J Obstetr Gynecol* 1996;175(3 Pt 1):724–729.
8. Moore CC. Congenital gastric outlet obstruction. *J Pediatr Surg* 1989;24(12):1241–1246.
9. Farrant P, Dewbury KC, Meire HB. Antenatal diagnosis of duodenal atresia. *B J Radiol* 1981;54:633–635.
10. Langer JC, Adzick NS, Filly RS, et al. Gastrointestinal tract obstruction in the fetus. *Arch Surg* 1989;124:1183–1186.
11. Kimble RM, Harding JE, Kolbe A. Does gut atresia cause polyhydramnios? *Pediatr Surg Int* 1998;13(2–3):115–117.
12. Ford EG, Senac MO Jr, Srikanth MS, et al. Malrotation of the intestine in children. *Ann Surg* 1992;215(2):172–178.
13. Stewart DR, Colodny AL, Daggett WC. Malrotation of the bowel in infants and children: a 15 year review. *Surgery* 1976;79(6):716–720.
14. Torres AM, Ziegler MM. Malrotation of the intestine. *World J Surg* 1993;17(3):326–331.
15. Clark DA. Times of first void and first stool in 500 newborns. *Pediatrics.* 1977;60(4):457–459.
16. Carty H, Brereton RJ. The distended neonate. *Clin Radiol* 1983;34: 367–380.
17. Hernanz-Schulman M. Imaging of neonatal gastrointestinal obstruction. *Radiol Clin North Am* 1999;37(6):1163–1186.

Meconium Syndromes and Cystic Fibrosis

Sonya R. Walker and Edward M. Barksdale, Jr.

The meconium syndromes encompass multiple gastrointestinal disorders leading to intestinal obstruction from meconium or foreign material. This group of diseases, including meconium ileus (MI; simple and complex), meconium peritonitis, meconium plug syndrome, and MI equivalent, share various overlapping aspects in pathophysiology, clinical presentation, diagnostic techniques, and management. The most common of these gastrointestinal meconium disorders, and their critical pathogenetic and molecular relationship to cystic fibrosis (CF), are discussed in this chapter.

MECONIUM ILEUS

History

First described by Landsteiner in 1905, MI is the newborn bowel obstruction caused by inspissated meconium, and associated with cystic degeneration and fibrosis of the pancreas. Pancreatic exocrine deficiency leading to the abnormal production of thick, viscous intestinal mucus was ultimately shown to be the primary cause of atypical meconium development (1–3). In 1936, Fanconi first reported CF, noting the association of pancreatic insufficiency and chronic pulmonary disease (4). Shortly thereafter in 1938, Anderson established the critical link between CF and MI, characterizing the histologic similarities between the bowel and pancreatic tissues (5). Evolution in surgical and medical therapies closely paralleled understanding of the pathophysiology of the disease. Prior to the mid-twentieth century, MI was generally fatal in newborns. In 1948, Hiatt and Wilson reported the first successful surgical treatment of MI using enterotomy and saline irrigation (6). Although several other surgical procedures were subsequently developed and significantly improved the survival for neonates with complicated MI, the concepts developed by Hiatt and Wilson are still today the basis of therapy for uncomplicated MI. In 1969, Noblett introduced a technique of nonoperative management of neonates with simple MI using hyperosmolar diatrizoate enema (7). Various modifications have been developed; however, the dilute water-soluble contrast enema remains the nonoperative standard of care for uncomplicated MI.

Epidemiology

Occurring primarily in white populations, the meconium syndromes are closely linked to CF. CF is one of the most common serious genetic diseases in whites. Approximately 5% to 6% of white individuals are carriers of the genetic defect (3,8). The incidence is about 1 in every 2,500 childbirths in the United States (9–11). CF is transmitted as an autosomal recessive trait, thus both parents must be heterozygotes for the gene in order to have an affected child. Each offspring has a one in four chance of developing the disease. MI will be the initial clinical manifestation of this disorder in 10% to 20% of affected infants. Ten to 30% of patients diagnosed with MI have a family history of CF. In families in which the first CF child has had MI, 29% of subsequent siblings with CF have MI, compared with 6% in families in which the first child with CF did not have MI (12,13). The number of males and females affected is almost equal. MI is uncommon in premature infants.

Genetics

Localization of the CF gene along with identification of the most prevalent genetic mutation was initially described in 1989 (14,15). Located on the long arm of chromosome 7, the gene has more than 800 known mutations at present (16,17). The most common mutation, ΔF508, a three base pair deletion from the gene, is responsible for approximately 70% of clinical cases (18,19). The gene encodes the cystic fibrosis transmembrane regulator (CFTR), which

Sonya R. Walker and Edward M. Barksdale, Jr.: Department of Surgery, University of Pittsburgh School of Medicine, Division of Pediatric Surgery, Children's Hospital of Pittsburgh, Pittsburgh, Pennsylvania 15213.

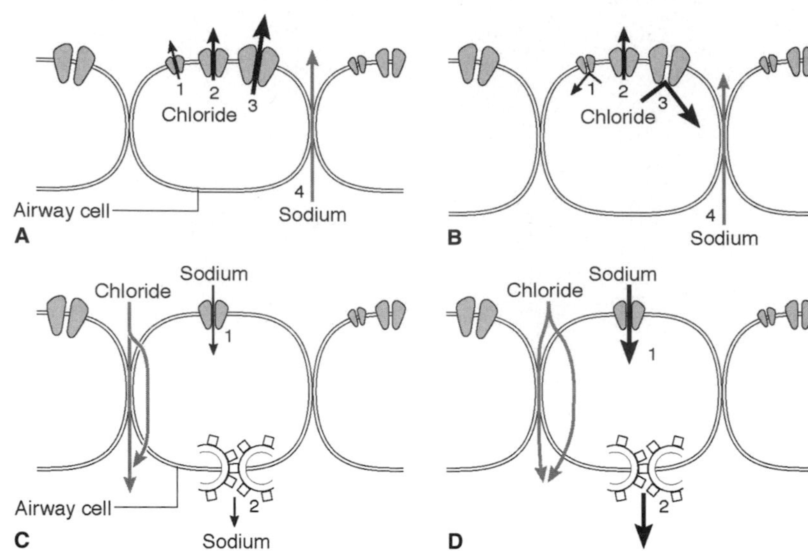

FIGURE 77-1. Chloride and sodium transport in normal and cystic fibrosis (CF) epithelial cells. **(A)** Epithelial cell (normal) with three types of chloride channels: 1, calcium dependent; 2, outwardly rectifying channel (ORCC); and 3, CF transmembrane regulator (CFTR), most important. Sodium passes between epithelial cells into the lumen. **(B)** CF epithelial cell with dysfunctional CFTR preventing chloride excretion. Calcium-dependent channel does not open, and the ORCC works minimally. **(C)** Epithelial cell (normal) sodium absorption. **(D)** CF epithelial cell with markedly upregulated sodium absorption.

is a cyclic adenosine monophosphate (cAMP)-induced chloride channel protein that resides in the apical membrane of epithelial cells (20). CFTR serves as a chloride channel activated by cAMP that regulates transepithelial fluid balance. Specifically, CFTR abrogates an amiloride-sensitive epithelial chloride channel, while inducing an alternate chloride channel (21) (Fig. 77-1). Mutations in this 1480 amino acid protein result in defective chloride transport in the apical membrane of epithelial cells of the respiratory, gastrointestinal, biliary, pancreatic, and reproductive systems. Types of defects fall into four or five major pathophysiologic categories that are based on how they disrupt CFTR synthesis and function (Table 77-1). CFTR synthesis occurs in the cell nucleus and undergoes folding and packaging in the endoplasmic reticulum prior to transport to the epithelial cell membrane. The membrane-bound CFTR regulates conductance through the chloride channels by responding to the appropriate signals (Fig. 77-2). The most common mutation, ΔF508, a class 2 defect, results in CFTR protein degradation in the endoplasmic reticulum prior to folding and trafficking. Patients who are homozygotes for this mutation typically develop significant pancreatic insufficiency, but may have variable pulmonary disease. The genetic basis of MI is unknown.

Pathogenesis

Cystic fibrosis is a systemic illness with diverse clinical presentations in various exocrine glands throughout the body. Abnormally thick and viscous mucous secretions may obstruct the bronchoalveolar tree, pancreatic ducts, and intestinal tract. Nasal mucus membranes, sweat and salivary glands, liver, and reproductive organs are also frequently affected. Common manifestations of this disease include pancreatic insufficiency in 90%, diabetes mellitus in 20%, obstructive biliary disease in 15–20%, and meconium ileus in 10–20% of all patients. Azoospermia occurs in nearly all affected males (22). Exocrine glands throughout the body are affected by this chloride transport defect. Abnormally thick and viscous mucus secretions obstructing the bowel, the pancreatic ducts, and air passages in the lung cause the most severe clinical manifestations.

The secretion of hyperviscous mucus and subsequent intestinal obstruction begins prenatally. The meconium

TABLE 77-1 CFTR Mutations and Their Role in Cystic Fibrosis Transmembrane Regulator Production and Function.[a]

Class 1 Production	*Class 2 Folding; Trafficking*	*Class 3 Regulation*	*Class 4 Conduction*	*Class 5 Reduced Production*
G542X	ΔF508	G551D	R117H	3849 + 10 kB C→T
W1282X	ΔI507	(ΔF508)	R347P	A455E???
3905insT	N1303K		R334W	
R553X	S549R			
	G480C			
	A455E???			

[a]Classifications are not exclusive; that is, ΔF508 has abnormal processing so little of it reaches the cell membrane, *and* the protein that does reach the cell membrane shows limited response to signals.

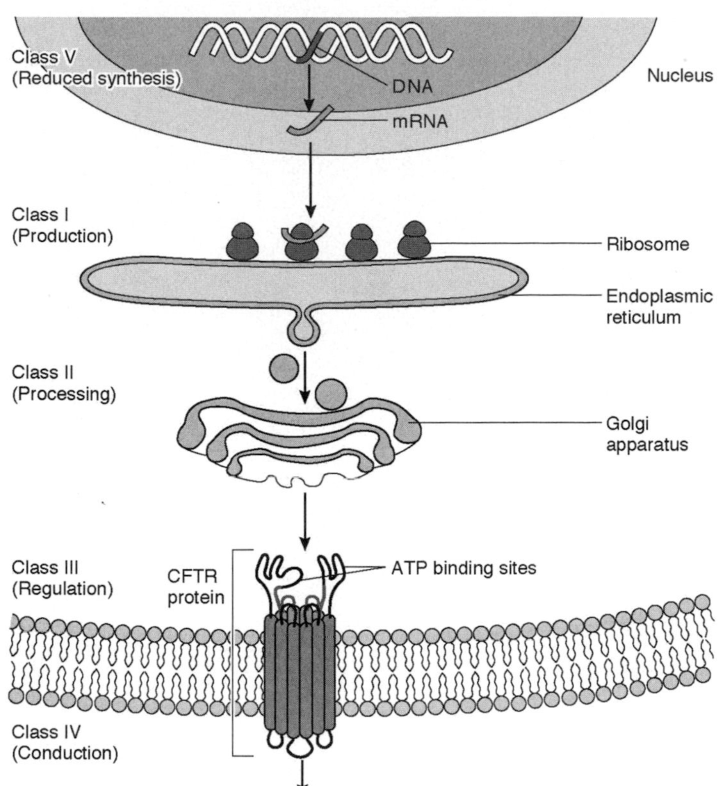

FIGURE 77-2. Cystic fibrosis gene and protein. CFTR, cystic fibrosis transmembrane regulator; ATP, adenosine triphosphate.

involved in MI is typically low in water content, minerals, and protein-bound carbohydrate and has several biochemical abnormalities, including elevated albumin, mucoprotein, and calcium, as well as low trypsin levels (23,24). The decreased carbohydrate and increased protein concentrations likely account for the hyperviscosity of the meconium (25,26). Neonates with MI and CF have a meconium protein content of 80% to 90%, compared with 7% in normal infants (27). Most of this extra protein has been shown to be albumin (28). The high viscosity and tenacity of the meconium result from a combination of a hyperviscous mucus secreted by abnormal intestinal glands, abnormal concentrating mechanisms of the proximal small intestine, and pancreatic exocrine deficiency in utero. Infants with MI and CF have severely affected intestinal glands, but mild pancreatic disease. It is believed that the intestinal glandular abnormality may be the primary precipitating factor for the development of meconium ileus, with the pancreatic disease playing a secondary role (29). The distal intestinal lumen becomes obstructed with meconium, leading to proximal bowel dilatation. Inspissated meconium located in the distal ileum and proximal colon develops into hard pellets due to the increased absorption of fluid from the stool. Disuse atrophy in utero results in a small-caliber colon or microcolon.

Pancreatic injury begins prenatally and continues throughout the lifetime of the individual. The progressive obstruction of pancreatic ducts leads to acinar atrophy, decreased exocrine secretions, and eventually, fibrosis and fatty changes of the exocrine gland (30,31). By early infancy, approximately 85% to 90% of CF patients have advanced pancreatic lesions that result in an absence of pancreatic enzymes in the duodenum (32). Autopsy studies have revealed that CF patients without MI have a pattern of progressive pancreatic involvement with age. In contrast, patients with MI generally have mild pancreatic involvement and more severe intestinal glandular disease (29). The glandular changes include dilation of the crypts of Lieberkuhn, accumulation of intraluminal secretions, and flattening of the epithelial lining cells.

At birth, the lungs are normal in CF patients. However, progressive and diffuse pulmonary disease develops as a result of mucus plugging of the small airways and secondary infection. The sweat sodium and chloride levels are elevated from birth. These levels are unrelated to the severity or distribution of organ involvement. The sweat electrolyte abnormality is caused by the impermeability of the epithelia to chloride ions. The chloride is unable to follow as the sodium is actively pumped out of luminal fluids. Sodium tends to be retained in the lumen of the apocrine glands by this mechanism (33) (Fig. 77-1).

Classification

Simple Meconium Ileus

MI is usually classified as either simple (uncomplicated) or complex (complicated). In simple cases, the distal ileum becomes obstructed by abnormal meconium as a result of a simple obturation. The proximal ileum is thickened, dilated, and packed with tarlike meconium. Distal to the site of obstruction, the bowel is collapsed and contains concrete, puttylike pellets of gray, inspissated meconium. The meconium in the distal bowel sometimes has a beadlike appearance. Due to the proximal obstructive disease, there is a microcolon, which is poorly developed and may contain small pellets of meconium. There is no classic histologic appearance for MI; however, tissue sections of the bowel may show intracellular inclusion bodies and intestinal crypts filled with inspissated meconium (Fig. 77-3).

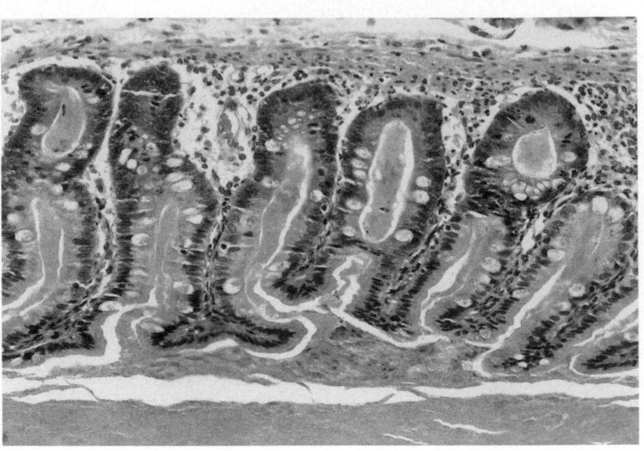

FIGURE 77-3. Inspissated mucus in meconium ileus. Histologic section of bowel showing dilated crypts filled with eosinophilic, inspissated mucus.

Complex Meconium Ileus

In utero, simple obturation obstruction of the bowel may progress to complicated MI. Intestinal necrosis or atresia, meconium peritonitis, pseudocyst, or all these conditions may occur in cases of complex MI. Most often, this is related to volvulus or ischemia of the dilated segment of the proximal ileum. Depending on the time at which the volvulus occurs and the in utero evolution of the process, the complicated form of this disease may result in intestinal atresia, perforation, or meconium peritonitis. Bacterial peritonitis results from postnatal volvulus and perforation, but occurs infrequently (Fig. 77-4).

Meconium Peritonitis

Meconium peritonitis was first reported by Morgagni in 1761 in *De Sedibus et Causis Morborum* as an aseptic, chemical, or foreign-body reaction resulting from prenatal spillage of meconium into the peritoneal cavity due to intestinal perforation (34,35). Ischemic necrosis and perforation result from the large meconium bolus located

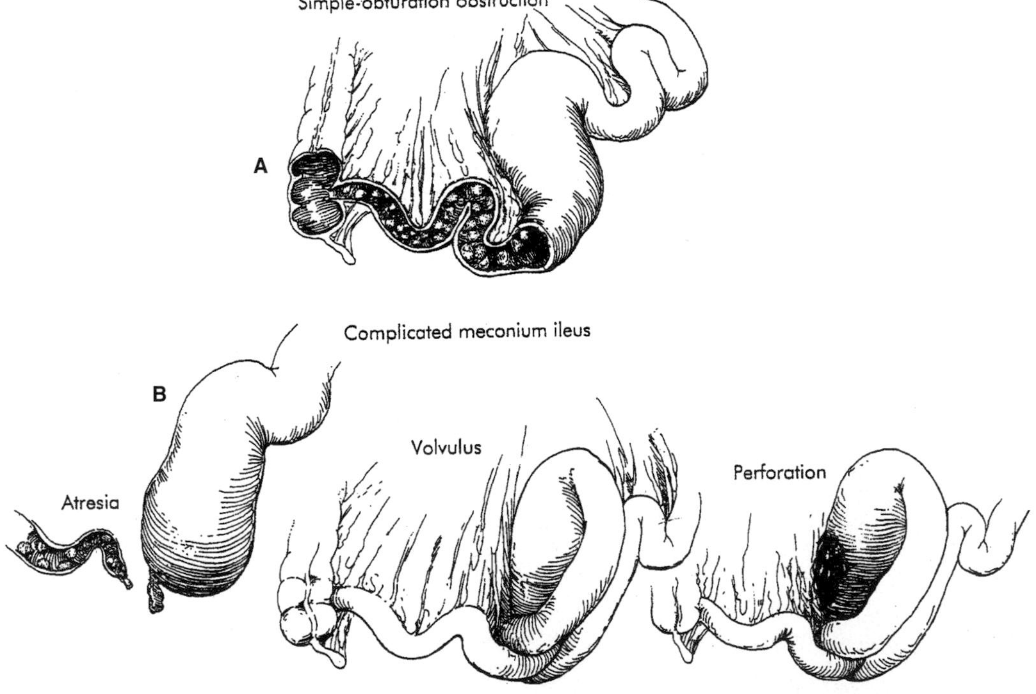

FIGURE 77-4. Complex meconium ileus (MI). **(A)** Simple MI with obstruction of the ileum by inspissated meconium pellets. The bowel proximal to the obstruction is dilated, in contrast to the small caliber of the colon distal to the obstruction. **(B)** Depiction of three variations of complex MI (atresia, volvulus, and perforation). (From Rescorla FJ, Grosfeld JL. Contemporary management of meconium ileus. *World J Surg* 1993;17:318, with permission.)

proximal to the obstruction. A segmental volvulus often occurs when the meconium-filled segment of redundant ileum twists. The narrow base of the volvulus may lead to ischemic necrosis of the bowel and result in isolated or multiple ileal atresias, formation of a stricture, or perforation. The perforation is typically secondary to segmental volvulus followed by gangrene with focal perforation (Fig. 77-4). Infants with complicated MI may present with intestinal perforation in the form of either free or encysted peritonitis. Three pathologic types of meconium peritonitis have been described, including generalized, fibroadhesive, and cystic (36). Generalized meconium peritonitis with ascites develops if the perforation and meconium extravasation occur in the late perinatal or early neonatal period. Diffuse distribution of meconium throughout the peritoneal cavity initiates the inflammatory process. However, due to the brief duration, no calcification occurs. The adhesions between bowel loops are more fibrinous, rather than fibrous, in generalized peritonitis. Most commonly, however, fibroadhesive meconium peritonitis occurs. When the perforation has occurred early enough prior to delivery, dense adhesions and calcification occur. Intraperitoneal meconium may form calcifications within 48 hours of perforation (37). The meconium contains digestive enzymes that induce an intense chemical peritonitis, initiated by the sterile meconium. Subsequently, dense, fibrous adhesions and agglutination of the bowel may result. The calcified and fibrous adhesions are often effective in sealing the site of perforation and frequently obscure identification of the site. When the fibroblastic reaction has not been effective in sealing the site of perforation, meconium may continue to leak into the peritoneal cavity, resulting in cystic meconium peritonitis. Segmental volvulus with ischemic necrosis of the bowel along with extravasation and liquefaction of meconium may lead to development of a pseudocyst. The pseudocyst consists of densely adherent, partially necrotic loops of intestine surrounding liquefied meconium. Frequently, a calcified fibrous peel or wall envelops this mass. This cyst may fill with air after birth and may then be called giant cystic meconium peritonitis (38). Colonic perforation distal to the obstruction may result from excessive intraluminal pressure from a contrast enema; however, this is not generally a difficult event to recognize and differentiate from the previous lesions.

Differential Diagnosis

MI must be differentiated from other forms of congenital distal intestinal obstruction, such as meconium plug syndrome, small left colon syndrome, colonic or ileal atresia, Hirschsprung's disease, and functional immaturity of the bowel. Many of these conditions may be distinguished from MI by diagnostic barium or water-soluble contrast enema. Ileal atresia may present similarly to MI, but generally does not have pellets in the ileum and usually has air–fluid levels in the small bowel. The plain film with MI often has a "ground glass" or hazy appearance reflecting the large amounts of air and inspissated meconium proximal, whereas ileal atresia has a clearer appearance with air contrast. Congenital aganglionosis, particularly total colonic Hirschsprung's disease, may mimic uncomplicated MI. If this is suspected, the patient's appendix may be sent at the time of laparotomy for histologic examination of ganglion cells. Congenital hypothyroidism, hypermagnesemia, hypocalcemia, and maternal narcotic use may produce a functional bowel obstruction that has a similar clinical presentation. Meconium peritonitis may be caused by various types of bowel obstruction that are not related to CF, including intussusception, internal hernia, volvulus, and atresia. However, it is often impossible to diagnose the cause for the peritonitis prior to exploration.

Clinical Presentation

Simple Meconium Ileus

Infants with MI are often small for gestational age, but are rarely premature. The in utero bowel obstruction may result in lower birth weights in neonates with MI due to the decreased absorption of amniotic fluid-derived nutrients. Often the first 24 hours of life are relatively normal for most neonates with simple MI, except that they may not pass meconium spontaneously. Following birth, progressive abdominal distension occurs as the proximal small intestine fills with air, feedings, and intestinal secretions. In the next 24 to 48 hours, bilious vomiting occurs and there is little or no passage of meconium. Distended, doughy loops of intestine that indent on palpation are frequently observed on abdominal physical examination. These are the proximal, meconium-filled loops of small bowel. The rectum and anus are often small in these infants, and this may be misinterpreted as anal atresia or stenosis. A classic finding on rectal examination is the presence of white mucous rather than meconium, reflecting the fact that an obstruction is interposed between the ampulla of Vater and the anus. Although more common with complex MI, a maternal history of polyhydramnios occurs in nearly 20% of infants with simple MI. Associated congenital anomalies are rarely present.

Complex Meconium Ileus

Complicated MI or meconium peritonitis commonly presents immediately (within 24 hours) after birth. In the case of antenatal pseudocyst formation, with or without calcification, prenatal ultrasound diagnosis is often established in contemporary practice. If distal obstruction is present without perforation, such as with distal ileal atresia or volvulus, the infant may tolerate feeds for the first day of life prior to developing symptoms of obstruction. Neonates with complicated MI are more severely ill compared with those with simple MI. Progressive abdominal distension occurs that may be associated with erythema and edema of the abdominal wall. Pneumoperitoneum and peritonitis may also present with these findings. The erythema and edema of the abdominal wall usually indicates an underlying pseudocyst or peritonitis. The abdomen may be very tense, and there may be a palpable mass usually secondary to a volvulus. Neonates with meconium peritonitis or giant cystic meconium peritonitis frequently have abdominal distension at birth and have bile-stained gastric aspirates. Respiratory compromise secondary to the abdominal distension may be present. Third-space losses may lead to hypovolemia that left untreated may progress to severe cardiovascular instability. Some patients with complex MI may also become septic late in their course.

Diagnosis

Cystic Fibrosis

The definitive diagnostic study for CF is the sweat test. Although reasonably accurate during the first few days of life, it may not be possible to collect an adequate volume of sweat until the infant is 4 to 6 weeks of age. The pilocarpine iontophoresis method yields a quantitative estimate of sodium and chloride levels on an accurately collected amount of uncontaminated sweat from the forearm, leg, or back of the infant (39). Pilocarpine, a cholinergic drug that stimulates the production of sweat, is placed topically and an electrical current (3 to 4 mA) is applied to facilitate cutaneous drug absorption. Filter paper secured to the skin, with an airtight binder to prevent evaporation, is used to collect sweat for the next hour. The CF diagnosis is confirmed with concentrations of sodium and chloride higher than 60 mEq per L if at least 100 mg of sweat has been collected. It is recommended that the test be performed after 4 to 6 weeks of life because normal infants may have elevated sweat electrolyte levels during the first few days of life. Many infants with MI are weak and debilitated postoperatively so it may not be possible to make the diagnosis of CF early. Although not diagnostic, the Boehringer-Mannheim test has occasionally been used as a screening test for CF. The test is based on the abnormal concentrating mechanisms of the proximal small intestine and demonstrates excessive levels of albumin in meconium. Rarely do normal infants have greater than 3 mg of albumin per gram of meconium. Infants with CF, in contrast, usually have as much as 80 mg of albumin per gram. This test is not specific, however, frequently yielding false-positive results.

Antenatal and neonatal genetic screening are routinely performed for patients or families with suspected or known CF. Likewise, certain states in the United States employ population-based newborn screens to detect occult CF. Although these are potentially quite helpful in detecting most cases, the large number of genotypes that produce the clinical CF phenotype makes all the genetic screening strategies less than 100% sensitive at present.

Prenatal (Radiologic)

Prenatal ultrasonography may be helpful in diagnosing MI. The presence of echogenic bowel after 20 weeks' gestation has been associated with MI (simple) and meconium peritonitis (40). This association is even stronger when screening fetuses with a family history of CF. Dilated bowel, intraabdominal calcification, or ascites are suggestive of complicated meconium ileus. Intrauterine intestinal perforation leading to intraperitoneal meconium causes calcifications in the abdomen or scrotum, whether the cause is MI or another event. Meconium peritonitis may be noted in utero, and the ultrasound usually demonstrates polyhydramnios, ascites, dilated fetal bowel, and intraabdominal echogenic masses (41,42). It is crucial to recognize that intraluminal calcified meconium is not associated with intestinal perforation and meconium peritonitis. This distinction may have a significant impact on the decision for and timing of surgical intervention.

Postnatal

A family history of CF supports the diagnosis of MI, but it is only present in approximately one-fourth of all cases. Maternal polyhydramnios is also an important clinical association to seek for MI. Generalized abdominal distension, bilious emesis, and failure to pass meconium within the first 48 hours after birth are the three cardinal signs of bowel obstruction from MI. Palpable loops of dilated bowel obstructed with meconium may be present. Plain abdominal radiographs may be extremely helpful. Radiologic features of simple MI include dilated intestinal loops of varying size, relative absence of air–fluid levels, and a characteristic "soap bubble" or "ground-glass" appearance of portions of the abdomen (Fig. 77-5). The soap bubble appearance, occurring as air passes into the intestine and mixes with thick meconium, frequently appears in the right lower quadrant and is also known as Neuhauser's sign (43). These findings are not specific for MI, but may also be seen with Hirschsprung's disease, ileal atresia, colon atresia, meconium plug syndrome, or small left colon syndrome. Air–fluid levels on decubitus radiographs, however, characterize many of these other distal bowel obstructions. The paucity of air–fluid levels in patients with MI is due to the bowel being completely filled with fluid or inspissated meconium. In cases of complicated MI such as ileal atresia or volvulus, more severe bowel distension, air–fluid levels, or a mass effect is usually seen. Scattered areas of calcification on abdominal plain films resulting from extravasated meconium in the peritoneal cavity is characteristic of neonates with perforation and meconium peritonitis. Giant cystic meconium peritonitis is illustrated by intraperitoneal calcification in addition to a cyst with air–fluid levels or ascites. A large dense mass with a

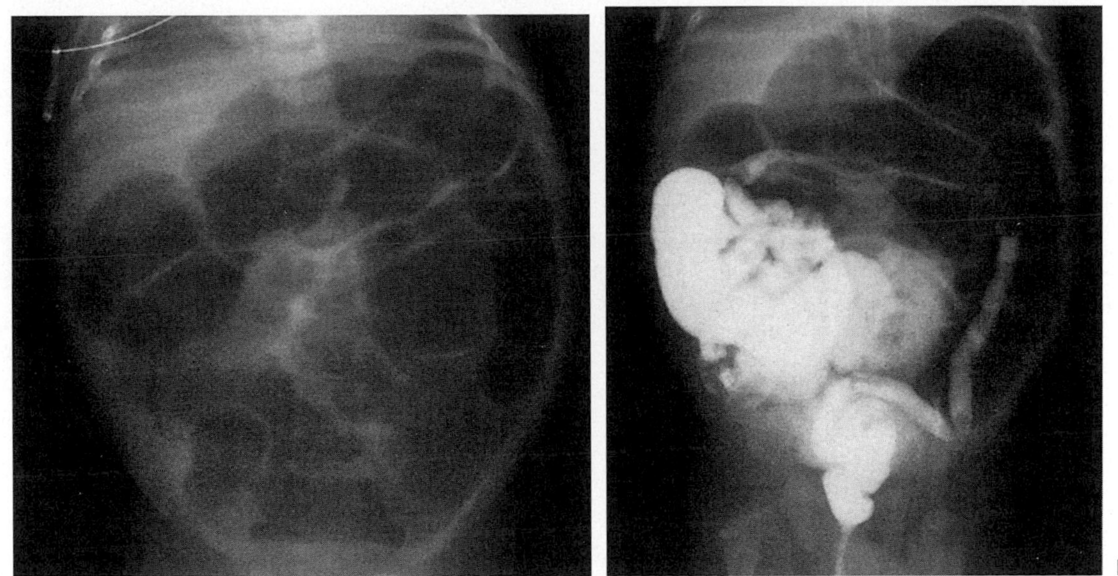

FIGURE 77-5. Abdominal radiographs of meconium ileus (MI). **(A)** Plain abdominal radiograph illustrating characteristic features of MI with dilated loops of intestine of varying size and relative absence of air–fluid levels. **(B)** Contrast radiograph showing dilated proximal bowel and the markedly small caliber of the distal bowel.

rim of calcification is suggestive of cystic meconium peritonitis.

An enema using water-soluble contrast material should be performed when simple MI is suspected. This condition is characterized by an empty microcolon with inspissated pellets outlined within the terminal ileum. The bolus of impacted meconium is outlined as a filling defect. Neonates with atresia also have a small-caliber terminal ileum with dilated intestine proximal to the atresia. With MI, the contrast material may then be used to wash out the obstructing plugs and inspissated meconium. When complicated MI is suspected, a contrast enema is used primarily to confirm the diagnosis, if necessary. In patients with complicated MI (calcification, cyst), a contrast enema study is not required routinely prior to laparotomy because the plain films are usually sufficient to indicate the diagnosis. Contrast material should not be given by mouth in suspected cases of MI due to the risk of aspiration. The diagnosis of an intestinal atresia is confirmed when the contrast material does not pass the atretic segment. Sometimes the symptoms of the complications of MI predominate and an associated atresia may be discovered incidentally at operation. The pathologist may also make the diagnosis of MI during examination of a resected surgical specimen or by postmortem evaluation.

Treatment

Nonoperative (Medical) Management

Patients with uncomplicated MI may be managed nonoperatively with one or more contrast enemas. Surgical intervention is also not required for asymptomatic patients with calcifications. Initial management includes naso- or orogastric tube decompression and intravenous fluids to replace preexisting deficits and ongoing losses. Blood cultures should also be obtained to rule out sepsis, and broad-spectrum antibiotics should be administered. The water-soluble enema is the nonoperative treatment of choice. The surgeon should examine the patient prior to the enema to rule out peritonitis or other contraindications to enema. Gastrografin, as used by Noblett, is a hyperosmolar (1,900 mOsm per L) aqueous solution of meglumine diatrizoate, containing a wetting agent, 0.1% polysorbate 80 (Tween 80), and 37% iodine. The hyperosmolality of this contrast media is believed to draw fluid into the intestinal lumen from plasma. The Tween 80 serves as an emulsifying agent, and this induces an osmotic diarrhea until the contrast has been passed. Most radiologists today do not use Tween 80 in the enema, and dilute the contrast to a lower concentration to decrease the osmolarity and potential complications (44,45). A straight, red rubber tube inserted in the rectum is used for administration of the enema under fluoroscopic observation. The solution is gently infused into the terminal ileum to mix with the inspissated meconium pellets and thick meconium in the dilated ileum. Resistance is encountered as the microcolon is filled. The large meconium cast is outlined as the contrast material reaches the terminal ileum. After the neonate has evacuated the contrast, a repeat enema is performed to clear any residual meconium. Upon returning to the neonatal unit, warm saline enemas containing 1% *N*-acetylcysteine are administered to facilitate complete evacuation. Careful observation of heart rate, blood pressure,

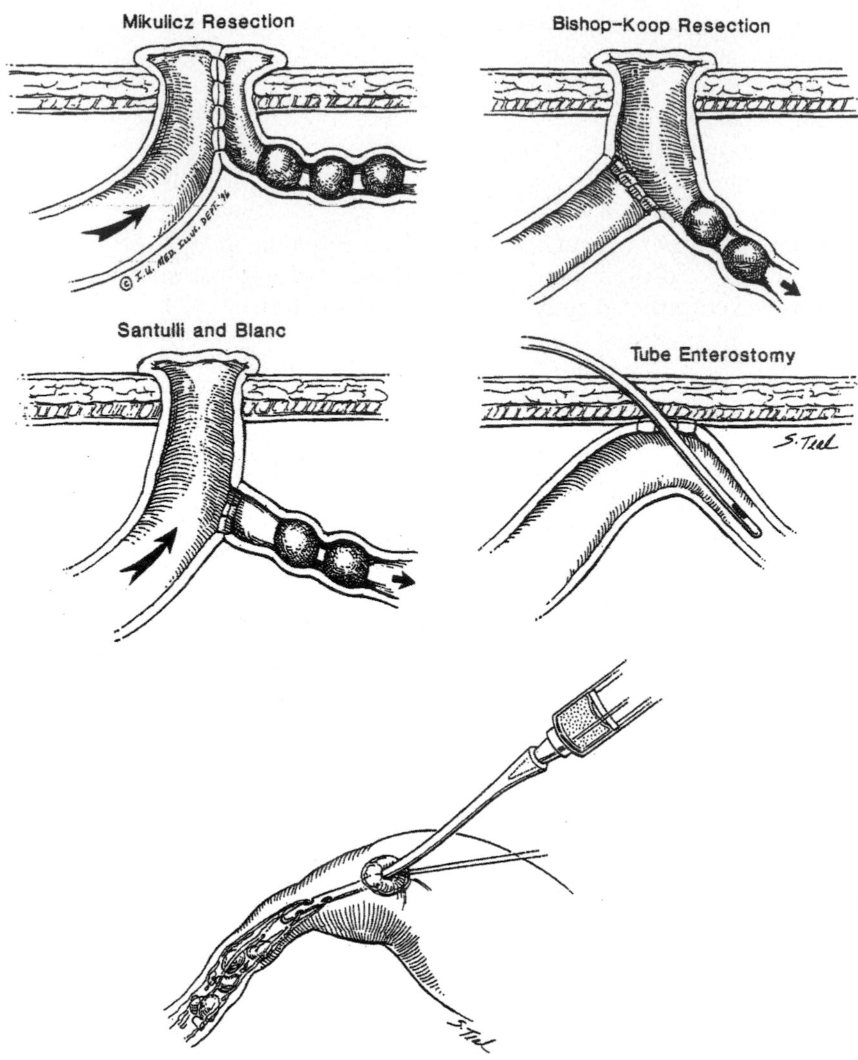

FIGURE 77-6. Surgical approaches to meconium ileus (MI). Various approaches to the surgical treatment of MI are depicted. The Mikulicz side-to-side anastamosis, the Bishop-Koop Roux-en-Y proximal end-to-distal side ileal anastamosis, the Santulli Roux-en-Y anastamosis with proximal "chimney" enterotomy (proximal to distal side-to-end anastamosis), and the tube enterostomy technique are commonly used for irrigation. The Hiatt-Wilson technique of enterotomy with irrigation is the current procedure of choice for simple MI (shown at the bottom). (From Rowe MI, O'Neill JA Jr, Grosfeld JL, et al. *Essentials of pediatric surgery*. St. Louis, MO: Mosby-Year Book,1995:611, with permission.)

and urine output are essential in the postprocedure management. Partially liquid meconium usually passes within the first 12 hours after the enema. It may be necessary to repeat the contrast enema when evidence of continued distention or persistent meconium obstruction is present. Five to 10 mL of 5% to 10% *N*-acetylcysteine per orogastric tube every 6 hours may aid in clearing the meconium. When the obstruction resolves, the orogastric tube is removed and the diet is advanced. Following relief of the bowel obstruction, the diagnosis of CF should be verified. Regardless of whether a diagnosis of CF has been confirmed in neonates with MI, appropriate therapy for CF should be initiated to avoid pulmonary complications.

Surgical Management

Intestinal obstruction is the most frequent indication for operation. Patients with clinical or radiologic evidence of complicated MI, including volvulus, intestinal gangrene, perforation, peritonitis, or small bowel atresia require immediate surgery. The exceptions are asymptomatic prenatally diagnosed infants in which the process resolves before delivery. This occasionally occurs with asymptomatic, extraluminal intraperitoneal, calcified meconium, or contained-free perforation. Surgical intervention is also required for simple MI patients who fail contrast enema treatment.

In 1948, Hiatt and Wilson reported the first survivors of surgical intervention with enterotomy and saline irrigation of obstructing meconium pellets (6). Subsequently, several operative techniques have been developed (Fig. 77-6). In 1953, Gross described relief of obstruction after resection of the dilated ileum and creation of Mikulicz side-by-side enterotomies (46). Intraoperative meconium evacuation was not required, and the exteriorized bowel loop could be opened after abdominal closure to avoid intraperitoneal contamination. A Mikulicz crushing clamp was then used to create a single lumen between the two limbs, and the stoma could be closed extraperitoneally. In 1957, Bishop and Koop advocated ileal resection,

Roux-en-Y proximal end-to-distal side ileal anastamosis, and distal ostomy for postoperative irrigation with pancreatic enzymes (47). This allowed minimization of contamination, anastamosis between appropriately sized bowel, access to distal bowel for decompression, and bedside stoma closure. Four years later, Santulli reported resection and Roux-en-Y anastamosis with proximal "chimney" enterotomy (48,49). A segment of the most dilated portion of ileum was resected, the proximal to distal side-to-end anastamosis was constructed, and an enterotomy with the end of the proximal bowel was created. The recommendation by Swenson in 1962 for resection, irrigation, and primary end-to-end anastamosis resulted in frequent leaks and was not widely used (50). All these procedures had the disadvantage of including an ileal resection in an infant with a disorder of intestinal function. However, in 1970, O'Neill repopularized the use of tube enterostomy placed at the junction of the proximal distended bowel and distal small-caliber intestine for postoperative irrigation, thus eliminating the need for a second procedure (51) (Fig. 77-6).

During the 1970s and 1980s, enterotomy with irrigation regained popularity and is currently the treatment of choice for uncomplicated MI that fails nonoperative management. A pursestring suture is placed on the antimesenteric border of the dilated ileum near the transition from large- to small-caliber intestine. A small soft catheter is inserted through an enterotomy and gently irrigated by manual mixing of the solution with the thick meconium and pellets. Several irrigating solutions have been used including 1% to 4% *N*-acetylcysteine, diatrizoate solution, hydrogen peroxide, pancreatic enzymes, and saline. Hydrogen peroxide is no longer used because of the potential for bowel perforation and gas embolism. Pancreatic enzymes were found to not be of value in liquefying the meconium in this circumstance. The meconium is removed through the enterotomy, and the pellets are either manually removed or flushed into the colon. Several irrigations may be required. The appendiceal stump has been used to instill hyperosmolar solution and evacuate meconium.

The goal of operative management is the complete evacuation of meconium and restoration of bowel continuity, if possible. It may be necessary to perform a variety of techniques such as enterotomy with irrigation or resection with or without a stoma. The actual procedure is dependent on the etiology and the operative findings. For complex MI, the dissection may be bloody and difficult because of dense vascular adhesions. Bowel that is severely distended, atretic, or nonviable must be resected. Resection, bowel irrigation, and primary end-to-end or end-oblique anastamosis, depending on the caliber of the bowel, are often sufficient for management of ileal atresia and volvulus. In MI cases with atresia, the 10- to 15-cm segment of dilated intestine proximal to the atretic segment is frequently atonic if left in place. These dilated segments can usually be sacrificed and still allow for adequate bowel length. Prevention of short gut syndrome by conservation of bowel is always a guiding principle. In cases of inadequate proximal bowel length and significant bowel dilation, consideration should be given to a tapering enteroplasty to preserve length. Some patients may require temporary diversion and gastrostomy for decompression and feeding. Ostomy closure is usually safe 4 to 6 weeks after initial laparotomy.

Antibiotics are administered for several days following surgery. It is usually recommended that the nasogastric drainage continue until the appearance of the drainage changes from bilious to clear and decreases in volume. Delay in oral intake is usually prolonged, and peripheral or central parenteral nutrition is usually required to meet the patient's nutritional needs. Normal bowel function usually returns in 5 to 10 days, and the diet can be advanced. This is also the time for initiating enteral exocrine pancreatic enzyme replacement. An elemental or semi-elemental diet can be substituted using a feeding tube if the patient has initial difficulty tolerating regular formula orally. In addition, vigorous pulmonary care is provided to aid in loosening bronchial secretions.

Complications

There are several potential complications involved in the treatment of CF and MI. Complications of hyperosmolar enemas include intestinal perforation, colonic mucosal and submucosal inflammation, necrotizing enterocolitis, hypovolemic shock, and death. A straight catheter, as opposed to a balloon catheter, is recommended for the enemas to prevent rectal perforation. Perforation of the ileum or cecum has been reported 12 to 48 hours after the enema is administered. Extreme bowel distention by the osmotic process or an injury to the intestinal wall by the contrast material are possible factors leading to this late perforation. Although surgical outcomes are quite favorable in simple MI, the reported operative mortality ranges between 10% and 20%. About 20% to 25% of simple MI patients will require operation for bowel obstruction from residual meconium obstruction. Other patients will have gastrointestinal complications, including malabsorption, biliary obstruction from inspissated bile and adhesive intestinal obstruction. Periodic atelectasis and pulmonary infections may occur as a complication of the underlying CF.

Long-term complications of MI and CF include the distal intestinal obstruction syndrome (which is discussed later in this chapter) (MI equivalent). About 10% of CF patients are affected. Intussusception, appendicitis, rectal prolapse, colon strictures, and gallbladder disease are also associated with CF. In the case of intussusception, the inspissated stool acts as a lead point. This complication is most commonly associated with MI equivalent.

The 4.9% incidence of appendicitis in CF patients is similar to that in the general population (52). Due to the chronic nature of CF and gradual obliteration of the appendiceal lumen with thick mucus, the presentation of appendicitis is often delayed. Patients may have abdominal pain and a right lower quadrant mass. Inflammation may be absent or delayed. In cases where inflammation does occur, it is usually the result of obstruction of the appendiceal orifice. This may progress to perforation and the formation of an abscess without a typical clinical appearance. Computed tomography scan may demonstrate the abscess if contrast material is in the cecum. Other patients may have symptoms of chronic, intermittent right lower quadrant pain and tenderness that resolve following appendectomy (53).

Rectal prolapse occurs in 11% to 30% of CF patients (54). This is typically prior to institution of adequate enzyme therapy, between 1 and 3 years of age. Any child presenting with rectal prolapse should have a sweat test because this may be the presenting sign of CF. Precipitating factors include frequent bowel movements, colonic distension, and elevated abdominal pressure from coughing. Enzyme therapy is usually successful, but occasionally patients may be resistant until 3 to 5 years of age. Rectal sclerotherapy or rectopexy may be necessary to treat persistent cases.

Colon stricture in children with CF is associated with high-dose enzyme therapy, and was originally described by Smyth in 1994 (55,56). A history of MI is present in 45% of these patients. Most cases occur in boys around 5 years of age. Clinical presentation almost always includes abdominal pain accompanied by either obstructive symptoms or diarrhea. Plain abdominal radiographs may or may not illustrate colon thickening and small bowel dilation. Barium enema is most reliable and demonstrates mucosal irregularity, nodular wall thickening, loss of haustral markings, and a stricture that may be located anywhere in the colon. Some patients require only decreased enzyme supplementation and observation. However, nearly all reported cases have required operative intervention with resection.

Fibrosing colonopathy (FC) is a rare, serious disorder occurring almost exclusively in only a small proportion of CF patients between the ages of 2 to 7 years (55,57–58). It is believed to result from prolonged exposure to high doses of pancreatic exocrine preparations. However, it has been reported in children who have not had any enzymatic therapy. It presents as a distal intestinal obstruction. The pathogenesis of FC is unknown. The most striking pathologic feature is dense submucosal fibrosis primarily of the ascending colon with possible pan colonic involvement (59–61). This results in a fusiform, long-segment luminal narrowing and shortening without significant reduction of the external diameter or focal stricture (62). Predisposing factors appear to be young age, history of colitis, previous intestinal surgery or MI, recurrent distal intestinal obstruction syndrome, use of recombinant human DNAse, laxatives, corticosteroids, and H_2-receptor blockers.

Biliary tract complications, such as a microgallbladder containing thick, colorless white bile with cystic duct occlusion or radiolucent gallstones (not cholesterol), are noted in 12% to 27% of CF patients (63). Approximately 4% of patients develop classic symptoms of cholecystitis. Cholecystectomy, preferentially laparoscopic, is the procedure of choice with symptomatic gallbladder disease.

MECONIUM PLUG SYNDROME

In 1956, Clatworthy first described a group of "plugged-up babies" with neonatal intestinal obstruction due to their colon's inability to discard the meconium residue from fetal life (64). The term meconium plug syndrome (MPS) was applied to this condition and, according to Clatworthy, was not an uncommon occurrence. MPS refers to a spectrum of clinical presentations that are characterized by transient obstruction of the neonatal colon. Various terms, including neonatal small left colon syndrome, left-sided microcolon, and functional colonic inertia of prematurity, have been used synonymously with MPS. It is believed that the normal "unplugging" process is impeded and the deflation of the gastrointestinal tract is retarded by either abnormal colonic motility or a meconium mass. Infants with MPS are generally healthy, although they may be born prematurely (64,65). Alternatively, some infants born to diabetic mothers, may be macrosomic or large for gestational age. The hypoglycemia in these infants of diabetic mothers is associated with increased endogenous glucagon production leading to hypoperistalsis (66).

The clinical presentation of neonates with MPS is identical to that of other conditions of distal intestinal obstruction. There is a significant degree of abdominal distension, bile-stained emesis, and failure to pass meconium during the first 24 to 48 hours of life. Although prenatal ultrasound examination during the third trimester has been reported for early diagnosis of MPS, typically this condition is diagnosed postnatally (67). A rectal examination in an infant with a distal bowel obstruction that reveals inspissated meconium is often diagnostic. Massive intestinal distension with multiple dilated loops of bowel along with air–fluid levels may be visualized on plain film. The plug may be revealed as a filling defect on contrast enema. Otherwise, a dilated colon proximal to an abrupt obstruction of the left colon with a distal microcolon may be seen on contrast enema.

Treatment often occurs simultaneously with diagnosis of MPS. The hypertonicity of the water-soluble contrast enema usually stimulates the passage of a long and thick plug of meconium. Occasionally, it may be necessary to repeat the contrast enema to evacuate any residual meconium. Alternatively, warm saline enemas given at the bedside may be used as a supplemental strategy to facilitate further evacuation. There are some reports of the use of amniocentesis and amniography with Urografin to relieve the obstruction. Following successful resolution of this obstruction, most infants can be fed and have an unremarkable course. Although rare, some infants will have underlying Hirschsprung's disease that presents with a meconium plug-like scenario. Suction biopsy is recommended in these infants. The likelihood of Hirschsprung's disease increases for children who become constipated following evacuation of the plugs. A diagnostic sweat test should also be completed in order to rule out cystic fibrosis and meconium ileus of the colon.

MECONIUM ILEUS EQUIVALENT/DISTAL INTESTINAL OBSTRUCTION SYNDROME

In 1941, Rasor and Stevenson first described mechanical intestinal obstruction due to inspissated stool in patients beyond the neonatal period (68). The term *meconium ileus equivalent* was initially applied to this condition due to its similarities with the neonatal disease. More recently, the term *distal intestinal obstruction syndrome* (DIOS) has been used to describe this condition that mimics MI, but presents in children, adolescents, and adults (69). The precise cause of this form of intestinal obstruction is unknown, but it is believed to be secondary to pancreatic exocrine insufficiency, decreased intestinal transit time, and abnormally thick intestinal mucus. The resulting fat and protein malabsorption accompanied by mucosal dysfunction leads to abnormally thick stool that is predisposed to obstruct the bowel. Precipitous episodes of dehydration or inadequate fluid replacement (particularly during warm weather), changes in diet, increased level of activity, abrupt cessation or decrease in pancreatic enzyme supplementation (especially in older adolescents and young adults) and acute respiratory CF exacerbations are among the most common precipitating factors implicated. DIOS has also been noted to occur following surgery for unrelated problems.

Patients with DIOS typically present with intestinal obstructive symptoms, including nausea, vomiting, colicky abdominal pain, abdominal distention, decreased stool frequency, and constipation. Physical exam findings may reveal an irregular right lower quadrant mass due to accumulation of abnormal fecal material. Chronic or recurrent symptoms are common.

Due to the similarities in presentation and the presence of a right lower quadrant mass, the diagnosis of DIOS may be difficult to distinguish from appendicitis and appendiceal abscess. This form of obturation obstruction can also be confused with constipation and intussusception, which are also common in patients with CF (70). Adhesive bowel obstruction, volvulus, opiate misuse, and Crohn's disease are other conditions that must be distinguished from DIOS. Typically, radiographic imaging techniques are useful in making this diagnosis. Small bowel dilatation and air–fluid levels are demonstrated on plain film radiographs of the abdomen. Large amounts of feculent material with a granular or "bubbly" appearance reminiscent of meconium ileus of the newborn period may be seen in these patients. Diagnosis is confirmed by water-soluble contrast study. In general, barium is contraindicated and should be avoided due to its propensity to exacerbate the obstruction.

Patients with DIOS usually respond well to nonoperative therapies. Initial management involves replacement of intravenous fluid deficits and gastric decompression in patients with copious vomiting. Significant bowel obstruction may be treated with antegrade (transileal) or retrograde (transrectal) tube irrigations followed by the instillation of a solution of 1% *N*-acetylcysteine and pulverized pancreazyme (70). Although *N*-acetylcysteine therapy is efficacious, it has poor palatability and potential toxicity. Because both oral and rectal use of this solution may induce liver injury, patients on prolonged *N*-acetylcysteine therapy must be monitored periodically for hepatic dysfunction (71). Intestinal lavage with a balanced salt solution (GoLytely or NuLytely) has also been a useful treatment for DIOS (72). These solutions are administered orally and are contraindicated in the presence of a complete bowel obstruction. Prokinetic agents have been used to decrease symptoms and decrease (not eliminate) the need for intestinal lavage for acute DIOS (73). When complete obstruction is present or with failure of antegrade solutions, contrast enemas should be used, both for diagnosis, but also for therapy. Water-soluble contrast can be administered orally or as an enema (74). Adequate enzyme replacement along with routine administration of stool softeners helps to prevent recurrence. Rarely is surgical intervention necessary to relieve DIOS.

DIOS may be complicated by volvulus, appendicitis, or intussusception. With an incidence of approximately 1% of CF patients, intussusception occurs at the average age of 9 years (75). Fecal material is believed to adhere to the mucosa and serve as a lead point. The most common location is ileocolic, but this may also be ileoileal and cecocolic. Abdominal pain and vomiting are the usual symptoms. A right lower quadrant mass with rectal bleeding is reported in one-fourth of patients. The diagnosis may be delayed in chronic cases. Ultrasound studies may not be reliable. Contrast enemas demonstrate a luminal defect and may be therapeutic. However, most patients require operative reduction or resection. The appendix should also be removed in this circumstance to prevent future problems.

ACKNOWLEDGMENTS

The authors thank the Department of Radiology and Dr. Ronald Jaffe of the Department of Pathology at Children's Hospital of Pittsburgh for supplying images. They also give special thanks to Dr. David Orenstein for his critical insights regarding CF and the care of patients with this disease.

REFERENCES

1. Landsteiner K. Darmverschluss durch eingedictes meconium pankreatitis. *Zentralbl Allg Pathol* 1905;16:903.
2. Brock D. A comparative study of microvillar enzyme activities in the prenatal diagnosis of cystic fibrosis. *Prenat Diagn* 1985;5:129.
3. Thomaidis TS, Arey JB. The intestinal lesions in cystic fibrosis of the pancreas. *J Pediatr* 1963;63:444.
4. Fanconi G, Uehlinger E, Knauer C. Das coeliakiesyndrome bei angeborener zystischer pancreasfibromatose und branchiektasien. *Wien Med Wochenschr* 1936;86:753.
5. Anderson DH. Cystic fibrosis of the pancreas and its relation to celiac disease: a clinical and pathologic study. *Am J Dis Child* 1938;56:344–449.
6. Hiatt RB, Wilson PE. Celiac syndrome: therapy of meconium ileus; report of eight cases with a review of the literature. *Surg Gynecol Obstet* 1948;87:317.
7. Noblett HR. Treatment of uncomplicated meconium ileus by Gastrografin enema: a preliminary report. *J Pediatr Surg* 1969;4:190.
8. Kerem BS, Rommens JM, Buchanan JA, et al. Identification of the cystic fibrosis gene: genetic analysis. *Science* 1989;245:1073.
9. Danks DM, Allan J, Anderson CM. A genetic study of fibrocystic disease of the pancreas. *Ann Hum Genet* 1965;28:323–356.
10. Kramm ER, Crane MM, Sirken MG, et al. A cystic fibrosis pilot survey in three New England states. *Am J Public Health* 1962;52:2041–2057.
11. Stephan U, Busch EW, Kollberg H, et al. Cystic fibrosis detection by means of a test strip. *Pediatrics* 1975;55:35–38.
12. Allan DL, Robbie M, Phelan PD, et al. Familial occurrence of meconium ileus. *Eur J Pediatr* 1981;135:291–292.
13. Kerem E, Corey M, Kerem B, et al. Clinical and genetic comparisons of patients with cystic fibrosis, with or without meconium ileus. *J Pediatr* 1989;114:767–773.
14. Rommens JM, Iannuzze MC, Kerem BS, et al. Identification of the cystic fibrosis gene: chromosome walking and jumping. *Science* 1989;245:1059.
15. Riordan J, Rommens JM, Kerem BS, et al. Identification of the cystic fibrosis gene: cloning and characterization of complimentary DNA. *Science* 1989;245:1066.
16. Knowlton RG, Cohen-Haguenauer O, Van Cong N, et al. A polymorphic DNA marker linked to cystic fibrosis is located on chromosome 7. *Nature* 1985;318:380.
17. Wainwright BJ, Scambler PJ, Schmidtke J, et al., Localization of cystic fibrosis locus to human chromosome 7 cen-q22. *Nature* 1985;318:384.
18. Estivill X, Ortigosa L, Perez-Frias J, et al. Clinical characteristics of 16 cystic fibrosis patients with missence mutation R334W, a pancreatic insufficiency mutation with variable age of onset and interfamilial clinical differences. *Hum Genet* 1995;95:331.
19. Worldwide survey of the ΔF508 mutation—report from the Cystic Fibrosis Genetic Analysis Consortium. *Am J Hum Genet* 1990;47:354.
20. Collins FS. Cystic fibrosis: molecular biology and therapeutic implications. *Science* 1992;256:774.
21. Riordan JR. The cystic fibrosis transmembrane conductance regulator. *Ann Rev Physiol* 1993;55:609.
22. Welsh MJ, et al., Cystic fibrosis. In: Scriver CR, Beaudet AL, Sly WS, et al. eds. *The metabolic and molecular basis of inherited disease,* 7th ed, New York: McGraw-Hill, 1994.
23. Di Sant' Agnese PA, Davis PB. Research in cystic fibrosis. *N Engl J Med* 1976;295:481–485.
24. Emery JL. Laboratory observations of the viscidity of meconium. *Arch Dis Child* 1954;29:34–37.
25. Buchanan DJ, Rapoport S. Chemical comparison of normal meconium and meconium from a patient with meconium ileus. *Pediatrics* 1952;9:304–309.
26. Di Sant' Agnese PA, Dische Z, Danikzen KA. Physicochemical differences of mucoproteins in duodenal fluid of patients with cystic fibrosis of pancreas and controls: clinical aspects. *Pediatrics* 1957;19:252–259.
27. Schutt WH, Isles TE. Protein in meconium from meconium ileus. *Arch Dis Child* 1968;43:178.
28. Green MN, Clarke JT, Shwachman H. Studies in cystic fibrosis of the pancreas: protein pattern in meconium ileus. *Pediatrics* 1958;21:635–641.
29. Thomaidis TS, Arey JB. The intestinal lesions in cystic fibrosis of the pancreas. *J Pediatr* 1963;63:444–453.
30. Farber SJ. Pancreatic function and disease in early life: pathologic changes associated with pancreatic insufficiency in early life. *Arch Pathol* 1944;37:238–250.
31. Anderson DH. Cystic fibrosis of the pancreas. *J Chron Dis* 1958;7:58–90.
32. Schwachmann H, Lebenthal E, Khaw KT. Recurrent acute pancreatitis in patients with cystic fibrosis with normal pancreatic enzymes. *Pediatrics* 1975;55:86–95.
33. Quinton PM, Bijman J. Higher bioelectric potentials due to decreased chloride absorption in the sweat glands of patients with cystic fibrosis. *N Engl J Med* 1983;308:1185–1189.
34. Boix-Ochoa J. Meconium peritonitis. *J Pediatr Surg* 1968;3:715–722.
35. Agerty HA. A case of perforation of the ileum in newborn infant with operation and recovery. *J Pediatr* 1943;22:233.
36. Lorimer WS, Ellis DH. Meconium peritonitis. *Surgery* 1966;60:470–475.
37. Rickham PP. Intraluminal intestinal calcifications in the newborn. *Arch Dis Child* 1975;32:31–34.
38. Moore TC. Giant cystic meconium peritonitis. *Ann Surg* 1963;157:566–572.
39. Gibson LE, Cooke RE. A test for concentration of electrolytes in sweat in cystic fibrosis of the pancreas utilizing pilocarpine by iontophoresis. *Pediatrics* 1959;23:545–549.
40. Caspi B, Elchalal U, Lancet M, et al. Prenatal diagnosis of cystic fibrosis: ultrasonographic appearance of meconium ileus in the fetus. *Prenat Diagn* 1988;8:379.
41. Estroff JA, Bromley B, Benacerraf BR. Fetal meconium peritonitis without sequelae. *Pediatr Radiol* 1992;22:277.
42. Foster MA, Nyberg DA, Mahony BS, et al. Meconium peritonitis: prenatal sonographic findings and their clinical significance. *Radiology* 1987;165:661.
43. Neuhauser EBD. Roentgen changes associated with pancreatic insufficiency in early life. *Radiology* 1946;46:319.
44. Kao SCS, Franken EA Jr. Nonoperative treatment of simple meconium ileus: a survey of the Society of Pediatric Radiology. *Pediatr Radiol* 1995;25:97.
45. Rescorla FJ, Grosfeld JL. Contemporary management of meconium ileus. *World J Surg* 1993;17:318.
46. Gross RE.Intestinal obstruction in the newborn resulting from meconium ileus. In: *The surgery of infancy and childhood*. Philadelphia: WB Saunders, 1953;1:175–191.
47. Bishop HS, Koop CE. Management of meconium ileus: resection, Roux-en-Y anastoomosis and ileostomy irrigation with pancreatic enzymes. *Ann Surg* 1957;145:410–414.
48. Santulli TV. Meconium ileus. In: Mustard WT, Ravitch MM, Snyder WH Jr, et al., eds. *Pediatric surgery,* 2nd ed. Chicago: Year Book, 1969:851–860.
49. Santulli TV, Blanc WA. Congenital atresia of the intestine: pathogenesis and treatment. *Ann Surg* 1961;154:939–948.
50. Swenson O. Meconium ileus and peritonitis. In: *Pediatric surgery,* 2nd ed. East Norwalk, CT: Appleton & Lange, 1962.
51. O'Neill JA, Grosfeld JL, Boles ET, et al. Surgical treatment of meconium ileus. *Am J Surg* 1970;119:99–105.
52. Holsclaw D, Hooboushe C. Occult appendiceal abscess complicating cystic fibrosis. *J Pediatr Surg* 1976;11:217.
53. Coughlin JP, Gauderer MW, Stern RC, et al. The spectrum of appendiceal disease in cystic fibrosis. *J Pediatr Surg* 1990;25:835.
54. Littlewood JM. Gastrointestinal complications. *Br Med Bull* 1992;48:847.
55. Smyth RL, van Velzen D, Smyth AR, et al. Strictures of ascending colon in cystic fibrosis and high-strength pancreatic enzymes. *Lancet* 1994;343:85.
56. Stevens J, Chong S, West K, et al. Colonic strictures in cystic fibrosis patients on very high-dose pancreatic enzyme supplementation. *Pediatr Pulmonol* 1994;10(suppl):275.

57. Lloyd-Still JD. Cystic fibrosis and colonic strictures. A new "iatrogenic" disease [Editorial]. *J Clin Gastroenterol* 1995;21:2–5.
58. Lloyd-Still JD, Uhing MR, Arango V, et al. The effect of intestinal permeability on pancreatic enzyme-induced enteropathy in the rat. *J Pediatr Gastroenterol Nutr* 1998;93:1171–1172.
59. Hasler WL. Pancreatic enzymes and colonic strictures with cystic fibrosis: a case-control study. *Gastroenterology* 1998;114:609–612.
60. Pawel BR, de Chadarevian JP, Franco ME. The pathology of fibrosing colonopathy of cystic fibrosis: a study of 12 cases and review of the literature. *Hum Pathol* 1997;28:385–389.
61. Reichard KW, Vinocur CD, Franco M, et al. Fibrosing colonopathy in children with cystic fibrosis. *J Pediatr Surg* 1997;32:237–241.
62. Smyth RL, Ashby D, O'Hea U, et al. Fibrosing colonopathy in cystic fibrosis: results of a case-control study. *Lancet* 1995;346:1247–1251.
63. Angelico M, Gandin C, Canuzzi P, et al. Gallstones in cystic fibrosis: a critical reappraisal. *Hepatology* 1991;14:768.
64. Clatworthy HW, Howard WHR, Lloyd J. The meconium plug syndrome. *Surgery* 1956;39:131–142.
65. Bughaighis AG, Emery JL. Functional obstruction of the intestine due to neurological immaturity. *Prog Pediatr Surg* 1971;3:37.
66. Stewart DR, Nixon GW, Johnson DG, et al. Neonatal small left colon syndrome. *Ann Surg* 1977;186:741–745.
67. Samuel N, Dicker D, Landman J, et al. Early diagnosis and intrauterine therapy of meconium plug syndrome in the fetus: risks and benefits. *J Ultrasound Med* 1986;5:425–428.
68. Rasor GB, Stevenson W. Meconium ileus equivalent. *Rocky Mount Med J* 1941;38:218–220.
69. Park RW, Grand RJ. Gastrointestinal manifestations of cystic fibrosis: a review. *Gastroenterology* 1981;81:1143.
70. Perman J, Breslow L, Ingall D. Nonoperative treatment of meconium ileus equivalent. *Am J Dis Child* 1975;129:1210–1211.
71. Bailey DJ, Andres JM. Liver injury after oral and rectal administration of *N*-acetylcysteine for meconium ileus equivalent in a patient with cystic fibrosis. *Pediatrics* 1987;79:281.
72. Cleghorn GJ, Forstner GG, Stringer DA. Treatment of distal intestinal obstruction syndrome in cystic fibrosis with a balanced intestinal lavage solution. *Lancet* 1986;1:8.
73. Koletzko S, Corey M, Ellis L, et al. Effects of cisapride in patients with cystic fibrosis and distal intestinal obstruction syndrome. *J Pediatr* 1990;117:815.
74. O'Halloran SM, Gilbert J, McKendrick OM, et al. Gastrografin in acute meconium ileus equivalent. *Arch Dis Child* 1986;1128.
75. Holsclaw D, Rocmans C, Shwachman H. Intussusception in patients with cystic fibrosis. *Pediatrics* 1971;48:51.

Chapter 78

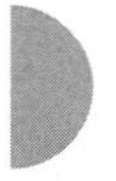

Jejunoileal Atresia

Milissa A. McKee

The evolution of the management of neonatal intestinal atresia parallels the development of pediatric surgery as a specialty and illustrates the necessity of surgeons dedicated to the care of children. Prior to 1950, the mortality rate in cases of atresia exceeded 90%. Since the mid-1960s, advances in surgical technique have allowed successful surgical treatment of this condition. Advances in general neonatal intensive care have been instrumental in further improving survival. The ability to provide total parenteral nutrition (TPN) as well as mechanical ventilation and general anesthesia to these vulnerable infants has reduced mortality to 1% to 10% in most series (1,2). Although the diagnosis of intestinal atresia or stenosis is a classic cause of neonatal intestinal obstruction, it remains a relatively rare occurrence. The estimated incidence ranges from 1 in 1,000 to 1 in 5,000 births in population-based studies (3). This incidence is similar to the overall incidence of duodenal atresia and far higher than colonic atresia. Knowledge of the diagnosis and treatment of these abnormalities continues to be essential to provide afflicted infants with the necessary treatment to achieve the expected successful outcome. The pediatric surgeon plays a central role in initial lifesaving surgical intervention, as well as in the recognition and management of the potential for long-term morbidity. Although most of these patients will recover over the initial hospitalization, a subset of these children will have prolonged needs related to malabsorption, short gut, TPN cholestasis, limited venous access, and infectious complications. Most cases are sporadic without specific etiologic agent or genetic pattern identified. There have been reports of familial cases and a higher incidence in twins. The ratio of males to females is equal. Associated extraintestinal anomalies are rare with a few notable exceptions, such as cystic fibrosis (4). As many as 20% of infants with one atresia will have multiple atresias (1).

Milissa A. McKee: Yale University School of Medicine, New Haven, Connecticut 06520.

ETIOLOGY

Normal development of the midgut is a complicated process (5). First recognizable by the third week in gestation, the midgut begins as a simple tubular structure. It then elongates considerably, herniating from the abdominal cavity where it undergoes rotation. It then returns to the abdomen and develops fixation to attain its normal configuration. Rapid epithelial proliferation between the fifth and eighth weeks may result in transient obliteration of the intestinal lumen. Somatic growth continues throughout gestation. Insults during this normal development are believed to result in the pathology seen in humans. The vast majority of patients demonstrate complete atresias with a smaller proportion (less than 10%). having stenosis or webs. These abnormalities may be seen anywhere in the jejunum or ileum.

There are many theories to explain the pathogenesis of jejunoileal atresia; however, no one concept has been universally accepted to account for the entire spectrum of anomalies seen in clinical practice. Figure 78-1 summarizes a variety of proposed theories. The best evidence to date implicates in utero vascular accidents resulting in intestinal atresia. In a seminal work by Louw and Barnard (6), the mesenteric vascular supply of fetal dogs was ligated late in gestation. The intestine was then examined after birth and noted to demonstrate the variety of anatomic defects seen in human clinical practice. Similar trials have been designed in many different animal models confirming the development of intestinal atresias in the setting of in utero mesenteric ischemia (7–9). The anatomic, functional, and pathologic findings are all strikingly similar to the clinical condition found in humans.

Additional observations in these models indicate that in utero intestinal perforation may heal with a variety of outcomes in the intestine, ranging from stenosis and atresia to normal appearance of involved segments with no evidence of injury. Furthermore, intestinal atresia has been noted to occur in association with a variety of insults that

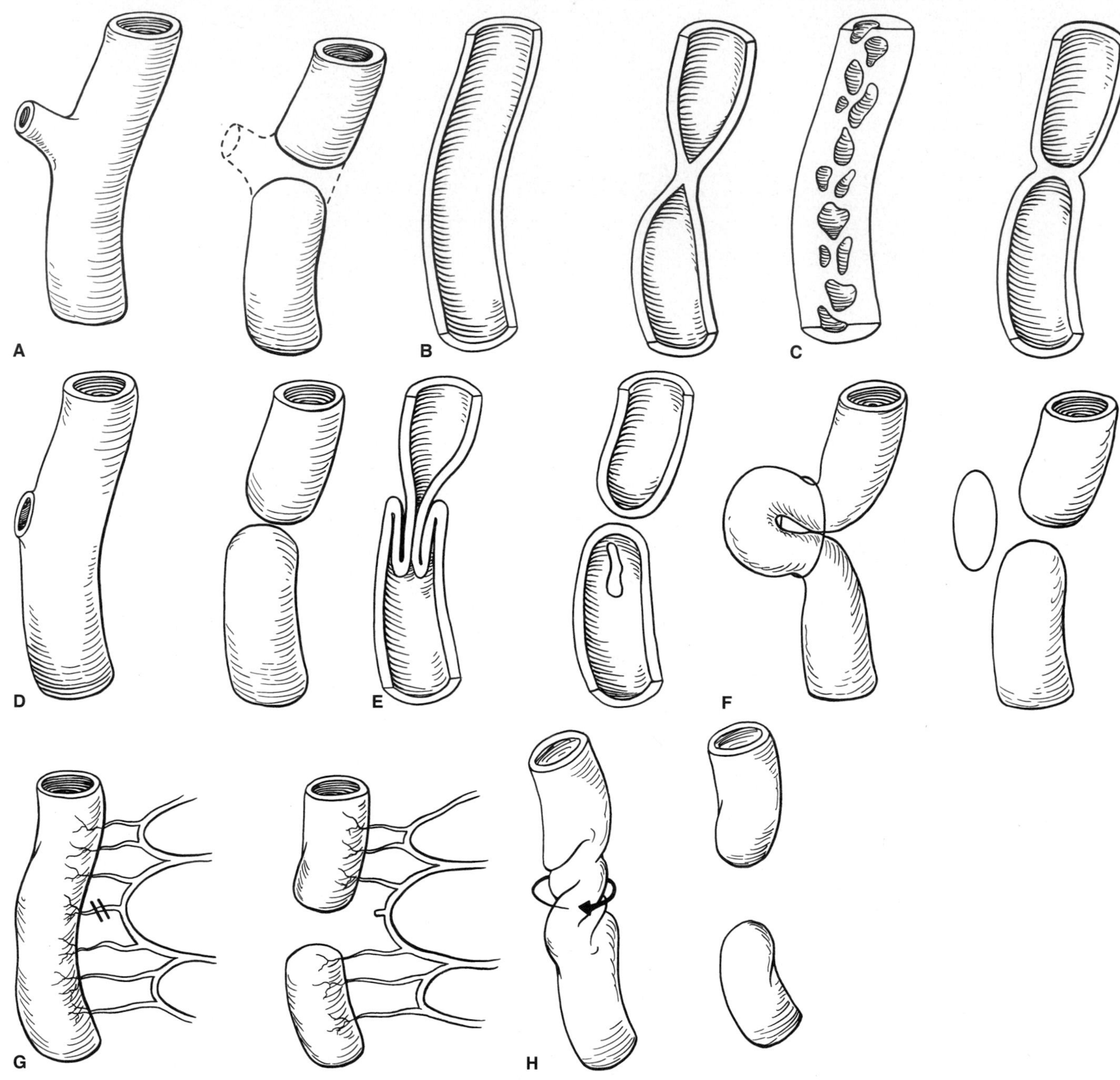

FIGURE 78-1. Abnormal organogenesis results in intestinal atresia or stenosis. Several possibilities are depicted in this illustration: **(A)** excessive resorption of Meckel's diverticulum; **(B)** attenuation, whereby cell proliferation fails to keep up with elongation (stenosis); **(C)** failure of complete recanalization (stenosis); **(D)** intestinal perforation in utero; **(E)** intussusception in utero; **(F)** entrapment of the intestine in the umbilical ring; **(G)** thrombosis of vascular supply, with local necrosis and closure of distal and proximal ends; and **(H)** segmental volvulus. (Adapted from Skandalakis JE, Gray SW, Ricketts R, et al. *Embryology for surgeons: the embryological basis for the treatment of congenital anomalies*. Baltimore: Williams & Wilkins, 1994:204.)

have in common mesenteric ischemia, such as volvulus, intussusception, internal hernia, and abdominal wall defects with constriction at the fascial defect (5,10).

Clinical evidence also supports the idea that atresia results from an insult late in gestation. It has been noted by many authors that bile, hair, and epithelial cells are commonly found distal to the atretic region, suggesting the lumen was patent at some time. Other extraabdominal anomalies are rare, likewise suggesting a late insult.

The main alternative theory is failure of recanalization. First hypothesized in 1900, this theory is a very plausible explanation for duodenal atresia, but is difficult to correlate with the previously mentioned clinical observations and the extensive evidence that mesenteric ischemia is involved in the pathogenesis of jejunoileal atresia.

Current research is ongoing to further elucidate the functional abnormalities associated with intestinal atresia. This will hopefully improve our understanding and management of these patients. Intestinal dysmotility (11), altered brush-border enzyme function, and malabsorption have all been noted in patients with atresia (12–14). Successful treatments for these abnormalities would be a tremendous step forward in the care of these patients with the potential to reduce long-term morbidity.

CLASSIFICATION

Jejujunoileal atresia is separated into four major groups, following the classification system revised by Grosfield into its current form (15). This classification is also summarized in Fig. 78-2.

Type I: Membranous atresia or web with intact mesentery The bowel and its mesentery remain in continuity to visual inspection. The proximal bowel dilates, depending on the degree of obstruction that may be partial if the web is fenestrated or complete. The web may be stretched for some distance within the lumen

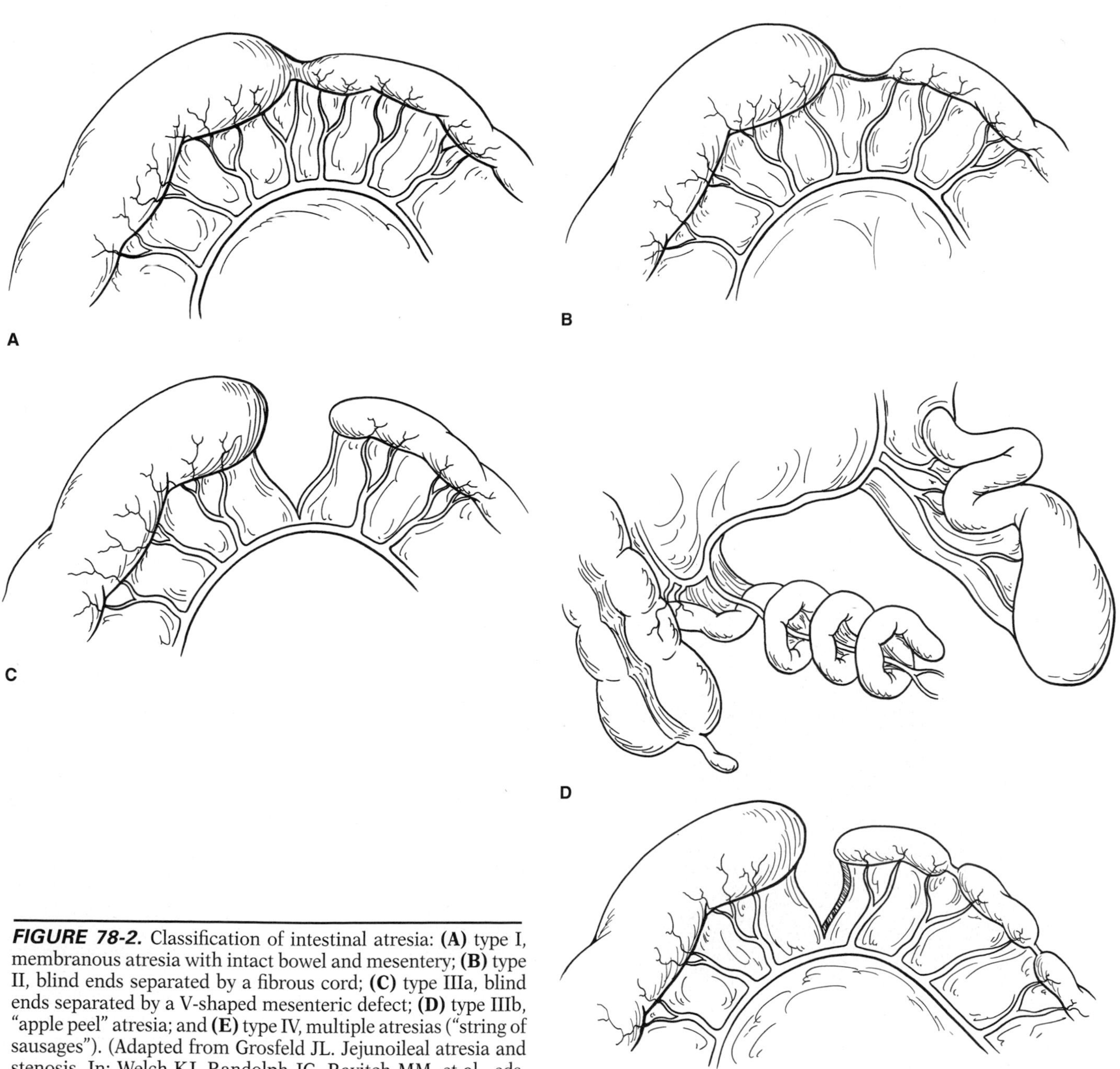

FIGURE 78-2. Classification of intestinal atresia: **(A)** type I, membranous atresia with intact bowel and mesentery; **(B)** type II, blind ends separated by a fibrous cord; **(C)** type IIIa, blind ends separated by a V-shaped mesenteric defect; **(D)** type IIIb, "apple peel" atresia; and **(E)** type IV, multiple atresias ("string of sausages"). (Adapted from Grosfeld JL. Jejunoileal atresia and stenosis. In: Welch KJ, Randolph JG, Ravitch MM, et al., eds. *Pediatric surgery*. Chicago: Year Book Medical, 1986:843.)

creating a windsock deformity. Overall, the bowel length is normal.

Type II: Blind ends of the bowel with intact mesentery The proximal and distal loops of bowel are blind ending, typically connected by a fibrous cord. The underlying mesentery remains intact, and the bowel length is again usually normal.

Type IIIa: Blind ending loops with mesenteric defect This form of atresia results in an often largely dilated blind proximal loop completely separated from a collapsed distal loop. There is an intervening mesenteric defect of variable size, and the total length of bowel may also be affected.

Type IIIb: Blind ending proximal loop, absent superior mesenteric artery, distal corkscrew bowel around marginal vessel, so-called "apple peel" atresia or Christmas tree deformity

This is a much more complex form of atresia likely related to a near catastrophic in utero vascular event, such as complete occlusion of the superior mesenteric artery based on thrombosis, embolic phenomena, or volvulus. The proximal bowel is dilated and bulbous in appearance, and ends blindly in a proximal location, often just past the ligament of Treitz or equivalent length. The distal bowel is quite small and wrapped around a marginal vessel from the ileocolic or right colic vessels, which is the entire blood supply to the midgut. This results in the typical appearance described as an "apple peel" atresia. An example of type IIIb atresia is shown in Fig. 78-3. In almost all cases, there is a significant loss of overall bowel length. Owing to both the large disparity in size between the proximal and distal bowel, as well as the tenuous vascular supply, the technical aspects of repair are challenging. These infants tend to be premature, small for gestational age, malrotated, and have a much higher potential for morbidity and mortality than other types of atresia. Also, in contrast to other forms of atresia, type IIIb atresias are believed to be associated with some form of genetic inheritance with a complex form of penetrance.

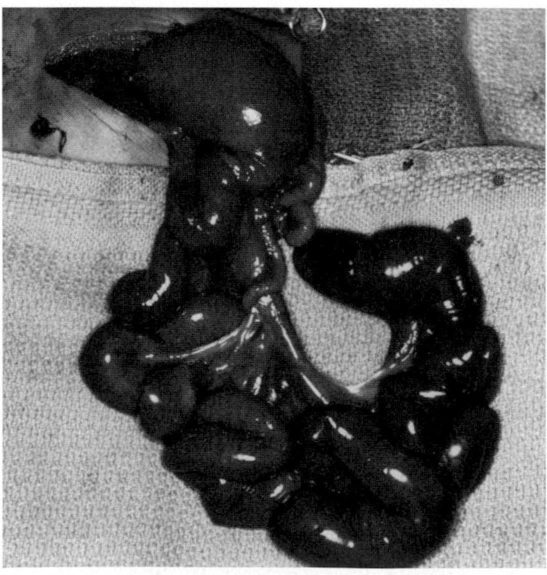

FIGURE 78-3. Operative photograph displaying characteristics of type IIIb atresia. Surgical correction presents problems owing to the technical considerations of poor blood supply.

Type IV: Multiple Atresias

This type of atresia involves a variable number of atretic segments, which may be any combination of the previously described types. Multiple atresias may be found in up to 20% of patients and should be looked for in all patients with intestinal atresia (1). Consideration should be given to immunodeficiency disorders in the setting of multiple atresias (16), and this type of atresia is more likely to be associated with other malformations (17).

DIAGNOSIS

The diagnosis of jejunoileal atresia may be made pre- or postnatally. In an increasing proportion of patients, prenatal ultrasonography raises the suspicion of bowel obstruction. Prenatal ultrasound remains more reliable at diagnosing duodenal atresia than jejunoileal atresia, but it is becoming increasingly useful. Findings on ultrasound include dilated loops of bowel (Fig. 78-4) and the associated finding of polyhydramnios related to lack of absorption of amniotic fluid in the obstructed bowel. The degree of

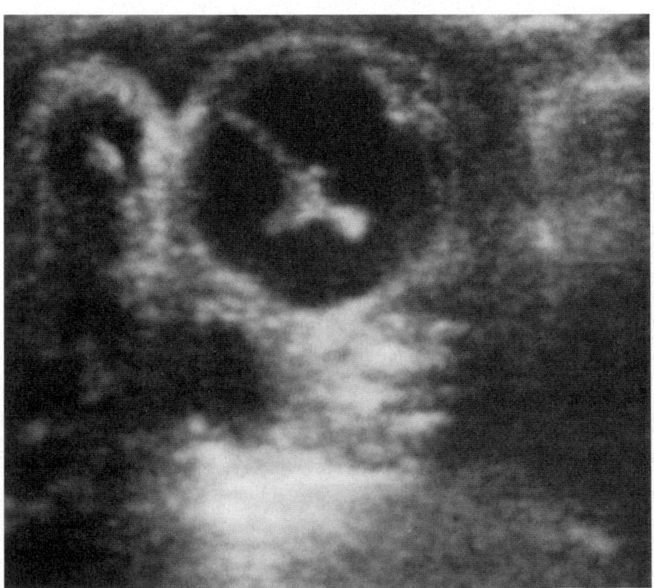

FIGURE 78-4. Prenatal ultrasound showing several dilated loops of fetal intestine. This infant proved to have jejunal atresia, although meconium ileus and other causes of neonatal obstruction create similar images.

polyhydramnios is, however, related to the location of the atresia and may not be present with more distal atresias. These findings, suggestive of obstruction, are not definitive for atresia and may be seen with other anomalies such as meconium ileus. Abnormal findings on prenatal ultrasound should prompt a referral for prenatal evaluation and counseling for the parents. Advance knowledge of a potential abnormality allows for anticipation of the potential perinatal needs of both mother and infant, as well as referral for delivery at a tertiary care center when indicated. The pediatric surgeon also plays an important role in education and reassurance of the family in a stressful situation.

A significant number of patients will not have the diagnosis of atresia suspected prenatally. Presentation in these cases will more likely demonstrate the classic symptoms of abdominal distension and bilious emesis early in the neonatal period. Often, intestinal obstruction will also result in the failure to pass meconium. The passage of a meconium stool does not rule out atresia because the time of onset for the obstruction during gestation may vary. Those that develop later in gestation may already have meconium present in the colon distal to the atresia, which will then pass postnatally. Vomiting is typically present. Examination of the abdomen will usually demonstrate distension and tympany. The degree of distension may vary, however, related to the location of intestinal obstruction. Proximal jejunal atresias may demonstrate very little distension, whereas distal ileal atresias will produce the more classic picture of impressive abdominal distension. Perforation would of course result in more significant findings, such as tenderness or abdominal wall erythema, as well as systemic signs of instability. Rectal examination is a necessary part of the exam with the most likely finding of white mucous material in the rectum. Jaundice is present in 20% to 30% of patients with intestinal atresia.

Jejunal atresia will produce symptoms of complete bowel obstruction early in life, therefore leading on the diagnosis fairly quickly. Incomplete obstructions of the basis of webs or intestinal stenosis may have a more insidious onset, presenting later in infancy or childhood. Ileal atresia results in a more delayed onset of symptoms, but still generally in the first few days of life. This more distal type of obstruction is not as easily recognized and, furthermore, must be differentiated from other causes of distal intestinal obstruction, such as meconium ileus and Hirschsprung's disease.

After appropriate clinical examination, plain abdominal films should be obtained. Typical findings include dilated loops of bowel with absence of distal gas (Fig. 78-5). The number of dilated, air-filled loops seen will once again depend on the level of intestinal atresia. Plain films may also demonstrate calcifications, a finding consistent with meconium peritonitis on the basis of prenatal perforation. It is not possible to differentiate reliably between small and large bowel loops in a newborn due to the lack of haustral markings. A contrast enema with water-soluble contrast material is the next step to evaluate these patients. This exam is useful for several reasons. The patency of the colon is established and its size demonstrated. Distal atresias commonly produce a microcolon (Fig. 78-6). The contrast study may demonstrate a transition zone consistent with Hirschsprung's disease or the findings of meconium ileus for which the exam may also be therapeutic. Furthermore, it is helpful to confirm the patency of the colon prior to laparotomy for small bowel atresia to rule out the possibility of additional unrecognized more distal atresias and prevent anastamosing bowel in the setting of distal obstruction. Upper gastrointestinal series is not necessary in the setting of complete obstruction, but may be useful in cases of partial obstruction.

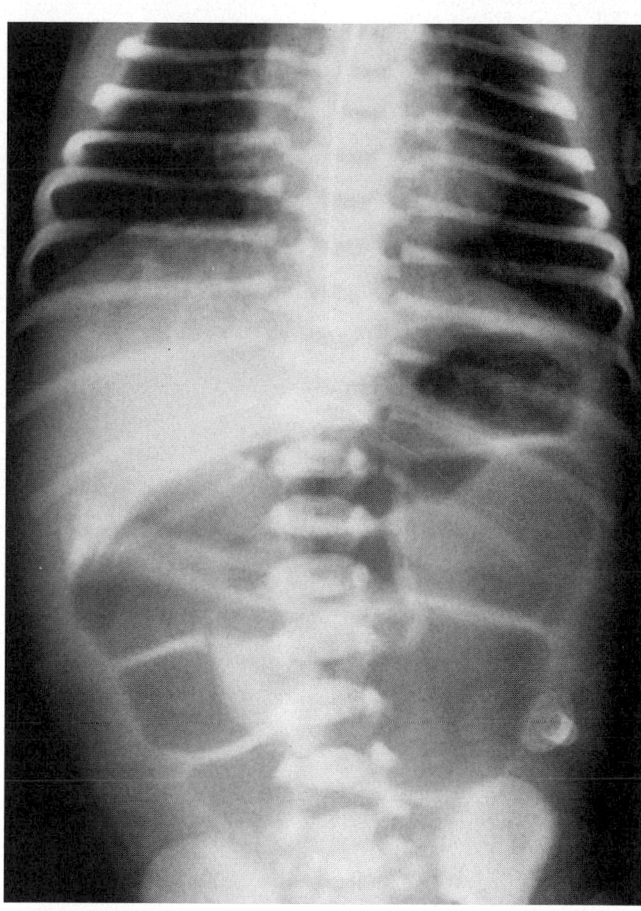

FIGURE 78-5. Abdominal radiograph showing dilated bowel loops indicative of obstruction. There is an absence of distal air. The level of the obstruction is difficult to determine from a plain film. This child has jejunoileal atresia.

The differential diagnosis in the setting of intestinal obstruction is extensive. Alternative diagnoses to intestinal atresia include meconium ileus, Hirschsprung's disease, malrotation with or without volvulus, duplication, internal hernia, and ileus from any source. In addition, some of these may be seen in conjunction with atresia, particularly, malrotation, meconium ileus, and meconium peritonitis.

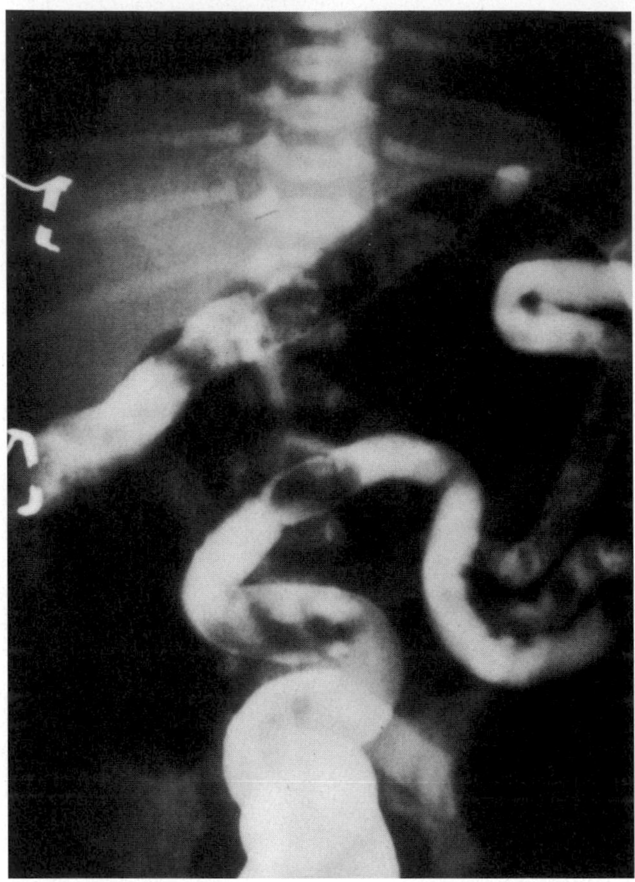

FIGURE 78-6. Contrast enema showing a small colon with dilated proximal air-filled loops in an infant with ileal atresia.

A contrast enema is invaluable in providing information to help differentiate between these causes. A family history of cystic fibrosis or Hirschsprung's disease would also be crucial in this scenario.

TREATMENT

The evaluation and treatment of an infant with signs of bowel obstruction should be expedient and concurrent with ongoing resuscitation. Intravenous access should be obtained if not already present and appropriate fluid and electrolyte repletion initiated. Orogastric decompression should be established with a tube of adequate caliber (10 F). Appropriate attention is required to maintain body temperature and avoid hypothermia. Broad-spectrum antibiotics are administered. Blood should be obtained for complete blood count, expanded electrolytes, bilirubin, blood gas, and blood type for cross-match. Any other findings or comorbidities on history or physical exam should be addressed. Complicating factors such as prematurity and congenital heart disease should be recognized and included in preoperative planning. All these issues must also be dealt with in the context of transport between hospitals or examination in the radiology suites.

After appropriate resuscitation and establishment of the diagnosis, prompt surgical exploration should be undertaken. Delay in diagnosis may result in ischemia or perforation of the obstructed segment, and in many cases, it is difficult to exclude malrotation with volvulus from the differential. When in the operating room, appropriate volume resuscitation, monitoring, and maintenance of temperature should be continued.

The abdomen is explored through a transverse upper abdominal incision, allowing access to the entire peritoneal cavity in an infant. The bowel is gently eviscerated and inspected. Any site of perforation, if present, is controlled, and the abdomen is irrigated with warmed saline until clear of debris. The entire intestine should be inspected thoroughly to determine the site of obstruction. Any coexisting abnormalities should be identified and addressed. The length of bowel present should be noted. At the site of atresia, the distal limb may be cannulated with a soft red rubber catheter and perfused with warm saline to demonstrate distal patency and eliminate the possibility of multiple atresias. This maneuver is potentiated by establishing the luminal continuity of the colon on preoperative contrast enema. Failure to identify a distal obstruction would have potentially disastrous consequences, including anastomotic breakdown, and may even be life threatening. Placement of a surgical gastrostomy was once considered essential, but is now rarely needed.

After identifying the site of atresia and establishing distal patency, the goal of the procedure shifts to the restoration of gastrointestinal continuity. The technique employed depends on the findings in each individual case and especially the length of bowel present. The underlying principle is to restore continuity while preserving intestinal length and maintaining function (18). The most common

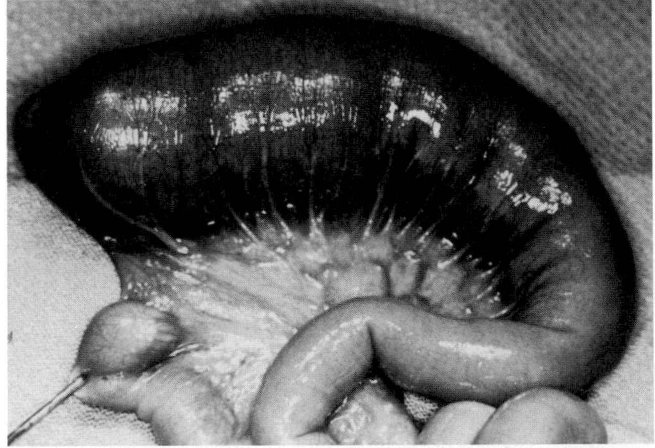

FIGURE 78-7. Characteristic appearance of dilated proximal jejunum and the diminutive bowel distal to the atresia. Limited resection of the thickened, dilated proximal segment permits a satisfactory anastomosis and restoration of intestinal continuity.

A B C

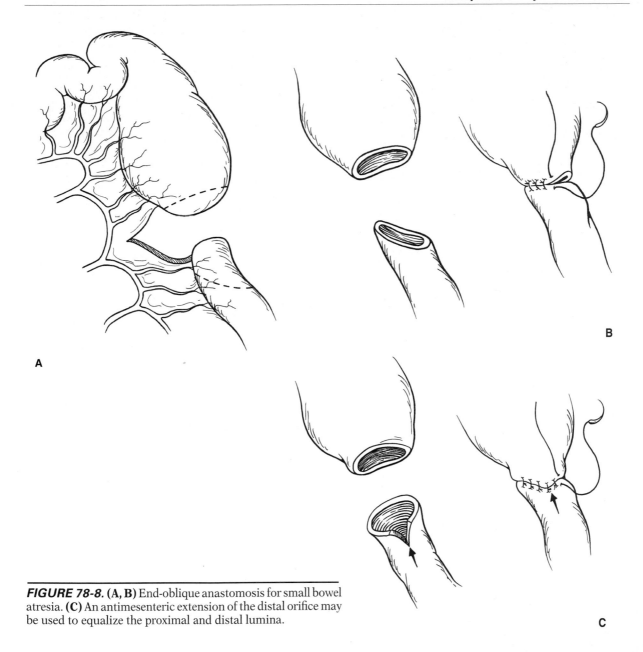

FIGURE 78-8. **(A, B)** End-oblique anastomosis for small bowel atresia. **(C)** An antimesenteric extension of the distal orifice may be used to equalize the proximal and distal lumina.

technique is primary anastomosis after resecting the dilated portion of the proximal loop (1,2). The proximal loop is usually quite bulbous and dilated, which may lead to ischemia and dysfunction. Leaving this portion in place will likely result in stasis and functional obstruction. In addition, the size mismatch between the proximal and distal limbs leads to technical difficulty in creating the anastomosis (Fig. 78-7). In cases where there is adequate bowel length, the bulbous proximal loop may be resected back to the more relatively normal diameter. This will still be larger than the distal limb, which may be beveled or opened on its antimesenteric border to make the two ends more equal (Figs. 78-8 and 78-9). A single-layer, full-thickness anastomosis with fine absorbable suture is most common. The mesenteric defect also may be a source of difficulty.

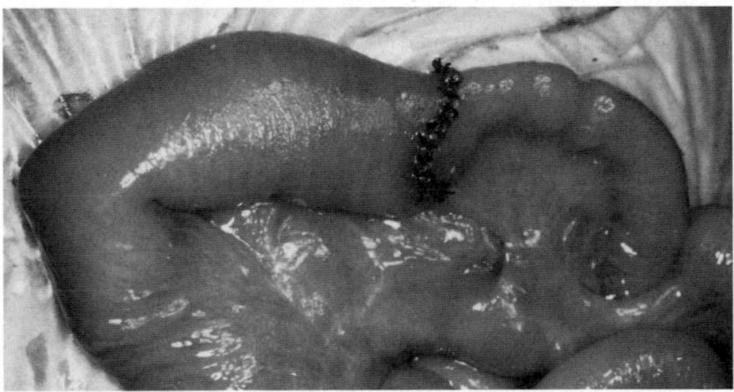

FIGURE 78-9. Operative photograph of a completed anastomosis for jejunoileal atresia with a large lumenal mismatch. This anastomosis may be at high risk for functional obstruction because of potential dysmotility of the proximal dilated segment.

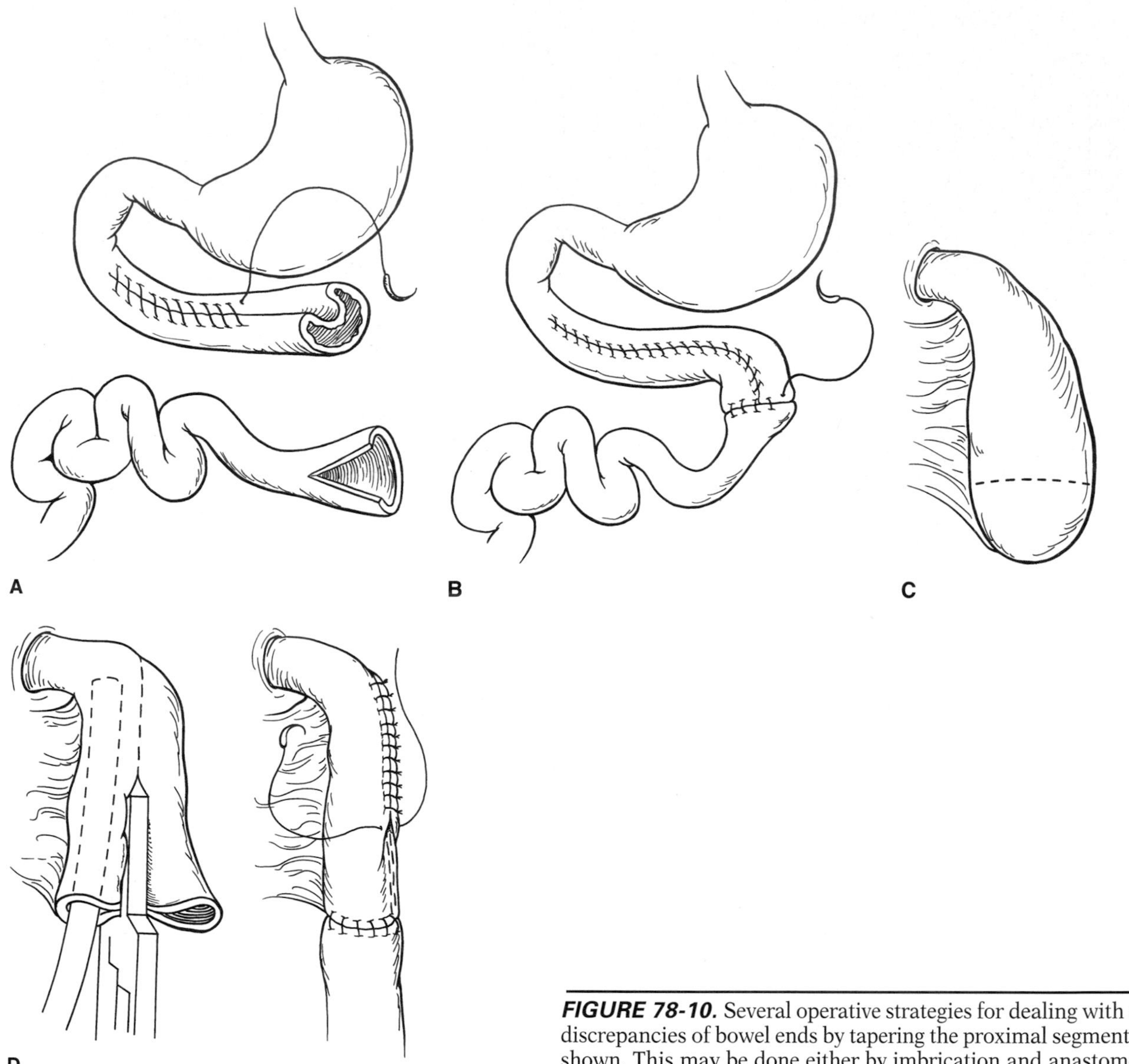

FIGURE 78-10. Several operative strategies for dealing with size discrepancies of bowel ends by tapering the proximal segment are shown. This may be done either by imbrication and anastomosis **(A,B)** or resection **(C, D, E)**.

Kinking of the anastomosis or of the mesentery is to be avoided, which is especially difficult in apple peel (type IIIB) atresias. Preserving the mesentery of the resected proximal bowel to provide a flap for closure of the mesenteric defect is a simple technique that may facilitate closure of larger defects (19). If the bowel length is questionable, as much bowel must be preserved as possible. This may be accomplished by a limited resection of the bulbous proximal tip with a tapering jejunoplasty on the antimesenteric surface of the bowel (Fig. 78-10) (20,21). An alternative technique is plication. This has been successfully used, but has a significant downside. In some cases the imbrication breaks down, resulting in recurrence of a large dilated loop of bowel causing functional obstruction. Primary anastomosis is the preferred technique with exteriorization of bowel reserved for those patients in whom intestinal viability is in question. Fortunately, this is rare.

Intestinal atresia in the setting of gastroschisis is a special problem. Recognition of the atretic segment may be difficult or impossible with the underlying thickening and inflammation of the bowel. The potential for an anastomosis to heal under these dubious conditions is also in doubt. Current opinion, in the absence of perforation, is to reduce the viscera into the abdominal cavity and to perform definitive repair on a delayed basis 4 to 6 weeks after closure when the acute inflammation has subsided (22).

Multiple atresias are also of special concern. If the atresias are grouped together and there is adequate bowel length, a single resection may be performed. Multiple anastamoses may be required in the setting of marginal intestinal length and multiple atresias.

POSTOPERATIVE CARE

Supportive care in the neonatal intensive care unit is provided for all major organ systems. Associated medical problems should be addressed. Mechanical ventilation if required, gastric decompression, fluid and electrolyte repletion, postoperative pain management, and appropriate antibiotic coverage are all routine. Parenteral nutrition should be initiated early and continued until bowel function has returned. Most patients with midgut atresia and adequate bowel length will recover within a few days and tolerate full enteral feedings within the first few weeks of life. The return of bowel function is, however, variable with more proximal anastomoses often taking weeks to begin functioning. In addition, a large discrepancy in bowel size or shorter intestinal length may result in lengthy hospitalization and prolonged feeding intolerance. These patients will require long-term nutritional support and slow deliberate feed advancement to achieve the ultimate goal of total enteral nutrition. Specific contributing factors include lactose intolerance, stasis with bacterial overgrowth, malabsorption, and exacerbations due to sepsis. In the event of marked delay in return of function or prolonged feeding intolerance, upper gastrointestinal series may be warranted. Persistently dilated proximal loops may suggest intestinal stasis, obstruction, and bacterial overgrowth. Extreme cases may require reexploration for anastomotic revision or tapering of the dilated loop.

The ability to eventually provide full enteral nutrition in difficult cases is enhanced by the use of elemental and hypoallergenic formulae. Weight gain should be monitored on a frequent basis and nutrition monitoring labs obtained weekly. Stool volume and frequency are also good indicators of feeding tolerance. Episodes of sepsis, especially related to the presence of a central line, are frequent complications. TPN cholestasis develops over time and is often acutely exacerbated by infectious episodes. Although the majority of patients with intestinal atresia no longer require gastrostomy tube placement at their original operation, it may be a consideration for those with marginal intestinal length. Infants who are expected to have short gut may have their care improved with a stable way to provide long-term continuous drip feedings. Given the higher incidence of cystic fibrosis in patients with intestinal atresia, appropriate evaluation and testing should be performed (4).

OUTCOME

The overall prognosis in cases of jejunoileal atresia is good. Since the mid-1970s, advances in neonatal care have allowed progressive reduction in mortality from a historical high of more than 90%. Many authors have now reported overall survival exceeding 90% (1,2). The most significant improvement over that time period has been the ability to provide long-term nutritional support, which is usually necessary for a period of weeks to months after the surgical repair. Type I, II, and IV atresia each account for about one-fourth of the patients with atresia. Less common but potentially more serious are the type IIIb atresias that comprise less than 10% of atresias seen, but have been associated with a disproportionate amount of the perioperative morbidity and mortality. Previous reports have suggested a mortality rate as high as 20% in the setting of type IIIb atresia. More recent data no longer show such a striking disparity, especially in early mortality (23,24). These patients do, however, have the potential to volvulize segments of bowel due to the tenuous blood supply, and simple overdistension of the proximal limb may cause necrosis. They are also more likely to have issues with short gut based on overall available intestinal length and malabsorption or mucosal dysfunction in the gut.

Operative mortality is quite low, typically less than 1%. In the early postoperative period, complications seen are most commonly infectious, such as pneumonia, peritonitis, and generalized sepsis. Early morbidity and mortality may also be related to comorbidities such as prematurity, congenital heart disease, and other associated problems. Late mortality is related to complications of short gut, namely, sepsis and liver disease. Specific surgical complications include small bowel obstruction due to adhesions, anastamotic dysfunction, and anastamotic leak. Anastomotic leak has been as high as 10% to 15% in older series, with more recent reports around 5%.

Infants with isolated atresia and with normal overall intestinal length should be expected to have an excellent outcome. Certainly, all patients undergoing major surgical intervention in the neonatal period are at some risk of early complications, such as anastamotic leak and infectious and respiratory complications. The mortality rate from early complication should be less than 1% to 2%. However, infants with significant loss of length are more complicated. In addition to the early potential morbidity, they are also subject to long-term complications of nutritional supplementation. Sepsis, multiorgan failure, cholestasis, and eventually liver failure may ensue with long-term TPN requirements. The absolute minimum bowel length required for survival is not clear. With advances in supportive care and elemental feedings, infants with ever-shorter lengths of bowel down to 10 to 20 cm have been reported survivors. In extreme cases, gut-lengthening procedures or even transplantation may be required.

Overall significant improvements in the care of infants with jejunoileal atresia have been recognized more recently. The majority of infants born with this condition can be expected to have a successful outcome and a relatively normal life. Future advances will likely be based on treatments designed to optimize intestinal function and adaptation.

REFERENCES

1. Dalla Vecchia LK, Grosfeld JL, West KW, et al. Intestinal atresia and stenosis: a 25-year experience with 277 cases. *Arch Surg* 1998;133:490–497.
2. Kumaran N, Shankar KR, Lloyd DA, et al. Trends in the management and outcome of jejuno-ileal atresia. *Eur J Pediatr Surg* 2002;12:163–167.
3. Cragan J, Martin M, Moore C, et al. Descriptive epidemiology of small intestinal atresia. *Teratology* 1993;48:441.
4. Roberts HE, Cragn JD, Cono J, et al. Increased frequency of cystic fibrosis among infants with jejunoileal atresia. *Am J Med Genet* 1998;78:446–449.
5. Skandalakis JE, Gray SW, Ricketts R, et al.The small intestines. In: *Embryology for surgeons: the embryological basis for the treatment of congenital anomalies.* Baltimore: Williams & Wilkins, 1994: 184–241.
6. Louw JH, Barnard CN. Congenital intestinal atresia: observations on its origin. *Lancet* 1955;2:1065.
7. Tovar JA, Sunol M, Lopez-Detorre B, et al. Mucosal morphology and experimental intestinal atresia: studies on the chick embryo. *J Pediatr Surg* 1991;26:184.
8. Touloukian RJ. Antenatal intestinal adaptation with experimental jejunoileal atresia. *J Pediatr Surg* 1978;13:468.
9. Trahair JS, Rodgers HS, Cool JC, et al. Altered intestinal development after jejunal ligation in fetal sheep. *Virchows Arch A* 1993;423:45.
10. Gornall P. Management of intestinal atresia complicating gastroschisis. *J Pediatr Surg* 1989;24:522.
11. Doolin J, Ormsbee HS, Hill JL. Motility abnormality in intestinal atresia. *J Pediatr Surg* 1987;22:320.
12. Serrano J, Zetterstrom R. Disaccharidase activities and intestinal absorption in infants with congenital intestinal obstruction. *J Pediatr Gastroenterol Nutr* 1987;6:238.
13. Tepas J, Wyllie RG, Shermeta DW, et al. Comparison of histochemical studies of intestinal atresia in human newborn and fetal lamb. *J Pediatr Surg* 1979;14:376.
14. Hamdy MH, Man DWK, Bain D, et al. Histochemical changes in intestinal atresia and its implications to surgical management: a preliminary report. *J Pediatr Surg* 1986;21:17.
15. Grosfeld JL. Jejunoileal atresia and stenosis. In: Welch KJ, Randolph JG, Ravitch MM, et al., eds. *Pediatric surgery.* Chicago: Year Book, 1986:838.
16. Walker MW, Lovell MA, Kelly TE, et al. Multiple areas of intestinal atresia associated with immunodeficiency and post-transfusion graft vs host disease. *J Pediatr* 1993;123:93.
17. Sweeney B, Surana R, Puri P. Jejunoileal atresia and associated malformations: correlation with the timing of in utero insult. *J Pediatr Surg* 2001;36:774–776.
18. Nixon HH, Tawes R. Etiology and treatment of small intestinal atresia: analysis of a series of 127 jejunal ileal atresias in comparison with 62 duodenal atresias. *Surgery* 1971;69:41.
19. Malcynski JT, Shorter NA, Mooney DP. The proximal mesenteric flap: a method for closing large mesenteric defects in jejunal atresia. *J Pediatr Surg* 1194;29:1607–1608.
20. Howard ER, Othersen HB. Proximal jejunoplasty in the treatment of jejunal atresia. *J Pediatr Surg* 1973;6:685.
21. Weber TR, Vane DW, Grosfeld JL. Tapering enteroplasty in infants with bowel atresia and shortgut. *Arch Surg* 1982;117:684.
22. Snyder CL, Miller KA, Sharp RJ, et al. Management of intestinal atresia in patients with gastroschisis. *J Pediatr Surg* 2001;36:1542–1545.
23. Festen S, Brevoord JC, Goldhoorn GA, et al. Excellent long-term outcome for survivors of apple peel atresia. *J Pediatr Surg* 2002;37: 61–65.
24. Waldhausen JH, Sawin RS. Improved long-term outcome for patients with jejunoileal apple peel atresia. *J Pediatr Surg* 1997;32:1307–1309.

Chapter 79

Necrotizing Enterocolitis

Shawn J. Rangel and R. Lawrence Moss

In the mid-1970s, necrotizing enterocolitis (NEC) emerged as the most common surgical emergency in the neonatal intensive care unit (NICU) (1,2). Almost three decades later, and despite a growing knowledge base supported by hundreds of laboratory and clinical research studies, NEC continues to pose a significant challenge to the pediatric surgeon with respect to its clinical management. At present, NEC remains the major cause of death for all neonates undergoing surgery, and the mortality from this disease is greater than from all congenital anomalies of the gastrointestinal (GI) tract combined (3).

NEC is almost exclusively a disease of prematurity. Little was known or documented about the disease in the first half of the twentieth century because survival was unlikely in the extremely premature. Subsequent advances, including development of modern neonatal respiratory care, allowed for the survival of babies of ever-decreasing gestational age and birth weight. A striking increase in the incidence of NEC was then observed, as these breakthroughs led to an increasing number of infants at risk for the disease.

The strength of epidemiologic evidence implicating prematurity as a risk factor for NEC is substantial. Premature infants comprise greater than 90% of all cases, and nearly 90% of these have birth weights less than 2,000 g (2,4). Prematurity is the only risk factor consistently identified in case-control studies, and the disease is relatively rare in countries where prematurity is uncommon (Japan and Sweden) (5). The incidence of NEC is estimated between 1% to 8% percent of NICU admissions (1 to 3 in 1,000 live births) (6,7). Incidence is higher in previously fed babies (15%) and in those weighing less than 1,500 g (10% to 15%) (8,9). NEC most commonly affects babies born between 30 and 32 weeks' gestation, and is diagnosed most often during the second week of life (10,11). Epidemiologic studies have characterized an inverse relationship between the degree of prematurity and the age of onset of NEC, with more premature infants developing NEC at relatively later postnatal ages (12).

The financial burden attributable to this disease is substantial. It has been estimated that the additional cost of treating NEC in a premature neonate ranges from $74,000 to $186,000 compared with age-matched controls without the disease (13). With current estimates of incidence rates, this translates into roughly onc-third of 1 billion per year in health care-related costs in the United States. The overall financial impact of this disease is likely to be much greater, however, because this estimate does not take into account the cost of caring for infants with lifelong morbidity from NEC.

Shawn J. Rangel and R. Lawrence Moss: Section of Pediatric Surgery, Yale University School of Medicine, New Haven, Connecticut 06520.

ANATOMY AND HISTOLOGY

NEC can affect any segment of the GI tract, from the stomach to the distal rectum. Injury most commonly involves both the small and large bowel together (40% to 45% of cases), followed by isolated lesions of the small intestine (30%) and colon (25%) (14). The ileocecal region is the most commonly affected area and is often the site of the most severe injury. Approximately 35% of patients will have focal disease at laparotomy, and a similar proportion will have multisegment disease localized to a relatively small length of bowel (14,15). In 15% to 20% of patients, exploration will reveal massive necrosis involving a considerable portion of the entire bowel. Such paninvolvement *(NEC totalis)* is often fatal.

Coagulation necrosis is the hallmark histologic finding in NEC and is present in more than 90% of pathology specimens (14). Coagulation necrosis is invariably associated with ischemic injury, suggesting the importance of diminished splanchnic perfusion in the pathogenesis of NEC. Bacterial overgrowth is found in approximately two-thirds of specimens. The depth of injury to the bowel can be variable, and areas of full- and partial-thickness necrosis may be found adjacent to frank perforation. In contrast to other causes of intestinal necrosis (infectious agents and ischemic necrosis), there is an exaggerated inflammatory response that extends to grossly normal areas of bowel. Pneumatosis intestinalis is found in approximately one-half of specimens and is considered pathognomonic for NEC. Mixed areas of acute and chronic inflammatory changes are common, and epithelial regeneration is found in more than one-half of specimens (14). These findings suggest the pathogenesis of NEC may involve a chronic process of injury and repair rather than a single critical insult, in contrast to a thromboembolic event.

PATHOGENESIS

Despite extensive clinical and laboratory investigation, a complete understanding of the pathogenesis of NEC remains elusive. The etiology of NEC has classically been attributed to a maladaptive response of the premature gut to the presence of feeding substrate and bacterial colonization. Although these risk factors are almost invariably present in documented cases of NEC, the overwhelming majority of premature babies who are exposed to these factors do not develop the disease. More contemporary models of pathogenesis have therefore placed greater emphasis on a multifactorial etiology, stressing the role of ischemia, reperfusion injury, and the complex cascade of inflammatory mediators. A synopsis of the laboratory and clinical evidence supporting current theories of pathogenesis is presented in the next section.

Ischemia and Reperfusion Injury

The role of ischemia and reperfusion injury in the pathogenesis of NEC has largely been characterized through neonatal animal models. The molecular events leading to cellular damage have been well characterized, although the factors initiating this process in the context of clinical NEC are still unknown. Hypoxia at the cellular level leads to a marked increase in the production of xanthine oxidase (XO). Upon reperfusion, XO converts hypoxanthine to xanthine and uric acid, releasing a host of reactive oxygen species in the process (hydroxyl, superoxide, and hydrogen peroxide radicals). These species can induce substantial damage to lipoprotein components of the cell membrane, increasing permeability and facilitating bacteria translocation. Even relatively brief periods of hypoxia can lead to prolonged and substantial changes in mucosal permeability through this mechanism (16).

The precise mechanism and temporal relationship for ischemic injury in the context of NEC remains unclear. Gross and histopathologic findings do not support a thromboembolic process or a generalized low-flow state as a primary mechanism of injury. In this regard, mesenteric infarction and low-output states (previously believed to be associated with NEC through umbilical artery catheter use and cardiogenic shock, respectively) appear to be distinct clinicopathologic entities. Increasing evidence suggests that ischemic injury associated with NEC may result from a maladaptive vascular response to early pathogenic events in the disease. As such, ischemia may play a role in the progression of NEC rather than serving as a critical precipitating factor.

Several theories have been proposed to explain the etiology of ischemia associated with NEC and prematurity. Hyperactive extrinsic vascular regulation (the so-called "diving" or "Herring-Breur" reflex) has been implicated because of its potential relevance to the neonate (17,18). Initially described in diving mammals, the reflex involves a preferential diversion of blood flow to the heart and brain during periods of severe hypoxia. This presumably occurs during the period of parturition. As such, this theory cannot adequately explain the clinical observation that NEC commonly occurs during the second week of life. Furthermore, significant episodes of hypoxia prior to bowel injury cannot be identified in most cases of NEC.

Other studies have attempted to characterize the vasoregulatory responses of the premature gut to hypoxia and prolonged sympathoadrenergic stimulation. Studies using neonatal pigs have identified a maladaptive response to these insults in the way of prolonged and exaggerated vasoconstriction (19). Such responses may exacerbate transient (and likely physiologic) episodes of hypoxia. Potential mechanisms include the presence of labile myogenic vascular reflexes, which may be particularly sensitive to changes in venous pressure (20). Such maladaptive vasoregulatory reflexes are not observed in the intestine of mature swine. Protection appears to be conferred through autoregulatory "escape" mechanisms, which are hardwired into the mature intestine (19). Future studies will need to further characterize how complex vasoregulatory mechanisms regulate the intestinal microcirculation, and how these may become dysfunctional in the premature infant.

Inflammatory Mediators

Several inflammatory mediators are elevated in the serum of premature neonates with NEC. These include tumor necrosis factor-alpha (TNF-α), platelet-activating factor (PAF), and the interleukins 6 and 8 (IL-6 and IL-8), among others (21–23). Intestinal cells of premature infants appear to elaborate higher concentrations of proinflammatory cytokines (particularly IL-8) in response to endotoxin and IL-1 compared with mature cells (21). The primary challenge has been to distinguish between those that play a pivotal role in the development and progression of NEC, and those that are nonspecific markers of inflammation. This is particularly challenging given the complexity and redundancy of the inflammatory cascade. Furthermore, many conditions associated with NEC can increase serum levels of inflammatory mediators through independent mechanisms (e.g., sepsis).

Data from animal models have identified PAF as a leading candidate for initiating the early pathogenic events in NEC. PAF is a potent vasoconstrictor of the mesenteric circulation and increases mucosal permeability (24). Infusion of PAF into the intestines of neonatal pigs leads to injury resembling NEC, and will also exacerbate the severity of injury in response to ischemia-reperfusion challenge (25,26). Pretreatment with PAF antagonists (WEB-2086) significantly attenuates injury in both models (27,28). These observations suggest that PAF may be integral to the pathogenic changes seen with ischemia-reperfusion injury. PAF may also influence the progression of NEC through secondary inflammatory pathways (particularly TNF-α) and as a potent chemokine for neutrophil activation (25,26). The propensity of NEC to involve the distal small bowel may reflect the relatively high concentration of PAF receptors in this area (29).

PAF-acetylhydrolase is the enzyme responsible for the metabolism of PAF, and serum levels of this enzyme are markedly attenuated in prematurity (30). Levels are even lower in premature neonates diagnosed with NEC. PAF-induced injury may therefore be due to an increase in functional activity rather than overproduction. The deleterious effects of PAF may be dependent on the presence of other factors, including bacterial endotoxin (31,32). Intestinal injury is not observed when PAF is given to germ-free rats (32). Furthermore, injury to mucosal cells in the presence of bacterial endotoxin may likewise be dependent on the presence of PAF. Pretreatment with PAF antibodies significantly reduces injury following the infusion of endotoxin (lipopolysaccharide) into the guts of neonatal pigs (33).

Nitric oxide (NO) has received much attention for its apparent protective function during ischemic stress. Endogenous NO is produced by three different isoforms of the enzyme nitric oxide synthase (NOS). Sources include endothelial cells, phagocytic cells in the circulation and tissues, and others. The protective effects of NO are mediated through vascular smooth muscle relaxation. This property may be important for counteracting the influence of vasoconstricting cytokines during periods of inflammation and ischemia. NO may also protect mucosal cells by directly modulating PAF activity and limiting neutrophil adhesion to the vascular endothelium (34).

Evidence for the protective role of NO is found in several observations from animal models: (1) The severity of mucosal injury is inversely related to the activity of NOS in tissue preparations; (2) inhibitors of NOS such as L-arginine significantly worsen PAF-induced intestinal necrosis; and (3) NO donors significantly reduce PAF-induced intestinal necrosis (35–37). These observations led to the postulate that the NOS regulatory pathway may be dysfunctional in premature neonates. However, the activity of NOS was found to be increased in premature neonates with documented NEC (38,39). It is possible that this observed increase could be inappropriately low when compared with a similar response in mature animals. However, more recent laboratory studies have suggested that the role of NO in the context of NEC may not always be protective. Higher activity levels of the inducible form of NOS have been correlated with increased severity of injury in the neonatal rat model (39). The reaction between NO and reactive oxygen species to generate even more reactive peroxynitrate compounds has been postulated as a potential mechanism for injury. These observations suggest that, much like molecular oxygen, the physiologic effects of NO may depend on the local cellular milieu. Further studies need to clarify the precise role of NO in the context of NEC, and how this protective mechanism may be exploited for potential therapeutic strategies.

Infectious Agents

Bacteria appear to be critical in the pathogenesis of NEC, given the observation that the disease does not occur before intestinal colonization is established. The degree of bacterial overgrowth in NEC appears to exceed that observed with other diseases associated with intestinal necrosis (14). Furthermore, the pathologic finding of pneumatosis in association with intestinal necrosis is exceedingly rare, except in the setting of NEC. Pneumatosis results from the accumulation of hydrogen gas in the intestinal wall due to fermentation of carbohydrates by intestinal flora. With stasis and significant bacterial loads, intraluminal pressure may increase to the point of impeding venous return, thereby promoting ischemia. However, the ability of colonizing bacteria to ferment lactose has not been correlated with the development of NEC. Furthermore, evidence for bacterial overgrowth is absent in up to one-third of pathology specimens (14).

These observations suggested that other bacterial factors may be important for initiating the pathogenic changes in NEC. Certain strains of *Escherichia coli* and *Clostridia* can cause intestinal necrosis directly by the elaboration of potent exotoxins (40). These organisms have been identified in relative "epidemics" of NEC affecting NICUs (41). Such epidemics have been halted with the implementation of organism-specific antibiotics and the appropriate hygiene measures. However, cultures obtained from blood, stool, and peritoneal aspirates in most cases of spontaneous NEC do not reveal pathogenic organisms. The most commonly isolated species include *E. coli, Klebsiella, Enterobacter, Pseudomonas, Clostridium*, and coagulase-negative *Staphylococci*, among others (42,43). This would suggest two different mechanisms of injury with a shared final common pathway. It is likely that, in true cases of NEC, normally nonpathogenic bacteria become functionally pathogenic due to changes in the mucosal barrier that occur early in the course of disease.

Physiology of the Premature Gut

Several physiologic deficiencies have been characterized in the gut of premature neonates (Fig. 79-1). Peristalsis and other aspects of intestinal motility can be substantially compromised, particularly when neonates are born prior to their eighth month of gestation (44). Clearance of bacteria may be impeded, potentially leading to stasis and bacterial overgrowth. Gut-associated immunity may also be affected. Relatively fewer functional B lymphocytes are present in the immature gut, and the ability to produce sufficient amounts of secretory IgA is reduced (45). This antibody is believed to protect mucosal cells by preventing the binding of pathogenic organisms. The production of pepsin, gastric acid, and mucus are also decreased in prematurity (46,47). These factors may have important secondary roles in limiting the proliferation of intestinal flora and their ability to bind to mucosal cells. Intestinal trefoil factor is a peptide that has recently been characterized in the mature rat intestine (48,49). The peptide appears to have several adaptive functions, including protecting the mucosal barrier from microbial invasion and limiting the production of reactive oxygen species during ischemic stress. Significantly lower levels of mRNA for this peptide have been found in the prenatal rat. In concert with potentially dysfunctional vasoregulatory mechanisms, these characteristics may collectively act to lower the threshold for NEC in premature infants.

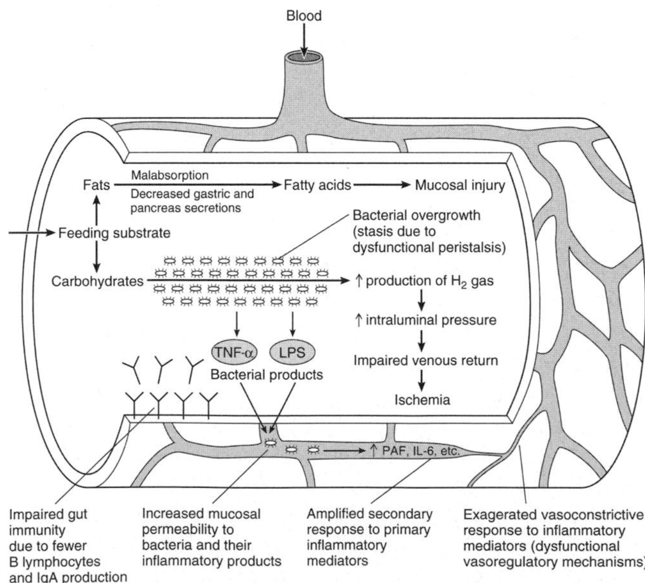

FIGURE 79-1. Characteristics of the premature gut that may increase the risk for developing necrotizing enterocolitis. TNF-α, tumor necrosis factor-alpha; LPS, lipopolysacharide; PAF, platelet-activating factor; IL-6, interleukin 6.

Role of Feeding

Epidemiologic studies have identified feeding as an important factor in the development of NEC. The majority of neonates who develop this disease have been previously fed, and the relative incidence of NEC is as much as 50% higher in this cohort (9). The relationship between feeding and NEC is complex, and appears to be dependent on the both the composition and quantity of substrate. Infusion of highly concentrated synthetic formulas leads to spontaneous endotoxemia and increased levels of PAF in healthy preterm infants (50,51). Other studies have demonstrated that high-osmolarity formulas can directly injure the villus border of mucosal cells (46). Malabsorption is common in premature neonates, and high concentrations of undigested fatty acids may also contribute to mucosal injury. Increased production of hydrogen gas from the fermentation of large carbohydrate loads may occur in the presence of stasis and bacterial overgrowth. Multiple clinical series have sought to determine whether the rate with which feedings are advanced in premature infants relates to the occurrence of NEC. Results have been inconclusive. Refer to the "Prevention" section later in this chapter.

Pharmacologic Agents and Other Risk Factors

Clinical and laboratory studies have identified a multitude of pharmacologic agents as possible risk factors for NEC. Case-control studies have shown an increased risk for NEC in neonates exposed to indomethacin both postnatally and prenatally (maternal tocolysis) (46,52,53). Indomethacin blocks prostaglandin synthetase and has been shown to impair mesenteric blood flow by increasing mesenteric vascular resistance (54). However, an association suggesting causality in the development of NEC has not held up in more rigorous clinical studies (55).

Other pharmacologic agents have been proposed to cause NEC through a variety of mechanisms. Methylxanthine compounds increase bacterial loads by altering gut motility and can damage enterocytes directly by their intraluminal metabolites (56). Vitamin E has been shown to interfere with intracellular bacterial killing in phagocytic cells (57). The hyperosmolarity of some drug preparations has been postulated to injure the villus border of mucosal cells (58). This potential mechanism is less plausible, however, given the relatively small volumes associated with clinical doses for most agents. Vasopressors and other agents used for hemodynamic support may exacerbate intestinal injury through their effects on the mesenteric circulation. Despite these potential mechanisms, no good clinical evidence exists to suggest that any of these agents play an important role in the initiation of NEC.

Case-control studies have identified relatively weak and inconsistent associations for other potential risk factors. These include hypoglycemia, premature rupture of membranes, chorioamnitis, hypercoagulable conditions, low-output states, prenatal cocaine exposure, and the use of umbilical catheters, among others (59–64). The intestinal injury associated with many of these "risk factors" is likely mediated through thromboembolic or vasoconstrictive mechanisms. Although clinically apparent injury may occur through the same final common pathway (ischemia and reperfusion), the initial pathogenic events for what we define as NEC may be quite different. This may suggest the misclassification of disease (and associated risk factors) in many earlier observational studies. Furthermore, the interpretation of existing clinical studies can be challenging for a number of other reasons. These include the frequent use of retrospective study designs, the frequency and severity of comorbid conditions, and difficulty with modeling the ever-increasing complexity of the neonate–NICU interaction, among others.

Unifying Concept of Pathogenesis

Our understanding of the pathophysiology of NEC is improving at a rapid pace. The experimental and clinical evidence outlined previously has led to a better understanding of the events that may be important for the initiation and progression of disease. Although the precise nature and temporal relationship of these events are yet to be determined, a unifying concept of pathogenesis is emerging from currently available data.

The initial insult leading to NEC may be a subclinical event such as a brief episode of perinatal hypoxia or postnatal infection. The injury from this event may not be clinically relevant in neonates with normally developed intestines. Upon colonization of the gut, bacteria may bind to injured mucosal cells and elicit a localized inflammatory response in reaction to endotoxin and other bacterial products. This may lead to further inflammation as the affected endothelial cells release proinflammatory cytokines, including TNF-α and PAF. In the presence of abnormal counterregulatory mechanisms (e.g., reduced PAF-acetylhydrolase), these factors may increase the permeability of mucosal cells leading to the translocation of bacteria and bacterial products. The inflammatory response is then further amplified, leading to the recruitment and activation of circulating neutrophils. Activation of neutrophils may further injure damaged mucosa through the release of secondary mediators and reactive oxygen species. A maladaptive vasoconstrictive response may then follow, further exacerbating injury through ischemia and reperfusion. The end result is a vicious cycle of positive feedback mechanisms that can ultimately lead to frank necrosis and perforation. This process may evolve over days, with injury and repair maintained in a fine balance. Other factors that may compromise mesenteric perfusion (sepsis) or increase oxygen demand (feeding) may tip the balance toward progressive and irreversible injury.

CLINICAL DIAGNOSIS

The diagnosis of NEC is dependent on the signs and symptoms characteristic of intestinal ischemia in the neonate. These may include gross or occult GI bleeding, high gastric residuals, feeding intolerance, diarrhea, and abdominal distension, among others. These signs have little predictive value for NEC as isolated clinical findings. However, NEC should be seriously considered when any of these manifest in a premature neonate with signs of evolving and unexplained sepsis. Specific to the physical exam, the finding of a fixed abdominal mass and erythema of the abdominal wall are the most predictive of NEC when present (near 100% specificity) (65). The diagnostic utility of these findings are limited by their poor sensitivities, however, being absent in as many as 90% of patients with documented disease. A sudden, unexplained need for increased ventilatory support in the premature neonate may also serve as a harbinger of NEC (66).

Symptoms can take on a fulminate course or remain remarkably insidious during this period. The neonate's inability to mount an effective inflammatory response and to develop physical signs of peritonitis may further complicate the clinical picture. These observations may make it difficult to differentiate NEC from other sources of neonatal sepsis. To aid in clinical diagnosis, Bell and colleagues devised a clinical staging system based on physical exam findings, laboratory data, and radiographic evidence of NEC (Table 79-1). Developed in 1978, the scale remains in wide use today for predicting the likelihood and severity of NEC (67).

Differential Diagnosis

NEC must be differentiated from other conditions associated with abdominal distention and sepsis. The most common challenge faced by the clinician is differentiating NEC from sepsis of a different etiology associated with ileus. Early NEC and sepsis with ileus can appear clinically indistinguishable. In many cases, differentiation between the two is only possible after observing the course of the disease in each patient.

The term *focal intestinal perforation* (FIP) has been applied to the surgical finding of a single isolated perforation occurring in a premature infant that is not associated with the radiographic finding of pneumatosis. Much debate has ensued as to whether FIP is simply a "mild" version of NEC or whether it is a distinct disease entity. Clinical studies have observed that perforations associated with FIP occur relatively earlier than NEC, and the lesions occur almost

TABLE 79-1 Clinical Staging System for Necrotizing Enterocolitis.

Stage	Systemic Signs	Gastrointestinal Signs	Radiographic Findings
I [Suspected necrotizing enterocolitis (NEC)]	Temperature instability, apnea, bradycardia	Poor feeding, increasing residuals, emesis, mild abdominal distension, occult gastrointestinal (GI) bleeding	Moderate abdominal distension with a mild ileus
II (Definite NEC)	Metabolic acidosis and thrombocytopenia in addition to the above	Marked abdominal distension, gross GI bleeding, in addition to the above	Significant ileus, pneumatosis, portal venous gas, "fixed" bowel loops
III (Advanced NEC)	Progressive deterioration of vital signs and evidence of septic shock (hypotension, neutropenia, disseminated intravarcular coagulation, etc.), in addition to the above	Evidence of generalized peritonitis, in addition to the above	Pneumoperitoneum, in addition to the above

From Bell MJ. Neonatal necrotizing enterocolitis. Therapeutic decisions based upon clinical staging. *Ann Surg* 1978;187:1–7, with permission.

invariably on the antimesenteric side of the distal ileum (68,69). Some reports have also described a different histologic profile associated with FIP, with coagulation necrosis and pneumatosis being notably absent in most specimens (68,69). The histology of NEC is very nonspecific, however, and early lesions may not exhibit the classic findings of well-established NEC (following secondary ischemic injury). Patients with FIP clearly have a better prognosis than those with NEC, although this may simply reflect the difference in the severity of bowel necrosis in the two cohorts. Ultimately, there may be little clinical relevance in distinguishing these processes, as the principles of management are the same for both.

Laboratory Studies

Laboratory parameters in patients with NEC are often nonspecific and generally indicate the presence of an inflammatory condition. Leukocyte and platelet counts may be elevated, normal, or low, depending on the severity of NEC and associated sepsis. Leukocytosis is the most common abnormality in NEC and is frequently accompanied by a refractory metabolic acidosis (65). Anemia may also be present if there is significant hemorrhage from the bowel wall. Severely depressed leukocyte and platelet counts have been associated with advanced disease and a worse overall prognosis (70,71). However, none of these individual parameters have sufficient sensitivity, specificity, or predictive accuracy to be of useful diagnostic value.

More recent efforts have attempted to identify novel serum markers for the earlier diagnosis and treatment of NEC. Neonates with confirmed stage II and III NEC were found to have significantly elevated serum levels of PAF compared with age-matched controls without the disease (72). However, only 3 of 11 (27%) patients in this case-control study had elevated levels prior to the onset of clinical signs. Furthermore, the lack of data regarding PAF levels in other causes of abdominal sepsis brings into question the specificity of this assay for NEC. Serum fatty acid-binding proteins have also been examined as a potential diagnostic marker for NEC. Similar to the PAF assay, levels were elevated in only a small proportion (12.5%) of patients with stage I disease (73). Further study is required to better define the diagnostic utility of these assays.

Imaging Studies

Plain abdominal films play a central role in the diagnosis of NEC. Radiographic findings commonly associated with NEC include generalized ileus, pneumatosis intestinalis, portal venous gas, pneumoperitoneum, and intraperitoneal fluid, among others (Fig. 79-2). Generalized ileus is the most common finding in documented cases of NEC (60% to 100% sensitivity), but is also associated with the least specificity (less than 10%) (74). The findings with the greatest positive predictive value include pneumatosis intestinalis, portal venous gas, and pneumoperitoneum (75). The diagnostic utility of these findings are limited by their moderately low sensitivities, however. Negative or equivocal radiographs in the context of other clinical evidence suggesting NEC should therefore be interpreted with extreme caution.

Pneumatosis intestinalis is pathognomonic for NEC, with a specificity of nearly 100% in most series (76,77). Pneumatosis is seen on X-ray as a collection of cystic or linear lucencies in the bowel wall, most often in the vicinity of the terminal ileum and ascending colon. This finding has moderate sensitivity for the purpose of diagnosis, being present in 50% to 70% of documented cases at laparotomy. Sensitivity may be relatively poor in patients who

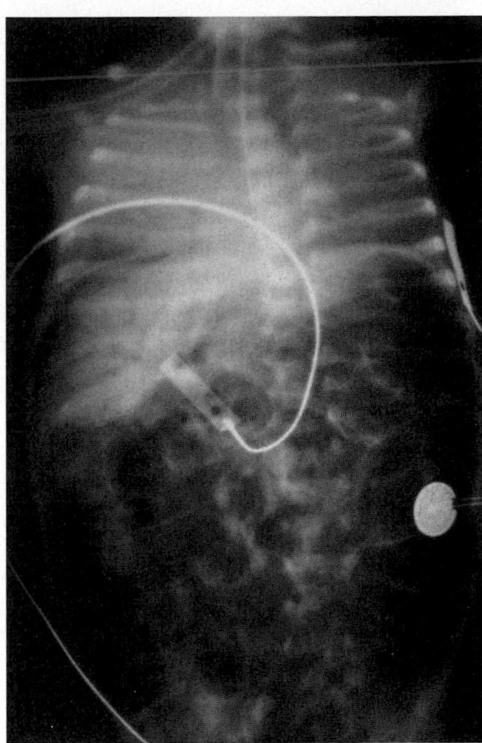

FIGURE 79-2. Abdominal radiograph demonstrating advanced necrotizing enterocolitis. Extensive pneumatosis can be seen throughout the bowel. Branching lucencies seen over the central portion of the liver indicate portal venous gas. The lucency lateral to the right edge of the liver is due to free intraperitoneal air.

have not been previously fed, however, because pneumatosis is dependent on the fermentation of carbohydrate substrate by intestinal flora (78).

Portal venous gas (PVG) appears as linear lucencies overlying the liver with branching patterns oriented to the portal venous circulation. Gas may arise directly from organisms within the portal system or from dissection of pneumatosis intestinalis into the venous circulation. The presence of PVG signifies severe disease and has been found to be a particularly poor prognostic finding. Mortality rates with NEC associated with PVG exceed 50% in some series, and may be as high as 93% in very low birth weight (VLBW) infants (65,79). However, it has been widely observed that many neonates with PVG recover without an operation, suggesting that PVG may be associated with other factors that affect prognosis. In a study of radiographic findings in 147 infants with NEC, PVG in association with severe pneumatosis was associated with an 80% probability of pannecrosis at laparotomy and an 86% mortality rate (65). From these observations, PVG in association with severe pneumatosis may constitute the only relatively strong indication for exploration based on radiographic findings alone.

Free air in the peritoneal cavity is fairly specific for NEC in cases when the pretest probability for NEC is moderately high (93% specificity) (75). False-positives in this cohort are usually due to focal intestinal perforation (if this is considered a distinct clinical entity), gastric perforation, or barotrauma from mechanical ventilation. Although free air is usually diagnostic of intestinal perforation, it is not uncommon to find a perforation in a patient undergoing exploration for suspected NEC in the absence of free air (40% sensitivity for NEC).

The role for other imaging modalities in the diagnosis of NEC is less clear. Contrast studies increase the risk of perforation and should not be considered in the acute phase of NEC. More recent studies have reported on the utility of ultrasound for identifying necrosis and PVG in the context of negative or equivocal plain films (80,81). A major limitation of this modality is the ability to accurately interpret exams in the presence of significant intraperitoneal fluid and bowel gas (common in NEC). Furthermore, it can be challenging to differentiate nonspecific inflammatory changes from frank necrosis, even in the best scanning conditions.

A more recent study examined the diagnostic value of magnetic resonance imagine (MRI) in a study of six patients with suspected NEC (82). In four of these patients, MRI characterized changes in the bowel wall that were qualitatively different from pneumatosis. All four of these patients were found to have necrotic bowel at exploration, leading to the conclusion that MRI may detect necrosis at an early stage. However, three out of the four patients had indications for exploration based on plain films alone. The diagnostic utility of MRI remains to be established, particularly given the risk of transporting these critically ill babies to the scanner.

Paracentesis

Paracentesis may be a useful diagnostic tool for identifying the occurrence of perforation in NEC, although there are no widely accepted guidelines for when it should be employed. Paracentesis has been used when the clinical suspicion for perforation or necrosis is high, but there is no obvious confirming radiographic evidence. Indications may include the presence of PVG, the presence of a fixed and dilated loop of bowel on sequential plain films, and the presence of cellulitis or a fixed abdominal mass on physical exam, among others. Paracentesis may be particularly useful in differentiating intestinal necrosis from barotrauma in mechanically ventilated patients.

A standard technique involves rotating the supine patient slightly to the right and advancing a 23-gauge butterfly needle gently and obliquely into the right lower quadrant while aspirating. At least 0.5 cc of free-flowing fluid should be obtained. A "positive" tap is evidenced by an aspirate containing bile or stool or one that reveals organisms on Gram stain. The most commonly identified organisms are *E. coli, Klebsiella*, coagulase-negative *staphylococci*, and yeast (65,83). A positive tap is invariably associated with perforation and is an indication for exploration. A negative tap may be followed with observation or by serial paracentesis until the neonate clinically improves or the tap becomes positive.

Paracentesis is a very accurate test with a reported specificity of 100% (84). Sensitivity has been reported to be somewhat less, ranging from 60% to 94%. As such, false-negatives can occur, and a negative tap does not reliably exclude perforation or gangrenous bowel. A negative tap should never be considered evidence against a decision to explore if other clinical signs are strongly suggestive of necrosis. It is noteworthy that the indications for paracentesis by some are considered clear indications for laparotomy by others. At present, there are no evidence-based guidelines to dictate when paracentesis should be performed. The decision to perform a paracentesis or proceed with exploration remains a judgment call by the surgeon, and this decision must carefully balance the risks of progressive necrosis with that of a negative laparotomy in a critically ill neonate.

MEDICAL MANAGEMENT

Once there is sufficient clinical evidence to suspect NEC, the principles of management include aggressive fluid resuscitation and hemodynamic support, bowel rest, broad-spectrum antibiotics, and close monitoring for the earliest signs of perforation. All neonates with suspected NEC should undergo pancultures and be started on antibiotics to cover the typical bowel pathogens, including gram-negative and anaerobic organisms. Common regimens may include ampicillin, gentamycin, and clindamycin, or vancomycin and a third-generation cephalosporin. Antibiotic coverage should be tailored to account for specific microbiology profiles in the NICU. Evidence from randomized trials has not supported earlier reports that enteral aminoglycosides decrease the risk of perforation (85). As many as one in six patients will develop secondary fungal infections when taking wide-spectrum antibiotics (86). This may be evidenced by persistent signs of sepsis or a refractory leukocytosis. Antifungal agents should be considered in this scenario while secondary cultures are pending.

Aggressive resuscitation and hemodynamic support are essential to optimize mesenteric perfusion and limit the progression of ischemia. Patients may require substantial fluid replacement due to massive interstitial fluid losses into the gut and peritoneum. Metabolic acidosis and electrolyte abnormalities are common and should be corrected aggressively. Vasoactive agents may be required for hemodynamic support in the presence of advanced sepsis. Dopamine is the initial agent of choice for this purpose due to its vasodilating effects on the mesenteric circulation (at low to moderate doses). Other vasopressors may also be required, but should be used with caution because they can exacerbate mesenteric ischemia.

All patients with suspected NEC should be made NPO and undergo gastric decompression to minimize intraluminal pressure. TPN provides the mainstay of nutrition during both the acute and healing phases of NEC, which in some neonates may last for weeks or even months. Serial abdominal examinations and plain radiographs should be performed periodically until there is clear clinical improvement or evidence of perforation. These radiographs must include both supine and dependent (left lateral decubitus, or cross-table lateral) views of the abdomen. Paracentesis may be useful in cases when perforation is suspected but radiographic findings are equivocal.

With adequate resuscitation and hemodynamic support, most children (60% to 70%) with NEC will improve without operative therapy (6). There are no consensus guidelines pertaining to the duration of support or to when feedings should be reinstated. It is generally recommended that antibiotics and NPO status be continued empirically for 7 to 10 days following the resolution of radiographic findings and abnormal laboratory parameters. Some have advocated a minimum of 2 weeks for neonates with stage II or III disease by Bell's criteria, although there is no good clinical evidence to support this practice. Feeding volumes should be advanced slowly, and the use of hyperosmolar formulas is to be avoided. As there is no good clinical evidence to support specific protocols, these are general guidelines and specific care should be tailored to the individual patient as appropriate.

Up to 20% of the patients who are successfully managed medically will ultimately develop signs of small bowel obstruction due to an intestinal stricture (1,17,87). Considerations in managing this complication are discussed in the next section.

OPERATIVE MANAGEMENT

Approximately 33% to 50% of patients with NEC will fail medical management and require an operation in the acute setting (88). Failure of medical therapy is more common in VLBW infants (79,89). Absolute indications for exploration include evidence of perforation on radiographs (most common indication) or by a positive peritoneal tap. Relative indications include the combined findings of PVG and extensive pneumatosis on plain film, or failure to improve with optimal medical therapy, among others. The desirable timing for exploration is after necrosis has developed, but before perforation has occurred. Unfortunately, no clinically effective method for identifying this period of opportunity exists.

Following adequate resuscitation, the principles of operative management include the excision of gangrenous bowel, exteriorization of viable proximal and distal stomas, and preservation of as much intestinal length as possible. Although resuscitation is essential prior to operative management, care should be taken not to volume overload because this may lead to hepatic congestion. The laparotomy is generally performed through a transverse supraumbilical incision, although an infraumbilical approach may be used to keep an engorged liver out of the operative field. Direct retraction of the liver should be avoided to reduce the risk of a potentially lethal subcapsular hematoma.

Peritoneal fluid should be sampled for Gram stain and culture. Affected bowel may appear dark gray, purple, or black, depending on the degree of ischemia and related inflammatory changes (Fig. 79-3). Subserosal gas and fibrinous exudates are commonly seen with advanced disease, whereas areas of transparent serosa may signify full-thickness necrosis and impending perforation. The bowel should be carefully examined from the stomach down to the distal rectum. Unless there is obvious proximal involvement, it is generally unnecessary to mobilize the retroperitoneal duodenum.

Resection of the involved segment(s) and formation of stomas comprise the standard of care for isolated disease. Previous reports have stressed the importance of preserving the ileocecal valve, but more recent data have suggested that outcome is more dependent on total intestinal length than presence of the valve (90). Attempts at preservation should never compromise the resection of all obviously nonviable bowel. Following resection, the peritoneal cavity is vigorously lavaged and the length of remaining bowel is measured. Stomas may be placed in the laparotomy wound, but many surgeons suggest placing them through separate incisions.

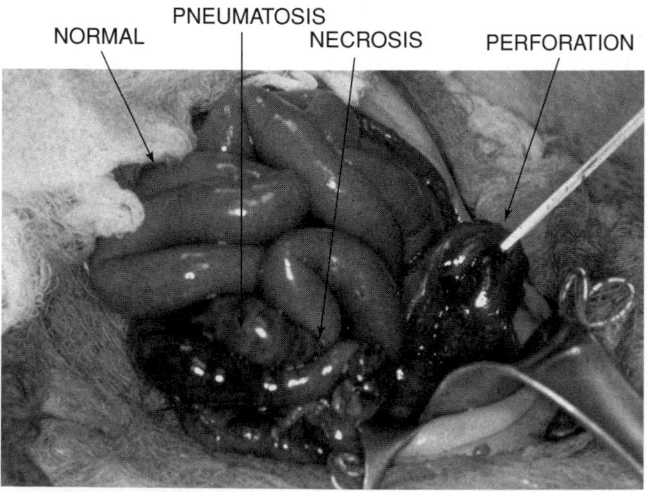

FIGURE 79-3. Gross findings at laparotomy for advanced necrotizing enterocolitis. Extensive areas of necrotic intestine with characteristic pneumatosis can be seen adjacent to grossly normal bowel.

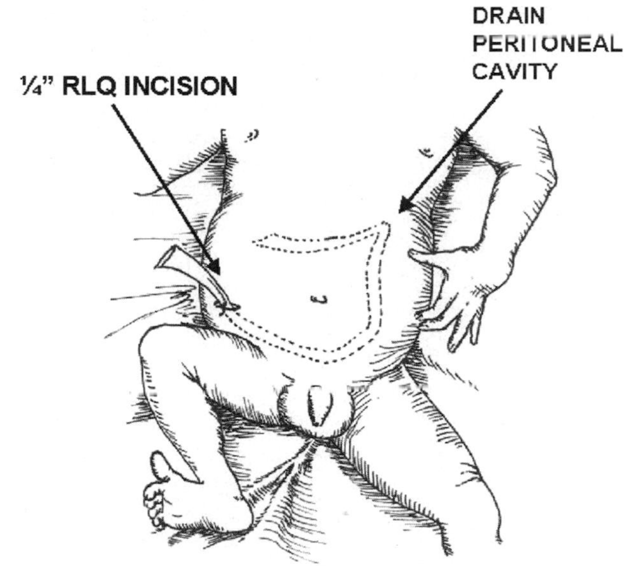

FIGURE 79-4. Schematic diagram of primary peritoneal drainage for perforated necrotizing enterocolitis. RLQ, right lower quadrant.

In 1977, Ein et al. first reported the use of primary peritoneal drainage (PPD) for perforation in VLBW infants (91). Peritoneal drainage involves making a right lower quadrant incision, irrigating the peritoneal cavity, and placing a small rubber drain in the abdomen (Fig. 79-4). The authors treated five patients between 760 g and 1,600 g described as septic and unstable with PPD. To the authors' surprise, three of these five "moribund" babies survived and the two that died of causes unrelated to NEC had intact GI tracts at autopsy. Although this report was anecdotal, the success of PPD was impressive compared with 35% to 55% mortality with conventional surgical treatment. Subsequently, this technique was widely criticized in the pediatric surgical community. This criticism led to a comment from the authors that PPD only should be used as a temporizing procedure in the "sickest" premature infants until formal laparotomy could be safely performed.

As experience with PPD increased, many babies treated with this "temporizing" procedure did not appear to need a subsequent laparotomy. The authors who first described the procedure reported their updated experience in 1980. They described 15 patients who underwent PPD with the intention of proceeding to laparotomy within 24 to 48 hours. Forty percent of these patients improved so markedly that laparotomy was not performed, and they completely recovered without further intervention.

PPD has never been studied in a controlled fashion or compared with laparotomy in a trial. In fact, every center using PPD reports selection bias in patient assignment. A more recent review of the published experience of the use of PPD for perforated NEC revealed that patients

TABLE 79-2 Comparison of Published Series Comparing Primary Peritoneal Drainage (PPD) and Laparotomy (LAP) for Perforated Necrotizing Enterocolitis.

	PPD				LAP			
Study	No.	GA[a] (wk)[b]	BW[a] (g)[b]	Survival (%)	No.	GA[a] (wk)[b]	BW[a] (g)[b]	Survival (%)
Cheu (135)	51	29	1,158	18 (35)	41	32	1,875	31 (76)
Takamatsu (136)	4	27	808	4 (100)	3	NA	NA	NA
Morgan (137)	29	27	994	23 (79)	20	32	1,854	18 (90)
Azarow (138)	44	28	1,100	27 (61)	42	31	1,700	24 (57)
Snyder (89)	12	29	1,134	3 (25)	91	31	1,628	52 (57)
Lessin et al. (139)	9	25	615	6 (67)	NA	NA	NA	NA
Ahmed (140)	23	27	910	10 (43)	22	35	2,271	19 (86)
Rovin (141)	18	28	1,118	16 (89)	10	29	1,274	9 (90)
Downard & Campbell (142)	24	26	794	19 (79)	9	30	1,510	7 (78)
Dimmitt et al. (143)	17	25	677	7 (41)	9	26	807	5 (56)
Total	231	27 (0.5)[c]	931 (63.2)[d]	133 (58%)[e]	244	31 (0.9)[c]	1,615 (155)[d]	165 (68%)[e]

[a]GA, gestational age; BW, birth weight.
[b]Means (SEM).
[c]$P = .0014$ for GA comparison.
[d]$P = .0004$ for BW comparison.
[e]$P = .03$ for survival rate comparison.

undergoing PPD were significantly smaller and more premature (Table 79-2) (92). Because of the marked selection bias and the lack of published information as to why patients were assigned to PPD versus laparotomy, the effectiveness of the two techniques could not be compared using meta-analysis techniques (92). The principal investigators from each institution used PPD in patients with a greater expected mortality. The fact that this "sicker" group of patients did better than predicted raises the question of whether PPD may be superior to laparotomy. This question is currently under assessment in randomized controlled trials in both the United States and the United Kingdom.

Resection and primary anastomosis has been advocated when there is limited involvement of adjacent bowel (93,94). There is no good evidence to suggest that this method is advantageous when compared with the traditional approach, and more extensive resection may be required to ensure the viability of anastomosed segments (95). Furthermore, some reports demonstrated higher complication rates (10%) in the way of anastomotic leaks and recurrent sepsis (94,95). The increased leak rate may be attributable to the unique histopathologic changes associated with NEC, where inflammation may extend well past grossly involved segments. From these clinical observations and histologic correlates, the authors strongly recommend against primary anastomosis as part of any operation for acute NEC. Simple suture closure of an isolated perforation is another intriguing approach. Reports of anecdotal success with this technique have emerged, but convincing evidence is lacking.

Several techniques have been described for the operative management of multisegment disease. Resection of all involved segments and the creation of multiple stomas is the traditional approach to preserve intestinal length. This approach can be technically challenging when many segments of bowel are involved, and the creation of a "high" jejunal stoma may lead to fluid and derangement and peristomal skin injury. With these considerations, several groups reported novel operative approaches to multisegment disease. In a more recent retrospective study of 83 cases of operatively treated NEC, mortality was compared between neonates undergoing primary anastomosis and those undergoing enterostomy for multisegment disease (90). The study found significantly lower mortality in the group receiving primary anastomosis (15% vs. 50%); however, it was not clear how patients were selected into the treatment groups. As the risk of anastomotic leakage in NEC is well known, the use of primary anastomosis may have been biased toward cases with less severe disease.

Moore advocated the "patch, drain, and wait" approach in the case of severe multisegment disease (96,97). The technique involves transverse single-layer closure of perforations rather than resection. Peritoneal drains are placed, the abdomen is closed, and long-term TPN support is provided. Nonhealing fistulas usually result and are subsequently repaired when inflammation resolves. This approach is potentially bowel sparing, but can be problematic in several ways. The operation does not remove the primary source of sepsis, and the peritoneal cavity can be difficult to drain. Attempting to suture edematous and acutely inflamed bowel may also be challenging. Finally, nonhealing fistulas must eventually be addressed in a potentially hostile abdomen.

There are few options available when massive intestinal necrosis is encountered at laparotomy (NEC totalis). Simple abdominal closure and supportive care is associated with a near 100% mortality rate (84). Extensive resection typically leads to severe short-gut consequences if the neonate survives. As a general rule, the surgeon should avoid resection of more than 70% of the total length of the small bowel. In the case where resection is clearly not feasible, the best approach may be decompression through a proximal stoma, abdominal closure, and a second-look laparotomy 24 to 48 hours later. Areas of hemorrhagic necrosis that may initially appear nonviable may improve considerably with decompression and continued resuscitation. A more limited resection may then be possible. Mortality and short-gut complication rates remain high, however, and further advances in the area of intestinal transplantation will be critical to the future survival of this cohort. In cases of clear-cut total necrosis of the intestine, the surgeon and family face the difficult decision of whether to declare the situation "unsalvageable" and provide comfort care versus proceeding with total intestinal resection in hopes of future transplantation.

POSTOPERATIVE MANAGEMENT

The principles of postoperative care include adequate hemodynamic support and close monitoring for recurrent disease. Gastric decompression is generally continued until the ileus has resolved and the stoma begins to function. Antibiotics are continued for 7 to 10 days following signs of clinical improvement and resolution of abnormal laboratory values. Meticulous stoma care is necessary to minimize skin breakdown and other complications at the stoma site. This is particularly important for high jejunal stomas, which may produce substantial volumes of caustic fluid. Frequent monitoring of serum electrolytes is also required for high-output stomas given the potentially significant loss of bicarbonate and sodium.

Recurrence of NEC following clinical resolution occurs in approximately 5% of cases (98). Contrary to initial reports, there appears to be no correlation between recurrent NEC and the initial site of disease, means of operative management, or timing of refeeding. Recurrent NEC presents an average of 5 weeks after the initial episode, and more than 70% of cases can be managed nonoperatively.

As with medically treated NEC, there are no consensus guidelines for reinstatement of enteral feedings after operative management. The risks of long-term TPN and feeding aversion must be carefully weighed against the risk of recurrent NEC. Enteral nutrition should not be attempted until there is clear evidence of stoma function and all signs and symptoms of sepsis have resolved. Protocols dictating mandatory periods of NPO status for 2 or more weeks are generally unnecessary and can lead to gut atrophy and bacterial translocation. Brief, self-limited periods of malabsorption are common following the resolution of NEC. Feeding regimens should therefore begin with small volumes of elemental-based formulas. Feedings should be advanced slowly to goal rate over 7 to 10 days, with stools frequently checked for reducing substances and occult blood. Many babies with ileal stomas will tolerate only a fraction of required calories via the enteral route and must be maintained on TPN until stoma closure.

Intestinal strictures arising from circumferential scarring commonly occur and will develop in 10% to 35% of patients (17,87). Predictive factors associated with the development of strictures have not yet been identified in epidemiologic studies. More than 70% of strictures are found in the colon, with the majority of these located in the sigmoid colon. A baby recovering from NEC treated medically who develops signs of a bowel obstruction should be evaluated for a stricture with GI contrast studies. A barium enema should be done first, followed by an upper GI series if the enema is normal. In operated patients, a stricture distal to a stoma will be clinically silent. Therefore, the distal GI tract should be studied with contrast prior to stoma closure.

There are no universally accepted guidelines regarding the timing of stoma takedown. The optimal timing for individual patients is a function of tolerance of enteral nutrition, stoma output, weight gain, and the time since operation. Although takedown should be performed as early as possible to restore continuity and minimize stoma-related complications, closure prior to 6 weeks may be technically demanding due to residual inflammation. Studies have not shown increased complication rates when closure is performed relatively early (weight less than 2,000 g) (99).

Other complications following the operative treatment of NEC are common. These include wound infection, dehiscence, enteric fistula, liver abscess, and stoma complications, among others. In a more recent prospective multicenter study, the complication rate for wound (infection and dehiscence) and stoma complications (stricture, prolapse, retraction, and necrosis) was 39% (100). Complications were significantly more frequent in babies born earlier than 28 weeks' gestation (49%).

PROGNOSIS

The prognosis for perforated NEC has steadily improved since the mid-1960s. This has been largely attributed to improvements in neonatal intensive care. The case–fatality rate has fallen from about 80% in the 1950s to its current estimate of 20% to 40% (1,2,87,101). The relatively wide variation in reported mortality is likely due to heterogeneous patient populations, particularly in the relative proportions of extremely low birth weight (ELBW) infants who continue to have excessively high mortality for stage III disease (50% to 60%). It can therefore be difficult to accurately compare mortality rates across different time periods, geographic areas, or even contemporary experiences.

Several studies have attempted to identify predictive factors for mortality in NEC. In a prospective cohort study of 91 patients with stage III disease, only intrauterine growth retardation and extent of bowel involvement were found to be predictive of mortality (102). Of note, gestational weight, age at operation, operative technique, and radiographic findings (including PVG and pneumoperitoneum) were not found to be significant in this study. In a retrospective analysis of 70 VLBW neonates with perforated NEC, no single comorbidity factor or combination of factors could be correlated with mortality, although the absolute number of predictors was found to be significant (103). In a series of 249 patients operated on for NEC over a 16-year-period, higher gestational age, age at operation, and birth weights were all associated with improved survival (11). Other studies have shown relatively increased mortality when NEC follows repair for congenital anomalies. This is particularly true when NEC follows the repair of abdominal wall or neural tube defects, where mortality approaches 50% to 70% in some series (104,105).

Approximately 10% of all neonates who survive NEC will experience some type of GI sequelae (106). Diarrhea is the most common GI complaint and is generally of the secretory or steatorrhea type (101). Bile-salt binders may be useful in managing these symptoms, particularly if the terminal ileum has been resected. Approximately 25% of all neonates who are managed operatively will require prolonged TPN support, and up to one-third of these will develop persistent short-gut syndrome (107). This is a devastating complication. Although some patients may ultimately be weaned from TPN after years of support, the majority are not so fortunate. Surgical options include bowel-lengthening procedures and intestinal transplantation. Bowel-lengthening procedures have yielded only sporadic and anecdotal success (108–111). The technique of small bowel transplantation remains challenging and experimental, although more recent results have been encouraging. In a retrospective study of 10 intestinal transplants performed for short-gut syndrome following NEC, the reported survival was 60% at a median follow-up time of 29 months (112). All survivors had been successfully weaned from TPN and had functioning grafts. Long-term data are not yet available.

An increasing amount of attention has been focused on assessing neurocognitive outcomes associated with NEC. Early reports documented significant growth retardation and neurocognitive deficits in as many of 50% of survivors (106). In a more recent retrospective study of 103 survivors with a mean follow-up of 7.5 years, more than 83% were found to be actively enrolled in school. However, 14.3% of those attending school were developmentally delayed and 28% required special education classes. This study may have underestimated the magnitude of neurocognitive problems because only 61% of parents responded to the study questionnaire. A more recent retrospective cohort study compared 20 NEC survivors with 40 controls matched on age and hospitalization timeline (113). The NEC cohort performed significantly worse on standardized psychomotor and neurodevelopmental test batteries, although somatic growth patterns were not significantly different between groups. A large follow-up study of 1,158 ELBW infants was more recently conducted by the National Institute of Child Health and Human Development (114). Using logistic regression techniques, the study attempted to identify risk factors that predicted poor performance on standardized neurocognitive test batteries. A history of NEC was found to be an independent predictor of poor performance on only one of four test batteries used in the study. The presence of grade III/IV intraventricular hemorrhage was associated with the highest increase risk for poor performance in all four tests, raising the question of potential confounding in the logistic model.

From these clinical observations, it is clear that survivors of NEC are at high risk for developmental delay and severe neurocognitive impairment. However, it is not possible from existing data to gauge whether the neurocognitive morbidity in NEC survivors is more severe (or qualitatively different) than that observed in neonates with similar comorbidity profiles. Prospective clinical studies using carefully matched controls are needed to better define the natural history of NEC in this context.

PREVENTION

Many strategies for the prevention of NEC have been implemented with varying degrees of success. These have included the use of prophylactic antibiotics, conditioning feeding protocols, breast milk-based diets, probiotic therapy, and enteral supplementation, among others. The utility of prophylactic antibiotics was more recently examined by the Cochrane Collaboration, an academic consortium dedicated to conducting high-quality systematic reviews (115). In a meta-analysis of five randomized trials, they found a 47% relative reduction in the risk of NEC and a 32% relative reduction in NEC-related mortality in the group receiving antibiotics. However, a statistically significant increase in the incidence of resistant organisms was also reported. The absolute reduction in the number of NEC cases was relatively small, and the authors concluded that the benefit of prophylaxis was unclear given the cost and potential long-term consequences of bacterial resistance. Although this strategy appears to be efficacious, the clinical utility of this approach will remain limited until we are better able to characterize risk factor profiles for the disease.

Several groups have examined the use of conditioning feeding protocols to reduce the risk of NEC. These protocols vary in their specific details, but generally involve the slow advancement of feedings during the first week of life to minimize hydrogen production and metabolic demands on the premature intestine. In a more recent retrospective study of 466 premature infants, an 84% reduction in NEC was found after implementation of a slow feeding protocol (20 mL per kg per day advancement) (116). These results were significant using a logistic regression model, although the comparison group was derived from historical controls. Several randomized studies have attempted to examine this further. In a more recent meta-analysis of available randomized data conducted by the Cochrane Collaboration, no significant difference in the risk of NEC was found between slow- and fast-advancing feeding protocols (117). However, the authors raised caution with the interpretation of their results due to the lack of standardization in feeding protocols across different studies. Furthermore, limitations of the pooled dataset precluded analysis of high-risk subgroups that may have benefited from slower feeding regimens (VLBW and ELBW infants).

Two well-designed randomized clinical trials have more recently been published that were not included in the Cochrane review. In the first study, premature infants weighing less than 1,500 g were randomized to receive either "slow" (15 mL per kg per day) or "fast" (35 mL per kg per day) feeding advancement (118). The authors found no difference in the incidence of NEC (13% in slow group, 9% in fast group), but observed that the fast group attained their birth weights more rapidly. In the second study, 141 premature infants born at gestational age less than 32 weeks were randomized to either "minimal" (20 mL per kg per day) or "advancing" (increasing 20 mL per kg per day to goal of 140 mL per kg per day) feeding protocols (119). The rate of NEC (primary outcome measure) was 7.5-fold higher in the rapidly advancing group (10.4% vs. 1.4%), and the study was terminated early due to significant treatment effect. Although the "minimal" group established full-enteral feeding volumes relatively later, there were no apparent complications from this. Specifically, there were no differences in the maturation of intestinal motor patterns, in late sepsis from all causes, or in the incidence of feeding intolerance. The results from these two contemporary trials seem to suggest that any degree of feeding advance, slow or rapid, may increase the risk of NEC after a certain threshold volume is reached.

Animal models of NEC have demonstrated a lower incidence and reduced severity of NEC-induced injury from breast milk feeding versus synthetic formula feeding. Breast milk appears to mediate its protective effects through several mechanisms. This includes the conferral of passive immunity through IgA, macrophages, and lactoferrin for binding iron (iron is required for *E. coli* growth) (120,121). Breast milk has also been shown to increase the diversity of bacterial species in the stools of ELBW infants. This may decrease the ability of potentially pathogenic organisms to colonize the gut. Several hormones, including erythropoietin, epidermal growth factor, and human growth hormone, have also been found in breast milk, suggesting that breast milk may exert trophic effects on the developing gut mucosa. Significantly higher levels of the antiinflammatory cytokines IL-10 and IL-12 have been found in animals fed breast milk compared with those receiving synthetic formula (122,123). Finally, breast milk may directly modulate inflammation through its high concentration of antioxidant compounds (primarily vitamin E) and PAF acetylhydrolase (124).

Although earlier observational studies have suggested a benefit for breast milk in reducing NEC in human infants, more recent data from randomized studies have been more difficult to interpret. In a more recent systematic review of six randomized clinical trials conducted by the Cochrane Collaboration, no significant differences were found in the incidence of NEC between infants fed breast milk and those who received formula feedings (125). The reviewers noted caution to their results, however, because only one of these trials focused on NEC as the primary outcome. Furthermore, the validity of pooled data was questioned due to the lack of standardization in feeding protocols.

Premature neonates have been shown to be deficient in native anaerobic flora (particularly *Lactobacillus* and *Bifidobacteria*) (126). This observation led to the hypothesis that oral supplementation with these probiotics may prevent NEC by limiting the colonization of potentially pathogenic organisms. In the neonatal rat model, enteral treatment with *Bifidobacterium infantis* reduced the incidence of intestinal damage following asphyxial stress by protecting against activation of the endotoxin-mediated inflammatory cascade (127). In a large nonrandomized clinical trial, all 1,237 patients admitted to a single NICU were given daily *Lactobacillus* and *Bifidobacteria* (250 million units per day for each organism) or placebo (128). A significant reduction in NEC was found when these infants were compared with historical controls from the previous year (6.6% vs. 2.8%). A critical analysis of the environmental and management factors that may have changed during that time period (and potentially confounded results) was not attempted, however. Furthermore, the annual variance in the incidence of NEC in their NICU was not reported. In a double-blind, randomized controlled trial (RCT) of 12 NICUs, 585 neonates with a gestational age less than 33 weeks or weight less than 1,500 g were randomized to receive daily *Lactobacillus* supplements or placebo (129). Although the incidence of NEC was not significantly different between groups, there was a strong trend toward protection in the probiotic group. Lack of significance may have been due to inadequate power given there were only 12 cases of NEC in the entire study. Furthermore, *Bifidobacter* and *Lactobacillus* may both be required to confer maximum protection against pathogenic colonization.

Supplementation of diet with oral IgA has been shown to reduce the severity of NEC in the neonatal rat model (121). However, a more recent Cochrane Collaboration review of three randomized trials including a total of 2,095 neonates did not show benefit for IgG or IgA + IgG therapy (130). There was no significant difference in the incidence of NEC, the need for surgery in documented cases, or NEC-related mortality. Arginine is a precursor for NO, and supplementation of this amino acid has been postulated to help maintain gut perfusion during periods of stress. In a more recent RCT of 152 premature neonates, supplementation with arginine (1.5 mmol per kg per day) was associated with a 75% relative reduction in NEC (131). The rate of NEC in the control group was 27%, however, suggesting there may be limitations to the generalizability of these results. Erythropoietin (EPO) is an endogenous hormone that appears to have trophic effects on gut mucosa. EPO receptors are upregulated in gut epithelium during periods of inflammatory stress and may protect against programmed cell death. In a retrospective study of 483 patients treated with EPO for anemia of prematurity, significantly fewer patients who received EPO developed NEC (10.8% vs. 4.6%) compared with age-matched controls (132). Development of NEC was not the primary outcome measure, however, and the comorbidity profiles of patients receiving EPO may have been quite different than those who did not. In the neonatal rat model, treatment with enteral polyunsaturated fatty acids (PFAs) has been shown to reduce mortality, endotoxemia, and PAF receptor expression (133). The mechanism for this protection is believed to occur through the modulation of PAF metabolism. The beneficial effects for PFA have also been demonstrated in human infants. In a double-blind RCT of diet and neurodevelopment as the primary outcome, significantly fewer patients who received egg-based formula developed NEC (17.6% vs. 2.9%) (134).

FUTURE DIRECTIONS

Over the past few decades, our knowledge base has substantially improved with respect to the pathogenesis and natural history of NEC. Despite these advances, however, NEC continues to pose significant challenges with respect to its prevention, diagnosis, and definitive treatment. Our ability to improve on current outcomes will hinge upon more rigorous clinical investigation and a better understanding of the earliest pathogenic events in NEC. Currently available animal models are limited in this latter regard because they suffer from conceptual and methodologic flaws in attempting to model the clinical factors associated with the onset of NEC. These models will certainly continue to evolve over time, and will eventually lead to the development of novel therapeutic and diagnostic strategies. More recent breakthroughs have led to the promise of a greater understanding of the developmental biology and physiology of the premature neonate's intestinal tract.

The use of rigorous clinical investigation is essential for translating continued advances in bench research to the surgical care of children. The majority of clinical evidence currently supporting the surgical care of NEC is founded on retrospective, often conflicting single-institutional case series data. Broader use of randomized trials and other high-quality prospective study designs is crucial if we are to identify the most efficacious therapy for NEC. Multicenter prospective databases will also be required if we are to accurately characterize the natural history of the disease, particularly with long-term neurocognitive outcomes. This could lead to earlier intervention strategies (e.g., focused special education), potentially resulting in decreased long-term morbidity and an improved quality of life for NEC survivors. With these continued efforts, the field of pediatric surgery is poised to make substantial strides toward improving the outcomes of this disease in the near future.

REFERENCES

1. Santulli TV. Acute necrotizing enterocolitis in infancy: a review of 64 cases. *Pediatrics* 1975;55:376–387.
2. Kliegman RM. Necrotizing enterocolitis. *N Engl J Med* 1984;310: 1093–1103.
3. Ricketts RR. Necrotizing enterocolitis. In: Ziegler, Weber, Azizkhan, eds. *Operative pediatric surgery.* New York: McGraw-Hill Professional; 2003. p. xxix, 1339.
4. Ryder RW. Necrotizing enterocolitis: a prospective multicenter investigation. *Am J Epidemiol* 1980;112:113–123.
5. Shimura K. Necrotizing enterocolitis: a Japanese survey. *NICU* 1990;3:5–7.
6. Holman RC. Necrotizing enterocolitis mortality in the United States, 1979–85. *Am J Public Health* 1989;79:987–989.
7. Kosloske AM. Epidemiology of necrotizing enterocolitis. *Acta Paediatr Suppl* 1994;396:2–7.
8. Book LS. Clustering of necrotizing enterocolitis. Interruption by infection-control measures. *N Engl J Med* 1977;297:984–986.
9. Kliegman RM. Necrotizing enterocolitis in neonates fed human milk. *J Pediatr* 1979;95:450–453.
10. Kliegman RM. Neonatal necrotizing enterocolitis: a nine-year experience. *Am J Dis Child* 1981;135:603–607.
11. Ladd AP. Long-term follow-up after bowel resection for necrotizing enterocolitis: factors affecting outcome. *J Pediatr Surg* 1998;33:967–972.
12. Teasdale F. Neonatal necrotizing enterocolitis: the relation of age at the time of onset to prognosis. *Can Med Assoc J* 1980;123:387–390.
13. Bisquera JA, Cooper TR, Berseth CL. Impact of necrotizing enterocolitis on length of stay and hospital charges in very low birth weight infants. *Pediatrics* 2002;109:423–428.
14. Ballance WA. Pathology of neonatal necrotizing enterocolitis: a ten-year experience. *J Pediatr* 1990;117:S6–13.
15. Grosfeld JL. Changing trends in necrotizing enterocolitis. Experience with 302 cases in two decades. *Ann Surg* 1991;214:300–306; discussion 306–307.

16. Parks DA, Bulkley GB, Granger DN. Role of oxygen-derived free radicals in digestive tract diseases. *Surgery* 1983;94:415–422.
17. Amoury RA. Necrotizing enterocolitis: a continuing problem in the neonate. *World J Surg* 1993;17:363–373.
18. Lloyd JR. The etiology of gastrointestinal perforations in the newborn. *J Pediatr Surg* 1969;4:77–84.
19. Ross G. Escape of mesenteric vessels from adrenergic and nonadrenergic vasoconstriction. *Am J Physiol* 1971;221:1217–1222.
20. Crissinger KD, Kvietys PR, Granger DN. Developmental intestinal vascular responses to venous pressure elevation. *Am J Physiol* 1988;254:G658–G663.
21. Nanthakumar NN. Inflammation in the developing human intestine: a possible pathophysiologic contribution to necrotizing enterocolitis. *Proc Natl Acad Sci USA* 2000;97:6043–6048.
22. Morecroft JA. Plasma cytokine levels in necrotizing enterocolitis. *Acta Paediatr Suppl* 1994;396:18–20.
23. Harris MC. Cytokine elevations in critically ill infants with sepsis and necrotizing enterocolitis [see comments]. *J Pediatr* 1994;124: 105–111.
24. Muguruma K, Gray PW, Tjoelker LW, et al. The central role of PAF in necrotizing enterocolitis development. *Adv Exp Med Biol* 1997;407:379–382.
25. Hsueh W. Platelet-activating factor, tumor necrosis factor, hypoxia and necrotizing enterocolitis. *Acta Paediatr Suppl* 1994;396:11–17.
26. Gonzalez-Crussi F. Experimental model of ischemic bowel necrosis. The role of platelet-activating factor and endotoxin. *Am J Pathol* 1983;112:127–135.
27. Caplan MS, Hedlund E, Adler L, et al. The platelet-activating factor receptor antagonist WEB 2170 prevents neonatal necrotizing enterocolitis in rats. *J Pediatr Gastroenterol Nutr* 1997;24:296–301.
28. Hu W, McNicholl IK, Choy PC, et al. Partial agonist effect of the platelet-activating factor receptor antagonists, WEB 2086 and WEB 2170, in the rat perfused heart. *Br J Pharmacol* 1993;110:645–650.
29. Hsueh W, Caplan MS, Qu XW, et al. Neonatal necrotizing enterocolitis: clinical considerations and pathogenetic concepts. *Pediatr Dev Pathol* 2003;6:6–23.
30. Caplan M. Serum PAF acetylhydrolase increases during neonatal maturation. *Prostaglandins* 1990;39:705–714.
31. Hsueh W, Gonzalez-Crussi F, Arroyave JL. Platelet-activating factor: an endogenous mediator for bowel necrosis in endotoxemia. *FASEB J* 1987;1:403–405.
32. Sun XM, MacKendrick W, Tien J, et al. Endogenous bacterial toxins are required for the injurious action of platelet-activating factor in rats. *Gastroenterology* 1995;109:83–88.
33. Hsueh W, Gonzalez-Crussi F, Arroyave JL. Platelet-activating factor-induced ischemic bowel necrosis. An investigation of secondary mediators in its pathogenesis. *Am J Pathol* 1986;122:231–239.
34. Moncada S, Higgs A. The L-arginine-nitric oxide pathway. *N Engl J Med* 1993;329:2002–2012.
35. Qu XW, Rozenfeld RA, Huang W, et al. Roles of nitric oxide synthases in platelet-activating factor-induced intestinal necrosis in rats. *Crit Care Med* 1999;27:356–364.
36. MacKendrick W. Endogenous nitric oxide protects against platelet-activating factor-induced bowel injury in the rat. *Pediatr Res* 1993;34:222–228.
37. Kubes P, McCafferty DM. Nitric oxide and intestinal inflammation. *Am J Med* 2000;109:150–158.
38. Ford H. The role of inflammatory cytokines and nitric oxide in the pathogenesis of necrotizing enterocolitis. *J Pediatr Surg* 1997;32:275–282.
39. Di Lorenzo M. Altered nitric oxide production in the premature gut may increase susceptibility to intestinal damage in necrotizing enterocolitis. *J Pediatr Surg* 2001;36:700–705.
40. Kosloske AM. Clostridial necrotizing enterocolitis. *J Pediatr Surg* 1985;20:155–159.
41. Rotbart HA. How contagious is necrotizing enterocolitis? *Pediatr Infect Dis* 1983;2:406–413.
42. Kosloske AM. A bacteriologic basis for the clinical presentations of necrotizing enterocolitis. *J Pediatr Surg* 1980;15:558–564.
43. Blakey JL. Enteric colonization in sporadic neonatal necrotizing enterocolitis. *J Pediatr Gastroenterol Nutr* 1985;4:591–595.
44. Takita S. Automaticity of the alimentary tract: observation on the fetal alimentary tract, the so-called ganglion-free intestine and the anastomosed organ. *Nippon Heikatsukin Gakkai Zasshi* 1970;6:79–86.
45. Udall JN Jr. Gastrointestinal host defense and necrotizing enterocolitis. *J Pediatr* 1990;117:S33–S43.
46. Hyman PE, Clarke DD, Everett SL, et al. Gastric acid secretory function in preterm infants. *J Pediatr* 1985;106:467–471.
47. Johnson LR. *Physiology of the gastrointestinal tract.* New York: Raven Press, 1981.
48. Lin J. Expression of intestinal trefoil factor in developing rat intestine. *Biol Neonate* 1999;76:92–97.
49. Tan XD, Chen YH, Liu QP, et al. Prostanoids mediate the protective effect of trefoil factor 3 in oxidant-induced intestinal epithelial cell injury: role of cyclooxygenase-2. *J Cell Sci* 2000;113(Pt 12):2149–2155.
50. Scheifele DW, Olsen E, Fussell S, et al. Spontaneous endotoxinemia in premature infants: correlations with oral feeding and bowel dysfunction. *J Pediatr Gastroenterol Nutr* 1985;4:67–74.
51. MacKendrick W. Increase in plasma platelet-activating factor levels in enterally fed preterm infants. *Biol Neonate* 1993;64:89–95.
52. Nagaraj HS, Sandhu AS, Cook LN, et al. Gastrointestinal perforation following indomethacin therapy in very low birth weight infants. *J Pediatr Surg* 1981;16:1003–1007.
53. Norton ME. Neonatal complications after the administration of indomethacin for preterm labor. *N Engl J Med* 1993;329:1602–1607.
54. Grosfeld JL, Kamman K, Gross K, et al. Comparative effects of indomethacin, prostaglandin E1, and ibuprofen on bowel ischemia. *J Pediatr Surg* 1983;18:738–742.
55. Gersony WM, Peckham GJ, Ellison RC, et al. Effects of indomethacin in premature infants with patent ductus arteriosus: results of a national collaborative study. *J Pediatr* 1983;102:895–906.
56. Robinson MJ, Clayden GS, Smith MF. Xanthines and necrotising enterocolitis. *Arch Dis Child* 1980;55:494–495.
57. Finer NN. Vitamin E and necrotizing enterocolitis. *Pediatrics* 1984;73:387–393.
58. Norris HT. Response of the small intestine to the application of a hypertonic solution. *Am J Pathol* 1973;73:747–764.
59. Kanto WP Jr. Perinatal events and necrotizing enterocolitis in premature infants. *Am J Dis Child* 1987;141:167–169.
60. De Curtis M. A case control study of necrotizing enterocolitis occurring over 8 years in a neonatal intensive care unit. *Eur J Pediatr* 1987;146:398–400.
61. Kliegman RM. Epidemiologic study of necrotizing enterocolitis among low-birth-weight infants. Absence of identifiable risk factors. *J Pediatr* 1982;100:440–444.
62. Martinez-Tallo E. Necrotizing enterocolitis in full-term or near-term infants: risk factors. *Biol Neonate* 1997;71:292–298.
63. Porat R. Cocaine: a risk factor for necrotizing enterocolitis. *J Perinatol* 1991;11:30–32.
64. Tyson JE, deSa DJ, Moore S. Thromboatheromatous complications of umbilical arterial catheterization in the newborn period. Clinicopathological study. *Arch Dis Child* 1976;51:744–754.
65. Kosloske AM. Indications for operation in necrotizing enterocolitis revisited. *J Pediatr Surg* 1994;29:663–666.
66. Dolgin SE. Alterations in respiratory status: early signs of severe necrotizing enterocolitis. *J Pediatr Surg* 1998;33:856–858.
67. Bell MJ. Neonatal necrotizing enterocolitis. Therapeutic decisions based upon clinical staging. *Ann Surg* 1978;187:1–7.
68. Pumberger W, Mayr M, Kohlhauser C, et al. Spontaneous localized intestinal perforation in very-low-birth-weight infants: a distinct clinical entity different from necrotizing enterocolitis. *J Am Coll Surg* 2002;195:796–803.
69. Buchheit JQ. Clinical comparison of localized intestinal perforation and necrotizing enterocolitis in neonates [see comments]. *Pediatrics* 1994;93:32–36.
70. Hutter JJ Jr. Hematologic abnormalities in severe neonatal necrotizing enterocolitis. *J Pediatr* 1976;88:1026–1031.
71. Ververidis M. The clinical significance of thrombocytopenia in neonates with necrotizing enterocolitis. *J Pediatr Surg* 2001;36:799–803.
72. Rabinowitz SS. Platelet-activating factor in infants at risk for necrotizing enterocolitis. *J Pediatr* 2001;138:81–86.
73. Edelson MB. Plasma intestinal fatty acid binding protein in

neonates with necrotizing enterocolitis: a pilot study. *J Pediatr Surg* 1999;34:1453–1457.

74. Daneman A. The radiology of neonatal necrotizing enterocolitis (NEC). A review of 47 cases and the literature. *Pediatr Radiol* 1978;7:70–77.
75. Kosloske AM. Necrotizing enterocolitis: value of radiographic findings to predict outcome. *AJR* 1988;151:771–774.
76. Kliegman RM. Neonatal necrotizing enterocolitis in the absence of pneumatosis intestinalis. *Am J Dis Child* 1982;136:618–620.
77. Engel RR, Virnig NL, Hunt CE. Origin of mural gas in necrotizing enterocolitis. *Pediatr Res* 1973;7:292–296.
78. Marchildon MB. Necrotizing enterocolitis in the unfed infant. *J Pediatr Surg* 1982;17:620–624.
79. Rowe MI. Necrotizing enterocolitis in the extremely low birth weight infant. *J Pediatr Surg* 1994;29:987–990; discussion 90-91.
80. Robberecht EA. Sonographic demonstration of portal venous gas in necrotizing enterocolitis. *Eur J Pediatr* 1988;147:192–194.
81. Lindley S. Portal vein ultrasonography in the early diagnosis of necrotizing enterocolitis. *J Pediatr Surg* 1986;21:530–532.
82. Maalouf EF. Magnetic resonance imaging of intestinal necrosis in preterm infants. *Pediatrics* 2000;105:510–514.
83. Mollitt DL. Does patient age or intestinal pathology influence the bacteria found in cases of necrotizing enterocolitis? *South Med J* 1991;84:879–882.
84. Ricketts RR. Neonatal necrotizing enterocolitis: experience with 100 consecutive surgical patients. *World J Surg* 1990;14:600–605.
85. Mimms GM. Oral gentamicin: prevention of necrotizing enterocolitis. *Pediatr Res* 1985;19:354.
86. Uauy RD. Necrotizing enterocolitis in very low birth weight infants: biodemographic and clinical correlates. National Institute of Child Health and Human Development Neonatal Research Network. *J Pediatr* 1991;119:630–638.
87. Horwitz JR. Complications after surgical intervention for necrotizing enterocolitis: a multicenter review. *J Pediatr Surg* 1995;30:994–998; discussion 98–99.
88. Kosloske AM. Necrotizing enterocolitis in the neonate. *Surg Gynecol Obstetr* 1979;148:259–269.
89. Snyder CL. Survival after necrotizing enterocolitis in infants weighing less than 1,000 g: 25 years' experience at a single institution. *J Pediatr Surg* 1997;32:434–437.
90. Fasoli L. Necrotizing enterocolitis: extent of disease and surgical treatment. *J Pediatr Surg* 1999;34:1096–1099.
91. Ein SH. Peritoneal drainage under local anesthesia for perforations from necrotizing enterocolitis. *J Pediatr Surg* 1977;12:963–967.
92. Moss RL, Dimmitt RA, Henry MC, et al. A meta-analysis of peritoneal drainage versus laparotomy for perforated necrotizing enterocolitis. *J Pediatr Surg* 2001;36:1210–1213.
93. Griffiths DM, Forbes DA, Pemberton PJ, et al. Primary anastomosis for necrotising enterocolitis: a 12-year experience. *J Pediatr Surg* 1989;24:515–518.
94. Harberg FJ. Resection with primary anastomosis for necrotizing enterocolitis. *J Pediatr Surg* 1983;18:743–746.
95. Cooper A. Resection with primary anastomosis for necrotizing enterocolitis: a contrasting view. *J Pediatr Surg* 1988;23:64–68.
96. Moore TC. Combination of "patch, drain, and wait" and home total parenteral nutrition for midgut volvulus with massive ischemia/necrosis. *Pediatr Surg Int* 1997;12:208–210.
97. Moore TC. Successful use of the "patch, drain, and wait" laparotomy approach to perforated necrotizing enterocolitis: is hypoxia-triggered "good angiogenesis" involved? *Pediatr Surg Int* 2000;16:356–363.
98. Stringer MD. Recurrent necrotizing enterocolitis. *J Pediatr Surg* 1993;28:979–981.
99. Musemeche CA. Enterostomy in necrotizing enterocolitis: an analysis of techniques and timing of closure. *J Pediatr Surg* 1987;22:479–483.
100. Chwals WJ. Surgery-associated complications in necrotizing enterocolitis: A multiinstitutional study. *J Pediatr Surg* 2001;36:1722–1724.
101. Patel JC. Neonatal necrotizing enterocolitis: the long-term perspective. *Am Surg* 1998;64:575–579; discussion 79–80.
102. de Souza JC. Prognostic factors of mortality in newborns with necrotizing enterocolitis submitted to exploratory laparotomy. *J Pediatr Surg* 2001;36:482–486.
103. Ehrlich PF. Outcome of perforated necrotizing enterocolitis in the very low-birth weight neonate may be independent of the type of surgical treatment. *Am Surg* 2001;67:752–756.
104. Oldham KT. The development of necrotizing enterocolitis following repair of gastroschisis: a surprisingly high incidence. *J Pediatr Surg* 1988;23:945–949.
105. Amoury RA. Necrotizing enterocolitis following operation in the neonatal period. *J Pediatr Surg* 1980;15:1–8.
106. Stevenson DK. Late morbidity among survivors of necrotizing enterocolitis. *Pediatrics* 1980;66:925–927.
107. Ricketts RR. Surgical treatment of necrotizing enterocolitis and the short bowel syndrome. *Clin Perinatol* 1994;21:365–387.
108. Bianchi A. Intestinal loop lengthening—a technique for increasing small intestinal length. *J Pediatr Surg* 1980;15:145–151.
109. Kim HB, Lee PW, Garza J, et al. Serial transverse enteroplasty for short bowel syndrome: a case report. *J Pediatr Surg* 2003;38:881–885.
110. Kim HB, Fauza D, Garza J, et al. Serial transverse enteroplasty (STEP): a novel bowel lengthening procedure. *J Pediatr Surg* 2003;38:425–429.
111. Thompson JS, Pinch LW, Young R, et al. Long-term outcome of intestinal lengthening. *Transplant Proc* 2000;32:1242–1243.
112. Vennarecci G. Intestinal transplantation for short gut syndrome attributable to necrotizing enterocolitis. *Pediatrics* 2000;105: E25.
113. Sonntag J. Growth and neurodevelopmental outcome of very low birthweight infants with necrotizing enterocolitis. *Acta Paediatr* 2000;89:528–532.
114. Vohr BR. Neurodevelopmental and functional outcomes of extremely low birth weight infants in the National Institute of Child Health and Human Development Neonatal Research Network, 1993–1994. *Pediatrics* 2000;105:1216–1226.
115. Bury RG, Tudehope D. Enteral antibiotics for preventing necrotizing enterocolitis in low birthweight or preterm infants [update of Cochrane Database Syst Rev 2000;(2):CD000405; PMID: 10796202]. *Cochrane Database Syst Rev* 2001;CD000405.
116. Kamitsuka MD. The incidence of necrotizing enterocolitis after introducing standardized feeding schedules for infants between 1250 and 2500 grams and less than 35 weeks of gestation. *Pediatrics* 2000;105:379–384.
117. Kennedy KA. Rapid versus slow rate of advancement of feedings for promoting growth and preventing necrotizing enterocolitis in parenterally fed low-birth-weight infants. *Cochrane Database Syst Rev* 2000;CD001241.
118. Rayyis SF, Ambalavanan N, Wright L, et al. Randomized trial of "slow" versus "fast" feed advancements on the incidence of necrotizing enterocolitis in very low birth weight infants. *J Pediatr* 1999;134:293–297.
119. Berseth CL, Bisquera JA, Paje VU. Prolonging small feeding volumes early in life decreases the incidence of necrotizing enterocolitis in very low birth weight infants. *Pediatrics* 2003;111:529–534.
120. Lucas A, Cole TJ. Breast milk and neonatal necrotising enterocolitis. *Lancet* 1990;336:1519–1523.
121. Barlow B, Santulli TV, Heird WC, et al. An experimental study of acute neonatal enterocolitis—the importance of breast milk. *J Pediatr Surg* 1974;9:587–595.
122. Dvorak B, Halpern MD, Holubec H, et al. Maternal milk reduces severity of necrotizing enterocolitis and increases intestinal IL-10 in a neonatal rat model. *Pediatr Res* 2003;53:426–433.
123. Nadler EP. Expression of inducible nitric oxide synthase and interleukin-12 in experimental necrotizing enterocolitis. *J Surg Res* 2000;92:71–77.
124. Hamosh M. Protective function of proteins and lipids in human milk. *Biol Neonate* 1998;14:163–176.
125. McGuire W, Anthony MY. Formula milk versus term human milk for feeding preterm or low birth weight infants. *Cochrane Database Syst Rev* 2001;CD002971.
126. Gewolb IH, Schwalbe RS, Taciak VL, et al. Stool microflora in extremely low birthweight infants. *Arch Dis Child Fetal Neonatal Ed* 1999;80:F167–F173.
127. Caplan MS. Bifidobacterial supplementation reduces the incidence

of necrotizing enterocolitis in a neonatal rat model [see comments]. *Gastroenterology* 1999;117:577–583.

128. Hoyos AB. Reduced incidence of necrotizing enterocolitis associated with enteral administration of *Lactobacillus acidophilus* and *Bifidobacterium* infantis to neonates in an intensive care unit. *Int J Infect Dis* 1999;3:197–202.
129. Dani C, Biadaioli R, Bertini G, et al. Probiotics feeding in prevention of urinary tract infection, bacterial sepsis and necrotizing enterocolitis in preterm infants. A prospective double-blind study. *Biol Neonate* 2002;82:103–108.
130. Foster J, Cole M. Oral immunoglobulin for preventing necrotizing enterocolitis in preterm and low birth-weight neonates. *Cochrane Database Syst Rev* 2001;CD001816.
131. Amin HJ, Zamora SA, McMillan DD, et al. Arginine supplementation prevents necrotizing enterocolitis in the premature infant [Comment]. *J Pediatr* 2002;140:425–431.
132. Ledbetter DJ. Erythropoietin and the incidence of necrotizing enterocolitis in infants with very low birth weight. *J Pediatr Surg* 2000;35:178–181; discussion 82.
133. Caplan MS. Effect of polyunsaturated fatty acid (PUFA) supplementation on intestinal inflammation and necrotizing enterocolitis (NEC) in a neonatal rat model. *Pediatr Res* 2001;49:647–652.
134. Carlson SE. Lower incidence of necrotizing enterocolitis in infants fed a preterm formula with egg phospholipids. *Pediatr Res* 1998;44:491–498.
135. Cheu HW. Peritoneal drainage for necrotizing enterocolitis. *J Pediatr Surg* 1988;23:557–561.
136. Takamatsu H. Treatment for necrotizing enterocolitis perforation in the extremely premature infant (weighing less than 1,000 g). *J Pediatr Surg* 1992;27:741–743.
137. Morgan LJ. Peritoneal drainage as primary management of perforated NEC in the very low birth weight infant. *J Pediatr Surg* 1994;29:30–34; discussion 314–315.
138. Azarow KS. Laparotomy or drain for perforated necrotizing enterocolitis: who gets what and why? *Pediatr Surg Int* 1997;12:137–139.
139. Lessin MS, Luks FI, Wesselhoeft CW Jr, et al. Peritoneal drainage as definitive treatment for intestinal perforation in infants with extremely low birth weight (<750 g). *J Pediatr Surg* 1998;33:370–372.
140. Ahmed T. The role of peritoneal drains in treatment of perforated necrotizing enterocolitis: recommendations from recent experience. *J Pediatr Surg* 1998;33:1468–1470.
141. Rovin JD. The role of peritoneal drainage for intestinal perforation in infants with and without necrotizing enterocolitis. *J Pediatr Surg* 1999;34:143–147.
142. Downard CT, Campbell T. *Peritoneal drainage for neonatal intestinal perforation.* Paper presented at the 33rd annual meeting of Pacific Association of Pediatric Surgeons, Las Vegas, NV, May 2000.
143. Dimmitt RA, Meier AH, Skarsgard ED, et al. Salvage laparotomy for failure of peritoneal drainage in necrotizing enterocolitis in infants with extremely low birth weight. *J Pediatr Surg* 2000;35:856–859.

Chapter 80

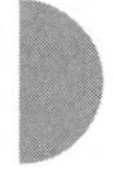

Appendix and Meckel's Diverticulum

Robert S. Sawin

APPENDIX

Anatomy

Embryology

The appendix develops from the cecum, which first appears during the fifth week as a ventral enlargement of the midgut. The appendix is first visible at 8 weeks, apparently the result of disproportionately slow growth of the terminal cecum compared with the rest of the hindgut. Although the appendix does continue to grow, its diameter is only 20% to 25% of the diameter of the cecum at birth. Absence of this expected asymmetric growth may explain the few documented patients with congenital absence of the appendix. The asymmetric growth of the appendix and cecum also causes the appendix to shift from the apex of the cecum to a more medial position near the ileocecal valve. The variability of this shift results in multiple possible positions of the appendix.

Gross Anatomy

In addition to the variable location of the tip of the appendix, its relationship to surrounding structures is protean. The appendix may lie across the psoas muscle or over the pelvic brim, resting on the pelvic fascia that overlies the obturator internus muscle. These positions account for the physical findings of pain on extension of the hip (psoas sign) or pain with flexion and internal rotation of the thigh (obturator sign). Additional variations in appendiceal position result from the abnormalities of midgut rotation. Because the attachment of the appendix to the base of the cecum is a constant, anomalies such as malrotation can lead to a left-sided appendix. The size and shape of the appendix also vary. It may be funnel shaped or cylindrical with a uniform caliber. The length can range from 0.3 to 33 cm, with appendices of males tending to be slightly longer than those of females. The diameter is typically less than or equal to 6 mm, and thus a measurement larger than that is one of the ultrasound criteria for diagnosis of appendicitis.

The arterial supply to the appendix is from the ileocolic artery, a branch of the superior mesenteric artery. One of four terminal branches of the ileocolic artery, the appendiceal artery passes posterior to the terminal ileum and gives off multiple short, straight branches to the appendix. The retroileal course of the appendiceal artery may predispose it to kinking with resultant ischemia and inflammation of the appendix. The venous drainage of the appendix is via the superior mesenteric vein to the portal vein, which accounts for the occasional findings of pylephlebitis or liver abscess following appendicitis (1).

Like the rest of the midgut, the appendix is innervated by branches of the splanchnic nerves that arise from the lower thoracic ganglia. Typically, the T10 ganglion is the one via which painful stimuli from the appendix are conducted to the dorsal nerve root, along the spinothalamic tract to the brain. Because the umbilical region of the abdominal wall develops from the same embryonic region, or dermatome, as the appendix, this explains in part why appendiceal pain initially localizes to the periumbilical region. This innervation is common to the kidney, upper ureter, and testicle, accounting for some of the organs that must be considered in the differential diagnosis of periumbilical pain.

Histology

Like the rest of the intestinal tract, the appendix has four layers. In both the mucosa and submucosa, germinal follicles and lymphoid pulp are prominent in infants and children. The lymphoid tissue gradually atrophies with age. Whether this lymphoid tissue predisposes children to appendicitis by luminal obstruction during periods of inflammation is unproved.

Robert S. Sawin: University of Washington, Children's Hospital and Regional Medical Center, Seattle, Washington 98105-0371.

Diseases

Appendicitis

Epidemiology

The risk of developing appendicitis has been estimated as 6% to 10% during an average lifetime. Residents of Third World countries have a substantially reduced risk of developing appendicitis compared with those in developed nations. A diet high in sugar, low in fiber content, and good hygiene with a resultant decreased exposure to enteric pathogens at an early age have all been hypothesized as risk factors for appendicitis. The epidemiologic literature, however, contains contradictory data. The risk of developing appendicitis is lowest in infancy, perhaps because of the relatively wide base of the appendix at that stage of development. Approximately 1% of all children younger than 15 years of age develop appendicitis with a peak incidence between 10 and 12 years of age (2).

The risk of developing appendicitis that progresses to perforation is greater in children than in adults. In published series of appendicitis from children's hospitals, the incidence of perforation is 20% to 76% but typically is approximately (3). This may be a consequence of the difficulty in making the diagnosis of acute appendicitis in the toddler or preschool-age child who cannot communicate as effectively as the older child. An additional factor is the unfortunate tendency of parents and physicians to attribute all childhood fevers and gastrointestinal symptoms to viral illnesses. There is also some evidence to suggest that easy access to health care providers may reduce the risk of perforation because managed care patients with private insurance have lower perforation rates than Medicaid or uninsured patients (4).

Pathophysiology

The pathologic sequence ending in appendicitis is believed to be analogous to that seen with cholecystitis. Although the causes of appendicitis and cholecystitis may be multiple, they often have in common obstruction of the proximal lumen. The role of obstruction in appendicitis was established by Wangensteen in an elegant experiment where the symptoms of appendicitis were replicated by ligating the base of an exteriorized appendix. Fecaliths are the most frequent example of obstructing appendiceal lesions and are present in approximately 30% to 50% of appendicitis patients (5). Other obstructing lesions may include lymphoid hyperplasia, foreign bodies, parasitic infections, or conditions that cause increased colonic pressure and decreased motility such as Hirschsprung's disease or meconium ileus. After the obstruction, the mucosa continues to secrete mucous, resulting in intraluminal pressure increases that lead to venous congestion and edema. The intramural pressure increases until ischemia and tissue acidosis of the appendiceal wall result. Finally, mucosal ulceration is followed by bacterial invasion leading to invasive infection of the appendix.

Although this orderly pathologic sequence is consistent with the progressive history and symptoms of appendicitis, the role of obstruction in the pathogenesis of appendicitis is somewhat equivocal. Likewise, the absence of fecaliths in 50% to 70% of the appendicitis patients supports the etiologic role of factors other than obstruction.

Microbiology

The possible role of viral infections in appendicitis has been implicated by the frequent prodrome of symptoms with which children with appendicitis may initially present. In addition, appendicitis has been described following *Varicella* infections. Cultures of mesenteric lymph nodes and resected appendices may grow *adenovirus* in children with appendicitis. It is hypothesized that the viral illness may result in lymphoid hyperplasia or lymphadenopathy, which can obstruct the lumen. In addition, the viral illness may result in dehydration leading to a higher likelihood of inspissated stool or mucous leading to fecalith formation and obstruction.

Enteric bacteria are the most common organisms associated with appendicitis. In the patients with perforation, *Escherichia coli*, *Enterococcus*, *Bacteroides*, and *Pseudomonas* are the species most frequently isolated from the abscess. Whether these are the main pathogens in nonperforated appendicitis is not known. Parasitic infections with *Enterobius* or *Ascaris* have also been reported in association with appendicitis. These organisms may cause a local inflammation or may contribute to luminal obstruction leading to bacterial invasion and supurative appendicitis.

Pathology

In the early stages of acute appendicitis, the appendix appears thickened and feels turgid, with increased serosal vascularity. The distal portion of the organ is often distended, especially when an obstructing lesion such as a fecalith is present. Histologically, the mucosa is ulcerated and infiltrated with inflammatory cells. As the bacterial invasion progresses, the inflammatory infiltrate progresses from the mucosa through the muscularis. Cloudy peritoneal fluid filled with polymorphonuclear cells but lacking bacteria may be seen as the inflammation progresses. Necrosis of all layers, or gangrenous appendicitis, may occur with or without perforation. If perforation has occurred, cloudy, foul-smelling peritoneal fluid is found. Usually, a polymicrobial flora can be cultured from this fluid. Microscopically dense sheets of polymorphonuclear leukocytes and erythrocytes are seen in the lumen, muscularis, and mesoappendix. The site of perforation may be difficult for the pathologist to identify, especially if the appendix is surrounded by the omentum.

TABLE 80-1 Symptoms of Appendicitis.

Symptom	Frequency (%)
Anorexia	95
Nausea/vomiting	85
Fever	60–80
Right lower quadrant pain	70
Diarrhea	10–30

Clinical Presentations

Acute Appendicitis

The child with appendicitis may present with many different symptoms, making appendicitis the most commonly misdiagnosed surgical lesion in the United States. The most frequent symptoms are listed in Table 80-1. The constellation of abdominal pain, fever, anorexia, and nausea is classically present in children with appendicitis. Unfortunately, fewer than one-half of the children with acute appendicitis present with this complete spectrum of symptoms. The orderly sequence of pathophysiologic events described previously usually causes a characteristic progression of symptoms. This sequence typically begins with vague abdominal pain apparently originating in the periumbilical region. This vague localization of pain is termed *referred pain*. The entire midgut shares the same T10 dermatome with the umbilicus so afferent pain stimuli are erroneously interpreted by the brain as originating in the umbilicus. Thus, any painful lesion or distension in the intestinal tract will cause a similar periumbilical pain. As the serosa of the appendix becomes inflamed, it begins to cause local inflammation of the adjacent peritoneum. With this peritoneal irritation, the pain is usually more localized to the right lower quadrant, thus manifesting itself as migration of pain to the right lower quadrant. As the inflammation and distention of the appendix progresses, the pain worsens. If the appendix is not removed at this time, then the swelling progresses and culminates in perforation. Thus, physical examination becomes especially important.

Examining the child with abdominal pain requires a calm, nonthreatening demeanor and careful observation. The child's appearance can be very revealing because the appendicitis patient will lie quietly, often with the knees drawn up, and resist movement in any way. Shaking of the bed or stretcher and having the patient cough may elicit wincing or complaint. Asking the child to get off the bed and walk can be informative. The child with early appendicitis may move reasonably comfortably, but will complain of pain when asked to walk on his or her heels or to jump to touch the examiner's hand held high. Having the child move from a supine to a sitting position or vice versa may also elicit discomfort.

Examination should begin with all other parts of the body. Auscultation of the lungs is important for pneumonia and can present as abdominal pain. Pain with external rotation of the thigh (obturator sign) or extension of the hip with the child in a left lateral decubitus position (psoas sign) indicates peritoneal irritation, often due to a retrocecal appendicitis. Before examining the abdomen, the examiner's hands should be warmed. Many surgeons ask the child to point with one finger to the spot that hurts the most. With the knees bent to relax the abdominal muscles, the examination should begin far away from the area of maximal tenderness. Younger children may be more willing to allow palpation if the examiner places the patient's hand or the stethoscope on the abdomen and palpates "through" these less threatening objects. Distraction by asking the child questions about their family, school, favorite activities, and so on, during the examination is very helpful. Close inspection of the facial expression is more discriminating than asking whether each maneuver hurts. If good relaxation can be accomplished, rectus muscle spasm can be appreciated. Sudden withdrawal of the palpating hand to check for rebound tenderness is startling for children, and therefore, not as reliable a physical sign as in adults. Palpation of the left lower quadrant eliciting right lower quadrant pain, termed *Rovsing's sign*, is a fairly specific sign for appendicitis. If diffuse tenderness and guarding are present, free perforation is likely, especially in children younger than 6 years of age. The rectal examination is considered most unpleasant by the patients and by some physicians, and is consequently often avoided. Although it should be deferred until last, it is occasionally one of the most important parts of the examination, particularly in the patient who does not have clear anterior abdominal wall tenderness, such as those with retrocecal appendicitis. The child should be gently advised that this exam will feel strange, but may not hurt. The left lateral decubitus position with the knees drawn to the chest works well. Once the discomfort of the examining finger is tolerated by the patient, the exam should begin away from the right pelvis, leaving it for last. Induration or focal tenderness in the right or midline pelvis are suggestive of appendicitis. If perforation has already occurred, a mass may be palpable on rectal exam, suggesting the option of operative transrectal drainage. It is also helpful to palpate posteriorly. This may differentiate pain due to peritoneal irritation from discomfort due to the examination alone.

Perforated Appendicitis

As mentioned previously, appendicitis leading to perforation is more common in children than in adults. The large diameter relative to the cecum and thin wall of the appendix in childhood may be contributing factors that predispose children to a more rapid progression of the disease. A more likely explanation of the higher perforation rates is the delay in presentation and the delay in diagnosis. Parents are prone to assuming that any gastrointestinal symptoms are related to "the flu" or to "something he or she ate," and thus are often slow to call the physician. Physicians frequently compound the problem with similar rationalization. Indeed, several studies have indicated that the major source of delays in making the diagnosis of appendicitis can be attributed to the health care provider (6).

The paradigm of the pathophysiologic sequence of appendicitis discussed previously is a convenient way to assist in making the diagnosis. It is reliable only if an accurate history is obtained and if the patient is examined sequentially. Because the goal is to make the diagnosis of acute appendicitis before perforation, the key period is the first 24 hours, for the risk of perforation within 24 hours of the onset of symptoms is less than 30%. Conversely, if symptoms have been present for more than 48 hours, the probability of perforation is greater than 70%. This paradigm is less useful in the children younger than 5 years of age because their disease history, physical signs, and symptoms are more difficult to assess and the diagnosis more difficult to make.

The symptoms of perforated appendicitis evolve from a transient decrease in the abdominal pain secondary to the release of pressure in the appendix, to a severe generalized abdominal pain, fever often higher than 38°C, worsening anorexia with nausea and vomiting, dehydration, and diarrhea (which can be misleading by suggesting the diagnosis of gastroenteritis). Occasionally, the child will progress through these symptoms and manage to localize the perforation by "walling off" the infection between the surrounding viscera and the omentum. This is particularly true of the retrocecal and retroileal appendices. Younger children with their veillike omentum are less capable of this localization and are more likely to have generalized peritonitis. The other physical findings in most children with perforated appendicitis are similar to those found in nonperforated appendicitis. The absence of bowel sounds or the presence of high-pitched, tinkling bowel sounds may suggest the presence of a small bowel obstruction, particularly in the children with retroileal appendicitis and those younger than age 6.

Appendiceal Mass

Appendicitis with a palpable mass is usually a consequence of perforation. The mass may be an abscess or a phlegmon, lacking frank pus and composed of omentum and matted loops of bowel. The management of patients who present with abdominal masses in the setting of appendicitis is controversial. Emergency surgery for such patients is seldom indicated because most will benefit from fluid resuscitation and initiation of broad-spectrum intravenous antibiotics before intervention. Laparotomy with drainage of the abscess, if present, and appendectomy has been the standard approach. Opponents of such an approach argue that the acute inflammation of the cecum and surrounding bowel can result in long, difficult operations with more blood loss, increased risk of bowel injury, and inability to safely perform a complete appendectomy.

Alternative approaches depend on whether the mass is an abscess or phlegmon, a distinction that may require ultrasonic or computed tomography (CT) scan imaging to resolve. Figure 80-1 shows an algorithm for the delayed laparotomy approach recommended by some pediatric surgeons. If the mass is determined to be a phlegmon, then intravenous antibiotics and volume resuscitation without immediate laparotomy is a safe and effective treatment, provided the patient shows clinical improvement with lower temperature spikes, decreasing leukocytosis, and decreasing abdominal tenderness. The elective interval appendectomy can be performed 6 to 8 weeks later. If clinical improvement does not occur after 12 to 24 hours of this nonoperative management, then laparotomy is indicated. If an abscess is identified, drainage by percutaneous, transvaginal, or transrectal routes is an effective treatment after resuscitation and intravenous antibiotics. Small abscesses (less than 2 cm in diameter) may be managed with antibiotics alone. As long as clinical improvement occurs, then antibiotic therapy is continued until the patient is afebrile, the white blood cell count is normal, and the abdominal tenderness is resolved. This postdrainage therapy can be completed as an outpatient, thus reducing the length of hospital stay. Interval appendectomy 6 to 8 weeks later is usually remarkably uncomplicated with a surprising absence of inflammatory adhesions and a postoperative hospital stay of 1 day. Whether this delayed operative therapy is superior to immediate appendectomy remains to be proven. One prosepective, nonrandomized study suggests that delayed surgical treatment is associated with a longer total length of stay and a higher morbidity rate (7). The question requires a controlled, randomized, prospective study.

Recurrent Appendicitis

There is some debate about the existence of recurrent or chronic appendicitis. If the paradigm of progressive pathophysiologic changes discussed earlier in this chapter is accepted, then it is difficult to reconcile the possibility of appendicitis resolving without some therapeutic intervention. Nonetheless, approximately one-fourth of patients with surgically proven acute appendicitis report a history of prior episodes of abdominal pain that are similar to the ones that prompted the appendectomy. Histopathology of resected appendices may show both chronic and acute inflammatory infiltrates and fibrosis, implicating prior episodes of acute appendicitis. In addition, as many as 60% of patients who are successfully treated in a nonoperative fashion for perforated appendicitis will have abdominal symptoms suggestive of recurrent appendicitis prior to the interval appendectomy. The histopathology of the interval appendectomy specimens may show acute, as well as the expected chronic, inflammation in such patients.

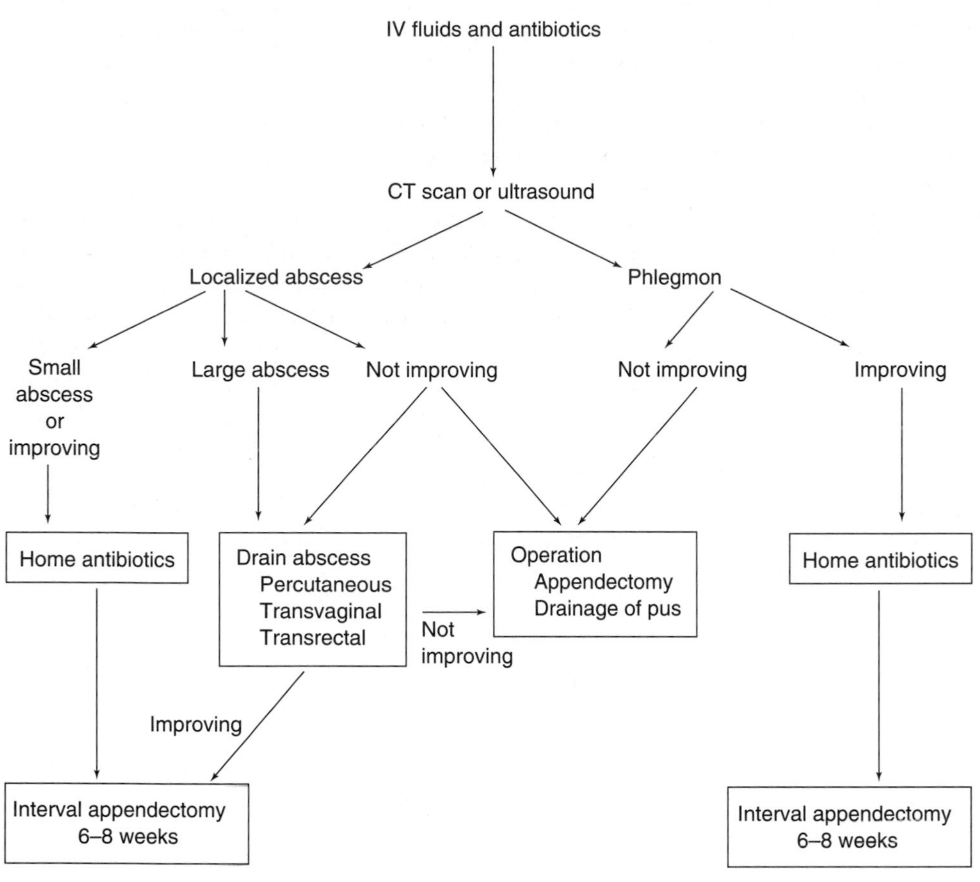

FIGURE 80-1. Algorithm for nonoperative management of perforated appendicitis. For children with a prolonged history, palpable mass, and no signs of systemic sepsis. IV, intravenous; CT, computed tomography.

A more uncommon entity is chronic appendicitis. Children with chronic abdominal pain are difficult to evaluate because many have no apparent pathologic cause for their pain. There are a small number of such children who undergo extensive diagnostic testing, including abdominal ultrasound and gastrointestinal contrast studies. Some of these patients have thickening of the appendix seen on ultrasound or no filling of the appendix seen on barium enema. These findings in the setting of chronic abdominal pain warrant an appendectomy and will frequently result in resolution of the symptoms. The diagnosis of chronic appendicitis is inferred, regardless of the absence of histopathologic confirmation. This absence of histologic verification prompts many physicians to attribute the symptomatic improvement to a placebo effect. Like postcholecystectomy syndrome and irritable bowel syndrome, chronic appendicitis may be difficult to define and diagnose, but there are patients whose disease appears to fit the diagnosis (8).

Special Considerations

Infants

Appendicitis in neonates is very uncommon and has a mortality rate of 50% to 80%. The diagnosis is often not recognized until postmortem. If identified in the neonatal period, appendicitis should be treated with emergent resection and rectal biopsies for frozen section diagnosis because Hirschsprung's disease is frequently the underlying cause. Colostomy at the level of ganglionated bowel is the only safe option in those patients with documented Hirschsprung's disease and appendicitis. Postoperative care in the neonatal intensive care unit with broad-spectrum antibiotics is typically warranted.

Appendicitis in children between 1 month and 1 year of age is unusual. These children are likely to present with perforated appendicitis and to manifest the complications of appendicitis, such as intestinal obstruction and systemic sepsis. It is indeed rare and fortuitous to make the diagnosis of acute appendicitis before perforation in this age group. This is a serious illness in infants and has a mortality rate as high as 10%.

Postpubertal Females

An accurate diagnosis of the source of abdominal pain in postpubertal girls is often difficult. In addition to appendicitis, ovarian pathology such as an ovarian cyst ruptured (or intact), ovarian torsion, pelvic inflammatory disease, and pain with ovulation, or mittelschmerz, can be common causes of severe lower abdominal pain. In most series, the rate of appendicitis resulting in perforation is no higher in this group of patients, but the rate of "negative appendectomies" (i.e., appendices lacking histologic evidence of inflammation) is reported to be as high as 40%. The liberal use of ultrasound examinations may result in lower negative appendectomy rates because ultrasound can be valuable to assess both the ovaries and the appendix. Diagnostic laparoscopy has been touted as an effective way to define the cause of lower abdominal pain in this age group. There is some debate, however, as to whether this avoids "unnecessary appendectomies" because many surgeons reason that the appendix should be removed during the laparoscopic procedure, regardless of its gross appearance.

Diagnostic Studies

Laboratory Tests

Although many different laboratory tests have been used to help discriminate appendicitis from other causes of abdominal pain, none are consistently reliable (9). The most reliable blood test is the white blood count (WBC) and differential because less than 5% of children with appendicitis have both a normal WBC and a differential count without a predominance of polymorphonuclear cells, or so-called "left shift." Unfortunately, nonsurgical illnesses such as gastroenteritis and ruptured ovarian cysts can also be associated with an elevated WBC and abnormal differential. Appendicitis resulting in perforation is almost always associated with leukocytosis and/or a marked left shift. However, a normal WBC in the setting of localized right lower quadrant tenderness or diffuse peritonitis should not dissuade one from operating for appendicitis. Plasma serotonin levels have been reported to be highly accurate in discriminating early appendicitis from other causes of abdominal pain, but this has not been confirmed on a large scale and is probably not practical in most clinical settings. Other serum tests, including c-reactive protein and erythrocyte sedimentation rate, have been touted as being helpful in diagnosing appendicitis. These tests are infrequently needed, have not been evaluated in large clinical trials, and merely add to the expense.

Urinalysis should be routinely performed on children with symptoms suggestive of appendicitis. An elevated urine-specific gravity and ketonuria are common findings in appendicitis, but are not diagnostic. The presence of leukocyte esterase, mild-to-moderate pyuria, or hematuria should raise the question of genitourinary tract pathology, but does not preclude the diagnosis of appendicitis because the inflammation of the appendix can cause irritation of the ureter or bladder. Marked pyuria with more than 25 WBCs per high-powered field is much more likely to be associated with pyelonephritis. An ultrasound may be helpful to assess the kidneys for inflammation and edema suggestive of pyelonephritis. In the absence of such ultrasound evidence or convincing flank tenderness, pyuria should not prevent the surgeon from performing an appendectomy.

Radiologic Examinations

Radiographic studies are frequently unnecessary in evaluating children with abdominal pain and should be reserved for the children whose symptoms are atypical or confusing. On plain films, findings such as an appendicolith, scoliosis, psoas shadow obliteration, a thickened flank stripe, and air–fluid level may be indicative of appendicitis. Of these, the finding of an appendicolith is the most compelling. If an appendicolith is identified in a child with localized abdominal pain, surgical exploration is indicated because almost all such patients will have acute appendicitis. The other features listed are occaionally helpful when evaluating patients with prolonged illness who may have retrocecal or walled-off appendicitis.

Ultrasonography

Advancements in ultrasound technology have resulted in its frequent application for the evaluation of patients with abdominal pain. The ultrasound image can detect the thickness of all layers of the bowel wall, luminal caliber, and whether the appendix is compressible. An edematous, distended (greater than 6 mm in diameter), or noncompressible appendix accurately predicts the presence of acute appendicitis, especially when its location corresponds to the point of maximal tenderness. The failure to identify these features of acute appendicitis, plus findings more suggestive of other diagnoses such as ovarian cysts or tumors; free pelvic fluid; thickened, edematous fallopian tubes; or thickened loops of small intestine may prevent an unnecessary emergency laparotomy. Multiple studies report sensitivities and specificities of 80% to 95% for the ultrasonic diagnosis of acute appendicitis. These studies vary significantly in the type of equipment used, the experience of the ultrasonographers, and the population of patients examined. Several factors predispose to false-negative results, including an obese habitus, recent perforation before the development of an abscess or phlegmon, and gaseous distention of the intestine. In addition, the reliability of the ultrasound study is clearly operator dependent. Thus, a surgeon must weigh the accuracy of the ultrasonographers in his or her own institution. The inability to identify the appendix over its entire length must be considered a nondiagnostic study and should not dissuade one from making the diagnosis of appendicitis in the appropriate clinical setting (10).

Computed Tomography

The use of CT scans to make the diagnosis of acute appendicitis in children has become common in some institutions (3).

There is considerable variation in the literature about the best method for CT imaging for the diagnosis of appendicitis. Although most radiologists routinely use intravenous contrast, some also recommend rectal contrast or oral contrast to opacify the bowel in the right lower quadrant. They argue that such contrast is necessary to differentiate unopacified or fluid-filled bowel from abscess. Other radiologists avoid enteral contrast to avoid obscuring the presence of a fecalith.

Although critics argue that CT is expensive and time-consuming, it may be useful in the atypical patient with an intraabdominal infection whose diagnosis is unknown or in whom a satisfactory ultrasound study is not possible. The utility of CT scanning for diagnosing appendicitis has not been verified in a large-scale, multiinstitutional prospective study. Although individual institution studies report a reduction in both negative appendectomies and the rate of perforated appendicitis and purport a reduction in unnecessary hospital admissions, a large-scale statewide database outcome study reported that appendectomy patients who had CT imaging tended to have more complicated and expensive hospital courses (11). Children who are obese, immunologically suppressed, or neurologically impaired, or who have a protracted illness and lack localizing physical findings, might be especially good candidates for CT imaging. CT scans may also be helpful in patients with perforated appendicitis for purposes of distinguishing phlegmon from abscess and planning percutaneous or transrectal drainage of an abscess (Fig. 80-2).

The normal appendix is ordinarily difficult to see with CT imaging. Appendicitis occasionally results in a target-shaped appearance of the appendix, which is a fairly specific finding. The inflammation associated with acute appendicitis causes edema and streaking of the surrounding fat. These findings are nonspecific and can be seen with other inflammatory lesions of the cecal region, such as neutropenic enterocolitis, inflammatory bowel disease (e.g., Crohn's disease), or bacterial enteritis. In small children who lack the same amount of intraabdominal fat as adults and older children, CT has limited utility unless a discrete abscess is seen.

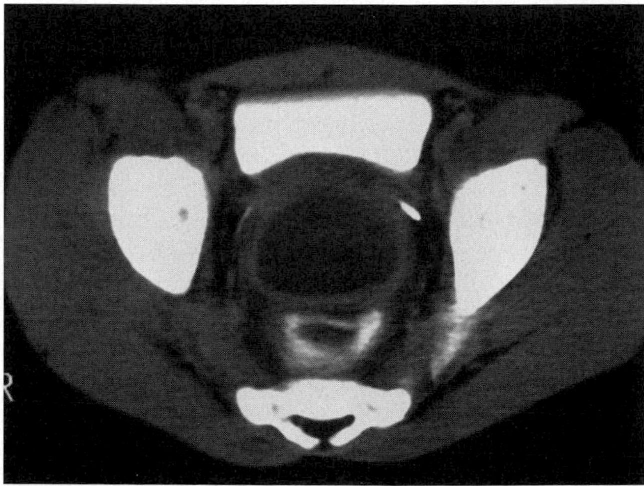

FIGURE 80-2. Computed tomography scan diagnosis of perforated appendicitis. This intraabdominal abscess developed after a several day history of abdominal pain, fever, and anorexia. The abscess was drained percutaneously and followed with an interval appendectomy 6 weeks later.

Barium Enema

Although several studies have supported the value of barium contrast enemas in making the diagnosis of appendicitis, this diagnostic study should also be used only in the atypical patient with a protracted acute illness or a history of chronic abdominal pain. Barium enema may be useful for such patients if the ultrasound and CT scan studies are nondiagnostic. The barium enema findings that suggest appendiceal pathology are nonfilling or incomplete filling of the appendix and extrinsic compression or distortion of the cecum. The incomplete filling of the appendix is consistent with the hypothesis that luminal obstruction is an important factor in the etiology of appendicitis. Unfortunately, as many as 20% of normal patients have nonfilling of the appendix and focal appendicitis of the distal tip may allow near complete filling, which appears deceptively normal. Like many other imaging studies, the use of barium enema for diagnosing appendicitis is operator dependent. When done with some regularity by experienced pediatric radiologists, barium enema can accurately detect appendicitis. Perhaps the best advantage of barium contrast studies is the feasibility of identifying other causes of right lower quadrant pain and tenderness, such as inflammation of the terminal ileum due to Crohn's disease, *Salmonella*, *Shigella*, or *Yersinia* infections.

Laparoscopy

The use of the laparoscope is gaining popularity in the management of children with abdominal pain consistent with possible appendicitis. The rationale for its use is that identification of some other cause of pathology or a normal appendix would obviate the need for a negative appendectomy with its incumbent risks. There are specific patient populations that have a high incidence of negative laparotomy, such as postpubertal girls. Laparoscopy has been especially advocated in that group of patients. Unfortunately, laparoscopy still requires a general anesthesia with its incumbent risks. Furthermore, some advocates of laparoscopy recommend that the appendix be removed via the laparoscope even if the appendix appears grossly normal, thus eliminating the stated advantage of reducing the negative appendectomy rate. However, if the cause of the pain is adnexal pathology, the laparoscope allows superior visualization of the pelvic organs compared with the typical appendectomy incision. For that reason, it seems laparoscopy may be most useful when the surgeon is suspicious of other causes of lower abdominal pain. Whether laparoscopic appendectomy is a technically better option in all patients is discussed later in the chapter.

Although WBC, radiographs, ultrasound or CT scans, or laparoscopy are sometimes helpful in making the diagnosis of appendicitis, particularly in postpubertal girls or children with prolonged illnesses, one can usually make the diagnosis without their use.

Surgical Treatment

Appendectomy

The only appropriate treatment for acute appendicitis is appendectomy. Nevertheless, patients are occasionally treated successfully for appendicitis when given antibiotics to treat presumed urinary tract infections or otitis media. Such patients will usually develop recurrent symptoms and require appendectomy in the future. The operation is best performed as soon as possible, provided the patient is satisfactorily prepared with fluid resuscitation and perioperative antibiotic treatment. Some authors have suggested that appendectomy for acute appendicitis can be deferred reasonably until regular working hours when a patient presents in the middle of the night. If one accepts the paradigm presented earlier that appendicitis is a progressive pathologic process and that the incidence of perforation increases with the duration of illness, then delaying the appendectomy may increase the risk of perforation. The concept of deferral for 6 to 12 hours is based on the premise that the pathologic process is slowed or arrested with systematic antibiotics. This remains a point of convergency. If the patient has clearly progressed to perforation already, then deferring the operation to maximize the time for resuscitation is prudent. The antibiotics of choice depend on whether perforation has occurred. For perioperative wound prophylaxis in patients with acute appendicitis without perforation, a broad-spectrum intravenous antibiotic such as a cephalosporin is adequate. For patients with suspected perforation, broad-spectrum coverage directed against gram-negative and anaerobic organisms is necessary. The combination of ampicillin, gentamicin, and metronidazole (or clindamycin) is the standard therapy against which all other antibiotic regimens are compared. Newer single agents have been used in several studies with apparently equal efficacy, although large studies in children with perforated appendicitis have not been reported.

Once the antibiotics, electrolyte, and volume resuscitation have been completed, laparotomy should be performed. Unless significant doubt about the diagnosis persists, the incision of choice is a right lower quadrant transverse incision placed directly over the point of maximal tenderness or the palpable mass. The incision should be lateral to the rectus muscle, but may be extended in a medial direction if greater exposure is needed during the operation. The external oblique is widely incised in the direction of its fibers, exposing the internal oblique, which is split in the direction of its fibers. The transversus abdominis and peritoneum can then be incised and cultures taken of any fluid found. In situations where the diagnosis is less certain, a lower midline incision or "incision of indecision" is made. Once the peritoneum is open, the operation is performed in the same fashion.

The cecum is identified first, usually by delivering the most lateral segment of bowel into the wound. If enlarged and inflamed, the appendix may be easily palpable. Otherwise, the appendix can be found consistently by following the taeniae coli to their confluence. If the appendix is retrocecal, encased in inflammatory adhesions, or immobile because of dense retroperitoneal attachments of the cecum, careful blunt dissection usually permits delivery into the wound. Occasionally, the incision needs to be extended to permit safe mobilization of the cecum or appendix. The appendix is mobilized by dividing the mesoappendix and then the organ is amputated at its base. Simple ligation of the base of the appendix is adequate in most cases, but many surgeons also imbricate the appendiceal stump using a pursestring or Z-stitch. The imbrication of too much tissue can lead to a mucocele or later result in a lead point for an intussusception. Mucoceles can be prevented by cauterization of the residual mucosa at the base of the appendix. After removal of the appendix, the wound is irrigated and the muscle layers are closed.

Failure to find an obviously inflamed appendix should prompt an exploration for other possible causes of abdominal tenderness. The list of differential diagnoses can be extensive, but in children, mesenteric adenitis; gynecologic pathology such as hemorrhagic ovarian cysts or torsion or infection; and inflammation of a Meckel's diverticulum and regional enteritis, both infectious and idiopathic, are the most common sources of this error in diagnosis. Consequently, examination of the distal small bowel, mesentery, fallopian tubes, and ovaries is necessary as a minimum. This can usually be accomplished through the same incision. If purulent or bloody fluid is seen in the peritoneal cavity, extension of the original incision or even a new midline incision is mandated to make a firm diagnosis. Some surgeons have proposed using a laparoscope through the partially closed original incision because this permits excellent visibility of all quadrants of the abdomen. Even if the appendix appears grossly normal, it should be removed, because the microscopy may reveal appendicitis, and such a patient with a right lower quadrant scar will be assumed to be without the appendix in the future. An exception should be made for patients with inflammatory bowel disease involving the cecum in the region of the base of the appendix. In such instances, the risk of a stump leak and subsequent fecal fistula from the cecum precludes a safe appendectomy.

For patients with suspected perforated appendicitis, broad-spectrum antibiotic therapy and nasogastric decompression are started before laparotomy. The operative technique for perforated appendicitis is essentially the same. Efforts to minimize the incision because of cosmetic concerns are ill advised because the inflammation and peritonitis make visibility more challenging. Peritoneal pus must be drained as completely as possible. Although it is common practice to culture the pus, the information gained is seldom used to alter the treatment. The organisms cultured and their sensitivities to antibiotics may only partially reflect the bacteriology of the intraabdominal infection, which is almost always polymicrobial. The antibiotic therapy should be kept broad enough to cover the most common gram-negative and anaerobic organisms, regardless of the culture results, and should not be discontinued until the fever, leukocytosis, and abdominal exam have all normalized.

Mobilization of the cecum and appendix can be much more difficult in patients with perforation, occasionally resulting in injury to the neighboring bowel. If the dissection and exposure of the appendix proves to be too difficult, placement of drains in the abscess cavities and closure of the abdomen is a safe option, albeit infrequently employed. This must be followed by an interval appendectomy to avoid a more than 50% risk of recurrent appendicitis.

Whether one should irrigate the pelvic and abdominal peritoneal cavity of patients with appendicitis is controversial. Some studies have suggested that irrigation interferes with normal macrophage function, yet a widely used protocol for pediatric perforated appendicitis includes irrigation with large amounts of saline and yields one of the lowest complication rates in the literature (12). Although many surgeons include antibiotics in the irrigation, there is no proven advantage over broad-spectrum intravenous antibiotics. There is considerably more debate regarding the use of peritoneal drains for these patients (13–15). Critics argue that no drain can effectively drain the peritoneal cavity, while proponents point to a very low rate of residual intraabdominal abscesses when drains are used. No randomized, controlled studies have been performed in the modern antibiotic era comparing the use of drains with no drains in perforated appendicitis. The major complication rates for the two approaches are similar. Wound closure in the face of gangrenous or perforated appendicitis is associated with an infection rate as high as 20%. If drains are not used, some surgeons recommend delayed primary closure, which can be facilitated by leaving widely spaced, nonabsorbable sutures in the skin at the completion of the operation. These sutures can be tied at 72 to 96 hours with a reasonable cosmetic result and a lower risk of wound infection. More recent series have reported wound infection rates of less than 5% with primary closure, even in perforated appendicitis patients. Alternatively, others believe that closure by secondary intention often has a very acceptable cosmetic result.

Laparoscopic appendectomy is gaining popularity, and many single institution studies suggest advantages when compared with open appendectomy. Larger meta-analyses or collective reviews verify that laparoscopic appendectomy slightly reduces the need for postop analgesia, may shorten hospital stays, and is associated with lower wound infection rates (16). However, laparoscopic appendectomy takes longer, costs more, and is associated with a higher rate of intraabdominal abscess in some studies (17). The excellent visibility of laparoscopy may be advantageous in larger or obese children in whom a very large incision would be necessary or in children with less certain diagnosis such as postpubertal females.

During laparoscopy, the mesoappendix can be divided by cautery by using stainless steel clips, or with an automatic stapler that fires two parallel sets of staples and cuts between them. The appendix is amputated using the stapler or by dividing the base of the appendix between three ligatures of absorbable sutures that are applied by "snaring" the appendix. Residual appendiceal mucosa can be carefully cauterized if necessary to prevent mucocele formation. The resected appendix is withdrawn through a port site. Irrigation of the pelvis and stump region is followed by suture closure of the port incisions. Although perforation was initially reported to be a contraindication for pediatric laparoscopic appendectomy, this is no longer the case.

Complications

The most common complications after appendectomy and their cumulative incidence in four recent studies involving 761 patients, include wound infection with 1% to 5% incidence in gangrenous or perforated appendicitis and small bowel obstruction, which occurs in approximately 1% to 2% of patients with perforation, but can also complicate the recovery of nonperforated patients, including those who undergo a negative appendectomy (18). Operative adhesiolysis is usually necessary. Intraabdominal or pelvic abscess with an incidence of approximately 2–8% is seen almost exclusively in children with perforated appendicitis. The abscess can be drained percutaneously by ultrasound or CT scan guidance, or may be drained through the rectum or vagina. Infertility in females has been attributed to a history of perforated appendicitis in several studies. However, in a more recent longitudinal study of women who had prepubertal perforated appendicitis, there was no difference in fertility rates compared with the general population (19). Finally, an enterocutaneous fistula occurs in 0.2% of cases.

Advancements in perioperative care and antibiotics have lowered the mortality rate for appendicitis (less than 1%), but have not eliminated it. Intraabdominal sepsis and multisystem organ failure have occurred in children who are typically younger (younger than 5 years old) or who have major illnesses prior to surgical intervention.

Tumors

Carcinoid tumors are uncommon in children, but may be identified in appendiceal specimens. Most of these appendices containing carcinoid are inflamed, often resulting in perforation, presumably because of the high-grade luminal obstruction. The histology of these tumors shows nests of small uniform cells invading the submucosa and muscularis, often extending to the serosa. These tumors are typically small and behave in a benign fashion, even if the lymph nodes contain tumor. Consequently, appendectomy alone without adjuvant therapy is sufficient treatment in children (20). Other more rare tumors include lymphoma, lymphosarcoma, and adenocarcinoid, a much more aggressive malignancy.

Incidental Appendectomy

There is significant debate about the wisdom of incidental appendectomy during other abdominal operations. Some advocates for incidental appendectomy maintain that it should be removed whenever the exposure allows for it because the appendix has no function and can potentially cause future morbidity. In addition, microscopy of incidental appendectomy specimens shows inflammation and fibrosis in as many as 20%. However, incidental appendectomy does potentially increase the operative morbidity, particularly for wound infections in otherwise clean operations. More recently described reconstructive procedures using the appendix have also challenged the wisdom of routine incidental appendectomy. The appendix is well suited as a conduit for urinary drainage (Mitrofanoff procedure) (21) and for biliary drainage. Thus, it should be preserved whenever possible in children with congenital biliary problems, neural tube defects, or genitourinary anomalies who may require reconstructive surgery in the future.

MECKEL'S DIVERTICULUM

Meckel's diverticulum is one of a constellation of congenital anomalies of the midgut that should more accurately be termed *omphalomesenteric duct-related anomalies*. The embryologic midgut is the open ventral portion of the archenteron that lies between the foregut and the hindgut. During the third week of gestation the midgut is opened into the yolk sac, which does not grow as rapidly as the rest of the embryo. Consequently, by the fifth week, the connection with the yolk sac becomes narrowed and is termed the *yolk stalk, vitelline duct,* or *omphalomesenteric duct*. Normally, this yolk stalk will disappear by the ninth gestational week, just prior to the midgut's return to the abdomen. Persistence of some portion of this omphalomesenteric duct results in many congenital anomalies, of which Meckel's (or omphaloileal) diverticulum is the most common.

Figure 80-3 shows the variety of omphalomesenteric duct remnants and their associated complications. Some are attached to the small intestine, and most are attached to the umbilicus. The location of those lesions attached to the bowel varies, with approximately 75% situated within 100 cm of the ileocecal valve. All attachments to the bowel are located on the antimesenteric side. Histologically, the omphalomesenteric diverticulum is a true diverticulum consisting of all four intestinal layers. The mucosa often contains ectopic gastric and pancreatic mucosa, especially in symptomatic patients. Those patients who develop hemorrhagic complications contain gastric mucosa alone or both pancreatic and gastric mucosa in more than 95% of the resected specimen (22). If Meckel's diverticula are resected from asymptomatic patients, variable incidence of ectopic mucosa have been described, ranging from 5% to 65% (22–24). The blood supply to the omphalomesenteric duct remnant is a vestige of the primitive vitelline artery, which usually arises directly from the mesentery and may be quite prominent, especially in patients with bleeding related to ectopic gastric mucosa.

Clinical Presentations

This lesion is found in approximately 2% of the population, often incidentally during laparotomy for other lesions or at the time of autopsy. Estimates of the probability of Meckel's diverticulum causing symptoms in a lifetime vary from 4% to 35%, depending on the age of the population studied (25). The risk of developing symptoms is lower than the incidence of ectopic mucosa as mentioned previously, suggesting that the mere presence of pancreatic or gastric mucosa does not necessarily predict development of symptoms. More than 60% of the patients who develop symptoms from this anomaly are younger than 2 years of age (22,23). The most common symptoms of this lesion are bleeding, intestinal obstruction, inflammation, and umbilical drainage. The incidence of each of these problems also varies with the age of the patients.

Bowel Obstruction

In infants, bowel obstruction is the most likely symptom of a Meckel's diverticulum. This can be due to either intussusception with the diverticulum as the lead point or to herniation of the bowel through a patent omphalomesenteric fistula. Occasionally, inversion of the diverticulum can cause obstruction without associated intussusception (26). Obstruction can also occur with volvulus around a fibrous remnant of the omphalomesenteric duct that is attached to Meckel's diverticulum or an internal hernia beneath the vestigial vitelline artery or fibrous remnant (23). If intussusception has occurred, the diagnosis can be made by barium or air contrast enema, CT scan, or ultrasonography (27). Enema reduction of the intussusception, however, is seldom successful. If the obstruction is due to prolapse of the intestine through the patent omphalomesenteric fistula, a characteristic "ram's horn" appearance

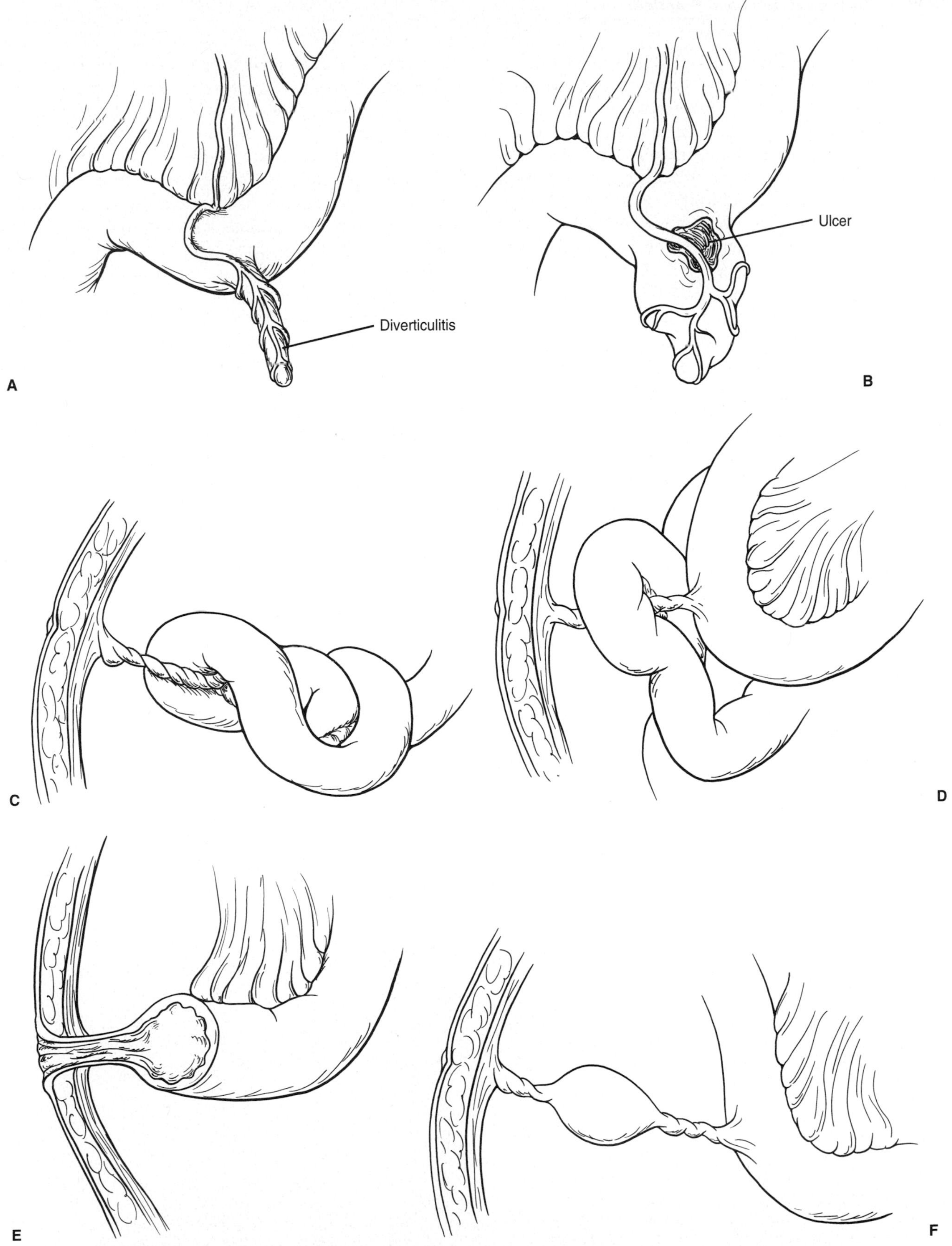

FIGURE 80-3. Omphalomesenteric remnants. **(A)** Meckel's diverticulum with diverticulitis. **(B)** Meckel's diverticulum with ulceration and hemorrhage. **(C, D)** Bowel obstruction from volvulus around attachment to the abdominal wall. **(E)** Patent omphalomesenteric duct. **(F)** Omphalomesenteric sinus and cyst.

may be seen. If obstruction occurs because of volvulus around a fibrous vitelline duct remnant that is not patent or because of an internal hernia beneath the vitalize artery, the diagnosis can be extremely difficult to make. The onset of pain is usually sudden and severe. In older children, the pain may be out of proportion to the physical findings, a characteristic of intestinal ischemia. Inspection of the umbilicus and barium enema will be of little help. Because the volvulus usually involves the distal small bowel and the obstruction is most often a closed loop, there may be little emesis until late in the course. The sequela of intestinal ischemia such as acidosis, peritonitis, and shock may occur first. In infants and toddlers, this can be a lethal lesion unless a high index of suspicion is maintained.

Bleeding

Hemorrhage is the most common complication of Meckel's diverticulum, occurring in approximately 50% of the symptomatic patients. The patients who develop bleeding are typically older with the mean age of approximately 2 years (22,23). The bleeding is usually painless, often massive, and frequently requires transfusion. Hemorrhage from Meckel's diverticulum is the most common cause of serious gastrointestinal bleeding in children. In the era prior to nuclear scintigraphy, children with massive, painless bleeding or children with unexplained chronic rectal bleeding were assumed to have Meckel's diverticulum and were taken to the operating room for a diverticulectomy after resuscitation. The diagnosis was usually correct, but other less common lesions were identified including juvenile retention polyps, hemangiomas, Peutz-Jeghers polyps, peptic ulcer disease, blood dyscrasias, and inflammatory bowel disease.

The bleeding associated with Meckel's diverticulum originates from ulceration of the ileal mucosa. This ulceration is presumably peptic in origin because the ectopic gastric mucosa contains parietal cells that secrete acid. The ileal mucosa is ill equipped to buffer the resulting acid secretion and thus is prone to ulceration. The site of ulceration is most often at the junction of the normal ileal mucosa and the ectopic gastric mucosa. A similar situation arises in patients with ectopic gastric mucosa in enteric duplication cysts. The remnant vitelline artery may be quite prominent in those patients who have bleeding from their Meckel's diverticulum.

The development of the technetium-99m pertechnetate isotope scan permits the visualization of the ectopic gastric mucosa, The isotope is taken up by the mucus-secreting cells of the ectopic gastric mucosa, as well as by those in the stomach. The remaining isotope is seen in the urinary bladder. Images are exposed every minute for 1 hour (Fig. 80-4). Failure to identify any ectopic gastric mucosa on scintigraphy is associated with only a 5% to 10% error rate. If rectal bleeding persists, a repeat scintigraphy scan is indicated. To enhance the sensitivity of the repeat scan, catheterization of the bladder and intravenous administration of pentagastrin and cimetidine are recommended by some authors. If the scan is still negative, CT scan and ultrasonography may be successful in identifying Meckel's diverticula (27). Other studies such as an isotope-labeled

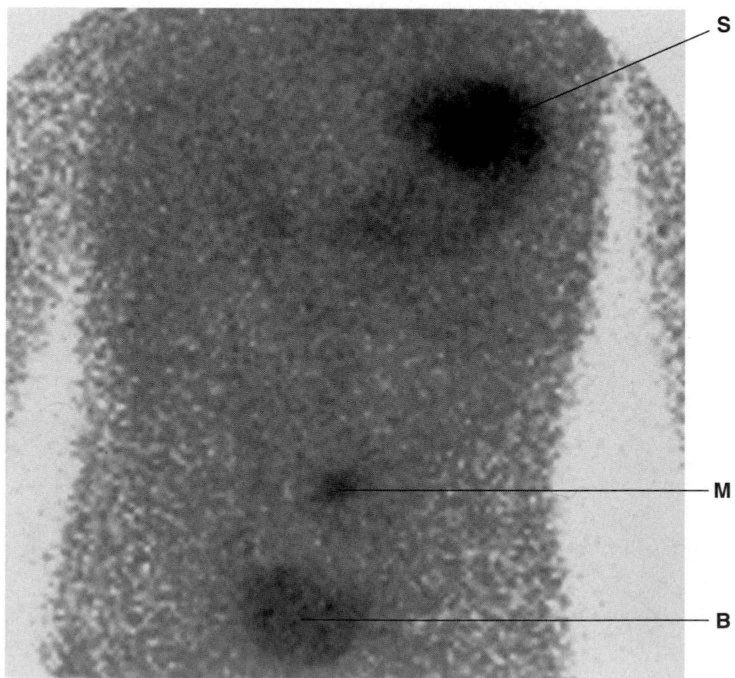

FIGURE 80-4. Technetium-99m pertechnatate scintigraphy of Meckel's diverticulum. Radionuclide signal is seen in the stomach **(S)**, bladder **(B)**, and Meckel's diverticulum **(M)**. Sensitivity of the scintigraphy can be enhanced by bladder catheterization and intravenous pentagastrin or cimetidine.

red blood cell scan or angiography may be considered, but are rarely needed in children. When no other source of gastrointestinal bleeding is identified by colonoscopy and gastroduodenoscopy, laparotomy or laparoscopy should be the next step.

Inflammation

Less commonly, Meckel's diverticula can become inflamed and result in diverticulitis that can present in a fashion similar to appendicitis. Like the appendix, the Meckel's diverticulum may become inflamed when the lumen is obstructed, resulting in increased pressure with decreased mural perfusion, tissue acidosis, and bacterial invasion of the wall. This can lead to progressive inflammation with tissue gangrene and perforation. The role of ectopic mucosa in this process is suggested by its high incidence in resected inflamed diverticula. It is possible that the gastric or pancreatic mucosa contributes to the luminal obstruction or that the gastric mucosa may lead to ileal mucosal ulceration first, which facilitates the bacterial invasion.

The symptoms of Meckel's diverticulitis are much like those of appendicitis. With both developing from the same dermatome, the symptoms begin with poorly localized periumbilical pain. Because the omphalomesenteric remnants are variable in their location and may be unattached to the umbilicus, the progressive inflammation of the Meckel's diverticulum may cause peritoneal irritation anywhere in the lower abdomen. Right lower quadrant or lower midline are the most common locations for the pain, owing to the distal ileal location of most Meckel's diverticula. As a result, patients with Meckel's diverticulitis are usually assumed to have appendicitis when taken to the operating room. Perforation of Meckel's diverticulum is potentially more serious than perforated appendicitis because it is more difficult to wall off due to its more mobile position. This may explain why perforated diverticulitis is more likely to result in diffuse peritonitis and pneumoperitoneum detectable on abdominal radiographs. For this reason, it is imperative to search carefully for other causes of peritonitis when a noninflamed appendix is discovered at the time of appendectomy.

Umbilical Drainage

Anomalies of the omphalomesenteric duct can also result in umbilical drainage. The quantity and character of the drainage may indicate the origin of the lesion. Clear or yellowish drainage signifies a probable urachal anomaly, whereas an omphalomesenteric duct remnant is manifest as feculent drainage. The most common umbilical lesion is probably an umbilical granuloma. This lesion may secrete a mucoid material that can be misleading by suggesting an intraabdominal communication. If the drainage persists despite cauterization of the presumed granuloma with silver nitrate or if the drainage is copious, catheterization of the lesion and injection with water-soluble contrast will allow radiographic assessment. If the contrast study demonstrates communication with the bladder or gastrointestinal tract, resection is necessary because the omphalomesenteric duct remnants that connect the ileum to the umbilicus can become the focal point of obstruction if not removed.

Treatment

Surgical resection of omphalomesenteric duct remnants must be preceded by volume resuscitation for all symptomatic patients, including blood transfusion for those who have hemorrhaged significantly. With the exception of those patients with intestinal obstruction and possible intestinal ischemia, laparotomy can be delayed until after the hematocrit is restored to near normal levels. Patients with obstructive symptoms should be resuscitated as rapidly as possible so relief of the obstruction can be expedited in order to obviate the need for ischemic bowel resection.

The incision chosen varies with the symptoms and the age of the patient. Infants with feculent umbilical drainage or a "ram's horn," indicating prolapse of the omphalomesenteric duct remnant, can be explored via a relatively small infraumbilical incision. Children with Meckel's diverticulitis are most often operated on via a Rockey Davis appendectomy incision, which may require medial extension to perform a resection of the involved ileum. A similar right lower quadrant incision works well for resection of a bleeding Meckel's diverticulum with ectopic mucosa. The patients with suspected intestinal obstruction should be explored via a generous transverse laparotomy incision to optimize exposure for intestinal decompression and resection of the necrotic sections of bowel in as rapid a fashion as possible.

When possible, omphalomesenteric duct anomalies can be resected without requiring removal of the ileum to which it is attached. Some surgeons use linear staplers applied to the base of the anomaly allowing complete amputation of the lesion without narrowing the lumen of the ileum. A V-shaped incision at the base of the remnant results in a defect of the antimesenteric wall of the ileum that can usually be closed in a transverse orientation to avoid a stenosis. This can be difficult when a large focus of ectopic mucosa or a resultant ulceration is present near the base of the diverticulum, or when the lesion has a very wide base. In those instances, a resection of the involved portion of ileum is required with an end-to-end anastomosis. Obstructing lesions such as an omphalomesenteric band should be excised, and the involved bowel can be salvaged. Unfortunately, the difficulty of promptly making the correct diagnosis often results in irreversibly ischemic intestine, which must be resected. In the absence of severe peritoneal soiling or hemodynamic instability, continuity of the small bowel can be safely restored. Meckel's diverticulitis, even in the face of perforation, can usually be managed by resection and primary anastomosis as well. The use of laparoscopy for resection of Meckel's diverticula has been described by several authors.

Incidental Finding

Controversy exists about what should be done when Meckel's diverticulum is encountered during a laparotomy for unrelated symptoms. The debate focuses on the probability of an omphaloileal diverticulum becoming symptomatic in the future contrasted with the complications associated with resection (25). Some generalizations may be helpful in making that intraoperative judgment. Lesions with palpable ectopic mucosa, a prominent vitelline artery or fibrous vitelline artery remnant, evidence of inflammation, or a narrow base may all be more prone to cause bleeding, obstruction, or diverticulitis, respectively, and should therefore be resected when discovered (24). It is also prudent to resect diverticula discovered in patients who present with abdominal pain. Any lesions with attachments to the umbilicus should be detached to prevent distal ileal volvulus. Because omphalomesenteric anomalies can become symptomatic at any age, the age of the patient at the time of laparotomy should not be a factor in the decision to resect the asymptomatic lesion. If the lesion is not resected, it is imperative to alert the patient's family and primary care physician about the presence of the lesion and its possible symptoms.

REFERENCES

1. McVay CB. Abdominal cavity and its contents. In: McVay CB, ed. *Surgical anatomy.* Philadelphia: WB Saunders, 1984:700–707.
2. Addiss DG, Shaffer N, Fowler BS, et al. The epidemiology of appendicitis and appendectomy in the United States. *Am J Epdidemiol* 1990;132:910–925.
3. Newman K, Ponsky T, Kittle K, et al. Appendicitis 2000: variability in practice, outcomes, and resource utilization at thirty pediatric hospitals. *J Pediatr Surg* 2003;38:372–379.
4. Braveman P, Schaaf VM, Egerter S, et al. Insurance related differences in the risk of ruptured appendicitis. *N Engl J Med* 1994; 331(7):444–449.
5. Jones BA, Demetriades D, Segal I, et al. The prevalence of appendiceal fecaliths in patients with and without appendicitis. A comparative study from Canada and South Africa. *Ann Sur* 1985;202(1):80–82.
6. Brender JD, Marcuse EK, Koepsell TD, et al. Childhood appendicitis: factors associated with perforation. *Pediatrics* 1985;76(2):301–306.
7. Samuel M, Hosie G, Holmes K. Prospective evaluation of nonsurgical versus surgical management of appendiceal mass. *J Pediatr Surg* 2002;37:882–886.
8. Gorenstin A, Serour F, Katz R, et al. Appendiceal colic in children: a true entity? *J Am Coll Surg* 1996;182:246–250.
9. Hoffmann J, Rasmussen OO. Aids in the diagnosis of acute appendicitis. *Br J Surg* 1989;76:774–779.
10. Lee JH, Jeong YK, Hwang JC, et al. Graded compression sonography with adjuvant use of a posterior manual compression technique in the sonographic diagnosis of acute appendicitis. *AJR* 2002;178(4):863–868.
11. Flum DR, Morris A, Koepsell T, et al. Has misdiagnosis of appendicitis decreased over time? A population-based analysis [see comment]. *JAMA* 2001;286(14):1748–1753.
12. Lund DP, Murphy EP. Management of perforated appendicitis in children: a decade of aggressive treatment. *J Pediatr Surg* 1994;29(8): 1130–1134.
13. Curran TJ, Muenchow SK. The treatment of complicated appendicitis in children using peritoneal drainage: results from a public hospital. *J Pediatr Surg* 1993;28(2):204–208.
14. Neilson IR, Laberge JM, Nguyen LT, et al. Appendicitis in children: current therapeutic recommendations. *J Pediatr Surg* 1990;25(11): 1113–1116.
15. Karp MP, Caldarola VA, Cooney DR, et al. The avoidable excesses in the management of perforated appendicitis in children. *J Pediatr Surg* 1986;21(6):506–510.
16. Sauerland S, Lefering R, Neugebauer EA. Laparoscopic versus open surgery for suspected appendicitis. *Cochrane Database Sys Rev* 2002;(1):CD001546.
17. Little DC, Custer MD, May BH, et al. Laparoscopic appendectomy: an unnecessary and expensive procedure in children? *J Pediatr Surg* 2002;37:310–317.
18. Lau WY, Fan ST, Yiu TF, et al. Negative findings at appendectomy. *Am J Surg* 1984;148(3):375–378.
19. Puri P, McGuinness EP, Guiney EJ. Fertility following perforated appendicitis in girls. *J Pediatr Surg* 1989;24(6):547–549.
20. Prommegger R, Obrist P, Ensinger C, et al. Retrospective evaluation of carcinoid tumors of the appendix in children. *World J Surg* 2002;26:1489–1492.
21. Sumfest JM, Burns MW, Mitchell ME. The Mitrofanoff principle in urinary reconstruction. *J Urol* 1993;150(6):1875–1877.
22. Vane DW, West K, Grosfeld JL. Vitelline duct anomalies: experience with 217 childhood cases. *Arch Surg* 1987;122:542–547.
23. St-Vil D, Brandt ML, Panic S, et al. Meckel's diverticulum in children: a 20 year review. *J Pediatr Surg* 1991;26(11):1289–1292.
24. Ludtke FE, Mende V, Kohler H, et al. Incidence and frequency of complications and management of Meckel's diverticulum. *Surg Gynecol Obstet* 1989;169:537–542.
25. Soltero JH, Bill AH. The natural history of Meckel's diverticulum and its relation to incidental removal. *Am J Surg* 1976;32:168–173.
26. Pantongrag-Brown L, Levine MS, Elsayed AM, et al. Inverted Meckel diverticulum: clinical, radiologic, and pathologic findings. *Radiology* 1996;199:693–696.
27. Daneman A, Lobo E, Alton DJ, et al. The value of sonography, CT and air enema for detection of complicated Meckel diverticulum in children with nonspecific clinical presentation. *Pediatr Radiol* 1998;28:928–932.

Chapter 81

Malrotation

Paul T. Stockmann

Malrotation is the term used to define the group of congenital anomalies resulting from aberrant intestinal rotation and fixation that occurs during the first 3 months of gestation. In 1932 and 1937, William Ladd reported a series of surgically treated infants with congenital duodenal obstruction, including malrotation (1,2). His operation, the Ladd procedure, included unrotating the midgut volvulus, mobilization of the duodenum and right colon by division of the congenital adhesive bands, and placement of the colon in the left side of the abdomen. This operation remains the standard treatment for this malformation.

"Bilious emesis in a newborn is a surgical emergency until proven otherwise" is a classic axiom in pediatric surgery. Due to the risk for significant adverse outcome, malrotation should be the first consideration in the differential diagnosis. The anomalies of intestinal rotation and fixation consist of a spectrum of anatomic defects with a wide range of clinical findings. Patients can be entirely asymptomatic or may be extremely ill, with an acute midgut volvulus and impending intestinal necrosis or death. Although patients may present at any age, most of these anomalies become apparent clinically during infancy and early childhood. Prompt recognition and treatment should result in a satisfactory outcome with low morbidity and mortality in the majority of cases. Conversely, diagnostic or therapeutic delay can result in death or permanent disability such as short bowel syndrome.

The true incidence of the malrotation variants is not known, but symptomatic lesions have an incidence of approximately 1 in 6,000 live births. Nonrotation, a common form of malrotation, has been noted in 0.5% of large autopsy series and in 0.2% of gastrointestinal (GI) contrast studies. Incomplete rotation is the most common form leading to early (i.e., neonatal) symptomatic disease and surgery, and nonrotation is the more common variant seen in asymptomatic cases. For surgically treated cases, 70% to 80% are classified as incomplete rotation, and 10% to 20% are nonrotation. Malrotation is more common in males than in females. It is estimated that this anomaly is the cause of 6% of all neonatal intestinal obstructions (3–5).

Paul T. Stockmann: Wayne State University, Children's Hospital of Michigan, Detroit, Michigan 48201.

EMBRYOLOGY

An understanding of the embryology of the intestinal tract in the first 3 months of fetal life is necessary to accurately identify and adequately treat the various types of malrotation (8). In the third week of gestation, the primitive alimentary tract is a simple tube lined with endoderm. It is divided into three distinct regions. The foregut is located within the headfold, and the hindgut is located within the tailfold. The midgut is the portion of bowel in between and is that part of the primitive GI tract that will herniate into the umbilical cord. This portion is supplied by the superior mesenteric artery (SMA) and will give rise to the alimentary tract extending from the duodenum to the transverse colon. The intestine returns into the abdomen by the twelfth week of gestation. Subsequently, a specific sequence of events occurs allowing rotation and fixation of the intestine and leading to the final position of the small and large bowel in postnatal life. Malrotation occurs when this dynamic sequence is incomplete or altered. This process is separated into three stages: herniation, return to the abdomen, and fixation.

Herniation

The midgut herniates into the yolk sac during the fifth week of gestation, led by the vitelline or omphalomesenteric duct at the apex. The SMA and its branches are centered within the primary loop and represent the axis for rotation. The proximal midgut is designated the duodenojejunal or prearterial limb, and the distal portion as the cecocolic or postarterial limb (Fig. 81-1A). The imaginary line of demarcation connects the omphalomesenteric duct and the origin of the SMA. Disproportionate growth and

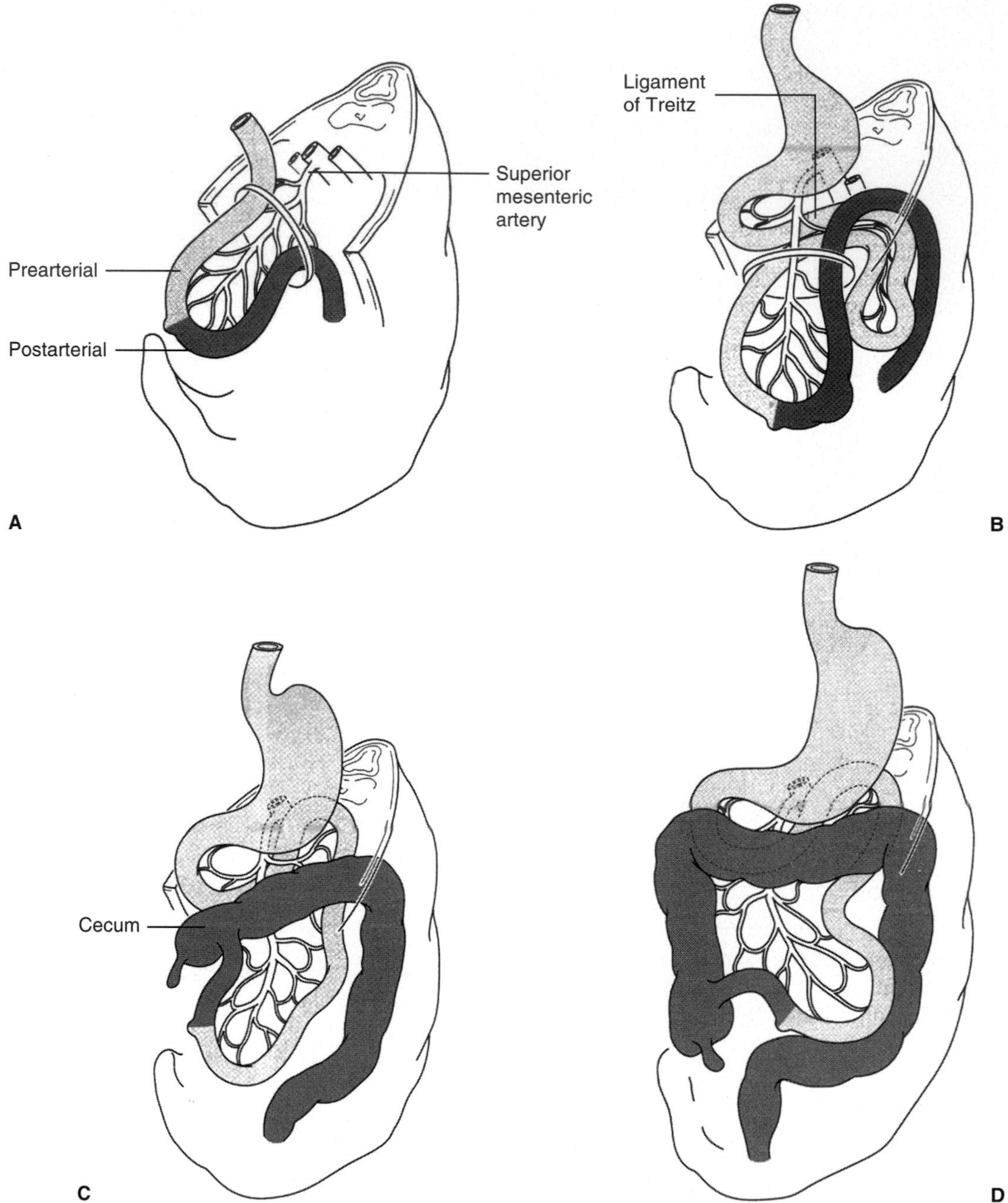

FIGURE 81-1. Normal midgut development, gestational week five through twelve (see text). **(A)** Fifth week: Midgut herniation into the umbilical cord. Superior mesenteric artery (SMA) is centered within the mesentery. **(B)** Tenth week: Duodenojejunal segment has rotated 270 degrees and posterior to the SMA and returned to the abdominal cavity. **(C)** Twelfth week: Entire midgut has returned to the abdominal cavity. Cecocolic segment (*dark shade*) completes counterclockwise rotation around and anterior to the SMA. **(D)** Complete rotation and fixation of midgut. The cecum is fixed in the iliac fossa, and the duodenojejunal junction is fixed in the left upper quadrant. (From Oldham KT. Pediatric abdomen. In: Greenfield LJ, Mullholland M, Oldham KT, et al., eds. *Surgery: scientific principles and practice*. Philadelphia: Lippincott, 1993, with permission.)

elongation of the duodenojejunal segment occurs with an initial 180-degree counterclockwise rotation of the limb to the right of the SMA (Fig. 81-1B). The proximal portion of the duodenojejunal limb will eventually rotate 270 degrees to become fixed in the retroperitoneum posterior and to the left of the SMA. The prearterial limb will ultimately give rise to the duodenum, the jejunum, and the majority of the ileum (Fig. 81-1C). The cecocolic segment undergoes reciprocal 180-degree counterclockwise rotation of the limb to the left of the SMA. The ileocecal junction, located within the postarterial limb, will eventually rotate 270 degrees (Fig. 81-1D), moving anterior to the SMA and descending into the retroperitoneal position in the right iliac fossa. The cecocolic limb will ultimately give rise to the terminal ileum, cecum, and right and proximal transverse colon.

Return to the Abdomen

The herniated midgut returns to the abdominal cavity between the tenth and twelfth week of gestation. Most of the important rotational anomalies are believed to occur due to altered or arrested development in this stage. The first segment to return to the abdomen is the duodenojejunal limb. During this process, the final 90 degrees of rotation occur to complete the 270-degree counterclockwise rotation around the SMA. The final configuration places the third portion of the duodenum posterior to the SMA and the ligament of Treitz in the left upper quadrant. The distal cecocolic limb returns next and also completes the terminal 90 degrees of the 270-degree rotation. The cecum and terminal ileum are the last portions of the midgut to return to the abdominal cavity. As a result, the transverse colon lies anterior to the SMA and the cecum is positioned in the right lower quadrant at level of the iliac fossa (Fig. 81-1E).

Fixation

The final stage in the process of development of the midgut is fixation of the duodenojejunal junction in the left upper quadrant and the ileocecal junction in the right lower quadrant. This process begins during the twelfth week of gestation and continues until after birth. Normal fixation can occur only if midgut rotation has been completed appropriately. The majority of the duodenum, as well as the ascending and descending colon, become fixed to the retroperitoneum. The jejunum, ileum, and transverse colon remain the mobile, intraperitoneal portions of the midgut. With normal intestinal rotation and fixation, the root of the mesentery of the small intestine stretches from two fixed, retroperitoneal structures—the ligament of Treitz in the left upper abdomen and the cecum in the right lower quadrant (Fig. 81-2). The normal, broad-based small bowel mesentery is not at risk to undergo axial rotation and form a midgut volvulus. Aberrant intestinal rotation and fixation produce anatomic variations prone to intestinal obstruction. Inadequate rotation and fixation result in the formation of an abnormal small bowel mesentery: The proximal and distal midgut may be fused together with a common mesentery encircling the SMA. This narrowed, mobile mesenteric pedicle is prone to clockwise rotation around the axis of the SMA, with subsequent compression and obstruction of both the intestinal tract and the mesenteric vessels. The end result can be an acute closed-loop intestinal obstruction with vascular occlusion. These anomalies are also known to cause extrinsic compression and obstruction of the duodenum secondary to anomalous peritoneal (Ladd's) bands. The bands extend from the retroperitoneum in the right upper quadrant and attach to the right colon, thus compressing the underlying duodenum.

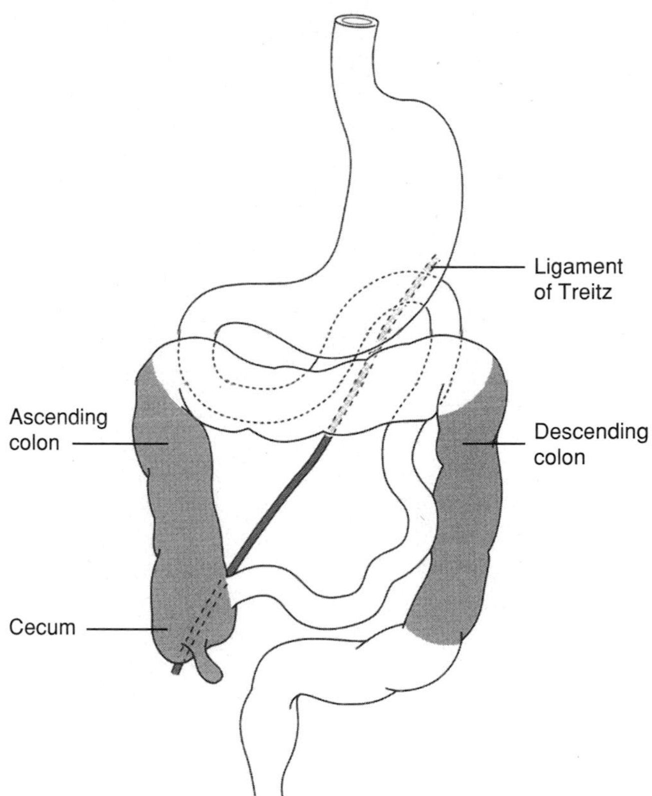

FIGURE 81-2. Normal midgut rotation and fixation. The broad mesenteric fixation extends obliquely from the ligament of Treitz to the cecum. The ascending and descending colon are fixed in the retroperitoneum (*shaded areas*). (From Oldham KT. Pediatric abdomen. In: Greenfield LJ, Mullholland M, Oldham KT, et al., eds. *Surgery: scientific principles and practice*. Philadelphia: Lippincott, 1993, with permission.)

CLASSIFICATION

Malrotation represents a spectrum of anomalies of intestinal rotation and fixation. The most common and clinically significant abnormalities include nonrotation and incomplete rotation. Less common and more variable malformations include mixed rotational and fixation anomalies, as well as mesocolic hernias.

Nonrotation

Nonrotation occurs as the result of failure of counterclockwise rotation of the midgut loop around the SMA. The duodenojejunal and cecocolic limbs undergo less than 90 degrees of counterclockwise rotation, and the cecocolic limb returns to the abdomen first instead of last. The duodenum does not rotate posterior to the SMA, and the ligament of Treitz fails to reach its normal position in the left upper quadrant. As a result, the colon resides in the left side of the abdomen with the cecum at or near the midline, and the small intestine rests in the right side of the abdomen (Fig. 81-3A). The duodenum can be compressed in the right upper quadrant by abnormal peritoneal bands. In addition, the normal C-shaped configuration is lost, and the duodenum may have a tortuous course along the right side of the abdomen. Portions of the duodenum and proximal jejunum are often fused to the ascending colon by anomalous peritoneal attachments. The midgut mesentery is narrow and highly mobile.

Patients with nonrotation have the anatomic risk factors for the development of acute midgut volvulus and extrinsic duodenal obstruction. Nonrotation is a common form of malrotation, reported to occur in approximately 0.5% of autopsies and in 0.2% of GI contrast studies (5). It is about twice as frequent in males as in females, and is commonly associated with both abdominal wall defects and diaphragmatic hernias. Affected individuals may be asymptomatic; others can present with symptomatic anomalies at any age, but most become evident in early childhood. Nonrotation is less commonly associated with obstruction and volvulus than incomplete rotation.

Incomplete Rotation

This variation of malrotation occurs as the result of partial rotation of the cecocolic and duodenojejunal limbs around the SMA. The counterclockwise rotation occurs only to approximately 180 degrees rather than the normal 270-degree rotation arc. As a result, there is abnormal positioning of the proximal small bowel and the cecum (Fig. 81-3B). The cecum and the first part of the ascending colon are located in the epigastrium against the third portion of the duodenum and override the superior mesenteric vessels. The configuration of the duodenum is abnormal, with the ligament of Treitz displaced inferiorly, to the right of the midline, and anterior to its normal position in the left upper quadrant. Retroperitoneal bands originating from the right upper quadrant to the cecum and ascending colon can compress the second portion of the duodenum. Incomplete rotation is a common variant of malrotation. The majority of patients present with symptomatic lesions during infancy. Incomplete rotation is the most common form of malrotation treated surgically.

The distinction between nonrotation and incomplete rotation is primarily arbitrary and based on the extent of inadequate midgut rotation and fixation rather than distinct pathologic entities. Approximately 90% of patients with symptomatic malrotation will have either nonrotation or incomplete rotation.

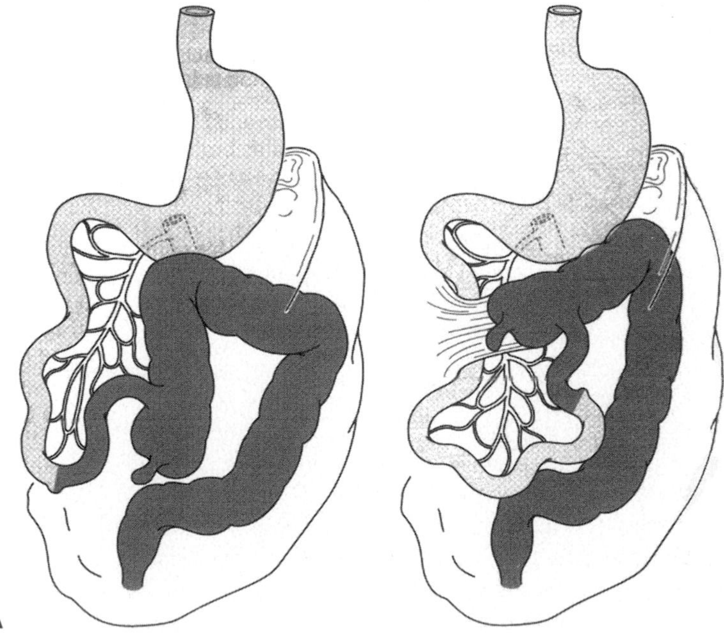

FIGURE 81-3. Malrotation: nonrotation and incomplete rotation. **(A)** Nonrotation: The duodenojejunal segment (*lightly shaded*) lies on the right side, and the cecocolic segments (*dark shaded*) lie on the left side of the abdomen. **(B)** Incomplete rotation: Partial rotation of both midgut segments with angulation and malposition of the duodenojejunal junction. Peritoneal (Ladd's) bands are adherent to the retroperitoneum, cecum, and duodenum, causing compression of the duodenum. (From Oldham KT. Pediatric abdomen. In: Greenfield LJ, Mullholland M, Oldham KT, et al., eds. *Surgery: scientific principles and practice*. Philadelphia; Lippincott: 1993, with permission.)

Mixed Rotational and Fixation Anomalies

The mixed anomalies are less common than nonrotation and incomplete rotation, and the anatomic variations are more diverse. These malformations result from arrested or aberrant rotation, or fixation of either the duodenojejunal limb or the cecocolic limb, or both. These anomalies also have a wide range of clinical presentations. Patients may be asymptomatic with trivial defects or develop intestinal obstruction resulting from a volvulus or extrinsic compression.

Reverse rotation is one type of mixed rotational anomaly (3). In this rare variant, midgut rotation occurs in a clockwise rather than a counterclockwise direction around the SMA axis so the duodenojejunal loop ultimately resides anterior rather than posterior to the SMA. If the cecocolic limb also undergoes reverse rotation, the transverse colon lies posterior to the SMA. Therefore, the anatomic arrangement is exactly reversed from normal. That is, the third portion of the duodenum is anterior to the SMA, which is anterior to the transverse colon. The clinical presentation is that of intestinal obstruction resulting from extrinsic compression of the transverse colon by the overriding superior mesenteric vessels or an ileocecal volvulus caused by inadequate fixation of the right colon. If reverse rotation of the duodenojejunal limb occurs in association with normal clockwise rotation of the cecocolic limb, a right mesocolic hernia will result. The hernia sac is formed by the mesentery of the right colon as it rotates to the right lower quadrant.

Another mixed anomaly occurs with incomplete rotation of the duodenojejunal limb, and normal rotation and fixation of the cecocolic limb. The ligament of Treitz is abnormally positioned inferiorly and to the right of the midline. The midgut mesentery is narrowed even though the ileocecal junction is fixed in the normal location in the right lower quadrant. Ladd's bands may be present and cause partial obstruction of the duodenum. These anomalies have a variable clinical presentation ranging from no symptoms to duodenal obstruction. The small bowel mesentery is somewhat narrow, but the risk of a volvulus is fairly low.

Another variation includes normal rotation and fixation of the duodenojejunal limb with nonrotation of the cecocolic limb, resulting in a malpositioned cecum in the epigastrium with Ladd's bands extending across the second portion of the duodenum. In this instance, the mesenteric pedicle is narrowed with the cecum and terminal ileum adjacent to the proximal jejunum. Therefore, patients with this malformation are at risk for a midgut volvulus.

Mesocolic Hernias

Mesocolic or paraduodenal hernias are another rare anomaly associated with abnormal development and fixation of the right or left mesocolon. Normally, the ascending and descending colons are fixed to the retroperitoneum. In mesocolic hernias, abnormalities in rotation and fixation lead to the development of potential spaces formed between the mesocolon and the retroperitoneum.

Right mesocolic hernias occur as a result of nonrotation (or reverse rotation) of the duodenojejunal segment combined with incomplete rotation and fixation of the cecocolic segment. The cecum has attachments to the retroperitoneum in the right upper quadrant, and the incompletely rotated small intestine becomes trapped within a hernia sac formed from the right mesocolon. The ligament of Treitz is absent, and the small bowel resides on the right side of the abdomen, posterior to the cecum and right colon.

A left mesocolic hernia occurs when the duodenojejunal segment rotates posterior and to the left of the SMA, but then invaginates into the left mesocolon posterior to the inferior mesenteric vein and into the retroperitoneum. The cecocolic segment rotates normally and becomes fixed in the retroperitoneum. The small bowel becomes trapped within a sac formed by the left mesocolon with the inferior mesenteric vein forming the anterior aspect of the neck of the sac. All mesocolic hernias are true internal hernias that can cause incarceration, obstruction, and strangulation of the intestine.

ASSOCIATED ANOMALIES

Rotational anomalies are associated with many other congenital malformations. Nonrotation is present in nearly all cases of congenital diaphragmatic hernia, gastroschisis, and omphalocele. In addition, 30% to 60% of patients with malrotation have other anomalies or conditions (6–10). The malformations involve the GI tract (50%), central nervous system (12%), cardiac (12%), respiratory (12%), and genitourinary (6%) systems. Atresia of the small bowel has an association with malrotation. In some cases, the cause of the atresia may be due to malrotation with antenatal midgut volvulus and intestinal ischemia, infarction, and resorption.

Other anomalies reported with malrotation include Meckel's diverticulum, duodenal web or stenosis, Hirschsprung's disease, imperforate anus, esophageal atresia with tracheoesophageal fistula, congenital short gut, biliary atresia, prune belly and megacystis-microcolon syndrome, cardiac anomalies, situs inversus, mesenteric cyst, pyloric stenosis, intussusception, and abnormalities of the biliary tree (11–16). A genetic basis has been proposed for a familial form of malrotation (17).

CLINICAL MANIFESTATIONS

Patients with malrotation may have one of several clinical presentations. The range includes the asymptomatic adult to the critically ill newborn with an abdominal catastrophe. Typical presentations involve newborns and infants with acute intestinal obstruction secondary to midgut volvulus or duodenal compression. Atypical presentations include older individuals with chronic or intermittent symptoms and less specific findings. Malrotation may be discovered incidentally during radiographic studies or operative exploration.

Approximately 66% of patients with malrotation become symptomatic during the first month of life, and nearly 90% present within the first year of life. Symptoms usually result from duodenal obstruction. The duodenum is the point of obstruction, and acute midgut volvulus with intestinal ischemia is the most significant and potentially life-threatening complication of malrotation. Although the majority of patients with acute midgut volvulus present within the first year of life, patients with malrotation are at risk to develop a volvulus at any age. Partial or complete duodenal obstruction also occurs from extrinsic compression from abnormal peritoneal (Ladd's) bands.

Atypical presentations are more common in older children and adults. The symptoms are more chronic and intermittent and result from partial or intermittent duodenal obstruction or a chronic midgut volvulus. These include abdominal pain and vomiting associated with weight loss or failure to thrive, and other nonspecific GI complaints (11,12).

Midgut Volvulus

Acute midgut volvulus is a true surgical emergency. Torsion of the narrow mesenteric pedicle produces an acute closed-loop intestinal obstruction and vascular insufficiency. Intestinal ischemia and necrosis may proceed rapidly unless treated promptly. Midgut volvulus is present in up to 50% of patients operated on for malrotation (7,9,11). The presentation of midgut volvulus commonly begins with the sudden onset of bilious vomiting in a previously healthy newborn. Bilious emesis is the cardinal feature of neonatal intestinal obstruction, and mandates urgent evaluation to exclude malrotation with volvulus. Although bilious vomiting may be due to nonsurgical disorders such as sepsis, intracranial hemorrhage, and electrolyte abnormalities, malrotation must be rapidly excluded from the differential diagnosis in order to prevent significant morbidity and mortality. Occult or gross blood in the stool may be due to intestinal ischemia and mucosal injury. Initially, the abdomen is nondistended, but persistent intestinal obstruction and vascular insufficiency leads to abdominal distention and tenderness with lethargy and other signs of shock. Abdominal radiographs initially may not be diagnostic. A high index of suspicion is important because the complications of vascular compromise can advance rapidly. Transmural intestinal necrosis and sepsis occur with hypotension, metabolic acidosis, respiratory and renal failure, and thrombocytopenia, all consistent with the abdominal catastrophe. If the history and physical findings are highly suspicious for acute midgut volvulus, urgent operative intervention is indicated without confirmatory radiographic studies. This is justified due to the disastrous consequences related to delayed treatment of this potentially correctable process.

A midgut volvulus may have an atypical presentation, primarily in older patients. The volvulus may be intermittent or incomplete and chronic. Common clinical findings include chronic abdominal pain, intermittent vomiting, weight loss, failure to thrive, malabsorption, and diarrhea (11,12). Vomiting is either bilious or nonbilious. Chronic volvulus causes partial vascular obstruction, resulting in mucosal malabsorption, protein loss, ischemia, or hemorrhage. Physical findings may be completely unremarkable, but blood in the stool may be detected. The diagnosis is confirmed radiographically by an upper GI series.

Duodenal Obstruction

Patients with malrotation more commonly present with duodenal obstruction in the absence of a midgut volvulus. Duodenal obstruction may be partial or complete, and manifested by bilious vomiting in an otherwise healthy child. The obstruction is due to either extramural compression of the duodenum by Ladd's bands, or caused by intrinsic kinking of the duodenum due to an irregular, tortuous course on the right side of the abdomen. The majority of patients present within the first year of life. In the absence of an associated midgut volvulus, the abdomen is usually neither distended nor tender. An intrinsic lesion, such as duodenal stenosis or atresia, is found in 6% to 12% of patients undergoing a laparotomy for malrotation (8,9). The search for, and correction of, an intrinsic duodenal obstruction is an essential component of the surgical management of malrotation. Patients lacking clinical evidence of acute midgut volvulus should undergo an urgent upper GI series. If midgut volvulus is diagnosed radiographically by evidence of duodenal obstruction with beaking, surgical treatment should proceed without delay. If malrotation is identified without evidence of volvulus, the child can be kept hydrated and operated on promptly, but not necessarily emergently.

Chronic partial duodenal obstruction can present at any age, but is most common in infants and young children (11). It may occur in association with intermittent or chronic volvulus or due to duodenal obstruction alone. Recurrent vomiting, frequently bilious, is characteristic. Intermittent, colicky abdominal pain and failure to thrive are common findings. Some patients may have evidence of early satiety due to the partial duodenal obstruction. Diarrhea and malabsorption occur if a concurrent volvulus is present. An upper GI series is diagnostic, and surgical correction is indicated. Malrotation may be discovered as an incidental finding during an operative procedure or a radiographic study for an unrelated problem. Asymptomatic patients with malrotation are at risk of developing acute midgut volvulus at any age (20). The complications associated with malrotation are based on anatomic factors that do not change with age.

Although midgut volvulus occurs most commonly in infants, catastrophic complications cannot be predicted based on age or clinical presentation. Patients identified to have rotational anomalies with high risk for midgut volvulus should undergo operative correction. The risk of significant morbidity and mortality for an elective Ladd procedure is very low, such that the benefits clearly exceed the risks for surgical therapy in these patients. Although most pediatric surgeons recommend surgical treatment for asymptomatic malrotation (9,11–13,19,21), some authors believe operative correction is necessary only in young children (22–24).

Malrotation occurs with virtually all abdominal wall defects (omphalocele and gastroschisis) and diaphragmatic hernia. Nonrotation is the most common variant. Most patients do not manifest extrinsic or intrinsic duodenal obstruction. Peritoneal adhesion formation following repair of the abdominal wall defect or diaphragmatic hernia is usually sufficient to prevent midgut volvulus (19).

DIAGNOSIS

The diagnosis of malrotation is based on clinical findings and radiographic studies. Prompt evaluation and surgical treatment is paramount for a satisfactory outcome. In the absence of strong clinical findings for midgut volvulus, the diagnosis is made preoperatively using plain and GI contrast radiographic studies.

Evaluation of an infant with bilious vomiting and suspected intestinal obstruction begins with plain abdominal radiographs. An obstructive series, including a supine and upright, or decubitus films are obtained. The definitive diagnosis of malrotation cannot be made on the basis of plain radiographs alone. These patients often have nonspecific findings on abdominal plain films that range from a normal bowel gas pattern to a complete small bowel obstruction with multiple dilated loops of bowel with air–fluid levels. Other findings associated with malrotation include gastric and proximal duodenal dilatation with a paucity of gas in the small intestine. Approximately 20% of patients will have a "double bubble" sign signifying duodenal obstruction. A "double bubble" sign with an absence of intestinal air beyond the duodenum indicates complete duodenal obstruction and may be seen with duodenal atresia. In this circumstance, no other imaging study is necessary, and surgery is indicated without further radiographic studies. Air noted in the distal intestine indicates partial duodenal obstruction and is more consistent with malrotation. Another important finding on plain films is a nearly gasless abdomen with a central mass effect due to an acute midgut volvulus. The combination of clinical and radiographic findings of an acute intestinal obstruction in a previously healthy young infant with a tender, distended abdomen suggesting intestinal compromise provides sufficient evidence to proceed with emergent operative exploration to prevent the potentially disastrous complications of intestinal necrosis.

The radiographic procedure of choice is an upper GI contrast study (25) performed by an experienced radiologist using fluoroscopic control. Barium or another water-soluble contrast may be used. Instillation of small amounts of contrast with multiple views of the area of interest will define the anatomy accurately. The upper GI diagnosis of malrotation is made on the basis of four findings: (1) incomplete duodenal obstruction, usually in the third portion; (2) the ligament of Treitz not to the left of the midline or at the level of the gastric antrum; (3) abnormal position of the proximal jejunal loops to the right of the midline; and (4) deformity of the duodenum with a "bird's beak," "corkscrew," or "coiled" configuration (Fig. 81-4). In malrotation, the duodenojejunal junction is located on the right side of the midline below the duodenal bulb and anterior to the vertebral bodies on the lateral projections. The proximal jejunum fills with contrast in the right side of the abdomen. Delayed films show the ileocecal junction not to be in the right lower quadrant.

The barium enema has been helpful in evaluating children with rotational and fixation anomalies; however, it has several limitations when compared with an upper GI series (18,26). Approximately 15% of individuals without malrotation will have a high and mobile cecum. Although consistent with malrotation, confirmation can be established only with an accurate description of the position of the ligament of Treitz. The colon in infants is quite redundant, causing difficulty in identifying the exact position and fixation of the cecum. Most important, malrotation may occur in the presence of a normally positioned cecum (26). Therefore, cecal position alone, as demonstrated by barium enema, cannot reliably confirm or exclude the diagnosis of malrotation. Despite these limitations, nonrotation and incomplete rotation have an abnormal position of the cecum and colon, usually high in the abdomen either on the right or left side (Fig. 81-4D). The barium enema can provide supportive anatomic detail in difficult and unusual cases.

Other imaging modalities such as abdominal ultrasound and computed tomography (CT) may demonstrate anatomic features consistent with malrotation (27–30). Both studies have been used to define the abnormal anatomic relationship between the SMA and vein. Normally, the SMA lies anterior and to the left of the superior mesenteric vein. In malrotation, the SMA is located either posterior to or to the right of the superior mesenteric

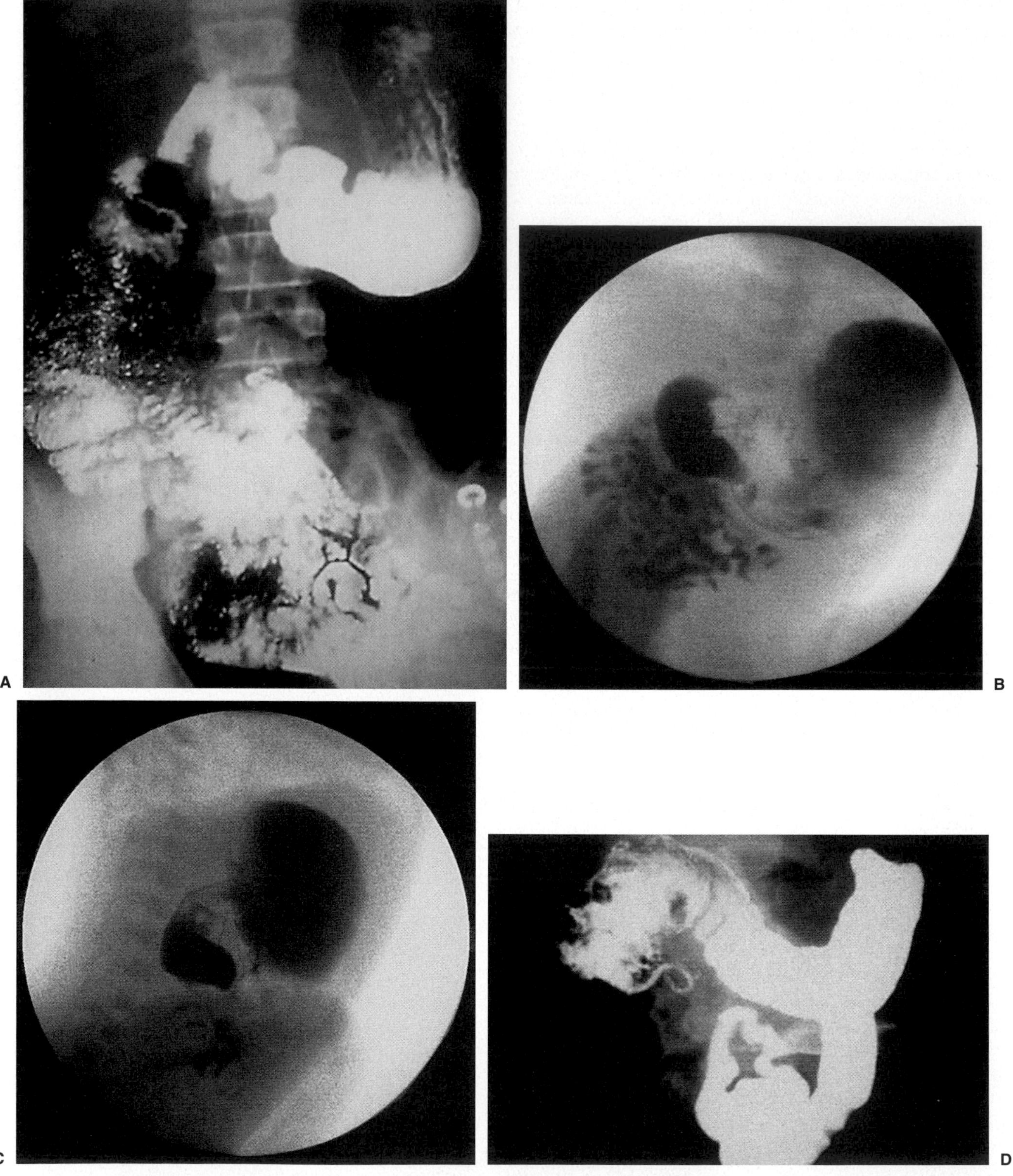

FIGURE 81-4. Malrotation: gastrointestinal contrast studies. **(A)** Upper gastrointestinal (UGI): nonrotation. Note the absence of the ligament of Treitz and the tortuous course of the malpositioned duodenum. The proximal jejunum lies on the right side. **(B, C)** UGI: incomplete rotation. Note the partial obstruction of the duodenum (third portion). The ligament of Treitz is displaced inferiorly, to the right, and anteriorly. The proximal jejunum lies on the right side. **(D)** Barium enema: incomplete rotation. Note the malpositioned cecum and ascending colon in the right upper quadrant.

vein. This reversed vascular relationship is consistent with, but not diagnostic for, malrotation. Furthermore, a normal SMA and vein relationship does not exclude malrotation. If the altered vascular relationship is demonstrated by ultrasound or CT, additional evaluation with an upper GI contrast study is necessary. Unfortunately, ultrasound has not been completely accurate with the diagnosis of malrotation based on vascular relationships. Currently, ultrasonography can provide supportive evidence in atypical cases of malrotation and during the evaluation of the vomiting child with possible pyloric stenosis.

TREATMENT

The treatment of symptomatic congenital anomalies of intestinal rotation and fixation is surgical. Neonates and young infants are at the greatest risk of developing the most catastrophic complications of malrotation—midgut volvulus with strangulation and intestinal necrosis. Avoiding errors and delays in diagnosis and treatment will prevent these potentially uncorrectable problems. The diagnosis, resuscitation, preoperative preparation, and operative management must be conducted in an orderly and expeditious manner. With acute midgut volvulus, delays of a few hours may result in irreversible intestinal necrosis (Fig. 81-5). The presence of midgut necrosis at the time of laparotomy is associated with a 50% mortality, and for those patients that survive, short bowel syndrome is a potentially permanent disability (11,31). Intestinal transplantation for short bowel syndrome is still in the developmental stage and is not considered a viable alternative for this complication.

The majority of patients with symptomatic malrotation have some degree of hypovolemia. Ideally, resuscitation begins before and during the evaluation process. This includes establishing reliable intravenous access, drawing specimens for blood products, instituting volume resuscitation, nasogastric decompression of the stomach, and Foley catheter drainage of the bladder for assessment of urinary output. Broad-spectrum antibiotic coverage is started prior to surgery. Measures should be taken to prevent hypothermia that can occur in the radiology suite and the operating room. Proper planning and communication allow for the child to be transported directly from the radiology suite to the operating room. Additional resuscitation efforts are completed in that setting.

Emergency surgical exploration is not necessary if signs of intestinal obstruction or volvulus are absent; however, an elective procedure should be carried out in a timely manner. Surgical correction is recommended for several reasons. First, the pathologic anatomy predisposes these patients to an acute midgut volvulus. Although this is most likely to occur in early infancy, patients with this anomaly are at risk of developing midgut volvulus at any age (20). Second, the diagnosis of malrotation is made by upper GI contrast studies. Because an upper GI is not commonly performed in asymptomatic patients, clearly many of these individuals have atypical symptoms resulting from the rotational anomaly. Many of these patients will benefit from

A
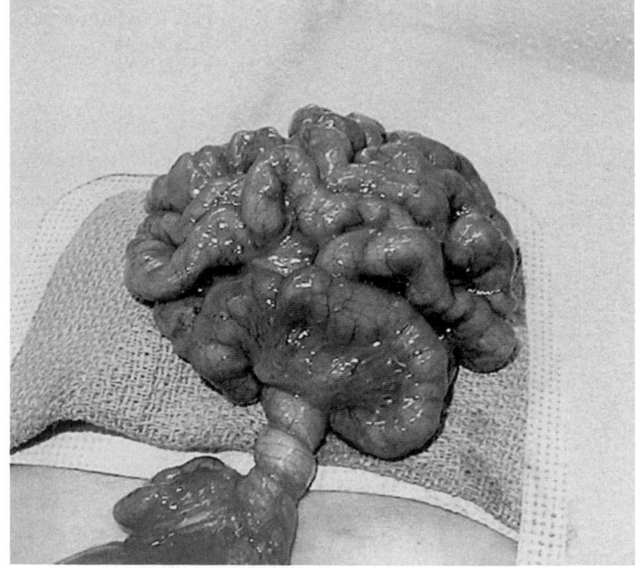
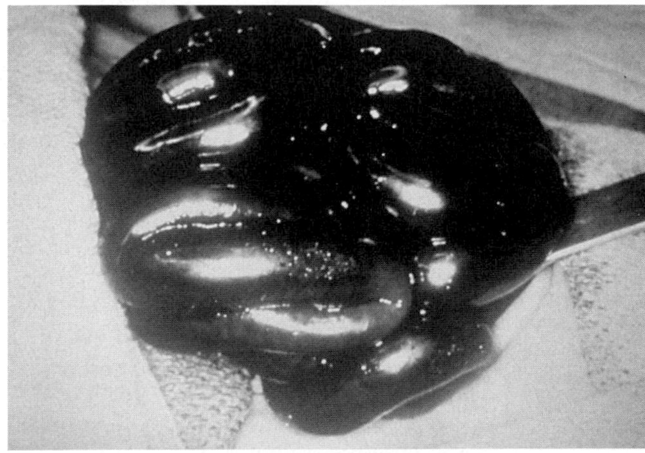
B

FIGURE 81-5. Malrotation and midgut volvulus. **(A)** Midgut volvulus without intestinal ischemia. Note the narrow mesenteric pedicle has rotated 720 degrees clockwise around the superior mesenteric artery. **(B)** Midgut volvulus with total intestinal infarction. This abdominal catastrophe is unsalvageable.

operative treatment with resolution or improvement in their abdominal symptoms. There are reports indicating that some patients with atypical and chronic symptoms do not benefit completely or substantially following correction of the malrotation. A portion of these patients have an intrinsic intestinal motility disorder (32,33). Occasionally, individuals have no apparent symptoms and the diagnosis is made during a diagnostic procedure or surgery for an unrelated problem. Surgical correction of the rotational anomaly is recommended in these cases, although some controversy still exists (19,21,22).

Patients with abdominal wall defects (gastroschisis and omphalocele) and diaphragmatic hernia deserve additional consideration. These patients usually have nonrotation without significant extrinsic duodenal compression or obstruction. Operative repair of the abdominal wall defect or diaphragmatic hernia commonly produces peritoneal adhesion formation that is usually sufficient to prevent midgut volvulus. A Ladd procedure is usually not necessary. Volvulus remains a rare possibility, and it should be considered in these patients if a postoperative intestinal obstruction occurs.

Minimally invasive surgical techniques have been used successfully to treat patients with rotational anomalies. Laparoscopic evaluation and operative correction of malrotation have been reported by several groups (34–37). A laparoscopic approach can be used for diagnostic purposes to evaluate equivocal cases of malrotation, and therapeutically to perform a Ladd procedure. Early results have been quite encouraging, with no significant postoperative complications. This technique has not been used in neonates with acute midgut volvulus. Currently, the use of laparoscopic techniques for treatment of malrotation has not achieved widespread acceptance. In centers where laparoscopic surgery is a major component of the pediatric surgical practice, laparoscopic correction of malrotation will become the treatment of choice in the near future.

OPERATIVE TECHNIQUE

The operation for correction of malrotation is referred to as the Ladd procedure (Fig. 81-6). The technique is named after Dr. William Ladd, who developed this operation in the early 20th century at the Boston Children's Hospital. The procedure consists of several important steps designed to correct the malformation and prevent recurrent obstruction or volvulus:

1. Recognition and reduction of acute midgut volvulus
2. Identification and correction of extrinsic and intrinsic duodenal obstruction

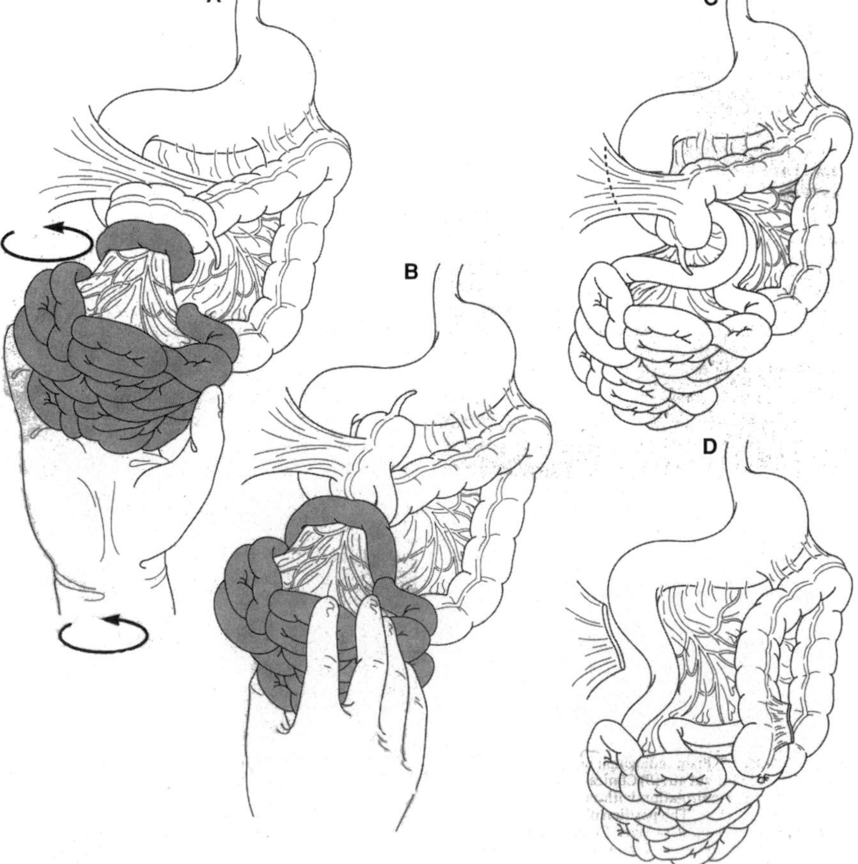

FIGURE 81-6. Ladd's procedure: operative correction of malrotation. **(A)** Evisceration and identification of the midgut volvulus and the twisted mesenteric pedicle. **(B)** Reduction of the volvulus by counterclockwise rotation of the intestinal mass. Complete reduction occurs when the duodenum (*right side*) and the cecum (*left side*) are parallel. **(C)** Identification and division of Ladd's peritoneal bands lateral to the duodenum. The duodenum is mobilized with a thorough Kocher maneuver. **(D)** Dissection and mobilization of the mesenteric pedicle. Additional peritoneal bands are divided to convert the pedicle into a wide plane. The superior mesenteric artery is visualized in the center of the mesentery. (From Oldham KT. Pediatric abdomen. In: Greenfield LJ, Mullholland M, Oldham KT, et al., eds. *Surgery: scientific principles and practice*. Philadelphia: Lippincott, 1993, with permission.)

3. Dissection and widening of the mesenteric pedicle to prevent recurrent midgut volvulus

A right upper quadrant transverse abdominal incision is preferred. The initial maneuver is rapid evisceration of the abdominal cavity to allow assessment for an acute midgut volvulus (Fig. 81-6). Adequate exposure and gentle manipulation are important. The entire midgut and root of the small bowel mesentery are quickly examined for an acute midgut volvulus, intestinal ischemia or infarction, and other anomalies such as intestinal atresia. The root of the mesentery is identified just below and behind the greater curvature of the stomach. At the root of the mesentery, the volvulus will become apparent. Initially, the colon is not easily identified because the ascending colon is wrapped around the root of the small bowel mesentery. Torsion always occurs in a clockwise rotation along the axis of the SMA.

Reduction of the volvulus is accomplished with careful rotation of the intestinal mass in a counterclockwise direction. Usually, one or two complete rotations are necessary to adequately untwist the volvulus. The root of the mesentery is examined, and reduction is complete when the duodenum and ascending colon are parallel and the duodenum is lateral to the ascending colon. Reduction of the volvulus corrects the closed-loop intestinal obstruction and vascular compromise to the midgut.

After the torsion has been reduced, the intestine is reevaluated for viability and adequacy of perfusion. This requires observation and support of the intestinal loops with warm, moist laparotomy sponges. After a waiting period of not more than 30 minutes, the effects of volvulus reduction should be apparent. Clearly necrotic intestine requires resection, whereas segments of marginal viability are preserved. Resection should be limited to small segments of intestine to preserve intestinal length as much as possible. An intestinal anastomosis or enterostomy is then performed as indicated by the gross pathologic findings. If there are large ischemic areas of questionable viability, no intestinal resection is performed, and a second-look procedure is planned within 24 to 48 hours. Overzealous excision of ischemic intestine in malrotation with midgut volvulus can lead to short bowel syndrome. Therefore, intestinal salvage techniques should be carried out whenever possible, specifically, resection of only clearly nonviable bowel with preservation of marginal tissue, diversion or closure of resected segments, and early reexploration. In some cases, a true abdominal catastrophe will be present with infarction of the entire midgut. This is an unsalvageable situation, and closure without resection is indicated. A thorough and frank discussion with the family should be carried out as soon as possible, and recommendations generally include comfort care measures only.

Following reduction of the midgut volvulus, the next step is the management of extrinsic duodenal obstruction. In most cases of malrotation, Ladd's peritoneal bands will be present. These bands produce extrinsic compression and distortion of the duodenum. These congenital adhesions are the retroperitoneal attachments of the cecum and the right colon that are normally present along the right paracolic gutter. With incomplete rotation and descent of the cecum and right colon, these bands extend from the right upper retroperitoneum over the duodenum to the right colon. Ladd's bands must be identified and carefully and completely divided to free the duodenum trapped underneath.

The initial step is to identify the pylorus, a constant landmark even in unusual and difficult cases. The first portion of the duodenum is noted, and the Ladd's bands are identified and divided close to the wall of the duodenum. Using sharp dissection, the duodenum is mobilized completely on its anterior, posterior, and lateral aspects with a generous and thorough Kocher maneuver. The entire length of the duodenum must be mobilized from the surrounding structures well into the first portion of the jejunum. This will change its configuration from one that is kinked and foreshortened to one without obstruction. It is important to stay near the serosa of the duodenum during this dissection to prevent a tear in the midgut mesentery.

Following complete mobilization of the duodenum to correct extrinsic compression, the next stage is focused on converting the narrow mesenteric pedicle to a broad, flat mesenteric plane. Dissection, mobilization, and widening of the midgut mesentery are performed to change the configuration of the mesentery and prevent a recurrent torsion and midgut volvulus. The root of the midgut mesentery may be distinctly abnormal and have the form of a thick cord. The mesentery is rolled up along the course of the SMA and vein. The vessels are trapped within this cord that is formed by the fusion of the duodenum on the right and the ascending colon on the left side.

Following division of the Ladd's bands that pass from the ascending colon over the duodenum to the retroperitoneum, additional peritoneal bands that approximate the duodenum and the ascending colon are identified and divided. This maneuver will allow the duodenum and ascending colon to be widely separated such that the base of the midgut mesentery will be converted from a narrow cord to a wide plane (Fig. 81-7). There may be adhesions between portions of the small bowel mesentery. These adhesions are divided, allowing the mesentery to widen. At least one, and often two, peritoneal bands are identified and divided in order to completely mobilize and widen the midgut mesentery. This process should encompass the entire midportion of the small bowel mesentery, extending upward to the junction of the superior mesenteric vessels and the neck of the pancreas. When successfully completed, the SMA and superior mesenteric vein will be clearly visible in the center of the mesentery. At this time, the midgut mesentery will be wide enough to place the duodenum in the right paracolic gutter, and the cecum and ascending colon into the left side of the abdominal cavity.

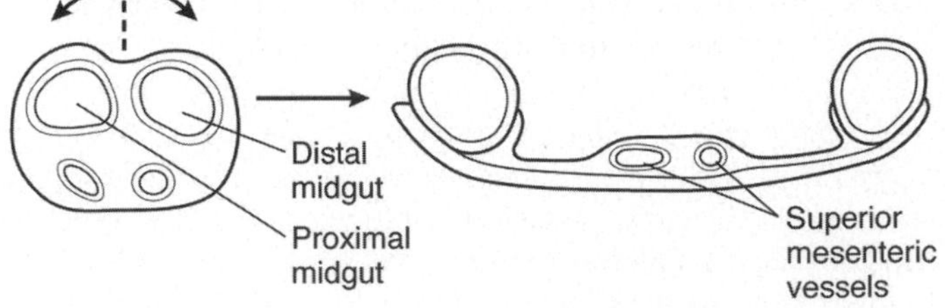

FIGURE 81-7. Dissection and mobilization of the narrow mesenteric pedicle. A cross section through the pedicle illustrates the approximation of the proximal midgut (duodenum), the distal midgut (colon), and the superior mesenteric vessels (posterior). Adequate dissection converts the narrow pedicle to a broad plane centered on the superior mesenteric artery.

The broad-based mesenteric root and the widely separated proximal and distal segments of the midgut are now at a low risk for volvulus.

Duodenal obstruction occurs in malrotation on the basis of more than one mechanism. It can result from acute midgut volvulus, but it also can occur as the result of extrinsic Ladd's bands and the tortuous course of the duodenum when it is not completely rotated. Following duodenal mobilization with the Kocher maneuver and division of all abnormal peritoneal bands, the duodenum should be widely patent unless an intrinsic lesion (i.e., duodenal stenosis, web) is present. After identification and treatment of the volvulus, division of all Ladd's bands, and broadening of the midgut mesentery have been completed, duodenal patency must be confirmed. Approximately 10% of malrotation cases have an associated duodenal stenosis or web.

A straightforward way to confirm luminal patency is to pass a no. 10 or no. 12 nasogastric tube through the patient's mouth or nose and into the stomach. The tube can be identified and gently guided through the pylorus and into the duodenum and proximal jejunum. This can be carried out promptly, and after duodenal patency has been verified, the tube can be pulled back into the stomach for postoperative nasogastric decompression. This method works well and is reliable. A gastrotomy and passage of a balloon catheter is not necessary. If the nasogastric tube cannot be easily passed into the jejunum, an intrinsic duodenal lesion is present. A duodenal atresia, stenosis, or web should be corrected at this point by a duodenoduodenostomy or excision of the web.

Surgically treated patients with malrotation will continue to have an abnormal position of the cecum postoperatively. During the mobilization and widening of the midgut mesentery, the cecum and right colon are dissected free and placed into the left side of the abdomen. The appendix, therefore, will be located either in the left upper or left lower quadrant of the abdomen. With this in mind, routine appendectomy is performed as part of the Ladd procedure. This eliminates acute appendicitis as a diagnostic possibility for the future. A standard or an inversion appendectomy are both acceptable alternatives. Following the appendectomy, the intestines are replaced into the peritoneal cavity. The duodenum and proximal small bowel are placed in the right paracolic gutter. The cecum and ascending colon are then placed into the left side of the abdomen so the duodenojejunal junction and the ileocecal junction are as far apart as possible. The midportion of the midgut is then replaced into the lower and midabdomen. During this process, it is helpful to verify that the midgut mesentery is flat, and the SMA and vein are visible in the bottom of the abdominal wound. Abdominal fixation of the midgut to theoretically prevent recurrent volvulus is not necessary.

Patients have an adynamic ileus usually for several days following a Ladd procedure in uncomplicated situations. Nasogastric drainage is maintained for several days after surgery. Broad-spectrum antibiotic therapy is continued postoperatively until the ileus has resolved.

Reverse Rotation

This rare anomaly results from midgut rotation in a clockwise direction around the SMA axis. The transverse colon lies behind the SMA, and the duodenum resides anterior to the SMA. Reverse rotation is usually seen in adults and is rarely reported in children. Symptoms of obstruction are generally due to extrinsic compression of the transverse colon by the superior mesenteric vessels or an ileocecal volvulus. Operative correction includes mobilization of the duodenum and the superior mesenteric vessels to allow the colon to be brought out laterally from beneath the SMA.

Mesocolic Hernias

Mesocolic hernias are rare rotational anomalies requiring surgical correction. Normally, the mesocolon of the ascending colon and the descending colon is fused to the retroperitoneum. In these cases, the mesocolon of either the right or the left colon forms a portion of the hernia sac. The sac usually contains a substantial portion of the midgut. Right mesocolic hernias frequently occur with incomplete rotation and fixation of the cecocolic segment such that the cecum is malpositioned into the right upper quadrant. A right mesocolic hernia is corrected by dividing the retroperitoneal attachments on the lateral aspect of the cecum and the ascending colon; the colon is then reflected to the left and mobilized with care taken to preserve the ascending mesocolon. The small bowel is freed from the hernia sac, and remains on the right side of the abdomen similar to a Ladd procedure. The midgut mesenteric pedicle is inspected, mobilized, and widened if not broad based. Left mesocolic hernias usually have normal rotation and fixation of the cecum and ascending colon. The left mesocolon forms the anterior aspect of the hernia sac, and the inferior mesenteric vein forms a portion of the neck of the sac. Surgical treatment may be difficult due to the location of the inferior mesenteric vein. The initial task includes reduction of the small intestine from the hernia sac, which may require mobilization of the inferior mesenteric vein. Then the neck of the sac is either closed or widely opened to eliminate the potential space for recurrent herniation.

COMPLICATIONS

Prompt recognition and surgical treatment of malrotation should result in a satisfactory outcome with few significant complications. The majority of serious and long-term complications are related to delays in diagnosis and treatment leading to intestinal ischemia and infarction. Complications specific to the surgical treatment of malrotation primarily include recurrent intestinal obstruction or short bowel syndrome due to intestinal necrosis.

Recurrent intestinal obstruction after a Ladd procedure results from (1) recurrent midgut volvulus, (2) adhesive bands, and (3) intestinal dysmotility.

Recurrent midgut volvulus has been reported in less than 5% of surgically treated cases of malrotation (7,10,11,18,19). Recurrent volvulus results from either inadequate adhesion formation and fixation of the midgut, or inadequate mesenteric dissection with a persistently narrowed midgut mesentery. Intestinal fixation has been advocated in the past to theoretically prevent recurrent volvulus (38). Long-term follow-up has not demonstrated any benefit from abdominal fixation (39). Adhesive intestinal obstruction is the most common complication and occurs in approximately 5% to 10% of patients following a Ladd procedure (7,10,11,18,19). Postoperative adhesion formation is expected and of benefit for successful surgical treatment of malrotation. Postoperative intussusception may occur following a Ladd procedure, or following other abdominal and thoracic procedures in children. Signs of persistent or recurrent postoperative intestinal obstruction necessitate prompt evaluation and treatment with a low threshold for operative intervention. A subset of patients successfully treated for malrotation has persistent GI symptoms. Intestinal motility disturbances have been identified in several cases of malrotation (32,33). Most patients are older than 1 year of age with long-standing symptoms. Manometric studies suggest a neuropathic defect due to abnormalities of the intrinsic enteric nervous system.

The most devastating complications result from intestinal necrosis secondary to midgut volvulus. Early complications include sepsis, shock, and multiple organ system failure caused by inflammatory and vasoactive mediators released into the circulation from devitalized tissue and microorganisms. Short bowel syndrome is the most important late complication following extensive intestinal resection. The incidence and severity generally correlate with the length of resection and the integrity of the remaining intestine. Intestinal adaptation may occur to allow eventual discontinuation of total parenteral nutrition. Midgut volvulus with intestinal necrosis represents approximately 18% of cases of short bowel syndrome in the pediatric population (40). Intestinal salvage strategies are strongly encouraged during surgical therapy to prevent short bowel syndrome. Expeditious diagnosis and treatment of malrotation with midgut volvulus remains the most significant factor in preventing this complication.

RESULTS

The contemporary results for the surgical treatment of malrotation are quite favorable. Survival with resolution of symptoms should be expected in the majority of cases. The current mortality rate for operative cases of malrotation is 3% to 9% (8,9,11,19,31). Mortality is increased in the presence of midgut volvulus, intestinal necrosis, age less than 1 month, and associated major anomalies (33). Death results secondary to midgut volvulus with intestinal infarction. Early deaths are due to overwhelming sepsis and multiple organ system failure, and late deaths occur as a result of the complications of short bowel syndrome. In patients who present with malrotation and midgut volvulus, 15% to 30% will have intestinal necrosis requiring resection. In the absence of intestinal necrosis, the mortality rate is 1%; however, in the presence of intestinal necrosis, mortality increases to 50%. The mortality risk has been correlated with the extent of intestinal necrosis such that the mortality rate is increased to 65% when greater than 75% of the intestine is necrotic (31).

The survival and outcome for patients treated surgically has improved significantly since the mid-1950s. Many factors have contributed to the favorable results. The most important is improved education and awareness of malrotation as a significant cause of intestinal obstruction. Enhanced neonatal and pediatric intensive care services, hyperalimentation, and enteral nutritional support have contributed to the improved survival and long-term outcome. Further improvements can occur, but these will be primarily due to contributions leading to earlier diagnosis and treatment.

In the absence of intestinal necrosis, the majority of patients treated with a Ladd procedure have a very satisfactory outcome. The symptoms of intestinal obstruction should resolve following surgery. Significant postoperative complications are infrequent. This is especially true in children less than 1 year of age with an acute presentation. In contrast, the long-term results are less than ideal in a subset of patients with malrotation who are older than 1 year of age and have chronic or intermittent symptoms. These individuals are more likely to have persistent symptoms of intestinal dysfunction following a successful Ladd procedure (41). In a number of cases, an intrinsic intestinal dysmotility disorder will be identified. Most patients with malrotation will benefit from surgical treatment with resolution or improvement in the presenting abdominal symptoms, and more important, the risk of a midgut volvulus and intestinal necrosis is markedly reduced.

REFERENCES

1. Ladd WE. Congenital obstruction of the duodenum in children. *N Engl J Med* 1932;206:277–283.
2. Ladd WE. Congenital duodenal obstruction. *Surgery* 1937;1:878–885.
3. Skandalakis JE, Gray SW, Ricketts R, et al. The small intestines. In: Skandalakis JE, Gray SW, eds. *Embryology for surgeons,* 2nd ed. Baltimore: Williams & Wilkins, 1994.
4. Byrne WJ. Disorders of the intestine and pancreas. In: Taeusch WH, Ballard RA, Avery ME, eds. *Diseases of the newborn*. Philadelphia: WB Saunders, 1991:685.
5. Estrada RL. *Anomalies of intestinal rotation and fixation*. Springfield, IL: Charles C Thomas, 1958.
6. Snyder WH, Chaffin L. Embryology and pathology of the intestinal tract: presentation of 40 cases of malrotation. *Ann Surg* 1954;130:368–380.
7. Stewart DR, Colodny AL, Daggett WC. Malrotation of the bowel in children: a 15 year review. *Surgery* 1976;79:716–720.
8. Ford EG, Senac MO, Srikanth MS, et al. Malrotation of the intestine in children. *Ann Surg* 1992;215:172–178.
9. Filston HC, Kirks DR. Malrotation—the ubiquitious anomaly. *J Pediatr Surg* 1981;16:614–620.
10. Smith IE. Malrotation of the intestine. In: Welch KJ, Randolph JG, Ravich MR, et al., eds. *Pediatric surgery,* 4th ed. Chicago: Yearbook Medical, 1986:882.
11. Powell DM, Othersen HB, Smith CD. Malrotation of the intestines in children: the effect of age of presentation and therapy. *J Pediatr Surg* 1989;24:777–780.
12. Spigland N, Brandt ML, Yazbeck S. Malrotation presenting beyond the neonatal period. *J Pediatr Surg* 1990;25:1139–1142.
13. Yanez R, Spitz L. Intestinal malrotation presenting outside the neonatal period. *Arch Dis Child* 1986;6e1:682–685.
14. Croitoru D, Neilson I, Guttman FM. Pyloric stenosis associated with malrotation. *J Pediatr Surg* 1991;26:1276–1278.
15. Brereton RJ, Taylor B, Hall CM. Intussusception and intestinal malrotation in infants: Waugh's syndrome. *Br J Surg* 1986;73:55–57.
16. Campbell KA, Sitzmann JV, Cameron JL. Biliary tract anomalies associated with intestinal malrotation in the adult. *Surgery* 1993;113:312.
17. Smith SL. Familial midgut volvulus. *Surgery* 1972;72:420.
18. Andrassy RJ, Mahour GH. Malrotation of the midgut in infants and children. *Arch Surg* 1981;116:158–160.
19. Rescorla FJ, Shedd FJ, Grosfeld JL, et al. Anomalies of intestinal rotation in childhood: analysis of 447 cases. *Surgery* 1990;108:710–716.
20. Wang CA, Welcj CE. Anomalies of intestinal rotation in adolescents and adults. *Surgery* 1963;54:839–855.
21. Prasil P, Flageole H, Shaw KS, et al. Should malrotation in children be treated differently according to age? *J Pediatr Surg* 2000;35(5):756–758.
22. Dilley AV, Pereira J, Shi EC, et al. The radiologist says malrotation: does the surgeon operate? *Pediatr Surg Int* 2000;16(1–2):45–49.
23. Silverman A, Roy C. *Pediatric clinical gastroenterology,* 3rd ed. St. Louis, MO: Mosby 1983;62–66.
24. Kullendorf CM, Mikaelsson C, Ivancev K. Malrotation in children with symptoms of gastrointestinal allergy and psychosomatic abdominal pain. *Acta Pediatr Scand* 1985;74:296–299.
25. Simpson AJ, Leonidas JC, Krasna IH, et al. Roentgen diagnosis of midgut malrotation: value of upper gastrointestinal radiographic study. *J Pediatr Surg* 1972;7:243–252.
26. Slovis TL, Klein MD, Watts FB. Incomplete rotation of the intestine with a normal cecal position. *Surgery* 1980;87:325–330.
27. Zerin JM, DiPietro MA. Superior mesenteric vascular anatomy at US in patients with surgically proved malrotation of the midgut. *Radiology* 1992;183:693.
28. Weinberger E, Winters WD, Liddell RM, et al. Sonographic diagnosis of intestinal malrotation in infants: importance of the relative positions of the superior mesenteric vein and artery. *Am J Radiol* 1992;159:825.
29. Zerin JM, DiPietro MA. Mesenteric vascular anatomy at CT: normal and abnormal appearance. *Radiology* 1991;179:739–742.
30. Shatzkes D, Gordon DH, Haller JO, et al. Malrotation of the bowel: misalignment in the superior mesenteric artery-vein complex shown by CT and MR. *J Comput Assist Tomogr* 1990;14:93–95.
31. Messineo A, MacMilan JH, Palder SB, et al. Clinical factors affecting mortality in children with malrotation of the intestine. *J Pediatr Surg* 1992;27:1343–1345.
32. Coombs RC, Buick RG, Gornall PG, et al. Intestinal malrotation: the role of small intestinal dysmotility in the cause of persistent symptoms. *J Pediatr Surg* 1991;26:553–556.
33. Devane SP, Smith VV, Bisset WM, et al. Persistent gastrointestinal symptoms after correction of malrotation. *Arch Dis Child* 1992;67:218.
34. Bass KD, Rothenberg SS, Chang JH. Laparoscopic Ladd's procedure in infants with malrotation. *J Pediatr Surg* 1998;33(2):279–281.
35. Mazziotti MV, Strasberg SM, Langer JC. Intestinal rotation abnormalities without volvulus: the rose of laparoscopy. *J Am Coll Surg* 1997;185(2):172–176.
36. Bax NM, van der Zee DC. Laparoscopic treatment of intestinal malrotation in children. *Surg Endosc* 1998;12(11):1314–1316.
37. Gross E, Chen MK, Lobe TE. Laparoscopic evaluation and treatment of intestinal malrotation in infants. *Surg Endosc* 1996;10(9):936–937.
38. Brennom WS, Bill AH. Prophylactic fixation of the intestine for midgut nonrotation. *Surg Gynecol Obset* 1974;138:181–184.
39. Stauffer UC, Herrmann P. Comparison of late results in patients with corrected intestinal malrotation with and without fixation of the mesentery. *J Pediatr Surg* 1980;15:9.
40. Warner BW, Ziegler MM. Management of the short bowel syndrome in the pediatric population. *Pediatr Clin North Am* 1993;40:1335–1350.
41. Mehall JR, Chandler JC, Mehall RL, et al. Management of typical and atypical intestinal malrotation. *J Pediatr Surg* 2002;37(8):1169–1172.

Chapter 82

Intussusception

Daniel P. Doody and Robert P. Foglia

Intussusception, the invagination of the intestine into an adjoining intestinal lumen, is among the most common causes of acute abdominal pain in children younger than 5 years of age. It is a disease primarily of infants and toddlers, although intussusception can occur in utero, in neonates, and in adults. Eighty percent to 90% of intussusception cases occur in children between 3 months and 3 years of age.

PATHOGENESIS

The pathogenesis of intussusception has been ascribed to an inhomogeneity of longitudinal forces along the intestinal wall. In the resting state, normal propulsive forces meet a certain resistance at any point. This stable equilibrium can be disrupted when a portion of the intestine does not appropriately promulgate peristaltic waves. Small perturbations provided by contraction of the circular muscle perpendicular to the axis of longitudinal tension result in a kink in the abnormal portion of the intestine, creating a rotary force (torque). Distortion may continue, in-folding the area of inhomogeneity and eventually capturing the circumference of the small intestine. This invaginated intestine then acts as the apex of the intussusceptum (1).

Intramural, intraluminal, or extramural processes may produce points of disequilibrium. Along with anatomic abnormalities, flaccid areas that follow a paralytic ileus can also create unstable segments because adjoining areas create discordant contractions with the return of bowel activity. Such a model offers an explanation as to the cause of postoperative intussusceptions, which are rarely found to have a surgical lead point, but can complicate any procedures that produce an ileus, including thoracotomies and cardiac procedures.

Daniel P. Doody: Department of Pediatric Surgery, Massachusetts General Hospital, Boston, Massachusetts 02114.

Robert P. Foglia: Department of Surgery, Washington University School of Medicine, St. Louis Children's Hospital, St. Louis, Missouri 63110.

PATHOLOGY

On sectioning, the tumor is composed of the internal layer, the returning middle layer, and the outer ensheathing layer (Fig. 82-1). The entering and returning layers, including the adjacent mesentery, are referred to as the *intussusceptum* and include any surgical lead point. The receiving or ensheathing layer is referred to as the *intussuscipiens*. With normal peristalsis, the length of the intussusception increases, and the cycle of venous congestion, lymphatic obstruction, and eventual arterial compromise is initiated. The vascular supply at the apex of the intussusceptum is the most compromised, and the mucosa of the apex experiences secondary sloughing. The combination of mucoid discharge from the bowel and vascular sloughing results in a currant jelly stool.

ETIOLOGY

The most common cause of intussusception is indeterminate and termed *idiopathic*. In a number of patients, particularly those younger than 3 years of age, there may be enlargement of Peyer's patch. These children may have had a viral illness as a prodrome 5 to 10 days earlier.

In 2% to 12% of all pediatric cases, the intussusception has an anatomically identifiable lead point. Children with intussusception secondary to surgical lead points usually require operative treatment because the intussusceptum is rarely reduced by pressure reduction. The frequency of lead points as the cause of intussusception increases with age. This is particularly true in children older than 4 years of age, in whom the prevalence of lead points complicating intussusception has been reported to be as high as 57% (2). In adults, the incidence of lead points associated with intussusception is as high as 97% (3). Meckel's diverticulum is the most common anatomic lead point identified in children. Other anatomic lead points include polyps of

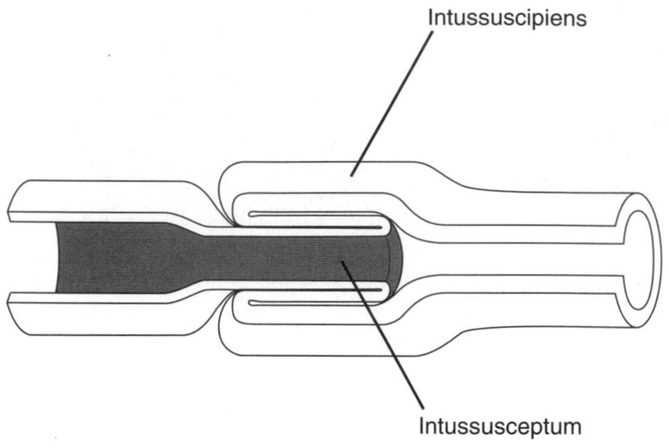

FIGURE 82-1. Diagrammatic representation of intussusception.

the ileum and colon; benign hamartomas associated with Peutz-Jeghers syndrome; submucosal hematomas associated with Henoch-Schönlein purpura; lymphoma; lymphosarcoma; enteric cysts; ectopic, pancreatic, and gastric rests; inverted appendiceal stumps; and anastomotic suture lines. In adults, about one-half of surgical lead points are malignant, and there is a higher incidence of colocolic intussusceptions.

Intussusception is a feature of the gastrointestinal (GI) problems associated with cystic fibrosis (CF) and Henoch-Schönlein purpura. Together, these medical processes account for 3% to 5% of cases of intussusception (4).

CLINICAL PRESENTATION

Although intussusception can occur at any age, it is convenient from the clinical perspective to divide these patients into those occurring in children younger than 3 years of age and those occurring in older children and adults. In children younger than 5 years of age, intussusception accounts for as many as 25% of abdominal surgical emergencies, exceeding the incidence of appendicitis. Therefore, the practitioner should always consider intussusception in the evaluation of young children and infants who present with acute abdominal pain.

The typical clinical history is that of a 6- to 9-month-old male infant who suddenly cries out, often drawing his or her knees up with the abdominal discomfort. Frequently, the child has emesis and often immediately evacuates. The child may appear diaphoretic during the crisis. The abdominal discomfort appears to last briefly, after which the infant is quiet and may appear well. The incident is repetitive, typically occurring in 15- to 30-minute intervals. As time passes, the child may become increasingly ill with abdominal distention, vomiting, and the eventual appearance of red currant jelly stools seen in approximately 30% of patients. With time, shock intervenes and cardiovascular collapse occurs.

At presentation, the infant is often exhausted and resting quietly. Occasionally and without stimulation, the child may arch and cry out. As the examination begins, the child appears irritable or diaphoretic. Tachycardia or hypotension can be found, even early in the illness, depending on the degree of bowel compromise. Pertinent physical findings are generally confined to the abdomen. A mass may be palpated in the right upper quadrant to midabdomen, but this finding may be difficult to appreciate because of the child's irritability.

Rarely, a cervixlike mass may be seen protruding through the anus. For prolapse of the intussusception to occur, the mesentery is lax, and the progression of the intussusceptum to the rectosigmoid is rapid. The distinction between intussusception and rectal prolapse, an uncommon finding in infants, can often be made by careful examination of the anal crypts at the dentate line. This anatomic landmark is everted in rectal prolapse, but is not seen with intussusception. An applicator that passes into the space between the apparent prolapse and the anus is also diagnostic of a prolapsed intussusceptum.

Although hematochezia is not always seen with intussusception, 60% to 90% of children with intussusception have gross or occult blood on rectal examination (5). Thirty percent of infants have passed mucoid, bloody stools (red currant jelly stools), and the remaining infants have occult blood on testing.

The differential diagnosis at presentation includes intestinal colic, gastroenteritis, intestinal duplication, appendicitis, incarcerated hernia, and more unusual forms of intestinal obstruction, such as internal hernia and volvulus.

RADIOGRAPHIC DIAGNOSTIC EVALUATION

Early in the course of the illness, supine and upright abdominal films show a normal or nonspecific bowel gas pattern. As the disease progresses, a more obvious pattern of small bowel obstruction with absence of gas in the colon is noted. The most predictive finding of the disease is the presence of a right upper quadrant soft-tissue density, found in 25% to 60% of cases (Fig. 82-2). The absence of bowel gas in the right lower quadrant (Dance's sign) may be identified in the patient with intussusception. Other radiographic findings include reduced amount of gas in the jejunum, lateralization of the ileum into the right iliac fossa, indiscernible cecal shadow, and reduced amount of feces in the colon (6). Even using these radiographic indicators, 50% to 66% of children who undergo a diagnostic enema for suspected intussusception do not have the disease (7).

Supine cross-table lateral (horizontal-beam) radiographs provide two additional findings that can be helpful in establishing the diagnosis of intussusception (8).

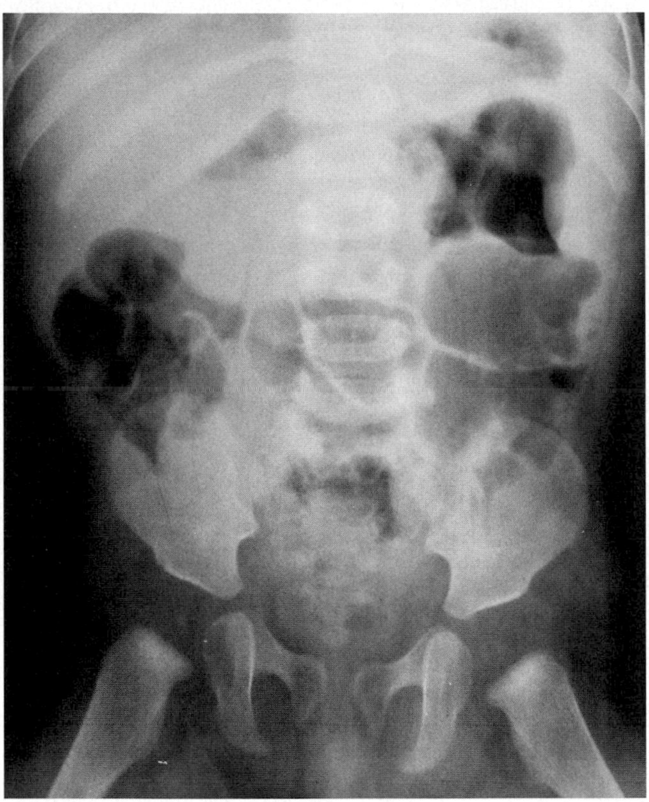

FIGURE 82-2. Supine abdominal radiograph showing soft-tissue density in right upper quadrant to midabdomen. Absence of normal cecal gas shadow can be seen in the right lower quadrant.

A homogeneous water-density anterior abdominal mass may displace upper abdominal gas inferiorly, or the mass may demonstrate craniocaudal separation into distinct upper and lower bowel gas patterns. One of these two radiographic findings was identified in 75% of intussusceptions in a small series. Other researchers have noted that the intussusceptum may be seen only in this projection and recommend this view as an additional indicator to decide if a diagnostic enema is indicated (9).

TREATMENT

Often with a clinically suggestive story and nonspecific findings on plain abdominal radiographs, contrast enemas are performed for diagnosis and therapy. Only in children who have clinical peritonitis or radiographic evidence of perforation is an attempt at pressure reduction absolutely contraindicated. Intravenous access should be obtained prior to a contrast enema. The enema can cause a showering of bacteria into the portal circulator and has approximately a 1% chance of bowel perforation. Patients should receive a broad-spectrum antibiotic to cover enteric organisms prior to the study.

Hydrostatic Reduction

Hydrostatic reduction was proposed by Hirschsprung in 1876 for the treatment of intussusception. The contrast study can be both diagnostic and therapeutic. The use of contrast enemas allows direct visualization of the reduction under fluoroscopic control and is reported to be successful in 65% to 70% of cases. In the hands of an experienced pediatric radiologist, the ratio of successful reduction approaches 85%.

A noninflatable rectal tube is inserted in the rectum, and the buttocks are taped to prevent loss of distending pressure. Contrast enters the rectosigmoid by gravity under fluoroscopic guidance. In the usual case, the contrast column meets a concave filling defect in the transverse colon that can be reduced in a retrograde fashion to the cecum (Fig. 82-3).

A radiographic "rule of threes" applies to hydrostatic reduction in intussusception to minimize the risk of perforation: (1) the barium contrast column should be no greater than 3 ft above the table (100 cm), (2) each attempt should persist until reduction of the intussusceptum fails to progress for a period of 3 to 5 minutes, and (3) a maximum of three attempts should be made. The rule of threes prevents the reduction of necrotic bowel, while optimizing the care of the infant. Experimentally, hydrostatic columns less than 3.5 ft are unable to reduce gangrenous bowel (10). At this height, a 60% weight per volume barium suspension generates an intraluminal

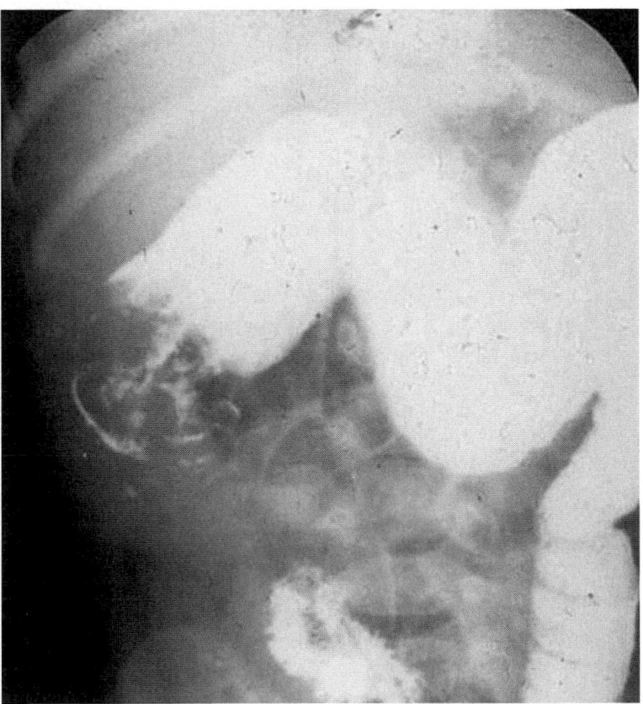

FIGURE 82-3. A barium contrast enema showing an intussusception at the hepatic flexure.

pressure of 120 mm Hg. Dilute water-soluble solutions require a greater height to generate the same intracolonic pressures. A 20% weight per volume meglumine sodium diatrizoate solution (Gastrografin) or 17.2% iothalamate meglumine solution (Cysto-Conray II) achieves an intraluminal pressure of 120 mm Hg at a height of 150 cm (5 ft) (11). Because most intussusceptions are reduced within the first two attempts, successful hydrostatic reduction after three attempts is unlikely (12). The attempted reduction should cease if a progressive reduction of the intussusceptum does not occur after 3 to 5 minutes of constant pressure because the intussusception is unlikely to reduce. In practice, if two attempts at radiographic reduction are not successful, operation is warranted. A radiographic finding often associated with irreducible intussusceptions is the dissection sign, which occurs when barium intercalates between the intussusceptum and the intussuscipiens (13) (Fig. 82-4). Although successful reductions of intussusceptions demonstrating this radiographic finding have been reported (14,15), this feature, coupled with a clinical history greater than 48 hours or radiographic evidence of a complete bowel obstruction, is often associated with intestinal gangrene. Surgery, rather than repeated attempts at hydrostatic reduction, is indicated in this circumstance.

As the intussusceptum is reduced through the ileocecal valve, contrast should reflux freely into the small intestine, a radiographic finding considered essential to document a successful reduction. Subtle radiographic features that may indicate an incomplete reduction are complete evacuation of barium without residual contrast in the small intestine and the persistence of small bowel meteorism.

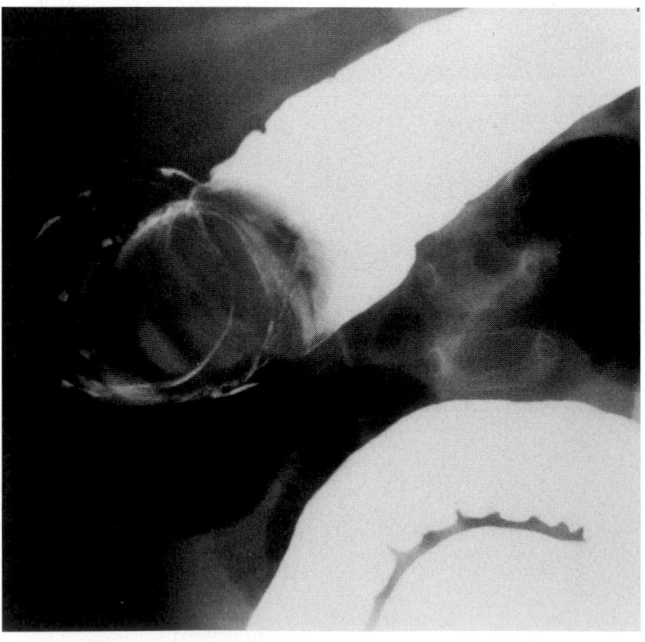

FIGURE 82-4. Partial reduction of intussusception demonstrating dissection sign. At surgery, the intussusceptum included a gangrenous Meckel's diverticulum as a surgical lead point.

On occasion, inability to reflux into the terminal ileum is ascribed to competency or edema of the ileocecal valve. Some authors propose that observation rather than laparotomy may be appropriate if contrast does not pass into the terminal ileum, but the infant becomes asymptomatic. These authors argue that 7% to 20% of intussusceptions are found at laparotomy to be reduced. By reevaluating the stable child after a short period of observation, the morbidity of surgery may be avoided (16–18). If it is uncertain whether the process has resolved completely, surgery is warranted. The counterargument to the roughly 10% to 15% reduction rate found at laparotomy is that this is comparable to an acceptable negative appendectomy rate and the potential sequelae of a missed intussusception is appreciably greater. In general, incomplete reduction requires operative intervention.

Ultrasound-guided Reduction

Ultrasound-guided hydrostatic reduction of intussusception can be performed (19). Diagnosis of intussusception is established by the ultrasonographic demonstration of target sign on transverse views (Fig. 82-5A) and pseudokidney sign on longitudinal views (Fig. 82-5B) of the intussusceptum. An enema consisting of saline and water-soluble contrast material (9:1 ratio) is used to reduce the intussusception, and the contrast confirms reflux into the terminal ileum on supine abdominal radiograph. The success rate is comparable to that for pneumatic reduction and may be higher than that for barium enema reduction. Radiographic exposure is lower with ultrasound-guided reduction, and with experienced ultrasonographers, this method may be preferable to fluoroscopically guided reduction. The technique may be limited in those infants with small bowel obstruction because the multiple air–fluid interfaces can interfere with accurate assessment of the reduction.

Pneumatic Reduction

Pneumatic reduction of intussusception has been used extensively in China and is now readily accepted in North America and Western Europe. The contraindications for hydrostatic reduction are equally applicable in evaluating children for pneumatic reduction. If a noninflatable balloon is used for pneumatic reduction, the buttocks are taped firmly to maintain a stable intracolonic pressure to reduce the intussusception. At an initial pressure of 80 mm Hg, air is delivered into the colon under fluoroscopic guidance. This pressure can be raised to a maximum of 120 mm Hg, equivalent to a 1-M column of barium suspension or a 1.5-M column of a 20% weight per volume meglumine sodium diatrizoate solution. Reflux of air into the terminal ileum signifies complete reduction of the intussusception. Higher rates of reduction are reported with air insufflation (87%) than with hydrostatic reduction

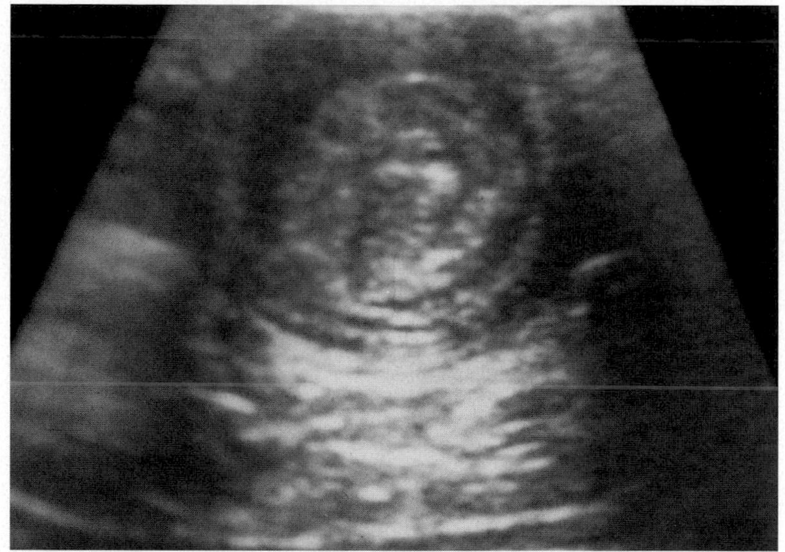

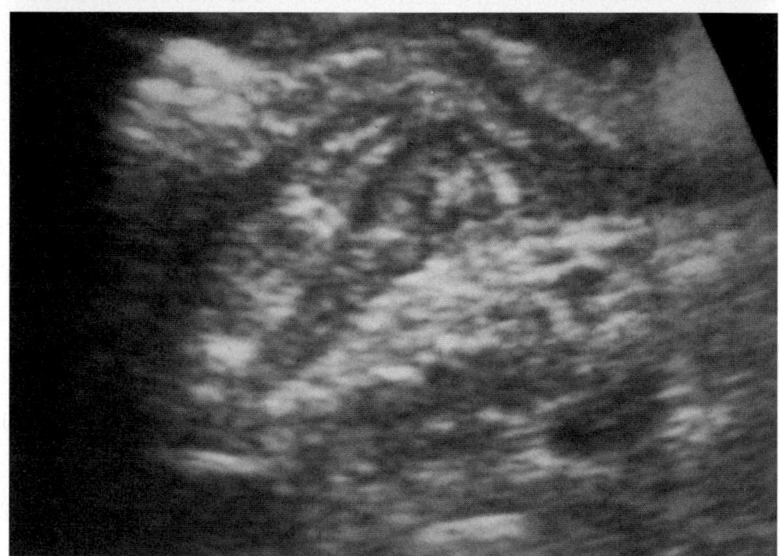

FIGURE 82-5. **(A)** Transverse view on ultrasound showing the concentric rings of the intussusceptum within the intussuscipiens (target sign). **(B)** Pseudokidney seen on longitudinal views of the intussusception.

(55% to 70%). As the intraluminal pressure is accurately monitored, a more effective mean intracolonic pressure is maintained and may explain the greater success rate with this method.

Technically, the use of air as a contrast medium can be challenging if a small bowel obstruction is present. An additional problem with air reduction is the phenomenon referred to as *pseudoreduction,* whereby air enters the small bowel before complete reduction of the intussusceptum. Greater success with hydrostatic or pneumatic reduction is found with ileocolic intussusception than with intussusception more proximal with the small intestine.

Operative Reduction

In children who have clinical evidence of peritonitis or radiographic evidence of perforation, and in those in whom pressure reduction is unsuccessful, surgery is indicated after initiating fluid resuscitation and starting broad-spectrum antibiotic therapy. A right transverse infraumbilical incision is made and carried down through the muscular layers, exposing the right lower quadrant. If necessary, the incision can be extended across the midline to perform a complete evaluation of the abdomen. The intussusception is reduced within the abdomen if possible. As the reduction becomes more difficult, the right colon to the hepatic flexure can be brought into the wound. Warm saline pads are placed around the intussusception, and compression is maintained for 1 to 2 minutes, reducing the tissue edema and facilitating the reduction. The intussusceptum is expressed from the intussuscipiens by placing gentle pressure at the apex of the lesion (Fig. 82-6). The intussusceptum never should be pulled from the intussuscipiens. Traction may disrupt the compromised bowel and force the surgeon to perform resection with anastomosis (Figs. 82-7A and 82-7B).

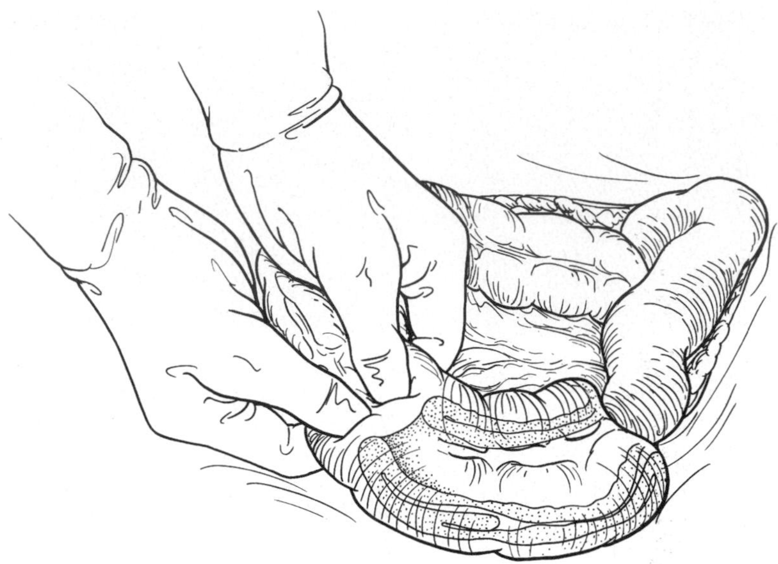

FIGURE 82-6. Manual reduction of ileocolic intussusception.

After the intestine is reduced, the bowel is inspected for viability and for surgical lead points. If vascular compromise is a concern, 10 to 15 minutes of observation in the operating theater is appropriate before performing a resection. In infants and young children, a large Peyer's patch or the ileocecal valve can mimic an intramural or intraluminal mass. Careful palpation of the intestine and awareness of these common findings should prevent unnecessary enterotomies. An incidental appendectomy may be performed if there is not significant edema and ecchymosis of the cecum.

Successful manual reduction can be expected in about 90% of pediatric patients, even if surgical lead points are present. These lead points, if identified, should be removed, and a primary enteroenterostomy should be performed. True irreducibility of the intussusception suggests that gangrenous intestine is present. Even in those instances, a primary resection and anastomosis is

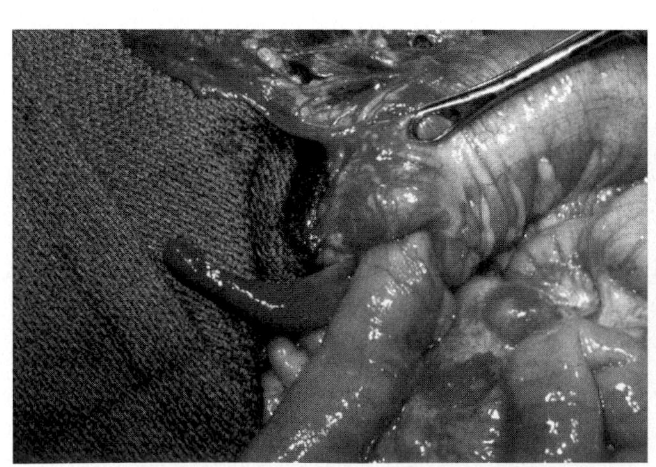

A

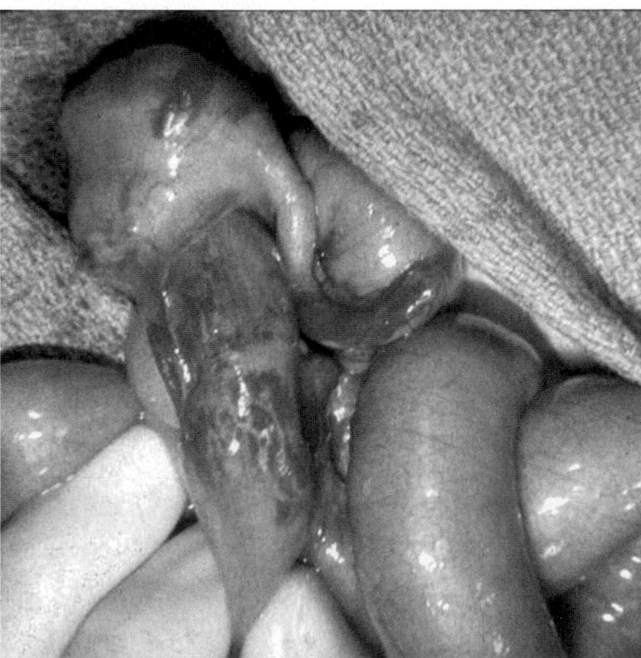

B

FIGURE 82-7. Operative reduction of an ileocolic intussusception. **(A)** Note the appendix partly within the intussusception. **(B)** Complete reduction. Note viable bowel and ecchymosis of the ileal wall and appendix from their being part of the intussusception.

appropriate unless the child is so seriously ill that resection and exteriorization are clinically indicated to expedite closure and lessen the anesthetic risk. The laparoscopic approach for operative treatment of intussusception is a reasonable option.

Ileocecopexy, suturing the last several centimeters of the terminal ileum to the ascending colon to prevent recurrent intussusception, has not been shown to be beneficial and is no longer recommended. There has been no proven advantage to the additional operative manipulation, and intussusception can occur after ileocecopexy.

Complications

Perforation with Pressure Reduction

In a large international survey (20), the cumulative incidence of perforation complicating hydrostatic reduction was 0.18%. It remains controversial whether pneumatic reduction is safer than hydrostatic reduction. The incidence of perforation has been higher with pneumatic reduction and varies between 1% and 2.8%. With increasing experience in pneumatic reduction, the incidence of perforation is decreasing.

A more intense inflammatory reaction occurs with the peritonitis complicating a perforation with barium than that seen with water-soluble contrast or air contrast enemas. The mixture of barium and feces can lead to a prolonged septic course. Infants younger than 6 months of age and children with symptoms for longer than 36 hours, or with evidence of bowel obstruction, are at greater risk for having gangrenous bowel complicating their intussusception. They are consequently at greater risk for perforation. If pressure reduction is attempted in these patients, a water-soluble solution or air contrast enema is the more appropriate medium.

Recurrent Intussusception

The rate of recurrent intussusception after successful hydrostatic reduction of intussusception varies between 5% and 11%. Recurrence after surgical reduction is comparable. The recurrence rate is lower in younger children due to the lack of a true anatomic lead point in many cases. In addition, in hyperplasia of Peyer's patch with lead point, this lymphatic enlargement is typically gone within 2 weeks. Thirty percent to 64% of recurrences occur within 72 hours of reduction, although recurrence may occur up to 36 months after successful reduction. Lead points are identified in fewer than 10% of the recurrent cases (21–23), and hydrostatic or pneumatic reduction is appropriate as the initial treatment.

Celiotomy is indicated for recurrent intussusception only when there is a reasonable expectation of finding a surgical lead point. Children whose presentations place them at greater risk of having an anatomic lead point include those who experience more than one recurrence without prior operation, children older than 3 years of age with recurrences after successful hydrostatic reduction, and children with known intestinal polyposis (24).

Mortality Rate

Although advances in treatment and increased awareness of the disease have led to a decreased death rate, misdiagnosis, inadequate fluid resuscitation, unrelenting sepsis, and delayed presentation continue to account for an intussusception-related case fatality rate of about 1% (25).

MEDICAL PROCESSES ASSOCIATED WITH INTUSSUSCEPTION

Cystic Fibrosis

Intussusception is among the many intestinal complications associated with CF and occurs in 1% of patients with mucoviscidosis (26). These children are older than children with idiopathic intussusception, with an average age of 9.75 years (range, 4 to 16 years). The cause of the intussusception is often ascribed to the thick, puttylike material that adheres to the intestinal mucosa. Many times, children with CF who have an intussusception have a chronic and indolent course, and distinguishing among distal intestinal obstruction syndrome (meconium ileus equivalent), an occult appendiceal abscess, and intussusception in a child with CF can be difficult.

Although hydrostatic reduction of intussusception in these patients is possible, operative reduction is required in most cases. Successful manual reduction at laparotomy is usually accomplished, and only rarely is surgical resection required.

Henoch-Schönlein Purpura

Sixty-five percent of patients with Henoch-Schönlein purpura have GI symptoms related to the underlying systemic vasculitis (27). Ninety-five percent of these children have cutaneous manifestations of the disease before the surgical process becomes evident (28). Abdominal pain and GI bleeding are common manifestations of intestinal vasculitis and may mask an intussusception, intestinal necrosis, or perforation. The severity of abdominal pain and the degree of leukocytosis are insignificantly different between patients who have abdominal manifestations of the intestinal vasculitis and those who have surgical complications of the disease.

Intussusception is the most common surgical complication of the disease and occurs in 3% of children with anaphylactoid purpura. In most, if not all, cases, a submucosal hematoma acts as a lead point. Sequential barium enema and upper GI series may establish the diagnosis of intussusception, although barium enema reduction is infrequently successful because the lesion is typically enteroenteric and not ileocolic. Surgical reduction of the intussusception is required in most cases.

POSTOPERATIVE INTUSSUSCEPTION

In series from large children's hospitals, postoperative intussusception accounts for 1.5% to 6% of all cases of intussusception (29,30). The incidence of postoperative intussusception after laparotomy is 0.08% to 0.5%, but this process may complicate cardiac, thoracic, and orthopedic procedures (31).

After the apparent return of intestinal peristalsis, postoperative intussusception is marked by the gradual appearance of an early bowel obstruction. Abdominal pain is a less prominent symptom, and the most common presenting signs are increasingly bilious nasogastric output and abdominal distention. Unlike adhesive bowel disease, which usually occurs more than 2 weeks after the procedure, obstruction from this form of intussusception occurs early in the postoperative course, on average, 8 to 11 days after surgery. The diagnosis of postoperative intussusception is infrequently established by contrast enema, and a contrast meal with small bowel films may identify the obstruction. The intussusception is most frequently located in the small intestine.

The cause of postoperative intussusception is believed to be altered peristalsis due to prolonged or excessive manipulation of the bowel, bruising of the intestine, anesthetic agents, or other neurogenic factors. The higher incidence of postoperative intussusception seen in children who have known dysmotility suggests that abnormal propulsion of the intestine may be an important factor. Lead points from anastomotic suture lines are rarely found.

NONISCHEMIC (CHRONIC) INTUSSUSCEPTION

About 15% of cases of intussusception in children may be described as subacute (symptoms of 4 to 14 days) or chronic (symptoms greater than 14 days) (32,33). Patients with nonischemic intussusception present with recurrent mild to moderate abdominal discomfort and other nonspecific GI complaints, including vomiting, diarrhea, rectal bleeding, and failure to thrive. Ischemic compromise of the intussusceptum is rarely found, and abdominal masses are infrequently appreciated in this group.

This nonspecific presentation and frequently normal abdominal examination lead to the common but erroneous diagnosis of gastroenteritis. The presence of a pink mucoid semiloose bowel movement may lead the examiner to suspect the diagnosis of chronic intussusception. Nonischemic intussusception should be included in the differential diagnosis of prolonged cases of vomiting and diarrhea, particularly if stools are positive for occult blood. Awareness of this entity will lead to correct diagnosis, and appropriate therapy can be initiated.

NEONATAL INTUSSUSCEPTION

Neonatal intussusception, with symptoms occurring in the first 30 days of life, is rare (34). Sixty percent to 75% of newborn infants with intussusception are found to have surgical lead points (Fig. 82-8). Once the diagnosis of neonatal intussusception is confirmed, surgery is the preferred treatment option. There is a high incidence of surgical lead points, a low rate of successful enema reduction in small infants (35,36), and a greater risk of bowel perforation in infants younger than 6 months of age undergoing pressure reduction (37). Repeated attempts at hydrostatic or pneumatic reduction are not indicated once the diagnosis is established.

INTUSSUSCEPTION IN ADULTS

Intussusception in adults is an unusual problem that may comprise 5% to 15% of all cases of intussusceptions in

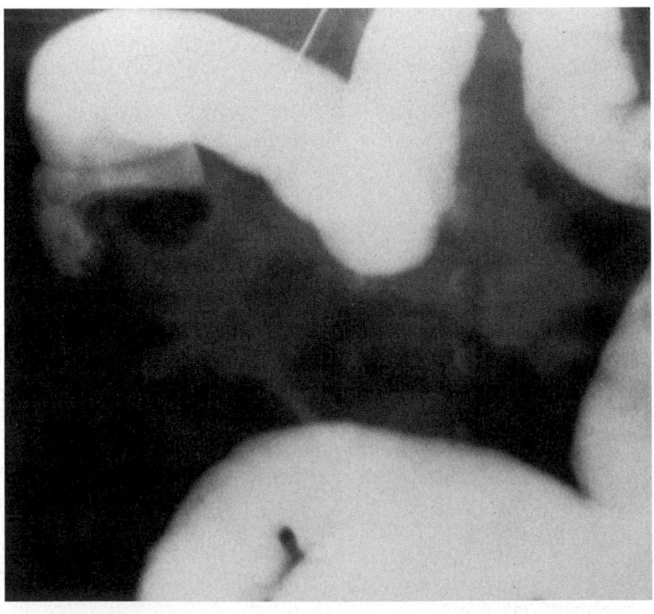

FIGURE 82-8. A 6-week-old patient who presented with failure to thrive, feces positive for occult blood, and intermittent symptoms of intestinal obstruction since the first week of life was found to have a nonreducible intussusception with persistent cecal filling defect on contrast enema. At exploration, the infant was found to have a cecal leiomyosarcoma as an intussusception lead point, which was resected.

large general hospitals (3,38). More than 90% of intussusceptions in adults have lead points, and almost one-half of these lead points are malignant neoplasms. Because of the high associated incidence of surgical lead points, intussusceptions in adults are generally not reducible by air contrast or hydrostatic enemas.

In adults, more than one-half of colocolic intussusceptions are associated with malignant neoplasms, and primary resection without manual reduction is recomm ended. Enteroenteric intussusceptions may be associated with postoperative intussusception, congenital anomalies, benign and malignant neoplasms, and enteric tubes passed for feeding. Manual reduction followed by more localized resection is appropriate because the incidence of carcinoma complicating intussusception of the small intestine is low.

In tropical countries, adults account for 40% to 50% of the reported cases of intussusception. Unlike in the United States and Great Britain, most intussusceptions in adults in tropical countries are idiopathic and not related to surgical lead points. This discrepancy has been ascribed to parasitic infestations, amebic ulcers, and diet, but the true cause of tropical intussusception is unknown.

REFERENCES

1. Reymond RD. The mechanism of intussusception: a theoretical analysis of the phenomenon. *Br J Radiol* 1972;45:1.
2. Ong NT, Beasley SW. The leadpoint in intussusception. *J Pediatr Surg* 1990;25:640.
3. Pang L-C. Intussusception revisited: clinicopathologic analysis of 261 cases, with emphasis on pathogenesis. *South Med J* 1989;82:215.
4. West KW, Stephens B, Vane DW, et al. Intussusception: current management in infants and children. *Surgery* 1987;102:704.
5. Losek JD, Fiete RL. Intussusception and the diagnostic value of testing stool for occult blood. *Am J Emerg Med* 1991;9:1.
6. Meradji M, Hussain SM, Robben SGF, et al. Plain film diagnosis in intussusception. *Br J Radiol* 1994;67:147.
7. Eklöf O, Thönell S. Conventional abdominal radiography as a means to rule out ileo-caecal intussusception. *Acta Radiol [Diagn] (Stockh)* 1984;25:265.
8. Johnson JF, Woisard KK. Ileocolic intussusception: new sign on the supine cross-table lateral radiograph. *Radiology* 1989;170:483.
9. White SJ, Blane CE. Intussusception: additional observations on the plain radiograph. *AJR* 1982;139:511.
10. Ravitch MM, McCune RM Jr. Reduction of intussusception by hydrostatic pressure: an experimental study. *Bull Johns Hopkins Hosp* 1948;82:550.
11. Kuta AJ, Benator RM. Intussusception: hydrostatic pressure equivalents for barium and meglumine sodium diatrizoate. *Radiology* 1990;175:125.
12. Mortensson W, Eklöf O, Laurin S. Hydrostatic reduction of childhood intussusception: the role of adjuvant glucagon medication. *Acta Radiol [Diagn] (Stockh)* 1984;25:261.
13. Fishman MC, Borden S, Cooper A. The dissection sign of nonreducible ileocolic intussusception. *AJR* 1984;143:5.
14. Stephenson CA, Seibert JJ, Strain JD, et al. Intussusception: clinical and radiographic factors influencing reducibility. *Pediatr Radiol* 1989;20:57.
15. Barr LL, Stansberry SD, Swischuk LE. Significance of age, duration, obstruction and the dissection sign in intussusception. *Pediatr Radiol* 1990;20:454.
16. Pierro A, Donnell SC, Paraskevopoulou C, et al. Indications for laparotomy after hydrostatic reduction for intussusception. *J Pediatr Surg* 1993;28:1154.
17. Ein SH, Palder SB, Alton DJ, et al. Intussusception: toward less surgery? *J Pediatr Surg* 1994;29:433.
18. Connolly B, Alton DJ, Ein SH, et al. Partially reduced intussusception: when are repeated delayed reduction attempts appropriate? *Pediatr Radiol* 1995;25:104.
19. Riebel TW, Nasir R, Weber K. US-guided hydrostatic reduction of intussusception in children. *Radiology* 1993;188:513.
20. Katz ME, Kolm P. Intussusception reduction 1991: an international survey of pediatric radiologists. *Pediatr Radiol* 1992;22:318.
21. Ein SH. Recurrent intussusception in children. *J Pediatr Surg* 1975;10:751.
22. Eklöf O, Reiter S. Recurrent intussusception: analysis of a series treated with hydrostatic reduction. *Acta Radiol [Diagn] (Stockh)* 1978;19:250.
23. Liu KW, MacCarthy J, Guiney EJ, et al. Intussusception: current trends in management. *Arch Dis Child* 1986;61:75.
24. Beasley SW, Auldist AW, Stokes KB. Recurrent intussusception: barium or surgery? *Aust N Z J Surg* 1987;57:11.
25. Stringer MD, Pledger G, Drakc DP. Childhood deaths from intussusception in England and Wales, 1984–9. *Br Med J* 1992;304:737.
26. Holsclaw DS, Rocmans C, Shwachman H. Intussusception in patients with cystic fibrosis. *Pediatrics* 1971;48:51.
27. Cull DL, Rosario V, Lally KP, et al. Surgical implications of Henoch-Schönlein purpura. *J Pediatr Surg* 1990;25:741.
28. Martinez-Frontanilla LA, Haase GM, Ernster JA, et al. Surgical complications in Henoch-Schönlein purpura. *J Pediatr Surg* 1984;19:434.
29. Ein SH, Ferguson JM. Intussusception: the forgotten postoperative obstruction. *Arch Dis Child* 1982;57:788.
30. Holcomb GW III, Ross AJ III, O'Neill JA Jr. Postoperative intussusception: increasing frequency or increasing awareness? *South Med J* 1991;84:1334.
31. West KW, Stephens B, Rescorla FJ, et al. Postoperative intussusception: experience with 36 cases in children. *Surgery* 1988;104:781.
32. Janik JS. Nonischemic intussusception. *J Pediatr Surg* 1977;12:567.
33. Shekhawat NS, Prabhakar G, Sinha DD, et al. Nonischemic intussusception in childhood. *J Pediatr Surg* 1992;27:1433.
34. Patriquin HB, Afshani E, Effman E, et al. Neonatal intussusception: report of 12 cases. *Radiology* 1977;125:463.
35. Jennings C, Kelleher J. Intussusception: influence of age on reducibility. *Pediatr Radiol* 1984;14:292.
36. Bettenay F, Beasley SW, de Campo JF, et al. Intussusception: clinical prediction of outcome of barium reduction. *Aust N Z J Surg* 1988;58:899.
37. Ein SH, Mercer S, Humphry A, et al. Colon perforation during attempted barium enema reduction of intussusception. *J Pediatr Surg* 1981;16:313.
38. Agha FP. Intussusception in adults. *AJR* 1986;146:527.

Chapter 83

Tumors of the Small Bowel

Nicholas A. Shorter

Tumors of the small bowel are uncommon at any age. Those occurring in children are almost all non-Hodgkin's lymphomas (NHL). The small intestine contains a mucosal epithelial layer, smooth muscle, connective tissue, and gut-associated lymphoid tissue, and each of these tissues can give rise to tumors. It is unknown why neoplastic transformation of the rapidly dividing mucosal cells is so infrequent. Primary smooth muscle tumors are also rare in all age groups, so this chapter focuses on the small bowel lymphomas of childhood.

CLASSIFICATION

Whereas most cases of NHL in adults arise in the lymph nodes, almost all cases in children are extranodal in origin and are histologically diffuse. The classification of the childhood tumors continues to evolve as more becomes known about the molecular biology of the different tumor cell types. The childhood NHL are currently divided into four groups (1,2):

1. Lymphoblastic lymphoma (indistinguishable from acute lymphoblastic leukemia)
2. The B-cell lymphomas, which include Burkitt's lymphoma (BL), the most common; Burkitt-like lymphoma (BLL); and large B-cell lymphoma (LBCL) (BL and BLL were previously called undifferentiated or small, noncleaved cell lymphoma)
3. Anaplastic large cell lymphoma
4. Other peripheral T-cell lymphomas

Most lymphoblastic tumors are of T-cell origin. BL, BLL, and LBCL arise from B cells and fall on a continuous spectrum of histologic appearance. The principal histologic difference between BL and BLL is the degree of cellular pleomorphism. Anaplastic large cell lymphomas are T-cell or null cell derived. It is controversial whether there is also a B-cell–derived form of large cell lymphoma. Without question, it will be possible to subdivide these tumors further and classify them more accurately on the basis of more precise molecular and genetic differences.

Nicholas A. Shorter: Pediatric Surgery, SUNY-Downstate Medical Center, Brooklyn, New York 11203.

EPIDEMIOLOGY

In the United States, lymphoma is the third most common childhood neoplasm and accounts for about 10% of childhood cancers (3). NHL is rare in children younger than 5 years of age, and the incidence increases with age throughout life (2). For unknown reasons, the incidence in white children is twice that in blacks, and boys are affected twice as frequently as girls (2). Thirty percent to 40% of the cases of childhood NHL originate in the abdomen (3). In about one-half of these, the primary site is in the intestinal tract, most commonly in the small bowel and usually the ileum, although a precise figure is difficult to obtain because in extensive abdominal disease it is often impossible to know where the tumor originated.

Etiologic factors are not yet well understood, and, for unknown reasons, the incidence of NHL has been increasing over the last several decades in all geographic areas and in all age groups (4). In children, the increase has been greatest in teenagers (2). NHL is more common in other parts of the world, and the incidence of the different subtypes varies in different countries. The association between endemic BL and the Epstein-Barr virus (EBV) is well known, but the specific role of this virus, if any, in the pathogenesis of this disease remains unclear, especially in light of the much lower rate of association seen in the sporadic form. A role for other viruses is unproven. The association of African BL with areas of holoendemic malaria is also well known (5) and may relate either to the immunosuppressive effect of malaria, which could increase the number of EBV-infected B cells, or to malaria-induced B-cell hyperplasia, which could predispose to chromosomal translocation. Immunodeficiency syndromes, including human immunodeficiency virus (HIV) infection, are associated with an increased incidence of NHL. Inherited genetic abnormalities may play a role, as evidenced by the identification in BL of mutations of the *p*53 gene and of members of the retinoblastoma family (6,7). The role of ionizing radiation alone is probably a small one. There is an increased risk for the development of NHL in patients who have been previously treated with combined modality therapy for Hodgkin's disease or with chemotherapy for other solid tumors (8,9).

CELL BIOLOGY

Almost all childhood lymphomas of the small bowel are of B-cell origin, either BL or BLL, and in the United States, 90% of these childhood lymphomas present in the abdomen (8). These tumors bear B-cell antigens, such as CD 19 and CD 20, as well as surface immunoglobulins, almost exclusively IgM (2). They are negative for terminal deoxynucleotidyl transferase, an enzyme that is almost invariably present in lymphoblastic lymphoma (2). B-cells first develop in the bone marrow, and immature B-cells then migrate to the periphery (lymph nodes, spleen, gut, liver) where maturation is completed (10). The small bowel lymphomas of childhood have the immmunophenotypic characteristics of a mature B cell, indicating that final malignant transformation occurs relatively late in the B-cell differentiation pathway.

In the majority of BL cases, the cells show a specific chromosomal translocation of a portion of the long arm of chromosome 8 to chromosome 14 (2,8). As a result of this molecular rearrangement, the *c-myc* oncogene from chromosome 8 comes to lie next to immunoglobulin heavy chain constant region sequences, resulting in abnormal *c-myc* activation. In a small proportion of cases, the translocation is from chromosome 2 or 22 to chromosome 8, which activates *c-myc* by putting it next to light chain constant region sequences (2,8). These translocations probably occur during the normal phase of immunoglobulin gene rearrangement. The subsequent inappropriate production of the c-myc protein presumably maintains the cell in a proliferating state rather than allowing it to enter a resting one [although normally this would lead to cell death via apoptosis (11), suggesting that other genetic modifications are also occurring]. Why these translocations occur is unknown, and it is also unclear whether they represent the primary or a secondary step in the development of the malignancy. A deficiency in DNA repair has been postulated to be a predisposing factor (8). The typical chromosome 8 break points are different in different regions of the world (2). Similar translocations may be seen in BLLs and LBCLs (2).

Mutations in the p53 tumor suppressor protein have been identified in about one-third of BLs, and the presence of mutation is independent of the geographic origin of the tumor, the 8;14 chromosomal break point locations, and the association of EBV (6,7). Mutations in members of the retinoblastoma family of proteins have also been reported (12). The exact role of the EBV in the development of BL is unknown (5). In 95% of African tumors and 40% to 80% of tumors in other developing countries, the cells carry the genome of this virus, but in North America only 15% of the tumors are positive. When EBV is present, it is unclear whether the virus plays an active, essential role in neoplastic transformation or merely predisposes to transformation by producing immortalized clones. The geographic differences in the rate of EBV association with NHL do not simply reflect the rate of exposure to the virus because even patients with negative tumors generally have serum antibodies to EBV (2). However, it may reflect the age of infection, which is typically much earlier in developing countries than it is in more affluent ones (2).

CLINICAL PRESENTATION, DIAGNOSIS, AND STAGING

Small bowel lymphomas typically present with abdominal pain, bowel obstruction, gastrointestinal (GI) bleeding, or perforation. Perforation has been associated with an extremely poor prognosis (13). There may be a palpable mass, most commonly in the right lower quadrant, and in extensive cases ascites may occur. The intramural tumor can act as the lead point of an intussusception. In most cases, symptoms have been present for only a short time, and constitutional symptoms such as fever and weight loss are uncommon (3). Rarely, with extensive disease, there can be ureteric obstruction, symptoms of venous obstruction, or neurological impairment due to neuroforaminal invasion and spinal cord compression.

More than one-half of the patients with abdominal tumors come to urgent exploration as a result of their presentation with an acute abdomen. The differential diagnosis usually does not include lymphoma, and the operative findings are usually unexpected (14). In another group—those with a palpable or radiologically identified mass but without acute symptomatology—the diagnosis is made at the time of a planned laparotomy and biopsy. If ascites are present, paracentesis may yield the diagnosis, and in some patients with extensive tumor spread, bone marrow sampling or superficial lymph node biopsy may be diagnostic. The role of laparoscopy will likely increase in the evaluation of a number of these patients. Diagnosis requires obtaining adequate tissue and proper handling of the specimens to ensure the necessary immunotyping and cytogenetic studies can be performed in addition to routine histologic examination. Some patients present only with chronic, often vague, abdominal pain. In the absence of a palpable mass or obstruction, diagnosis of a small bowel lesion can be difficult. A filling defect may be visible on a small bowel barium study, or a small mass may be identified on a computed tomography scan using oral contrast. However, when only nonspecific symptoms are present, even if studies are obtained, the diagnosis may prove elusive until other symptoms appear as a result of further disease progression.

It is recognized that all cases of childhood NHL are systemic from the onset and require chemotherapy. Thus, staging plays a different role in NHL than it does in Hodgkin's disease. The goal is to evaluate overall tumor burden, which is the single most important prognostic factor (2). Serum lactate dehydrogenase levels correlate with tumor burden and can be used both as a prognostic factor and to monitor response to therapy (15). The most widely used staging system is the St. Jude staging system for NHL (Table 83-1). The major shortcoming of this staging system is that stage III includes patients with a wide range of tumor burdens (2).

Most patients with small bowel tumors will have a laparotomy, either for diagnosis alone or to treat an acute abdominal process. In addition to obtaining adequate material for diagnosis, a full exploration should be performed at that time to evaluate the extent of intraabdominal disease. For staging purposes, patients with disease localized to the bowel and its mesentery must be distinguished from those with extensive intraabdominal spread. Disease should be looked for in the liver, spleen, kidneys, pancreas, peritoneal surfaces, ovaries, and retroperitoneum (16). In most cases involvement can be determined grossly, with sampling of suspect nodes or lesions. A splenectomy is not performed, even if the spleen is involved, and routine liver biopsies are not indicated unless they are requested as part of an ongoing protocol. Staging laparotomy is not indicated in those patients in whom the diagnosis of an intraabdominal NHL has been made in some other way, such as via bone marrow sampling.

Further routine studies include chest radiographs, bone scans, bone marrow sampling, and lumbar puncture. Other studies are obtained on an individual basis. Gallium scans are a useful whole body screen because the lymphoma cells avidly take up the isotope. Bone marrow involvement at presentation is seen in about 20% of patients and may be occult in another 20% (8). Central nervous system (CNS) involvement at presentation is uncommon, but spread frequently occurs in the absence of prophylactic therapy (8).

TABLE 83-1 St. Jude Staging System for Non-Hodgkin's Lymphoma.

Stage	Description
Stage I	A single tumor (extranodal) or single anatomic area (nodal), with the exclusion of mediastinum or abdomen
Stage II	A single tumor (extranodal) with regional node involvement
	Two or more nodal areas on the same side of the diaphragm
	Two single (extranodal) tumors with or without regional node involvement on the same side of the diaphragm
	A primary gastrointestinal tract tumor with or without involvement of associated mesenteric nodes only
Stage III	Two single tumors (extranodal) on opposite sides of the diaphragm
	Two or more nodal areas above and below the diaphragm
	All primary intrathoracic tumors (mediastinal, pleural, thymic)
	All extensive primary intraabdominal disease
	All paraspinal or epidural tumors, regardless of other tumor sites
Stage IV	Any of the above with initial central nervous system or bone marrow involvement

TREATMENT

Most small bowel lymphomas are discovered at the time of laparotomy. If the disease is restricted to the bowel, it should be resected (only short resections are necessary because extensive bowel involvement is not seen in the absence of widespread intraabdominal disease), with grossly negative margins and with resection of the associated mesentery (14,16,17). Resection in this setting correlates with a favorable prognosis (which may reflect the small volume of disease rather than a therapeutic effect of the resection itself), is associated with minimal complications, and has the additional benefits of eliminating the risk of tumor lysis syndrome and the chance of bowel perforation or GI hemorrhage in that segment after the initiation of chemotherapy (14). With more extensive disease, attempts at tumor resection are not justified because even extensive debulking does not improve survival. Such procedures can lead to complications such as acute renal failure and hemorrhage and can result in a delay in the initiation of chemotherapy (14,16). Biopsy only is indicated. In this setting, however, a segmental bowel resection may still be necessary to treat the presenting acute abdominal process.

In the setting of an emergent abdominal exploration, intraoperative decision making should be straightforward. Frozen sections may be able to confirm the diagnosis of lymphoma (although not the subtype), but, when negative, cannot be relied on. With extensive disease, the diagnosis is usually self-evident from the gross appearance. In disease limited to the bowel, the diagnosis may be suspected by the experienced eye, but sometimes is not confirmed until the permanent sections are examined. In the latter group, the need for resection is usually obvious from the need to treat the acute abdominal process. On occasion, it may not be possible intraoperatively to distinguish between a nonobstructing inflammatory intestinal mass and a lymphoma. In that situation, resection is justified on clinical suspicion alone. The importance of proper handling of lymphoma specimens cannot be overemphasized. It is mandatory in cases of diagnostic uncertainty to alert the pathologist to the possibility of lymphoma. Inadequate processing of the material results in the loss of critical diagnostic information, which has important therapeutic significance.

Chemotherapy is the mainstay of modern treatment of childhood NHL. Radiation has little if any role because it has been shown to increase toxicity without providing any therapeutic advantage (2,18,19). Because these tumors grow rapidly, treatment should begin quickly. Any significant delay can worsen prognosis because of the increase in the patient's overall tumor burden. Patients with extensive intraabdominal spread may have significant biochemical abnormalities (elevated uric acid levels, hyperphosphatemia, hyperkalemia) that should be corrected rapidly before the initiation of therapy (2,3,8). These children are at risk during therapy for the tumor lysis syndrome, with development of urate nephropathy and renal failure, sometimes requiring dialysis. Adequate hydration, the maintenance of high urine flow, and allopurinol or urate oxidase administration are vital to prevent this (2,3,8,20).

A number of chemotherapy protocols are effective in treating the childhood B-cell lymphomas (2). Risk stratification based on tumor burden is key to the goal of providing adequate treatment while minimizing the risk of toxicity (15,18). Patients with limited abdominal disease (i.e., completely resected intestinal tumors) require less intensive treatment than those with more extensive disease. CNS prophylactic intrathecal chemotherapy is mandatory, except in some patients with completely resected abdominal disease. Short courses of very intensive therapy appear as effective as more prolonged treatment. Refinements are continually being made in all protocols in an attempt to decrease the morbidity of treatment. Local abdominal recurrence is rare as the sole site of disease; therefore, second-look surgical procedures are rarely indicated (16).

OUTCOME

Survival from intestinal lymphoma has improved dramatically since the 1970s (2). A survival rate greater than 95% is now expected in children with totally resected small bowel disease. For more extensive disease, cure rates range between 70% and 90% in those patients without bone marrow or CNS involvement. Although initial bone marrow and CNS involvement have correlated with a worse prognosis, refinements in treatment are now leading to improved survival even in these groups. Recurrence is usually associated with a poor prognosis, although some salvage therapies involving autologous bone marrow transplants appear to show better results, but only with documented chemotherapy-sensitive tumors (2). As treatment has improved, recurrent disease has become rare and is almost never observed beyond 1 year from the initiation of therapy (2). Most treatment failures are now due either to primary resistance of the tumor or to toxic death (2).

OTHER TUMORS

Although rare, numerous benign tumors have been reported in the small bowel, including neurofibromas, hemangiomas, juvenile polyps (rare sporadic lesions or in the setting of a juvenile polyposis syndrome), adenomatous polyps (in familial polyposis or Gardner syndrome), hamartomas (especially in Peutz-Jeghers syndrome), inflammatory pseudotumor, and intestinal fibromatosis (nearly exclusively in newborns) (21). When symptomatic, these tumors commonly present with intestinal obstruction or bleeding, and, at times, may cause intussusception. Appropriate therapy is resection.

Carcinoid tumors are found rarely in the small intestine (22,23). These tumors contain argentaffin cells derived from endocrine cells of the bowel. There is a female predominance in childhood (23,24). Carcinoids have been reported to occur throughout the alimentary tract, but arise most commonly in the appendix or in the ileum. In rare cases, small bowel carcinoid may be multicentric (25). Most carcinoids are benign, but malignancy can occur. The carcinoid syndrome is very rare. In tumors restricted to the bowel, resection is curative. Even with metastases, prolonged survival is possible because of the indolent nature of many of these tumors (26). An unexplained association has been noted between carcinoid tumor and colonic adenocarcinoma (23).

Small intestinal smooth muscle tumors, leiomyomas and leiomyosarcomas, are very rare in children, but pediatric leiomyosarcomas occur most commonly in the GI tract (27,28). Intestinal obstruction is the most common clinical presentation, and there is often a palpable mass. Bowel perforation is not uncommon and may occur with either benign or malignant lesions (29). GI leiomyosarcomas are slightly more common in girls, and about one-third present in the first month of life. The differentiation between the benign and the malignant forms can be difficult, and is based on the mitotic rate, tumor size, and extent of necrosis. For benign lesions, resection alone is adequate. In the malignant form, a favorable outcome is associated with low grade and complete surgical excision (27). Malignant leiomyosarcomas tend to be locally invasive, and local recurrence is most frequent. Chemotherapy and radiation therapy do not seem to improve survival. There may be differences between the behavior of leiomyosarcoma in children and adults; that is, younger patients, especially infants, tend to have a better outcome (29,30). Infantile intestinal leiomyosarcoma has an excellent prognosis with resection alone regardless of tumor grade, suggesting a different disease process from that seen in adults and older children (30). An unexplained association has been noted between smooth muscle tumors in children and immune deficiency states, including HIV infection. Some of the AIDS- linked tumors may be associated with the EBV (31). There are some data suggesting that irradiation may predispose to the development of leiomyosarcoma, but this is far from being proven (28,32). A 12;14 translocation has been identified in a childhood leiomyosarcoma that is similar to one seen in adults, suggesting a pathogenic role for this genetic rearrangement (28,32). A role has also been postulated for the retinoblastoma gene because leiomyosarcomas have been reported in patients with bilateral retinoblastoma, both within and outside the radiation field, and mutations at the RB1 locus have now been reported in sporadic leiomyosarcomas (28).

Adenocarcinoma of the small bowel can occur in association with the Peutz-Jeghers syndrome (33). Patients with familial polyposis, Gardner syndrome, and small bowel Crohn's disease are also at risk for progression to small bowel malignancy (26). Metastatic lesions from other tumors can be seen in the small intestine, either as a result of hematogenous spread or direct peritoneal implantation.

REFERENCES

1. Harris NL, Jaffe ES, Diebold J, et al. World Health Organization classification of neoplastic diseases of the hematopoietic and lymphoid tissues. *J Clin Oncol* 1999;17:3835.
2. Magrath IT. Malignant non-Hodgkin's lymphomas in children. In: Pizzo PA, Poplack DG, eds. *Principles and practice of pediatric oncology*, 4th ed. Philadelphia: Lippincott Williams & Wilkins, 2002:661.
3. Link MP. Non-Hodgkin's lymphoma in children. *Pediatr Clin North Am* 1985;32:699.
4. Hartge P, Devesa SS, Fraumeni JF. Hodgkin's and non-Hodgkin's lymphomas. *Cancer Surv* 1994;19-20:423.
5. Facer CA, Playfair JHL. Malaria, Epstein-Barr virus, and the genesis of lymphomas. *Adv Cancer Res* 1989;53:33.
6. Bhatia KG, Gutierrez MI, Huppi K, et al. The pattern of p53 mutations in Burkitt's lymphoma differs from that of solid tumors. *Cancer Res* 1992;52:4273.
7. Gaidano G, Ballerini P, Gong JZ, et al. p53 mutations in human lymphoid malignancies: association with Burkitt lymphoma and chronic lymphocytic leukemia. *Proc Natl Acad Sci U S A* 1991;88:5413.
8. Magrath I. Malignant non-Hodgkin's lymphomas in children. In: Pizzo PA, Poplack DG, eds. *Principles and practice of pediatric oncology.* Philadelphia: JB Lippincott, 1993:537.
9. Zarrabi MH, Rosner F. Second neoplasms in Hodgkin's disease: current controversies. *Hematol Oncol Clin North Am* 1989;3:303.
10. Nairn R, Helbert M. *Immunology.* New York: Mosby, 2002.
11. Prendergast GC. Mechanisms of apoptosis by c-myc. *Oncogene* 1999;18:2967.
12. Cinti C, Leoncini L, Nyongo A, et al. Genetic alterations of the retinoblastoma-related gene RB2/p130 identify different pathogenetic mechanisms in and among Burkitt's lymphoma subtypes. *Am J Pathol* 2000;156:751.
13. Yanchar NL, Bass J. Poor outcome of gastrointestinal perforations associated with childhood abdominal non-Hodgkin's lymphoma. *J Pediatr Surg* 1999;34:1169.
14. LaQuaglia MP, Stolar CJH, Krailo M, et al. The role of surgery in abdominal non-Hodgkin's lymphoma: experience from the Children's Cancer Study Group. *J Pediatr Surg* 1992;27:230.
15. Reiter A. Schrappe M, Tiemann M, et al. Improved treatment results in childhood B-cell neoplasms with tailored intensification of therapy: a report of the Berlin-Frankfurt-Munster group trial NHL-BFM 90. *Blood* 1999;94:3294.
16. Shamberger RC, Weinstein HJ. The role of surgery in abdominal Burkitt's lymphoma. *J Pediatr Surg* 1992;27:236.
17. Attarbaschi A, Mann G, Dworzak M, et al. The role of surgery in the treatment of pediatric B-cell non-Hodgkin's lymphoma. *J Pediatr Surg* 2002;37:1470.
18. Link MP, Shuster JJ, Donaldson SS, et al. Treatment of children and young adults with early-stage non-Hodgkin's lymphoma. *N Engl J Med* 1997;337:1304.
19. Link MP, Donaldson SS, Berard CW, et al. Results of treatment of childhood localized non-Hodgkin's lymphoma with combination chemotherapy with or without radiotherapy. *N Engl J Med* 1990; 322:1169.
20. Wossman W, Schrappe M, Meyer U, et al. Incidence of tumor lysis syndrome in children with advanced stage Burkitt's lymphoma/leukemia before and after introduction of prophylactic use of urate oxidase. *Ann Hematol* 2003;82:160.
21. Dahms BB.The gastrointestinal tract. In: Stocker JT, Dehner LP, eds. *Pediatric pathology.* Philadelphia: JB Lippincott, 1992:653.
22. Grundy R, Pritchard J. Carcinomas and other rare tumors. In: Voute PA, Barrett A, Lemerle J, eds. *Cancer in children.* Berlin: Springer-Verlag, 1992:339.
23. Spunt SL, Pratt CB, Rao BN, et al. Childhood carcinoid tumors: the St. Jude Children's Research Hospital experience. *J Pediatr Surg* 2000;35:1282.
24. Bethel CAI, Bhattacharyya N, Hutchinson C, et al. Alimentary tract malignancies in children. *J Pediatr Surg* 1997;32:1004.
25. Ford EG.Gastrointestinal tumors. In: Andrassy RJ, ed. *Pediatric surgical oncology.* Philadelphia: WB Saunders, 1998:289.
26. Leichtner AM. Intestinal neoplasms. In: Walker WA, Durie PR, Hamilton JR, et al., eds. *Pediatric gastrointestinal disease.* Philadelphia: BC Decker, 1991:771.
27. Angel CA, Gant LL, Parham DM, et al. Leiomyosarcomas in children: clinical and pathologic characteristics. *Pediatr Surg Int* 1992;7:116.
28. Miser JS, Pappo AS, Triche TJ, et al. Other soft tissue sarcomas of childhood. In: Pizzo PA, Poplack DG, eds. *Principles and practice of pediatric oncology*, 4th ed. Philadelphia: Lippincott Williams & Wilkins, 2002:973.
29. Goh DW, Raafat F, Gornall P, et al. Intestinal leiomyoma in neonates. *Pediatr Surg Int* 1990;5:208.
30. Simpson BB, Reynolds EM, Kim SH, et al. Infantile intestinal leiomyosarcoma: surgical resection (without adjuvant therapy) for cure. *J Pediatr Surg* 1996;31:1577.
31. McClain KL, Leach CT, Jenson HB, et al. Association of Epstein-Barr virus with leiomyosarcomas in children with AIDS. *N Engl J Med* 1995;332:55.
32. Miser JS, Pritchard DJ, Triche TJ, et al. The other soft tissue sarcomas of childhood. In: Pizzo PA, Poplack DG, eds. *Principles and practice of pediatric oncology.* Philadelphia: JB Lippincott, 1993:823.
33. Cordts AE, Chabot JR. Jejunal carcinoma in a child. *J Pediatr Surg* 1983;18:180.

Chapter 84

Crohn's Disease

Thomas T. Sato and Subra Kugathasan

INTRODUCTION

Inflammatory bowel disease includes the similar but distinct entities of Crohn's disease, ulcerative colitis, and in some cases, indeterminate colitis. Inflammatory bowel disease is characterized by chronic, idiopathic gastrointestinal (GI) inflammation with typical onset in late childhood or adolescence (1). Although inflammatory bowel disease is relatively rare in the pediatric population, the effects of the disease can be quite serious and its treatment is lifelong. The surgeon's role in the management of inflammatory bowel disease is evolving as significant new therapeutic interventions are being introduced into clinical use (2).

Although the term *inflammatory bowel disease* is used for a variety of chronic idiopathic inflammatory bowel disorders, Crohn's disease and ulcerative colitis comprise the vast majority of observed pediatric cases. Crohn's disease is characterized by a transmural inflammatory process that can involve any region of the GI tract, whereas ulcerative colitis is a mucosal inflammatory process limited to the colon. Although there are several similarities in the manifestations of inflammatory bowel disease in children compared with adults, there are also substantial differences and unique issues that arise in the pediatric population. In particular, Crohn's disease is more common than ulcerative colitis in children, and when ulcerative colitis is diagnosed during childhood, the finding of extensive pancolitis is not unusual. In addition, children with inflammatory bowel disease may experience significant growth impairment, pubertal delay, and difficulty with psychosocial adjustment during adolescence and early adulthood. Ulcerative colitis is discussed in detail in Chapter 87.

Thomas T. Sato: Medical College of Wisconsin, Division of Pediatric Surgery, Children's Hospital of Wisconsin, Milwaukee, Wisconsin 53201.

Subra Kugathasan: Medical College of Wisconsin and Inflammatory Bowel Disease Program, Division of Pediatric Gastroenterology, Children's Hospital of Wisconsin, Milwaukee, Wisconsin 53201.

Epidemiology

The highest disease rates for inflammatory bowel disease are in western countries. Epidemiologic data are consistent with a gradual increase in the incidence of Crohn's disease and ulcerative colitis since the mid-1950s (3,4). Both genetic and environmental factors appear to interact to make specific individuals susceptible to the disease (5).

Retrospective European studies and a prospective, population-based study in Great Britain have demonstrated that the incidence of inflammatory bowel disease has increased since the mid-1970s (6–8). Generally, there has been greater increase in the incidence of Crohn's disease than ulcerative colitis in Europe. An initial, systematic, population-based epidemiologic study in North America has recently been completed. All children younger than 18 years of age newly diagnosed with inflammatory bowel disease in the state of Wisconsin over a 2-year period were evaluated. The incidence of inflammatory bowel disease was 7 per 100,000 children, with equivalent incidence across ethnic groups and population density. Urbanization and population density did not appear to be related to a change in the incidence of the disease. Only 11% of the patients had a family history of inflammatory bowel disease, suggesting that the pathogenesis of inflammatory bowel disease is multifactorial (9).

Etiology of Inflammatory Bowel Disease

The etiology of inflammatory bowel disease remains unknown. The chronic nature of the inflammatory process in both Crohn's disease and ulcerative colitis suggests that there is both an initiating event, as well as factors that allow perpetuation of the GI inflammatory response. Despite the fact that Crohn's disease and ulcerative colitis are distinct clinical entities, they are both characterized by an inflammatory response that may overlap and make definitive clinical diagnosis difficult. A widely accepted hypothesis to explain the observed clinical manifestations of inflammatory bowel disease is that an environmental trigger induces an inflammatory response in genetically susceptible individuals (10). Following establishment of the inflammatory response, it is speculated that host genetic factors play a substantial role in the trajectory of the inflammatory process. Given the broad clinical spectrum of inflammatory bowel disease, it is likely that there are several genetic loci that lead to host susceptibility, as well as different patterns in the host inflammatory response.

There is substantial evidence that specific genes may influence the development and the progression of inflammatory bowel disease. The NOD2/CARD15 gene is associated with Crohn's disease. In particular, mutations of the NOD2/CARD15 gene may contribute to the phenotypic expression of inflammatory bowel disease in children with early onset of disease and/or with a strong family history of Crohn's disease (observed in the Ashkenazi Jewish population) (11,12). As many as 17% to 40% of patients with Crohn's disease may have mutation(s) in the NOD2 gene, which is believed to regulate the inflammatory response to exposure to bacterial lipopolysaccharide (13). Genetic predisposition to an altered or deficient response to bacterial lipopolysaccharide in the intestinal lumen may be one mechanism that makes specific individuals more susceptible for the development of Crohn's disease. The use of genetic information may allow estimation of an unaffected person's risk of developing inflammatory bowel disease, the expected disease progression of an already affected individual, and specific targeting of therapy based on pharmacogenetic principles.

The triggering event or agent that initiates inflammatory bowel disease in a genetically susceptible individual is of considerable interest. The GI mucosal barrier is a highly regulated and immunologically active surface with constant inflammatory challenge from bacteria. Involved colonic mucosa from patients with established inflammatory bowel disease has been observed to permit significantly more bacterial adhesion compared with specimens from healthy subjects (14). Intact mucosa in adjacent areas of bowel appears to maintain barrier function against bacterial invasion, suggesting that mucosal changes in inflammatory bowel disease may compromise the barrier function. Once this barrier is compromised, expansion of the gut-associated lymphoid tissue, including the gut intraepithelial lymphocytes, occurs rapidly. Although the host inflammatory response is essential in the regulation of the GI tract, uncontrolled or persistent activation of the intestinal inflammatory response by elements of normally occurring bacterial flora may, in part, be responsible for the manifestations of the disease. Several studies have failed to identify a single infectious agent that is responsible for the initiation and establishment of the disease. In addition, there are currently no compelling data to suggest that selective decontamination of the GI tract is an effective preventive strategy for inflammatory bowel disease.

DIAGNOSIS

Clinical Presentation

A detailed history and physical examination remain the most important aspects in the evaluation of an adolescent with abdominal pain suspected of having inflammatory bowel disease. The clinical presentation of Crohn's disease varies with the anatomic location(s) of involvement, which can occur in any region of the GI tract. In comparison, the clinical presentation of ulcerative colitis is relatively uniform given that the primary disease is limited to the colon. Table 84-1 summarizes the presenting clinical symptoms and signs in Crohn's disease and ulcerative colitis in children. In general, the severity of GI inflammation reflects the severity of the clinical presentation.

Abdominal Pain

The most common presenting complaint of children and adolescents with inflammatory bowel disease is abdominal pain (2,15). Most children and adolescents ultimately diagnosed with inflammatory bowel disease do not present with the acute onset of abdominal pain; however, upon careful review, there is usually a history of recurrent or persistent pain over time. The pain may not be specific or

TABLE 84-1 Presenting Clinical Symptoms and Signs of Children Diagnosed with Crohn's Disease and Ulcerative Colitis.

	Crohn's Disease (%)	*Ulcerative Colitis (%)*
Abdominal pain	62–95	33–71
Diarrhea	66–77	67–90
Weight loss	80–92	39–43
Rectal bleeding	14–60	52–90
Growth impairment	30–33	6
Perirectal disease	25	0
Extraintestinal manifestation	15–25	2–16

Compiled from Refs. 2, 9, and 15–19.

well localized. Establishment of a diagnosis on the basis of symptoms and abdominal examination may be difficult. Given the pathophysiology, a high index of suspicion must be maintained when a child presents with a history of subacute or chronic abdominal pain. Abdominal pain associated with Crohn's disease tends to be severe and persistent, and may either awaken the adolescent from sleep or interfere with normal eating patterns. Involvement of the terminal ileum or ileocecal region with Crohn's disease is associated with a history of chronic or recurrent right lower quadrant abdominal pain that may mimic acute appendicitis in all aspects except symptom duration. A palpable mass may be present in the right lower quadrant secondary to an inflammatory phlegmon. In 10% of pediatric patients with Crohn's disease, odynophagia and dysphagia may be observed with esophageal involvement (15).

Diarrhea

The vast majority of children and adolescents with inflammatory bowel disease present with diarrhea at some point in their clinical course (15). Whether from Crohn's disease or ulcerative colitis, involvement of the colon may often be associated with grossly bloody diarrhea. With distal colonic involvement, the diarrhea may be characterized by urgency, tenesmus, and incontinence, and is often nocturnal. Crohn's disease involving only the small bowel may also present with episodic diarrhea (16,17). In conjunction with abdominal pain, children with significant, persistent diarrhea may become more socially isolated, particularly in school where frequent trips to the restroom are either discouraged or embarrassing.

Hematochezia

The presence of hematochezia suggests colonic involvement. Adolescents with Crohn's disease of the small intestine are less likely to present with rectal bleeding than individuals with ulcerative colitis (18,19). As many as one-half of all children with inflammatory bowel disease present with relatively mild symptoms, characterized by less than four stools per day and intermittent hematochezia (20). Stools may have only streaks of blood, or they may only be hemoccult positive. Approximately 30% of children with either Crohn's disease or ulcerative colitis are moderately ill, presenting with gross hematochezia associated with frequent diarrhea. In 10% to 15% of cases of pediatric inflammatory bowel disease, patients present with acute, fulminant disease characterized by greater than six episodes of diarrhea per day with copious hematochezia that may require red blood cell transfusion. Fulminant colitis is a potentially life-threatening event that may occur in Crohn's colitis, ulcerative colitis, or indeterminate colitis. Clinical presentation of fulminant colitis includes abdominal pain, nausea, anorexia, and bloody diarrhea associated with systemic manifestations of tachycardia, hypotension, and diffuse abdominal distention and tenderness. Toxic megacolon, although rare in the pediatric age group, is a complication of inflammatory bowel disease that is a surgical emergency requiring prompt total abdominal colectomy and end ileostomy (21).

Weight Loss and Growth Impairment

As many as 80% of children and adolescents with Crohn's disease will have weight loss prior to definitive diagnosis (15,22). Weight loss is a more common finding in Crohn's disease than in ulcerative colitis in the pediatric population. In some children with Crohn's disease, the presenting clinical finding is linear growth deceleration (23). Deviation from growth velocity curves and height for age curves may precede the diagnosis of Crohn's disease, even in the absence of proven nutrient malabsorption or reduced caloric intake. In children with established Crohn's disease, the resting energy expenditure is generally normal (24). It is unknown why growth impairment occurs, although lack of adequate caloric intake secondary to abdominal pain, diarrhea, or anorexia may reflect active inflammatory disease, growth hormone resistance, or medication effects. Because the pubertal growth spurt accounts for approximately 16% of the adult height, disease onset in prepubertal children prior may have a substantial impact on total linear growth. Overall, the prevalence of significant growth impairment during childhood and adolescence in pediatric patients with inflammatory bowel disease is approximately 13% to 58% (18,25).

Delayed Puberty

Similar to deceleration of linear growth, the presence of inflammatory bowel disease in prepubertal children is associated with significant delay in puberty (26,27). Delayed or prolonged duration of puberty is more common in children with Crohn's disease than ulcerative colitis, particularly in children who have active disease without a history of remission, or in children with frequent disease exacerbations during the prepubertal period. Prepubertal onset of Crohn's disease has been reported to be associated with a delay in menarche until 16 years of age or older in 73% of girls; in comparison, girls with ulcerative colitis in this same study achieved puberty at age 14 years or younger (27). The delay in sexual maturation is multifactorial and is believed, in part, to reflect malnutrition. In some children with active Crohn's disease associated with growth arrest, supplemental caloric intake may be useful to promote puberty onset and increased growth velocity (28). Adequate caloric intake alone does not guarantee appropriate progression through puberty and increased growth velocity for all children with active inflammatory bowel disease, suggesting that there are other factors contributing to delayed sexual maturation. In adolescents with delayed puberty secondary to active Crohn's disease, intestinal resection of the active inflammatory bowel has been associated with progression of puberty within 1 year of operative intervention (29). It is unknown why intestinal resection leads to progression of puberty in this population, but it is speculated that the inhibitory effects of inflammatory mediators such as tumor necrosis factor-alpha and interleukin-1 are reduced with removal of the inflammatory focus. Because both nutritional and inflammatory mediators can exert effects on the hypothalamic-pituitary-gonadal axis, decreased caloric intake and reduced body weight are associated with decreased activity of the hypothalamic neurons that produce gonadotropin releasing hormone. This can lead to delayed gonadal maturation and subsequent delay in puberty as observed in prepubertal children or adolescents with inflammatory bowel disease.

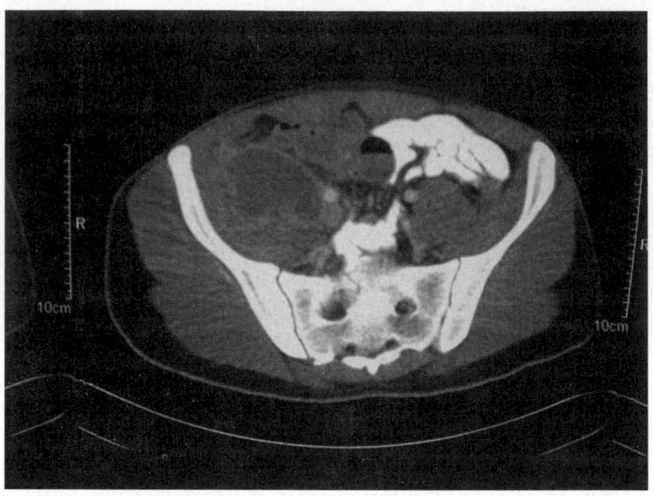

FIGURE 84-1. Computed tomography imaging of ileocecal Crohn's disease with enteric fistula to the right psoas muscle, leading to abscess formation. The abscess was drained percutaneously prior to operative intestinal resection.

Perirectal Disease and Fistula

Perirectal and perianal disease, along with fistula formation, are unique findings in Crohn's disease. In children with Crohn's disease and perianal or perirectal disease, approximately 25% to 30% will have multiple anal skin tags, nonhealing anal fissures, perianal or perirectal fistulas, or perirectal abscess (30). Perirectal pain is unusual unless there is an abscess present, and suspicion for an abscess should be high in the presence of erythema, tenderness, and swelling in association with systemic symptoms such as fever. Crohn's disease should be considered in any child with recurrent, multiple, or persistent perianal abscesses or fistulas. In addition, Crohn's disease should be suspected in children with a history of weight loss, abdominal pain, diarrhea, and perianal disease. Rarely, perianal or perirectal involvement secondary to chronic granulomatous disease or tuberculosis may be encountered (31,32). A small percentage of adolescents may have aggressive and highly destructive perianal Crohn's disease as their predominant symptom (33), although multiple perianal and perineal fistula observed in adults with a "watering can" perineum are fortunately rare in the pediatric population. Significant perianal involvement with Crohn's disease in the pediatric population may be clinically misdiagnosed as nonaccidental traumatic injury secondary to sexual assault (34).

The most common fistulas encountered in Crohn's disease are enterocutaneous and comprise at least 80% of the clinical fistulas observed. Fistulas may occur between small and large intestine, vagina, bladder, and abdominal

TABLE 84-2 Clinical Features Distinguishing Crohn's Disease and Ulcerative Colitis.

Clinical Features	*Crohn's Disease*	*Ulcerative Colitis*
Age at onset	Childhood to adolescence	Adolescence to early adulthood
Distribution	Entire gastrointestinal (GI) tract	Colon only
	Skip lesions	Continuous proximal involvement from rectum
Weight loss	Common	Uncommon
Hematochezia	Uncommon	Common
Obstruction	Common	Uncommon
Fistula	More common	Uncommon
Perianal disease	More common	Uncommon
Risk of cancer	Controversial	Escalates with duration of disease
Radiology	Entire GI tract, particularly terminal ileum	Colon only
	Fistulas, strictures	Colitis
Pathology	Transmural inflammation	Mucosal inflammation
	Granulomas	Nongranulomatous inflammation

wall. Fistulas may present as localized drainage of enteric contents from the abdominal wall, perineum, or operative wound. Enteroenteric or enterocolic fistulas may present with malnutrition secondary to malabsorption. Patients with Crohn's disease presenting with a newly diagnosed intraabdominal, pelvic, or psoas abscess should be assumed to have a transmural fistula (Fig. 84-1).

Clinical features distinguishing Crohn's disease from ulcerative colitis are listed in Table 84-2.

EXTRAINTESTINAL MANIFESTATIONS

Established inflammatory bowel disease is often (25% to 35%) accompanied by diverse extraintestinal manifestations that can affect virtually any anatomic systems. The most common extraintestinal findings in children are involvement of the dermatologic, rheumatologic, ocular, and hepatobiliary systems. Severity of the extraintestinal manifestation is not necessarily related to the severity of inflammatory bowel disease, and it is uncommon for an extraintestinal manifestation to be the singular presenting event in children. These manifestations are observed in both Crohn's disease and ulcerative colitis.

Arthritis/Arthralgia

Symptoms related to arthritis, including ankylosing spondylitis or sacroilitis, and peripheral arthropathy (knees, ankle, hips, wrists, and elbows) have been well-described as coexisting or even preceding the development of GI symptoms of inflammatory bowel disease (35). Arthritis is more commonly observed with colonic involvement, and the severity of arthritic symptoms may be independent of the extent or severity of the inflammatory bowel disease. Arthritic symptoms may be transient and migratory in presentation. Clubbing of the fingers in children with Crohn's disease reflects the progression of hypertrophic osteoarthopathy of the distal finger joints.

Skin and Oropharyngeal Mucosa

A characteristic dermatologic finding in children or adolescents with inflammatory bowel disease is erythema nodosum or pyoderma gangrenosum. Erythema nodosum is an inflammatory lesion characterized by a raised, erythematous, painful nodule occurring over the tibia, lower leg, ankle, or extensor surfaces of the arms. Pyoderma gangrenosum is a small, painful skin pustule that coalesces into a larger, sterile abscess, forming a necrotic, deep, transdermal ulcer. The association between these skin lesions and the presence of inflammatory bowel disease is significant enough that children diagnosed with either skin lesion should undergo a complete GI workup even in the absence of GI symptoms (15).

Examination of the mouth and oropharynx is important in children and adolescents suspected of having inflammatory bowel disease. Aphthous ulcerations of the mouth or gums may accompany intestinal disease. In Crohn's disease, granulomatous inflammation of the lips, gums, and face have been described (36).

Ocular

Eye findings are uncommon in pediatric inflammatory bowel disease and can rarely be the sole presenting extraintestinal manifestation of disease. Uveitis, episcleritis, and iritis have been described and generally require ophthalmologic examination with a slit lamp.

Hepatobiliary/Pancreatic

Clinically significant hepatic involvement in association with inflammatory bowel disease is uncommon in the pediatric population, potentially reflecting a shorter duration of underlying disease. However, up to 14% of children diagnosed with inflammatory bowel disease may have abnormal serum aminotranferases at some point in their treatment. Chronic hepatitis or sclerosing cholangitis have been associated with long-standing inflammatory bowel disease and are generally observed in older age groups. However, when these abnormalities persist, further workup is necessary to rule out associated conditions, such as sclerosing cholangitis or chronic hepatitis. In children with primary sclerosing cholangitis associated with inflammatory bowel disease, intrahepatic disease predominates; common bile duct strictures appear to be less common (37). Therefore, primary sclerosing cholangitis should be suspected in any child or adolescent with chronic liver disease associated with inflammatory bowel disease despite normal serum alkaline phosphatase levels.

There are isolated reports of pancreatitis occurring in children with both ulcerative colitis and Crohn's disease (38). Duodenal involvement with Crohn's disease may occur, but is not a prerequisite for pancreatitis observed with inflammatory bowel disease.

Other

Abnormalities of the urethra, hydronephrosis, or hydroureter may be observed in established inflammatory bowel disease. Renal calculi and amyloidosis may also be present. Despite the tendency for hematochezia to be more common with inflammatory bowel disease of the colon, the presence of a microcytic, hypochromic iron-deficiency anemia is more common during the initial presentation of Crohn's disease than ulcerative colitis (9).

DIAGNOSTIC APPROACH

The diagnosis of inflammatory bowel disease is often delayed in children because the symptoms tend to be nonspecific and the index of suspicion for inflammatory bowel disease is relatively low among primary care physicians. The definitive diagnosis of inflammatory bowel disease is based on clinical, laboratory, radiologic, endoscopic, and pathologic evaluation. The differential diagnosis of chronic abdominal pain and diarrhea associated with weight loss includes viral and bacterial gastroenteritis, irritable bowel syndrome, parasitic infections, celiac disease, and cystic fibrosis. In the presence of hematochezia, the exclusion of intestinal infections by enteric pathogens such as *Salmonella, Shigella, Campylobacter, Yersinia, Escherichia coli* 0157/H7, and *Clostridium difficile* is necessary. Henoch-Schönlein purpura, Behçet's disease, hemolytic-uremic syndrome, or GI involvement from vasculitis should also be considered in the older child or adolescent presenting with abdominal pain and hematochezia. The differential diagnosis of abdominal pain and diarrhea in the acute setting should also include appendicitis, cholecystitis, pancreatitis, or intraabdominal abscess secondary to intestinal or gynecologic conditions. The presence of an intraabdominal abscess associated with chronic or subacute abdominal pain in a child should raise suspicion of a transmural intestinal process (perforated appendicitis, trauma, Crohn's disease).

Table 84-3 outlines a suggested initial diagnostic evaluation in a child or adolescent with clinical features consistent with inflammatory bowel disease. Pediatric patients with active inflammatory bowel disease typically present with a microcytic, hypochromic, heterogenous anemia; hypoalbuminemia (serum albumin 2.0 to 3.5 g per dL); elevated erythrocyte sedimentation rate (above 20 mm per hour); and a mild thrombocytosis (platelets greater than 400,000 mm^3). Routine laboratory tests in conjunction with a history of abdominal pain and hematochezia generally have enough sensitivity to identify patients who should undergo endoscopy for tissue diagnosis.

TABLE 84-3 Diagnostic Evaluation of the Pediatric Patient with Suspected Inflammatory Bowel Disease.

Laboratory studies
Complete blood cell count with differential
Reticulocyte count, serum iron, ferritin
Erythrocyte sedimentation rate
Total protein and serum albumin
Aminotransferases, alkaline phosphatase, bilirubin
Stool cultures
Enteric pathogens, ova, and parasites
Clostridium difficile toxin and culture
Radiological studies
Upper gastrointestinal series with small bowel follow-through
Computed tomography scan abdomen and pelvis (if abscess suspected)
Endoscopy/laparoscopy
Esophagogastroduodenoscopy with biopsies
Colonoscopy and terminal ileoscopy with biopsies
Diagnostic laparoscopy with biopsies

Additional diagnostic adjuncts include commercially available serologic panels used to examine for the presence of antibodies directed against host antigenic targets (38). Currently available tests evaluate for the presence of host antibodies to neutrophil proteins (perinuclear anticytoplasmic antibodies or pANCA) and microbial antigens, including *Saccharomyces cerevisiae* (ASCA) and *E. coli* outer-membrane porin (anti-OmpC). In general, serologic tests for inflammatory bowel disease have high specificity, whereas routine laboratory tests have high sensitivity (39). A retrospective review of serologic testing in children diagnosed with inflammatory bowel disease found a sensitivity of 68% and specificity of 92% with combined pANCA and ASCA serology (40). Therefore, although the utility of serologic testing as a screening tool for inflammatory bowel disease is relatively low, some clinicians may find it useful in confirming the need for endoscopic evaluation in children with GI symptoms and signs consistent with inflammatory bowel disease.

Endoscopic Evaluation

Children suspected of having inflammatory bowel disease should undergo further diagnostic testing to establish a definitive diagnosis. The use of fiberoptic endoscopy by pediatric gastroenterologists and surgeons is a safe and efficacious method for visual and diagnostic tissue sampling. Endoscopic evaluation and mucosal biopsy not only provides tissue diagnosis, but can also allow for accurate localization of the disease. Endoscopic findings may also be useful in differentiating Crohn's disease from ulcerative colitis and in diagnosing the extent and severity of the inflammatory process.

Children with suspected inflammatory bowel disease should undergo both upper endoscopy and colonoscopy. Significant oropharyngeal, gastric, and duodenal endoscopic findings have been reported in as many as 65.1% of children with Crohn's disease in the absence of upper GI symptoms (19,41). Endoscopic findings consistent with Crohn's disease include the presence of small bowel disease, visualization of aphthous ulcers, inflammatory lesions with intervening areas of normal intestine (skip lesions), rectal sparing, or the presence of granulomas on histologic examination. Aphthous ulcers are small, oval lesions in the intestinal mucosa that reflect a friable mucosa overlying superficial lymphoid aggregates. In contrast, the inflammatory process in ulcerative colitis will always involve the rectum and is continuous to variable levels of

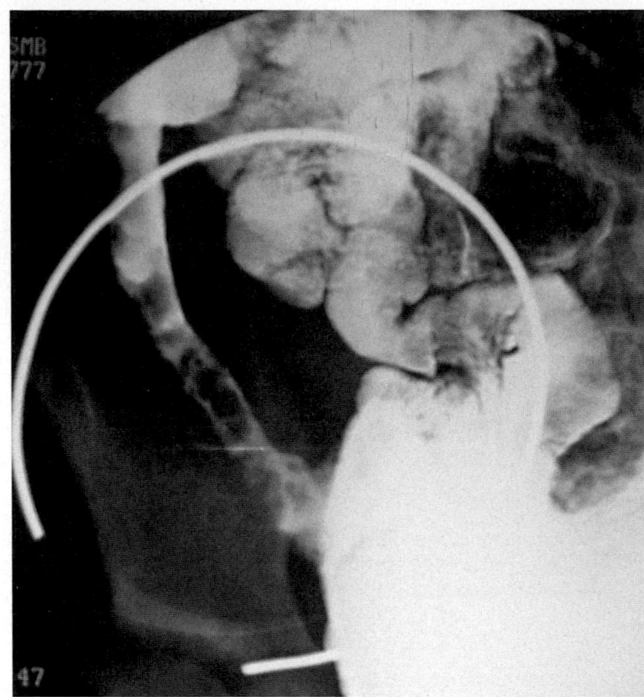

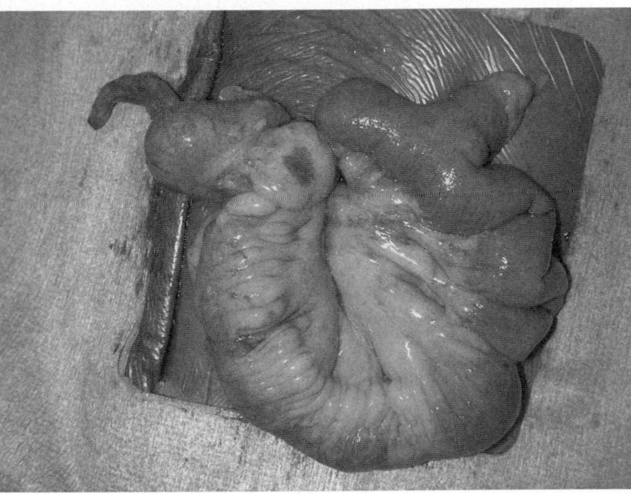

A B

FIGURE 84-2. **(A)** Upper gastrointestinal series with small bowel follow-through demonstrating strictured terminal ileum secondary to Crohn's disease. **(B)** Intraoperative findings of same patient demonstrating mesenteric thickening and fat-wrapping of the ileum. The patient also has a Meckel's diverticulum.

the proximal colon. The inflammatory process may involve the distal terminal ileum (backwash ileitis). The diagnosis of Crohn's disease is generally confirmed with the clinical findings of small bowel involvement or perirectal disease, or the presence of granulomas on biopsy. When the inflammatory process is limited to the colon, approximately 10% to 15% of the cases are clinically and histologically indistinguishable; therefore, a diagnosis of Crohn's colitis versus ulcerative colitis cannot be definitively made. These children are considered to have indeterminate colitis.

Radiologic Evaluation

In children with upper GI symptoms, a contrast upper GI series with small bowel follow-through may be useful in the identification and localization of abnormalities. Inflammatory bowel disease involving the small bowel may lead to mucosal ulceration, stenosis, obstruction, or fistula (Fig. 84-2). Because Crohn's disease tends to affect the terminal ileum in children, particular attention should be directed toward the distal small bowel. Computed tomography (CT) scan imaging of the abdomen and pelvis is useful in the presence of symptoms suggestive of in intraabdominal abscess or concern with a fistula. Radiolabeled leukocyte scintigraphy has been reported to be useful in diagnostic workup for inflammatory bowel disease; recent data discourage the use of leukocyte scintigraphy as a screening test for pediatric inflammatory bowel disease because false-negative results are common, and it may be unreliable for detecting disease in the proximal intestine (42).

MEDICAL MANAGEMENT

The contemporary management of children and adolescents diagnosed with inflammatory bowel disease requires a multidisciplinary approach involving the primary care physician, the pediatric gastroenterologist, pediatric surgeon, nutritionist, psychologist, and social worker. Given the systemic nature of inflammatory bowel disease, additional pediatric subspecialists, including ophthalmologists, rheumatologists, dermatologists, and endocrinologists, must also be readily available.

Medical management of inflammatory bowel disease is directed toward inducing and maintaining a quiescent state of remission for inflammatory bowel disease patients, while preserving the best attainable quality of life. In children, restoring or improving normal growth and development through puberty is an important secondary goal of treatment. To measure the activity of inflammatory bowel disease and its response to treatment, the Pediatric Crohn's Disease Activity Index (PCDAI) was developed. It is a validated, clinically useful tool (43). The PCDAI permits

HISTORY (Recall, 1 wk)

Abdominal pain

None	______ (0)
Mild—brief, does not interfere with activities	______ (5)
Moderate to severe—daily, longer lasting, affects activites, nocturnal	______ (10)

Stools (per day)

0–1 liquid stools, no blood	______ (0)
Up to 2 semiformed with small blood, or 2–5 liquid	______ (5)
Gross bleeding, or ≥6 liquid, or nocturnal diarrhea	______ (10)

PATIENT FUNCTIONING, GENERAL WELL-BEING (Recall, 1 wk)

No limitation of activities, well	______ (0)
Occasional difficulty in maintaining age-appropriate activities, below par	______ (5)
Frequent limitation of activity, very poor	______ (10)

LABORATORY

HCT (%)

<10 y:	>33	______ (0)	11–14 y M:	>35	______ (0)
	28–32	______ (2.5)		30–34	______ (2.5)
	<28	______ (5)		<30	______ (5)
11–19 y F:	≥34	______ (0)	15–19 y M:	≥37	______ (0)
	29–33	______ (2.5)		32–36	______ (2.5)
	<29	______ (5)		<32	______ (5)

ESR (mm/hr)	<20	______ (0)
	20–50	______ (2.5)
	>50	______ (5)
Albumin (g/dL)	≥3.5	______ (0)
	3.1–3.4	______ (5)
	≤3	______ (10)

EXAMINATION

Weight

Weight gain or voluntary weight stable/loss	______ (0)
Involuntary weight stable, weight loss 1%–9%	______ (5)
Weight loss ≥10%	______ (10)

Height

At diagnosis

<1 channel decrease	______ (0)
1–2 channel decrease	______ (5)
>2 channel decrease	______ (10)

or

Follow-up

Height velocity ≥–1 SD	______ (0)
Height velocity <–1 SD, >–2 SD	______ (5)
Height velocity ≤–2 SD	______ (10)

Abdomen

No tenderness, no mass	______ (0)
Tenderness or mass without tenderness	______ (5)
Tenderness, involuntary guarding, definite mass	______ (10)

Perirectal disease

None, asymptomatic tags	______ (0)
1–2 indolent fistulas, scant drainage, no tenderness	______ (5)
Active fistula, drainage, tenderness, or abscess	______ (10)

Extraintestinal Manifestations

(Fever ≥38.5 for 3 d over past week, definite arthritis, uveitis, *E. nodosum*, *P. gangrenosum*)

0	______ (0)
1	______ (5)
≥2	______ (10)

TOTAL SCORE ______________

FIGURE 84-3. Pediatric Crohn's disease activity index. HCT, hematocrit; ESR, erythrocyte sedimentation rate; SD, standard deviation. (From Hyams JS, Ferry GD, Mandel FS, et al. Development and validation of a pediatric Crohn's disease activity index. *J Pediatr Gastroenterol Nutr* 1991;12:439–447, with permission).

calculation of a numeric score ranging from 0 to 100 based on a child's well-being, degree of abdominal pain, number of bowel movements with or without blood, weight changes, linear growth, physical examination findings, and laboratory abnormalities (hematocrit, sedimentation rate, and serum albumin) (Fig. 84-3). Currently, there is not an equivalent activity index available for pediatric patients with ulcerative colitis. The IMPACT 35 questionnaire, an outcome measurement tool that evaluates the quality of life in children older than 10 years of age with either Crohn's disease or ulcerative colitis, has also been validated (44).

Medications

Medical therapy for pediatric inflammatory bowel disease has evolved rapidly since the mid-1980s. With novel pharmacologic agents aimed at modulating the immune response, it is possible to induce and maintain remission in most children with inflammatory bowel disease. From a surgical perspective, virtually all children with diagnosed inflammatory bowel disease will have received medical therapy, whether in the acute setting or in the form of maintenance therapy prior to surgical intervention. Therefore, it is important to understand the rationale for specific medical therapies, as well as the risks, complications, and potential issues that may arise in the surgical patient.

Corticosteroids

Despite many novel agents for use in inflammatory bowel disease, corticosteroids remain the initial treatment choice for acute therapy in moderate to severe Crohn's disease and ulcerative colitis. At appropriate dosage, either oral or intravenous corticosteroids have potent antiinflammatory activity and will generally induce rapid improvement in disease activity. However, there are no data supporting the use of corticosteroids for maintenance therapy. A retrospective review examining the historical use of corticosteroids for Crohn's disease from 1970 to 1993 demonstrated that 80% of treated patients were in disease remission after 30 days of therapy, but by 1 year, 38% had undergone operative intervention and 28% were corticosteroid dependent for disease control (45). Reversible short-term side effects of corticosteroid therapy include weight gain, hirsutism, acne, glucose intolerance, and mood changes. Long-term side effects that tend to be nonreversible include growth retardation, osteopenia, avascular osteonecrosis, skin changes, and cataracts. For many young children and adolescents, the side effects of corticosteroid use are particularly undesirable.

Attempts to reduce the systemic effects of corticosteroids have led to the development of drugs with high first-pass hepatic metabolism. Budesonide is a highly potent controlled-release corticosteroid formulation reported to be efficacious in inducing remission in children with Crohn's disease limited to the terminal ileum and right colon (46). Systemic effects are more limited with Budenoside than with corticosteroids lacking high first-pass metabolism. Given the emergence of more effective therapies, the lack of evidence of efficacy for maintenance therapy, and the serious adverse side effects, current guidelines recommend the use of corticosteroids only for acute, short-term treatment in pediatric inflammatory bowel disease. Most pediatric gastroenterologists and pediatric surgeons are in agreement that the duration of corticosteroid therapy in a child or adolescent with an acute episode of inflammatory bowel disease should be limited to less than 3 months. Significant corticosteroid-related side effects or complications are generally considered indications for operative management.

Aminosalicylates

Aminosalicylates are the drug of choice for initial therapy for mild to moderate ulcerative colitis (47). These compounds are related to aspirin, and the prototype is sulfasalazine. This drug has a 5-aminosalicylate (5-ASA) moiety bound to sulfapyridine, which is cleaved by colonic bacteria. The active component, 5-ASA, acts locally in the colon to decrease mucosal inflammation. Many of the side effects related to sulfasalazine are related to the sulfapyridine component, and therefore, newer drugs have become available with different delivery systems. Most of the newer 5-ASA drugs are generally well tolerated, with the most common side effects being headache and rashes. Less frequent but more severe adverse effects include hypersensitivity reactions, hepatitis, pancreatitis, and decreased sperm count. The role of 5-ASA compounds in initial and maintenance therapy of Crohn's disease involving the colon remains controversial.

Azathioprine and 6-Mercaptopurine

Azathioprine and its metabolite, 6-mercaptopurine (6-MP), are immunosuppressive agents that have been used in the treatment of steroid-refractory Crohn's disease since the 1980s. These drugs may take 3 to 6 months to achieve maximal effect at disease control, and the majority of both adult and pediatric patients with Crohn's disease will have disease remission (48). In a multicenter, placebo-controlled clinical trial, newly diagnosed children with moderate to severe Crohn's disease treated with 6-MP in addition to corticosteroids had significant reduction of corticosteroid therapy (both duration and dosage), as well as significant reduction in disease relapse rate (49). These data have led many pediatric gastroenterologists to begin 6-MP either initially or very early in the treatment of moderate to severe Crohn's disease. Side effects include an idiosyncratic allergic reaction consisting of fever, pancreatitis, and myalgia. Long-term side effects include myelosuppression, infection, and elevation of hepatocellular enzymes. Pharmacogenetic analysis for thiopurine methyl transferase activity allows identification of patients with slow metabolism of azathioprine/6-MP who are at greater risk for myelosuppression (50). In addition, patients on azathioprine or 6-MP can be monitored for 6-thioguanine nucleotide levels for dosage adjustment based on drug metabolism.

Methotrexate

Methotrexate is reported to be effective in inducing remission and decreasing corticosteroid dosage in adults with chronic, active, steroid-refractory Crohn's disease (51). The largest pediatric experience with the immunosuppressive agent methotrexate is in children and adolescents with juvenile rheumatoid arthritis. More recently, an open-label study of children with Crohn's disease refractory to 6-MP reported a response rate of approximately 50% to methotrexate (52). The long-term effectiveness of methotrexate, as well as other potent immunosuppressive agents such as cyclosporine, remains unclear, and therefore, pediatric experience with these agents is limited. Adverse side effects of methotrexate include myelosuppression, mucositis, pneumonitis, hepatitis, and infection.

Antibiotics

The most commonly used antibiotic in the treatment of inflammatory bowel disease is metronidazole, an imidazole derivative with substantial coverage for anaerobic organisms. Although metronidazole has not been shown to directly treat intestinal inflammation, it has been used effectively to treat both intraabdominal and perineal Crohn's disease, particularly disease complicated by fistula or abscess (53). A controlled trial using metronidazole following ileal resection for Crohn's disease in adults demonstrated decreased recurrence rate in treated patients, although nearly 75% experienced relapse if they discontinued the antibiotic (54). Small, uncontrolled trials using antibiotics such as trimethoprim-sulfamethoxazole and ciprofloxacin have reported efficacy in the adult population. In the absence of established infection, the safety and efficacy of antibiotic treatment in pediatric inflammatory bowel disease remains unknown.

Biologic Agents

Greater insight into the pathophysiology of inflammatory bowel disease has led to recognition of the distinct roles that proinflammatory cytokines play in initiating and maintaining an inflammatory state in the intestine. Modulation of the local host inflammatory response using therapies directed against cytokines, such as tumor necrosis factor alpha (TNF-α), represent the translation of basic science into clinical practice. The strategy of using inflammatory mediator blockade in the treatment of inflammatory bowel disease is best characterized by current use of Infliximab (Remicade, Centocor, Inc., Malvern, PA), a commercially available, chimeric human-mouse monoclonal antibody directed against human TNF-α. Blockade of TNF-α inhibits the inflammatory process and allows for mucosal healing in inflammatory bowel disease (55). Experimental data demonstrate that anti-TNF-α therapy may also downregulate intestinal epithelial cell apoptosis, allowing for a net decrease in chronic intestinal inflammation (56). Infliximab has been demonstrated to be clinically effective in treating pediatric patients with Crohn's disease that is otherwise resistant to corticosteroids and 6-MP (57,58). Infliximab also has emerging clinical utility in the treatment of perianal or enterocutaneous fistulous Crohn's disease by reducing the inflammatory response and allowing fistula closure (59).

Novel therapies aimed at selective blockade of the detrimental mucosal immune response are under current investigation, including the use of monoclonal antibodies targeted to modulate endothelial cell–leukocyte adhesion molecule interactions.

Nutritional Therapy

Many children with inflammatory bowel disease will have underlying nutritional deficiency. Initial diagnosis of the pediatric patient with inflammatory bowel disease will often lead to recognition of malnutrition at the onset of treatment. In the acute setting, treatment strategies using corticosteroids along with bowel rest are commonly employed to allow the intestinal inflammation to decrease. To maintain caloric and micronutrient intake, either total parenteral nutrition or enteral nutrition is required. In the absence of intestinal obstruction or symptoms that prevent oral intake, the enteral route is the preferred nutritional method. Primary enteral nutrition typically uses elemental and/or polymeric formulas that are relatively unpalatable, and therefore, elemental nutritional formulas are often given by nasoenteric or gastric feeding tubes. The use of primary nutritional therapy via bowel rest and controlled enteral feeding has been used successfully in Canada and Europe with remission rates of 50% to 80% reported in Crohn's disease (60). Inflammatory bowel disease controlled by primary nutritional therapy usually relapses after a normal diet is resumed, making this strategy limited in long-term management.

The more common scenario in surgical practice is to use nutritional therapy for supplemental caloric and micronutrient intake to improve perioperative weight gain, growth, and wound healing. Supplemental nutritional therapy is generally employed when a child or adolescent is unable to fully take recommended daily allowances for energy expenditure. In the child with less than adequate oral daytime intake, supplemental nocturnal nasoenteric feeding may be useful, particularly in children with disease relapse associated with growth failure.

Psychological Support

Children and adolescents have age-specific psychological needs and issues. The diagnosis of a chronic and lifelong condition such as inflammatory bowel disease in childhood has substantial ramifications for both parents and children. The medical and surgical management of pediatric inflammatory bowel disease may have profound effects on body image and appearance. In particular, cosmetic effects of corticosteroid use, frequent diarrheal stools, nasogastric or gastrostomy tubes, and enterostomies make many children with inflammatory bowel disease feel inadequate. Therefore, a number of children with inflammatory bowel disease benefit from professional psychological support.

Because adolescence is generally a period of transitional self-image, the development of normal self-esteem in a teenager with inflammatory bowel disease may become markedly altered. The psychosocial aspects of chronic inflammatory bowel disease are intensified as many activities are focused on school participation. The effects of delayed growth, short stature, and delayed puberty associated with inflammatory bowel disease may become dramatically apparent. The need to take multiple medications per day, sometimes in excess of 10 to 15 tablets, is a substantial limitation in quality of adolescent life, and compliance with medication is a source of conflict.

Psychological counseling by a professional familiar with inflammatory bowel disease can be helpful to assist adolescents in adjusting and adapting to life with a chronic disease. Most regional centers caring for children and adolescents with inflammatory bowel disease offer access to counseling in addition to peer support groups for both parents and patients.

SURGICAL MANAGEMENT

Although both Crohn's disease and ulcerative colitis are idiopathic inflammatory conditions of the GI tract, each disease has distinctly different clinical features that allow surgical intervention to be discussed separately. However, common to both diseases, the aim of medical management is to induce and maintain clinical remission using methods with proven safety, efficacy, and minimal adverse side effects. The adolescent age group is a particularly vulnerable population for delay in growth and puberty secondary to recurrent or persistent disease, and in some cases, long-term use of corticosteroids. Therefore, most pediatric gastroenterologists with specific interest in inflammatory bowel disease maintain a low threshold for treatment escalation with immunomodulating drugs and 83 agents. Despite the best medical efforts, there is a significant subgroup of pediatric patients with inflammatory bowel disease who will require operative intervention. Common indications for surgical management are listed in Table 84-4.

SURGERY FOR CROHN'S DISEASE

Regional ileitis was described in 1932 by Crohn and colleagues (61). Observation of an identical, transmural inflammatory process occurring in a discontinuous manner throughout the entire small intestine led to the term *regional enteritis*. Upon recognition that the same inflammatory process occurred in the colon, the term *Crohn's disease* was applied to describe the regional inflammatory intestinal condition, and it was recognized that any site in the GI tract could be affected (62).

Indications for operative intervention in Crohn's disease include the failure of maximal medical management (including complications of medical therapy), in addition to specific complications of the disease. These complications are hemorrhage, intestinal perforation with or without abscess, bowel obstruction from intestinal stricture, or symptomatic fistulas. Substantial growth failure or delay in puberty in the presence of segmental, active disease despite medical management should be considered a relative indication for operative resection. In addition, quality of life should be considered, including subjective pain symptoms, level of physical activity, attendance at school, and self-esteem.

A few consistent principles guide the operative management of Crohn's disease in the pediatric population. First, surgical treatment must recognize that, because there is currently no cure for Crohn's disease, any operative procedure must have as its goal the effective relief of symptoms or complications, while preserving as much intestinal length as possible. Second, the vast majority of children with established inflammatory bowel disease will be on corticosteroids and/or immunomodulating drugs, and potential drug effects must be accounted for in the perioperative period. Multidisciplinary management of children with Crohn's disease is necessary in that all patients will require long-term management by a pediatric gastroenterologist and a primary care physician. Finally, surgical intervention in the emergent setting for Crohn's disease is unusual, but may be required for intestinal perforation, toxic megacolon, or GI hemorrhage.

Prior to any operative procedure for Crohn's disease, accurate localization of the involved segment(s) of intestine is essential. Review of the clinical and endoscopic history of the patient, as well as careful evaluation of the diagnostic imaging studies, will generally provide the necessary anatomic data. In the acute setting, CT scan imaging of the abdomen and pelvis with intravenous and oral contrast has become a rapid, accurate method of localizing disease and its potential complications (intestinal obstruction, abscess, fistula). Surgical procedures for Crohn's disease must be tailored to the anatomic location and extent of the disease encountered.

Acute intestinal obstruction in the setting of Crohn's disease results from the transmural inflammatory process causing local edema and narrowing of the intestinal lumen. When the inflammatory process becomes chronic, fibrosis of the intestinal wall may occur, causing an irreversible intestinal stricture. Initial intestinal obstruction may be incomplete in the early course of disease, and symptoms of intermittent, crampy abdominal pain associated with occasional emesis may be reported. It is this early

TABLE 84-4 Indications for Operative Management in Inflammatory Bowel Disease.

Failure of medical management
Growth failure
Delayed puberty
Complications of drug therapy
Lack of compliance to medical regimen
Persistent active disease despite maximal medical therapy
Complications of the disease
Hemorrhage
Intraabdominal abscess
Intestinal perforation or impending perforation (toxic megacolon)
Intestinal stricture, obstruction, or fistula
Persistent perianal disease (Crohn's)
Mucosal dysplasia (ulcerative colitis)
Psychosocial factors
Quality of life (persistent school absence, >12 stools per day, etc.)

phase of the inflammatory response that is reversible with corticosteroid therapy. Chronic progression of the inflammatory process leading to collagen deposition and fibrotic stricture is generally heralded by exacerbation and persistence of abdominal pain and emesis. In some children, terminal ileal disease will remain active with persistence of symptoms despite maximal medical therapy. In others, induction of an initial clinical response and remission may be followed by relapse, leading to recurrent inflammation and subsequent healing with fibrosis and stricture.

A palpable right lower quadrant mass in a child with suspected or known Crohn's disease is usually secondary to an inflammatory phlegmon. It is not uncommon for the mass to be composed of involved terminal ileum with deep, penetrating ulcers or internal fistulas from walled-off intestinal perforation into adjacent bowel, mesentery, or body wall (63). An abscess may be present either retroperitoneal in the adjacent soft tissues or within the peritoneum. In the acute setting, this can be confused with perforated appendicitis. Children undergoing exploration for suspected appendicitis who are found to have Crohn's disease should be referred to a pediatric gastroenterologist for complete workup. An appendectomy can safely be performed in this setting if the cecum is not involved with inflammation. That is, the major risk for enterocutaneous fistula arises from the diseased terminal ileum or small bowel, not the appendiceal stump in an otherwise normal cecum.

Given disease distribution, ileocecal resection is the most commonly performed operation in children and adolescents with Crohn's disease. Contemporary surgical management dictates that any intestinal resection for Crohn's disease should be limited to the grossly involved intestinal segment. Data do not support the use of frozen section analysis for identification of clear microscopic margins because this does not result in a reduced complication rate or lower disease recurrence (64). For symptomatic small bowel disease, segmental resection with primary anastomosis is the preferred option. There are currently no data demonstrating superiority of hand sewn versus stapled anastomosis techniques in the surgical management of pediatric Crohn's disease. In the presence of a preoperatively diagnosed intraabdominal abscess, percutaneous drainage of the abscess and treatment of established intraabdominal infection with intravenous antibiotics may be useful to reduce the local inflammatory response prior to exploration and bowel resection. The use of laparoscopic-assisted bowel resection in the management of pediatric Crohn's disease has been reported to be successful in reducing the length of stay and potentially decreasing the need for postoperative parenteral narcotics (65,66).

When fistulous disease is encountered, the tracts should be carefully identified and divided. Typically, the diseased intestinal segment is resected, and the adjacent normal hollow viscus is closed primarily. Patients with a fistula between the small intestine and the sigmoid colon have been reported to have a significant probability (greater than 50%) of also having an enterovesical fistula, mandating careful interrogation of the bladder and pelvis in this setting (67).

For isolated small intestinal obstruction resulting from well-established, fibrotic stricture, or in a child with multiple small bowel strictures, stricturoplasty may be preferred to resection and anastomosis for preservation of bowel length (Fig. 84-4). Stricturoplasty is limited to the chronically inflamed, fibrotic segments of intestine and is generally not advisable in acutely inflamed, edematous intestine. Data suggest that stricturoplasty can be performed safely to treat fibrotic stricture without a higher rate of suture line leak, infection, or ultimately, disease recurrence in pediatric patients with Crohn's disease (68). Intestinal bypass procedures are generally avoided in Crohn's disease, with the exception of gastric outlet obstruction secondary to severe duodenal stricture. In this unusual situation, gastrojejunostomy may be required.

In patients with Crohn's colitis, the extent of resection is dependent on the extent of disease involvement. Surgical options include segmental colectomy, subtotal colectomy with ileorectal anastomosis, or total proctocolectomy with ileostomy. Colonic and/or perineal involvement is common in children presenting with Crohn's disease 5 years of age and younger and is associated with failure to thrive more commonly than ulcerative colitis (69). Accurate diagnosis is desirable in that the surgical treatment for ulcerative colitis differs considerably.

For segmental colonic disease, there is a growing surgical trend to perform segmental colectomy with anastomosis (70). Relatively high recurrence rates with segmental colectomy in previous studies predate current medical management with aggressive immunomodulatory and 83 agents. However, typical colonic involvement with Crohn's disease is multifocal, and therefore, subtotal colectomy is generally required for intractable disease. A more recent study reviewing 118 adults undergoing subtotal colectomy with ileorectal anastomosis for Crohn's colitis reported an 86% rectal preservation rate, despite disease recurrence rates of 58% and 83% at 5 and 10 years, respectively (71). The absence of ileal disease, lack of extraintestinal manifestations, and prophylactic treatment with 5-ASA were considered positive factors influencing rectal preservation in this report.

Children with intractable pancolitis from Crohn's disease are generally well treated with either subtotal colectomy or total proctocolectomy with Brooke ileostomy. Subtotal colectomy with ileostomy as a primary procedure has been reported to be successful for disease control with only minor problems involving the retained rectal stump (72). The results of sphincter-saving ileoanal pouch procedures and continent ileostomies performed in pediatric patients with a primary diagnosis of Crohn's colitis have been

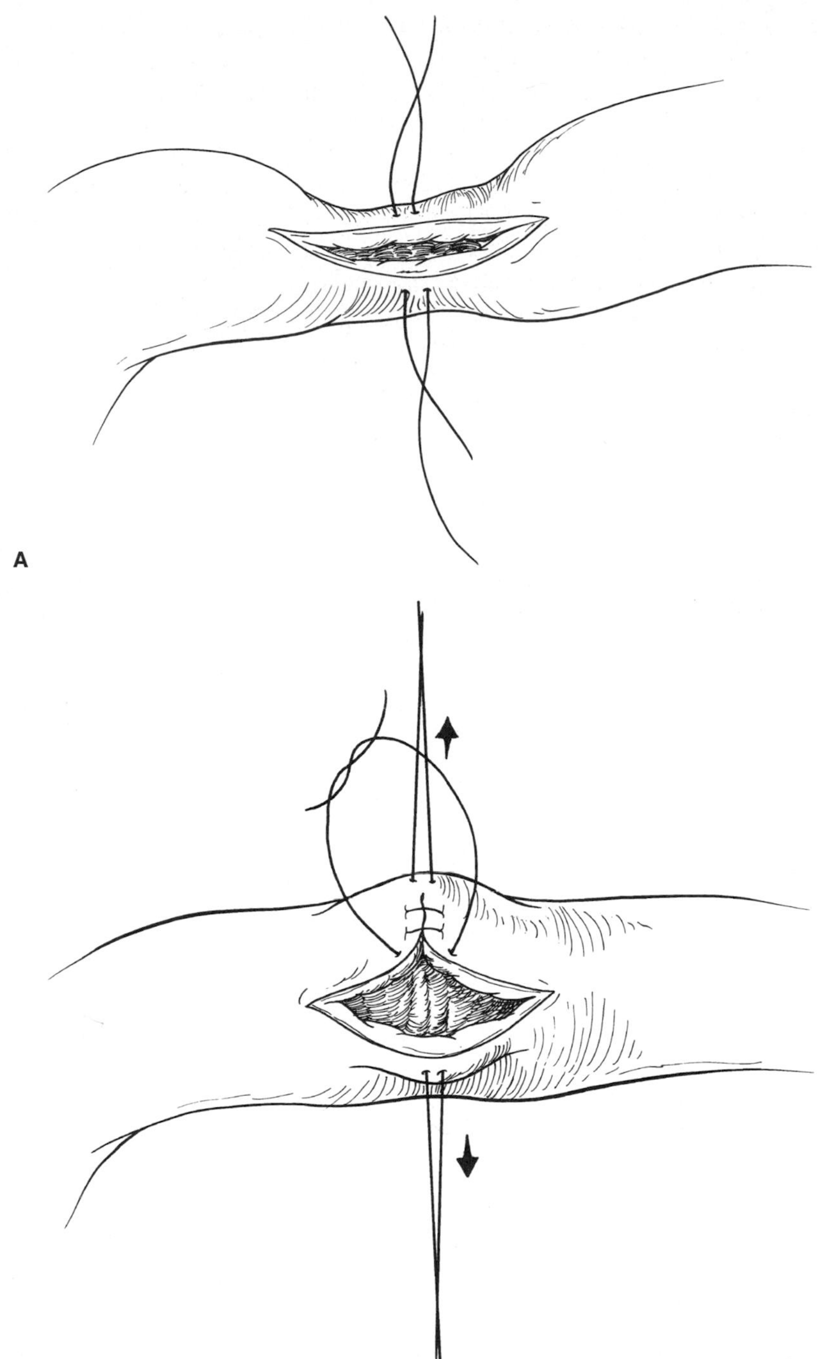

FIGURE 84-4. Stricturoplasty for Crohn's disease involving the small bowel. The bowel is incised longitudinally across the stricture **(A)** and closed transversely **(B)**.

discouraging in terms of complication rate, probability of recurrent disease, and need for reoperation (73). Patients with an unexpected, secondary diagnosis of Crohn's disease following restorative ileoanal pouch reconstruction for colitis have been reported to have good functional outcome and quality of life (74). Patients with a secondary diagnosis of Crohn's disease represent a group in whom a primary diagnosis of Crohn's colitis was elusive or indeterminate. In fact, it is speculated that these individuals may have less virulent disease. Some investigators advocate consideration of ileal pouch-anal anastomosis as an option in nongranulatomatous colitis or in Crohn's colitis in the absence of small bowel or perianal disease (75). Because current data do not allow for accurate preoperative selection of this subgroup in children, ileal-pouch-anal anastomosis in pediatric Crohn's colitis is not widely accepted or recommended. Along with a clear understanding of the potential risks and complications by patients and parents, restorative pouch procedures for pediatric Crohn's disease should therefore be considered the exception rather than the rule.

Approximately 13% of pediatric patients with Crohn's disease will have clinically significant perianal disease (30,63). Perianal fistulous disease may be complex, with deep fissures and tracts that may traverse the sphincter. Diagnostic imaging with fistulograms or CT scanning of the pelvis with rectal contrast may be extremely useful in delineating the extent of disease and in identifying perirectal abscess. If a perirectal abscess is found, incision and drainage is required. Anal stricture secondary to chronic inflammatory fibrosis may also be encountered. Severe and intractable perianal Crohn's disease in children is usually accompanied by rectal or colonic disease, and in rare cases, rectosigmoid resection with colostomy or proctocolectomy with ileostomy may be required for symptom control. In this setting, fecal diversion with a defunctioning ileostomy has been observed to be relatively ineffective at allowing the excluded segment of involved bowel to heal. Whether contemporary use of aggressive immunomodulatory agents and 83 modifiers leads to reduction of intractable perianal Crohn's disease remains unclear.

Outcome (Complications, Recurrence, and Quality of Life)

With directed therapy and coordinated medical and surgical management of Crohn's disease, the overall surgical outcome is generally good. Many adolescents are able to return to activity and school, and there may be significant postoperative improvement in weight for age, height for age, weight for height, and resting energy expenditure in this age group (29,76). However, patients and their parents must be educated that, because surgical intervention is largely directed at complications of a lifelong disease, continued medical treatment is required and a high likelihood of future operative procedures exists.

Complications following operation for Crohn's disease in children are common. In one large series, 94 children with Crohn's disease underwent 124 surgical procedures, with 29 children experiencing 37 complications (77). The most common complications observed were postoperative small bowel obstruction and abdominal or pelvic abscess. Operations for Crohn's disease must also anticipate that further surgical intervention will likely be required. Clinical recurrence rates of symptomatic disease following operative intervention have been reported to be 17% at 1 year, 38% at 3 years, and as high as 60% at 5 years (78). Recurrence is more common with colonic disease and with more severe, aggressive disease (as measured by the PCDAI and/or the preoperative use of 6-MP) at the time of operation. Therefore, postoperative maintenance drug therapy appears essential for adequate disease remission. Given the emergence of newer drug therapies since the mid-1990s, the natural history of disease recurrence may change substantially.

Long-term follow-up of children with Crohn's disease has demonstrated that a majority (80%) of patients consider their health to be good to excellent (79). Assessment of health-related quality-of-life issues in children with inflammatory bowel disease requires an age- and disease-specific tool (80). Specifically, absence from school, inability to participate in physical activities, and concern with taking vacations and staying at friends' homes are significant issues that impact lifestyle in this age group (81).

CONCLUSION

Inflammatory bowel disease remains an infrequent but important surgical problem in the pediatric population. Current clinical diagnostic techniques have improved differentiation between Crohn's disease and ulcerative colitis in most cases. Both diseases are currently treatable with conventional and biologic treatment regimens aimed at controlling the intestinal inflammatory response and improving the quality of life. Surgical management of inflammatory bowel disease in children and adolescents is directed toward disease and complication control. Surgical decisions must also account for age-specific issues such as growth arrest and delayed puberty. Operative management in Crohn's disease can dramatically improve the quality of life for many children and adolescents, but they will require continued medical management to maintain disease remission. In contrast, definitive cure and cessation of medical therapy is possible with surgical management of ulcerative colitis. The contemporary treatment of pediatric inflammatory bowel disease is a model for the multidisciplinary management of potentially lifelong disorders.

REFERENCES

1. Shashinder H, Integlia MJ, Grand RJ. *Clinical manifestations of pediatric inflammatory bowel disease,* 5th ed. Philadelphia: WB Sanders, 2000.
2. Shanahan F. Inflammatory bowel disease: immunodiagnostics, immunotherapeutics, and ecotherapeutics. *Gastroenterology* 2001;120: 622–635.
3. Calkins BM, Lilienfeld AM, Garland CF, et al. Trends in incidence rates of ulcerative colitis and Crohn's disease. *Dig Dis Sci* 1984;29:913–920.
4. Sonnenberg A, McCarty DJ, Jacobsen SJ. Geographic variation of inflammatory bowel disease within the United States. *Gastroenterology* 1991;100:143–149.
5. Cho JH. Update on the genetics of inflammatory bowel disease. *Curr Gastroenterol Rep* 2001;3:458–463.
6. Armitage E, Drummond HE, Wilson DC, et al. Increasing incidence of both juvenile-onset Crohn's disease and ulcerative colitis in Scotland. *Eur J Gastroenterol Hepatol* 2001;13:1439–1447.
7. Barton JR, Gillon S, Ferguson A. Incidence of inflammatory bowel disease in Scottish children between 1968 and 1983: marginal fall in ulcerative colitis, three-fold rise in Crohn's disease. *Gut* 1989;30:618–622.

8. Sawczenko A, Sandhu BK, Logan RF, et al. Prospective survey of childhood inflammatory bowel disease in the British Isles. *Lancet* 2001;357:1093–1094.
9. Kugathasan S, Binion DG, Hoffmann GF. Highest worldwide incidence of pediatric inflammatory bowel disease in Wisconsin: results of the Wisconsin pediatric IBD alliance, a population based prospective study of epidemiology, clinical patterns and natural history of pediatric IBD. *J Invest Med* 2003;51:S92.
10. Fiocchi C. Inflammatory bowel disease: etiology and pathogenesis. *Gastroenterology* 1998;115:182–205.
11. Zhou Z, Lin XY, Akolkar PN, et al. Variation at NOD2/CARD15 in familial and sporadic cases of Crohn's disease in the Ashkenazi Jewish population. *Am J Gastroenterol* 2002;97:3095–3101.
12. Bonen DK, Cho JH. The genetics of inflammatory bowel disease. *Gastroenterology* 2003;124:521–536.
13. Ogura Y, Bonen DK, Inohara N, et al. A frameshift mutation in NOD2 associated with susceptibility to Crohn's disease. *Nature* 2001;31:603–606.
14. Swidsinski A, Ladhoff A, Pernthaler A, et al. Mucosal flora in inflammatory bowel disease. *Gastroenterology* 2002;122:44–54.
15. Baldassano RN, Piccoli DA. Inflammatory bowel disease in pediatric and adolescent patients. *Gastroenterol Clin North Am* 1999;28:445–458.
16. Gryboski JD. Crohn's disease in children 10 years old and younger: comparison with ulcerative colitis. *J Pediatr Gastroenterol Nutr* 1994;18:174–182.
17. Hyams JS, Davis P, Grancher K, et al. Clinical outcome of ulcerative colitis in children. *J Pediatr* 1996;129:81–88.
18. Motil KJ, Grand RJ, Davis-Kraft L, et al. Growth failure in children with inflammatory bowel disease: a prospective study. *Gastroenterology* 1993;105:681–691.
19. Ruuska T, Vaajalahti P, Arajarvi P, et al. Prospective evaluation of upper gastrointestinal mucosal lesions in children with ulcerative colitis and Crohn's disease. *J Pediatr Gastroenterol Nutr* 1994;19:181–186.
20. Hyams JS, Davis P, Grancher K, et al. Clinical outcome of ulcerative colitis in children. *J Pediatr* 1996;129:81–88.
21. Katz JA. Medical and surgical management of severe colitis. *Semin Gastrointest Dis* 2000;11:18–32.
22. Griffiths AM, Nguyen P, Smith C, et al. Growth and clinical course of children with Crohn's disease. *Gut* 1993;34:939–943.
23. Stephens M, Batres LA, Ng D, et al. Growth failure in the child with inflammatory bowel disease. *Semin Gastrointest Dis* 2001;12:253–262.
24. Azcue M, Rashid M, Griffiths A, et al. Energy expenditure and body composition in children with Crohn's disease: effect of enteral nutrition and treatment with prednisolone. *Gut* 1997;41:203–208.
25. Sentongo TA, Semeao EJ, Piccoli DA, et al. Growth, body composition, and nutritional status in children and adolescents with Crohn's disease. *J Pediatr Gastroenterol Nutr* 2000;31:33–40.
26. Ferguson A, Sedgwick DM. Growth failure in pediatric IBD. *J Pediatr Gastroenterol Nutr* 1994;18:504–505.
27. Ferguson A, Sedgwick DM. Juvenile onset inflammatory bowel disease: height and body mass index in adult life. *BMJ* 1994;308:1259–1263.
28. Ballinger AB, Savage MO, Sanderson IR. Delayed puberty associated with inflammatory bowel disease. *Pediatr Res* 2003;53:205–210.
29. Sentongo TA, Stettler N, Christian A, et al. Growth after intestinal resection for Crohn's disease in children, adolescents, and young adults. *Inflamm Bowel Dis* 2000;6:265–269.
30. Tolia V. Perianal Crohn's disease in children and adolescents. *Am J Gastroenterol* 1996;91:922–926.
31. Isaacs D, Wright VM, Shaw DG, et al. Chronic granulomatous disease mimicking Crohn's disease. *J Pediatr Gastroenterol Nutr* 1985;4:498–501.
32. Chung CC, Choi CL, Kwok SP, et al. Anal and perianal tuberculosis: a report of three cases in 10 years. *J R Coll Surg Edinburgh* 1997;42:189–190.
33. Markowitz J, Grancher K, Rosa J, et al. Highly destructive perianal disease in children with Crohn's disease. *J Pediatr Gastroenterol Nutr* 1995;21:149–153.
34. Sellman SP, Hupertz VF, Reece RM. Crohn's disease presenting as suspected abuse. *Pediatrics* 1996;97:272–274.
35. Cabral DA, Malleson PN, Petty RE. Spondyloarthropathies of childhood. *Pediatr Clin North Am* 1995;42:1051–1070.
36. Dupuy A, Cosnes J, Revuz J, et al. Oral Crohn disease: clinical characteristics and long-term follow-up of 9 cases. *Arch Dermatol* 1999;135:439–442.
37. Wilschanski M, Chait P, Wade JA, et al. Primary sclerosing cholangitis in 32 children: clinical, laboratory, and radiographic features, with survival analysis. *Hepatology* 1995;22:1415–1422.
38. Kugathasan S, Halabi I, Telega G, et al. Pancreatitis as a presenting manifestation of pediatric Crohn's disease: a report of three cases. *J Pediatr Gastroenterol Nutr* 2002;35:96–98.
39. Ruemmele FM, Targan SR, Levy G, et al. Diagnostic accuracy of serological assays in pediatric inflammatory bowel disease. *Gastroenterology* 1998;115:822–829.
40. Khan K, Schwarzenberg SJ, Sharp H, et al. Role of serology and routine laboratory tests in childhood inflammatory bowel disease. *Inflamm Bowel Dis* 2002;8:325–329.
41. Sharif F, McDermott M, Dillon M, et al. Focally enhanced gastritis in children with Crohn's disease and ulcerative colitis. *Am J Gastroenterol* 2002;97:1415–1420.
42. Grahnquist L, Chapman SC, Hvidsten S, et al. Evaluation of 99mTc-HMPAO leukocyte scintigraphy in the investigation of pediatric inflammatory bowel disease. *J Pediatr* 2003;143:48–53.
43. Hyams JS, Ferry GD, Mandel FS, et al. Development and validation of a pediatric Crohn's disease activity index. *J Pediatr Gastroenterol Nutr* 1991;12:439–447.
44. Otley A, Smith C, Nicholas D, et al. The IMPACT questionnaire: a valid measure of health-related quality of life in pediatric inflammatory bowel disease. *J Pediatr Gastroenterol Nutr* 2002;35:557–563.
45. Faubion WA Jr, Loftus EV Jr, Harmsen WS, et al. The natural history of corticosteroid therapy for inflammatory bowel disease: a population-based study. *Gastroenterology* 2001;121:255–260.
46. Kundhal P, Zachos M, Holmes JL, et al. Controlled ileal release Budesonide in pediatric Crohn disease: efficacy and effect on growth. *J Pediatr Gastroenterol Nutr* 2001;33:75–80.
47. Sutherland L, Roth D, Beck P, et al. Oral 5-aminosalicylic acid for maintenance of remission in ulcerative colitis. *Cochrane Database Syst Rev* 2002;4.
48. Kirschner BS. Safety of azathioprine and 6-mercaptopurine in pediatric patients with inflammatory bowel disease. *Gastroenterology* 1998;115:813–821.
49. Markowitz J, Grancher K, Kohn N, et al. A multicenter trial of 6-mercaptopurine and prednisone in children with newly diagnosed Crohn's disease. *Gastroenterology* 2000;119:895–902.
50. Dubinsky MC, Lamothe S, Yang HY, et al. Pharmacogenomics and metabolite measurement for 6-mercaptopurine therapy in inflammatory bowel disease. *Gastroenterology* 2000;118:705–713.
51. Feagan BG, Rochon J, Fedorak RN, et al. Methotrexate for the treatment of Crohn's disease. The North American Crohn's Study Group Investigators. *N Engl J Med* 1995;332:292–297.
52. Mack DR, Young R, Kaufman SS, et al. Methotrexate in patients with Crohn's disease after 6-mercaptopurine. *J Pediatr* 1998;132:830–835.
53. Sutherland L, Singleton J, Sessions J, et al. Double blind, placebo controlled trial of metronidazole in Crohn's disease. *Gut* 1991;32:1071–1075.
54. Rutgeerts P, Hiele M, Geboes K, et al. Controlled trial of metronidazole treatment for the prevention of Crohn's recurrence after ileal resection. *Gastroenterology* 1995;108:1617–1621.
55. Hanauer SB, Feagan BG, Lichtenstein GR, et al. Maintenance infliximab for Crohn's disease: the ACCENT I randomized trial. *Lancet* 2002;359:1541–1549.
56. Marini M, Bamias G, Rivera-Nieves J, et al. TNF-alpha neutralization ameliorates the severity of murine Crohn's-like ileitis by abrogation of intestinal epithelial cell apoptosis. *Proc Natl Acad Sci U S A* 2003;100:8366–8371.
57. Hyams JS. Use of infliximab in the treatment of Crohn's disease in children and adolescents. *J Pediatr Gastroenterol Nutr* 2001;33:S36–S39.
58. Stephens MC, Shepanski MA, Mamula P, et al. Safety and steroid-sparing experience using infliximab for Crohn's disease at a pediatric

inflammatory bowel disease center. *Am J Gastroenterol* 2003;98:104–111.

59. Present DH, Rutgeerts P, Targan S, et al. Infliximab for the treatment of fistulas in patients with Crohn's disease. *N Engl J Med* 1999;340:1398–1405.
60. Griffiths AM, Ohlsson A, Sherman PM, et al. Meta-analysis of enteral nutrition as a primary treatment of active Crohn's disease. *Gastroenterology* 1995;108:1056–1067.
61. Crohn BB, Ginzburg L, Oppenheimer GD. Regional ileitis: a pathological and clinical entity. *JAMA* 1984;251:73–79.
62. Lockhart-Mummery HE, Morson BC. Crohn's disease of the large intestine. *Gut* 1964;5:493–509.
63. Telander RL, Schmeling DJ. Current surgical management of Crohn's disease in childhood. *Semin Pediatr Surg* 1994;3:19–27.
64. Heimann TM, Greenstein AJ, Lewis B, et al. Prediction of early symptomatic recurrence after intestinal resection in Crohn's disease. *Ann Surg* 1993;218:294–298.
65. Diamond JR, Langer JC. Laparoscopic-assisted versus open ileocolic resection for adolescent Crohn's disease. *J Pediatr Gastroenterol Nutr* 2001;33:543–547.
66. von Allmen D, Markowitz JE, York A, et al. Laparoscopic-assisted bowel resection offers advantages over open surgery for treatment of segmental Crohn's disease in children. *J Pediatr Surg* 2003;38(6):963–965.
67. Schraut WH, Chapman C, Abraham VS. Operative treatment of Crohn's ileocolitis complicated by ileosigmoid and ileovesical fistulae. *Ann Surg* 1984;207:48–51.
68. Oliva L, Wyllie R, Alexander F, et al. The results of stricturoplasty in pediatric patients with multifocal Crohn's disease. *J Pediatr Gastroenterol Nutr* 1994;18:306–310.
69. Mamula P, Telega GW, Markowitz JE, et al. Inflammatory bowel disease in children 5 years of age and younger. *Am J Gastroenterol* 2002;97:2005–2010.
70. Andersson P, Olaison G, Bodemar G, et al. Surgery for Crohn colitis over a twenty-eight-year period: fewer stomas and the replacement of total colectomy by segmental resection. *Scand J Gastroenterol* 2002;37:68–73.
71. Cattan P, Bonhomme N, Panis Y, et al. Fate of the rectum in patients undergoing total colectomy for Crohn's disease. *Br J Surg* 2002;89:454–459.
72. Davies G, Evans CM, Shand WS, et al. Surgery for Crohn's disease in childhood: influence of site of disease and operative procedure on outcome. *Br J Surg* 1990;77:891–894.
73. Alexander F, Sarigol S, DiFiore J, et al. Fate of the pouch in 151 pediatric patients after ileal pouch anal anastomosis. *J Pediatr Surg* 2003;38:78–82.
74. de Oca J, Sanchez-Santos R, Rague JM, et al. Long-term results of ileal pouch-anal anastomosis in Crohn's disease. *Inflamm Bowel Dis* 2003;9:171–175.
75. Morphugo E, Petras R, Kimberling J, et al. Characterization and clinical behavior of Crohn's disease initially presenting predominantly as colitis. *Dis Colon Rectum* 2003;46:918–924.
76. Varille V, Cezard JP, de Lagausie P, et al. Resting energy expenditure before and after surgical resection of gut lesions in pediatric Crohn's disease. *J Pediatr Gastroenterol Nutr* 1996;23:13–19.
77. Patel HI, Leichtner AM, Colodny AH, et al. Surgery for Crohn's disease in infants and children. *J Pediatr Surg* 1997;32:1063–1068.
78. Baldassano RN, Han PD, Jeshion WC, et al. Pediatric Crohn's disease: risk factors for postoperative recurrence. *Am J Gastroenterol* 2001;96:2169–2176.
79. Castile RG, Telander RL, Cooney DR, et al. Crohn's disease in children: assessment of the progression of disease, growth, and prognosis. *J Pediatr Surg* 1980;15:462–469.
80. Griffiths AM, Nicholas D, Smith C, et al. Development of a quality-of-life index for pediatric inflammatory bowel disease: dealing with differences related to age and IBD type. *J Pediatr Gastroenterol Nutr* 1999;28:S46–S52.
81. Akobeng AK, Suresh-Babu MV, Firth D, et al. Quality of life in children with Crohn's disease: a pilot study. *J Pediatr Gastroenterol Nutr* 1999;28:S37–S39.

Chapter 85

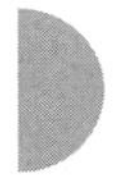

Intestinal Duplications

John J. Aiken

Enteric duplications and mesenteric, omental, and retroperitoneal cysts are rare developmental anomalies that frequently present a diagnostic as well as therapeutic challenge to the clinician and surgeon. These lesions vary greatly in appearance, size, location, and presentation. Although most enteric duplications are symptomatic and present at an early age, some remain undiagnosed into adulthood. These lesions can present with severe and even life-threatening complications, and some have been demonstrated to harbor malignancy. They are frequently misdiagnosed as more common intestinal conditions and are not suspected until encountered intraoperatively. The goals of surgical management are to relieve symptoms, to preserve intestinal function, and to prevent future complications. Due to the potentially complex anatomy and a shared blood supply between intestinal duplications and the native intestine, appropriate management requires familiarity with the anatomic and clinical characteristics of this entity. This chapter reviews the incidence, anatomic location, theories of disordered embryology likely to give rise to these lesions, modes of clinical presentation, and general principles of diagnosis and treatment of intestinal duplications and mesenteric, omental, and retroperitoneal cysts.

INTESTINAL DUPLICATIONS

Intestinal duplications are rare congenital developmental abnormalities that can occur anywhere from the mouth to the anus (1). The first report of an intestinal duplication was by Calder in 1733 (2). The medical literature describes a wide variety of lesions, and the nomenclature includes terms such as enteric cyst, enterogenous cyst, diverticula, giant diverticula, ileum duplex, jejunal duplex, inclusion cyst, unusual Meckel's diverticula, and others (3). Ladd is credited with unifying the nomenclature in 1937 when he suggested the term *duplication of the alimentary tract* be used to encompass this constellation of abnormalities (4). Ladd's inclusive terminology emphasized that these lesions were congenital developmental anomalies that shared several characteristics: (1) the presence of a well-developed smooth muscle component, (2) the epithelial lining represents some portion of the alimentary tract, and (3) most duplications are intimately attached to some portion of the gastrointestinal (GI) tract. In modern practice, the defining characteristics of intestinal duplications are their location in close proximity to the alimentary tract and a common muscular wall and shared blood supply with the adjacent intestine. The usual location is dorsal to the normal intestine—that is, related to the mesenteric aspect, in contrast to vitelline duct remnants, such as Meckel's diverticula, which lie on the antimesenteric aspect of the bowel (5). They may be either cystic or tubular in shape. Because these are rare lesions, there are few large patient series reported (Table 85-1) (1,6–14). The epithelial lining is variable, but most often reflects the epithelium of the adjacent intestine. Multiple mucosal types have been identified in the same lesion and the presence of heterotopic tissue of diverse origins, including thyroid stroma, lymphoid aggregates resembling Peyer's patches, ciliated bronchial epithelium, lung tissue, and cartilage, has been reported (3). Communication with the normal GI tract may also occur, although this is not common. A critical feature of as many as one-third of intestinal duplications is the presence of ectopic gastric mucosa, predisposing the cyst to ulceration, bleeding, and perforation if communication with the native bowel exists. In addition, alimentary tract duplications are frequently associated with vertebral abnormalities and other congenital malformations. In 10% to 20% of cases, multiple duplications are present in a single individual. Intestinal duplications are named for the associated GI structures rather than for the type of mucosa lining the cyst. The most common location for an intestinal duplication is the small intestine, in particular, the ileocecal region. Thoracic duplications are the most frequent duplications to be

John J. Aiken: Department of Surgery/Pediatric Surgery, Children's Hospital of Wisconsin, Milwaukee, Wisconsin 53226.

TABLE 85-1 A Summary of Several Reports of Enteric Duplications.

Investigators	Total Number of Patients	Location								
		Cervical	Mediastinal	Thoraco-Abdominal	Gastric	Duodenal	Jejunal and Ileal	Colonic	Rectal	Other
Gross (1)	68	1	13	3	2	4	32	9	4	
Sieber (6)	25		5		4	2	16	5		
Houston & Lynn (7)	8		1	1			6			
Basu et al. (8)	28		7		1	3	16	4	2	
Mellish & Koop (9)	38	1	6	2	1		18	6	4	
Grosfeld et al. (10)	20		4	2	1		9	4		
Favara et al. (11)	37	3	4		3	4	20	4		
Wrenn (5)	25		3	2	1	2	12	3	4	
Holcomb et al. (12)	96	1	20	3	8	2	47	20		
Ildstad et al. (3)	20		6		1		13			
Bower et al. (13)	78		16		7	5	34	10	2	2
Hudson (14)	90		10		6	8	59	3	3	1
Total	530	6 (1%)	95 (18%)	13 (2%)	35 (7%)	30 (6%)	282 (53%)	68 (13%)	19 (4%)	3 (0.5%)

associated with vertebral abnormalities and may communicate with the spinal canal, or transdiaphragmatically with the abdominal cavity.

The symptoms and clinical presentation of intestinal duplications vary greatly depending on size, location, presence of gastric mucosa, and communication with the normal bowel. A mass discovered on physical examination or radiographic examination of the chest or abdomen is a common mode of discovery. Specific symptoms are often related to the location of the duplication. Cervical and thoracic duplications may cause respiratory symptoms or dysphagia, or may be an incidental finding on chest radiograph (15,16). Gastric and duodenal duplications may present as a palpable abdominal mass or due to symptoms of gastric outlet obstruction. Pain is the most common symptom and may be caused by distension of the duplication or result from a complication such as intestinal obstruction, peptic ulceration, or perforation. Intestinal obstruction may result from compression of the adjacent bowel lumen or due to the mass effect of the duplication leading to volvulus or intussusception. GI bleeding is also a common complication of enteric duplications. The bleeding can be acute and severe, presenting as hematemesis, melena, or hematochezia, depending on location and magnitude of bleeding. Chronic occult bleeding may present as anemia. The cystic lesions most often do not communicate with the normal intestine. These may achieve a large size and create a mass effect on plain radiographs or be noted as a palpable mass on physical exam. The tubular duplications of the small intestine more frequently communicate with the native bowel and have a high incidence of heterotopic gastric mucosa (17,18). Peptic ulceration can lead to perforation and free intraperitoneal hemorrhage or fistulization into adjacent structures. The majority of alimentary tract duplications that cause clinical symptoms are diagnosed in infancy (greater than 80% before 2 years of age) (19). Older infants and children with intestinal duplications may experience indolent and vague abdominal complaints over prolonged periods or intermittent GI bleeding and anemia. Colonic or presacral duplications typically present due to obstruction, constipation, or prolapse through the anus. Enteric duplications are frequently associated with vertebral abnormalities such as spina bifida or missing, fused, or hemivertebrae. Rarely, there may be an intraspinal component causing neurologic symptoms from spinal cord compression. Myelomeningocele is associated with some enteric duplications, especially in the thoracic cavity. Some duplications remain silent and persist into adulthood (20). Neoplastic changes have been reported in duplications diagnosed in adulthood—most in duplications of the colon and rectum (21,22). Hindgut duplications may be associated with splitting of the lower vertebrae and sacrum and severe urogenital abnormalities, such as doubling of the external genitalia or other perineal abnormality.

Intestinal duplications are often difficult to diagnose preoperatively. Common intestinal conditions, such as appendicitis, pyloric stenosis, intussusception, or malrotation, are frequent misdiagnoses when the duplication is found at laparotomy. In cases of large lesions, the diagnosis may be suspected by the finding on plain radiographs of a chest or abdominal mass with displacement of adjacent structures. This finding in the abdomen may prompt GI contrast studies, which may demonstrate the impression of a mass lesion on normal bowel (Fig. 85-1) and possibly communication with the lumen of the native bowel (Fig. 85-2), which is diagnostic of an intestinal duplication. Ultrasound has proven to be an excellent diagnostic modality

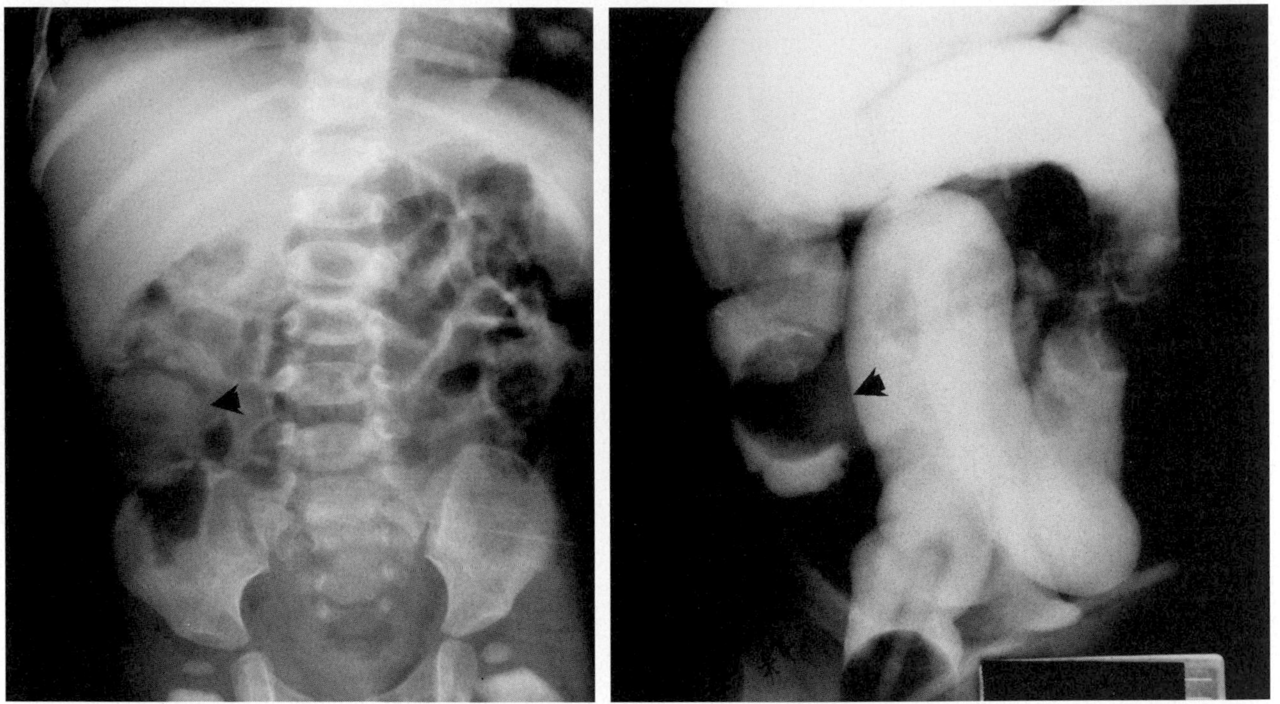

FIGURE 85-1. **(A)** A circular mass *(arrow)* in the cecum suggests the presence of a lesion. **(B)** Subsequent contrast enema demonstrates an intramural duplication cyst *(arrow)* in this 14-month-old with intermittent obstructive symptoms.

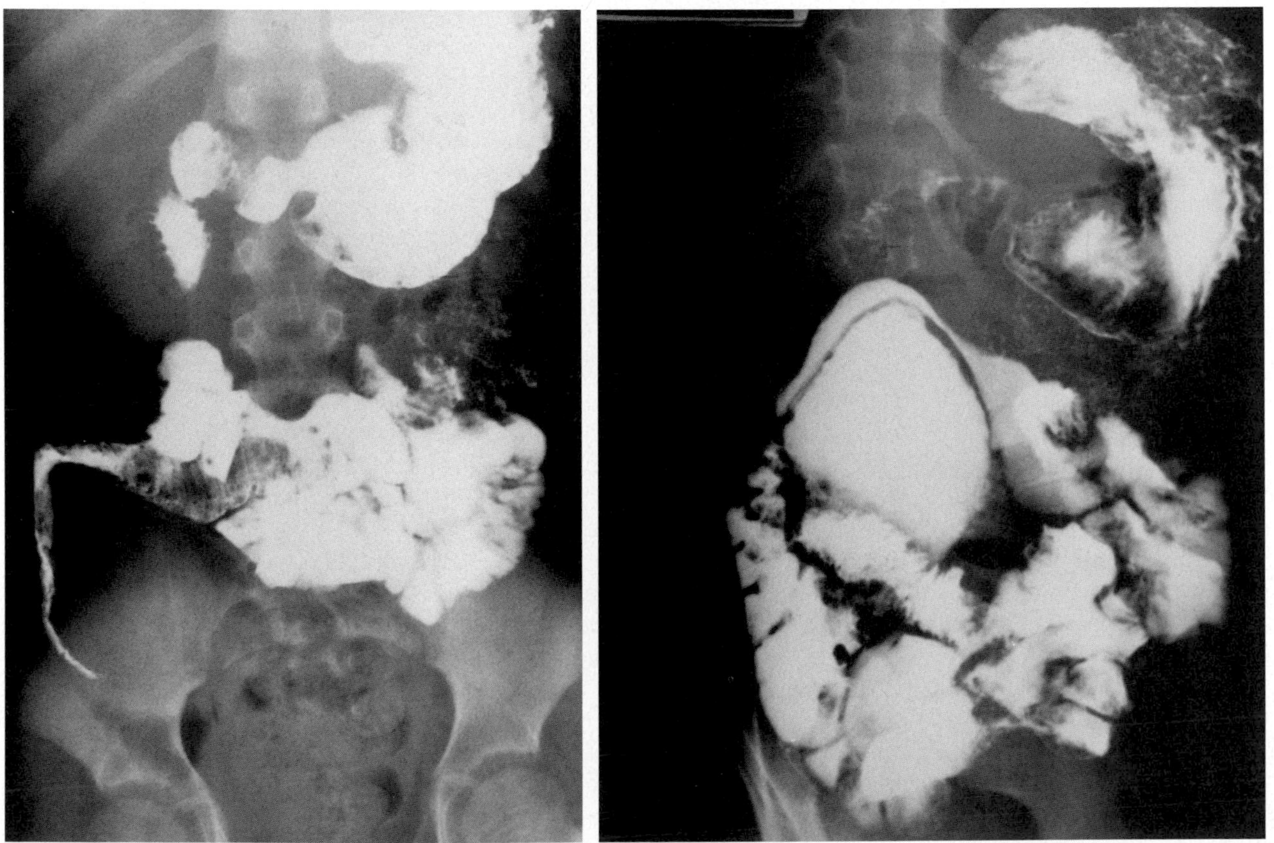

FIGURE 85-2. A rare example of a communicating cystic duplication is found in this 10-year-old who presented with bleeding and a mass effect on abdominal flat plate. Upper gastrointestinal contrast study shows an extrinsic mass impression on the bowel **(A)**, whereas a later film **(B)** demonstrates filling of the duplication cavity.

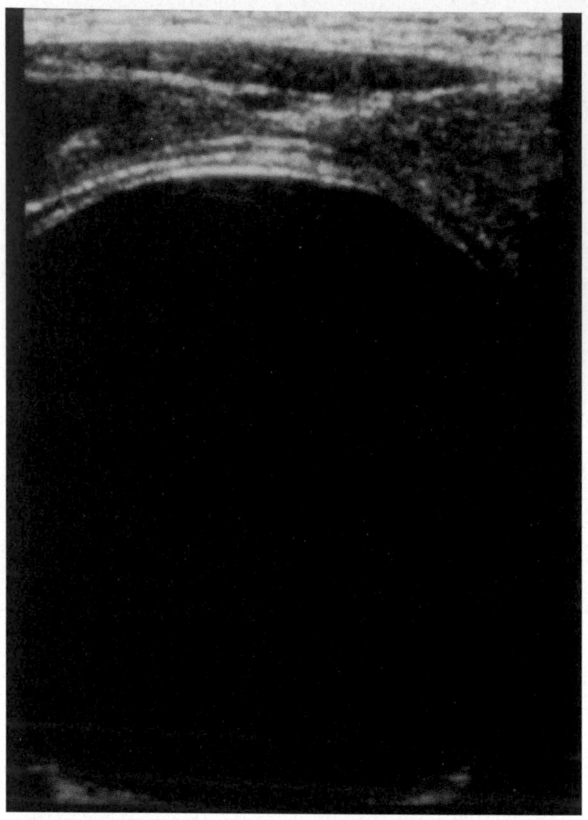

FIGURE 85-3. Ultrasound study of a patient with gastric duplication demonstrating the classic findings of triple layering.

for enteric duplications, and the classic triple-layer image (Fig. 85-3) is pathoneumonic of intestinal duplications (23). Ultrasound is also useful to evaluate for possible associated genitourinary anomalies in cases of hindgut duplications and should be done routinely. Thoracic duplications are often apparent on routine chest radiography. Axial imaging with contrast-enhanced computed tomography (CT) scan or magnetic resonance imaging (MRI) are also good tests to demonstrate thoracic duplication cysts and their relationship to adjacent structures, and are particularly helpful in evaluating for possible associated vertebral abnormalities or central nervous system (CNS) lesions. In cases that present with GI bleeding, radionuclide technetium scanning can be very helpful in diagnosing and localizing duplications in the thorax, small bowel, and hindgut (24). Enteric duplications have been diagnosed on prenatal ultrasound examinations (25).

Duplications in the pediatric population are benign lesions, and therefore, the surgical therapy should aim primarily to eliminate symptoms, preserve function, and prevent future complications and recurrence. There have been a small number of case reports of an intestinal duplication harboring malignancy, almost exclusively adenocarcinoma in adult patients (16). Mortality due to bleeding or sepsis from perforation is related to delay in diagnosis and definitive treatment. Although some of these lesions are technically challenging, morbidity and mortality should be rare in modern practice.

INCIDENCE

Enteric duplications are rare lesions and their exact incidence is difficult to determine. They are reported in 1 of every 4,500 autopsies (26). They appear to be most often seen in white males; the exception being complex hindgut duplications, which are more common in females. There does not appear to be a familial incidence. Alimentary tract duplications are most commonly located in the small intestine and mediastinum (posterior), whereas rectal, duodenal, gastric, and thoracoabdominal locations are extremely rare. Synchronous duplications are reported in as many as 15% of patients.

ASSOCIATED ANOMALIES

Associated anomalies are common with alimentary tract duplications. Most important is an association between thoracic and thoracoabdominal duplications and vertebral anomalies, such as missing, bifid, or fused vertebrae (12,27). Esophageal duplications are seen in association with other esophageal malformations, such as esophageal atresia and tracheoesophageal fistula, and pulmonary agenesis. Small intestine cystic duplications have been reported with coexisting intestinal atresias and malrotation (11,13). Tubular hindgut duplications are an extremely complex and diverse group of anomalies frequently associated with genitourinary and other severe malformations (28,29).

EMBRYOLOGY

The embryogenesis of intestinal duplications is not known. There are many theories, but none adequately explains the origin of all lesions in this diverse constellation of anomalies, suggesting that more than one pathogenic possibility may be necessary to explain the anatomic variability. The following is a brief discussion of the more common theories of disordered embryogenesis resulting in intestinal duplications.

Split Notochord Theory

Bentley and Smith proposed the "split notochord syndrome" in an attempt to explain the frequent association between developmental anomalies of the skin, spine, CNS, and the GI tract (30). The dorsal location and relatively frequent (15%) association of enteric duplications with vertebral abnormalities provide support for this theory. The notochord is formed during the third week of the gestation when a proliferation of cells from the primitive streak of the ectoderm develops as a midline structure separating the lining of the yolk sac (primitive endoderm) from the lining of the amniotic cavity (primitive ectoderm). A transient opening, the neurenteric canal, appears and connects the neural ectoderm with the GI endoderm. The notochord is at first in intimate association with the endodermal cells, but normally it later migrates and separates from them as part of the process of cephalic growth of the ectoderm and notochord mesoderm. Persistence of the neurenteric canal causes the notocord to split as it migrates, resulting in the development of spina bifida or other vertebral anomalies and anterior and posterior meningomyelocele. If the notochord fails to detach from the endoderm, adherent endodermal cells may be pulled anterior and cephalad as the tissues separate. These endodermal cells, detached from the roof of the developing gut, may form an intestinal duplication. If they remain attached to the notochord, they may also act as a local barrier to the later fusion of the vertebral mesoderm, resulting in vertebral abnormalities. Beardmore and Wigglesworth (31) proposed that there was adherence of the ectoderm and endoderm in the neural plate that caused the notochord to "split" as it grew. The splitting of the notochord by the persistent neurenteric canal as it migrates may result in a vertebral anomaly (Fig. 85-4). The resulting tubular structure may extend through the diaphragm, connecting abdominal viscera to the thoracic or cervical spine. If the connection is lost, an isolated mediastinal duplication or an intramesenteric abdominal diverticulum may result, and the vertebral anomaly may resolve. Failure of regression of the neurenteric canal and persistent attachment to the notochord may prevent closing of the vertebral bodies, resulting in a spectrum of neurenteric pathology, including occult anterior spina bifida, intraspinal enteric cyst, dorsal enteric sinus, neurenteric cyst, diastematomyelia, or a complete dorsal enteric fistula. The absence of spinal defects in many alimentary tract duplications makes the split notochord theory less tenable as a unifying model of origin for alimentary tract duplications (32).

A second theory suggests that failure of the normal regression of *embryonic diverticula* may occur. Diverticula are common in the developing human GI tract (33). Their finding at numerous sites around the circumference of the gut wall provides a potential explanation for small cystic duplications noted in the intestinal wall, and for enteric cysts located in the presacral space. However, this theory does not explain the propensity for the location of enteric cysts within the leaves of the bowel mesentery, or the finding of multiple types of mucosa lining the wall of some enteric duplications.

The theory of *median septum formation* suggests that the walls of adjacent fetal bowel may be flattened by extrinsic compression with subsequent adherence and fusion resulting in doubling of the lumen. Although this would explain the occurrence of adjacent or side-by-side tubular duplications, there is no embryonic evidence for this theory.

The association of complex tubular duplications of the colon and rectum with urogenital anomalies and doubling of other body parts may best be explained by the theory of *partial or abortive twinning* (5,9,28,29,34–38). This theory suggests that the axial structures in hindgut duplications are "twinned" because of a split in the primitive streak, resulting in two notochords, separated at their caudal ends, which later fuse during cranial elongation of the embryo. This would result in the duplication of structures derived from the hindgut, including distal ileum, colon, rectum, and anus. With this anomaly, doubling of the genitalia and of the bladder and urethra, exstrophy of the bladder, spina bifida, omphalocele, and other lesions are observed with extraordinary frequency. It is speculated that twinning early in the hindgut's caudal growth may result in duplication of other pelvic organs, including genital structures, whereas later twinning may result only in colorectal duplication. Doubling of the anus, vagina, bladder, lower trunk, and extremities (dipygus) all have been described and can be associated with rare cases of double spines and two heads.

It has also been proposed that intestinal duplications may result from environmental stresses exerted on the embryo during fetal development. Mellish and Koop theorized that trauma or hypoxia could induce duplications and twinning in lower orders (9). Based on the work of Louw, they concluded that vascular insufficiency could lead to some types of duplications seen in humans. In addition, intestinal duplications are often seen in association with intestinal atresia, and intrauterine vascular accidents are known precipitants of intestinal atresias (38).

CERVICAL DUPLICATIONS

Cervical esophageal duplications are rare, with fewer than 10 cases reported in the literature (39). The majority present at a young age, most at younger than 1 year (15,39,40,41). Cervical duplications are typically spherical cysts that do not communicate with the lumen of the associated native esophagus. They may be appreciable as a neck mass on physical examination. Their intimate attachment to the esophagus may serve to differentiate them from cysts of branchial origin. These cysts tend to compress adjacent structures, causing dysphagia, vomiting, or respiratory distress. Because the newborn or infant airway is easily compressible, respiratory compromise associated with cervical duplication cysts can be life threatening, making rapid diagnosis and treatment critically important. Ventilatory support may be necessary perioperatively. When a cervical duplication is suspected,

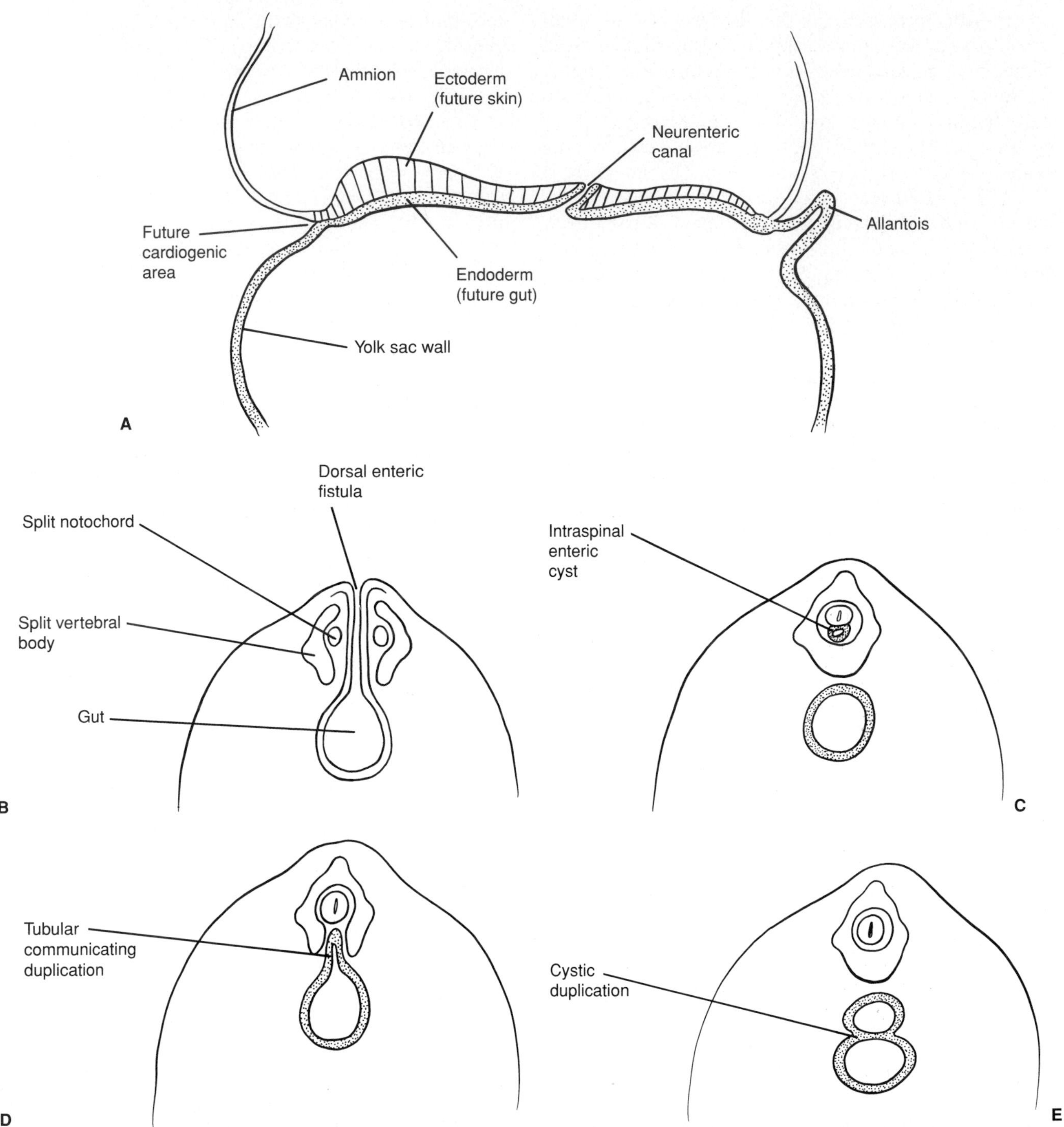

FIGURE 85-4. Diagrammatic representation of the split notochord theory of duplication development. **(A)** A sagittal view of the developing embryo illustrating the neurenteric canal. During spinal organogenesis, gastrointestinal endoderm is entrapped, forming a traction diverticulum as the separation begins. A persistent neurenteric canal results in dorsal enteric fistula **(B)**, enteric cysts **(C)**, tubular communicating duplication **(D)**, cystic duplication **(E)**, spina bifida, and other vertebral anomalies.

further evaluation can be obtained by ultrasound or CT. Axial imaging with either CT or MRI scans is optimal to delineate anatomic relationships with other structures and also permit evaluation of the vertebral column, although no patients have presented with neurologic symptoms.

Total excision is the preferred treatment for cervical duplications. This is achieved by dissecting the cyst and common wall away from the native esophagus. In cases where total excision may compromise the native esophagus or adjacent vital structures, partial excision and removal or stripping of the cyst mucosal lining should also be curative and prevent future complications. The remaining seromuscular cyst wall is simply oversewn in this instance (35).

THORACIC AND THORACOABDOMINAL DUPLICATIONS

Thoracic duplication cysts represent up to 15% of cases in some series, whereas thoracoabdominal lesions are rare, making up only approximately 2% (42,43). As many as one-third of these thoracic lesions will have a second or third duplication cyst located below the diaphragm (12,41,44,45). Thoracic duplications appear to be more common on the right side and have the highest incidence of associated vertebral anomalies, including anterior or posterior spina bifida, hemivertebrae, or myelomeningocele. Rarely, they may have an associated intraspinal mass lesion or CNS involvement. Thoracoabdominal lesions communicate with the intestinal tract below the diaphragm, most often through the esophageal hiatus and generally connect to the duodenum or jejunum after passing behind the stomach and pancreas. The likely presentation in an infant or neonate is respiratory distress as a result of accumulation of fluid and debris within the cyst. These duplications commonly contain gastric mucosa, and older patients may present with symptoms of "heartburn" or severe hemorrhage from peptic ulceration. Thoracic duplications have been reported in association with other esophageal malformations, such as esophageal atresia and tracheoesophageal fistula, and with other anomalies, including lung agenesis, omphalocele, and pericardial defects (46–49). The term *neurenteric cyst* has been used for thoracic duplications associated with vertebral anomalies (48). Ulceration of a thoracic duplication into the adjacent esophagus or bronchus may result in melena, hematemesis, or hemoptysis (5). Thoracic duplications may also be discovered as an incidental finding on chest radiographs. They typically appear as a well-defined posterior mediastinal shadow. Axial imaging using CT or MRI is imperative in cases of thoracic or thoracoabdominal duplications to evaluate for possible communication to the spinal canal and should also include the abdomen due to the high incidence of associated abdominal duplications (41). The typical finding on CT is a well-circumscribed, homogeneous mass with an enhancing rim. The lack of enhancement of the central core of the mass lesion distinguishes the duplication cyst from neurogenic tumors (50). Myelography may be helpful in carefully selected cases. A severe form of this malformation is the dorsal enteric fistula, a mucosa-lined fistula tract leading from the alimentary tube to the skin of the back, passing through a bifid spinal cord and vertebral column (51–53).

The preferred treatment of thoracic and thoracoabdominal duplications is complete excision. This is generally straightforward for the noncommunicating type, but can be a technically challenging and formidable task in the more complex lesions. The need for evaluation for possible connection to the spinal canal and careful monitoring for development of neurologic symptoms has been emphasized. In cases with spinal canal involvement, a combined surgical approach with an experienced neurosurgical team should be employed. To avoid compromise of the esophageal lumen, the technique of partial cyst excision combined with mucosal stripping is an alternative to total excision. Thoracoabdominal duplications are often extensive lesions and can be managed by staged excision. In this setting, generally the portion of the cyst causing symptoms is excised first. It is important to note that following excision of the abdominal portion, the thoracic component may suddenly increase in size due to increased secretions or lack of drainage, leading to acute respiratory symptoms. The surgeon must be prepared for this possibility, and for this reason, most thoracoabdominal duplications are excised using a single extended procedure. Separate chest and abdominal incisions are generally used. The abdominal portion of thoracoabdominal duplications is often tubular and may require surgical management by internal drainage and mucosal stripping to avoid extensive intestinal resection.

GASTRIC DUPLICATIONS

Enteric cysts associated with the stomach comprise only approximately 5% to 7% of cases (Fig. 85-5). They are typically cystic, located on the greater curvature or posterior wall, and have no communication with the stomach (54,55). Gastric duplications are variable in size from small lesions almost certain to be asymptomatic to large cysts causing obvious abdominal distension and a readily palpable mass on physical exam (Fig. 85-6). They are more common in boys than girls and typically present early in the first year of life due to vomiting, poor feeding and weight gain, or abdominal distension. When located at or near the pylorus, these lesions typically cause gastric outlet obstruction leading to projectile vomiting in infancy and thus may mimic pyloric stenosis (56,57). The cyst mucosal lining is often gastric and poor drainage and inadequate neutralization of acid secretions can lead to local inflammation (pain), ulceration (bleeding), and even perforation with free air and intraperitoneal hemorrhage (58). Patients may present with melena, hematemesis, and anemia. Penetrating ulceration with erosion into the stomach, colon, and pancreas and through the abdominal wall has been reported. Pancreatitis caused by erosion into the pancreas has been reported as an unusual presentation of a gastric duplication (59). Gastric duplications have also been reported to erode through the diaphragm, presenting with chest symptoms such as hemoptysis and respiratory distress from lung compression and parenchymal erosion. Rarely, gastric duplications may be completely separate

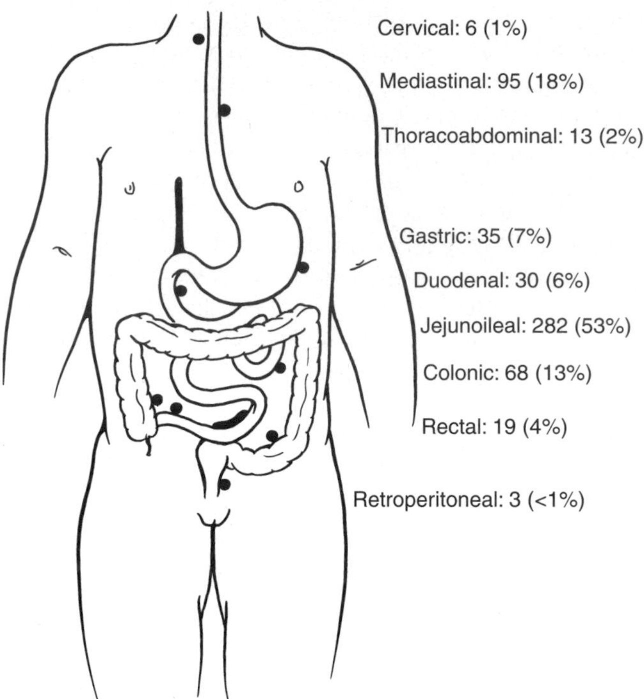

FIGURE 85-5. An anatomic representation of the incidence and location of enteric duplications taken from the studies listed in Table 85-1.

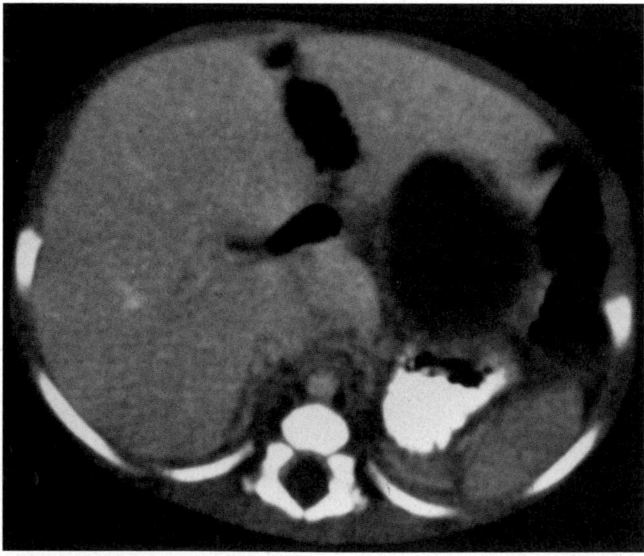

FIGURE 85-6. A 1-month-old presented with vomiting and an upper gastrointestinal bleed. A CT scan demonstrates displacement of abdominal viscera by a gastric duplication (no contrast) that does not communicate with the stomach (filled with contrast). (Courtesy of Dr. Francis Blankenburg, Department of Radiology, Packard Children's Hospital at Stanford University, Palo Alto, CA.)

from the stomach and are located in the retroperitoneum (60).

Gastric duplications are often confused with more common GI conditions, such as pyloric stenosis, malrotation, and duodenal atresia or stenosis. A gastric duplication should be suspected when plain radiographs demonstrate a mass effect, displacing the stomach in an infant or child. Further evaluation should proceed with an ultrasound or upper GI contrast study. Intestinal duplications have a classic appearance on ultrasound examination with an inner echogenic mucosal layer and an outer hypoechoic muscular rim. The contrast study may demonstrate an extrinsic compression defect. Endoscopic ultrasound, CT scan, and MRI scan may provide useful information in selected cases. Technetium scanning can demonstrate gastric mucosa in a gastric duplication, but the normal stomach uptake can lead to false-negative tests. Complications associated with undiagnosed gastric duplications occur frequently, with bleeding and perforation being most common.

The preferred treatment of gastric duplications is complete resection by dissecting the common wall with the stomach. Entry into the stomach during resection is simply closed, and gastric resection is generally not necessary. Wedge resection of small portions of the gastric wall can also be performed. Because of the presence of gastric mucosa and potential for penetrating ulceration and bleeding, management of gastric duplications by internal drainage is associated with a high complication rate. In situations in which removing the entire cyst would result in significant anatomic risk and place the child in nutritional jeopardy, partial resection should be performed combined with mucosal stripping and oversewing of the remaining wall, as described earlier. The important principle is to not leave mucosa behind that is at risk for ulceration, bleeding, recurrent cyst formation, or neoplastic changes.

DUODENAL DUPLICATIONS

Duodenal duplications comprise approximately 6% of enteric cysts of the alimentary tract (Fig. 85-5). They are typically located on the posteromedial aspect of the second or third portion of the duodenum and lined with duodenal or distal small bowel mucosa. Most duodenal duplications are cystic and about 25% communicate with the lumen of the native duodenum (16). A primary concern for patients with a duodenal duplication is the potential for involvement of the biliary tract or other adjacent vital structures. Only about 15% of duodenal duplications contain gastric mucosa.

Duodenal duplications are often difficult to diagnose because the symptoms can be intermittent, vague, and nonspecific. Patients typically present with signs and symptoms of intermittent upper intestinal obstruction, such as colicky abdominal pain and vomiting. Plain radiographic findings are often minimal, but may demonstrate a dilated proximal duodenum or an upper abdominal mass effect. These cases are less likely to be discovered during infancy and the mean age of diagnosis is approximately 3 years. Some are diagnosed in adults (61). The complications associated with undiagnosed duodenal duplications are similar to those of other enteric duplications and include peptic ulceration, bleeding, anemia, and fistulization. Duodenal duplications tend to be cystic, and proximity to the biliary tree and pancreas can result in compression of the bile or pancreatic duct resulting in jaundice or pancreatitis (62). There are rare reports of enteric duplications arising from the biliary tree or pancreas (63). Associated vertebral anomalies or transdiaphragmatic erosion and respiratory complications are rare with duodenal duplications.

Duodenal duplications may be discovered on upper GI contrast study in evaluation for vomiting and signs and symptoms of upper intestinal obstruction. The findings suggestive of duodenal duplication on contrast study include complete obstruction or narrowing of the duodenal lumen, a widened C-loop, or an intraluminal filling defect of the duodenum. When discovered, the differential diagnosis for cystic lesions in this area includes choledochal cyst, cystic lymphangioma, congenital hepatic or pancreatic cyst, and pancreatic pseudocyst. Ultrasound and contrast-enhanced CT scan are both helpful studies to confirm the diagnosis, investigate the biliary tree, and delineate relationships of the duplication cyst with adjacent structures.

The preferred treatment for duodenal duplications is complete excision with the attached segment of duodenum, but this is rarely possible because of proximity to the ampulla of Vater and the potential for injury to the biliary tree and pancreatic duct, particularly with any inflammatory changes. Cholangiography, either preoperatively or intraoperatively, is important to assess the relation to the biliary and pancreatic ductal systems. If complete excision is not technically possible, marsupialization or internal drainage to the duodenum or jejunum (Roux-en-Y) are acceptable alternatives provided the duplication cyst does not contain gastric mucosa. If gastric mucosa is present, excision of the free portion of the cyst wall and mucosal stripping from the remaining portion is the recommended surgical management. Mucosal stripping may be associated with significant intraoperative bleeding and appropriate preoperative planning should include type and cross-matching of blood. Endoscopic drainage of duodenal duplications has been reported (64,65).

SMALL INTESTINE DUPLICATIONS

The small intestine, and particularly the ileocecal region, is the most common location for enteric duplications, accounting for approximately 50% of cases in most reported series (10,12,13). Intestinal duplications of the ileum are differentiated from Meckel's diverticulum by their mesenteric location and shared blood supply and muscular wall with the native bowel (Fig. 85-7). Duplications of the small intestine can be cystic or tubular and vary greatly

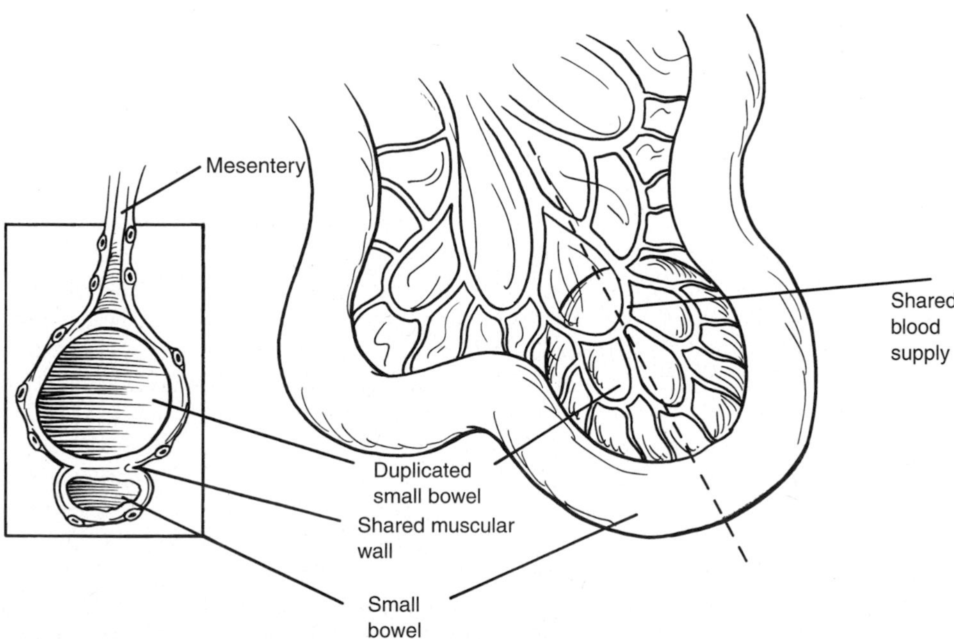

FIGURE 85-7. A small bowel duplication in cross section, demonstrating the common wall, shared blood supply, and intramesenteric location.

in size, from small spherical lesions measuring only a few centimeters to tubular lesions extending the entire length of the small bowel. The classic ileal duplication cyst is spherical, located on the mesenteric border, shares a muscularis with the associated bowel, and does not communicate with the lumen of the associated bowel. These cysts may cause abdominal pain from distension or lead to obstruction, volvulus, or intussusception. Recurrent or chronic intussusception has also been reported as a rare presentation of duplication cysts of the small intestine. Newborns with associated intestinal atresia make up 15% of patients presenting with ileal duplications, with the presumed etiology being in utero volvulus leading to a mesenteric injury resulting in atresia. Rarer are the tubular duplications of the small intestine, and these can be particularly difficult to diagnose and manage. The tubular duplications can be quite extensive and frequently communicate with the lumen of the adjacent bowel (18). The communication can be anywhere along the common wall with the native bowel: proximally, distally, or at multiple sites. The tubular duplications that have a proximal communication with the native bowel are most likely to become dilated due to accumulation of intestinal fluid and secretions, and to create an abdominal mass that can result in intestinal obstruction by compression of the adjacent intestine, or lead to volvulus or perforation (Fig. 85-8). Tubular duplications with a distal communication with the native bowel generally drain satisfactorily. Tubular duplications, particularly jejunal, have a high incidence of heterotopic gastric mucosa and complications from peptic ulceration, such as perforation, melena, and hematochezia are highest in this location (66–68).

Duplications of the small intestine can present acutely in the neonatal period, present after a prolonged period of indolent and vague abdominal symptoms, or remain asymptomatic. The acute presentation is generally due to complications of intestinal obstruction, volvulus, or GI bleeding. Duplications of the small intestine are mobile and less likely than gastric or duodenal duplications to be appreciated as an abdominal mass on physical exam. Ileal duplications are frequently diagnosed at laparotomy for more common intestinal conditions, such as appendicitis, Hirschsprung's disease, or intussusception, whereas jejunal duplications are confused with Meckel's diverticulum, peptic ulcer disease, malrotation, or atresia when the presentation occurs in the neonatal period.

The preferred treatment for duplications of the small intestine is resection of the duplication with the associated native bowel and primary anstamosis. This is generally straightforward for small cystic or short tubular duplications. Long tubular duplications pose much more of a technical challenge surgically. Surgical resection is not possible if the length of resection will place the patient at risk for malabsorption, nutritional deficiencies, or short-gut syndrome (Fig. 85-9). Long tubular duplications can be managed with internal drainage by creating a window in the common wall into the native intestinal lumen at the end of the duplication to avoid extensive intestinal resection. This approach should be accompanied by stripping of the mucosa through counterincisions along the common wall to avoid complications associated with retained gastric mucosa. Alternatively, some reports have described a potential dissection plane between the native bowel and the duplication that may allow excision of the duplication without having to remove the associated intestine (69,70). Others have used the approach described by Bianchi (71) for bowel-lengthening procedures (72). This technique involves dissection and separation of the leaves of the mesentery, preserving the posterior vascular arcade to the native intestine, and thus may permit resection of the duplication without removing the associated intestine. Internal drainage of the distal end of the duplication to the stomach is an alternative surgical approach described and has been performed successfully to manage this difficult problem (68).

DUPLICATIONS OF COLON AND RECTUM

Enteric duplications of the hindgut comprise the most complex group of duplications and account for approximately 20% of cases. The spectrum of hindgut duplications is remarkably variable, ranging from small intramural colonic duplications to complex lesions often associated with lower vertebral and complex urogenital abnormalities. These lesions may be isolated cysts in the abdomen or pelvis or tubular structures that may have an external fistula to the perineum, an internal fistula to the urinary tract, or a communication with the normal colon (28,34,35). The incidence of neoplastic change in hindgut duplications, predominantly adenocarcinoma, is higher than in any other location (22). Hindgut duplications generally contain normal colonic epithelium. The tubular form of duplication is more common in the colon and may communicate with the rectum distally or have a separate perineal opening near the anus (73). An unusual variety, most likely a result of *partial twinning,* is a complete duplication of the colon and rectum with separate anal orifices and often associated with genitourinary system anomalies. Rectal duplications may be seen as part of the "Currarino triad." This syndrome, inherited in an autosomal dominant manner, consists of a presacral tumor, anorectal stenosis, and sacral bony abnormalities (74). An association has been noted between complete duplication of the colon and extrapulmonary sequestration with esophageal communication (75).

Constipation, obstruction, and volvulus are the most common presenting symptoms in patients with hindgut duplications. Complications as a result of peptic ulceration

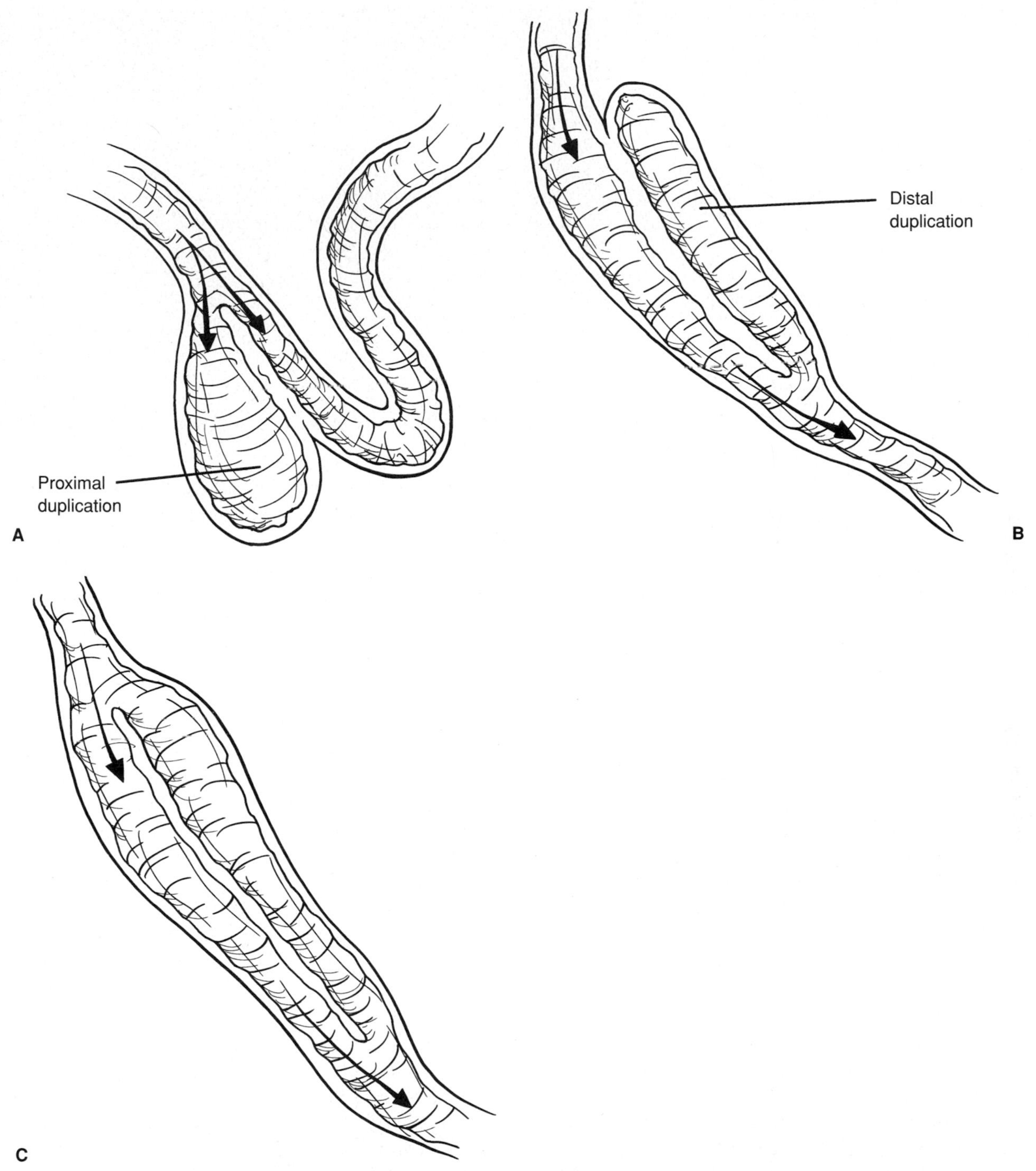

FIGURE 85-8. Schematic depiction of the various forms of communicating tubular duplications. Duplication communicating proximally, forming bulbous mass **(A)**; duplication communicating distally, remaining clinically asymptomatic **(B)**; duplication communicating proximally and distally **(C)**.

are rare because ectopic gastric mucosa is uncommon in hindgut duplications. Although hindgut duplications are a diverse and complex group of lesions, several unifying types are described: midline duplications, cystic remnants of the tailgut, and bilateral tubular duplications of the colon and rectum.

Midline duplications are typically cystic in nature and lie in the mesentery, posterior to the colon or rectum (19). Tubular duplications are distinctly uncommon in this location. These lesions typically have the classic characteristics of enteric duplications in other locations, including dorsal location and a shared common wall and blood supply

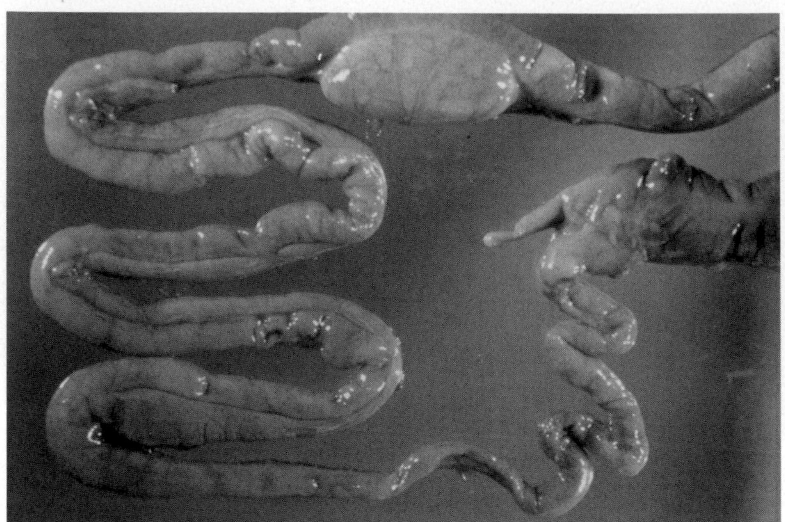

FIGURE 85-9. An autopsy specimen showing a tubular small bowel duplication involving a portion of the ileum and much of the jejunum. (Courtesy of Dr. Carlos Abramowsky, Department of Pathology, Egleston Children's Hospital at Emory University, Atlanta, GA.)

with the associated bowel. They are predominantly presacral and may be asymptomatic or can cause obstruction or prolapse of the rectum or anus. Because of the shared blood supply and common wall, these cysts may require an extensive resection for definitive therapy. If attached to the rectum, consideration should be given to protection with a temporary diverting colostomy.

The second general type of hindgut duplication is the *tail-gut cyst,* a cystic structure located between the anus and the coccyx that contains enteric epithelium. In contrast to the *midline duplication*, it does not have a shared blood supply or common wall and is generally excised easily without resection of the associated rectum. The *tail-gut cyst* is considered to be a remnant of the opening between the ectoderm and endoderm at the posterior end of the neural tube. Most midline defects have been attributed to this persistent developmental structure. Presacral tumors with enteric epithelium should probably be considered remnants of this tail-gut abnormality. Obstruction and constipation are the most common presenting signs in infants with midline duplications and tail-gut cysts (76). The recommended treatment is excision. As is true with sacrococcygeal teratomas, resection of the lesion with the coccyx is recommended.

The third type of hindgut duplication is the most complex anomaly with complete duplication of hindgut structures, possibly with separate anal orifices. This form of duplication is typically located "side-by-side" to the normal bowel, rather than within the leaves of the mesentery. The association of colon duplication in conjoined and incomplete twinning has been reported, and this anomaly may represent an attempt at partial twinning (77). These patients often have major associated urogenital anomalies. The entire hindgut, including distal ileum, cecum, appendix, and entire colon, may be double and drain through a single anal orifice or through separate ones. Both lumens may be unobstructed and function normally or there may be imperforate anus distally involving one or both lumens, and the ventrally positioned colon may end as a rectovesical, rectourethral, or rectovaginal fistula. When the distal opening is inadequate, that part of the colon may become massively distended, compressing and possibly obstructing the associated bowel, or it may rupture. Paired or septated bladder and uteri, duplicated external genitalia, and major renal anomalies have all been reported in association with extensive hindgut duplications (78,79). The caudal spinal cord has also been found to have anomalies that range from an anterior meningomyelocele to complete duplication of an otherwise normal cord. Some fully developed cases have demonstrated complete duplication of all caudal intestinal structures, beginning at Meckel's diverticulum, and include two bladders and two vaginas that communicate with two unicornate uteri and open into separate vulvas. In boys, a bifid penis and scrotum have been reported, and the lumbar vertebrae and the sacrum may be doubled or bifid. The uterus and vagina are not derived from the hindgut, but are commonly doubled in severe cases. This failure of fusion of the mullerian-derived structures is considered secondary to the doubling of the urogenital sinus, to which their distal ends attach.

Most of these complex hindgut duplications are found in girls (70%). Duplications involving the complete hindgut or colorectum are found in 70%, whereas 10% to 30% have more complex caudal twinning with double bladders, urethras, vaginas, and uteri and abnormal genitals. The evaluation and management of these complex hindgut duplications must be individualized. The duplicated external genitalia are considered to have normal function and are often left in place in female patients. Reports of women with this hindgut abnormality successfully giving vaginal birth to infants from both vaginas have been published. Boys with a duplicated penis are usually treated surgically to attempt a more normal perineal appearance. The absence of reflux or obstruction allows urologic procedures to be performed electively in these patients with completely duplicated caudal twinning. However, obstructive symptoms may require early urologic intervention. Patients who present with doubled genitals typically have a communication either internally with the normal colon or externally to the perineum that allows the duplication to empty, and they do not develop obstructive symptoms. However, patients with normal external anatomy and a duplicated hindgut often present with obstruction, with the normal colon being compressed by the blind end of the abnormal obstructed colon. These colons are often densely adherent and share the same blood supply, requiring a drainage procedure to preserve the normal bowel. Colonic duplications may masquerade as a perirectal abscess or fistula in ano and persistent perineal excoriation associated with a fistula tract should raise suspicion to the possibility of a duplication with gastric mucosa within the fistula tract (80).

The surgical management of complex hindgut duplications associated with perineal and genitourinary malformations is often a formidable undertaking. The presenting complaints in patients with severe abnormalities of the hindgut include obstruction of adjacent bowel by the dilated duplication or complications from the obstruction. Information contributing to the diagnosis can be obtained from barium studies when there are two obvious anal orifices (Fig. 85-10). When only one anus exists, the situation is difficult to diagnose before surgery. If the duplication is a long segment, blind-ending, and fused with a normal rectum and perineal anus, a transanal connection can be made with the duplication by excising part of the common rectal wall. Any connection to the genitourinary system must be repaired, if present. Alternative approaches to these difficult cases include excising the lesion along with the normal colon, enlarging existing communications with the normal bowel, or excising a portion of the common wall of the cyst and the normal colon at their distalmost area of attachment. In addition, staged excision has been used. The first step is a temporary diverting colostomy of the colon and duplication followed by excision of the duplication, or as much as possible, and anastamosis of the distal end of the duplication to the colon so both drain through a single anal orifice. If the colon and duplication both end above the perineum a similar anastamosis has to be followed by a pull-through type procedure. The posterior sagital approach of Peña has been recommended and used successfully.

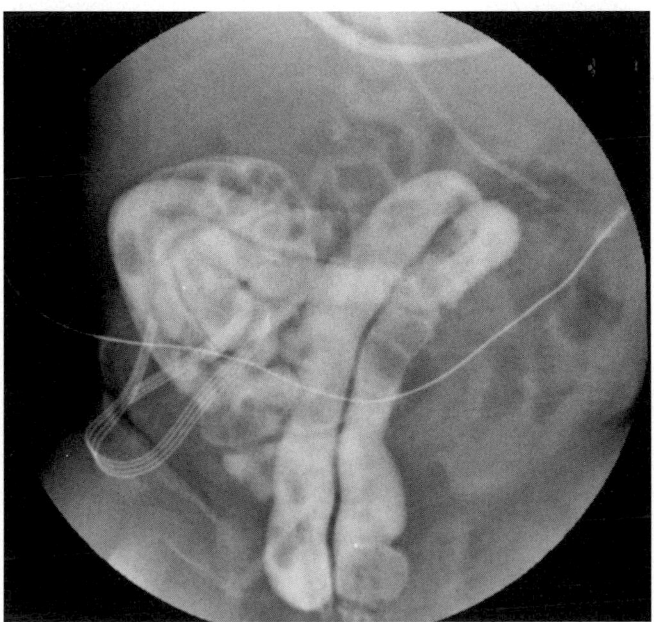

FIGURE 85-10. A contrast enema of an infant presenting with doubled anal orifices at birth in addition to other abdominal wall abnormalities.

MESENTERIC, OMENTAL, AND RETROPERITONEAL CYST

Cysts of the, mesentery, omentum, or retroperitoneum are uncommon, having an incidence of approximately 1 per 100,000 hospital admissions in most series. These lesions are benign unilocular or multilocular endothelium-lined cysts that contain either chyle, with its characteristic high triglyceride content and high lymphocyte count, or serous fluid (81). They occasionally contain bloody fluid as a result of hemorrhage into the cyst. In contrast to intestinal duplications, these cysts are typically thin-walled and smooth and the cyst wall is comprised of fibrous connective tissue lined by endothelial cells. Dilated lymphatics are often associated with the cyst, and there may be calcification in the wall. Most omental cysts and colonic mesenteric cysts have serous contents, whereas mesenteric cysts located in the small bowel and retroperitoneum are equally divided between serous and chylous (82,83).

Mesenteric, omental, and retroperitoneal cysts are considered together because of the shared embryologic origin of the structures from which they originate (84,85). The most probable explanation of embryogenesis, first proposed by Gross, is that they represent a congenital, developmental abnormality of the lymphatic system, which results in ectopic lymphatic tissue that proliferates and collects fluid owing to a lack of communication with the central lymphatic system (86–88). This developmental theory could account for their occurrence in the newborn. Other proposals attribute these cysts to obstructions of the lymphatic system or to a failure of the mesenteric leaves to fuse during development (89). The concept of lymphatic obstruction seems less likely because attempts to create lymphatic obstruction in animal models have failed to produce cystic lesions. Furthermore, lymphangiography has failed to demonstrate the presence of obstructed lymphatics in cases of mesenteric, omental, or retroperitoneal cysts (90).

Mesenteric cysts are seen in all age groups, with about 25% to 40% reported in children. Mesenteric cysts appear to be more common than omental cysts by a factor of 3 to 1, and retroperitoneal cysts are the least common, representing only about 5% of mesenteric cysts (91).

MESENTERIC CYSTS

Mesenteric cysts may be found anywhere in the mesentery from the duodenum to the rectum, with the most common location being the small intestine. They are easily confused with enteric duplications because both are located on the mesenteric side of the bowel and are closely associated with the adjacent intestine. The two lesions may be differentiated in that a bowel duplication will have a well-defined mucosal layer and will share a common blood supply and muscular layer with the adjacent bowel. These features are lacking in mesenteric cysts. The natural history is generally one of slow growth, and this may explain their relative lack of symptoms until presentation in older age groups. They appear to be equally divided between males and females.

In studies of both adults and children, these lesions are difficult to diagnose because they are often large and soft in consistency. They are often mobile and easily missed on physical examination. Mesenteric cysts appear more likely than omental and retroperitoneal cysts to become symptomatic at an early age because of their close proximity to the bowel. The complaint at presentation is commonly abdominal pain due to hemorrhage, obstruction, or volvulus. Rapid enlargement of mesenteric cysts may occur from hemorrhage, and patients may present with an "acute abdomen" with peritonitis or with pain characteristic of an acute, mechanical small bowel obstruction. In children, presentation is typically acute as a result of intestinal obstruction from compression of adjacent bowel or volvulus, whereas adults are more likely to present with chronic abdominal complaints (92). In addition, acute abdominal distension from hemorrhage or bowel infarction, or chronic, progressive abdominal distension can also occur. Rare complications include cystic torsion or rupture, malignant degeneration, and obstruction of the urinary system. Large cysts may mimic ascites or cause biliary tract compression with resultant jaundice (93,94). There are reported cases of mesenteric or retroperitoneal cysts presenting as an inguinal hernia (95). The jejunum is the most common location of mesenteric cysts.

Plain abdominal radiographs are nonspecific, but may show a homogenous, gasless structure displacing loops of bowel. This appearance can mimic ascites. Fine calcifications in the wall of the cyst may be present. Abdominal ultrasound is the diagnostic procedure of choice in the case of a suspected mesenteric cyst. The mesenteric cyst appears as a well-circumscribed cystic structure with thin walls and often contains septae. There may be internal echoes from hemorrhage, debris, or infection. CT scans with contrast can add helpful information in selected cases to define the extent of the cyst and to confirm that the cyst is not originating from the pancreas, kidney, or ovary.

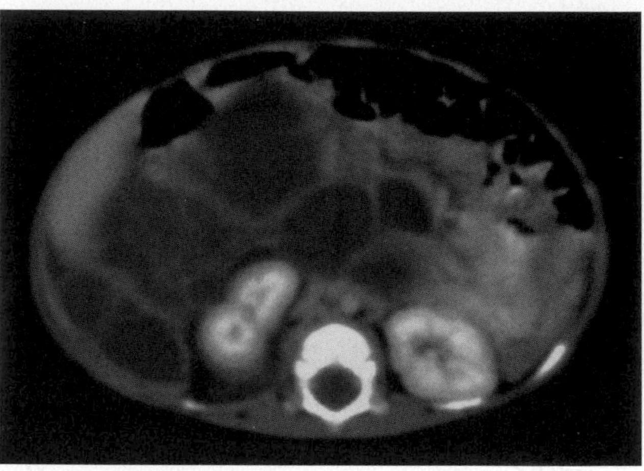

FIGURE 85-11. Computed tomography scan of an infant with abdominal distention and a large diffuse mesenteric cyst involving the enteric retroperitoneum. The cysts were marsupialized and drained with closed suction drains without recurrence. (Courtesy of Dr. Barry Shandling, Hospital for Sick Children, Toronto, Ontario, Canada.)

The preferred treatment for these cysts is complete surgical excision. This is generally technically straightforward for omental cysts, but may require simultaneous bowel resection in cases of mesenteric cysts due to the intimate relationship between the cyst and the intestine (96). This appears to be necessary in approximately 50% of cases of mesenteric cysts. In patients in whom simple enucleation of the cyst is not possible and excision with the associated bowel would require an extensive bowel resection and place the patient at risk for nutritional deficiencies or short-gut syndrome, marsupialization of the cyst is an alternative approach. This technique involves partial cyst excision, breakdown of any loculations or septations within the cyst, and the temporary placement of drains to avoid early recurrence (Fig. 85-11). Other techniques to minimize recurrence include sclerosing the cyst lining with 10% glucose solution, electrocautery, or iodine. Marsupialization can also be performed for extensive cysts of the retroperitoneum.

OMENTAL CYSTS

Lymphatic malformations of the omentum occur less frequently than in the mesentery. They most commonly present due to nonspecific abdominal pain, superinfection

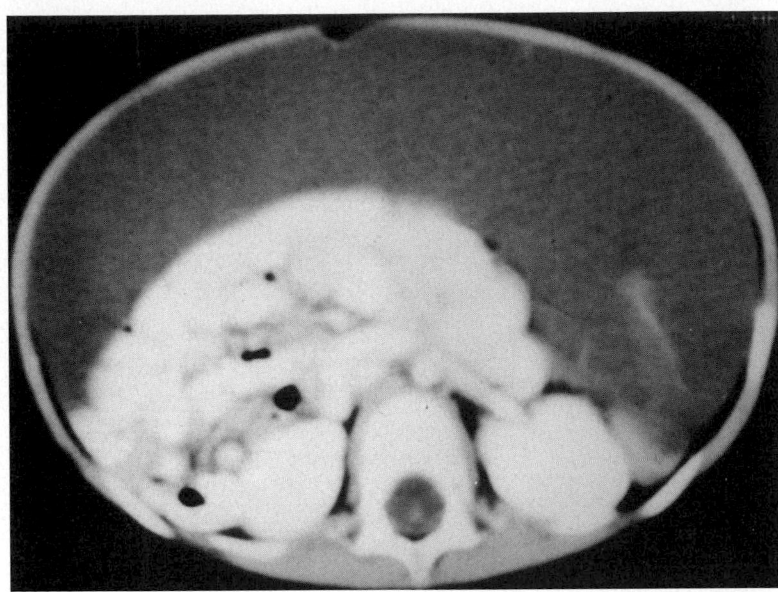

FIGURE 85-12. Computed tomography scan of a large omental cyst in a 3-year-old boy with abdominal distention.

of the cyst fluid, or as an asymptomatic abdominal mass. Omental cysts tend to be freely mobile in both the transverse and cephalad to caudad planes, and cause posterior or cephalad displacement of the stomach (Fig. 85-12) (90).

Ultrasound evaluation typically shows a thin-walled cystic mass, often with fine internal septae located anteriorly. The preferred treatment is complete surgical excision. Bowel resection is rarely necessary and recurrence is rare.

RETROPERITONEAL CYSTS

Retroperitoneal cysts are the least common of abdominal lymphatic malformations. They can be located anywhere in the retroperitoneum, but are most commonly reported beneath the lateral peritoneal reflections (97). Ultrasound characteristics are not different from previously described for mesenteric and omental cysts. Their proximity to major blood vessels and vital structures makes them difficult to completely excise, and for this reason, the incidence of recurrence for retroperitoneal cysts is higher than with other forms of cysts.

REFERENCES

1. Gross RE. *The surgery of infancy and childhood.* Philadelphia: WB Saunders, 1953:221.
2. Calder J. *Med Essays Observ* 1733;1:205.
3. Ildstad ST, Tollerud DJ, Weiss RG, et al. Duplications of the alimentary tract. Clinical characteristics, preferred treatment, and associated malformations. *Ann Surg* 1988;208:184–189.
4. Ladd WE. Duplications of the alimentary tract. *South Med J* 1937;30:363–371.
5. Wrenn EL. Alimentary tract duplications. In: Ashcraft KW, Holder TM, eds. *Pediatric surgery,* 2nd ed. Philadelphia: WB Saunders, 1993:421–433.
6. Sieber WK. Alimentary tract duplication. *Arch Surg* 1956;73:283.
7. Houston HE, Lynn HB. Duplication of the small intestine in children. *Mayo Clin Proc* 1966;41:246.
8. Basu R, Forshall I, Rickham PP. Duplication of the alimentary tract. *Br J Surg* 1960;47:477.
9. Mellish RWP, Koop CE. Clinical manifestations of duplication of the bowel. *Pediatrics* 1961;27:397.
10. Grosfeld JL, O'Neill JA, Clatworthy HW. Enteric duplications in infancy and childhood: an 18-year review. *Ann Surg* 1970;172:83.
11. Favara BE, Franciosi RA, Akers DR. Enteric duplications, thirty-seven cases: a vascular theory of pathogenesis. *Am J Dis Child* 1971;122:501.
12. Holcomb GW III, Gheissari A, O'Neill JA. Surgical management of alimentary tract duplications. *Ann Surg* 1989;209:167.
13. Bower RJ, Sieber WK, Kiesewetter WB. Alimentary tract duplications in children. *Ann Surg* 1978;188:669.
14. Hudson HW. Giant diverticula or reduplications of the intestinal tract. *New Engl J Med* 1935;213:1123.
15. Winslow RE. Duplication of the cervical esophagus. An unrecognized cause of respiratory distress in infants. *Ann Surg* 1984;50:506.
16. Bond SJ, Groff DB. Gastrointestinal duplications. In: O'Neill JA Jr, Rowe MI, Grosfeld JL, et al., eds. *Pediatric surgery,* 5th ed. St. Louis, MO: Mosby–Year Book, 1998:1257–1267.
17. Stringer MD, Spitz L, Abel R, et al. Management of alimentary tract duplication in children. *Br J Surg* 1995;82:74–78.
18. Wrenn EL Jr. Tubular duplication of the small intestine. *Surgery* 1962;52:494.
19. Heiss K. Intestinal duplications. In: Oldham KT, Colombani PM, Foglia RP, eds. *Surgery of infants and children: scientific principles and practice.* Philadelphia: Lippincott–Raven, 1997.
20. Anderson MC, et al. Duplications of the alimentary tract in the adult. *Arch Surg* 1962;85:110.
21. Crowley LV, Page HG. Adenocarcinoma arising in a presacral enterogenous cyst. *Arch Pathol* 1960;69:64.
22. Orr MM, Edwards AJ. Neoplastic change in duplication in duplication of the alimentary tract. *Br J Surg* 1975;62:264.
23. Kangarloo H, et al. Ultrasonic evaluation of abdominal gastrointestinal tract duplication in children. *Radiology* 1979;131:191.
24. Praturi R, Nance RW Jr, Stevens JS. Technetium pertechtenate scintigraphy in an ileal duplication of the stomach and duodenum. *J Nucl Med* 1993;34:294.
25. Bidewell JK, Nelson A. Prenatal ultrasound diagnosis of congenital duplication of the stomach. *J Ultrasound Med* 1986;10:589.

26. Potter EL. *Pathology of the fetus and newborn.* Chicago: Year Book Medical, 1961.
27. Pang D. Split cord malformation: part II: clinical syndrome. *Neurosurgery* 1992;31:481.
28. Ravitch MM. Hind gut duplication: doubling of colon and genital urinary tracts. *Ann Surg* 1953;137:588.
29. Smith ED. Duplication of the anus and genitourinary tract. *Surgery* 1969;66:909–921.
30. Bentley JFR, Smith JR. Developmental posterior enteric remnants and spinal malformations. *Arch Dis Child* 1960;35:76–86.
31. Beardmore HE, Wigglesworth FW. Vertebral anomalies and alimentary duplications. *Pediatr Clin North Am* 1958;5:457.
32. Iyer CP, Mahour GH. Duplications of the alimentary tract in infants and children. *J Pediatr Surg* 1995;30:1267–1270.
33. Lewis FT, Thyng FW. Regular occurrence of intestinal diverticula in embryos of pig, rabbit, and man. *Am J Anat* 1908;7: 505–519.
34. Beach PD, et al. Duplication of the primitive hindgut of the human being. *Surgery* 1969;66:205.
35. Brunschwig A, et al. Duplication of the entire colon into a vaginal anus. *Surgery* 1948;24:1010.
36. Rowe MI, Ravitch MM, Ranninger K. Operative correction of caudal duplication (dipygus). *Surgery* 1968;63:840.
37. VanZwallenburg BR. Doublecolon. *Am J Roentgenol Radium Ther Nucl Med* 1952;68:22.
38. Louw JH. Congenital intestinal atresia and stenosis in the newborn. *Ann Royal Coll Surg Engl* 1959;25:209.
39. Gans SL, et al. Duplication of the cervical esophagus in infants and children. *Surgery* 1968;63:852.
40. Borcar J, Hughes CF. Duplications of the cervical esophagus in adults. *Aust N Z J Surg* 1988;58:746.
41. Pokorny WJ, Goldstein IR. Enteric thoracoabdominal duplications in children. *J Thorac Cardiovasc Surg* 1984;87:821.
42. Superina RA, Ein SH, Humphreys RP. Cystic duplications of the esophagus and neurenteric cysts. *J Pediatr Surg* 1984;19: 527.
43. Gross RE, et al. Thoracic duplications which originate from the intestine. *Ann Surg* 1950;131:363.
44. Olsen L, et al. Multiple intestinal duplications in a child with thoracic meningomyelocele and hydrocephalus. *Eur J Pediatr Surg* 1992;2:45.
45. Wolf YG. Thoraco-abdominal enteric duplication with meningocele, skeletal anomalies and dextrocardia. *Eur J Pediatr Surg* 1990;149:786.
46. Falon M, Gordon ARG, Lendrum AC. Mediastinal cysts of foregut origin associated with vertebral anomalies. *Br J Surg* 1954;41:520–533.
47. Narashimharao KL, Mitra SK. Esophageal atresia associated with esophageal duplication cyst. *J Pediatr Surg* 1987;22:984–985.
48. Alrabeeah A, et al. Neurenteric cyst–a spectrum. *J Pediatr Surg* 1988;23:752.
49. Murakami A, Kobayashi S, Moriyasu K, et al. A case of esophageal duplication cyst associated with a total left pericardial defect. *Kyobu Geka* 1991;4:334–336.
50. Mahboubi S, Finkelstein M, Afshani E. Esophageal duplication in children: a report of three cases evaluated by computerized tomography. *Pediatr Emerg Care* 1985;1:90.
51. Bremer JL. Dorsal intestinal fistula: accessory neurenteric canal; diastematomyelia. *Arch Pathol* 1952;54:132.
52. Dines J, et al. Dorsal herniation of the gut: a rare manifestation of the split notocord syndrome. *J Pediatr Surg* 1967;2:359.
53. Singh A, Singh R. Split notocord syndrome with dorsal enteric fistula. *J Pediatr Surg* 1982;17:412.
54. Batels RJ. Duplication of the stomach: case report and review of the literature. *Ann Surg* 1967;33:747.
55. Kremer RM, Kephoff RB Jr. Duplication of the stomach. *J Pediatr Surg* 1970;5:360.
56. Ramsey GS. Enterogenous cyst of the stomach simulating hypertrophic pyloric stenosis. *Br J Surg* 1957;4:632.
57. Grosfeld JL, et al. Duplication of pylorus in the newborn—a rare cause of gastric outlet obstruction. *J Pediatr Surg* 1970;5:365.
58. Kleinhaus S, Boley SJ, Winslow P. Occult bleeding from a perforated gastric duplication in an infant. *Arch Surg* 1981;116:122.
59. Hoffman M, et al. Gastric duplication cyst communicating with aberrant pancreatic duct: a rare cause of recurrent acute pancreatitis. *Surgery* 1987;101:369.
60. Curran JP, et al. Ectopic gastric duplication cyst in an infant. *Clin Pediatr* 1984;23:50.
61. Inouge WY, et al. Duodenal duplication: case report and literature review. *Ann Surg* 1965;162:910.
62. Lavine JE, Harrison M, Heyman MB. Gastrointestinal duplication causing relapsing pancreatitis in children. *Gastroenterology* 1989;97:1556.
63. Akers DR, et al. Duplications of the alimentary tract: report of three unusual cases associated with bile and pancreatic ducts. *Surgery* 1972;71:817.
64. Al Traif I, Khan MH. Endoscopic drainage of a duodenal duplication cyst. *Gastrointest Endosc* 1992;38:64.
65. Lang T, et al. Treatment of recurrent pancreatitis by endoscopic drainage of a duodenal duplication. *J Pediatr Gastroenterol Nutr* 1994;18:494.
66. Wardell S, Vidican DE. Ileal duplication cyst causing massive bleeding in a child. *J Clin Gastroenterol* 1990;12:681.
67. Jewett TC Jr. Duplication of the entire small intestine with massive melena. *Ann Surg* 1958;147:239.
68. Jewett TC Jr, Walker AB, Cooney DR. A long-term follow-up on a duplication of the small intestine treated by gastroduplication. *J Pediatr Surg* 1983;18:185.
69. Bar-Maor JA, et al. Tubular duplication of the jejunum and ileum lined entirely by gastric mucosa. *J Pediatr Gastroenterol Nutr* 1985;4:303.
70. Schwartz DL, et al. Tubular duplication with autonomous blood supply: resection with preservation of adjacent bowel. *J Pediatr Surg* 1980;15:341.
71. Bianchi A. Intestinal loop lengthening—a technique for increasing small intestine length. *J Pediatr Surg* 1980;15:145.
72. Norris R, et al. A new surgical approach to duplications of the intestine. *J Pediatr Surg* 1986;21:167.
73. Soper RT. Tubular duplication of the colon and distal ileum. *Surgery* 1968;63:998.
74. Currarino G, Coln D, Votteler T. Triad ofanorectal, sacral, and presacral anomalies. *AJR Am J Roentgenol* 1981;137:395.
75. Flye MM, Izant RJ. Extrapulmonary sequestration with esophageal communication and complete duplication of the colon. *Surgery* 1972;71:744.
76. Perry CL, Merritt JW. Presacral enterogenous cyst. *Ann Surg* 1949;129:881.
77. O'Neill JA Jr, et al. Surgical experience with thirteen conjoined twins. *Am Surg* 1988;208:299.
78. Ravitch MM, Scott WW. Duplication of the entire colon, bladder, and urethra. *Surgery* 1953;34:843.
79. Smith ED, Stephens FD. Duplication and vesicointestinal fissure. *Birth Defects* [original article series] 1988;24:551.
80. LaQuaglia MP, et al. Rectal duplications. *J Pediatr Surg* 1990;25:980.
81. Colodny AH. Mesenteric and omental cysts. In: Welch K, et al., eds. *Pediatric surgery.* Year Book Medical, 1986.
82. Kutz RJ, Heimann TM, Beck AR, et al. Mesenteric and retroperitoneal cysts. *Ann Surg* 1986;203:109.
83. Chung MA, Brandt ML, St-Vil D, et al. Mesenteric cysts in children. *J Pediatr Surg* 1991;26:1306.
84. Okur H, Kucukaydin M, Ozukotan BH, et al. Mesenteric, omental, and retroperitoneal cysts in children. *Eur J Surg* 1997;163: 673–677.
85. Vanek VW, Phillips AK. Retroperitoneal, mesenteric, and omental cysts. *Arch Surg* 1984;119:838–842.
86. Takiff H, Calabria R, Yin L, et al. Mesenteric cysts and intra-abdominal cystic lymphangiomas. *Arch Surg* 1985;120:1266–1269.
87. Egozi EI, Ricketts RR. Mesenteric and omental cysts in children. *Am Surg* 1997;63:287–290.
88. Ricketts RR.Mesenteric and omental cysts. In: O'Neill JA, Rowe MI, Grosfeld JL, et al., eds, *Pediatric surgery,* 5th ed. St. Louis, MO: Mosby–Year Book, 1998.

89. Hardin WJ, Hardy JD. Mesenteric cysts. *Am J Surg* 1970;119:640–645.
90. Bliss DP, Coffin CM, Bower RJ, et al. Mesenteric cysts in children. *Surgery* 1994;115:571–577.
91. Chirathivat S, Shermeta D. Recurrent retroperitoneal mesenteric cyst. *Gastroenterol Radiol* 1979;4:191–193.
92. Molitt DL, Ballantine TVN, Grosfeld JL. Mesenteric cysts in infancy and childhood. *Surg Gynecol Obstet* 1978;147:182–184.
93. Klin B, Lotan G, Efrati Y, et al. Giant omental cyst in children presenting as pseudoascites. *Surg Laparasc Endosc* 1997;7:291–293.
94. Perrielo VA, Flemma RJ. Lymphangiomatous omental cyst in infancy masquerading as ascites. *J Pediatr Surg* 1969;4:227–230.
95. Mohanty SK, Bal RK, Maudar KK. Mesenteric cyst—an unusual presentation. *J Pediatr Surg* 1998;33:792–793.
96. Hebra A, Brown MF, McGeehin KM, et al. Mesenteric, omental, and retroperitoneal cysts in children: a clinical study in 22 cases. *South Med J* 1993;86:173–176.
97. Burkett JS, Pickleman J. The rationale for surgical treatment of mesenteric and retroperitoneal cysts. *Am Surg* 1994;60: 432–435.

PART E

Colon

Chapter 86

Hirschsprung's Disease

Jacob C. Langer

Hirschsprung's disease occurs in approximately 1 in 5,000 live-born infants. The disease is characterized by absence of ganglion cells in the myenteric and submucosal plexuses of the intestine, which results in absent peristalsis in the affected bowel. Without normal peristalsis, these children develop a form of functional intestinal obstruction.

The first description of a child with Hirschsprung's disease appeared in the eighteenth century by Domenico Battini, whose description of a typical child with congenital megacolon was published after Battini's death in 1800 (1). In 1886, Harald Hirschsprung, a Danish pathologist, described several cases of the condition that ultimately bore his name (2). During subsequent years, surgeons were taught to resect the grossly abnormal colon and perform an anastomosis to the rectum (which rarely worked) or a colostomy. In his textbook on pediatric surgery published in 1926, Fraser said:

> This is an obscure disease of the large intestine, in which the essential features are an inability of the colon to part with its contents. . . . The only curative treatment which the pathology and clinical course of the affection show to be applicable is that of excision of the affected bowel with the union of unaffected gut above to the upper end of the rectum below (3).

Between the turn of the nineteenth century and the 1940s, a number of papers were published that observed abnormalities in the innervation of the colon, but the absence of ganglion cells that we now consider to be the sine quo non of Hirschsprung's disease was not widely recognized until 1948, when Whitehouse and Kernohan summarized the literature and presented a series of cases of their own (4). Shortly thereafter, Swenson confirmed that aganglionosis was the cause of obstruction in these children and recommended rectosigmoidectomy as the optimal treatment of this disease (5). Although initially this operation was performed without decompressing colostomy in most children (6), technical difficulties in small infants and the debilitated and malnourished state in which many children presented caused most surgeons to adopt a multistaged approach with colostomy as the initial step. In more recent years, advances in surgical technique and earlier diagnosis have resulted in an evolution toward one-stage and minimal access procedures for the treatment of this disease.

Jacob C. Langer: University of Toronto, Pediatric General Surgery, Hospital for Sick Children, Toronto, Ontario M5G 1X8, Canada

ETIOLOGY

Abnormalities in Neural Crest Cell Migration

Early work in the chick embryo by Le Douarin and Teillet suggested that normal ganglion cells originate in the vagal neural crest and migrate from there into the embryonic intestine (7). Subsequent work in several strains of mice that develop congenital aganglionosis suggested there is a delay or arrest in this migration, which results in the neural crest cells failing to reach the distal bowel (8). Later work by other investigators suggested that neural crest cells actually originate in both vagal and sacral sites and migrate toward the middle of the intestine (9,10). This raised the possibility that the neural crest cells get to their destination, but then fail to survive, proliferate, or differentiate due to abnormalities in their microenvironment. Evidence has accumulated of differences in extracellular matrix proteins (11,12), abnormal cell–cell interactions (13), and absence of neurotrophic factors (14) in aganglionic bowel when compared with normal bowel, all of which support the concept that abnormalities in the microenvironment may play a role in producing the distal aganglionosis that is characteristic of Hirschsprung's disease.

TABLE 86-1 Syndromes and Genetic Abnormalities Commonly Associated with Hirschsprung's Disease.

Syndrome	*Identified Genetic Basis*
Down syndrome	Trisomy 21
Neurocristopathy syndromes	Endothelin and SOX-10
Waardenberg-Shah syndrome	
Yemenite deaf-blind-hypopigmentation	
Piebaldism	
Other hypopigmentation syndromes	
Goldberg-Shprintzen syndrome	SIP1?
Multiple endocrine neoplasia 2	RET
Congenital central hypoventilation syndrome (Ondine's curse)	?

Genetic Abnormalities in Hirschsprung's Disease

It has long been recognized that Hirschsprung's disease may have a genetic basis (15). Approximately 10% of children have a positive family history, especially those with longer segment disease. Children with Down syndrome and other genetic abnormalities also have a higher incidence of Hirschsprung's disease, and the incidence of associated congenital anomalies is approximately 20%. There are a number of clearly defined syndromes that are known to be associated with Hirschsprung's disease (Table 86-1).

Since the early to mid-1990s, a number of investigators have focused on the genetics of Hirschsprung's disease (16), and there are now several gene families recognized as being clearly associated with this condition. These include the RET protooncogene, the endothelin family of genes, and several others that are currently under investigation.

The RET protooncogene encodes a tyrosine kinase receptor. Mutations in this gene are known to be involved in the etiology of multiple endocrine neoplasia syndromes type 2, and more recently, different mutations have been associated with some cases of Hirschsprung's disease. These mutations have been found in 17% to 38% of children with short-segment disease, and in 70% to 80% of those with long-segment involvement (17). Mice in whom the RET protooncogene has been knocked out exhibit absence of renal development and panintestinal aganglionosis (18). There are also a number of other genes that encode for RET ligands, including glial cell line-derived neurotrophic factor (GDNF) and neurturin. Mice in whom either GDNF or neurturin have been knocked out develop ganglion cell abnormalities (19,20), and both GDNF and neurturin mutations have also been found in association with RET abnormalities in a small number of patients with Hirschsprung's disease (21,22).

The endothelin family of genes was first suspected of being involved in the development of Hirschsprung's disease during investigation of a large kindred of Mennonites. The endothelin-B receptor and its most important ligand, endothelin-3, are vital to the development of the enteric nervous system, as well as many other neural crest-derived cells. The combination of aganglionosis and piebaldism (caused by melanocyte abnormalities) are present in naturally occurring and endothelin knockout mice (23). This combination, in addition to congenital deafness, is seen in the Waardenburg-Shah syndrome in humans, which has been shown to be due to abnormalities in the endothelin system (24). It is estimated that approximately 3% to 7% of cases of Hirschsprung's disease are related to this family of genes. Another candidate gene that has more recently been identified is SOX-10, a transcriptional modulator. This gene was found to be mutated in another spontaneous mouse model of aganglionosis, the Dom mouse, and mutations of this gene have subsequently been found in a small number of children with the Waardenburg-Shah syndrome (25).

One additional gene that has been described in a small number of children with Hirschsprung's disease is SIP1, which encodes for the transcription factor Smad interacting protein 1. These children have a syndrome that includes mental retardation, microcephaly, and distinct facial features (26).

How Do the Genetic Abnormalities Result in Abnormal Neural Crest Cell Migration?

It is unclear exactly how these genetic abnormalities cause abnormal neural crest cell migration and result in the phenotype of Hirschsprung's disease. It is clear that this is a complex process and that development of the disease is a multigenic phenomenon that can occur at any number of stages during the normal process of neural crest cell migration, differentiation, and survival. There is evidence from animal models that some mutations, particularly those in the endothelin and SOX-10 genes, may produce early maturation or differentiation of neural crest cells, which decreases the number of available progenitor cells and prevents the neural crest cells from migrating further (27,28). There is also evidence that mutations in the RET protooncogene and its related genes likely act by depriving the migrating neural crest cells of an adequately supportive microenvironment (29). Both pathways may also involve apoptosis of migrating neural crest cells (30,31).

CLINICAL PRESENTATION

There are three ways that Hirschsprung's disease characteristically presents—neonatal bowel obstruction, chronic constipation, and enterocolitis. In addition, some children have associated anomalies or a recognized syndrome that is associated with an increased risk of Hirschsprung's disease.

Neonatal Bowel Obstruction

Approximately 50% to 90% of children with Hirschsprung's disease present during the neonatal period with abdominal distention and bilious vomiting; there has been a tendency in more recent decades for patients to be recognized earlier. Typically, there is a delay in the passage of meconium; whereas 95% of normal term infants pass meconium in the first 24 hours of life, less than 10% of children with Hirschsprung's disease have passed meconium during that time. A prenatal history suggestive of intestinal obstruction is rare, except in children with total colonic disease (32). Occasionally, the distal colonic obstruction is so severe that it results in cecal perforation (33). Plain radiographs usually show dilated bowel loops throughout the abdomen. The differential diagnosis of this picture includes all causes of neonatal distal intestinal obstruction, such as jejuno-ileal atresia, meconium ileus or meconium plug syndrome, congenital band, and high anorectal malformation.

Chronic Constipation

Some children are able to manage through the neonatal period and present later with chronic constipation. Commonly, the onset of the constipation is around the time of weaning from breast milk. Although most children who present after the neonatal period have short-segment disease, this history may also be found in those with longer segment or even total colonic involvement, particularly if the child has been exclusively breastfed.

Because constipation is frequently seen in childhood, it may be difficult to differentiate Hirschsprung's disease from the other, more common causes of constipation. Clinical features that point to this diagnosis include failure to pass meconium in the first 48 hours of life, failure to thrive, gross abdominal distention, and dependence on enemas without significant encopresis. Although many clinicians look for "tightness" of the anal sphincter on rectal examination, this finding is unreliable. Children with functional megacolon often exhibit "stool-holding" behavior and usually date the onset of the constipation to the time of initiation of bowel training.

Enterocolitis

Enterocolitis is characterized by fever, abdominal distention, and diarrhea, and may be life threatening. Approximately 10% of children with Hirschsprung's disease have enterocolitis as part of the presentation, and because this disease is usually thought of as causing constipation, the diagnosis may therefore be missed. In most cases, the suspicion of Hirschsprung's disease will be raised if on careful history failure to pass meconium and intermittent obstructive episodes are elicited.

Associated Anomalies and Syndromes

Hirschsprung's disease may be associated with a wide range of other anomalies, such as malrotation, genitourinary abnormalities, congenital heart disease, limb abnormalities, cleft lip and palate, hearing loss, mental retardation, and dysmorphic features. In addition, it may be part of a large number of recognized syndromes, some of which have an identifiable chromosomal or genetic basis (Table 86-1). Hirschsprung's disease should therefore be suspected in any child with constipation or neonatal obstruction who is known to have one of these syndromes. In addition, a diagnosis of Hirschsprung's disease should alert the clinician to the increased possibility of other problems.

DIAGNOSIS

The appropriate diagnostic approach may vary, depending on the age of the patient and the presenting clinical picture. After a careful history and physical examination, the diagnostic steps may include radiographic studies, anorectal manometry, and rectal biopsy.

Radiographic Studies

The first step in the diagnostic pathway for a newborn with a distal bowel obstruction is a water-soluble contrast enema, which can usually rule out intestinal atresia and meconium ileus, the two most common of these diagnoses in addition to Hirschsprung's disease. In children with Hirschsprung's disease, the contrast enema may demonstrate a transition zone between the normal and aganglionic bowel (Fig. 86-1). However, because only about 75% of neonates with Hirschsprung's disease will demonstrate a transition zone (34), the absence of a transition zone does not rule out the diagnosis. In older children with Hirschsprung's disease, the absence of a transition zone is less common, but may still be present due to a very short aganglionic segment. Other findings on the contrast enema that suggest the diagnosis of Hirschsprung's disease include a rectosigmoid index (the ratio of rectal diameter/sigmoid diameter) less than 1.0 and retention of barium on a 24-hour postevacuation film.

Anorectal Manometry

Anorectal manometry aids in the diagnosis of Hirschsprung's disease through identification of the rectoanal inhibitory reflex, which is present in normal individuals but absent in the vast majority of children with Hirschsprung's disease (Fig. 86-2) (35). Although

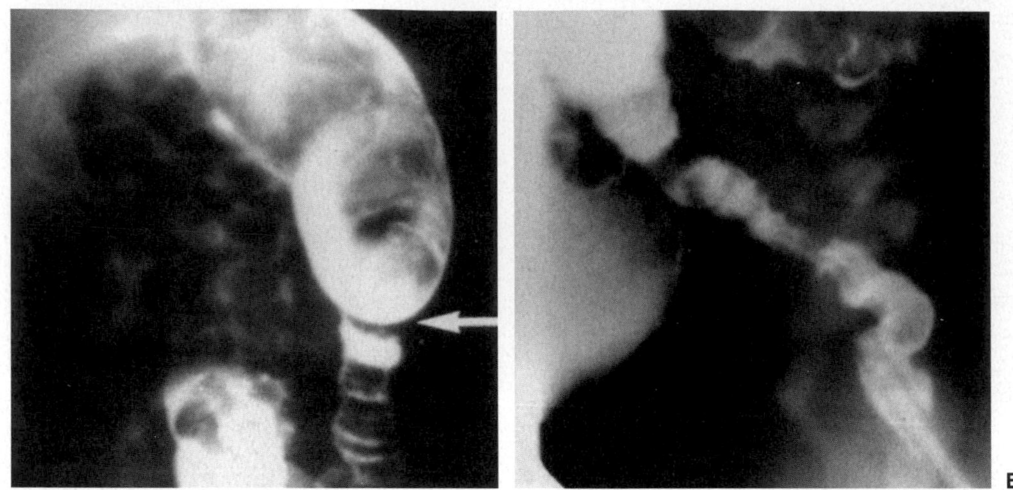

FIGURE 86-1. **(A)** Contrast enema demonstrating a classic rectosigmoid transition zone in Hirschsprung's disease. **(B)** Lateral view of rectum illustrates typical distal spasm of rectim. (Adapted from Sato T, Oldham K. Pediatric abdomen. In: Greenfield LJ. *Surgery: scientific principles and practice,* 3rd ed. Philadelphia: Lippincott Williams & Wilkins, 2001:2001, with permission.)

anorectal manometry is possible in newborns, it is not widely available for this age group and may be unreliable. In older children, the test is technically easier, but false-positive results may occur due to masking of the relaxation response by contraction of the external sphincter.

Rectal Biopsy

Definitive diagnosis of Hirschsprung's disease is based on histologic evaluation of a rectal biopsy, looking for the presence or absence of ganglion cells and the finding of hypertrophied nerve trunks (Fig. 86-3). The biopsy is usually taken 1–2 cm above the dentate line; going too distally may result in a false-positive diagnosis of Hirschsprung's disease because ganglion cells may normally be absent in this area. The most common technique for rectal biopsy is a suction device that samples mucosa and underlying submucosa. Many pathologists believe that a suction rectal biopsy lacking ganglion cells is consistent with (but is not diagnostic) of Hirschsprung's disease. Evaluation of suction biopsies may be enhanced by staining for acetylcholinesterase, which has a characteristic staining pattern in the submucosa and mucosa (36). Other stains, such as glial fibrillary acidic protein, have also been described for the diagnosis of Hirschsprung's disease, but have not been widely adopted (37). Punch biopsies or full-thickness biopsies, which may provide more tissue and deeper levels, may be needed if the suction biopsy sample is inadequate. Some surgeons prefer these techniques as the first choice.

PREOPERATIVE PREPARATION

Once the diagnosis of Hirschsprung's disease has been established, there are a number of priorities prior to surgical management. Children with dehydration or sepsis must be stabilized and resuscitated using intravenous fluids and antibiotics. Those with intestinal obstruction require a nasogastric tube. Enterocolitis may be relatively mild or may be life threatening. The degree of colonic obstruction can allow for the overgrowth of bacteria, thus leading to diarrhea. If enterocolitis is present, aggressive fluid resuscitation, broad-spectrum antibiotic therapy, nasogastric decompression, and attempts to decompress the obstruction should be instituted quickly.

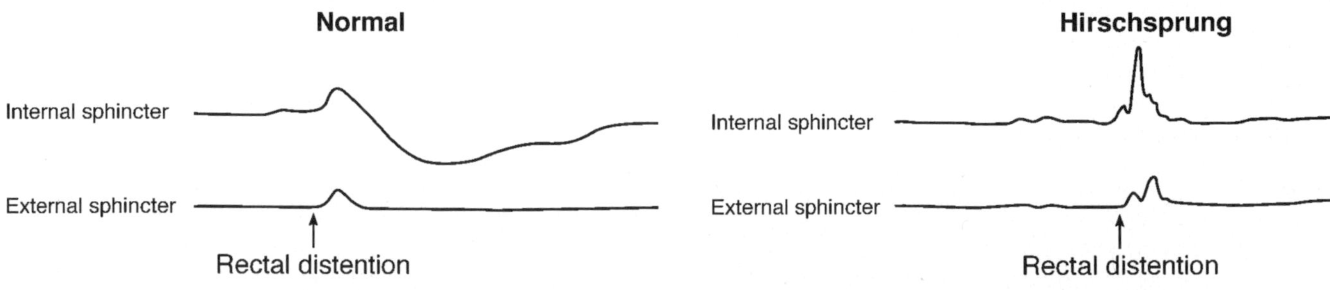

FIGURE 86-2. The anorectal inhibitory reflex. Distension of the rectum with a balloon results in a reflex relaxation of the internal anal sphincter in a normal individual. In a child with Hirschsprung's disease, there is no reflex relaxation.

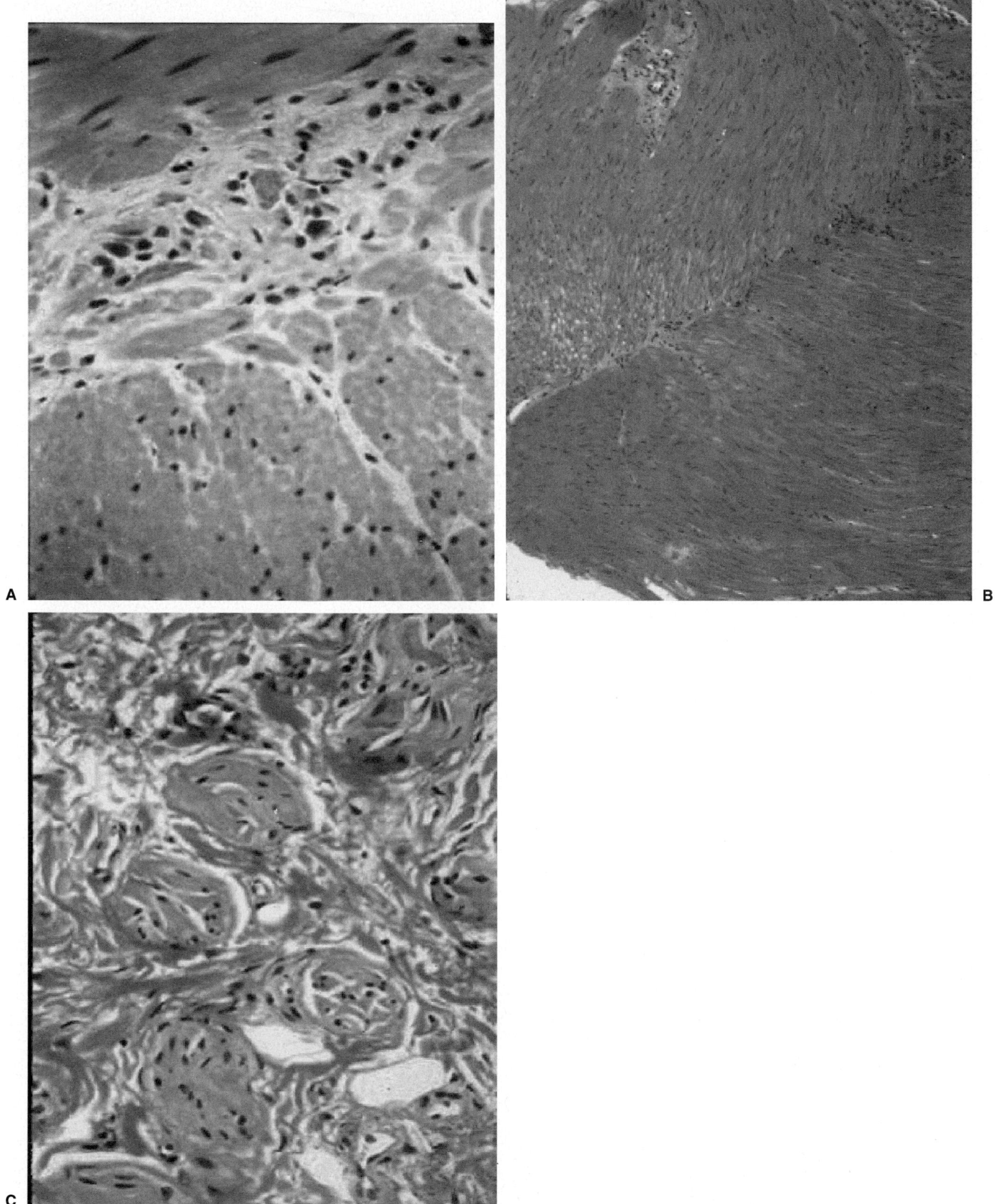

FIGURE 86-3. Histology of Hirschsprung's disease. **(A)** Normal ganglion cells in the myenteric plexus. **(B)** Myenteric plexus without any ganglion cells. **(C)** Hypertrophied nerve cells that are typical of Hirschsprung's disease.

Once a child has been stabilized, surgery can be performed semielectively. While waiting for surgery, most children can be fed breast milk or an elemental formula in combination with rectal stimulations or irrigations. Those that do not tolerate oral or nasogastric feeding can be nourished with parenteral nutrition. In the older child with an extremely dilated colon, weeks or months of irrigations may permit the colon to come down to a more normal size prior to definitive surgery.

SURGICAL OPTIONS

The goals of surgical management for Hirschsprung's disease are to remove the aganglionic bowel and reconstruct the intestinal tract by bringing the normally innervated bowel down to the anus, while preserving normal sphincter function. There have been many operations devised to accomplish these goals, but the most commonly performed at the present time are the Swenson, Duhamel, and Soave procedures (Fig. 86-4). There are no prospective controlled series comparing surgical treatments of Hirschsprung's disease. It is therefore difficult to determine if there are any significant advantages to one over the others. It is probably true that surgeons will get the best results doing the operation they have been trained to do and do with some frequency.

The Swenson procedure (Fig. 86-5) is essentially a low anterior resection of the rectum with an end-to-end anastomosis performed by prolapsing the rectum and pulled-through bowel outside the anus. A number of publications have documented excellent results from this approach, including a more recent long-term follow-up of a large group of patients, including some of Swenson's original patients (38).

Duhamel described a technique in which the native rectum is left in situ and the normally innervated colon is brought behind the rectum in the presacral space. An end-to-side anastomosis is then performed, and the two lumens are joined. Originally, this was accomplished by placing several clamps and cutting between them, but in more recent years most surgeons use a linear stapler for this (Fig. 86-6). The Duhamel procedure has also been widely used around the world, and excellent long-term results have been published (39).

The Soave procedure (or endorectal pull-through) was designed to avoid injury to pelvic vessels and nerves, which are theoretically at risk with the aforementioned procedures, particularly the Swenson procedure. The operation consists of a mucosal proctectomy with preservation of the rectal muscular cuff, and the normally innervated colon is pulled through the muscular cuff and anastomosed just above the dentate line. In the original description, the pulled-through bowel was left hanging out for several weeks, and was then amputated and the anastomosis was completed. Boley's modification, in which the anastomosis is performed primarily, is the technique usually employed today (40) (Fig. 86-7).

Other approaches that are performed more frequently outside North America include the Rehbein procedure and the use of long myectomy without resection. The Rehbien operation involves a somewhat higher anastomosis than the previously mentioned operations, although long-term follow-up suggests very good results in experienced hands (41). For children with short-segment Hirschsprung's disease, some surgeons have employed a simple myectomy,

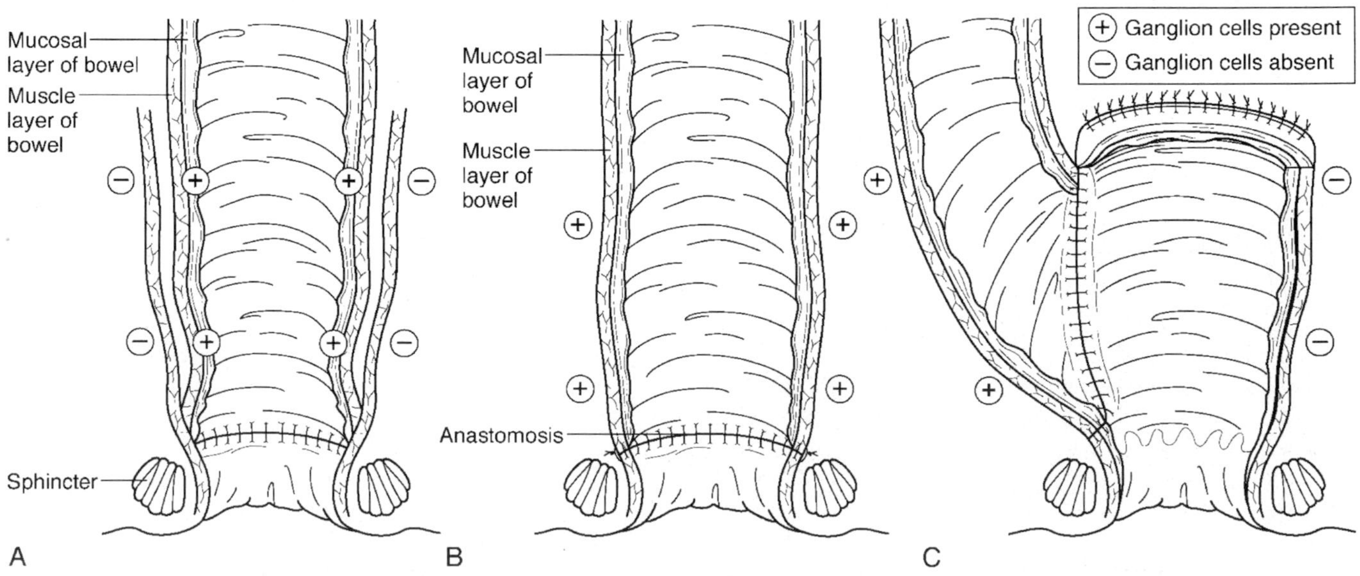

FIGURE 86-4. Common operations for Hirschsprung's disease: **(A)** the Soave procedure, **(B)** the Swenson procedure, and **(C)** the Duhamel procedure.

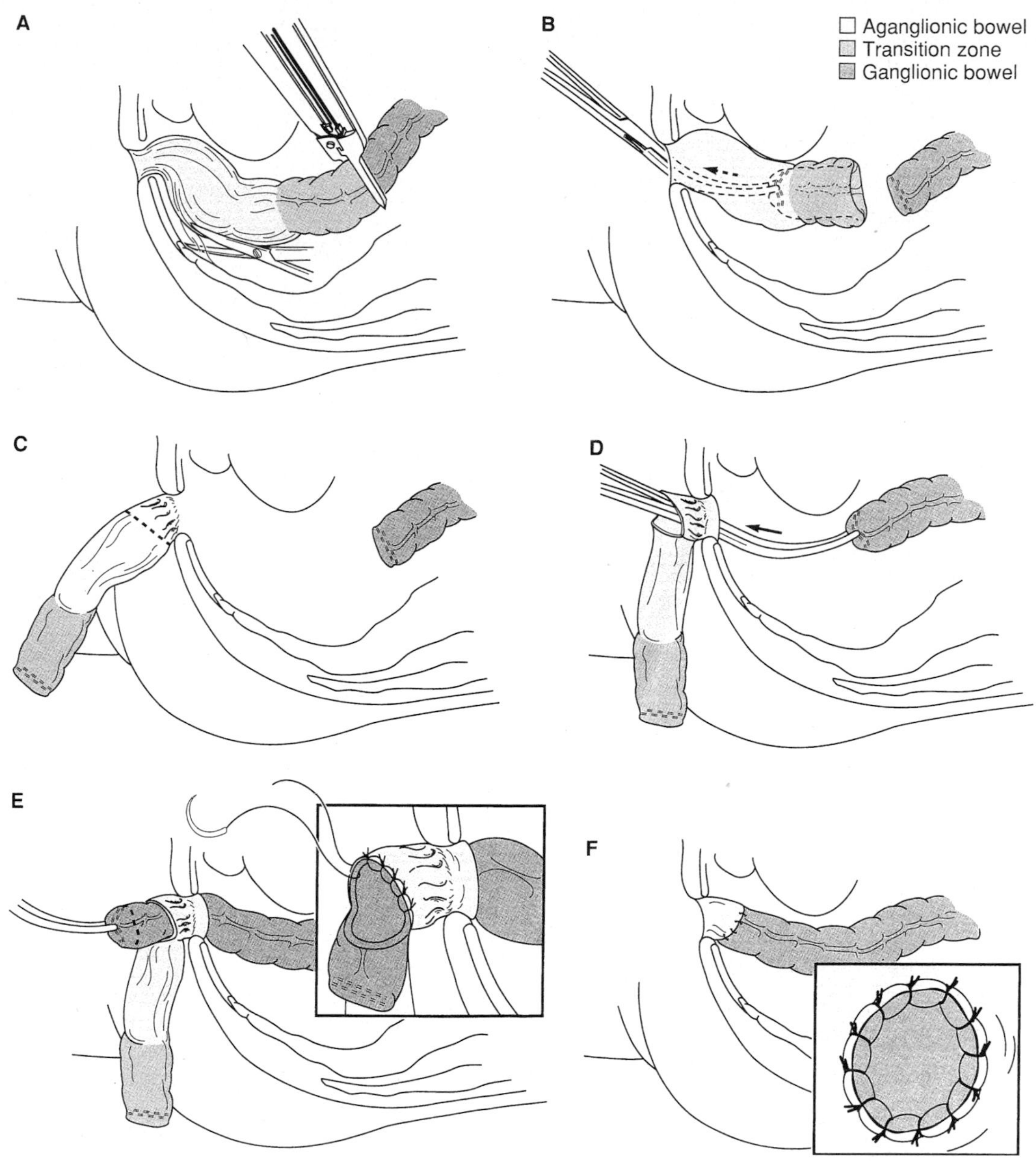

FIGURE 86-5. Swenson procedure. **(A)** Extramural rectal dissection. **(B, C)** Eversion of aganglionic segment and full-thickness rectum. **(D)** Pull-through of normal, ganglionic bowel. **(E)** Colorectal anastomosis. **(F)** Completed procedure. (From Sato T, Oldham K. Pediatric abdomen. In: Greenfield LJ. *Surgery: scientific principles and practice,* 3rd ed. Philadelphia: Lippincott Williams & Wilkins, 2001:2005, with permission.)

going proximally up to 5 or 6 cm. This can be performed transanally or through a posterior approach. Although good results have been reported in some series, long-term outcomes have not been reported and this approach has not been widely adopted in North America.

Since the earliest descriptions of surgery for Hirschsprung's disease, most authors have advocated a preliminary colostomy. This allows for definitive pathology and colonic decompression followed by a period of growth and a subsequent reconstructive operation. There are a number of options for the approach to creation of the stoma. Some surgeons prefer to create a transverse loop colostomy as the first stage, followed by a laparotomy with "leveling" biopsies to determine the transition zone and a pull-through at the same time. The colostomy is then closed in a third stage. This approach is problematic if the transition zone is near the splenic flexure because there may not be enough length to perform the pull-through. More commonly, surgeons do a laparotomy with biopsies as the first stage, and bring the colostomy out just above the transition zone. The second stage usually involves using the colostomy to pull through, and only using a

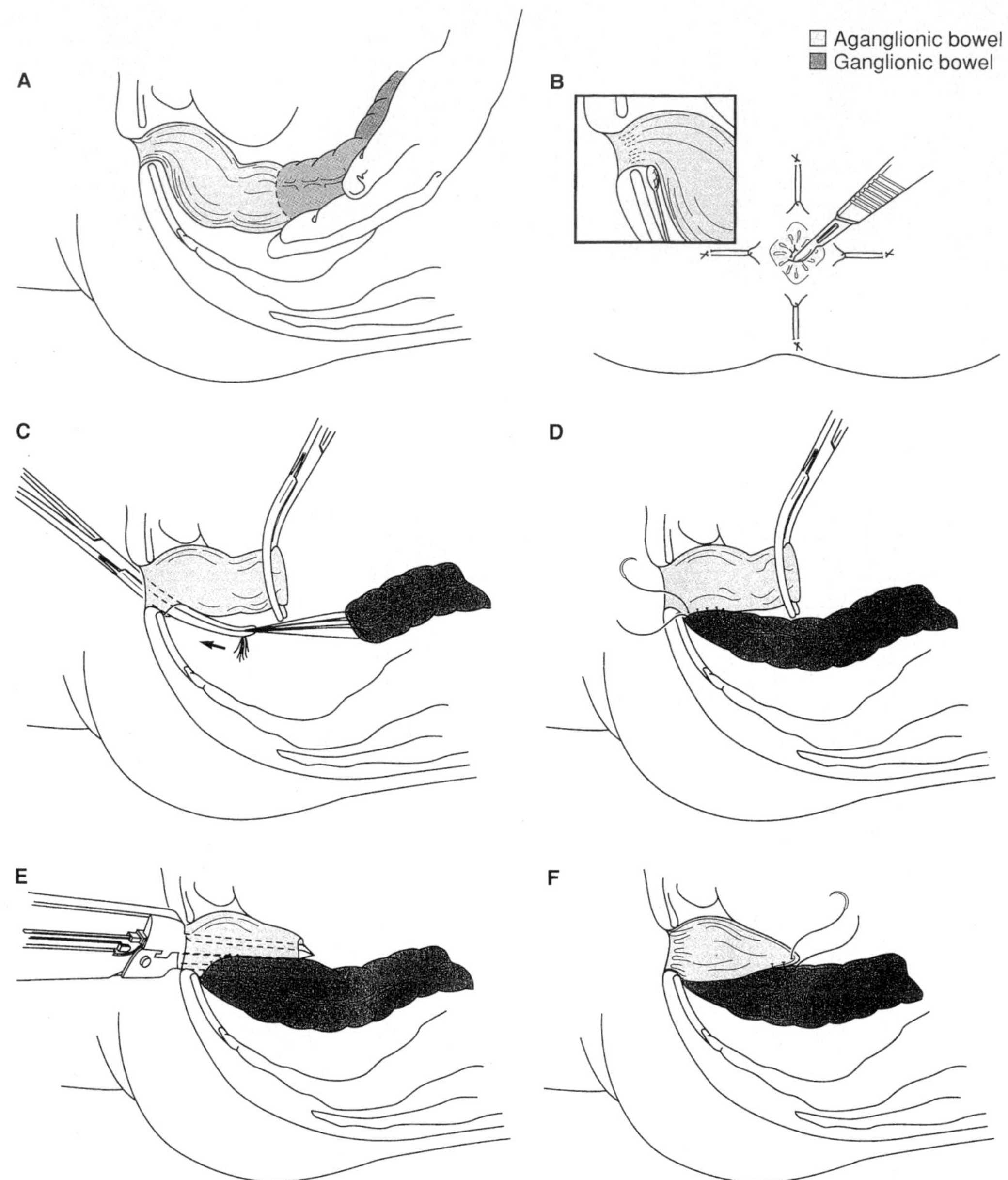

FIGURE 86-6. Duhamel procedure (Martin modification). **(A)** Blunt retrorectal dissection. **(B)** Incision in the posterior wall of the aganglionic rectum. **(C)** Rectorectal pull-through after resection of the proximal aganglionic segment. **(D)** End-to-side colorectal anastomosis preserving aganglionic rectum (as originally described). **(E)** Stapled conversion of anastomosis into an extended side-to-side colorectal anastomosis (Martin modification). **(F)** Completed procedure. (From Sato T, Oldham K. Pediatric abdomen. In: Greenfield LJ. *Surgery: scientific principles and practice,* 3rd ed. Philadelphia: Lippincott Williams & Wilkins, 2001:2003, with permission.)

more proximal colostomy in cases where the anastomosis is difficult or tenuous. An ileostomy may occasionally be required for cases in which cecal perforation has occurred or in cases of total colonic disease.

Single-stage Pull-through

In the early days of surgery for Hirschsprung's disease, most children presented with malnutrition, severe enterocolitis, or an extremely dilated colon, and a colostomy was performed as a lifesaving procedure. In addition, there was a sense that performing a reconstructive operation in a small neonate was technically difficult and that results could be improved by waiting until the child was bigger. The standard approach was therefore to routinely perform a colostomy as the first step, and then do a definitive pull-through around 1 year of age. Over the years, as surgical techniques and magnification techniques improved, many surgeons began to do the definitive operation at earlier ages. However, the use of a routine stoma remained the

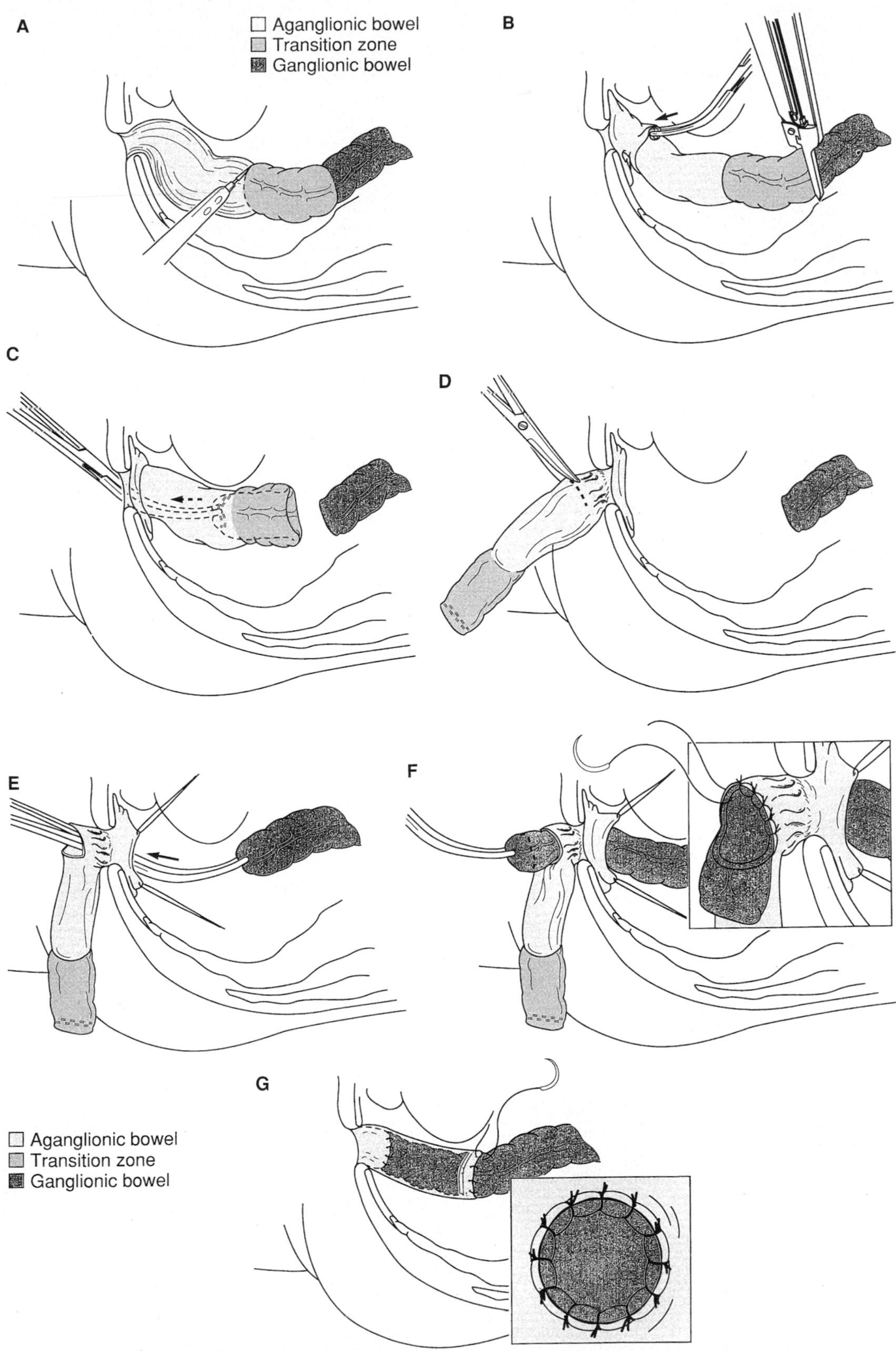

FIGURE 86-7. Soave endorectal procedure. **(A)** Endorectal dissection initiated. **(B)** Endorectal dissection complete. **(C)** Eversion of the aganglionic segment and rectal mucosal tube. **(D)** Incision of everted rectal tube. **(E)** Endorectal pull-through. **(F)** Colorectal anastomosis. **(G)** Completed procedure. (From Sato T, Oldham K. Pediatric abdomen. In: Greenfield LJ. *Surgery: scientific principles and practice,* 3rd ed. Philadelphia: Lippincott Williams & Wilkins, 2001:2004, with permission.)

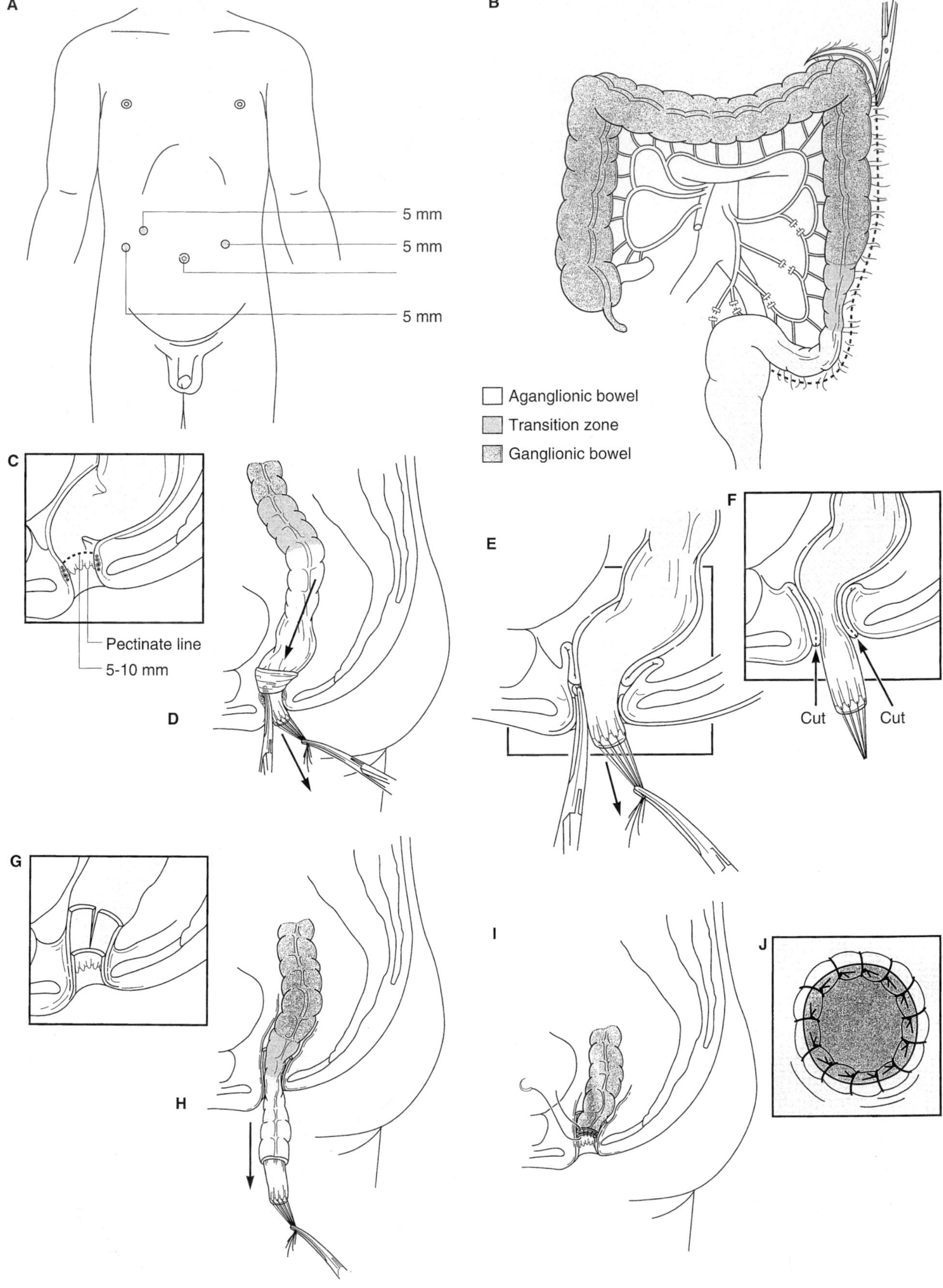
A
5 mm
5 mm
5 mm
B
Aganglionic bowel
Transition zone
Ganglionic bowel
C
Pectinate line
5-10 mm
D
E
F
Cut
Cut
G
H
I
J

practice of most pediatric surgeons, except for some children who presented at an older age and did not have extremely dilated proximal colons.

In the 1980s, a number of surgeons began to report one-stage pull-through procedures without the use of a defunctioning colostomy, even in smaller children (42). During the early to mid-1990s, one-stage operations became increasingly popular, and many reports documented the safety of this approach (43). Some studies suggested that there were advantages to avoiding the known morbidity of stomas in infants (44) and that a one-stage approach was more cost effective (45). Despite the move toward one-stage surgery for Hirschsprung's disease, it is still universally accepted that a stoma may be indicated for children with severe enterocolitis, perforation, malnutrition, or massively dilated proximal bowel, and in situations where there is inadequate pathology support to reliably identify the transition zone on frozen section.

Minimal Access Surgery

With the popularity of laparoscopic surgery in the early 1990s, many pediatric surgeons began to include these techniques in their practices. Georgeson was the first to describe a laparoscopic approach to surgery for Hirschsprung's disease, which is a modification of the Soave procedure. His operation involves laparoscopic biopsy to identify the transition zone, laparoscopic mobilization of the rectum below the peritoneal reflection, and a short mucosal dissection from below (Fig. 86-8). The rectum is then prolapsed through the anus and the anastomosis is performed from below. This procedure is associated with a shorter time in hospital, and the early results appear to be equivalent to those reported for the open procedures (46). Laparoscopic approaches have been also described for the Duhamel and Swenson operations, with excellent short-term results reported.

The transanal Soave procedure uses the same mucosal dissection from below as the Georgeson operation, but without the intraabdominal mobilization of the rectum (47,48). The rectal muscle is incised circumferentially several centimeters above the dentate line, and the dissection is continued on the rectal wall, dividing the vessels right on the rectum. The entire rectum and part of the sigmoid colon can be delivered through the anus. The transition zone is identified, and the anastomosis is performed from below (Fig. 86-9). This operation has been shown to be safe and associated with a short hospital stay, early feeding, and minimal analgesia requirements, particularly when compared with the open Soave operation (49,50). The transanal approach can be used in a patient with a preexisting colostomy and has the advantage that it can be performed by any pediatric surgeon, including those without advanced laparoscopic skills.

There is controversy surrounding the need to determine the level of the transition zone prior to beginning the anal dissection, both for the laparoscopic and the transanal pull-through. Options for accessing the proximal bowel in order to do the biopsy include laparoscopy or a small umbilical incision. These approaches can also be used to mobilize the splenic flexure in children with higher transition zones. Proponents of biopsy point to the inaccuracy of the contrast enema in predicting the level of aganglionosis. This is particularly important if the predicted transition zone is in the distal colon and the true transition zone is in the proximal colon because many surgeons prefer a different surgical approach to long-segment disease. A more recent study suggests that 8% of children with a rectosigmoid transition zone on contrast study have a more proximal pathological transition zone, data that support this approach (51). However, there is no particular benefit to surgeons who prefer to use a straight Soave pull-through for long-segment disease. One large multicenter review of patients undergoing the transanal pull-through demonstrated no difference in terms of postoperative pain, feeding, and hospital stay between those who had a preliminary biopsy to determine the pathological transition zone and those who did not (52).

LONG-SEGMENT HIRSCHSPRUNG'S DISEASE

Long-segment Hirschsprung's disease is usually defined as a transition zone that is proximal to the midtransverse colon. Most of these children actually have total colonic disease, which also usually includes some of the distal ileum. In rare cases, most of the entire small bowel is also

FIGURE 86-8. Laparoscopically assisted pull-through for Hirschsprung's disease. **(A)** Sites for operative trocar placement. **(B)** Division of colon and rectal mesentery with mobilization of proximal colon. **(C)** Circumferential incision in rectal mucosa 5 to 10 mm cephalad to the pectinate line. **(D)** Mucosal traction sutures to facilitate further dissection from rectal muscular cuff. **(E)** Transanal submucosal dissection is continued cephalad to meet the caudal extent of the transperitoneal rectal dissection. **(F)** Circumferential incision of rectal muscular cuff. **(G)** Rectal muscular cuff is split posteriorly to accommodate the pull-through segment (the pull-through segment is not shown here to clarify this maneuver). **(H)** Rectum and sigmoid colon are pulled through the rectal muscular cuff to the anastomotic site. **(I)** Colon is transected at appropriate site with confirmation of ganglion cells by frozen section. **(J)** Transanal, end-to-end single-layer colorectal anastomosis. (From Sato T, Oldham K. Pediatric abdomen. In: Greenfield LJ. *Surgery: scientific principles and practice,* 3rd ed. Philadelphia: Lippincott Williams & Wilkins, 2001:2006, with permission.)

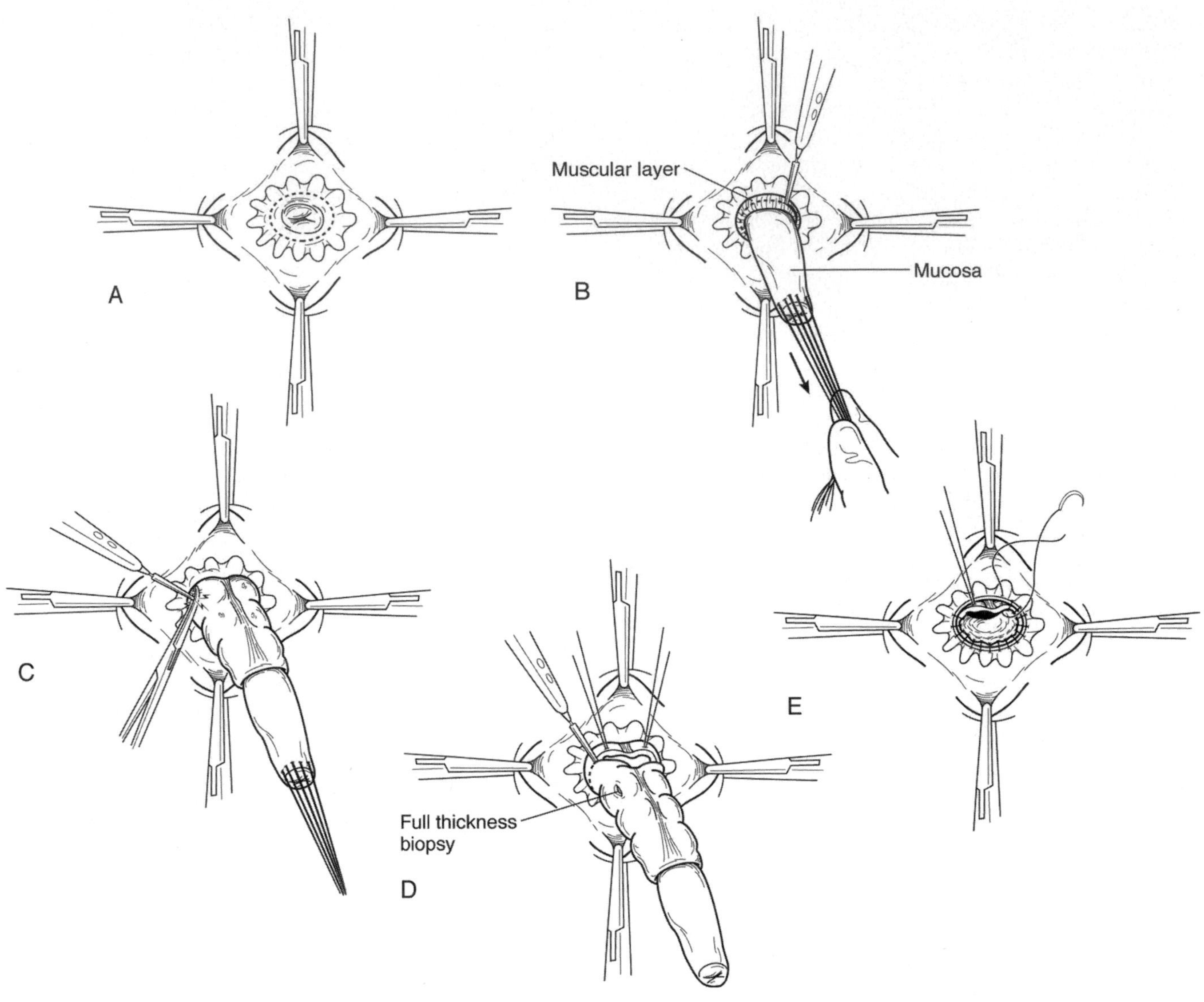

FIGURE 86-9. The transanal Soave pull-through.

involved. Children with long-segment disease have some unique issues, both with respect to management options and long-term results (53). Outcome for these children appears to be related to the length of the aganglionic segment (54).

Diagnosis

Long-segment disease is more common in girls than is short-segment disease, and there is more often a positive family history. Prenatal ultrasound may show evidence of dilated bowel loops and polyhydramnios suggestive of intestinal obstruction. Most children with long-segment disease present in the neonatal period with a picture of small bowel obstruction. Contrast enema will show a small colon that is often foreshortened (the "question mark" sign, shown in Fig. 86-10), but is usually not as narrow as the microcolon seen in meconium ileus and intestinal atresia. Enterocolitis is very common in this group of children. The diagnosis can be confirmed by rectal biopsy. In some cases, especially in children who are breastfed, the child may not develop fulminant symptoms until formula or solid food is introduced.

Management

As with short-segment disease, the child should be resuscitated using a nasogastric tube, intravenous fluid administration, and antibiotics. A laparotomy should be performed and biopsies obtained for frozen section identification of the transition zone. Although initial biopsies can be focused to an obvious area of size discrepancy, the pathological transition zone may differ from what the surgeon sees grossly. Some surgeons have started with an appendectomy, assuming that lack of ganglion cells in the appendix is diagnostic of total colonic disease. However, there may be patients in whom the appendix appears aganglionic in the face of shorter segment disease (55).

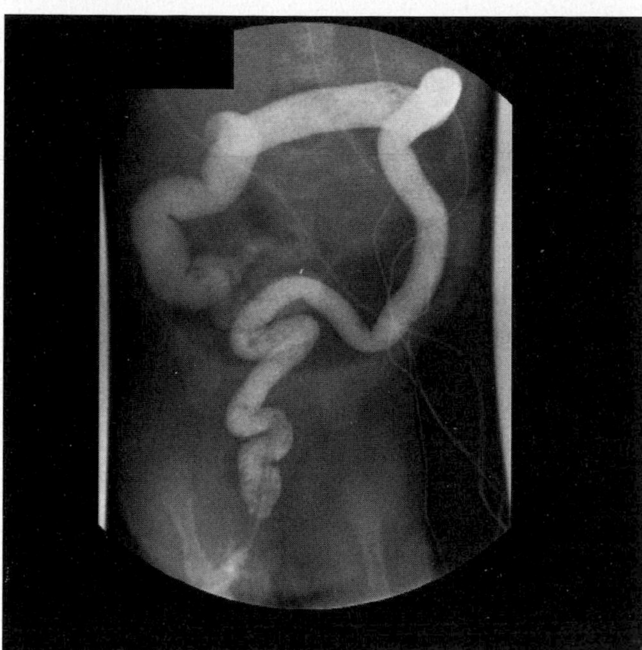

FIGURE 86-10. Barium enema in a child with total colonic Hirschsprung's disease. Note the "question mark" appearance of the colon.

Once the level of aganglionosis has been identified, most surgeons bring out a proximal stoma, with a plan to wait for the permanent sections and to perform a definitive reconstructive procedure at several months to 1 year of age. However, there have been reports of primary pull-through without ileostomy for total colonic disease, with good short-term results (43). This approach requires a high degree of confidence in the pathologist because it requires doing a total colectomy on the basis of frozen sections alone.

The options for reconstruction of children with long-segment Hirschsprung's disease can be divided into three main categories: straight pull-through, colonic patch, and J-pouch construction. Straight pull-throughs can be performed using any one of the standard techniques (i.e., Swenson, Duhamel, or Soave), and can be performed open or laparoscopically. The concept of a colon patch is to do a side-to-side anastomosis between normally innervated small bowel and aganglionic colon, using the small bowel for motility and the colon for water absorption. The first such operation was described by Martin, and consisted of a long Duhamel reconstruction involving the entire left colon (56). More recently, Kimura described using the right colon, which theoretically has greater water absorption capacity, but that requires a staged approach in order to bring the right colon into the pelvis (57). Several authors have published modifications of Kimura's operation. Although the colon patch procedures should permit decreased stool output from better water absorption, the aganglionic colon gradually tends to dilate and many of these patients develop severe enterocolitis that requires removal of the patch (58). The J-pouch procedure is the same as that performed commonly for children and adults with ulcerative colitis and polyposis. Although it has been used by a small number of surgeons for Hirschsprung's disease, there has been little written about the results of this approach (59).

NEAR-TOTAL INTESTINAL HIRSCHSPRUNG'S DISEASE

Children with total or near-total intestinal aganglionosis present a difficult challenge for the surgeon because they do not have adequate nutrient absorptive capacity and therefore rely on total parenteral nutrition (TPN). The extent of aganglionosis should be established at the time of the first laparotomy, and a stoma should be brought out at that point using normally innervated bowel. Some surgeons prefer to bring out a stoma further downstream from the transition zone in the hope that stomal output will be lower and there will be fewer problems with fluid and electrolyte loss; however, this approach may increase the risk of persistent intestinal obstruction and bacterial overgrowth. A central venous catheter should be inserted for parenteral nutrition, and a gastrostomy should be considered for continuous feeding of breast milk or elemental formula. The use of "trophic" feeds may help to prevent the inevitable development of TPN-induced cholestasis (60). In addition, some children will experience enough adaptation to eventually get off TPN and nourish themselves entirely enterally, which is the optimal goal of therapy.

There are several surgical options available for the management of near-total intestinal aganglionosis, particularly for those in whom there is not enough absorptive capacity and inadequate adaptation. For those children who develop significant proximal dilatation of the normally innervated bowel, tapering, imbrication, or bowel-lengthening procedures, such as the Bianchi operation, may be used (61). Zeigler popularized a technique known as "myectomy-myotomy," in which a length of aganglionic small bowel distal to the transition zone undergoes myectomy (Fig. 86-11) (62). The concept is that the normal bowel will provide a "running start" to the enteric contents, which will then passively traverse the myectomized segment where further absorption will occur. Although a few successful cases using this technique have been reported, most surgeons have not found it to be highly successful. For children with ongoing liver failure due to TPN-induced cholestasis, small bowel transplantation may offer the only chance for survival (63).

INTRAOPERATIVE AND EARLY POSTOPERATIVE COMPLICATIONS

The complications of surgery for Hirschsprung's disease include the general group of complications of any abdominal surgery, including bleeding, infection, injury to

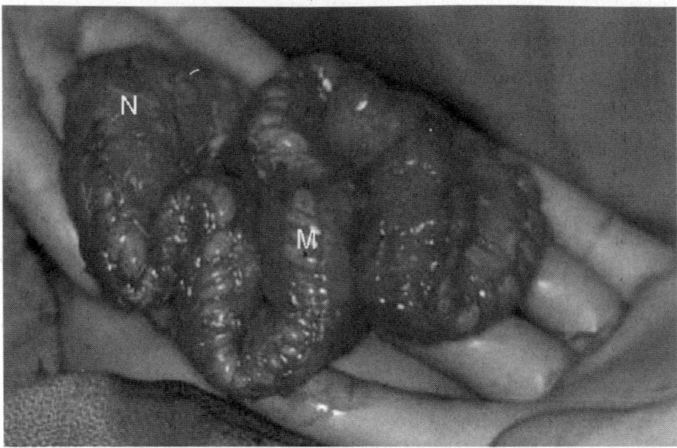

FIGURE 86-11. Long myectomy for a child with near-total intestinal Hirschsprung's disease, involving 10 cm of innervated jejunum and aganglionosis of the remaining intestinal tract. N, normal proximal jejunum; M, myectomy in aganglionic jejunum.

TABLE 86-2 Potential Causes of Late Complications Following a Pull-through.

Persistent obstructive symptoms
Mechanical obstruction
Persistent or acquired aganglionosis
Colonic motility disorder
Internal sphincter achalasia
Stool-holding behavior
Incontinence
Abnormal sphincter function
Abnormal sensation
"Overflow" incontinence due to constipation
Enterocolitis
Obstruction
Genetic or immunologic predisposition
Abnormal mucin

adjacent organs, and the risks of anesthesia. Those children who undergo a staged procedure with a preliminary stoma may experience stoma-specific complications such as stricture, retraction, prolapse, and skin breakdown (64).

Anastomotic complications, although uncommon, can be seen after any of the standard pull-through procedures. Anastomotic leak occurs infrequently, and can be avoided by close attention to adequate blood supply of the pulled-through bowel and to minimizing tension on the anastomosis. Although it has never been studied in a prospective fashion, the incidence of anastomotic leak in series of laparoscopic and transanal pull-throughs appears to be lower than that reported in the older literature of open pull-throughs. Strictures and retraction of the pull-through may also occur as a result of poor blood supply and tension, and appear to be less common with the Duhamel procedure.

LATE COMPLICATIONS

The long-term problems in children with Hirschsprung's disease include ongoing obstructive symptoms, incontinence, and enterocolitis. Quite often, an individual child may have a combination of problems. The incidence of these problems varies in the literature, but ranges up to 50% in some series. More recent publications report higher numbers, likely due to increasing recognition of these problems.

Obstructive Symptoms

Obstructive symptoms may take the form of abdominal distension, bloating, vomiting, or ongoing severe constipation. Many of these children have symptomatology postoperatively that is identical to the symptoms of Hirschsprung's disease with which they initially presented. In some cases, the child will have a good response to surgery and then develop obstructive symptoms later; in other cases, the child will not have any improvement postoperatively.

There are five major reasons for persistent obstructive symptoms after a pull-through (Table 86-2). These include mechanical obstruction, recurrent or acquired aganglionosis, a colonic or proximal small bowel motility disorder, internal sphincter achalasia, or functional megacolon caused by stool-holding behavior (65). Mechanical obstruction may be the result of a stricture (more commonly seen after the Swenson or Soave procedure) or a retained aganglionic spur from a Duhamel procedure that may fill with stool and obstruct the pulled-through bowel. The Duhamel procedure may also be complicated by a kink that causes obstruction. These complications can be identified using simple digital rectal examination and a barium enema. Although some strictures can be managed using repeated dilatations, many require revision of the pull-through. Duhamel spurs can be resected from above or managed by extending the staple line from below, with or without laparoscopic visualization.

Although rare, some children may have persistent aganglionosis. This may be due to pathologist error (66), or a transition zone pull-through (67), and in some cases there may be ganglion cell loss after a pull-through (68). It is imperative to perform a rectal biopsy to determine whether there are normal ganglion cells present, and if there are not, most children should undergo a repeat pull-through. This can be done using either a Soave or a Duhamel approach (69,70).

It is well recognized that children with Hirschsprung's disease may have associated motility disorders, which may be focal (usually involving the left colon) or diffuse. In some cases, these abnormalities may be associated with histologic abnormalities such as intestinal neuronal dysplasia (71). In children who have been shown not to have a mechanical obstruction and who have normal ganglion cells on rectal biopsy, an investigation for motility disorder should be performed. This can include a radiologic shape study, colonic manometry (72), and laparoscopic biopsies looking for intestinal neuronal dysplasia (73). If a focal abnormality is found, consideration should be given to resection and repeat pull-through using normal bowel. If the abnormality is diffuse, the appropriate treatment is bowel management and the use of prokinetic agents.

Internal sphincter achalasia refers to the nonrelaxation of the internal anal sphincter that is present in all children with Hirschsprung's disease. However, in some children it may result in persistent obstructive symptoms. Traditionally, the treatment for this was internal sphincterotomy or myectomy, which is still recommended by many surgeons (74). Other authors have suggested the use of intrasphincteric botulinum toxin (75) or the application of nitroglycerin paste (76), both of which relax the sphincter in a reversible fashion.

There remains a group of children that do not have an identifiable cause for their symptoms and that do not respond to surgical or medical relaxation of the sphincter. Most of these children suffer from stool-holding behavior, and are best treated using a bowel management regimen consisting of laxatives, enemas, and behavior modification, including support for the child and family. In some severe cases of obstructive symptoms, the child may be best served by use of a cecostomy (77) and administration of antegrade enemas, or even by the creation of a proximal stoma.

An algorithm for the investigation and management of the child with obstructive symptoms is shown in Fig. 86-12.

Incontinence

There are three main reasons for a child to be incontinent after a pull-through: abnormal sphincter function, abnormal sensation, or "overflow" incontinence due to constipation (Table 86-2). Abnormal sphincter function may be due to sphincter injury during the pull-through or to a previous myectomy or sphincterotomy. A number of techniques exist for identifying this kind of injury, including anorectal manometry and anal sonography. Abnormal sensation may take the form of either lack of sensation for a full rectum (which can also be identified using anorectal manometry) or injury to the transitional epithelium, which permits differentiation between gas, liquid, and solid stool. This injury may occur during a pull-through, especially if the anastomosis is performed too low.

Most children with incontinence after a pull-through have overflow of stool because of ongoing constipation. Once sphincter injury and a problem with sensation have been ruled out, the child should be worked up and treated for obstructive symptoms as described in the previous section.

Enterocolitis

As mentioned previously, enterocolitis may be a presenting feature of Hirschsprung's disease. However, it may also occur after surgical correction of the disease. Although the clinical features of enterocolitis are generally agreed upon (fever, abdominal distention, and diarrhea), a precise definition has not been developed. There is therefore wide

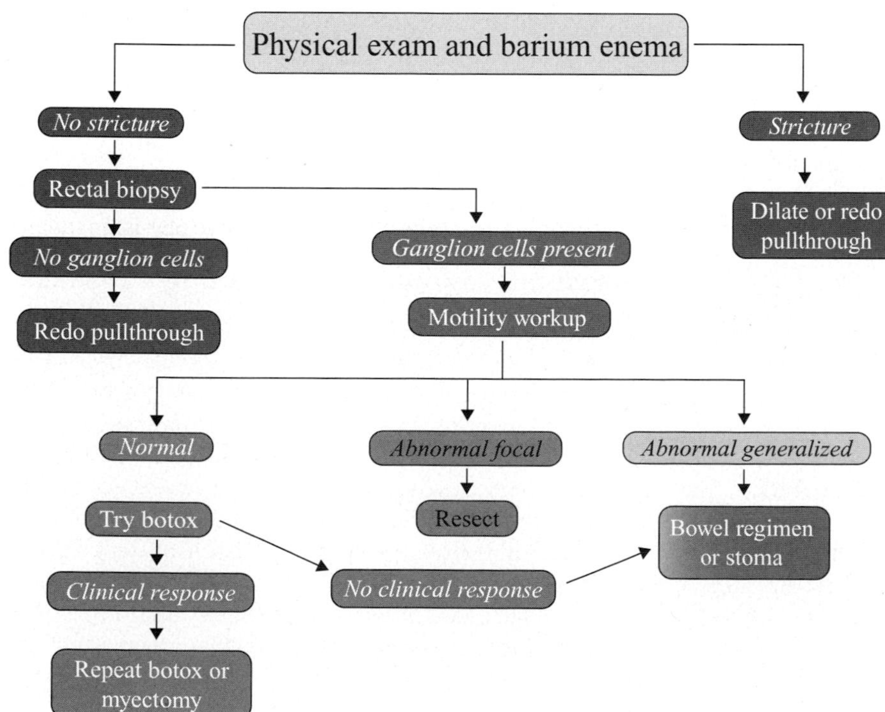

FIGURE 86-12. Algorithm for the investigation and management of the child with obstructive symptoms following a pull-through.

variation in the reported incidence of this problem postoperatively, with estimates ranging from 17% to 50% (78).

The etiology of enterocolitis is also controversial. It is generally agreed that situations that cause obstruction and stasis will predispose children to developing enterocolitis. Particular infectious agents such as *Clostridium difficile* or rotavirus have been postulated as causative, but there are few data to support a specific pathogen (79). There is also evidence that inherent abnormalities in the mucosal immune system may predispose some children to develop this complication (80,81). In addition, the problem also seems to be more common in children with longer segment disease and those with trisomy 21 (82). Finally, there may be genetically controlled abnormalities in mucin production or composition that may also play a role in the development of this problem (83).

The treatment of enterocolitis is largely symptomatic, and involves nasogastric drainage, intravenous fluids, broad-spectrum antibiotics, and decompression of the rectum and colon using rectal stimulation or irrigations. Minimization of the risk of enterocolitis can be accomplished by using preventive measures such as routine irrigations (84) or chronic administration of metronidazole, particularly in those who are believed to be at higher risk for this complication based on clinical or histologic grounds (85). Because enterocolitis is the most common cause of death in children with Hirschsprung's disease and can occur postoperatively even in children who did not have it preoperatively (86), it is extremely important that the surgeon educate the family about the risk of this complication and urge early return to the hospital if the child should develop any concerning symptoms.

LONG-TERM OUTLOOK

Despite the relatively common occurrence of postoperative problems, there is evidence from long-term follow-up studies that most children with Hirschsprung's disease overcome these issues and do very well (87). These studies suggest that obstructive symptoms and incontinence seem to resolve with time, and that the risk of enterocolitis, in the absence of an ongoing obstructive cause, is almost eliminated after the first 5 years of life. Sexual function, social satisfaction, and quality of life all appear to be relatively normal in the vast majority of patients.

"VARIANT" HIRSCHSPRUNG'S DISEASE

"Variant" Hirschsprung's disease is a term that has been used to describe conditions that resemble Hirschsprung's disease in their presentation and course, but that are not characterized by absence of ganglion cells on rectal biopsy (88). There remains much controversy about the definitions, features, and even the existence of many of these conditions.

Intestinal Neuronal Dysplasia

Intestinal neuronal dysplasia (IND) was first described by Meier-Ruge. Two types of IND are usually described (89). Type A is much less common, and is characterized by diminished or absent sympathetic nerves and hyperplasia of the myenteric plexus. Type B consists of dysplasia of the submucous plexus with thickened nerve fibers and giant ganglia, and identification of ectopic ganglion cells in the lamina propria. Type B is often present in children who also have Hirschsprung's disease, although it may also occur on its own. Intestinal neuronal dysplasia may be either diffuse or focal.

Despite multiple publications on the topic of IND, there is still much controversy about the incidence of this condition and whether it exists at all (90). Much of the controversy revolves around the difficulty in establishing clear criteria for the diagnosis among pathologists, and there is also concern that some cases may in fact be secondary to obstruction rather than the cause of it. Until a clear consensus is developed, the apparent incidence of this problem will continue to vary considerably from one center to another.

Hypoganglionosis

This is a rare form of dysganglionosis, which is characterized by sparse and small ganglia, usually in the distal bowel. There may also be abnormalities in cholinesterase distribution. The appropriate treatment is to resect the abnormal colon and perform a pull-through procedure, much as one would do for a child with Hirschsprung's disease. It is important to differentiate this condition from immature ganglia, which is seen in preterm children who may present with a picture of distal intestinal obstruction. The latter condition is self-limited and should not be treated surgically.

Internal Sphincter Achalasia and Ultrashort-segment Hirschsprung's Disease

As mentioned previously, all children with Hirschsprung's disease lack the rectoanal inhibitory reflex. However, there are some children with ganglion cells present on rectal biopsy who also lack the inhibitory reflex and may therefore develop obstructive symptoms that resemble those of Hirschsprung's disease. This condition has been termed *internal sphincter achalasia* (91), and some authors have also called this ultrashort-segment Hirschsprung's disease (although others reserve the latter term for children with a documented aganglionic segment of less than 1 to 2 cm). The diagnosis is made using anorectal manometry and rectal biopsy. These children should be managed initially with a bowel management regimen. If this is unsuccessful, some surgeons advocate anal sphincter myectomy, and others have had success with temporary sphincter-relaxing measures such as botulinum toxin (92) or nitroglycerin paste. The latter choices have some appeal due to the likelihood that the symptoms will improve significantly over time in most of these children.

Desmosis Coli

This is a condition that has more recently been described by Meier-Ruge and that is characterized by total or focal lack of the connective tissue net of the circular and longitudinal muscles and the connective tissue layer of the myenteric plexus, without any abnormality of the enteric nervous system (93). Patients with this condition present with chronic constipation. One family has been described in which Hirschsprung's disease and desmosis coli coexisted (94), although in most cases they are completely separate entities.

REFERENCES

1. Fiori MG. Domenico Battini and his description of congenital megacolon: a detailed case report one century before Hirschsprung. *J Peripher Nerv Syst* 1998;3:197–206.
2. Jay V. Legacy of Harald Hirschsprung. *Pediatr Devel Pathol* 2001;4:203–204.
3. Fraser J. *Surgery of childhood.* New York: William Wood and Company, 1926.
4. Whitehouse FR, Kernohan JW. The myenteric plexus in congenital megacolon. *Arch Int Med* 1948;82:75.
5. Swenson O, Rheinlander HF, Diamond I. Hirschsprung's disease: a new concept in etiology-operative results in 34 patients. *N Engl J Med* 1949;241:551.
6. Gross RE. Congenital megacolon (Hirschsprung's disease). In: Gross RE, ed. *The surgery of infancy and childhood.* Philadelphia: WB Saunders, 1953:330–347.
7. Le Douarin NM, Teillet M-A. The migration of neural crest cells to the wall of the digestive tract in avian embryo. *J Embryol Exp Morph* 1973;30:31–48.
8. Webster W. Embryogenesis of the enteric ganglia in normal mice and in mice that develop congenital aganglionic megacolon. *J Embryol Exp Morphol* 1973;30:573–585.
9. Gershon MD, Epstein MC, Hegstrand L. Colonization of the chick gut by progenitors of enteric serotogenic neurons: distribution, differentiation and maturation within the gut. *Dev Biol* 1980;77:41–51.
10. Tam PKH, Lister J. Developmental profile of neuron-specific enolase in human gut and its implications in Hirschsprung's disease. *Gastroenterology* 1986;90:1901–1906.
11. Parikh DH, Tam PK, Lloyd DA, et al. Quantitative and qualitative analysis of the extracellular matrix protein, laminin, in Hirschsprung's disease. *J Pediatr Surg* 1992;27:991–995; discussion 995–996.
12. Parikh DH, Tam PK, Van Velzen D, et al. Abnormalities in the distribution of laminin and collagen type IV in Hirschsprung's disease. *Gastroenterology* 1992;102:1236–1241.
13. Langer JC, Betti PA, Blennerhassett MG. Smooth muscle from aganglionic bowel in Hirschsprung's disease impairs neuronal development in vitro. *Cell Tiss Res* 1994;276:181–186.
14. Hoehner JC, Wester T, Pahlman S, et al. Alterations in neurotrophin and neurotrophin-receptor localization in Hirschsprung's disease. *J Pediatr Surg* 1996;31:1524–1529.
15. Amiel J, Lyonnet S. Hirschsprung disease, associated syndromes, and genetics: a review. *J Med Genet* 2001;38:729–739.
16. Parisi MA, Kapur RP. Genetics of Hirschsprung disease. *Curr Opin Pediatr* 2000;12:610–617.
17. Seri M, Yin L, Barone V, et al. Frequency of RET mutations in long- and short-segment Hirschsprung disease. *Hum Mutat* 1997;9:243–249.
18. Schuchardt A, D'Agati V, Larsson-Lomberg L, et al. Defects in the kidney and enteric nervous system of mice lacking the tyrosine kinase receptor Ret. *Nature* 1994;367:380–383.
19. Sanchez MP, Silos-Santiago I, Frisen J, et al. Renal agenesis and the absence of enteric neurons in mice lacking GDNF. *Nature* 1996;382:70–73.
20. Heuckeroth RO, Enomoto H, Grider JR, et al. Gene targeting reveals a critical role for neurturin in the development and maintenance of enteric, sensory, and parasympathetic neurons. *Neuron* 1999;22:253–263.
21. Angrist M, Bolk S, Halushka M, et al. Germline mutations in glial cell line-derived neurotrophic factor (GDNF) and RET in a Hirschsprung disease patient. *Nat Genet* 1996;14:341–344.
22. Hofstra RM, Osinga J, Buys CH. Mutations in Hirschsprung disease: when does a mutation contribute to the phenotype. *Eur J Hum Genet* 1997;5:180–185.
23. Hosoda K, Hammer RE, Richardson JA, et al. Targeted and natural (piebald-lethal) mutations of endothelin-B receptor gene produce megacolon associated with spotted coat color in mice. *Cell* 1994;79:1267–1276.
24. Edery P, Attie T, Amiel J, et al. Mutation of the endothelin-3 gene in the Waardenburg-Hirschsprung disease (Shah-Waardenburg syndrome). *Nat Genet* 1996;12:442–444.
25. Pingault V, Bondurand N, Kuhlbrodt K, et al. SOX10 mutations in patients with Waardenburg-Hirschsprung disease. *Nat Genet* 1998;18:171–173.
26. Wakamatsu N, Yamada Y, Yamada K, et al. Mutations in SIP1, encoding Smad interacting protein-1, cause a form of Hirschsprung disease. *Nat Genet* 2001;27:369–370.
27. Paratore C, Eichenberger C, Suter U, et al. Sox10 haploinsufficiency affects maintenance of progenitor cells in a mouse model of Hirschsprung disease. *Hum Mol Genet* 2002;11:3075–3085.
28. Gershon MD. Endothelin and the development of the enteric nervous system. *Clin Exp Pharmacol Physiol* 1999;26:985–988.
29. Gershon MD. Lessons from genetically engineered animal models. II. Disorders of enteric neuronal development: insights from transgenic mice. *Am J Physiol* 1999;277:G262–G267.
30. Kapur RP. Early death of neural crest cells is responsible for total enteric aganglionosis in Sox10(Dom)/Sox10(Dom) mouse embryos. *Pediatr Dev Pathol* 1999;2:559–569.
31. Bordeaux MC, Forcet C, Granger L, et al. The RET proto-oncogene induces apoptosis: a novel mechanism for Hirschsprung disease. *EMBO J* 2000;19:4056–4063.
32. Belin B, Corteville JE, Langer JC. How accurate is prenatal sonography for the diagnosis of imperforate anus and Hirschsprung's disease? *Pediatr Surg Int* 1995;10:30–32.
33. Soper RT, Opitz JM. Neonatal pneumoperitoneum and Hirschsprung's disease. *Surgery* 1962;51:527–533.
34. Smith GHH, Cass D. Infantile Hirschsprung's disease—is barium enema useful? *Pediatr Surg Int* 1991;6:318–321.
35. Tobon F, Reid NCRW, Talbert JL, et al. Nonsurgical test for the diagnosis of Hirschsprung's disease. *N Engl J Med* 1968;278:188–194.
36. Schoefield DE, Devine W, Yunis EJ. Acetylcholinesterase-stained suction rectal biopsies in the diagnosis of Hirschsprung's disease. *J Pediatr Gastroent Nutr* 1990;11:221–228.
37. Kawana T, Nada O, Ikeda K, et al. Distribution and localization of glial fibrillary acidic protein in colons affected by Hirschsprung's disease. *J Pediatr Surg* 1989;24:448–452.
38. Sherman JO, Snyder ME, Weitzman JJ, et al. A 40-year multinational retrospective study of 880 Swenson procedures. *J Pediatr Surg* 1989;24:833–838.
39. Stockmann PT, Philippart AI. The Duhamel procedure for Hirschsprung's disease. *Semin Pediatr Surg* 1998;7:89–95.
40. Weinberg G, Boley SJ. Endorectal pull-through with primary anastomosis for Hirschsprung's disease. *Semin Pediatr Surg* 1998;7:96–102.
41. Fuchs O, Booss D. Rehbein's procedure for Hirschsprung's disease. An appraisal of 45 years. *Eur J Pediatr Surg* 1999;9:389–391.
42. So HS, Schwartz DL, Becker JM, et al. Endorectal "pull-through"

without preliminary colostomy in neonates with Hirschsprung's disease. *J Pediatr Surg* 1980;15:470–471.

43. Teitelbaum DH, Cilley RE, Sherman NJ, et al. A decade of experience with the primary pull-through for Hirschsprung disease in the newborn period: a multicenter analysis of outcomes. *Ann Surg* 2000;232:372–380.
44. Langer JC, Fitzgerald PG, Winthrop AL, et al. One vs two stage Soave pull-through for Hirschsprung's disease in the first year of life. *J Pediatr Surg* 1996;31:33–37.
45. Bufo AJ, Chen MK, Shah R, et al. Analysis of the costs of surgery for Hirschsprung's disease: one-stage laparoscopic pull-through versus two-stage Duhamel procedure. *Clin Pediatr* 1999;38:593–596.
46. Georgeson KE, Cohen RD, Hebra A, et al. Primary laparoscopic-assisted endorectal colon pull-through for Hirschsprung's disease: a new gold standard. *Ann Surg* 1999;229:678–683.
47. Langer JC, Minkes RK, Mazziotti MV, et al. Transanal one-stage Soave procedure for infants with Hirschsprung disease. *J Pediatr Surg* 1999;34:148–152.
48. De la Torre-Mondragon L, Ortega-Salgado JA. Transanal endorectal pull-through for Hirschsprung's disease. *J Pediatr Surg* 1998;33:1283–1286.
49. Langer JC, Seifert M, Minkes RK. One-stage Soave pullthrough for Hirschsprung disease: a comparison of the transanal vs open approaches. *J Pediatr Surg* 2000;35:820–822.
50. De la Torre L, Ortega A. Transanal versus open endorectal pull-through for Hirschsprung's disease. *J Pediatr Surg* 2000;35:1630–1632.
51. Proctor ML, Traubici J, Langer JC, et al. Correlation between radiographic transition zone and level of aganglionosis in Hirschsprung's disease: implications for surgical approach. *J Pediatr Surg* 2003;38:775–778.
52. Langer JC, Durrant AC, de la Torre ML, et al. One-stage transanal Soave pullthrough for Hirschsprung disease: a multicenter experience with 141 children. *Ann Surg* 2004;238:569–576.
53. Tsuji H, Spitz L, Kiely EM, et al. Management and long-term follow-up of infants with total colonic aganglionosis. *J Pediatr Surg* 1999;34:158–162.
54. Fouquet V, De Lagausie P, Faure C, et al. Do prognostic factors exist for total colonic aganglionosis with ileal involvement? *J Pediatr Surg* 2002;37:71–75.
55. Anderson KD, Chandra R. Segmental aganglionosis of the appendix. *J Pediatr Surg* 1986;21:852–854.
56. Martin L. Surgical management of total colonic aganglionosis. *Ann Surg* 1972;176:343–346.
57. Nishijima E, Kimura K, Tsugawa C, et al. The colon patch graft procedure for extensive aganglionosis: long-term follow-up. *J Pediatr Surg* 1998;33:215–219.
58. Hoehner JC, Ein SH, Shandling B, et al. Long-term morbidity in total colonic aganglionosis. *J Pediatr Surg* 1998;33:961–965.
59. Rintala RJ, Lindahl HG. Proctocolectomy and J-pouch ileo-anal anastomosis in children. *J Pediatr Surg* 2002;37:66–70.
60. Amii LA, Moss RL. Nutritional support of the pediatric surgical patient. *Curr Opin Pediatr* 1999;11:237–240.
61. Vernon AH, Georgeson KE. Surgical options for short bowel syndrome. *Semin Pediatr Surg* 2001;10:91–98.
62. Ziegler MM, Royal RE, Brandt J, et al. Extended myectomy-myotomy. A therapeutic alternative for total intestinal aganglionosis. *Ann Surg* 1993;218:504–509.
63. Park BK. Intestinal transplantation in pediatric patients. *Prog Transplant* 2002;12:97–113.
64. Nour S, Beck J, Stringer MD. Colostomy complications in infants and children. *Ann Royal Coll Surg Engl* 1996;78:526–530.
65. Langer JC. Persistent obstructive symptoms after surgery for Hirschsprung disease: development of a diagnostic and therapeutic algorithm. *J Pediatr Surg* (*in press*).
66. Shayan K, Smith D, Langer JC. Reliability of intraoperative frozen sections in the management of Hirschsprung disease. *J Pediatr Surg* (*in press*).
67. White FV, Langer JC. Circumferential distribution of ganglion cells in the transition zone of children with Hirschsprung disease. *Pediatr Dev Pathol* 2000;3:216–222.
68. Cohen MC, Moore SW, Neveling U, et al. Acquired aganglionosis following surgery for Hirschsprung's disease: a report of five cases during a 33-year experience with pull-through procedures. *Histopathology* 1993;22:163–168.
69. Langer JC. Repeat pullthrough surgery for complicated Hirschsprung disease: indications, techniques, and results. *J Pediatr Surg* 1999;34:1136–1141.
70. Teitelbaum DH, Coran AG. Reoperative surgery for Hirschsprung's disease. *Sem Pediatr Surg* 2003;12:124–131.
71. Schmittenbecher PP, Sacher P, Cholewa D, et al. Hirschsprung's disease and intestinal neuronal dysplasia—a frequent association with implications for the postoperative course. *Pediatr Surg Int* 1999;15:553–558.
72. Di Lorenzo C, Solzi GF, Flores AF, et al. Colonic motility after surgery for Hirschsprung's disease. *Am J Gastroenterol* 2000;95:1759–1764.
73. Mazziottti MV, Langer JC. Laparoscopic full-thickness intestinal biopsies in children. *J Pediatr Gastroenterol Nutr* 2001;33:54–57.
74. Abbas Banani S, Forootan H. Role of anorectal myectomy after failed endorectal pull-through in Hirschsprung's disease. *J Pediatr Surg* 1994;29:1307–1309.
75. Minkes RK, Langer JC. A prospective study of botulinum toxin for internal anal sphincter hypertonicity in children with Hirschsprung's disease. *J Pediatr Surg* 2000;35:1733–1736.
76. Millar AJ, Steinberg RM, Raad J, et al. Anal achalasia after pull-through operations for Hirschsprung's disease—preliminary experience with topical nitric oxide. *Eur J Pediatr Surg* 2002;12:207–211.
77. Chait PG, Shlomovitz E, Connolly BL, et al. Percutaneous cecostomy: updates in technique and patient care. *Radiology* 2003;227:246–250.
78. Teitelbaum DH, Coran AG. Enterocolitis. *Sem Pediatr Surg* 1998;7:162–169.
79. Wilson-Storey D, Scobie WG, McGenity KG. Microbiological studies of the enterocolitis of Hirschsprung's disease. *Arch Dis Child* 1990;65:1338–1339.
80. Wilson-Storey D, Scobie WG. Impaired gastrointestinal mucosal defense in Hirschsprung's disease: a clue to the pathogenesis of enterocolitis? *J Pediatr Surg* 1989;24:462–464.
81. Imamura A, Puri P, O'Briain DS, et al. Mucosal immune defence mechanisms in enterocolitis complicating Hirschsprung's disease. *Gut* 1992;33:801–806.
82. Caniano DA, Teitelbaum DH, Qualman SJ. Management of Hirschsprung's disease in children with trisomy 21. *Am J Surg* 1990;159:402–404.
83. Mattar AF, Coran AG, Teitelbaum DH. MUC-2 mucin production in Hirschsprung's disease: possible association with enterocolitis development. *J Pediatr Surg* 2003;38:417–421.
84. Marty TL, Seo T, Sullivan JJ, et al. Rectal irrigations for the prevention of postoperative enterocolitis in Hirschsprung's disease. *J Pediatr Surg* 1995;30:652–654.
85. Elhalaby EA, Teitelbaum DH, Coran AG, et al. Enterocolitis associated with Hirschsprung's disease: a clinical histopathological correlative study. *J Pediatr Surg* 1995;30:1023–1026; discussion 1026–1027.
86. Marty TL, Matlak ME, Hendrickson M, et al. Unexpected death from enterocolitis after surgery for Hirschsprung's disease. *Pediatrics* 1995;96:118–121.
87. Yanchar NL, Soucy P. Long term outcomes of Hirschsprung's disease: the patients' perspective. *J Pediatr Surg* 1999;34:1152–1160.
88. Puri P. Variant Hirschsprung's disease. *J Pediatr Surg* 1997;32:149–157.
89. Ryan DP. Neuronal intestinal dysplasia. *Sem Pediatr Surg* 1995;4:22–25.
90. Csury L, Pena A. Intestinal neuronal dysplasia: myth or reality? *Pediatr Surg Int* 1995;10:441–446.
91. Davidson M, Bauer CH. Studies of distal colonic motility in children IV: achalasia of the distal rectal segment despite presence of ganglia in the myenteric plexuses of this area. *Pediatrics* 1958;21:746–761.
92. Messineo A, Codrich D, Monai M, et al. The treatment of internal anal sphincter achalasia with botulinum toxin. *Pediatr Surg Int* 2001;17:521–523.
93. Meier-Ruge WA. Desmosis of the colon: a working hypothesis of primary chronic constipation. *Eur J Pediatr Surg* 1998;8:209–303.
94. Marshall DG, Meier-Ruge WA, Chakravarti A, et al. Chronic constipation due to Hirschsprung's disease and desmosis coli in a family. *Pediatr Surg Int* 2002;18:110–114.

Chapter 87

Ulcerative Colitis

Terry L. Buchmiller-Crair

Ulcerative colitis (UC) is an idiopathic inflammatory process limited to the colorectal mucosa that is characterized by intestinal inflammation and alteration in bowel function. The overall incidence of UC ranges from 3.5 to 8.0 per 100,000, and is typically seen in adults with a bimodal distribution during the third and eighth decades. The incidence falls to 1.5 to 2.0 per 100,000 for the last two to three decades of life (1). UC is a relatively rare disease in childhood, with only 15% to 20% of patients being diagnosed prior to 16 years of age (2).

The pediatric presentation of UC, however, can portend an ominous clinical course. The principles of medical management parallel those of adults, with the addition of meticulous attention to growth, nutrition, and psychological impact (1). Children with a history of UC for 10 years have an increased risk of developing colon cancer. However, UC is a curable disease if all colorectal mucosa is surgically removed. This initially involved the performance of a total colectomy, proctectomy, and placement of a permanent end ileostomy. However, patient, parental, and surgeon dissatisfaction with the commitment to a lifetime ileostomy led to the development of many contemporary anal-sparing options based on the principle of ileal reservoir creation. The addition of minimally invasive options in the surgeon's armamentarium has made the surgical treatment of UC an even more attractive option for both the parents of young children, and the body-conscious teenager.

HISTORICAL PERSPECTIVE

Diarrheal disease was described in the early writings of Hippocrates (c. 400 BC) as a significant health problem (4). Bailey, a British pathologist who lived from 1761 to 1823, first reported diarrheal disease attributed to what would later be termed *ulcerative colitis* (5). He described autopsy reports of intestinal pathology, suggesting that UC was responsible for mortality in the late eighteenth century. It was not until the nineteenth century that a differentiation emerged between the more common infectious diarrhea and UC. Crohn (6), in his historical treatise on UC from 1962, noted autopsy descriptions of 200 cases of diarrhea and dysentery from the Union Army during the Civil War. These cases were likely attributed to UC, and herald the time when the term "ulcerative colitis" was first applied. Wilks and Moxon published their classic anatomic description of UC 16 years later in 1875, differentiating it from dysentery (6). In 1907, Lockhart-Mummery (7) first reported an increased incidence of colon carcinoma in 7 of 36 UC patients. Kirsner (8) later recommended chronic surveillance of UC patients with an illuminated proctosigmoidoscope.

Medical management in this early era consisted mainly of dietary restrictions and homeopathic medications. The original surgical therapy was a sigmoid colostomy described by Pennel in 1850 (9). Subsequently, an irrigation appendicostomy was described in 1902, followed by the use of a completely diverting ileostomy in 1913. These diversions were later used in conjunction with partial resection of the diseased colon with antegrade irrigations initiated either through the appendicostomy or ileostomy.

Total colectomy, with or without a proctectomy, and an end ileostomy were considered definitive therapy in the 1940s. The resultant high-output ileostomy was associated with significant peristomal complication rates until Brooke described surgical maturation of the stoma in 1952 (10). Brooke's technique permitted effective appliance application, therefore abrogating many of these local complications.

The modern era of surgical therapy for UC was heralded by a novel anus-saving technique using a rectal mucosectomy and intestinal pull-through procedure reported by Ravitch and Sabiston in 1947 (11). However, the resultant acute and chronic postoperative complications

Terry L. Buchmiller-Crair: Children's Hospital of New York Presbyterian, Weill Medical College of Cornell University, New York, New York 10021.

rendered this technique initially unacceptable, being favored by the subsequently developed Kock continent ileostomy. The Koch pouch permitted reasonable fecal continence via the catheterized stoma and potential freedom from a chronic appliance (12). However, a stoma was still necessary, and the procedure was accompanied by significant complications.

This undesirable situation led to a reevaluation of the intestinal pull-through procedure initially described by Ravitch and Sabiston. A modification of the Soave technique commonly used for the correction of Hirschsprung's disease was proposed for the treatment of UC by Martin and LeCoultre (13). Emphasizing extensive preoperative preparation, precise operative technique, and the addition of a temporary diverting ileostomy, this modification resulted in an acceptable complication rate and functional results. However, significant postoperative morbidity persisted with an undesirable high stool frequency rate and nighttime incontinence following ileostomy closure (14).

These complications prompted the further addition of several types of surgically constructed ileal reservoirs or pouches that could be used in conjunction with the endorectal ileal pull-through procedure (ERIPT) (15–19). Indeed, pediatric surgeons were leaders in developing the contemporary surgical options now used in the management of UC. The addition of a pouch offered faster postoperative recovery, less frequent stooling, and facilitated an earlier return to a more normal pattern of daily living. The introduction of an ileal pouch had its negative effect, however, creating a new entity of reservoir inflammation termed *pouchitis*. Pouchitis manifests as diarrhea, bleeding, and pain, and requires chronic antibiotic therapy in 26% to 40% of patients (18–21). Pouch use is still debated, because outcomes following the ERIPT with or without a pouch are relatively equivalent after the first year. This has prompted some pediatric surgeons to avoid pouch use in the younger pediatric patients who seem to have less morbidity in the early postoperative period.

ETIOLOGY

The etiology of UC remains undetermined. UC occurs with an equal gender distribution and is four times more frequent in the white population. The incidence of UC is increased in the United States and Europe, especially in Scandinavia and England, demonstrating regional variation (22–24). UC also occurs four times more frequently in Jewish populations (25), with a higher incidence in Jewish immigrants to North America and Europe compared with Jews living in Israel. There is a lower incidence in Mediterranean regions, Africa, and Asia. These variations suggest a strong genetic risk for UC coupled with potential environmental and/or socioeconomic factors. Although the incidence of UC exceeded that of Crohn's disease in the first half of the twentieth century, these inflammatory bowel diseases (IBDs) are now equivalent.

The etiology of IBD has been related to environmental factors, but no conclusive evidence implicates diet, as previously suggested. The effect of cigarette smoking on the incidence of IBD has been widely studied. Harries and colleagues first linked a lower incidence of UC with smoking in 1982 (26). Although smoking doubles one's risk for Crohn's disease, the incidence of UC is reduced by 50%. At least one adult case has shown remission of UC related to the use of nicotine gum. The risk of UC remains increased in former smokers as compared with those who have never smoked (27).

Appendectomy appears to protect against the development of UC (28). Patients having undergone prior appendectomy developed symptoms of UC at a significantly later age. However, there was no impact on the extent of disease, disease course, use of immunosuppressive therapy, or ultimate need for surgical treatment. Prior appendectomy is also associated with the development of primary sclerosing cholangitis. The performance of an appendectomy is unlikely to be of benefit in cases of established UC (28).

Genetic Predisposition

A genetic predisposing factor would help explain the geographic, racial, and cultural distribution of UC. Approximately 15% of UC patients have one or more family members with a form of IBD. The relative risk for UC in siblings is 16.6 with a high degree of concordance for disease characteristics (29).

Patients with UC complicated by idiopathic ankylosing spondylitis and uveitis have an increased incidence of the major antigen type HLA-W27 (30). Several other potential candidate genes have been suggested with an association of specific HLA-DRB1 alleles (31) and C3435T MDR1 gene polymorphism (32). Antineutrophilic cytoplasmic antibodies have been detected in healthy family members of UC patients (33). Abnormal plasma polyunsaturated fatty acid patterns are noted during periods of both active and inactive IBD, in both UC and Crohn's disease (34). Mucin abnormalities have been suggested as a predisposing factor in UC related either to secondary infection or toxin invasion (35).

A two-stage genomewide search for susceptibility loci in IBD was performed involving 186 affected siblings with loci on chromosomes 2 and 6 linked to UC (29). Global gene expression profiles of inflamed colonic tissue by DNA microarray analysis has identified 170 genes with differing expression profiles for IBD (36). Fine mapping may ultimately lead to specific gene identification for UC.

Infectious

A specific infectious organism was originally suspected in IBD. The role of bacteria or viruses as primary pathogens versus secondary invaders remains unclear. The development of Crohn's disease may be related to *Mycobacterium paratuberculosis* (37), although conclusive evidence is still lacking (38). Despite extensive investigation, no specific relationship between an infectious bacterial or viral etiologic factor and UC has been demonstrated.

Immunologic

The immunologic response of the colonic mucosa to either a chemical or bacterial antigen is the most attractive contemporary theory of UC. The clinical spectrum of disease, histological appearance, and changes in immune system function all suggest that an underlying immunocellular response produce the mucosal changes seen in IBD (39). Potential pathogenic factors (dietary, genetic, environmental, and microbiologic) may individually, or jointly, be critical in inciting this immune response. The specific effector cell (plasma cells, T cells, macrophages, or neutrophils), and the role of their secreted products (antibodies, eicosanoids, cytokines, and oxygen radicals) have yet to be fully delineated.

Most investigation has focused on the mucosal T cell, with directed efforts toward elucidating the mechanism of antigen processing by T-cell receptors. The response of the trimolecular complex to the presenting antigen with varying utilization of the α- and β-chain regions of the T-cell receptor and human leukocyte antigen (HLA) surface molecules is being defined. Colonic T cells in the lamina propria produce increased interleukin 5 (IL-5) in UC patients (40). Abnormal utilization of the T-cell receptor has been identified in UC with decreased expression of the $V\beta 2$ genes in the lamina proprial T cells and the $V\delta 3$ genes in intraepithelial lymphocytes (41,42). It is hypothesized that restricted or predominant antigens trigger a specific T-cell response in IBD.

The soluble mediators released by cells during the IBD inflammatory response are being comprehensively studied. Fiocchi (43) provided a review of the complex intestinal mucosal cytokine network in IBD. Interleukin 6 (IL-6) levels are elevated in Crohn's disease, but not in UC (44). Interleukin 1 (IL-1), a proinflammatory cytokine, and its receptor antagonist (Il-lra), an antiinflammatory protein, show imbalance in the mucosa of IBD patients (45). Tumor necrosis factor-alpha (TNF-α) is increased in both the blood and stool of pediatric IBD patients (46,47). Mediator profiles could potentially be used to differentiate UC from Crohn's disease. It is hypothesized that correction of mediator imbalance could ultimately have therapeutic implications in IBD (39).

Nonimmune cells, including epithelial, endothelial, muscle, and intestinal fibroblasts, also have a putative role in the pathogenesis of IBD. These nonimmune cells function during antigen presentation and immune regulation, and as secretors of soluble mediators. Gut epithelial cells display and present class II (HLA-DR) antigen (48,49). Epithelial cells produce platelet-activating factor, a potent proinflammatory lipid mediator that occurs in excess in UC (50). Intestinal muscularis mucosa cells and mucosal fibroblasts proliferate in response to immune-derived cytokines, including IL-1, IL-6, and TNF-α (51). It appears, therefore, that the intestinal immune response in IBD involves a complex interaction between immune cells, cytokines, fibroblasts, and epithelial, mesothelial, and endothelial cells. Defining this interaction may hold the key to selective therapeutic ablation of the intestinal IBD response.

PATHOLOGIC AND HISTOLOGIC CHARACTERISTICS

UC and Crohn's disease are distinct entities with a significantly different clinical prognosis that can be difficult to differentiate using anatomic and histologic criteria. UC is a chronic mucosal inflammation of the large intestine invariably involving the rectum, and extending proximally in continuity to involve all or part of the colon. Children are most likely to develop pancolitis, with the rectosigmoid remaining the most severely involved area. In 10%, there is mild terminal ileal inflammation and edema. This *backwash ileitis* is a misnomer because no evidence supports the etiologic reflux of luminal contents (52).

Crohn's disease, in distinction to UC, is a transmural granulomatous disease that typically involves the small intestine. The seldom seen Crohn's colitis can, however, be initially confused with UC. Frank distal ileal involvement should implicate Crohn's disease. Cases of indeterminate colitis should be thoroughly investigated prior to undertaking surgical treatment, when possible.

Gross Pathology

The inflammatory response of UC is limited to the colonic mucosa and submucosa. Grossly, the colonic mesentery becomes shortened, with increased superficial vascularity and fat deposition. Endoscopic examination of the lumen reveals a hypervascular and friable mucosa with superficial ulcers that undermine the submucosa in mild, active disease. Advanced disease leads to mucosal fissures with islands of bridging mucosa resulting in the typical "cobblestone" appearance with pseudopolyp formation. These mucosal changes can revert to a more normal nonpolypoid appearance during periods of remission (53). UC typically develops in a circumferential mucosal pattern in contrast to Crohn's disease that manifests as mesenteric linear ulcerations.

Histology

As noted previously, typical UC manifests as a mucosal-submucosal process, but can appear microscopically to

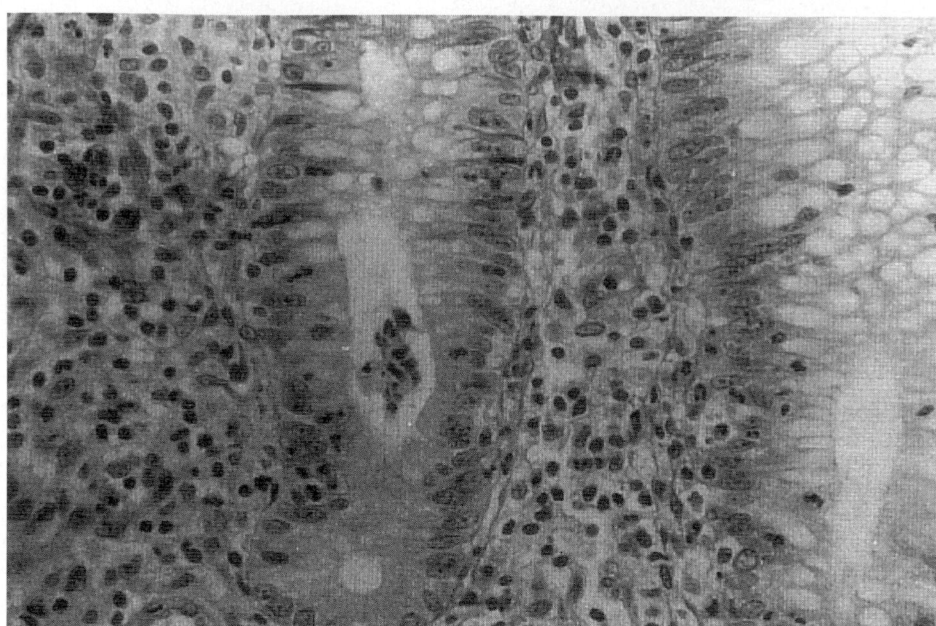

FIGURE 87-1. Micrograph of intestinal crypt with diminished goblet cells and a characteristic crypt abscess.

involve deeper layers. The histologic appearance of UC, unfortunately, cannot always be fully differentiated from infectious and inflammatory conditions, such as shigellosis, amebiasis, and gonorrheal colitis (53). Early, acute UC appears as an infiltrate of round cells and polymorphonuclear leukocytes into the crypts of Lieberkuhn at the mucosal base with resultant characteristic crypt abscesses (Fig. 87-1). The overlying epithelial cells stain poorly and are vacuolated. The ulcerated areas contain collections of collagen and granulation tissue that descend to, but rarely through, the muscularis. Transmission electron microscopy demonstrates swollen mitochondria with widened interstitial spaces, and a broadened endoplasmic reticulum. During periods of remission the mucosa may revert to normal.

With chronic inflammation, the muscularis becomes thickened and fibrotic, with gross flattening of haustral folds. Full thickness intestinal wall inflammation occurs only in fulminant UC and toxic megacolon (30). Chronically inflamed mucosa may become atrophic and is predisposed to dysplasia in long-standing disease. Biopsy confirms UC and assists the clinical picture in assessing disease activity.

CLINICAL PRESENTATION

UC is typically diagnosed in young adults, although 18% of cases present between 10 and 20 years of age, and 4% in children younger than 10 years of age (52). Symptoms associated with pediatric UC are listed in Table 87-1. Presentation is usually insidious, with persistent diarrhea and rectal bleeding, commonly with pus or mucous. In 15% of children, however, the onset is fulminant with profuse bloody diarrhea, severe crampy abdominal pain, fever, and occasionally sepsis. The distribution of UC in children is usually more extensive compared with adults and indices

TABLE 87-1 Clinical Presentation of Pediatric Ulcerative Colitis.

Presenting symptoms
Abdominal pain
Lower abdominal cramping
Tenesmus
Diarrhea
Mucous
Purulent exudate
Rectal bleeding
Anorexia
Weight loss
Chronic fatigue
Growth retardation
Extracolonic manifestations
Esophagitis and gastritis
Arthralgia
Arthritis
Anemia
Uveitis
Skin lesions
Oral ulcerations
Pyoderma gangrenosum
Erythema nodosum
Liver disease
Nephrolithiasis
Osteoporosis
Mental depression

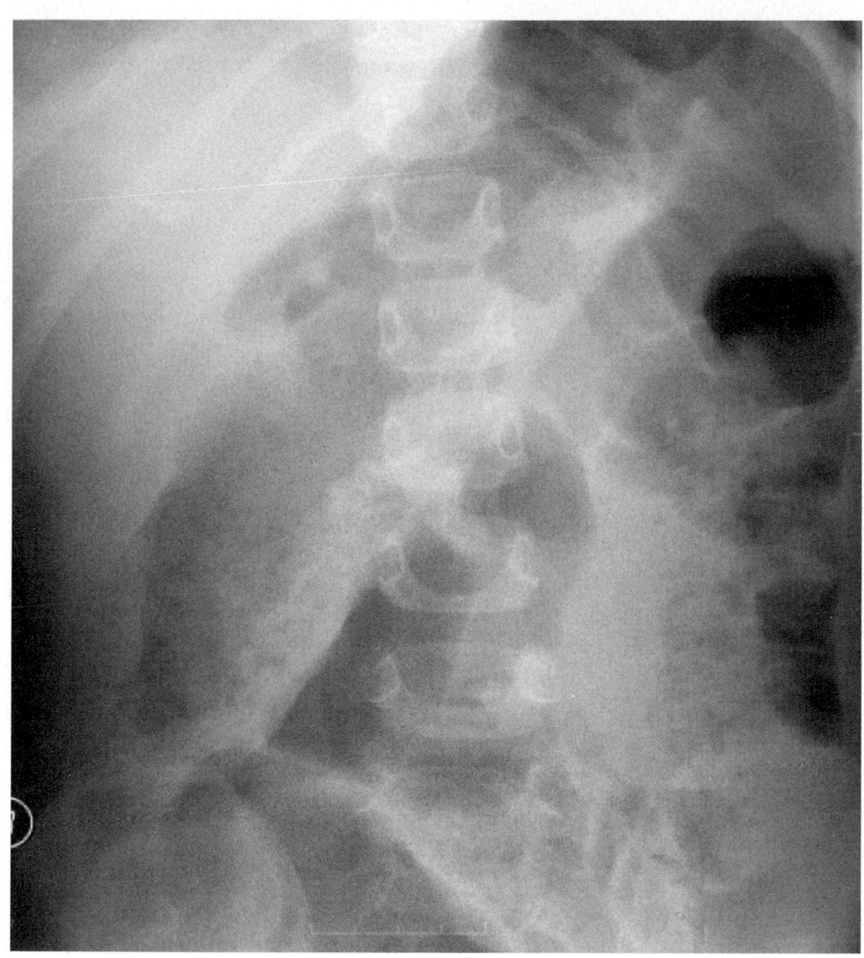

FIGURE 87-2. Plain radiograph of severe ulcerative colitis with toxic megacolon.

of disease severity can be unreliable. Most children respond to the initiation of medical therapy, but 5% will develop toxic megacolon (Fig. 87-2) necessitating emergent surgery.

The significant rectal bleeding that occurs is predictable when the gross and microscopic picture of UC is considered. The mucosal edema and ulcerations combined with the exuberant granulation tissue preclude normal colonic absorption. The resultant diarrhea irritates and produces further disruption of the friable mucosa. Crampy lower abdominal pain or tenesmus can be presenting symptoms, but tend to occur more commonly with chronic disease. Other chronic symptoms include anemia, anorexia, weight loss, growth retardation, and chronic fatigue. Often, these chronic symptoms manifest in children as the lack of desire to participate in social and athletic activities.

Growth retardation is predominantly related to the degree of intestinal inflammation and resultant poor nutrition in combination with the side effects of medical therapy (54). Approximately 14% of pediatric UC patients have decreased height at the time of diagnosis (55). Many more manifest decreased growth velocity, as well as delayed sexual maturation (56). Short stature UC patients have normal growth hormone levels, but lower urinary gonadotropins (57). There is a linear relationship between growth and disease activity, which is independent of steroid use (54). This growth delay persists throughout puberty and is not reversed after surgery, implicating that growth failure is a "prepatterned" manifestation of IBD (54).

Most children develop quiescent colitis punctuated by periodic exacerbations, often precipitated by stress or infections. Although not causative, psychological factors and stress do play a role in relapse rates. Permanent remission after a single attack occurs in fewer than 10% of children with UC. Many progress to chronic colitis with shorter and less frequent remissions. Nearly 50% of those diagnosed in childhood will need a colectomy before the age of 18 (58) as will nearly one-half of all children with pancolitis. Predictive factors for colectomy also include steroid use. Nearly 77% of those who are refractory to medical management came to operation within 3 years. Falcone and colleagues provide a review on predicting the need for colectomy in the pediatric UC patient (58).

Colorectal carcinoma is reported in 3% of children with UC patients within 10 years of disease presentation and increases by 10% to 15% with each subsequent decade (3).

Cancer risk is associated with pancolitis, earlier symptom development, and frequent flares. Dysplasia on endoscopic biopsy indicates a high risk for subsequent carcinoma. Colonoscopic surveillance may be associated with a decreased risk from death from colorectal carcinoma in patients with long-standing UC (59). As the time to dysplasia in IBD may be accelerated, earlier consideration for definitive surgery is encouraged (60).

Extracolonic Manifestations

Extracolonic manifestations of UC are listed in Table 87-1 and occur in up to 60% of children. Esophagogastroduodeoscopy (EGD) reveals esophagitis and mild to moderate gastritis in 50% of children (61). Gastroduodenal biopsy can show ulcerations, villous atrophy, and increased intraepithelial lymphocytes (62,63). Focally enhanced gastritis, classically considered a marker of Crohn's disease, also occurs in 20% of patients with UC (61). Liver disease, as manifest by abnormal liver function tests (LFTs), can result from either fatty infiltration or sclerosing cholangitis (64). Although primary sclerosing cholangitis occurs in 15% of adults, it is very uncommon in children (60).

Arthralgia and arthritis occur in 30% of patients and may be the presenting symptom of UC. Joints commonly affected include the wrists, knees, and ankles. Symptoms often respond to systemic steroids, but tend to recur upon medication withdrawal. Symptoms are often independent from the course of underlying colitis.

Skin lesions (65) include both erythema nodosum and pyoderma gangrenosum. Erythema nodosum occurs mainly on the trunk and occasionally limbs and is characterized by tender, red subcutaneous nodules. Pyoderma gangrenosum, a chronic deep ulceration of the skin, occurs most often on the lower limbs. Less than 5% of lesions are resistant to local and systemic therapy. Unlike the arthritides, resistant skin lesions resolve with the remission of colitis or with surgical extirpation of disease.

Children with IBD have decreased bone mineral density that manifests as osteoporosis and osteomalacia. These bone mineralization disorders are predicted by both the cumulative corticosteroid dose and overall nutritional status, especially in girls (66,67). Chronic recurrent osteomyelitis in IBD is very rare (68). Additional conditions include nephrolithiasis in 8% of children, likely related to chronic fluid loss and poor oral intake (30), anemia from hematochezia, uveitis (less than 2%), stomatitis, peripheral thrombotic events, and the rare, acute cerebrovascular accident (69).

Chronic and severe UC can produce emotional changes with feelings of inferiority and depression in the pediatric patient. Although emotional stress has never been established as an etiologic factor in UC, disease exacerbation can occur in association with episodes of severe emotional stress. Care providers should be cognizant of these occasionally subtle changes, and seek professional help for both the child and family.

DIAGNOSIS

Clinical Examination

Children with UC in remission or with only mild active disease may have a normal physical examination. Those with an acute flare may have fever, signs of dehydration, and systemic toxicity. Abdominal tenderness may be elicited on palpation of the left lower quadrant over the sigmoid; abdominal distension is variable. External hemorrhoids may result from frequent defecation due to diarrhea. Digital rectal examination may reveal grossly bloody or heme-positive stool. Anal fissures, fistula, and abscesses are exceedingly rare and would cause one to reconsider the diagnosis in favor of Crohn's disease. Patients with chronic UC may have decreased height, delayed sexual characteristics, anemia, pallor, and Cushingoid features from chronic steroid use. As the symptoms and physical findings of new-onset UC can be nonspecific, stool specimens should be obtained to exclude a specific responsible infectious pathogen. Screening should include *Salmonella, Shigella*, and *Campylobacter* cultures, and analyses for *Clostridium difficile* toxin and *Entamoeba histolytica*.

Laboratory Data

Acute flares of UC may result in electrolyte imbalances, specifically hyponatremia and hypokalemia from diarrheal losses. Anemia is present in two-thirds. Leukocytosis is variable and the sedimentation rate is elevated. With chronic disease, the prothrombin time may be prolonged and the serum albumin decreased.

An accurate serologic or stool assay would be desirable for the diagnosis of UC, particularly in the pediatric population, allowing invasive endoscopic procedures to be minimized. Currently, no such routine test exists, but several listed as follows show promise. Peripheral blood intracellular cytokine analysis in children is being assessed for pattern expression in IBD (70). Serum IL-6 levels in pediatric UC patients are markers of microscopic intestinal inflammation with a sensitivity of 82% and specificity of 100% (71). Levels of lamina propria IL-6 from colonic biopsies demonstrate significant correlation with the severity of histologic inflammation (71). Both serum hepatocyte growth factor levels in children and young adults (72) and fecal calprotectin, a stable neutrophil protein (73,74), show positive correlation with disease activity.

Autoantiboides are present in UC, the most common being perinuclear antineutrophil cytoplasmic antibody (pANCA) (75,76). pANCA is 92% specific for UC and is absent in controls (77). pANCA is not related to disease location, duration, activity, complications, or treatment, and remains positive after colonic resection (77). Serodiagnostic testing using pANCA for both the definitive diagnosis of UC and for monitoring disease progression is under evaluation (78).

Radiographic

Plain radiographs range from normal to grossly abnormal with signs of toxic megacolon (Fig. 87-1) or perforation. Contrast enemas are used sparingly because they can stimulate a UC flare. When obtained in acute UC, contrast enemas show an irregular serrated border from mucosal ulcerations. In chronic UC, extensive pseudopolyps are seen, and the colon may become narrow and foreshortened with the loss of haustral markings, the so-called rigid or "lead pipe" colon. An upper gastrointestinal series obtained in a quiescent state in a patient with suspected IBD can rule out small bowel involvement from Crohn's disease.

Experience is evolving using gadodiamide-enhanced magnetic resonance imaging (MRI) in UC, showing loss of haustral markings, and colonic wall thickening with contrast enhancement (79). MRI fails to recognize Crohn's disease, but is 100% specific for UC (80), and parallels findings on colonoscopy. Last, the use of 18F-fluorodeoxyglucose positron emission scanning is under investigation (81).

Endoscopy

The accurate diagnosis and assessment of disease extent in a child with UC is dependent on endoscopic examination with biopsy of the rectum and colon. Sigmoidoscopy suggests UC by the visualization of a friable, edematous colonic mucosa covered with a thin purulent exudate, often containing superficial ulcers. Colonoscopy is used to monitor disease progression and to screen for dysplasia and carcinoma. The presence of toxic megacolon is a contraindication for the use of both contrast enemas and full colonoscopic evaluation due to the risk of colonic perforation.

MEDICAL MANAGEMENT

Less than 10% of children who develop acute UC will recover without a future relapse. Pediatric UC is classified as mild, moderate, or severe disease (Table 87-2) and forms the basis for treatment strategies (82). The preexisting use of complementary or alternative medicines in children can include megavitamins, dietary supplements, and herbals in up to 19% (83). As many have potential for adverse side effects and drug interactions, use should be assessed by a thorough medical history (83).

Maintenance medical therapy for UC is largely based on antiinflammatory and immunosuppressive regimens. Mild to moderate disease is treated as an outpatient with oral forms of 5-ASA such as sulfasalazine, olesalazine, balsalazide, or mesalamine. Topical steroid or nonsteroidal enemas may be used (84). Oral antibiotics such as metronidazole and tobramycin have been used during acute UC flares, but their efficacy remains unproven (85).

TABLE 87-2 Clinical Classification of Ulcerative Colitis.

Mild ulcerative colitis (UC) (<6 stools/d)
No fever
Normal hemoglobin
Normal serum albumin
Moderate UC (>6 stools/d)
Fever >38°C
Anemia, hypoalbuminemia, or both
Severe UC (>8 stools/d)
Severe abdominal tenderness
High fever
Anemia
Leukocytosis
Toxic megacolon

Moderate disease often involves the addition of oral steroids to maintain remission. The hesitancy to use long-term steroids in the pediatric population has led to a mounting experience using combinations of 6-mercaptopurine and azathioprine (86,87). Steroids were discontinued in up to 87% of patients acutely, with two-thirds achieving permanent freedom (87,88). Side effects (commonly increased LFTs) were minimal and reversible in the majority, and responded to dose reduction (88). Eighteen percent of patients required cessation of therapy due to persistent side effects, including fever, pancreatitis, GI intolerance, and recurrent infection (88). No long-term sequelae have been documented.

Severe UC usually mandates inpatient management as complete bowel rest is indicated. Also, because a poor nutritional state is frequently present, total parenteral nutrition (TPN) is an important adjunct to medical therapy, particularly in the child who may require urgent operation. TPN use in severe UC, however, does not achieve the same high remission rate as noted in Crohn's disease (89,90). Systemic intravenous corticosteroids have formed the cornerstone of treatment of severe UC for more than 40 years. Short-term immunosuppression is added in resistant cases (91). The use of Infliximab (anti-TNF-α antibody) in children with severe UC has shown efficacy for up to 2 months, with 66% being able to discontinue steroid use (92,93).

Acute, fulminant UC is the presenting symptom in nearly 15% of pediatric cases of UC. These children have profuse bloody diarrhea, abdominal cramps, fever, and often sepsis. Approximately 3% to 5% will acutely develop toxic megacolon. This most fulminant form of UC is heralded by abdominal distention and pancolonic dilatation on abdominal x-ray (Fig. 87-2). Urgent treatment mandates the addition of broad-spectrum parenteral antibiotics, TPN, and close observation in a monitored setting because perforation is not uncommon. If perforation occurs, rapid preoperative fluid resuscitation, the continued use of broad-spectrum antibiotics, and emergent colectomy is required.

SURGICAL MANAGEMENT

Surgery for UC is indicated for the failure of medical management, hemorrhage, perforation, toxic megacolon, sepsis, and cancer risk (Table 87-3). As many as 50% of children with UC will require surgical resection within 10 years of diagnosis (94). Acute UC should respond to medical management within the first few weeks of therapy; otherwise, an unacceptable complication rate ensues.

Failure of chronic medical management includes the persistence of diarrhea, hematochezia, abdominal pain, anemia, and hypoproteinemia. The long-term side effects of chronic steroid therapy must be closely monitored, particularly in the pediatric patient (57). Growth failure, delayed sexual maturation, and chronic poor nutrition are indications for early surgery, particularly before epiphyseal closure and the pubertal growth spurt to allow potential recovery.

Long-term active disease can result in colonic mucosal aneuploidy, leading to histologic dysplasia and possible neoplastic transformation (95), justifying routine endoscopic surveillance. As previously noted, children have a 10% to 20% colon cancer risk per decade after 10 years of active UC (3). Because UC is limited to the colon, as opposed to Crohn's disease, surgical colectomy is curative. Also, because reconstructive ERIPTs are contraindicated in Crohn's disease, the diagnosis must be certain (96).

Preoperative Preparation

Careful preoperative preparation for elective or urgent surgical procedures is paramount. Often, children are debilitated and malnourished from receiving long-term steroid and/or immunosuppressive therapy. With the exception of emergent surgery for toxic megacolon, adequate preoperative therapy includes restoration of metabolic balance and nutritional repletion. Adjunctive TPN is occasionally required for 2 to 6 weeks. The reduction of immunosuppressive medications and/or corticosteroids is attempted, and blood transfusions are judiciously used.

A mechanical bowel preparation is administered the day prior to surgery. A balanced hyperosmotic oral solution such as Golytely is routinely administered, followed by enteral neomycin and erythromycin. In small children, a nasogastric tube may be needed for solution administration. Caution must be exercised to prevent intravascular volume depletion during bowel preparation by the provision of maintenance intravenous fluid.

The future right lower quadrant ileostomy site is marked preoperatively with the child awake, with consideration for clothing, body habitus, and cosmesis. Broad-spectrum intravenous antibiotics are started just prior to the surgical procedure. A preoperative dose of hydrocortisone is given if there was recent steroid dependence. Corticosteroids are tapered during the recovery period, returning to preoperative dosages within 5 to 7 days.

TABLE 87-3 Indications for Surgical Management of Ulcerative Colitis.

Acute
Hemorrhage
Intestinal perforation or impending perforation (i.e., toxic megacolon)
Chronic
Failed medical management (i.e., socially or physically dysfunctional)
Growth failure
Delayed sexual maturation
Histologic dysplasia

Surgical Procedures

Emergent Procedures

Severe attacks of UC have a 40% prevalence in children, with one-half requiring emergent surgery (97). An emergent operation for toxic megacolon, fulminant UC, or perforation demands aggressive preoperative intravascular resuscitation with Foley catheter placement, judicious transfusion, intravenous broad-spectrum antibiotic coverage, and steroid replacement. An expeditious subtotal abdominal colectomy is performed, with distal staple closure of the retained sigmoid colon as a Hartmann pouch. An end ileostomy is created.

Elective Procedures

The choice of surgical procedure used in conjunction with a child's total colectomy is dependent on the child's preoperative condition and the family's wishes (Table 87-4). Many historical options now have rare contemporary use and are detailed as follows for completeness.

Total Proctocolectomy and Permanent Ileostomy

In extremely rare cases, the child or parents will elect to have placement of a permanent Brooke ileostomy. A midline laparotomy affords excellent exposure with the incision distanced from the premarked ileostomy site to facilitate good appliance placement. The colon is mobilized routinely and divided at the level of the midsigmoid with a

TABLE 87-4 Surgical Options for Ulcerative Colitis Patients.

Pancolectomy with
Brooke ileostomy
Kock (continent) ileostomy
Abdominal colectomy with ileorectostomy (not appropriate for pediatric patients)
Abdominal colectomy with rectal mucosectomy
With ileoanal anastomosis (no reservoir)
With ileal pouch-anal anastomosis
J-pouch (two ileal loops)
S-pouch (three ileal loops plus spout)
Lateral reservoir (two ileal loops plus spout)
W-pouch (four ileal loops plus spout)

stapler. The mesenteric vessels are ligated and divided. The pelvic dissection begins by opening the peritoneal reflection at the rectum. Careful cautery dissection and division of the vessels near the bowel wall minimize interruption of the sacral parasympathetic nerves, with the potential for bladder or sexual dysfunction. The dissection proceeds extramurally to within 4 to 5 cm of the dentate line. The open rectum is irrigated with either a dilute iodine solution or a nonabsorbable antibiotic solution.

An incision encircling the anus is made approximately 1 cm distal to the dentate line and dissection is carried proximally to join the previous dissection, again staying extramural and on the bowel wall maintaining meticulous hemostasis. After removal of the colon and rectum, the pelvis is again irrigated and the muscles approximated with absorbable sutures. The perineal skin is closed loosely with nonabsorbable sutures.

The permanent ileostomy is constructed by removing the skin, subcutaneous tissue, and underlying fascial disc at the premarked ileostomy site. The distal ileum is cleared of its mesenteric vessels for approximately 3 to 5 cm. The ileum is brought through the stoma site and sutured to the surrounding fascia with absorbable sutures. Although some surgeons prefer not to mature the stoma, a carefully performed Brooke ileostomy with interrupted seromuscular, full-thickness, and dermal sutures afford the best appliance fit in the early postoperative period. A temporary stoma appliance is applied following incision closure.

Continent Ileostomy

A continent Kock ileostomy is another rarely used option, which involves the construction of an ileal reservoir with a nipple valve for catheterization and the maintenance of continence (98). The mechanical complication rate, high incidence of reservoir inflammation, and visible stoma with its required maintenance, however, render this an undesirable primary choice for most children and their families. Its current use is relegated primarily to patients who have already had a proctocolectomy with Brooke ileostomy and now desire a continent stoma.

The operation proceeds as above for the total proctocolectomy. To form a continent ileostomy, approximately 45 to 50 cm of distal ileum is required depending on patient size. The proximal 30 to 35 cm is used to create a double-loop pouch to serve as the reservoir. The distal end of the outflow loop is intussuscepted and sutured in place to produce a nipple valve. The remaining protruding distal ileum is sutured to the fascia with the distal "spout" sutured flush to the skin. The pouch maintains continence, and is catheterized to release the ileal effluent.

Colectomy with Ileorectal Anastomosis

A total abdominal colectomy with an ileorectal anastomosis has been occasionally used in adult UC patients. However, the potential complications of UC recurrence and malignant transformation of the retained rectal mucosa make this an inappropriate choice for the pediatric UC patient.

Endorectal Ileal Pull-through Procedure: Overview

The most commonly used contemporary procedure that offers improved stool continence without a permanent abdominal wall stoma is a modification of the pull-through technique first described by Ravitch and Sabiston (11) and later refined by Martin and Le Coultre (13). The total abdominal colectomy is combined with a rectal mucosectomy and an ERIPT, with or without a pouch procedure to aid in initial stool storage capacity. These variations are addressed in the following sections.

The ERIPT can also be performed in stages for severe UC (low hemoglobin, low serum albumin, or high steroid requirement) (99) with an initial subtotal colectomy and temporary ileostomy as described previously. A second-stage rectal mucosectomy and ileoanal anastomosis with diverting ileostomy (ERIPT) is performed several months later after full recovery, nutritional restoration, and cessation of systemic steroids and immunosuppressives. After complete healing of the ileoanal anastomosis is verified by contrast study and endoscopy, the ileostomy is closed as the third procedure.

Straight Endorectal Ileal Pull-through Procedure (Without Pouch) The child is anesthetized and placed in lithotomy, with meticulous attention paid to position and padding to prevent peroneal nerve palsy or lower-extremity vascular compression. The abdomen and perineum are prepped as a single sterile field. A total abdominal colectomy is performed as described previously. The ileum is mobilized to the origin of the superior mesenteric artery and should reach the perineum without tension. The rectum is mobilized distally, opening the peritoneum as previously described, and dissecting extramurally along the bowel wall. This dissection proceeds distally to a point approximately 4 to 5 cm above the anus.

Following rectal stump irrigation, the mucosectomy may be performed from above (Soave technique), below, or by a combination of the two. To begin the Soave endorectal dissection, the rectal wall is infiltrated with a 1:100,000 dilution of epinephrine in saline both to minimize bleeding and emphasize the submucosal plane. An incision is made in the rectal muscle, and the circumferential submucosal dissection is carried distally. If the child has a history of severe rectal disease, even if quiescent, this approach is frequently impractical. In this case, the rectum is divided and the submucosal dissection is begun from the perineum near the dentate line and extended proximally. This requires digital rectal dilatation and the placement of a self-retaining retractor. Traction sutures are placed distal to the dentate line and the submucosa is injected with the dilute epinephrine solution. The dentate line is visualized and a proximal circumferential incision is made with cautery. It is essential that all rectal mucosa be removed to prevent chronic pelvic infection, draining fistulae, recurrence of UC, and future risk of malignancy. The Mayo Clinic reported that 4 of 29 resected pouches contained rectal mucosa (100).

The ileum is brought down through the muscular sleeve maintaining proper orientation and verifying the absence of tension. The staple line is removed, and the ileum is meticulously sutured to the dentate line using absorbable, interrupted sutures with mucosal apposition (Fig. 87-3A). The muscular sleeve is divided longitudinally from the abdomen in the posterior midline to avoid stenosis. The proximal abdominal edge of the sleeve is loosely sutured to the contiguous ileal wall to roughly reconfigure the sphincter muscle. Pelvic drains may occasionally be used, but are withdrawn on postoperative day 4 or 5.

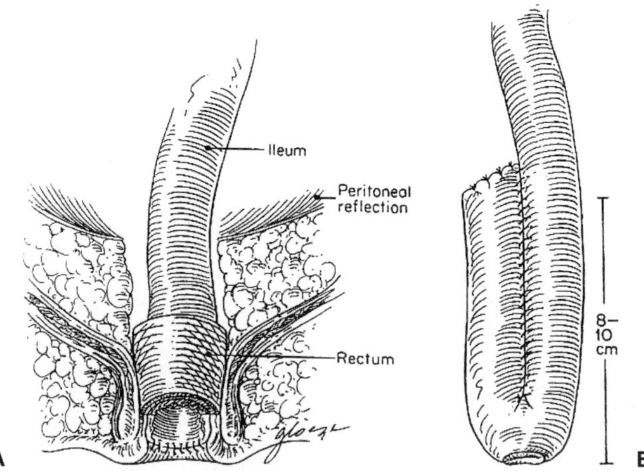

FIGURE 87-3. Comparison of **(A)** straight endorectal ileal pull-through and the **(B)** J-pouch reservoirs used most frequently in children. (Reprinted from the graphic collection of EW Fonkalsrud, with permission.)

A diverting ileostomy is recommended independent of pouch creation to minimize the risk of pelvic sepsis if there is an anastomotic leak. A 12.5% late diversion rate was reported when an initial ileostomy was not used (101). A retrospective review evaluating an end versus a loop ileostomy favored the completely diverting, end stoma with a lower wound infection rate, less peristomal skin irritation, reduced appliance cost, and increased patient satisfaction (102). The shortened operative time required for closure of the loop ileostomy was outweighed by its increased cost and complication rate (102).

A completely diverting, end ileostomy is constructed by dividing the bowel 15 to 20 cm proximal to the ileoanal anastomosis with a stapler. The proximal end is brought through the preoperatively marked site in the right lower abdomen. The distal ileal stump can be loosely sutured alongside the abdominal wall to facilitate identification during ileostomy reversal and to minimize the chance of an internal hernia.

Endorectal Ileal Pull-through Procedure: With Reservoir The initial diarrhea, urgency and nighttime incontinence encountered with the straight ERIPT have encouraged the addition of an ileal reservoir to increase initial stool storage capacity. There are four major types of pouches: the J-pouch (Fig. 87-3B) and lateral reservoir with two loops, the S-pouch with three loops, and the W-pouch with four loops. The lateral reservoir and S- and W-pouches require a spout that may contribute to potential complications such as poor vascularity, ileoanal stenosis, and poor emptying if too long. The S- and W-pouches require up to 60 cm of distal ileum for construction, potentially contributing to malabsorption. In these pouches, the terminal ileum is folded on itself and the contiguous loops are joined after opening up the adjacent common walls. The multiple-loop pouches are more difficult to construct and have a higher postoperative leak and infection rate than the straight pull-through or J-pouch. The J-pouch is the most popular reservoir used in pediatric UC surgery, but some surgeons prefer the lateral reservoir (19).

The J-pouch is formed by doubling the distal ileum back on itself and anastomosing the two communicating loops together over a 15 cm distance. A stapling instrument is used to construct the pouch through the opening at the distal end (Fig. 87-4). The loop is pulled though the pelvis, and the distal opening is meticulously anastomosed to the anus as described previously (Fig. 87-5). A double-stapling technique using a circular stapler for the ileoanal anastomosis is occasionally used in the larger adult patient. More recently, Geiger used this technique in pediatric patients with a low early complication rate (103). However, the surgeon must ensure the removal of all rectal mucosa in the pediatric patient to make the double-stapling technique a feasible option. A completely diverting ileostomy is placed as described previously.

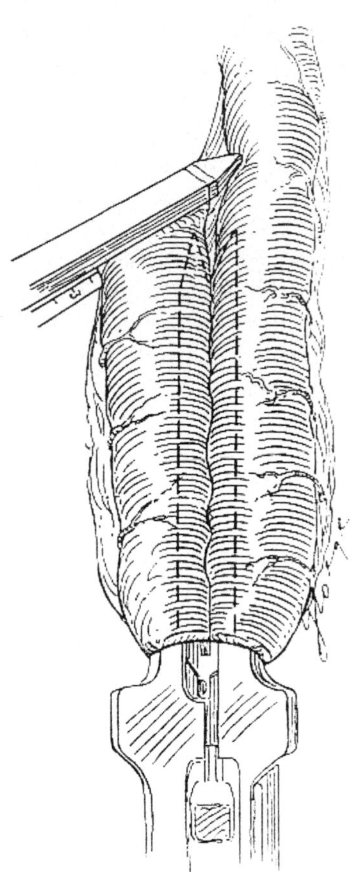

FIGURE 87-4. Stapled J-pouch. The end of the distal ileum is looped back on itself and an apical incision is made. The antimesenteric sides are approximated, and a long anastomosis is constructed with the stapler. The upper open end of the reservoir is stapled closed. (Reprinted from the graphic collection of EW Fonkalsrud, with permission.)

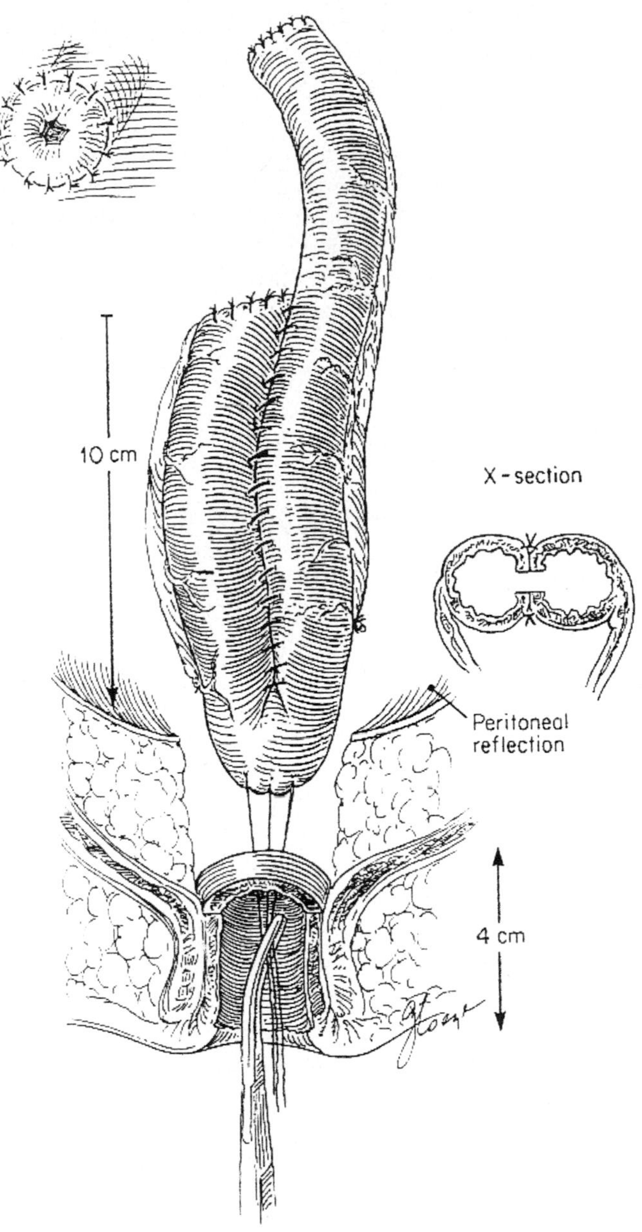

FIGURE 87-5. Pull-through of the J-pouch. The looped end is opened after a tension-free pull-through, and the ileoanal anastomosis is hand sewn. (Reprinted from the graphic collection of EW Fonkalsrud, with permission.)

POSTOPERATIVE CARE

Intravenous antibiotics are continued for several days until the patient is taking an oral diet. Oral metronidazole is commonly started and used for approximately 3 weeks. The ileoanal anastomosis is evaluated at 3 weeks either in the office or under sedation in the operating room, depending on patient tolerance. No rectal medications or manipulations are permitted prior to this examination. Home rectal dilatations using an appropriately sized smooth dilator are initiated twice a day (BID) (adult size is approximately equal to Hegar no. 19). Weekly or biweekly office visits are required until stoma closure to ensure proper healing of the ileoanal anastomosis and to wean medications as tolerated. Complete anastomotic healing is evaluated not only by physical examination, but also by outpatient contrast enema prior to ileostomy closure.

The ileostomy is typically closed in 2 to 4 months if there is no significant anastomotic stricture. Prophylactic application of stoma skin preparation to the perianal area for the week prior to ileostomy closure seems to improve the perianal rash that can complicate the postoperative period. Rigid endoscopy under anesthesia at the time of ileostomy closure is suggested as a final check of the anastomosis and pouch, if present.

A constipating diet is recommended once the patient commences oral intake and should be continued for the first several weeks following ileostomy closure. Judicious use of antidiarrheal medications (Imodium or Lomotil) is often required in the early postoperative period, particularly if a reservoir was not used. Caution should be exercised to avoid inducing stasis enteritis. Rectal dilations are weaned after proper healing of the ileoanal anastomosis is assured.

Patients are examined every 3 months during the first year, then annually if asymptomatic. An endoscopic examination of the pull-through segment is performed with biopsy as indicated. The use of Metamucil or other bulk-forming agents is helpful in maintaining proper stool consistency. Chronic antidiarrheal use for loose stools is only undertaken after evaluation has excluded pouchitis or anatomic concerns.

ERIPT RESULTS

A review of 812 adult and pediatric UC patients from the Cleveland Clinic report an overall complication rate of 62.7%, with ultimate pouch removal required in only 4.5% of the patients (104). Many authors have provided extensive reviews of outcomes after ERIPT, both with and without a pouch, in the pediatric population (101,105–110). Complications include minor wound infection (2% to 3%), steroid withdrawal mimicking intestinal obstruction, rare anastomotic leaks, pelvic sepsis, rectovaginal or anal fistulas (0% to 2%), ileoanal strictures (14%), adhesive bowel obstruction (8% to 35%) necessitating lysis of adhesions (7%), stomal revision, and reclassification into Crohn's disease (less than 1%). Major complications are more common in patients on steroid treatment (107). Less than 5% of patients with or without a reservoir become dissatisfied and elect to have a permanent ileostomy constructed (110). Antidiarrheal medications may be used with caution, but only after endoscopy and mucosal biopsy of the pouch have ruled out pouchitis.

Straight Endorectal Ileal Pull-through Procedure

Coran reported on 79 UC pediatric and adult patients undergoing a straight ERIPT for UC (110). All had a diverting ileostomy and there were no anastomotic leaks. Six had mild anastomotic narrowing that responded to dilations. There is an initial high stool frequency (15 to 20 per day) with loose diarrhea during the period of adaptation. This results in a higher rate of early morbidity with nighttime incontinence, a perianal rash, mild sleep deprivation, and an altered lifestyle for the child and family. The family must be prepared for this period of adaptation to minimize frustration. The straight pull-through segment progressively dilates over the first 2 years, demonstrating a "normal" appearance on barium enema, suggesting attainment of normal rectal capacity (111). The mean stool frequency improves to 12 per day at 3 months (110), and even further to 3 to 8 per day at 3 years, achieving equivalence to the pouch procedures (108).

All patients have daytime continence. Nocturnal soiling occurred in 11% of patients at 1 year and disappeared by 3 years. Bowel obstruction requiring operation occurred in 7%. Only 3% chose to return to an end ileostomy due to a high stool frequency. Episodes of "pouchitis" range from 0% to 40% (108,110), but appear to be much less frequent. This has a particular benefit in the younger pediatric patients who seem to have less morbidity during the early postoperative adaptive period. Annual or semiannual biopsies of the pull-though ileum have not shown significant inflammation (110). A pouch may later be constructed in patients having undergone a straight ERIPT after the period of adaptation if stool frequency remains high, or if incontinence and urgency persist, with favorable results in 50% (112).

Endorectal Ileal Pull-through Procedure with Pouch

Several authors provide large reviews of the ileoanal pouch procedure in the pediatric patient (105,107,109,113). The addition of a pouch reduces the stool frequency to 4 to 6 per day within the month following ileostomy closure and has the primary advantage of returning the child to their daily activities much sooner than those without a pouch (6 weeks vs. 3 months). Nighttime incontinence is also significantly decreased (20).

In 10-year follow-up, all patients have daytime continence, and the majority can delay defecation up to 1.5 hours. More than 84% can always sense stool from flatus. Fifty percent of patients experience minimal fecal soiling (less than 1 tsp) less than once per week (108), whereas only 5% experience occasional nighttime soiling and wear a protective pad (105). Several researchers have found better functional outcomes in children with a J-pouch as compared with those with a more complex pouch or straight ERIPT (108,109). Results are comparable to major adult series (109).

Warner and colleagues reported surgical outcomes in the very young pediatric UC patient. The average age at diagnosis was 4 years and most had severe pancolitis. ERIPT with a pouch was performed at a mean age of 6.8 years with a 9-year follow-up. Results were comparable to adolescents and young adults with a slightly higher rate of nighttime incontinence (106).

The major chronic reservoir complication is *pouchitis,* which occurs in 16% to 69% of all pediatric patients (105–108,114) and is defined as either acute (less than 3 months) or chronic (greater than 3 months) (114). Symptoms include diarrhea, urgency, and excessive nighttime stooling. Pouchitis is suspected by clinical presentation, but is ultimately confirmed by endoscopy and mucosal biopsy. The Heidelberg Pouchitis Activity Score and clinical management algorithms based on primary versus secondary causes are available to assist the clinician (114).

Oral metronidazole, with the occasional addition of steroid enemas, is the cornerstone of treatment. It is critical to determine if pouchitis is due to an underlying anatomic reason, such as an ileoanal stricture because 87% respond to surgical revision. Replacement of a temporary or permanent ileostomy may be required in severe cases (115). Long-term complications of pouchitis in the pediatric patient are unknown.

Chronic pouch stasis manifests as progressive diarrhea, frequency, urgency, and soiling, and is related to the creation of larger, more complex pouches from the early UC experience (116). Stasis is often associated with pouch enlargement, an elongated efferent limb, and obstruction to outflow, which mandate surgical revision (117). Options for revision include transanal resection of the elongated spout, abdominoperineal mobilization of the pouch with partial resection and tapering, pouch removal and reconstruction, and conversion to a permanent ileostomy (117). Fonkalsrud et al. provided an extensive analysis of patients requiring revisional surgery, including reconstruction of large pouches and conversions from the straight pull-through due to increased stool frequency (105). Most patients require revision within 2 years of their initial operation. In long-term follow-up, excellent function in reported in 95% (105). Pouch removal was only required in 3% with end ileostomy placement (117). One-half of these instances occurred in patients ultimately reclassified as having Crohn's disease (105).

LAPAROSCOPIC PROCEDURES

Many small retrospective series are reporting the use of laparoscopic techniques to perform virtually all elective surgical procedures listed previously in the pediatric patient (105,118,119). Although longer operating room times are required, perioperative outcomes demonstrate similar length of stay (LOS) and narcotic use, earlier return of bowel function, and improved cosmesis in the laparoscopic cohorts (119). The long-term effect on bowel obstruction remains unknown. The use of laparoscopic surgery in the pediatric population with fulminant UC has yet to be defined, but adult series show an equivalent complication rate with decreased LOS (120). Full details of laparoscopic techniques in adult UC patients are available (121,122).

LONG-TERM FOLLOW-UP

The use of health-related, quality-of-life (QOL) measurements is encouraged, particularly in the pediatric population. QOL measurements clearly show reduced functioning in the physical, psychological, and social functioning domains in pediatric UC patients (123). A specific questionnaire for the child and adolescent IBD patient was developed at The Hospital for Sick Children in Toronto, Canada (124). Bowel symptoms were more troubling and disabling for children with UC compared with those with Crohn's disease, whereas the systemic symptoms, body image concerns, and ability to function in school and leisure activities were improved (124). Many children with UC demonstrate emotional responses of unfairness, frustration, anger, and embarrassment, with very few disparities between age groups (124).

Pediatric UC patients expressed greater long-term satisfaction after pouch reconstruction compared with the straight ERIPT (108). Parental anxiety still remains high following ERIPT, although not vastly different from population norms (113). The presence of chronic pouchitis and nocturnal incontinence negatively affects both the physical summary scores and the overall QOL (113). The majority, however, have a QOL, physical functioning, mental health, and self-esteem equivalent to peers (113). The vast majority of pediatric ERIPT patients is quite satisfied and has accommodated to their stooling habits by maximizing dietary, medicinal, and lifestyle changes.

Many women with UC are in childbearing years. In those managed medically, relapse rates of UC do not increase in pregnancy (125). Women with UC also appear to have normal fecundity before surgical treatment (126). The effects of the pouch procedure on fertility remain unknown or nonspecific due to pelvic surgery (127). Infertility issues are more common after the surgical treatment of UC, and there is increased incidence of dyspareunia and ovarian cysts in 7.4% of women. Spontaneous vaginal delivery appears quite safe without perineal complications. The role of vaginal delivery versus cesarean section in women after the surgical treatment of UC is still being defined (127).

ACKNOWLEDGMENTS

The author wants to thank Dr. David Dudgeon, the author of this chapter in the original edition of this textbook, for providing the foundation of this updated version.

REFERENCES

1. Ferguson A. Assessment and management of ulcerative colitis in children. *Eur J Gastroenterol Hepatol* 1997;9(9):858–863.
2. Farmer RG, Easley KA, Rankin GB. Clinical patterns, natural history, and progression of ulcerative colitis. A long-term follow-up of 1116 patients. *Dig Dis Sci* 1993;38(6):1137–1146.
3. Devroede GJ, Taylor WF, Saver WG, et al. Cancer risk and life expectancy of children with ulcerative colitis. *N Engl J Med* 1971; 285(1):17–21.
4. Adams F. *The genuine works of Hippocrates*. Baltimore: Williams & Wilkins, 1939.
5. Morson B. Current concepts of colitis: the 1970 Lettsomian lectures. *Trans Med Soc Lond* 1970;86:159.
6. Crohn B. An historical note on ulcerative colitis [Letter]. *Gastroenterology* 1962;42:366.

7. Lockhart-Mummery J. The causes of colitis: with special reference to its surgical treatment, with an account of 36 cases. *Lancet* 1907;1:1638.
8. Kirsner JB. Historical aspects of inflammatory bowel disease. *J Clin Gastroenterol* 1988;10(3):286–297.
9. Goligher J, De Dombal FT, Watts JM, et al. *Ulcerative colitis.* Baltimore: Williams & Wilkins, 1968.
10. Brooke BN. The management of an ileostomy including its complications. 1952. *Dis Colon Rectum* 1993;36(5):512–516.
11. Ravitch M, Sabiston DC. Anal ileostomy with preservation of the sphincter: a proposed operation in patients requiring total colectomy for benign lesions. *Surg Gynecol Obstet* 1947;84:1095.
12. Koch N. Historical perspective. In: Dozois RR, ed. *Alternatives to conventional ileostomy.* Chicago: Year Book Medical, 1985:133.
13. Martin LW, LeCoultre C. Technical considerations in performing total colectomy and Soave endorectal anastomosis for ulcerative colitis. *J Pediatr Surg* 1978;13(6D):762–764.
14. Becker JM. Anal sphincter function after colectomy, mucosal proctectomy, and endorectal ileoanal pull-through. *Arch Surg* 1984;119(5):526–531.
15. Parks AG, Nicholls RJ. Proctocolectomy without ileostomy for ulcerative colitis. *Br Med J* 1978;2(6130):85–88.
16. Utsunomiya J, Iwama T, Imajo M, et al. Total colectomy, mucosal proctectomy, and ileoanal anastomosis. *Dis Colon Rectum* 1980;23(7):459–466.
17. Wong WD, Rothenberger DA, Goldberg SM. Ileoanal pouch procedures. *Curr Probl Surg* 1985;22(3):1–78.
18. Nicholls RJ, Pezim ME. Restorative proctocolectomy with ileal reservoir for ulcerative colitis and familial adenomatous polyposis: a comparison of three reservoir designs. *Br J Surg* 1985;72(6):470–474.
19. Fonkalsrud EW, Stelzner M, McDonald N. Experience with the endorectal ileal pullthrough with lateral reservoir for ulcerative colitis and polyposis. *Arch Surg* 1988;123(9):1053–1058.
20. McIntyre PB, et al. Comparing functional results one year and ten years after ileal pouch-anal anastomosis for chronic ulcerative colitis. *Dis Colon Rectum* 1994;37(4):303–307.
21. Lobo AJ, et al. Carriage of adhesive *Escherichia coli* after restorative proctocolectomy and pouch anal anastomosis: relation with functional outcome and inflammation. *Gut* 1993;34(10):1379–1383.
22. Kildebo S, et al. The incidence of ulcerative colitis in Northern Norway from 1983 to 1986. The Northern Norwegian Gastroenterology Society. *Scand J Gastroenterol* 1990;25(9):890–896.
23. Stowe SP, et al. An epidemiologic study of inflammatory bowel disease in Rochester, New York. Hospital incidence. *Gastroenterology* 1990;98(1):104–110.
24. Yoshida Y, Murata Y. Inflammatory bowel disease in Japan: studies of epidemiology and etiopathogenesis. *Med Clin North Am* 1990;74(1):67–90.
25. Burakoff R. Update on the epidemiology of IBD. *Prog Inflamm Bowel Disc* 1994;15:1.
26. Harries AD, Baird A, Rhodes J. Non-smoking: a feature of ulcerative colitis. *Br Med J (Clin Res Ed)* 1982;284(6317):706.
27. Jick H, Walker AM. Cigarette smoking and ulcerative colitis. *N Engl J Med* 1983;308(5):261–263.
28. Selby WS, et al. Appendectomy protects against the development of ulcerative colitis but does not affect its course. *Am J Gastroenterol* 2002;97(11):2834–2838.
29. Satsangi J, et al. Genetics of inflammatory bowel disease. *Clin Sci (Lond)* 1998;94(5):473–478.
30. Fonkalsrud EW. Inflammatory bowel disease. In: Ashcraft K, ed. *Pediatric surgery,* 2nd ed. Philadelphia: WB Saunders, 1993:440.
31. Bouma G, et al. Genetic markers in clinically well defined patients with ulcerative colitis (UC). *Clin Exp Immunol* 1999;115(2):294–300.
32. Schwab M, et al. Association between the C3435T MDR1 gene polymorphism and susceptibility for ulcerative colitis. *Gastroenterology* 2003;124(1):26–33.
33. Shanahan F, et al. Neutrophil autoantibodies in ulcerative colitis: familial aggregation and genetic heterogeneity. *Gastroenterology* 1992;103(2):456–461.
34. Esteve-Comas M, et al. Abnormal plasma polyunsaturated fatty acid pattern in non-active inflammatory bowel disease. *Gut* 1993;34(10):1370–1373.
35. Tysk C, et al. Colonic glycoproteins in monozygotic twins with inflammatory bowel disease. *Gastroenterology* 1991;100(2):419–423.
36. Lawrance IC, Fiocchi C, Chakravarti S. Ulcerative colitis and Crohn's disease: distinctive gene expression profiles and novel susceptibility candidate genes. *Hum Mol Genet* 2001;10(5):445–456.
37. Prantera C, et al. Antimycobacterial therapy in Crohn's disease: results of a controlled, double-blind trial with a multiple antibiotic regimen. *Am J Gastroenterol* 1994;89(4):513–518.
38. Sanderson JD, et al. Mycobacterium paratuberculosis DNA in Crohn's disease tissue. *Gut* 1992;33(7):890–896.
39. Fiocchi C. The immune system in inflammatory bowel disease. *Acta Gastroenterol Belg* 1997;60(2):156–162.
40. Fuss IJ, et al. Disparate CD4+ lamina propria (LP) lymphokine secretion profiles in inflammatory bowel disease. Crohn's disease LP cells manifest increased secretion of IFN-gamma, whereas ulcerative colitis LP cells manifest increased secretion of IL-5. *J Immunol* 1996;157(3):1261–1270.
41. Duchmann R, Strober W, Fiocchi C, et al. TCR V(beta)2 gene expression is selective in control but not in IBD lamina propria lymphocytes. *Gastroenterology* 1992;102:A617.
42. Landau S, Balk SB, Yan L, et al. T-cell receptor (TCR) delta variable region utilization is altered in ulcerative colitis. *Gastroenterology* 1992;102:A650.
43. Fiocchi C. Cytokines. In MacDermott RP and Stinson W, ed. *Inflammatory bowel disease.* New York: Elsevier, 1992:137.
44. Mahida YR, Kurlac L, Gallagher A, et al. High circulating concentrations of interleukin-6 in active Crohn's disease but not ulcerative colitis. *Gut* 1991;32(12):1531–1534.
45. Cominelli F, Fiocchi C, Eisenberg SP, et al. Imbalance of IL-1 and IL-1 receptor antagonist in the intestinal mucosa of Crohn's disease and ulcerative colitis patients. *Gastroenterology* 1992;100:A3.
46. Murch SH, et al. Serum concentrations of tumour necrosis factor alpha in childhood chronic inflammatory bowel disease. *Gut* 1991;32(8):913–917.
47. Braegger CP, et al. Tumour necrosis factor alpha in stool as a marker of intestinal inflammation. *Lancet* 1992;339(8785):89–91.
48. Mayer L, et al. Expression of class II molecules on intestinal epithelial cells in humans. Differences between normal and inflammatory bowel disease. *Gastroenterology* 1991;100(1):3–12.
49. Mayer L, Eisenhardt D. Lack of induction of suppressor T cells by intestinal epithelial cells from patients with inflammatory bowel disease. *J Clin Invest* 1990;86(4):1255–1260.
50. Ferraris L, et al. Intestinal epithelial cells contribute to the enhanced generation of platelet activating factor in ulcerative colitis. *Gut* 1993;34(5):665–668.
51. Strong S, West GA, Klein, JS, et al. Inflammatory cytokines stimulate proliferation of intestinal mucosa mesenchymal cells. *Gastroenterology* 1992;102:A701.
52. Sloan WP Jr, Bargen JA, Gage RB. Life histories of patients with chronic ulcerative colitis: a review of 2,000 cases. *Gastroenterology* 1968;54(4):S819–S822.
53. Becker J, Moody FG. Ulcerative colitis. In: Sabiston J, ed. *Textbook of surgery.* Philadelphia: WB Saunders, 1986:1011.
54. Motil KJ, et al. Growth failure in children with inflammatory bowel disease: a prospective study. *Gastroenterology* 1993;105(3):681–691.
55. Markowitz J, Daum F. Growth impairment in pediatric inflammatory bowel disease. *Am J Gastroenterol* 1994;89(3):319–326.
56. Saha MT, et al. Growth of prepubertal children with inflammatory bowel disease. *J Pediatr Gastroenterol Nutr* 1998;26(3):310–314.
57. McCaffery TD, et al. Severe growth retardation in children with inflammatory bowel disease. *Pediatrics* 1970;45(3):386–393.
58. Falcone RA Jr, Lewis LG, Warner BW. Predicting the need for colectomy in pediatric patients with ulcerative colitis. *J Gastrointest Surg* 2000;4(2):201–206.
59. Karlen P, et al. Increased risk of cancer in ulcerative colitis: a population-based cohort study. *Am J Gastroenterol* 1999;94(4):1047–1052.
60. Faubion WA Jr, et al. Pediatric "PSC-IBD": a descriptive report of associated inflammatory bowel disease among pediatric patients with psc. *J Pediatr Gastroenterol Nutr* 2001;33(3):296–300.
61. Sharif F, et al. Focally enhanced gastritis in children with Crohn's

disease and ulcerative colitis. *Am J Gastroenterol* 2002;97(6):1415–1420.

62. Tobin JM, et al. Upper gastrointestinal mucosal disease in pediatric Crohn disease and ulcerative colitis: a blinded, controlled study. *J Pediatr Gastroenterol Nutr* 2001;32(4):443–448.
63. Kaufman SS, et al. Gastroenteric inflammation in children with ulcerative colitis. *Am J Gastroenterol* 1997;92(7):1209–1212.
64. Lagercrantz R, Winberg J, Zetterstrom R. Extracolonic manifestations in chronic ulcerative colitis. *Acta Paediatr Scand* 1958;47:675.
65. Edwards F, Truelove SC. The course and prognosis of ulcerative colitis. III. Complications. *Gut* 1964;5:1.
66. Gokhale R, et al. Bone mineral density assessment in children with inflammatory bowel disease. *Gastroenterology* 1998;114(5):902–911.
67. Boot AM, et al. Bone mineral density and nutritional status in children with chronic inflammatory bowel disease. *Gut* 1998;42(2):188–194.
68. Bousvaros A, et al. Chronic recurrent multifocal osteomyelitis associated with chronic inflammatory bowel disease in children. *Dig Dis Sci* 1999;44(12):2500–2507.
69. Keene DL, et al. Cerebral vascular events associated with ulcerative colitis in children. *Pediatr Neurol* 2001;24(3):238–243.
70. Mack DR, et al. Peripheral blood intracellular cytokine analysis in children newly diagnosed with inflammatory bowel disease. *Pediatr Res* 2002;51(3):328–332.
71. Brown KA, et al. Lamina propria and circulating interleukin-6 in newly diagnosed pediatric inflammatory bowel disease patients. *Am J Gastroenterol* 2002;97(10):2603–2608.
72. Srivastava M, et al. Elevated serum hepatocyte growth factor in children and young adults with inflammatory bowel disease. *J Pediatr Gastroenterol Nutr* 2001;33(5):548–553.
73. Bunn SK, et al. Fecal calprotectin as a measure of disease activity in childhood inflammatory bowel disease. *J Pediatr Gastroenterol Nutr* 2001;32(2):171–177.
74. Bunn SK, et al. Fecal calprotectin: validation as a noninvasive measure of bowel inflammation in childhood inflammatory bowel disease. *J Pediatr Gastroenterol Nutr* 2001;33(1):14–22.
75. Pikarsky A, Zmora O, Wexner SD. Immunosuppressants and operation in ulcerative colitis. *J Am Coll Surg* 2002;195(2):251–260.
76. Dubinsky MC, et al. Clinical utility of serodiagnostic testing in suspected pediatric inflammatory bowel disease. *Am J Gastroenterol* 2001;96(3):758–765.
77. Ruemmele FM, et al. Diagnostic accuracy of serological assays in pediatric inflammatory bowel disease. *Gastroenterology* 1998;115(4):822–829.
78. Mamula P, et al. Inflammatory bowel disease in children 5 years of age and younger. *Am J Gastroenterol* 2002;97(8):2005–2010.
79. Nozue T, et al. Assessment of disease activity and extent by magnetic resonance imaging in ulcerative colitis. *Pediatr Int* 2000;42(3):285–288.
80. Durno CA, et al. Magnetic resonance imaging to distinguish the type and severity of pediatric inflammatory bowel diseases. *J Pediatr Gastroenterol Nutr* 2000;30(2):170–174.
81. Skehan SJ, et al. 18F-fluorodeoxyglucose positron tomography in diagnosis of paediatric inflammatory bowel disease. *Lancet* 1999;354(9181):836–837.
82. Kirschner B. *Chronic inflammatory bowel disease: ulcerative colitis and Crohn's disease*. Norwalk, CT: Appleton & Lange; 1987;933.
83. Heuschkel R, et al. Complementary medicine use in children and young adults with inflammatory bowel disease. *Am J Gastroenterol* 2002;97(2):382–388.
84. Mantzaris GJ, et al. Intermittent therapy with high-dose 5-aminosalicylic acid enemas maintains remission in ulcerative proctitis and proctosigmoiditis. *Dis Colon Rectum* 1994;37(1):58–62.
85. Mantzaris GJ, et al. Intravenous tobramycin and metronidazole as an adjunct to corticosteroids in acute, severe ulcerative colitis. *Am J Gastroenterol* 1994;89(1):43–46.
86. Fraser AG, et al. Long-term risk of malignancy after treatment of inflammatory bowel disease with azathioprine. *Aliment Pharmacol Ther* 2002;16(7):1225–1232.
87. Kader HA, et al. Experiences with 6-mercaptopurine and azathioprine therapy in pediatric patients with severe ulcerative colitis. *J Pediatr Gastroenterol Nutr* 1999;28(1):54–58.
88. Kirschner BS. Safety of azathioprine and 6-mercaptopurine in pediatric patients with inflammatory bowel disease. *Gastroenterology* 1998;115(4):813–821.
89. Elson CO, et al. An evaluation of total parenteral nutrition in the management of inflammatory bowel disease. *Dig Dis Sci* 1980;25(1):42–48.
90. Dickinson RJ, et al. Controlled trial of intravenous hyperalimentation and total bowel rest as an adjunct to the routine therapy of acute colitis. *Gastroenterology* 1980;79(6):1199–1204.
91. Lichtiger S, et al. Cyclosporine in severe ulcerative colitis refractory to steroid therapy. *N Engl J Med* 1994;330(26):1841–1845.
92. Serrano MS, et al. Use of infliximab in pediatric patients with inflammatory bowel disease. *Ann Pharmacother* 2001;35(7–8):823–828.
93. Mamula P, et al. Infliximab as a novel therapy for pediatric ulcerative colitis. *J Pediatr Gastroenterol Nutr* 2002;34(3):307–311.
94. Sedgwick DM, et al. Population-based study of surgery in juvenile onset ulcerative colitis. *Br J Surg* 1991;78(2):176–178.
95. Befrits R, et al. DNA aneuploidy and histologic dysplasia in long-standing ulcerative colitis. A 10-year follow-up study. *Dis Colon Rectum* 1994;37(4):313–319; discussion 319–320.
96. Deutsch AA, et al. Results of the pelvic-pouch procedure in patients with Crohn's disease. *Dis Colon Rectum* 1991;34(6):475–477.
97. Barabino A, et al. Severe attack of ulcerative colitis in children: retrospective clinical survey. *Dig Liver Dis* 2002;34(1):44–49.
98. Ein SH. A ten-year experience with the pediatric Kock pouch. *J Pediatr Surg* 1987;22(8):764–766.
99. Nicholls RJ, Holt SD, Lubowski DZ. Restorative proctocolectomy with ileal reservoir. Comparison of two-stage vs. three-stage procedures and analysis of factors that might affect outcome. *Dis Colon Rectum* 1989;32(4):323–326.
100. O'Connell PR, et al. Does rectal mucosa regenerate after ileoanal anastomosis? *Dis Colon Rectum* 1987;30(1):1–5.
101. Dolgin SE, et al. Restorative proctocolectomy in children with ulcerative colitis utilizing rectal mucosectomy with or without diverting ileostomy. *J Pediatr Surg* 1999;34(5):837–839; discussion 839–840.
102. Fonkalsrud EW, Thakur A, Roof L. Comparison of loop versus end ileostomy for fecal diversion after restorative proctocolectomy for ulcerative colitis. *J Am Coll Surg* 2000;190(4):418–422.
103. Geiger JD, et al. A new operative technique for restorative proctocolectomy: the endorectal pull-through combined with a double-stapled ileo-anal anastomosis. *Surgery* 2003;134(3):492–495.
104. Fazio VW, et al. Ileal pouch-anal anastomoses complications and function in 1005 patients. *Ann Surg* 1995;222(2):120–127.
105. Fonkalsrud EW, Thakur A, Beanes S. Ileoanal pouch procedures in children. *J Pediatr Surg* 2001;36(11):1689–1692.
106. Robb BW, et al. Restorative proctocolectomy with ileal pouch-anal anastomosis in very young patients with refractory ulcerative colitis. *J Pediatr Surg* 2003;38(6):863–867.
107. Rintala RJ, Lindahl HG. Proctocolectomy and J-pouch ileo-anal anastomosis in children. *J Pediatr Surg* 2002;37(1):66–70.
108. Telander RL, et al. Long-term follow-up of the ileoanal anastomosis in children and young adults. *Surgery* 1990;108(4):717–723; discussion 723–725.
109. Durno C, et al. Outcome after ileoanal anastomosis in pediatric patients with ulcerative colitis. *J Pediatr Gastroenterol Nutr* 1998;27(5):501–507.
110. Coran AG. A personal experience with 100 consecutive total colectomies and straight ileoanal endorectal pull-throughs for benign disease of the colon and rectum in children and adults. *Ann Surg* 1990;212(3):242–247; discussion 247–248.
111. Bank ER, White SJ, Coran AG. The radiographic appearance of the endorectal pull-through. *Pediatr Radiol* 1986;16(3):216–221.
112. Fonkalsrud EW, Stelzner M, McDonald N. Construction of an ileal reservoir in patients with a previous straight endorectal ileal pull-through. *Ann Surg* 1988;208(1):50–55.
113. Stavlo PL, et al. Pediatric ileal pouch-anal anastomosis: functional outcomes and quality of life. *J Pediatr Surg* 2003;38(6):935–939.
114. Heuschen UA, et al. Long-term follow-up after ileoanal pouch procedure: algorithm for diagnosis, classification, and management of pouchitis. *Dis Colon Rectum* 2001;44(4):487–499.

115. Fonkalsrud EW. Update on clinical experience with different surgical techniques of the endorectal pull-through operation for colitis and polyposis. *Surg Gynecol Obstet* 1987;165(4):309–316.
116. Nicholls J, et al. Restorative proctocolectomy with a three-loop ileal reservoir for ulcerative colitis and familial adenomatous polyposis. Clinical results in 66 patients followed for up to 6 years. *Ann Surg* 1984;199(4):383–388.
117. Fonkalsrud EW, Bustorff-Silva J. Reconstruction for chronic dysfunction of ileoanal pouches. *Ann Surg* 1999;229(2):197–204.
118. Santoro E, et al. Laparoscopic total proctocolectomy with ileal J pouch-anal anastomosis. *Hepatogastroenterology* 1999;46(26):894–899.
119. Proctor ML, et al. Is laparoscopic subtotal colectomy better than open subtotal colectomy in children? *J Pediatr Surg* 2002;37(5):706–708.
120. Bell RL, Seymour NE. Laparoscopic treatment of fulminant ulcerative colitis. *Surg Endosc* 2002;16(12):1778–1782.
121. Hasegawa H, et al. Laparoscopic restorative proctocolectomy for patients with ulcerative colitis. *J Laparoendosc Adv Surg Tech A* 2002;12(6):403–406.
122. Kienle P, et al. Laparoscopically assisted colectomy and ileoanal pouch procedure with and without protective ileostomy. *Surg Endosc* 2003;17(5):716–720.
123. Koot HM, Bouman NH. Potential uses for quality-of-life measures in childhood inflammatory bowel disease. *J Pediatr Gastroenterol Nutr* 1999;28(4):S56–S61.
124. Griffiths AM, et al. Development of a quality-of-life index for pediatric inflammatory bowel disease: dealing with differences related to age and IBD type. *J Pediatr Gastroenterol Nutr* 1999;28(4):S46–S52.
125. Hudson M, et al. Fertility and pregnancy in inflammatory bowel disease. *Int J Gynaecol Obstet* 1997;58(2):229–237.
126. Ording Olsen K, et al. Ulcerative colitis: female fecundity before diagnosis, during disease, and after surgery compared with a population sample. *Gastroenterology* 2002;122(1):15–19.
127. Counihan TC, et al. Fertility and sexual and gynecologic function after ileal pouch-anal anastomosis. *Dis Colon Rectum* 1994;37(11):1126–1129.

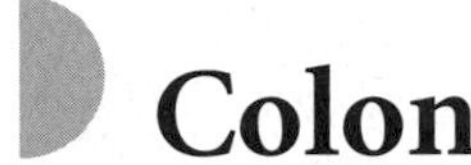

Colon

James D. Geiger

ANATOMIC CONSIDERATIONS

Embryology

The primitive gut, which is divided into the foregut, the midgut, and the hindgut, develops during the fourth week of gestation. The midgut develops into the small intestine (beginning at the entrance of the common bile duct), and the large intestine develops proximal to the midtransverse colon. This intestinal segment receives blood from the superior mesenteric artery. The hindgut develops into the large bowel distal to the midtransverse colon, as well as the proximal anus and the lower urogenital tract, and receives its main blood supply from the inferior mesenteric artery.

The developing midgut migrates out of the abdominal cavity during the sixth week of pregnancy. During the ensuing 4 weeks, the midgut rotates 270 degrees in a counterclockwise direction about the superior mesenteric artery before assuming its final anatomic position in the abdominal cavity, which leaves the cecum positioned in the right side of the abdomen.

Anatomy

The colon is a tubular structure approximately 30 to 40 cm in length at birth that reaches 1.5 m in length in the adult. It is continuous with the small intestine at the ileocecal valve proximal and ends distally at the anal verge. The external appearance of the colon is differentiated from the small bowel because of differences in their musculature. Although both organs have inner circular and outer longitudinal muscle layers, the colonic longitudinal muscle fibers coalesce into three discrete bands, termed *teniae*, located at 120-degree intervals about the colonic circumference. The teniae start at the base of the appendix and run continuously to the proximal rectum and are important for identification of the colon during surgery. Outpouchings of the colon (haustra) separate the teniae. The folds between the haustra have a semilunar appearance when viewed from within the colon. On the outside of the colon are fatty-filled sacs of peritoneum called *appendices epiploicae* or *omental appendices;* these are more prominent in older children and in children with obesity.

The first portion of the colon, the cecum, lies in the right iliac fossa, and is slightly dilated compared with the rest of the colon. The cecum is more mobile in neonates, even with normal rotation, and may be located toward the right upper abdomen. The vermiform appendix is a blind outpouching of the cecum that begins inferior to the ileocecal valve. The ascending colon extends cranially from the cecum along the right side of the peritoneal cavity to the undersurface of the liver. In most individuals, the mesentery of the ascending colon has fused with the parietal peritoneum, making this segment of the colon a retroperitoneal structure. At the hepatic flexure, the colon turns medially and anterior to emerge into the peritoneal cavity as the transverse colon,which supports the greater omentum. The transverse colon can be quite mobile on its mesentery, even dropping below the pelvic brim before reaching its attachment to the diaphragm at the splenic flexure. The descending colon travels posterior and then inferior in the retroperitoneal compartment to the pelvic brim. There it reemerges into the peritoneal cavity as the sigmoid colon. This is an S-shaped segment of variable length. Its mobility and tortuosity can be a challenge during endoscopy, also causing it to be susceptible to volvulus.

The arterial supply to the colon is derived from the superior and inferior mesenteric arteries. The superior mesenteric artery provides the blood supply to the colon from the ileocecal area to the distal third of the transverse colon. The cecum is supplied by the anterior and posterior cecal arteries, the ascending colon by the ileocolic and right colic branches, and the transverse colon by the middle colic artery. The distal transverse colon, descending colon, and sigmoid colon are all supplied by the superior and inferior

James D. Geiger: University of Michigan, C.S. Mott Children's Hospital, Ann Arbor, Michigan 48109–0245.

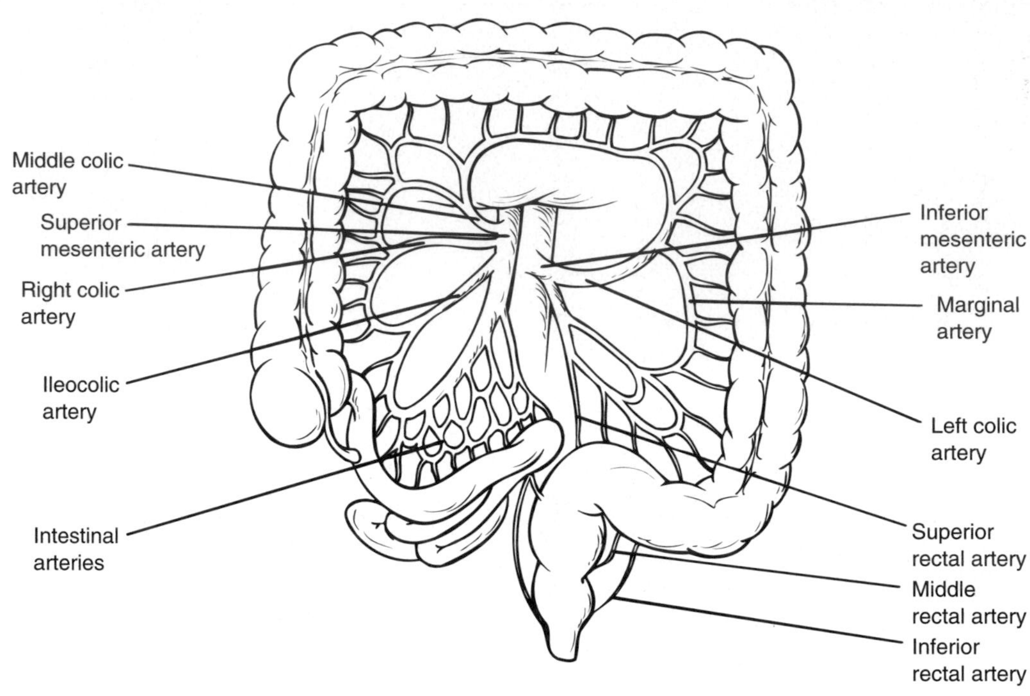

FIGURE 88-1. The anatomy and blood supply of the colon.

left colic branches of the inferior mesenteric artery. There is communication among arterial branches through the marginal arteries, which extend from the ileocolic junction to the distal sigmoid colon (Fig. 88-1).

ANATOMIC CONGENITAL ANOMALIES

Colonic Atresia

Of the gastrointestinal (GI) tract atresias, only gastric atresia is more uncommon than colonic atresia. Acquired obstruction of the colon, usually secondary to necrotizing enterocolitis, is significantly more common than congenital atresia. Isolated colonic atresia may be associated with ophthalmologic defects, skeletal anomalies, jejunal atresia, aganglionosis, and abdominal wall defects. Colonic atresia presents as distal intestinal obstruction in the neonate, with abdominal distention, bilious emesis, and absent passage of meconium (1,2). It must be differentiated from other causes of ileal or colonic obstruction. Contrast enema is useful in the evaluation of these neonates, revealing a distal microcolon with incomplete colonic filling. Importantly, in neonates with clinically apparent small bowel atresia, either a contrast enema or intraoperative evaluation of the colon must be completed to rule out a concurrent more distal obstruction such as colonic atresia (Fig. 88-2). Failure to establish distal patency produces a predictable postoperative failure.

Optimal management techniques are determined by the location of the colon atretic segment, as well as other medical problems. Generally, simple atresia of the colon is managed by limited segmental resection of the dilated proximal segment and with primary end-oblique anastomosis. Rarely, exteriorization as a colostomy with distal mucous fistula is employed because of prohibitive luminal discrepancy, if there are concerns about abnormalities in vascularity or innervation adjacent to the atretic segment, or if the patient has other confounding medical risks.

ROTATIONAL ANOMALIES

Abnormalities of intestinal rotation represent a spectrum of incomplete or nonrotation of either (or both) the duodenojejunal or cecocolic intestinal limb and are discussed in detail elsewhere (see Chapter 87). With reverse rotation, the duodenum and jejunum lie anterior to the superior mesenteric vessels, which may then obstruct the posteriorly placed transverse colon. This can result in chronic colonic obstruction, which requires reflection of the colon and reversal of the rotation. Cecal volvulus, with associated obstruction and distention, results from lax fixation of the right colon and cecum in the retroperitoneum, leading to a freely mobile cecum. Ninety percent of patients with cecal volvulus have a full axial volvulus; 10% have a cecal bascule (cecum folded on itself in an anterior cephalad direction). Treatment includes reduction of the volvulus, followed generally by resection and possibly by fixation.

Sigmoid volvulus is the most common form of colonic volvulus and typically results from acquired redundancy of

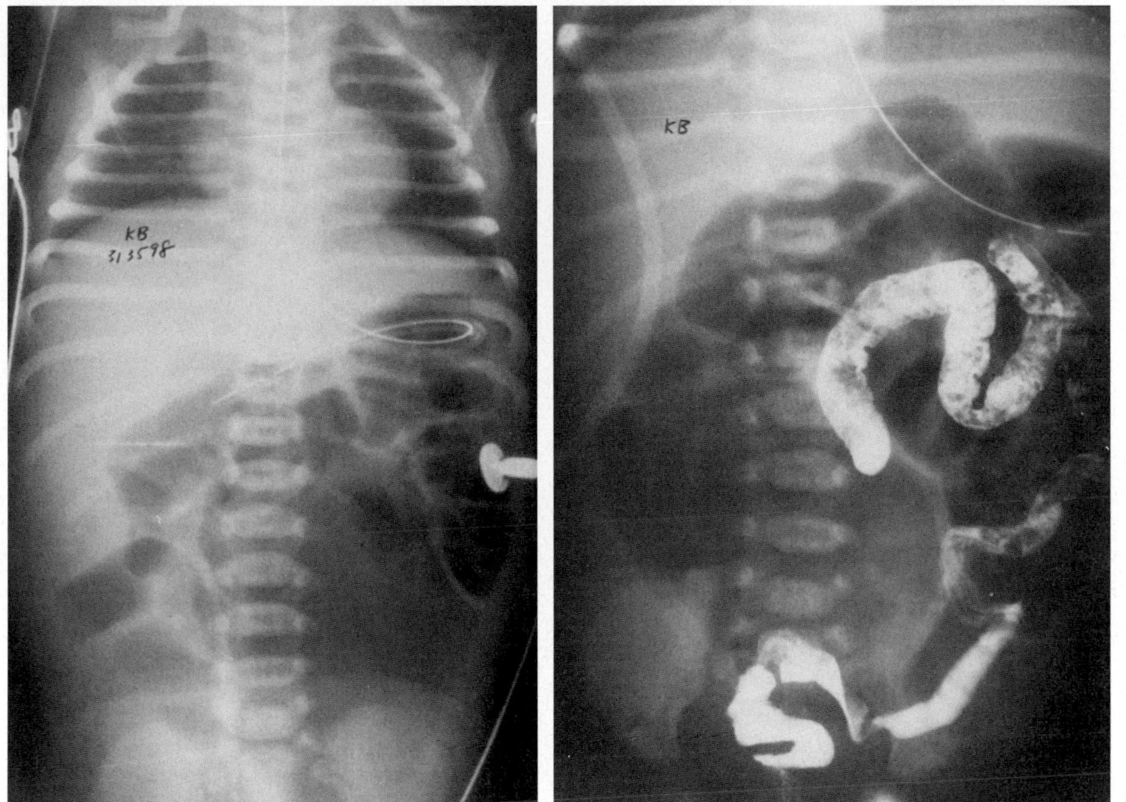

FIGURE 88-2. **(A)** Plain abdominal radiograph of an infant with colonic atresia. **(B)** Radiograph after barium enema in the same patient. Note the contrast-filled distal microcolon and the cut-off in the midtransverse colon.

the sigmoid colon mesentery in children with chronic constipation and neurologic disorders such as cerebral palsy. Plain abdominal radiographs may be diagnostic. The dilated sigmoid appears as an inverted dilated U-shaped, sausagelike intestinal loop. Water-soluble contrast enema may be diagnostic, but should not be performed on patients with suspected colonic necrosis. Reduction of the volvulus may occur during the examination. If necrosis or perforation is suspected, reduction should not be attempted, and the patient should undergo emergency laparotomy. If peritonitis is not apparent, rigid or flexible sigmoidoscopy should be performed in an attempt to reduce the volvulus. Unsuccessful detorsion, bloody discharge, or evidence of mucosal ischemia indicates strangulation or necrosis, and the patient should undergo emergency exploration.

PHYSIOLOGY

The colon is much more than a receptacle and conduit for the end products of digestion. It absorbs water, sodium, and chloride, and secretes potassium, bicarbonate, and mucus. In addition, it is the site of digestion of certain carbohydrates and proteins and provides the environment for the bacterial production of vitamin K.

Water and Electrolyte Exchanges. The major absorptive function of the colon is the final regulation of water and electrolyte balance in the intestine. The colon reduces the volume of enteric contents by absorbing greater than 90% of the water and electrolytes presented to it.

Sodium and Potassium. The colon is able to absorb sodium against very high concentration gradients, especially the distal colon, which shares many basic cellular mechanisms of sodium and water transport with the distal convoluted tubule of the kidney, including the ability to respond to aldosterone. A patient with an ileostomy loses this absorptive capacity and may not tolerate increased sodium losses or decreased sodium intake (3). Potassium transport in the colon is mainly passive, along an electrochemical gradient generated by the active transport of sodium.

Chloride and Bicarbonate. Chloride, like sodium, is actively absorbed across the colonic mucosa against a concentration gradient. Chloride and bicarbonate are exchanged at the luminal border. Chloride absorption is facilitated by an acidic environment, and the secretion of bicarbonate is enhanced by increased concentration of luminal chloride.

Short-chain Fatty Acids. Although active absorption of nutrients is minimal, the colon can passively absorb short-chain fatty acids (SCFAs) formed by intraluminal bacterial fermentation of unabsorbed carbohydrates, particularly fiber. The absorbed SCFAs butyrate, acetate, and propionate are the major fuel sources of the colonic epithelium. They provide the energy required for active sodium transport, and altered SCFA metabolism or SCFA deficiency may result in impaired colonic sodium absorption. There is evidence that SCFA metabolism is impaired in patients with ulcerative colitis and that intraluminal infusion of SCFAs can be of benefit in patients with colitis. SCFAs have also been shown to be effective in treating diversion colitis (which can occur after a diverting ileostomy or colostomy) (4).

Diarrhea. A number of agents can stimulate fluid and electrolyte secretion in the colon, including bacteria, enterotoxins, hormones, neurotransmitters, and laxatives. Gut hormones, particularly vasoactive intestinal polypeptide, have been shown to have significant effects on colonic absorption and secretion. Prostaglandins play a role in the pathogenesis of diarrhea associated with ulcerative colitis and several laxatives. Bile salt malabsorption after terminal ileal resection and long-chain fatty acid malabsorption in steatorrhea are clinically important examples of secretory diarrhea induced by colonic mucosal inflammation. The colonic mucus and fluid are high in potassium and may result in potassium depletion in chronic cases.

Colonic Microflora. The human colon is sterile at birth, but is colonized within a matter of hours from the environment in an oral to anal direction. *Bacteroides*, destined to be the dominant bacteria in the colon, is first noted at about 10 days after birth. By 3 to 4 weeks after birth, the characteristic stool flora is established and persists into adult life. The large intestine harbors a dense microbial population, with bacteria accounting for approximately one-third of the dry weight of feces. Each gram of feces contains 10^{11} to 10^{12} bacteria, with anaerobic bacteria outnumbering aerobic organisms by a factor of 10^2 to 10^4. *Bacteroides* species are the most common colonic organisms, present in concentrations of 10^{11} to 10^{12} organisms per milliliter of feces. The complex and important symbiotic relationship between humans and colonic bacteria is not completely defined, but it is recognized that endogenous colonic bacteria suppress the emergence of pathogenic microorganisms, play an important role in the breakdown of carbohydrates and proteins that escape digestion in the small bowel, participate in the metabolism of numerous substances that are salvaged by the enterohepatic circulation (including bilirubin, bile acids, estrogen, and cholesterol), and produce certain beneficial elements such as vitamin K (5).

CHRONIC IDIOPATHIC INTESTINAL PSEUDOOBSTRUCTION

Chronic idiopathic intestinal pseudoobstruction (CIP) is a clinical syndrome defined by the presence of signs and symptoms characteristic of intestinal obstruction in the absence of anatomic obstruction (6). Patients most frequently present with abdominal pain and distention, failure to thrive, and vomiting and constipation. Most cases are congenital and of either myopathic or neuropathic origin (rarely both). Most are sporadic, with no obvious family history. Histologic findings can include muscle fibrosis, vacuolar degeneration and disorganization of myofilaments, maturational arrest of myenteric plexuses, neuronal intestinal dysplasia, or a completely normal intestinal wall. In addition to these idiopathic cases, pseudoobstruction can be seen in association with Down syndrome, neurofibromatosis, multiple endocrine neoplasia type 2B, Russell-Silver syndrome, Duchenne muscular dystrophy, acute viral gastroenteritis, and extreme prematurity.

The clinical presentation is one of abdominal distention and vomiting (Fig. 88-3). More than one-half of affected infants develop symptoms within a few days of birth. Of these, about 40% have associated malrotation. Some less severely affected infants present with vomiting and failure to thrive within the first few months of life. Notably, more than three-fourths of affected infants present during the first year of life. Although laparotomy for biopsy alone is not indicated, many of these children undergo surgery for treatment of malrotation or evaluation of intestinal obstruction. When this scenario develops a full-thickness, biopsy of bowel wall should be obtained. The tissues should be processed for conventional histology, appropriate histochemistry, electron microscopy, and silver stains to evaluate for myopathic or neuropathic processes.

Although CIP is a clinical diagnosis, manometric studies can be useful in documenting abnormalities in amplitude or coordination of contractions. Esophageal, antroduodenal, colonic, and anorectal manometry can help determine the site and type of pseudoobstruction and assist in evaluating the response to therapy. Contemporary prokinetic drugs may be helpful, but are not sufficient in most affected children. Erythromycin is not effective for generalized motility disorders or those with isolated colonic involvement, but can bring relief in neuropathic gastroparesis. Nutritional support is vital because the clinical course is often characterized by unpredictable remissions and exacerbations, and malnutrition can result. Most

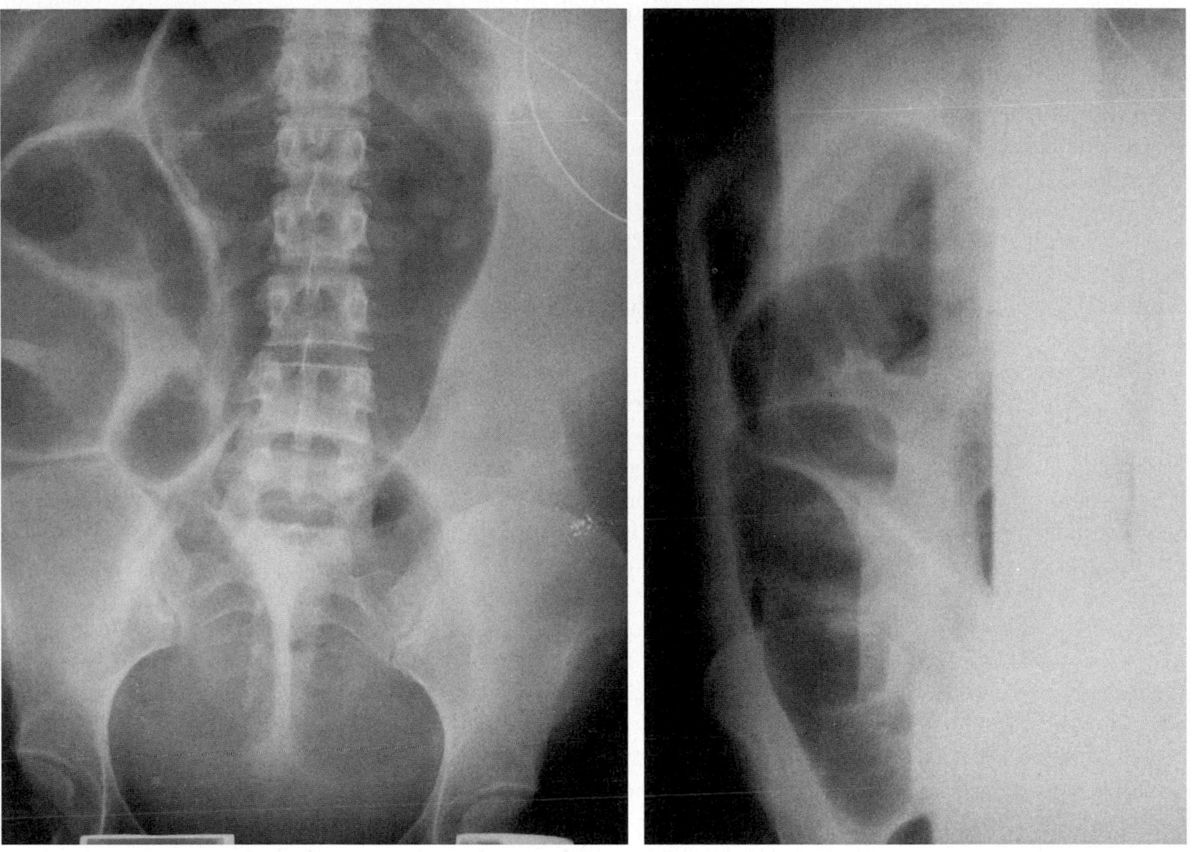

FIGURE 88-3. Supine **(A)** and decubitus **(B)** abdominal radiographs of a child with chronic idiopathic intestinal pseudoobstruction demonstrate marked bowel distension.

children tolerate all or some of their nutrition enterally, and this is desirable because it is less morbid than parenteral nutrition. Surgery should play a limited role in the long-term treatment of CIP, although one or more laparotomies are common prior to establishing the diagnosis. Even though gastrostomy tube placement can be useful in allowing a convenient access for long-term tube feeding or venting, other procedures, such as fundoplication, pyloroplasty, or gastrojejunostomy, have proved less useful. Colectomy has been helpful in a few children with isolated colonic pseudoobstruction (7). Prolonged postoperative ileus is to be expected in these patients, and the development of adhesions makes evaluation of future episodes of acute pseudoobstruction increasingly difficult. Almost all mortality is related to complications of total parenteral nutrition (8).

A relatively well-defined subset of CIP patients includes neonates with megacystis-microcolon intestinal hypoperistalsis syndrome. This rare cause of functional neonatal intestinal obstruction is associated with hypoperistalsis, malrotation, dilated proximal ileum, narrow distal ileum and colon, and bladder distention. The cause of this syndrome is unknown, but possible mechanisms include visceral myopathy, imbalance in gut peptides, defective autonomic inhibitory neuroeffector activity, and destruction of hollow viscus smooth muscle and neural network by an in utero intramural inflammatory process with resultant fibrosis. This disorder appears to be autosomal recessive and is usually lethal; most deaths occur within the first year of life. Mortality is primarily related to complications of total parenteral nutrition, including sepsis, liver disease, and catheter complications. Prenatal ultrasound diagnosis allows counseling in subsequent pregnancies in affected families (9,10).

COLITIS

Pseudomembranous Colitis

Although more than 60% of neonates may be colonized with *Clostridium difficile,* it is usually asymptomatic due to immaturity of the neonatal intestine receptor sites for *C. difficile* toxins (11). Pseudomembranous colitis is the most common clinical presentation and is almost invariably caused by toxin-producing *C. difficile* infection after antibiotic usage. Toxigenic *Clostridium perfringens* type C and *Shigella dysenteriae* type 1 may also be responsible for the development of pseudomembranous colitis. Nearly all antimicrobial agents have been implicated in the disorder, including antifungal, antiviral, and antimicrobial agents to which *C. difficile* is susceptible, including vancomycin and metronidazole. Pseudomembranous colitis has also been reported in infants whose only exposure to antibiotics was through breast milk. The risk of development appears unrelated to the dose or duration of antibiotic treatment. The protection against *C. difficile* proliferation provided by normal intestinal flora can be disrupted by antibiotic usage, increasing susceptibility to pseudomembranous colitis (12,13).

The pathogenicity of *C. difficile* is due to its production of toxins. Toxin A is an enterotoxin that binds to receptors on the mucosal epithelial surface, resulting in severe inflammation and fluid secretion. Toxin B is a cytotoxin that induces alterations in cell shape and causes diffuse enterocyte cell damage. Although the production of toxin is necessary for the development of colitis, the titer of toxin found in a patient's stool does not necessarily correlate with the severity of disease. Extraintestinal circulation of toxin after mucosal and submucosal invasion may be responsible for the shock state and sudden death that infrequently accompany severe disease.

Pseudomembranous colitis most frequently presents with mild to moderate, watery, nonbloody diarrhea beginning 7 to 10 days after the initiation of antibiotics, although the spectrum of disease can vary widely. Some patients present with fulminant disease and an acute abdomen with signs of toxic megacolon or perforation, even in the absence of preceding diarrhea. It is frequently among the potential diagnoses in patients evaluated for surgical disease, so it is essential for surgeons to be knowledgeable of its clinical features. In unrecognized and untreated catastrophic disease, mortality rates are as high as 20%. The diagnosis should also be considered in any child with a severe, protracted course of debilitating diarrhea, especially after antibiotic treatment. The diagnosis can be established by visualizing classic yellowish white, plaquelike pseudomembranes on endoscopy. More frequently, the diagnosis is made noninvasively in the appropriately suspicious clinical setting. Plain films of the abdomen may reveal "thumbprinting," reflecting a markedly edematous colonic wall. Computed tomography of the abdomen may demonstrate colonic wall thickening and inflammation. The most sensitive method to establish a diagnosis of pseudomembranous colitis is by *C. difficile* toxin detection. The most accurate method of toxin detection remains the cytotoxin tissue culture assay. The latex agglutination test is less reliable, although it can be used as a rapid screening test (14).

Patients who have mild pseudomembranous colitis, typically with fever, mild abdominal pain, and diarrhea, may respond to discontinuation of the implicated antibiotic. In more severe disease, treatment should include oral vancomycin, 40 mg per kg per day in three divided doses, or metronidazole, 20 to 30 mg per kg per day in three divided doses, continued for 7 to 10 days. The addition of this specific therapy allows for continued treatment with the inducing antibiotic, if necessary. Enteral administration of these therapeutic antibiotics, including by rectal or stomal irrigation if the oral route is unavailable, is much more effective than intravenous administration in reaching effective intraluminal concentrations. When parenteral therapy must be given, as with severe ileus, intravenous metronidazole achieves therapeutic fecal concentrations; intravenous vancomycin is less effective and does not reach adequate intraluminal concentrations. Relapse after treatment occurs in 10% to 20% of patients and is most often due to sporulation of *C. difficile.* These spores are resistant to treatment, and either longer courses of treatment or pulsed doses of antibiotics may be effective (12,15).

Children who have undergone definitive surgical treatment for Hirschsprung's disease, have significantly prolonged carriage of *C. difficile* and may develop "post pull-through enterocolitis." The cause of this increased sensitivity to pseudomembranous colitis is unclear. Because the clinical picture of *C. difficile*-associated pseudomembranous colitis can be indistinguishable from that of Hirschsprung's enterocolitis, with fever, abdominal pain, and diarrhea, empiric but specific therapy should be started while awaiting results of stool evaluation in patients who are seriously ill (16,17).

ENTERIC INFECTIONS

Viral gastroenteritis is the second most common illness in the United States, where it accounts for 300 to 400 annual childhood deaths (18). Worldwide, viral gastroenteritis is responsible for more than 4 million childhood deaths per year. Rotavirus is responsible for more cases of diarrheal disease in infants and children than any other single cause. Norwalk virus and enteric adenoviruses are other relatively common viral pathogens that cause acute gastroenteritis. Rotavirus accounts for the winter peak in childhood gastroenteritis, whereas the enteric adenoviruses are responsible for the summer peak. Both tend to affect children younger than 2 years of age, are accompanied by significant diarrhea, and not uncommonly result in dehydration. Treatment is supportive; oral rehydration solutions are extremely useful and are often lifesaving in cases of dehydration.

Whereas viral agents invade villus enterocytes along the entire span of the small intestine, infecting bacterial agents often act in the colon. Several bacterial virulence mechanisms act specifically on the colon, causing cytotoxin injury, direct epithelial cell invasion, and enteroadhesive activity. *Salmonella* sp is the most common cause of bacterial diarrhea in children in the United States, and the incidence of this disease appears to be increasing. Because of the invasiveness of this organism, infection can result in colitis and bacteremia, especially in patients with lymphoproliferative diseases and sickle cell anemia. Antibiotic treatment, with ampicillin or trimethoprim-sulfamethoxazole, is recommended in patients at high risk for the development of disseminated disease, those who appear septic, neonates, and those with complicated cases of gastroenteritis (19). *Shigella* sp is the second most common pathogen identified in cases of bacterial diarrhea in children and is an especially common cause of outbreaks of diarrhea in day-care settings. Although *Shigella* sp most frequently causes a mild, self-limited diarrhea, antibiotics are sometimes appropriate for patients who are severely ill to shorten the course of disease and to decrease the period of shedding of the organism. Nonpathogenic strains of *Escherichia coli* are among the most common bacteria in the normal flora of the human intestine, but pathogenic strains are an important cause of diarrheal disease. Enterohemorrhagic *E. coli* can occur in sporadic cases and in food-borne outbreaks. These bacteria produce a range of symptoms from watery diarrhea to hemorrhagic colitis. Verotoxic serotype 0157:H7 is implicated in the development of the hemolytic-uremic syndrome, characterized by microangiopathic hemolytic anemia, uremia, and thrombocytopenia. It is the most common cause of acute renal failure in children. Antibiotic treatment does not hasten resolution of this disease, but aggressive, supportive measures are required because hemolytic-uremic syndrome is associated with high morbidity and mortality rates (20). Significant medical complications include encephalopathy, pancreatitis, cardiomyopathy, hypertension, and seizures. Most patients can be treated successfully nonoperatively, but surgery may be required to support dialysis or for treatment of the acute abdomen with colonic microvascular injury leading to inflammation or necrosis. Acidosis, peritonitis, or obvious perforation or obstruction are reported and may require emergent colonic resection with or without diversion. Resection for late stenosis after resolution of the acute illness has also been reported (21).

GI manifestations of AIDS are often like bacterial colitis, with abdominal pain and bloody diarrhea. Cytomegalovirus is the most common associated colonic pathogen and can cause necrotizing lesions that can lead to hemorrhage or perforation. Treatment with ganciclovir is often effective, although relapses are common (22).

Polyps and Polypsosis Syndromes

Juvenile Polyp

Solitary polyps of the colon are common during childhood, usually presenting with painless rectal bleeding. These lesions, known as juvenile polyps, are most commonly hamartomas; solitary adenomas are extremely rare. More than one polyp is found 40% to 50% of the time (23). The typical clinical presentation is intermittent, involving painless rectal bleeding or perianal polyp protusion between 2 and 5 years of age (24–27). The differential diagnosis of rectal bleeding is broad and includes anal fissure, Meckel's diverticulum, vascular malformations, allergic enteropathy, colitis, and trauma. Juvenile polyps can be found throughout the colon, but are most common in the rectosigmoid region.

The natural history of juvenile polyps is unclear. It is believed that some polyps outgrow the blood supply and "autoamputate." Although this has never been proven, it appears to occur with some clinical frequency. Histologically, the typical juvenile polyp has a single layer of colonic epithelium. The main body of the polyp has a distinctive cystic architecture, with mucous-filled glands, a prominent lamina propria, and dense infiltration with inflammatory cells. The pathogenesis of the common juvenile polyp is unknown. The large number of inflammatory cells suggests a contribution from inflammatory mediators. Genetic mutations, aneuploidy, and tumor suppressor genes have not been identified in sporadic juvenile polyps (27,28).

Although the risk of development of malignancy in a solitary juvenile polyp is very small (29), such polyps should be removed, even when discovered incidentally. The preferred method for diagnosis and treatment is pancolonoscopy with polypectomy. Multiple juvenile polyps are associated with a small but increased risk of colon neoplasia; however, the degree of risk is unknown. Three or more sporadic juvenile polyps, or any number of polyps occurring in the context of a family history of juvenile polyps or colon cancer, are believed to increase the risk of developing cancer, but the evidence for this, especially in young children, is tenuous. Patients with multiple polyps or recurrent polyps should be considered for surveillance colonoscopy, and young patients with any polyps showing adenomatous histology should be evaluated for a genetic polyposis syndrome (30,31). Molecular genetic diagnosis offers a prospect for development of more precise criteria for cancer risk in children and adults with juvenile polyps so clearer screening recommendations can be defined.

Juvenile Polyposis Syndrome

Juvenile polyposis syndrome (JPS) is a rare autosomal dominant disorder defined by multiple hamartomatous polyps primarily in the colon, but occasionally throughout the GI tract (Table 88-1). The diagnostic criteria for JPS require three or more juvenile polyps of the colon, polyposis involving the entire GI tract, or any number of polyps in a proband with a known family history of juvenile polyps.

Patients generally come to medical attention late in childhood or early adolescence with rectal bleeding. In cases of diffuse polyps, patients may present with failure to thrive, anemia, hypoalbuminemia, and abdominal pain

TABLE 88-1 Hamartomatous Polyposis Syndromes.

Syndrome	Phenotype	Mutant Gene[a]
Peutz-Jeghers syndrome	Perioral pigmentations, pigmentations of fingers, upper and lower gastrointestinal (GI) hamartomatous lesions, extraintestinal malignancies include pancreatic, breast, ovarian, testicular, and adenoma malignum, a well-differentiated multicystic adenocarcinoma of the uterus	*LKB1* (*STK11*) (45–47)
Familial juvenile polyposis	GI hamartomatous polyps, increased risk of GI cancer (stomach, colorectum)	*Smad4* (*DPC4*) (27) *BMPRIA*35
Cowden's disease[b]	Colonic hamartomatous polyps, benign and malignant neoplasms of the thyroid, breast, uterus, and skin (multiple trichilemmomas)	*PTEN* (*MMAC1, DEP1*) (82)
Bannayan-Riley-Ruvalcaba syndrome	Microcephaly, fibromatosis, hamartomatous polyposis, hemangiomas, speckled penis	*PTEN* (79,80)

[a]Alternative names are given in parentheses.
[b]The diagnosis is made only when pathognomonic features of the other syndromes are not present.

early in life, even in infancy (32,33). The polyps are usually between 50 and 200 in number, most commonly in the rectosigmoid region and vary between 5 and 60 mm in size.

JPS was initially believed to be associated with mutation of in the PTEN (*p*hosphatase with *ten*sin homology) gene, but this mutation is now linked to Cowden syndrome. More recently, it has been shown that germ-line mutations in the SMAD-4 gene (18q21) account for approximately 50% of the reported familial cases of the syndrome (26,34,35). Mutation in the SMAD-4 gene presumably leads to a loss of heteromeric complex formation, growth inhibition, and neoplastic progression (36). Larger polyps are more likely to have epithelial dysplasia and are more likely to develop invasive malignancy (37).

Management and surveillance recommendations for these individuals are derived from their significantly increased risk of upper and lower GI malignancies (38). Proband and first-degree relatives should be screened starting at age 12 years, by upper and lower endoscopy. If negative, surveillance endoscopy should be repeated every 3 years (34,39,40). If a small number of polyps are found on the initial screen, endoscopic polypectomy with follow-up may suffice. When there are numerous polyps or symptoms such as bleeding or diarrhea persist, prophylactic colectomy should be considered after adolescence. There are insufficient data to support the use of prophylactic colectomy with ileorectal anastomosis solely for the risk of colorectal cancer. Cyclooxygenase inhibitors have been advocated for these patients, but their use in pediatric JPS is unclear.

Peutz-Jeghers Syndrome

Peutz-Jeghers syndrome (PJS) is a rare autosomal-dominant condition with variable penetrance in which GI polyps occur in association with macular melanin pigmentation (41). Polyps arise primarily in the proximal small bowel and, to a lesser extent, in the colon and stomach. The usual initial presentation of a patient with PJS is intestinal obstruction with polyp intussusception or GI bleeding (42,43). Melanin deposition occurs in most, although not all, patients. It is seen most frequently on the lips and buccal mucosa, and occasionally on the hands, feet, and eyelids.

The typical histopathology of PJS polyp demonstrates hypertrophy or hyperplasia of the smooth muscle layer that extends in a treelike manner into the superficial epithelial layer. As the smooth muscle extends upward toward the epithelial layer, invagination of the epithelium will result in islands of epithelial cells trapped within the underlying smooth muscle.

Genetic alterations in the LKB1/STK (19p13) gene that encode for a multifunctional serine-threonine kinase, which is important in signal transduction, are responsible for approximately 50% of cases of PJS (44–46). The genetics of PJS are complex and alterations in particular genes, along with environmental and epigenetic influences, all play some part in the ultimate clinical phenotype.

There is an increased risk of colorectal cancer and extraintestinal malignancy in patients with PJS. In some series, nearly 50% of patients developed invasive malignancies (47). Extraintestinal malignancies associated with PJS include pancreatic, breast, ovarian, testicular, and adenoma malignum, a well-differentiated multicystic adenocarcinoma of the uterus (47).

Management of GI polyposis is mandated by symptoms and abnormalities on surveillance examination, including any diagnosis of invasive malignancy. Polyps that are symptomatic or greater than 1.5 cm in size should be excised by enteroscopic polypectomy or exploratory laparotomy, and a complete intraoperative small bowel endoscopy should be completed (48). Extensive small bowel resections should not be done in order to avoid

TABLE 88-2 Familial Adenomatous Polyposis Syndromes.

Syndrome	Gene	Clinical Feature	Cancer Risk
Familial adenomatous polyposis (FAP)	Adenomatous polyposis coli (APC)	Gastrointestinal (GI) polyposis, congenital hypertrophy of the retinal pigment epithelium	Colon 100%, periampullary, thyroid hepatoblastoma, other
Gardner's syndrome	APC	Colon adenomas, desmoids, dental anomalies, osteomas, epidermal cyst	As for FAP above
Attenuated FAP	APC	Reduced adenoma numbers, right-sided polyps, few desmoids	Colon, generally later onset, fewer tumors
Turcot's syndrome	APC	GI adenomas, central nervous system tumors	Colon, medulloblastoma

the risk of short bowel syndrome. All patients with PJS should be screened for extraintestinal malignancies beginning in adolescence. Specific recommendations have been published by the St. Mark's Polyposis Registry (49) and include blood counts, pelvic ultrasound in girls, testicular ultrasound in boys, and pancreatic ultrasound in all individuals. Every 2 years, a complete evaluation of the GI tract should be completed. Patients should be screened for breast cancer according to the clinical recommendations for other high-risk individuals (i.e., patients with BRCA1 or BRCA2 mutations). Pap smears should be done at least every 3 years.

Familial Adenomatous Polyposis

Familial adenomatous polyposis (FAP) is the most common genetic polyposis syndrome, with an estimated prevalence between 1:5,000 and 1:17,000. The inheritance pattern is autosomal dominant, although spontaneous mutations account for approximately 30% of cases. Patients with FAP typically develop multiple adenomas throughout the colon, usually more than 100 and sometimes more than 1,000 (Table 88-2). Polyps may begin to appear in childhood and usually do so during adolescence. These increase in number with age (Fig. 88-4). Progression to colorectal cancer is considered inevitable by the fifth decade of life in patients with FAP, and there are reports of cancer occurring in children younger than 10 years of age (50). Adenomas can also occur in other regions of the GI tract (e.g., stomach and duodenum), leading to periampullary carcinoma in about 5% of patients (51,52). The condition is caused by mutations in the adenomatous polyposis coli (APC) gene at 5q21, which encodes a protein of 2,843 amino acids. The APC protein may be regarded as a tumor suppressor; its major functions include regulation of cell growth and migration, signal transduction, and control of chromosome stability. Central to the development of adenomas is APC-mediated regulation of β-catenin, a cytoplasmic protein and nuclear transcription factor involved in stimulation of cell growth. Mutational inactivation of APC leads to the accumulation of β-catenin, uncontrolled cell proliferation, and tumor formation. Interestingly, an acquired mutation of APC is found in most sporadic colorectal cancers.

Extraintestinal manifestations of FAP include desmoid tumors, epidermoid cysts, osteomas, fibromas, lipomas, and congenital hypertrophy of the retinal pigment epithelium. These benign conditions may signal the presence of FAP in at-risk patients. The presence of congenital hypertrophy of the retinal pigment epithelium is predictive of FAP (53–55), but should be supplemented with genetic

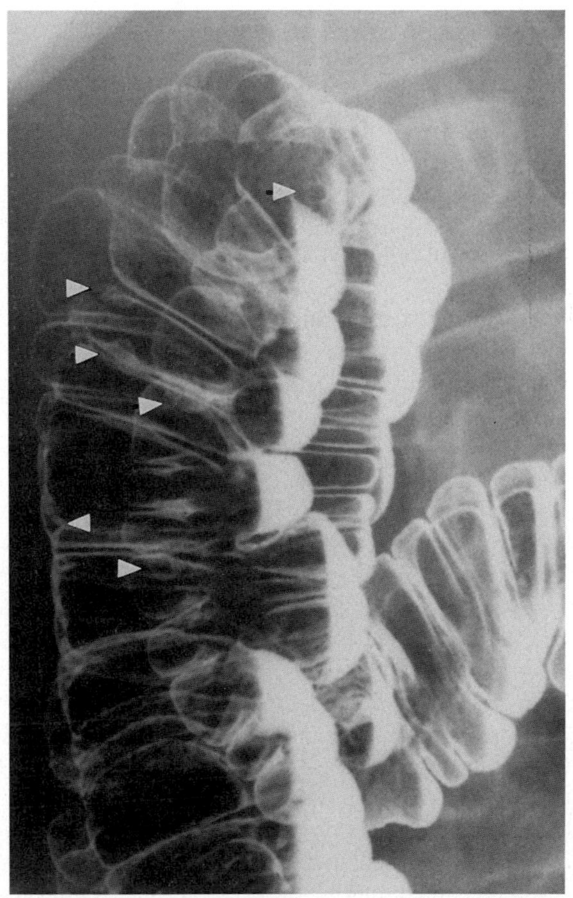

FIGURE 88-4. Radiograph after an air-contrast barium enema demonstrates multiple adenomatous polyps *(arrows)* in a patient with familial adenomatous polyposis.

testing. Gardner's syndrome is a phenotypic variant of FAP, which includes desmoid tumors, exostoses, and other extracolonic manifestations, as outlined previously. The occurrence of brain tumors in FAP is known as Turcot's syndrome. Hepatoblastoma occurs in 1.6% of children born to a parent with FAP, a relative risk approximately 850 times that of the general population. Screening of at-risk children with α-fetoprotein levels and hepatic ultrasonography between 0 and 6 years of age should be considered (30,56). Other less common tumors that may occur in families with FAP include papillary thyroid cancers, sarcomas, pancreatic carcinomas, and medulloblastomas.

There has been a large amount of data collected on APC mutations in FAP that has made it possible to correlate type and location of mutations with clinicopathologic features of the disease. There is wide variability in the clinical presentation in terms of age at disease onset, as well as number and distribution of adenomatous polyps. Mutations of the APC gene at the 5′ end and toward the 3′ end of the gene are associated with a form of FAP characterized by relatively low numbers of polyps and later-onset disease, designated as attenuated APC (57–59). On the contrary, the most frequent APC germ-line mutation, localized at codon 1309, is associated with a very severe form of FAP, characterized by hundreds to thousands of polyps that occur at an earlier age (60,61).

FAP can be diagnosed by the presence of colon adenomas in families with known FAP. Genetic diagnosis can be achieved by the detection of APC mutations in peripheral blood lymphocyte DNA using a commercially available protein truncation assay or by direct DNA sequencing. Genetic counseling should be provided by a genetic counselor or a medical geneticist before DNA is collected and at the time of disclosure of test results (62,63). In a family with a known APC gene mutation, genetic testing of relatives can discriminate between affected and unaffected individuals with a high degree of certainty. Formal recommendations for the timing of genetic testing in children have not been proposed, but considering the current known risk, waiting until about age 10 is reasonable (64). Genetic testing has limitations, and negative results should not alter cancer surveillance in patients with adenomatous polyposis and a negative family history of FAP. Early diagnosis and treatment of FAP is essential because of the 100% risk of cancer. Screening and surveillance is performed to identify a mutant APC allele of GI adenomas. A child with negative genetic testing in a family with an identified APC gene mutation has the same risk of colorectal cancer as the general population. Children with indeterminate genetic testing or with positive results should have flexible sigmoidoscopy annually beginning at 10 years of age. Surveillance upper endoscopy using a side-viewing scope is indicated beginning in the third decade of life. Recommendations are modified for kindreds with attenuated FAP. As further understanding of the genetic nuances of this disease is gleaned, it may be possible to individualize timing of surveillance studies and specific studies to evaluate for extraintestinal disease.

Prophylactic total proctocolectomy remains the preferred treatment for patients with FAP (65,66). Most experts suggest colectomy soon after polyps are identified. Chemoprevention has been investigated primarily with nonsteroidal antiinflammatory drugs (NSAIDs) with mixed results. Patients with FAP who were treated with 400 mg of celocoxib, a selective inhibitor of cyclooxygenase-2, twice a day for 6 months had a 28% reduction in the mean number of colorectal polyps, as compared with patients in the placebo group (67). In another study, 8 patients treated with refecoxib 25 mg each day demonstrated a 70% to 100% reduction in the rate of polyp formation, and no patients developed colon cancer during the short follow-up period (68). However, polyps may return while the patient is taking NSAIDs. In one study, regression of colonic adenomas occurred in all patients after 6 months of sulindac (200 mg per day) (69). However, after 2 years, the number and size of polyps increased and sulindac did not influence the progression of polyps toward a malignant pattern (69). There is still hope that these agents may decrease the need or at least delay surgery, and a number of chemoprevention trials will hopefully better define the role of antiinflammatory agents in FAP (70).

Desmoid Disease

Desmoids, also referred to as aggressive fibromatoses, are locally infiltrating growths of fibrous tissue that occur in musculoaponeurotic tissues. These tumors arise most often in the abdominal wall and mesentery, but can also occur in the extremities and trunk (71). Although they do not metastasize, desmoids are locally invasive and have a high rate of recurrence. Associated etiologic factors include the germ-line mutation, estrogens, and surgical trauma. Desmoid tumors are rare in the sporadic form of FAP, but occur in approximately 10% of individuals affected with familial FAP. A relationship between specific APC mutations and increased risk for desmoids has been identified (72–74). These lesions can progress rapidly, but have also resolved spontaneously. Desmoids are the second most common cause of death after colorectal cancer in these patients (75,76). Attempted surgical resection carries a high morbidity and mortality, and may stimulate further tumor growth. Medical treatments such as NSAIDs, antiestrogens, and cytotoxic chemotherapy have been tried with limited success (71). Children who present with extraintestinal desmoid tumors should be evaluated for possible FAP (77).

Other Polyposis Syndromes

Turcot's syndrome is characterized by concurrence of a primary brain tumor and multiple colorectal adenomas.

Patients with a polyposis syndrome and neurologic symptoms should undergo a detailed neurologic examination, including imaging for a possible brain tumor. The management of colonic polyps in Turcot's syndrome is the same as for FAP.

Juvenile polyposis may rarely occur as part of the Bannayan-Riley-Ruvalcaba (also known as Ruvalcaba-Myrhe-Smith syndrome) characterized by macrocephaly, juvenile polyposis, pigmentation of the genitalia, psychomotor delay, and occasionally lipid storage myopathy (78,79).

Cowden disease is the association of multiple hamartomas of the stomach, small intestine, or colon with macrocephaly, fibrocystic disease, breast cancer, nontoxic goiter, and thyroid cancer. Germ-line mutations in the tumor suppressor gene PTEN have been identified in both polyposis syndromes (80).

Gorlin's syndrome is an autosomal dominant condition consisting of upper GI hamartomas and pink or brown macules of the hands and face. In addition, these patients may have frontal bossing, hypertelorism, skeletal abnormalities, and intracranial calcification. Infants should be screened by ultrasound for medulloblastoma (81).

In most patients with polyposis, a clear-cut diagnosis can be made histologically; however, in rare cases, patients may be classified as has having a mixed polyposis syndrome.

Cancer

Colorectal cancer in young patients (age younger than 21 years) is rare and accounts for less than 1% of all colorectal cancers reported for all ages, but the incidence in young patients appears to be increasing (82). Patients usually present in their late teen years with advanced stage and frequently have a very aggressive, often fatal course (83–85).

Familial adenomatous polyposis, inflammatory bowel disease, and hereditary nonpolyposis colorectal cancer (HNPCC) will account for a small number of the cases of colorectal cancer in young patients; the majority is sporadic in nature. Microsatellite instability, a characteristic pattern of genetic instability seen in microsatellite DNA that occurs in most cases of HNPCC (86), has also been described in nearly 50% of young patients with colorectal cancer (87).

As compared with cancers without microsatellite instability, these cancers are not associated with distinct clinical, histologic, or familial features. They appear to have a low rate of K-*ras* mutations and loss of heterozygosity at 17p or 18q (87). However, the exact genetic and developmental factors that account for the aggressive nature and poor prognosis of these tumors are yet to be elucidated.

The signs and symptoms of colon carcinoma, abdominal pain, vomiting, constipation, weight loss, and melena or hematochezia are similar in children and adults. The rarity of carcinoma in childhood, however, leads to the expectation of alternative diagnoses and often delays the diagnosis of colorectal cancer.

The most important prognostic factor in patients with colorectal cancer is the depth of invasion of the primary tumor. The first practical staging system to incorporate this observation was the Dukes classification. It was originally designed for the classification of rectal tumors, but has been expanded with modification to allow the classification of colon carcinoma.

MODIFIED DUKES CLASSIFICATION

Stage A—extension of the lesion from the mucosa through the muscularis propria without serosal involvement

Stage B—extension of the lesion from the mucosa through the serosa into the perirectal or pericolonic fat

Stage C_1—extension of the lesion from the mucosa through the serosa to involve extracolonic tissues and lymph nodes

Stage C_2—extension of the lesion from the mucosa through the serosa to involve extracolonic tissues and lymph nodes as high as the point of ligature of the major vessels at the aorta

Stage D—evidence of distant organ (hematogenous) involvement

This staging system is usually combined with the tumor, node, metastasis (TNM) classification to complete the staging. Several significant differences can be found in the nature of the colon carcinomas found in children and adults. Although mucinous adenocarcinoma is seen in only about 5% of adults, this more poorly differentiated aggressive carcinoma accounts for about 50% of cases in children. There is also a shift from the pattern of left-sided lesions seen in adults to a more even distribution of tumors throughout the colon in children. Because of these differences, and the frequent delay in diagnosis, children and adolescents tend to present with more advanced disease than adults. Most patients have modified Dukes stage C or D disease at presentation, with involvement of regional lymph nodes and distant metastases preventing curative resection. Incomplete tumor removal is associated with an extremely poor prognosis and few long-term survivors. Young adults and children have a significantly lower overall 5-year survival rate than do older patients, owing to the increased incidence of advanced disease at presentation (82–84).

The goal of surgery for colon carcinoma is to maximize the chance for cure through en bloc removal of tumor and lymph node basins with adequate margins. The most significant factors affecting prognosis reflect the stage of disease at the time of presentation and the aggressiveness of the tumor. The results of adjuvant therapy to prevent dissemination of disease at the time of surgery and to control distant disease have been disappointing. No adjuvant therapy is recommended for Dukes stage A lesions, therapy in defined clinical trials is recommended for Dukes stage B lesions, and either treatment with levamisole plus 5-fluorouracil or entry into clinical trial is indicated for Dukes stage C lesions. The rare tumor division of the Children's Oncology Groups is working to create a registry for this unusual tumor in children so diagnosis and therapy may be improved.

REFERENCES

1. Oldham KT. Atresia, stenosis and other obstructions. In: O'Neill JA Jr, Rowe MI, Grosfeld JL, et al., eds. *Pediatric surgery*, 5th ed. St. Louis, MO: Mosby-Year Book, 1998.
2. El Ghoneimi A, Valla JS, Limonne B, et al. Laparoscopic appendectomy in children: report of 1379 cases. *J Pediatr Surg* 1994;29:786.
3. Sacher P, Hirsig J, Gresser J, et al. The importance of oral sodium replacement in ileostomy patients. *Prog Pediatr Surg* 1989;24:226–231.
4. Edwards CM, George B, Warren B. Diversion colitis—new light through old windows. *Histopathology* 1999;34:1–5.
5. Guarner F, Malagelada JR. Gut flora in health and disease. *Lancet* 2003;361:512–519.
6. DiLorenzo C, Hyman PE. Gastrointestinal motility in neonatal and pediatric practice. *Gastroenterol Clin North Am* 1996;25:203–224.
7. Heneyke S, Smith VV, Spitz L, et al. Chronic intestinal pseudo-obstruction: treatment and long term follow up of 44 patients. *Arch Dis Child* 1999;81:21–27.
8. Mousa H, Hyman PE, Cocjin J, et al. Long-term outcome of congenital intestinal pseudoobstruction. *Dig Dis Sci* 2002;47:2298–2305.
9. Anneren G, Meurling S, Olsen L. Megacystis-microcolon-intestinal hypoperistalsis syndrome (MMIHS), an autosomal recessive disorder: clinical reports and review of the literature. *Am J Med Genet* 1991;41:251–254.
10. White SM, Chamberlain P, Hitchcock R, et al. Megacystis-microcolon-intestinal hypoperistalsis syndrome: the difficulties with antenatal diagnosis. Case report and review of the literature. *Prenat Diagn* 2000;20:697–700.
11. McFarland LV, Brandmarker SA, Guandalini S. Pediatric *Clostridium difficile*: a phantom menace or clinical reality? *J Pediatr Gastroenterol Nutr* 2000;31:220–231.
12. Yassin SF, Young-Fadok TM, Zein NN, et al. *Clostridium difficile*-associated diarrhea and colitis. *Mayo Clin Proc* 2001;76:725–730.
13. Farrell RJ, LaMont JT. Pathogenesis and clinical manifestations of *Clostridium difficile* diarrhea and colitis. *Curr Topics Microbiol Immunol* 2000;250:109–125.
14. Markowitz JE, Brown KA, Mamula P, et al. Failure of single-toxin assays to detect *Clostridium difficile* infection in pediatric inflammatory bowel disease. *Am J Gastroenterol* 2001;96:2688–2690.
15. Morris AM, Jobe BA, Stoney M, et al. *Clostridium difficile* colitis: an increasingly aggressive iatrogenic disease? *Arch Surg* 2002;137:1096–1100.
16. Hardy SP, Bayston R, Spitz L. Prolonged carriage of *Clostridium difficile* in Hirschsprung's disease. *Arch Dis Child* 1993;69:221–224.
17. Bagwell CE, Langham MR Jr, Mahaffey SM, et al. Pseudomembranous colitis following resection for Hirschsprung's disease. *J Pediatr Surg* 1992;27:1261–1264.
18. King CK, Glass R, Bresee JS, et al. Managing acute gastroenteritis among children: oral rehydration, maintenance, and nutritional therapy. *MMWR Recomm Rep* 2003;52:1–16.
19. Alam NH, Ashraf H. Treatment of infectious diarrhea in children. *Paediatr Drugs* 2003;5:151–165.
20. Brandt J, Wong C, Mihm S, et al. Invasive pneumococcal disease and hemolytic uremic syndrome. *Pediatrics* 2002;110:371–376.
21. Brandt ML, O'Regan S, Rousseau E, et al. Surgical complications of the hemolytic-uremic syndrome. *J Pediatr Surg* 1990;25:1109–1112.
22. Ukarapol N, Chartapisak W, Lertprasertsuk N, et al. Cytomegalovirus-associated manifestations involving the digestive tract in children with human immunodeficiency virus infection. *J Pediatr Gastroenterol Nutr* 2002;35:669–673.
23. Cynamon HA, Milov DE, Andres JM. Diagnosis and management of colonic polyps in children. *J Pediatr* 1989;114:593–596.
24. Gupta SK, Fitzgerald JF, Croffie JM, et al. Experience with juvenile polyps in North American children: the need for pancolonoscopy. *Am J Gastroenterol* 2001;96:1695–1697.
25. Corredor J, Wambach J, Barnard J. Gastrointestinal polyps in children: advances in molecular genetics, diagnosis, and management. *J Pediatr* 2001;138:621–628.
26. Entius MM, Westerman AM, van Velthuysen ML, et al. Molecular and phenotypic markers of hamartomatous polyposis syndromes in the gastrointestinal tract. *Hepatogastroenterology* 1999;46:661–666.
27. Hoffenberg EJ, Sauaia A, Maltzman T, et al. Symptomatic colonic polyps in childhood: not so benign. *J Pediatr Gastroenterol Nutr* 1999;28:175–181.
28. Wu TT, Rezai B, Rashid A, et al. Genetic alterations and epithelial dysplasia in juvenile polyposis syndrome and sporadic juvenile polyps. *Am J Pathol* 1997;150:939–947.
29. Kapetanakis AM, Vini D, Plitsis G. Solitary juvenile polyps in children and colon cancer. *Hepato-Gastroenterology* 1996;43:1530–1531.
30. Giardiello FM, Offerhaus JG. Phenotype and cancer risk of various polyposis syndromes. *Eur J Cancer* 1995;31A:1085–1087.
31. Wirtzfeld DA, Petrelli NJ, Rodriguez-Bigas MA. Hamartomatous polyposis syndromes: molecular genetics, neoplastic risk, and surveillance recommendations. *Ann Surg Oncol* 2001;8:319–327.
32. Albuquerque C, Cravo M, Cruz C, et al. Genetic characterisation of patients with multiple colonic polyps. *J Med Genet* 2002;39:297–302.
33. Stiff GJ, Alwafi A, Jenkins H, et al. Management of infantile polyposis syndrome. *Arch Dis Child* 1995;73:253–254.
34. Allen BA, Terdiman JP. Hereditary polyposis syndromes and hereditary non-polyposis colorectal cancer. *Best Pract Res Clin Gastroenterol* 2003;17:237–258.
35. Bevan S, Woodford-Richens K, Rozen P, et al. Screening SMAD1, SMAD2, SMAD3, and SMAD5 for germline mutations in juvenile polyposis syndrome. *Gut* 1999;45:406–408.
36. Huang SC, Chen CR, Lavine JE, et al. Genetic heterogeneity in familial juvenile polyposis. *Cancer Res* 2000;60:6882–6885.
37. Desai DC, Murday V, Phillips RK, et al. A survey of phenotypic features in juvenile polyposis. *J Med Genet* 1998;35:476–481.
38. Howe JR, Mitros FA, Summers RW. The risk of gastrointestinal carcinoma in familial juvenile polyposis. *Ann Surg Oncol* 1998;5:751–756.
39. Dunlop MG, British Society for Gastroenterology Association of Coloproctology for Great Britain Ireland. Guidance on gastrointestinal surveillance for hereditary non-polyposis colorectal cancer, familial adenomatous polypolis, juvenile polyposis, and Peutz-Jeghers syndrome. *Gut* 2002;51:V21–V27.
40. Agnifili A, Schietroma M, Mattucci S, et al. [Clinical assessment of juvenile polyposis with particular reference to the risk of neoplastic malignancy. Analysis of 412 patients reported in the international literature]. *Chirurgia Italiana* 2000;52:393–404.
41. Entius MM, Keller JJ, Westerman AM, et al. Molecular genetic alterations in hamartomatous polyps and carcinomas of patients with Peutz-Jeghers syndrome. *J Clin Pathol* 2001;54:126–131.
42. Sasaki T, Fukumori D, Sato M, et al. Peutz-Jeghers syndrome associated with intestinal intussusception: a case report. *Int Surg* 2002;87:256–259.
43. Oncel M, Remzi FH, Church JM, et al. Course and follow-up of solitary Peutz-Jeghers polyps: a case series. *Int J Colorectal Dis* 2003;18:33–35.
44. Lim W, Hearle N, Shah B, et al. Further observations on LKB1/STK11 status and cancer risk in Peutz-Jeghers syndrome. *Br J Cancer* 2003;89:308–313.
45. Baas AF, Boudeau J, Sapkota GP, et al. Activation of the tumour suppressor kinase LKB1 by the STE20-like pseudokinase STRAD. *EMBO J* 2003;22:3062–3072.
46. Smith DP, Rayter SI, Niederlander C, et al. LIP1, a cytoplasmic protein functionally linked to the Peutz-Jeghers syndrome kinase LKB1. *Hum Mol Genet* 2001;10:2869–2877.

47. Giardiello FM, Brensinger JD, Tersmette AC, et al. Very high risk of cancer in familial Peutz-Jeghers syndrome. *Gastroenterology* 2000;119:1447–1453.
48. Edwards DP, Khosraviani K, Stafferton R, et al. Long-term results of polyp clearance by intraoperative enteroscopy in the Peutz-Jeghers syndrome. *Dis Colon Rectum* 2003;46:48–50.
49. Spigelman AD, Murday V, Phillips RK. Cancer and the Peutz-Jeghers syndrome. *Gut* 1989;30:1588–1590.
50. Church JM, McGannon E, Burke C, et al. Teenagers with familial adenomatous polyposis: what is their risk for colorectal cancer? *Dis Colon Rectum* 2002;45:887–889.
51. Groves CJ, Saunders BP, Spigelman AD, et al. Duodenal cancer in patients with familial adenomatous polyposis (FAP): results of a 10 year prospective study. *Gut* 2002;50:636–641.
52. Offerhaus GJ, Entius MM, Giardiello FM. Upper gastrointestinal polyps in familial adenomatous polyposis. *Hepatogastroenterology* 1999;46:667–669.
53. Valanzano R, Cama A, Volpe R, et al. Congenital hypertrophy of the retinal pigment epithelium in familial adenomatous polyposis. Novel criteria of assessment and correlations with constitutional adenomatous polyposis coli gene mutations. *Cancer* 1996;78: 2400–2410.
54. Pang CP, Fan DS, Keung JW, et al. Congenital hypertrophy of the retinal pigment epithelium and APC mutations in Chinese with familial adenomatous polyposis. *Ophthalmologica* 2001;215:408–411.
55. Pang CP, Lam DS. Differential occurrence of mutations causative of eye diseases in the Chinese population. *Hum Mutat* 2002;19:189–208.
56. King JE, Dozois RR, Lindor NM, et al. Care of patients and their families with familial adenomatous polyposis. *Mayo Clin Proc* 2000;75: 57–67.
57. Friedl W, Meuschel S, Caspari R, et al. Attenuated familial adenomatous polyposis due to a mutation in the 3' part of the APC gene. A clue for understanding the function of the APC protein. *Hum Genet* 1996;97:579–584.
58. Soravia C, Berk T, Madlensky L, et al. Genotype-phenotype correlations in attenuated adenomatous polyposis coli. *Am J Hum Genet* 1998;62:1290–1301.
59. Su LK, Barnes CJ, Yao W, et al. Inactivation of germline mutant APC alleles by attenuated somatic mutations: a molecular genetic mechanism for attenuated familial adenomatous polyposis. *Am J Hum Genet* 2000;67:582–590.
60. Ficari F, Cama A, Valanzano R, et al. APC gene mutations and colorectal adenomatosis in familial adenomatous polyposis. *Br J Cancer* 2000;82:348–353.
61. Crabtree MD, Tomlinson IP, Hodgson SV, et al. Explaining variation in familial adenomatous polyposis: relationship between genotype and phenotype and evidence for modifier genes [Comment]. *Gut* 2002;51:420–423.
62. Jarvinen HJ. Genetic testing for polyposis: practical and ethical aspects. *Gut* 2003;52:ii19–ii22.
63. Grady WM. Genetic testing for high-risk colon cancer patients. *Gastroenterology* 2003;124:1574–1594.
64. Giardiello FM, Brensinger JD, Petersen GM, et al. The use and interpretation of commercial APC gene testing for familial adenomatous polyposis [Comment]. *N Engl J Med* 1997;336:823–827.
65. Coffey JC, Winter DC, Neary P, et al. Quality of life after ileal pouch-anal anastomosis: an evaluation of diet and other factors using the Cleveland Global Quality of Life instrument. *Dis Colon Rectum* 2002;45:30–38.
66. Coran AG. A personal experience with 100 consecutive total colectomies and straight ileoanal endorectal pull-throughs for benign disease of the colon and rectum in children and adults. *Ann Surg* 1990;212:242–247; discussion 247–248.
67. Steinbach G, Lynch PM, Phillips RK, et al. The effect of celecoxib, a cyclooxygenase-2 inhibitor, in familial adenomatous polyposis. *N Engl J Med* 2000;342:1946–1952.
68. Hallak A, Alon-Baron L, Shamir R, et al. Rofecoxib reduces polyp recurrence in familial polyposis. *Dig Dis Sci* 2003;48:1998–2002.
69. Tonelli F, Valanzano R, Messerini L, et al. Long-term treatment with sulindac in familial adenomatous polyposis: is there an actual efficacy in prevention of rectal cancer? *J Surg Oncol* 2000;74:15–20.
70. Mathers JC, Mickleburgh I, Chapman PC, et al. Can resistant starch and/or aspirin prevent the development of colonic neoplasia? The Concerted Action Polyp Prevention (CAPP) 1 Study. *Proc Nutr Soc* 2003;62:51–57.
71. Dormans JP, Spiegel D, Meyer J, et al. Fibromatoses in childhood: the desmoid/fibromatosis complex. *Med Pediatr Oncol* 2001;37:126–131.
72. Bertario L, Russo A, Sala P, et al. Genotype and phenotype factors as determinants of desmoid tumors in patients with familial adenomatous polyposis. *Int J Cancer* 2001;95:102–107.
73. Caspari R, Olschwang S, Friedl W, et al. Familial adenomatous polyposis: desmoid tumours and lack of ophthalmic lesions (CHRPE) associated with APC mutations beyond codon 1444. *Hum Mol Genet* 1995;4:337–340.
74. Wallis YL, Morton DG, McKeown CM, et al. Molecular analysis of the APC gene in 205 families: extended genotype-phenotype correlations in FAP and evidence for the role of APC amino acid changes in colorectal cancer predisposition. *J Med Genet* 1999;36:14–20.
75. Arvanitis ML, Jagelman DG, Fazio VW, et al. Mortality in patients with familial adenomatous polyposis. *Dis Colon Rectum* 1990; 33:639–642.
76. Bertario L, Presciuttini S, Sala P, et al. Causes of death and post-surgical survival in familial adenomatous polyposis: results from the Italian Registry. Italian Registry of Familial Polyposis Writing Committee. *Semin Surg Oncol* 1994;10:225–234.
77. Wehrli BM, Weiss SW, Yandow S, et al. Gardner-associated fibromas (GAF) in young patients: a distinct fibrous lesion that identifies unsuspected Gardner syndrome and risk for fibromatosis. *Am J Surg Pathol* 2001;25:645–651.
78. Zigman AF, Lavine JE, Jones MC, et al. Localization of the Bannayan-Riley-Ruvalcaba syndrome gene to chromosome 10q23. *Gastroenterology* 1997;113:1433–1437.
79. Lowichik A, White FV, Timmons CF, et al. Bannayan-Riley-Ruvalcaba syndrome: spectrum of intestinal pathology including juvenile polyps. *Pediatr Dev Pathol* 2000;3:155–161.
80. Negoro K, Takahashi S, Kinouchi Y, et al. Analysis of the PTEN gene mutation in polyposis syndromes and sporadic gastrointestinal tumors in Japanese patients. *Dis Colon Rectum* 2000;43:S29–S33.
81. Raffel C, Jenkins RB, Frederick L, et al. Sporadic medulloblastomas contain PTCH mutations. *Cancer Res* 1997;57:842–845.
82. O'Connell JB, Maggard MA, Liu JH, et al. Rates of colon and rectal cancers are increasing in young adults. *Am Surg* 2003;69:866–872.
83. Cusack JC, Giacco GG, Cleary K, et al. Survival factors in 186 patients younger than 40 years old with colorectal adenocarcinoma. *J Am Coll Surg* 1996;183:105–112.
84. Rodriguez-Bigas MA, Mahoney MC, Weber TK, et al. Colorectal cancer in patients aged 30 years or younger. *Surg Oncol* 1996;5:189–194.
85. Recalde M, Holyoke ED, Elias EG. Carcinoma of the colon, rectum, and anal canal in young patients. *Surg Gynecol Obstet* 1974;139:909–913.
86. Lynch HT, de la Chapelle A. Hereditary colorectal cancer. *N Engl J Med* 2003;348:919–932.
87. Datta RV, LaQuaglia MP, Paty PB. Genetic and phenotypic correlates of colorectal cancer in young patients [Comment]. *N Engl J Med* 2000;342:137–138.

Chapter 89

Rectum and Anus

Charles N. Paidas, Marc A. Levitt, and Alberto Peña

For more than 100 years, surgeons around the world have been grappling with the morphologic consequences of events involving the caudal end of the embryo that occur between the fourth and eighth weeks of gestation. The anomalies are known as anorectal malformations (ARMs). As the embryologic and genetic sequencing of events continue to unfold, the questions of how and why these caudal defects occur are to be answered. For the time being, the pediatric surgeon is consulted for antenatal counseling, postnatal and perioperative opinions, and definitive operative correction of ARMs. Ultimately, the pediatric surgeon should manage the sequelae of these defects, including constipation, fecal and possibly urinary incontinence, and sexual inadequacies, regardless of how impeccable the initial operative correction. As many females with ARMs have approached childbearing age, the pediatric surgeon is frequently consulted by obstetricians. General surgeons also call on the pediatric surgeon for clarification of anatomy in patients with ARMs.

For centuries, an anal orifice was blindly created by making an incision in the perineum of children with imperforate anus. Many of these children did well, probably because these were defects with an anus located very close to the skin of the perineum (low defects). In contrast, most children with higher defects did not survive. In Paris in 1835, Amussat (1) actually performed the first surgical anoplasty by suturing the wall of the rectum to the skin edges without a colostomy. This procedure became the standard for what we now call a low imperforate anus. Until 1953, a key recommendation for the repairs of high imperforate anus was to stay close to the sacrum to avoid damage to the urinary tract during the dissection. Cadaveric dissections by Stephens (2) led him to use a combined sacral and abdominoperineal approach, whereby he pulled the rectum down as close to the genitourinary tract as possible in an effort to preserve the puborectalis sling. In contrast to pre-1953, preservation of the puborectalis sling became the theme for many subsequent operative approaches to ARMs (3–5). As more was learned about ARMs, not only the existence of the puborectalis sling, but also the role (if any) such a muscle might play in bowel continence was questioned.

A posterior sagittal approach to ARMs was introduced in 1982 (6,7). Through a wide posterior sagittal incision and with electrical stimulation of muscle, the surgeon can more correctly identify a spectrum of anorectal anomalies and tailor the reconstruction of the perineum. The posterior sagittal anorectoplasty (PSARP) approach to ARMs hopefully facilitates correlations of the anatomy of these malformations to the clinical results obtained for each type of male and female defect.

EMBRYOLOGY

Since the mid-1990s, the science of embryology has evolved from the mere study of isolated events in development to a two-stage process that links the formation of the body plan with the organs and tissues that belong in the respective regions of this body plan. We now know that there are a set of genes that "pattern" the embryo so organs and tissues appear where they are spatially meant to be and that an additional set of genes are responsible for the actual formation of these organs and tissues (8). As a result of a process called *gastrulation*, this body plan is set up by the end of the third week of gestation. There is substantial literature identifying the genes responsible for the patterning of the cranial region of the embryo and the tissues these genes specify (9). However, there is a paucity of data describing patterning of the caudal region of the embryo (10–14). What we have learned about caudal region human embryology is that there is an intimate relationship among muscle, bone, and nerves at the caudal end of

Charles N. Paidas: Department of Surgery, Johns Hopkins University School of Medicine, Johns Hopkins Hospital, Baltimore, Maryland 21287.

Marc A. Levitt, and Alberto Peña: Department of Pediatric Surgery, Schneider Children's Hospital, Long Island Jewish Medical Center, New Hyde Park, New York 11042.

the embryo, demanding a clinical management algorithm that considers this embryologic trio.

Anomalies of the anorectum have been previously explained on the basis of an arrest of the caudal descent of the urorectal septum toward the cloacal membrane during the fourth week and ending by the eighth week of gestation (15). The urorectal septum is composed of mesoderm. The growth, migration, and differentiation of this mesoderm constitute a critical pathway for normal descent of the urorectal septum, as well as other mesodermally derived tissues in its vicinity. For example, formation of the muscular and skeletal systems also derives from mesoderm. Furthermore, it is quite likely that embryonic induction of a specific developmental pathway in one group of cells (i.e., movement of the urorectal septum) may induce adjacent tissue (i.e., sacral somites) to transform into muscle, bone, and skin. Substances that might alter this induction of organs or disrupt cell–cell interaction following specification by a genetic code include proteins of the extracellular matrix (laminin, fibronectin, and collagen types I and IV) (16,17) and growth factors. Activation of a sequential family of genes or intracellular biochemical changes may further affect the induction of these tissues. Such is the case for expression of sonic hedgehog (Shh) gene and its secreted protein signaling pathway (18). Transcription factors responsive to Shh, such as Gli2 and Gli3, may also be equally important in the genesis of ARMs and normal caudal region embryology (19). Shh signaling is essential for normal development of the caudal region of the embryo in mice. Mutations in the Shh signaling pathway have produced a spectrum of anorectal anomalies similar to those found in humans (20). Thus, in addition to the spectrum of anorectal anomalies that results from dysmorphogenesis of the mesodermally derived urorectal septum, important consideration must be given to the induction of the caudal regional triad of muscle, bone, and nerve in weeks three through eight of gestation (Table 89-1).

In general, ARMs are not related to either the preimplantation or fetal period, but instead are related to the embryonic period of gestation (2 to 8 weeks). During the third week of embryogenesis, the process of gastrulation transforms the bilaminar germ disk into a trilaminar disk by ingress of epiblasts into the hypoblasts in an area called the *primitive streak*. Three definitive layers of the newly formed trilaminar germ disk are called ectoderm, endoderm, and mesoderm. The trilaminar germ disk forms the basis for the body plan, both cranially and caudally (21,22). Gastrulation then is synonymous with formation of mesoderm, and thus, the body plan. The implication of dysmorphogenesis this early in gestation is that patterning of the embryo is altered. Also, if something abnormal occurs this early in gestation, we should look regionally for other anomalies. There are, however, some malformations that almost never have associated defects (see "Anatomy, Classification, and Description of Defects"). This has clinical relevance because we know that with ARMs there is a 40% to 50% overall incidence of associated malformations (23,24).

TABLE 89-1 Timetable of Embryologic Events Leading to Formation of the Anorectum.

Week	*Event*
3	Gastrulation and formation of caudal eminence
4	Mesoderm forms somites; neural crest migration; formation of lumbosacral spinal nerves
4–6	Cloaca forms; somites differentiate
5	Sclerotome cells migrate around neural tube
6	Tourneux and Rathke mesoderm form and migrate; septation of cloaca into urogenital sinus and anorectal canal; caudal end of embryo develops from caudal eminence
7	Sacrum and caudal spinal cord completely formed
7–8	Striated muscle of perineum (levator ani, external sphincter) formed
8	Fusion of anal membrane (ectoderm) and the superior two-thirds (mesoderm) of anorectal canal give rise to dentate line and canalization of anus

At either end of the embryo, the ectoderm and endoderm fuse, excluding the mesoderm in these areas, and give rise to a cranial buccopharyngeal and caudal cloacal membrane. It is believed that the cloacal membrane fuses and canalizes in humans by the eighth week to give rise to the anus and distal urethra. However, formation of the cloacal membrane and an anal opening from the dorsal segment of the cloacal membrane has been identified as early as 10 days postcoitus in mice. Absence of any of the dorsal part of the developing cloaca and its membrane (as opposed to the urorectal septum) seems to give rise to a spectrum of fistulas or communications of the hindgut with the urogenital tract (25,26). These findings lend credence to the notion that the events leading to formation of ARMs can be ascribed to a much earlier time in gestation (i.e., gastrulation) and are not solely the result of the movement of the urorectal septum. Although these early embryologic errors were observed in a mutant mouse strain (Sd mouse), it is quite possible that this early sequence of dysmorphogenesis can also occur in humans (27). Further examination of the Sd mouse reveals that it has an abnormal notochord, resulting in reduced number of caudal vertebrae and abnormal cloaca and caudal gastrointestinal and genitourinary pathology (28). In ethylene-thiourea–treated rat embryos, ARMs were found in association with abnormalities of notochord development in the lumbosacral area and the cloaca, suggesting a relationship between the notochord, cloaca, and ARMs (29,30). These data suggest that there are very early links in the genetic code of the caudal body plan and the set of genes that subsequently form organs.

During the third week of embryogenesis as gastrulation proceeds, the primitive streak regresses caudally. In the caudal region of the embryo, the streak disappears, giving rise to a mass of mesoderm cells called the *caudal eminence*. The caudal eminence gives rise to two very intimately related areas, including the caudal somites of the body and the caudal end of the neural tube. Mesoderm inferior to the second sacral level fuses with the more cranial neural tube. The caudal region of the body plan is dependent on the formation, differentiation, and migration of the caudal eminence and its derivatives. This process is complete by 6 weeks of development.

In the latter part of the third week of embryogenesis, the mesoderm cells on either side of the regressing primitive streak give rise to paraxial, intermediate, and lateral plate mesoderm. Paraxial mesoderm yields axial skeleton, voluntary muscle, and skin dermis. The intermediate mesoderm produces the urinary system and elements of the genital anatomy. The ventral layer of the lateral plate mesoderm gives rise to visceral mesoderm, and the dorsal layer of the lateral plate gives rise to parietal mesoderm, parts of the limbs, and most of the dermis.

Paraxial mesoderm gives rise to somitomeres, all during the third and fourth weeks, starting in the cranial end and terminating caudally. In humans, somitomeres form somites numbering 39 pairs in a cranial–caudal direction. Somites give rise to axial skeleton, vertebral columns, skull bones, voluntary muscles (i.e., levator muscle complex, external sphincter), and dermis (perineal skin) (31). They also give rise to the segmental pattern within the body wall that eventually gives rise to other structures, such as blood vessels and nerves. The five pairs of sacral somites form the sacrum and associated musculature of the pelvis (levator ani group and external sphincter). The three pairs of coccygeal somites form the coccyx and probably contribute to induction of paraxial mesoderm in the perineum.

Somites subdivide into three types of mesoderm: myotomes, dermatomes, and mesenchymal sclerotomes. Sclerotomes (ventral portion of the somite) develop first and differentiate into vertebrae at all levels of the developing embryo. The adhesion molecule, N-cadherin, has been reported to be important for dissolution of the somite and formation of the sclerotome (32). Along the ventral surface of the body, myotomes are called *hypomeres*. These hypomeres migrate into lateral plate mesoderm, along with their respective dermatome and spinal nerves (33). The muscles of the perineal region differentiate from hypomeres of the sacral and coccygeal regions of the embryo. As expected, dermatomes and spinal nerves also migrate along with the hypomeres, giving rise to the levator ani musculature, external anal sphincter, and voluntary muscles of the external genitalia and their corresponding nerves (34). Thus, in the caudal region of the developing embryo, like in the cranial region of the body plan, organization and migration of these mesodermally derived somites give rise to the triad of muscle, bone, and nerve.

Regionalization of the postgastrulation mesoderm in the area of the sacrum and coccyx is probably regulated by pattern formation. In the case of the anorectum, pattern formation facilitates localization of the urinary tract anterior to the rectum, as well as a series of migrations that culminate in separate genital, urinary, and gastrointestinal tracts. In addition, the correct position of muscle with respect to the bones of the perineum is also probably dependent on pattern formation. This process is believed to be controlled in part by a class of genes called *homeobox genes* (35–39) and other families of homeotic genes, all of which are genes that regulate the expression of other genes by producing transcriptional factors. The pharyngeal arches in the cranial region of the embryo are a prototype of patterning regulated by homeobox genes (40). The homeobox or *Hox* gene expression may specify a code for postgastrulation mesoderm differentiation, such as the paraxial mesoderm, and simultaneously all three germ layers surrounding this area (41,42).

During the fourth week, the neural plate folds into the neural tube by a process called *neurulation*. Special subpopulations of cells that arise from the lateral regions of the developing neural tube are called *neural crest cells*. These specialized detached cells give rise to a variety of components of the peripheral nervous system that ultimately innervate the developing gut (including the hindgut). In fact, peripheral sensory neurons and parasympathetic and sympathetic peripheral motor neurons are all *neural crest derivatives*. An important neurologic milestone related to ARMs, during the fourth week of embryogenesis, is the formation of the spinal nerves from sacral levels 2, 3, and 4, which contributes to the peripheral parasympathetic nervous system. In contrast to the failure of migration and thus absence of ganglion cells observed in Hirschsprung's disease, abnormal matrix, cell-to-cell communication, or an abnormal induction pathway of neural crest development may be the basis for rectosigmoid proprioceptive and motility problems associated with ARMs. In the absence of any gross anatomic abnormality, the clinical manifestations of such a molecular embryologic phenomenon may include postoperative complaints of constipation and incontinence.

The caudal end of the neural plate (flanked by somites) gives rise to the lower end of the spinal cord. Secondary neurulation takes place once the neural plate has closed (primary neurulation) over a period of 7 weeks and is defined as the formation of the spinal cord at the caudal limit or tail bud of the embryo (43). The tail bud contributes to the sacral and coccyx levels of the spinal cord. The caudal eminence also induces both spinal cord and other paraxial mesoderm cells so ultimately this area forms the nervous system of the caudal part of the body. Defects in the caudal eminence give rise to sacral agenesis and the fatal dysmorphogenic caudal regression syndrome of Duhamel (44) (Fig. 89-1). Muscle, bone, and nerve pathology is associated with this lethal condition that may be the result of abnormal gastrulation in a very specific area of the primitive streak. It is possible that defects in the derivatives of the mesodermally derived caudal eminence are caused by

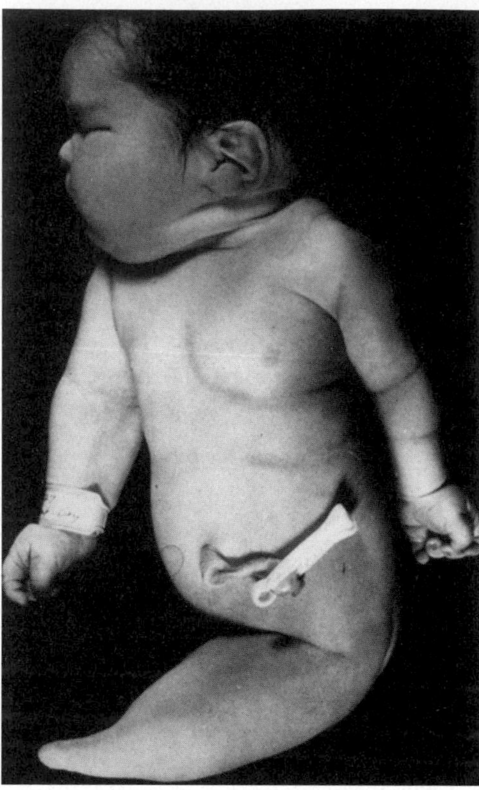

FIGURE 89-1. Sirenomelia, the most severe form of the Duhamel caudal regression or dysplasia syndrome, is characterized by a constellation of congenital anomalies that includes muscle, bone, and nerve derived from the caudal eminence.

macromolecules of the extracellular matrix (16). In addition, cell surface glycoproteins and cell adhesion molecules (N-CAM) participate in the transformation of the caudal eminence (45). These disturbances may have a multifactorial etiology and include both genetic and environmental causes.

It is widely held, but has never been proved, that between weeks four and six the primitive gut tube at the level of the cloacal membrane gets canalized and partitioned into an anterior urogenital sinus and a posterior anorectum by the cranial caudal growth of a mesodermally derived partition called the *urorectal septum* (Fig. 89-2). Ultimately, the urorectal septum fuses with the cloacal membrane, and the fusion site is called the *perineal body*.

Overgrowth of the cloacal membrane prevents the lateral mesoderm from forming the anterior abdominal wall and the cloaca ruptures. If the cloacal membrane ruptures after complete descent of the urorectal septum, exstrophy of the bladder occurs, whereas rupture before descent of the septum yields cloacal exstrophy.

The urorectal septum is a composite of two mesoderm structures: the midline Tourneux fold and two lateral Rathke folds (Fig. 89-2). In contrast to the superior two-thirds of the anal canal, the inferior one-third is derived from ectoderm called the *anal pit* or *proctodeum*. The anal membrane resorbs by the eighth week, and this area when fused with the descending mesoderm of the hindgut is called the *pectinate* or *dentate line*. Some authors believe that proof of this process of septation of the cloaca or caudal migration of a septum is lacking and the partitioning of the cloaca is the result of normal dorsal–ventral

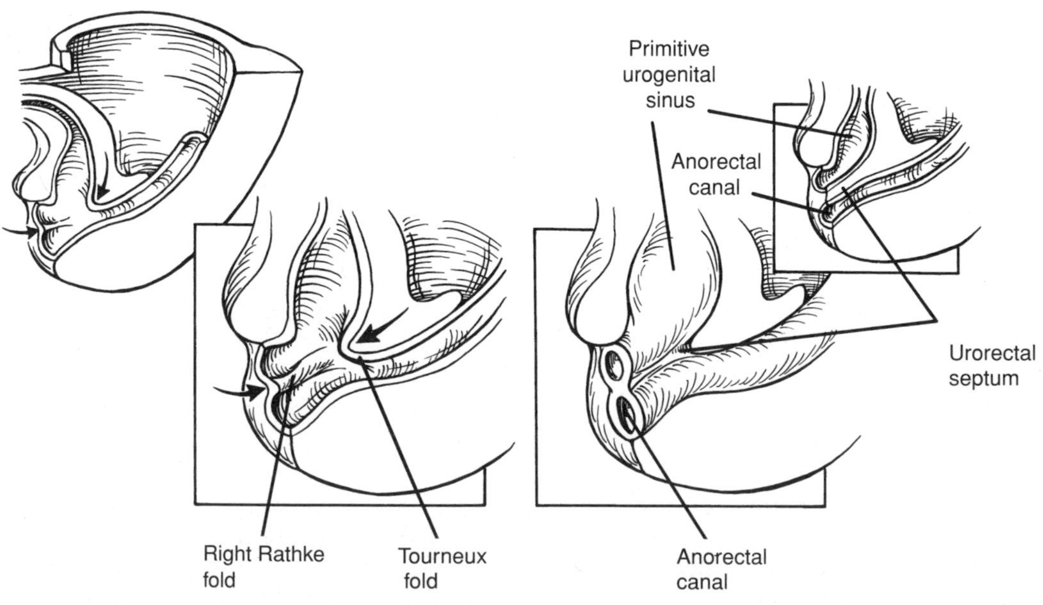

FIGURE 89-2. Septation of the cloacal membrane by the urorectal septum. Craniocaudal and lateral mesoderm of the urorectal septum partition the cloaca into an anterior urogenital sinus and posterior anorectum.

cloacal development (25,26,46). In fact, in three-dimensional image reconstruction of human embryos, the urogenital sinus and anorectum form early and are separated by the urorectal septum as a passive structure (47). The catenoidal geometric shape of the urorectal septum, like the tracheoesophageal septum, also suggests this is a passive structure (48).

The failure of Rathke folds to develop results in arrest of the inferior part of the urorectal septum, and thus, rectourethral (prostatic) fistulas in the male and a common channel (cloaca) for the urethra, vagina, and rectum in the female.

In females, the distal end of the urogenital sinus forms the vestibule and distal third of the vagina. The proximal vagina and uterus are formed following fusion of the paramesonephric ducts (müllerian ducts) and union of these structures with the proximal urogenital sinus. It is believed that formation of the uterus, vagina, and fallopian tubes requires the absence of antimüllerian hormone or müllerian-inhibiting substance (49).

The arrest of Rathke folds usually takes place just below the paramesonephric ducts, but a slightly more caudal failure of Rathke folds could result in a high rectovaginal fistula in the female.

The failure of both Tourneux and Rathke folds could result in rectobladder neck fistulas in both males and females, however, we suspect that this is not true because we have not seen a rectovesical fistula in a female with normal genitalia. Instead, failure of both folds is more likely to be a cloacal anomaly in the female. In the female, failure of formation of both folds can also result in duplicated vaginas and uteruses that empty into one bladder. This concept is consistent with what we find in the spectrum of cloacal anomalies.

Malalignment of Tourneux and Rathke folds may result in formation of a rectourethral (bulbar) fistula in males and a low vaginal or vestibular fistula in females.

Imperforate anus without fistula results from the anal pit not forming. Mesodermally derived Tourneux and Rathke folds are aligned, but the ectodermally derived anal pit has not fused with the mesoderm. Thus, the result is an imperforate anus, but no fistula to the skin.

Formation of the anal pit and failure of the anal membrane to resorb or resorb incompletely results in rectal atresia or anal stenosis, respectively. This fusion defect consists of cloacal ectoderm and descending rectal mesoderm.

Fusion of the genital folds gives rise to a covered anus. This does not happen in females because in the absence of testosterone there is no fusion of the genital folds, but instead they remain separate to form the labia. Defects in the mesoderm at the level of the perineal body where fusion of the ectoderm and endoderm is taking place result in a perineal fistula that by definition is an opening with no surrounding external anal sphincter.

In the next few years, it should not be surprising to find genetic literature linking the formation of the body plan (gastrulation) with postgastrulation organ formation in the caudal region of the embryo. Ultimately, these data should give rise to the regionalized phenomenon of caudal patterning of muscle, bone, and nerve. The Sd mouse and the Shh knockout are excellent models to study ARMs and may be used in the future to probe the two-stage process involving the origin, fate, and interaction of mesoderm (the body plan) and regional organ formation.

GENETICS

As early as 1950, records were compiled about congenital anomalies, their incidence, and their overall contribution to maternal and fetal morbidity and mortality. More than 90% of congenital anomalies develop in the first 8 weeks of gestation and more than one-half of these occur in the first 4 weeks or just after gastrulation (50). As for ARMs, the overall incidence approaches 1 in 5,000 live births (51), and the risk for future pregnancies in a mother of a patient with ARMs is 1 in 100 or 1% (52). Relative to all types of caudal regression anomalies, ARMs are much more common if one separates the incidence of persistent cloaca (1:40,000 to 50,000) and cloacal exstrophy (1:400,000) (53). Yet, we suspect that the real incidence of persistent cloaca is much higher based on the fact that so many alleged rectovaginal fistulas are cloacas. In general, males slightly outnumber females by about three to one, and there seems to be no ethnic predilection.

The genetic basis of ARMs is multifactorial, meaning there is no one single cause (54). ARMs can be caused by a sporadic or an inherited event. Sporadic events are isolated and probably induced by an unknown genetic or environmental cause. It is unclear if a sporadic case is inherited. If, however, another sibling or descendent has an ARM, then one can infer that the malformation is inherited either as an isolated event or as part of a syndrome. The patterns of ARM inheritance include the mendelian disorders (autosomal dominant, recessive, etc.), chromosomal abnormalities (i.e., cat eye syndrome), or environmental teratogens (i.e., maternal diabetes). Some syndromes that include ARMs can be inherited as a result of multiple gene mutations, hence, the term *heterogeneous causation*. The actual incidence of sporadic versus inherited ARMs is unknown despite literature quotes supporting a higher incidence of isolated ARMs (55). Based on the fact that there is a reported range of associated anomalies between 22% and 72%, it is very possible that sporadic cases are in fact part of a syndrome (24). Granted we have multiple examples of hindgut dysmorphogenesis that can account for these associations, and it is compelling to consider a syndromic etiology as advances in molecular genetics occur. There is some evidence, albeit scant, that isolated low anal malformations (perineal fistula, covered anus) may be inherited, whereas isolated high ARM lesions are likely to be sporadic embryologic events with little to no risk of familial recurrence (56,57). Similar to the sporadic ARMs, the familial-related ARMs carry a 50% incidence of associated malformations (58).

Both from a reproductive counseling perspective and for postnatal care, the potential for inheriting an ARM must be considered. Because it is nearly impossible to make an antenatal diagnosis of the more common ARMs, detailed family pedigree may provide a clue to potential hereditary mechanisms. Risks of recurrence within a family can then be based on the pattern of inheritance. For example, if an autosomal dominant condition is identified, it carries a 50% incidence of recurrence, whereas a recessive condition occurs in 25% of offspring. Family genetic counseling about ARMs should also include the potential for association with other system anomalies and chromosomal defects. A prenatal karyotyping should be performed in all cases in which there is a family history of ARMs.

Postnatal physical examination should alert physicians to the possibility that the baby has a syndrome. Table 89-2 is a helpful guide for the extraanal anomalies associated with ARMs. The Mendelian inheritance in man (MIM) number is an online computerized database (59) that can be accessed for a more complete update of each diagnosis. The vertebral, anal, tracheoesophageal, renal, and radial limb anomalies (VATER) (60,61) or vertebral, anal, cardiac, tracheoesophageal, renal, and nonradial limb anomalies (VACTERL) (62,63) associations should not be the sole extraanal associations ruled out when evaluating a patient with an ARM. This is especially important from an embryologic perspective when we consider that the mesoderm involved in the VATER and VACTERL associations as well as all components of the other anomalies listed in Table 89-2 are present by the fifth week of gestation. Likewise, if a baby has skeletal, visceral, or neurologic anomalies, one should look for the constellation of bowel, bladder, or bone anomalies (64).

ANATOMY, CLASSIFICATION, AND DESCRIPTION OF DEFECTS

In general, the frequency of ARMs is slightly higher in males compared with females, and this also includes the potential for associated anomalies. A rectourethral (bulbar and prostatic urethra) fistula is the most frequent defect in newborn males followed by a perineal fistula. Higher defects, such as the rectobladder neck fistula, occur in less than 10% of male series (65,66).

In females, by far the most frequent defect is an imperforate anus with a rectovestibular fistula followed in frequency again by the perineal fistula. Most cases of rectovaginal fistulas are probably misdiagnosed rectovestibular fistulas or cloacas because in Peña's series of more than 1,600 cases, rectovaginal fistulas were virtually nonexistent. The common cloaca comprises about 10% of the defects in females and ranks third in frequency (65,66).

Imperforate anus without a fistula occurs in less than 5% of cases in both sexes and has a high association with Down syndrome (65,66).

Although there is a long history of proposed classifications for ARMs, the 1984 Wingspread classification (67) of high, intermediate, and low defects has been used extensively (68,69). With respect to therapy and prognosis, however, the classification falls short of implications and utility. A therapy-oriented classification is shown in Table 89-3. This proposed categorization combines diagnosis and treatment, and therefore, should facilitate more homogeneous communication about specific malformations among pediatric surgeons.

Male Defects

Perineal Fistula

Perineal fistula is a low defect (Fig. 89-3). The lowest part of the rectum opens on the perineum anterior to the center of the external sphincter. The more proximal rectum remains within the muscles of the sphincter. A subepithelial rectoperineal fistula can be found along the midline raphe from the base of the scrotum or penis (Fig. 89-4). Occasionally, a skin tag is encountered (bucket handle deformity) (Fig. 89-4B), below which meconium may be seen coming from the fistulous tract. Male and female patients with a perineal fistula have a well-developed midline groove and anal dimple, normal sacrum, ample sphincter musculature, normal rounded contour of their buttocks, and minimal urinary and neurologically associated anomalies.

Rectourethral Fistula

The rectourethral fistula defect (Fig. 89-5) is characterized by the rectum communicating with the posterior part of the urethra at its lower (bulbar, Fig. 89-5) or upper segment (prostatic, Fig. 89-5). In general, the patients with a bulbar fistula have a substantial sphincter mechanism, normal sacrum, prominent midline groove, and well-defined anal dimple. In contrast, those males with a rectoprostatic urethral fistula have a more flat contour buttock, poor sphincter mechanism, abnormal sacrum, and poorly defined anal dimple. Most males fit these observations, but there are exceptions such that a rectoprostatic fistula can be associated with a normal sacrum, defined anal dimple, and good muscle.

Above the rectourethral fistula, the rectum and urethra share a common wall. As expected, the common wall is longer in cases of a bulbar fistula in contrast with a prostatic fistula. The rectum in both types of rectourethral

TABLE 89-2 Anorectal Malformations (ARMs) in Association with Extraanal Anomalies.

Syndrome	Prominent Features	Causation[a,b]
Arm alone		
Isolated imperforate anus	None	Heterogeneous, AR, XLR, and AD
Arm and neurologic anomalies		
Anosacral defect	Anterior sacral meningocele, teratoma, or cyst	Heterogeneous, AD (176450), XLD (312800)
FG syndrome	Macrocephaly, broad forehead, frontal hair upswept, hypotonia, mental retardation	XL (305450)
Arm and skeletal anomalies		
Baller-Gerold	Craniosynostosis, radial defect, short stature	AR (218600)
IVIC syndrome	Radial defects, strabismus, thrombocytopenia, deafness	AD (147750)
Jarcho-Levin	Rib and vertebral defects, respiratory failure in infancy	AR (277300)
Presacral teratoma	Sacral dysgenesis	AD (176450)
Saldino-Noonan	Short ribs, short limbs, postaxial polydactyly, visceral abnormalities, lethality	AR (263530)
Say	Preaxial polydactyly, malformed vertebral bodies and ribs (may be the same as PIV syndrome)	Sporadic
Thanatophoric dysplasia	Micromelia, platyspondyly, early death	Sporadic (187600)
Townes-Brocks	Deafness, triphalangeal thumbs, overfolded helices, flat feet	AD (107480)
Arm and chromosomal anomalies		
Cat eye	Ocular coloboma; ear, cardiac, and renal anomalies; variable mental retardation	Heterogeneous; have an extra small metacentric chromosome, possibly rearranged chromosome 2
Tetrasomy 12p	Coarse face, sparse anterior scalp hair, hypertelorism, epicanthus, hypotonia, hypomelanotic spots, severe mental retardation	Chromosomal anomaly
Arm and cardiovascular anomalies		
Fuhrmann	Polydactyly, heart defect	Uncertain
Arm and urogenital anomalies		
Hypertelorism-hypospadias	Hypertelorism, hypospadias (may be the same as Opitz G syndrome)	XLR (313600)
Opitz BBB	Hypertelorism, hypospadias, swallowing defects	
Opitz G	Hypertelorism, hypospadias, swallowing defects	AD (145410)
Arm and multiple anomalies		
Ankyloblepharon filiforme	Fused eyelids and normal globe endocardial cushion defects, fused digits, cleft lip and palate, esophageal atresia	AD (106250)
Adnatum		Chromosomal anomaly
ASP association	Anal anomalies, sacral defect, presacral mass (ASP) (teratoma, cyst, or meningomyelocele)	AD (176450)
Axial mesodermal defect	Sacral dysgenesis; dysfunction of lower limbs, bladder, and bowel; aphalangy, spinal, and rib abnormalities	AR
Caudal regression	Dysgenesis of lower spine; variable dysfunction of bladder, bowel, and lower limbs	Heterogeneous, maternal diabetes mellitus in some cases AD (182940)
Christian skeletal dysplasia	Metopic ridge, cervical fusion, dysplastic spine, abducens palsy, mental retardation	XLR (309620)
Cryptophthalmos	Palate, ear, renal, laryngeal, genital, digital, and eye malformations	AR (219000)
Diabetes, maternal	Fetal overgrowth; increased incidence of neural tube defects, cardiac anomalies, caudal dysgenesis, and renal defects	Exposure of abnormal glucose metabolism during pregnancy

(continued)

TABLE 89-2 *(Continued)*

Syndrome	Prominent Features	Causation[a,b]
Johanson-Blizzard	Hypoplastic alae nasi, exocrine pancreatic insufficiency, deafness, hypothyroidism	AR (243800)
Kaufman-McKusick	Congenital heart defects, polydactyly, hydrometrocolpos	AR (236700)
Lowe	Sensorineural deafness, nephritis	AD
Meckel	Encephalocele, polydactyly, cystic kidneys	AR (249000)
OEIS	Omphalocele, exstrophy of the bladder, imperforate anus, spinal defects (OEIS)	Uncertain, may have vascular causation
Pallister-Hall	Hypothalamic hamartoblastoma, hypopituitarism, postaxial polydactyly	Sporadic (146510)
Pallister: ulnar-mammary	Ulnar ray defects, delayed puberty, oligodactyly or polydactyly, hypoplasia of apocrine glands and breasts, genital anomalies	AD (181450)
PIV	Polydactyly, imperforate anus, vertebral anomalies (PIV)	Sporadic (174100)
Potter variant	Renal, lung, thymic, parathyroid, dysplasia	AR (?), chromosomal anomaly
Rieger	Ocular anterior chamber anomalies, hypodontia	AD (180500)
Sirenomelia	Single, lower limb, renal agenesis, genital agenesis	Sporadic, based on vascular steal
Vacterl (vertebral, anal, cardiac tracheoesophageal, renal, and radial limb defects)	Vertebral, anal, cardiac, tracheoesophageal, renal, and radial limb defects	Sporadic (19235)

[a]Number in parentheses represents the Online Mendelian Inheritance in Man (OMIM) classification (51) online database.
[b]D, autosomal dominant; AR, autosomal recessive; ASP, anal anomalies, sacral defect, presacral mass; PIV, polydactyly, imperforate anus, vertebral anomalies; XL, X-linked; XLR, X-linked recessive; XLD, X-linked dominant. (114,144)

fistulas is usually surrounded by the funnel-shaped voluntary striated muscle mechanism innervated by the sacral plexus (sacral levels 2, 3, and 4).

Rectobladder Neck Fistula

In the case of rectobladder neck fistula defect (Fig. 89-6), the rectum opens at the bladder neck in a T configuration. In contrast with a rectourethral fistula common wall, patients with a bladder neck fistula do not share a common wall. In these defects, the rectum is located above the funnel-shaped levator musculature. Ectopic ureters usually open into the bladder close to the site of the fistula. The perineum is usually flat, there is a paucity of perineal muscle, and the sacrum is dystrophic and frequently absent. This ARM has a high frequency of associated anomalies.

Imperforate Anus Without Fistula

In the imperforate anus without fistula defect, the rectum ends approximately 2 cm from the perineal skin. The sphincter mechanism, muscles, and sacrum are usually present, and thus, bowel function is predictably good. Even

TABLE 89-3 Proposed Classification of Defects.

Male		Female	
No Colostomy	*Colostomy*	*No Colostomy*	*Colostomy*
Rectoperineal (cutaneous) fistula	Rectourethral fistula (bulbar, prostatic) Rectobladder neck Imperforate anus without fistula Rectal atresia and stenosis	Rectoperineal (cutaneous) defects Rectovestibular fistula (determined by surgeon's experience)	Vestibular fistula (determined by surgeon's experience) Rectovaginal fistula (extremely unusual) Persistent cloaca Imperforate anus without fistula Rectal atresia and stenosis

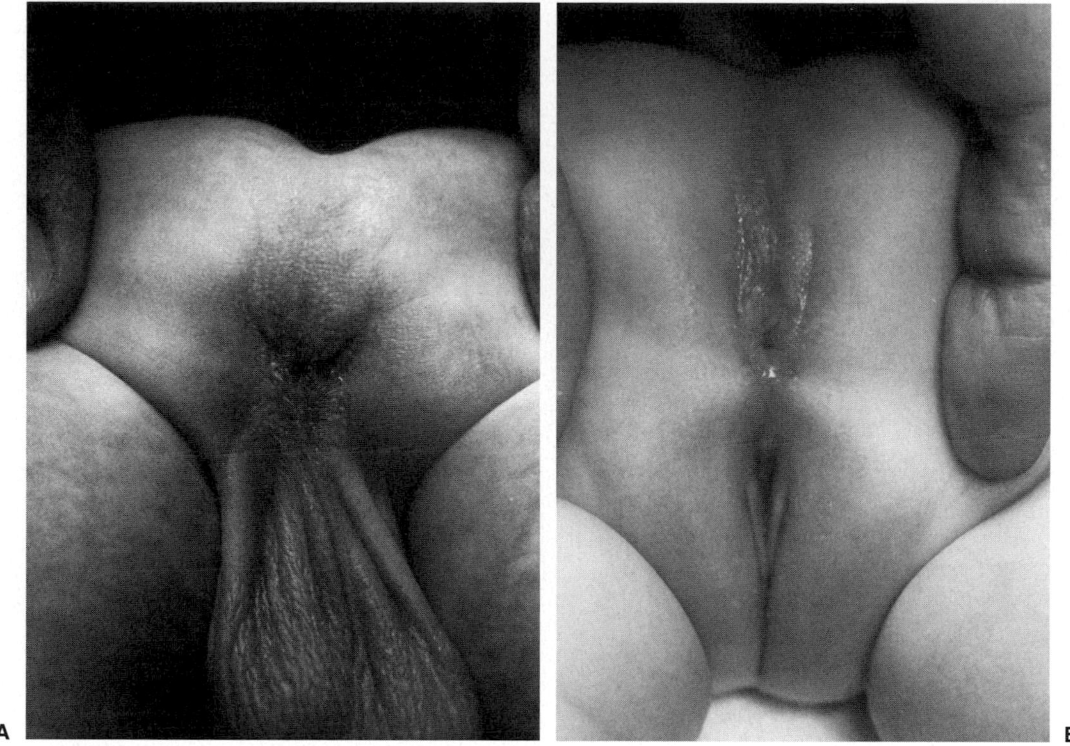

FIGURE 89-3. Perineal fistula in (**A**) male and (**B**) female. Electrical stimulation of perineal skin shows that the anal opening is anterior to the external sphincter muscle.

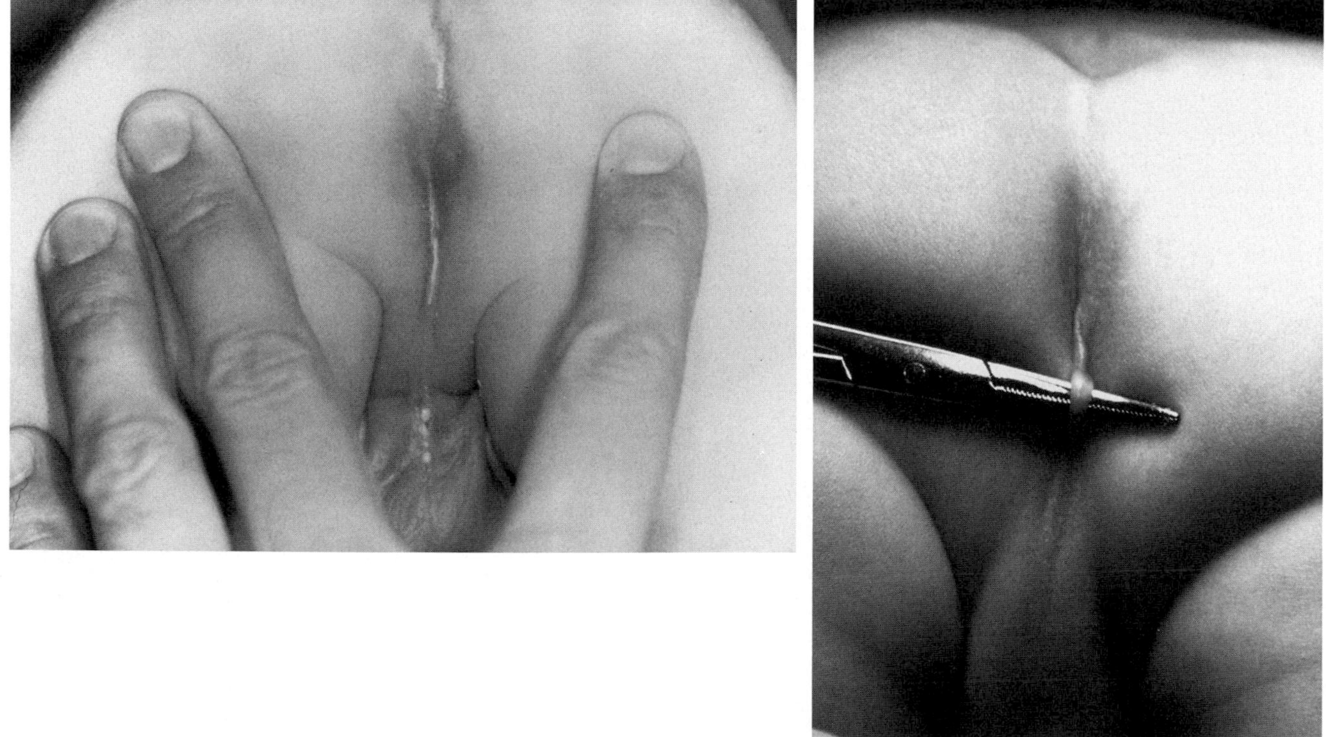

FIGURE 89-4. (**A**) Subepithelial rectoperineal fistula. (**B**) Bucket handle deformity.

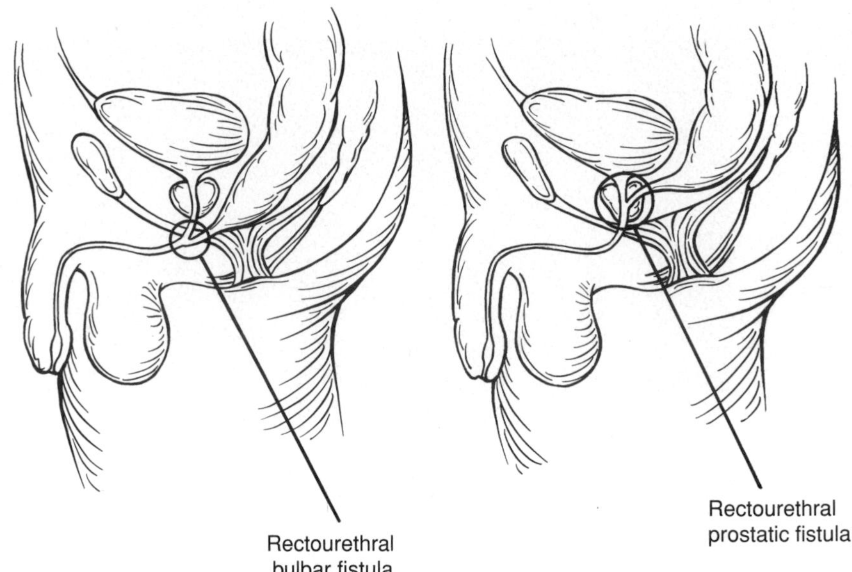

FIGURE 89-5. (**A**) Rectourethral bulbar fistula. (**B**) Rectourethral prostatic fistula.

though there is no direct communication between the urethra and anus, there is a very thin common wall between these structures.

Rectal Atresia and Stenosis

In the cases of rectal atresia and stenosis, the rectum ends blindly (atresia) or partially communicates with the distal anal canal (stenosis). Typically, these patients have a normal-looking anus that ends blindly 1 to 2 cm above the perineal skin. The atresia or stenosis occurs at the embryologic junction of the anal canal with the rectum. These two structures are separated by a thin membrane or fibrous band. Following repair, continence and sensation are usually excellent. Voluntary muscles, sacrum, and perineum are nearly normal.

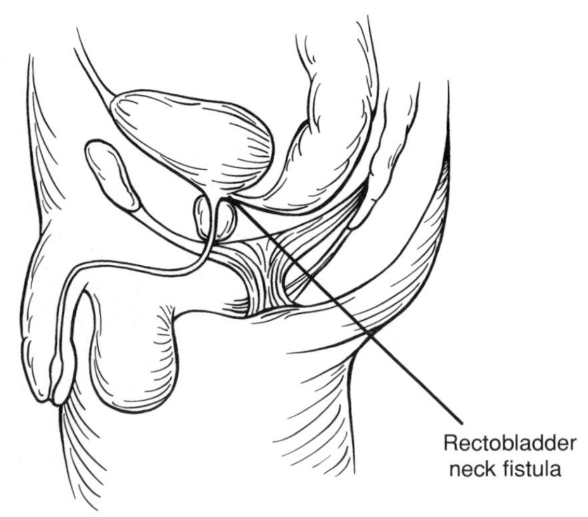

FIGURE 89-6. Rectobladder neck fistula.

Female Defects

Rectoperineal Fistula

The rectoperineal fistula malformation is the equivalent to the low-lying male cutaneous fistula because it is also surrounded by skin. The anus opens onto the perineal body anterior to the external sphincter, yet the opening is posterior to the vestibule of the vagina. These patients have an excellent anal dimple and buttock contour. The sacrum in this defect is normal, as is the presence of the levator musculature. Rectum and vagina are also well separated, and thus, there is no shared common wall.

Rectovestibular Fistula

The rectovestibular fistula ARM is characterized by the rectum opening immediately behind the hymen within the vestibule of the vagina (Fig. 89-7). This defect is frequently erroneously diagnosed as a rectovaginal fistula. Just above the fistula, the rectum and vagina are separated by a thin common wall. Yet, these patients usually have excellent musculature, normal sacrum, and anal dimple.

Imperforate Anus Without Fistula and Rectal Atresia and Stenosis

The imperforate anus without fistula and rectal atresia and stenosis malformations has similar anatomic, diagnostic, therapeutic, and prognostic implications in males and females. Imperforate anus without a fistula has a slightly higher incidence in females compared with males.

Persistent Cloaca

The persistent cloaca (Fig. 89-8) defect is characterized by fusion of the rectum, vagina, and urethra into a single

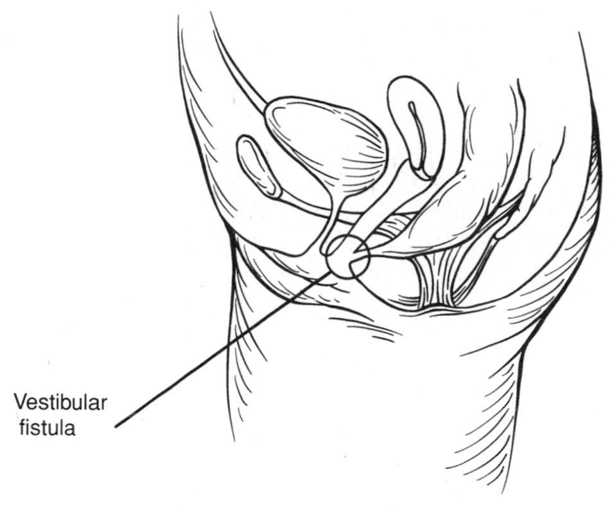

FIGURE 89-7. Rectovestibular fistula in parasagittal plane and introitus. The fistula is anterior to the hymenal ring, yet within the introitus. We do not consider this a low defect and as such bring up a colostomy prior to definitive repair.

common channel (70). The length of the common channel varies between 1 and 10 cm. A short common channel is usually defined as shorter than 3 cm, whereas common channels longer than 3 cm are considered long-channel malformations. Figure 89-8A is the perineum in a female baby with imperforate anus, small genitalia, and single perineal orifice. Figure 89-8B shows a child with cloaca who has a common channel of approximately 3 cm. In contrast, Figure 89-8C shows a case in which the common channel is much longer. In this situation, separation and mobilization of the three structures, creating two walls out of each common wall between the urethra and the vagina, as well as between the vagina and the rectum, is difficult and most likely requires some form of vaginal replacement and probable laparotomy. Urinary function may be compromised in these long-channel defects. The perineum is usually well developed, and musculature, sacrum, and innervations are adequate in cases of short common channels. Frequently, the vagina in cases of persistent cloaca is distended and full of secretions (hydrocolpos). In some series, the incidence of a hydrocolpos approaches 40% (69,70). The hydrocolpos may compress the trigone of the bladder and interfere with drainage of the ureters. In addition, the vagina and uterus frequently suffer from different degrees of septation or even complete separation of two hemivaginas or two hemiuteruses. Patients with persistent cloaca have a high incidence of associated anomalies.

ANATOMY AND PHYSIOLOGY

For the pediatric surgeon, pertinent aspects of the anatomy and physiology of the anorectum should include knowledge of the normal process of defecation and continence and how these processes can be affected by the spectrum of ARMs. With respect to both defecation and continence, we must focus on the sphincter mechanism, anorectal sensation, proprioception, and finally, rectosigmoid motility. These areas comprise the functional elements of normal defecation and fecal continence. It is incumbent on the surgeon to realize how defecation and fecal continence can exist, given a spectrum of ARMs, a spectrum of anatomy, physiology.

Anatomy of Normal Children

Sphincter Mechanism

In normal children, the muscle groups of the sphincter mechanism include the voluntary striated muscles of the external sphincter and the levator musculature, and the involuntary, smooth muscle, internal sphincter (Fig. 89-9).

The striated external sphincter follows a circular path around the anus and is organized into three parts: subcutaneous, superficial, and deep (71) (Fig. 89-9). It is believed that the external sphincter is in a tonic state of contraction at rest. Because it can both relax and augment its baseline state of contraction at rest, it is possible that the striated muscle composition of the external sphincter is not homogeneous. This concept of differing cell types of striated muscle within the external sphincter, however, has not as yet been elucidated. The external sphincter is innervated by the pudendal nerve and the autonomic nervous system. The pudendal nerve is derived from the sacral plexus roots S2 to S4. This nerve is both motor to the external sphincter and sensory to the skin around the anus. Autonomic innervation of the external sphincter is via the nervi erigentes, derived from segments S2 to S4 of the spinal cord. This parasympathetic pelvic splanchnic nerve provides afferent information about the degree or magnitude of rectal fullness. Sympathetic innervation of the external sphincter probably exists, but no studies have yet identified its specific role.

The levator ani muscle is a series of striated muscle groups composed of ischiococcygeus, ileococcygeus, pubococcygeus, and puborectalis. The levator ani muscle extends from the pubic bone, the lowest portion of the sacrum, and the middle of the pelvis downward and medial to join with the external sphincter (71). This muscle group is usually depicted as a funnel-shaped sling. In contrast with the innervation of the external sphincter, the motor innervation of the levator musculature is from only S3 and S4. It is also innervated by the autonomic system (both sympathetic and parasympathetic).

The internal sphincter has been described as a continuation of the circular smooth muscle inner layer of the muscularis propia of the bowel wall (Fig. 89-9). The internal sphincter is under sympathetic (resting tone) and parasympathetic (relaxation) control (72).

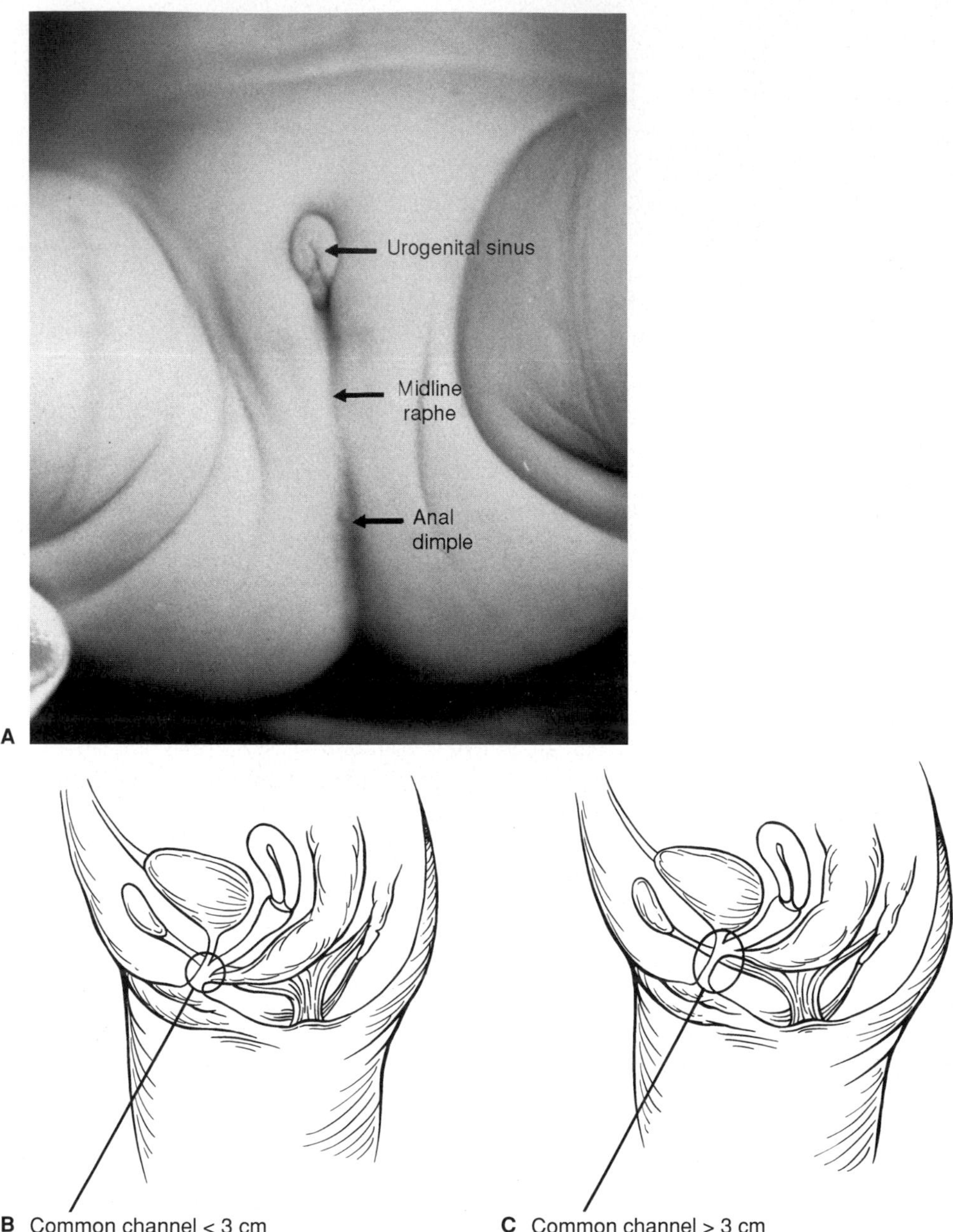

FIGURE 89-8. (**A**) Persistent cloaca, external topography. (**B**) Common channel cloaca shorter than 3 cm. (**C**) Common channel cloaca longer than 3 cm.

Pain, touch, temperature, and pressure are felt through sensory afferents located in the anal mucosa, including a zone slightly more than 1 cm above the dentate line (73). The rectum is devoid of these sensory afferents except for pacinian corpuscles, which are pressure receptors located in the rectum between internal and external sphincters and in the presacral space and submucosa of the anal canal (74).

These anal mucosa sensory afferents traverse the spinal cord and then travel to the cortex, all with the feelings of fullness and ultimately a desire to defecate. Each sensory nerve ending is responsible for one kind of stimulus. Proprioceptive stretch receptors exist within the muscle spindles of the voluntary striated muscle mechanism. These receptors carry afferent impulses stimulated in response to rectal distention. These sensory afferents are derived from the neural crest in contrast with the mesoderm origin of the caudal eminence muscle, bone, and nerve (73,75).

Anatomy of Children with Anorectal Malformations

Children with ARMs challenge the traditional concept of the gross anatomy of the sphincter mechanism. After many years using the posterior sagittal approach to repair ARMs, it is our concept that the external sphincter runs in a paramedian direction rather than a circular direction. In addition, the muscular boundaries of the external sphincter are

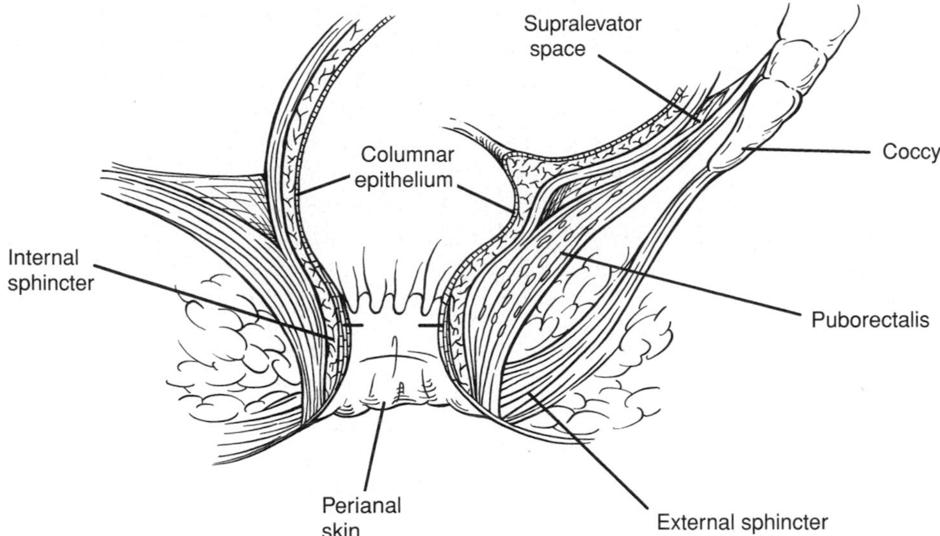

FIGURE 89-9. Normal parasagittal anatomy of the perineal musculature. Voluntary striated muscle includes the external sphincter (parasagittal fibers) and levator musculature. The internal sphincter is composed of involuntary smooth muscle.

fused; thus, we are unable to distinguish the components of the external sphincter.

During a posterior sagittal dissection, the junction of levator musculature with external sphincter is defined by a vertical group of striated muscle fibers called the *muscle complex* (76) (Fig. 89-10). Electrical stimulation of the upper end of the levator group pulls the rectum forward. Stimulation of the muscle complex (vertical fibers) elevates the anus, and the paramedian fibers of the external sphincter close the anus.

Furthermore, in children with ARMs, there are varying degrees of striated muscle development from almost normal-looking striated muscle to virtually no muscle seen at operation. In very high defects, the rectum may rest at the upper part of the funnel-shaped voluntary striated muscle; in lower defects, the rectum may traverse the base of the muscular funnel.

Once again, the internal sphincter is said to be a continuation of the outer circular smooth muscle of the bowel wall. In children with ARMs, however, we have never seen what is referred to as the limits or, for that matter, the actual internal sphincter. Instead, if surgeons biopsy a segment of the wall of the rectum during an operative dissection for ARMs, they obtain histologic reference to smooth muscle. When subjected to electrical stimulation and drugs, this type of biopsy seems to respond as though it was, in fact, a bowel sphincter-type of smooth muscle; however, there has been no clear evidence for a definable internal sphincter in patients with ARMs (77).

Physiology of Normal Children

Continence in the normal child requires intact sphincter function, anal canal sensation and proprioception, and coordinated colonic and rectosigmoid motility. Unfortunately, much of the mechanism that underlies these events is unclear. Moreover, the movement of stool from the rectosigmoid down to the anus—namely, the process of

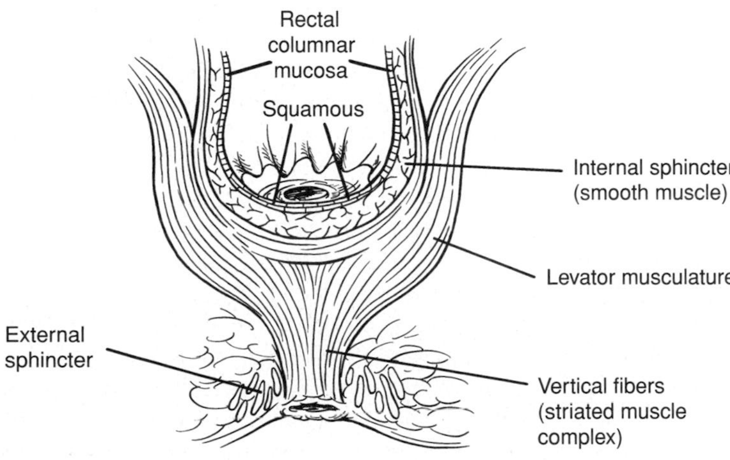

FIGURE 89-10. The muscle complex. The muscle complex consists of vertical striated muscle fibers connecting the external sphincter with the levator muscle. In patients with imperforate anus, there are varying degrees of loss of the funnel-shaped striated muscle.

defecation—is even less well defined. As such, it is difficult to provide answers to pathologic conditions when normal physiology has not been elucidated.

Sphincter Function

The two normally present types of sphincters include the voluntary external sphincter and the involuntary internal sphincter. Rectal manometric studies assume the internal sphincter provides the majority of resting pressure in the rectum by virtue of its near maximal contraction in the basal state (78). In response to rectal distention, during manometry, there is a fall in the pressure of the lower rectum and the anal canal that is called the *relaxation reflex* (79). It is assumed that relaxation of the internal sphincter provokes this fall in the intraluminal pressure. Relaxation is followed by a brief increase in pressure that is interpreted as a contraction of the external sphincter. This rectoanal inhibitory reflex (RAIR) is a manometric finding and may not be entirely extrapolated to defecation. In view of the fact that both structures (internal and external sphincters) are superimposed anatomically (Fig. 89-9), we do not understand how these conclusions were reached. In other words, how can we say that it is the internal or the external sphincter relaxing when they are both superimposed?

Nitric oxide has emerged as the neurotransmitter that mediates the RAIR. It has been assumed that the nonadrenergic, noncholinergic parasympathetic nerves in the wall of the internal sphincter produce relaxation of the sphincter in response to rectal distention. The inhibitory nerve cell bodies lie in the rectal myenteric ganglia, and their processes pass to the sphincter (80). The RAIR does not require connection to the spinal cord, but instead is transmitted via the ganglion cells in the internal sphincter's intermuscular plexus of Auerbach. This reflex is classically absent in patients with Hirschsprung's disease and variably present in patients with a high imperforate anus who have undergone operative correction (81).

In adults, anal endosonography provides definition of the voluntary striated external sphincter and involuntary smooth muscle internal sphincter (82). It is also possible to determine the status of the pudendal nerve by using electroneurography (83). These techniques may have future benefit for postoperative evaluation of incontinence following repair of ARMs.

Sensation and Proprioception

It is believed that in normal children, innervation of the anus and anal skin is not present at birth, but is acquired as the child learns to defecate and, therefore, toilet train (84). These receptors are not necessary for keeping the external sphincter contracted because normal newborns have an external sphincter reflex (85). The presence or absence of these receptors and the status of the voluntary muscle in newborns has not been elucidated. Furthermore, it is difficult to assume that innervation of the anus and anal skin is not present early in life, as evidenced by the facial grimaces that these children use when wanting to defecate. Moreover, there are many additional unanswered questions about the role of and presence of sensory nerve endings in the newborn, as well as the contribution, if any, of the anal mucosa to continence and defecation.

Colonic and Rectosigmoid Motility

It is well known that it takes between 3 and 6 hours for the gastric content to transit the small bowel. The intestinal content reaches the cecum in a liquid state. It then takes about 20 to 24 hours for that fecal material to reach the rectum and become formed (solid). The rectosigmoid acts as a reservoir and keeps the fecal material for variable periods of time. The anal canal (below the pectinate line); however, is usually empty because of the action of the surrounding sphincteric mechanism. Occasionally, however, there are peristaltic waves that push the fecal material toward the anus. The voluntary sphincter can be voluntarily relaxed, allowing sampling to occur. The rectal content moves distally and touches the exquisitely sensitive tissue of the anal canal, providing the individual with valuable information related to the nature of the rectal content (gas, solid, liquid). Depending on the surrounding social circumstances, the individual may let the rectal content escape or may contract the sphincteric mechanism, pushing stool or gas back into the rectum. The distention of the rectum produces a vague sensation of fullness or even a colicky pain (proprioception), but does not provide specific information concerning the physical characteristic of the content.

We know very little about the mechanism that triggers the peristalsis of the rectosigmoid to defecate, but certainly we know that the degree of rectal fullness has a definite role. Thus, when the time comes, the rectosigmoid generates waves of peristalsis aiming to empty the lumen. Individuals can restrain this temporarily by using the voluntary sphincter. With a voluntary decision to allow the stool to come out, the sphincter is relaxed and the individual waits for the next peristaltic wave. Normal defecation allows a massive emptying of the rectosigmoid followed by another resting period of about 24 hours, during which the rectosigmoid acts again as a reservoir.

The importance of rectosigmoid motility has been highly underestimated in the past for a variety of reasons, not the least of which are a suitable animal model and proper equipment for the study of children. Tonic, phasic, and high-amplitude propagated contractions (HAPCs, those greater than 80 mm Hg) and rectal motor complexes (RMCs) are the hallmarks of normal colonic motility in children, but they are not necessarily representative of rectosigmoid motility. These responses are intrinsic to the bowel wall and are derived from brain–gut connections (86). With age in normal children, the number of HAPCs falls and parallels the decrease in daily bowel movements (87). The RMC is the only colonic activity that occurs distal to the rectosigmoid (88). Colonic motility as defined by both the HAPCs and the RMCs should be stimulated after eating. This colonic response to food is diagnostic of normal colonic motility and forms the basis for future studies of abnormal colonic motility in children with pseudoobstruction (89). None of these colonic motility studies evaluate the propagation of a wave through to the anal canal. Most of these studies stop at the rectosigmoid, which is the area where most HAPCs stop. Furthermore, the role of the more distal RMCs is unknown.

Physiology of Children with Anorectal Malformations

Sphincter Function

Some studies suggest that for children with high imperforate anus, nerve cell numbers in the medial ventral horn of the spinal cord, corresponding to the external anal sphincter and muscle complex, are reduced (90).

In contrast to the spectrum of voluntary striated muscle abnormalities in children with ARMs, the status of the smooth muscle does not seem to affect prognosis. Some authors suggest the internal sphincter is crucial for bowel control. Although postoperative manometry in some patients with ARMs shows that there is occasional preservation of the RAIR, there is no evidence that absolutely links the presence or absence of the internal anal sphincter to normal bowel control.

Sensation and Proprioception

Children born with ARMs have a spectrum of sensation and proprioception. Agenesis of these nerve endings, such as occurs in high imperforate anus, may mean that for whatever spectrum of voluntary striated musculature is present there may also be a defect in sensation and proprioception. In children with ARMs, a feeling of fullness (proprioception) may be accompanied by a spectrum of exquisite or rudimentary sensation to no sensation at all. Thus, when dealing with a high imperforate anus, it is imperative to appreciate all the musculature and its symmetry in an effort to relocate the neoanus between the fibers of the voluntary striated mechanism (74). Only in this optimally relocated anatomic scenario can distention and proprioception help the child have fecal continence. In these children, sensation is a consequence of distention of the neoanus. They cannot rely on an intact voluntary striated muscle mechanism because by definition there is a paucity of this muscle mass and its innervation. Therefore, many of these children cannot hold stool nor have a normal bowel movement when liquids are present in their neoanus. Solid feces will distend the rectum, but liquid stools do not; thus, liquid stools must be avoided at all costs.

Colonic and Rectosigmoid Motility

Children with ARMs have a spectrum of rectosigmoid motility disorders. Children with ARMs subjected to surgical techniques that preserve rectosigmoid suffer from constipation. Constipation, one of the most important functional sequelae of ARMs, is probably the result of hypomotility of the rectosigmoid. The hypomotility is self-perpetuating and self-aggravating to the point that, if left untreated, megasigmoid develops (91). In extreme cases, children may develop fecal impaction and encopresis or overflow pseudoincontinence. Analysis of results after PSARP shows that constipation is worse in the lower defects (see "Results"). Knowing this and the fact that hypomotility can begin a vicious cycle leading to megasigmoid, it is incumbent on the pediatric surgeon to avoid the cycle of hypomotility, constipation, and megasigmoid. In fact, aggressive patient follow-up using dietary, mechanical, and pharmacologic treatment prevents this cycle. Usually, suppositories, enemas, or colonic irrigations suffice. Constipation from functional, postoperative, and neurologic etiologies has been treated with the prokinetic agent cisapride (92,93). It stimulates the smooth muscle of the entire gastrointestinal tract by releasing acetylcholine, shortening transit time, and causing improved sensitivity to distention. What cannot be overemphasized is the concept that constipation, especially for the lower ARM defects is expected, and thus, all precautions should be taken to avoid aggravating this problem.

In contrast with the problem of constipation secondary to hypomotility, children with ARMs who for whatever reason have lost their rectosigmoid suffer from the exact opposite (i.e., tendency for diarrhea). These children have no reservoir capacity, are highly sensitive to fruits and vegetables, and worst of all suffer from incontinence. They have a spectrum of hypermotility dysfunction with the most severe complaints in children with no colon.

Unfortunately, there is a paucity of data in the literature concerning the normal mechanism of rectosigmoid motility and even less information in patients with ARMs. The clinical findings in children treated for constipation and incontinence, however, are compelling for the importance of rectosigmoid motility.

ASSOCIATED ANOMALIES

Because arrest of migration of mesoderm within the caudal eminence and abnormal resorption of the cloacal membrane are likely embryologic causes of ARMs, it follows that other mesodermally derived tissues should be affected. These tissues include derivatives of the paraxial and lateral plate mesoderm that consist of the genitourinary, skeletal, muscular, and gastrointestinal systems. The incidence of associated malformations depends on the type of anorectal defect, but a specific type of associated malformation does not seem to correlate with a specific ARM.

Genitourinary System

The most common associated malformations are derivatives of the genitourinary system, with an incidence in the range of 20% to 54% (94–96). They include the following:

- Absent, dysplastic, or horseshoe kidneys
- Vesicoureteral reflux
- Hydronephrosis
- Hypospadias
- Bifid scrotum

The triad of penile agenesis, complete absence of the median raphe, and imperforate anus is incompatible with life (97).

In general, the higher the ARM, the greater the likelihood of an associated genitourinary anomaly. For example, patients with a persistent cloaca or a rectobladder neck fistula have a 90% chance of associated genitourinary anomaly. Rectourethral or rectovestibular fistulas have an associated incidence of 30%, but a child with a perineal fistula has less than a 10% chance of an associated genitourinary anomaly (96). This information is important for the neonatal management of these children. Therefore, it should be mandatory for all newborns with an ARM to undergo an abdominopelvic ultrasound. If hydronephrosis is found, a voiding cystourethrogram (VCUG) should be performed before the colostomy is created (98). In so doing, appropriate additional decompression of bladder, vagina, or both may be performed when indicated along with the colostomy under a single episode of anesthesia. Patients with a rectobladder neck fistula (flat bottom) and patients with cloacas represent potential urologic emergencies and should not undergo colostomy without a prior urologic diagnosis. Deteriorating renal function from hydronephrosis, urosepsis, or uncorrectable metabolic acidosis is the most frequent cause of morbidity and mortality in patients with ARMs. Associated genitourinary reflux should be treated with suppressive antibiotics.

Patients with symptomatic voiding pathology (vesicoureteral reflux) usually have a high imperforate anus (rectourinary fistulas) and bony sacral and spinal cord anomalies (44%). Yet, these may exist in the absence of sacral agenesis. However, patients without voiding symptoms tended to have a low imperforate anus and minimal or no bone anomalies (8%) (99).

Skeletal System

In general, the higher the ARM, the more likely there is an associated skeletal anomaly. Such anomalies include the following:

- Partial or complete lumbosacral agenesis
- Hemivertebrae
- Agenesis of thoracic vertebrae
- Scoliosis
- Hemisacrum or scimitar sacrum
- Asymmetric sacrum
- Posterior protruding sacrum
- Agenesis of the coccyx

As many as 45% of patients with ARMs have sacral abnormalities (100). There appears to be an excellent correlation between the degree of skeletal sacral anomaly and the functional prognosis of the newborn with an ARM. Absence of one of the five sacral vertebrae does not seem to correlate with function or outcome (101). Two or more absent vertebrae, however, have been shown to represent a poor prognostic sign of bowel function (102). Many times it is difficult to actually count the number of sacral vertebrae. Thus, the sacral ratio technique seems to be a useful method to help the surgeon predict functional prognosis. In addition, sometimes children have five sacral vertebrae, yet the sacrum may be very short and looks obviously abnormal. As a result, a more accurate way to evaluate the sacrum was perfected. After placing the newborn either in an anteroposterior or a lateral position, three lines are drawn (Fig. 89-11). Line A extends across the uppermost portion of the iliac crest; line B unites the inferior–posterior iliac spines; and line C runs parallel to lines A and B and passes through the lowest sacral point visible on the radiograph. Normal children have an average sacral ratio (BC:AB) of 0.7:0.8, in contrast to children with severe ARMs whose ratio may be as low as zero. Low ratios correlate with poor functional prognosis (i.e., incontinence). The sacral ratio seems to be a predictor of functional outcome when comparing types of ARMs.

Absence of any portion of the spine from the midthoracic level or higher is probably not compatible with intrauterine life. The absence of the coccyx is invariably asymptomatic, but absence of any lumbosacral vertebrae may have associated anomalies such as the limbs and genitourinary system in addition to ARMs (103). The Currarino triad is an example of a specific anomaly of the sacrum instead of agenesis that is found in association with two other anomalies (104). The triad consists of a scimitar sacrum, anal stenosis, and presacral mass (i.e., lipoma, lipomeningocele) (Fig. 89-12). All children with anal stenosis and an ARM should have a lumbosacral spine X-ray to rule out this triad. If indeed a scimitar sacrum is found, then an ultrasound of the pelvis or a magnetic resonance

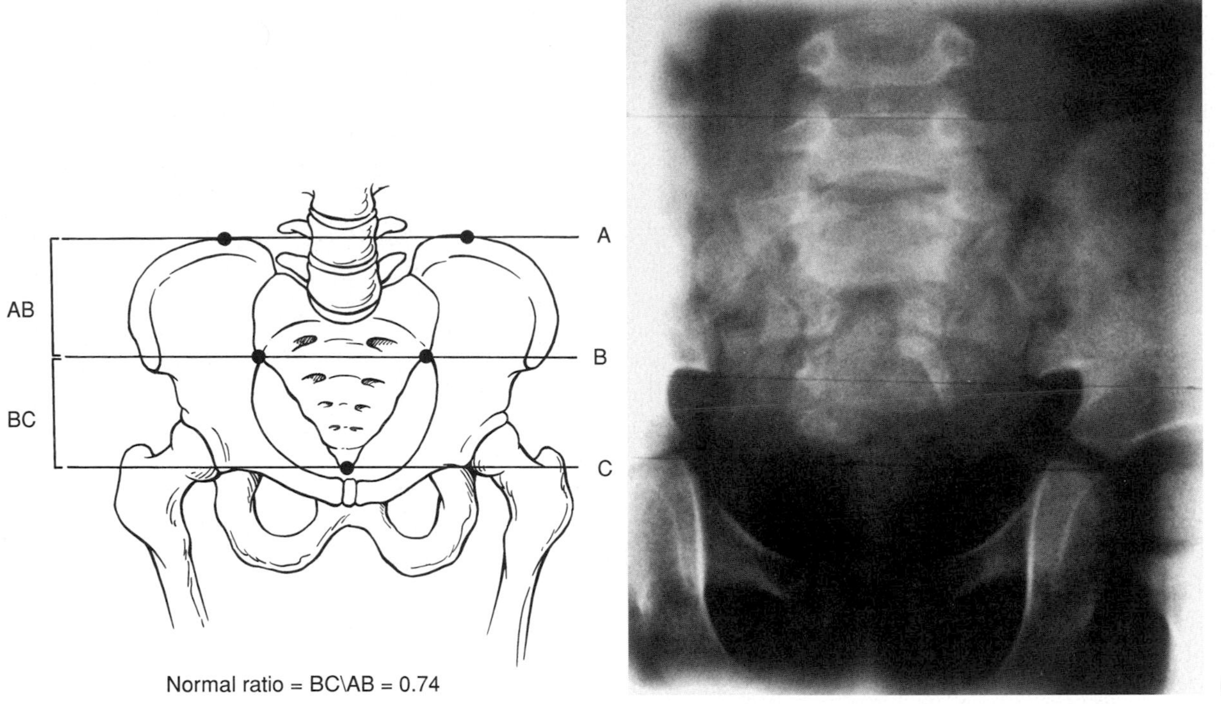

FIGURE 89-11. (**A**) Sacral ratio. Three lines are drawn in either the anteroposterior or lateral position. Line A extends across the uppermost portion of the iliac crest. Line B unites the inferior–posterior iliac spines, and line C is parallel to lines A and B and passes through the lowest sacral point visible on radiograph. (**B**) Actual radiograph showing an abnormal ratio of 0.31.

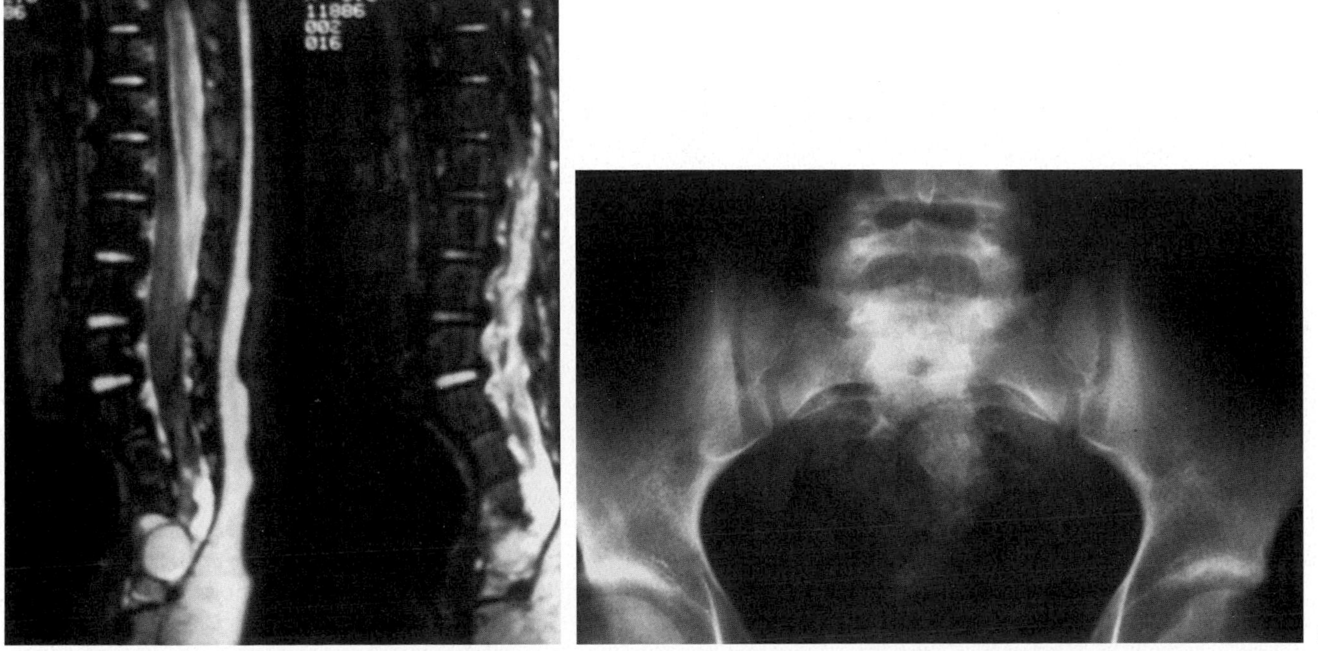

FIGURE 89-12. The Currarino triad. These children have anal stenosis, presacral masses, and scimitar sacrum. (**A**) Magnetic resonance scan shows the presacral mass, which in this case is a lipomeningocele. (**B**) The plain radiograph is a scimitar sacrum.

(MR) scan of the spine should be obtained to exclude a presacral mass.

Factors that may influence the normal development of the vertebral column include insulin-dependent maternal diabetes, trauma to the fetus, and prolonged fever during pregnancy (105). Overall causes of sacral anomalies like the etiology of ARMs are multifactorial and include both environmental and hereditary factors. Interestingly, characteristics of patients with isolated lumbosacral deformities are similar to those with ARMs. These similarities include flattening of the buttocks, shortening of the intergluteal cleft, loss of perineal muscle mass, and motor deficits of the levator (S2 to S5) and gluteal muscles (L5 to S1). Sensation is derived from dorsal root ganglia and peripheral sensory nerves, both of which are derived from neural crest tissue. In contrast with isolated ARMs, where we find abnormalities not only in motor ability, but also in neural crest–derived perineal sensation, sensation in children with lumbosacral agenesis is relatively unaffected (106). When compared with abnormalities of the sacrum alone or sacrum and limb deformities, sacral agenesis associated with any visceral anomalies (e.g., ARMs) constitutes the worst functional prognosis (107).

Nervous System

A study performed on 94 patients with all forms of ARMs showed a 38% incidence of spinal anomalies (108). Given the paucity of data in the literature, however, the frequency of spinal anomalies with ARMs is at best an approximation. In addition, it is difficult to speculate who should or should not undergo screening for spinal anomalies. As such, all patients with ARMs should have their lumbosacral spine evaluated with plain radiographs. Screening with an MR scan should be *mandatory* for some children and *recommended* for others (Table 89-4) (109). There are no data to support the notion that spinal dysraphism (i.e., tethered cord), except in severe cases, is directly linked to the functional outcome in patients with ARMs. It appears, however, that the higher the ARM the more likely it is for the child to have associated neurologic and skeletal problems. Therefore, it is mandatory for all patients with ARMs to undergo a pelvic ultrasound to rule out the possibility of spinal dysraphism (110). Magnetic resonance imaging (MRI) may also be used, including in the neonate, as the sole study to evaluate potential associated anomalies (111). Radiologists claim they can make the diagnosis of a tethered cord with ultrasound in patients younger than 3 months of age; older patients require MRI. The MR scan is difficult in babies because it requires remote anesthesia services for deep sedation and sometimes intubation to keep the baby immobile. In addition, the baby is relatively inaccessible for the duration of the scan, which makes monitoring cumbersome. We recommend going directly to an MR scan for the evaluation of the postoperative patient with constipation, incontinence, or bladder dysfunction that cannot be explained by the nature, type, and height of the original ARM (112).

TABLE 89-4 Indications for Screening for Tethered Cord with ARMs.

Mandatory
Myelodysplasia
Abnormal sacral ratio (AP $<$ 0.4 or LAT $<$ 0.6)[a]
Complex defect
Cloacal exstrophy
Recommended
Rectobladder neck fistula
Persistent cloaca (common channel $>$3 cm)
Presacral mass
Hemivertebrae
Genitourinary anomaly
Poor result despite good prognosis

[a] AP, anteroposterior; LAT, lateral.

Various associated spinal anomalies have been reported:

- Tethered cord
- Dural sac stenosis
- Narrow spinal canal
- Diastematomyelia
- Myelomeningocele, meningocele
- Intraspinal teratoma
- Neurogenic bladder

Prevention of rostral migration of the spinal cord during development because of an abnormal point of fixation secondary to bony deformities results in a shortened cauda equina and low-lying conus medullaris. During an axial growth spurt, the spine grows faster than the cord and this may provoke stretching, traction, and eventual infarction of the cord above the point of fixation. Normally, the conus is at the level of L3 at birth, ascends to the upper border of L2 by age 5, and remains there through adulthood. Detecting the conus below L3 suggests tethering. Although metrizamide computed tomography (CT) scans have been used in the past, the MR scan for definitive diagnosis and ultrasound for screening (in patients younger than 3 months of age) are used today (113). Knowledge of the presence of a tethered cord instead of operation for correction should be the standard of care. On the other hand, there is clear benefit from untethering a spinal cord in patients with progressive symptoms. As the vertebral column lengthens with age, symptoms are usually radicular pain, myelopathies, and foot deformities. Postoperative constipation or fecal incontinence as isolated symptoms has not been shown to be associated with a tethered cord (109). If a pelvic ultrasound, performed when the infant is younger than 3 months of age, detects any abnormalities of the spinal canal or the vertebrae, then an MR scan should be performed to rule out any possibility of an associated neural abnormality.

Gastrointestinal and Cardiovascular Systems

Gastrointestinal anomalies are probably fourth in the frequency of potential anomalies associated with ARMs, followed by intracardiac defects. The following associated anomalies can occur separately or as VATER and VACTERL associations:

- Esophageal atresia
- Duodenal atresia
- Ventricular or atrioseptal defects
- Tetrology of Fallot
- Hirschsprung's disease

Keep in mind that none of these associated gastrointestinal and cardiac anomalies have contributed to the overall prognosis of the ARM. These associations, however, have made it mandatory for an echocardiogram to be performed and an orogastric tube to be inserted. If bilious drainage is discovered in the newborn period, a contrast study should be performed. Likewise, if the orogastric tube does not pass, there should be a high index of suspicion for esophageal atresia.

Concerning the possible association of Hirschsprung's disease and ARMs, one can submit a piece of the pulled-through bowel at the time of definitive repair or perform a suction rectal biopsy of the distal limb of the colostomy at any time (114). The authors, however, have never seen a child with concurrent ARMs and enterocolitis from Hirschsprung's disease, yet there are many children with ARMs and constipation who probably have been misdiagnosed with associated Hirschsprung's disease.

PRENATAL DIAGNOSIS

In general, gastrointestinal anomalies occur as isolated in utero events in 65% to 70% of cases, and multiple organ systems are involved in the remaining 30% to 35% (115). In cases of lower gastrointestinal tract anomalies such as ARMs, the incidence of associated anomalies approaches 50% (23,24). In contrast with the most gastrointestinal anomalies, few if any ARM cases are diagnosed prenatally. Although this is a shortcoming, ARMs should not be included in a list of congenital anomalies that cause major long-term disability or death (116). Antenatal diagnosis of ARMs is at best included in a list of possible diagnoses. This problem is operator dependent, limited technically, and finally nonspecific, unless dramatic in presentation (i.e., sirenomelia). Nonspecific prenatal ultrasound findings include the following (117):

- Dilatated, U-shaped colon in the lower abdomen or pelvis
- Highly distended vagina
- Calcified intraluminal meconium or enterolithiasis
- Normal or diminished amniotic fluid volume (associated bilateral renal disorders)
- Absence of a circular rim of hypoechogenicity in perineum with a central linear echo running sagittally
- Absent kidney
- Absent radius
- Hydronephrosis
- Septated, cystic pelvic mass, oligohydramnios, and impaired fetal growth in girls, in the case of cloaca

Prenatal anal ultrasonography has identified the normal anal canal by the presence of a circular rim of hypoechogenic tissue in the perineum, together with a central linear echogenic stripe. The absence of these findings is suggestive but not as yet pathognomonic for ARMs (118). Caudal regression syndromes (119) ranging from lumbosacral agenesis to the mermaidlike caudal features in association with ARM, genitourinary, central nervous system, and cardiorespiratory anomalies are easier to identify in contrast with isolated ARMs.

Dilated colon is gestational age dependent (usually not seen prior to 24 to 26 weeks) and nonspecific because it can also be associated with meconium plug syndrome, Hirschsprung's disease, small left colon syndrome, or atresia (120). Dilated colon in the lower abdomen or pelvis has a long list of differential diagnoses, including ovarian cyst, hydrometrocolpos, obstructive uropathy, megacystis-microcolon intestinal hypoperistalsis syndrome, urachal cyst, and ARMs such as a cloacal malformation. In general, effort should be made to identify kidneys, liver, spleen, and bladder before considering a sonolucent pelvic mass to be an ARM.

Polyhydramnios implies either a misdiagnosis or an additional anomaly such as esophageal atresia. In fact, 1 of 15 healthy pregnancies with polyhydramnios is associated with proximal instead of distal gastrointestinal tract obstruction (121). Polyhydramnios then should not imply a hindgut anomaly.

Microvillar disaccharidase activity is diminished, presumably because like most intestinal atresias there is an obstruction to the passage of colonic contents (122–124). These intestinal enzymes may be present in amniotic fluid in response to desquamation of intestinal cells in utero. Fetal intestinal disaccharidases (α- and β-glucosidase, β-galactosidase) within amniotic fluid are detectable during the tenth week of gestation, peaking by the seventeenth week, and finally are found at very low levels by the twenty-second week (125). Reasons for this evolution are unclear, but may be related to the formation and recanalization of the intestinal tract and its patency, both in the cranial and caudal axes. As amniotic fluid volume increases during the third trimester, the enzymes may be diluted or the disaccharidases may be cleared by fetal swallowing. In general, institutions using the intestinal enzyme activity as an aid to the diagnosis of bowel obstruction restrict their sampling to a gestational age of 14 to 21 weeks (126).

The diagnosis of a cloacal malformation has been established by identifying a septated cystic mass in the pelvis, no evidence of bladder, oligohydramnios, and hydronephrosis by ultrasound (127).

NEONATAL DIAGNOSIS AND MANAGEMENT OF ANORECTAL MALFORMATIONS

Male Algorithm

As for clinical evaluation, the patient with an ARM should not present as an intestinal obstruction; instead, the diagnosis should be made during clinical examination of the newborn (128) (Fig. 89-13).

Performing a diverting colostomy and managing any life-threatening–associated anomalies (e.g., cardiac and urinary tract) are the two most important issues in the newborn period, regardless of gender. Inspection of the male perineum should allow a diagnosis, and thus, direct the need for a diverting colostomy in 80% to 90% of cases. Questionable cases rely on the presence of meconium in the urine, and cross-table lateral radiograph The cross-table lateral radiograph can pinpoint the bowel as close as 5 mm from the skin provided the radiograph is performed after 18 hours of life. The cross-table lateral film has replaced the traditional invertogram. A cross-table lateral radiograph is taken with the baby in the prone position and the pelvis elevated (129). If the rectum is located less than 1 cm from the perineal skin, this is considered a low-lying ARM. In such cases, in retrospect, most likely a perineal fistula was missed during the examination of the perineum. All lesions higher than 1 cm are high ARMs and require a diverting colostomy.

It usually takes 16 to 24 hours for the newborn intestine to pass meconium through a fistula communicating with the skin or the urethra. Thus, decisions about performing a diverting colostomy should not be made before 24 hours of life. In the interim, gauze can be placed on the tip of the penis looking for filtered meconium, and an ultrasound of the abdomen must be performed to rule out kidney pathology and hydronephrosis (130). An echocardiogram should also be performed if a heart murmur or cyanosis is present.

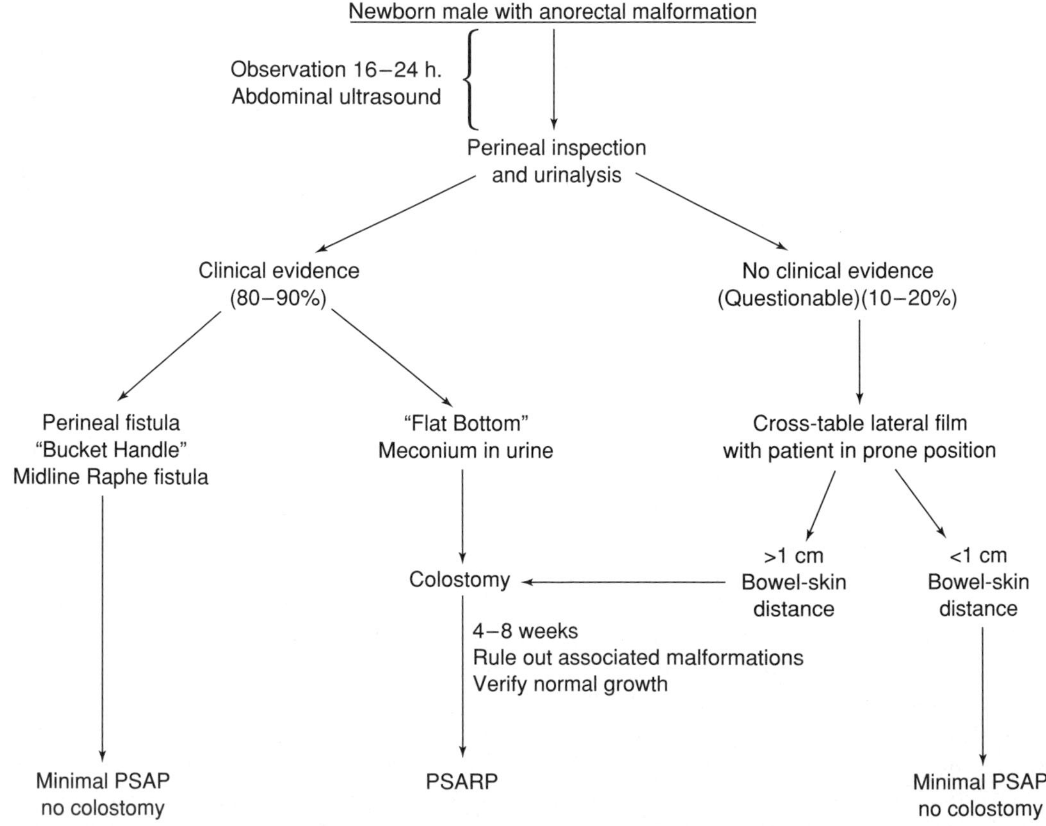

FIGURE 89-13. Algorithm for the neonatal management of anorectal malformations in a male. PSAP, posterior sagittal anoplasty; PSARP, posterior sagittal anorectoplasty.

Low defects include subepithelial midline passage of meconium through fistula or prominent skin tag (bucket handle deformity) (Fig. 89-4). These ARMs are usually treated with a perineal anoplasty either via a posterior sagittal approach or via dilitations if the baby is ill, with a minimal posterior sagittal approach deferred for a future time.

Higher defects on inspection are characterized by a very flat bottom, meconium in the urine, or air in the bladder. All high defects require a diverting descending colostomy in the newborn period and definitive repair usually by 3 months of age provided there has been consistent weight gain and associated malformations have been managed. Prior to creation of the colostomy in the newborn period, the need for urinary diversion should be ruled out because, if indicated, this procedure can be performed simultaneously.

Female Algorithm

Simple perineal inspection provides the diagnosis in virtually 90% of ARMs in females (Fig. 89-14). For example, cutaneous and vestibular fistulas are readily identified during a perineal exam. One must immobilize the baby's legs and use good lighting. A rectovestibular fistula orifice can usually be identified just outside the hymen. A rectovaginal fistula is identified by meconium coming from inside the vagina through the hymen, but this is an exceedingly rare malformation. A perineal (cutaneous) fistula has the same prognostic and therapeutic significance as in males. A vestibular fistula tends to be competent and to remain patent with serial dilatations, which can be performed if the infant is ill. Depending on the surgeon's experience, a primary repair in the newborn period can be undertaken. The safest approach is always a colostomy with a future repair that avoids potential infection and dehiscence, which have occurred with newborn repair of rectovestibular fistulae. Passage of stool through this fistula for prolonged periods of time can induce varying degrees of megacolon and potential constipation. A single perineal orifice means the baby has a persistent cloaca. In most of these cases, there is an associated urologic emergency that requires prompt evaluation. Thus, these babies will most likely receive a colostomy, a vaginostomy or vesicostomy, or any other urinary diversion. A midline, lower abdominal mass in these newborns is pathognomonic for a hydrocolpos. It is imperative for pediatric surgeons dealing with cloacas to be aware of the fact that a very dilated vagina is a significant problem for these newborn babies. During the neonatal period, the baby should not be taken to the operating room until the urinary tract is adequately evaluated and the presence of a hydrocolpos has been ruled out. If

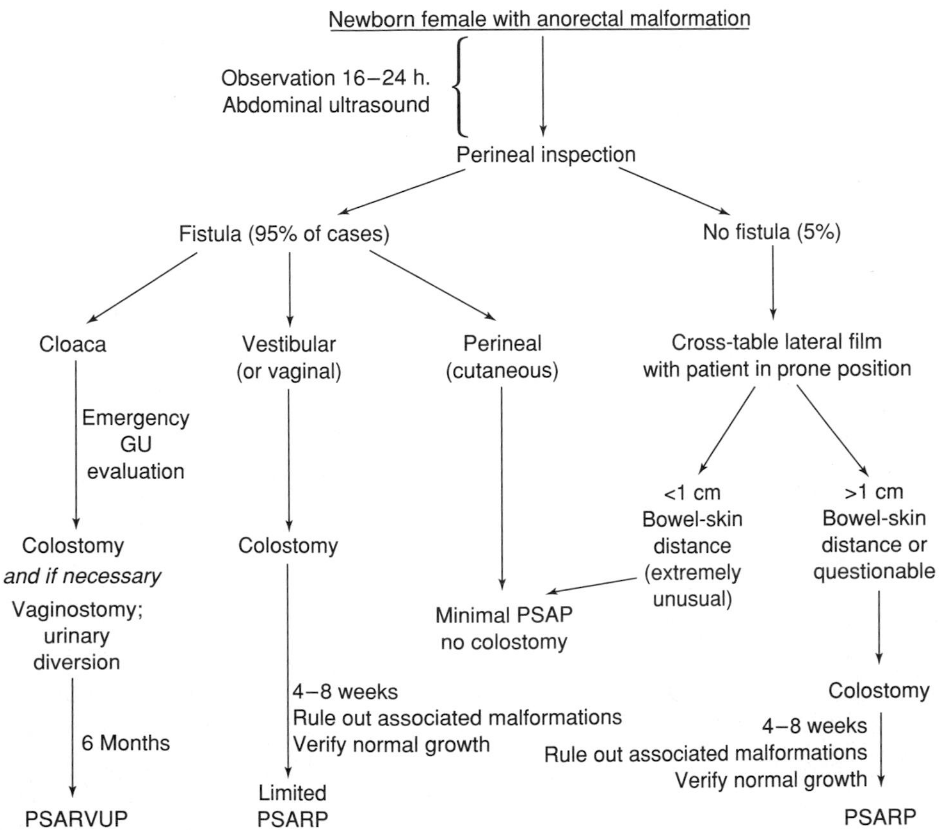

FIGURE 89-14. Algorithm for the neonatal management of anorectal malformations in a female. GU, genitourinary; PSAP, posterior sagittal anoplasty; PSARP, posterior sagittal anorectoplasty; PSARVUP, posterior sagittal anorecto vagino urethroplasty.

the baby has a hydrocolpos, it is mandatory for the surgeon not only to open a colostomy, but also to insert tubes into the dilated vagina or vaginas to decompress them and thus prevent complications, such as pyocolpos or ureteral obstruction.

If a female does not pass meconium in the first 16 to 24 hours of life, then again a cross-table lateral radiograph is indicated. In addition, an abdominal ultrasound to evaluate the kidneys and ureters is also required.

Perineal Fistula

Special consideration is given to this variant of ARM because it is frequently discovered in the pediatrician's office for the workup of constipation (131,132). Usually, the sphincteric mechanism is present and functioning. The anal orifice, however, is well forward of the muscles and a posterior shelf and pocket or cul-de-sac is palpable during rectal examination. The clinical picture is remarkably consistent. Chronic constipation persists despite all medical management using formula changes, laxatives, and stimulants. The referral to pediatric surgeons is usually to rule out Hirschsprung's disease, and in most of these patients, there is no aganglionic bowel. These patients need a thorough physical examination that includes the anus. In fact, the diagnosis can be suspected merely by inspection. The anus should normally be positioned at the midpoint of a line drawn between the base of the vagina or scrotum and the tip of the coccyx. The perineal fistula is anterior to this midpoint position and thus outside some, if not all, of the external anal sphincter. Not all these patients require repositioning operatively. Those who fail medical treatment with stool softening and have recurrent urinary tract infections should probably undergo anoplasty. Our recommendation is reconstruction using a minimal posterior sagittal approach that facilitates exposure of the external sphincter and its junction with the muscle complex. An anterior operative approach can also be performed. Restoration of the perineal body and positioning of the anus within these structures is all that is required. A colostomy is not indicated. In newborns, no bowel preparation is required. However, in older patients a very strict bowel preparation is mandatory, along with 5 to 7 days of nothing-by-mouth status that usually means peripheral alimentation.

Anoplasty

The indication for some form of anoplasty includes cases of male and female perineal fistulas (Fig. 89-15). Regardless of the type of operation performed, the goal is to restore the anus to its normal anatomic position within the external sphincter. Because postnatal bacteria flora usually takes 3 days to be present in the baby's stool, no bowel preparation is necessary if the anoplasty is performed during this time period. Prophylactic antibiotics are given, and in males a Foley catheter in the bladder is mandatory. The most frequent complication is urethral injury because, even in the low defects, the rectum and urethra are intimately attached. The operation is a minimal posterior sagittal anoplasty (Fig. 89-15).

The minimal posterior sagittal anoplasty not only uses the nerve stimulator, but also takes advantage of the direct visualization of the external sphincter from anterior to posterior. Multiple 6–0 traction sutures are placed around the perineal orifice, and then a dissection is performed circumferentially around the rectum. The sphincters should

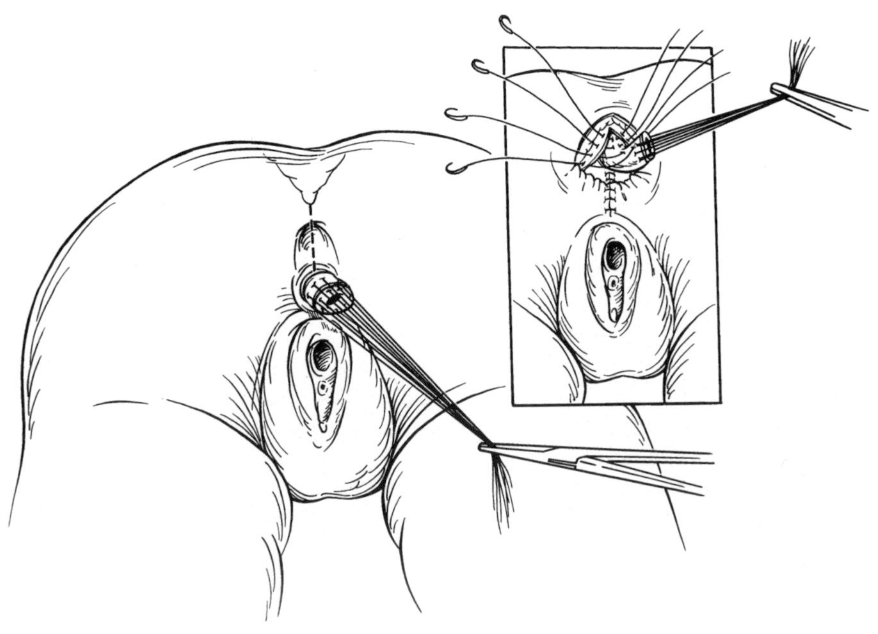

FIGURE 89-15. The minimal posterior sagittal anoplasty.

TABLE 89-5 Anal Dilatations Recommended with Sizes and Schedule.

Age	Dilator Size (mm)
1–3 mo	12
4–8 mo	13
9–12 mo	14
1–3 y	15
4–14 y	16
≥14 y and older	17
Schedule	
Once a day for 1 mo	
Every third day for 1 mo	
Twice a week for 1 mo	
Once a week for 1 mo	
Once a week for 3 mo	

not be mobilized. It is the bowel that is to be dissected. Just enough bowel is mobilized to allow placement of the neoanus within the confines of the sphincter. In females, there is little to no morbidity with this procedure. Maintaining a plane immediately beyond the anus and not traveling beyond these limits facilitates protection of the bulbar urethra. Prior to the neoanoplasty, the perineal body should be restored using interrupted absorbable suture material. Two weeks after the minimal PSARP, a schedule of dilatations is begun (Table 89-5).

Colostomy

A descending colostomy is the procedure of choice for ARMs (133). In general, a completely diverting descending colostomy should be created in a newborn with a high ARM. Complete diversion is difficult, if not impossible, with a loop colostomy, and thus, the potential for continued communication between rectum and urinary tract is high. Also, a loop colostomy in contrast to a completely diverting colostomy predisposes the child to urinary tract infections. The propensity for continued overflow into the distal bowel and consequent abnormal bowel distention can compromise the definitive repair and bowel motility. Postoperative constipation can be associated with megarectum, secondary to fecal impaction, created by this overflow into the distal bowel. If a loop colostomy is created too loosely, there is the potential for prolapse of the proximal stoma. The most common error is opening the colostomy too distally, leaving one with an incomplete length of bowel for the definitive repair, and thus forcing the surgeon to gain length by performing a laparotomy.

The descending colon double-barrel colostomy is our procedure of choice. Both types of stomas should be created through an oblique left lower quadrant incision using two layers of long-term absorbable sutures, one incorporating the posterior sheath and the second layer using the anterior sheath. Either stoma should be created so the distal stoma is narrow to avoid prolapse. The distal stoma (mucous fistula) should be irrigated with warm saline in the operating room so the distal bowel is cleared of meconium. A loop colostomy leads to megarectosigmoid and continued fecal contamination of the urinary tract (134).

Preoperative Colostography

A preoperative colostogram is usually performed 3 to 4 weeks following creation of the stoma. It is commonly performed on an outpatient basis because the baby has likely been discharged from the hospital. The purpose of the colostogram is to define the anatomy of the distal bowel and establish the site of fistulous connection with the urinary tract. Thus, the procedure is called a *distal colostogram*. In a retrospective review of boys with ARM, the risk of urologic injury was increased in those males who did not undergo a properly performed distal colostogram to define the level of the fistula (135). The single most important limitation to an adequate study is the fact that the distal rectum is surrounded by the sphincteric mechanism, which even in patients with ARMs exerts enough tone to collapse the rectum. For adequate filling of the distal bowel, enough hydrostatic pressure must be exerted to overcome the resting muscle tone and ultimately fill the distal bowel and fistula site. Therefore, we recommend injection of contrast material into the distal bowel using a Foley catheter with 2- to 3-mL inflation of the balloon. The lumen of the mucous fistula is occluded by pulling on the catheter and hand injecting a radiopaque water-soluble contrast using fluoroscopy. The anal dimple is marked with a piece of lead. In the anteroposterior position, the first piece of information to be obtained is the measurement of available length of distal bowel. Next, in the lateral projection, the fistula site is determined again by injection of contrast. The contrast material that passes into the urethra usually goes into the bladder. To complete the study, contrast should distend the bladder and the patient should be seen voiding (136). A VCUG is not necessary because the distal colostogram, if performed as outlined, provides the essential information. The bladder, urethra sacrum, and anal dimple should be visualized in all projections. Failure of a colostogram is frequently the result of lack of back pressure while injecting the contrast or muscle action around the distal rectum.

In patients with a common cloaca, contrast should be injected through the common channel on the perineum, the distal colostomy, and the vesicostomy and vaginostomy when present (Fig. 89-16). A VCUG in children with cloacas is very difficult to obtain, except in those with a cystostomy or vesicostomy.

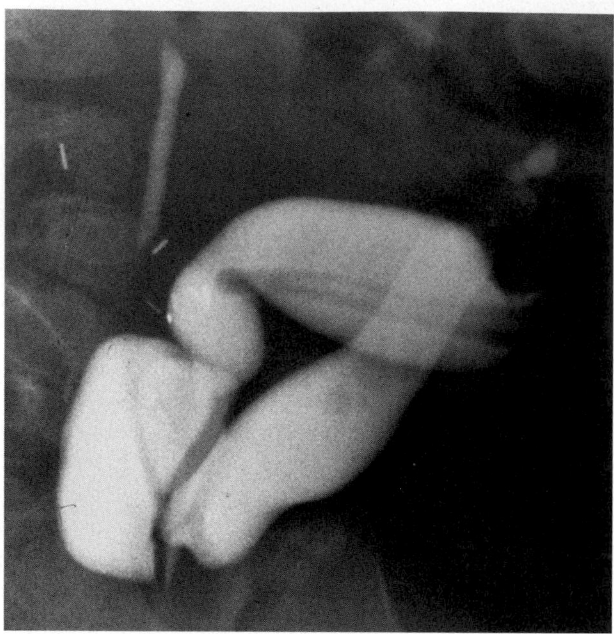

FIGURE 89-16. Distal colostogram of cloaca showing connection between bladder, vagina, and bowel. The length of the common channel is determined during cystoscopy.

DEFINITIVE REPAIR

General Concepts

The indications for definitive repair of an imperforate anus include all patients with nonlife-threatening–associated anomalies and nonlife-threatening chromosomal defects. Myelomeningocele, high cloaca, and absent sacrum are not contraindications to definitive repair. Absence of the colon, however, is a contraindication to PSARP.

Although a variety of abdominoperineal approaches have been advocated for the repair of ARMs, the authors recommend the posterior sagittal approach for all defects. In cases of a rectobladder neck fistula, a laparotomy or laparoscopy is required to find and mobilize the distal rectum (137). In a patient with persistent cloaca with a common channel longer than 3 cm, a laparotomy may also be required.

Patient Positioning

The prone position with the pelvis elevated is the optimal position for the posterior sagittal approach to ARMs. A Foley catheter is inserted into the bladder prior to positioning the patient. It is not uncommon for the catheter to follow the fistula tract into the rectum and end up in the field during the operation. It should be redirected once the rectum has been opened.

Electrical Stimulation

Although the patient is paralyzed, electrical stimulation of the perineum can be conducted through a series of reflex arcs directly via muscle. Stimulation facilitates maintaining symmetry of muscle during the dissection. When stimulating on the skin, 100 to 200 mA may be required, whereas current of 20 to 40 mA is all that should be required directly on muscle.

Incision

A midline incision facilitates keeping the sphincter mechanism symmetrically about the midline. Direct regional periodic electrical stimulation of the sphincteric mechanism ensures equal distribution of the voluntary striated muscle. There have been no published reports of nerves and vessels crossing the midline in this part of the body. Thus, staying in the midline raphe that seems to divide whatever spectrum of muscle is present is a prudent maneuver. Exposure using a sharp, self-retaining retractor should only be performed in a superficial plane.

Anatomy

From the posterior sagittal approach, the anatomy of a normal child is different compared with the potential paucity of muscle in children with ARMs (Figs. 89-9 to 89-11). One should be able to identify an external sphincter (parasagittal fibers), vertical fibers of the striated muscle complex, and the levator. Smooth muscle, but no discrete internal sphincter, has been identified.

Posterior Sagittal Anorectoplasty

Operative Approach for Males

Rectourethral Fistula (Bulbar and Prostatic)

The incision for the rectourethral fistula procedure usually extends from just above the coccyx through to and including the center of the anal dimple and perineal body (Fig. 89-5). The *parasagittal fibers* of the external sphincter are meticulously divided in their parallel course to the midline. This dissection is facilitated by electrical stimulation of these fibers, which usually run anteriorly and posteriorly to the anal dimple. Remember that ARMs are a spectrum of defects; thus, a spectrum of this voluntary striated muscle density will be encountered.

Medial to the parasagital fibers and running perpendicular to them is the *muscle complex* composed of voluntary striated fibers. This muscle is really the distal (caudal) continuum of the levator muscle (Fig. 89-17).

Deep to the parasagittal fibers is ischiorectal fat. If the surgeon does not stay in the midline, a small hernia of this fat can protrude into the operative field. The midline raphe in this area is very thin, and thus, the potential for this fat

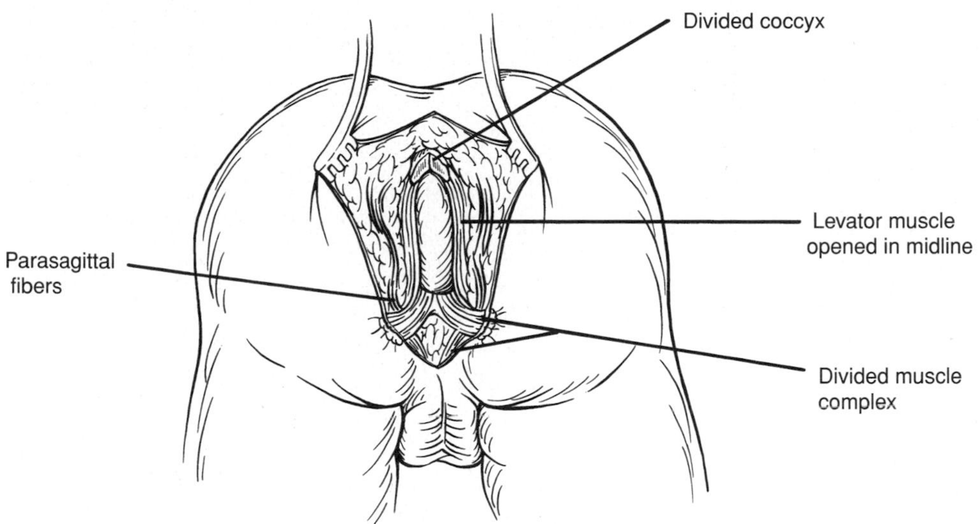

FIGURE 89-17. Exposure of parasagittal fibers, muscle complex, and levator muscle via the posterior sagittal approach.

to herniate is common. As the dissection continues deep to the ischiorectal fat, the midline *levator musculature* comes into the field (Fig. 89-18). The levator fibers run parallel to the skin incision.

Electrical stimulation of all three groups of muscle produces distinctive contraction of the anal dimple. For example, stimulation of the levator muscle contracts the anus in a forward motion. Stimulation of the muscle complex moves the anal dimple up toward the pelvis. The parasagittal fibers circumferentially contract the anus. Suture markers can be placed at the junction of the muscle complex and parasagittal fibers because these points form the posterior and anterior limits of the neoanus.

At this point in the procedure, the surgeon needs to have a sense of how extensive a dissection must be performed to find the rectum. Distal colostography provides the most valuable information to delineate the anatomic position of the bowel to ultimately approach the fistula.

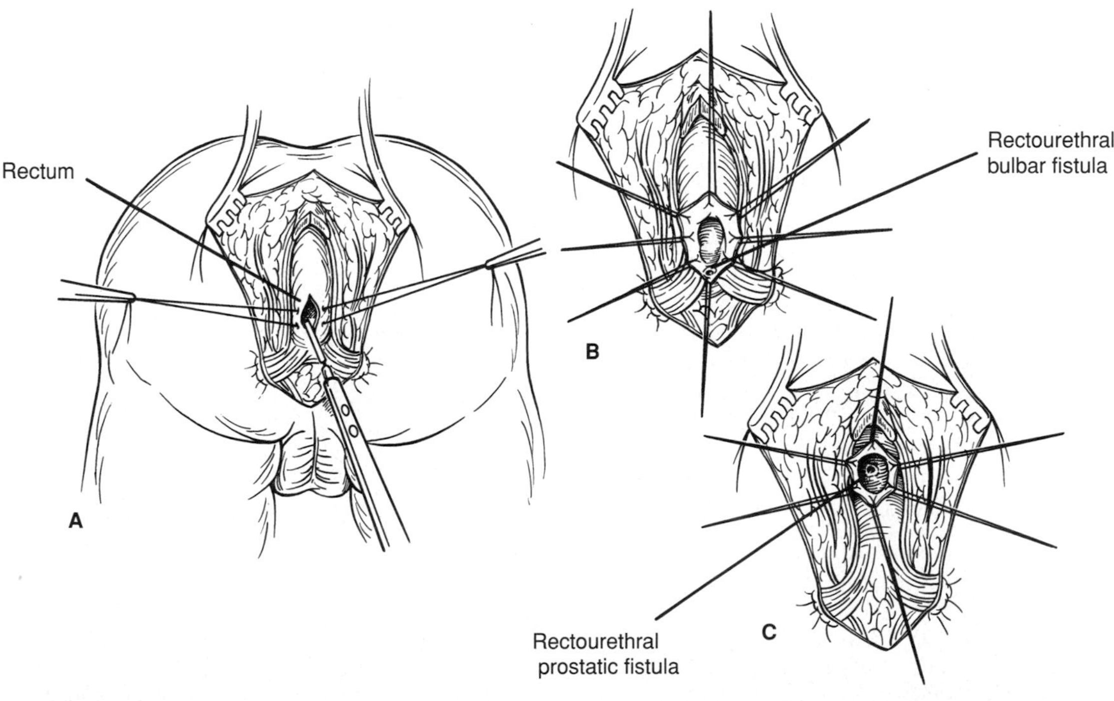

FIGURE 89-18. Locating the fistula via the posterior sagittal anorectoplasty approach. (**A**) Stay sutures on either side of the rectum facilitate opening the rectum. In cases of bulbar fistula (**B**) and prostatic urethral fistula (**C**), the stay sutures provide access to the fistula opening.

Thus, for example, the location of the rectum in a rectourethral bulbar fistula should be evident distally in the operative field after the levator muscle has been divided, whereas in cases of a prostatic fistula the bowel is located much higher in the field. Based on distal colostography, one can readily appreciate that the rectum in a bladder neck fistula cannot be seen or reached from a posterior sagittal approach; therefore, it must be found and mobilized through the abdomen, either with an abdominal incision or with laparoscopy. Once the rectum is identified, a series of posterior stay sutures facilitate opening the rectum in the midline. The rectal incision is extended until the fistula site, usually anterior in location, is found (Fig. 89-18).

Above the fistula, there is no plane of dissection between the urethra and rectum. Therefore, a submucosal dissection must be performed separating these two structures. Silk stay sutures will facilitate this dissection. Uniform traction can be exerted on these stay sutures while dissecting between rectum and urethra for a distance of 6 to 8 mm above the fistula (Fig. 89-19). A plane is encountered that independently separates the urethra and rectum. The urethral fistula is sutured with interrupted absorbable sutures. At this point in the procedure, circumferential dissection of the rectum is performed to mobilize and gain enough length to reach the perineum. Nerves, fascia, and blood vessels outside the circular outer wall layer of the rectum must be divided to gain adequate length. The consequences of this denervation are unclear. Recall that the rectum has an excellent intramural blood supply, and therefore, the rectal wall must remain intact to avoid devascularization of the rectum. If the rectum is entered at multiple sites, however, the potential for ischemia and fibrosis is increased. A tension-free neoanoplasty must be assured after an adequate mobilization. The size of the rectum, the available space, and the limits of the external sphincter dictate the need for a posterior tapering of the rectum. In general, this tapering is not necessary; however, if the rectum cannot be tailored to rest within the limits of the sphincteric mechanism, then tapering should be performed. The tapering is always done from the posterior rectal wall so the suture line does not lie against the suture line of the closed urinary fistula.

After the rectum is dissected and placed in its new position, the fistula is closed, and all bleeding is cauterized, the reconstruction can proceed. The perineal body is first created by reapproximating the tissue anterior to and including the anterior limits of the external sphincter. Electrical stimulation should facilitate localizing this anterior limit. Next, the levator musculature behind the rectum is reapproximated from the cut edge of the coccyx to the posterior limit of the muscle complex. The rectal wall is not included in these bites. The posterior limit of the muscle complex is sutured together with the posterior wall of the

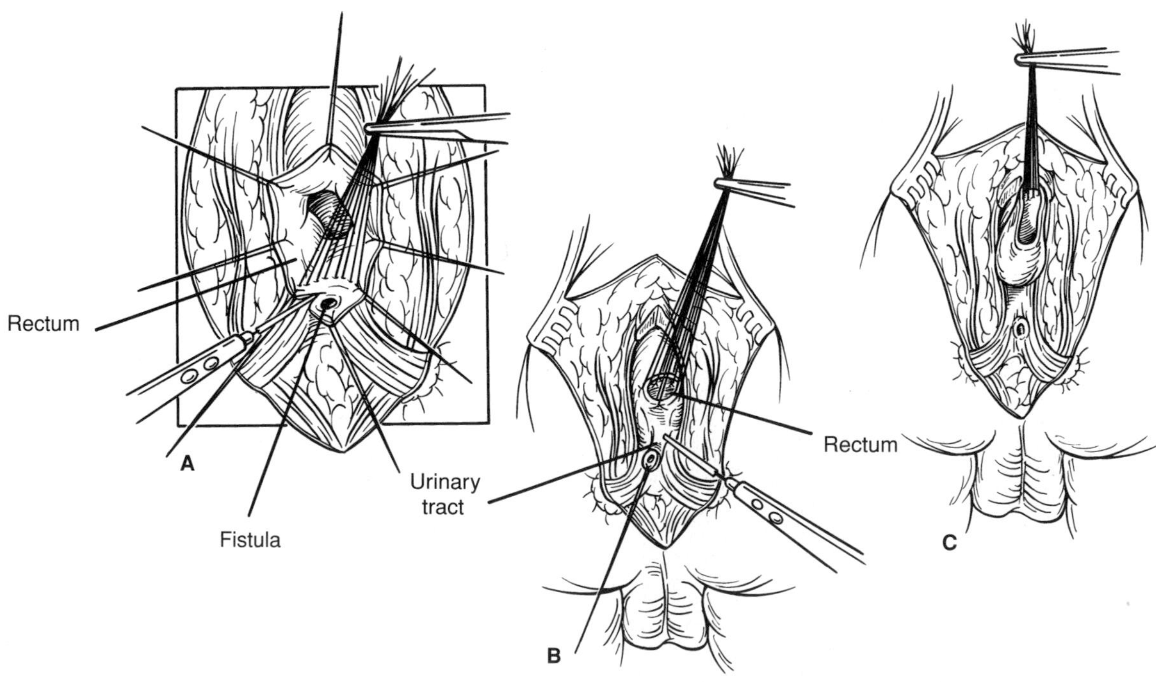

FIGURE 89-19. Separation of rectum and urethral fistula via the posterior sagittal anorectoplasty approach. Traction sutures are used to begin a submucosal dissection (**A**) that ultimately separates the rectum (**B**) from the urinary tract (**C**).

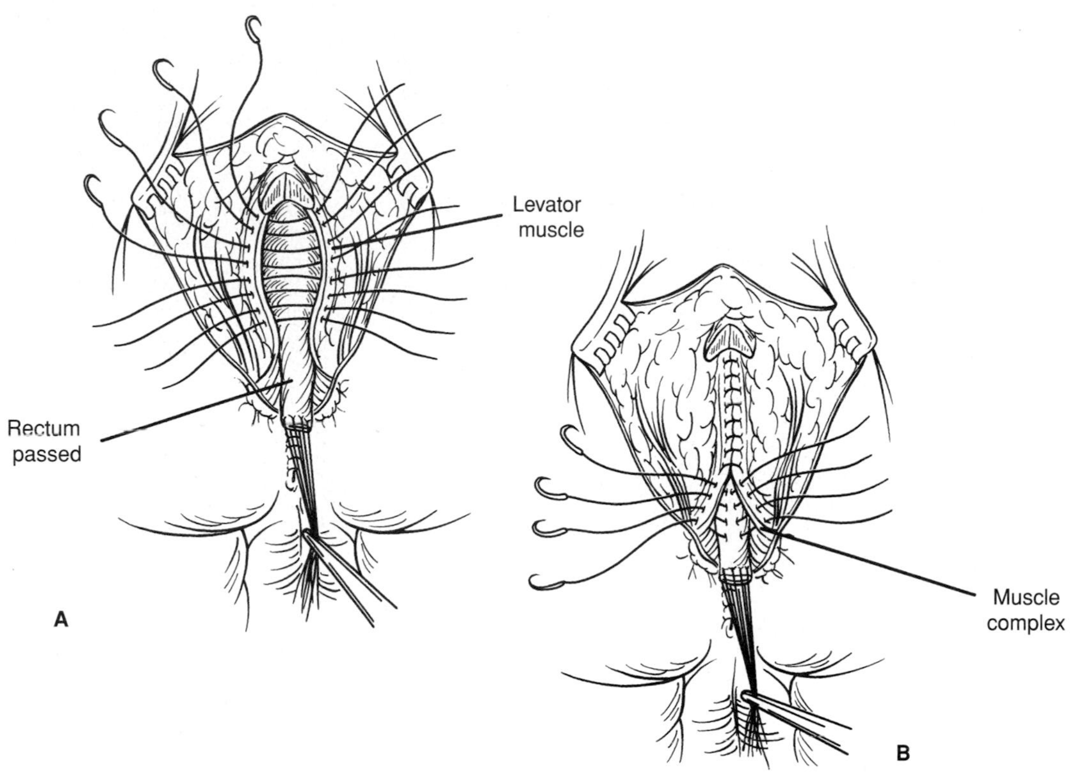

FIGURE 89-20. Suturing the voluntary striated muscle mechanism. (**A**) The levator muscle is reapproximated from the coccyx to the posterior limit of the muscle complex. (**B**) The posterior limit of the muscle complex is sutured to the posterior rectal wall.

rectum (Fig. 89-20). This maneuver usually prevents prolapse of the rectum. The ischiorectal fat and subcutaneous tissue are sutured with careful attention to avoid any dead space. Skin is closed using a subcuticular stitch or interrupted absorbable sutures. Ultimately, the anoplasty is performed using 16 absorbable 5–0 sutures in a circumference that incorporates skin and full-thickness bowel within the boundaries set forth by stimulation of the muscle complex and external sphincter (Fig. 89-21).

Rectobladder Neck Fistula

In the case of a rectobladder neck fistula, a laparotomy or laparoscopy (137), along with a posterior sagittal approach, is required (Fig. 89-6). Therefore, we recommend a total body preparation extending from the nipples, including both the anterior and posterior body walls through to and including both lower extremities. The operation begins by posteriorly dividing the sphincter mechanism in the midline as detailed previously. A red rubber catheter is useful as a marker and should be positioned in front of the levator muscles and in the presacral space, simulating the desired position of the rectum (Fig. 89-22). The surgeon can then elect to reconstruct the perineal musculature, the levator muscle, and muscle complex, and to close the wound as in the case of the rectourethral fistula around the rubber catheter. The patient can then be turned and the abdominal component begun. The sigmoid colon is identified and the dissection proceeds to the bladder neck. In general, the junction of the bladder neck and the sigmoid colon is at most 2 cm below the peritoneal reflection. Usually, there is no requirement for an endorectal dissection. It is important to stay as close to the rectal wall as possible because any lateral dissection runs the risk of damage to the vas deferens and ureters. The rectosigmoid usually narrows as it approaches the bladder and ultimately inserts in a T fashion into the trigone. The rectum is divided, and the bladder is closed with two to three absorbable sutures. Next, the red rubber catheter is found in the retroperitoneum and is anchored to the bowel (Fig. 89-23). If there is significant disparity in the size of the bowel so it appears that the bowel cannot be pulled onto the perineum, then a posterior tapering of the rectum can be performed. In addition, if the mobilization of the rectum is limited by the vasculature, the necessary length can be obtained by dividing the peripheral branches of the inferior mesenteric vessels. The major blood supply to the rectum is via its intramural blood supply. Once the bowel is pulled through the presacral space to the perineum, an anoplasty can be performed as previously described.

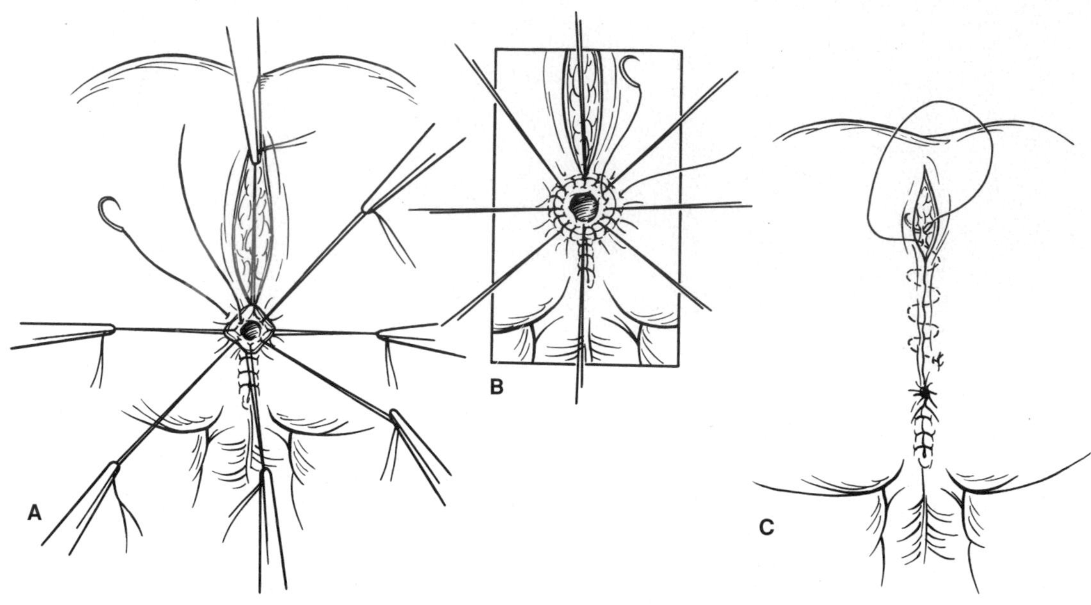

FIGURE 89-21. Anoplasty. The anoplasty incorporates full-thickness bowel to skin and is located within the boundaries of the muscle complex and external sphincter fibers.

Imperforate Anus Without Fistula

In the case of imperforate anus without fistula, the rectum is usually located at the level of a bulbar urethral fistula. Here the rectum is intimately associated with the posterior urethra, and meticulous dissection to separate the two must be performed. The remainder of the operative procedure follows the techniques described for rectourethral fistula defects.

Rectal Atresia and Stenosis

We recommend a posterior sagittal approach for the rectal atresia and stenosis defect. The distal end of the anal canal must be sutured end to end to the blind-ending rectum (Fig. 89-24). In general, the two structures are usually separated by, at most, a distance of 1 cm. Minimal mobilization is required because the upper rectum usually lies very close to the anal canal. A strict protocol of bowel

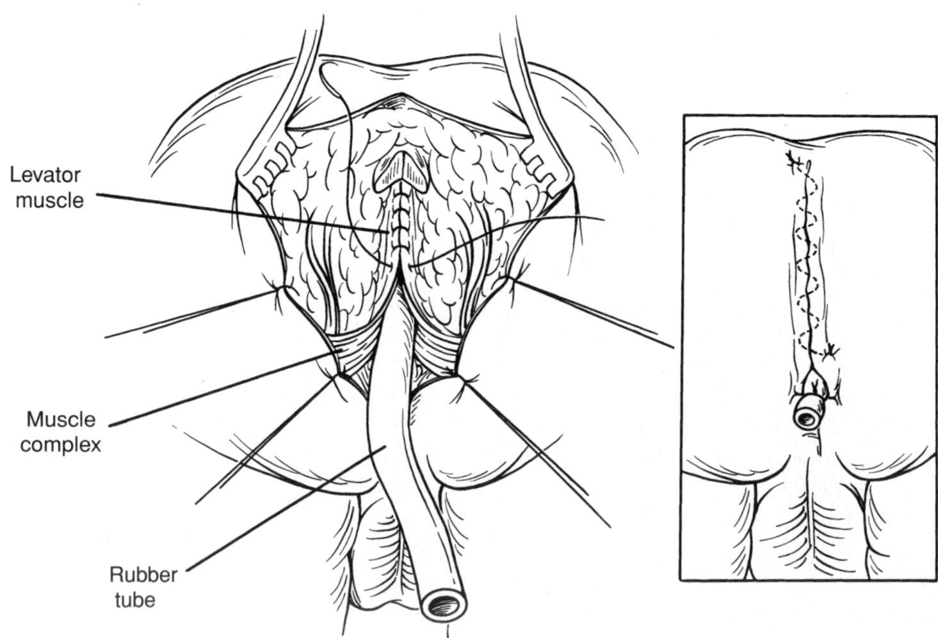

FIGURE 89-22. Posterior sagittal anorectoplasty approach for recto-bladder neck fistula. A catheter can be positioned in front of the levator musculature into the presacral space. The musculature can then be reconstructed, the wound closed, and the child turned for the abdominal portion of the procedure.

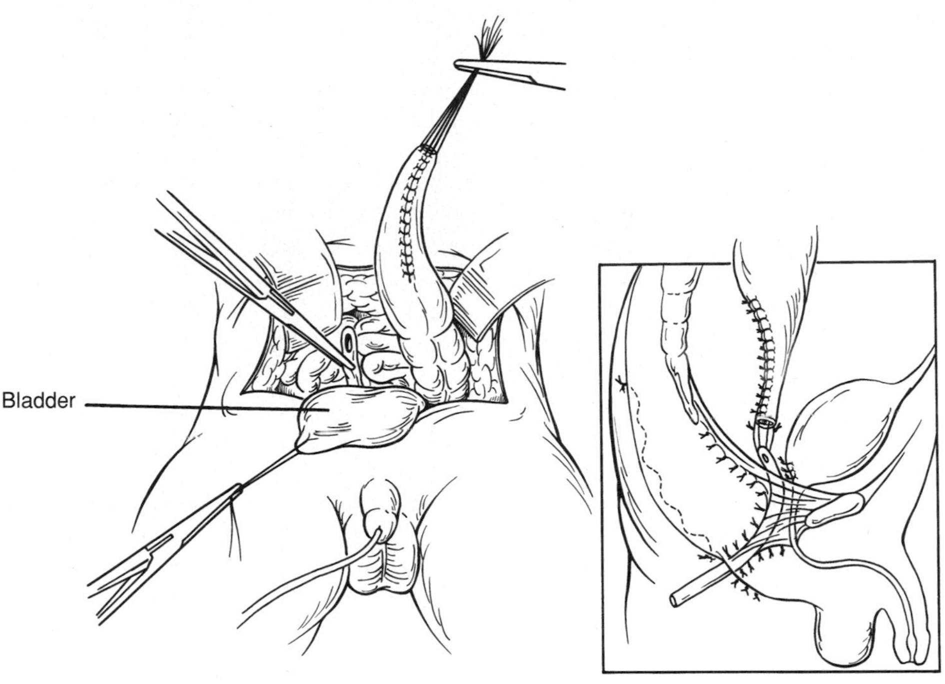

FIGURE 89-23. Posterior sagittal anorectoplasty completion and bladder neck repair. The rectosigmoid usually enters the bladder at the level of the trigone. After dividing the rectum and closing the bladder, the rectum can be anchored to the catheter and pulled through the presacral space.

dilatation must be followed to avoid a stricture because one must remember that after the operation the anastomosis is going to be constantly compressed by an almost normal sphincteric mechanism.

An anterior perineal approach has been described for those malformations requiring colostomy at birth (Table 89-3) (138). In these cases, the entire operation is carried out with the child in lithotomy position. Proponents of this anterior approach contend that visualization of the membranous and bulbar urethra, as well as anterior fibers of the levator muscle, is easily perceived. Tubularization of perineal skin is invaginated through the external anal

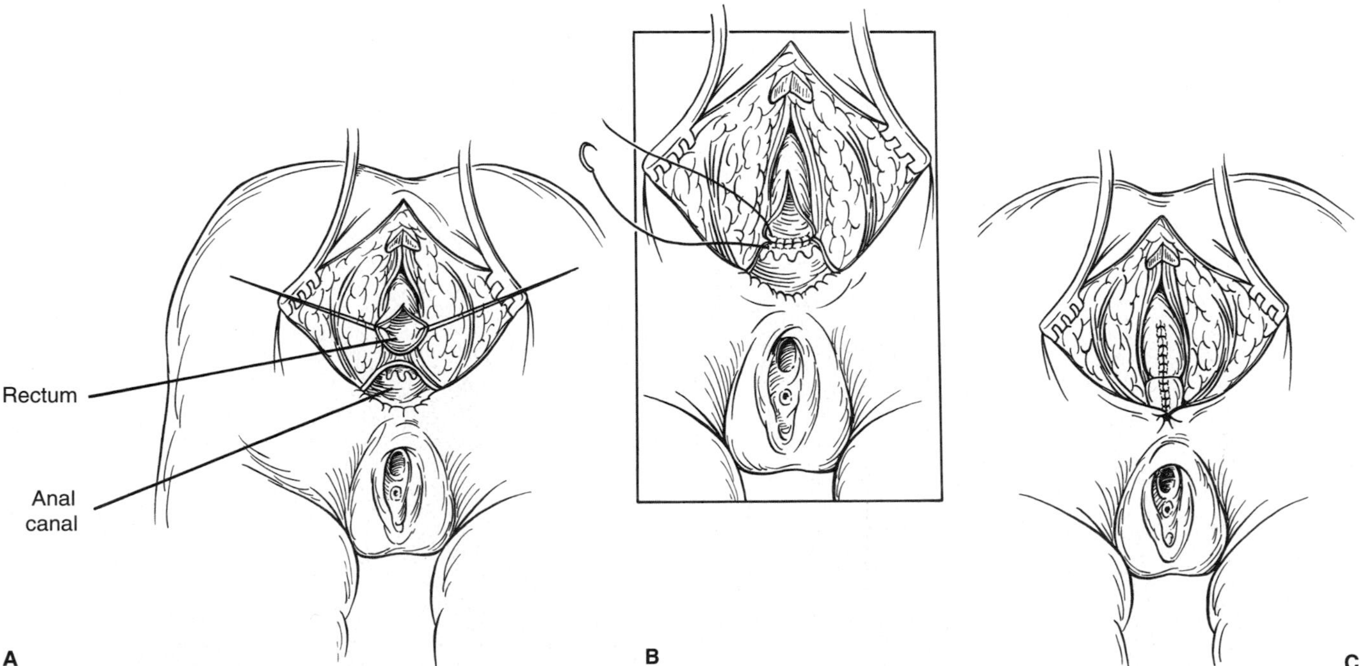

FIGURE 89-24. Posterior sagittal anorectoplasty repair of rectal atresia. The distal end of the bowel is sutured end-to-end to the blind-ending rectum (**A, B**), and then the rectum is closed (**C**).

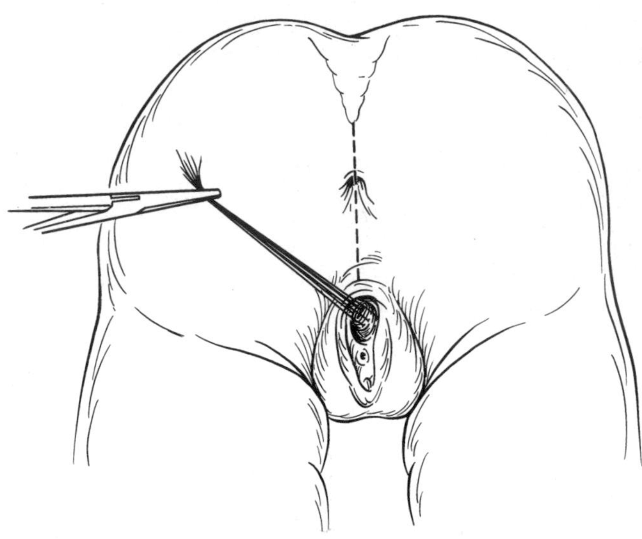

FIGURE 89-25. Posterior sagittal anorectoplasty repair of rectovestibular fistula. This procedure should begin with control of the fistula using traction sutures.

sphincter, and rectocutaneous anastomosis performed. Suture through rectum, levator, external anal sphincter, and subcutaneous tissue anchors the anastomosis.

Operative Approach for Females

Rectovestibular Fistula

There is an obvious disagreement in the pediatric surgical literature concerning the appropriate management of the rectovestibular fistula (139–141) (Fig. 89-7). In part, this is because of a fundamental underestimation of the complexity of the defect. There is no question that this ARM can be repaired without a colostomy, but the functional prognosis should be excellent. Yet, in the absence of a protective colostomy, the repair of the vestibular fistula carries a significant morbidity characterized by wound dehiscence and infection that can jeopardize the final functional prognosis. Therefore, a protective colostomy is advised if the surgeon is not experienced with this meticulous dissection. A PSARP is performed at 1 month of age provided the baby is otherwise healthy.

A limited posterior sagittal anoplasty incision begins anterior to the coccyx and is continued to and around the fistula in the vestibule anterior to the hymen (Fig. 89-25). Multiple 6–0 sutures are placed around the fistula site to exert a uniform traction, and this parachute technique is used to facilitate dissection of the rectum. The posterior wall of the rectum is identified, and the dissection proceeds laterally. Inferior hemorroidal vessels are cauterized as the dissection proceeds laterally. Separation of the rectum and vagina is facilitated by pulling on the stay sutures surrounding the fistula (Fig. 89-26). Anteriorly, there is an extensive common wall between the rectum and vagina, but two walls must be created until complete separation into a definable rectal and vaginal wall plane develops. Tension resulting from too small a dissection predisposes to dehiscence.

Using electrical stimulation, the limits of the neoanus are identified and marked with sutures (see "Operative Approach for Males, Rectourethral Fistula"). A perineal body is restored with one or two layers of tissue separating the rectum and vagina, and including the anterior limits of the muscle complex (Fig. 89-27). The muscle complex is reconstructed by incorporating the posterior edge of bowel in the midline (Fig. 89-27). The levator muscle is usually not

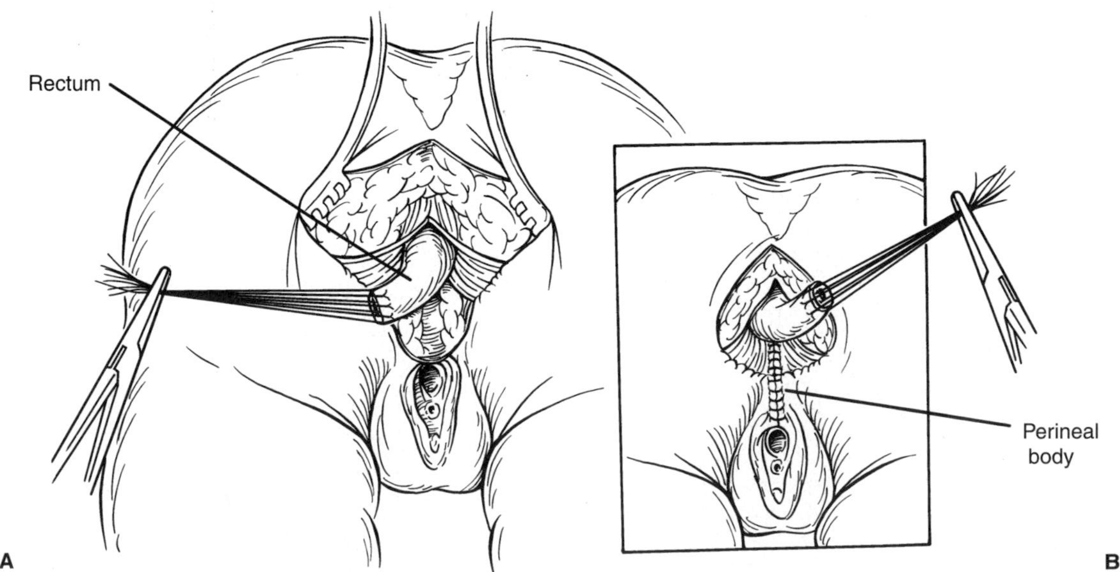

FIGURE 89-26. Separation of rectum from vagina. (**A**) The rectum is separated from the vagina until two common walls exist. (**B**) The perineal body is reconstructed.

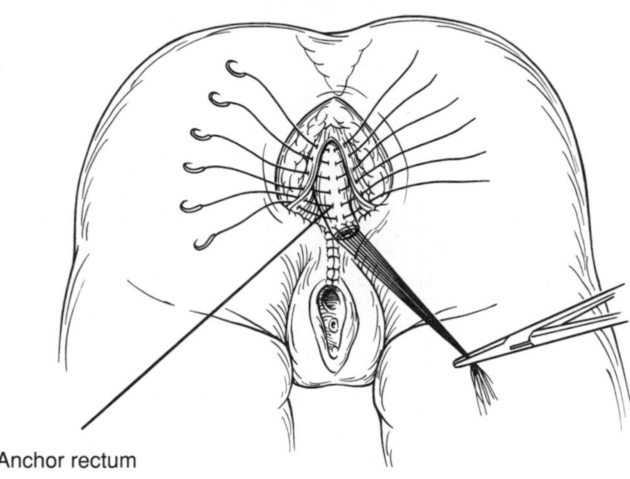

FIGURE 89-27. Reconstruction of the voluntary striated muscle. In these cases, the levator is usually not exposed, instead the muscle complex must be reapproximated and anchored to the rectum.

exposed. An anoplasty and a skin closure are performed as previously described (see "Operative Approach for Males, Rectourethral Fistula").

In cases of the rare vaginal fistula, the dissection is similar, except here the levator is divided because the rectum must be mobilized to reach the perineum.

Persistent Cloaca

The repair of persistent cloaca is the most technically challenging of all types of ARMs (Fig. 89-8). The common channel represents the confluence of urinary tract, vagina, and rectum. The operative procedure begins with a long midsagittal incision extending from the middle of the sacrum through the perineum and into the common single opening. A midsagittal incision is performed, and parasagittal fibers of the external sphincter, then the muscle complex, and finally the levator muscle are divided as mentioned previously.

During the initial experience with this malformation, a posterior sagittal operation, with or without a laparotomy, depending on the complexity of the defect, was used. The rectal wall is opened in the midline distally and held open with stay sutures. The rectum is separated from the vagina (Fig. 89-28), and then the vagina must be separated from the urinary tract (Fig. 89-29). Ultimately, all structures should reach the perineum. The rectum and vagina have a common wall, as described in cases of vestibular fistula. A more complex relation is the attachment of the vagina and urethra; in fact, the separation of these structures is the most difficult part of the operation. The vagina and urinary tract have a more extensive common wall such that the vagina surrounds the posterior urethra about 270 degrees, ultimately creating two cul-de-sacs on either side of the urethra (Fig. 89-29). The neourethra should be reconstructed using two layers of interrupted sutures (Fig. 89-30A). Then the vagina must be mobilized and placed behind the urethra so there are no facing suture lines (Fig. 89-30B). The vagina can be rotated 90 degrees to avoid this. Likewise, any damaged urethral wall should be repaired and again suture lines should not be in opposition. A perineal body should be created after the urethra and

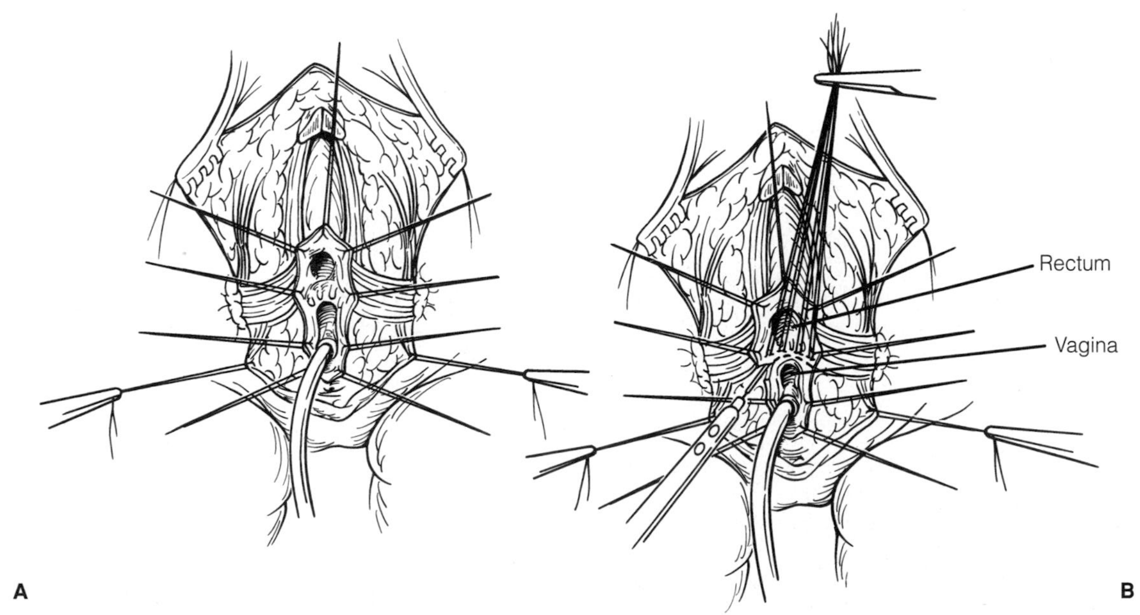

FIGURE 89-28. Separation of rectum from vagina in cloaca. (**A**) Opening the cloaca. (**B**) Separation of rectum from vagina.

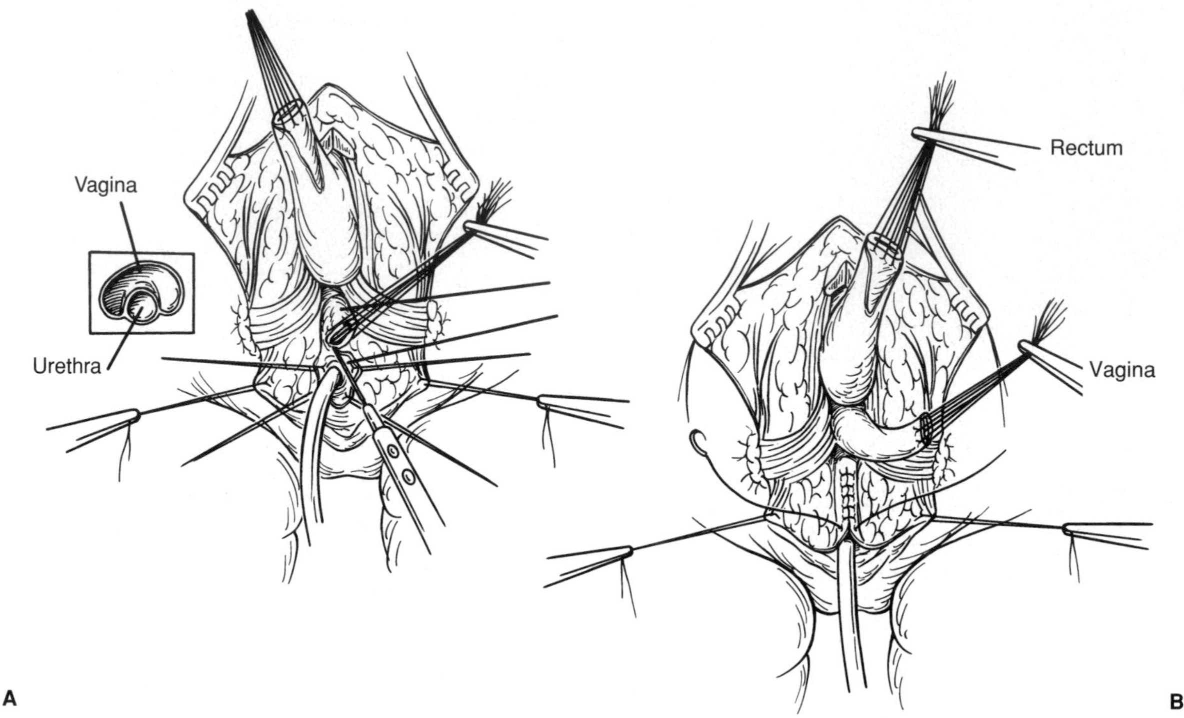

FIGURE 89-29. Separation of vagina from urethra and urethral reconstruction. (**A**) Separation of vagina from urethra. Note how the vagina surrounds the posterior half of the urethra. (**B**) Urethral reconstruction.

vagina have been reconstructed, and the rectum should be situated within the limits of the sphincter and muscle complex, as previously described.

More recently, a maneuver called *total urogenital mobilization* has been employed (142). With this technique, the rectum is separated as previously done, but then the vagina and the urethra are mobilized together as a unit down to the perineum. (Fig. 89-31) This maneuver shortened the operative time by 50% to 70%. The complications of urethral and vaginal strictures were eliminated because the blood supply of these two structures when kept together was excellent, the cosmetic result was better, and the

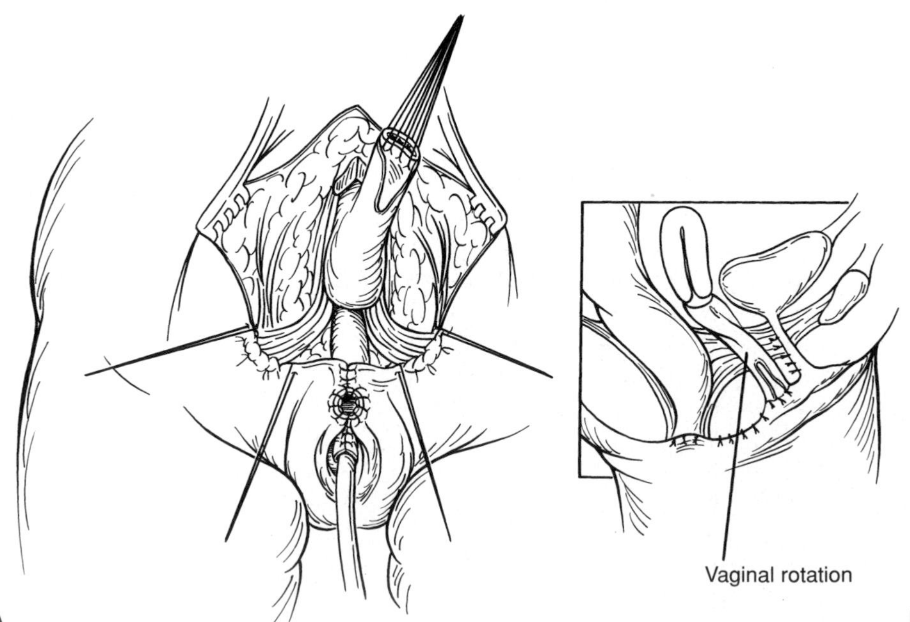

FIGURE 89-30. Neourethra and vagina reconstructed. (**A**) Reconstruction of both urethra and vagina and the limits of the neoanus identified. (**B**) To avoid suture lines facing each other, the vagina is rotated 90 degrees before reconstruction.

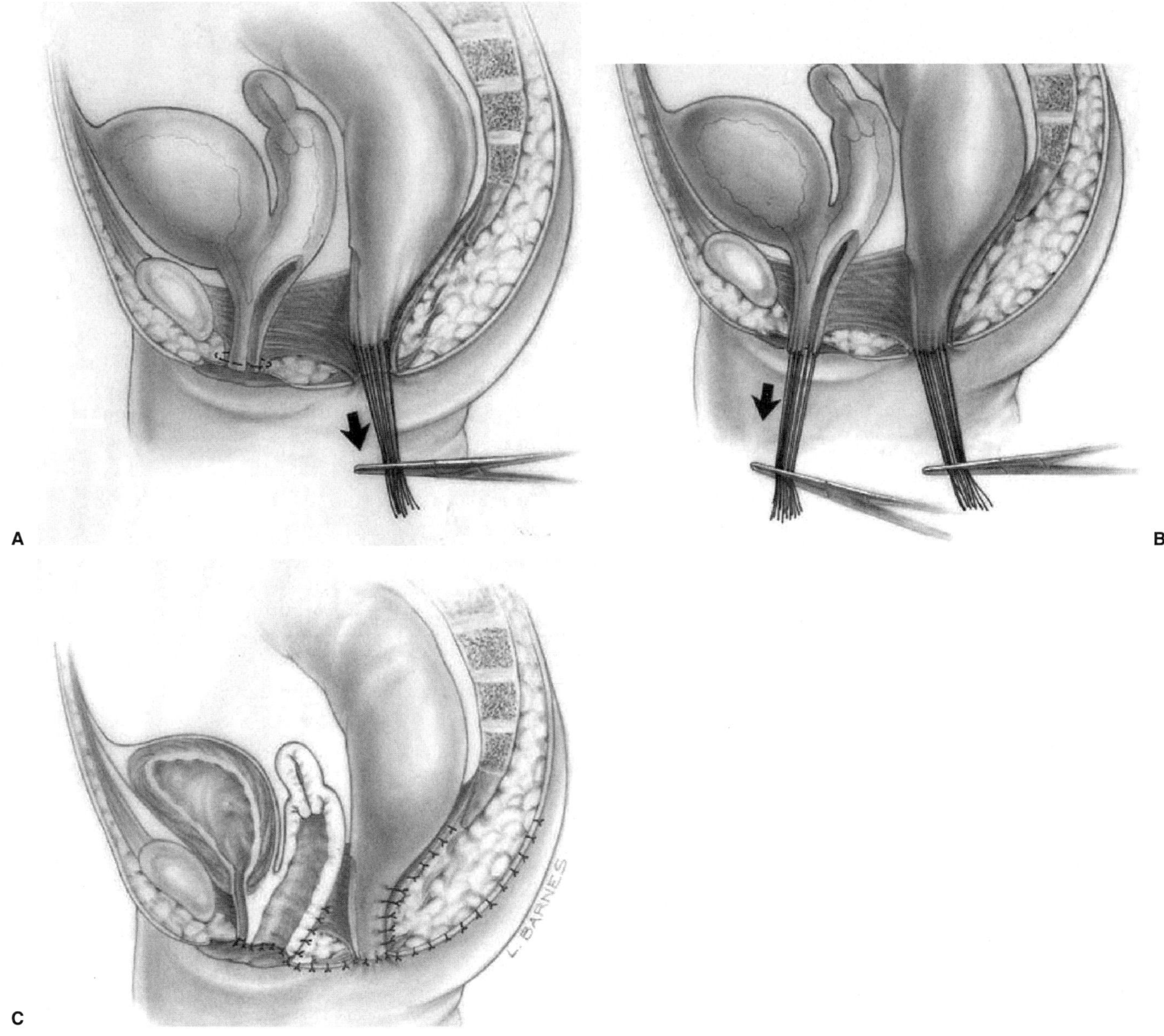

FIGURE 89-31. Total urogenital mobilization. From a posterior sagittal approach, the rectum is separated as previously described, but vagina and urethra are mobilized as a unit (**A, B**). Reconstruction involves suturing the urogenital sinus component and neoanus to perineum (**C**).

functional results were similar to the results obtained with the previous technique.

When a patient has a common channel longer than 3 cm, the likelihood of repairing the entire defect via a posterior sagittal approach alone decreases significantly. Under these circumstances, it is usually mandatory to open the abdomen to complete the repair of the malformation. Once the surgeon opens the abdomen, he or she becomes involved in a complex decision-making algorithm to repair these complex defects. The bladder must be opened, and ureteral catheters must be introduced into each ureter to avoid damage to them because the common wall that separates the bladder from the vagina involves a significant portion of both ureters. The vagina must be separated from the urinary tract, which is one of the most tedious and delicate maneuvers in the repair of these defects, and requires a meticulous technique, finesse, patience, and dedication. At this point, the surgeon must look at the characteristics of the vagina, as well as its size, to determine the best way to repair the genital component of the malformation.

In cases of two large hemivaginas, bilateral hydrocolpos, and two hemiuteruses, the potential for ischemic injury during the attempt to mobilize the vaginas is high. If the horizontal length of the vaginas is longer than the

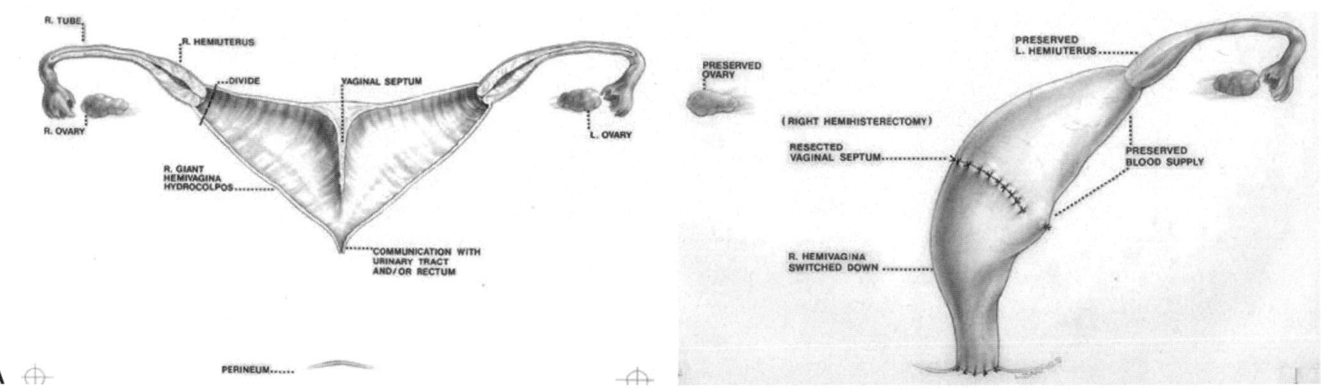

FIGURE 89-32. The vaginal switch maneuver. If the horizontal length of the vaginas is longer than the vertical length, the blood supply of one hemivagina is sacrificed and the hemiuterus on the same side is excised (**A**). Next, the common septum separating both hemivaginas is excised and the vaginas are tubularized into a single vagina that is switched onto the perineum (**B**).

vertical length, the blood supply of one hemivagina is sacrificed and the hemiuterus on the same side is excised. Next, the common septum separating both hemivaginas is excised and the vaginas are tubularized into a single vagina that is switched onto the perineum. This is called the *vaginal switch* maneuver (Figs. 89-32A and B). A vaginal dome flap can be created in those instances where the vagina is very large. This flap off the dome of the vagina can be tubularized to reach the perineum. It is important for the surgeon to have enough experience to determine which maneuver is appropriate for which vaginal anatomy (143).

When the patient has very short vaginas, located very high in the pelvis, then it is necessary to perform some sort of vaginal replacement that can be done with the rectum, colon, or a small bowel, depending on the specific anatomic situation. If the patient has a wide rectum, one can replace a vagina with a portion of it, longitudinally separating the neovagina and preserving its blood supply.

For cases involving vaginal atresia or a small vagina, a piece of small intestine or colon can be used to obtain enough length for the vagina to be situated behind the urethra and reach the perineum (144–146). A laparotomy is performed and a piece of bowel is chosen with a fairly long mesentery so its vascular arcades can be manipulated through the pelvis posterior to the neourethra. The fate of the upper end of the replacement depends on the anatomy. It is either sewn shut as a blind pouch in cases of vaginal atresia or is sewn to the atretic portion of the vagina. The main disadvantage in using bowel to replace the vagina is excess mucus secretions. Skin flaps for any type of vaginal reconstruction should be avoided because of the high incidence of fibrosis, retraction, and scar formation.

When the patient has a colostomy that interferes with the use of the colon or if the patient has a tendency to suffer from diarrhea, then one has to use the small bowel to replace the vagina. On the most extreme end of this spectrum of malformations, one can find patients that have two hemivaginas attached to the bladder neck. In addition, the rectum may also open into the bladder neck. When one separates these structures, the patient is left with no bladder neck. At that point, the pediatric surgeon and/or urologist must decide whether that bladder neck is worth reconstructing, or if the patient would do better with a permanent closure of the bladder neck and opening of a temporary vesicostomy. In the latter situation, the patient will eventually require some sort of continent diversion that usually includes a bladder augmentation, reimplantation of the ureters, and a creation of a Mitrofanoff type of conduit (143).

In a small group of patients with a 1-cm common channel, it is better to repair the rectal component and to perform only a vaginoplasty or introitoplasty without separating the vagina from the urinary tract and,without total urogenital mobilization. The patient is left with a slight female hypospadias, which is clinically irrelevant.

The duration of the operation of the main repair in cloaca patients varies, depending on the length of the common channel and the complexity of the malformation. In patients with a common channel shorter than 3 cm, the operation may last approximately 3 hours, the patient stays in the hospital for 2 days, and the functional results are very good. When the common channel is longer than 3 cm, the patient has a complex malformation with associated defects such as bilateral hydrocolpos, or vaginas implanted in the bladder neck, megaureters, vesicoureteral reflux, hydronephrosis, ectopic ureters, and/or atretic müllerian structures. These operations usually last from 6 to 12 hours (143).

It is extremely important to follow these patients on a long-term basis because of their many potential problems. The patients may suffer from constipation that must be treated aggressively because we know that constipation produces overflow pseudoincontinence. Also, the patients always have the potential to suffer from urinary tract infections. The patients that received some sort of continent urinary diversion are patients for life. They require supervision concerning the metabolic problems inherent to a continent diversion, evaluation of renal function, stone formation, potential development of vesicoureteral reflux, and urinary tract infections.

The patients must also be followed closely looking for gynecologic and obstetric problems. We already detected a significant number of patients who reached adolescence and suffered from the incapacity to drain the menstrual flow. They developed large collections of menstrual blood trapped in the peritoneum due to different types of atresias of the müllerian system (147). We now try to detect these atresias early in life. We intubate and irrigate the fallopian tubes to ensure they are patent. We do this as soon as we have the opportunity to be inside the abdomen in one of these patients either during the main repair or during the colostomy closure (147).

The pediatric surgeon should try to endoscopically measure the length of the common channel as early as possible to try to establish the functional prognosis for the patient, which will help the parents adjust their expectations. From a therapeutic point of view, this will help the surgeon determine whether the patient is going to be treated by him or her alone, in conjunction with a pediatric urologist, or whether the patient should go to a referral center that specializes in pediatric colorectal problems.

POSTOPERATIVE MANAGEMENT

Postoperative ARM children have little pain, except for those who undergo laparotomy. Patient-controlled anesthesia instead of epidural pain control is advisable. In cases of rectourethral or bladder neck fistula, the Foley catheter remains for 4 to 5 days. After a cloacal repair, the Foley catheter remains for 10 to 14 days. Suprapubic drainage may be indicated in cases of cloacas with a common channel longer than 3 cm. Perioperative intravenous antibiotics are given for 2 to 3 days, and a topical antibiotic ointment can be used for the wound. Sitz baths are usually started by postoperative day 3 to 4.

Timing the Colostomy Closure

In general, anal dilatations are started 2 weeks after repair. The operating surgeon should perform the first one, then twice-daily dilatations should be performed by the family or health care worker. Each week the dilator can be advanced by 1 mm in caliber until the desired size is reached. Once the desired size is achieved, the stoma can be closed. Dilatations, however, must be continued twice daily until the dilator can be passed easily. Then dilatations proceed once daily for a month followed by every third day for the next month, twice a week for 1 month, once a week for 1 month, and finally once a month for 3 months. A systematic program of postoperative anal dilatation to avoid anal strictures cannot be overemphasized (Table 89-5).

After closure of the colostomy, children may suffer from a diaper rash secondary to multiple daily bowel movements. A typical paste used for the diaper rash consists of vitamin A and D ointment, aloe, neomycin, Desitin, and Mylanta. Nystatin is added if the rash is the result of yeast. We encourage the use of a constipating diet to add bulk to the stool. The surgeon, however, must be cognizant of the fact that these children were born with no anus and some element of rectal atresia; thus, the major postoperative physiologic problem is a hypomotility disorder of the pulled-through bowel. In the unfortunate situation in which the rectum and colon were resected, hypermotility and intractable diarrhea may be the chief postoperative complaint.

Bowel Training Program

We encourage families of children about 2 years of age with a good prognosis type of ARM to begin a bowel training program (BTP) of using the potty after each meal. If the family is unsuccessful in toilet training by the time the child is ready to attend school, then we recommend delaying the start of school and continuing with the BTP or beginning a bowel management program (BMP) for the temporary period of 1 year. We do not recommend that children with repaired ARMs be allowed to suffer in diapers at school while their peers are toilet trained.

Bowel Management Program

The BMP is designed to keep artificially clean all those children who suffer temporary or permanent fecal incontinence. Therefore, the BMP is usually indicated in children with high defects and poor anatomy. Obviously, children with ARMs have a spectrum of defects, and thus, we should expect a spectrum of results regardless of how impeccable an operation. The basic principle of this program involves cleaning the colon once a day and keeping the colon quiescent (i.e., no motility or little motility) for 24 hours. This is conducted using enemas (Fleet) and colonic irrigations (via Foley catheter using Fleet enema or saline), as well as dietary manipulation and medications (i.e., Lomotil or Imodium). Once the child desires more independence, a Malone appendicostomy can be created (148–151).

RESULTS

The single most important concept in analyzing a series of results is that each ARM has its own set of postoperative problems and outcome. Thus, the authors must stress that expectations of continence in a child with a perineal fistula compared with a bladder neck fistula must be different. In general, results can and should focus on voluntary bowel movements, degree of soiling, and incidence of constipation. Some authors believe that the posterior sagittal approach has not changed the prognosis of children with anorectal malformations (138,152–154). The senior author of this chapter has critically reviewed his ARM patients ages 3 and older and who are at least 6 months postoperative from closure of their stoma (66).

Table 89-6 shows the number of patients who achieved a voluntary bowel movement in each type of defect. Children with a perineal fistula and rectal atresia or stenosis had the best results, followed by repair of the vestibular fistula. Children who had an ARM without a fistula had better rates of voluntary bowel movements compared with those with a bulbar fistula. Ascending to the level of a prostatic fistula resulted in less voluntary bowel movements when compared with the bulbar-urethral fistula. The short channel cloaca is more likely to have a voluntary bowel movement compared with the long channel. The poorest prognosis for a voluntary bowel movement is seen in children with a bladder neck fistula (66).

Children who soil are again related to type of defect. Soiling was not a problem for children with rectal atresia or perineal fistula. It is typically described as a nondisturbing event and is considered normal by parents. Instead, children with high ARMs such as bulbar and prostatic, bladder neck, cloaca, and vaginal fistulas had the highest incidence.

Children who are totally free of soiling and have a voluntary bowel movement are called *totally continent*. Children with perineal fistula, rectal atresia, or vestibular fistula have a higher percentage of total continence compared with bladder neck fistulas.

Constipation is most frequent in children with perineal fistula, rectal atresia, vestibular fistulas, and bulbar urethral fistulas and less so in cloaca, vaginal, or bladder neck fistulas. This is in contrast to the percentage of soiling that is highest in children with cloaca, vaginal, or bladder neck fistulas.

Thus, in general, children with a perineal fistula, rectal atresia, or stenosis (the low ARM) should have a voluntary bowel movement and be nearly totally continent, yet have a high incidence of constipation. In contrast, the bladder

TABLE 89-6 Global Functional Results.

	Voluntary Bowel Movement		*Soiling*		*Totally Continent*		*Constipated*	
	No. of Patients	***%***	***No. of Patients***	***%***	***No. of Patients***	***%***	***No. of Patients***	***%***
Perineal fistula	39/39	100	3/43	20.9	35/39	89.7	30/53	56.6
Rectal atresia or stenosis	8/8	100	2/8	25	6/8	75	4/8	50
Vestibular fistula	89/97	91.8	36/100	36	63/89	70.8	61/100	61
Imperforate anus without fistula	30/35	85.7	18/37	48.6	18/30	60	22/40	55
Bulbar-urethral fistula	68/83	81.9	48/89	53.9	34/68	50	52/81	64.2
Prostatic fistula	52/71	73.2	67/87	77.1	16/52	30.8	42/93	45.2
Cloaca—short common channel	50/70	71.4	50/79	63.3	25/50	50	34/85	40
Cloaca—long common channel	18/41	43.9	34/39	87.2	5/18	27.8	17/45	34.8
Vaginal fistula	3/4	75	4/5	80	1/3	33.3	1/5	20
Bladder neck fistula	8/44	18.2	39/43	90.7	1/8	12.5	7/45	15.6

	Urinary Incontinence	
	No. of Patients	***%***
Rectal atresia or stenosis	0/8	0
Perineal fistula	0/38	0
Bulbar-urethral fistula	2/85	2.4
Imperforate anus without fistula	1/37	2.7
Prostatic fistula	7/85	8.2
Bladder neck fistula	7/38	18.4
Cloaca—short common channel	5/18	27.8
Vaginal—fistula	1/5	20
Cloaca—long common channel	37/48	77.1

neck, cloaca, or vaginal fistulas (the high defects) have the lowest incidence of voluntary bowel movement and constipation and highest frequency of soiling.

Urinary incontinence seems to be most frequent in children with poor sacrums and a persistent cloaca (66). In general, excluding the persistent cloaca, if a child has a normal sacrum and an isolated ARM, we should expect relatively normal urinary function.

COMPLICATIONS

Table 89-7 lists the complications following PSARP. They can be divided into early and late problems. They should not be confused with functional sequelae of the original ARM, but instead are operator dependent. Early complications include infection and dehiscence secondary to ischemia from damage of the intramural blood supply of the bowel. A neurogenic bladder can be the result of not staying in the midline during the dissection. In cases of long-channel cloacas (greater than 3 cm), a neurogenic bladder may be an unavoidable sequela of the anomaly. Other early complications include transient femoral nerve palsy from defective cushioning of the child's groin. Additional complications include intraoperative injury to the urethra and vas deferens and complete necrosis of a mobilized vagina in the case of a cloaca.

Late complications include vaginal and neoanus anastomotic strictures, narrow introitus (cloaca), urethrovaginal fistula (cloaca), persistent rectourethral fistula, and prolapse of the pulled-through bowel. Postoperative complications following cloacal repair have been markedly reduced with the introduction of the total urogenital mobilization technique. A posterior urethral diverticulum found post-operatively on a VCUG may represent retained rectum. This complication has never been seen following a PSARP. It may cause urinary dribbling despite a normally reconstructed anus and takedown of the fistula. This late complication has been seen after the abdominoperineal type of pull-through procedure.

TABLE 89-7 Complications.

Early
Infection
Dehiscence
Neurogenic bladder
Transient femoral nerve palsy
Intraoperative injury to urethra, vas deferens
Complete necrosis of the mobilized vagina
Late
Anastomotic stricture
Neoanus
Vagina
Narrow introitus
Urethrovaginal fistula
Persistent rectourethral fistula
Prolapse of bowel
Retained rectum

EVALUATION, MANAGEMENT, AND RECOMMENDATIONS FOR POSTOPERATIVE FUNCTIONAL DISORDERS

Problems Following Posterior Sagittal Anorectoplasty

After an ARM is repaired, the goal is fecal continence of the patient. Most normal children become toilet trained between the ages of 2.5 to 3 years of age. Prior to this age in children with ARMs, there are some signs that indicate the possibility for toilet training. Good prognostic signs include 1 to 3 bowel movements per day and no soiling in between, evidence for sensation when passing stool (e.g., pushing or making faces), good quality sacrum, well-formed and contoured buttocks, and urinary control. Early postoperative signs of poor prognosis include constant soiling of stool, absence of any sensation during defecation, dribbling or urinary incontinence, flat bottom, and poor quality sacrum (more than two sacral vertebrae missing).

The most common postoperative sequelae seen in children with imperforate anus following PSARP include constipation, soiling, and absence of voluntary bowel movements.

Constipation

Constipation occurs a few days or even weeks after the colostomy is closed. These children are not close to toilet-training age, so this problem is not associated with continence. Constipation should be diagnosed and treated very early in the postoperative care of a child with ARMs. After PSARP, constipation should be expected, especially with the lower defects (see "Results"), and therefore prevented. Most doctors or parents make the diagnosis of constipation if a child does not have a bowel movement in 4 to 48 hours. However, constipated children frequently have multiple small loose tiny bowel movements during the day, which confuses the parents and physicians. In reality, these children never empty their rectosigmoid colon and may be suffering from fecal impaction. Postoperative constipation is believed to be caused by a hypomotility disorder of the ectatic rectum. Iatrogenic causes of postoperative constipation following PSARP include loop and transverse colostomies that allow passage of stool into the distal segment of bowel, as well as delays in definitive PSARP repair (i.e., operation 1 year after creation of the colostomy). If untreated, hypomotility results in incomplete emptying of the rectosigmoid colon, constipation, and impaction.

Denervation of the rectal pouch, provoked by its dissection and mobilization, and tapering of the rectum have been invoked as causes of constipation. This proved not to be the case in our series, however (66,91). Instead, we have seen post-PSARP constipation associated with lower defects (by definition minimal dissection and no tapering). By contrast, patients with higher defects (by definition more dissection) suffer from less constipation.

Post-PSARP constipation is treated with laxatives. We have found that each child suffers from a different degree of constipation; therefore, the amount and type of laxative regimen must be individualized. In general, we first start with dietary awareness (benefits of fresh fruit and vegetables) and proceed from natural fiber-based laxatives (pear and prune juices, bran) to active medication such as stimulants (lactulose, polyethylene glycol, mineral oil) and cathartics (senna). If by the end of the day the child has not had a bowel movement, enemas are introduced as a last resort. The amount of laxative must be increased daily until we find the appropriate dose for the child, but in the meantime the rectum must be emptied every day by the use of an enema. Once we can provoke a bowel movement using the laxatives, then the child no longer needs to use enemas.

The literature is replete with the use of behavior modification and biofeedback techniques to help keep the colon clean, but these have not been used in cases of constipation after repair of ARM (155,156). The authors have no personal experience with the use of these techniques for ARMs. Biofeedback is dependent on rectal sensation, but because the child must be able to make a response, age is crucial. Anal manometry is helpful for biofeedback techniques (157). Children who are in the process of toilet training, having two to three bowel movements per day and soiling in between, may also benefit from behavior modification techniques.

Soiling

Soiling is either associated with voluntary or involuntary bowel movements. Soiling associated with a voluntary bowel movement should be viewed as a symptom of constipation. Children with a defect that has a good prognosis may soil between bowel movements. This sign must alert the clinician to the presence of chronic impaction. Thus, this type of soiling is usually treated and eliminated with laxative therapy. Generally, these children will respond successfully. Children with involuntary bowel movements and soiling should be considered totally incontinent. In children with a poor prognosis, soiling indicates incontinence and is expected. Because of their original poor prognosis, we recommend a trial of BMP. If this is not successful, we offer the child a permanent diversion or a continent appendicostomy.

No Voluntary Bowel Movements

In children with a poor prognosis, having no voluntary bowel movements, despite a good PSARP repair, this is expected and signifies incontinence. These children can be helped with the BMP (see "Postoperative Management"). In children with a good prognosis, lack of voluntary bowel movements may represent overflow pseudoincontinence secondary to constipation or real incontinence resulting from poor operative technique. Treating these children with laxatives will elucidate the differential problem.

Problem of Fecal Incontinence After ARM Repair

The pediatric surgeon is frequently called in consultation for a child suffering from fecal incontinence after an operation for ARMs performed at another institution. The initial evaluation should consist of a detailed history (including a review of the actual X-rays and pathology), knowledge of the type of operation performed (endorectal, rectosigmoid resection), and physical examination. Accuracy of classification of the original defect facilitates a more realistic appraisal of the prognosis. A physical examination should verify that the rectum is in proper position to describe the contour of the buttocks. Radiographs of the lumbosacral spine should be evaluated for abnormalities, and the sacral ratio should be calculated (see "Associated Anomalies"). A contrast enema identifies a megasigmoid colon and shows exactly how much colon is remaining after the pull-through procedure. The postevacuation film gives an idea of the type of motility that the patient has. An MRI study determines the position of the anus in relation to the voluntary striated mechanism and identifies a tethered cord (158,159). Voiding cystourethrography and kidney ultrasound examination should be performed even if there are no associated complaints or urinary incontinence. This is done because sometimes children have asymptomatic urethral and bladder problems as a consequence of an ARM repair. Finally, a rectal exam should be performed.

A decision-making algorithm for postoperative fecal incontinence is shown in Fig. 89-33. After the children have been evaluated as described, they fall into four major categories.

Incontinence with Bad Prognosis (Not Operable)

The first group consists of patients who have a bad prognosis, and thus, they would not benefit from any type of reoperation. In this group are children with a poor sacrum (more than two sacral vertebrae missing), flat bottom, paucity of muscle, high defects, absence of perineal sensation, poor bowel movement pattern, and possibly associated urinary incontinence. A further reason for not

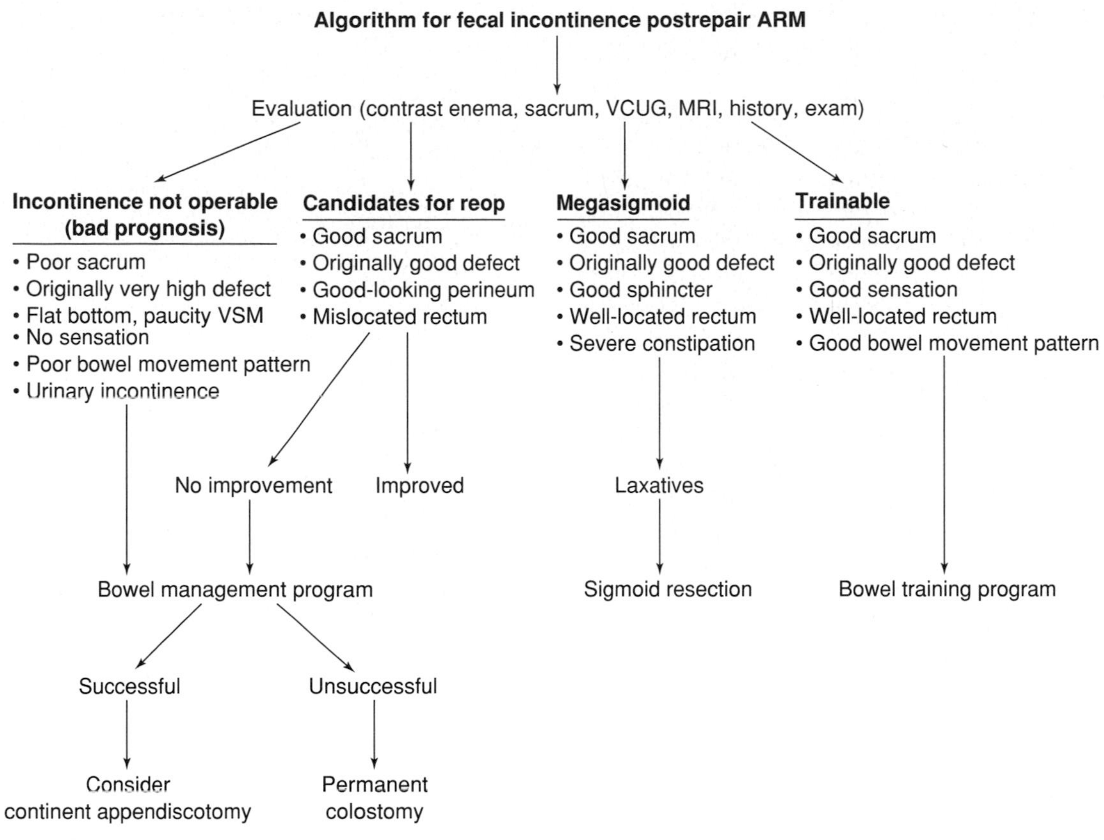

FIGURE 89-33. Algorithm for fecal incontinence postrepair of anorectal malformations. ARM, anorectal malformation; VCUG, voiding cystourethrogram; MRI, magnetic resonance imaging; VSM, voluntary skeletal muscle.

reoperating on a child with postoperative incontinence is the problem of a short colon (i.e., children missing the rectosigmoid colon for whatever reason), which is verified with a contrast study. Children with short colons have an inability to form solid stool, and thus, regardless of the status of their voluntary muscle mechanism, never gain bowel control. This bad prognosis, nonoperable group of children can be helped by a BMP. This program involves teaching the parents to clean the child's colon once daily through the use of enemas or colonic irrigations. The goal is to keep the colon quiescent between enemas.

If the child is incontinent and also suffers from constipation, he or she probably requires only large-volume enemas to remain completely clean for 24 hours. If, however, the child is incontinent and suffers from episodes of diarrhea (resulting from a lost rectosigmoid colon, as occurs in children who undergo an endorectal pull-through procedure), we recommend both a constipating diet and medication to slow the colon. Again, the goal is to keep the colon clean between enemas.

The BMP is successful in 95% of these cases. If the BMP is successful, but children are dissatisfied with the enemas given in the BMP, they may be candidates for a continent appendicostomy as they get older (148,149). In contrast, if the BMP is unsuccessful, as in the case of nonmanageable diarrhea, which occurs in approximately 5% of cases, a permanent colostomy should be recommended.

Candidates for Reoperation

The second group of patients with postoperative fecal incontinence includes children who are candidates for reoperation. These are children with a well-formed sacrum, good-looking perineum, good muscles, and sensation, with a mislocated rectum after repair of a rectourethral fistula in males or a rectovestibular fistula in females. Relocating the neoanus within the limits of the voluntary striated mechanism allows many of these children to become toilet trained. If, however, there is no postoperative improvement, a BMP should be instituted.

Megasigmoid

The third category of patients with postoperative fecal incontinence is characterized by those children with severe constipation and fecal impaction resulting in a megasigmoid colon. This is a very specific group of children who are characterized by a properly located rectum and good sphincters and sacrum, but troubled by severe constipation and subsequent incontinence. The surgeon is consulted for fecal incontinence in spite of the fact that the child should be continent.

Because these patients originally had a good prognosis, there is a strong suspicion that the child is not really incontinent, but instead is continent while suffering from overflow pseudoincontinence. How do we know that a child such as this is indeed continent? Perhaps the child is constipated and suffers from fecal incontinence. These children should first be managed using laxatives. Enemas should be avoided because they will obscure your ability to determine if the patient is continent. If these children are continent, laxative therapy should work and be titrated to avoid impaction. If the child becomes continent, the child and family then have two options. The child may continue laxative therapy for life (provided this keeps the child continent) or undergo a sigmoid resection and thus eliminate or diminish the need for laxatives altogether (91). The resection of the sigmoid (with preservation of the rectum because the child had a good operation and one does not want to eliminate the patient's reservoir) cures or alleviates a great deal of the constipation and makes the child continent. If diarrhea is a problem after sigmoid resection, then we recommend small-volume enemas to keep the colon clean and a constipating diet to decrease colonic motility.

If the child remains fecally incontinent despite resolving the constipation, he or she suffers from real incontinence. In this situation, we take advantage of the fact that the child is constipated (has hypomotility of the rectum), and discontinue all laxatives and use large-volume enemas. Under these circumstances, by keeping the rectosigmoid clean using daily enemas, the child should stay clean because he or she is constipated.

Trainable

The final category includes those children who are deemed trainable. These are children who were born with a good prognosis type of defect and underwent a good, uncomplicated operation. All indications are that they will have bowel control, but they are slightly delayed in becoming toilet trained; therefore, a BTP is indicated.

REFERENCES

1. Amussat JZ. Gustiure d'une operation d'anus artificial practique avec succes par un nouveau procede. *Gaz Med Paris* 1835;3:735.
2. Stephens FD. Imperforate anus: a new surgical approach. *Med J Aust* 1953;1:202.
3. Kiesewetter WB. Imperforate anus II: the rationale and technique of sacroabdominoperineal operation. *J Pediatr Surg* 1967;2:106.
4. Louw JH, Cywes S, Cremin BJ. The management of anorectal agenesis. *S Afr J Surg* 1971;9:21.
5. Rehbein F. Imperforate anus: experiences with abdomino-perineal and abdomino-sacro-perineal pull-through procedures. *J Pediatr Surg* 1967;2:99.
6. Peña A, DeVries P. Posterior sagittal anorectoplasty: important technical considerations and new applications. *J Pediatr Surg* 1982;17:796.
7. DeVries PA, Peña A. Posterior sagittal anorectoplasty. *J Pediatr Surg* 1982;5:638.
8. Carlson B. *Human embryology.* St. Louis, MO: Mosby, 1994.
9. Larsen WJ. *Human embryology.* London: Churchill Livingstone, 1993:369.
10. Duhamel B. Embryology of exomphalos and allied malformations. *Arch Dis Child* 1963;38:142.
11. Hartwig N, Steffelaar JW, van de Kaa C, et al. Abdominal wall defect associated with persistent cloaca: the embryologic clues in autopsy. *Am J Clin Pathol* 1991;96:640.
12. Shenefelt RE. Morphogenesis of malformations in hamsters caused by retinoic acid: relation to dose and stage at treatment. *Teratology* 1972;5:103.
13. Chen Y, Huang L, Russo AF. Retinoic acid is enriched in Hensen's node and is developmentally regulated in the early chicken embryo. *PNAS* 1992;89:10056.
14. Cohen AR. The mermaid malformation: cloacal exstrophy and occult spinal dysraphism. *Neurosurgery* 1991;28:834.
15. Carlson BM. Human embryology and developmental biology, 3rd edition. Mosby: Philadelphia, 2004;363–364.
16. Griffith CM, Sanders E. Effects of extracellular matrix components on the differentiation of chick embryo tail bud mesenchyme in culture. *Differentiation* 1991;47:61.
17. Spemann H. *Embryonic development and induction.* New York: Hafner, reprinted in 1938.
18. Tabin CJ, McMahon AP. Recent advances in Hedgehog signaling. *Trends Cell Biol* 1997;7:442–446.
19. Kimmel SG, Mo R, Hui CC, et al. New mouse models of congenital anorectal malformations. *J Pediar Surg* 2000;35(2):227–231.
20. Mo R, Kim JH, Zhang J, et al. Anorectal malformations caused by defects in sonic hedgehog signaling. *Am J Pathol* 2001;159(2):765–774.
21. Rosa F, Roberts AB, Danielpour D, et al. Mesoderm induction in amphibians: the role of TGF-BZ like factors. *Science* 1988;239:783.
22. Faust C, Magnuson T. Genetic control of gastrulation in the mouse. *Curr Opin Genet Dev* 1993;3:491.
23. Santulli TV, Schullinger JN, Kiesewetter WB, et al. Imperforate anus: a survey from the members of the surgical section of the American Academy of Pediatrics. *J Pediatr Surg* 1971;6:484.
24. Hasse W. Associated malformations with anal and rectal atresia. *Prog Pediatr Surg* 1976;9:99.
25. Kluth D, Hillen M, Lambrecht W. The principles of normal and abnormal hindgut development. *J Pediatr Surg* 1995;30:1143.
26. Paidas CN, Morreale RF, Holoski KM, et al. Septation and differentiation of the embryonic human cloaca. *J Pediatr Surg* 1999;34(5):877–884.
27. Kluth D, Lambrecht W, Reich P, et al. SD-mice: an animal model for complex anorectal malformations. *Eur J Pediatr Surg* 1991;1:183.
28. Danforth CH, Sd. Danforth's short tail, semidominant. In: Lyon MF, Searle AG, eds. *Genetic variants and strains of the laboratory mouse,* 2nd ed. New York: Oxford University Press, 1989:324.
29. Qi BQ, Beasley SW, Frizelle FA. Clarification of the processes that lead to anorectal malformations in the ETU-induced rat model of imperforate anus. *J Pediatr Surg* 2003;37(9):1305–1312.
30. Qi BQ, Beasley SW, Frizelle FA. Evidence that the notochord may be pivotal in the development of sacral and anorectal malformations. *J Pediatr Surg* 2003;38(9):1310–1316.
31. Christ B, Wilting J. From somites to vertebral column. *Ann Anat* 1992;174:23.
32. Duband JL, Durfour S, Hatta K, et al. Adhesion molecules during somitogenesis in the avian embryo. *J Cell Biol* 1987;104:1361.
33. Hamilton WJ, Boyd JD, Mossman HW. *Human embryology,* 3rd ed. Baltimore: Williams & Wilkins, 1962:414.
34. Patten BM. *Human embryology,* 3rd ed. New York: McGraw-Hill, 1968:248.
35. Scott MP. Vertebrate homeobox gene nomenclature. *Cell* 1992; 71:551.
36. Gamer L, Wright C. Murine Cdx-4 bears striking similarities to the Drosophila caudal gene in its homeodomain sequence and early expression pattern. *Mech Dev* 1993;43:71.
37. Krumlauf R. Hox genes in vertebrate development. *Cell* 1994;78:191.
38. Zhou X, Sasaki H, Lowe L, et al. Nodal is a novel TGF-B-like

gene expressed in the mouse node during gastrulation. *Nature* 1993;361:543.
39. Takada S, Stark K, et al. Wnt-3a regulates somite and tailbud formation in the mouse embryo. *Genes Dev* 1994;8:174.
40. Hunt P, Gulisano M, Cook M, et al. A distinct Hox code for the branchial region of the vertebrate head. *Nature* 1991;353:861.
41. Joly J, Maury M, Joly C, et al. Expression of a zebrafish caudal homeobox gene correlates with the establishment of posterior cell lineages at gastrulation. *Differentiation* 1992;50:75.
42. Joly JS, Joly C, Schulte-merkel, et al. The ventral and posterior expression of the zebrafish homeobox gene evel is perturbed in dorsalized and mutant embryos. *Development* 1993;119:1261.
43. O'Rahilly R, Muller F. Neurulation in the human embryo: neural tube defects. *Ciba Symp* 1994;181:70.
44. Duhamel B. From the mermaid to anal imperforation: the syndrome of caudal regression. *Arch Dis Child* 1961;36:152.
45. Griffith CM, Wiley MJ, Sanders E. The vertebrate tail bud: three germ layers from one tissue. *Anat Embryo* 1992;185:101.
46. Van der Putte SCJ. E. Normal and abnormal development of the anorectum. *J Pediatr Surg* 1986;21:434.
47. Kluth D, Llambrecht W. Current concepts in the embryology of anorectal malformations. *Semin Pediatr Surg* 1997;6(4):180–186.
48. Rogers DS, Paidas CN, Morreale RF, et al. Septation of the anorectal and genitourinary tracts in the human embryo: crucial role of the catenoidal shape of the urorectal sulcus. *Teratology* 2003;66(2):144–152.
49. Larsen WJ, ed. Development of the urogenital system. In: *Human embryology.* New York: Churchill Livingstone, 1993:235.
50. Stevenson SS, Worcester J, Rice RG. 677 Congenitally malformed infants and associated gestational characteristics. I. General considerations. *Pediatrics* 1950;6:37.
51. Stephens FD, Smith ED. *Anorectal malformations in children.* Chicago: Year Book Medical Publishers, 1971.
52. Anderson RC, Read SC. The likelihood of recurrence of congenital malformations. *Lancet* 1954;74:175.
53. Jones KL. *Smith's recognizable patterns of human malformations,* 4th ed. Philadelphia: WB Saunders, 1988.
54. Fraser FC. Causes of congenital malformations in human beings. *J Chron Dis* 1959;10:97–110.
55. Stevenson RE. In: Stevenson RE, Hall JG, Goodman RM, eds. *Rectum and anus in human malformations and related anomalies,* vol 2. New York: Oxford University Press, 1993:chap. 20.
56. Reid IS, Turner G. Familial anal abnormality. *J Pediatr* 1976;88:992.
57. Cozzi F, Wilkinson AW. Familial incidence of congenital anorectal anomalies. *Surgery* 1968;64:669.
58. Murken JD, Albert A. Genetic counseling in cases of anal and rectal atresia. *Prog Pediatr Surg* 1976;9:115.
59. Center for Medical Genetics, Johns Hopkins University (Baltimore, MD), and National Center for Biotechnology Information, National Library of Medicine (Bethesda, MD). Online Mendelian Inheritance in Man, OMIM™, 1996. Available: http//www3.ncbi.n1m.nih.gov/omim/
60. Quan S. The VATER association: a spectrum of associated defects. *J Pediatr* 1973;82:104.
61. Temtamy M. Extending the scope of the Vater association. *J Pediatr* 1974;85:345.
62. Kaufman RL. Birth defects and oral contraceptives. *Lancet* 1973;1:1396.
63. Nora A, Nora L. A syndrome of multiple congenital anomalies associated with teratogenic exposure. *Arch Environ Health* 1975;30: 17–21.
64. Blumel J, Evans EB. Partial and complete agenesis or malformation of the sacrum with associated anomalies. *J Bone Joint Surg* 1959;41:497.
65. Peña A. Results in the management of 322 cases of anorectal malformations. *Pediatr Surg Int* 1988;3:105.
66. Peña A. Anorectal malformations. *Semin Pediatr Surg* 1995;4:35.
67. Stephens FD, Smith ED. Classification, identification and assessment of surgical treatment of anorectal anomalies. *Pediatr Surg Int* 1986;1:200.
68. Anorectal anomalies. In: Raffensperger JG, ed. *Swenson's pediatric surgery,* 5th ed. Norwalk, CT: Appleton & Lange, 1990:583.
69. Templeton JM, O'Neill JA. Anorectal malformations. In: Welch KJ, Randolph JG, Ravitch MM, et al., eds. *Pediatric surgery.* Chicago: Yearbook Medical, 1986:1022.
70. Peña A. The surgical management of persistent cloaca: results in 54 patients treated with a posterior sagittal approach. *J Pediatr Surg* 1989;24:590.
71. Gardner E, Gray DJ, O'Reilly R. *Anatomy,* 3rd ed. Philadelphia: WB Saunders, 1966:506.
72. Devroede G, Lamarche J. Functional importance of extrinsic parasympathetic innervation to the distal colon and rectum in man. *Gastroenterology* 1974;66:273.
73. Duthie HL, Gairns FW. Sensory nerve-endings and sensation in the anal region of man. *Br J Surg* 1960;47:585.
74. Li L, Li Z, Hou H-S, et al. Sensory nerve endings in the puborectalis and anal region: normal findings and changes in anorectal anomalies. *J Pediatr Surg* 1990;25:658.
75. Boemers TM, van Gool JD, de Jong TP, et al. Urodynamic evaluation of children with the caudal regression syndrome. *J Urol* 1994;151:1038.
76. Peña A. Figure of muscle complex. In: *Atlas of surgical management of anorectal malformations.* New York: Springer-Verlag, 1989:2.
77. Peña A, Hedlund H. Does the distal rectal muscle in anorectal malformations have the functional properties of a sphincter? *J Pediatr Surg* 1990;25:985.
78. Orr WC, Schuster MM.Clinical applications of anorectal manometry. In: Barkin J, O'Phelan CA, eds. *Advanced therapeutic endoscopy.* New York: Raven Press, 1990:147.
79. Schuster MM, Hendrix TR, Mendelhoff AI. The internal anal sphincter response: manometric studies on its normal physiology, neural pathways, and alteration in bowel disorder. *J Clin Invest* 1963;42:196.
80. O'Kelly TJ, Davies JR, Brading AF, et al. Distribution of nitric oxide synthase containing neurons in the rectal myenteric plexus and anal canal. *Dis Colon Rectum* 1994;37:350.
81. Meunier P, Louis D, Jaubert de Beaujeu M. Physiologic investigations of primary constipation in children: comparison with the barium enema study. *Gastroenterology* 1984;87:1351.
82. Alexander AA, Miller CS, He L, Chen JX, et al. High-resolution endoluminal sonography of the anal sphincter complex. *J Ultrasound Med* 1994;13:281.
83. Jost W, Schimrigk K. *Dis Colon Rectum* 1994;37:697.
84. Zheng L, Hong shen L, et al. Sensory nerve endings in the puborectalis and anal region of the fetus and newborn. *Dis Colon Rectum* 1992;35:552.
85. Ming Y, Zheng L. Electromyography of external anal sphincters in the child. *Chin J Pediatr Surg* 1988;9:31.
86. Altschuler SM. Neurology of the gut. In: Wylie R, Hyams JS, eds. *Pediatric gastrointestinal disease pathophysiology: diagnosis management.* Philadelphia: WB Saunders, 1993:74.
87. Weaver LT. Bowel habits from birth to old age. *J Pediatr Gastroenterol Nutr* 1988;7:637.
88. Orkin BA, Hanson RB, Kelly KA. The rectal motor complex. *J Gastrointest Motil* 1989;1:5.
89. DiLorenzo C. Pediatric gastrointestinal motility. In: Hyman P, ed. New York: Academic Professional Information Services, 1994:215.
90. Li L, Li Z, Wang LY, et al. Anorectal anomaly: neuropathological changes in the sacral spinal cord. *J Pediatr Surg* 1993;28:880.
91. Peña A, El Behery M. Megasigmoid: a source of pseudoincontinence in children with repaired anorectal malformations. *J Pediatr Surg* 1993;18:199.
92. Staiano A, Cucchiara S, Andreotti MR, et al. Effect of cisapride on chronic idiopathic constipation in children. *Dig Dis Sci* 1991; 36:733.
93. Staiano A, DelGuidice E. Colonic transit and anorectal manometry in children with severe brain damage. *Pediatrics* 1994;94:169.
94. Belman BA, King LR. Urinary tract abnormalities associated with imperforate anus. *J Urol* 1972;108:823.
95. Parrott TS. Urologic implications of anorectal malformations. *Urol Clin North Am* 1985;12:13.
96. Rich MA, Brock WA, Peña A. Spectrum of genitourinary malformations in patients with imperforate anus. *Pediatr Surg Int* 1988;3:110.
97. Gilbert J, Clark R, Koyle M. Penile agenesis: a fatal variation of an uncommon lesion. *J Urol* 1990;143:338.
98. Sheldon C. Occult neurovesical dysfunction in children with imperforate anus and its variants. *J Pediatr Surg* 1991;26:49.

99. Kakizaki H, Noromura K, Asano Y, et al. Preexisting neurogenic voiding dysfunction in children with imperforate anus: problems management. *J Urol* 1994;151:1041.
100. Greenfield F. Urodynamic evaluation of the patient with an imperforate anus: a prospective study. *J Urol* 1991;146:539.
101. Peña A. Posterior sagittal anorectoplasty: results in the management of 332 cases of anorectal malformations. *Pediatr Surg Int* 1988;3:94.
102. Peña A. Imperforate anus and cloacal malformations. In: Ashcraft K, Holder T, eds. *Pediatric surgery.* Philadelphia: WB Saunders, 1993: 372.
103. Freedman B. Congenital absence of the sacrum and coccyx: report of a case and review of the literature. *J Surg* 1950;37:299.
104. Currarino G, Coln D, Votteler T. Triad of anorectal, sacral and presacral anomalies. *Am J Roentgenol* 1981;137:395.
105. Sarnat HB, Case ME, Graviss R. Sacral agenesis. *Neurology* 1976;26:1124.
106. Pang D, Hoffman HJ. Sacral agenesis with progressive neurologic deficit. *Neurosurgery* 1980;7:118.
107. Banta JV, Banta JV, Nichols O, et al. Sacral agenesis. *J Bone Joint Surg* 1969;51A:693.
108. Denton J. The association of congenital spinal anomalies with imperforate arus. *Clin Orthop* 1982;162:91.
109. Levitt MA, Patel M, Rodriguez G, et al. The tethered spinal cord in patients with anorectal malformations. *J Pediatr Surg* 1997;32(3):462–468.
110. Karrer FM, Flannery AM, Nelson MD, et al. Anorectal malformations: evaluation of associated spinal dysraphic syndromes. *J Pediatr Surg* 1988;23:45.
111. Davidoff AM, Thompson CV, Grimm JM, et al. Occult spinal dysraphism in patients with anal agenesis. *J Pediatr Surg* 1991;26:1001.
112. Sachs T, Applebaum H, Touran T, et al. Use of MRI in evaluation of anorectal anomalies. *J Pediatr Surg* 1990;25:817.
113. Carson JA, Barnes PD, et al. Imperforate anus: the neurologic implication of sacral abnormalities. *J Pediatr Surg* 1984;19:838.
114. Watanatittan S, Suwatanaviroj A, Limprutithum T, et al. Association of Hirschsprung's disease and anorectal malformations. *J Pediatr Surg* 1991;26:192.
115. Barss VA, Benacerraf BR, Frigoletto FD. Antenatal sonographic diagnosis of fetal gastrointestinal malformations. *Pediatrics* 1985;76:445.
116. Morrison I. Perinatal mortality: basic considerations. *Semin Perinatol* 1985;9:144.
117. Nyberg, DA, Mahony BS, Pretorius DH. *Diagnostic ultrasound of fetal anomalies: text and atlas.* Chicago: Year Book, 1990:chap 10.
118. Guzman E, Ranzini A, Day-Salvatore D. The prenatal ultrasonographic visualization of imperforate anus in monoamniotic twins. *J Ultrasound Med* 1995;14:547.
119. Loewy, JA, Richards DG, Toi A. In-utero diagnosis of the caudal regression syndrome: report of three cases. *J Clin Ultrasound* 1987;15:469.
120. Harris RD, Nybeerg DA, Mack LA, et al. Anorectal atresia: prenatal sonographic diagnosis. *Am J Roentgenol* 1987;149:395.
121. Duenholter JH, et al. Prenatal diagnosis of gastrointestinal tract obstruction. *Obstet Gynecol* 1976;47:618.
122. Rudd N, Klimek ML. Familial caudal dysgenesis: evidence for a major dominant gene. *Clin Genet* 1990;38:170.
123. Pinsky L. The syndromology of anorectal malformation (atresia, stenosis, ectopia). *Am J Med Genet* 1978;1:461.
124. Benzie RJ, Doran TA. The fetoscope: a new clinical tool for prenatal genetic diagnosis. *Am J Obstet Gynecol* 1975;121:460.
125. Potier M, Dallaire L, Melancon SB. Occurrence and properties of fetal intestinal glycosidases in human amniotic fluid. *Biol Neonate* 1975;27:141.
126. Romero R, Pili G, Jeanty P, et al. *Prenatal diagnoses of congenital anomalies.* Norwalk, CT: Appleton & Lange, 1988:233.
127. Landle IM, Hamilton EF. The antenatal sonographic visualization of cloacal dysgenesis. *J Ultrasound Med* 1986;5:275.
128. Carty H, Brereton RJ. The distended neonate. *Clin Radiol* 1983;34:367.
129. Narasimharao KL, Prasad GR, Katariya S. Prone cross table lateral view: an alternative to the invertogram in imperforate anus. *Am J Roentgenol* 1983;140:227.
130. Donaldson J, Black CT, Reynolds M, et al. Ultrasound of the distal pouch in infants with imperforate anus. *J Pediatr Surg* 1989;24:465.
131. Leape LL, Ramenofsky ML. Anterior ectopic anus: a common cause of constipation in children. *J Pediatr Surg* 1978;13:627.
132. Hendren H. Constipation caused by anterior location of the anus and its surgical correction. *J Pediatr Surg* 1978;13:505.
133. Peña A. *Atlas of surgical management of anorectal malformations.* New York: Springer-Verlag, 1990:19.
134. Wilkins S, Peña A. The role of colostomy in the management of anorectal malformations. *Pediatr Surg Int* 1988;3:105.
135. Hong AR, Acuna MF, Peña L, et al. Urologic injuries associated with repair of anorectal malformations in male patients. *J Pediatr Surg* 2002;37(3):339–344.
136. Gross GW, Wolfson, PJ, Peña A. Augmented-pressure colostogram in imperforate anus with fistula. *Pediatr Radiol* 1991;21:56.
137. Georgeson KE, Inge TH, Albanese CT. Laparoscopically assisted anorectal pull-through for high imperforate anus—a new technique. *J Pediatr Surg* 2000;35(6):927–931.
138. Mollard P, Soucy P, Louis D, et al. Preservation of infralevator structures in imperforate anus repair. *J Pediatr Surg* 1989:24:1023–1027.
139. Bliss DP, Tapper D, Anderson JM, et al. Does posterior sagittal anorectoplasty in patients with high imperforate anus provide superior fecal continence? *J Pediatr Surg* 1996;31:26.
140. Zivkovic SM, Kristie ZD, Vukanic DV. Vestibular fistula: the operative dilemma—cutback, fistula transplantation or posterior sagittal anorectoplasty? *Pediatr Surg Int* 1991;6:111.
141. Moore TC. Advantages of performing the sagittal anoplasty operation for imperforate anus at birth. *J Pediatr Surg* 1990;25:276.
142. Peña A. Total urogenital mobilization—an easier way to repair cloacas. *J Pediatr Surg* 1997;32(2):263–268.
143. Peña A, Levitt MA, Hong A, et al. Surgical management of cloacal malformations: a review of 339 patients. *J Pediatr Surg.* 2004;39: 470.
144. Peña A. The surgical management of persistent cloaca: results in 54 patients treated with a posterior sagittal approach. *J Pediatr Surg* 1989;24:590.
145. Hendren WH. Further experience in reconstructive surgery for cloacal anomalies. *J Pediatr Surg* 1982;17:695.
146. Hendren WH. Repair of cloacal anomalies. *Curr Tech J Pediatr Surg* 1986;21:1159.
147. Levitt MA, Stein DM, Peña A. Gynecological concerns in the treatment of teenagers with cloaca. *J Pediatr Surg* 1998;33(2):188–193.
148. Malone PS, Ransley PG, Kiely EM. Preliminary report: the antegrade continence enema. *Lancet* 1990;336:1217.
149. Levitt MA, Soffer SZ, Peña A. Continent appendicostomy in the bowel management of fecal incontinent children. *J Pediatr Surg* 1997;32(11):1630–1633.
150. Paidas CN. Fecal incontinence in children with anorectal malformations. *Semin Pediatr Surg* 1997;6(4):228–234.
151. Peña A, Guardino K, Torilla JM, et al. Bowel management for fecal incontinence in patients with anorectal malformations. *J Pediatr Surg* 1998;33(1):133–137.
152. Langemeijer RATM, Molenaar JC. Continence after posterior sagittal anorectoplasty. *J Pediatr Surg* 1991;26:587.
153. Brain AJL, Kiely EM. Posterior sagittal anorectoplasty for reoperation in children with anorectal malformations. *Br J Surg* 1989;76:57.
154. Smith D. The bath water needs changing but don't throw out the baby: an overview of anorectal malformations. *J Pediatr Surg* 1987;22:335.
155. Loening-Baucke V. Functional constipation. *Semin Pediatr Surg* 1995;4:26.
156. Berquist WE. Biofeedback therapy for anorectal disorders. *Semin Pediatr Surg* 1995;4:48.
157. Orr W, Schuster MM. *Clinical applications of anorectal manometry: advanced therapeutic endoscopy.* New York: Raven Press, 1990:147.
158. Taccone A, Martucciello G, Dodero P, et al. New concepts in preoperative imaging of anorectal malformations. *Pediatr Radiol* 1992;22:196.
159. Sato Y, Pringle KC, Bergman RA, et al. Congenital anorectal anomalies: MR imaging. *Radiology* 1988;168:157.
160. Stevenson R. *Rectum and anus in human malformations and related anomalies,* vol 2. New York: Oxford University Press, 1993:chap 20.

PART F

Liver, Biliary Tract, and Pancreas

Chapter 90

Liver Physiology and Pathophysiology

Edward P. Tagge, Patrick B. Thomas, and Derya U. Tagge

The liver serves a key role in many critical metabolic pathways. As the first organ to receive a nutrient-enriched blood supply from the portal system, it is strategically situated to perform a large number of diverse metabolic functions. In addition, the unique vascular structure of the liver provides unparalleled access to nutrients and xenobiotics absorbed from the intestinal lumen. Processing, redistribution, and storage of metabolic fuels such as glucose and fatty acids are a major responsibility of the liver. Protein production, particularly albumin and the coagulation factors, is an extremely important function of the liver. The liver also contains a host of biochemical pathways for the modification and detoxification of compounds absorbed from the small intestine.

ANATOMY

Morphogenesis

The liver and the biliary system originate from the primitive foregut. The hepatic anlage appears during the fourth week of gestation as a duodenal diverticulum. The hepatic lobules are identifiable at the sixth gestational week, and the cystic duct and the gallbladder are fully recanalized by the seventh to eighth week. The liver reaches a peak relative size of about 10% of fetal weight at the ninth week, dropping to 5% of body weight at birth and eventually 2% in an adult. Early in gestation, hematopoietic cells outnumber functioning hepatocytes in the hepatic anlage. Near term, the hepatocytes dominate the organ, and hematopoiesis is virtually absent by the second postnatal month in full-term infants.

Fetal hepatic blood flow is derived from the hepatic artery and from the portal and umbilical veins, which form the portal sinus. The portal venous inflow is directed mainly to the right lobe of the liver; and umbilical flow is directed primarily to the left. The ductus venosus shunts blood from the portal and umbilical veins to the hepatic vein, bypassing the sinusoidal network. Because the oxygen saturation is lower in portal than in umbilical venous blood, the right hepatic lobe has lower oxygenation and greater hematopoietic activity than the left hepatic lobe. The ductus venosus obliterates when oral feedings are initiated, ensuring all blood traverse the hepatic vascular sinusoidal system.

Ultrastructure

The fundamental unit in the liver is the hepatic acinus, which can be envisioned as a wheel, with the central vein comprising the hub and four to six portal triads representing the rim. The transport and metabolic activities of the liver are facilitated by the structural arrangement of liver cell cords, which are formed by rows of hepatocytes, separated by sinusoids that converge toward the tributaries of the central vein. This relationship establishes the patterns of flow for substances to and from the liver. Plasma proteins and other plasma components are secreted by the liver. Absorbed and circulating nutrients arrive through the portal vein or the hepatic artery, pass through the sinusoids where they are modified by the hepatocytes, and are

Edward P. Tagge, Patrick B. Thomas, and Derya U. Tagge: Medical University of South Carolina, Department of Surgery, Divisions of Pediatric Surgery and General Surgery, Charleston, South Carolina 29425.

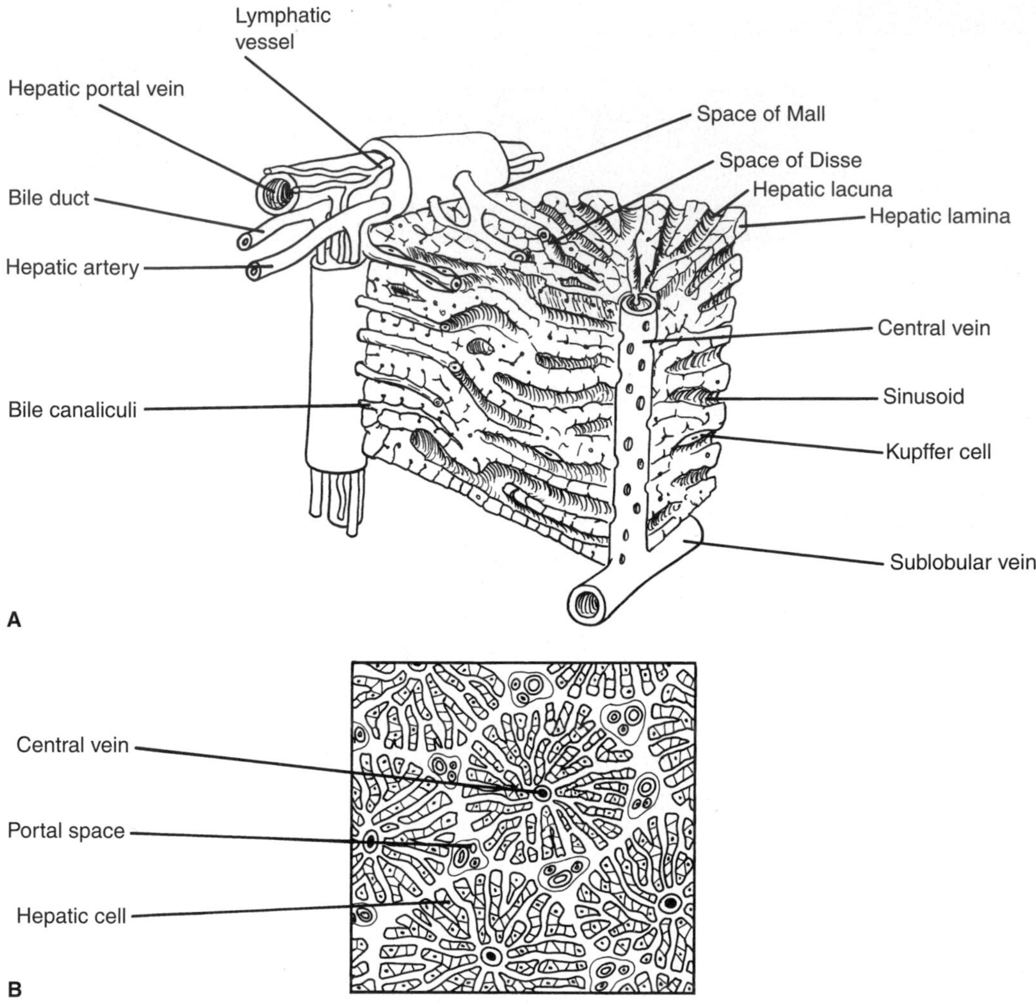

FIGURE 90-1. Liver lobule. (Adapted from Anatomical Charts, Co.)

returned to the systemic circulation at the central vein. Biliary components are transported via the series of enlarging channels from the bile canaliculi through the bile ductule to the common bile duct.

Our understanding of the ultrastructural anatomy of the hepatocyte has been made possible through electron microscopy and cell fractionation techniques (Fig. 90-1). Hepatocytes are epithelial cells that are bounded by three separate membrane domains: (1) the basolateral membrane, which abuts the sinusoidal space; (2) the apical membrane, which circumscribes the canaliculus; and (3) the lateral hepatic membrane between adjacent hepatocytes (1). The liver's unique sinusoidal structure is well suited for the bidirectional transfer of a variety of solutes, including macromolecules, across the sinusoidal membrane. The low pressure allows blood to percolate slowly through the sinusoids and hepatic acinus. Fenestrae within the sinusoidal endothelium and the absence of a basement membrane permit direct contact of the portal blood with the hepatic sinusoidal surface in the space of Disse. Canalicular membranes of adjacent hepatocytes form bile canaliculi, which are bounded by tight junctions preventing transfer of secreted compounds back into the sinusoid. There are abundant mitochondria, which are the sites of substrate metabolism, of key processes in gluconeogenesis, and of storage and release of energy. An extensive endoplasmic reticulum is the site of protein and triglyceride synthesis and drug metabolism. The prominent golgi apparatus is active in protein packaging and possibly in bile secretion.

There are a variety of nonparenchymal cells in the liver, which serve other important physiologic roles. The sinusoidal space houses macrophage-derived Kupffer cells, which are phagocytic cells. These cells are important mediators of the hepatic inflammatory response. The lipocyte, identified phenotypically by its high lipid content, is the major site for vitamin A storage. It is also the major cell type responsible for synthesis of extracellular collagen, and is a critical component of the fibrogenic response to liver injury.

METABOLIC FUNCTIONS

A major responsibility of the liver is to provide a continual source of energy for the body. The liver regulates nutrient flux during periods of nutrient absorption, digestion, and modification for storage. It also makes nutrients available systemically during periods of fasting. The regulation of these metabolic pathways involves complex interactions among the nutrient content of the blood, end products of nutrient metabolism, and hormonal regulation.

Carbohydrate Metabolism

Glucose is the central component of all metabolic pathways because it can be converted to amino acids, fatty acids, or glycogen (the major storage form of glucose). Maintaining adequate circulating levels of glucose is essential for the central nervous system. The brain normally uses glucose as its major metabolic fuel, and hepatic glycogen is the main storage site for the glucose-dependent brain, erythrocytes, retina, and renal medulla (2). The liver serves a key role in maintaining total carbohydrate stores because of its ability to store glycogen and synthesize glucose from precursors (3). Glycogen constitutes approximately 10% of liver weight. The liver can store approximately a 2-day supply of glucose in the form of glycogen before gluconeogenesis occurs. By gluconeogenesis, the liver is able to produce up to 240 g of glucose a day, which is approximately twice the metabolic needs of the retina, red blood cells, and brain.

Immediately after birth, an infant is dependent on hepatic glycogenolysis; thereafter, an infant is capable of both glycogenolysis and gluconeogenesis. The fluctuations in serum glucose concentration in preterm infants are due in part to the fact that efficient regulation of the synthesis, storage, and degradation of glycogen develops only near the end of full-term gestation.

Fatty Acids Metabolism

The liver plays a central role in regulating the body's total fatty acid needs. Oxidation of fatty acids to carbon dioxide and water yields the highest adenosine triphosphate (ATP) production of any metabolic fuel. Fatty acids are thus the most efficient long-term storage form of energy. Fatty acid oxidation particularly provides a major source of energy in early life, complementing glycogenolysis and gluconeogenesis. Newborn infants are relatively intolerant of prolonged fasting, owing in part to a restricted capacity for hepatic ketogenesis. Rapid maturation of the ability of the liver to oxidize fatty acid occurs during the first few days of life. Because milk provides the major source of calories in early life, this high-fat, low-carbohydrate diet mandates active gluconeogenesis to maintain blood sugar levels. When the glucose supply is limited, ketone body production from endogenous fatty acids provides substrate for hepatic gluconeogenesis and an alternative fuel for brain metabolism. Excess glucose can be converted to fatty acid for future use and stored in distal sites such as adipose tissue.

Fatty acids are also involved in various physiologic functions. For instance, fatty acids are constituent parts of various cellular structural components such as membranes. Furthermore, they are involved in regulatory functions in intracellular communication, golgi function, and anchoring of membrane proteins. The liver serves a central role in the synthesis of fatty acid for storage in distal sites and the trafficking of lipids within the body. For lipids to be transferred between different locations, the liver synthesizes a large number of apolipoproteins.

Lipids may be stored temporarily in the liver as fat droplets, excreted directly into bile, or metabolized into bile acids. The liver is the major site of sterol excretion from the body and is the site of bile acid synthesis. The production and metabolism of sterols require complex regulation of multiple enzymatic pathways, and bile acids play a critical role in modulating these enzyme activities. Bile acids are recirculated 20 to 30 times per day via a unique enterohepatic circulation that requires specific active transport processes (4) (Fig. 90-2). In the terminal ileum, a unique sodium-dependent bile acid transporter prevents loss of bile acids in the stool (5), and in the liver the activity of specific transmembrane transporters and intracellular binding proteins are required to capture and recirculate the bile acids. Bile acids also play an important role in micellization of fats for intestinal absorption.

Protein Metabolism

Formation of plasma proteins is a vital function of the liver (Table 90-1). Because protein metabolism is such an important part of liver function, the synthetic capability of the liver is routinely assessed by measurement of specific serum proteins it produces. The liver synthesizes blood coagulation proteins factor II (prothrombin), factor VII, factor IX, factor X, protein C, and protein S. All these proteins undergo a unique, vitamin K-dependent gamma-carboxylation of specific glutamic acid residues, which is essential for normal activity.

More than 95% of serum α_1-antitrypsin (α_1-AT), a member of the serine protease inhibitor family, is synthesized by the liver. Absent or reduced α_1-AT activity is manifested clinically by destruction of the lung parenchyma with the early onset of emphysema. The liver also synthesizes carrier proteins albumin and alpha-fetoprotein (AFP). Albumin functions as a nonspecific carrier protein that binds fatty acids, bile acids, and numerous other compounds, as well as providing serum oncotic pressure that opposes hydrostatic pressure. AFP serves a similar function in the

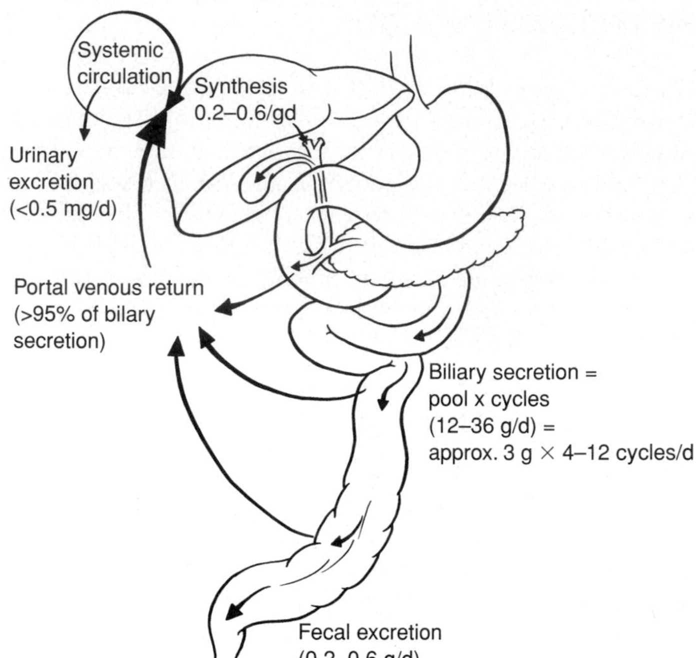

FIGURE 90-2. Enterohepatic circulation of bile acids. (From Carey MC. The enterohepatic circulation. In: Arias IM, Popper H, Schacter D, et al., ed. *The liver: biology and pathobiology*. New York: Raven Press, 1982:430, with permission.)

TABLE 90-1 Important Proteins Produced by the Liver.

Category	*Protein*	*Function*
Coagulation proteins	Fibrinogen (factor 1)	Forms fibrin
	Prothrombin (factor II)	Converts fibrinogen to fibrin
	Factors V, VII, IX, X, XI, and XII	Serves as extrinisic and intrinsic pathway
	Plasminogen	Forms plasmin
	Antithrombin III	Acts as protease inhibitor
	Protein S	Acts as protein C cofactor
	Protein C	Acts as anticoagulant
Transport proteins	Albumin	Acts as carrier protein, provides oncotic pressure
	Transferrin	Transports iron
	Ceruloplasmin	Transports copper
	Haptoglobin	Transports free hemoglobin
	Thyroxin-binding globulin	Transports thyroid hormone
	Retinol-binding protein	Transports vitamin A
	Vitamin D-binding protein	Transports vitamin D
Acute-phase reactants	α_2-Macroglobulin	Binds endopeptidases
	α_1-Antitrypsin	Inhibits serine proteases
	C-reactive protein	Modifies inflammation
Lipoprotein metabolism	Apolipoprotein AI and AII	Acts as Lecithin cholesterol acyltransferase (LCAT) cofactors
	Apolipoprotein CI, CII, and CIII	Inhibits binding to liver
	Apolipoprotein E	Recognizes receptor
	Apo B100	Synthesizes and secretes very low-density lipoprotein

developing organism. Synthesis of albumin appears at approximately the seventh and eighth gestational week and increases in inverse proportion to that of AFP, which is a dominant fetal protein. By the third and fourth month of gestation, the fetal liver is able to produce each of the major protein classes, at concentrations considerably below those achieved at maturity. AFP is entirely replaced by serum albumin at the end of the first year of life. During liver regeneration, as in acute viral hepatitis, and in liver tumors such as hepatoblastoma and hepatocellular carcinoma, serum AFP levels may be elevated.

Biotransformation

The liver plays a major role in the biotransformation of drugs, particularly those poorly excreted in the urine. This occurs in two phases. Phase I uses microsomal enzymes such as the cytochrome P450 enzymes to make the drugs more polar. In phase II, the drugs are conjugated with other moieties to facilitate their excretion in bile or urine. Newborn infants have a decreased capacity to metabolize metabolic byproducts and detoxify certain drugs, owing to underdevelopment of these hepatic enzyme systems. For example, newborn infants have decreased activity of uridine diphosphate (UDP)-glucuronyl transferase (rate-limiting enzyme in bilirubin excretion), which converts unconjugated bilirubin to the readily excreted glucuronide conjugate. Microsomal activity can be stimulated by the administration of phenobarbital or other inducers of cytochrome P450.

Hepatic Excretory Function

Bile acids are the major product of degradation of cholesterol, and their secretion is the major determinant of bile flow. Incorporation of bile acids into micelles with cholesterol and phospholipid creates an efficient vehicle for solubilization and intestinal absorption of lipophilic compounds, such as dietary fats and fat-soluble vitamins. The primary bile acids, cholic acid and chenodeoxycholic acid, are synthesized in the liver. In response to a meal, contraction of the gallbladder delivers bile acids to the intestine. After mediating fat digestion, the bile acids enter the enterohepatic recirculation as described previously. Bile acids are reabsorbed from the terminal ileum and returned to the liver via portal blood, where they are taken up by liver cells and reexcreted in bile. In an adult, this enterohepatic circulation involves 90% to 95% of the circulating bile acid pool. Bile acids that escape ileal reabsorption reach the colon, where the bacterial flora, through dehydroxylation and deconjugation, produces the secondary bile acids, deoxycholate and lithocholate.

Neonates have inefficient ileal reabsorption and a low rate of hepatic clearance of bile acids from portal blood. The latter results in elevated serum concentrations of bile acids in healthy newborns, often to levels that would suggest liver disease in older individuals. The size of the bile acid pool in a neonate is about one-half that of an adult, and the bile acid concentration in the proximal intestinal lumen is similarly decreased to levels that are frequently below the concentration required for micelle formation (2 mM); accordingly, absorption of dietary fats and fat-soluble vitamins is reduced, but not sufficiently to produce malabsorption. Transient phases of "physiologic cholestasis" and "physiologic steatorrhea" have a role in the nutrition of low birth weight infants, but are otherwise of minor importance.

CLINICAL MANIFESTATIONS OF LIVER DISEASE

Acute or chronic liver injury can reduce the metabolic and synthetic capabilities of the liver, thereby resulting in diverse clinical disorders and a variety of clinical presentations. Liver enlargement, although not pathognomonic, is one of the more common presentations of liver disease. In a newborn infant, extension of the liver edge more than 3.5 cm below the costal margin in the midclavicular line suggests hepatic enlargement. In children, the normal liver edge can be felt up to 2 cm below the right costal margin. The downward displacement of the liver by the diaphragm or thoracic organs can create an erroneous impression of hepatomegaly. Examination of the liver should note the consistency, contour, tenderness, or the presence of any masses or bruits, as well as assessing splenic size. Ultrasonography can often help in evaluating unexplained hepatomegaly.

Jaundice becomes clinically apparent in children and adults when the serum concentration of bilirubin reaches 2 to 3 mg per dL. Bilirubin occurs in four forms: (1) unconjugated bilirubin tightly bound to albumin, (2) free or unbound bilirubin (the form responsible for kernicterus), (3) conjugated bilirubin, and (4) delta fraction (bilirubin covalently bound to albumin). Jaundice may reflect accumulation of either unconjugated or conjugated bilirubin. An increase in unconjugated bilirubin may indicate increased production, hemolysis, reduced hepatic removal, or altered metabolism of bilirubin. Significant accumulations of conjugated bilirubin (more than 20% of total) reflect decreased excretion by damaged hepatic parenchymal cells or disease of biliary tract. Cholestasis is a more general term, defined as accumulation in serum of substances normally excreted in bile, such as bilirubin, cholesterol, bile acids, and trace elements.

Cirrhosis is an advanced form of liver disease, and may result from hepatitis, toxic injury, or chronic biliary obstruction. Cirrhosis is defined histologically by the presence of bands of fibrous tissue linking portal areas, thus forming parenchymal nodules. Cirrhosis may be macronodular, with nodules of various sizes (up to 5 cm) separated by broad septa, or micronodular, with nodules of uniform size (less than 1 cm) separated by fine septa. The progressive scarring of cirrhosis leads to altered hepatic blood flow, further impairing liver cell function and causing the development of portal hypertension (PH).

PH is defined as an increase in portal venous pressure to greater than 20 mm Hg. Because the portal vein drains the splanchnic area into the hepatic sinusoids, pressure is normally slightly higher (5 to 10 mm Hg) in the portal vein than in other venous systems in order to overcome the resistance of the sinusoidal system. However, in liver disease, a combination of increased hepatic resistance and increased circulating blood volume can lead to hypertension in the portal system, manifesting as gastrointestinal (GI) bleeding at points of portosystemic collaterals.

Ascites is a common manifestation of end-stage liver disease. In patients with significant hepatic disease, sinusoidal blockade caused by cirrhosis increases hydrostatic pressure and transudation of fluid.

Metabolic abnormalities may complicate acute or chronic liver disorders, leading to encephalopathy. This neuropsychiatric disturbance can present in a variety of ways, including restless, altered mentation, varying levels of consciousness, or even coma. With chronic liver disease, hepatic encephalopathy may be recurrent, precipitated by bleeding, infection, drugs or electrolyte and acid–base disturbances.

There is a close relationship between hepatic and renal dysfunction. Systemic disease may affect both organs individually and/or simultaneously, or parenchymal liver disease may produce secondary impairment of renal function. Hepatorenal syndrome is defined as renal failure in a patient with cirrhosis and no other demonstrable cause of renal failure. The pathophysiology is poorly defined, but seems to involve altered hormonal metabolism that leads to abnormalities of renal blood flow.

EVALUATION OF LIVER DISEASE

Adequate evaluation of a child with suspected liver disease starts with an accurate history and a careful physical examination. Further evaluation is aided by judicious selection of diagnostic tests, followed by imaging studies and potentially a liver biopsy. Any single biochemical assay provides limited information, which must be placed in the context of the entire clinical picture.

Biochemical Liver Tests

The liver performs a diverse array of biochemical, synthetic, and excretory functions, and as a result, no single biochemical test is capable of providing an accurate assessment of hepatic function. Biochemical liver tests have limited sensitivity and specificity, and do not all reflect liver function as the common misnomer "liver function tests" implies (6).

The aminotransferases include aspartate aminotransferase (AST, formerly SGOT) and alanine aminotransferase (ALT, formerly SGPT). These enzymes are elevated in many forms of liver disease, especially those that are associated with significant hepatocyte necrosis, such as seen in ischemic injury. Although ALT is relatively liver specific, AST is also found in skeletal and cardiac muscle, kidney, brain, pancreas, and blood cells. Lactate dehydrogenase (LDH) is a very nonspecific assay, as elevated levels are seen with skeletal or cardiac muscle injury, hemolysis, stroke, and renal infarction, in addition to acute and chronic liver disease.

Alkaline phosphatase (AP) comprises a group of enzymes present in a large variety of tissues, particularly bone and liver. Elevation of AP in the setting of liver disease results from increased synthesis and from release of the enzyme into serum, rather than from impaired biliary secretion. Levels of AP up to three times normal are relatively nonspecific. Because marked elevations of AP can be seen with both infiltrative hepatic disorders and biliary obstruction (intra- or extrahepatic), the level of AP cannot be used to distinguish between them. Elevation of AP is commonly seen in neonatal liver disease of various causes. Hepatic gamma glutamyl transpeptidase (GGTP) is derived from hepatocytes and biliary epithelia. Like AP, GGTP is found in the liver and many extrahepatic tissues, including the kidney and pancreas. However, it is not found in appreciable quantities in bone, and it is thus helpful in confirming the hepatic origin of an elevated AP level. The normal serum GGTP level is significantly higher in infants than in adults. Benign recurrent intrahepatic cholestasis and Byler's syndrome, both rare cholestatic liver diseases that often present in infancy, are characterized by elevation of the serum AP without an elevated GGTP.

Bilirubin is an organic anion that is derived primarily from the catabolism of hemoglobin. Serum bilirubin consists of two major forms, a water-soluble, conjugated, "direct" fraction and a lipid-soluble, unconjugated, "indirect" fraction. The serum bilirubin level is normally almost entirely unconjugated, reflecting a balance between the rates of production and hepatobiliary excretion. Unconjugated hyperbilirubinemia (i.e., indirect bilirubin fraction greater than 85% of the total serum bilirubin) results from either increased bilirubin production (most likely by hemolysis) or from defects in hepatic uptake or conjugation. Conjugated hyperbilirubinemia (i.e., direct bilirubin fraction greater than 50% of the total serum bilirubin) occurs as a result of a defect in hepatic excretion, with subsequent regurgitation of conjugated bilirubin from hepatocytes into the serum. This impaired biliary excretion occurs in both parenchymal liver disease and biliary tract obstruction (7). Thus, measurement of the conjugated fraction does not reliably distinguish biliary obstruction from parenchymal liver disease. Because conjugated bilirubin is cleared by the kidney, serum concentrations of bilirubin rarely exceed 30 mg per dL in the absence of hemolysis or renal failure.

The liver plays a crucial role in hemostasis. All major coagulation factors except factor VIII are synthesized in hepatocytes (see Chapter 16, Fig. 16-2) The prothrombin time (PT) measures the rate of conversion of prothrombin to thrombin and reflects the activity of several of the factors involved in the extrinsic coagulation pathway, including factors II, V, VII, and X. Vitamin K is required for the gamma-carboxylation of factors II, VII, IX, and X, which is essential for the normal function of these factors. Prolongation of the PT may occur in decompensated liver disease with hepatocellular dysfunction and in chronic cholestatic disease with fat malabsorption and concomitant vitamin K deficiency.

Approximately 10 g of albumin is synthesized and secreted by hepatocytes each day. With progressive parenchymal liver disease, albumin synthetic capacity decreases. Thus, albumin concentrations are believed to reflect one of the important synthetic functions of the liver. However, the serum albumin concentration reflects a variety of extrahepatic factors, including nutritional and volume status, vascular integrity, catabolism, hormonal factors, and loss in the urine or stool. Therefore, a low serum albumin level is not specific for liver disease.

Liver Biopsy

Because the morphologic features of specific hepatic diseases are frequently distinctive, liver biopsy combined with clinical data can suggest an etiology. Tissue obtained by percutaneous liver biopsy can be used for histologic examination, for enzyme analysis to detect inborn errors of metabolism, and for analysis of stored material (e.g., iron, copper). In infants and children, needle biopsy of the liver is easily accomplished through the percutaneous approach. The procedure can be performed safely in infants as young as 1 week, and patients usually require only sedation and local anesthesia. The risk of development of a complication such as hemorrhage, hematoma, creation of an arteriovenous fistula, pneumothorax, or bile peritonitis is very small. In patients with significant liver disease, correction of any associated coagulopathy is strongly encouraged prior to percutaneous liver biopsy. If the coagulopathy is not correctable, liver biopsy under direct visualization is a relatively straightforward procedure.

Imaging Procedures

Various techniques help define the size, shape, and architecture of the liver, as well as the anatomy of the biliary system. A plain roentgenographic study may suggest hepatomegaly. Calcifications or collections of gas may be evident within the liver, biliary tract, or portal circulation.

Ultrasonography provides extremely useful information about the size, composition, and blood flow of the liver. Ultrasound is particularly useful in children because it can be done at the bedside without the need for sedation or general anesthesia. Even in neonates, ultrasonography can assess gallbladder size, visualize gallstones, detect dilatation of the biliary tract, and define a choledochal cyst. In patients with PH, ultrasonography can evaluate patency of the portal vein or demonstrate collateral circulation. Small amounts of ascitic fluid can be easily seen on ultrasound, as can mass lesions as small as 1 to 2 cm.

Computed tomography (CT) scanning provides more detailed information, but is less suitable for use in younger patients because of the small size of structures and the paucity of intraabdominal fat for contrast. When a hepatic tumor is suspected, CT scanning is the best method to define anatomic extent, solid or cystic nature, and vascularity. Either CT scanning or ultrasonography may be used to guide percutaneously placed fine needles for biopsies or aspiration of specific lesions.

Occasionally, direct visualization of the intrahepatic and extrahepatic biliary tree may be required in some patients to evaluate the cause, location, or extent of biliary obstruction. Gastroduodenoscopy with endoscopic retrograde cholangiopancreatography (ERCP) has been performed in children for more than 20 years (8). The technique has been quite successful in managing children with a large number of biliary disorders (9,10). More recently ERCP has even been used in some centers to delineate the extrahepatic ductal anatomy in infants, and has been successful in making a differential diagnosis of neonatal hepatitis from extrahepatic biliary atresia (BA) (11,12). Occasionally, percutaneous transhepatic cholangiography has been used to outline the biliary ductal system in infants and young children. Magnetic resonance imaging (MRI) is receiving increasing attention as an alternative imaging technology; magnetic resonance cholangiopancreatography can be of value in differentiating biliary tract lesions (13).

Radionuclide scanning relies on selective uptake of a radiopharmaceutical agent. Commonly used agents include (1) technetium 99m-labeled sulfur colloid, which undergoes phagocytosis by Kupffer cells and (2) ^{99m} Tc-iminodiacetic acid agents, which are taken up by hepatocytes and excreted into bile. The ^{99m} Tc-sulfur colloid scan may detect focal lesions (e.g., tumors, cysts, or abscesses) greater than 2 to 3 cm in diameter. The ^{99m} Tc-substituted iminodiacetic acid dyes may differentiate intrahepatic cholestasis from extrahepatic obstruction in neonates. Imaging results are best when scanning is preceded by a 5- to 7-day period of treatment with phenobarbital to stimulate bile flow.

Selective angiography of the celiac, superior mesenteric, or hepatic artery may be used to visualize the hepatic or portal circulation. Angiography is occasionally used to define the blood supply of tumors before surgery and is useful in the study of patients with known or presumed PH. The patency of the portal system, the extent of collateral circulation, and the caliber of vessels under consideration for a shunting procedure can be evaluated. MRI and variations on CT scanning can now provide similar information.

CHOLESTASIS

Neonatal Cholestasis

Neonatal cholestasis must always be considered in a newborn who is jaundiced for more than 14 to 21 days; measurement of the serum total and conjugated bilirubin in these infants is mandatory (14). Conjugated hyperbilirubinemia, dark urine, and pale stools are pathognomonic of the neonatal hepatitis syndrome that should be investigated urgently. This neonatal hepatitis syndrome has many causes—infectious, genetic, metabolic, or miscellaneous. These abnormalities give rise either to mechanical obstruction of bile flow or to functional impairment of hepatic excretory function and bile secretion (Table 90-2). Neonatal cholestasis may be divided into extrahepatic and intrahepatic disease. The most important condition in the differential diagnosis is BA because these infants require expeditious surgical drainage. However, differentiation among extrahepatic BA, idiopathic neonatal hepatitis, and intrahepatic cholestasis is often particularly difficult.

The clinical features of infants with neonatal cholestasis provide very few clues about etiology (15). The initial step is prompt recognition of any specific or treatable primary causes of cholestasis, such as sepsis, an endocrinopathy (hypothyroidism or panhypopituitarism), nutritional hepatotoxicity caused by a specific metabolic illness (galactosemia), or other metabolic diseases (tyrosinemia). Recognition of such entities allows institution of appropriate therapy and may possibly prevent further injury. Hepatobiliary disease may be the initial manifestation of homozygous α_1-AT deficiency or of cystic fibrosis. Neonatal liver disease may also be associated with congenital syphilis and specific viral infections, notably echo virus, herpes virus, and the hepatitis viruses. Additional cholestatic disorders include neonatal iron storage disease and inborn errors of bile acid biosynthesis.

BA is a disorder of the infant liver in which there is obliteration or discontinuity of the extrahepatic biliary system, resulting in obstruction of bile flow. Untreated, the resulting cholestasis leads to progressive conjugated hyperbilirubinemia, cirrhosis, hepatic failure, and subsequent death within 2 years. The natural history of BA has been favorably altered by the Kasai portoenterostomy; approximately one-fourth of patients who undergo a Kasai portoenterostomy will survive more than 10 years without liver transplantation, one-fourth drain bile but develop cirrhosis, and the remaining one-half of patients never experience adequate bile flow (16). The portoenterostomy should be performed before there is irreversible sclerosis of the intrahepatic bile ducts; this is before the child reaches 3 months of age (17). BA represents the most common indication for pediatric liver transplantation (18–20).

No single biochemical test or imaging procedure can clearly differentiate clearly infants with BA from those with neonatal hepatitis. Ultrasonography should be carried out because it may detect a choledochal cyst, common bile duct stone, or another unusual cause of dilatation of the biliary tract. Hepatobiliary scintigraphy using iminodiacetic acid analogs after phenobarbital stimulation can be helpful to differentiate BA from neonatal hepatitis (21). Liver biopsy can occasionally provide reliable discriminatory evidence because BA is characterized by bile duct proliferation, whereas neonatal hepatitis has diffuse hepatocellular disease and giant cell transformation. However, unless another disease is clearly diagnosed with these tests, the child should undergo expeditious exploratory laparotomy and intraoperative cholangiogram by a surgeon who has experience doing the Kasai portoenteostomy.

Cholestasis in the Older Child

Acute viral hepatitis accounts for most cases of cholestasis after the neonatal period, although many of the conditions causing neonatal cholestasis may also cause chronic cholestasis in older patients. An adolescent with conjugated hyperbilirubinemia should be evaluated for acute and chronic hepatitis, α_1-AT deficiency, Wilson's disease, liver disease associated with inflammatory bowel disease, and the syndromes of intrahepatic cholestasis (with or without bile duct paucity). Other causes include cholelithiasis (22) and abdominal tumors.

INHERITED METABOLIC DISORDERS

Inborn errors of metabolism encompass a vast variety of maladies with varied presentations and pathophysiology. Metabolic liver disease may present as an acute, life-threatening illness in the neonatal period or may be manifested as chronic liver disease in adolescence, progressing to liver failure, cirrhosis, or hepatocellular carcinoma.

α_1-Antitrypsin Deficiency

Deficiency of α_1-AT is the most common metabolic disease affecting the liver, affecting 1 in 2,000 live births in the U.S. white population. It is also associated with chronic liver disease and hepatocellular carcinoma in adults, and is a well-known cause of pulmonary emphysema. It is transmitted in an autosomal recessive fashion with codominant expression. α_1-AT binds with and promotes the degradation of serine proteases, most important, neutrophil elastase, which are responsible for triggering inflammatory

TABLE 90-2 Causes of Neonatal Cholestasis Syndrome.

Surgically correctable obstructive lesions		
	Extrahepatic biliary atresia	
	Choledochal cyst	
	Spontaneous bile duct perforation	
Surgically noncorrectable obstructive lesion		
	Alagille's syndrome	
Inborn errors of metabolism		
	Disorders of carbohydrate metabolism	
		Galactosemia
		Hereditary fructose intolerance
		Fructose-1,6 diphosphatase deficiency
		Glycogen storage disease (Ia, Ib, III, IV, VI)
	Disorders of amino acid and protein metabolism	
		Tyrosinemia
		Carbamoyl phosphate synthetase (CPS) deficiency
		Ornithine transcarbamylase (OTC) deficiency
		Citrullinemia
		Argininosuccinic aciduria
	Disorders of lipid metabolism	
		Gaucher disease
		Niemann-Pick type C
	Disorders of bile acid metabolism	
		Isomerase deficiency
		Reductase deficiency
		Zellweger syndrome
	Disorders of metal metabolism	
		Wilson's disease
		Perinatal hemochromatosis
	Disorders of bilirubin metabolism	
		Crigler-Najjar syndrome
		Gilbert disease
		Dubin-Johnson rotor syndrome
Congenital infections		
	Cytomegalovirus	
	Rubella virus	
	Herpes virus	
	Hepatitis B virus	
	Echovirus 14, 19	
	Coxsackievirus B	
	Toxoplasmosis	
	Syphilis	
Miscellaneous		
	Idiopathic giant cell hepatitis	
	Cystic fibrosis	
	Hemolytic disease	
	Neonatal hypopituitarism	
	Inspissated bile syndrome	

cascades and activating complement. α_1-AT is normally responsible for more than 90% of antielastase activity in alveolar lavage fluid. Eight percent to 12% of newborns and 3% to 7% of older children with α_1-AT deficiency (PiZZ) present with cholestasis (23). Emphysema develops in all persons with null α_1-AT phenotypes by age 20 to 30 years. Although emphysema is due to uninhibited proteolytic destruction of the connective tissue matrix of the lung, liver disease is believed to result from the toxic effects of the mutant α_1-AT molecule retained within the endoplasmic reticulum of liver cells (24). The prognosis of patients with liver disease presenting in infancy secondary to α_1-AT deficiency is variable; not all patients progress to end-stage liver disease.

Presenting symptoms of neonatal hepatic involvement can include jaundice, slow weight gain, irritability, lethargy, acholic stools, or a bleeding diathesis. Later presentation can include abdominal distention, hepatosplenomegaly, ascites, or an upper GI bleed secondary to esophageal varices. The initial treatment of the patient with α_1-AT deficiency is symptomatic. It has been suggested that breastfeeding until the end of the first year of life may decrease the manifestations of cholestatic liver disease, as may administration of ursodeoxycholic acid. The importance of the use of fat-soluble vitamins, adequate nutrition, and counseling regarding the avoidance of second-hand smoke cannot be overemphasized. Although treatment of α_1-AT deficiency-associated liver disease is mostly supportive, orthotopic liver transplantation (OLT) has been employed as a treatment for patients who have progressed to end-stage liver disease; α_1-AT deficiency is the most common metabolic liver disease for which transplantation is performed. In addition to replacing the injured organ, transplantation corrects the metabolic defect, thereby avoiding progression of systemic disease (25).

Glycogen Storage Disease

More than ten distinct disorders of glycogen metabolism have been described in the literature. The overall incidence of glycogen storage disease (GSD) is estimated to range from 1 in 50,000 to 1 in 100,000. GSD type I, resulting from the deficiency of glucose-6-phosphatase activity, is the most common of the errors in glycogen metabolism. Most patients present in infancy with hypoglycemic seizures and growth failure. Physical signs invariably include hepatomegaly (secondary to vastly increased glycogen storage), short stature, and adiposity. These patients demonstrate mild elevations in serum aminotransferase levels, but generally do not progress to cirrhosis or liver failure. By age 15, most patients develop hepatic adenomas, although adenomas have been described in patients as young as 3 years of age.

Medical therapy includes a formula that does not contain fructose or galactose, with frequent daytime feedings and continuous nocturnal administration (26). As solids are introduced, high-carbohydrate foods should be emphasized. These patients require special attention during acute illnesses that may affect intake or metabolism because they can become hypoglycemic quickly. Liver transplantation has successfully corrected the metabolic error in patients with GSD type I and allowed catch-up growth, even into the third decade. As survival is extended, these patients may demonstrate signs of other systemic complications, such as progressive kidney disease, cardiovascular disease, and malignancy (27).

Tyrosinemia

There are four known human diseases involving enzymatic deficiencies in the catabolic pathway for the amino acid tyrosine: alkaptonuria and hereditary tyrosinemia types I, II, and III. Only hereditary tyrosinemia type I (HTI) leads to progressive liver dysfunction. HTI is an autosomal recessive-transmitted disease with a worldwide incidence of about 1 in 100,000 (28). The enzymatic defect in patients with tyrosinemia has been identified as a deficiency of fumarylacetate hydrolase (FAH). FAH deficiency leads to accumulation of the upstream metabolites fumarylacetoacetate and maleylacetoacetate, which are then converted to the toxic intermediates succinylacetoacetate and succinylacetone (SA). Patients with HTI can present acutely with liver failure or with chronic disease and hepatocellular carcinoma. In the *acute* form, patients manifest liver disease in the first 6 months of life, with hypoglycemia, ascites, jaundice, and a bleeding diathesis. The acute form of HTI is usually fatal within the first 2 years of life due to recurrent bleeding and liver failure (35 of 47 deaths); however, hepatocellular carcinoma (7 of 47) and neurologic crisis (3 of 47) accounted for some deaths (29). Patients with the *chronic* form of HTI classically show similar but milder symptoms, presenting after 1 year of age with hepatomegaly, rickets, nephromegaly, and growth retardation. These patients also are likely to have neurologic problems and hepatocellular carcinoma.

The diagnosis of tyrosinemia should be suspected in any child with neonatal liver disease or a bleeding diathesis or in any child older than 1 year of age with undiagnosed liver disease or rickets. Elevated serum and urine succinylacetone (SA) and urine δ-aminolevulinic acid (ALA) levels are regarded as pathognomonic for tyrosinemia, although the diagnosis can be confirmed with an assay for FAH using lymphocytes, erythrocytes, or liver tissue.

Historically, the treatment of tyrosinemia has been dietary management, based on the restriction of tyrosine and phenylalanine. Dietary restriction has been shown to reverse the renal damage and improve the metabolic bone disease; however, the liver disease progresses. Nevertheless, an adequate intake of these amino acids is necessary to ensure normal growth and development. OLT has become a mainstay therapy for patients with tyrosinemia (30).

Porphyrias

This diverse group of metabolic derangements stems from errors in the synthesis of heme, with many forms associated with primary expression in the liver or direct hepatic toxicity. The porphyrias are usually classified either by the site of major biochemical abnormality or by the clinical features. In five of the porphyrias, the liver is the major site of expression, and in two others, both the liver and bone marrow are involved. The porphyrias are divided clinically into those that are acute, with dramatic and potentially life-threatening neurologic symptoms, and those with only cutaneous symptoms.

The term *acute porphyria* refers to the nature of the neurologic attacks, which are recurrent, dramatic, and life threatening. Abdominal pain is present in more than 90% of patients, followed in frequency by tachycardia and dark urine in about 80% of patients (31). Acute intermittent porphyria is the most common of the acute porphyrias, occurring in approximately 1 in 10,000 people, and in as many as 1 in 500 patients with psychiatric disorders. Hepatic involvement is variable; elevated serum aminotransferase and bile acids levels may be seen, and patients are at increased risk of developing hepatocellular carcinoma (32). The overall survival for patients with acute porphyria is good. Treatment is based on avoidance of drugs and other precipitating factors. Intravenous administration of hematin, a congener of heme, can have a dramatic effect on the neurologic symptoms, especially if given early in an attack (33). OLT has been attempted for several of the porphyrias, with mixed results (34).

Wilson's Disease

Wilson's disease, a disorder of copper metabolism, is a progressive neurologic disease with chronic liver disease and a corneal abnormality, the Kayser-Fleischer ring. Wilson's disease is an autosomal recessive disorder resulting from the dysfunction of a copper ATPase responsible for transporting copper into the secretory pathway for incorporation into ceruloplasmin and excretion into the bile. The incidence is approximately 1 in 30,000. In Wilson's disease, inadequate biliary copper excretion leads to copper accumulation in the liver, brain, kidney, and cornea. Copper, a component of several essential enzymes, is toxic to tissues when present in excess.

The clinical presentation of Wilson's disease is extremely variable. The age at onset of symptoms is usually between 5 and 35 years. The presentation may be as chronic or fulminant liver disease, a progressive neurologic disorder without hepatic dysfunction, isolated acute hemolysis, or psychiatric illness. The hepatic presentation of Wilson's disease is more common in children than in adult patients. Wilson's disease should be considered as a possible diagnosis in any child with hepatomegaly, persistently elevated serum aminotransferase levels, or evidence of fatty liver. Recurrent bouts of hemolysis may predispose to the development of gallstones, and thus children with unexplained cholelithiasis should be tested for Wilson's disease. Unlike other types of chronic liver disease, Wilson's disease is rarely complicated by hepatocellular carcinoma. In patients who have predominantly hepatic disease, evidence of subtle neurologic involvement can often be found. Changes in school performance, dexterity, and even handwriting may be seen. A soft whispery voice (hypophonia) is another early feature of neurologic involvement.

Because a diagnosis of Wilson's disease has not usually been made, fulminant viral hepatitis is usually the working diagnosis. Slit-lamp examination may reveal Kayser-Fleischer rings, copper deposition in Descemet's membrane in the cornea; however, Kayser-Fleischer rings may be absent in 15% to 50% of patients with exclusively hepatic involvement. The laboratory diagnosis of Wilson's disease is confirmed by decreased serum ceruloplasmin, increased urinary copper content, and elevated hepatic copper concentration. Molecular genetic analysis is complex because more than 100 unique mutations have been identified, and most individuals are compound heterozygotes. These patients may respond to chelation treatment with penicillamine (35). For those with irreversible liver failure, hepatic transplantation is curative.

Cystic Fibrosis

Liver disease can be the presenting symptom of cystic fibrosis (CF) in the newborn, and CF-associated liver disease has been associated with meconium ileus syndrome (36). The diagnosis should be considered in any infant with neonatal cholestasis, although only 2% of such patients have CF. Liver disease may become more prevalent as the mean age of survival for patients with CF increases; however, liver involvement is not universal and seems to peak during the adolescent years. The diagnosis of significant liver disease in this patient population can be difficult because the presenting signs are subtle. Hepatomegaly, present in approximately 30% of patients, has been shown to correlate well with the presence of cirrhosis and is often the first finding of liver disease. Liver biochemical test results may remain relatively normal despite histologic evidence of cirrhosis.

Treatment of patients with CF with ursodeoxycholic acid improves the biochemical indices of liver injury; however, conclusive evidence that the drug halts the progression to cirrhosis is not yet available (37). Portosystemic shunts can be effective treatment for patients with PH. Liver transplantation has been performed successfully for patients with decompensating liver and stable pulmonary function (38).

VIRAL HEPATITIS

Six viruses have been identified that produce liver disease as their major clinical manifestation: five are RNA viruses (hepatitis A, C, D, E, and G) and hepatitis B is a DNA virus.

Hepatitis A Virus

Hepatitis A virus (HAV) is an RNA virus that infects per the oral route. Once absorbed in the intestine, the virus reaches the liver, where replication takes place in the hepatocyte cytoplasm. Antigenic detection is possible 1 to 2 weeks after inoculation and persists up to 8 weeks. New virions are excreted via bile to the intestine, where it is shed into the stool in high titers. Because it is relatively resistant to degradation by environmental conditions, the virus is spread easily within a population, with a very high attack rate (80% of those exposed become infected).

HAV results in acute infection only, and the clinical spectrum of disease ranges from silent asymptomatic infection to fulminant hepatitis. Prodromal symptoms include fatigue and weakness, anorexia, nausea and vomiting, and abdominal pain. The development of jaundice and dark urine occurs within 1 to 2 weeks of the onset of prodromal symptoms, although anicteric infections are three times more likely than icteric infections in children (39). Although more than 90% of children younger than the age of 5 are asymptomatic, 70% to 80% of adults are symptomatic. Overall, HAV is typically a benign, self-limited infection, with the majority of patients exhibiting complete recovery within 2 months of the onset of disease.

Hepatitis B Virus

Hepatitis B virus (HBV) is a partially double-stranded DNA that is predominantly hepatotropic. In contrast to classical retroviruses such as HIV, HBV transcripts are synthesized entirely from episomal DNA. Integration of HBV DNA does occur in chronic infection and may be important for hepatic carcinogenesis. In the United States, approximately 1.25 million people are chronically infected with HBV and spread of infection is predominantly by horizontal routes. Adults and adolescents are at greatest risk of infection in the United States because of acquisition from sexual activity, injection drug use, and blood transfusion (40). Although only 1% to 3% of all reported cases of HBV infection in the United States are believed to occur in children, 20% to 30% of all chronic HBV infections in the United States occur in children younger than age 5 years. Infants born to HBeAg-positive mothers with high viral loads have an 80% risk of perinatal acquisition in the absence of interventions. Interestingly, children of HBsAg-positive mothers who are not infected at birth remain at high risk, as 60% become infected by the age of 5 years (41). The mechanism of this later infection is unknown, although breastfeeding is not believed to be an important mode of transmission.

Clinical observations suggest that the immune response of the host is more important than viral factors in the pathogenesis of liver injury caused by HBV. For instance, infants with immature immune systems who acquire HBV infection at birth typically have only mild liver injury. Conversely, HBV-induced fulminant hepatic failure is associated with a vigorous immune response, low serum levels of virus, and massive hepatocellular necrosis. The incubation period of hepatitis B varies from 1–6 months. Clinical presentation varies from asymptomatic infection to liver failure.

Current serologic assays for the diagnosis of acute and chronic HBV infection are both sensitive and specific. In acute infection, HbsAg, indicating active HBV infection, becomes detectable approximately 6 weeks after inoculation, before the onset of clinical symptoms or biochemical abnormalities. Biochemical abnormalities usually coincide with the prodromal phase of the acute illness and may persist for several months. The serum ALT level is typically higher than the serum AST level, and levels of both aminotransferases are usually 500 U per L or greater. Bilirubin elevations are usually modest (5 to 10 mg per dL). With the onset of symptoms, IgM anti-HBc becomes detectable. IgM anti-HBc may persist for many months, and IgG anti-HBc may persist for many years, if not a lifetime. Anti-HBs is the last serologic test to become positive and is a marker of resolving infection.

Treatment of acute HBV infection is largely supportive. The most profound complication of acute HBV infection is fulminant hepatic failure, defined as the onset of hepatic encephalopathy within 8 weeks of the onset of symptoms. Although this complication is infrequent (occurring in less than 1% of cases), the prognosis is poor. If clinical symptoms of hepatic failure develop, patients should be referred for consideration of liver transplantation. Chronic HBV infection is usually defined as detectable HPV surface antigenemia for a period of 6 months or more. The risk of chronicity after neonatally acquired infection is extremely high (up to 90%), and the risk of developing hepatocellular carcinoma (HCC) is markedly increased in those patients. Patients with chronic HBV appear to derive long-term benefit from interferon (42), although patients with PH, variceal bleeding, or hepatorenal syndrome should be referred for liver transplantation. Because of many improvements in the treatment of HPV after transplantation, orthotopic liver transplantation is now the standard of care for patients with decompensated HBV-induced liver disease (43).

Hepatitis C Virus

Hepatitis C virus (HCV) is an important public health problem because it is a major cause of chronic hepatitis, cirrhosis, and HCC. The most striking feature of this virus is its ability to induce persistent infection in at least 85% of infected persons, despite a vigorous humoral and cellular host immune response. HCV is a single-stranded RNA virus. Its modes of transmission can be divided into percutaneous (blood transfusion and needle stick inoculation) and nonpercutaneous (sexual contact, perinatal exposure). Perinatal transmission occurs exclusively from mothers who are HCV RNA positive at the time of delivery (44); the risk posed to the infant from breastfeeding is minimal. In contrast to the high efficiency of perinatal transmission of HBV, the efficiency of perinatal transmission of HCV is low (0% to 10%).

Acute infection is rarely seen in clinical practice because the majority of patients experience no clinical symptoms. Jaundice may develop in 25% of these patients, whereas

10% to 20% may present with nonspecific symptoms such as fatigue, nausea, and vomiting. Infection with HCV, once established, persists in the vast majority of patients. Disease progression is largely silent, and patients often are identified only on routine biochemical screening or blood assay.

The primary goal of therapy for HCV infection is to eradicate the infection early in the course of the disease to prevent progression to end-stage liver disease and eventually to HCC. Interferon-α–based regimens constitute the cornerstone of current antiviral therapies (42). Several trials have shown that treatment with a combination of interferon-α plus ribavirin (an oral antiviral agent with activity against DNA and RNA viruses) results in a higher frequency of sustained biochemical and virologic response than does treatment with interferon alone (45). New formulations of interferon, pegylated interferons, have been developed more recently, which are able to sustain more uniform plasma levels and consequently enhance viral suppression (46,47).

PORTAL HYPERTENSION AND VARICEAL BLEEDING

PH, defined as an elevation of portal pressure higher than 10 to 12 mm Hg, is a major cause of morbidity and mortality in children with liver disease. Although there have been considerable advances in treatment since the mid-1990s, the complications of PH—GI hemorrhage, ascites, and encephalopathy—continue to pose difficult challenges.

Etiology

The causes of PH are conventionally classified according to the localization of the site of maximal resistance to portal flow. The three major categories of PH are prehepatic, intrahepatic, and posthepatic. Portal vein obstruction is the major cause of prehepatic PH in childhood. Umbilical infection secondary to umbilical vein catherization spreads to the left branch of the portal vein, which then leads to formation of thrombus in the portal vein. Fibroblasts transform the clot into a firm, collagenous plug in which tortuous venous channels develop, the so-called *cavernous transformation*. Pressure rises in the portal vein remnant, transforming usually small venous collaterals into esophageal, gastric, duodenal, and jejunal varices. Portal vein thrombosis has also been associated with neonatal dehydration, intraabdominal infections, inflammatory bowel disease, sclerosing cholangitis, and hypercoagulable states, such as factor V Leiden deficiency or protein C and protein S deficiencies. At least one-half of reported cases have no defined cause.

The intrahepatic causes of PH are numerous, with the site of resistance conventionally divided into presinusoidal, sinusoidal, and postsinusoidal. Presinusoidal hypertension can be caused by increased flow, as a result of an arteriovenous fistula or by obstruction to flow, as in congenital hepatic fibrosis. Cirrhosis is the predominant cause of sinusoidal PH and is related to obstruction of blood through the portal vein. There are numerous causes of childhood cirrhosis, including BA, α1-AT deficiency, Wilson's disease, GSD, and CF.

Postsinusoidal causes also occur in childhood. The Budd-Chiari syndrome involves obstruction to hepatic vein drainage, and can occur anywhere between the efferent hepatic veins and the right atrium. Venoocclusive disease seen after total body irradiation and/or chemotherapy is the most frequent cause of hepatic vein obstruction in children.

Pathophysiology

The initial hemodynamic abnormality in PH is increased resistance to portal blood flow. Curiously, despite the development of significant collaterals diverting portal blood into systemic veins, increased portal pressures are maintained by an overall increase in portal venous flow. Clinically, a hyperdynamic circulation is achieved by tachycardia, an increase in cardiac output, and decreased systemic vascular resistance. The increase in portal blood flow is related to the contribution of hepatic and collateral flow; the actual portal blood flow reaching the liver is reduced.

Normal, uncorrected pressure in the portal vein ranges from 5 to 10 mm Hg. Portal pressure is usually expressed as a portal pressure gradient (ΔP) and is most often determined in patients with cirrhosis as the hepatic venous pressure gradient (HVPG). A pressure measurement is made via a catheter wedged into a hepatic vein; this measurement is termed the *wedged hepatic venous pressure* (WHVP). After withdrawal of the catheter tip into the hepatic vein, a free hepatic vein pressure (FHVP) is obtained. The HVPG is obtained by subtracting the value of the WHVP from the FHVP.

Anatomic Sites of Collateral Formation

Spontaneous portosystemic collaterals develop in a number of anatomic sites: (1) squamocolumnar junctions of the GI tract, (2) recanalized umbilical vein, (3) retroperitoneum, (4) and sites of previous abdominal surgery or intraabdominal trauma (Fig. 90-3). Esophageal varices are the most important site of bleeding in PH and are supplied mainly by an enlarged coronary (left gastric) vein and the short gastric veins. They generally achieve their greatest prominence 2 to 3 cm above the gastroesophageal junction and in time may extend cephalad to the midesophagus. The next most common site for the formation of clinically significant varices is the stomach, either in obvious continuity with esophageal varices or as free-standing gastric varices. These superficial submucosal collaterals are prone to rupture and bleed. In addition to varices, the vascularity of the stomach is also abnormal, demonstrating prominent

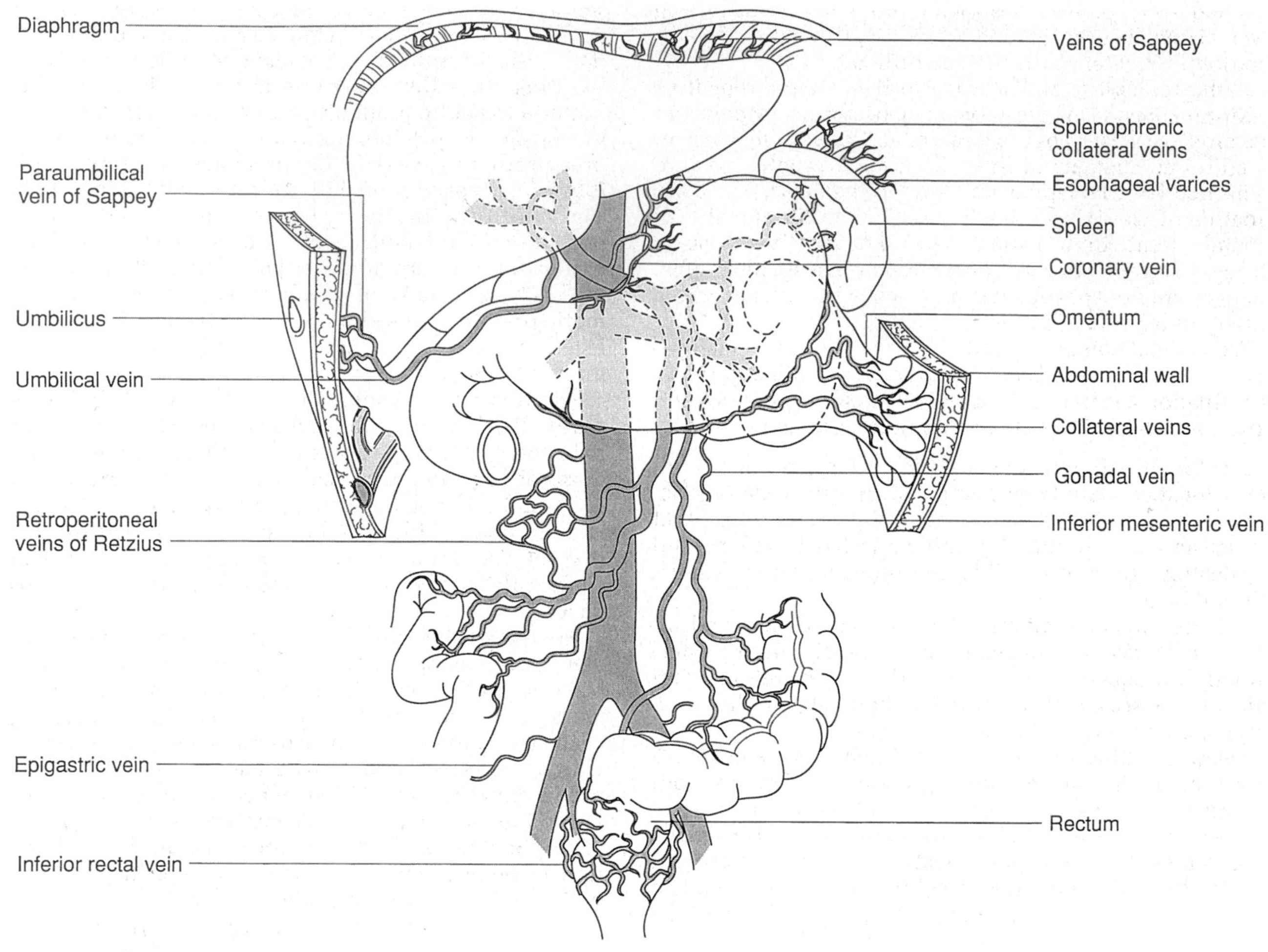

FIGURE 90-3. Potential venous collaterals that develop with portal hypertension. The veins of Sappey drain portal blood through the base areas of the diaphragm and through paraumbilical vein collaterals to the umbilicus. The veins of Retzius form in the retroperitoneum and shunt portal blood from the bowel and other organs to the vena cava. (From Marvin MR, Emond JC. Cirrhosis and portal hypertension. In: Greenfield LJ, Mulholland MW, Oldham KT, et al., eds. *Surgery: scientific principles and practice,* 3rd ed. Philadelphia: Lippincott Williams & Wilkins, 2001, with permission.)

submucosal arteriovenous communications. The resulting vascular ectasia has been called *congestive gastropathy* and contributes to a significant risk of bleeding from the stomach.

Diagnosis

Children with PH, regardless of the underlying cause, may have recurrent bouts of life-threatening hemorrhage. Variceal bleeding accounts for approximately one-fifth to one-third of all deaths in cirrhotic patients. The most important determinant of survival is the patient's level of hepatic function; prognosis is generally much better in patients without significant liver impairment, such as those with portal vein thrombosis.

Physical examination may show hepatomegaly, jaundice, palmar erythema, ascites, and periumbilical vascularity, a *caput medusae*. However, GI bleeding, either as melena or hematemesis, is the most frequent manifestation of PH.

Doppler flow ultrasonography can demonstrate the patency of the portal vein and flow within the portal system, in addition to detecting the presence of esophageal varices. An upper GI can also diagnose esophageal varices. Selective arteriography of the celiac axis, superior mesenteric artery, and splenic vein can map the involved vascular anatomy and measure portal pressure. However, endoscopy is the most reliable method for detecting esophageal varices. Endoscopy is undertaken after initial hemodynamic resuscitation and is essential for the precise diagnosis because only 60% to 80% of bleeding episodes in these patients are from esophageal varices. Once a diagnosis of PH has been established, several endoscopic features of esophageal varices may predict a risk for hemorrhage: variceal size and the presence of so-called *red signs*. Red signs, including cherry red spots and red wale markings (longitudinal, raised, red streaks), are usually associated with the most advanced grade of varices and are believed to represent focal weaknesses in the variceal wall (48).

Treatment

The management of children with PH has substantially changed more recently, owing to the good results and broader application of both endoscopic sclerotherapy and orthotopic liver transplantation (49). The therapy of PH consists of emergency treatment of potentially life-threatening hemorrhage and prophylaxis directed at prevention of initial or subsequent bleeding. Prompt and appropriate hemodynamic resuscitation should be followed by implementation of measures aimed at arresting and preventing the recurrence of bleeding. The major therapies available for the achievement of these goals rely on one of two fundamental approaches: lowering of portal pressure or local obliteration of the varices.

Treatment of patients with variceal hemorrhage must initially focus on fluid resuscitation and blood transfusion, as needed. Correction of coagulopathy by administration of vitamin K, platelets, or fresh frozen plasma transfusion is essential. A nasogastric tube should be placed to document the presence of blood within the stomach and to monitor for ongoing bleeding. An H_2 receptor blocker such as ranitidine should be given intravenously to reduce the risk of bleeding from gastric erosions.

Pharmacologic therapy to decrease portal pressure may be considered in patients who do not stop bleeding spontaneously. Propanolol has been used to directly decrease portal pressures. Vasopressin or one of its analogs is commonly used, due to its ability to increase splanchnic vascular tone and thus decrease portal blood flow. Vasopressin is administered initially with a bolus of 0.33 U per kg followed by a continued infusion, but its use is occasionally limited by its vasoconstrictive side effects. The somatostatin analog octreotide decreases splanchnic blood flow with fewer side effects. Although studies in adults are promising, its use and efficacy in children have not been well evaluated.

Balloon tamponade, using Sengstaken-Blakemore or Minnesota tubes, has been used for many years to diminish variceal flow and control bleeding by compressing the varices. These balloons can control active bleeding in more than 90% of cases. However, there is a high rate of rebleeding when the balloon is deflated, and thus balloon tamponade is considered a temporizing measure in patients who have active, life-threatening hemorrhage. Other potential serious complications include esophageal perforation and aspiration pneumonia. Thus, patients should be intubated for airway protection before insertion of the tube, and the position of the gastric balloon should be confirmed radiographically before being fully inflated.

Endoscopy is the cornerstone of the management of GI hemorrhage, as both a diagnostic and a therapeutic modality. Treatment options include injection sclerotherapy and variceal band ligation (50). Injections may be directed into the veins (intravariceal injection) or adjacent to the variceal channels (paravariceal injection); different sclerosants are available, including 5% sodium morrhuate, 1% to 3% sodium tetradecyl sulfate, 5% ethanolamine oleate, and absolute alcohol. Although bleeding may be controlled acutely in most cases, further sessions of sclerotherapy are required and treatments can be associated with further bleeding, esophageal ulceration, and stricture formation. These complications led to the development of an alternative endoscopic therapy referred to as *variceal banding*, based on the principles of hemorrhoidal banding. However, the use of banding in the actively bleeding patient is a technically challenging procedure and experience with the technique in children is limited.

Until the early 1980s, the treatment of choice of bleeding esophageal varices was based on two main types of open surgery: portosystemic shunts and devascularization procedures (49,51–53). Shunt operations have traditionally been classified as total, partial, or selective, on the basis of their intended impact on portal blood flow. Total shunts divert all portal blood flow into the inferior vena cava; end-to-side portacaval shunt is the best example. The side-to-side portacaval shunt differed in that theoretically only part of the portal stream was diverted into the vena cava. However, in reality, not only did the side-to-side portacaval shunt allow total diversion of portal blood flow, but it also facilitated diversion of part of the hepatic arterial blood backward into the vena cava, leading to hepatic encephalopathy and liver failure. Other nonselective shunts have used large diameter portacaval prosthetic H grafts, small diameter grafts, and mesocaval shunts. Selective shunts, a shunt engineered to decompress variceal flow while preserving prograde portal blood flow, were designed to avoid the encephalopathy seen with total shunts. The Warren or distal splenorenal shunt, the best example of a selective shunt, decompresses varices through the splenic vein to the left renal vein and disconnects other potential portosystemic connections (Fig. 90-4). This procedure yielded good results in children, even when applied in toddlers (49,54). Direct surgical devascularization of the varices offers the potential for control of bleeding without the shunt-related complication of encephalopathy and can be applied when the anatomy is unfavorable for a shunt. Improved long-term control of bleeding has been reported with the Sugiura operation, a more extensive procedure consisting of transthoracic paraesophageal devascularization, esophageal transection, splenectomy, esophagogastric devascularization, pyloroplasty, and vagotomy (53). However, since the introduction of

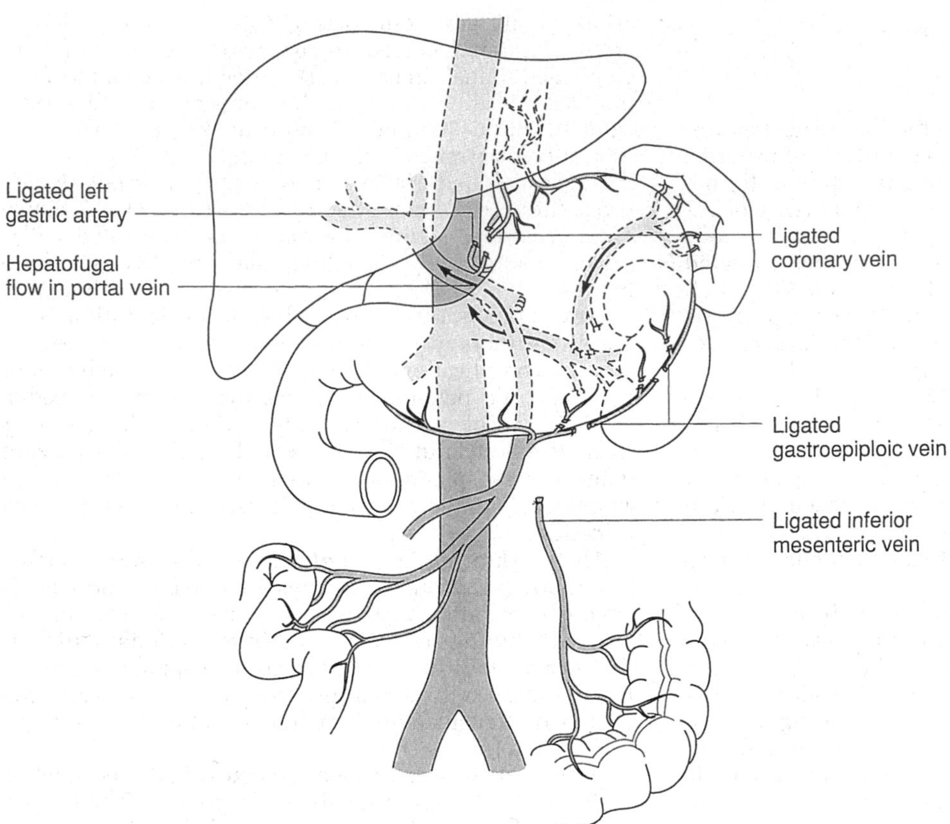

FIGURE 90-4. Distal splenorenal Warren shunt. The splenic vein is divided near its junction with the superior mesenteric vein. The distal end of the splenic vein is anastomosed to the renal vein. Varices are selectively decompressed through the stomach and short gastric veins into the splenic vein and then into the vena cava through the renal vein. Portal hypertension is maintained in the portal and superior mesenteric veins to provide enough pressure to drive portal blood through the diseased liver. (From Marvin MR, Emond JC. Cirrhosis and portal hypertension. In: Greenfield LJ, Mulholland MW, Oldham KT, et al., eds. *Surgery: scientific principles and practice,* 3rd ed. Philadelphia: Lippincott Williams & Wilkins, 2001, with permission.)

sclerotherapy for the treatment of bleeding esophageal varices, the number of surgical procedures has sharply decreased.

As noted previously, all surgical options have the potential for significant morbidity and mortality. Attempts to devise a less invasive approach to portal decompression led to the development of a nonsurgical shunt, the transjugular intrahepatic portosystemic shunt (TIPS) (Fig. 90-5). TIPS is a percutaneous method of creating a side-to-side portacaval shunt by the deployment of an expandable metallic stent placed by an interventional radiologist (55). The potential advantages of this technique include avoidance of general anesthesia, decreased procedural morbidity and mortality rates, and avoidance of surgery in the region of the hepatic hilum, which may be important in potential liver transplantation candidates. However, the TIPS procedure is prone to thrombosis, particularly in younger children, and may precipitate the hepatic arterial steal phenomenon known to cause hepatic encephalopathy.

Orthotopic liver transplantation represents the definite therapy for PH (56,57). A prior portosystemic shunting operation does not preclude a successful liver transplantation, although it does make the operation technically more difficult. However, liver transplantation is expensive, requires lifelong immunosuppression, and is limited by a significant donor shortage. Thus, there remains the need for managing PH in patients who are awaiting transplantation or who are not considered transplantation candidates.

ASCITES AND SPONTANEOUS BACTERIAL PERITONITIS

Ascites

Ascites is an accumulation of serous fluid within the peritoneal cavity. There are multiple causes of ascites; hepatic, renal, and cardiac disease are the most common causes in children (Table 90-3). The clinical hallmark of ascites is abdominal distention, although considerable intraperitoneal fluid may accumulate before ascites is detectable by the classic physical signs of bulging flanks, shifting dullness, and a fluid wave. The course, prognosis, and treatment of ascites depend entirely on the cause. Patients with any type of ascites are at increased risk for spontaneous bacterial peritonitis.

Chylous ascites can result from obstruction or injury to the intraabdominal portion of the lymphatic system. Causes include lymphangiomatosis, congenital malformations, tumors, enlarged lymph nodes, previous abdominal surgery, or trauma. Because of loss of serum proteins (and thus oncotic pressure), not only will the child present with abdominal distension, but he or she may also have

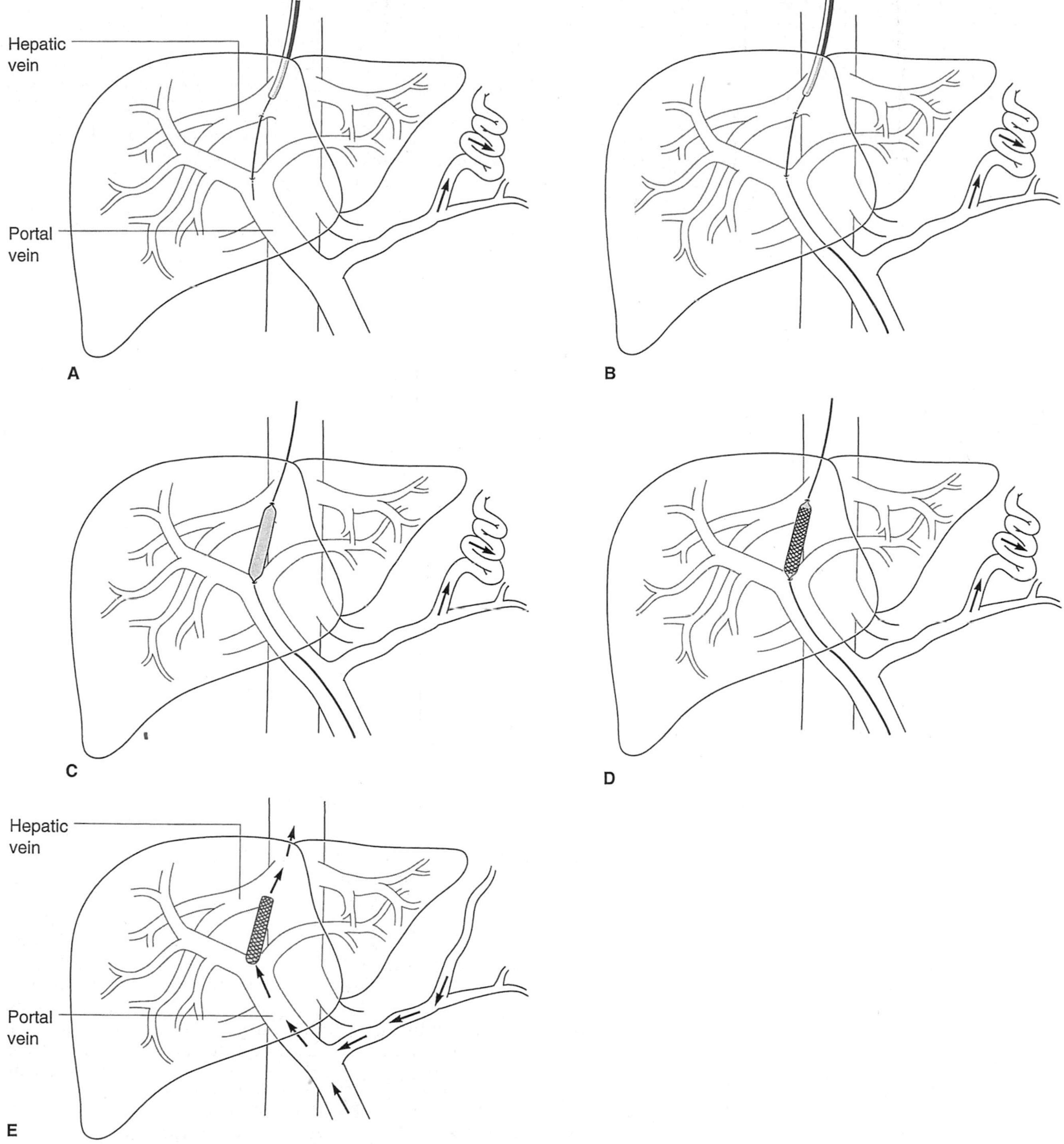

FIGURE 90-5. Schematic representation of the creation of a transjugular intrahepatic portosystemic shunt. **(A)** Needle is advanced from supraheptic vena cava into portal vein using fluoroscopy. **(B)** Wire is advanced through needle into the superior mesenteric vein. **(C)** The tract between hepatic and portal vein is dilated with andioplasty balloon catheter. **(D)** Balloon-expandable stents are placed in the tract between hepatic and portal vein. **(E)** Final appearance of stent, with intrahepatic shunt from portal vein to hepatic vein. (From Zemel G, Katzen BT, Becker GJ, et al. Percutaneous transjugular portosystemic shunt. *JAMA* 1991;266:390, with permission.)

TABLE 90-3 Causes of Childhood Ascites.

Serous ascites	
	Cirrhosis
	Nephrosis
	Right-sided heart failure
	Budd-Chiari syndrome
	Postop (venous pressure shunt, peritoneal dialysis)
Biliary ascites	
	Neonatal bile duct perforation
	Hepatitis
	Cystic fibrosis
Chylous ascites	
	Malrotation with volvulus
	Lymphangioma
	Small bowel obstruction
	Trauma
Urinary ascites	
	Posterior urethral valves
	Bladder perforation
	Ureterocele
Pancreatic ascites	
	Acute pancreatitis
	Pancreatic pseudocyst
Ovarian ascites	
	Cyst (torsion, rupture)
	Tumors
Malignant ascites	
	Any intraperitoneal neoplasm

peripheral edema. Diagnosis of chylous ascites depends on paracentesis. If the patient has not eaten, the fluid will appear serous; however, if the child has recently had a fat-containing meal, it will be milky. Fluid analysis will disclose a high cell count that is predominantly lymphocytic, an elevated triglyceride level, and high protein content. Serum hypoalbuminemia and lymphopenia are commonly seen. Treatment includes feedings of a high-protein, low-fat diet supplemented with medium-chain triglycerides (absorbed directly into the portal circulation). Parenteral alimentation may be necessary to decrease lymph flow to facilitate sealing of the leak. Laparotomy may be indicated to search for the site of the leak if a trial of dietary management has been unsuccessful, particularly in cases secondary to trauma or previous surgery.

The presence of ascites in conjunction with palmar erythema and/or abdominal wall collateral veins is suggestive of parenchymal liver disease. In ascites secondary to liver disease, vasopressin, renin-aldosterone, and sympathetic nervous systems are activated (58,59). These changes lead to renal vasoconstriction and subsequent sodium and water retention. Fluid then weeps from the congested hepatic sinusoids as ascites.

The mainstay of therapy for children with cirrhotic ascites is dietary sodium restriction and diuretics. Fluid loss and weight change are related directly to sodium balance. In the presence of avid renal retention of sodium, sodium intake is limited to 1 to 2 mEq per kg per day. Aggressive restriction of fluid is inappropriate, except for patients with severe hyponatremia. Diuresis may be maintained by the use of agents such as furosemide alone or in combination with spironolactone (3 to 5 mg per kg day in four doses). Importantly, patients with ascites without peripheral edema are at risk for reduced plasma volume, and thus diuretic doses and dietary sodium intake must be carefully adjusted to achieve weight loss and negative sodium balance.

Refractory ascites is defined as ascites unresponsive to a sodium-restricted diet and high-dose diuretic treatment. Refractoriness may be manifested by minimal weight loss despite diuretics, diuretic complications, or the development of tense ascites (60). Tense ascites alters renal blood flow and systemic hemodynamics, and requires urgent therapy. In the 1960s, portacaval shunts were used to treat refractory ascites, but operative hemorrhagic complications and portosystemic encephalopathy led to the abandonment of this approach. Presently, treatment options for refractory ascites include serial therapeutic paracenteses, peritoneovenous shunts, TIPS, and liver transplantation. Large-volume paracentesis and intravenous albumin infusion may improve hemodynamics, renal perfusion, and symptoms (61). TIPS is now considered the second-line treatment for these patients (62–64). A more recent randomized trial in diuretic-resistant patients has demonstrated a survival advantage for TIPS compared with serial paracenteses (65). Although there was initial enthusiasm for peritoneovenous shunting, high complication and failure rates, as well as randomized trials demonstrating no survival advantage, have led to the relegation of this procedure to third-line therapy. Finally, for patients with no psychosocial or medical contraindications, evaluation for liver transplantation is essential once ascites has become diuretic resistant.

Spontaneous Bacterial Peritonitis

Spontaneous bacterial peritonitis (SBP) is the most common cause of inflammation of ascitic fluid. Spontaneous forms of ascitic fluid infection are believed to be the result of overgrowth of a specific organism in the gut, "translocation" of that microbe from the gut to mesenteric lymph nodes, and resulting spontaneous bacteremia and subsequent colonization of susceptible ascitic fluid (66). The diagnosis of SBP is made when there is a positive ascitic fluid culture and an elevated ascitic fluid absolute polymorphonucleocyte count, without evidence of an intraabdominal surgically treatable source of infection. The most common bacterial infection of ascitic fluid is monomicrobial, with a low bacterial concentration (median colony count of only 1 organism per milliliter). Thus, the decision to begin empiric antibiotic treatment is not routinely based on culture, but on the cell count and differential.

Although SBP is approximately six times as common as surgical peritonitis in a patient with ascites, secondary peritonitis should be considered in any patient with neutrocytic ascites because clinical symptoms and signs will not distinguish between them. Ascitic fluid total protein, glucose, and LDH can be of some value in distinguishing SBP from intestinal perforation. Patients who meet two of the following three criteria are likely to have surgical peritonitis: total protein greater than 1 g per dL, glucose less than 50 mg per dL, and LDH greater than the upper limit of normal for serum. The most apparent difference between the spontaneous forms of ascitic fluid infection and the secondary forms is that the former are always monomicrobial and the latter are usually polymicrobial.

Escherichia coli, streptococci (mostly pneumococci), and *Klebsiella* cause most episodes of SBP. Timely diagnosis requires a high index of suspicion and a low threshold for performing a paracentesis because the symptoms and signs of infection are often subtle. A slight change in mental status, fever, or abdominal pain in a patient with ascites should raise the suspicion of infection and prompt a paracentesis. Cefotaxime or a similar third-generation cephalosporin appears to be the treatment of choice for suspected SBP. Anaerobic coverage is not needed, nor is coverage for *Pseudomonas* or *Staphylococcus*. Less than 5% of patients die of infection if appropriate antibiotics are administered in a timely fashion. However, spontaneous ascitic fluid infection is a good marker of end-stage liver disease and has been proposed as an indication for liver transplantation.

ACUTE LIVER FAILURE

Acute liver failure (ALF) arises from loss of hepatic parenchyma or severe functional impairment that may result from a variety of insults to the liver. ALF has been defined by three criteria: (1) rapid development of hepatocellular dysfunction, (2) encephalopathy, and (3) absence of a prior liver disease. The clinical features of ALF result directly from loss of critical hepatocellular functions (protein synthesis, intermediary metabolism, and detoxification). The disorder usually evolves over a very short period.

Etiology

ALF is a rare condition in the pediatric population. Patients who present with severe failure of liver synthetic function have a high mortality with medical therapy alone. The main causes of death are cerebral edema, hemorrhage, renal failure, and sepsis. The etiology of ALF is age specific, with a significant number due to inborn errors of metabolism, especially in neonates and infants. Treatment of children with ALF is supportive, aimed at preventing and managing associated complications until the native liver recovers or until liver transplantation. Sedation should not be administered unless a decision for artificial ventilation has been made. Because all children are potential transplant candidates, transfer to and management in a liver transplant centre is recommended. Prognostic criteria for mortality are less well defined compared with the adult population, although a significantly elevated international normalized ratio (INR) greater than or equal to 4 carries a high chance of death, and liver transplantation should be considered at this stage. Auxiliary transplantation is an attractive option in selected individuals and provides the chance to stop immunosuppression if sufficient hepatic regeneration occurs. The use of various liver assist devices and hepatocyte transplantation as a bridge to liver transplantation show promise, although when used in isolation, they do not have an impact on overall patient survival (67).

Fulminant hepatic failure is most commonly a complication of viral hepatitis, and there is a high risk of fulminant hepatic failure in young people with combined hepatitis B and D infections. A large number of other viruses, including but not exclusively Epstein-Barr virus, adenovirus, and cytomegalovirus, may produce fulminant hepatitis in children. Various hepatotoxic drugs and chemicals may also cause acute fulminant hepatic failure. Acetaminophen is directly hepatotoxic and predictably produces hepatocellular necrosis with an overdose. Even recommended therapeutic dosages of acetaminophen can sometimes result in ALF in patients who are fasting or who chronically use alcohol or drugs that induce cytochrome oxidases. Predictable liver injury may occur after exposure to Amanita mushrooms or carbon tetrachloride. Idiosyncratic damage may follow the use of drugs such as halothane or sodium valproate. Ischemia and hypoxia may produce liver failure. A large number of metabolic disorders can rarely be associated with hepatic failure, including Wilson's disease, galactosemia, tyrosinemia, neonatal iron storage disease, and deficiencies of mitochondrial electron transport.

The mechanisms that lead to fulminant hepatic failure are poorly understood. It is unknown why only about 1% to 2% of patients with viral hepatitis experience liver failure, but it is speculated that a hyperimmune response to the virus underlies the massive liver necrosis. Whatever the initial cause of hepatocyte injury, various factors may contribute to the pathogenesis of liver failure, including impaired hepatocyte regeneration, endotoxemia, and decreased hepatic reticuloendothelial function.

Clinical Presentation

The initial presentation of ALF may include nonspecific complaints such as nausea, vomiting, and fatigue. However, hepatocellular injury soon leads to impaired elimination of bilirubin, depressed synthesis of coagulation factors (I, II, V, VII, IX, and X), diminished glucose synthesis, and increased lactate levels. Coagulopathy increases the risk of GI and intracranial hemorrhage, hypoglycemia contributes to brain injury, and acidosis can produce cardiovascular dysfunction.

Encephalopathy is a defining criterion for ALF. In infants, irritability, poor feeding, and a change in sleep rhythm may be the only findings. Patients are often somnolent or combative on arousal, and may rapidly progress to deeper stages of coma in which extensor responses and decerebrate and decorticate posturing appear. A staging system has been developed to help monitor change and identify potential transplantation candidates. This system consists of stage 1—subtle changes in affect, stage 2—drowsiness and asterixis, stage 3—marked somnolence and extensor reflex rigidity, and stage 4—frank coma. Progressive cerebral edema will produce intracranial hypertension, which can impair cerebral perfusion, leading to irreversible neurologic damage or even uncal herniation and death.

Infections develop in as many as 80% of patients with ALF, and respiratory failure and renal failure are commonly associated with ALF. A potential consequence of ALF is the syndrome of multiple organ failure, which manifests clinically as hypotension, pulmonary edema, acute tubular necrosis, and disseminated intravascular coagulation. Multiple organ failure is a significant contributor to patient mortality.

Laboratory Findings

Initially, serum aminotransferase activities may be markedly elevated, followed by elevation of the direct and indirect bilirubin levels. The blood ammonia concentration is usually increased, and PT is always prolonged and often does not improve after parenteral administration of vitamin K. Hypoglycemia can occur, particularly in infants, as can metabolic acidosis or respiratory alkalosis. Liver biopsy reveals confluent massive necrosis of hepatocytes. Bridging necrosis may be seen, and a particular zonal pattern of necrosis may be observed with certain insults (e.g., centrilobular damage is associated with acetaminophen hepatotoxicity or with circulatory shock).

Treatment

Patients with ALF fall into two broad categories: (1) those in whom intensive medical care enables recovery of hepatic function, and (2) those who require liver transplantation to survive. Thus, it is critical to rapidly determine to which group a particular patient belongs. The following characteristics have been demonstrated to be associated with a poor outcome: negative serology for hepatitis A or B, younger age (younger than 10 years) or older age (older than 40 years), markedly elevated serum bilirubin level, marked prolongation of the prothrombin time, acidosis, and an elevated serum creatinine level. Among patients with a cause of ALF other than acetaminophen toxicity, the presence of any single adverse prognostic characteristic was associated with a mortality rate of 80%, and the presence of three adverse characteristics was associated with a mortality rate of more than 95%. Because these mortality rates vastly exceed those associated with liver transplantation, the presence of any single indicator of a poor prognosis should prompt serious consideration for liver transplantation.

The initial management of ALF should include an attempt to identify the cause of ALF because a small number of causes of ALF can be treated specifically. For example, acetaminophen toxicity can be treated with *N*-acetylcysteine, and herpes-induced fulminant hepatitis has been reported to respond to intravenous acyclovir. Otherwise, management of fulminant hepatic failure is supportive because no therapy is known to reverse hepatocyte injury or to promote hepatic regeneration. Intensive medical care is warranted in all patients with ALF. Patients with profound encephalopathy (i.e., stage 3 and stage 4) should undergo endotracheal intubation to prevent aspiration, to reduce cerebral edema by hyperventilation, and to facilitate pulmonary toilet. Intracranial pressure monitoring and treatment with osmotherapy and barbiturates are two options for treating intracranial hypertension, although cerebral edema is an extremely serious complication that responds poorly to those measures. GI hemorrhage, infection, and hypovolemia may precipitate encephalopathy and should be identified and corrected. Protein intake should be restricted or eliminated. Lactulose should be given every 2 to 4 hr orally or by nasogastric tube in doses (10 to 50 mL) sufficient to cause diarrhea. Oral or rectal administration of a nonabsorbable antibiotic such as neomycin may reduce enteric bacteria responsible for ammonia production. Because clinical recognition of infection may be difficult, surveillance cultures in patients with ALF are extremely helpful. If renal failure is present, measurement of central pressures provides a direct guide to fluid therapy. Because patients with ALF have a propensity to develop adult respiratory distress syndrome, early measurement of central venous or pulmonary arterial pressure in oliguric patients is preferable to empiric administration of fluid boluses. If oliguria persists in the face of adequate central filling pressures, continuous arteriovenous hemofiltration should be initiated.

Liver transplantation has improved the outcome for some patients with ALF. Before the era of liver transplantation, less than one-half of patients with ALF survived. In contrast, survival rates for patients with ALF who undergo liver transplantation have been substantially higher, with an overall survival rate greater than 70% in some centers. Reduced-size allografts and living donor transplantation have been important advances in the treatment of infants with hepatic failure (68). Partial auxiliary orthotopic or heterotopic liver transplantation has also been successful in a small number of children, allowing regeneration of the native liver and eventual withdrawal of immunosupression. However, transplantation is not always successful. In one series, patients who presented with multisystem organ failure had 100% mortality rate, despite liver transplantation (69). Another series noted that ALF during the first year of life is a severe condition with poor prognosis, despite the advent of liver transplantation (70). Many patients with irreversible ALF never have the chance to undergo transplantation because of medical contraindications or the unavailability of donor livers. More recent advances in the experimental therapy of ALF have been limited. Treatment strategies, such as charcoal hemoperfusion and administration of prostaglandin E_1, which showed early promise, have not been shown to be superior to standard care.

Prognosis

Children with hepatic failure may fare somewhat better than adults, but overall mortality exceeds 70%. The prognosis may vary considerably with the cause of liver failure and stage of hepatic encephalopathy. With intensive medical support, survival rates of 50% to 60% occur with hepatic failure complicating acetaminophen overdose and with fulminant HAV or HBV infection. In contrast, recovery can be expected in only 10% to 20% of patients with liver failure caused by non-A, non-B, or non-C hepatitis, or an acute onset of Wilson's disease. Survival of 50% to 75% is being achieved in patients with the poorest prognosis after orthotopic liver transplantation.

REFERENCES

1. LeBlanc GA. Hepatic vectorial transport of xenobiotics. *Chem Biol Interact* 1994;90:101–120.
2. McGarry JD, Kuwajima M, Newgard CB, et al. From dietary glucose to liver glycogen: the full circle round. *Ann Rev Nutr* 1987;7:51–73.
3. Alonso MD, Lomako J, Lomako WM, et al. A new look at the biogenesis of glycogen. *FASEB J* 1995;9:1126–1137.
4. Bahar RJ, Stolz A. Bile acid transport. *Gastroenterol Clin North Am* 1999;28:27–58.
5. Wong MH, Oelkers P, Craddock AL, et al. Expression cloning and characterization of the hamster ileal sodium-dependent bile acid transporter. *J Biol Chem* 1994;269:1340–1347.
6. Rosenthal P. Assessing liver function and hyperbilirubinemia in the newborn. National Academy of Clinical Biochemistry. *Clin Chem* 1997;43:228–234.
7. Rosenthal P, Henton D, Felber S, et al. Distribution of serum bilirubin conjugates in pediatric hepatobiliary diseases. *J Pediatr* 1987;110:201–205.
8. Cotton PB, Laage NJ. Endoscopic retrograde cholangiopancreatography in children. *Arch Dis Child* 1982;57:131–136.
9. Ashida K, Nagita A, Sakaguchi M, et al. Endoscopic retrograde cholangiopancreatography in paediatric patients with biliary disorders. *J Gastroenterol Hepatol* 1998;13:598–603.
10. Tagge EP, Tarnasky PR, Chandler J, et al. Multidisciplinary approach to the treatment of pediatric pancreaticobiliary disorders. *J Pediatr Surg* 1997;32:158–164.
11. Guelrud M, Jaen D, Mendoza S, et al. ERCP in the diagnosis of extrahepatic biliary atresia. *Gastrointest Endosc* 1991;37:522–526.
12. Ohnuma N, Takahashi T, Tanabe M, et al. The role of ERCP in biliary atresia. *Gastrointest Endosc* 1997;45:365–370.
13. Ng KK, Wan YL, Lui KW, et al. Three-dimensional magnetic resonance cholangiopancreatography for evaluation of obstructive jaundice. *J Formosan Med Assoc* 1997;96:586–592.
14. McKiernan PJ. Neonatal cholestasis. *Semin Neonatol* 2002;7: 153–165.
15. Trauner M, Meier PJ, Boyer JL. Molecular pathogenesis of cholestasis. *N Engl J Med* 1998;339:1217–1227.
16. Bates MD, Bucuvalas JC, Alonso MH, et al. Biliary atresia: pathogenesis and treatment. *Semin Liver Dis* 1998;18:281–293.
17. Tagge DU, Tagge EP, Drongowski RA, et al. A long-term experience with biliary atresia. Reassessment of prognostic factors. *Ann Surg* 1991;214:590–598.
18. Laurent J, Gauthier F, Bernard O, et al. Long-term outcome after surgery for biliary atresia. Study of 40 patients surviving for more than 10 years. *Gastroenterology* 1990;99:1793–1797.
19. Ryckman F, Fisher R, Pedersen S, et al. Improved survival in biliary atresia patients in the present era of liver transplantation. *J Pediatr Surg* 1993;28:382–385.
20. Whitington PF, Balistreri WF. Liver transplantation in pediatrics: indications, contraindications, and pretransplant management. *J Pediatr* 1991;118:169–177.
21. Lin WY, Lin CC, Changlai SP, et al. Comparison technetium of Tc-99m disofenin cholescintigraphy with ultrasonography in the differentiation of biliary atresia from other forms of neonatal jaundice. *Pediatr Surg Int* 1997;12:30–33.
22. Tagge EP, Othersen HB Jr, Jackson SM, et al. Impact of laparoscopic cholecystectomy on the management of cholelithiasis in children with sickle cell disease. *J Pediatr Surg* 1994;29:209–212.
23. Mowat AP. Alpha 1-antitrypsin deficiency (PiZZ): features of liver involvement in childhood. *Acta Paediatr Suppl* 1994;393:13–17.
24. Perlmutter DH. Alpha-1-antitrypsin deficiency. *Semin Liver Dis* 1998;18:217–225.
25. Vennarecci G, Gunson BK, Ismail T, et al. Transplantation for end stage liver disease related to alpha 1 antitrypsin. *Transplantation* 1996;61:1488–1495.
26. Goldberg T, Slonim AE. Nutrition therapy for hepatic glycogen storage diseases. *J Am Diet Assoc* 1993;93:1423–1430.
27. Lee PJ, Leonard JV. The hepatic glycogen storage diseases—problems beyond childhood. *J Inherited Metab Dis* 1995;18:462–472.
28. Grompe M. The pathophysiology and treatment of hereditary tyrosinemia type 1. *Semin Liver Dis* 2001;21:563–571.
29. van Spronsen FJ, Thomasse Y, Smit GP, et al. Hereditary tyrosinemia type I: a new clinical classification with difference in prognosis on dietary treatment. *Hepatology* 1994;20:1187–1191.
30. Mohan N, McKiernan P, Preece MA, et al. Indications and outcome of liver transplantation in tyrosinaemia type 1. *Eur J Pediatr* 1999;158. Suppl 2:S49–54.
31. Elder GH, Hift RJ, Meissner PN. The acute porphyrias. *Lancet* 1997;349:1613–1617.
32. Andant C, Puy H, Bogard C, et al. Hepatocellular carcinoma in patients with acute hepatic porphyria: frequency of occurrence and related factors. *J Hepatol* 2000;32:933–939.
33. Badminton MN, Elder GH. Management of acute and cutaneous porphyrias. *Int J Clin Pract* 2002;56:272–278.
34. Polson RJ, Lim CK, Rolles K, et al. The effect of liver transplantation in a 13-year-old boy with erythropoietic protoporphyria [Comment]. *Transplantation* 1988;46:386–389.
35. Loudianos G, Gitlin JD. Wilson's disease. *Semin Liver Dis* 2000;20:353–364.
36. Lykavieris P, Bernard O, Hadchouel M. Neonatal cholestasis as the presenting feature in cystic fibrosis. *Arch Dis Child* 1996;75:67–70.
37. Sokol RJ, Durie PR. Recommendations for management of liver and biliary tract disease in cystic fibrosis. Cystic Fibrosis Foundation Hepatobiliary Disease Consensus Group. *J Pediatr Gastroenterol Nutr* 1999;28.
38. Noble-Jamieson G, Barnes N, Jamieson N, et al. Liver transplantation for hepatic cirrhosis in cystic fibrosis. *J Roy Soc Med* 1996;27:31–37.
39. Romero R, Lavine JE. Viral hepatitis in children. *Semin Liver Dis* 1994;14:289–302.

40. Alter MJ, Mast EE. The epidemiology of viral hepatitis in the United States. *Gastroenterol Clin North Am* 1994;23:437–455.
41. Beasley RP, Hwang LY. Postnatal infectivity of hepatitis B surface antigen-carrier mothers. *J Infect Dis* 1983;147:185–190.
42. Fishman LN, Jonas MM, Lavine JE. Update on viral hepatitis in children. *Pediatr Clin North Am* 1996;43:57–74.
43. Shouval D, Samuel D. Hepatitis B immune globulin to prevent hepatitis B virus graft reinfection following liver transplantation: a concise review. *Hepatology* 2000;32:1189–1195.
44. Ohto H, Terazawa S, Sasaki N, et al. Transmission of hepatitis C virus from mothers to infants. The Vertical Transmission of Hepatitis C Virus Collaborative Study Group [Comment]. *N Engl J Med* 1994;330:744–750.
45. Poynard T, Marcellin P, Lee SS, et al. Randomised trial of interferon alpha2b plus ribavirin for 48 weeks or for 24 weeks versus interferon alpha2b plus placebo for 48 weeks for treatment of chronic infection with hepatitis C virus. International Hepatitis Interventional Therapy Group (IHIT). *Lancet* 1998;352:1426–1432.
46. Zeuzem S, Feinman SV, Rasenack J, et al. Peginterferon alfa-2a in patients with chronic hepatitis C. *N Engl J Med* 2000;343:1666–1672.
47. Heathcote EJ, Shiffman ML, Cooksley WG, et al. Peginterferon alfa-2a in patients with chronic hepatitis C and cirrhosis. *N Engl J Med* 2000;343:1673–1680.
48. North Italian Endoscopic Club for the study and treatment of esophageal varices. Prediction of the first variceal hemorrhage in patients with cirrhosis of the liver and esophageal varices. A prospective multicenter study. The North Italian Endoscopic Club for the Study and Treatment of Esophageal Varices. *N Engl J Med* 1988;319:983–989.
49. Maksoud JG, Goncalves ME. Treatment of portal hypertension in children. *World J Surg* 1994;18:251–258.
50. de Franchis R, Primignani M. Endoscopic treatments for portal hypertension. *Semin Liver Dis* 1999;19:439–455.
51. Alvarez F, Bernard O, Brunelle F, et al. Portal obstruction in children. II. Results of surgical portosystemic shunts. *J Pediatr* 1983;103:703–707.
52. Shun A, Delaney DP, Martin HC, et al. Portosystemic shunting for paediatric portal hypertension. *J Pediatr Surg* 1997;32:489–493.
53. Shah SR, Nagral SS, Mathur SK. Results of a modified Sugiura's devascularisation in the management of "unshuntable" portal hypertension. *HPB Surg* 1999;11:235–239.
54. Renard TH, Andrews WS, Rollins N, et al. Use of distal splenorenal shunt in children referred for liver transplant evaluation. *J Pediatr Surg* 1994;29:403–406.
55. Heyman MB, LaBerge JM. Role of transjugular intrahepatic portosystemic shunt in the treatment of portal hypertension in pediatric patients. *J Pediatr Gastroenterol Nutr* 1999;29:240–249.
56. Reyes J, Iwatsuki S. Current management of portal hypertension with liver transplantation. *Adv Surg* 1992;25:189–208.
57. Knechtle SJ, Kalayoglu M, D'Alessandro AM, et al. Portal hypertension: surgical management in the 1990s. *Surgery* 1994;116:687–693.
58. Schrier RW. Pathogenesis of sodium and water retention in high-output and low-output cardiac failure, nephrotic syndrome, cirrhosis, and pregnancy (1). *N Engl J Med* 1988;319:1065–1072.
59. Schrier RW. Pathogenesis of sodium and water retention in high-output and low-output cardiac failure, nephrotic syndrome, cirrhosis, and pregnancy (2). *N Engl J Med* 1988;319:1127–1134.
60. Arroyo V, Gines P, Gerbes AL, et al. Definition and diagnostic criteria of refractory ascites and hepatorenal syndrome in cirrhosis. International Ascites Club. *Hepatology* 1996;23:164–176.
61. Kramer RE, Sokol RJ, Yerushalmi B, et al. Large-volume paracentesis in the management of ascites in children. *J Pediatr Gastroenterol Nutr* 2001;33:245–249.
62. Nazarian GK, Bjarnason H, Dietz CA Jr, et al. Refractory ascites: midterm results of treatment with a transjugular intrahepatic portosystemic shunt. *Radiology* 1997;205:173–180.
63. Sergent G, Gottrand F, Delemazure O, et al. Transjugular intrahepatic portosystemic shunt in an infant. *Pediatr Radiol* 1997;27:588–590.
64. van Buuren HR, Cheng KH, Pieterman H, et al. Transjugular intrahepatic portosystemic shunt. Requiem for the surgical portosystemic shunt? *Scand J Gastroenterol Suppl* 1993;200:48–52.
65. Rossle M, Ochs A, Gulberg V, et al. A comparison of paracentesis and transjugular intrahepatic portosystemic shunting in patients with ascites. *N Engl J Med* 2000;342:1701–1707.
66. Runyon BA, Squier S, Borzio M. Translocation of gut bacteria in rats with cirrhosis to mesenteric lymph nodes partially explains the pathogenesis of spontaneous bacterial peritonitis. *J Hepatol* 1994;21:792–796.
67. Aw MM, Dhawan A. Acute liver failure. *Indian J Pediatr* 2002;69:87–91.
68. Miwa S, Hashikura Y, Mita A, et al. Living-related liver transplantation for patients with fulminant and subfulminant hepatic failure. *Hepatology* 1991;30:1521–1526.
69. Nicolette L, Billmire D, Faulkenstein K, et al. Transplantation for acute hepatic failure in children. *J Pediatr Surg* 1998;33:998–1002.
70. Durand P, Debray D, Mandel R, et al. Acute liver failure in infancy: a 14-year experience of a pediatric liver transplantation center. *J Pediatr* 2001;139:871–876.

Chapter 91

Surgical Liver Disease

Max R. Langham, Jr. and Alan W. Hemming

Surgical procedures form the basis of current treatment for a number of disorders affecting the liver. The pathophysiology of many of these disorders is incompletely understood, and effective medical therapy for most has not become a reality. Until such treatments are developed, resection of discrete lesions or replacement of the entire liver for diffuse disease will remain the cornerstone of effective treatment in conjunction with procedures designed to lessen the impact of portal hypertension. Improved operative techniques, coupled with significant advances in preoperative imaging, anesthesia, and intensive care, have created a golden age in liver surgery. This chapter briefly reviews the surgical anatomy of the liver and relevant hepatic physiology, and discusses technical aspects of liver resection, emphasizing preoperative and intraoperative decision making and postoperative care.

HISTORY

The history of surgical therapy for liver disease in children is short. Ladd and Gross only devoted slightly more than a page for the entire subject of liver tumors in their seminal text entitled *Abdominal Surgery of Infancy and Childhood* (1). Surgical exploration was advised with resection of benign lesions, but only one of the nine patients described had such a resection. Willis Potts, in his text *The Surgeon and the Child* (2) published in 1959, did not even mention liver resections. In 1974, Exelby and others surveyed the Surgical Section of the American Academy of Pediatrics and reported 227 children with malignant liver lesions (3). Fifty-two percent were resected for cure, with a 19% operative mortality. This compared favorably with the 33% operative mortality he had previously reported from a single institution (4). Operative mortality has fallen sharply since the 1980s, with several large contemporary series reporting operative mortality of 5% or less (5,6). This dramatic improvement is due to improved anesthesia support, coupled with a better understanding of the segmental anatomy of the liver, with subsequent abandonment of most nonanatomic resections.

In the 1970s, cure rates with resection alone and no chemotherapy were 60% for hepatoblastoma and 33% for hepatocellular carcinoma. King has nicely outlined the advent in the late 1970s of multiinstitutional cooperative studies of chemotherapy for these lesions (7). Preoperative chemotherapy became increasingly popular during the 1980s for children with potentially unresectable lesions (8–12). Initially reported as a method to improve resection rates for stage III or IV tumors, some authors now advocate preoperative chemotherapy for potentially resectable lesions (13,14). No properly controlled data have been reported that compare preoperative with postoperative chemotherapy for resectable lesions. Perioperative morbidity, mortality, cure rates, and long-term quality of life would be appropriate outcome measures of such a study. A series of more recent trials has confirmed improved cure rates for hepatoblastoma (5,15), but not hepatocellular carcinoma (16,17) with chemotherapy either before or after resection. Finally, since the 1990s, a resurgent interest has been seen in liver transplantation for malignant hepatic tumors (18,19).

ANATOMY

The liver is approximately 5% of total body weight in neonates and young infants (20), declining to 2% of total body weight in adolescents and adults. The anatomy of the liver has been described using various and different methods; however, surgical anatomy is based on the segmental nature of vascular and bile duct distribution (21–24).

The liver receives a dual blood supply from both the portal vein and the hepatic artery that run, along with the bile duct, within the Glissonian sheath or main portal pedicle.

Max R. Langham, Jr.: Division of Pediatric Surgery, University of Florida, Gainesville, Florida 32610-0286.

Alan W. Hemming: Division of Transplantation, University of Florida, Gainesville, Florida 32610-0286.

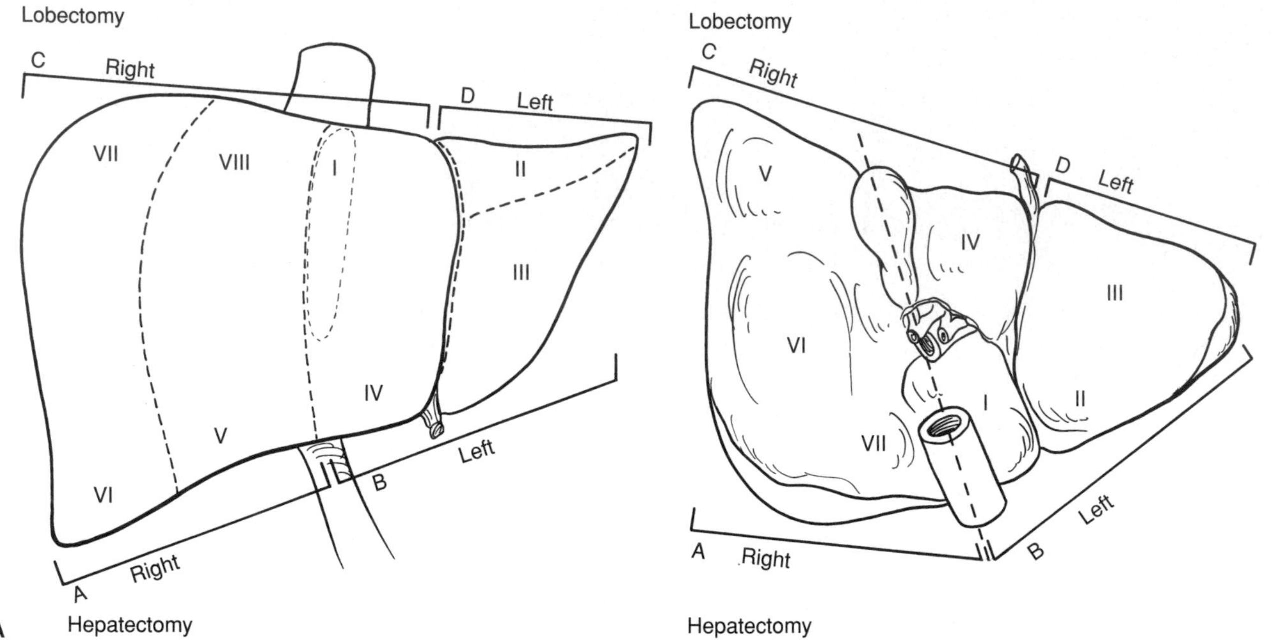

FIGURE 91-1. Segmental anatomy of the liver. Historically in the United States, the surgical anatomy of the liver was based on a division into the right and left hemilivers along Cantlies line. With improved understanding of the segmental anatomy of the liver and its variations, this has become oversimplified and should be abandoned. Obvious sources of confusion include the diagrammed terminology listing a right hepatectomy as including segments V, VI, VII, and VIII, whereas a right lobectomy includes these segments and segments I and IV [in common usage a right trisegmentectomy, although this terminology has also been criticized by Strasberg and others (23).]

The portal pedicle divides into right and left branches and then supplies the liver in a segmental fashion. Venous drainage is via the hepatic veins, which drain directly into the inferior vena cava. Hepatic segmentation is based on the distribution of the portal pedicles and their relation to the hepatic veins. Most historic depictions of the anatomy accurately locate the segments on the surface of the liver, but fail to provide a three-dimensional appreciation of the vascular anatomy, which is critical to the surgeon (Fig.91-1). More recent depictions of the anatomy have emphasized these relationships and are therefore much more useful (Fig. 91-2). The three hepatic veins run in the portal scissurae and divide the liver into four sectors, which are in turn divided by the portal pedicles running in the hepatic scissurae. The liver is divided into right and left hemilivers by the middle hepatic vein. The right hepatic vein divides the right hemiliver into anterior and posterior sectors. The plane of the portal pedicle divides the anterior sector into an inferior segment 5 and a superior segment 8, and the posterior sector into an inferior segment 6 and a superior segment 7. The left hemiliver lies to the left of the middle hepatic vein and is divided into anterior and posterior sectors by the left hepatic vein. The anterior sector is divided by the umbilical fissure into segment 4 medially and segment 3 laterally. The segment posterior to the left hepatic vein is segment 2. The plane of the portal pedicle divides segment 4 into a superior segment 4a and an inferior segment 4b. Segment 1 is the caudate lobe, which lies between the inferior vena cava and the hepatic veins. The caudate lobe has variable portal venous, hepatic arterial, and biliary anatomy, and is essentially independent of the portal pedicle divisions and hepatic venous drainage. Segmental anatomy is important in considering hepatic resection because essentially any segment or combination of segments can be resected if attention is paid to maintaining vascular and biliary continuity to remaining segments, and to preserving an adequate residual mass of functional liver.

LIVER PHYSIOLOGY

Protecting and preserving a minimum of two segments of normal liver is necessary to preserve the liver's central role in homeostasis. If parenchymal liver disease is present, a careful evaluation of the disease severity is imperative because resection of relatively small volumes of liver can result in morbidity, which is most commonly related to disruption of several of the wide variety of vital physiologic functions served by the liver. Complications and mortality are related more to the amount of functional liver left behind than to the amount resected. In normal liver, total hepatic function is related to the volume of

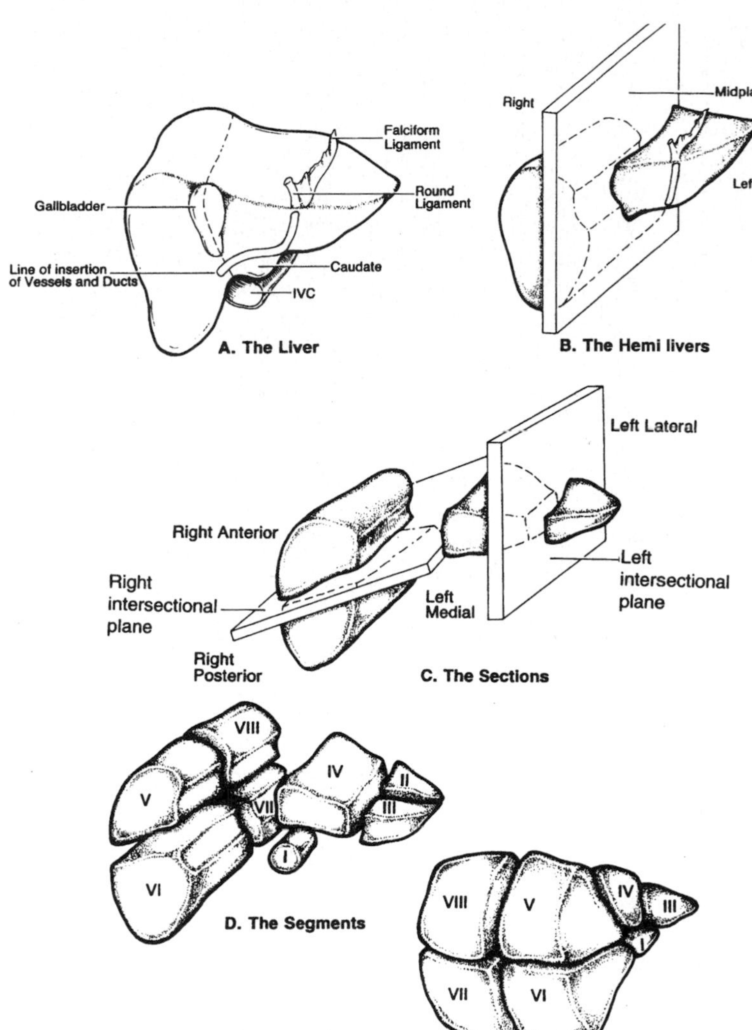

FIGURE 91-2. Surgical anatomy of the liver. **(A)** Important surface anatomy includes Cantlies line (interrupted line from the inferior vena cava through the gallbladder and extending to the middle hepatic vein superiorly. Segment 1 is below the vessels and ducts to segments 2 and 3 that also divide the left hemi liver vertically into 2 sections, the left medial section (segment 4) and the left lateral section (segments 2 and 3). **(B)** In this depiction, the liver is divided into right and left hemi livers along Cantlies line as in older drawings. **(C)** The right hemi liver is divided into anterior (segments V and VIII) and posterior sections (VI and VII) based on the branching of the right portal pedicle and venous drainage that is not depicted. The left hemi liver is divided vertically as described in A. **(D)** An exploded view of the individual segments. Isolated segmentectomy may in some instance require vascular reconstruction. An example would be a segment VII resection if venous drainage of segment VI is dependent on the right hepatic vein.

liver. Unfortunately, in patients with cirrhosis the histologic severity does not correlate with liver function. A variety of methods have been used to assess the function and correlate this with the amount of liver that can be safely resected (25–27). Indocyanine green clearance (ICG) is the best method tested in cirrhotic adults. An ICG residual at 15 minutes (ICG R_{15}) of less than 15% suggests adequate function to allow safe hepatectomy, whereas a value of more than 25% suggests that no resection will be tolerated (28). The vital metabolic and physiologic role of the liver is discussed briefly as it relates to surgical resection.

Arterial flow to the liver supplies 25% of the blood flow, but more than 50% of the oxygen delivery to the organ, and provides the sole blood supply to the major bile ducts (29). Ligation or embolization of the hepatic artery rarely causes hepatic necrosis in humans. Thrombosis of the artery after liver transplantation may cause an ischemic cholangiopathy (30–32) that can also be seen after devascularization of the bile duct during laparoscopic cholecystectomy (33). Hepatic arterial flow is regulated by both sympathetic and parasympathetic fibers derived from the vagus nerves, the celiac plexus, the lower thoracic ganglia, and the right phrenic nerves (34). Hepatic blood flow and metabolic function appear normal even after complete denervation of the liver associated with orthotopic liver transplantation (35). The impact of partial hepatic resection and hilar dissection on functions mediated by these neural plexi is largely unknown. A number of pharmacologic agents that may alter hepatic blood flow are currently being used after hepatic resection to improve liver regeneration. These include prostaglandin E1, *N*-acetyl cysteine, and others (36–39). There is little evidence that supports their use, and the precise mechanisms of action of the drugs are not well understood. However, we continue to use these agents in patients with marginal liver function after resection.

Venous blood flows from the gut and spleen via the portal vein into the liver, supplying about 75% to 80% of the total hepatic blood flow. There is usually little resistance to flow in this system, with the portal vein pressure within 5 mm Hg of that measured in the hepatic veins. Visceral nerves and enteric hormones regulate splanchnic blood flow, which increases during digestion (40,41), but large changes in blood flow to the gut typically produce little or no change in total blood flow to the normal liver (42) because of regulation of hepatic arterial flow. There is some evidence that cirrhosis can disrupt this autoregulation, contributing to elevation in portal pressures (43).

Acute portal hypertension is uncommon after uncomplicated anatomic liver resections, which usually result in a rise in portal pressure of only 2 to 3 mm Hg. Major hepatic resections in the face of preexisting portal hypertension are contraindicated because further increase in portal pressure causes congestion of the intestine and increased intraabdominal pressure, and can be associated with hepatorenal syndrome or bowel necrosis (44). Patients with long-standing portal hypertension are less likely to develop intestinal necrosis, but are at risk for variceal bleeding in the early postoperative period. Portal hypertension may negatively affect hepatic regeneration, with some experimental evidence suggesting that partial portal vein ligation before resection increases hepatic ornithine decarboxylase activity and thymidine kinase activity after resection (45). Separate studies suggest that portosystemic shunting may improve survival in rats after massive hepatectomy (46). Portal hypertension can be inferred preoperatively based on liver biopsy and physical examination, and can be definitely determined using hepatic vein wedge pressures, splenic pulp pressures, or transhepatic portal vein cannulation. There is no widely accepted method of predicting postresectional portal pressures preoperatively. Judgment even of an experienced hepatobiliary surgeon is unreliable. In children, we have frequently performed liver resections in the face of some portal hypertension with limited mortality, but significant morbidity. Results of total hepatectomy and liver transplantation in children with significant hepatic parenchymal disease are excellent, making it preferred to major hepatic resection in such children.

The effects of limited portal vein blood flow on the liver have been less well characterized. Portal vein stenosis or thrombosis is a serious postoperative problem that may lead to acute hepatic necrosis and death. Chronic partial obstruction of portal venous flow, such as that seen in cavernous transformation of the portal vein may be associated with inhibition of hepatic growth that may be reversible by establishing more normal portal flow with a Rex shunt (superior mesenteric vein or portal vein collateral shunted for intrahepatic left portal vein). Portal vein stenosis after complex hepatic resections may be associated with impaired hepatic regeneration through similar mechanisms, but paucity of data renders this observation speculative.

Liver regeneration after partial hepatectomy appears to be dependent on tumor necrosis factor alpha (TNF-α). Animals treated with anti TNF-α antibodies do not regenerate their liver after partial hepatectomy (47). Regenerative liver failure occurs in mice lacking type 1 TNF receptors (48). Cellular signaling begins rapidly with increased expression of the antiapoptotic transcription factor, nuclear factor kB (NF-kB), in a TNF-α–dependent manner within 15 minutes of partial hepatectomy (48,49). In healthy animals, DNA synthesis is detectable 24 hours after partial hepatectomy and reaches a peak within 72 hours posthepatectomy (50). Poor nutritional status, sepsis, and chemotherapy may negatively affect hepatic regeneration after resection, which is in part regulated by insulin (51,52). Ischemic preconditioning has been proposed as a way to make use of these cellular changes to improve tolerance to hepatic ischemia during resection.

Bile is produced by active transport across the canalicular membranes of the hepatocyte. Bile flow is in part dependent on bile salts secreted by the hepatocytes and in part independent of this secretion, and related to glutathione and bicarbonate secretion (53,54). The composition of bile is altered in the bile ductules and ducts. Both hormones and second messengers regulate bile flow in response to various stimuli. Preoperative cholestasis in children who are candidates for liver resection is most often seen in patients with chronic hepatitis, and is relatively rare in children living in the United States. Obstruction of the bile ducts due to tumors is also uncommon in children, but has been reported in patients with non-Hodgkin's lymphoma (55), neuroblastoma (56), rhabdomyosarcoma (57), and pancreatoblastoma (58), and from benign inflammatory masses (59,60). Significant preoperative cholestasis should be carefully evaluated before any major liver resection because it implies diminished hepatic function and an increased risk of complications or death.

Cholestasis may complicate liver resection and may be due to an inadequate residual functional liver mass, devascularization of the bile duct during resection, decreased hepatic perfusion, sepsis, mechanical obstruction of the bile ducts, or a bile leak. Although bilirubin commonly increases slightly after an uncomplicated resection, any sustained increase in serum bilirubin should prompt an evaluation of the hepatobiliary tree. Cholestasis is hepatotoxic and is a potent stimulant of hepatic fibrosis. This may rapidly become clinically important, emphasizing the necessity of prompt intervention (61,62).

The liver produces a large volume of lymph, estimated in normal adults to be as high as 1 to 3 L per day. Increased sinusoidal pressure seen in cirrhosis or Budd Chiari syndrome may cause dramatic increases in lymphatic flow (63). The effect of hepatic resection on lymph flow has not been studied to our knowledge. Ascites formation after liver resection may be due to increased sinusoidal pressure as portal pressures rise. Lymph leaks due to complete or incomplete node dissections are usually self-limited. Treatment of ascites in either case is dependent on reducing sodium intake and limiting total daily fluids and the use of diuretics.

The liver plays a central role in glucose homeostasis. Hepatic glycogen is a primary substrate for glucose production via glycogenolysis during fasting and is a major site of gluconeogenesis. Net glucose production by the liver is stimulated by catecholamines, glucagon, and parasympathetic (64) stimulation. Insulin inhibits hepatic production of glucose. After a major liver resection, serum glucose should be monitored. Hypoglycemia, although unusual, occurs more commonly in children than adults undergoing equivalent liver resections. This is particularly true in children younger than 2 years of age because hepatic glycogen stores are small. Profound hypoglycemia suggests significant hepatic insufficiency and is an ominous finding.

Acute hepatic failure results in a stereotypical neurohormonal response that leads to water and sodium retention that also occurs after major resectional liver surgery and represents the most common fluid and electrolyte problem the hepatobiliary surgeon faces in practice. Sodium retention occurs due to an increased reabsorption of sodium in the proximal and distal tubules (65). This is mediated by the renin, angiotensins, and aldosterone system with possible contribution of the sympathetic nervous stimulation, but not atrial natriuretic factor (66). It results in ascites and edema. Occasionally, the ascites and fluid overload will be severe enough to result in respiratory difficulty, pulmonary edema, and pleural effusions. Concomitant retention of free water and an exaggerated antidiuretic hormone response after surgery frequently results in hyponatremia that can be profound. Water retention can be linked to (1) reduced delivery of filtrate to the ascending limb of the loop of Henle, (2) reduced renal synthesis of prostaglandins, and (3) increased secretion of arginine vasopressin (67). Failure to recognize sodium retention as one of the causes of the water retention can be problematic. Hyponatremia in these patients is almost always due to excess water retention and is not due to sodium depletion. Administration of sodium in this setting makes matters worse, not better. Those patients with severely compromised liver function and portal hypertension can suffer renal artery vasoconstriction and acute tubular necrosis (hepatorenal syndrome) (68).

Severe liver disease or massive hepatic resection can affect the child's ability to metabolize narcotics and other drugs. In the setting of a major liver resection, the half-life of these drugs is likely to be prolonged, although specific data of clinical relevance is difficult to find. The surgeon should be aware that drug toxicity may be increased after liver resection; thus, drug levels should be monitored where appropriate, and drug doses modified if necessary.

LIVER PATHOLOGY AND PREOPERATIVE EVALUATION

Primary tumors of the liver constitute the most common indication for liver resection in children. A more complete discussion of these tumors is presented in Chapter 38. Table 91-1 lists the pathologic type of liver tumors reported by Weinberg and Finegold (69) as well as those seen at our institution. Malignant hepatic lesions are more common than benign liver tumors in children. In children, approximately two-thirds of liver masses are malignant with hepatoblastoma accounting for 65%, hepatocellular carcinoma 25%, and sarcomas 10% (69). Benign lesions comprise about one-third of hepatic masses in children and include hemangiomas, hemangioendotheliomas, mesenchymal hamartomas, inflammatory pseudotumors, and adenomas. Focal nodular hyperplasia is rare, but has been reported in children (71,72). A number of points present in the history, and physical examination can be helpful in appropriately evaluating a child with a mass in the liver.

Malignant neoplasms are more likely to be asymptomatic. Hepatoblastomas are usually very large masses that present in the first few years of life. More than one-half of the 213 children enrolled in POG P 9645 (73) presented before their second birthday. Children with hepatocellular

TABLE 91-1 Pathologic Types of Primary Liver Tumors in Children.[a]

	n		%	
Tumor	***UF/Shands***	***Weinberg et al.***	***UF/Shands***	***Weinberg et al.***
Hepatoblastoma	17	532	28	43
Hepatocellular Carcinoma	14	284	23	23
Sarcoma	6	79	10	6
Benign vascular tumor	6	166	10	13
Mesenchymal hamartoma	11	75	18	6
Adenoma	2	22	3	2
Focal nodular hyperplasia	0	22	0	2
Miscellaneous	4	57	7	5

[a]Weinberg and Finegold's large collected series of liver tumors in children (69) is probably the best benchmark against which to compare smaller series, such as the authors' at Shands Children's Hospital at the University of Florida (UF/Shands) (70). The overall incidence of malignant tumors in children varies between 61% in the smaller series and 72% in the larger series. We suspect that the true incidence of benign lesions in children is higher because of a referral bias to both treating institutions.

carcinomas are typically school age or older and usually have had preexisting liver disease (74,75). Important exceptions are those children with tyrosinemia who may develop hepatocellular carcinoma in the first few years of life if not treated with 2-(2-nitro-4-trifluoromethylbenzoyl)-1, 3-cyclohexanedione (76,77). Children with sarcomas are also older and more likely to present with right upper quadrant pain or other symptoms. Benign lesions present in a bimodal age distribution with most vascular lesions, mesenchymal hamartomas present in infancy or early childhood, and most adenomas present in adolescence.

A careful physical exam demonstrates an abdominal mass in the majority of patients. Often this can be seen if the patient is observed in a relaxed state with a tangential light shining across the abdomen. In children with liver malignancies, serum α-fetoprotein is usually elevated at the time of presentation, often dramatically in those patients with hepatoblastoma and less impressively in hepatocellular carcinoma (78). Radiographic imaging is critical early in the initial evaluation, before any biopsy is performed. The two best studies are triple-phase computed tomography (CT) or magnetic resonance imaging (MRI) (79,80). These studies have largely displaced angiography. Some authors have challenged the accuracy of these studies in determining resectability with one group citing a 20% error rate (80). Newer generation scanners have improved to the extent that such errors should be rare. If resectability is questionable a repeat study should be done at an institution with expertise in pediatric hepatobiliary problems. General anesthesia is needed in some children to obtain optimal imaging. However, multiarray CT scanners can obtain complete images often in less than 10 seconds. Software allows for three-dimensional reconstruction and greatly improves the information derived compared with CT scans a decade ago. The importance of obtaining the best possible anatomic understanding of the tumor and its relationship to the segmental anatomy of the liver cannot be overstated (Figs. 91-3 to 91-5). If malignancy is suspected, evaluation of the chest is critical in order to identify possible pulmonary metastases (Fig. 91-6).

More recent advances in liver imaging have in large part eliminated the need for biopsy in preresection planning. With current use of triphasic CT scanning, gadolinium- and ferrite-enhanced MRI, and positron emission topography scanning, the majority of liver tumors can be diagnosed accurately without liver biopsy. Biopsy should be reserved for situations in which the results would alter disease management. The most common such scenarios include very large lesions, those that are deemed unresectable, and those with evidence of metastatic disease (81). In these situations, both the Children's Oncology Group and the International Society of Pediatric Oncology, Liver Tumor Study Group (SIOPEL), recommend biopsy with preresection chemotherapy (82). It is imperative that the biopsy is planned with the subsequent liver resection in mind. We favor needle biopsy of hepatic lesions through normal liver, which will be subsequently included in the resection. This diminishes the chance of tumor spillage and upstaging a malignant lesion (Fig. 91-7). Transvenous biopsy should be avoided because of the possibility of vascular spread of the lesion.

Benign lesions of the liver in children can represent special challenges. Luks et al. reported a series of 22 such patients treated with a 96% survival (83). Twenty such children were treated in our unit between 1968 and 1998 with an 80% survival (70). Fourteen of these children were resected with one death (7%). This child had a large hemangioendothelioma being treated under an Institutional

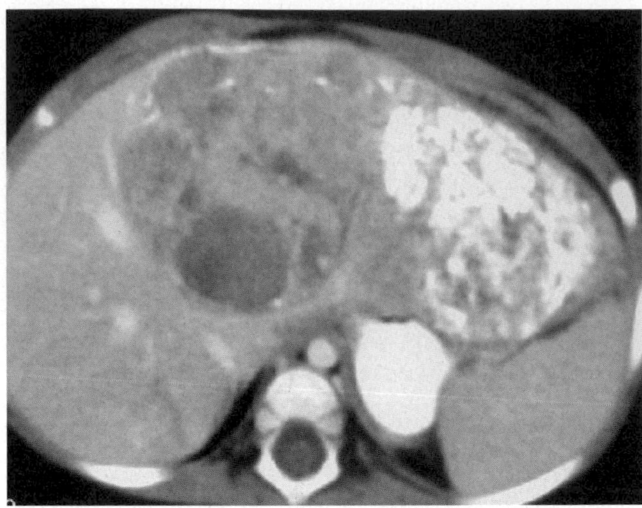

FIGURE 91-3. A computed tomography scan showing hepatoblastoma with calcification involving both lobes of the liver.

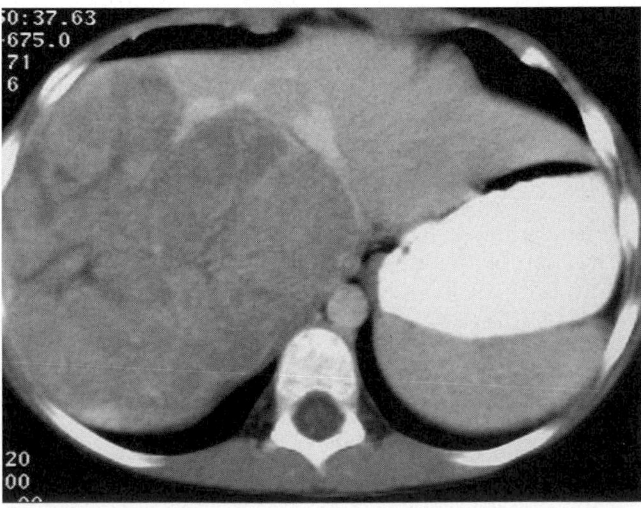

FIGURE 91-4. A computed tomography scan showing a hepatoblastoma as a hypovascular mass in the right lobe.

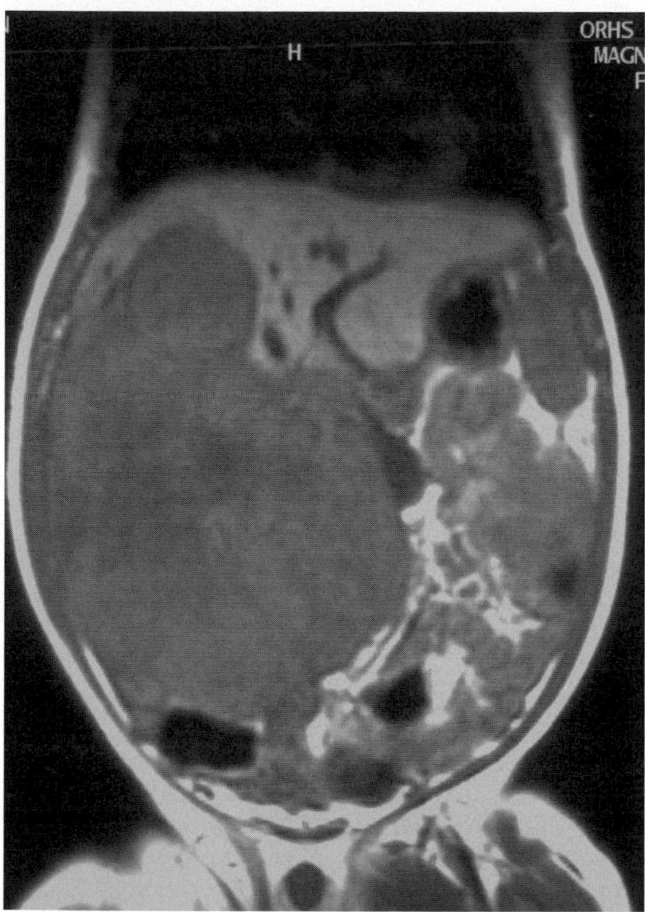

FIGURE 91-5. Preoperative imaging of liver tumors in children. A preoperative magnetic resonance imaging of a body with a hepatoblastoma that extends around the portal pedicle in the hilum and has resulted in some biliary dilation on the right side. This child requires preoperative chemotherapy in hopes of making anatomic resection possible.

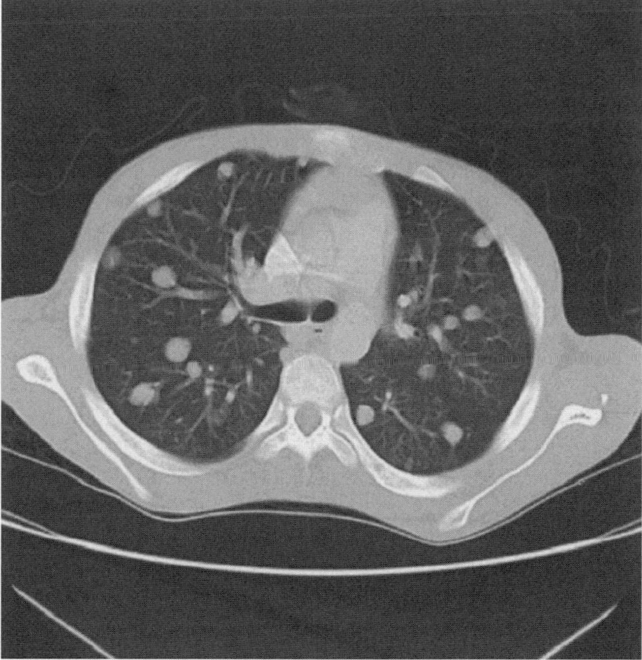

FIGURE 91-6. Evaluation for metastatic disease in children with liver tumors. A computed tomography (CT) image of the chest in a child with mestastatic hepatocellular carcinoma. Accurate staging disease is critical in planning the management of children with hepatic neoplasms. Although these metastases were visible on plain chest radiographs, discovery by CT scanning of isolated small metastasis is common.

Review Board (IRB)-approved protocol with alpha 2 interferon. She decompensated and subsequently died after an emergent liver transplant done while she was hemodynamically unstable. Six (30%) other children, including three with hemangiomas, were not resected and one-half died within 6 months from complications of their massive tumor. In this limited experience, infantile hemangiomas are often diffuse and may not be resectable due to anatomic problems. A variety of treatments for such infants have been proposed, including hepatic artery ligation, steroids, interferon, chemotherapy, and radiation therapy (84). Transplantation is probably safer and more effective than these treatments but, as pointed out above, cannot be depended on as a salvage treatment after a patient becomes unstable. Due to the logistics involved, it is important to begin the transplant process early. Most nonvascular benign tumors, even very large ones, are resectable. Indications for resection include their potential for bleeding and malignant degeneration (85–88). Adenomas are most common in postadolescent women on birth control pills and may be initially observed while withdrawing the hormonal stimulus. The potential for treatment using cytosolic hormone receptors in liver disease is debatable (89), as is the treatment of multiple adenomas with tamoxifen. Multiple hepatic adenomas may occur in patients with glycogen storage disease and requires careful follow-up because of reported development of hepatocellular carcinoma (90–92).

With these aforementioned exceptions, the prognosis of children with both benign and malignant lesions depends on surgical resection. In this context, staging liver masses based on resectability is appropriate. Historically, in the United States staging was done after abdominal exploration and depended primarily on the resectability of the tumor (Table 91-2). More recently, SIOPEL has developed a pretreatment tumor extension system (PRETEX), which is being used to study response to preoperative chemotherapy. This system focuses on the number of involved sectors of the liver at presentation. Use of such a system adds clarity to decision making in the treatment of both benign and malignant lesions. In general, children with PRETEX numbers 1 to 3 may be candidates for curvative resection, whereas children with PRETEX 4 lesions will require alternative therapy, possibly including complete hepatectomy and transplantation.

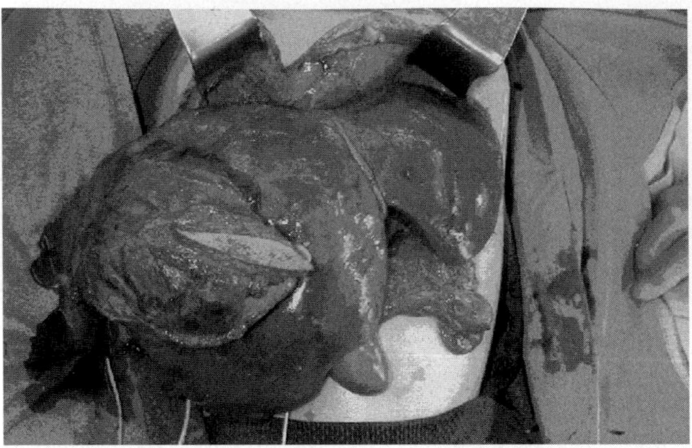

FIGURE 91-7. Tumor extension into abdominal wall after biopsy of hepatoblastoma. An open biopsy of this hepatoblastoma resulted in an exophytic tumor growing into the child's abdominal incision. En bloc resection as part of the hepatectomy combined with adjuvant therapy has resulted in long-term cure. Our preference is to biopsy this type of lesion using a needle passed through a portion of normal liver that will be removed with the ultimate resection. This can be done either open or percutaneously, depending on the anatomy, and decreases tumor spillage or extension dramatically.

PRERESECTION TREATMENT OF HEPATIC NEOPLASMS

Hepatoblastoma is chemosensitive, and treatment with adjuvant or neoadjuvant chemotherapy is recommended. The intergroup study by the Children's Cancer Study Group and the Pediatric Oncology Group contained 182 evaluable patients with hepatoblastoma of whom 59 had stage 1 or 2 (32%) disease and underwent resection followed by chemotherapy, whereas 123 children with stage 3 or 4 tumors were treated with chemotherapy prior to resection. Regimens and results are listed in Table 91-3. In the preresection phase, response to chemotherapy can be assessed by serial CT scans and alpha fetoprotein levels.

The importance of microscopically negative margins is debatable. Results of SIOPEL 1 and 2 suggest that microscopically positive margins do not adversely affect survival in hepatoblastoma treated with chemotherapy (93). Collected data suggest that patients with isolated but "unresectable" hepatoblastoma treated with orthotopic liver transplantation have a 5-year survival rate of more than 80% (94). Transplantation in the face of recurrent or distant disease has resulted in a much lower survival (30% to 40%). The role of hepatic transplantation in patients with multifocal disease confined to the liver is less clear, but aggressive multimodal therapy including transplantation has resulted in survival of 16 of 19 highly selected patients in two series (94,95).

Treatment of hepatocellular carcinoma or sarcomas is nearly totally dependent on surgical resection. Randomized trials have not shown benefit of adjuvant or neoadjuvant therapy for adults with resectable hepatocellular carcinoma (96,97). Preresection treatment of children with hepatocellular carcinoma using cisplatin and doxorubicin has resulted in partial response in one-half of children, but survival remains poor (98). The most common site of recurrences after resection is in the liver, underscoring the need for effective adjuvant therapy (99). Therapies proposed for advanced hepatocellular carcinoma in adults include pre- or postoperative chemotherapy (100), isolated hepatic perfusion after cytoreductive surgery (101), thalidomide (102), tamoxifen (103), interferon (104), I^{131} (105), and retinoids. These therapies have been used in limited series with variable results. No controlled trials have shown survival benefit for any of these therapies.

Dependence on resection as the essential component of therapy for hepatic malignancies, as well as the realization that complications result from inadequate mass of residual liver, have stimulated interest in methods to augment the normal parenchyma before resection. Preoperative portal vein embolization was first described by Kinoshita et al. (106) and later used by Makuuchi et al. in the setting of hepatic resection of hilar cholangiocarcinomas (107). The underlying concept is that occlusion of portal venous flow to the side of the liver ipsilateral to the lesion will cause hypertrophy of the contralateral side and increase the size of the future liver remnant. In adults, we currently consider preoperative portal vein embolization for patients without cirrhosis who require an extended hepatectomy that will leave a predicted liver volume after resection less than 25% of the preresection liver volume. Liver volume is assessed using three-dimensional CT volumetry. The portal vein ipsilateral to the tumor is embolized with coils or cyanoacrylate, and the contralateral side allowed to hypertrophy over 4 to 6 weeks. In adults, portal vein embolization has been demonstrated to increase the volume of the remnant liver by up to 30% and reduce the incidence of postoperative liver dysfunction and complications (108). The value of portal vein embolization in children has not been established.

TABLE 91-2 Intergroup (Pediatric Oncology Group–Childrens Cancer Group) Staging System.

Stage I	Complete resection with negative margins
Stage IIA	Complete resection following chemotherapy or radiation therapy
Stage IIB	Total resection with microscopically positive margins or preoperative rupture
Stage IIIA	Unresectable primary or gross residual disease after resection
Stage IIIB	Disease in regional lymph nodes
Stage IV	Metastatic disease

TABLE 91-3 Results of Intergroup Study of Hepatoblastoma by Stage.[a]

Stage	n	Chemotherapy	5-Year Event-free Survival (%)	5-Year Survival (%)
IFH[b]	9	Adriamycin (four courses)	100	100
IUH[b]	43	Randomized[c]	91	98
II	7	Randomized[c]	100	100
III	83	Randomized[c]	64	69
IV	40	Randomized[c]	25	37

[a]Treatment and results by stage for combined therapy of hepatoblastoma. (Ortega JA, Douglass EC, Feusner JH, et al. Randomized comparison of cisplatin/vincristine/flurouracil and cisplatin/continuous infusion doxorubicin for treatment of pediatric hepatoblastoma: a report from the Children's Cancer Group and the Pediatric Oncology Group. *J Clin Oncol* 2000;18(14):2665–2675.)
[b]FH, favorable histology; UH, unfavorable histology.
[c]Randomized: cisplatin, vincristine, and 5-flurouracil versus cisplatin and adriamycin (continuous infusion).

TECHNICAL ASPECTS OF LIVER RESECTION

The application of hepatic resection for the management of primary and secondary liver malignancies has increased in the last decade. Advances in patient selection, surgical technique, and perioperative management have resulted in increased safety. Most series of hepatic resections from experienced centers report operative mortality less than 5% in all patients and mortality of approximately 1% in patients with no underlying cirrhosis (109–112). Extended hepatectomy defined as resection of five or more hepatic segments as described by Couinaud (113) is still associated with increased mortality (109,114). The increased morbidity and mortality seen with extended resections are largely due to postoperative hepatic insufficiency associated with complications such as cholestasis, coagulation abnormalities, fluid retention, and hepatic synthetic dysfunction. Hepatic insufficiency becomes an even more formidable problem when complex biliary or vascular reconstructions are required in addition to the extended hepatectomy. More recently, there has been an emphasis on linking complications after extended hepatic resection to the amount or volume of liver left after the resection rather than to the amount of liver resected (115).

An intimate knowledge of the segmental anatomy of the liver and the detailed anatomy of the portal pedicles, hepatic veins, and vena cava, and their variations is essential to safely operating on the liver (21,113). Terminology used to describe the different resections has varied in the past, with recent attempts to standardize terminology among liver surgeons (23).

VASCULAR CONTROL

Because complications of liver resection are often related to excessive blood loss, a number of techniques have been developed to achieve preresection vascular control and decreased bleeding (116).

Division or occlusion of the vascular structures supplying the segment(s) of liver to be removed can establish selective inflow control. This technique has the advantage of preserving blood flow to the segment of the liver being preserved and is our preferred technique. Isolation of the vascular structures of the segments to be removed can be achieved either within the Glissonian sheath by separately dissecting and dividing the hepatic artery, portal vein, and bile duct, or alternatively by an extra Glissonian technique whereby the bile plate is lowered and the entire portal pedicle is isolated, clamped, and divided en mass (Fig. 91-8). Total inflow occlusion (Pringle maneuver) clamps the entire inflow of the liver and has been shown to reduce blood

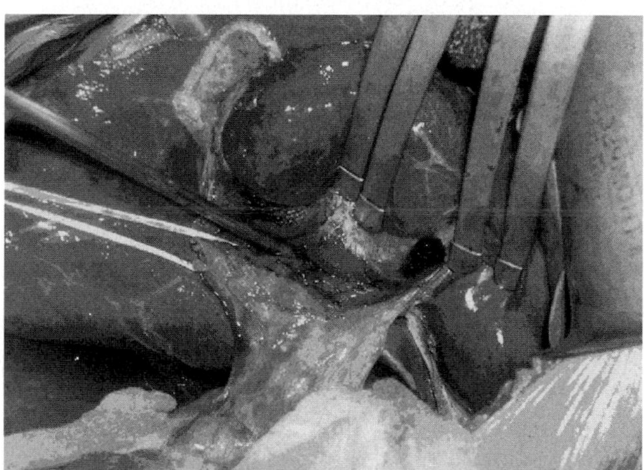

FIGURE 91-8. Techniques of segmental resection: isolation of portal pedicle to segments 5 and 8 after dropping the bile plate. The right portal pedicle has been encircled with a vessel loop after making an incision in the peritoneal reflection above the bifurcation of the porta hepatis. Dissecting the portal pedicles as a single entity reduces operative time and biliary injuries. Isolated clamping of the pedicle provides inflow occlusion to the segments to be resected and allows accurate parenchymal dissection.

loss during the parenchymal transection phase of the resection (117). Although there is some concern regarding warm ischemic injury, there is abundant data showing that the normal liver can tolerate inflow occlusion for up to 1 hour, and there are reports suggesting that some cirrhotic livers can safely tolerate 60 minutes of inflow occlusion as well (118). We use total inflow occlusion when selective occlusion provides insufficient control. Clamp times are expected to be less than 30 minutes for formal right or left hepatectomies, but may be higher for more complex parenchymal transsections. In such cases, total occlusion is carried out in 25- to 30-minute increments with 10-minute reperfusion intervals. More recently, we have begun applying the principle of ischemic preconditioning to the liver with an initial portal cross-clamp of 10 minutes early in the procedure prior to parenchymal transection followed by 15 minutes of reperfusion before beginning to transect the parenchyma. Ischemic preconditioning has been shown to protect the liver against subsequent episodes of more prolonged ischemia and to reduce hepatocellular apoptosis postreperfusion (119). Total vascular isolation of the liver with both inflow occlusion and occlusion of the supra- and infrahepatic vena cava can be useful for technically demanding cases where the vena cava or proximal hepatic veins are involved with tumor. Total isolation has been shown to be safe for up to 60 minutes in normal liver, but can be accompanied by varying degrees of hemodynamic instability (120). In cases where this is required, we carry out as much of the operation as possible prior to isolation of the liver to reduce the ischemic time and the period of hemodynamic instability (121,122). In unusual cases, where both portal and hepatic veins are involved with tumor, resection can occasionally still be performed using ex vivo liver resection techniques, where the liver is completely removed and flushed with cold preservation solution. The resection and reconstruction of portal and hepatic venous structures can then be undertaken on the back bench in a controlled, bloodless field, and the remnant liver then reimplanted into the patient using standard liver transplantation techniques (123,124). Others have advocated hypothermic circulatory arrest (125,126) for larger tumors that may require vascular reconstruction. Our experience suggests that this technique be reserved for tumors that have intracardiac extension via the hepatic veins and inferior vena cava.

Central Venous Pressure and Circulating Volume Control

The most troublesome bleeding during liver resection is usually from hepatic vein branches. Maintaining the central venous pressure (CVP) below 5 torr during the period of hepatic transection minimizes this bleeding. Cooperation of the anesthetist in limiting volume loading and occasionally using pharmacologic agents to reduce CVP is essential. However, if total vascular isolation is to be used, volume loading prior to caval clamping is required to avoid an acute decrease in cardiac output at the time the clamps are applied.

Parenchymal Transection

Meticulous technique is required in dividing the hepatic parenchyma to identify and ligate, clip, or coagulate all vessels and ducts. This can be accomplished with an instrument such as a Kelly clamp, but there is accumulating evidence that the ultrasonic dissector can increase the speed of the operation and reduce blood loss. More recently, other tools for parenchymal transection have been introduced into the armamentarium of the liver surgeon, including the water jet and tissue link devices. Although these newer devices have their proponents, they have not yet been proven to be better than the ultrasonic dissector. The use of drains following liver resection is optional based on the surgeon's preference. A policy of draining only those patients with specific indications has resulted in a very low complication rate (127).

Laparoscopy

Laparoscopy has been used for staging hepatic tumors for more than a decade and, more recently, has been extended to encompass the hepatic resection itself. Laparoscopic marsupialization of large hepatic cysts is relatively straightforward. The use of endoscopic vascular staplers to resect the cyst wall has simplified the procedure and reduces the risk of biliary leaks from compressed biliary radicles against the cyst wall. In experienced hands, laparoscopic left lateral segment resections or resections of the anterior segments of the liver can be performed with comparable results to the same procedure performed via an open approach (128). A complication peculiar to laparoscopic liver resection is CO_2 embolism. Transecting even small hepatic veins while there is positive pressure CO_2 pneumoperitoneum can lead to significant CO_2 embolism, but this can be minimized by both meticulous parenchymal transections along with the use of lower insufflation pressures.

Most reports to date, however, have focused on the use of laparoscopic liver resection for benign liver lesions. The suitability of laparoscopic resection for malignant disease has not been adequately addressed. Whether laparoscopic ultrasound provides similar sensitivity in detecting additional lesions in the liver as compared with open combined manual and intraoperative ultrasound assessment of the liver is not known. The ability to achieve comparable oncologic margins with laparoscopic liver resection as with open resection is debatable. The use of laparoscopic liver resection for malignant disease should only be expanded if comparable long-term results can be achieved.

ALTERNATE TREATMENTS OF HEPATIC MASSES

Transarterial chemoembolization (TACE) has been used in children with hepatoblastoma as an adjunct to resection (129) and for recurrent or progressive disease (130). Malogolowkin et al. have used the technique for unresectable hepatocellular carcinoma, as well as progressive or recurrent hepatoblastoma, with some good tumor response in nine children, three of whom have survived long term (131). A large randomized trial of TACE (CCG 8961) was halted when the material used for the embolization was removed from the market. There is a clear need for such a trial as salvage therapy.

Local ablation techniques, such as cryoablation or radiofrequency ablation (RFA), have been commonly used in adults with liver tumors (132–134). The role of these techniques is currently in flux. Local ablation techniques have not been proven to be of equal efficacy to surgical resection, and care must be taken in selecting patients for these techniques. For either cryo- or radiofrequency ablation, a probe is directed with imaging guidance into the tumor. The tumor, along with a surrounding 1-cm margin of normal liver, is destroyed either by freezing or by the application of radiofrequency energy and subsequent heat generation. Cryoablation in general requires an open procedure and has been largely replaced in North America with RFA. RFA can be performed percutaneously, laparoscopically, or as open procedure. Either technique is limited to tumors 4 to 5 cm in largest diameter. Occasionally, multiple tumors within the liver preclude resection alone because of concerns about inadequate residual parenchymal mass. In these cases, it may be useful to resect a lesser amount of liver and use radiofrequency to ablate any remnant tumor. This preserves liver function and allows a possibly curative approach. To date, however, there is no definitive proof that this aggressive approach to liver malignancy alters disease progression. Several ongoing trials are currently underway in adults to answer the question of whether this combined approach is reasonable therapy. The use of these techniques has not been reported in children and cannot currently be recommended outside an appropriate research setting.

POSTOPERATIVE CARE AND COMPLICATIONS

Nonanatomic resections of the liver for malignancy have been shown to result in a higher probability of histologically positive margins (135). They also result in a higher incidence of other complications and therefore should be abandoned.

Following resection of one or two segments of the liver, postoperative care should be straightforward. If blood loss has not been a problem and inflow occlusion has not been used, the child can be managed with age-appropriate intravenous fluids, with expectation of early return of bowel function and resumption of a regular diet. Standard postoperative pain management should be used without need for significant adjustment of doses. Patient-controlled analgesia is routinely used in patients older than 4 years. A low dose of continuous fentanyl for the first day or two is used in infants and toddlers. We have not used epidural analgesia either during or after hepatic surgery because of the risk of intrathecal bleeding.

More extensive resections (three to four segments) may cause early problems with glucose homeostasis, fluid retention, and need to adjust medications metabolized by the liver. Radical resections (five to six segments) routinely cause these problems, and may result in transient hepatic insufficiency requiring support of the coagulations system and aggressive nutritional support. Some of these patients will have significant fluid retention, hyponatremia, and renal dysfunction requiring fluid and salt restriction with the use of diuretics, and in severe cases, temporary renal replacement therapy. Serum phosphate levels should be monitored and hypophosphatemia treated (136). Drugs metabolized by the liver must be used with adjusted doses. This is particularly true for narcotics, which remain the preferred analgesics in this population. Hepatic encephalopathy, a frequent complication of liver failure, is uncommon after resection. However, even modest doses of narcotics can lead to stupor or coma following extensive resections if there is reduced hepatocellular reserve. In the setting of coagulopathy and thrombocytopenia, nonsteroidal antiinflammatory medications should be avoided altogether, as should acetaminophen. A pediatric intensive care unit with a nursing staff familiar with support of children with liver failure is a key resource to provide care for children undergoing extensive liver resections.

Postoperative complications increase with complexity of resection, amount of blood loss, length of ischemia, and are related to the amount of functional liver left after resection (137). Bleeding has been discussed and is most problematic in patients with coagulopathy following surgery. Preexisting liver disease is often associated with an accentuated stress response (138). Marked elevations of portal pressures postoperatively, with an attendant increase in risk of bleeding can create challenges postoperatively. Because oliguria and ascites often complicate massive liver resections, urine output and abdominal girth may not accurately predict bleeding. Monitoring of heart rate, central venous pressure, serial hematocrits, and drain output is helpful, but involvement of the operating surgeon with first-hand knowledge of the patient's anatomy is crucial in making the judgments necessary to successfully manage patients during this period. Reoperation should be performed promptly if needed to control bleeding.

In those children undergoing vascular reconstruction or prolonged vascular exclusion, thrombosis of either the portal vein or hepatic artery may occur, although this is seen infrequently. These events are usually related to injury to the portal triads of the remaining segments or to obstruction of the hepatic veins draining those segments, and may result in hepatic necrosis or further impair hepatic function resulting in liver failure and death. Doppler ultrasound examinations done at the bedside are reasonably accurate in evaluating the hepatic vessels and are part of the routine postoperative care following vascular reconstruction. Emergency evaluation and, if indicated, emergent reexploration should be carried out in any patient with suspected thrombosis of the hepatic artery or portal vein.

Small bile leaks occur after 5% to 10% of hepatic resection and are usually of little consequence. They are more common and frequently more serious after extensive resections. The incidence of bile leak may be related to technique of parenchymal transection (139,140). A bile leak should be suspected in any patient with a fever or jaundice after a liver resection. CT scans are usually diagnostic. Commonly, collections may be drained percutaneously. If a biliary reconstruction has not been done, an endoscopic retrograde cholangiopancreatogram should be performed to determine whether the leak is central or peripheral. A concomitant sphincterotomy with or without stent placement decreases the intrabiliary pressure and will aid in resolution of most peripheral leaks. Persistent central bile leaks or obstruction of the biliary tree are rare complications, but may require operative reconstruction of the biliary system (141).

Infectious complications following liver resections occur in 8% to 28% of patients (142), particularly in those patients with some aspect of hepatic insufficiency. Intraabdominal sepsis is most commonly associated with biliary complications, which need to be corrected in order to successfully treat the sepsis. In the setting of portal hypertension and liver failure, sepsis may rapidly lead to systemic inflammatory response syndrome with a high mortality. Line sepsis, pneumonia, and urinary tract infections may present with an increased bilirubin level and transaminase elevations.

The effect of chemotherapy on liver growth is not clear in adults, and data in children are almost nonexistent. In adults without chemotherapy, the liver has regenerated to 70% to 80% of original size by 6 weeks and takes up to 1 year to grow to a final size of about 90% of normal, never regenerating to full size. The liver's central role in growth and development argues that better understanding of the interaction of resection and chemotherapy on liver regeneration will be important in optimizing therapy for hepatoblastoma.

CONCLUSION

Surgery plays a central role in control and treatment of both benign and malignant diseases of the liver that occur in children. Technical progress in hepatic surgery has occurred rapidly since the 19[illegible] [illegible] field is still in a stage of rapid change. Improve[illegible] in preoperative patient selection and therapy, and in the management of patients both during and after surgery will continue to allow improved results. The specific roles of liver resection and orthotopic liver transplantation for both benign and malignant lesions in children continue to evolve at this time. Pre- and postoperative chemotherapy for malignant lesions is of crucial importance in hepatoblastoma. Effective treatments for hepatocellular carcinoma and sarcomas are not currently available, leaving surgical resection as the patient's only real hope for cure. For these patients, improved understanding of mechanisms which regulate liver regeneration may allow resectional therapy that is not currently safe. The next decade promises rapid progress in this arena.

REFERENCES

1. Ladd WE, Gross RE. *Abdominal surgery in infancy and childhood.* Philadelphia: WB Saunders, 1941.
2. Potts WJ. *The surgeon and the child.* Philadelphia: WB Saunders, 1959.
3. Exelby PR, Filler RM, Grosfeld JL. Liver tumors in children in the particular reference to hepatoblastoma and hepatocellular carcinoma: American Academy of Pediatrics Surgical Section Survey—1974. *J Pediatr Surg* 1975;10:329.
4. Exelby PR, El-Domeri A, Huvos AG, et al. Primary malignant tumors of the liver in children. *J Pediatr Surg* 1971;6:272.
5. Fuchs J, Rydzynski J, Von Schweinitz D, et al. Pretreatment prognostic factors and treatment results in children with hepatoblastoma: a report from German Copperative Pediatric Liver Tumor Study HB 94. *Cancer* 2002;95(1):172–182.
6. Schnater JM, Aronson DC, Plaschkes J, et al. Surgical view of the treatment of patients with hepatoblastoma: results from the first prospective trial of the International Society of Pediatric Oncology Liver Tumor Study Group. *Cancer* 2002;94(4):1111–1120.
7. King DR. Liver tumors. In: O'Neill JA, Rowe MI, Grosfeld JL, et al., eds. *Pediatric surgery,* 5th ed. St. Louis: Mosby, 1998:426–428.
8. Weinblatt ME, Siegel SE, Siegel MM, et al. Preoperative chemotherapy for unresectable primary hepatic malignancies in childern. *Cancer* 1982;50:1061–1064.
9. Andrassy RJ, Brennan LP, Siegel MM, et al. Preoperative chemotherapy for hepatoblastoma in children: report of six cases. *J Pediatr Surg* 1980;15:517–522.
10. Champion J, Greene AA, Pratt CB. Cisplatin (DDP): an effective therapy for unresectable or recurrent hepatoblastoma. *J Am Soc Clin Oncol* 1982;671:173.
11. Black CY, Cangir A, Choroszy M, et al. Marked response to preoperative high-dose cisplatinum in children with unresectable hepatoblastoma. *J Pediatr Surg* 1991;26:1070–1073.
12. Filler RM, Ehrlich PJ, Greenberg ML, et al. Preoperative chemotherapy in hepatoblastoma. *Surgery* 1991;110:591–597.
13. Stringer MD. Liver tumors. *Semin Pediatr Surg* 2000;9(4):196–208.
14. Brown J, Perilongo G, Shafford E, et al. Pretreatment prognostic factors for children with hepatoblastoma—results from the International Society of Pediatric Oncology (SIOP) Study SIOPEL-1. *Eur J Cancer* 2000;36:1418–1425.

15. Katzenstein HM, Longdong WB, Douglass EC, et al. Treatment of unresectable and metastatic hepatoblastoma: a pediatric oncology group phase II study. *J Clin Oncol* 2002;20(16):3438–3444.
16. Czauderna P, Mackinlay G, Perilongo G, et al. Hepatocellular carcinoma in children: results of the first prospective study of the International Society of Pediatric Oncology Group. *J Clin Oncol* 2002;20(12):2798–2804.
17. Katzenstein HM, Krailo MD, Malogolowkin HM, et al. Hepatocellular carcinoma in children and adolescents: results from the Pediatric Oncology Group and the Children's Cancer Group intergroup study. *J Clin Oncol* 2002;20(12):2789–2797.
18. Reyes JD, Carr B, Dvorchik I, et al. Liver transplantation and chemotherapy for hepatoblastoma and hepatocellular carcinoma in childhood and adolescence. *J Pediatr* 1996;136:795–804.
19. Superina R, Bilik R. Results of liver transplantation in children with unresectable liver tumors. *J Pediatr Surg* 1996;31:835–839.
20. Jonas MM, Perez AR. Liver disease in infancy and childhood. In: *Schiff's diseases of [illegible]er,* 9th ed. Philadelphia: Lippincott Williams & Wilkins, 200[illegible]
21. Bismuth H, Cas[illegible]ng [illegible], Garden OJ. Segmental surgery of the liver. *Surgery annual,* 1938;20:291–310.
22. McCluskey DA III, Skandalakis LJ, Colburn GL, et al. Hepatic surgery and hepatic surgical anatomy: historical partners in progress. *World J Surg* 1997;21:330–342.
23. Strasberg SM. Terminology of liver anatomy and liver resections: coming to grips with hepatic Babel. *J Am Coll Surg* 1997;184:413–434.
24. Couinaud C. Surgical anatomy of the liver. Several new aspects. *Chirurgie* 1986;112:337–342.
25. Kokudo N, Vera DR, Tada K, et al. Predictors of successful hepatic resection: prognostic usefulness of hepatic asialoglycoprotein receprot analysis. *World J Surg* 2002;26(11):1324–1347.
26. Ercolani G, Grazi GL, Calliva R, et al. The lidocaine (MEGX) test as an index of hepatic function: its clinical usefulness in liver surgery. *Surgery* 2000;127(4):464–471.
27. Zoedler T, Ebener C, Necker H, et al. Evaluation of liver function tests to predict operative risk in liver surgery. *HPB Surgery* 1995;9(1):13–18.
28. Fan ST. Methods and related drawbacks in estimation of surgical risks in cirrhotic patients undergoing hepatectomy. *Hepatogastroenterology* 2002;49(43):17–20.
29. Northover JM, Terblanche J. A new look at the arterial supply of the bile duct in man and its surgical implications. *Br J Surg* 1979;66(6):379–384.
30. Peclet MH, Ryckman FC, Pederson SH, et al. The spectrum of bile duct complications in pediatric liver transplantation. *J Pediatr Surg* 1994;29(2):214–219.
31. Egawa H, Uer[illegible] S, In[illegible] Y, et al. Biliary complications in pediatric living r[illegible]p[illegible]ntation. *Surgery* 1998;124(5):901–910.
32. Yamanaka, [illegible] TH, et al. Surgical complications and long-term c[illegible] pediatric liver transplantation. *Hepatogastroenterology* [illegible](35):1371–1374.
33. Mathisen O, Soreide O, Bergan A. Laparoscopic cholecystectomy: bile duct and vascular injuries: management and outcome. *Scand J Gastrocenterol* 2002;37(4):476–481.
34. Bhathal P, Grossman HJ. Nerve supply and nervous control of liver function. In: Bircher J, ed. *Oxford text book of clinical hepatology,* 2nd ed. Oxford, Oxford University Press, 1999.
35. Lindfeldt J, Balkan B, Vandijk G, et al. Influence of peri-arterial hepatic denervation on the glycemic response to exercise in rats. *J Autonom Nerv Syst* 1993;44:45–52.
36. Shimada M, Matsumata T, Taketomi A, et al. The role of prostaglandins in hepatic resection. *Prostaglandins Leukot Essent Fatty Acids* 1994;50(2):65–68.
37. Tsukada K, Sakaguchi T, Aono T, et al. Indocyanine green disappearance enhanced by prostaglandin E1 in patients with hepatic resection. *J Surg Res* 1996;66(1):64–68.
38. Orii R, Sugawara Y, Hayashida M, et al. Effects of amrinone on ischaemia-reperfusion injury in cirrhotic patients undergoing hepatectomy: a comparative study with prostaglandin E1. *Br J Anaesth* 2000;85(3):389–395.
39. Sato T, Yasui O, Kurokawa T, et al. Appraisal of intra-arterial infusion of prostaglandin E1 in patients undergoing major hepatic resection in four cases. *Tohoku J Exp Med* 2001;195(2):125–133.
40. Norryd C, Dencker H, Lunderquist A, et al. Superior mesenteric blood flow in man studied with a dye dilution technique. *Acta Chir Scand* 1975;141:109.
41. Norryd C, Dencker H, Lunderquist A, et al. Superior mesenteric blood flow during digestion in man. *Acta Chir Scand* 1975;141:197.
42. Lautt WW, Greenway CV. Conceptual review of the hepatic vascular bed. *Hepatology* 1987;7:952.
43. Vorobioff J, Bredfeldt JE, Groszmann RJ. Increased blood flow through the portal system in cirrhotic rats. *Gastroenterology* 1984;87(5):1120–1126.
44. Bruix J, Catells A, Bosch J, et al. Surgical resection of hepatocellular carcinoma in cirrhotic patients:prognostic valve of preoperative portal pressure. *Gastroenterology* 1996;111(4):1018–1022.
45. Kanh D, Kajani M, Zeng Q, et al. Effect of partial portal vein ligation on hepatic regeneration. *J Invest Surg* 1988;1(4):267–276.
46. Koyama S, Sato Y, Hatakeyama K. The subcutaneous splenic transposition prevents liver injury induced by excessive portal pressure after massive hepatectomy. *Hepatogastroenterology* 2003;50(49):37–42.
47. Ackerman P, Cote P, Yang SQ, et al. Antibodies to tumor necrosis factor alpha inhibit liver regeneration after partial hepatectomy. *Am J Physiol* 1992;263:579–585.
48. Yamada Y, Kirillova I, Peschon JJ, et al. Initiation of liver growth by tumor necrosis factor: deficient liver regeneration in mice lacking type I tumor necrosis factor receptor. *Proc Natl Acad Sci U S A* 1997;94:1441–1446.
49. Cressman DE, Greenbaum LE, Haber BA, et al. Rapid activation of PHF/NF kappa B in hepatocytes, a primary response in the regenerating liver. *J Biol Chem* 1994;269.
50. Zajicek G, Arber N, Schwartz-Arad D. Streaming liver VIII: cell production rates following partial hepatectomy. *Liver Transpl Surg* 1991;11:347–351.
51. Starzl TE, Porter KA, Kashiwagi N. Portal hepatatrophic factors, diabetes mellitus and acute liver atrophy, hypertrophy and regeneration. *Surg Gynecol Obstet* 1975;141(6):843–858.
52. Bucher ML, Swaffield MN. Regulation of hepatic regeneration in rats by synergistic action of insulin and glucagon. *Proc Natl Acad Sci U S A* 1975;72(3):1157–1160.
53. Boyer JL. Bile secretion: models, mechanisms, and malfunctions: a perspective on the development of modern cellular and molecular concepts of bile secretion and cholestasis. *J Gastroenterol* 1996;31:475–481.
54. Erlinger S. Review article: new insights into the mechanism of hepatic transport and bile secretion. *J Gastroenterol Hepatol* 1996;11:575–579.
55. Ravindra KV, Stringer MD, Prasad KR, et al. Non-Hodgkin lymphoma presenting with obstructive jaundice. *Br J Surg* 2003;90(7):845–849.
56. Okada T, Yoshida H, Matsunaga T, et al. Endoscopic internal biliary drainage in a child with malignant obstructive jaundice caused by neuroblastoma. *Pediatr Radiol* 2003;33(2):133–135.
57. Ruymann FB, Raney RB, Crist WM, et al. Rhabdomyosarcoma of the biliary tree in childhood. A report from the Intergroup Rhabdomyosarcoma Study. *Cancer* 1985;56(3):575–581.
58. Klimstra DS, Wenig BM, Adair CF, et al. Pancreatoblastoma. A clinicopathologic study and review of the literature. *Am J Surg Pathol* 1995;19(12):1371–1389.
59. Heneghan MA, Kaplan CG, Priebe CJ Jr, et al. Inflammatory pseudotumor of the liver: a rare cause of objective jaundice and portal hypertension in a child. *Pediatr Radiol* 1984;14(6):433–435.
60. Choi BY, Kim WS, Cheon JE, et al. Inflammatory myofibroblastic tumour of the liver in a child: CT and MR findings. *Pediatr Radiol* 2003;33(1):30–33.
61. Negi SS, Sakhuja P, Malhotra V, et al. Factors predicting advanced hepatic fibrosis in patients with postcholecystectomy bile duct strictures. *Arch Surg* 2004;139(3):299–303.
62. Jackson CC, Wu Y, Chenren S, et al. Bile decompression in children with histopathological evidence of pre-existing liver cirrhosis. *Ann Surg* 2002;68(9):816–819.
63. Dumont AE, Mulholland JH. Flow rate and composition of thoracic-duct lymph in patients with cirrhosis. *N Engl J Med* 1960;263:471.

64. Pilkis SJ. Hepatic gluconeogenesis/glycolysis: regulation and structure/function relationships of substrate cycle enzymes. *Ann Rev Nutr* 1991;11:465–515.
65. Jalan R, Hayes PC. Hepatic encephalopathy and ascites. *Lancet Oncol* 1997;350(9087):1209–1215.
66. Panos MZ, Anderson JV, Forbes A, et al. Human atrial natriuretic factor and renin-aldosterone in paracetamol induced fulminant hepatic failure. *Gut* 1991;32(1):85–89.
67. Arroyo V, Claria J, Salo J, Jiminez W, et al. Antidiuretic hormone and the pathogenesis of water retention in cirrhosis with ascites. *Semin Liver Dis* 1994;14:44–58.
68. Colle I, Moreau R, Pessione F, et al. Relationships between haemodynamic alterations and the development of ascites in patients with cirrhosis. *Eur J Gastroenterol Hepatol* 2001;13(3):251–256.
69. Weinberg AG, Finegold MJ. Primary hepatic tumors of childhood. *Hum Pathol* 1983;14(6):512–537.
70. Josephs MD, Langham MR Jr, Lauwers G, et al. *Evidence based strategy for improving outcome of children with liver tumors.* Abstract data presented at the meeting of International Society of Pediatric Surgical Oncology, Lake Buena Vista, Florida, May 2000.
71. Reymond D, Plaschkes J, Luthy AR, et al. Focal nodular hyperplasia of the liver in children: review of follow-up and outcome. *J Pediatr Surg* 1995;30(11):1590–1593.
72. Hung PL, Huang SC, Kuo HW, et al. Hepatic focul nodular hyperplasia in children: report of three cases. *Chang Gung Med J* 2001;24(10):657–662.
73. Katzenstein HM. Study Committee Progress Report POG P 9645 Phase III Protocol for the Treatment of Children with Hepatoblastoma. Available: www.cog.org/
74. Esquivel CO, Gutierrez C, Cox KL, et al. Hepatocellular carcinoma and liver dysplasia in children with chronic liver disease. *J Pediatr Surg* 1994;29(11):1465–1469.
75. Chan KL, Fan ST, Tam PK, et al. Paediatric hepatoblastoma and hepatocellular carcinoma: retrospective study. *Hong Kong Med J* 2002;8(1):13–17.
76. Russo PA, Mitchell GA, Tanquay RM. Tyrosinemia: a review. *Pediatr Dev Pathol* 2001;4(3):212–221.
77. Mohan N, McKiernan P, Preece MA, et al. Indications and outcome of liver transplantation in tyrosinaemia type 1. *Eur J Pediatr* 1999;158(Suppl 2):S49–S54.
78. Gregory JJ, Finlay JL. Alpha-fetoprotein and beta-human chorionic gonadotropin: their clinical significance as tumour markers. *Drugs* 1999;57(4):463–467.
79. Rummency E, Weissleder R, Stark DD, et al. Primary liver tumors: diagnosis by MRI imaging. *AJR Am J Roentgenol* 1989;152(1):63–72.
80. King SJ, Babyn PS, Greenberg ML, et al. Value of CT in determining the resectability of hepatoblastoma before and after chemotherapy. *AJR Am J Roentgenol* 1993;160(4):793–798.
81. Von Schwinitz D, Burger D, Mildenberger H. Is laparotomy the first step in treatment of childhood liver tumors? The experience from the German Cooperative Pediatric Liver Tumor Study HB-89. *Eur J Pediatr Surg* 1994;4(2):82–86.
82. Schnater JM, Aronson DC, Plaschkes J, et al. Surgical view of the treatment of patients with hepatoblastoma: results from the first prospective trial of the International Society of Pediatric Oncology Liver Tumor Study Group. *Cancer* 2002;94(4):1111–1120.
83. Luks FI, Yasbeck S, Brandt ML, et al. Benign liver tumors in children: a 25-year experience. *J Pediatr Surg* 1991;26(11):1326–1330.
84. Iyer CP, Stanley P, Mahour GH. Hepatic hemangiomas in infants and children: a review of 30 cases. *Am Surg* 1996;62(5):356–360.
85. Lauwers GY, Grant LD, Donnelly WH, et al. Hepatic undifferentiated (embryonal) sarcoma arising in a mesenchymal hamartoma. *Am J Surg Pathol* 1997;10:1248–1254.
86. Corbally MT, Spitz L. Malignant potential of mesenchymal hamartoma: an unrecognized risk. *Pediatr Surg Int* 1992;7:321–322.
87. DeChadarevian JP, Pawel BR, Faerber EN, et al. Undifferentiated (embryonal) sarcoma arising in conjunction with mesenchymal hamartoma of the liver. *Mod Pathol* 1994;7:490–493.
88. Ramanujam TM, Ramesh JC, Goh DW, et al. Malignant transformation of mesenchymal hamartoma of the liver: case report and review of the literature. *J Pediatr Surg* 1999;34:1684–1686.
89. Porter LE, Elm MS, Van Thiel DH, et al. Hepatic estrogen receptor in human liver disease. *Gastroenterology* 1987;92(3):735–745.
90. Lerut JP, Ciccarelli O, Sempoux C, et al. Glycogenosis storage type I diseases and evolutive adenomatosis: an indication for liver transplantation. *Transpl Int* 2003;16(12):879–884.
91. Matern D, Seydewitz HH, Bali D, et al. Glycogen storage disease type I: diagnosis and phenotype/genotype correlation. *Eur J Pediatr* 2002;161(Suppl 1):S10–S19.
92. Labrune P, Trioche P, Duvaltier I, et al. Hepatocellular adenomas in glycogen storage disease type I and III: a series of 43 patients and review of the literature. *J Pediatr Gastroenterol Nutr* 1997;24(3):276–279.
93. Brugieres L, Phillips A, Rondelli R, et al. Hepatoblastoma with microscopic residual disease after surgery: data from SIOPEL 1 and 2 studies. *Med Pediatr Oncol* 2000;35(177).
94. Otte JB, Pritchard J, Aronson DC, et al. Liver transplantation for hepatoblastoma: results of the International Society of Pediatric Oncology (SIOP) Study SIOPEL-1 and review of the world experience. *Pediatr Blood Cancer* 2004;42:74–83.
95. Srinivasan P, McCall J, Pritchard J, et al. Orthotopic liver transplantation for unresectable hepatoblastoma. *Transplantation* 2002;74:652–655.
96. Schwartz JD, Schwartz M, Mandeli J, et al. Neoadjuvant and adjuvant therapy for resectable hepatocellular carcinoma: review of randomized clinical trials. *Lancet Oncol* 2002;3(10):593–603.
97. Kwok PC, Lam TW, Lam PW, et al. Randomized controlled trial to compare the dose of adjuvant chemotherapy after curative resection of hepatocellular carcinoma. *J Gastroenterol Hepatol* 2003;18(4):450–455.
98. Czauderna P. Adult type vs. childhood hepatocellular carcinoma—are they the same or different lesions? Biology, natural history, prognosis and treatment. *Med Pediatr Oncol* 2002;39(5):519–523.
99. Cha C, Fong Y, Jarnagin WR, et al. Predictors and patterns of recurrence after resection of hepatocellular carcinoma. *J Am Coll Surg* 2003;197(5):753–758.
100. Mathurin P, Raynard B, Dharancy S, et al. Meta-analysis: evaluation of adjuvant therapy after curative liver resection for hepatocellular carcinoma. *Aliment Pharmacol Ther* 2003;17(10):1247–1261.
101. Ku Y, Iwasaki T, Tominaga M, et al. Reductive surgery plus percutaneous isolated hepatic perfusion for multiple advanced hepatocellular carcinoma. *Ann Surg* 2004;239(1):53–60.
102. Wang TE, Kao CR, Lin SC, et al. Salvage therapy for hepatocellular carcinoma with thalidomide. *World J Gastroenterol* 2004;10(5):649–653.
103. Engstrom PF, Levin B, Moertel CG, et al. A phase II trial of Tamoxifen in hepatocellular carcinoma. *Cancer* 1990;65(12):2641–2643.
104. Tabor E. Interferon for preventing and treating hepatocellular carcinoma associated with hepatitis B and C viruses. *Dig Liver Dis* 2003;35(5):297–305.
105. Raoul JL, Messner M, Boucher E, et al. Preoperative treatment of hepatocellular carcinoma with intra-arterial injection of ^{131}I-labelled lipiodol. *Br J Surg* 2003;90(11):1379–1383.
106. Kinoshita H, Sakai K, Hirohashi K, et al. Preoperative portal vein embolization for hepatocellular carcinoma. *World J Surg* 1986;10(5):803–808.
107. Makuuchi M, Thai BL, Takayasu K, et al. Preoperative portal embolization to increase safety of major hepatectomy for hilar duct carcinoma: a preliminary report. *Surgery* 1990;107(5):521–527.
108. Hemming AW, Reed AI, Howard RJ, et al. Preoperative portal vein embolization for extended hepatectomy. *Ann Surg* 2003;237(5):686–693.
109. Belghiti J, Hiramatsu K, Benoist S, et al. Seven hundred forty-seven hepatectomies in the 1990's: an update to evaluate the actual risk of liver resection. *J Am Coll Surg* 2000;191(1):38–46.
110. Jarnagin WR, Gonen M, Fong Y, et al. Improvement in perioperative outcome after hepatic resection: analysis of 1,803 consecutive cases over the past decade. *Ann Surg* 2002;236(4):406–407.
111. Choti MA, Bowman HM, Pitt HA, et al. Should hepatic resections be performed at high-volume referral centers? *J Gastrointest Surg* 1998;2(1):11–20.
112. Hemming AW, Sielaff TD, Gallinger S, et al. Hepatic resection of non-colorectal nonneuroendocrine metastases. *Liver Transpl Surg* 2000;6(1):97–101.

113. Couinaud C. Le foie: etudes anatomicales et chirurgicales. Paris: Masson and Cie, 1957:187–208.
114. Melendez J, Ferri E, Zwillman M, et al. Extended hepatic resection: a 6-year retrospective study of risk factors for perioperative mortality. *J Am Coll Surg* 2001;192(1):47–53.
115. Shirabe K, Shimada M, Gion T, et al. Postoperative liver failure after major hepatic resection for hepatocellular carcinoma in the modern era with special reference to remnant liver volume. *J Am Coll Surg* 1999;188(3):304–309.
116. Takenaka K, Kanematsu T, Fuzawa K, et al. Can hepatic failure after surgery for hepatocellular carcinoma in cirrhotic patients be prevented? *World J Surg* 1990;14:123–127.
117. Man MB, Fan ST, Ng I, et al. Prospective evaluation of Pringle maneuver in hepatectomy for liver tumors by a randomized study. *Ann Surg* 1997;6:704–713.
118. Nagasue N, Yukaya H, Suehiro S, et al. Tolerance of the cirrhotic liver to normothermic ischemia. A clinical study of 15 patients. *Am J Surg* 1984;147:772–775.
119. Clavien PA, Yaclav S, Sindram D, et al. Protective effects of ischemic preconditioning for liver resection performed under inflow occlusion in humans. *Ann Surg* 2000;232:155–162.
120. Huguet C, Addario-Chieco P, Gavelli A, et al. Technique of hepatic vascular exclusion for extensive liver resection. *Am J Surg* 1992;163: 602–605.
121. Hemming AW, Reed AI, Langham MR, et al. Hepatic vein reconstruction for resection of hepatic tumors. *Ann Surg* 2002;235(6): 850–858.
122. Hemming AW, Langham MR, Reed AI, et al. Resection of the inferior vena cava for hepatic malignancy. *Am Surg* 2001;67(11):1081–1087.
123. Hemming AW, Cattral MS. Ex-vivo liver resection with replacement of the inferior vena cava and hepatic vein replacement by transposition of the portal vein. *J Am Coll Surg* 1999;189:523–526.
124. Hemming AW, Chari RS, Cattral MS. Ex vivo liver resection. *Can J Surg* 2000;43(3):222–224.
125. Ein SH, Shandling B, Williams WG, et al. Major hepatic tumor resection using profound hypothermia and circulation arrest. *J Pediatr Surg* 1981;16(3):339–342.
126. Oldhafer KJ, Fuchs J, Steinhoff G, et al. Extended liver resection in small children under circulatory arrest and "low flow" cardiopulmonary bypass. *Chirurgie* 2000;71(6):692–695.
127. Burt BM, Brown J, Jarnagin W, et al. An audit of results of a nodrainage practice policy after hepatectomy. *Am J Surg* 2002;184(5): 441–445.
128. Lesurtel M, Cherqui D, Laurent A, et al. Laparoscopic versus open left lateral hepatic lobectomy: a case control study. *J Am Coll Surg* 2003;196(2):236–242.
129. Han YM, Park HH, Lee JM, et al. Effectiveness of pre-operative transarterial chemoembolization in presumed inoperable hepatoblastoma. *J Vasc Interv Radiol* 1999;10(9):1275–1280.
130. Oue T, Fukuzawa M, Kusafuka T, et al. Transcatheter arterial chemoembolization in the treatment of hepatoblastoma. *J Pediatr Surg* 1998;33(12):1771–1775.
131. Malagolowkin MH, Stanley P, Steele DA, et al. Feasibility and toxicity of chemoembolization for children with liver tumors. *J Clin Oncol* 2000;18(6):1279–1284.
132. Erce C, Parks RW. Interstitial ablative techniques for hepatic tumours. *Br J Surg* 2003;90(3):272–289.
133. Lam CM, Ng KK, Poon RT, et al. Impact of radiofrequency ablation on the management of patients with hepatocellular carcinoma in a specialized centre. *Br J Surg* 2004;91(3):334–338.
134. Curley SA, Marra P, Beaty K, et al. Early and late complications after radiofrequency ablation of malignant liver tumors in 608 patients. *Ann Surg* 2004;239(4):450–458.
135. Fuchs J, Rydzynski J, Hecker H, et al. The influence of preoperative chemotherapy and surgical technique in the treatment of hepatoblastoma—a report from the German Cooperative Liver Tumour Studies HB 89 and HB 94. *Eur J Pediatr Surg* 2002;12(4):255–261.
136. Smyrniotis V, Kostopanagiotou G, Katsarelias D, et al. Changes of serum phosphorus levels in hepatic resections and implications on patients' outcomes. *Int Surg* 2003;88(2):100–104.
137. Wei AC, Tung-Ping, Poon R, et al. Risk factors for perioperative morbidity and mortality after extended hepatectomy for hepatocellular carcinoma. *Br J Surg* 2003;90(1):33–41.
138. Lan AK, Luk HN, Goto S, et al. Strees response to hepatectomy in patients with a healthy or a diseased liver. *World J Surg* 2003;27(7):761–764.
139. Nakayama H, Masuda H, Shibata M, et al. Incidence of bile leakage after three types of hepatic parenchymal transection. *Hepatogastroenterology* 2003;50(53):1517–1520.
140. Kim J, Ahmad SA, Low AM, et al. Increased biliary fistulas after liver resection with the harmonic scalpel. *Am Surg* 2003;69(9):815–819.
141. Tanaka S, Hirohashi K, Tanaka H, et al. Incidence and management of bile leakage after hepatic resection for malignant hepatic tumors. *J Am Coll Surg* 2002;195(4):484–489.
142. Towu E, Kiely E, Pierro A, et al. Outcome and complications after resection of hepatoblastoma. *J Pediatr Surg* 2004;39(2):199–202.

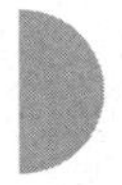

Biliary Atresia

Peter W. Dillon and Thomas F. Tracy, Jr.

Biliary atresia is one of the most serious digestive disorders of infants and young children (1). It is a process of uncertain pathogenesis that leads to fibrosis and obliteration of the extrahepatic ductal system resulting in obstruction to bile flow and cholestasis. Progressive injury to intrahepatic ductular structures and surrounding hepatic parenchyma through a destructive inflammatory process ultimately leads to cirrhosis and hepatic failure. If left untreated, the prognosis for biliary atresia patients is extremely poor with death usually occurring within 2 years. Since the introduction of the Kasai portoenterostomy in the 1960s, the treatment for biliary atresia has been surgical. With continued improvement in hepatic transplantation, the prognosis for infants with this disorder has improved dramatically. The strategy of sequential surgical therapy initially involving a portoenterostomy procedure followed by liver transplantation if needed is widely accepted. However, both surgical therapies serve only to palliate the disease process, and there are no specific therapeutic interventions targeted to influence the pathologic endogenous inflammatory process itself. For that matter, little is known about the etiology, pathologic mechanisms, or even possible treatment strategies for this disorder.

SURGICAL HISTORY

Burns described an infant with jaundice and acholic stools in 1817; this was the first recorded case of biliary atresia in the English language (2). In 1892, John Thompson, a physician in Edinburgh, described the clinical course and autopsy results of 49 patients with congenital obliteration of the bile ducts (3). J.B. Holmes, a pediatrician and pathologist at Johns Hopkins, reported 82 autopsy cases in 1916 and predicted the feasibility of a biliary-enteric anastomosis. His work served as the basis for the subsequent development of the classification of the disease process into "correctible" and "noncorrectable" types. Reports of surgical success with the "correctable" form of biliary atresia were published by Ladd in 1928 and Gross in 1940 (4,5). However, results from institutions elsewhere in the United States and in Europe were otherwise dismal, and the only surviving patients were in the "correctable" forms of biliary atresia, where an anastomosis could be made to a biliary cyst external to the liver surface. Results were so poor with "noncorrectable" forms of atresia that few patients were operated on or even actively treated until the mid-1960s. During this time, many surgical procedures were attempted with little success. These operations included partial hepatic resection with drainage, placement of intrahepatic drains, and drainage of hepatic lymph through the thoracic duct (6–8). At that time, it was the opinion of most surgeons in the United States that direct reconstruction of the extrahepatic biliary tract for noncorrectable atresia was futile. If surgery was to be considered, it was believed that delaying the procedure as long as possible was desirable in the hope that spontaneous resolution of the obstructive process would occur. There was concern that surgery would increase the postoperative mortality of neonatal hepatitis or cirrhosis. Even the operative procedures were conservative in nature because all attempts were made to preserve ductal structures so they would have a chance to reopen spontaneously in the postoperative period.

In Japan, Kasai's work with biliary atresia patients began to challenge these concepts. In 1955, he noted that when the extrahepatic biliary tract was excised to the hilum, bile flow from the porta hepatis occurred. Over the next several years, he devised and perfected a procedure in which the structures in the porta hepatis were drained via a Roux-en-Y jejunal limb. Although his operation has since undergone numerous modifications, Kasai's lasting contribution to the surgical treatment of biliary atresia was the

Peter W. Dillon: Department of Surgery, Penn State College of Medicine, Penn State Children's Hospital, Milton S. Hershey Medical Center, Hershey, Pennsylvania 17033.

Thomas F. Tracy, Jr.: Department of Surgery and Pediatrics, Brown Medical School, Hasbro Children's Hospital, Providence, Rhode Island 02903.

realization that the occluded extrahepatic ductal system could be isolated and dissected to the porta hepatis and that a functional enteric anastomosis could potentially be constructed to drain the remnant porta hepatis.

EPIDEMIOLOGY

Biliary atresia has a worldwide incidence of 1 in 8,000 to 17,000 live births, and it is more common in girls than in boys (9,10). Epidemiologic studies suggest that racial and environmental factors may play a role in its pathogenesis. In the United States, the incidence of this disorder is almost two times greater in African American than in white infants, and it is more common in Chinese than Japanese infants (11,12). Although several cases have been reported in families, the disease does not have a familial incidence, and twins have been reported to be both affected and only one affected (13–16).

Maternal factors relating to the disease process have been inadequately studied, but maternal age and parity appear to have no relationship (11). Infants tend to be of low birth weight and are usually full term as the disease is rarely seen in stillborns or premature infants. However, in a more recent study from Sweden biliary atresia was found with higher incidence in infants less than or equal to 32 weeks' gestational age or when maternal age was greater than or equal to 35 years or parity was 4 or greater (17).

Several regional studies have shown an increased incidence of biliary atresia at certain times of the year leading some to suggest an infectious etiology. However, these data are conflicting and contradictory. An increased incidence of the disease was noted in Texas from 1972 to 1980 in late summer and fall, but in Atlanta from 1968 to 1993 winter and early spring clustering was reported (11,18). However, studies from Michigan and multiple countries in Europe have failed to demonstrate significant regional variation, seasonal variation, or space–time clustering (19–24). These conflicting reports may support a growing belief that biliary atresia is not a single disease but the result of complex processes yielding a common final inflammatory pathway targeting and ultimately destroying the extrahepatic bile ducts.

PATHOGENESIS

One of the greatest handicaps in dealing with biliary atresia is the fact that the etiology of this disease remains unknown. As a result of both clinical and experimental investigations, several general mechanisms have been proposed as potential causes of biliary atresia; however, no single theory has elicited a consensus. Potential initiating events include occult viral infection, environmental toxin exposure, a defect in ductal morphogenesis, a disorder of the immunologic or inflammatory system, and a defect in the fetal hepatic circulation (25).

The possibility that a viral infection in the pre- or perinatal period is the cause of biliary atresia has been a focus of clinical research efforts. Multiple lines of evidence in animal models have been developed suggesting that viruses are involved. It has been noted that liver specimens from biliary atresia patients exhibit pathologic findings consistent with viral infection including upregulation of Fas ligand, biliary epithelial apoptosis, and mononuclear cell activation within the portal tracts (26). The related hypothesis is that destruction of the intra- and extrahepatic bile ducts subsequently results from an immunologic reaction triggered by viral-induced neoantigens on the biliary epithelium. Specific viruses proposed as potential pathogens in this scenario include reovirus 3, cytomegalovirus (CMV), rotavirus C, human papillomavirus, and retroviruses. At present, however, the data remain inconclusive.

In the 1980s, it was found that a number of infants with biliary atresia demonstrated serologic reactivity to reovirus type 3 when compared with controls, and reovirus 3 particles were detected in the extrahepatic ductal tissue of an infant with biliary atresia (27–29). These studies were subsequently supported by molecular investigations in which RNA specific to reovirus was demonstrated in extrahepatic biliary tissue from biliary atresia patients (30). However, subsequent studies have failed to detect the presence of reovirus 3 in the disease (31,32). Investigations of other viruses have yielded similar conflicting results. Evidence of CMV infection has been found in a number of infants with biliary atresia, but not in others (33–35). Reports focused on rotavirus C and human papillomavirus have yielded similar contradictory results (36–39). More recently, possible retrovirus infection has also been reported (40). No association with biliary atresia has been found for one important group of hepatic viral infections, hepatitis A, B, and C (41,42). Although many investigators believe an infectious mechanism is likely, there are no definitive data implicating a specific agent as a causative factor. It is possible that a virus could initiate or contribute to this disorder depending on the presence of specific cofactors or conditions. Finally, it must be noted that these infections are relatively common and may be incidental and unrelated.

Environmental toxin exposure during pregnancy is a potential cause of biliary atresia, although there is no current evidence implicating a specific teratogen or environmental factor. Investigators have noted several studies reporting a time–space clustering of cases, possibly consistent with toxin or environmental exposure. One report suggests that farming or pesticide exposure and maternal infectious illness during the last trimester of gestation increased the risk of developing biliary atresia (10).

Primary pathology of the immune system, either congenital or acquired, could possibly result in an "autoimmune" process in which biliary epithelium and ductal structures are targeted. Circulating autoantibodies, including antineutrophil cytoplasmic antibodies (ANCA), have been detected in biliary atresia patients (43). Additional support for this theory is derived from serologic studies of human leukocyte antigen (HLA) expression in affected infants, as well as from pathologic similarities to the adult processes of primary sclerosing cholangitis and primary biliary cirrhosis. An increase in the frequency of the HLA-B12 allele expression was noted in infants with biliary atresia as compared with controls (44). A subsequent study was unable to confirm these observations (45). An increased frequency of HLA-B8 expression has also been reported—an observation that is important given the association of this HLA allele with other autoimmune disorders (46). It is now recognized that HLA genotypes are not alone in their association with autoimmune disease processes, and that these can be more accurately defined by determining the variation in expression of a number of genes encoding immune regulatory proteins (47). Most important among these genes are those encoding the proinflammatory cytokines tumor necrosis factor alpha (TNF-α), interleukin 1 (IL-1), and the immunoregulatory cytokine interleukin 10 (IL-10). Using DNA genotyping, no association of biliary atresia has been demonstrated for HLA class I or II gene expression or for the common polymorphisms of the genes encoding IL-1, TNF-α, and IL-10. At present, it appears that biliary atresia is not an HLA-associated disease (48).

When first described, biliary atresia was believed to represent a defect in the morphogenesis of the biliary tract, hence the name. As many as 30% of infants with biliary atresia have coexisting anatomic anomalies including visceral organ asymmetry, offering support to the concept of abnormal embryogenesis as an etiology. Indirect support for this cause is found in more recent investigations of the *inv* mouse. Mutations in the inversin gene in homozygous mutants result in *situs inversus* with mirror image left–right inversions of stomach, liver, and spleen (49,50). Some of these animals have polysplenia, preduodenal portal vein, and intestinal malrotation—clinical findings associated with biliary atresia. These mice become progressively jaundiced after birth with marked abnormalities of the intrahepatic bile ducts and a histologic picture that resembles biliary atresia (51). The potential involvement of this gene in patients with biliary atresia and situs anomalies is an area of current research. Abnormalities in the morphogenesis and differentiation of intrahepatic bile ducts have been described in the livers of some infants with biliary atresia (52–54). It has been proposed that interruption of the normal remodeling process of the primitive ductal plate may result in persistence of this structure and inadequate bile duct lumen formation. Histologic evidence of ductal plate malformation has been observed in cases of extra- and intrahepatic atresia of the bile ducts and has also been associated with abnormalities in the hepatic artery (55,56). Elucidation of the molecular regulatory factors potentially responsible for such an abnormality may come from ongoing investigations in a murine knockout model. In the mouse, it has been found that ductal plate malformations occur in the absence of the transcription factors hepatocyte nuclear factor-6 (HNF-6) and hepatocyte nuclear factor 1B (HNF-1b) (57,58). Other signaling pathways such as Jagged-1/Notch, deficient in Alagille syndrome, may also be important in bile duct morphogenesis (59).

The concept that local ischemia during fetal hepatobiliary development may contribute to the pathogenesis of biliary atresia has been the focus of renewed interest. The close relationship between the development of the hepatic vasculature and the biliary system is well recognized. During the course of normal biliary development, the epithelial ductal plates of the developing intrahepatic bile ducts induce vasculogenesis in the portal mesenchyme resulting in development of hepatic artery branches. These structures in turn influence development of the embryonic bile ducts in the portal mesenchyme (56). Arteriopathy resulting in abnormal vascular–ductal interactions is a possible mechanism in the development of biliary atresia. Thickened, hyperplastic arterioles with medial hypertrophy and concentric fibrosis have been found in resected ductal specimens (60,61). These findings may indicate the presence of ductal ischemia during development, but whether they represent a primary or secondary event in the development of biliary atresia remains to be determined.

Because a rational argument can be made for a number of the hypotheses, the current concept among most experts is that biliary atresia is the late clinical manifestation of complex and heterogeneous processes that can likely be initiated by a number of different events (62).

Regardless of initial etiology, a contributing factor to the progression of bile duct destruction may be extravasation of bile into tissues. Extravasated bile has been detected in excised bile duct specimens (63). The inflammatory response triggered by the presence of extraluminal bile may perpetuate ductal destruction and, ultimately, obstruction. Progressive cholestasis is associated with hepatic parenchymal accumulation of toxic, hydrophobic bile acids linked in turn to hepatocyte necrosis and apoptosis. The mechanisms of bile acid-induced apoptosis include oxidative stress with cellular depletion of adenosine triphosphate (ATP), mitochondrial injury, stimulation of caspase 8, and activation of caspase 9 and 3 (64). Antioxidant therapy may modify these apoptotic mechanisms and protect cellular structures (65).

EMBRYOLOGY OF THE BILIARY SYSTEM

The human liver and its accompanying biliary ducts begin visible development in the third week of gestation (66). The hepatic diverticulum develops as a bud from the ventral surface of the foregut and invades the mesenchymal tissue of the septum transversum. The septum transversum is the mesenchymal tissue plate that separates the developing embryonic thoracic and abdominal cavities. By the seventh week of gestation, primitive portal tracts are established following the ingrowth of a sinusoidal vascular network from the vitelline vein. Interactions with surrounding mesenchyme yield mature portal venous structures. The intrahepatic ductal system forms from hepatoblasts adjacent to the mesenchyme in the portal tracts beginning in the eighth week of gestation. These hepatoblasts differentiate into biliary epithelial cells and form the ductal plate—first a single and then a double layer of cells surrounding the portal tract. Lumena develop within the two layers of the ductal plate and coalesce into tubular structures. By the eleventh week of gestation, these structures have become centrally located within the portal tract, whereas the remaining ductal plate components resorb. Subsequent maturation of the developing biliary tree takes place from the porta hepatis outward through the liver. Maturation of the entire intrahepatic biliary tree continues through birth and for several weeks thereafter.

Development of the extrahepatic system is not as well elucidated. The gallbladder and extrahepatic ductal system arise from the caudal portion of the hepatic diverticulum, whereas the cranial portion of the diverticulum fuses with the septum transversum (67). Throughout development, the intrahepatic and extrahepatic biliary systems maintain their patency and continuity, and at no time during normal gestation has a solid phase been identified in ductal system formation (68).

A number of complex and redundant interactions occur in the genetic control of hepatic and biliary system organogenesis (69). In early gestation, the domain-specific expression of the Foxa (forkhead box a; formerly Hnf3, hepatocyte nuclear factor-3) proteins in the endoderm control the initial stages of hepatic development. The foxa proteins regulate almost all the liver-specific genes as well as genes in the lung and pancreas. A subclass of the GATA zinc-finger transcription factors has also been found to regulate liver-specific gene expression as well as endoderm-specific signals from bone morphogenic proteins (Bmps) (69,70). Bmps appear to be strongly expressed in the septum transversum mesenchyme. Other known regulatory factors include fibroblast growth factor (Fgf), hepatocyte growth factor (Hgf), vascular endothelial growth factor receptor 2 (Vegfr-2), and transcription factors such as haematopoietically expressed homeobox (Hex), prospero-related homeobox 1 (Prox1), and c-Met (Hgf receptor). A number of factors are required for tissue growth and generation of hepatic structures including Kras (Kirsten rat sarcoma oncogene), c-Jun, Sek1, and nuclear factor-6β pathway components (NF-6β).

At present, regulation of biliary tract morphogenesis is not fully understood; however, hepatic nuclear factor 6 (Hnf6) is expressed in embryonic liver tissue, hepatic ducts, and the gallbladder. Along with Hnf1b, it exerts control over biliary duct development (57). Expression of the forkhead transcription factor Foxf1 in the septum transversum mesenchyme has also been shown to regulate development of the extrahepatic ductal system including the gallbladder (71). In addition, Jagged 1 (JAG 1), a notch ligand, expression has been localized to the ductal plate tissues starting in the fourteenth week of gestation with subsequent expression on biliary epithelium in postnatal liver (72). Mutations in Jagged 1 expression have been associated with Alagille syndrome and may be associated with biliary atresia (73,74). Further studies will elucidate the roles of these factors in the development of this disease process.

Fetal studies have shown that bile formation begins at approximately 12 weeks gestational age and increases in volume until birth. However, in the full-term neonate bile formation is markedly low compared with adult levels (75). A number of factors are responsible for this age-dependent difference. Decreased bile salt uptake by the immature liver contributes to a smaller neonatal bile acid pool as compared with adults. In addition, ileal transport of bile acids is decreased in the neonatal period resulting in higher losses of bile salts in the stool and therefore decreased recirculation (76). Because bile acids are the primary stimulus for bile secretion, the smaller size of the bile salt pool and the immature enterohepatic system combine to limit the rate of bile formation (77).

Immaturity of the bile acid system is also associated with the presence of atypical bile acids in the meconium and stool of neonates. These atypical bile acids consist of multiple hydroxylated species and may be hepatotoxic (78,79). Their presence during development in a cholestatic process such as ductal obstruction may contribute to the associated inflammatory reaction.

PATHOLOGY

Characteristic pathologic findings in biliary atresia include portal tract edema, bile duct proliferation, portal and periductalar inflammation, and associated areas of hepatic cell injury (Fig. 92-1). Additional histologic findings within the liver parenchyma include bile duct plugs, giant cell proliferation, haemosiderin deposition, and increased hematopoietic activity. Longitudinal studies have shown the progressive nature of these processes even with surgical therapy (80). Macroscopic examination of the involved extrahepatic ductal system usually shows fibrous obliteration of the common and hepatic ductal structures with an absent or atretic gallbladder. The gallbladder may contain "white bile"—clear mucous—with no pigment. In severe cases, the liver is dark green in color, congested, and large and firm in texture. Nodular changes in the hepatic capsule consistent with the development of cirrhosis may be

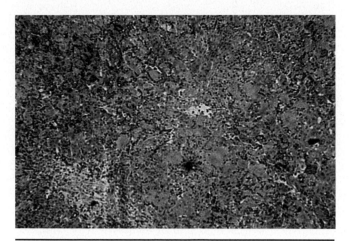

FIGURE 92-1. Histologic characteristics of biliary atresia in a liver biopsy include bile duct plugs, bile duct proliferation, and portal and periportal inflammation. The presence of bridging fibrosis between the portal tracts indicates the development of early cirrhosis.

evident. Histologic examination of livers with advanced disease shows evidence of progressive micronodular cirrhosis with bridging fibrosis between portal tracts, as well as portal destruction. Beyond 6 months of age, the ductular proliferation in the portal tracts disappears and is replaced by collagen deposition.

Histologic studies of resected extrahepatic ductal specimens have shown that ductal involvement with the disease process is quite variable (81,82). In some cases, the common bile duct will be completely obliterated with a fibrotic reaction and very little evidence of inflammation. In other patients, there may be one or more ductlike structures patent within the fibrous tract to the porta hepatis. The lumens of these structures are variable in size, often 30 to 80 μm in diameter. The epithelial cell lining is usually destroyed in this circumstance, and inflammatory cell infiltrates are present in the surrounding connective tissue. A third group consists of specimens in which microscopic ductular structures with lumens greater than 100 μm in diameter are found. The epithelial cell lining may be partially intact, but the surrounding tissues demonstrate fibrosis and mononuclear cell infiltrates. Ductal size and structure have been reported to correlate with bile flow following surgical correction, but this has been a point of considerable controversy and questionable clinical import (83).

Extensive proliferation of the bile ductules within the portal tracts is one of the crucial pathognomonic findings for biliary atresia. However, this can also be seen in other hepatic disease processes. The origin of these newly formed bile ductules appears to be from hepatocytes positioned around the ductal plate (84). Increased and unregulated cell proliferation of the bile ducts is believed to be responsible for this observation. Abnormal biliary epithelial cell expression of Fas ligand and other markers of apoptosis cell proliferation have been noted in liver specimens from patients with biliary atresia (85,86). In addition to the proliferation of bile ductules, abnormalities of the larger intrahepatic bile ducts are found. Specifically, a paucity of interlobular ducts or ductopenia is reported (87–89). Cytokeratin immunostaining for CK 7 and CK 19 subtypes may help in the identification of these ductal structures (90).

Histologic differentiation of other hepatic disease processes and biliary atresia based on a liver biopsy specimen alone is difficult. Mononuclear cell infiltrate within the hepatic parenchyma, giant cell transformation, ductular proliferation, and ductopenia are also seen in neonatal hepatitis, alpha-1 antitrypsin deficiency, TPN-induced cholestasis, and the syndromic and nonsyndromic forms of intrahepatic bile duct paucity (Alagille's syndrome).

The original classification of biliary atresia into correctable and noncorrectable forms has been refined by the Japanese Society of Pediatric Surgeons into three types (91). This morphologic classification system is based on gross findings and operative cholangiograms:

Type I—atresia of the common bile duct
Type II—atresia of the common hepatic ducts
Type III—atresia of the right and left hepatic ducts (i.e., the porta hepatis)

Two additional subclassifications are described according to the patterns of the distal extrahepatic bile ducts and ductular structures at the porta hepatis. Almost 90% of all cases were found to be type III.

IMMUNOLOGY OF BILIARY ATRESIA

The pathology of ductal destruction is not unique to biliary atresia. Bile ductules are also preferentially destroyed in liver allograft rejection, drug-induced ductopenia, and primary biliary cirrhosis (92). Biliary epithelial cells express a number of ligands in both healthy and diseased states that are important in controlling or initiating various immune and inflammatory reactions. Cell surface proteins such as the ABO blood group determinants, major histocompatibility complex (MHC) class I determinants, and integrin receptors are constitutively expressed on biliary epithelial cells. The expression of MHC class II glycoproteins and the adhesion molecules—intercellular adhesion molecule-1 (ICAM-1), LFA-3, NCAM, and CD-51—can be induced by cytokine stimulation. Thus, it appears biliary epithelial cells are active participants in the immunologic and inflammatory events associated with their destruction.

The basis for understanding the potential role of the inflammatory response in biliary atresia was established by Landing in his observations on the nature of the process he termed *infantile obstructive cholangiopathy* (93). He proposed that the disease resulted from an acquired inflammatory process and offered the following observations:

1. No laboratory data will be wholly able to differentiate neonatal hepatitis from biliary atresia.
2. Liver biopsy and cholangiograms are the most effective ways of differentiating the diagnosis.
3. No surgical mode of therapy will cure a significant fraction of infants with biliary atresia because the disease process actually destroys intrahepatic bile ducts as well. Biliary atresia is more in need of preventive or prophylactic measure than of new surgical procedures.
4. Because the obliterative process can resolve, even if not usually completely, surgical procedures of the Kasai type (portoenterostomy) should be considered for all infants.

Since these observations of Landing, a significant amount of information has accrued regarding immunologic events associated with biliary atresia. MHC expression on hepatic and ductal structures has been found to be quite variable in cases of biliary atresia. Class I determinants are constitutively expressed on all nucleated cells within the liver, and no differences have been detected between control and diseased livers (94). Variable expression of the class II determinant HLA-DR on biliary epithelial cells, Kuppfer cells, sinusoidal lining cells, and hepatocytes has been reported (80,94–98). It has been proposed that HLA-DR expression may be related to the severity and time course of the disease with strongest expression linked to progressive bile duct and hepatic parenchymal destruction (99).

Adhesion molecule expression is believed to play an important role in the immune-mediated destruction of ductal structures and surrounding hepatic parenchyma. ICAM-1 appears to be the most important adhesion molecule, and its expression has been demonstrated on intra- and extrahepatic ductal structures including proliferating bile ductules and interlobular ducts (97,98,100). Hepatocytes and sinusoidal lining cells in areas of active inflammation also express ICAM-1. Variable expression of vascular cell adhesion molecule-1 (VCAM-1) has been demonstrated on bile duct structures and sinusoidal lining cell membranes in areas of active inflammation. E-selectin expression has been detected on sinusoidal endothelium but not on any ductal structures.

In contrast, bile ducts in livers with cholestatic injury or with hepatitis fail to express ICAM-1, and no other cause of cirrhosis has been found to induce ICAM-1 expression on ductal structures. The only other hepatic disease processes known to be associated with increased ductal expression of ICAM-1 are primary biliary cirrhosis and primary sclerosing cholangitis. Thus, it appears that, in those diseases where ductal destruction is central to the pathologic process, ductal ICAM-1 expression is a unique and important finding.

The inflammatory cell infiltrates associated with biliary atresia result from specific pathways of immunologic activation. Lymphocyte infiltration of portal areas and lymphocytes within the biliary epithelial layer have been reported (101). Mononuclear cell populations with demonstrated involvement in the pathogenesis of biliary atresia include macrophages, natural killer (NK) cells, B cells, and T cells (80,97,98,102,103). In both portal and parenchymal infiltrates, all lymphocytes have been found to express lymphocyte function-associated antigen-1 (LFA-1)—the ligand for ICAM-1—and HLA-DR determinants. In terms of T-cell populations, CD4+ lymphocytes significantly outnumber CD8+ cells in areas of portal and parenchymal infiltration, and those CD8+ present in the portal region appear to have their cytotoxic activity downregulated (104). Expansion of the hepatic macrophage population has also been demonstrated and may correlate with the severity of the disease process (98,99,102). Macrophage activation with the upregulation of CD14—the lipopolysaccharide (LPS) receptor—occurs as part of the inflammatory process (102,105). These activated macrophages are a potential source of cytokine generation, a process known to stimulate the inflammation, fibrosis, and ultimately cirrhosis (106).

Proinflammatory peptides, including the chemokines RANTES, IP-10, MIP-1α, MIP-1β, and IL-8 as well as the growth factor TGF-β1, have been detected in the livers of biliary atresia patients (107,108). Increased gene expression of the proinflammatory cytokines osteopontin and interferon (IFN)-γ has also been reported (109). These data indicate a commitment to lymphocyte-mediated inflammation through a number of different pathways including T_H1-like cytokines, but whether these are primary pathogenic events or secondary to a self-perpetuating inflammatory process is not known.

However, elevated serum levels of several cytokines are reported in biliary atresia patients. These may reflect the stage of the disease or response to therapy. Both IL-1B and IL-6 levels were elevated in patients with failed Kasai procedures, but normal in those with a successful operation (110). Interferon-inducible protein-10—a chemokine produced in response to lipopolysaccharide, IFN-γ, IL-1β, or TNF-α—is also elevated in the sera of biliary atresia (111). Elevated levels of IL-18—a cytokine with the capacity to stimulate IFN-γ production from activated T cells and NK cells and induce ICAM-1 expression—have also been detected (106). Although inflammatory cytokines are clearly involved, serum levels of these cytokines cannot be used as reliable indicators of disease activity.

A number of other serum moieties have been proposed as markers of disease severity. Hyaluronic acid levels have been found to be elevated in patients with biliary atresia and have a direct relationship to the severity of hepatic fibrosis (112). Normally cleared by hepatic sinusoidal endothelial cells, hyaluronic acid levels in serum are elevated if progressive hepatic destruction sufficiently impairs uptake. However, this process is not specific to biliary atresia. In known biliary atresia patients, high serum concentrations may identify infants with significant hepatic compromise and a poor prognosis (113). Plasma endothelin-1 levels also correlate with the severity of liver cirrhosis and portal hypertension in biliary atresia patients (114). Low levels of serum insulin-like growth factor-1 (IGF-1) have been reported in patients with biliary atresia, and the lowest levels noted are in infants requiring hepatic transplantation (115). Soluble ICAM-1 and VCAM-1 are also elevated in the serum of biliary atresia infants (116,117). These may be as useful for monitoring the degree of active inflammation in biliary atresia patients as they are for other conditions (118).

Although the etiology of biliary atresia remains unclear, the pathologic findings of ductal and parenchymal destruction clearly reflect immune-mediated processes. With the recruitment of various mononuclear cell populations capable of inducing either cytotoxic or apoptotic responses, bile duct destruction occurs with secondary involvement of periductular and hepatic parenchymal cells. Progressive cellular destruction triggers a cascade of events leading to chronic liver injury including fibrosis and cirrhosis.

ANIMAL MODELS

Research efforts in biliary atresia have been handicapped by the lack of a suitable animal model for experimentation. No other animal species is known to develop a similar biliary process (119,120). As a result, a number of different animal models based on infectious, inflammatory and, more recently, developmental etiologies have been proposed. However, none of them have been able to replicate all the pathologic characteristics of the disease process seen in infants.

Investigators have attempted to reproduce biliary atresia by ligating the hepatic artery in fetal sheep (121). Common bile duct damage results, but the histologic findings in the liver are inconsistent with biliary atresia. Direct ligation of the common bile duct usually results in ductal dilatation, but in certain rat species it can result in ductal proliferation, fibrosis, and cirrhosis (122,123). This rat model has served as a tool for investigating mechanisms of chronic liver injury. Other models have attempted to induce a condition resembling biliary atresia by triggering an inflammatory reaction against either the extra- or intrahepatic ductal systems. Murine extrahepatic bile duct segments have been engrafted beneath the renal capsule of allogeneic recipients, thereby eliciting an immune response (124). The inflammatory response involves both class I and class II histocompatibility antigen expression and results in the rejection of the tissue. Nonspecific inflammation of the biliary tract resulting in a histologic picture of cholangitis has been elicited in hamsters by the constant infusion of phorbol myristate acetate, a potent chemotactic agent, into the biliary system (125). The nonphysiologic conditions required have limited the applicability of this model.

Because of the strong belief that biliary atresia can be triggered by certain viral infections in the perinatal period, a number of experimental models have investigated the effects of viruses on the hepatobiliary system in young mice. Initial studies found that reovirus type 3 induced a reaction in the biliary tree resembling extrahepatic biliary atresia (126). Subsequent studies have shown that, although the biliary tract may be a target for viral infection, the lesions in this model are transient or segmental and do not cause obstruction to bile flow (127). Rotavirus administration to weanling mice has also been shown to cause a condition resembling biliary atresia (128–131). The effects on the liver and biliary system were noted when the virus was administered to the pups immediately after birth because administration to the mother prenatally was ineffective. This model has been used to investigate potential therapeutic interventions (132).

With the development of molecular biology techniques, a number of mouse strains with selective genetic alterations have enabled investigations into the mechanisms of biliary tract development. The transgenic *inv* mouse has a recessive deletion of the inversin gene, resulting in situs inversus and jaundice as noted previously (51). The liver in these mice develops a histologic picture resembling extrahepatic biliary obstruction, although there is minimal hepatic inflammation or necrosis. In another murine model, hepatocyte nuclear factor-6 (HNF-6) gene expression has been found to play a crucial role in the morphogenesis of the intrahepatic bile ducts (57). In HNF-6 knock-out mice, ductal plate malformations with absent intrahepatic bile ducts were noted. Unfortunately, until the cause or causes of biliary atresia are identified, none of these provides an entirely suitable animal model.

ASSOCIATED CONDITIONS

Associated anomalies have been reported in 10% to 25% of patients with biliary atresia and occur in the *fetal* or *embryonic* form of the disease (133–137). Commonly known as the *polysplenia syndrome*, the anomalies reported in these infants include polysplenia, intestinal malrotation, absent inferior vena cava with azygous continuation, symmetric bilobed liver, situs inversus, preduodenal portal vein, bilobed right lung, and cardiac malformations. As a result of an analysis of the segregation patterns of these anomalies, two major groups have been proposed (10). Approximately one-third of patients are in a group that is labeled the *laterality sequence* or *developmental field complex*. This group consists of various combinations of anomalies in the polysplenia syndrome of left–right asymmetry. These include cardiovascular malformations, polysplenia, abdominal situs inversus, intestinal malrotation, and malformations of the portal vein and hepatic artery apparently involving disruption of left–right asymmetry. More recent experimental work in the *inv* mouse supports these observations (see "Animal Models"). The second group of patients, consisting of more than one-half of the study population, is composed of nonsyndromic anomalies. These usually consist of isolated anomalies of the heart, kidneys, or gastrointestinal (GI) tract. Most of the GI malformations were Meckel's diverticula, but midgut volvulus and intestinal atresias have also been reported.

DIAGNOSIS

Following birth, almost every infant experiences some degree of hyperbilirubinemia. This is generally physiologic and resolves over time. However, if jaundice is detected beyond 2 weeks of age, diagnostic evaluation is warranted, and the detection of conjugated hyperbilirubinemia always indicates the presence of significant hepatobiliary disease. Because clinical differentiation among the various causes of neonatal cholestasis is impossible, diagnostic evaluations must identify anatomic or obstructive causes of jaundice such as biliary atresia, choledochal cyst, or spontaneous bile duct perforation. Nonsurgical causes of neonatal jaundice are numerous and include infections, metabolic, genetic, and toxic etiologies beyond the scope of this chapter (Table 92-1).

Clinically, the signs of biliary atresia are jaundice, dark urine, pale stools, and hepatomegaly. Jaundice is occasionally present at birth and becomes more pronounced with time. Stools may not be completely acholic but have a pale green or light yellow color. Total serum bilirubin levels are typically in the range of 6 to 12 mg per dL, with a direct component of 50% or more of the total. However, hyperbilirubinemia greater than 2 mg/DL or with a direct component greater than 20% of the total should be investigated. Serum transaminases can be moderately elevated, and both the alkaline phosphatase and γ-glutamyl transpeptidase levels are elevated with biliary atresia. Additional serologic tests in the differential diagnosis of neonatal cholestasis include the hepatitis serologies, TORCH titers (toxoplasmosis, rubella, cytomegalovirus, and herpesvirus), and alpha-1-antitrypsin levels to rule out these possibilities. Unfortunately, serologic tests alone are incapable of differentiating biliary atresia from other causes of cholestasis.

Ultrasonography is useful in the initial evaluation of neonatal cholestasis, although it is not diagnostic for biliary atresia. The classic finding in patients with biliary atresia is a shrunken, nondistended gallbladder without a visible common duct structure. Precise identification of the porta hepatis and the fibrous cone of the scarred common hepatic ducts can be done with high-resolution ultrasonography and is reported to be a specific finding for biliary atresia (138). Abnormalities in the shape, wall thickness, and morphology of the gallbladder can also be detected with biliary atresia (139). In the differential diagnosis of cholestasis, ultrasonography is important in evaluating the common bile duct for choledochal cyst abnormalities or choledocholithiasis, and in determining the presence of polysplenia syndrome.

Nuclear imaging or hepatobiliary scintigraphy is commonly employed to differentiate obstructive from parenchymal causes of jaundice. After intravenous injection of the ^{99m}technetium-labeled iminodiacetic acid tracer, it is taken up in the liver and subsequent visualization of the isotope in the intestine excludes biliary atresia. Phenobarbital administration for up to 5 days is used to enhance the sensitivity of the test. Lack of appearance of the isotope in the intestine has a specificity for biliary atresia of only 50% to 75% because severe intrahepatic cholestasis and paucity syndrome may yield similar nonvisualization results (140).

A number of other diagnostic tests have been studied, but remain clinically impractical or difficult to carry out. Magnetic resonance cholangiopancreatography (MRCP) has been done, but decreased bile flow in cases of severe cholestasis undermines the ability of the test to identify extrahepatic bile ducts and thereby diagnose biliary atresia (141,142). Endoscopic retrograde cholangiopancreatography (ERCP) has also been used to diagnose biliary atresia (143,144). However, it remains clinically impractical because of the specialized equipment and training required to perform the procedure successfully. Finally, duodenal intubation for 24 hours has been shown to effectively rule out the possibility of biliary atresia if bile is detected in the aspirates (145).

The most definitive test for establishing the diagnosis of biliary atresia is a liver biopsy obtained percutaneously as part of the initial evaluation of the jaundiced infant or at the time of abdominal exploration in conjunction with an operative cholangiogram. With an experienced pathologist, a percutaneous liver biopsy has a diagnostic accuracy of greater than 90% (146). If the liver biopsy is obtained at the time of laparotomy, frozen section analysis of the specimen is required. The differential diagnosis includes alpha-1-antitrypsin deficiency, Alagille syndrome, nonsyndromic paucity of interlobular bile ducts, cystic fibrosis, and total parenteral nutrition (TPN)-induced cholestasis—all of which may have similar-appearing hepatic histology on frozen section analysis. If the diagnosis is uncertain on frozen section biopsy and the cholangiogram is nondiagnostic, the operation should be terminated. A definitive portoenterostomy procedure can be performed subsequent if and when the diagnosis is confirmed with permanent sections and special staining studies if necessary (Fig. 92-2).

TABLE 92-1 Causes and Associated Syndromes of Neonatal Jaundice.

Hepatic		
Congenital infections		
	Cytomegalovirus	Echovirus
	Rubella virus	Coxsackievirus
	Herpes virus	Reovirus
	Hepatitis virus B	Varicella virus
	Toxoplasmosis	Syphilis
	Tuberculosis	Listeriosis
Metabolic disorders		
	Galactosemia	Tyrosinemia
	Hereditary fructose intolerance	
	Alpha-1 antitrypsin deficiency	
	Cystic fibrosis	
	Hypopituitarism	
	Bile acid synthesis defects	
	Citrin deficiency	
Storage disorders		
	Gaucher's disease	Wolman's disease
	Niemann-Pick disease	Glycogen storage disease 4
	Neonatal iron storage disease	
Genetic disorders		
	Alagille syndrome	Turner syndrome
	Down syndrome	Zellweger syndrome
	Aagenaes syndrome	
Familial cholestatic disorders		
	Byler syndrome	FIC1 deficiency
	BSEP deficiency	MDR3 deficiency
Idiopathic disorders		
	Idiopathic neonatal hepatitis	
	Nonsyndromic paucity of interlobular bile ducts	
Miscellaneous disorders		
	Congenital hepatic fibrosis	Histiocytosis X
	Inspissated bile syndrome	Sepsis
	Total parenteral nutrition-associated cholestasis	
	Ischemia-reperfusion injury	
	Caroli's syndrome	
Extrahepatic		
Biliary atresia		
Choledochal cyst		
Spontaneous perforation of the common bile duct		
Choledocholithiasis		
Neonatal sclerosing cholangitis		
Bile duct stenosis/extrinsic bile duct compression (tumor)		

MEDICAL MANAGEMENT

The treatment of biliary atresia has changed little since Kasai demonstrated the efficacy of the hepatoportoenterostomy as a surgical intervention. There still is no specific therapeutic intervention targeted to influence the pathologic process directly.

Medical therapies in the postoperative period following a portoenterostomy procedure include treatments designed to augment bile flow and to suppress the risk of cholangitis. More controversial is the role of antiinflammatory therapy to improve native liver function and modify the disease process.

A number of pharmaceutical agents have been used to improve bile flow following surgery. All have limited efficacy. Neither cholestyramine nor phenobarbital has been effective in improving bile flow or decreasing cholestasis in these patients (147). Administration of ursodeoxycholic acid has been shown to lower serum bilirubin levels and improve other biochemical indices of hepatic function, as

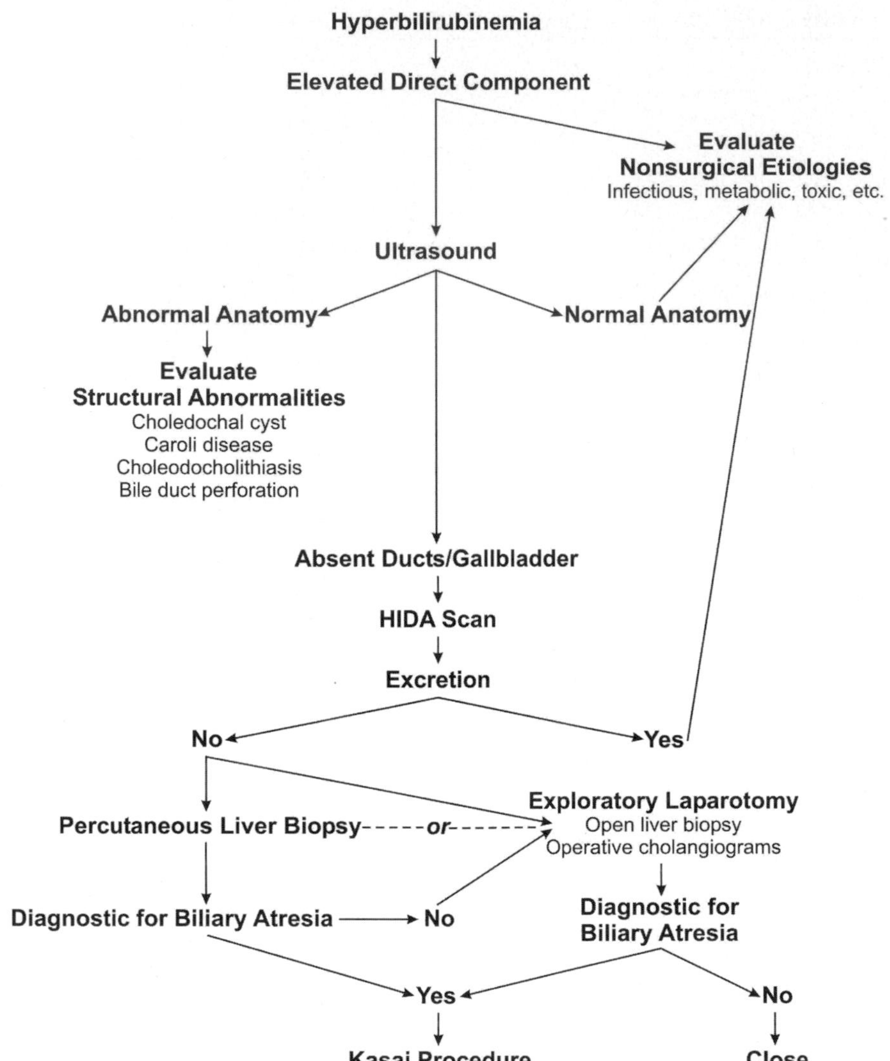

FIGURE 92-2. Diagnostic algorithm for jaundiced neonate with suspected biliary atresia. Iminodiacetic acid (IDA).

well as relieve the pruritis associated with elevated bile salt deposition (148–150). Its use in liver disease is based on the concept that the accumulation of endogenous and toxic bile salts leads to hepatocellular and biliary tract injury. By competing for intestinal absorption of endogenous bile acids, ursodeoxycholic acid alters the bile salt pool principally through a reduction in the levels of chenodeoxycholic acid. It has also been shown to facilitate the excretion of bilirubin and bile acids into the bile through the liver and decrease bile viscosity and sludging in the biliary tree (151). Ursodeoxycholic acid may also have immunomodulatory effects, as it has been shown to decrease MHC class I expression on biliary epithelial cells in patients with biliary cirrhosis. However, despite the improvements in clinical and biochemical indices, this therapy has not changed the clinical outcome for biliary atresia patients.

Medical therapy with corticosteroids has been an area of significant clinical investigation since the mid-1990s. Corticosteroids were initially proposed in conjunction with broad-spectrum antibiotics to treat episodes of acute cholangitis following surgery (152–154). Short-term, high-dose blast therapy was also employed to augment bile flow in cases where a previously functioning portoenterostomy developed evidence of decreasing bile excretion (155). Repetitive pulse administration of corticosteroids was then reported by pediatric surgeons in Japan with encouraging results (156,157). More recently, high-dose, long-term corticosteroid therapy similar to that used in treatment protocols for hepatic transplantation has proven successful in improving jaundice-free survival status following surgery and decreasing the requirement for liver transplantation in the first 5 years of life (158,159). Such therapy resulted in a jaundice-free status in more than 70% of treated infants compared with less than 20% in historical controls. The mechanisms by which corticosteroids influence the clinical course of biliary atresia remain unclear. At present, a federally funded multicenter prospective trial of preoperative glucocorticoid therapy is underway in the United States. Although their immunosuppressive and antiinflammatory properties are well known, corticosteroids also promote bile salt-independent bile flow within the liver (160). It is clear that surgery on the extrahepatic bile ducts alone is inadequate to treat biliary atresia, and it is likely that more specific pharmacologic strategies will develop.

SURGERY

At present, the surgical procedure of choice for biliary atresia is the hepatic portoenterostomy that was first described by Kasai in 1959 (161). There have been numerous subsequent modifications, but the success of this operation remains critically dependent on a meticulous dissection of the porta hepatis and its subsequent anastomosis to a Roux-en-Y limb of jejunum.

The operation is initiated by entering the abdomen through a right subcostal incision that can be extended to the left side, if necessary. A midline incision also affords acceptable access. If a percutaneous liver biopsy had not been performed as part of the preoperative evaluation, the first stage of the operation involves a liver biopsy and cholangiogram to confirm the diagnosis. After having determined the diagnosis, some surgeons then perform a complete mobilization of the liver with division of both left and right triangular ligaments. Although such an approach provides excellent visualization of the hilum, it is not necessary and may compromise surgical access to the right upper quadrant if a liver transplantation is required in the future. To approach the portal tract, the gallbladder is mobilized from the hepatic bed while maintaining the continuity of the cystic duct to the fibrotic remnants of the common bile duct. The peritoneum overlying the portal tract is incised, the cystic artery is ligated, and the hepatic artery is identified. The fibrotic common bile duct is mobilized from the anterior surface of the portal vein, and divided and ligated distally just cephalad to the duodenum. Using the gallbladder as a point of traction, the fibrous ductal structures are carefully dissected proximally to the portal plate. The left and right hepatic arteries frame the field of dissection laterally and medially, whereas the bifurcation of the portal vein defines the inferior boundary. Several small branches from the portal vein may be encountered during the dissection, particularly at the level of the bifurcation. The fibrotic porta hepatis is sharply divided flush with the liver parenchyma at this level. A Roux-en-Y limb of proximal jejunum is fashioned and anastomosed to the porta as an end-to-end or end-to-side anastomosis. The length of this limb is most often reported 10 to 40 cm, with some evidence that subsequent drug absorption of immunosuppressive agents is impaired with longer defunctionized limbs. Either a running or interrupted technique with absorbable suture can be used to construct the anastomosis. Meticulous attention must be paid to suture placement along the cut edge of the porta hepatis in order to minimize the risk of compromising the microductular structures (Fig. 92-3).

A number of modifications to Kasai's original procedure have been described. The Roux limb can be exteriorized as a double-barreled stoma and then closed 1 to 2 months later (162). This diversion allowed for the daily quantification of bile output and offered the ability to monitor postoperative status. However, the presence of a stoma required the bile drainage to be refed, either down the distal limb or via gastrostomy, making management difficult. The incidence of postoperative complications, including bleeding from parastomal varices and the risk of dehydration and electrolyte abnormalities, was quite high. This technique is presently seldom used.

Several other modifications remain controversial in the conduct of biliary atresia surgery. To prevent cholangitis, the incorporation of an antireflux valve within the Roux limb has been proposed. This is achieved by intussuscepting a portion of the bowel upon itself. Although a number of different techniques are available to construct such a valve, their effectiveness in preventing cholangitis is questionable, and both obstruction and failure have been reported (163–165). In addition, there is controversy regarding the extent of dissection of the fibrous portal plate at the hepatic hilum. Extensive dissection of the hilum deep into the liver parenchyma until the secondary portal branches are encountered has been proposed (166,167). It is currently unknown if such techniques serve to improve bile drainage and the long-term effectiveness of the portoenterostomy procedure. Finally, the role of reoperative surgery following an initial portoenterostomy is poorly defined. In patients with a functioning portoenterostomy and stable disease, the sudden onset of jaundice and acholic stools should prompt an extensive review for a process amenable to medical or surgical intervention. Potential causes of such dysfunction include the accumulation of scar and granulation tissue at the anastomosis or a mechanical complication with the Roux limb itself (168). In such cases, reexploration of the anastomosis has been reported to be successful in one-third of the patients (169). However, the results for reoperative surgery for insufficient bile drainage following an initial portoenterostomy have been dismal, and there is little support for redo surgery in these patients (170–173). These infants should be evaluated for transplantation rather than reexploration.

A concern of transplant surgeons has been the effect of multiple surgical procedures on the outcome of hepatic transplantation in these patients. Initial studies showed a

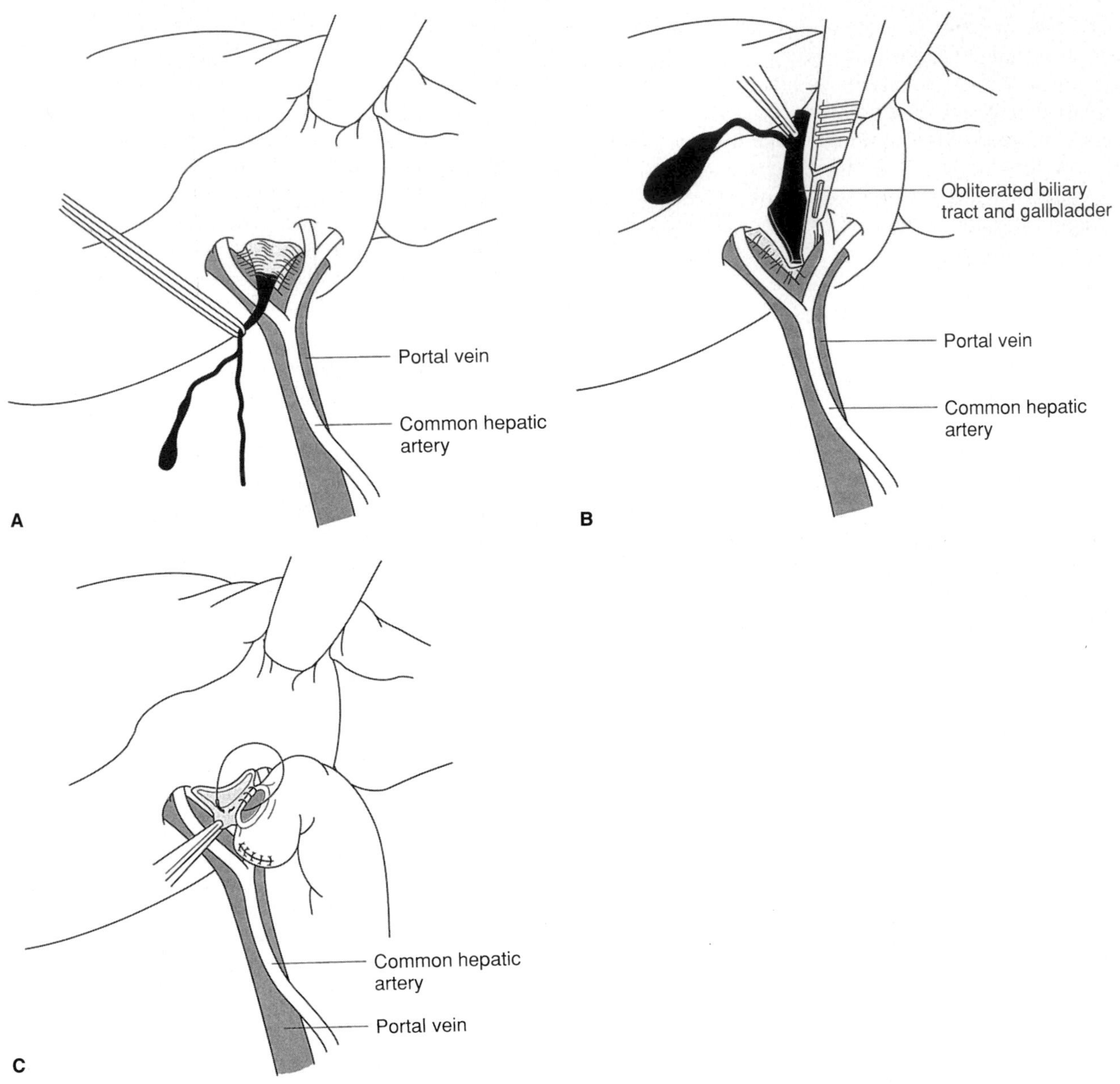

FIGURE 92-3. Surgical steps involved in the Kasai hepatoportoenterostomy: **(A)** mobilization of the gallbladder and cystic duct in continuity with the fibrotic common duct, **(B)** transection of the fibrotic porta hepatis at the level of the hepatic parenchyma, and **(C)** anastomosis of the jejunal roux limb to the porta. (From Greenfield LJ. *Surgery, scientific principles and practice,* 3rd ed. Philadelphia: Lippincott Williams & Wilkins, 2001:2029, with permission.)

higher rate of complications with a transplant procedure following multiple pretransplant procedures, although the continued evolution of transplant experience suggests that such concerns are no longer valid (174–178).

In a small number of patients, a patent gallbladder, cystic duct, and common bile duct will permit the construction of a portoenterostomy (179). Unfortunately, the gallbladder often functions poorly as a conduit, and this is rarely used in contemporary practice.

OUTCOMES

The importance of the hepatopo[illegible]ostomy in the surgical treatment of biliary atre[illegible] [illegible]ghlighted by the marked improvement in surviv[illegible] [illegible] the 1960s in a number of large series (91,18[illegible] [illegible] measures of success following portoenterost[illegible] [illegible] [illegible] with a native liver and the [illegible] [illegible] of a jaundice-free clinical state. Results, howev[illegible] [illegible] quite varied with

TABLE 92-2 Long-term Outcomes in Biliary Atresia Patients.[a]

Surgery	
Jaundice-free status	26%–80%
5-Year survival (with native liver)	48%–60%
10-Year survival (with [illegible]	20%–53%
Surgery with adjuvan[illegible]	
Jaundice-free status	> 71%
4- to 5-Year survival (with native liver)	71%–85%
Complications	
Cholangitis	40%–100%
Varices	40%–80%
Hemorrhage	10%–60%
Liver transplantation	50%–70%

[a]Adapted from Refs. 91, 156–159, 180, 183–187, 189-193, 198, 199, 211–213, 222, and 223.

reasons such as age of the patient at the time of surgery and the experience of the surgeon and institution cited as important factors (181) (Table 92-2).

If untreated, the anticipated life expectancy of an infant with biliary atresia is approximately 1 year, and survival to 3 years of age is quite rare (182). Following a Kasai procedure, 5-year survival rates with a native liver have ranged between 48% and 60%. Although 10-year survival rates as high as 71% have been reported at some institutions in Japan, most studies have indicated that such long-term survival ranges between 20% and 45% (91,180,183–186) Table 92-2. The latest data from the Japanese Biliary Atresia Registry includes more than 1,000 patients from many institutions and shows an average 5-year survival rate of 60% and a 10-year rate of 53% (187). Currently, even if the portoenterostomy procedure fails, overall survival rates greater than 80% can be expected due to advancements in pediatric liver transplantation (188).

The goal of a successful hepatoportoenterostomy is the establishment of enteric bile flow and the attainment of a jaundice-free state. Unfortunately, the surgical restoration of bile flow does not necessarily lead to a normalization of bilirubin levels. In experienced hands, the efficacy of a portoenterostomy in achieving bile flow varies between 72% and 90% (91,189,190). The number of patients who subsequently become anicteric is much lower. In several Japanese studies, jaundice clearance has been reported in 70% to 80% of patients (91,191,192). Other studies have not been as favorable with the achievement of jaundice-free status between 27% to 60% (91,180,189,190,193). Even with jaundice-free status, the long-term efficacy of the operation in preserving hepatic function is limited. In Japan, a nationwide study of patients with biliary atresia surviving more than 10 years showed that only 8% remained jaundice free (189).

Ultimately, the clinical success of a portoenterostomy procedure is judged by the requirement for hepatic transplantation. With overall survival rates greater than 80% in a number of studies, many groups have championed sequential therapy of biliary atresia with a portoenterostomy followed by transplantation when needed (190,194–197). Liver transplantation is required in 50% to 70% of biliary atresia patients with most occurring in the first 2 years of life (180,198). The probability of failure of a portoenterostomy resulting in death or transplantation was 33% at 1 year and 55% at 5 years (199). Predicting which patients will ultimately require liver transplantation remains difficult (200,201).

A number of prognostic variables and their relationship to clinical outcomes have been reported in infants with biliary atresia including age, microscopic appearance of the resected ductal tissue, microscopic appearance of the liver, extrahepatic anomalies, and bilirubin excretion. Of these, age of the patient at the time of surgery and the histologic characteristics of the resected extrahepatic ductal tissue appear most important. Kasai made the initial observations on the importance of age of the patient at surgery in determining outcome (202). In general, infants who undergo an hepatoportoenterostomy in the first 2 to 3 months of life have the best prognosis (185,203). More specifically, a large, multivariate analysis has shown that after 10 weeks of age, the risk of failure increases significantly (199). However, performance of a Kasai procedure in patients who are diagnosed at a late age may still be beneficial (204). Extrahepatic ductal histology also correlates with surgical outcome. The most widely studied ductal characteristics have been the diameter and number of residual ducts in the resected tissue of the porta hepatis. Biliary ductules with diameters greater than 150 μm were associated with a greater surgical success rate when compared with smaller ductules, and the findings of few or absent ductal remnants and no portal inflammation were predictors of poor prognosis (199,203,205). The establishment of adequate enteric bile flow may be the most important prognostic factor in predicting the outcome following surgery, for without it there will be no success. As previously noted, even establishing bile flow is no guarantee of a positive outcome. When the Roux-en Y limbs were routinely exteriorized as part of the portoenterostomy, daily bilirubin excretion greater than 6 to 10 mg per day was associated with the clinical clearance of jaundice and improved long-term survival (191,206,207). Levels of bile excretion less than this resulted in disease progression over time, and ultimately, liver failure.

Although satisfactory bile drainage can often be obtained with a portoenterostomy, the biliary atresia disease process tends to be progressive with gradual deterioration in hepatic function over time (80). As a result, fewer than 10% of patients currently survive 25 years with a functional native liver (208). These results will undoubtedly improve with time as the current cohort of patients ages, but the fact remains that surgery seldom cures biliary atresia. However, when successful, the quality of life for long-term survivors following a hepatoportoenterostomy can compare favorably with the normal population (209,210).

COMPLICATIONS

A number of complications can occur following surgical therapy for biliary atresia, and these may have dramatic effects on native liver function and survival. Clinical problems include technical issues of creating an enteric anastomosis directly to the biliary system, nutritional deficiencies caused by chronic cholestasis, and associated liver dysfunction. These complications highlight the progressive nature of this disease process and the requirement for life-long meticulous follow-up and management.

The most important complication in the postoperative period is cholangitis. This occurs with an incidence ranging from 40% to 100% (180,211–213). One important reason for the variable incidence reports is that the definition is purely clinical, e.g., fever, increased jaundice, and possibly evidence of decreased bile flow. Proper management of this complication is essential because it has been shown that repeated episodes of cholangitis have a detrimental impact on the prognosis of infants with biliary atresia (207,214). It is presumed that the development of this complication results from an ascending bacterial infection from the small bowel conduit as a result of the direct anastomosis between the bowel and the abnormal biliary tree, but this is unproven. In extreme cases, the infant can present with sepsis. The diagnosis should be suspected any time clinical deterioration is detected following surgery. Although it is most common in the time period immediately following surgery, such events can occur 2 or more years later (181). Multiple pathogens have been implicated in this complication including *Escherichia coli, Klebsiella, Psuedomonas, Staphylococcus, Enterobacter, Streptococcus faecalis, Bacteroides, Clostridia,* and *Candida.* Therefore, broad-spectrum antibiotic coverage with biliary penetration is considered standard therapy. Current recommendations are to consider administration of imipenem/cilastin or one of the third-generation cephalosporins and an aminoglycoside (215). If liver function fails to improve as evidenced by return of stool pigments and improvement in serum bilirubin and other liver function assays, short-term pulse therapy with corticosteroids should be initiated. The most common practice is to administer a 5-day course of methylprednisolone at a dose of 10 mg per kg on day 1, 5 mg per kg on day 2, 2.5 mg per kg on day 3, 1 mg per kg on day 4, and 0.5 mg per kg on day 5. Oral prednisone therapy at 1 mg per kg for 2 to 4 weeks can also be administered. Infants with intractable or chronically recurring cholangitis should be evaluated for anatomic obstruction or high resistance to bile flow within the Roux-en-Y limb with ultrasound, hepatic nuclear scintigraphy, or percutaneous contrast injection. Lengthening of the Roux limb or the construction of an intussuscepted valve within the conduit have been successful surgical strategies for intractable cholangitis though the proper role of reoperative surgery is not well defined (216).

Even with a functioning portoenterostomy, several complications may result. As a consequence of cholestasis, retention of bile salts within the hepatocytes occurs. This increase in cellular bile salt concentration is also associated with an increase in the serum levels of bile salts, reduced bile salts in the enterohepatic circulation, and a decrease in the total bile salt pool. Elevated bile salt levels within the hepatic parenchyma may lead to continued liver damage and contribute to disease progression through mechanisms of cellular membrane destabilization and destruction. The resulting injury serves to further hepatic fibrosis and the subsequent development of cirrhosis.

One of the common clinical issues associated with chronic cholestasis is pruritis. The relationship of pruritis to bile salt levels within the tissues is debated, but therapeutic interventions to reduce pruritis usually have an effect on serum bile salt concentrations as well (217–219). Bile salts act on peripheral pain afferent nerves to produce the sensation of itching through opiate-mediated pathways. Opiate antagonists can be administered to minimize these sensations. Unremitting pruritis can be an indication for liver transplantation (220,221).

Because biliary atresia is associated with liver injury and hepatic fibrosis even when diagnosed early, almost all patients have some degree of portal hypertension. Clinically, the presence of portal hypertension is manifested by the presence of esophageal or gastric varices, hypersplenism, and ascites. Esophageal varices are found in 40% to 80% of biliary atresia infants by 5 years of age, and GI hemorrhage occurs in 10% to 60% of patients (181,222,223). Prophylactic sclerotherapy of esophageal varices resulted in an increased incidence of bleeding from gastric varices and portal hypertensive gastropathy with no effect on the overall incidence of GI hemorrhage or survival after such an event (224). There is little information on the efficacy of medical management with selective beta blockade or vasodilator therapy in children. For patients with active GI hemorrhage, treatment includes aggressive hemodynamic stabilization, reversal of coexistent coagulopathy, somatostatin, vasopressin, and endoscopic variceal sclerotherapy or banding (225,226). If hemorrhage continues, treatment options include either a surgical or radiologic portosystemic shunt, a gastric devascularization procedure, or hepatic transplantation. Hypersplenism leading to severe leukopenia or thrombocytopenia is rare and has been treated with partial splenic embolization (227).

Fat malabsorption, including the fat-soluble vitamins A, D, E, and K, is a predictable nutritional consequence of biliary atresia. Recognized complications resulting from deficiencies in these vitamins include keratopathy (vitamin A deficiency), rickets (vitamin D deficiency), ataxic neuropathy (vitamin E deficiency), and coagulopathy (vitamin K deficiency). In addition, essential fatty acid deficiency and abnormalities in prostaglandin metabolism have been documented (228). Although proper supplementation can correct these abnormalities, nutritional management of these infants can be difficult. In addition to malabsorption, another determinant of malnutrition in biliary atresia is the increased oxygen consumption and hypermetabolism associated with chronic liver disease. Resting energy expenditure is elevated compared with normal infants, and protein metabolism is significantly impaired (229). Increased protein catabolism may result in a negative nitrogen balance and depletion of body mass. Energy and nitrogen balance studies may serve to facilitate the long-term nutritional management of these infants.

ACKNOWLEDGMENTS

This work was supported by The Friends of Mia Fund.

REFERENCES

1. Balistreri WF, Grand R, Hoofnagle JH, et al. Biliary atresia: current concepts and research directions. *Hepatology* 1996;23:1682–1692.
2. Mowatt AP. Biliary atresia into the 21st century: a historical perspective. *Hepatology* 1996;23:1682–1692.
3. Hays DM, Kimura K. *Biliary atresia: the Japanese experience.* Cambridge, MA: Harvard University Press, 1980.
4. Ladd WE. Congenital atresia and stenosis of the bile ducts. *JAMA* 1928;91:1082–1185.
5. Ladd WE, Gross RE. Surgical anastomoses between the biliary and intestinal tracts of children. *Ann Surg* 1940;112:51–63.
6. Longmire WP, Sanford MC. Intrahepatic cholangiojejunostomy with partial hepatectomy for biliary obstruction. *Surgery* 1948;24:264–271.
7. Sterling JA. Artificial bile ducts in the management of congenital biliary atresia. *J Int Coll Surg* 1961;36:293–298.
8. Absolon MD, Rikkers H, Aust JB. Thoracic duct lymph drainage in congenital biliary atresia. *Surg Gynecol Obstet* 1965;120:123.
9. Balistreri WF. Neonatal cholestasis. *J Pediatr* 1985;106:171–184.
10. Carmi R, Magee CA, Neill CA, et al. Extrahepatic biliary atresia and associated anomalies: etiologic heterogeneity suggested by distinctive patterns of associations. *Am J Med Genetics* 1993;45:683–693.
11. Yoon PW, Bresee JS, Olney RS, et al. Epidemiology of biliary atresia: a population-based study. *Pediatrics* 1997;99:376–382.
12. Shim WKT, Kasai M, Spence MA. Racial influence on the incidence of biliary atresia. *Prog Pediatr Surg* 1974;6:53–62.
13. Sweet LK. Congenital malformation of the bile ducts: a report of three cases in one family. *J Pediatr* 1932;1:496–501.
14. Smith BM, Laberge JM, Schreiber R, et al. Familial biliary atresia in three siblings including twins. *J Pediatr Surg* 1991;26:1331–1333.
15. Werlin SL. Extrahepatic biliary atresia in one of twins. *Acta Paediatr Scand* 1981;70:943–944.
16. Hyams JS, Glaser JH, Lecihtner AM, et al. Discordance for biliary atresia in two sets of monozygotic twins. *J Pediatr* 1985;107:420–422.
17. Fischler B, Haglund B, Hjern A. A population based study on the incidence and possible pre- and perinatal etiologic risk factors of biliary atresia. *J Pediatr* 2002;141:217–222.
18. Strickland AD, Shannon K. Studies in the etiology of extrahepatic biliary atresia: time space clustering. *J Pediatr* 1982;100:749–753.
19. Ayas MF, Hillemeier AC, Olson AD. Lack of evidence for seasonal variation in extrahepatic biliary atresia during infancy. *J Clin Gastroenterol* 1996;22:292–294.
20. Houwen RH, Kerremans I, van Steensel-Moll HA, et al. Time space distribution of extrahepatic biliary atresia in The Netherlands and West Germany. *Z Kinderchir* 1988;43:68–71.
21. Chardot C, Carton M, Spire-Bendelac N, et al. Epidemiology of biliary atresia in France: a national study 1986–1996. *J Hepatol* 1999;31:1006–1013.
22. Heriksen NT, Drablos PA, Aagenaes O. Cholestatic jaundice in infancy. The importance of familial and genetic factors in aetiology and prognosis. *Arch Dis Child* 1981;56:622–627.
23. McKiernan PJ, Hbaker AJ, Kelly DA. The frequency and outcome of biliary atresia in the UK and Ireland. *Lancet* 2000;355:25–29.
24. Davenport M, Dhawan A. Epidemiologic study of infants with biliary atresia. *Pediatrics* 1998;101:729–730.
25. Sokol RJ, Mack C, Narkewicz MR, et al. Pathogenesis and outcome of biliary atresia: current concepts. *J Pediatr Gastroenterol Nutr* 2003;37:4–21.
26. Sokol RJ, Mack C. Etiopathogenesis of biliary atresia. *Semin Liver Dis* 2001;21:517–524.
27. Morecki R, Glaser JH, Cho S, et al. Biliary atresia and reovirus type 3 infection. *N Engl J Med* 1982;307:481–484.
28. Glaser JH, Morecki R. Reovirus type 3 and neonatal cholestasis. *Semin Liver Dis* 1987;7:100–107.
29. Morecki R, Glaser JH, Johnson AB, et al. Detection of reovirus type 3 in the porta hepatis of an infant with extrahepatic biliary atresia: ultrastructural and immunocytochemical study. *Hepatology* 1984;4:1137–1142.
30. Tyler TL, Sokol RJ, Oberhaus SM, et al. Detection of reovirus RNA in hepatobiliary tissues from patients with extrahepatic biliary atresia and choledochal cysts. *Hepatology* 1998;27:1475–1482.
31. Brown WR, Sokol RJ, Levin MJ, et al. Lack of correlation between infection with reovirus 3 and extrahepatic biliary atresia or neonatal hepatitis. *J Pediatr* 1988;113:670–676.
32. Steele MI, Marshall CM, Lloyd RE, et al. Reovirus 3 not detected by reverse transcriptase-mediated polymerase chain reaction analysis of preserved tissue from infants with cholestatic liver disease. *Hepatology* 1995;21:697–702.
33. Fishler B, Ehrnst A, Forsgren M, et al. The viral association of neonatal cholestasis in Sweden: a possible link between cytomegalovirus infection and extrahepatic biliary atresia. *J Pediatr Gastroenterol Nutr* 1998;27:57–64.
34. Chang MH, Huang JJ, Huang ES, et al. Polymerase chain reaction to detect human cytomegalovirus in livers of infants with neonatal hepatitis. *Gastroenterology* 1992;103:1022–1025.
35. Jevon GP, Dimmick JE. Biliary atresia and cytomegalovirus infection: a DNA study. *Pediatr Dev Pathol* 1999;2:11–14.
36. Riepenoff-Talty M, Gouvea V, Evans MJ, et al. Detection of group C rotavirus in infants with extrahepatic biliary atresia. *J Infect Dis* 1996;174:8–15.
37. Bobo L, Ojeh C, Chiu D, et al. Lack of evidence for rotavirus by polymerase chain reaction/enzyme immunoassay of hepatobiliary samples from children with biliary atresia. *Pediatr Res* 1997;41:229–234.
38. Drut R, Drut RM, Gomez MA, et al. Presence of human papillomavirus in extrahepatic biliary atresia. *J Pediatr Gastroenterol Nutr* 1998;27:530–535.
39. Domiati-Saad R, Dawson DB, Margraf LR, et al. Cytomegalovirus and human herpesvirus 6, but not human papillomavirus, are present in neonatal giant cell hepatitis and extrahepatic biliary atresia. *Pediatr Dev Pathol* 2000;3:367–373.
40. Mason A, Nair S. Primary biliary cirrhosis: new thoughts on pathogenesis and treatment. *Curr Gastroenterol Rep* 2002;4:45–51.
41. Balistreri WF, Tabor E, Gerety RJ. Negative serology for hepatitis A and B viruses in 18 cases of neonatal cholestasis. *Pediatrics* 1980;66:269–271.

42. A-Kader HH, Nowicki MJ, Kuramoto KI, et al. Evaluation of the role of hepatitis C virus in biliary atresia. *Pediatr Infect Dis J* 1994;13:657–659.
43. Vasiliauskas E, Targan S, Cobb L, et al. Biliary atresia: an autoimmune disorder? *Hepatology* 1995;22:87.
44. Silveira TR, Salzano FM, Donaldson PT, et al. Association between HLA and extrahepatic biliary atresia. *J Pediatr Gastroenterol Nutr* 1993;16:114–117.
45. Jurado A, Jara P, Camarena C, et al. Is extrahepatic biliary atresia an HLA-associated disease? *J Paediatr Gastroenterol Nutr* 1997;22:557–558.
46. A Kader HH, El-Ayyouti M, Hawas S, et al. HLA in Egyptian children with biliary atresia. *J Pediatr* 2002;141:432–433.
47. Donaldson PT, Manns MP. Immunogenetics of liver disease. In: Benhamou JP, McIntyre N, Rizetto M, et al., eds. *Oxford textbook of clinical hepatology.* Oxford: Oxford University Press, 1999:173–188.
48. Donaldson PT, Clare M, Constantini PK, et al. HLA and cytokine gene polymorphisms in biliary atresia. *Liver* 2002;22:213–210.
49. Yokoyama T, Copeland NG, Jenkins NA, et al. Reversal of left–right asymmetry: a situs inversus mutation. *Science* 1993;260:679–682.
50. Morgan D, Turnpenny L, Goodship J, et al. Inversin, a novel gene in the vertebrate left–right axis pathway, is partially deleted in the *inv* mouse. *Nat Genet* 1998;20:149–156.
51. Mazziotti MV, Willis LK, Heuckeroth RO, et al. Anomalous development of the hepatobiliary system in the *inv* mouse. *Hepatology* 199;30:372–378.
52. Desmet VJ. Cholangiopathies: past, present, and future. *Semin Liver Dis* 1987;7:67–76.
53. Desmet VJ. Congenital diseases of intrahepatic bile ducts: variation on the theme "ductal plate malformation." *Hepatology* 1992;16:1069–1083.
54. Jorgensen MJ. The ductal plate malformation. *Acta Pathol Microbiol Scand* 1977;257:1–88.
55. Desmet VJ. Intrahepatic bile ducts under the lens. *J Hepatol* 1985;1:545–549.
56. Libbrecht L, Cassiman D, Desmet V, et al. The correlation between portal myofibroblasts and the development of intrahepatic bile ducts and arterial branches in human liver. *Liver* 2002;22:252–258.
57. Clotman F, Lannoy VJ, Reber M, et al. The one-cut transcription factor HNF6 is required for normal development of the biliary tract. *Development* 2002;129:1819–1828.
58. Coffinier C, Gresh L, Fiette L, et al. Bile system morphogenesis defects and liver dysfunction upon targeted deletion of HNF1beta. *Development* 2002;129:1829–1838.
59. Emerick KM, Rand EB, Goldmuntz E, et al. Features of Alagille syndrome in 92 patients: frequency and relation to prognosis. *Hepatology* 1999;29:822–829.
60. Ho CW, Shioda K, Shirasaki K, et al. The pathogenesis of biliary atresia: a morphological study of the hepatobiliary system and the hepatic artery. *J Pediatr Gastroenterol Nutr* 1993;16:53–60.
61. Desmet V. *Vascular pathogenesis.* Paper presented at the American Association for the Study of Liver Diseases: Biliary Atresia, December 6–8, 2002, Atlanta, Georgia.
62. Perlmutter DH, Shepherd RW. Extrahepatic biliary atresia: a disease or a phenotype? *Hepatology* 2002;35:1297–1304.
63. Tan CEL, Driver M, Howard ER, et al. Extrahepatic biliary atresia: a first trimester event. Clues from light microscopy and immunohistochemistry. *J Pediatr Surg* 1994;29:808–814.
64. Sokol RJ, Straka MS, Dahl R, et al. Role of oxidant stress in the permeability of transition induced in rat hepatic mitochondria by hydrophobic acids. *Pediatr Res* 2001;49:519–531.
65. Yerushalmi B, Dahl R, Gumpricht E, et al. Bile acid induced rat hepatocytes apoptosis is inhibited by anti-oxidants and blockers of the mitochondrial permeability transition. *Hepatology* 2001;33:616–626.
66. Crawford JM. Development of the intrahepatic biliary tree. *Semin Liver Dis* 2002;22:213–226.
67. Lemaigre FP. Development of the biliary tract. *Mech Develop* 2003;120:81–87.
68. Tan CEL, Moscoso GJ. The developing human biliary system at the porta hepatis level between 29 days and 8 weeks of gestation: a way to understanding biliary atresia. Part 1. *Pathol Int* 1994;44:587–599.
69. Zaret KS. Regulatory phases of early liver development: paradigms of organogenesis. *Nature Rev Genet* 2002;3:499–512.
70. Boussard P, Zaret KS. GATA transcription factors as potentiators of gut endoderm differentiation. *Development* 1998;125:4909–4917.
71. Kalinichenko VV, Zhou Y, Bhattacharyya D, et al. Haploinsufficiency of the mouse forkhead box F1 gene cause defects in gallbladder development. *J Biol Chem* 2002;277:12369–12374.
72. Louis AA, Van Exken P, Haaber BA, et al. Hepatic jagged 1 expression studies. *Hepatology* 1999;30:1269–1275.
73. Piccoli DA, Spinner NB. Alagille syndrome and the jagged 1 gene. *Semin Liver Dis* 2001;21:525–534.
74. Kohsaka T, Yuan ZR, Guo SX, et al. The significance of human jagged 1 mutations detected in severe cases of biliary atresia. *Hepatology* 2002;36:904–912.
75. Balistreri WF, Heubj JE, Suchy FJ. Immaturity of the enterohepatic circulation in early life: factors predisposing to "physiologic" maldigestion and cholestasis. *J Pediatr Gastroenterol Nutr* 1983;2:346–354.
76. deBelle RC, Vaupshas V, Vitullo BB, et al. Intestinal absorption of bile acids: immature development in the neonate. *J Pediatr* 1979;79:472–477.
77. Emeerick KB, Whitington PF. Molecular basis of neonatal cholestasis. *J Pediatr Gastroenterol Nutr* 2002;49:221–235.
78. Back PW. Developmental pattern of bile acid metabolism as revealed by bile acid analysis of meconium. *Gastroenterology* 1980;78:671–676.
79. Strandvik BW. Tetrahydroxylated bile acids in the healthy newborn. *Eur J Clin Invest* 1982;12:301–305.
80. Nietgen GW, Vacanti JP, Perez-Atayde AR. Intrahepatic bile duct loss in biliary atresia despite portoenterostomy: a consequence of ongoing obstruction? *Gastroentology* 1992;102:2126–2133.
81. Miyano T, Suruga K, Tsuchiya H, et al. A histological study of the remnant of extrahepatic bile duct in so-called uncorrectable biliary atresia. *J Pediatr Surg* 1977;12:19–25.
82. Chandra RS, Altman RP. Ductal remnants in extrahepatic biliary atresia: a histopatholoci study with clinical correlation. *Pediatrics* 1978;93:196–200.
83. Ohi R, Shikes RH, Stellin GP, et al. In biliary atresia duct histology correlates with bile flow. *J Pediatr Surg* 1984;19:467–470.
84. Thung SN. The development of proliferating ductular structures in liver disease. *Arch Pathol Lab Med* 1990;114:407–411.
85. Funaki N, Sasano H, Shizawa S, et al. Apoptosis and cell proliferation in biliary atresia. *J Pathol* 1998;186:429–433.
86. Liu C, Chiu JH, Chin T, et al. Expression of Fas ligand on bile ductule epithelium in biliary atresia—a poor prognostic factor. *J Pediatr Surg* 200;35:1591–1596.
87. Raweily EA, Gibson AA, Burt AD. Abnormalities of intrahepatic bile ducts in extrahepatic biliary atresia. *Histopathology* 1990;17:521–527.
88. Desmet VJ. Congenital diseases of intrahepatic bile ducts: variations on the theme "ductal plate malformations." *Hepatology* 1992;16:1069–1083.
89. Nio M, Ohi R, Chiba T. Morphology of intrahepatic bile ducts in jaundice-free patient with biliary atresia. *Biliary Atresia* 1991;1:7–10.
90. Treem WR, Krymowski GA, Cartun RW, et al. Cytokeratin immunohistochemical examination of liver biopsies in infants with Alagille syndrome and biliary atresia. *J Pediatr Gastroenterol Nutr* 1992;15:73–80.
91. Ohi R, Ibrahim M. Biliary atresia. *Semin Pediatr Surg* 1992;1:115–124.
92. Demetris AJ. Immunopathology of the human biliary tree. In: Sirica AE, Longnecker DS, eds. *Biliary and pancreatic ductal epithelia.* New York: Marcel Dekker, 1997:127–180.
93. Landing BH. Considerations of the pathogenesis of neonatal hepatitis, biliary atresia and choledochal cyst—the concept of infantile obstructive cholaniopathy. *Prog Pediatr Surg* 1975;6:113–139.
94. Dillon PW, Belchis D, Minnick K, et al. Differential expression of the major histocompatibility antigens and ICAM-1 on bile duct epithelial cells in biliary atresia. *Tohoku J Exp Med* 1997;181:33–40.

95. Nakada M, Nakada K, Kawaguchi F, et al. Immunologic reaction and genetic factors in biliary atresia. *Tohoku J Exp Med* 1997;181:41–47.
96. Muraji T, Hashimoto K, Ifuku H, et al. Increased expression of HLA-DR antigens on biliary epithelial cells in biliary atresia. *J Jpn Soc Pediatr Surg* 1988;24:793–796.
97. Borrme U, Nemeth A, Hultcrantz R, et al. Different expression of HLA-DR and ICAM-1 in livers from patients with biliary atresia and Byler's disease. *J Hepatol* 1997;26:857–862.
98. Davenport M, Gonde C, Redkar R, et al. Immunohistochemistry of the liver and biliary tree in extrahepatic biliary atresia. *J Pediatr Surg* 2001;36:1017–1025.
99. Kobayashi H, Puri P, O'Brian S, et al. Hepatic overexpression of mhc class II antigens and macrophage-associated antigens (CD68) in patients with biliary atresia of poor prognosis. *J Pediatr Surg* 1997;32:590–593.
100. Dillon PW, Belchis D, Tracy T, et al. Increased expression of intercellular adhesion molecules in biliary atresia. *Am J Pathol* 1994;145:263–267.
101. Ohya T, Fujimoto T, Shimomura H, et al. Degeneration of intrahepatic bile duct with lymphocyte infiltration into biliary epithelial cells in biliary atresia. *J Pediatr Surg* 1995;30:515–518.
102. Tracy TF, Dillon PW, Fox ES, et al. The inflammatory response in pediatric biliary disease: macrophage phenotype and distribution. *J Pediatr Surg* 1996;31:121–126.
103. Chen K, Gavaler JS, Van Thiel DH, et al. Phenotypic characterization of mononuclear infiltrate present in liver of biliary atresia. *Dig Dis Sci* 1989;34:1564–1570.
104. Ahmed AF, Ohtani H, Nio M, et al. CD8+ T cells infiltrating into bile ducts in biliary atresia do not appear to function as cytotoxic T cells: a clinicopathological analysis. *J Pathol* 2001;193:383–389.
105. Ahmed AF, Nio M, Ohtani H, et al. In situ CD14 expression in biliary atresia: comparison between early and late stages. *J Pediatr Surg* 2001;36:240–243.
106. Urushihara N, Iwagaki H, Yagi T, et al. Elevation of serum interleukin-18 levels and activation of Kupffer cells in biliary atresia. *J Pediatr Surg* 2000;35:446–449.
107. Krams SM. *Cell mediated immunity.* Paper presented at The American Association for the Study of Liver Diseases Pediatric Single Topic Conference: Biliary Atresia, December 6–8, 2002, Atlanta, Georgia.
108. Rosenweig RN, Omori M, Pate K, et al. Transforming growth factor-B1 in plasma and liver of children with liver disease. *Pediatr Res* 1998;44:402–409.
109. Bezerra JA, Tiao G, Ryckman FC, et al. Genetic induction of proinflammatory immunity in children with biliary atresia. *Lancet* 2002;360:1653–1659.
110. Rosenthal P, Cochin J, Frankland M, et al. Monitoring serum cytokine levels in children with acute and chronic liver disease. *Hepatology* 1992;16:486A.
111. Kobayashi H, Narumi S, Tamatani T, et al. Serum IFN-inducible protein-10: a new clinical prognostic predictor of hepatocytes death in biliary atresia. *J Pediatr Surg* 1999;34:308–311.
112. Hasegawa T, Sasaki T, Kimura T, et al. Measurement of serum hyaluronic acid as a sensitive marker of liver fibrosis in biliary atresia. *J Pediatr Surg* 2000;35:1643–1648.
113. Dhawan A, Trivedi P, Cheeseman P, et al. Serum hyaluronic acid as a early prognostic marker in biliary atresia. *J Pediatr Surg* 2001;36:443–446.
114. Hasegawa T, Kimura T, Sasaki T, et al. Plasma endothelin-1 level as a marker reflecting the severity of portal hypertension in biliary atresia. *J Pediatr Surg* 2001;36:1609–1612.
115. Yoshida S, Nio M, Hayashi Y, et al. Serum insulinlike growth factor-I in biliary atresia. *J Pediatr Surg* 2003;38:211–215.
116. Minnick KE, Kreisberg R, Dillon PW. Soluble ICAM-1 (sICAM-1) in biliary atresia and its relationship to disease activity. *J Surg Res* 1998;76:53–56.
117. Kobayashi H, Horikoshi K, Long L, et al. Serum concentration of adhesion molecules in postoperative biliary atresia patients: relationship to disease activity and cirrhosis. *J Pediatr Surg* 2001;36:1297–1301.
118. Rope BO, Heidenthal E, deVries RR, et al. Circulating adhesion molecules in disease. *Immunol Today* 1993;14:506–512.
119. Harper P, Plant JW, Linger DB. Congenital biliary atresia and jaundice in lambs and calves. *Aust Vet J* 1990;67:18–22.
120. Rosenberg DP, Morecki R, Lollini LO, et al. Extrahepatic biliary atresia in a rhesus monkey. *Hepatology* 1983;3:577–581.
121. Pickett LK, Briggs HC. Biliary obstruction secondary to hepatic vascular ligation in fetal sheep. *J Pediatr Surg* 1969;4:95–100.
122. Spitz L. Ligation of the common bile duct in the fetal lamb: an experimental model for the study of biliary atresia. *Pediatr Res* 1980;14:740–748.
123. Aldana PR, Goeke ME, Carr SC, et al. The expression of regenerative growth factors in chronic liver injury and repair. *J Surg Res* 1994;57:711–717.
124. Schreiber RA, Kleinman RE, Barksdale EM Jr, et al. Rejection of murine congenic bile ducts: a model for immune-mediated bile duct disease. *Gastroenterology* 1992;102:924–930.
125. Schmeling DJ, Oldham KT, Guice KS, et al. Experimental obliterative cholangitis: a model for the study of biliary atresia. *Ann Surg* 1991;213:350–355.
126. Philips PA, Keast D, Paradimitriou JM, et al. Chronic obstructive jaundice induced by reovirus type 3 in weanling mice. *Pathology* 1969;1:193–203.
127. Organ EL, Rubin DH. Pathogenesis of reovirus gastrointestinal and hepatobiliary disease. *Curr Top Microbiol Immunol* 1998;233:67–83.
128. Riepenhoff-Talty M, Schaekel K, Clark F, et al. Group A rotaviruses produce extrahepatic biliary obstruction in orally inoculated newborn mice. *Pediatr Res* 1993;33:394–399.
129. Petersen C, Biermanns D, Kuske M, et al. New aspects in a murine infectious model for extrahepatic biliary atresia. *J Pediatr Surg* 1997;32:1190–1195.
130. Peterson C, Grasshoff S, Luciano L. Diverse morphology of biliary atresia in an animal model. *J Hepatol* 1998;28:603–607.
131. Qiao H, DeVincentes A, Alashari M, et al. Pathogenesis of rotavirus-induced bile duct obstruction (a model for biliary atresia) in normal BALB/C and CB 17 scid mice with severe combined immunodeficiency (SCID). *Pediatr Res* 1999;45:116A.
132. Petersen C, Bruns E, Kuske M, et al. Treatment of extrahepatic biliary atresia with interferon-alpha in a murine infectious model. *Pediatr Res* 1997;42:623–628.
133. Chandra RS. Biliary atresia and other structural anomalies in the congenital polysplenia syndrome. *J Pediatr* 1974;85:649–655.
134. Dimmick JE, Bove KE, McAdams AJ. Extrahepatic biliary atresia and polysplenia syndrome. *J Pediatr* 1975;86:644–645.
135. Maksem JA. Polysplenia syndrome and splenic hypoplasia associated with extrahepatic biliary atresia. *Arch Pathol Lab Med* 1980;104:212–214.
136. Paddock RJ, Arensman RM. Polysplenia syndrome: spectrum of gastrointestinal congenital anomalies. *J Pediatr Surg* 1982;17:563–566.
137. Miyamoto M, Kajimoto T. Associated anomalies in biliary atresia patients. In: Kasai M, ed. *Biliary atresia and its related disorders.* Amsterdam: Excerpta Medica, 183:13–19.
138. Choi SO, Park WH, Lee HJ, et al. "Triangular cord": a sonographic finding applicable in the diagnosis of biliary atresia. *J Pediatr Surg* 1996;31:363–366.
139. Farrant P, Meire HB, Mieli-Vergani G. Improved diagnosis of extrahepatic biliary atresia by high frequency ultrasound of the gallbladder. *Br J Radiol* 2001;74:952–954.
140. Gilmour SM, Hershkop M, Reifen R, et al. Outcome of hepatobiliary scanning in neonatal hepatitis syndrome. *J Nucl Med* 1997;38:1279–1282.
141. Guibaud L, Lachaud A, Touraine R, et al. MR cholangiography in neonates and infants: feasibility and preliminary applications. *Am J Roentgenol* 1998;170:27–31.
142. Norton KI, Glass RB, Kogan D, et al. MR cholangiography in the evaluation of neonatal cholestasis: initial results. *Radiology* 2002;222:687–691.
143. Guelrud M, Jaen D, Mendoza S, et al. ERCP in the diagnosis of extrahepatic biliary atresia. *Gastrointest Endosc* 1991;37:522–526.
144. Iinuma Y, Narisawa R, Iwafuchi M, et al. The role of endoscopic retrograde cholangiopancreatography in infantile cholestasis. *J Pediatr Surg* 2000;35:545–549.

145. Meisheri LV, Kasat LS, Kumar A, et al. Duodenal intubation and test for bile—a reliable method to rule out biliary atresia. *Pediatr Surg Int* 2002;18:392–395.
146. Zerbini MC, Gallucci SD, Maezono R, et al. Liver biopsy in neonatal cholestasis: a review on statistical grounds. *Mod Pathol* 1997;10:793–799.
147. Vajro P, Couturier M, Lemonnier F, et al. Effects of postoperative cholesytramine and phenobarbital administration on bile flow restoration in infants with extrahepatic biliary atresia. *J Pediatr Surg* 1986;21:362–365.
148. Nittono H, Tokita A, Hayashi M, et al. Ursodeoxycholic acid therapy in the treatment of biliary atresia. *Biomed Pharmacother* 1989;43:37–41.
149. Yamishiro Y, Ohtsuke Y, Shimizu T, et al. Effects of ursodeoxycholic acid treatment on essential fatty acid deficiency in patients with biliary atresia. *J Pediatr Surg* 1994;29:425–428.
150. Ryckman FC, Alonso MA, A-Kader H, et al. *The effect of ursodeoxycholic acid (udca) therapy in biliary atresia: a randomized, double blind, controlled trial.* Paper presented at Biliary Atresia: New Clues from Etiology to Therapy Interdisciplinary Symposium, July 2–3, 1999, Hannover, Germany.
151. Kitani K, Kanai S. The choleretic effect of ursodeoxycholate in the rat. *Life Sci* 1982;31:1973–1978.
152. Kasai M, Suzuki H, Ohashi E, et al. Technique and results of operative management of biliary atresia. *World J Surg* 1978;2:571–580.
153. Altman RP, Anderson KD. Surgical management of intractable cholangitis following successful Kasai procedure. *J Pediatr Surg* 1982;17:894–900.
154. Ohi R, Hanamatsu M, Mochizuki I, et al. Progress in the treatment of biliary atresia. *World J Surg* 1985;9:285–293.
155. Karrer FM, Lilly JR. Corticosteroid therapy in biliary atresia. *J Pediatr Surg* 1985;20:693–695.
156. Muraji T, HigashimotoY. T, The improved outlook for biliary atresia with corticosteroid therapy. *J Pediatr Surg* 1997;32:1103–1107.
157. Muraji T, Nishijima E, Higashimoto Y, et al. Biliary atresia: current management and outcome. *Tohoku J Exp Med* 1997;181:155–160.
158. Dillon PW, Owings E, Cilley RE, et al. Immunosuppression as adjuvant therapy for biliary atresia. *J Pediatr Surg* 2001;36:80–85.
159. Meyers RL, Book LS, O'Gorman MA, et al. High dose steroids, ursodeoxycholic acid, and chronic intravenous antibiotics improve bile flow after Kasai procedure in infants with biliary atresia. *J Pediatr Surg* 2003;38:406–411.
160. Miner RB, Gaito JM. Bile flow in response to pharmacologic agents. *Biochem Pharm* 1979;28:1063–1066.
161. Kasai M, Suzuki M. A new operation for "noncorrectable" biliary atresia: hepatic portoenterostomy. *Shujitsu* 1959;13:733–739.
162. Kasai M, Suzuki H, Ohashi E, et al. Technique and results of operative management of biliary atresia. *World J Surg* 1978;571–580.
163. Nakajo T, Hashizume K, Saeki M, et al. Intussusception-type antireflux valve in the Roux-en-Y loop to prevent ascending cholangitis after hepatic portojejunostomy. *J Pediatr Surg* 1990;25:311–314.
164. Saeki M, Nakano M, Hagane K, et al. Effectiveness of an intussusceptive antireflux valve to prevent ascending cholangitis after hepatic portojejunostomy in biliary atresia. *J Pediatr Surg* 1991;26:800–803.
165. Muraji T, Nishijima E, Higashimoto Y, et al. Biliary atresia: current management and outcome. *Tohoku J Exp Med* 1997;181:155–160.
166. Toyosake A, Okamoto E, Okasora T, et al. Extensive dissection at the porta hepatis for biliary atresia. *J Pediatr Surg* 1994;29:896–899.
167. Schweizer P, Kirschner H, Schittenhelm C. Anatomy of the porta hepatis as a basis for extended hepatoporto-enterostomy for extrahepatic biliary atresia—a new surgical technique. *Eur J Pediatr Surg* 2001;11:15–18.
168. Levy J, Martin EC, DeFelice A, et al. Obstruction of the roux limb after portoenterostomy for biliary atresia: a delayed complication. *J Pediatr Surg* 1990;25:1264–1265.
169. Ibrahim M, Miyano T, Ohi R, et al. Japanese biliary atresia registry, 1989 to 1994. *Tohoku J Exp Med* 1997;181:85–95.
170. Hasegawa T, Kimura T, Ssaki T, et al. Indication for redo hepatic portoenterostomy for insufficient bile drainage in biliary atresia: re-evaluation in the era of liver transplantation. *Pediatr Surg Int* 2003;19:256–259.
171. Altman RP. Results of reoperations for correction of extrahepatic biliary atresia. *J Pediatr Surg* 1979;14:305–309.
172. Freitas L, Gauthier F, Valayer J. Second operation for repair of biliary atresia. *J Pediatr Surg* 1987;22:857–860.
173. Hata Y, Uchino J, Kasai Y. Revision of portoenterostomy in congenital biliary atresia. *J Pediatr Surg* 1985;20:217–220.
174. Cuervas-Mons V, Rimola A, Van Thiel DH, et al. Does previous abdominal surgery alter the outcome of pediatric patients subjected to orthotopic liver transplantation? *Gastroenterology* 1986;90:853–857.
175. Mius JM, Brems JJ, Hiatt JR, et al. Orthotopic liver transplantation for biliary atresia. *Arch Surg* 1988;123:1237–1239.
176. Starzl TE, Gordon RD, Iwatsuki R. Liver transplantation in children—a solution for biliary atresia? *Proc Am Coll Surg Ann Clin Congress* 1985;71:17–18.
177. Beath S, Pearmain G, Kelly D, et al. Liver transplantation in babies and children with extrahepatic biliary atresia. *J Pediatr Surg* 1993;28:1044–1047.
178. Goss JA, Shackleton CR, Scvenson K, et al. Orthotopic liver transplantation for congenital biliary atresia. An 11-year, single center experience. *Ann Surg* 1996;224:276–287.
179. Karrer FM, Lilly JR, Stewart BA, et al. Biliary atresia registry, 1976 to 1989. *J Pediatr Surg* 1990;25:1076–1080.
180. Davenport M, Kerker N, Mieli-Vergani G, et al. Biliary atresia: the King's College hospital experience (1874–1995). *J Pediatr Surg* 1997;32:479–485.
181. Mowatt AP. Extrahepatic biliary atresia and other disorders of the extrahepatic bile ducts presenting in infancy. In: Mowatt, AP *Liver disorders in childhood,* 3rd ed. Oxford, England: Butterworth-Heineman, 1998.
182. Adelman S. Prognosis of uncorrected biliary atresia: an update. *J Pediatr Surg* 1978;13:389–392.
183. Karrer FM, Lilly JR, Stewart BA, et al. Biliary atresia registry, 1976 to1989. *J Pediatr Surg* 1990;25:1076–1081.
184. Howard ER.Biliary atresia: aetiology, management and complications. In: Howard ER, ed. *Surgery of liver disease in infancy.* London: Butterworth, 1991:39–59.
185. Schweizer P, Lunzmann K. Extrahepatic bile duct atresia: how efficient is the hepatoporto-enterostomy? *Eur J Pediatr Surg* 1998;8:150–154.
186. Matsuo S, Suita S, Kubota M, et al. Long-term results and clinical problems after portoenterostomy in patients with biliary atresia. *Eur J Pediatr Surg* 1998;8:142–145.
187. Nio M, Ohi R, Miyano T, et al. Five and 10 year survival rates after surgery for biliary atresia: a report from the Japanese Biliary Atresia Registry. *J Pediatr Surg* 2003;38:997–1000.
188. Diem HU, Eurard V, Vinh HT, et al. Pediatric liver transplantation for biliary atresia: results of primary grafts in 328 recipients. *Transplantation* 2003;75:1692–1697.
189. Miyano T, Fujimoto T, Ohya T, et al. Current concept of treatment of biliary atresia. *World J Surg* 1993;17:332–336.
190. Maksoud JG, Fauza DO, Silva MM, et al. Management of biliary atresia in the liver transplantation era: a 15 year, single center experience. *J Pediatr Surg* 1998;33:115–118.
191. Ohi R, Hanamatsu M, Mochizuki I, et al. Progress in the treatment of biliary atresia. *World J Surg* 1985;9:285–293.
192. Kobayashi A, Tabashi F, Ohbe Y, et al. Long-term prognosis in biliary atresia after hepatic portoenterostomy: analysis of 35 patients who survived beyond 5 years of age. *J Pediatr* 1984;105:243–249.
193. Lopez-Santamaria M, Gamez M, Murcia J, et al. Long-term follow up of patients with biliary atresia successfully treated with hepatic portoenterostomy. The importance of sequential treatment. *Pediatr Surg Int* 1998;13:327–330.
194. Ryckman FC, Alonso MH, Bucuvalas JC, et al. Biliary atresia—surgical management and treatment options as they relate to outcome. *Liver Transplant Surg* 1998;4:S24–S33.
195. Otte JB, de Ville de Goyet J, Reding R, et al. Sequential treatment of biliary atresia with Kasai portoenterostomy and liver transplantation: a review. *Hepatology* 1994;20:41S–48S.
196. Wood RP, Langnas AN, Stratta RJ, et al. Optimal therapy for patients with biliary atresia: portoenterostomy ("Kasai" procedures) versus primary transplantation. *J Pediatr Surg* 1990;25:153–162.
197. Aronson DC, de Ville de Goyet J, Francois D, et al. Primary

management of biliary atresia: don't change the rules. *Br J Surg* 1995;82:672–673.

198. Volpert D, White F, Finegold MJ, et al. Outcome of early hepatic portoenterostomy for biliary atresia. *J Pediatr Gastroenterol Nutr* 2001;32:265–269.
199. Altman RP, Lilly JR, Greenfield J, et al. A multivariable risk factor analysis of the portoenterostomy (Kasai) procedure for biliary atresia. *Ann Surg* 1997;226:348–355.
200. Jiang CP, Lee HC, Yeung CY, et al. A scoring system to predict the need for liver transplantation for biliary atresia after Kasai portoenterostomy. *Eur J Pediatr (in press)*.
201. Shinka M, Ohhama Y, Take H, et al. Evaluation of the PELD risk score as a severity index of biliary atresia. *J Pediatr Surg* 2003;38:1001–1004.
202. Kasai M, Kimura S, Asakura Y, et al. Surgical treatment of biliary atresia. *J Pediatr Surg* 1968;3:665–675.
203. Davenport M, Howard ER. Macroscopic appearance at portoenterostomy—a prognostic variable in biliary atresia. *J Pediatr Surg* 1996;31:1387–1390.
204. Chardot C, Carton M, Spire-Bendelal N, et al. Is the Kasai operation still indicated in children older than 3 months diagnosed with biliary atresia? *J Pediatr* 2001;138:224–228.
205. Tan CE, Davenport M, Driver M, et al. Does the morphology of the extrahepatic biliary remnants in biliary atresia influence survival? A review of 205 cases. *J Pediatr Surg* 1994;29:1459–1464.
206. Stewart BA, Hall RJ, Karrer FM, et al. Long-term survival after Kasai's operation for biliary atresia. *Pediatr Surg Int* 1990;5:87–93.
207. Houwen R, Zweirstra R, Soverijner R, et al. Prognosis of extrahepatic biliary atresia. *Arch Dis Child* 1989;64:214–218.
208. Okazaki T, Kobayashi H, Yamataka A, et al. Long-term postsurgical outcome of biliary atresia. *J Pediatr Surg* 1999;34:312–315.
209. Howard ER, MacLean D, Nio M, et al. Survival patterns in biliary atresia and comparison of quality of life of long-term survivors in Japan and England. *J Pediatr Surg* 2001;36:892–897.
210. Kuroda T, Saeki M, Nakano M, et al. Biliary atresia, the next generation: a review of liver function, social activity, and sexual development in the late postoperative period. *J Pediatr Surg* 2002;37:1709–1712.
211. Howard ER, Mowatt AP. Hepatobiliary disorders in infancy: hepatitis; extrahepatic biliary atresia; intrahepatic biliary hypoplasia. In: Thomas HC, McSween RNM, eds. *Recent advances in hepatology.* London: Churchill Livingstone, 1984:153.
212. Ernest van Heurn LW, Saing H, Tam PK. Cholangitis after hepatic portoenterostomy for biliary atresia: a multivariate analysis of risk factors. *J Pediatr* 2003;142:566–571.
213. Ohi R. Surgery for biliary atresia. *Liver* 2001;21:175–182.
214. Lunzmann K, Schweizer P. The influence of cholangitis on the prognosis of extrahepatic biliary atresia. *Eur J Pediatr Surg* 1999;9:19–23.
215. Sokol RJ, Mack C, Narkewicz MR, et al. Pathogenesis and outcome of biliary atresia: current concepts. *J Pediatr Gastroenterol Nutr* 2003;37:4–21.
216. Muraji T, Tsugawa C, Nishijima E, et al. Surgical management for intractable cholangitis in biliary atresia. *J Pediatr Surg* 2002;37:1713–1715.
217. Jones EA, Bergasa NV. The pruritis of cholestasis: from bile acids to opiate agonists. *Hepatology* 1990;11:884–887.
218. Jones EA, Bergasa NV. The pruritis of cholestasis and the opioid system. *JAMA* 1992;268:3359–3362.
219. Whitington PF. Chronic cholestasis of infancy. *Pediatr Clin N Am* 1996;43(1):1–26.
220. Bergassa NV, Jones EA. Management of the pruritis of cholestasis: potential role of opiate antagonists. *Am J Gastroenterol* 1991;86:1404–1412.
221. Whitington PF, Balistreri WF. Liver transplantation in pediatrics: indications, contraindications, and pretransplant management. *J Pediatr* 1991;118:169–177.
222. Ohi R, Mochizuk I, KoMatsu K, et al. Portal hypertension after successful hepatic portoenterostomy in biliary atresia. *J Pediatr Surg* 1986;21:271–274.
223. Miga D, Sokol RJ, Mackenzie T, et al. Survival after first esophageal variceal hemorrhage in patients with biliary atresia. *J Pediatr* 2001;139:291–296.
224. Goncalves ME, Cardoso SR, Maksoud JG. Prophylactic sclerotherapy in children with esophageal varices: long-term results of a controlled prospective randomized trial. *J Pediatr Surg* 2000;35:401–405.
225. Karrer FM, Markewicz MR. Esophageal varices: current management in children. *Semin Pediatr Surg* 1999;8:193–201.
226. Sasaki T, Hasegawa T, Nakajima K, et al. Endoscopic variceal ligation in the management of gastroesophageal varices in postoperative biliary atresia. *J Pediatr Surg* 1998;33:1628–1633.
227. Harned RK II, Thompson HR, Kumpe DA, et al. Partial splenic embolization in five children with hypersplenism: effects of reduced volume embolization on efficacy and morbidity. *Radiology* 1998;209:803–806.
228. Miyano T, Yamiasahiro Y, Shimizu T, et al. Essential fatty acid deficiency in congenital biliary atresia: successful treatment to reverse deficiency. *J Pediatr Surg* 1986;21:277–281.
229. Pierro A, Koletzko B, Carnielli V, et al. Resting energy expenditure is increased in infants and children with extrahepatic biliary atresia. *J Pediatr Surg* 1989;24:534–538.

Chapter 93

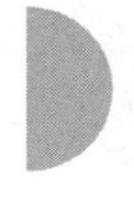

Disorders of the Gallbladder and Biliary Tract

Mark D. Stringer

DEVELOPMENT OF THE BILIARY SYSTEM

The liver develops from an endodermal bud in the ventral floor of the foregut at about 22 days' gestation. One type of endodermal cell in the cranial portion of the liver diverticulum serves as a common precursor for both hepatocytes and the intrahepatic and hilar bile ducts. Immature hepatocytes, or *hepatoblasts,* are derived from these early cells and retain the potential to differentiate into either hepatocytes or intrahepatic ducts. These cells may persist as a facultative stem cell and can be stimulated to proliferate and differentiate under certain pathologic conditions.

At about 2 months' gestation, primitive intrahepatic bile ducts can be distinguished from early hepatocytes by their tendency to form a sleeve around portal venous branches and associated mesenchyme. This sleeve is termed the *ductal plate.* Portions of the sleeve are duplicated, forming small linear tubules that differentiate into bile ducts. This process begins at the liver hilum and extends peripherally into the segmental distribution of the developing liver. At the hilum, connection is made to the extrahepatic bile ducts. Formation of the major branches of the biliary tree is completed by 10 to 12 weeks' gestation, but the peripheral branches continue developing throughout gestation.

The development of the distal common bile duct and pancreaticobiliary junction is particularly relevant to pediatric surgeons. During the fifth week of gestation, the dorsal and ventral pancreatic buds appear. The dorsal bud forms the body of the pancreas and empties through what will become the accessory pancreatic duct (Santorini) into the duodenum. The ventral bud arises from the distal common bile duct, rotates dorsally to join the body of the pancreas as the uncinate process, and empties through the main pancreatic duct (Wirsung) into the common bile duct. During normal development, the junction between the main pancreatic duct and the common bile duct migrates distally through the duodenal wall to unite within the sphincter of Oddi at the ampulla (Fig. 93-1). Abnormalities in this process account for a variety of anatomically based biliary disorders of childhood.

Mark D. Stringer: Children's Liver and GI Unit, St. James's University Hospital, Leeds LS9 7TF, United Kingdom.

Physiologic Maturation

The hepatocyte performs a multitude of essential physiologic tasks. These include production of plasma proteins, gluconeogenesis and glycogenolysis, biotransformation of toxins and chemicals, bile acid metabolism and cholesterol regulation, and bilirubin excretion. During gestation, many of these functions are performed for the fetus through placental transport and maternal hepatic function. Many of the excretory functions of the fetal liver mature only after birth. The physiologic immaturity of the newborn liver undoubtedly contributes to the pathophysiology of several neonatal diseases characterized by abnormal bile composition or flow.

Bile acids are formed in the liver by stereospecific additions and modifications of cholesterol. Bile acid metabolism is a critical determinant of cholesterol regulation and intestinal absorption of dietary fat.

The enterohepatic circulation maintains the bile acid pool by recycling excreted bile acids. This occurs through a sodium–bile acid cotransport system present on the ileal brush border. The bile acids then return to the liver through the portal circulation, where they are actively secreted by a second sodium–bile acid cotransporter across the hepatocyte canalicular membrane. Bacteria present in the jejunum and ileum metabolize a portion of the primary bile acids to secondary bile acids (deoxycholic acid, ursodeoxycholic acid, and lithocholic acid), which are passively absorbed in the colon and reenter the hepatic circulation. Lithocholate can be hepatotoxic and may contribute to

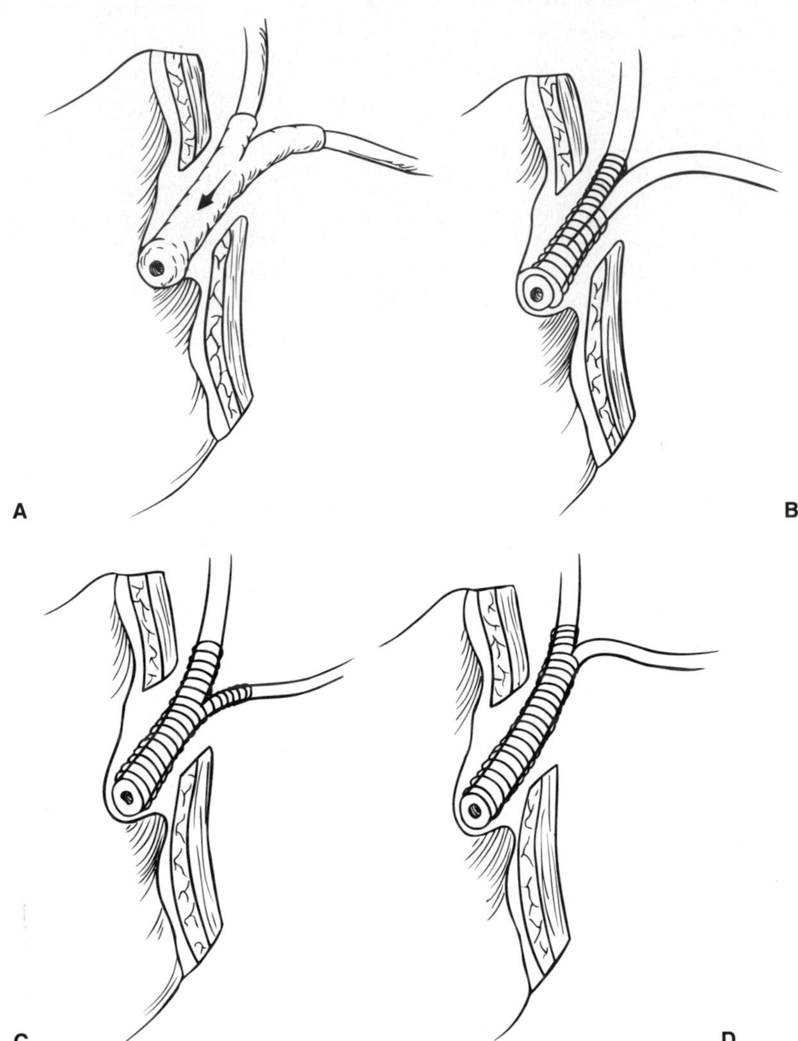

FIGURE 93-1. **(A, B)** Normal embryologic development of the pancreaticobiliary junction before 8 weeks' gestation, with migration of the junction through the duodenal wall and no disturbance of mesenchymal differentiation of the ampullary sphincter complex. **(C, D)** Incomplete migration of the junction, with secondary long, common channel and abnormal development of the sphincter complex.

the liver damage associated with various types of cholestasis.

Bile acids are first detected in human fetuses at about 14 weeks' gestation. The bile acid pool increases in late gestation, but remains relatively smaller in children than adults. Despite decreased bile acid pool size and diminished intestinal absorption, serum bile acids remain elevated in human infants younger than 6 months of age, implying ineffective hepatic clearance. Thus, the newborn infant is relatively predisposed to cholestasis.

Most bilirubin is the product of heme degradation derived from effete erythrocytes. Erythrocyte half-life is shorter in the fetus and neonate; therefore, production of unconjugated bilirubin is relatively greater than in the adult. Most pigment is transferred unaltered across the placenta to the maternal circulation. Bilirubin uridine 5′-diphosphate (UDP)-glucuronyltransferase, which conjugates bilirubin, is first detected at about 20 weeks' gestation, but its activity remains low until after birth. The serum bilirubin concentration normally peaks on the third to fifth day of life in full-term newborns and gradually declines to adult levels thereafter. Bacterial flora responsible for the conversion of conjugated bilirubin to urobilin are absent or reduced in the newborn gut, which allows the enzyme β-glucuronidase to deconjugate the accumulated bilirubin. This results in the absorption of a significant load of unconjugated bilirubin from the newborn intestine and accounts for the increased jaundice seen when there is delayed passage of meconium or intestinal obstruction.

THE GALLBLADDER

The gallbladder develops from the fourth week of gestation as an outgrowth from the caudal part of the hepatic endodermal diverticulum of the foregut. It stores and concentrates hepatic bile. Its motility and absorptive capacity are influenced by circulating hormones (e.g., cholecystokinin, secretin, gastrin, and pancreatic polypeptide) and by the enteric nervous system.

Congenital Anomalies

Various morphologic abnormalities of the number, shape, position, and mucosal lining of the gallbladder have been recorded. Most cases of agenesis of the gallbladder are incidental findings at autopsy or laparotomy. Estimated incidence is about 1 in 3,000 to 6,000 (1). Agenesis may be an isolated finding or it may be associated with multiple congenital malformations. An intrahepatic gallbladder can be excluded by ultrasound scan. Duplications may occur. Variations include bilobed and completely duplicated gallbladders (2). The latter have either a Y-shaped cystic duct or two separate cystic ducts, and they may be surrounded by a common serosal coat or lie in separate but adjacent fossae. It is uncertain whether duplication predisposes to cholelithiasis (3).

The gallbladder may lie to the left of the falciform ligament, and the cystic duct either enters the hepatic duct from the left or, more commonly, the common duct from the right (2,4). The condition is usually without clinical sequelae.

Gallbladder septa can be congenital or acquired, longitudinal or transverse, and single or multiple. Some are composed of fibrous tissue whereas others contain smooth muscle fibers (3). Incomplete septa predispose to cholelithiasis (5).

Ectopic gastric mucosa within the extrahepatic biliary tree is well described. The gallbladder is affected more often than the bile ducts (6). Most cases are incidental findings, but abdominal pain, cholecystitis, hemobilia, and/or obstructive jaundice have been reported.

Cholelithiasis

The prevalence of gallstones in children varies according to geography and age. Ultrasound studies provide the following estimates: 0.5% of neonates in Germany (7), 0.13% to 0.2% of infants and children in Italy (8), and less than 0.13% of children in Japan (9). Most studies show a bimodal distribution with a small peak in infancy and a steadily rising incidence from early adolescence onward (10). In early childhood, boys are affected at least as often as girls, but a clear female predisposition emerges during adolescence. In Western children, there has been a consistent increase in both the prevalence of gallstones and the frequency of cholecystectomy for cholelithiasis since the mid-1970s (11–15). This may reflect improved detection from the widespread use of diagnostic ultrasonography and/or a genuine increase in the incidence of cholelithiasis.

Gallstone Composition

There are four major types of gallstone in adults (16), and an additional variety has been characterized in children (17) (Table 93-1). Mixed cholesterol stones develop as a result of cholesterol supersaturation of bile; they are the most common variety in adults and are also found in adolescent girls. Noncholesterol components of these calculi include calcium salts (bilirubinate, carbonate, phosphate, fatty acids) and proteins. In young children, black pigment stones are most frequent. They are formed from the supersaturation of bile with calcium bilirubinate, the calcium salt of unconjugated bilirubin. Black pigment stones are typical of hemolytic disorders and are also found in association with total parenteral nutrition (TPN) (18). Brown pigment stones develop from biliary stasis and bacterial infection, and occur more often in the bile ducts than in the gallbladder. Calcium carbonate stones were previously considered rare and reported largely in association with milky bile (19), but they are now known to be more common (17).

Biliary sludge is sonographically echogenic but, unlike a gallstone, does not cast an acoustic shadow (20). It consists of mucin, calcium bilirubinate, and cholesterol crystals. Gallbladder sludge may complicate TPN/fasting,

TABLE 93-1 Major Varieties of Gallstones in Children.

Type	*Mixed Cholesterol*	*Pure Cholesterol*	*Black Pigment*	*Brown Pigment*	*Calcium Carbonate*
Composition	Cholesterol + calcium salts	Cholesterol	Pigment polymer + calcium bilirubinate	Calcium bilirubinate + calcium salts of fatty acids	Calcium carbonate polymorphs
Shape	Round or faceted	Round, smooth	Spiky or faceted	Ovoid or irregular	Irregular surface, round or faceted
Color	Brown pigment in rings or specks	Yellow-white	Black	Brown, soft	Brown or white
Number	Multiple	Usually single	Multiple	Single or multiple	Usually single
Microbiology	Sterile	Sterile	Sterile	Infected	Sterile
Major risk factors	Female gender, obesity	Female gender, obesity	Hemolysis	Cholangitis, strictures	Children, gallbladder obstruction

pregnancy, sickle cell disease, treatment with Ceftriaxone or Octreotide, and bone marrow transplantation. Spontaneous resolution or progression to gallstone formation is possible. Sludge itself may cause biliary complications.

Etiology

The predominant factors in gallstone formation are biliary stasis, excess bilrubin pigment, and lithogenic bile. Numerous predisposing conditions have been identified.

Hemolytic disorders such as sickle cell anemia, hereditary spherocytosis, and thalassemia major create excess bilirubin pigment. The prevalence of pigment gallstones in affected children increases with age (21–23). In sickle cell disease, cholelithiasis is present in approximately 10% to 15% of children younger than 10 years of age, but in 40% or more of older children (21,24). Other hemolytic disorders, such as hemolytic uremic syndrome, ABO or rhesus incompatibility, and cardiac valve replacement, may also be complicated by pigment stones.

The association between TPN and biliary sludge/cholelithiasis is well established (25). Fasting and TPN promote biliary stasis by impairing both the enterohepatic circulation of bile acids and cholecystokinin-induced gallbladder contraction (26). Limited data suggest that TPN-associated calculi are either pigment stones with a high calcium bilirubinate content (18,27) or calcium carbonate stones (17). Premature infants are particularly susceptible to this complication (28).

Ileal resection/disease is a risk factor for cholelithiasis (27,29). Even a limited ileal resection (less than 50 cm) in the neonate, particularly when associated with a period of parenteral nutrition, predisposes to gallstones (30). Symptomatic gallstones occur in 10% to 20% of children with short bowel syndrome (31). Children with Crohn' s disease affecting the terminal ileum are also at risk of cholelithiasis. Pathogenesis is probably related to disturbances of the enterohepatic circulation of bile salts (10).

In adolescents, gallstones are typically composed of cholesterol and associated with an adult pattern of risk factors (i.e., female gender, obesity, pregnancy, and a positive family history) (13,32). Estrogens increase cholesterol secretion and progesterone slows gallbladder emptying (33). Biliary stasis from mechanical obstruction (e.g., choledochal cyst or cystic duct anomalies) or functional impairment of gallbladder emptying is an additional risk factor. An excessive bilirubin load in the presence of an immature bilirubin excretion mechanism may predispose to pigment stone formation. Thus, polycythemia, multiple blood transfusions, and phototherapy (which stimulates biliary excretion of unconjugated bilirubin) have been implicated as etiologic factors in the newborn.

Many other conditions have been associated with an increased incidence of cholelithiasis in children (10). Examples include cystic fibrosis, Down syndrome, childhood cancer, bone marrow transplantation, cardiac transplantation, spinal surgery, dystrophia myotonica, and chronic intestinal pseudoobstruction.

The contribution of each etiologic factor in different series of children with cholelithiasis will vary with institutional referral patterns, age distribution, method of detection of gallstones, and the era under study (11,14,15,32). In prepubertal children, black pigment stones often predominate, but from adolescence onward cholesterol stones become increasingly frequent.

Clinical Features

The presenting features of cholelithiasis are age dependent. Most reported cases of fetal gallstones resolve spontaneously (34).

Reports of infants with gallstones have increased in more recent years. Premature babies are at greatest risk because of poor gallbladder contractility in response to enteral feeding (35), repeated blood transfusions, furosemide therapy, reduced bile acid output (36), ileal resection, and systemic or biliary infection (37,38). Gallstones are often asymptomatic in this age group, but may cause poor feeding or vomiting. Complications such as acute cholecystitis, choledocholithiasis with obstructive jaundice, and/or cholangitis are uncommon, and biliary perforation is rare (37,38).

Older children with symptomatic gallstones tend to complain of abdominal pain localized to the right upper quadrant or epigastrium, associated with nausea and vomiting. Some present with obstructive jaundice or pancreatitis.

Fatty food intolerance, biliary colic, and acute or chronic cholecystitis are well described in most adolescent patients with symptomatic stones. In acute cholecystitis, there may be fever, right upper quadrant tenderness, and occasionally a palpable mass. Jaundice and/or pancreatitis may complicate a common duct stone.

Diagnosis

Cholelithiasis is readily diagnosed by ultrasound scan (US) in a fasted patient. Gallstones are usually mobile, may be solitary or multiple, and cast an acoustic shadow. Stone size rather than calcium content determines the presence or absence of acoustic shadowing (39). Gallbladder wall thickness, the diameter of the common bile duct, the liver, and the remaining biliary tree should also be assessed. Between 20% and 50% of gallstones in children are radiopaque. Radioisotope studies with ^{99m}Tc diisopropyl iminodiacetic acid (DISIDA) is a sensitive and specific investigation for acute cholecystitis; nonvisualization of the gallbladder in an otherwise patent biliary system usually indicates acute cholecystitis. Magnetic resonance cholangiography (MRC) and endoscopic ultrasound are helpful in the diagnosis of choledochlithiasis. Endoscopic retrograde cholangiography (ERC) is more invasive, but has the additional advantage that it may be therapeutic.

Management of Cholelithiasis

Gallstones in infants occasionally resolve spontaneously as a result of dissolution and/or passage through the biliary tree (38–41). Early surgery can be deferred in the asymptomatic infant with gallbladder calculi, provided there is no other evidence of biliary tract disease. Acute calculous cholecystitis generally requires cholecystectomy, although in neonates a brief period of conservative management may be worthwhile (42).

Management of asymptomatic gallbladder calculi in older children is controversial. There is a good argument for elective cholecystectomy in selected children with hemolytic disorders. For other children, a conservative policy has been recommended (43). However, cholecystectomy in experienced centers is generally safe, the chance of spontaneous resolution of gallstones in older children is low, and a child with cholelithiasis is at risk of complications for life.

Gallbladder sludge frequently resolves spontaneously once the precipitant is removed. Thus, biliary sludge associated with TPN usually disappears after enteral feeding has been resumed. For infants who remain dependent on TPN, cholecystokinin and/or ursodeoxycholic acid can be helpful in clearing sludge (44) and rendering the bile less hepatotoxic.

Dissolution therapy for gallstones in children is of little value. Despite prolonged treatment, low dissolution rates and high recurrence rates have been observed in adults with cholesterol stones. Calcified and pigment stones and calculi within a nonfunctioning gallbladder are not amenable to treatment. Extracorporeal shock wave lithotripsy has rarely been used for gallstones in children (45).

Surgery

Cholecystectomy is the standard treatment for *symptomatic* or *complicated* gallbladder stones. Rarely, in a severely ill child, cholecystostomy may be a safer initial option.

In the hemolytic disorders, *asymptomatic* gallstones deserve special consideration.

Cholecystectomy is indicated for hereditary spherocytosis patients with asymptomatic calculi undergoing splenectomy for hematologic indications (22). Cholecystotomy and stone extraction is associated with an unacceptable incidence of recurrent calculi (46). Prophylactic cholecystectomy at the time of splenectomy is not indicated in children without gallstones (47).

Opinion is divided about patients with sickle cell anemia, but many authors favor elective cholecystectomy for asymptomatic gallstones. This is for several reasons: the increasing risk of complications with age (48), the increased morbidity of emergency surgery for gallstone complications (49), and the difficulty of distinguishing cholecystitis from a sickle cell abdominal crisis (50). Laparoscopic cholecystectomy is probably advantageous (51) and, using this approach, a selective preoperative transfusion policy is appropriate (52).

Cholecystectomy is recommended for thalassemia major children with asymptomatic cholelithiasis undergoing splenectomy (53).

Cholecystectomy

Before surgery, routine blood tests and a recent biliary tract ultrasound scan should be available. Awareness of normal variants of biliary anatomy is important. Minicholecystectomy via a small right upper quadrant incision and laparoscopic cholecystectomy are both associated with minimal morbidity. However, the latter is associated with a reduced stress response and analgesic requirement, more rapid recovery, earlier discharge, and improved cosmesis (54). In adults, there is a slightly higher incidence of common bile duct injury with laparoscopic compared with open cholecystectomy (0.2% to 0.5% vs. 0.1% to 0.2%) (55).

The technique of laparoscopic cholecystectomy has been well described (10,56). An operative cholangiogram can be used to clarify anatomy and/or identify a common bile duct stone, but the latter is unlikely if the caliber of the common duct is normal and there is no history of jaundice, pancreatitis, or abnormal liver function. Cholangiography can be carried out with a Kumar clamp and sclerotherapy needle (57).

Holcomb et al. recorded no major complications and no conversions in 100 laparoscopic cholecystectomies (the smallest patient was 10 kg) (56). Prasad et al. described a cystic duct stump leak diagnosed by ERC and treated successfully by external drainage, antibiotics, and endoscopic insertion of a nasobiliary catheter (58).

Choledocholithiasis

Common bile duct stones are uncommon, but are relatively more frequent in children with sickle cell disease (59) and in infants (15,38). Obstructive jaundice, cholangitis, and/or pancreatitis are typical presenting features in symptomatic cases. Although US (conventional or endoscopic), MRC (Fig. 93-2), and computed tomography (CT) may be helpful in diagnosis, endoscopic retrograde cholangiopancreatography (ERCP) offers the possibility of both diagnosis and treatment. ERCP and sphincterotomy with stone retrieval can be performed before or after laparoscopic cholecystectomy (60,61). Early ERCP is recommended for common duct stones associated with obstructive jaundice (bilirubin greater than 100 (μmol/L) and/or cholangitis, but not for most cases of gallstone pancreatitis because the stone usually passes spontaneously. Laparoscopic cholecystectomy with intraoperative cholangiography is usually undertaken a few weeks after the episode of gallstone pancreatitis (56).

Choledocholithiasis can be treated by open exploration of the common bile duct, laparoscopic common duct exploration (56), or ERCP, sphincterotomy, and stone extraction. In some centers, percutaneous techniques are used (62). In small infants, cholecystotomy and irrigation may be successful. An initial short period of observation may be worthwhile if the infant is well without evidence of sepsis or progressive obstruction because some stones will pass spontaneously (37,40).

Acquired Disorders of the Gallbladder

If the gallbladder is suspended by a peritoneal fold from the under surface of the liver, it is at risk of torsion. Presentation is with acute abdominal pain and vomiting, and a mobile tender mass may be palpable in the right hypochondrium (63). Cholecystectomy is curative.

Severe acute distention of the gallbladder (acute hydrops) may progress to acalculous cholecystitis if infection, ischemia, or chemical inflammation supervene. This is seen most often in children who are critically ill for other reasons (Table 93-2) (64,65). A multifactorial etiology is likely, involving dehydration, biliary stasis, infection, and gallbladder ischemia. In Kawasaki disease, vasculitis is the probable cause. In tropical countries, *Salmonella typhi* infection and ascariasis should be considered (66). Clinical features include abdominal pain, vomiting, fever, localized tenderness, and, in 50% of cases, a palpable right upper quadrant mass. Laboratory investigations reveal a leukocytosis, raised inflammatory markers, hyperbilirubinemia, and mild hyperamylasemia. Ultrasound shows a markedly distended gallbladder. Initial management is with antibiotics and intravenous fluids. Cholecystectomy is indicated if there is progressive clinical deterioration, a persistent tender mass, and/or increasing gallbladder distension on US. Tube cholecystostomy is an option if the gallbladder is viable.

TABLE 93-2 Conditions Associated with Acalculous Cholecystitis.

- Sepsis
- Hypovolemic shock
- Burns
- Trauma
- Postcardiac surgery
- Gastroenteritis
- Total parenteral nutrition
- Kawasaki disease
- Typhoid fever

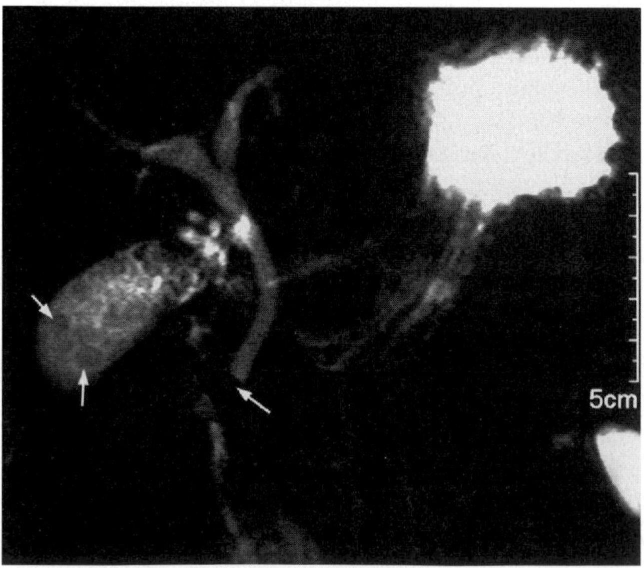

FIGURE 93-2. Magnetic resonance cholangiogram showing a mildly dilated common bile duct with an obstructing gallstone *(longer arrow)* and stones in the gallbladder *(shorter arrows)*.

An aggressive variant of chronic calculous cholecystitis is xanthogranulomatous cholecystitis, in which there is dense inflammation of the gallbladder wall extending into adjacent tissues (67). It may be confused with malignancy. On cut section, the gallbladder wall has multiple yellow nodules containing foamy histiocytes.

Impaired gallbladder contractility (dyskinesia) in the absence of cholelithiasis is a rare cause of chronic abdominal pain in children (68). US shows a normal gallbladder, and the diagnosis rests on demonstrating impaired gallbladder contraction in response to an injection of cholecystokinin during a DISIDA scan. Treatment is by cholecystectomy.

Polypoid lesions of the gallbladder are rare in childhood. They may occur as a manifestation of metachromatic leukodystrophy, Peutz-Jeghers syndrome, or pancreaticobiliary malunion. Other, idiopathic polyps have a variable histology (adenoma, gastric heterotopia, cholesterol polyp, and epithelial hyperplasia) (69). Cholecystectomy is recommended for idiopathic polyps if there are biliary symptoms or if the polyp is greater than or equal to 1 cm in size.

THE BILE DUCT

Congenital Bile Duct Dilatation (Choledochal Cysts)

Congenital bile duct dilatation is a better term for this spectrum of anomalies known traditionally as choledochal cysts. Choledochal cysts may cause symptoms at any age, but typically present with obstructive jaundice and/or abdominal pain in infants and children. Although rare, they are more common in females (about 3 to 4:1) and in Oriental races.

Classification

Choledochal cysts can be categorized according to their anatomic appearance into five types (Fig. 93-3): type I—cystic (Ic) or fusiform (If), type II—diverticulum, type III—choledochocele (dilatation of the terminal common bile duct within the duodenal wall), type IV—multiple extra- and intra-hepatic duct cysts (IVa) or multiple extrahepatic duct cysts (IVb), and type V—intrahepatic duct cysts (single or multiple). In large series, type I cysts account for at least 75% of all cases, and type IVa cysts account for most of the remainder; other varieties are rare (70,71). Pancreaticobiliary malunion may occur without choledochal dilatation, and this has been termed a *forme fruste* choledochal cyst (72).

Pathology

In more than 75% of patients with a choledochal cyst (particularly type I and IV cysts), there is an anomalous junction between the distal common bile duct and the pancreatic duct; the ducts unite outside the duodenal wall some distance proximal to the ampulla of Vater. This is termed *pancreaticobiliary malunion* (PBM). This common channel often exceeds 5 to 10 mm in length (73), and it is not surrounded by the normal sphincter mechanism (74). Consequently, pancreatic juice refluxes into the biliary tree. This has been confirmed by dynamic magnetic resonance cholangiopancreatography (MRCP) after secretin stimulation (75). High concentrations of pancreatic enzymes are frequently found in bile within cysts (76). This may produce chronic inflammation of the cyst and predispose to later malignant degeneration. Isolated PBM without choledochal dilatation has been implicated in the pathogenesis of gallbladder cancer in adults (77).

A common channel also predisposes to reflux of bile into the pancreatic duct, which may precipitate pancreatitis.

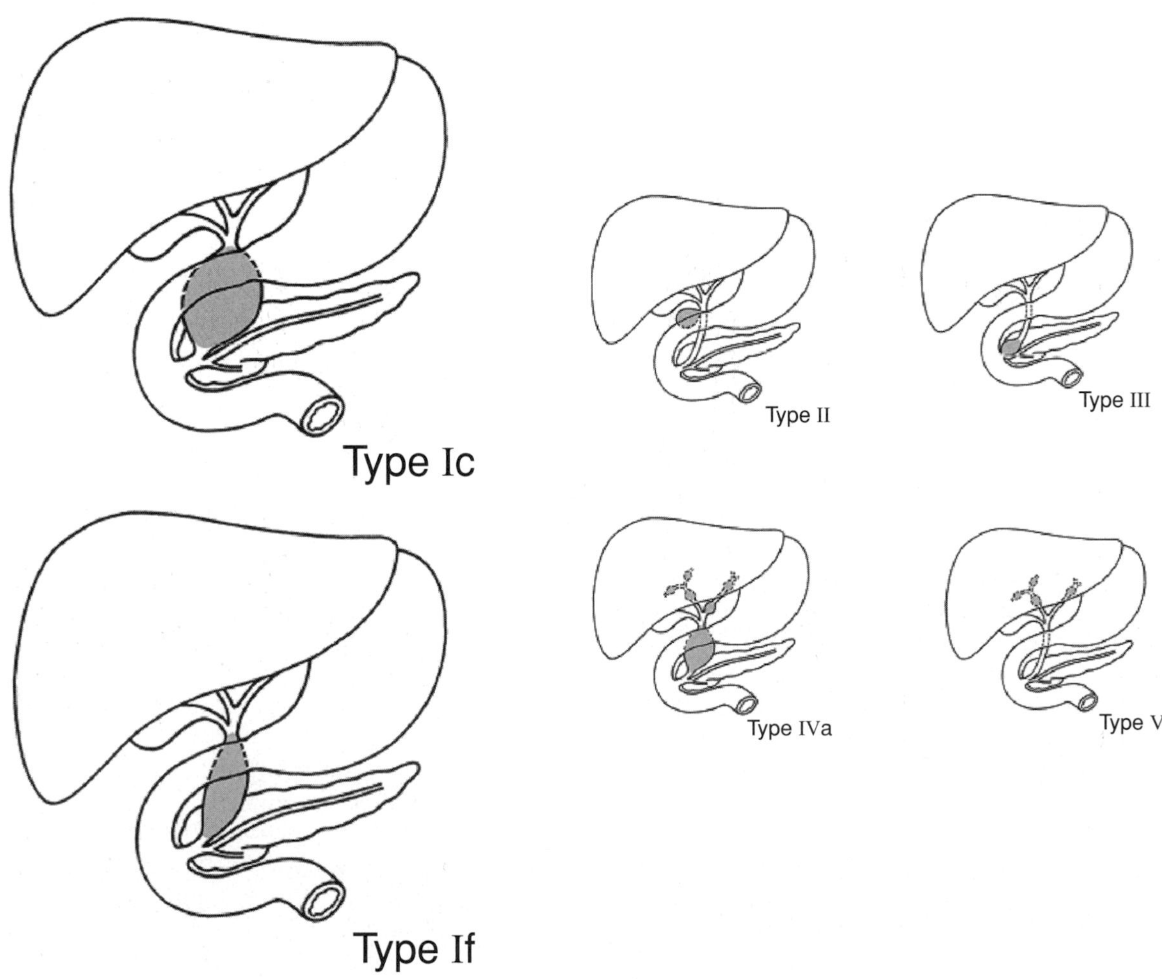

FIGURE 93-3. Classification of congenital bile duct dilatation (choledochal cysts).

In some patients, the common channel is dilated and the type of union very complex (78). PBM is not present in all choledochal cysts, and Lilly suggested that it should be regarded as only one manifestation of a disordered embryology that affects the whole of the extrahepatic biliary tree (79).

Type I cysts typically extend from just below the common hepatic duct bifurcation to the duodenum. The gallbladder is usually normal or only slightly dilated. Hilar duct strictures may be found with type IVa cysts (80). The duodenal papilla is frequently located distal to the mid-descending duodenum (81). Other biliary abnormalities are rare, but multiseptate gallbladder (82), accessory bile ducts (83), and biliary tract duplications have been reported.

In older children, the wall of the choledochal cyst is thickened and composed of fibrous tissue with occasional elastin and smooth muscle fibers. The biliary epithelial lining may be ulcerated. The degree of histologic damage and the rate of epithelial metaplasia and dysplasia are related to the age of the patient (84). Liver histology varies from mild inflammation of the portal tracts, with some periportal fibrosis through to cirrhosis.

Choledochal cysts are congenital. Two main etiologic theories have been proposed. An acquired weakness of the wall of the bile duct associated with PBM was first suggested by Babbitt, who contended that reflux of pancreatic juice damages and weakens the common bile duct causing dilatation (85). However, PBM is not found in all patients with congenital choledochal dilatation, and it can occur with a normal caliber bile duct. In addition, choledochal cysts have been detected as early as 15 weeks' gestation, a time when acinar development of the pancreas is rudimentary, which argues against a significant role for pancreaticobiliary reflux in such cases. An alternative and more plausible explanation is obstruction of the distal common bile duct. Ligation of the distal bile duct in newborn lambs causes cystic choledochal dilatation; however, in mature sheep, the gallbladder distends selectively, suggesting that the timing of obstruction is critical (86). A stenosis is often seen just below a type Ic cyst, but whether this is congenital or acquired is uncertain (87). A distal obstruction could be functional rather than mechanical, and occur as a result of PBM and an abnormal sphincter of Oddi.

A genetic predisposition to choledochal cysts seems likely in view of the female preponderance and geographic distribution. Familial examples have been reported (88), but twin studies have not shown a classical pattern of inheritance.

Clinical Features

The majority of choledochal cysts are diagnosed before 10 years of age, but they can present at any age. Type Ic choledochal cysts have been detected by routine prenatal sonography as early as 15 weeks' gestation (71). Differential diagnosis includes duodenal atresia, an ovarian cyst, a duplication cyst, and cystic biliary atresia. Progressive enlargement of the cyst during gestation (89) and the presence of dilated intrahepatic ducts on postnatal scan (90) are indicative of a choledochal cyst rather than biliary atresia, but it may be difficult to distinguish these two conditions. Postnatally, if the infant is otherwise well, early surgery is recommended, particularly if there is conjugated hyperbilirubinemia. This excludes cystic biliary atresia. Early surgery also avoids the risk of biliary or hepatic complications, which can develop rapidly after prenatal detection of a choledochal cyst (91). The results of surgical treatment at this age are generally excellent (71,92).

Infants typically present with obstructive jaundice with or without vomiting and an abdominal mass. Even in those with PBM, biliary amylase concentrations are low because of pancreatic immaturity; significant levels are only reached after 1 year of age (76).

Recurrent abdominal pain is the dominant presenting feature in older children, but intermittent jaundice may occur (71). The classic triad of jaundice, pain, and a right hypochondrial mass is found in fewer than 10% of patients (70,71). Plasma and/or biliary amylase levels are elevated in most patients with abdominal pain secondary to congenital choledochal dilatation. However, pancreatitis is only confirmed radiologically or at surgery in a small proportion. The hyperamylasemia is secondary to either diffusion of pancreatic amylase through the denuded epithelium of the cyst wall or to cholangiovenous reflux of amylase-rich fluid induced by a high intracholedochal pressure (93). A choledochal cyst should always be considered in the differential diagnosis of obstructive jaundice or pancreatitis. In such cases, an abdominal ultrasound scan typically shows a persistently dilated common bile duct, but this can be subtle in type If dilatations, measuring only 5 to 10 mm. Healthy children have a common bile duct diameter of less than 3.5 mm and infants less than 2 mm (94).

Malformations outside the biliary tree are rare. Urinary tract anomalies and intestinal malrotation have been described (95,96).

Complications

Choledochal cysts are prone to complications (Fig. 93-4). Perforation is rare, typically occurring in preschool children. Spontaneous perforation may affect any part of the cyst and is not directly related to cyst size. Intraperitoneal rupture causes biliary peritonitis, whereas retroperitoneal rupture is less dramatic (97). Abdominal pain and distension, vomiting, fever, mild jaundice, and progressive biliary ascites are typical features. Definitive surgery may be possible at diagnosis (98), but if the inflammation is severe or the anatomy uncertain, preliminary

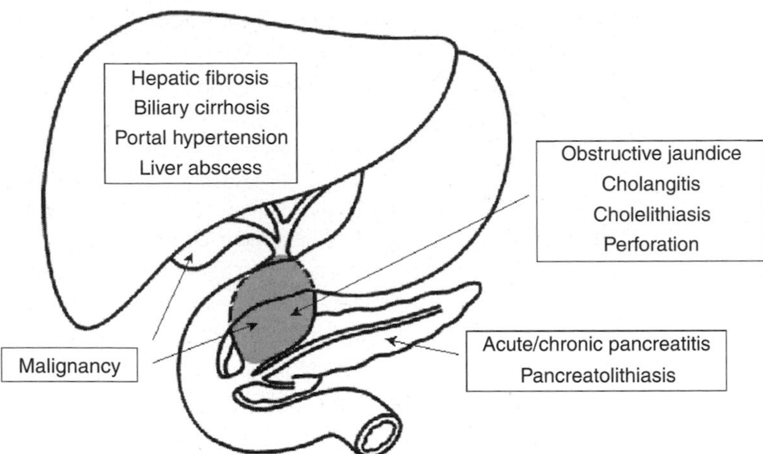

FIGURE 93-4. The complications of choledochal cysts.

T-tube drainage of the choledochal cyst and delayed surgery is a safe option (71,97). Choledochal cysts may be complicated by recurrent pancreatitis. Protein plugs and calculi forming in a dilated common channel exacerbate this tendency. Gallstones are relatively uncommon. Yamaguchi reported an 8% prevalence in 1,433 Japanese cases (99).

Portal hypertension may develop in older children because of portal vein obstruction from cyst compression or secondary biliary cirrhosis, or in association with Caroli' s disease.

Malignancy risk is age related and has been estimated to be 0.7% in the first decade, 7% in the second decade, and 14% after 20 years of age (100,101). Iwai et al. reported the youngest case, a 12-year-old girl with adenocarcinoma complicating a type IVa cyst with a long common channel (102). Malignancy may develop in the cyst wall or gallbladder. PBM is associated with an increased biliary epithelial turnover and is a predisposing factor (103). Stasis and chronic inflammation are also important. The risk of malignancy is greatest in patients who have been treated by internal drainage of a choledochal cyst (cystenterostomy) (104). However, even after cyst excision, malignancy may affect residual extrahepatic ducts or dilated intrahepatic ducts, indicating the need for lifelong surveillance (105). Histology usually shows cholangiocarcinoma or adenocarcinoma (100,101). The prognosis of these malignant tumors is poor.

Investigations

Biochemical liver function tests may be normal or reflect obstructive jaundice. Hyperamylasemia is often present during episodes of abdominal pain. The prothrombin time may be prolonged with cholestasis. A detailed US is the initial investigation of choice. The size, contour, and position of the cyst, the appearance of the proximal bile ducts, the vascular anatomy, and the hepatic echotexture are assessed. Percutaneous transhepatic cholangiography and ERCP give excellent visualization of ductal anatomy, including the pancreaticobiliary junction, but both investigations are invasive and associated with a small risk of complications, such as pancreatitis and biliary sepsis. ERCP should be avoided during an episode of acute pancreatitis. MRCP is noninvasive and can be performed without the use of contrast agents or irradiation (106). Bile and pancreatic juices have a high signal intensity on T2-weighted images (Fig. 93-5). Definition of the pancreatic duct and common channel may be suboptimal in small children (107). In uncomplicated cases, a detailed US supplemented by intraoperative cholangiography provide sufficient anatomic detail. Contrast-enhanced CT may be useful in patients with complications such as pancreatitis, cyst rupture, or suspected malignancy.

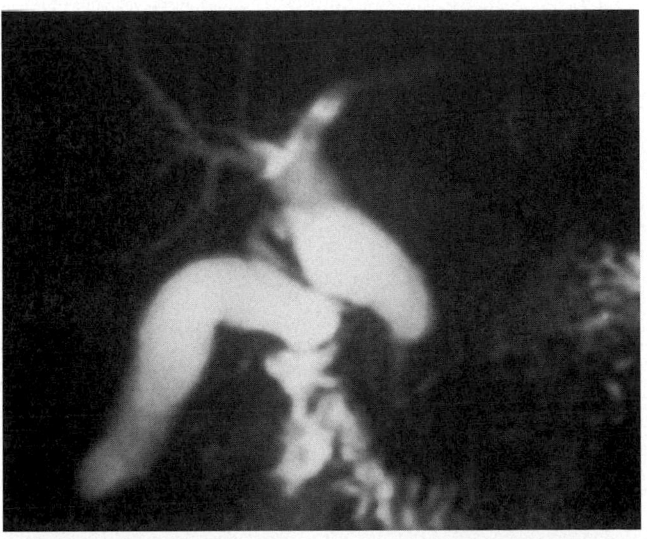

FIGURE 93-5. Magnetic resonance cholangiopancreatography demonstrating a type I choledochal cyst with pancreaticobiliary malunion.

Surgery

Radical cyst excision and reconstruction by hepaticoenterostomy is the optimum treatment for the common types of choledochal cyst. In experienced centers, the procedure can be performed safely at all ages with no mortality and minimal morbidity. Cystenterostomy has a prohibitive long-term morbidity (cholangitis, cholelithiasis, pancreatolithiasis, anastomotic stricture, biliary cirrhosis, and malignancy), and patients treated previously in this way should undergo revisional surgery (108).

Any preoperative coagulopathy is corrected and prophylactic intravenous broad-spectrum antibiotics are given on induction of anesthesia and continued postoperatively for 5 days if there is a history of cholangitis. A high transverse or oblique incision gives excellent exposure. The appearance of the liver, spleen, and pancreas is noted. If the anatomy of the choledochal cyst is in doubt, an operative cholangiogram should be performed; the cyst, pancreaticobiliary junction, and intrahepatic ducts need to be demonstrated. A sample of bile is aspirated from the cyst for culture and pancreatic enzyme estimation.

The cyst is dissected, keeping close to its wall, and the gallbladder is mobilized. Large cysts may require initial decompression. The bile duct is freed circumferentially and encircled just above the superior border of the pancreas (Fig. 93-6). Operative cholangiography provides a guide to the distal level of bile duct transection. The distal common bile duct is divided just within the pancreas and oversewn with absorbable sutures. The common hepatic duct is transected at the level of the bifurcation, where it should be healthy and well vascularized. Dilated proximal intrahepatic ducts and/or a dilated common channel are cleared of debris using heparinized saline irrigation, biliary balloon catheters, and/or a cystoscope (109). Transduodenal sphincteroplasty can be considered if the common channel contains large amounts of debris. A 30–40 cm retrocolic Roux loop of jejunum is anastomosed to the hepatic duct bifurcation at the hilum using fine interrupted monofilament absorbable sutures. An intussusception valve in the Roux loop is unnecessary. The anastomosis must be wide, and this can be achieved by extension onto the extrahepatic portion of the left hepatic duct. Hepaticoduodenostomy is an alternative technique, but hepatico-appendico-duodenostomy should be avoided because of a high incidence of late obstructive complications (110). A liver biopsy is performed before closing the abdomen. Abdominal drainage is unnecessary in straightforward cases.

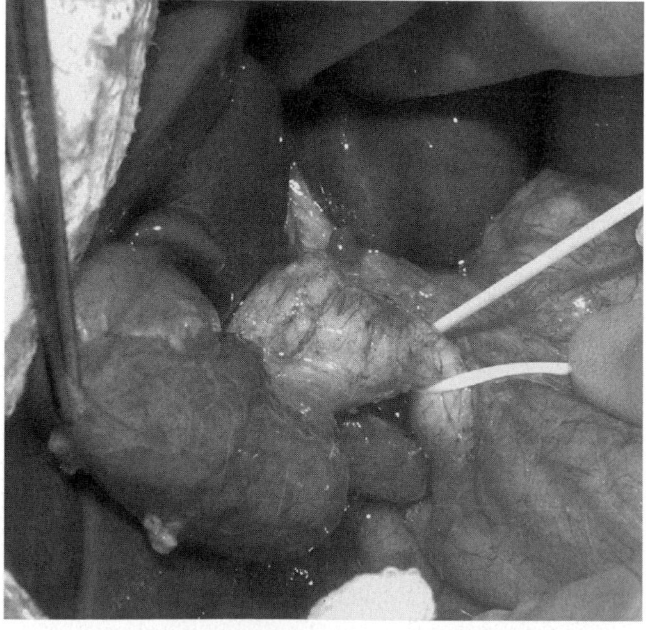

FIGURE 93-6. Operative view of a choledochal cyst. A sling has been placed around the distal common bile duct to assist further proximal and distal dissection.

Laparoscopic excision and reconstruction is feasible (111), but it remains to be determined whether long-term outcomes are comparable to open surgery. Preliminary external drainage via a T-tube may be helpful in patients with cyst rupture or uncontrolled cholangitis. Cyst excision can be performed subsequently. Intramural resection of the posterior wall of the cyst (excising the mucosa and inner wall of the cyst) may help to avoid damage to the portal vein and hepatic arteries if there is dense inflammation or portal hypertension (112). Unless there is a wide connection to the common bile duct, type II cysts can be treated by local excision of the diverticulum (113). Large choledochoceles (type III cysts) can be excised transduodenally. Smaller lesions have been treated by deroofing and sphincteroplasty or by endoscopic sphincterotomy (114). A type V cyst confined to one side of the liver can be treated by hepatic lobectomy. More diffuse varieties are complicated by recurrent cholangitis and stone formation, and liver transplantation may be necessary.

Results and Complications

Radical cyst excision and hepaticojejunostomy yields consistently good results, even in small infants (115). Successful treatment can lead to regression of hepatic fibrosis and even early biliary cirrhosis. Early postoperative complications such as anastomotic leakage and intestinal obstruction are rare. Hepaticoduodenostomy may cause transient duodenal obstruction/ileus. Late complications are uncommon, but include cholangitis, anastomotic stricture, intrahepatic and common channel calculi, pancreatitis, adhesive bowel obstruction and, very rarely, malignancy. In a large Japanese series of 200 children followed up for a mean period of 11 years, complications developed in 18 (9%) (116). Strictures and calculi are more likely complications after resection of a type IVa cyst or after enteric anastomosis to the common hepatic duct.

Pancreatitis may develop years after cyst excision in patients with a dilated or complex common channel. ERCP is useful for the investigation and treatment of such patients.

Caroli's Disease

In this condition, there is congenital segmental saccular dilatation of the intrahepatic bile ducts, which may be localized or diffuse. Intrahepatic biliary stasis predisposes to recurrent cholangitis. Intrahepatic abscess and/or stone formation complicate the disease. Most cases present as young adults, but some children are affected (117).

In 1968, Caroli classified these intrahepatic cysts into type 1, which is rarer and presents with recurrent cholangitis, and type 2 (Caroli's syndrome), where cholangitis is associated with congenital hepatic fibrosis, portal hypertension, and renal disease (118). These two subtypes have become less distinct as experience has accumulated. Caroli's disease has a variable pattern of inheritance.

Prophylactic antibiotics may reduce the frequency of cholangitis. Liver abscesses require drainage. Localized forms of the disease can be treated by hepatic resection, whereas liver transplantation may be required for more diffuse varieties associated with complications. Biliary malignancy is a risk in adults.

BENIGN EXTRAHEPATIC BILE DUCT OBSTRUCTION

The major causes of bile duct obstruction in infants and children are summarized in Table 93-3 (119–130). Most of these conditions require surgical management. Two conditions warrant particular attention.

Inspissated bile within the distal common bile duct may cause obstructive jaundice in newborns. Early reports identified hemolysis as an important precipitant, but subsequent associations have included diuretic therapy, parenteral nutrition, prematurity, and cystic fibrosis. Inspissated bile plug syndrome may be difficult to distinguish from biliary atresia. In both conditions, there may be jaundice and acholic stools, conjugated hyperbilirubinemia, and no biliary excretion on a radionuclide scan. However, US usually reveals dilated proximal bile ducts and inspissated bile.

Spontaneous resolution may occur (40). Treatment with ursodeoxycholic acid may help. More persistent obstruction can be cleared by percutaneous, transhepatic irrigation of the bile ducts, ERC and retrograde irrigation, or cholecystectomy and bile duct irrigation. Occasionally, transduodenal sphincteroplasty may be required to remove an impacted mass of material or stones (131).

TABLE 93-3 Causes of Bile Duct Obstruction in Infants and Children.

Intraluminal
Biliary atresia
Gallstones/biliary sludge
Choledochal cyst
Inspissated bile plug syndrome
Hemobilia
Ascariasis/hydatid disease
Strictures
■ Inflammatory stricture:
Pancreaticobiliary malunion
Idiopathic (119)
Postradiotherapy (120)
Sclerosing cholangitis
- Primary, which may be associated with inflammatory bowel disease (121)
- Neonatal
- Secondary to Langerhans cell histiocytosis or congenital immunodeficiencies
Recurrent pyogenic cholangitis (122)
After spontaneous biliary perforation (123)
Gastric heterotopia (124)
Mirizzi syndrome
■ Traumatic stricture:
Blunt abdominal trauma (accidental and nonaccidental)
Iatrogenic injury
■ Ischemic stricture: (e.g., after liver transplant)
■ Neoplastic (benign) stricture: (e.g., inflammatory pseudotumor)
Extramural
Lymph nodes (including leukemia and lymphoma) (125–127)
Duodenal malformation
Pancreatic tumor
Neuroblastoma (128)
Intestinal malrotation with volvulus
Choledochal varices
Pancreatitis (including fibrosing pancreatitis) (129)
Miscellaneous
Cystic fibrosis (130)
Congenital bile duct malformations

Infection with the roundworm, *Ascaris lumbricoides*, is common in Africa, Asia, and Central America. Adult roundworms live within the small bowel. Eggs are passed in the feces and ingested by humans. Swallowed ova hatch in the duodenum of the new host, and their larvae penetrate the gut wall and migrate to the pulmonary circulation via the portal venous system and liver. Further maturation in the lungs is followed by larval migration into the trachea and esophagus before further maturation in the small bowel. Adult worms can reach up to 30 cm in length. Migration up the common bile duct may cause complications such as pyogenic cholangitis, bile duct perforation, cholecystitis, pancreatitis, and liver abscess (132).

In uncomplicated cases, jaundice is not usually present, although the gallbladder may be palpable. Ascariasis can be diagnosed by examination of the stools. Ultrasound confirms the biliary distension, and endoscopy may show worms within the duodenum and across the ampulla.

Conservative treatment of uncomplicated cases initially consists of analgesia, antispasmodics, intravenous fluids, and nasogastric decompression, which results in worms returning to the duodenum in most affected children. Anthelmintics are then administered. ERCP and worm extraction is recommended if symptoms persist. If this fails or is not possible, surgical extraction of worms via a choledochotomy may be necessary (133); a T-tube enables postoperative cholangiography and irrigation.

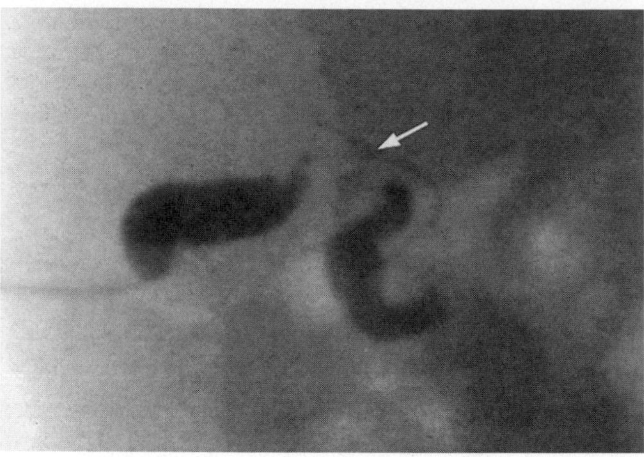

FIGURE 93-7. Operative cholangiogram in a 3-week-old baby with spontaneous perforation of the bile duct. The arrow indicates the typical site of perforation at the junction of the cystic and common bile duct.

SPONTANEOUS BILIARY PERFORATION

Spontaneous perforation of the extrahepatic bile ducts should always be considered in a young infant who develops obstructive jaundice after an initial period of good health or who presents with progressive ascites. The majority of infants present subacutely within 3 months of birth with mild, fluctuating, obstructive jaundice and slowly progressive biliary ascites. An acute presentation with abdominal distension and tenderness is rare.

The typical site of bile duct perforation is at the junction of the cystic and common bile ducts. The cause is unknown, but biliary obstruction from inspissated bile in the distal common bile duct or from ampullary stenosis may account for some cases. The differential diagnosis includes bile duct perforation secondary to trauma, choledochal cyst, or necrotizing enterocolitis (134).

Abdominal ultrasonography may show a complex loculated collection of bile around the common bile duct (which may be mistaken for a choledochal cyst) and within the lesser sac and/or generalized ascites. A hepatobiliary radionuclide scan confirms intraabdominal extravasation of bile.

Historically, nonoperative management was frequently fatal (135) and surgical exploration is now recommended. Operative cholangiography via the gallbladder will confirm the site of perforation and assess the patency of the common bile duct (Fig. 93-7). Definitive treatment is dictated by the findings (136). Cholecystectomy is sufficient for rare instances of cystic duct perforation, but for the usual site of perforation, tube cholecystostomy, and simple drainage is appropriate if there is free flow of contrast into the duodenum. If there is distal common bile duct obstruction, catheter irrigation may clear inspissated bile, but drainage should be combined with cholecystostomy. If a distal bile duct stricture is demonstrated, hepaticojejunostomy is indicated.

EXTRAHEPATIC BILE DUCT TUMORS

Extrahepatic bile duct tumors are extremely rare and, with the exception of rhabdomyosarcoma, are limited to case reports (137).

Rhabdomyosarcoma affecting the biliary tree accounts for only 0.8% of all rhabdomyosarcomas (138). The median age at presentation is 3.5 years (139). Presentation is typically with obstructive jaundice, which may be accompanied by abdominal pain, distension, and fever. Preoperatively, the tumor may be misdiagnosed as a choledochal cyst if the presence of solid tissue within dilated bile ducts is not recognized (Fig. 93-8). US, CT, and

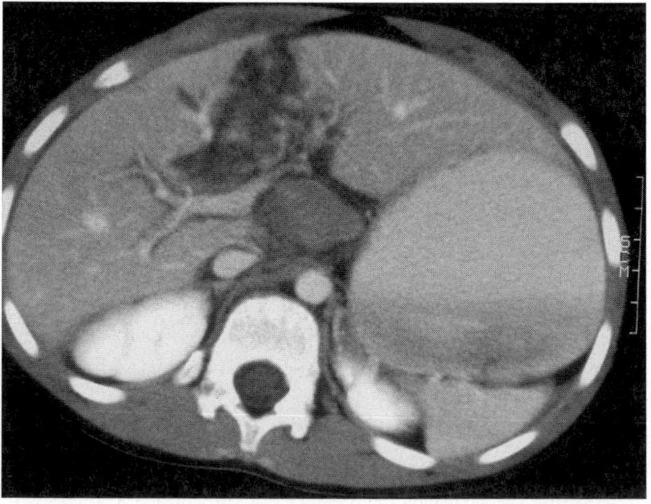

FIGURE 93-8. Computed tomography scan of a 3-year-old child with a biliary rhabdomyosarcoma. The child had undergone an exploratory procedure prior to referral following an erroneous diagnosis of a choledochal cyst.

magnetic resonance imaging (MRI) are useful in assessing the tumor, but may overlook intraabdominal nonnodal metastases. About 30% of cases have local or distant metastatic spread at the time of presentation (138,139). Potential sites of tumor spread include regional lymph nodes, omentum, peritoneum, lung, liver, and bones.

Macroscopically, these tumors have a polypoid appearance. They infiltrate proximally beneath the bile duct epithelium into the liver. Invasion of adjacent organs also occurs. Microscopically, biliary rhabdomyosarcomas are either embryonal or botryoid. The tumor probably arises from mesenchymal rests beneath the epithelium of the common bile or hepatic ducts.

In more recent years, significant advances in treatment have been made by the Intergroup Rhabdomyosarcoma Study Group in the United States. Spunt et al. analyzed the outcome of 25 cases treated between 1972 and 1998 (139). Overall estimated 5-year survival was 66%. After exclusion of patients with distant metastatic disease, all of whom died, the 5-year survival rate was 78%. This was despite the fact that only 6 (24%) of the children had undergone attempted complete tumor resection and only 2 had clear surgical margins. The authors concluded that surgery is critical only for diagnosis and accurate staging, but complete resection is rarely possible even with radical surgery. Thus, chemotherapy with or without endoscopic stent placement may be more appropriate than radical surgery in the treatment of obstructive jaundice secondary to rhabdomyosarcoma. The role of radiotherapy is less well defined.

CHOLESTATIC SYNDROMES

The fundamental defect in progressive familial intrahepatic cholestasis (PFIC) is impaired bile acid secretion. PFIC was originally described in Amish families descended from Jacob Byler (Byler's disease). However, it is now recognized that there are three distinct phenotypes, each corresponding to a specific gene defect in the FIC1, BSEP, and MDR3 genes (140). The disorder causes severe intrahepatic cholestasis that typically begins in early infancy and progresses inexorably to cirrhosis. Severe pruritus, jaundice, hepatomegaly, and growth failure are characteristic. Persistent cholestasis and fat-soluble vitamin deficiencies cause rickets and osteopenia, coagulopathy, and neuropathy. Cirrhosis may be complicated by hepatocellular carcinoma.

Pruritus is relatively resistant to medical therapy. Liver transplantation is used successfully to treat patients with intractable symptoms or end-stage cirrhosis and, more recently, hepatocyte transplantation is offering promise to newly diagnosed infants. Partial biliary diversion has been proposed as a means of ameliorating symptoms and delaying liver damage from the retention of hepatotoxic bile salts. Several techniques have been tried, but the most reliable and effective is partial external biliary diversion. A short jejunal conduit is anastomosed to the gallbladder and exteriorized as a stoma in the right iliac fossa. Potential surgical complications include hemoperitoneum, stomal herniation, and intestinal obstruction (141). The procedure is contraindicated in children with severe hepatic fibrosis or cirrhosis.

Several studies have analyzed the results of partial external biliary diversion in both PFIC and Alagille syndrome, a similar genetic disorder of cholestasis. At least 75% of patients with PFIC experience significant improvement in pruritus and biochemical liver function, and a smaller proportion have improved growth (141–143). Early diversion may also delay the progression of the liver disease in PFIC. In Alagille syndrome, pruritus and xanthomas respond well, but there is no effect on growth (144).

REFERENCES

1. Bennion RS, Thompson JE, Tompkins RK. Agenesis of the gallbladder without extrahepatic biliary atresia. *Arch Surg* 1988;123:1257–1260.
2. Gross RE. Congenital anomalies of the gallbladder. A review of 148 cases, with report of a double gallbladder. *Arch Surg* 1936;32:131–162.
3. Harlaftis N, Gray SW, Skandalakis JE. Multiple gallbladders. *Surg Gynecol Obstet* 1977;145:928–934.
4. Newcombe JF, Henley FA. Left-sided gallbladder. *Arch Surg* 1964;88:494–497.
5. Esper E, Kaufman DB, Crary GS, et al. Septate gallbladder with cholelithiasis: a cause of chronic abdominal pain in a 6-year-old child. *J Pediatr Surg* 1992;27:1560–1562.
6. Lamont N, Winthrop AL, Cole FM, et al. Heterotopic gastric mucosa in the gallbladder: a cause of chronic abdominal pain in a child. *J Pediatr Surg* 1991;26:1293–1295.
7. Wendtland-Born A, Wiewrodt B, Bender SW, et al. Prevalence of gallstones in the neonatal period. *Ultraschall Med* 1997;18:80–83.
8. Palasciano G, Portincasa P, Vinciguerra V, et al. Gallstone prevalence and gallbladder volume in children and adolescents: an epidemiological ultrasonographic survey and relationship to body mass index. *Am J Gastroenterol* 1989;84:1378–1382.
9. Nomura H, Kashiwagi S, Hayashi J, et al. Prevalence of gallstone disease in a general population of Okinawa, Japan. *Am J Epidemiol* 1988;128:598–605.
10. Stringer MD. Gallbladder disease and cholelithiasis. In: Howard ER, Stringer MD, Colombani PM, eds. *Surgery of the liver, bile ducts and pancreas in children,* 2nd ed. London: Arnold Publishers, 2002:189–208.
11. Bailey PV, Connors RH, Tracy TF Jr, et al. Changing spectrum of cholelithiasis and cholecystitis in infants and children. *Am J Surg* 1989;158:585–588.
12. Friesen CA, Roberts CC. Cholelithiasis. Clinical characteristics in children. *Clin Pediatr* 1989;7:294–298.
13. Grosfeld JL, Rescorla FJ, Skinner MA, et al. The spectrum of biliary tract disorders in infants and children: experience with 300 cases. *Arch Surg* 1994;129:513–520.
14. Waldhausen JHT, Benjamin DR. Cholecystectomy is becoming an increasingly common operation in children. *Am J Surg* 1999;177:364–367.
15. Kumar R, Nguyen K, Shun A. Gallstones and common bile duct calculi in infancy and childhood. *Aust N Z J Surg* 2000;70:188–191.

16. Lafont H, Ostrow JD. Calcium salt precipitation in bile and biomineralization of gallstones. In: Afdhal NH, ed. *Gallbladder and biliary tract diseases*. New York: Marcel Dekker, 2000:317–360.
17. Stringer MD, Taylor DR, Soloway RD. Gallstone composition: are children different? *J Pediatr* 2003;142:435–440.
18. O'Brien CB, Berman JM, Fleming CR, et al. Total parenteral nutrition gallstones contain more calcium bilirubinate than sickle cell gallstones. *Gastroenterology* 1986;90:1752(A).
19. Wu SS, Casas AT, Abraham SK, et al. Milk of calcium cholelithiasis in children. *J Pediatr Surg* 2001;36:644–647.
20. Ko CW, Sekijima JH, Lee SP. Biliary sludge. *Ann Intern Med* 1999;130:301–311.
21. Sarnaik S, Slovis TL, Corbett DP, et al. Incidence of cholelithiasis in sickle cell anemia using the ultrasonic gray-scale technique. *J Pediatr* 1980;96:1005–1008.
22. Croom RD III, McMillan CW, Sheldon GF, et al. Hereditary spherocytosis. Recent experience and current concepts of pathophysiology. *Ann Surg* 1986;203:34–39.
23. Chittmittrapap S, Buachum V, Dharmklong-at A. Cholelithiasis in thalassemic children. *Pediatr Surg Int* 1990;5:114–117.
24. Bond LR, Hatty SR, Horn MEC, et al. Gall stones in sickle cell disease in the United Kingdom. *Br Med J* 1987;295:234–236.
25. Whitington PF, Black DD. Cholelithiasis in premature infants treated with parenteral nutrition and furosemide. *J Pediatr* 1980; 97:647–649.
26. Jawaheer G, Pierro A, Lloyd DA, et al. Gallbladder contractility in neonates: effects of parenteral and enteral feeding. *Arch Dis Child* 1995;72:F200–F202.
27. Roslyn JJ, Berquist WE, Pitt HA, et al. Increased risk of gallstones in children receiving total parenteral nutrition. *Pediatrics* 1983;71:784–789.
28. Matos C, Avni EF, Van Gansbeke D, et al. Total parenteral nutrition (TPN) and gallbladder diseases in neonates. Sonographic assessment. *J Ultrasound Med* 1987;6:243–248.
29. Pellerin D, Bertin P, Nihoul-Fekete CI, et al. Cholelithiasis and ileal pathology in childhood. *J Pediatr Surg* 1975;10:35–41.
30. Davies BW, Abel G, Puntis JWL, et al. Limited ileal resection in infancy: the long term consequences. *J Pediatr Surg* 1999;34:583–587.
31. Georgeson K, Brown P. Short bowel syndrome. In: Stringer MD, Oldham KT, Mouriquand PDE, et al., eds. *Pediatric surgery and urology: long term outcomes*. Philadelphia: WB Saunders, 1998:237–242.
32. Reif S, Sloven DG, Lebenthal E. Gallstones in children. Characterization by age, etiology, and outcome. *Am J Dis Child* 1991;145:105–108.
33. Afdhal NH. Epidemiology, risk factors, and pathogenesis of gallstones. In: Afdhal NH, ed. *Gallbladder and biliary tract diseases*. New York: Marcel Dekker, 2000:127–146.
34. Stringer MD, Lim P, Cave M, et al. Fetal gallstones. *J Pediatr Surg* 1996;31:1589–1591.
35. Lehtonen L, Svedstrom E, Kero P, et al. Gallbladder contractility in preterm infants. *Arch Dis Child* 1993;68:43–45.
36. Halpern Z, Vinograd Z, Laufer H, et al. Characteristics of gallbladder bile of infants and children. *J Pediatr Gastroenterol Nutr* 1996;23:147–150.
37. Jonas A, Yahav J, Fradkin A, et al. Choledocholithiasis in infants: diagnostic and therapeutic problems. *J Pediatr Gastroenterol Nutr* 1990;11:513–517.
38. Debray D, Pariente D, Gauthier F, et al. Cholelithiasis in infancy: a study of 40 cases. *J Pediatr* 1993;122:385–391.
39. Good LI, Edell SL, Soloway RD, et al. Ultrasonic properties of gallstones. Effect of stone size and composition. *Gastroenterology* 1979;77:258–263.
40. Keller MS, Markle BM, Laffey PA, et al. Spontaneous resolution of cholelithiasis in infants. *Radiology* 1985;157:345–348.
41. Jacir NN, Anderson KD, Eichelberger M, et al. Cholelithiasis in infancy: resolution of gallstones in three of four infants. *J Pediatr Surg* 1986;21:567–569.
42. Ghose SI, Stringer MD. Successful non-operative management of neonatal acute calculous cholecystitis. *J Pediatr Surg* 1999;34:1029–1030.
43. Bruch SW, Ein SH, Rocchi C, et al. The management of nonpigmented gallstones in children. *J Pediatr Surg* 2000;35:729–732.
44. Rintala RJ, Lindahl H, Pohjavuori M. Total parenteral nutrition-associated cholestasis in surgical neonates may be reversed by intravenous cholecystokinin: a preliminary report. *J Pediatr Surg* 1995;30:827–830.
45. Sokal EM, DeBilderling G, Clapuyt P, et al. Extracorporeal shock-wave lithotripsy for calcified lower choledocholithiasis in an 18-month-old boy. *J Pediatr Gastroenterol Nutr* 1994;18:391–394.
46. De Caluwe D, Akl U, Corbally M. Cholecystectomy versus cholecystolithotomy for cholelithiasis in childhood: long-term outcome. *J Pediatr Surg* 2001;36:1518–1521.
47. Sandler A, Winkel G, Kimura K, et al. The role of prophylactic cholecystectomy during splenectomy in children with hereditary spherocytosis. *J Pediatr Surg* 1999;34:1077–1078.
48. Lachman BS, Lazerson J, Starshak RJ, et al. The prevalence of cholelithiasis in sickle cell disease as diagnosed by ultrasound and cholecystography. *Pediatrics* 1979;64:601–603.
49. Stephens CG, Scott RB. Cholelithiasis in sickle cell anemia: surgical or medical management. *Arch Intern Med* 1980;140:648–651.
50. Ariyan S, Shessel FS, Pickett LK. Cholecystitis and cholelithiasis masking as abdominal crises in sickle cell disease. *Pediatrics* 1976;58:252–258.
51. Tagge EP, Othersen HB, Jackson SM, et al. Impact of laparoscopic cholecystectomy on the management of cholelithiasis in children with sickle cell disease. *J Pediatr Surg* 1994;29:209–213.
52. McDermott EWM, AlKhalifa K, Murphy JJ. Laparoscopic cholecystectomy without exchange transfusion in sickle cell disease. *Lancet* 1993;342:1181.
53. Pappis CH, Galanakis S, Moussatos G. Experience of splenectomy and cholecystectomy in children with chronic hemolytic anemia. *J Pediatr Surg* 1989;24:543–546.
54. Kim PC, Wesson D, Superina R, et al. Laparoscopic cholecystectomy versus open cholecystectomy in children: which is better? *J Pediatr Surg* 1995;30:971–973.
55. Savassi-Rocha PR, Almeida SR, Sanches MD, et al. Iatrogenic bile duct injuries. *Surg endosc* 2003;17:1356–1361.
56. Holcomb GW III, Morgan WM III, Neblett WW III, et al. Laparoscopic cholecystectomy in children: lessons learned from the first 100 patients. *J Pediatr Surg* 1999;34:1236–1240.
57. Holzman MD, Sharp K, Holcomb GW, et al. An alternative technique for laparoscopic cholangiography. *Surg Endosc* 1994;8:927–930.
58. Prasad H, Poddar U, Thapa BR, et al. Endoscopic management of post laparoscopic cholecystectomy bile leak in a child. *Gastrointest Endosc* 2000;51(1):506–507.
59. Bhattacharyya N, Wayne AS, Kevy SV, et al. Perioperative management for cholecystectomy in sickle cell disease. *J Pediatr Surg* 1993;28:72–75.
60. Guelrud M, Mendoza S, Jaen D, et al. ERCP and endoscopic sphincterotomy in infants and children with jaundice due to common bile duct stones. *Gastrointest Endosc* 1992;38:450–453.
61. Gholson CF, Grier JF, Ibach MB, et al. Sequential endoscopic/laparoscopic management of sickle hemoglobinopathy-associated cholelithiasis and suspected choledocholithiasis. *South Med J* 1995;88:1131–1135.
62. Pariente D, Bernard O, Gauthier F, et al. Radiological treatment of common bile duct lithiasis in infancy. *Pediatr Radiol* 1989;19:104–107.
63. Levard G, Weil D, Barret D, et al. Torsion of the gallbladder in children. *J Pediatr Surg* 1994;29:569–570.
64. Ternberg JL, Keating JP. Acute acalculous cholecystitis: complicaton of other illnesses in childhood. *Arch Surg* 1975;110:543–547.
65. Tsakayannis DE, Kozakewich HP, Lillehei CW. Acalculous cholecystitis in children. *J Pediatr Surg* 1996;31:127–130.
66. Ameh EA. Cholecystitis in children in Zaria, Nigeria. *Ann Trop Paediatr* 1999;19:205–209.
67. Byard RW, Thorner PS, Cutz E, et al. Xanthogranulomatous cholecystitis and cholecystoduodenal fistula formation associated with total parenteral nutrition in a six year old child. *Pathology* 1990;22:239–241.
68. Gollin G, Raschbaum GR, Moorthy C, et al. Cholecystectomy for suspected biliary dyskinesia in children with chronic abdominal pain. *J Pediatr Surg* 1999;34:854–857.
69. Stringer MD, Ceylan H, Ward K, et al. Gallbladder polyps in children—classification and management. *J Pediatr Surg* 2003;38: 1680–1684.

70. Miyano T, Yamataka A, Kato Y, et al. Hepaticoenterostomy after excision of choledochal cyst in children: a 30-year experience with 180 cases. *J Pediatr Surg* 1996;31:1417–1421.
71. Stringer MD, Dhawan A, Davenport M, et al. Choledochal cysts: lessons from a 20-year experience. *Arch Dis Child* 1995;73:528–531.
72. Miyano T, Ando K, Yamataka A, et al. Pancreatobiliary maljunction associated with non-dilatation or minimal dilatation of the common bile duct in children: diagnosis and treatment. *Eur J Pediatr Surg* 1996;6:334–337.
73. Guelrud M, Morera C, Rodriguez M, et al. Normal and anomalous pancreaticobiliary union in children and adolescents. *Gastrointest Endosc* 1999;50:189–193.
74. Iwai N, Yanagihara J, Tokiwa K, et al. Congenital choledochal dilatation with emphasis on pathophysiology of the biliary tract. *Ann Surg* 1992;215:27–30.
75. Matos C, Nicaise N, Deviere J, et al. Choledochal cysts: comparison of findings at MR cholangiopancreatography and endoscopic retrograde cholangiopancreatography in eight patients. *Radiology* 1998;209:443–448.
76. Davenport M, Stringer MD, Howard ER. Biliary amylase and congenital choledochal dilatation. *J Pediatr Surg* 1995;30:474–477.
77. Yamauchi S, Koga A, Matsumoto S, et al. Anomalous junction of pancreaticobiliary duct without congenital choledochal cyst: a possible risk factor for gallbladder cancer. *Am J Gastroenterol* 1987;82:20–24.
78. Todani T, Watanabe Y, Fujii T, et al. Anomalous arrangement of the pancreatobiliary ductal system in patients with a choledochal cyst. *Am J Surg* 1984;147:672–676.
79. Lilly JR. Surgery of coexisting biliary malformations in choledochal cyst. *J Pediatr Surg* 1979;14:643–647.
80. Todani T, Watanabe Y, Toki A, et al. Co-existing biliary anomalies and anatomical variants in choledochal cyst. *Br J Surg* 1998;85:760–763.
81. Li L, Yamataka A, Yian-Xia W, et al. Ectopic distal location of the papilla of Vater in congenital biliary dilatation: implications for pathogenesis. *J Pediatr Surg* 2001;36:1617–1622.
82. Tan CEL, Howard ER, Driver M, et al. Non-communicating multiseptate gallbladder and choledochal cyst: a case report and review of publications. *Gut* 1993;34:853–856.
83. Duh Y-C, Lai H-S, Chen W-J. Accessory hepatic duct associated with a choledochal cyst. *Pediatr Surg Int* 1997;12:54–56.
84. Komi N, Tamura T, Tsuge S, et al. Relation of patient age to premalignant alterations in choledochal cyst epithelium: histochemical and immunohistochemical studies. *J Pediatr Surg* 1986;21:430–433.
85. Babbitt DP. Congenital choledochal cysts: new etiological concept based on anomalous relationships of common bile duct and pancreatic bulb. *Ann Radiol* 1969;12:231–240.
86. Spitz L. Experimental production of cystic dilatation of the common bile duct in neonatal lambs. *J Pediatr Surg* 1977;12:39–42.
87. Ito T, Ando H, Nagaya M, et al. Congenital dilatation of the common bile duct in children. The etiologic significance of the narrow segment distal to the dilated common bile duct. *Zeitschrift für Kinderchirurgie* 1984;39:40–45.
88. Lane GJ, Yamataka A, Kobayashi H, et al. Different types of congenital biliary dilatation in dizygotic twins. *Pediatr Surg Int* 1999;15:403–404.
89. Matsubara H, Oya N, Suzuki Y, et al. Is it possible to differentiate between choledochal cyst and congenital biliary atresia (type I cyst) by antenatal ultrasonography? *Fetal Diagn Ther* 1997;12:306–308.
90. Kim WS, Kim IO, Yeon KM, et al. Choledochal cyst with or without biliary atresia in neonates and young infants: US differentiation. *Radiology* 1998;209:465–469.
91. Lugo-Vincente HL. Prenatally diagnosed choledochal cysts: observation or early surgery? *J Pediatr Surg* 1995;30:1288–1290.
92. Suita S, Shono K, Kinugasa Y, et al. Influence of age on the presentation and outcome of choledochal cyst. *J Pediatr Surg* 1999;34:1765–1768.
93. Stringel G, Filler RM. Fictitious pancreatitis in choledochal cyst. *J Pediatr Surg* 1982;17:359–361.
94. Hernanz-Schulman M, Ambrosino MM, Freeman PC, et al. Common bile duct in children: sonographic dimensions. *Radiology* 1995;195:193–195.
95. Samuel M, Spitz L. Choledochal cyst: varied clinical presentations and long-term results of surgery. *Eur J Pediatr Surg* 1996;6:78–81.
96. Sugimoto T, Yamagiwa I, Obata K, et al. Choledochal cyst and duodenal atresia: a rare combination. *Pediatr Surg Int* 2002;18:281–283.
97. Ando K, Miyano T, Kohno S, et al. Spontaneous perforation of choledochal cyst: a study of 13 cases. *Eur J Pediatr Surg* 1998;8:23–25.
98. Karnak I, Tanyel FC, Buyukpamukcu N, et al. Spontaneous rupture of choledochal cyst: an unusual cause of acute abdomen in children. *J Pediatr Surg* 1997;32:736–738.
99. Yamaguchi M. Congenital choledochal cyst. Analysis of 1433 patients in the Japanese literature. *Am J Surg* 1980;140:653–657.
100. Voyles CR, Smadja C, Shands WC, et al. Carcinoma in choledochal cysts: age-related incidence. *Arch Surg* 1983;118:986–988.
101. Bismuth H, Krissat J. Choledochal cystic malignancies. *Ann Oncol* 1999;10(suppl 4):S94–S98.
102. Iwai N, Deguchi E, Yanagihara J, et al. Cancer arising in a choledochal cyst in a 12-year-old girl. *J Pediatr Surg* 1990;12:1261–1263.
103. Kaneko K, Ando H, Watanabe Y, et al. Pathologic changes in the common bile duct of an experimental model with pancreaticobiliary maljunction without biliary dilatation. *Pediatr Surg Int* 2000;16:26–28.
104. Todani T, Watanabe Y, Toki A, et al. Carcinoma related to choledochal cysts with internal drainage operations. *Surg Gynecol Obstet* 1987;164:61–64.
105. Kobayashi S, Asano T, Yamasaki M, et al. Risk of bile duct carcinogenesis after excision of extrahepatic bile ducts in pancreaticobiliary maljunction. *Surgery* 1999;126:939–944.
106. Kim SH, Lim JH, Yoon HK, et al. Choledochal cyst: comparison of MR and conventional cholangiography. *Clin Radiol* 2000;55:378–383.
107. Lam WWM, Lam TPW, Saing H, et al. MR cholangiography and CT cholangiography of pediatric patients with choledochal cysts. *Am J Roentgenol* 1999;173:401–405.
108. Kaneko K, Ando H, Watanabe Y, et al. Secondary excision of choledochal cysts after previous cystenterostomies. *Hepatogastroenterology* 1999;46:2772–2775.
109. Yamataka A, Segawa O, Kobayashi H, et al. Intraoperative pancreatoscopy for pancreatic duct stone debris distal to the common channel in choledochal cyst. *J Pediatr Surg* 2000;35:1–4.
110. Delarue A, Chappuis JS, Esposito C, et al. Is the appendix graft suitable for routine biliary surgery in children? *J Pediatr Surg* 2000;35:1312–1316.
111. Tanaka M, Shimizu S, Mizumoto K, et al. Laparoscopically assisted resection of choledochal cyst and Roux-en-Y reconstruction. *Surg Endosc* 2001;15:545–551.
112. Lilly JR. Total excision of choledochal cyst. *Surg Gynecol Obstet* 1978;146:254–256.
113. Iuchtman M, Martins MS, Scheidemantel RE. Congenital diverticulum of the choledochus: report of a case. *Int Surg* 1971;55:280–282.
114. Dohmoto M, Kamiya T, Hunerbein M, et al. Endoscopic treatment of a choledochocele in a 2-year-old child. *Surg Endosc* 1996;10:1016–1018.
115. Miyano T, Yamataka A, Kato Y, et al. Hepaticoenterostomy after excision of choledochal cyst in children: a 30-year experience with 180 cases. *J Pediatr Surg* 1996;31:1417–1421.
116. Yamataka A, Ohshiro K, Okada Y, et al. Complications after cyst excision with hepaticoenterostomy for choledochal cysts and their surgical management in children versus adults. *J Pediatr Surg* 1997;32:1097–1102.
117. Pinto RB, Lima JP, da Silveira TR, et al. Caroli's disease: report of 10 cases in children and adolescents in southern Brazil. *J Pediatr Surg* 1998;33:1531–1535.
118. Caroli J. Diseases of intrahepatic bile ducts. *Isr J Med Sci* 1968;4:21–35.
119. Bowles MJ, Salisbury JR, Howard ER. Localized, benign, non-traumatic strictures of the extrahepatic biliary tree in children. *Surgery* 2001;130:55–59.
120. Cherqui D, Palazzo L, Piedbois P, et al. Common bile duct stricture as a late complication of upper abdominal radiotherapy. *J Hepatol* 1994;20:693–697.
121. El-Shabrawi M, Wilkinson ML, Portmann B, et al. Primary sclerosing cholangitis in childhood. *Gastroenterology* 1987;92:1226–1235.
122. Saing H, Tam PKH, Choi TK, et al. Childhood recurrent pyogenic cholangitis. *J Pediatr Surg* 1988;23:424–429.

123. Davenport M, Saxena R, Howard ER. Acquired biliary atresia. *J Pediatr Surg* 1996;31:1721–1723.
124. Martinez-Urrutia MJ, Vasquez Estevez J, Larrauri J, et al. Gastric heterotopy of the biliary tract. *J Pediatr Surg* 1990;25:356–357.
125. Jaing TH, Yang CP, Chang KW, et al. Extrahepatic obstruction of the biliary tract as the presenting feature of acute myeloid leukemia. *J Pediatr Gastroenterol Nutr* 2001;33:620–622.
126. Pietsch JB, Shankar S, Ford C, et al. Obstructive jaundice secondary to lymphoma in childhood. *J Pediatr Surg* 2001;36:1792–1795.
127. Ravindra KV, Stringer MD, Prasad KR, et al. Non-Hodgkin lymphoma presenting with obstructive jaundice. *Br J Surg* 2003;90:845–849.
128. Gow KW, Blair GK, Phillips R, et al. Obstructive jaundice caused by neuroblastoma managed with temporary cholecystostomy tube. *J Pediatr Surg* 1995;30:878–882.
129. Sylvester FA, Shuckett B, Cutz E, et al. Management of fibrosing pancreatitis in children presenting with obstructive jaundice. *Gut* 1998;43:715–720.
130. Bilton D, Fox R, Webb AK, et al. Pathology of common bile duct stenosis in cystic fibrosis. *Gut* 1990;31:236–238.
131. Heaton ND, Davenport M, Howard ER. Intraluminal biliary obstruction. *Arch Dis Child* 1991;66:1395–1398.
132. Davies MRQ, Rode H. Biliary ascariasis in children. *Progr Pediatr Surg* 1982;15:55–74.
133. Wani NA, Chrungoo RK. Biliary ascariasis—surgical aspects. *World J Surg* 1992;16:976–979.
134. Ibanez DV, Vila JJ, Fernandez MS, et al. Spontaneous biliary perforation and necrotizing enterocolitis. *Pediatr Surg Int* 1999;15:401–402.
135. Lilly JR, Weintraub WH, Altman RP. Spontaneous perforation of the extrahepatic bile ducts and bile peritonitis in infancy. *Surgery* 1974;75:664–673.
136. Howard ER. Spontaneous biliary perforation. In: Howard ER, Stringer MD, Colombani PM, eds. *Surgery of the liver, bile ducts and pancreas in children,* 2nd ed. London: Arnold Publishers, 2002:169–174.
137. Howard ER. Tumors of the extrahepatic bile ducts. In: Howard ER, Stringer MD, Colombani PM, eds. *Surgery of the liver, bile ducts and pancreas in children,* 2nd ed. London: Arnold Publishers, 2002:209–216.
138. Ruymann FB, Raney RB, Crist WM, et al. Rhabdomyosarcoma of the biliary tree in childhood. A report from the Intergroup Rhabdomyosarcoma Study. *Cancer* 1985;56:575–581.
139. Spunt SL, Lobe TE, Pappo AS, et al. Aggressive surgery is unwarranted for biliary tract rhabdomyosarcoma. *J Pediatr Surg* 2000;35:309–316.
140. Jacquemin E. Progressive familial intrahepatic cholestasis. Genetic basis and treatment. *Clin Liver Dis* 2000;4:753–763.
141. Emond JC, Whitington PF. Selective surgical management of progressive familial intrahepatic cholestasis (Byler's disease). *J Pediatr Surg* 1995;30:1635–1641.
142. Ismail H, Kalicinski P, Markiewicz M, et al. Treatment of progressive familial intrahepatic cholestasis: liver transplantation or partial external biliary diversion. *Pediatr Transplant* 1999;3:21–24.
143. Melter M, Rodeck B, Kardorff R, et al. Progressive familial intrahepatic cholestasis: partial biliary diversion normalizes serum lipids and improves growth in non-cirrhotic patients. *Am J Gastroenterol* 2000;95:3522–3528.
144. Emerick KM, Whitington PF. Partial external biliary diversion for intractable pruritus and xanthomas in Alagille syndrome. *Hepatology* 2002;35:1501–1506.

PART G

Spleen

Chapter 94

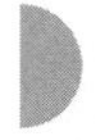

Pediatric Spleen Surgery

Henry E. Rice

ANATOMY

The spleen arises as a condensation within the dorsal mesogastrium at 5 to 6 weeks' gestation. With continued growth, the spleen is carried into the left upper quadrant of the abdomen. The convex smooth surface of the spleen faces superiorly, posteriorly, and to the left in relation to the abdominal surface of the diaphragm. The costodiaphragmatic recess of the pleura extends down as far as the inferior border of the normal-size spleen.

At birth, the spleen normally weighs between 10 and 12 g, and its growth parallels body weight. The normal spleen size and weight vary somewhat between children, and closely correlate with the size of the child (1). One rule of thumb is for assessing normal splenic size is that the spleen and left kidney are the same length as measured by ultrasonography. Using two standard deviations above the mean as a guide, the upper limit of normal for the spleen/kidney ratio is 1.25 (1).

The visceral relationships of the spleen are with the greater curvature of the stomach, the tail of the pancreas, the left kidney, and the splenic flexure of the colon. The parietal peritoneum is firmly adhered to the splenic capsule, except at the splenic hilum. The peritoneum extends superiorly, laterally, and inferiorly to form the suspensory ligaments of the spleen. The splenorenal ligament extends from the anterior left kidney to the hilum of the spleen and contains the splenic vessels. These layers continue superiorly to the greater curvature of the stomach to form the two leaves of the gastrosplenic ligament through which the short gastric arteries and veins course.

The splenic artery arises from the celiac trunk and courses along the superior border of the pancreas. The branches of the splenic artery include the pancreatic branches, short gastric arteries, left gastroepiploic artery, and terminal splenic branches. The splenic artery divides into several branches within the splenorenal ligament before entering the splenic hilum, where they branch again into these trabeculae as they enter the splenic pulp (Fig. 94-1). Two variations of the splenic vasculature exist, as described by Michels in 1942(2). In the *distributed* pattern, multiple branches arise from the main trunks approximately 2 to 3 cm from the hilum. In the *magistral* pattern, the pedicle formed by the artery and vein enters the hilum as a compact bundle.

As small arteriolar branches branch into the spleen, their adventitial coat becomes replaced by a sheath of lymphatic tissue. It is these lymphatic sheaths that comprise the white pulp of the spleen and that are interspersed along the arteriolar vessels as lymphatic follicles. The interface between the white pulp and the red pulp is known as the *marginal zone*. As the arterioles lose their sheaths of lymphatic tissue, they traverse the marginal zone and enter the red pulp, which is composed of large branching, thin-walled blood vessels called *splenic sinuses and sinusoids*.

The venous sinusoids empty into the veins of the red pulp, and these veins drain back along the trabecular veins that empty into major tributaries, ultimately joining to form the splenic vein. The splenic vein runs inferior to the artery and posterior to the pancreatic tail and body. The splenic vein joins the superior mesenteric vein behind the neck of the pancreas to form the portal vein. The inferior mesenteric vein often empties into the splenic vein; it may also empty into the superior mesenteric vein at or near the confluence of the splenic vein and superior mesenteric vein.

VARIANTS OF NORMAL ANATOMY

Congenital asplenia (Ivemark syndrome) arises from a failure of normal organogenesis and is a consequence of

Henry E. Rice: Division of Pediatric Surgery, Duke University Medical Center, Durham, North Carolina 27710.

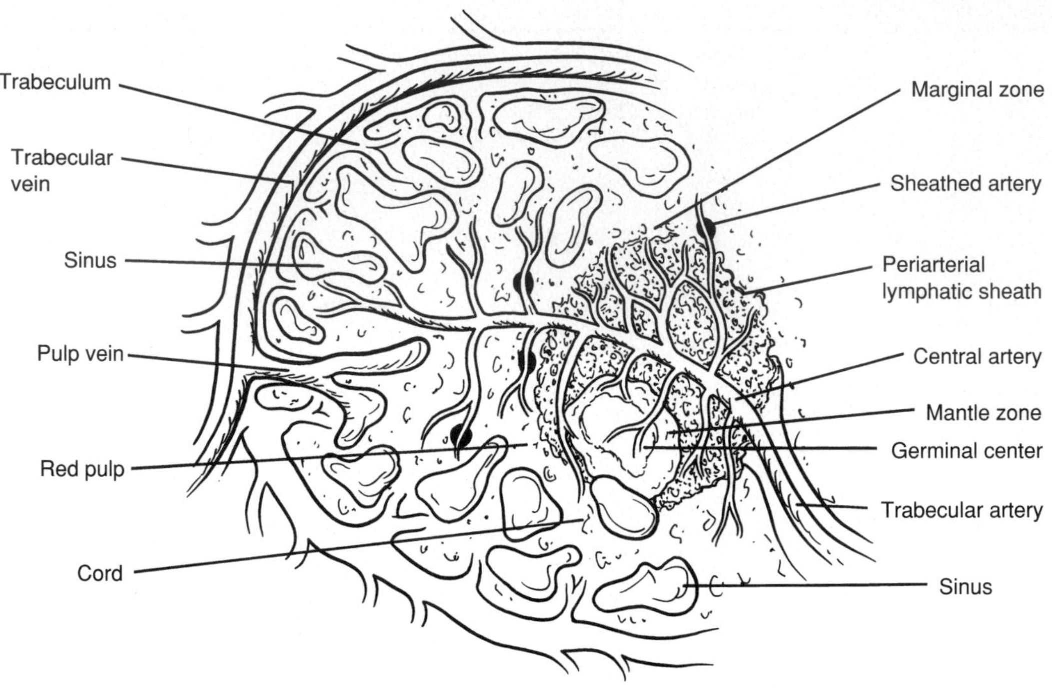

FIGURE 94-1. Microscopic anatomy of the spleen.

bilateral right-sidedness. It can be associated with bilateral trilobed lungs and a centrally located isomeric liver. It is often associated with heterotaxy syndromes, and the stomach is often located in the right side of the abdomen. Asplenia has a high rate of association with complex congenital heart disease, with the most common combinations including total anomalous pulmonary venous return, common atrium, atrioventricular canal, double outlet right ventricle, and pulmonary stenosis or atresia (3). Functional asplenia can be diagnosed by the presence of Howell-Jolly bodies on a peripheral blood smear.

Congenital polysplenia occurs with multiple spleens located along the greater curvature of the stomach. Similar to asplenia, it is often associated with *situs inversus* and cardiac defects. Importantly, polysplenia can be associated with other surgical conditions, such as biliary atresia and preduodenal portal vein. Despite the numerous splenic remnants, splenic immune function is generally normal.

A wandering spleen (splenic ectopia) refers to the spleen being mobile and present anywhere in the abdomen other than the left upper quadrant. Although its etiology is not well defined, it is probably the result of failure of the fusion of the dorsal mesogastrium to form the suspensory ligaments of the spleen. It generally presents with the sudden onset of abdominal pain related to torsion, although chronic or intermittent pain can also occur. Therapy is individualized based on the presence or absence of perfusion to the spleen at the time of presentation and exploration—if the spleen has torsed and is nonviable, splenectomy is indicated. If functional splenic tissue remains, splenopexy in the normal anatomic position is required.

SPLENIC FUNCTION

The spleen has important hematopoietic functions during early fetal development, and along with the liver, is a major site of red and white blood cell production. By the fifth month of gestation, the bone marrow assumes the predominant role in hematopoiesis, and normally there is no significant hematopoietic function left in the spleen. The spleen continues to function throughout gestation and after birth for blood filtration, removal of intracellular material, and immunologic defense.

The filtration functions of the spleen are closely linked to its unique vascular anatomy. The arteries flow through the white pulp (lymphoid tissues), after which most of the blood flow enters the macrophage-lined reticular meshwork and the blood flows back to the venous circulation through the venous sinuses. Blood elements must pass through slits in the lining of the venous sinuses; if they cannot pass, they are trapped in the spleen and ingested by splenic phagocytes. Experimental animal studies have demonstrated that an intact splenic arterial system is necessary for optimal control of infection (4).

The mechanical filtration of the spleen is essential for the processing of immature and senescent erythrocytes.

Normal red blood cells (RBCs) are biconcave and deform relatively easily to facilitate passage through the microvasculature. As immature RBCs pass through the spleen, they undergo several types of repair, including removal of nuclei and excessive cell membranes, converting them from a spherical nucleated to a biconcave mature morphology. In cases of anatomic or functional asplenia, there are characteristic alterations in the morphologic appearance of the peripheral RBCs. These include the presence of target cells (immature cells), Howell-Jolly bodies (nuclear remnant), Heinz bodies (denatured hemoglobin), Pappenheimer bodies (iron granules), stippling, and spur cells. Aged RBCs that have lost membrane plasticity are trapped and destroyed in the spleen.

In children with various congenital hemolytic anemias, abnormal erythrocytes are trapped by the splenic filtering mechanism, resulting in worsening anemia, symptomatic splenomegaly, and splenic infarction. In autoimmune hemolytic anemias, IgG bound to the cell membrane targets the RBCs for splenic destruction by splenic macrophages. A similar IgG-dependent mechanism is involved in platelet destruction in immune thrombocytopenic purpura (ITP). The mechanical filtration of the spleen is important for the clearance of circulating pathogens that reside within erythrocytes, such as malarial parasites or bacteria such as *Bartonella* species. Mechanical filtration by the spleen is also essential for the removal of unopsonized, noningested bacteria from the circulation, and may be particularly important for clearing microorganisms for which the host has no specific antibody.

Finally, the spleen is a major site of production for the opsonins properdin and tuftsin, and removal of the spleen results in decreased serum levels of these factors. Properdin can initiate the alternative pathway of complement activation to produce destruction of bacteria, as well as foreign and abnormal cells. Tuftsin is a tetrapeptide that enhances the phagocytic activity of both polymorphonuclear leukocytes and mononuclear phagocytes. The spleen is the major site of cleavage of tuftsin from the heavy chain of IgG, and circulating levels of tuftsin are suppressed in asplenic subjects (5). Moreover, neutrophil function is decreased in asplenic patients, and the defect appears to result from the absence of a circulating mediator (6).

These immune functions of the spleen contribute to the maintenance of normal host defenses against certain types of infectious agents. It is well established that people lacking a spleen are at a significantly higher risk for overwhelming postsplenectomy infection (OPSI) with fulminant bacteremia, pneumonia, or meningitis, as compared with those with normal splenic function (7). Major pathogens in OPSI include organisms such as *Streptococcus pneumoniae,* in which polysaccharide capsules requiring both antibody and complement are important in host defense against these organisms. Asplenic subjects have defective activation of complement by the alternative pathway, leaving them more susceptible to infection.

OVERWHELMING POSTSPLENECTOMY SEPSIS

OPSI is among the more devastating sequelae associated with functional or anatomic asplenia, and is the most common fatal late complication of splenectomy (7–11). The association between removal of the spleen and sepsis has been recognized since 1919, although attention was refocused on this condition by King and Shumaker in 1952 (9). They reported sepsis in five infants who had undergone splenectomy, and subsequent reports have confirmed the association of overwhelming sepsis with functional or anatomic asplenia.

The exact incidence of OPSI has been difficult to determine, and the incidence of infection in postsplenectomy patients is likely underreported. However, the risk of fatal OPSI appears to be greater in young children (younger than 4 years of age), and may be as high as up to 1 per 300 to 350 patient-years follow-up (7–11). Although the risk of overwhelming postsplenectomy sepsis is reduced by use of immunizations to *S. pneumoniae*, *Meningococcus*, and *Haemophilus influenzae,* as well as postoperative antibiotic prophylaxis, its risk is never eliminated (10). Moreover, concerns persist of incomplete protection by pneumococcal vaccinations, antibiotic resistance, and poor compliance with antibiotic prophylaxis (10,11).

OPSI typically begins with a prodromal phase characterized by fever and chills and nonspecific symptoms, including sore throat, malaise, myalgias, diarrhea, and vomiting. Patients may have had symptoms for 1 to 2 days before seeking appropriate medical treatment. Pneumonia and meningitis may be present, but many cases have no identifiable focal site of infection and present with high-grade primary bacteremia. Progression of the illness can be quite rapid, with the development of hypotension, disseminated intravascular coagulation, respiratory distress, coma, and death within hours of presentation. The mortality rate is between 50% and 70% for fully developed OPSI, and this high mortality persists despite current use of broad-spectrum antibiotics and intensive care. Survivors of severe OPSI often have a long and complicated recovery, with severe sequelae such as extremity gangrene, deafness from meningitis, mastoid osteomyelitis, bacterial endocarditis, and cardiac valvular destruction.

The spleen is important for generating responses to thymus-independent antigens. Prior to a planned elective splenectomy, immunizations against *Pneumococcus*, *Meningococcus*, and *H. influenzae* should be administered whenever possible (Fig. 94-2). The American Academy of

The heptavalent pneumococcal conjugate vaccine (PCV7), Prevnar (Lederle Laboratories, Pearl River, NY; Wyeth-Ayerst Pharmaceuticals, Marietta, PA), is recommended for children 24 to 59 months old who are at high risk for invasive pneumococcal infection, including children with asplenia. The following schedules are recommended by the American Academy of Pediatrics for these children who are 24 to 59 months of age and who may have received previous doses of 23-valent pneumococcal polysaccharide (23PS) vaccine or PCV7 (12,51):

1. *For high-risk children who have received four doses of PCV7, a dose of 23PS vaccine is recommended at 24 months of age, to be given at least 6 to 8 weeks after the last dose of PCV7.*
2. *For high-risk children who have received one to three doses of PCV7 before 24 months of age, a single additional dose of PCV7 should be given at least 6 to 8 weeks after the last dose of PCV7. This should then be followed by a dose of 23PS vaccine at least 6 to 8 weeks later. An additional dose of 23PS vaccine should be given no earlier than 3 to 5 years after the initial dose of 23PS vaccine.*
3. *For high-risk children 24 to 59 months old who have received only a single previous dose of 23PS vaccine, there are minimal data regarding the safety of subsequent doses of pneumococcal conjugate vaccines. However, two doses of PCV7 are recommended, to be given at an interval of 6 to 8 weeks. Administration of the PCV7 immunization series should begin no earlier than 6 to 8 weeks after the last dose of 23PS vaccine. An additional dose of 23PS vaccine is recommended 3 to 5 years after the first dose of 23PS vaccine.*
4. *For high-risk children 24 to 59 months old who have received no previous doses of either 23PS vaccine or PCV7, two doses of PCV7 are recommended, to be given at an interval of 6 to 8 weeks, followed by a single dose of 23PS vaccine no less than 6 to 8 weeks after the last dose of PCV7. An additional dose of 23PS vaccine is recommended 3 to 5 years after the last dose.*

Immunization against *Haemophilus influenzae* type b infections should be initiated at 2 months of age, as recommended for otherwise healthy young children and for all previously unimmunized children with asplenia.

Quadrivalent meningococcal polysaccharide vaccine should also be administered to asplenic children 2 years of age and older. No known contraindication exists to giving these vaccines at the same time in separate syringes at different sites.

FIGURE 94-2. Recommendations of the American Academy of Pediatrics for the immunization of children undergoing splenectomy (12,51).

Pediatrics has recommended that the immunization precede splenectomy by at least 2 weeks (12). In cases of trauma requiring splenectomy in which presplenectomy immunizations are not possible, immunizations should be administered to patients prior to discharge from the hospitalization in which their splenectomy occurred, rather than waiting until a follow-up visit. Many of these patients become lost to follow-up, and clinical studies have demonstrated adequate antibody response to immediate immunization (13). Simultaneous immunization with *H. influenzae* type b, *Meningococcus*, and polyvalent pneumococcal vaccine is both immunogenic and well tolerated.

ANTIBIOTIC PROPHYLAXIS

Postoperative antibiotic prophylaxis is generally recommended for all young children after splenectomy, and some authorities have advocated this form of prophylaxis in older children and adults, although data showing the efficacy of this treatment are lacking (14). Several clinical trials have supported the use of antibiotic prophylaxis in specific populations of young children who are increased risk for pneumococcal infection, such as those with sickle cell disease. For example, antibiotic prophylaxis efficacy against invasive *pneumococcal* infections has been demonstrated in children with sickle cell disease in a prospective multicenter, randomized, double-blind trial of penicillin administration (125 mg of penicillin VK, administered orally twice daily to 3 years of age, and 250 mg twice daily thereafter) (15). A 84% decrease was observed in the incidence of pneumococcal infection in the antibiotic prophylaxis group.

Problems with the use of orally administered penicillin in children have included reports of breakthrough invasive infections and low compliance (16). In addition, several investigators have demonstrated an increase in penicillin-resistant strains of pneumococci in children with sickle cell disease (17). The specific effect of antibiotic prophylaxis on reduction of infection risk, compliance with prophylaxis, and effects on nasopharyngeal colonization with *pneumococci* have not been studied specifically in children after surgical splenectomy (14).

The exact length of time to continue antibiotic prophylaxis for children after splenectomy is unclear. A multicenter study of children with sickle cell disease examined the safety of discontinuing penicillin prophylaxis after 5 years of age (18). Children who had received at least 2 years of penicillin prophylaxis before their fifth birthday and one dose of *pneumococcal* polysaccharide vaccine were randomized to receive continued prophylaxis or placebo. There was no difference in the rate of invasive pneumococcal infection among the children receiving penicillin prophylaxis and those receiving placebo—4 cases (2%) and 2 cases (1%), respectively. The small numbers of enrolled children and the low incidence of pneumococcal disease limit the interpretation of these data. In general, most young children continue antibiotic prophylaxis for several years after splenectomy, although the ideal duration for continued prophylaxis is unclear.

Available data do not support the practice of long-term penicillin prophylaxis in asplenic adults. Another approach that appears rational is to provide the asplenic patient with a supply of oral antibiotics, with instructions to begin taking the medication at the onset of rigor or a febrile illness if appropriate medical evaluation is not immediately available. Fever and rigor in an asplenic patient should prompt immediate aggressive empirical treatment with antibiotic coverage, even in the absence of culture data.

DISORDERS OF THE SPLEEN

Hereditary Spherocytosis and Other Erythrocyte Membrane Disorders

Hereditary spherocytosis (HS) is caused by a defect in the RBC membrane that affects the spectrin component (19). The characteristic finding is increased numbers of spherocytes in the peripheral blood. HS is the most common cause of hemolytic anemia in people of Northern European heritage, with a prevalence of 1 in 5,000. The defect in the RBC membrane is not uniform and may affect one or more membrane components. In the classic autosomal dominant form, the defect may be in beta spectrin, ankyrin, or protein 3. In the recessive form, the defect is in either the alpha spectrin or protein 4.2.

The cardinal features of HS are anemia, jaundice, and splenomegaly. Some patients may be asymptomatic and are detected only on family screening. Anemia is the most common presentation (50% of cases); each of the other clinical features may be present at diagnosis in 10% to 15% of cases. During the course of the illness, about 50% of patients develop jaundice, and 50% develop a palpable spleen in the first year of life. Anemia is much more likely to be severe in early childhood than later in life. The reticulocyte count is elevated generally, and the peripheral smear may show spherocytes in up to 80% of cases and occasionally nucleated RBCs. The definitive diagnostic test is the incubated osmotic fragility test, which shows a pattern of increased fragility in HS.

Splenectomy decreases the rate of hemolysis and usually leads to resolution of the anemia (20). Classic indications for splenectomy in HS are severe anemic crises and repeated transfusion requirements. It is generally recommended that the operation be delayed until after the fourth or fifth year of life to preserve immunologic function of the spleen in young children who are most at risk for OPSI (20).

Other anemias associated with erythrocyte structural abnormalities include hereditary elliptocytosis, hereditary pyropoikilocytosis, hereditary xerocytosis, and hereditary hydrocytosis. These conditions result in abnormalities of the erythrocyte cellular membrane and increased RBC destruction. Splenectomy is indicated for severe anemia that commonly occurs in these conditions.

Erythrocyte Enzyme Deficiencies

Pyruvate kinase (PK) deficiency and glucose-6-phosphate dehydrogenase (G6PD) deficiency are the two RBC enzyme defects associated with hemolytic anemia (19). These deficiencies result in abnormal glucose metabolism, leading to increased hemolysis. PK deficiency is an autosomal recessive condition in which there is decreased RBC deformability resulting in increased hemolysis (21). These patients often have splenomegaly, and splenectomy has been shown to decrease their transfusion requirements. G6PD deficiency is an X-linked hereditary condition that is most frequently seen in people of African, Middle Eastern, or Mediterranean ancestry. Hemolytic anemia occurs in most patients after exposure to certain drugs or chemicals. Splenectomy is rarely indicated in patients with G6PD deficiency.

Thalassemia Syndromes

Thalassemia syndromes are caused by a defect in hemoglobin synthesis that leads to abnormal erythrocytes and splenic sequestration and destruction. The most common thalassemia syndromes are characterized by diminished or absent production of normal alpha-globin polypeptides (alpha-thalassemias) or beta-globin chains (beta-thalassemias) (22). The decreased globin synthesis causes a microcytic anemia, the severity of which depends on the remaining number of functional alpha and beta genes; however, because nonthalassemic globin chains are produced at a normal rate, the resulting imbalance of globin chain production also can contribute to the pathophysiology. Progressive splenic sequestration in the thalassemia syndromes leads to splenomegaly, increasing transfusion requirements, and splenic infarcts. Splenectomy may be helpful in managing severe hemolytic anemias.

Sickle Cell Anemias Syndromes

The term *sickle cell disease* encompasses a variety of disorders with varied clinical manifestations (23). Homozygous sickle cell disease (Hgb SS) accounts for 60% to 70% of sickle cell disease in the United States. Other sickle cell disorders are caused by coinheritance of a sickle gene with a gene for beta-thalassemia or for hemoglobin C, $D_{\text{Los Angeles}}$, E, Lepore, O_{Arab}, C_{Harlem}, or Quebec-Chori. These disorders are characterized by chronic hemolysis and vasoocclusion of varying severity. Although Hgb SS disease tends to have more severe clinical manifestations than Hgb SC disease and other less common variants, a great deal of individual heterogeneity exists in severity for each disorder. For example, some children with Hgb SC have frequent episodes of pain and/or recurrent episodes of acute chest syndrome, whereas others are essentially asymptomatic. In contrast, sickle cell trait is a benign carrier state, important principally for its genetic counseling implications.

The spleen is susceptible to damage by sickle erythrocytes because its slow microcirculation provides an environment conductive to the polymerization of sickle hemoglobin. Splenic injury in children with Hgb SS disease begins as early as 3 to 6 months of life, with intense congestion of the red pulp by sickled erythrocytes (23). Such congestion lead to functional asplenia, which predisposes to infection with *S. pneumoniae, H. influenzae* type b, *Salmonella* sp, *Klebsiella* sp, and other bacteria. At early stages, the spleen is often enlarged and palpable, and patients are increased risk for acute splenic sequestration. With the passage of years, the spleen becomes smaller and the splenic pulp is completely replaced by fibrous tissue, a process often termed *autosplenectomy*. The importance of the early development of splenic dysfunction in patients with sickle cell disease is underscored by the observation that bacterial infection is the leading cause of death in children with sickling disorders. In addition, some episodes of splenic sequestration are life threatening when rapid splenic enlargement causes a precipitous fall in the hemoglobin level.

As with other congenital hemolytic anemias, the development of splenic dysfunction varies among different forms of sickle cell disease. The problem is most severe in children with Hgb SS, in whom early functional asplenia can be documented by demonstrating the absence of reticuloendothelial function with a radionuclide spleen scan. Similarly, the percentage of pocked or pitted red cells correlates well with splenic function as assessed by liver–spleen scan (24). The Cooperative Study for Sickle Cell Disease has demonstrated that the proportion of children with Hgb SS who are functionally asplenic is 14% at 6 months of age, 28% at 1 year, 58% at 2 years, 78% at 3 years, and 94% at 5 years (25). Thus, most patients with Hgb SS are at risk for fulminant septicemia and death during the first 3 years of life, and splenectomy carries greater risk during the period before the onset of functional asplenia.

Indications for Splenectomy in Congenital Hemolytic Anemias

In all congenital hemolytic anemias, children can develop symptoms related to both acute life-threatening splenic sequestration and hypersplenism. In these conditions, there may be rapid splenic enlargement, resulting in severe pain, anemic crises, and need for both acute as well as chronic requirement for blood transfusions. In addition to acute splenic sequestration, these patients may suffer from massive splenomegaly causing discomfort and interfering with daily activities. Classic indications for splenectomy in these children patients include acute splenic sequestration crisis, hypersplenism, and splenic abscess. Children with some congenital hemolytic anemias may have less acute symptoms such as failure to thrive and poor growth; these conditions may be improved after splenectomy as the result of decreased whole-body total protein turnover and decreased resting metabolic rate. Splenic abscesses may also occur in children with congenital hemolytic anemias, and are characterized by fever, abdominal pain, and a tender, enlarged spleen.

Immune Thrombocytopenic Purpura

Immune thrombocytopenic purpura (ITP) is one of the most common bleeding disorders during childhood. In most cases, it is acute and self-limited, and the outcome, defined as normalization of the platelet count and absence of serious clinical bleeding, is very favorable. Approximately 80% of the patients will recover a normal platelet count (greater than 150,000 to l) by 6 months after diagnosis following drug treatment or observation alone. Patients with persistent thrombocytopenia beyond the arbitrary endpoint of 6 months are defined as having chronic ITP (26).

Children with ITP have polyclonal and monoclonal antibodies directed a variety of platelet membrane receptors. The main antigenic targets are epitopes in the receptor for fibrinogen, glycoprotein IIb-IIIa (GP IIb-IIIa), also called α_{2b} β_3, and the receptor for von Willebrand factor, the glycoprotein Ib-IX-V complex (GP Ib-IX-V) (26). When platelets coated with antibodies enter the spleen, they are sequestered from the circulation by mononuclear phagocytes via the Fc receptor. This has been confirmed by the fact that patients with refractory ITP may respond to an investigational preparation of anti-FcγR antibodies with a rise in the platelet count (27).

Splenectomy is not required generally for the treatment of acute ITP. Management varies in children with chronic ITP according to the severity of the thrombocytopenia. Patients who are asymptomatic and maintain platelet counts higher than 50,000 per mm^3 may simply be followed with no specific treatment. Children with platelet counts between 30,000 and 50,000 per mm^3 may also be observed without treatment; however, careful follow-up is essential in these patients because they are at risk for more severe thrombocytopenia. Medical treatment for chronic ITP is generally based on the use of glucocorticoids, gamma globulin, and anti-D immunoglobulin (26).

The removal of the spleen in children with chronic ITP produces a normal platelet count in 75% of cases (28). Although splenectomy is a common procedure in adults with chronic ITP who do not respond to therapy, its application in young children is far less frequent due to concerns of postsplenectomy sepsis. Because the rate of spontaneous remission in children with ITP is high, the benefit of splenectomy should be carefully weighed against the risks. There is a general consensus that children with persistent disease 12 months after diagnosis who have clinical bleeding or with considerable quality-of-life impairment are candidates for splenectomy (26,29).

MALIGNANCIES

Hodgkin's Disease

Hodgkin's disease typically affects young adults in their late teens to early 30s. Historically, staging laparotomy for Hodgkin's disease with splenectomy provided diagnostic information that was necessary to select appropriate therapy. The purpose of staging laparotomy is to stage pathologically the extent of disease below the diaphragm. However, advances in imaging techniques, with widespread availability of dynamic helical computed tomography (CT) scan and fluorodeoxyglucose positron emission tomography imaging, have improved nonoperative staging of Hodgkin's disease. This improved nonoperative staging, along with the use of less toxic systemic chemotherapeutics for earlier stages of Hodgkin's disease, has led to the virtual elimination of need for staging laparotomy. Currently, staging laparotomy and splenectomy are indicated only for highly selected patients with an early clinical stage of disease (stage IA or IIA) in whom radiographic staging remains unclear, and in whom pathologic staging of the abdomen will significantly influence the therapeutic management. When indicated, staging laparotomy for Hodgkin's disease should include a thorough abdominal exploration, splenectomy with splenic hilar lymphadenectomy, bilateral liver biopsies, retroperitoneal lymphadenectomy, iliac crest bone marrow biopsy, and, in premenopausal women, oophoropexy.

Non-Hodgkin's Lymphoma

Children with non-Hodgkin's lymphoma (NHL) may present with isolated splenic disease, and the most common primary splenic neoplasm is NHL. Children can develop NHL as a secondary malignancy after treatment for a number of cancers, particularly Hodgkin's disease (30). Splenectomy occasionally plays an important role in the diagnosis and staging of older children and adults with NHL, although its role in younger children is unclear. Children with diffuse NHL can develop splenomegaly, and splenectomy is indicated when the bulk of the spleen contributes to abdominal pain, fullness, and early satiety. Splenectomy may also be effective in the treatment of patients who develop hypersplenism with associated anemia, thrombocytopenia, and neutropenia (31).

NHL that appears clinically confined to the spleen has been called *malignant lymphoma with prominent splenic involvement.* There is frequent involvement of the splenic hilar lymph nodes, extrahilar nodes, bone marrow, and liver in these patients, and about 75% exhibit clinical evidence of hypersplenism. In a series of 59 adults with this form of NHL, 40 underwent splenectomy, and 82% of the cytopenic patients who underwent splenectomy had correction of their hematologic abnormalities postoperatively (32). For those with low-grade NHL who had spleen-predominant features, survival was significantly improved after splenectomy than after otherwise similar treatment without splenectomy.

Nonlymphoid Tumors of the Spleen

The spleen is a site of metastatic tumor in up to 7% of autopsies of cancer patients. The primary solid tumors that most frequently metastasize to the spleen are carcinomas of the breast, lung, and melanoma; however, virtually any primary malignancy may metastasize to the spleen. Metastases to the spleen are often asymptomatic, but may be associated with symptomatic splenomegaly or even spontaneous splenic rupture. Splenectomy may provide effective palliation in carefully selected symptomatic patients with splenic metastasis.

Vascular neoplasms are the most common primary splenic tumors of childhood. They include both benign hemangiomas and malignant angiosarcomas (or hemangiosarcomas). Children with splenic malignancies may present with splenomegaly, hemolytic anemia, ascites, and pleural effusions, or with spontaneous splenic rupture. These are highly aggressive tumors that have a poor prognosis. Spleen lymphangiomas may become symptomatic by causing splenomegaly. Although these tumors can be diagnosed in many cases without the use of splenectomy, a splenectomy may be required for the treatment or palliation of these tumors.

Splenic Cysts

Splenic cysts are classified as true cysts, which may be either nonparasitic or parasitic, and pseudocysts. True cysts are characterized by a squamous epithelial lining, and many are congenital. These cysts are benign and apparently do not have malignant potential greater than any other native tissue. Most splenic cysts in children in North America are in fact pseudocysts without an epithelial lining, and are secondary to either previously recognized or unrecognized trauma.

When symptomatic, patients with splenic cysts may complain of upper abdominal fullness, early satiety, pleuritic chest pain, left shoulder pain, or renal symptoms from compression of the left kidney. The presence of symptoms is often related to the size of the cysts, and cysts smaller than 8 cm are rarely symptomatic (33). Rarely, these cysts may present with acute symptoms related to rupture, hemorrhage, or infection. The diagnosis of splenic cyst is made with both sonography and CT imaging. Operative intervention is indicated for symptomatic cysts and for large cysts. Either total or partial splenectomy may provide successful treatment, and the advantage of partial splenectomy is the potential for preservation of splenic function. More recent reports describe successful experience with partial splenectomy, cyst wall resection, or partial decapsulation, which may be accomplished with either an open or a laparoscopic approach (33).

Most splenic parasitic cysts occur in areas of endemic hydatid disease (*Echinococcus* species). Radiographic imaging may reveal cyst wall calcifications or daughter cysts. Although hydatid cysts are uncommon in North America, this diagnosis should always be excluded before the performance of invasive diagnostic or therapeutic procedures that may risk spillage of cyst contents. Serologic tests for *Echinococcus* species are often helpful in verifying the presence of parasites. Spillage of cyst contents may precipitate an anaphylactic shock and risk intraperitoneal dissemination of infective scolices. In cases of large cysts, splenectomy is the treatment of choice, and great care should be taken to avoid rupture of the cysts intraoperatively. The cysts may be sterilized by injection of a 3% sodium chloride solution, alcohol, or 0.5% silver nitrate.

Pseudocysts account for 70% to 80% of all nonparasitic cysts of the spleen. A history of prior trauma can usually be elicited. Most splenic pseudocysts are unilocular, and the cysts are smooth and thick walled. Small asymptomatic splenic pseudocysts (less than 4 cm) do not require treatment and may undergo involution over time. When the pseudocysts are symptomatic, patients often present with left upper quadrant and referred left shoulder pain. Symptomatic pseudocysts should be treated surgically. A partial splenectomy offers effective therapy. If technically difficult, a total splenectomy should be performed. Other options include percutaneous drainage, although there is little data on the long-term efficacy of this approach in children.

Splenic Abscess

Splenic abscess is an uncommon but severe and potentially fatal illness. Predisposing illnesses include immunodeficiencies, malignancies, polycythemia vera, endocarditis, previous trauma, and hemoglobinopathies (34). Most splenic abscesses result from hematogenous spread of infecting organism from another location. Gram-positive cocci, such as *Staphylococcus, Streptococcus,* or *Enterococcus* species, and gram-negative enteric organisms are often the infectious agents. Splenic abscesses may also be caused by other fastidious organisms, including *Mycobacterium tuberculosis, Mycobacterium avium,* and *Actinomyces* species. Immunosuppressed patients may develop multiple fungal abscesses, typically from *Candida* species infection.

The presentation of splenic abscess is often nonspecific and insidious, including abdominal pain, fever, peritonitis, and pleuritic chest pain. The abdominal pain may be localized in the left upper quadrant, but may be vague and ill defined. The diagnosis is made generally by CT or with ultrasonography. Unilocular abscesses may be amenable to CT-guided drainage, and this approach, along with systemic antibiotic administration, has a success rate that of 75% to 90% in adults (35), although there is little experience in children with this approach. Failure of a prompt clinical response to percutaneous drainage should lead to splenectomy without delay. Multilocular abscesses should be treated by total splenectomy, with antibiotic administration.

Splenic Trauma

The care of a child with an injured spleen is addressed in Chapter 26.

TECHNICAL ISSUES

Laparoscopic Splenectomy

Many surgeons prefer to use the laparoscopic approach for most elective splenectomies. The technique of laparoscopic splenectomy was first described in adults, and now has been extended to large series of children (36,37). In experienced hands, laparoscopic splenectomy can be performed as safely and effectively as open splenectomy, particularly when the spleen size is normal or only slightly enlarged. Early experiences with laparoscopic splenectomy have demonstrated many similarities to the early days of laparoscopic cholecystectomy. The procedure offers the advantages of more rapid postoperative recovery and shorter duration of hospital stay (37).

Technique

Various techniques have been described for laparoscopic splenectomy. We prefer to position the patient in a supine position, although others prefer the right lateral decubitus position. Appropriate patient positioning is of paramount importance to the successful completion of a laparoscopic splenectomy. The patient is positioned so the table may be flexed to create a wider working space. The patient is placed in a reverse Trendelenburg position to facilitate gravity retraction of the viscera away from the left upper quadrant. A nasogastric tube and a urinary catheter are inserted, and pneumatic compression stockings are applied.

In the supine approach, the surgeon and first assistant both stand to the right of the patient (Fig. 94-3). Pneumoperitoneum with carbon dioxide is created using an open Hasson cannula insertion and maintained at 10 to 15 mm Hg, and we use this port for a 30-degree telescope. The position of the telescope is chosen carefully because

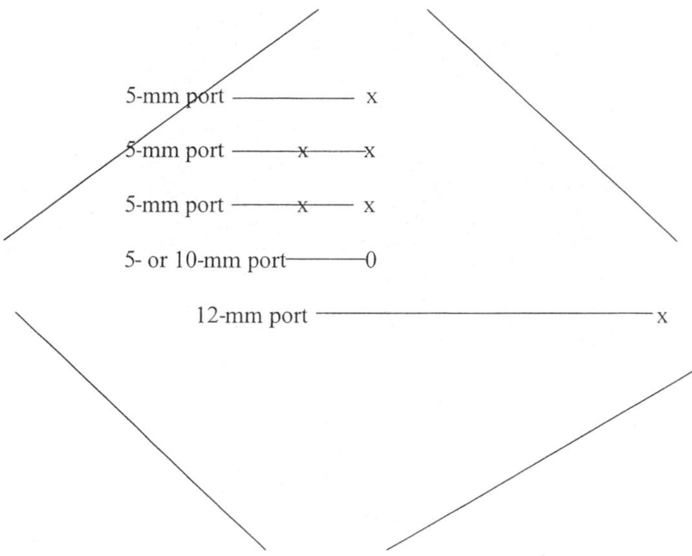

FIGURE 94-3. Patient position and trochar placement for laparoscopic splenectomy. Our preference is to position both the operating surgeon and assistant on the right side of the table. The working ports are placed in the upper and lower right flanks, and the camera and assisting ports are placed in the umbilicus and left flank, respectively. [Adapted from Rothenberg SS. Laparoscopic splenectomy in children. *Semin Laparosc Surg* 1998;5(1):19–24, with permission.]

a low insertion of the trocar hampers a direct view during dissection. Two or three additional 5-mm trocars are inserted, and a 12-mm trocar is inserted in the left anterior axillary line at the level of the umbilicus. If the distance between the umbilicus and the left costal margin after creation of the pneumoperitoneum exceeds the width of the hand, the position of this trocar is moved superiorly toward the left costal margin. We prefer to use the left two ports to use as working trocars, and the fourth 5-mm trocar is placed in subxyphoidal position for the first assistant. The subxiphoid trocar is oriented to the right side through the falciform ligament and the table tilted to the left.

Careful abdominal exploration in search of accessory spleens is performed before the initiation of the dissection. The stomach is retracted to the right and the gastrosplenic ligament is inspected, followed by the splenocolic ligament, greater omentum, and phrenosplenic ligament. On opening the gastrosplenic ligament, the splenic pedicle behind the pancreatic tail is inspected. The dissection proceeds in five stages: (1) division of the splenocolic ligament, (2) ligation of the inferior polar vessels, (3) division of the short gastric vessels, (4) hilar control, and (5) division of the phrenic attachments of the spleen. We prefer the use of harmonic shears for the majority of dissection. The splenocolic ligament is divided, leaving connective tissue on the spleen to be grasped to avoid direct manipulation of the spleen. Dissection proceeds medially and superiorly toward the splenorenal ligament. The inferior polar branches are divided using clips or the harmonic shears. Gentle retraction of the mobilized inferior pole exposes the hilar groove, and the vascular distribution of the hilum is evaluated.

Once the hilum has been controlled, we usually employ a stapling device to divide the hilar vessels. The remaining short gastric vessels at the superior pole of the spleen and the phrenic attachments are divided, and the specimen is then turned onto its convex surface. The left lateral port is removed, and a puncture-resistant retrieval bag (Cook Surgical, Inc. Indianapolis, Indiana) is introduced. The bag is directed toward the diaphragm and is held open facing the telescope. The patient is placed in a Trendelenburg position to facilitate the introduction of the spleen into the bag. The end of the closed bag is brought out through the left flank trocar, and the spleen is morcellated with ring forceps and removed in large fragments. During all manipulations, caution is used to avoid spillage of splenic fragments between the sac and the umbilical incision. The fascias of all port sites are closed.

Results

Results of laparoscopic splenectomy for benign hematologic diseases are comparable with open splenectomy, which is generally associated with a mortality rate of less than 1% and a morbidity rate of 10% to 20%. The incidence of conversion to open splenectomy is between 0% and 20% in most series. Most of the conversions are caused by intraoperative bleeding, but lack of surgical experience, extensive adhesions, and massive splenomegaly have been cited as contributory factors (37–39). In two large series of adults undergoing laparoscopic splenectomy, the mean operative time ranged from 88 to 261 minutes, with an open conversion rate ranging from 0% to 30% (40,41). The perioperative morbidity rates averaged 8% and 12%, respectively (range, 0% to 30%), and the mortality rate was 0.7% (0% to 6%). Postoperative recovery after laparoscopic splenectomy is surprisingly fast. Most patients are able to return to full activities within 1 week if their underlying hematologic disorder allows. Most important, the hematologic response and long-term cure rates for most hematologic diseases appear to be comparable between laparoscopic and open splenectomy.

Partial Splenectomy

For children with congenital hemolytic anemias, a partial splenectomy has been proposed as an alternative to total splenectomy, with the goal of removing enough spleen to gain a desired hematologic effect while preserving splenic immune function (42–44). The use of total splenectomy in children is restricted by concern of OPSI (7,9). However, the application of partial splenectomy is limited because of technical difficulties and concerns of splenic regrowth (43,45–47).

More recently, our group and others have renewed an interest in partial splenectomy in children (43–45,48). The objective of a partial splenectomy is to remove 80% to 90% of splenic volume. Our technique involves partial devascularization of the spleen to maintain flow either from the short gastric arcades to the upper pole or from the left gastroepiploic artery or the splenic artery to the lower pole (Fig. 94-4). We transect the parenchyma using a TA surgical stapler® (with 4.5-mm staples (U.S. Surgical Corporation, Norwalk, CT) (Fig. 94-3B). Bleeding from the splenic bed is controlled with an Argon beam coagulator® (Conmed Corp., Utica, NY), suture ligation, or topical hemostatic agents. In the case of a narrow vascular pedicle, the splenic remnant is fixed to the abdominal wall. The postoperative stay is 3 to 4 days, and children are kept at activity restrictions for 6 weeks to minimize the risk of bleeding. All children receive preoperative immunizations, as well as antibiotic prophylaxis with penicillin for at least 1 year postoperatively.

We have followed children with congenital hemolytic anemias who underwent partial splenectomy. In our experience, no child has required subsequent conversion to total splenectomy, although conversion has been required for other groups (44). Using ultrasonography, we have found little early regrowth of the splenic remnant following partial splenectomy. In several patients, there is later regrowth, although this rate is quite variable and does not appear to be associated with recurrent hemolysis, a finding supported by others (43,44). The reasons for the discrepancy between splenic regrowth and hematologic status are unclear, although it may be due to altered blood flow or parenchymal remodeling after partial resection.

In the children with hereditary spherocytosis (HS), there appears to be sustained control of hemolysis after partial splenectomy. Mean hemoglobin concentrations increased by at least 2 gm per dL, and this difference has persisted throughout 4 to 6 years of follow-up (Fig. 94-5). Reticulocyte counts and serum bilirubin levels decreased after partial splenectomy, and there was a reduction in signs and symptoms of hypersplenism. For children without HS, a partial splenectomy did not significantly affect hemoglobin levels, although these children had reduced symptoms of hypersplenism and control of splenic sequestration.

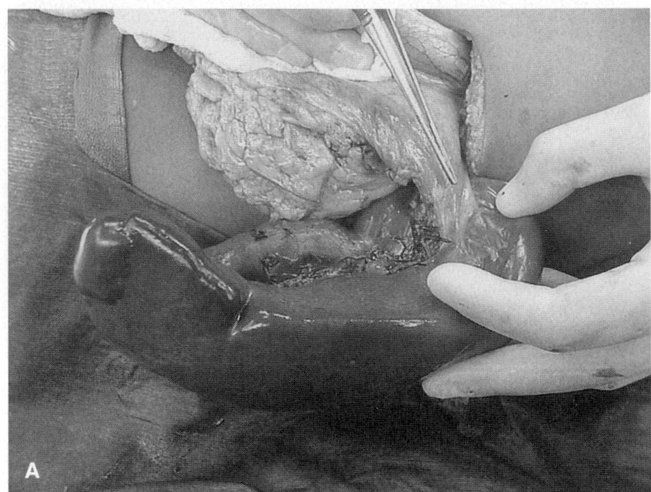

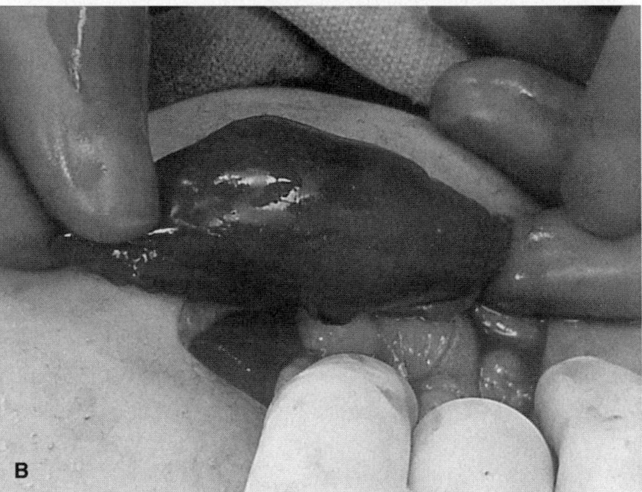

FIGURE 94-4. **(A)** Intraoperative photograph of the spleen following devascularization of the lower pole and major splenic vessels. The upper pole of the spleen is perfused by the short gastric vessels.**(B)** The spleen is transected at the transition between ischemic and perfused tissue with the use of a TA surgical stapler (see text). Hemostasis is supported by use of argon beam coagulator and topical hemostatic agents.

Classical indications for splenectomy in children with HS include repeated transfusions or anemic crises (49). However, many children have less severe symptoms of hemolysis, including fatigue, cholelithiasis, and growth failure (43,49). For children with milder symptoms of hemolysis, a total splenectomy has been difficult to justify, and a partial splenectomy may offer some benefit. More recent innovations for total splenectomy in children include the use of laparoscopy, which may decrease operative morbidity compared with an open approach (36).

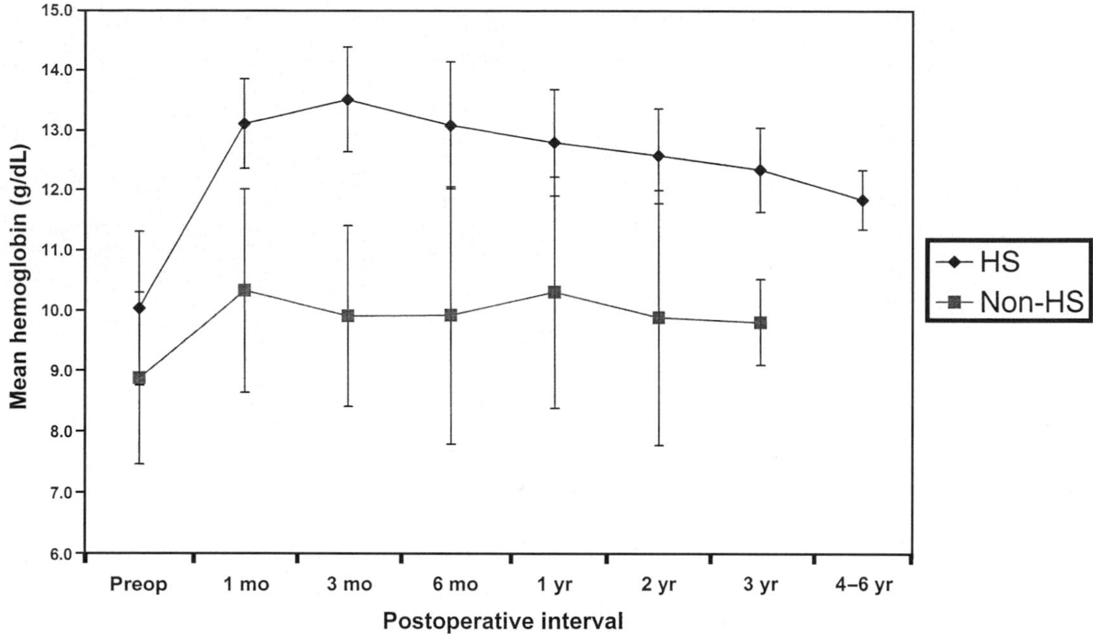

FIGURE 94-5. Mean hemoglobin levels after partial splenectomy for children with hereditary spherocytosis (HS) ($n = 15$) or for children without HS ($n = 8$). Diagnoses for children without HS include pryuvate kinase deficiency, congenital nonspherocytotic hemolytic anemia of unknown etiology, Hgb SS, Hgb SC, Hgb CC, HgbS-beta thalassemia. For children with HS, hemoglobin levels increased compared with preoperative values throughout 4 to 6 years of follow-up ($p < 0.05$ by paired Student's t-test). For children without HS, there was no change in hemoglobin levels after partial splenectomy. Error bars show the standard deviation within each study group. (In: Rice HE, Oldham KT, Hillery CA et al. Clinical and hematologic benefits of partial splenectomy for congenital hemolytic anemias in children. *Ann Surg* 2003;237(2):281–288.)

The role for partial splenectomy in children with other congenital hemolytic anemias is quite different than in children with HS. In sickle hemoglobinopathies, a partial splenectomy appears to control symptoms of hypersplenism and splenic sequestration, but does not always preserve long-term splenic function. In contrast to sickle hemoglobinopathies, it appears that hemolysis from PK deficiency is readily controlled by partial splenectomy. Our experience with PK deficiency shows both reduced hemolysis and retained splenic function following partial splenectomy, in contrast to the experience of Sandoval et al. (50)

REFERENCES

1. Loftus WK, Metreweli C. Ultrasound assessment of mild splenomegaly: spleen/kidney ratio. *Pediatr Radiol* 1998;28:98–100.
2. Michels NA. The variational anatomy of the spleen and the splenic artery. *Am J Anat* 1942;70:21–72.
3. Macartney FJ, Zuberbuhler JR, Anderson RH. Morphological considerations pertaining to recognition of atrial isomerism. Consequences for sequential chamber localisation. *Br Heart J* 1980;44:657–667.
4. Chadburn A. The spleen: anatomy and anatomical function. *Semin Hematol* 2000;37:13–21.
5. Bohnsack JF, Brown EJ. The role of the spleen in resistance to infection. *Annu Rev Med* 1986;37:49–59.
6. Foster PN, Bolton RP, Cotter KL, et al. Defective activation of neutrophils after splenectomy. *J Clin Pathol* 1985;38:1175–1178.
7. Lynch AM, Kapila R. Overwhelming postsplenectomy infection. *Infect Dis Clin North Am* 1996;10:693–707.
8. Leonard AS, Giebink GS, Baesl TJ, et al. The overwhelming postsplenectomy sepsis problem. *World J Surg* 1980;4:423–432.
9. King H, Shumacker HB Jr. Susceptibility to infection after splenectomy performed in infancy. *Ann Surg* 1951;136:239–242.
10. Brigden ML, Pattullo AL. Prevention and management of overwhelming postsplenectomy infection—an update. *Crit Care Med* 1999;27:836–842.
11. Gold HS, Moellering RCJ. Antimicrobial drug resistance. *N Engl J Med* 1996;335:1445–1453.
12. American Academy of Pediatrics. *Policy statement: recommendations for the prevention of pneumococcal infections, including the use of pneumococcal conjugate vaccine (Prevnar), pneumococcal polysaccharide vaccine, and antibiotic prophylaxis (RE9960). J Pediatr* 2000;106:362–366.
13. Rutherford EJ, Livengood J, Higginbotham M, et al. Efficacy and safety of pneumococcal revaccination after splenectomy for trauma. *J Trauma* 1995;39:448–452.
14. Overturf GD. Diseases TCoI: Technical report: prevention of pneumococcal infections, including the use of pneumococcal conjugate and polysaccharide vaccines and antibiotic prophylaxis (RE9960). *Pediatrics* 2000;106:367–376.
15. Gaston MH, Verter JI, Woods G, et al. Prophylaxis with oral penicillin in children with sickle cell anemia: a randomized trial. *N Engl J Med* 1986;314:1593–1599.
16. Buchanan GR, Smith SJ. Pneumococcal septicemia despite pneumococcal vaccine and prescription of penicillin prophylaxis in children with sickle cell anemia. *Am J Dis Child* 1986;140:428–432.
17. Norris CF, Mahannah SR, Smith-Whitley K, et al. Pneumococcal colonization in children with sickle cell disease. *J Pediatr* 1996;129:821–827.
18. Falletta JM, Woods GM, Verter JI, et al. Discontinuing penicillin

prophylaxis in children with sickle cell anemia: Prophylactic Penicillin Study II. *J Pediatr* 1995;127:685–690.
19. Sackey K. Hemolytic anemia: part 1. *Pediatr Rev* 1999;20:152–158.
20. Delaunay J. Genetic disorders of the red cell membrane. *Crit Rev Oncol Hematol* 1995;19:79–110.
21. Miwa S, Fujii H. Pyruvate kinase deficiency. *Clin Biochem* 1990;23:155–157.
22. Glader BE, Look KA. Hematologic disorders in children from Southeast Asia. *Pediatr Clin North Am* 1996;43:665–681.
23. Lane PA. Sickle cell disease. *Pediatr Clin North Am* 1996;43:639–664.
24. Pearson HA, Gallagher D, Chilcote R, et al. Developmental pattern of splenic dysfunction in the sickle cell disorders. *Pediatrics* 1985;76:392–397.
25. Brown AK, Sleeper LA, Miller ST, et al. Reference values and hematologic changes from birth to 5 years in patients with sickle cell disease. *Arch Pediatr Adolesc Med* 1994;148:796–804.
26. Di Paola JA, Buchanan GR. Immune thrombocytopenic purpura. *Pediatr Clin North Am* 2002;49:911–928.
27. Clarkson SB, Bussel JB, Kimberly RP, et al. Treatment of refractory immune thrombocytopenic purpura with an anti-Fc gamma-receptor antibody. *N Eng J Med* 1986;314:1236–1239.
28. Mantadakis E, Buchanan GR. Elective splenectomy in children with idiopathic thrombocytopenic purpura. *J Pediatr Hematol Oncol* 2000;22(2):148–153.
29. Medeiros D, Buchanan GR. Idiopathic thrombocytopenic purpura: beyond consensus. *Curr Opin Pediatr* 2000;12:4–9.
30. Prósper F, Robledo C, Cuesta B, et al. Incidence of non-Hodgkin's lymphoma in patients treated for Hodgkin's disease. *Leuk Lymph* 1994;14:457–462.
31. Brodsky J, Abcar A, Styler M. Splenectomy for non-Hodgkin's lymphoma. *Am J Clin Oncol* 1996;19:558–561.
32. Morel P, Dupriez B, Gosselin B, et al. Role of early splenectomy in malignant lymphomas with prominent splenic involvement (primary lymphomas of the spleen). *Cancer* 1993;71:207–215.
33. Tsakayannis DE, Mitchell K, Kozakewich HP, et al. Splenic preservation in the management of splenic epidermoid cysts in children. *J Pediatr Surg* 1995;30:1468–1470.
34. Smith MD Jr, Nio M, Camel JE, et al. Management of splenic abscess in immunocompromised children. *J Pediatr Surg* 1993;28:823–826.
35. Gleich S, Wolin DA, Berbsman H. A review of percutaneous drainage of splenic abscess. *Surg Gynecol Obstet* 1988;167:211–216.
36. Farah RA, Rogers ZR, Thompson WR, et al. Comparison of laparoscopic and open splenectomy in children with hematologic disorders. *J Pediatr* 1997;131:41–46.
37. Cusick RA, Waldhausen JH. The learning curve associated with pediatric laparoscopic splenectomy. *Am J Surg* 2001;181:393–397.
38. Friedman RL, Hiatt JR, Korman JL, et al. Laparoscopic or open splenectomy for hematologic disease: which approach is superior? *J Am Coll Surg* 1997;185:49–54.
39. Friedman RL, Fallas MJ, Carroll BJ, et al. Laparoscopic splenectomy for ITP. *Surg Endosc* 1996;10:991–995.
40. Gigot JF, Jamar F, Ferrant A, et al: Inadequate detection of accessory spleens and splenosis with laparoscopic splenectomy: a shortcoming of the laparoscopic approach in hematologic diseases. *Surg Endosc* 1998;12:101–106.
41. Katkhouda N, Hurwitz MB, Rivera RT, et al. Laparoscopic splenectomy: outcome and efficacy in 103 consecutive patients. *Ann Surg* 1998;228:568–578.
42. Tchernia G, Gauthier F, Mielot F, et al. Initial assessment of the beneficial effect of partial splenectomy in hereditary spherocytosis. *Blood* 1993;81:2014–2020.
43. Tchernia G, Bader-Meunier B, Berterottiere P, et al. Effectiveness of partial splenectomy in hereditary spherocytosis. *Curr Opin Hematol* 1997;4:136–141.
44. Bader-Meunier B, Gauthier F, Archambaud F, et al. Long-term evaluation of the beneficial effect of subtotal splenectomy for management of hereditary spherocytosis. *Blood* 2001;97:399–403.
45. Tchernia G, Gauthier F, Mielot F, et al. Initial assessment of the beneficial effect of partial splenectomy in hereditary spherocytosis. *Blood* 1993;81:2014–2020.
46. Svarch E, Vilorio P, Nordet I, et al. Partial splenectomy in children with sickle cell disease and repeated episodes of splenic sequestration. *Hemoglobin* 1996;20:393–400.
47. Guzzetta PC, Ruley EJ, Merrick HFW, et al. Elective subtotal splenectomy—indications and results in 33 patients. *Ann Surg* 1990; 211:34–42.
48. Freud E, Cohen IJ, Mor C, et al. Splenic "regeneration" after partial splenectomy for Gaucher disease: histological features. *Blood Cells Molecules Dis* 1998;24:309–316.
49. Delaunay J. Genetic disorders of the red cell membrane. *Crit Rev Oncol Hematol* 1995;19:79–110.
50. Sandoval C, Stringel G, Weisberger J, et al. Failure of partial splenectomy to ameliorate the anemia of pyruvate kinase deficiency. *J Pediatr Surg* 1997;32:641–642.
51. American Academy of Pediatrics. Asplenic children. In: Pickering LK, ed. *2000 red book: report of the Committee on Infectious Diseases.* Grove Village, IL: American Academy of Pediatrics, 2000:66–67.

PART H

Urinary and Genital Systems

Chapter 95

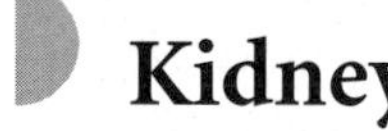

Kidney

Michael A. Keating and Mark A. Rich

INTRODUCTION

The paired kidneys are crucial to the well-being of every child. As the organs of hematologic cleansing and urinary excretion, they play a central role in fluid, electrolyte, and acid–base balance. In addition, they also provide endocrine function, with known roles in vitamin D metabolism and the production of erythropoietin and renin.

ANATOMY

Familiarity with renal anatomy establishes the basis for understanding and managing many diseases of the kidney, regardless of whether they are surgical, medical, traumatic, or neoplastic.

Gross Anatomy

Location, Size, and Orientation

The kidneys of children share many characteristics with those of adults, although certain differences having clinical implications exist. Positioned slightly above the level of the umbilicus and located on either side of the vertebral column, these paired, bean-shaped organs are well protected in the retroperitoneum. The right kidney usually is more dependently positioned as a consequence of its displacement by the liver. Medially, the organs are buttressed by the paraspinous muscles. Posteriorly, their upper poles are shielded by the lower ribs. However, the underdeveloped abdominal musculature of children and their softer ribs offer the anterolateral surface less effective protection against trauma. Here, an intimate association with several adjacent organs readily explains the high incidence of associated visceral injuries when the kidneys themselves are traumatized (1,2).

Each kidney and its adjacent adrenal gland are contained within a thin condensation of connective tissue, the perirenal or Gerota's fascia. This fascial envelope is circumferentially intact, with the exception of an inferior hiatus that allows for exit of the ureter. Although it does not provide mechanical protection, Gerota's fascia is an important anatomic barrier against the extension of primary renal tumors—including Wilms' tumor—to adjacent organs. It also effectively contains and controls the hemorrhage of most blunt trauma. Variable amounts of fat also surround the kidneys in either a perinephric (within the fascia) or paranephric (outside of the fascia) position, buttressing them in the retroperitoneum. Unfortunately, the paucity of fat in most children makes the organ extremely mobile and more susceptible to contrecoup, flexion, and deceleration injuries.

The kidneys of the child, especially at an early age, are larger with respect to overall body size than those of an adult. This results in a relative abdominal projection that, again, makes them more susceptible to injury. Nomograms have been developed that estimate normal renal size with respect to age, although correlations should be made with overall size. As a general rule, the length of a normal kidney equals that of the adjacent two and one half vertebral bodies. The absence of growth on serial examination should prompt an investigation into cause. In addition to size, the axis of the pediatric kidney provides a clue to abnormal development. Normally, each upper pole is distinctly medial to the lower pole, and lines drawn along the longitudinal

Michael A. Keating and Mark A. Rich: Department of Surgery, Division of Urology, University of South Florida School of Medicine, Nemours Children's Clinic, Orlando, Florida 32806.

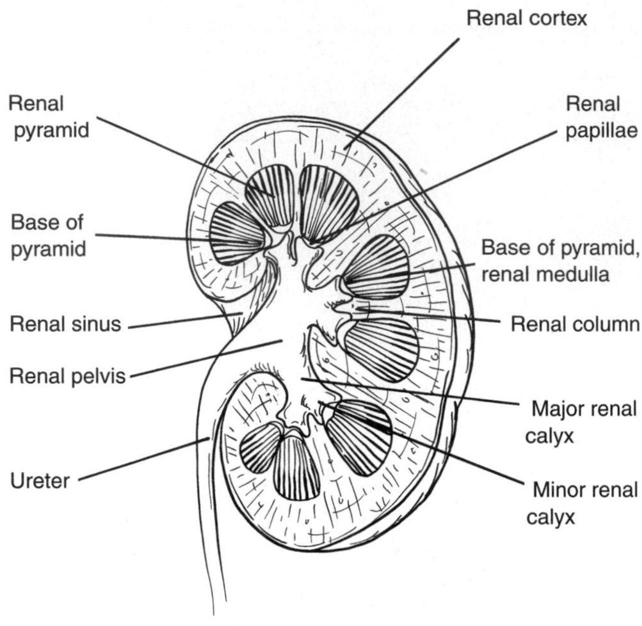

FIGURE 95-1. Macroanatomy of kidney on sagittal section.

axis of the kidneys typically intersect at the 10th thoracic vertebrae. Vertical or laterally displaced axes can be caused by the upper pole hydronephrosis of a duplex collecting system, tumors of the kidney or adrenal glands, or renal ectopia from incomplete migration or rotation during embryogenesis (see below).

Parenchyma and Collecting System

Sagittal sectioning allows an appreciation of the kidney's macroanatomy (Fig. 95-1). A thick fibrous capsule that adheres to its entire surface maintains the integrity of the renal parenchyma. The capsule is used whenever possible to reinforce the closure of renal wounds because the soft friable parenchyma, like liver, lacks the consistency needed to hold sutures without tearing. Immediately beneath the capsule lies the contiguous outer layer of the kidney, the *cortex*, which contains the glomeruli, proximal and distal tubules, and collecting ducts. Deep to this lies the central renal medulla, composed of straight portions of the tubules, loops of Henle, the vasa recta, and terminal collecting ducts. The *medulla* is divided into discrete pyramid-shaped structures that have their base along the corticomedullary junction and are called, appropriately enough, the renal *pyramids*.

The concavity of the medial surface of each kidney is called the *hilum*. Here the renal vein, artery, and pelvis are positioned in an anterior-to-posterior direction. The fat-filled space surrounding the renal pelvis and overlying kidney is called the *renal sinus*. The renal pelvis typically branches into two or three major *calyces* as it enters the substance of the kidney. Further divisions result in two or three minor calyces. Each renal pyramid (and hence renal lobe) empties into a minor calyx at the papilla, which accounts for the convex impressions seen on pyelography.

Vasculature

There can be significant variation in renal vascularity. Normally, the blood supply to each kidney comes from a single main artery that branches off the aorta, just inferolateral to the superior mesenteric artery. Auxiliary arteries from the aorta and adrenal or gonadal arteries frequently supply the superior and inferior poles, especially to the left kidney. These vessels cross the collecting system and are sometimes implicated in obstructions of the ureteropelvic junction.

Within the renal sinus, the main artery gives off a posterior branch that supplies that segment of the kidney exclusive of the poles. Its anterior limb divides into four branches that feed the apical, upper, middle, and lower segments. Despite any variations that might occur with arterial origins and distribution, there is no collateral blood supply between the individual segments. Each segmental artery is an end artery. Brodel's line defines a plane between the anterior and posterior branches that, in theory, allows a relatively avascular surgical approach to the center of the kidney.

Unlike its arterial supply, the venous drainage of the kidney freely crosses segmental boundaries. After entering the ascending vasa rectae, venous blood drains into the interlobular veins, and then retraces the arterial path to the main renal vein. Like its arterial counterpart, the renal vein exhibits a great deal of variation. In most cases, the left renal vein, which is the longer of the two, has lumbar, gonadal, and adrenal branches. In contrast, the right renal vein is notoriously short and has no collaterals because the comparable right-sided collateral veins drain directly into the vena cava. This difference in collateral drainage gives the left kidney far more resiliency after ligation or thrombosis of its main vein.

Microanatomy and Functional Correlates

At the microscopic level, the kidney becomes a marvel of the interplay between function and structure. The basic unit of function, the *nephron*, is composed of a vascular capillary tuft, the true glomerulus, and the glomerular or Bowman's capsule. In common usage, however, the term *glomerulus* refers to the combination of capillary tuft and capsule (Fig. 95-2). Each kidney is comprised of about 1 million nephrons whose formation is complete at birth. The kidney is not a resilient organ and the organ's functional reserve is limited.

Blood flows to the glomerulus by way of the afferent arteriole and exits through the efferent arteriole. Both vessels enter the glomerulus at the vascular pole or hilum directly

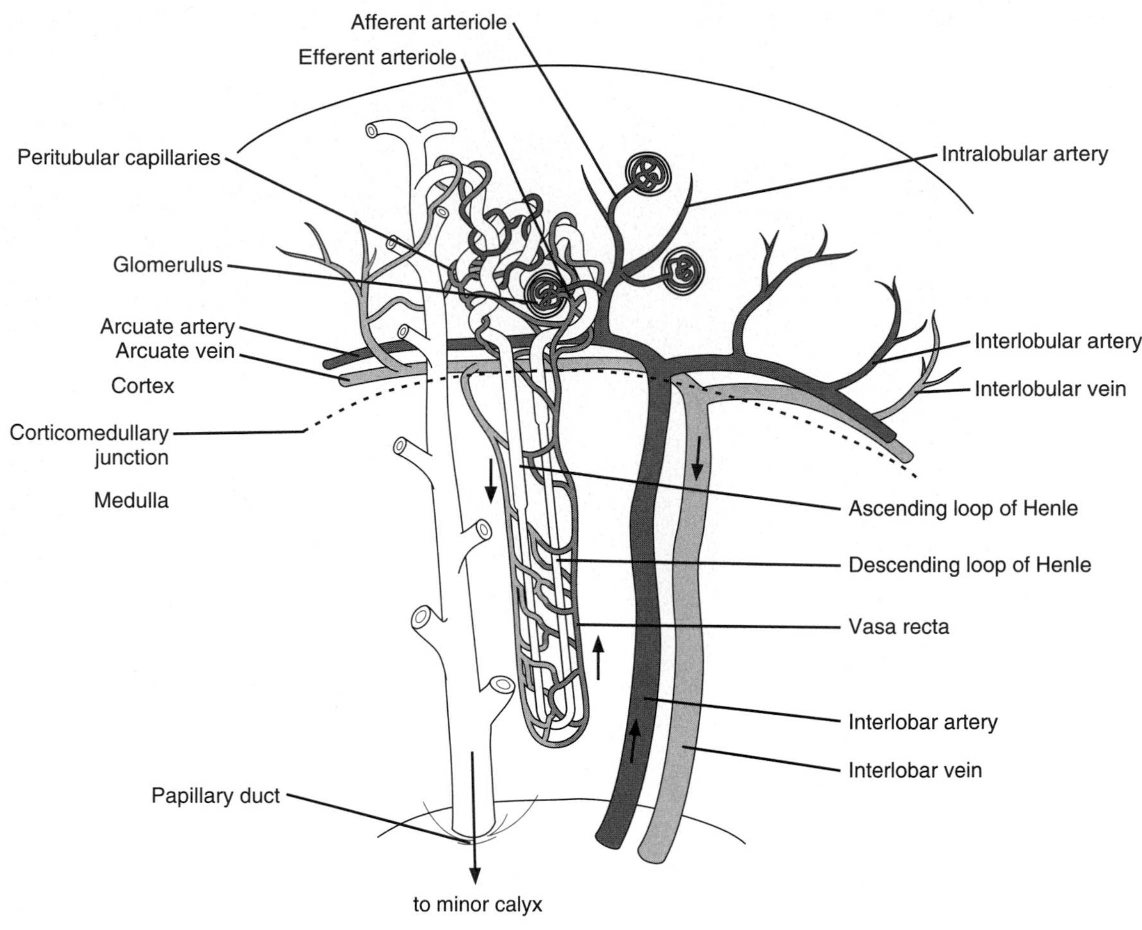

FIGURE 95-2. Nephron microanatomy and relation to intrarenal vasculature.

opposite the proximal renal tubule at the urinary pole. The glomerulus invaginates the blind-ending renal tubule and the fenestrated epithelial lining of its capillaries, and initiates the ultrafiltration of plasma. Urine ultimately results. The principal driving force regulating glomerular filtration is hydrostatic pressure, a consequence of systemic blood pressure. Glomerular filtration pressure is progressively opposed until ultrafiltration ceases by the hydrostatic pressure in Bowman's space and colloid osmotic pressure of the arteriole.

The epithelial component of Bowman's capsule, which surrounds the glomerular tuft and is continuous with the epithelium of the proximal tubule, has both a visceral (lining the capillary tuft) and a parietal (comprising the wall of capsule itself) component. Varying degrees of hematuria, proteinuria, and renal insufficiency result, depending on the severity.

Within the proximal convoluted tubule, the longest portion of the nephron, about 65% of the ultrafiltrate is isotonically reabsorbed. Sodium is actively transported into the peritubular space, and chloride and water passively follow. After passing through the proximal tubule, the ultrafiltrate enters the descending (thin) portion of the loop of Henle accompanied by the adjacent vasa recta. Many loops extend through the medulla to the tips of the papilla with the collecting ducts. Here, a *countercurrent multiplier* acts to increase the osmotic concentration of the medullary interstitium by actively reabsorbing salt. On its upward swing, ultrafiltrate hypotonicity results because the ascending (thick) loop is impermeable to water, yet salts are actively reabsorbed along their elevated osmotic gradients (Fig. 95-3). The distal tubule and collecting ducts ultimately course back through this same hypertonic medullary interstitium, where water reabsorption is mediated largely under the influence of antidiuretic hormone. Final sodium handling also occurs here, influenced partly by aldosterone.

Henle's loop ascends to the distal convoluted tubule, which courses alongside the glomerulus of origin. The two are functionally linked by the tubule's macula densa, a modified group of cells believed to influence the release of renin by the juxtaglomerular apparatus. Multiple collecting tubules drain into individual collecting ducts that run through the medulla and out to the renal papilla, where other collecting ducts are gathered to give the papilla a porous appearance.

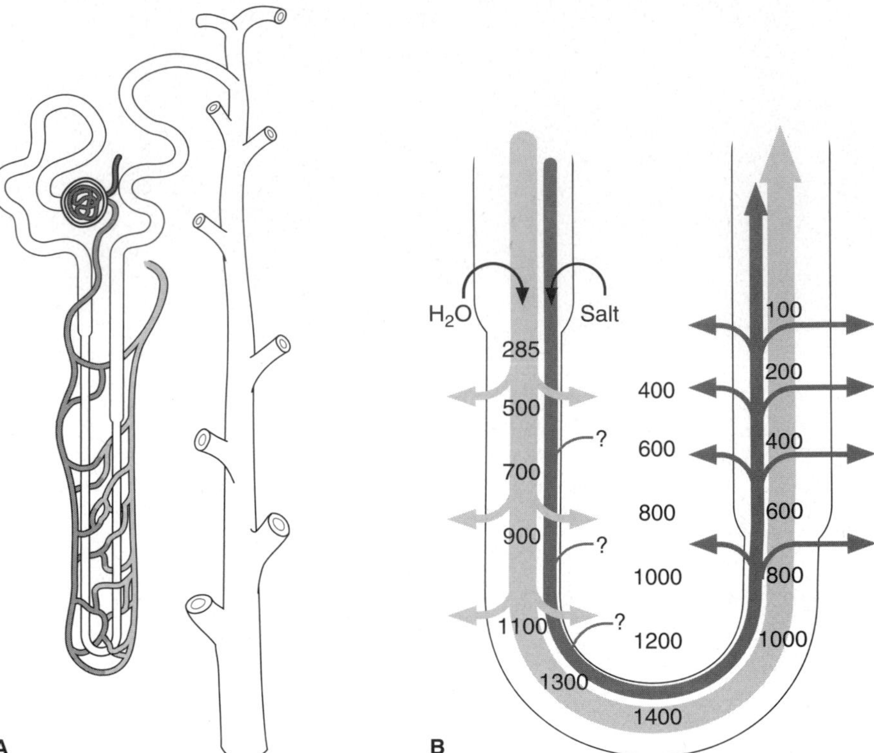

FIGURE 95-3. **(A)** "Countercurrent multiplier" of the loop of Henle. **(B)** The active transport of salt out of the ascending limb increases medullary osmotic concentration. Water is then reabsorbed by osmotic force if distal tubular and collecting duct permeability, under the influence of antidiuretic hormone, allows.

EMBRYOLOGY

Congenital anomalies of the urinary tract are common in otherwise normal children, with a rate as high as 3% cited in asymptomatic infants screened with ultrasound (3,4). A significant number of these will require surgical intervention. In addition, because it is synchronously developing with other organs, the urinary tract is often adversely influenced by the same teratogenic, chromosomal, and nonspecific influences that result in syndromes.

The mature kidney evolves through three developmental phases. The pronephros, mesonephros, and metanephros are derived from intermediate mesoderm, which coalesces adjacent to the second through sixth somites. The superior portion of the primordial anlage or nephrogenic cord is composed of primitive tubules known as the *pronephros*. This appears by the third week of gestation and involutes by week 5.

The medially positioned *mesonephros* is induced from the mesoderm by the descending mesonephric duct, the wolffian duct, which extends caudally to communicate with the anterior cloaca. The union of duct with mesoderm creates about 40 pairs of mesonephric nephrons, which produce urine between the fifth and tenth weeks of development. Although the mesonephros gradually involutes, vestigial tubules can be found in both genders near the reproductive tracts. The mesonephric duct persists as the vas deferens in males. In females, remnants persist as Gartner's duct along the anteromedial vaginal wall.

Formation of the mature kidney depends on reciprocal inductive effects of the caudal portion of the nephrogenic cord or *metanephros* and the ureteral bud. The ureteral bud begins to project from the caudal end of the mesonephric (wolffian) duct during the fourth and fifth weeks of gestation. After the bud unites with the metanephric blastema, its ampulla is induced to repetitively branch for 15 generations. Nephrogenesis is completed by birth, although renal maturation with proximal tubule convolution, collecting tubule elongation, and Henle's loop extension into the medulla continue afterward. Each nephron follows a sequential order of maturation in segmentation of glomerulus, proximal tubule, and distal tubule.

Nephrogenesis does not occur if the bud is absent or unable to come into close contact with the metanephrogenic blastema. When the tissues are separated enough to prevent epithelial–mesenchymal interaction, differentiation does not occur. After its initial induction by contact, proliferation and morphogenesis of the metanephros continues under the influence of growth factors, extracellular matrix, and proteins.

Abnormalities in the interplay of the ureteral bud and metanephros are implicated in a number of congenital abnormalities of the kidney. For example, ectopic ureters or severely refluxing ureters positioned off the trigone are commonly associated with renal dysplasia or hypoplasia, findings that are rarely associated with a normal ureter. Calyceal diverticula, some cystic variants, megacalycosis, and renal ectopia also undoubtedly have an embryonic basis where problems with ampullary branching, segmentation of the nephron, or renal ascent can occur. Nevertheless, etiologies are difficult to prove.

ANOMALIES OF NUMBER AND POSITION

Renal Agenesis

Unilateral

Unilateral renal agenesis is a fairly common anomaly (1 per 1,100 in autopsy series and 1 per 1,500 in radiographic reviews). The 2:1 male predominance seen with renal agenesis probably results from the delicate interplay required of the ureteral bud and the wolffian duct. The timing of the error in embryogenesis determines its effects on the urinary tract and associated organ system anomalies (Table 95-1). The most common organ systems involved include cardiovascular (30%), gastrointestinal (25%), and musculoskeletal (14%) (5). As many as one-half of patients with one kidney still have a rudimentary ureter on the affected side, an indication that the problem occurred after the ureteral bud has extended from the wolffian duct, which remains normal. The other one-half of affected males have an absence of the ureter and ipsilateral hemitrigone of the bladder, as well as absence of the wolffian structures (ejaculatory duct, seminal vesicle, and vas deferens) as indicators of an earlier insult in development. In both instances, the ipsilateral gonad is usually normal.

Similar errors in embryogenesis also affect females for apparently the same reasons. Other than giving off the ureteral bud before they involute, the wolffian ducts play a crucial role in the development of the internal genitalia by guiding the müllerian ducts into position along the urorectal septum. It is easy to implicate abnormalities of this sequence with a unicornuate uterus, where the müllerian duct is never properly positioned, or in uterine didelphys, where the normal fusion and canalization of the two ducts is somehow deterred. Not surprisingly, both anomalies are commonly associated with renal agenesis in female patients. For the same reasons, complete absence or hypoplasia of the vagina is also frequently associated with renal agenesis (the so-called *Mayer-Rokitansky-Kuster-Hauser syndrome*).

Unilateral renal agenesis is occasionally discovered during the evaluation children with multiple organ system anomalies [e.g., syndrome of vertebral defects, imperforate anus, tracheoesophageal fistula, and radial and renal dysplasia (VATER)], serendipitously or in concert with an associated symptomatic genital abnormality such as hydrocolpos. They are most often diagnosed by antenatal ultrasound. After delivery, renal scintigraphy can be used to confirm the diagnosis. Parents are also made aware of the possible genital implications of the finding. Ultrasound can be used to confirm the presence of a cervix and uterus in infants and young girls. Some clinicians have also recommended screening the siblings of affected children, in whom a 10% rate of asymptomatic renal anomalies has been reported.

Until more recently, it was believed that children with solitary kidneys experienced no increased nephrologic risk. Compensatory hypertrophy of the single moiety occurs, and life expectancy is assumed to be normal. However, concerns have been raised about the hyperfiltration load assumed by the remaining kidney.

TABLE 95-1 Common Associations with Renal Agenesis.

	Unilateral	*Bilateral*
Urologic	Ureteral absence or atresia Asymmetric or hemitrigone Contralateral renal ectopia, malrotation	Ureteral atresia Absent or hypoplastic bladder

Genital	Male
	  Absent vas deferens, seminal vesicle
	Female
	  Unicornuate or didelphic uterus
	  Duplicate or absent vagina
		Male
		  Hypospadias
		  Penile agenesis
		  Undescended testes
		Female
		  Rudimentary, anomalous, or absent uterus, vagina
		  Hypoplastic or absent ovaries

Pulmonary	—	Pulmonary hypoplasia
Cardiovascular	Septal, valvular defects	Present
Gastrointestinal	Imperforate anus Esophageal stricture, atresia	Imperforate anus
Orthopedic	Vertebral, phalangeal anomalies	Club feet Spina bifida
Other	Syndromes: VATER,[a] Poland, Turner's	Characteristic (Potter) facies

[a]VATER, syndrome of vertebral defects, anorectal anomalies, tracheoesophageal fistula, and radial and renal dysplasia.

Bilateral

Bilateral renal agenesis is less common than its unilateral counterpart (1 in 4,800 births). Male patients are more commonly affected (75%), although the wolffian derivatives are usually normal. Failure of the ureteral bud is typically implicated because an absent or atretic ureter is found in nearly 90% of cases. An increased incidence of imperforate anus and spina bifida suggests a regional disturbance of the cloaca in some children. In the remainder, a 10% incidence of testicular agenesis in the presence of intact wolffian structures points to a dual insult to the renal and gonadal anlagen in the dorsal coelom.

Anhydramnios or oligohydramnios during pregnancy is usually the harbinger of bilateral renal agenesis. Antenatal ultrasound confirms absence of the kidneys and no evidence of bladder filling after a prolonged examination. Although false-positive results have been reported, consideration is given to termination of pregnancy because of the poor prognosis. Intrauterine compression of the fetus results in the classic stigmata of Potter syndrome (clubbed feet, bowed legs, loose skin, and prominent epicanthal fold of the cheek) and severe pulmonary hypoplasia. Stillbirths result in one-half of the cases, whereas the remaining infants die during the first day of life from pulmonary distress. Anuria and gradual renal failure are predictable for the occasional child who remains alive for a slightly longer period of time. Normal newborns should void during the first 24 hours. Anuria is occasionally prolonged by tocolytic agents given the mother or by spinal flexion from traumatic birth. Renal agenesis is suggested by more prolonged anuria, especially without a distended bladder. Ultrasound is usually diagnostic, although renal scintigraphy can also be performed for confirmation. The risk of similar involvement in subsequent pregnancies has been estimated at 2% to 5%, underscoring the need for an autopsy of any baby believed to have this diagnosis.

RENAL FUSIONS AND ECTOPIA

Early errors in development can adversely affect the ascent and rotation of the metanephros and result in an impressive array of anomalies in position and configuration (6). Despite their distorted configurations, most of these renal anomalies never become clinically significant. However, they should serve as a caution to clinicians because affected children often have abnormalities of other organs.

Horseshoe Kidney

Horseshoe kidneys are the most common fusion anomaly, with an incidence of 1 in 400. A 2:1 male prevalence exists. Girls with Turner's (45XO) syndrome (60%) and children with trisomy 18 (21%) are also prone to this anomaly. Fusion of the lower poles is found in more than 90% of cases. An isthmus of functioning renal tissue is usually found anterior to the great vessels, just below the inferior mesenteric artery. Renal vasculature is highly variable, and only 30% of horseshoe kidneys have a single renal artery. The remainder receives additional branches from the aorta or the hypogastric, middle sacral, and common iliac arteries.

Most ectopic and fused kidneys are malrotated. The ureters are anteriorly directed and draped over the inferior poles and isthmus of the anomaly. Variable degrees of hydronephrosis are the rule, but full-blown obstruction exists in one-third or less of patients. Stasis does present a problem, however, and calculi ultimately develop in about 20% of patients. When symptoms do occur, vague abdominal pain, a palpable mass, or urinary infections are common presenting signs. A renal scan or intravenous pyelogram (IVP) is diagnostic.

Long-term survival is unaffected by the presence of a fusion or ectopia. However, these kidneys are more prone to trauma and can be difficult to operate on because of their highly variable vasculature. Depending on the pelvic or renal surgery that is planned, arteriography can provide information about the blood supply to the kidney that may be crucial to success. Voiding cystourethrography is also indicated in any symptomatic child with a horseshoe kidney. Vesicoureteral reflux is seen in one-half of these children, and presents a risk factor for infection and upper tract damage in an already abnormal kidney. In addition, for reasons that remain unclear, there is an increased incidence of nephroblastomas and Wilms' tumor in horseshoe kidneys.

Crossed Renal Ectopia

Crossed renal ectopia is less common than horseshoe kidney (1 in 1,000) and also preferentially affects male patients (2:1). Four categories lend order to what is sometimes bizarre anatomy. In decreasing order of frequency, these include crossed fused (Fig. 95-4A), crossed nonfused (Fig. 95-4B), solitary crossed (Fig. 95-4C), and bilateral crossed (Fig. 95-4D). Crossed fusions constitute 90% of the variants seen, and the left kidney is the ectopic moiety 75% of the time. In most cases, the orthotopic kidney and ureter are normally positioned. Its lower pole, however, is fused to the upper pole of the crossed ectopic kidney, whose ureter is normally inserted in the bladder on the contralateral side. In less well-defined cases, the ureteral origins remain unchanged, but both kidneys meld together on one side.

Other Renal Ectopias

Whenever a kidney occupies an abnormal position, it is classified as ectopic. A compilation of series suggests an overall occurrence of about of 1 in 900. *Pelvic ectopia*, in

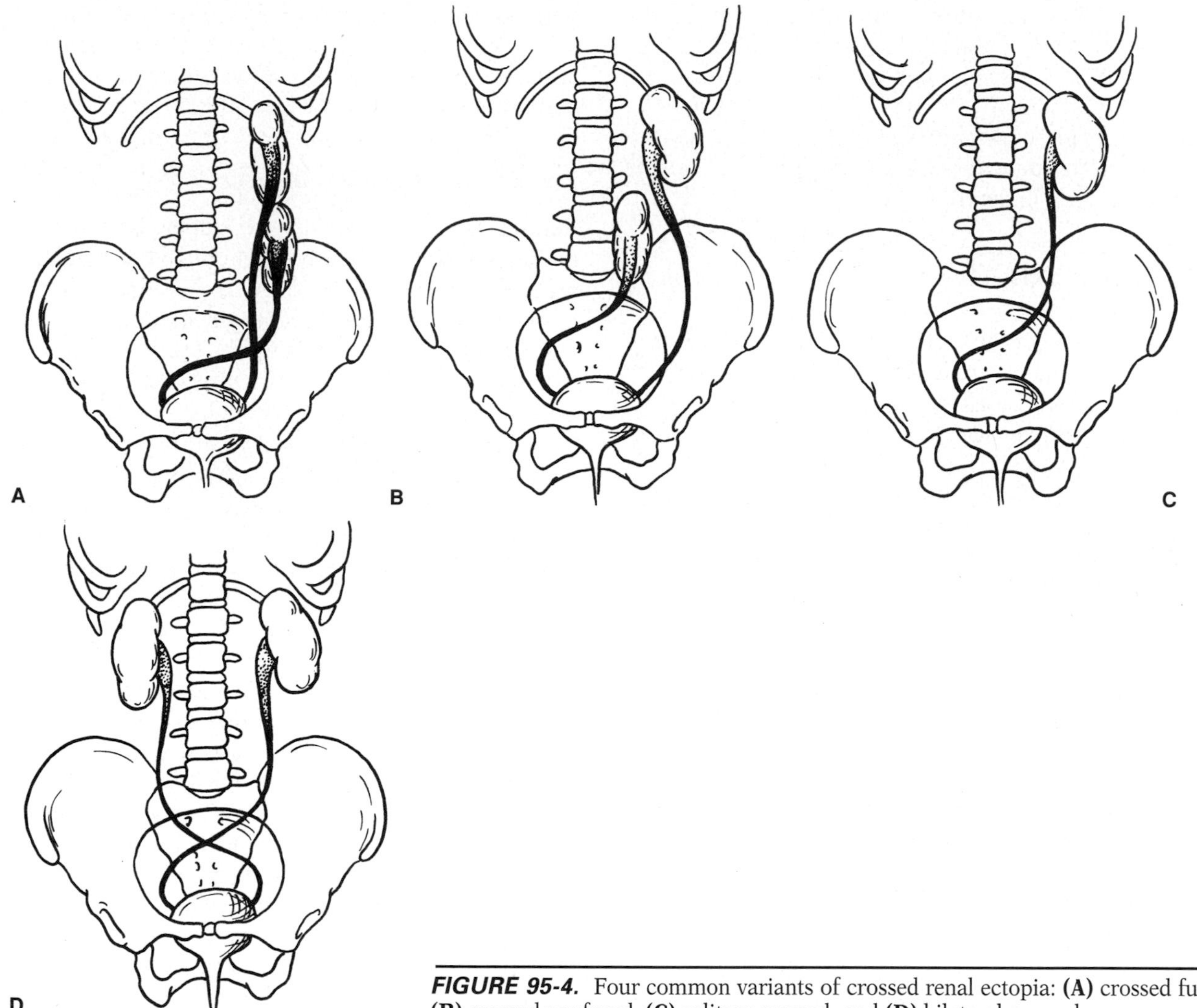

FIGURE 95-4. Four common variants of crossed renal ectopia: **(A)** crossed fused, **(B)** crossed nonfused, **(C)** solitary crossed, and **(D)** bilateral crossed.

which the kidney is opposite the sacrum, is the most common type (1 per 3,000). Additional ascent yields *lumbar* (near the sacral promontory) and *abdominal* (above the iliac crest) variants. Because of its different embryologic origin, the adrenal gland is normally positioned, regardless of the position of the kidney.

Ectopic kidneys often are dysmorphic and smaller than normal, yet most are asymptomatic despite their abnormal location. Vascularity typically emanates from anomalous branches of the adjacent great vessels. Presentations include hydronephrosis, obstruction, calculi, infection, vague abdominal pain, and posttraumatic hematuria. Moieties positioned over the sacrum may be difficult to visualize. Renal scintigraphy, computed tomography (CT), and ultrasonography are other options in imaging that can be used to make the diagnosis.

Other anomalies (up to 85%) commonly occur with ectopic kidneys (Table 95-2). Because ipsilateral vesicoureteral reflux is a frequent finding (70%), voiding cystourethrography is recommended to complete the workup

TABLE 95-2 Common Associations with Ectopic Kidney.

Musculoskeletal
Vertebral, rib anomalies
Cranial asymmetry
Absent bones
Urologic
Vesicoureteral reflux
UPJ[a] obstruction
Contralateral agenesis
Genital
Male patients:
Undescended testis
Hypospadias
Urethral duplication
Female patients:
Uterine or vaginal anomalies, atresia, agenesis
Other
Cardiovascular, gastrointestinal

[a]UPJ, ureteral pelvic junction.

of affected children. In addition, the contralateral kidney is abnormal in as many as 50% of patients, causing some investigators to implicate a teratogen in the etiology. Finally, the high incidence of müllerian malformations in girls (45%), including duplications of the vagina and a unicornuate or bicornuate uterus, suggests a problem with the ureteral bud early in development.

CYSTIC DISEASES

The nomenclature of the more common cystic diseases of the kidney can lead to confusion (Table 95-3). The terms *polycystic* and *multicystic* are not synonymous. Instead, polycystic kidney disease (PKD) refers to one of three conditions, two of which are genetically determined and the third acquired. In contrast, the designation of multicystic kidney denotes a histologically distinct entity that is not heritable and generally is devoid of accompanying systemic manifestations.

Polycystic Kidney Disease

Although differing in many ways, the three variants of PKD share the common denominator of cystic development. Theories abound for their appearance, although each remains unproven. Contributions of epithelial proliferation, reversal of the normal secretory–absorptive polarity of tubule cells, and basement membrane abnormalities and nephrotoxins—both exogenous and from endogenous errors of metabolism—all have been implicated by ongoing work.

Although general patterns do exist, the manifestations of PKD comprise a spectrum that can occur across the ages. As a result, its subclassifications (autosomal recessive, autosomal dominant, and acquired) are typically based on modality of acquisition rather than cystic type, their distribution, or the age at presentation (7).

TABLE 95-3 Cystic Disease of the Kidney.

Genetic
Autosomal recessive (infantile) polycystic kidneys
Autosomal dominant (adult) polycystic kidneys
Juvenile nephronophthisis–medullary cystic disease complex
Juvenile nephronophthisis (autosomal recessive)
Medullary cystic disease (autosomal dominant)
Congenital nephrosis (autosomal recessive)
Familial hypoplastic glomerulocystic kidney disease (autosomal dominant)
Cysts associated with multiple malformation syndromes
Nongenetic
Multicystic kidney (multicystic dysplasia)
Multilocular cyst (multilocular cystic adenoma)
Simple cyst
Medullary sponge kidneys (less than 5% inherited)
Sporadic glomerulocystic kidney disease
Acquired renal cystic disease
Calyceal diverticulum (pyelogenic cyst)

Autosomal Recessive Disease

Autosomal recessive polycystic kidney disease (ARPKD) is typically diagnosed during childhood, although it can present in adolescence. The terms *infantile* or *juvenile* have been discouraged because the dominantly transmitted variant, or so-called "adult" PKD, can also occur in children. ARPKD is an uncommon condition whose incidence ranges from 1 in 6,000 to 1 in 40,000 in different series. In keeping with its pattern of transmission, 25% of the offspring of carriers are expected to be homozygous and manifest the disease. An alternative diagnosis should be entertained if either parent reports having a "cystic kidney." There is no gender predilection. Most cases appear to be due to a defect in a gene localized to chromosome 6p.

Clinical Features

ARPKD is uniformly accompanied by liver abnormalities, ranging from biliary ductal ectasia to periportal fibrosis with portal hypertension and its sequelae. The severity of one organ's involvement is usually inversely related to that of the other. Renal involvement predominates in recessive disease that is diagnosed during the perinatal period, whereas hepatic dysfunction usually accounts for detection in later childhood. The clinical presentations follow accordingly (8).

When the diagnosis is made in utero, fetal kidneys are typically enlarged and diffusely hyperechoic. In some cases, they become large enough to impede labor, making vaginal delivery difficult. Some degree of oligohydramnios is usually present and results in pulmonary hypoplasia. Most perinatal mortality is caused by respiratory failure rather than the sequelae of renal involvement. Neonates who survive present with oliguria, abdominal masses, and some degree of pulmonary compromise. Infants who live past the first month of life generally do satisfactorily, although hypertension is almost universal.

Congenital hepatic fibrosis is usually detected later in development. A third pattern can affect persons at any age and represents a composite of the presentations typical of the newborn and older child. Here, both the liver and kidneys are significantly affected, and the prognosis is uniformly bleak.

Evaluation and Differential Diagnosis

The antenatal diagnosis of ARPKD is suspected when bilateral hyperechoic, enlarged kidneys are seen by ultrasound. Included in the differential diagnosis are multicystic dysplastic kidneys, although they usually show more significant cystic dilatation. There are no known genetic markers for the disease, and its variable presentation can lead to confusion and undue concern. For example, some cases of antenatally diagnosed hyperechoic kidneys demonstrate normal echogenicity and function postnatally. Conversely, fetuses with normal ultrasonic findings early in gestation may demonstrate hyperechoic kidneys typical for ARPKD later in development. In both instances, the presence of oligohydramnios is an ominous prognostic sign.

The kidneys of the neonate with ARPKD are easily palpable, smooth, firm flank masses that are often visible through the anterior abdominal wall. Unlike kidneys affected by massive hydronephrosis, these do not transilluminate because of the small size of the cysts. They also maintain their reniform shape, despite being as much as 10 times normal size. Newborns affected by oligohydramnios may also exhibit Potter facies, including abnormal ears, beaked nose, and recessed chin.

Ultrasound in affected newborns shows bilateral renal enlargement with dense echogenicity. The cysts are tiny and do not usually contain enough fluid to appear cystic, but their ubiquity and interface with solid parenchyma give rise to the signature echo-dense pattern of the disease.

In older children, the discovery of renal disease is usually made during the evaluation of hepatic dysfunction. Ultrasonography provides the best screen of the urinary tract. The kidneys generally are large for age, although there may be some shrinkage from their impressive neonatal size. Their sonographic appearance resembles that of the neonate, but there are often several larger discrete cysts. Medullary streaking is characteristic of PKD when an excretory urogram (IVP) is obtained. CT and magnetic resonance imaging (MRI) may differentiate between the cystic diseases by demonstrating other organ involvement more typical of the dominant variant.

Pathology

The pathologic features of ARPKD mirror its clinical presentation. Regardless of its degree, renal involvement uniformly affects the distal collecting duct of the nephron. Cortical involvement is uniformly severe and gives the parenchyma a bubblelike texture if the renal capsule is stripped away. Older children have less pronounced cortical changes and a tendency to have larger cysts (2 cm).

Nonobstructive biliary ductal ectasia (a mimic of Caroli disease) is present in some degree in every child with ARPKD from birth, although the amount of periportal fibrosis increases with age. This progression probably accounts for the predominance of liver-related symptoms in older patients.

Autosomal Dominant Disease

Autosomal dominant polycystic kidney disease (ADPKD) is far more common than its recessive counterpart and occurs in 1 in 1,000 live births. The mechanisms of renal injury probably begin in utero in more severe cases, and the disease is occasionally diagnosed in younger children. More typically, renal involvement becomes apparent at approximately 40 years of age.

Variable expression occurs among members of the same family. Progeny with the trait have an 80% chance of developing cystic degeneration by their mid-20s. Patients with ADPKD have only a 50% chance of developing end-stage renal disease by their seventieth birthday, even if the disease is diagnosed at an early age (9).

Clinical Features

The diagnosis of ADPKD is made in adults 90% of the time. However, the condition is being recognized more frequently in children as awareness increases and imaging techniques improve. There are differences in the pattern of childhood ADPKD compared with that diagnosed in adults, who usually present with hypertension or flank pain. A comparison of ARPKD and ADPKD is shown in Table 95-4.

Although the disease is more commonly discovered during screening of affected families, antenatal diagnosis is also possible. Perinatal ultrasound findings can mimic ARPKD, with bilaterally enlarged, echo-dense kidneys. Children and adolescents with symptomatic disease may present with hematuria, abdominal masses or urinary infection. With the onset of cystic degeneration, concentrating defects of the urine often precede the gradual rises in blood urea nitrogen and creatinine that occur. Rapidly progressive renal failure, hypertension, proteinuria, and hematuria are also common.

Cystic involvement of other organs is common with ADPKD, but cases that become clinically apparent do so at a later age. These can include cysts of the spleen, thyroid, ovary, endometrium, epididymis, and seminal vesicle and diverticula of the colon. Simple cysts of the liver develop in 30% to 50% of patients, although secondary hepatic dysfunction is rare. Berry aneurysms of the circle of Willis present a more serious threat to affected individuals and are found in 10% to 40% of adults. The hypertension that accompanies the condition further increases the risk of intracranial hemorrhage.

Evaluation and Differential Diagnosis

Early ultrasound screening in affected children usually shows normal kidneys, and renal cysts in fetuses or young children are rarely due to ADPKD. With the onset of the disease, both kidneys typically become enlarged. Multiple, variably sized echo-free cysts are seen, and the kidneys lose their reniform shape, unlike the hyperechoic kidneys of the recessive variant. The picture can be confused with multicystic dysplasia, which is usually unilateral, or with other syndromes that feature cysts of the kidneys.

TABLE 95-4 Comparison of Autosomal Recessive and Dominant Polycystic Kidney Disease.[a]

	ARPKD	ADPKD
Incidence	1 in 6,000–40,000	1 in 1,000
Inheritance	Autosomal recessive	Autosomal dominant, 100% penetrance, variable expression
Age at diagnosis	0–late adolescence	0–35 yr
Imaging	US: Enlarged kidneys with increased echogenicity IVP: Poor function, contrast streaks extend to cortex CT: Evaluate other organ involvement	US: Multiple large, echolucent cysts IVP: Poor function, distorted collecting system CT: Evaluate other organ involvement
Other organs affected	Liver: congenital hepatic fibrosis (with late onset)	Cysts: liver, spleen, thyroid, ovary, endometrium, epididymis, seminal vesicle Vascular: circle of Willis aneurysms
Presentation	Younger: renal failure Older: liver disease	Renal failure
Histologic features	Kidney: collecting duct ectasia Liver: periportal fibrosis	Any portion of nephron involved; multiple cysts of varying size

[a]ARPKD, autosomal recessive polycystic kidney disease; ADPKD, autosomal dominant polycystic kidney disease; US, ultrasound; IVP, intravenous pyelogram; CT, computed tomography.

CT or MRI can be used to assess function and other organ involvement. The cysts of the kidneys appear as radiolucent areas, creating a "Swiss cheese" appearance, and puddling of contrast is seen on delayed films. Retrograde studies risk infection and should be avoided.

Acquired Cystic Disease

Patients in end-stage renal failure often develop acquired cystic kidney disease (ACKD) (10). Uremic toxins have been implicated in cyst growth because bilateral involvement is the rule, and cystic regression is noted after successful transplantations. Because of the 3:1 male predominance, a role for a sex-related endogenous growth factor is postulated.

The incidence of ACKD ranges from 35% to 60% of patients with end-stage renal failure. Cystic degeneration is generally related to the duration of renal failure and length of treatment. Common presentations include fever with infection, flank pain from an intracystic bleed, or hematuria and retroperitoneal hemorrhage, especially in hemodialysis patients on anticoagulants. Cysts develop predominantly in the cortex and reach variable sizes, although most are 0.5 to 1.0 cm in diameter. These cysts can have a lining with hyperplastic epithelial cells having irregular nuclei with prominent nucleoli. These may represent the cellular precursors of renal tumors that arise in as many as 25% of patients with ACKD. Tumors usually are multiple, bilateral, and small (less than 2.5 cm in diameter). Because of their size, they receive the designation of benign adenoma. Larger lesions (greater than 3.0 cm) believed to be renal cell carcinomas (RCCs) are rare.

Multicystic Dysplastic Kidney

Multicystic dysplastic kidney (MCK) is the most common cystic disease of the kidney in newborns and infants. With an incidence of 1 in 4,300 live births, this disease represents about 10% of all fetal uropathies. Unlike their polycystic counterparts, MCKs are not genetically transmitted but, instead, seem to result from an early error in embryogenesis. It is plausible that obstruction alone could account for the insult. Some investigators believe that MCKs represent one end of the spectrum of ureteropelvic junction obstruction. Similar to ectopic kidneys, there is a 2:1 male predominance. Bilateral dysplasia is extremely rare and incompatible with life.

Clinical Features

MCK is the most common abdominal mass in newborns, and until more recently, surgical removal was almost uniformly recommended. With ultrasonography, most MCKs are discovered prenatally and the number of children with MCKs has increased in more recent years. This has altered the understanding of the anomaly's natural history and, in turn, its management. In its initial report, the Multicystic Kidney Registry noted that 54% of 260 MCKs became radiographically undetectable when followed for more than 5 years (11). As cyst fluid is resorbed, the tissue–fluid interface disappears and the kidney progressively decreases in size, which explains why ultrasonic detection is lost. This type of involution is probably responsible for many patients found serendipitously with solitary kidneys before the era of ultrasound.

The risks posed by MCKs that do not involute or by dysplastic renal tissue devoid of its cystic fluid is not fully defined. Urinary infections occur in 2.5%, and hypertension occurs in less than 1% of patients. Nephrogenic rests are more common in MCDK, but the risks for Wilms' tumor are not significantly elevated. It seems reasonable to follow most MCKs serially (every 3 to 6 months during the first year and once a year thereafter) until involution occurs. Afterward, periodic checks of the blood pressure and urine are appropriate. Nephrectomy is reserved for the uncommon cases that are symptomatic because of size, infection, and hypertension or that enlarge or show atypical cystic changes on ultrasonic follow-up.

Evaluation and Differential Diagnosis

Ultrasound usually is diagnostic, although differentiation from obstructive hydronephrosis can be difficult. In contrast to hydronephrosis, which usually manifests with one large central sonolucent area (the pelvis) in communication with multiple smaller peripheral cysts (the calyces), MCKs show multiple cysts of varying sizes that fail to communicate. Typically, there is no identifiable renal parenchyma or centrally located renal pelvis and no uptake of radionuclide on the affected side. When function is seen, the kidney probably is obstructed rather than dysplastic. In poorly functioning kidneys, the decision to reconstruct rather than remove is sometimes not made until the parenchyma can be assessed at exploration. Another option with marginal function is to place a nephrostomy tube to see whether any recovery from obstruction occurs. A voiding cystourethrogram is also obtained to complete the evaluation of the urinary tract. Reflux is found in 30% of contralateral solitary kidneys. In addition, contralateral hydronephrosis is fairly common and places the patient at risk if obstruction is present.

Other Cystic Conditions

Juvenile Nephronopthisis—Medullary Cystic Disease

Juvenile nephronophthisis (JN) and medullary cystic disease (MCD) were initially described separately, but generally are designated as a "complex" because of their anatomic and clinical similarities. Whereas about 300 cases have been reported, the two differ mainly in age at presentation and mode of transmission. An etiology of the complex remains unclear, but a primary defect of the tubular basement membrane may be at fault.

Clinical Features

The diagnosis of MCD is typically made after the third decade of life and is transmitted in an autosomal dominant pattern. In contrast, JN presents before 20 years of age and is passed in an autosomal recessive fashion. Although less common, JN accounts for 10% to 20% of adolescent renal failure. Consanguineous mating is often recognized in affected families. JN is also more frequently involved in syndromes such as *renal–retinal dysplasia*, where retinitis pigmentosa accompanies the cystic changes of the kidney. Other common extrarenal manifestations include liver fibrosis, mental retardation, cerebellar ataxia, and skeletal abnormalities.

Despite these differences, both conditions share several clinical characteristics. Concentrating defects are predictable and occur in more than 80% of cases. Not surprisingly, polyuria and polydipsia are the usual presenting symptoms. Although less severe than true nephrogenic diabetes insipidus, vasopressin resistance exists and sodium replacement often becomes necessary. Infection, calculi, and hypertension are all uncommon.

Evaluation

The diagnosis of JN-MDC is sometimes one of exclusion, especially early in the disease process, when renal imaging results are usually normal. An index of suspicion should be raised by the clinical picture and family history. Later in the course of the condition, multiple small medullary cysts can be appreciated by ultrasound. Other studies are of little value in the face of marginal renal function. As with ultrasonography, renal biopsy findings may be normal early on, although most patients eventually develop interstitial nephritis and atrophic tubular dilatation from the distal convolutions and collecting tubules.

Prognosis

Progression to end-stage renal disease is predictable, and dialysis is usually required within 5 to 10 years after making the diagnosis. In the interim, therapy is supportive. Renal transplantation is an option, provided related donors are well screened to rule out the presence of the same condition in a transplanted kidney.

Medullary Sponge Kidney

Medullary sponge kidneys are affected by *collecting duct ectasia*. As a result, numerous small cysts are found at the papillary tips of the renal pyramids. Unlike JN-MDC, however, medullary sponge kidneys are not an inherited disorder. The disease, whose etiology is unknown, is usually bilateral. Although renal function remains stable throughout life, symptoms are common. Most are discovered after 20 years of age, but childhood disease does occur. Microlithiases form in 60% of patients with sponge kidneys because of stasis, mild acidification defects, and hypercalcuria (30%). Renal colic from their passage is the most common presentation of the condition. Hematuria and urinary infection can also occur.

The cystic dilatations that result are usually too small (1 to 5 mm) to be appreciated by ultrasound, although hyperechogenicity from small calculi may be seen. Instead, excretory urography remains the mainstay of diagnosis. A "shotgun pellet" distribution of calcification on the plain film and contrast puddling in dilated tubules is pathognomonic for the disease. Surgery is rarely indicated, and medical management is directed at prevention of calculi and urinary infections.

Simple Cysts

The management of simple cysts in children has changed dramatically because of increased recognition and a better understanding of their natural history. In the past, surgery was the accepted therapy for the entity. It is now understood that true simple cysts can occur in children of any age, including neonates, and that their incidence increases with age.

Most simple cysts are found during the workup of some other urologic problem. The average age at presentation is 4 years. Other cysts occasionally present as an abdominal mass or with hypertension. Simple cysts are usually single and unilateral. Multiple or bilateral cystic changes suggest a different diagnosis such as PKD.

Ultrasound alone is usually diagnostic. Simple cysts should be smooth walled and filled with anechoic fluid. Exceptions to these criteria should cause concern. The most important differential to exclude is a cystic Wilms' tumor variant. Multilocular cysts and calyceal diverticula can also resemble simple cysts. An upper pole location raises the possibility of a duplicated system associated with an ureterocele or ectopic ureter. Excretory urography can help rule out collecting system anomalies. CT, needle aspiration, and even open exploration are sometimes necessary to confirm a diagnosis if the criteria of simple cyst is not met. When the diagnosis is made in a child, periodic surveillance is all that is necessary to rule out significant change.

Calyceal Diverticulum

A calyceal diverticulum is a cystic cavity peripherally located and connected to an otherwise normal minor calyx. Most are in the upper pole, but they can occur anywhere in the kidney. Multiple diverticula are uncommon. Many are also associated with reflux in children. An acquired form of the anomaly is described, which may result from inflammation, obstruction, or trauma. Calyceal diverticula are rare anomalies found at a rate of about 0.03%. Most are usually discovered incidentally. They are prone to leave affected patients more susceptible to urinary infections, calculi, and hematuria as a consequence of stasis.

HYPOPLASIA

Small kidneys having a reduced number of nephrons are termed *hypoplastic*. Anatomically, the reduction can be global or segmental (the Ask-Upmark kidney). Inadequate ureteral bud branching and an aberrant interaction with the renal blastema are the presumed etiology. The differential diagnosis includes renal dysplasia and scarring from pyelonephritis.

The unilateral hypoplastic kidney is usually asymptomatic and incidentally discovered. Bilateral maldevelopment is rare. Renal failure results if there are insufficient nephrons to maintain metabolic homeostasis. Hypertension is uncommon with hypoplasia and, in the unilateral setting, more often is indicative of reflux nephropathy.

TUMORS

Most primary renal tumors in childhood are Wilms' tumors. These are discussed in detail in Chapter 35. Renal cell carcinoma (RCC) accounts for less than 10% of childhood renal tumors. The median age at presentation (11 years) is older than that of Wilms' tumor, although RCC occasionally occurs during the first few years of life. During the second decade, the incidence of RCC gradually exceeds that of Wilms' tumor. Most cases are sporadic, but a familial variant caused by a translocation of chromosomes 3 and 8 has been described.

The presentation in children is similar to that in adults, with the exception of the absence of paraneoplastic syndromes often seen with RCC in older age groups. Abdominal or flank pain with gross hematuria typically occur. Fever, weight loss, and failure to thrive are also common. Ultrasonography demonstrates a solid renal mass and provides the best assessment of renal vein and caval involvement. CT provides better anatomic resolution of the extent of the tumor. The metastatic workup evaluates for pulmonary and skeletal disease and includes a chest CT and bone scan.

Prognosis is related to the stage of disease and age at presentation. Localized tumors (stage I) and children younger than 11 years of age have the most favorable outcome. Like adult disease, grade and histopathologic characteristics are less reliable indicators of outcome. Surgery is the mainstay of therapy in children, and an estimated 50% can be cured by radical nephrectomy. Chemotherapy or hormonal manipulation has been ineffective, whereas the benefits of immunotherapy remain unproven. Radiation is used to provide palliation, particularly for bony metastases.

Other Renal Tumors

Other primary malignant tumors of the kidney in children are even less common than RCC. Rhabdomyosarcoma and leiomyosarcoma have been described, and neuroblastoma may involve the kidney primarily. Transitional cell carcinomas of the collecting system are rare in children, although benign fibroepithelial polyps are common. Hematuria and urinary obstruction result. Other benign tumors also arise from fibrous, lymphatic, and vascular elements of the kidney. One example is hemangiopericytoma, a rare renin-secreting tumor that occasionally causes juvenile hypertension.

Secondary renal involvement also occurs, especially with the lymphoproliferative disorders. Lymphoblastic leukemia and non-Hodgkin's lymphoma are common tumors. Bilateral or diffuse multinodular infiltration of the kidneys strongly suggests this diagnosis. Recognition is important because treatment in these cases is nonsurgical.

VASCULAR CONDITIONS

Renal Vein Thrombosis

Renal vein thrombosis (RVT) in newborns and children results from low-flow vascular states (12). Common causes include maternal diabetes, severe dehydration, nephrotic syndrome, trauma, hypercoagulable states, and perinephric inflammation.

The prognosis for the kidney depends on the acuteness of the thrombosis and the response of its secondary venous outflow. On occlusion of its main renal vein, the left kidney is more resilient than the right because the adrenal, ureteral, gonadal, and lumbar veins vent the elevated renal vein pressure. On the contralateral side, these same veins drain into the vena cava, leaving the right kidney a relatively isolated organ. When the onset is acute, hemorrhagic infarction results from venous congestion and obstruction. Fortunately, RVT is usually unilateral and renal failure is rare, although some degree of uremia and acidosis is seen in most patients.

The classic presentation of RVT in the newborn is gross hematuria with a palpable mass. RVT accounts for 20% of neonatal hematuria. Red blood cells (RBCs), platelets, and fibrin are destroyed in the evolving clot, and thrombocytopenia, anemia, and increased fibrin split products are commonly seen. Other findings at any age can include proteinuria, varicocele, pedal edema if the vena cava is involved, and pulmonary embolism. Ultrasonography is the diagnostic test of choice. In the acute setting, this shows an enlarged kidney without hydronephrosis and distorted internal architecture. Doppler study and renal scintigraphy document significantly decreased blood flow. Excretory urography should be avoided because further dehydration can result from contrast load, and venography is rarely necessary to confirm the diagnosis.

Treatment is directed at correcting metabolic imbalances, azotemia, and dehydration. Prompt diagnosis and correction of these abnormalities is the key to limiting the progression of thrombosis and avoiding bilateral involvement. The prognosis in most cases of RVT is excellent, although the function of many kidneys is impaired, especially when thrombosis affects the right renal vein. The literature is scattered with reports of surgery for RVT. However, the place of surgery, for what is typically small vessel disease, is difficult to defend in the acute setting. Medical management and supportive treatment assume priority. When renovascular hypertension persists, a nephrectomy may become necessary. The use of anticoagulants such as heparin or thrombolytic therapy with agents such as streptokinase or urokinase remains controversial.

Renal Artery Thrombosis

Renal artery thrombosis (RAT) affects two distinct populations of children (13). The first and more common are neonates with umbilical artery catheters. Mechanical factors such as catheter tip location above the renal arteries and prolonged or traumatic placement are associated with an increased incidence of thrombosis, as is the use of hyperosmolar (i.e., radiographic contrast) or sclerosing agents. Systemic conditions such as low perfusion states and sepsis also increase the tendency to thrombosis. Secondary embolization through a patent ductus arteriosus is another common etiology in newborns.

RAT is suspected in any neonate with hematuria who has had a recent umbilical artery catheter or who has a heart murmur. Small cortical infarcts may not result in other symptoms, but larger ones can cause proteinuria, decreased renal function, leukocytosis, and fever. Hypertension can initiate congestive heart failure if the condition goes unrecognized. Ultrasonography may show a decrease in size of the affected kidneys, whereas high-resolution color Doppler study is gradually replacing umbilical artery angiography and radionuclide perfusion studies as the diagnostic study of choice.

Because the neonate poorly tolerates hypertension and congestive failure, supportive medical treatment must be aggressive and initiated promptly. This includes immediate removal of the offending catheter. Fortunately, most thromboses affect only one kidney and the outcome is usually good. Renal recovery is related to the extent of arterial compromise and the degree of intrarenal collateral circulation. Dialysis may be required if renal failure is present in the rare case of bilateral thromboses. Surgery or thrombolytic agents have been of equivocal value and are avoided for unilateral conditions. Nephrectomy is a last resort when medical management fails.

The second group affected by RAT is older children with preexisting conditions, such as heart disease (particularly after cardiac catheterization) or fibromuscular dysplasia of the renal arteries. In addition, the pediatric kidney is particularly susceptible to vascular trauma with sudden deceleration because of its relative mobility. The resultant shear forces can raise intimal flaps that lead to thrombosis.

Because hematuria may be absent, a high index of suspicion is important. Treatment is surgical, although renal viability depends on early recognition of the condition.

Arteriovenous Malformations

Renal arteriovenous (AV) malformations can be either congenital or acquired, with the latter accounting for about 75% of the cases. Trauma accounts for most, and usually results in a solitary communication between a vein and artery. In contrast, congenital anomalies are tortuous vascular collections having multiple communications within the vascular supply. Symptoms depend on location and size. Most patients have an abdominal bruit, and large fistulas can cause cardiac failure or hypertension from progressive renal ischemia.

Management depends on clinical significance. Most AV malformations are asymptomatic and never come to attention. Others may be responsible for minute amounts of microscopic hematuria or sporadic bouts of gross hematuria. Vascular instability or posttraumatic massive blood loss warrant more immediate attention. If time allows, contrast angiography is the diagnostic test of choice. Embolization is usually effective, although partial or total nephrectomy is sometimes necessary.

HEMATURIA

Hematuria is a common problem, with 3% to 5% of children expected to have at least one episode in their lifetime (14,15). Although hematuria can be the harbinger of a serious nephrologic or urologic problem, most workups yield negative results.

Etiology

There are more than 100 causes of hematuria, most of which are medical in origin. Two major designations based on the morphologic features of RBCs can be assigned without reviewing the individual entities. *Glomerular hematuria* distorts cellular morphologic features and tends to be nephrologic in origin, whereas intact RBCs typically accompany *nonglomerular* etiologies. These are largely urologic and related to the collecting system and tubules. Common causes are listed in Table 95-5.

TABLE 95-5 Common Causes of Hematuria in Childhood.

Mimics
Porphyrins
Beets, blackberries, red food dye
Pyridium
Hematologic
Coagulopathies
Renal vein and artery thrombosis
Sickle cell disease
Glomerular diseases
Hemolytic-uremic syndrome
IgA nephropathy
Poststreptococcal glomerulonephiritis
Postinfectious nephritis
Stones and hypercalcuria
Anatomic abnormalities and tumors
Trauma
Exercise

Glomerular Hematuria

Glomerular injury can result from immunologic, inherited, or coagulation disorders. Immunologic injury is the most common and results from the localization of circulating antibody–antigen immune complexes or interaction of antibody with in situ antigen. The process is called *glomerulonephritis* to typify the resulting inflammation of the glomerular capillaries. The pathologic manifestations range from transient proliferation of the glomerular endothelial and mesangial cells caused by immune complex and matrix accumulation, to full-blown fibrin deposition in Bowman's space (crescents) and glomerular sclerosis.

IgA Nephropathy (Berger's Disease)

Berger's disease is perhaps the most common nephrologic cause of pediatric hematuria. The disease usually presents with recurrent painless hematuria after exercise, respiratory virus, or fever. The bleeding typically resolves and has a favorable prognosis. Biopsy confirmation yields IgA deposits within the glomerular mesangium. Crescentic glomerular changes, later age at presentation, proteinuria, and hypertension are less favorable signs.

Poststreptococcal Glomerulonephritis

Poststreptococcal glomerulonephritis is extremely common and occurs 7 to 30 days after bouts of impetigo or acute pharyngitis caused by group A β-hemolytic *streptococci*. Tea-colored urine containing red cell casts and heavy proteinuria result. Malaise, hypertension, and edema from hypoalbuminemia also can be present. Antistreptolysin O titers often are nonspecifically elevated, whereas a depressed complement (C3) is more indicative of an active or recent infection. A complete recovery is expected in more than 95% of case with supportive treatment alone. Most proteinuria subsides within a few weeks. That which persists warrants an in-depth nephrologic workup.

Hemolytic-uremic Syndrome

The hemolytic-uremic syndrome is composed of the triad of renal failure, hemolytic anemia, and thrombocytopenia, and is believed to be autoimmune in origin. It usually follows a prodrome of intestinal flu-like illness in young children. This is the single most common cause of hematuria among young children. Dialysis may be required to treat the consequent renal failure, although many patients fully recover.

Nonglomerular Hematuria

Tubulointerstitial Disorders

Patients with tubulointerstitial disorders, including the infantile PKD and MCDs discussed earlier, occasionally present with hematuria. Congenital abnormalities of tubular uptake or excretion, including renal tubular acidosis (type 1), cystinuria, and oxalosis, can also be implicated. Acquired tubular disorders have numerous causes that include nephrotoxic agents (aminoglycosides, penicillin derivatives, cimetidine, lithium, and cyclosporine), radiation nephritis, infections, or immune rejection in transplanted kidneys. Nonsteroidal antiinflammatory agents are a particular problem in this regard and cause hematuria in one-third of patients who abuse the medication. The term *interstitial nephritis* refers to inflammation between the glomeruli in the areas surrounding the tubules. The pathogenesis remains poorly understood, although hypersensitivity and an immune response may initiate the inflammatory changes seen. In addition to hematuria, proteinuria and urinary concentration defects result.

Hypercalcuria

Hypercalcuria is an increasingly detected cause of microscopic hematuria. The site of bleeding remains undefined. Patients affected with the disorder may be prone to urolithiasis in later life, which is also included in the differential diagnosis. Furosemide (Lasix) increases calcium excretion. Infants who receive this medication for treatment of pulmonary conditions are prone to hypercalcuria and secondary calcium phosphate stone formation.

Vascular Causes

Vascular causes include sickle cell disease, RVT, RAT, and AV malformations. Patients with bleeding disorders and coagulopathies are also prone to bleeds of the urinary tract.

Urinary Tract Infection

Urinary tract infection (UTI) is the most common urologic cause of hematuria.

Other Common Causes

Other causes of nonglomerular hematuria include tumors, trauma, urinary calculi, nephropathy resulting from vesicoureteral reflux, and upper urinary tract obstruction with hydronephrosis. Lower tract anomalies include a variety of urethral abnormalities, including valves, polyps, stricture, prolapse, and meatal stenosis. Perineal irritation and diaper rash are sometimes implicated. A common cause is *urethrorrhagia*, a nonspecific inflammation of the bulbar urethra that causes spotting in the underwear of prepubertal boys. Culture results are negative, and the condition is self-limited in most cases. Toilet dysfunction and retentive behavior have been implicated as a possible cause. In theory, the high voiding pressures generated by the bladder, after prolonged durations between voiding, result in irritation of the urethra immediately below the urinary sphincter. Urethroscopy is reserved for boys whose spotting lasts more than 6 months, unless another cause is suspected. In rare cases, urethral stricture can result from the inflammation.

Evaluation

Gross hematuria in the newborn period is regarded as an emergency because renal vein thrombosis and renal arterial thrombosis represent potentially life-threatening conditions. Seen later in life, it often suggests a urologic cause and demands further evaluation, although "pseudohematuria" from urinary pigments and other causes of bloody diapers should be ruled out. Some RBCs are expected in normal urine as the body rids itself of more than 1 million corpuscles each day. More than five RBCs per high-power field in two or three samples warrant further evaluation. Tea-colored urine or microscopic hematuria usually implicates a nephrologic cause. Concomitant proteinuria or cellular casts are more worrisome findings that suggest renal disease. Urinary tumors, the most common cause of hematuria in adults, are uncommon in children. As a result, the diagnostic approach differs markedly in children, where cystoscopy is rarely indicated (Fig. 95-5).

A thorough history and physical examination are performed in every child and may aid in the diagnosis. Otherwise, the microscopic and dipstick analysis of the urine is the cornerstone of the evaluation. Additional laboratory and radiographic testing is directed at differentiating the few serious entities from the remainder, which have no long-term sequelae. Although some variability exists, a urine culture, blood urea nitrogen, creatinine, streptozyme (antistreptozyme O titer), serum complement, and serum protein studies are usually obtained. A spot calcium–creatinine ratio is also used to rule out hypercalcuria, with a ratio of greater than 0.21 deserving further quantification with a 24-hour urine collection.

Ultrasonography provides the best screen of the urinary tract. This noninvasive inexpensive test can provide a wealth of information. The bladder, in addition to the kidneys, should be evaluated. Ultrasound is normal in most instances of uncomplicated hematuria. When the screening is abnormal, other studies (e.g., CT, voiding cystourethrography, renal scintigraphy, excretory urography) become necessary. Pathologic diagnosis can be instrumental to directing therapy of some disease processes, and renal biopsies are used to evaluate persistent

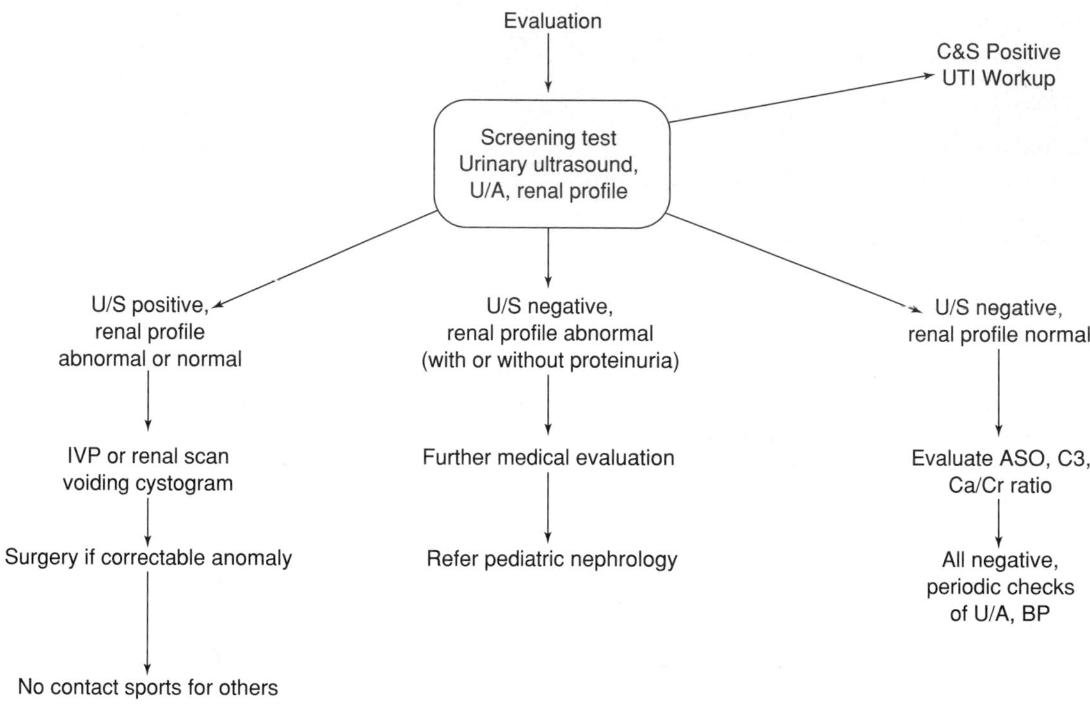

FIGURE 95-5. Algorithm for evaluation of hematuria in children. U/A, urinalysis; U/S, ultrasound; IVP, intravenous pyelogram; C&S, culture and sensitivity; UTI, urinary tract infection; ASO, antistreptolysin O; C3, third component of complement; Ca/Cr, calcium/creatinine; BP, blood pressure.

hematuria, associated significant proteinuria, or decreasing renal function that occur in the absence of a known cause.

PROTEINURIA

Small amounts (up to 150 mg per 24 hours) of protein can be found in the urine of otherwise healthy children. Dipsticks are sensitive for albumin, but may miss lower weight proteins, including Bence Jones protein and γ-globulins. As a consequence, persistent proteinuria should be quantified with a timed urine collection.

Etiology

Nonpathologic proteinuria is usually serendipitously found. The most common cause is orthostatic, generally considered a benign condition. The diagnosis is established by finding normal protein excretion in a supine urine collection, but increased protein excretion while upright. First-voided specimens are compared with those from later in the day after activity. If both specimens contain protein, further evaluation is necessary. Other benign causes include fever in excess of 38.3°C and exercise, which can also increase hemoglobin and RBCs in the urine of some patients. *Pathologic proteinuria* can be caused by either tubular or glomerular disease. Glomerulonephritis is the most common and is usually nonselective in its protein loss.

Nephrotic Syndrome (Nephrosis)

The most serious form of proteinuria manifests as the nephrotic syndrome, characterized by the appearance of edema, proteinuria, hypoalbuminemia, and hyperlipidemia (16). Most cases are idiopathic and are accompanied by minimal changes in the glomeruli. The remaining cases are attributed to some form of glomerulonephritis. The loss of albumin can cause a decrease in plasma oncotic pressure. Edema appears when serum albumin levels fall below 2.5 g per dL and protein losses generally exceed 2 g per 24 hours. Lipid elevations result from increased liver synthesis in the face of hypoproteinuria and diminished levels of lipoprotein lipase, which normally clears lipid from the plasma.

The diagnosis of nephrotic syndrome is made on the basis of the 24-hour urine collection and evaluation of serum albumin, cholesterol, and triglyceride levels. Most idiopathic disease responds to steroids. Renal biopsy is indicated in patients who do not respond and in older children, who more commonly have glomerulonephritis. In addition to steroids and sodium restriction, diuretics, intravenous albumin, antihypertensive agents, and cyclophosphamide are occasionally necessary for fulminant cases or those that continue to cause serious relapses. Fortunately, most children respond to steroids and have no residual renal dysfunction, although recurrent episodes are common until the second decade of life.

URINARY TRACT INFECTION

Clinical Presentation

Most patients with a UTI have symptoms that suggest a specific diagnosis. In contrast, symptoms of newborns are typically nonspecific. Failure to thrive and lethargy are worrisome findings, whereas high fevers are uncommon. Infants and younger children arrive with the more classic signs of fever, malodorous urine, dysuria, urinary frequency, lethargy, and gastrointestinal symptoms, including nausea and vomiting. Pyelonephritis usually causes vague abdominal discomfort rather than localized flank pain. Even without infection, children with vesicoureteral reflux, the most common cause of UTIs, may describe abdominal or flank discomfort. When reflux has gone undetected and renal scarring has occurred from significant infection, children can arrive at any age with renal insufficiency, hypertension, and impaired somatic growth.

A urinalysis should be included in the evaluation of any patient who presents with fever or malaise. Unfortunately, urinary infections often are overlooked, and their ill-defined presentations are mistakenly attributed to otitis media, viral gastroenteritis, respiratory infections, or fever of undetermined origin. Until a proper diagnosis is made, severe renal damage can continue, especially if reflux is present. If fever is present, the likelihood of having vesicoureteral reflux or some other anatomic abnormality (and presumably, pyelonephritis) is greatly increased. Lower tract infections alone (e.g., cystitis) rarely cause serious systemic complaints or symptoms.

Verification

When a UTI is suspected from the clinical history, a culture becomes essential to making the diagnosis. Microscopic study alone might not provide a valid assessment of the urine, although the combined used of dipsticks increases sensitivity.

Evaluation

Some studies suggest that most (80% to 95%) children who have one UTI are highly likely to have another. As a consequence, it seems reasonable to rule out an anatomic abnormality as early as possible in children who are susceptible to infections. When no anatomic anomaly is present, the tendency to infections is usually related to retentive urinary behavior and improper toilet hygiene. However, the diagnostic yield is significant. For example, vesicoureteral reflux is found in 29% to 50% of children with a UTI. About 30% of these patients already have some evidence of renal parenchymal scarring. Unfortunately, there are no reliable clinical features of their infections that distinguish children with reflux or other anatomic abnormalities from those without. Even in the absence of fever, renal scarring can occur after only a single UTI. These data amplify the need for a thorough evaluation of any child believed to have a urinary infection.

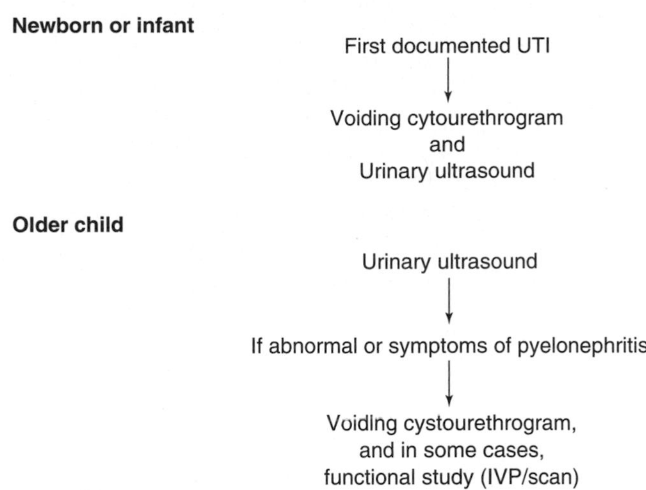

FIGURE 95-6. Algorithm for evaluation of urinary tract infection (UTI) in children. IVP, intravenous pyelogram.

The evaluation of a child believed to have reflux is tailored to the individual according to the age, gender, and clinical history (17,18). Any child younger than 5 years of age with a valid, clearly documented UTI should be evaluated for reflux. Children with a UTI and fever, regardless of age, should also be evaluated. In addition, boys of any age with a UTI should be assessed radiographically for the presence of reflux, unless they are sexually active or have a history of urologic disease. An algorithm for evaluation is shown in Fig. 95-6. Although this can be tailored somewhat for age and symptom complex, the combination of a voiding cystourethrogram and ultrasonography provides the best screen. In the past, invasive studies such as a voiding cystourethrogram were postponed until the urine culture result is negative. However, there are children who reflux only when they are infected, and some clinicians have begun to test soon after an infection is diagnosed.

Treatment

Treatment is directed at the offending organism based on culture and sensitivity results. Infections should be treated for 7 to 10 days regardless of severity, especially because the distinction between upper and lower tract infections is sometimes difficult to make. Studies show that the incidence and severity of renal scarring can be decreased by prompt identification and treatment of pyelonephritis. Radiographic evaluation is usually deferred until the acute phases of the infection have waned. Treatment of the individual entities that might be associated with UTIs, including vesicoureteral reflux, is discussed elsewhere in this text.

REFERENCES

1. Guerriero WG. Etiology, classification and management of renal trauma. *Surg Clin North Am* 1989;68:1071.
2. Blankenship JC, Cox CE, Chauhan R, et al. Prognostic value of renal trauma grading system and importance of follow-up imaging studies for blunt renal trauma. *J Urol* 1999;161(suppl):14A.
3. Arger PH, Coleman BG, Mintz MC, et al. Routine fetal genitourinary tract screening. *Radiology* 1986;156:485.
4. Steinhart JM, Kuhn JP, Eisenberg B, et al. Ultrasound screening of healthy infants for urinary tract abnormalities. *Pediatrics* 1988;82:609.
5. Emanuel B, Nachman R, Aronson N, et al. Congenital solitary kidney: a review of 74 cases. *Am J Dis Child* 1974;127:17.
6. Cook WA, Stephens FD. Fused kidneys: morphologic study and theory of embryogenesis. *Birth Defects* 1977;13:327.
7. Anderson GA, Degroot D, Lawson RK. Polycystic renal disease. *Urology* 1993;42:358.
8. Gang Kaplan BS, Fay J, Shaw V, et al. Autosomal recessive polycystic kidney disease. *Pediatr Nephrol* 1989;3:43.
9. Gabow PA. Autosomal dominant polycystic kidney disease. *N Eng J Med* 1992;339:332.
10. Querfeld U, Schneble F, Wradzidlo W, et al. Acquired cystic kidney disease before and after renal transplantation. *J Pediatr* 1992;121:61.
11. Wacksman J, Phipps L. Report of the multicystic kidney registry: preliminary findings. *J Urol* 1993;150:1870.
12. Keating MA, Althausen AF. The clinical spectrum of renal vein thrombosis. *J Urol* 1985;133:938.
13. Kavaler E, Hensle TW. Renal artery thrombosis in the newborn infant. *Urology* 1997;50:282.
14. Schroeder PL, Francisco LL. Evaluating hematuria in children. *Postgrad Med* 1990;88:171.
15. Diven SC, Travus LB. A practical primary care approach to hematuria in children. *Pediatr Nephrol* 2000;14:65–72.
16. Kelsch R, Sedman AB. Nephrotic syndrome. *Pediatr Rev* 1993;14:30–38.
17. AAP Committee on Quality Improvement. Practice parameter: the diagnosis, treatment and evaluation of the initial urinary tract infection in febrile infants and children. *Pediatrics* 1999;103:843.
18. Koff SA, Wagner TT, Jayanthi VR. The relationship among dysfunction elimination syndromes, primary vesicoureteral reflux and urinary tract infections in children. *J Urol* 1998;160:1019.

Chapter 96

Upper Urinary Tract

John S. Wiener

The upper urinary tract has the sole function of transporting urine from its origin (the nephrons within the kidney) to its storage organ (the bladder). Alteration of this transport of urine can be congenital or acquired. Maldevelopment of the upper urinary tract is relatively common and results in numerous congenital anomalies that are increasingly being detected prior to birth. Acquired diseases of the upper urinary tract are less common in children than in adults, but include urolithiasis and neoplasia. Manifestation of upper urinary tract pathology is usually related to obstruction and may be silent or painful, can be detrimental to the kidney and its multiple functions, and may promote infection secondary to stasis of urine. Infection of the urinary tract is typically localized to the bladder (*cystitis*) or renal parenchyma (*pyelonephritis*); the upper urinary tract may act as a conduit, allowing bacteria to ascend from the former to the latter. Retrograde flow of urine from the bladder into the upper urinary tract (*vesicoureteral reflux*), thus, can increase the likelihood of pyelonephritis.

ANATOMY OF THE UPPER URINARY TRACT

The upper urinary tract begins where the collecting ducts of the nephrons within each renal pyramid coalesce at a papilla and empty into a *calyx*. There are typically eight or nine calyces in each kidney, and these are usually grouped in sets in the upper, mid, and lower segments of the kidney (1). The *renal pelvis* fills most of the renal sinus in the center of the kidney and funnels medially and downward into the ureter across the *ureteropelvic junction*. The normal renal pelvis is usually wholly contained within the renal sinus, but can extend medially beyond the renal contour (termed an *extrarenal pelvis*.)

The *ureter* is intimately related to the peritoneum, psoas major muscle, and numerous blood vessels and nerves as it courses through the retroperitoneum from the ureteropelvic junction to the *ureterovesical junction*. The ureter contains a rich vascular plexus fed from multiple sources, including the renal artery, aorta, gonadal arteries, iliac arteries, and superior and inferior vesical arteries (1). Venous and lymphatic drainage are similar. Nervous input comes from multiple plexuses, including renal, aortic, superior hypogastric, and pelvic. Visceral pain caused by distention or irritation of the ureter is referred to somatic distribution along corresponding spinal segments and may manifest as pain in the flank, abdomen, groin, or scrotum and labia (2,3). Surgical anatomy of the ureter is simply divided into *upper ureter* (renal pelvis to upper sacral border), *middle ureter* (across the sacroiliac bony landmarks), and *lower ureter* (lower sacral border to bladder). The ureter passes through the muscularis layer of the bladder in an oblique tunnel normally of sufficient length to prevent retrograde flow of urine from the bladder back into the ureter. The ureter opens into the bladder at one of the lateral corners of the *trigone*—the triangular-shaped base of the bladder defined by the points of the two ureteral orifices and the internal urethral orifice.

PHYSIOLOGY OF THE UPPER URINARY TRACT

The muscles of the ureter contract in response to stretch from urine filling, and these contractions transport boluses of urine from the kidney to the bladder. This peristalsis can be seen radiographically on intravenous pyelograms or computed tomography (CT) scans as distinct small boluses of contrast-containing urine within the ureter. Complete opacification of the entire length of the ureter on such studies is not normal and would suggest distal obstruction. Ureteral peristalsis originates with electrical activity in pacemaker cells found in the calyces and is conducted distally via junctions between smooth muscle cells (4). Resting ureteral pressure is only 0 to 5 cm H_2O and rises to 20 to 80 cm H_2O with contraction. This is usually

John S. Wiener: Departments of Surgery and Pediatrics, Duke University, Section of Pediatric Urology, Duke University Medical Center, Durham, North Carolina 27710.

higher than intravesical bladder pressure in the normal state, allowing passage of the urine bolus into the bladder (1,3,5). Obstruction of the flow of urine dilates the walls of the ureter, preventing adequate coaptation and propulsion of the urine distally. This, in turn, stretches the renal pelvis and capsule and may be manifested clinically as renal colic.

EMBRYOLOGY OF THE UPPER URINARY TRACT

At the end of the fourth week of embryonic life, the *ureteral bud* begins as an outgrowth from the *mesonephric (wolffian) duct* near its insertion into the cloaca. The ureteral bud then grows cephalad until it encounters the *metanephros* (Fig. 96-1). A complex interplay between the distal ureteral bud and *metanephric blastema* is responsible for branching of the ureteral bud and its induction of renal development. A multitude of genes have been linked to this process of nephrogenesis, and genetic alterations can result in congenital anomalies of the ureters and kidneys (6,7). Ectopic branching of the ureteral bud can impact the metanephros ectopically, resulting in renal maldevelopment encountered in some congenital upper urinary tract malformations, such as *obstructive uropathies* and *vesicoureteral reflux*. The normal ureteral bud will eventually branch 15 times as it grows radially into the metanephros, forming the renal pelvis, infundibula, and calyces (1). Distally, the ureteral bud and mesonephric duct are incorporated into the cloaca to form the trigone of the bladder and intramural portion of the ureter. The ureteral orifice migrates cranially and laterally, whereas the mesonephric ducts move distally and medially toward the bladder neck and urethra. The distal end of the latter structure becomes the epididymis, vas deferens, seminal vesicle, and ejaculatory duct in males and Gartner's ducts on the anterior vaginal wall in females.

The ureteral bud is initially patent, but becomes obliterated in the sixth week. Two weeks later, recanalization begins in the midureter and extends caudally and cranially so the entire ureter should be patent again by the ninth or tenth week. Timing is critical because urine production commences by the eight to ninth week and will comprise more than 90% of the amniotic fluid by the early second trimester. Delayed recanalization at either end of the ureter can lead to obstruction and altered renal development and may explain why the two most common sites of congenital obstruction are at the ureteropelvic junction (UPJ) and ureterovesical junction (UVJ), respectively. Abnormal early branching of the ureteral bud is fairly common and leads to duplication anomalies of the upper urinary tract. It is estimated that 1 in 125 individuals have partial ureteral duplication (two ureters joining above the bladder with only a single distal ureter entering the bladder), and 1 in 500 have complete ureteral duplication (two separate ureters with separate orifices within the bladder) (8). It should be noted that this does not imply supranumerary kidneys, but merely two separate pelvises and ureters in one kidney on one or both sides. In complete duplication, the ureters cross so the upper pole ureter inserts medially and caudally, and the lower ureteral orifice is more lateral and cranial. The upper pole ureter may insert too far distally (termed *ectopic*) and be obstructed by its opening into the bladder neck, urethra, or mesonephric duct remnants (the reproductive ductal structures in males or Gartner's duct in females). In rare cases in females with complete duplication, continuous lifelong urinary incontinence can occur due to an insertion of the upper pole ureter into the urethra or vagina. The lower pole ureter in completely duplicated systems may reflux due to insufficient muscular backing of the intramural ureter in its far lateral position.

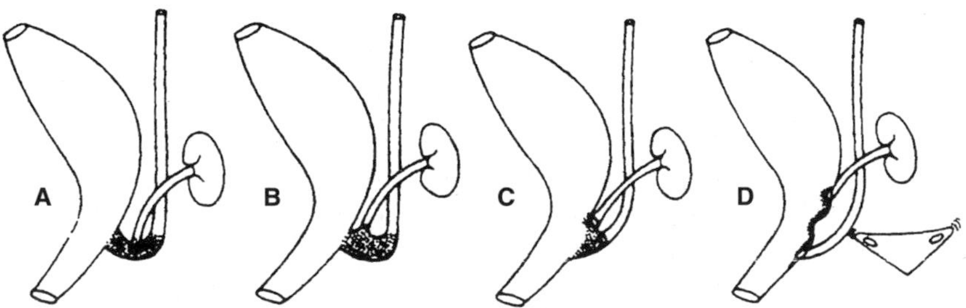

FIGURE 96-1. Embryologic rearrangement and migration of the orifices of the ureteric bud and ureters from the wolffian duct to the urinary tract and formation of the trigone. A single ureter arises from a normal position on the duct **(A)** and migrates to the lateral corner of the trigone **(D)**. **B** and **C** show the expansion of the common excretory duct and wolffian duct into the urethra and bladder. (From Ravitch MM, et al. *Pediatric surgery*, 3rd ed. Chicago: Year Book, 1979:1189, with permission.)

PATHOLOGY OF THE UPPER URINARY TRACT

Pathology of the upper urinary tract is easily classified. Most pathology is due to obstruction, and most *obstructive uropathies* in childhood are congenital. Obstruction during fetal development of the urinary tract may alter development of the ureter and kidney, and compromise ultimate renal function. Acquired obstruction is unusual in childhood, but may be related to iatrogenic causes, neoplasms, or *urolithiasis*. Primary neoplasms of the ureter and renal collecting system in children are exceedingly rare. Finally, *vesicoureteral reflux* is a pathologic entity of the upper urinary tract that facilitates bacterial ascent up into the kidney and can result in recurrent pyelonephritis. In rare cases, reflux and obstruction can be present in the same ureter.

OBSTRUCTIVE UROPATHY

Pathophysiology

Obstruction of the upper urinary tract is usually partial, but can be complete. Complete obstruction destroys renal function eventually; partial obstruction may impair function, but the degree of impairment is dependent on timing of its onset (during prenatal development), chronicity, and degree of obstruction. Most of our knowledge regarding the effects of obstruction stems from research focused on acute obstruction in postnatal models. The classic model of acute unilateral obstruction demonstrates a triphasic response: ureteral pressure and renal blood flow initially increase simultaneously, blood flow then decreases while ureteral pressure remains elevated, and finally both parameters decline (9). As obstruction becomes chronic, the decreased blood flow leads to irreversible declines in glomerular filtration rates and other components of renal function (10,11). Early studies of unilateral ureteral obstuction in a fetal lamb model found that obstruction in the first half of gestation resulted in renal dysplasia, whereas obstruction in the latter half of gestation only caused dilation of the pelvis and calyces (*pelvicaliectasis*) with preservation of histologic appearance (12). In the latter group, the degree of parenchymal atrophy was proportional to the period of obstruction. In other fetal models, it appears that increased pressure in the renal pelvis may not alter renal development; however, reduction of renal blood flow is likely deleterious (10). The fetal ureter may be able to undergo a greater degree of dilation and elongation in response to obstruction than the adult ureter, and this may dampen the pressure effects of obstruction (11). Further complexity in assessing the effects of fetal obstruction exists because normal and hydronephrotic kidneys may function similarly at normal rates of urine production, but diuresis may knock the partially obstructed kidney out of equilibrium (10). What is clear is that higher degrees and longer periods of obstruction are more deleterious to the kidney and that early fetal obstruction can affect renal development.

Prenatal Diagnosis

A generation ago, most uropathies presented with urinary tract infection (UTI) or a palpable mass on physical examination. Hydronephrosis was previously considered the most common cause of abdominal masses in neonates (13). The advent of routine prenatal sonography beginning in the mid-1980s has dramatically changed the presentation of upper urinary tract anomalies in children, so that today abnormal prenatal sonogram is the most common presentation of uropathies (14). Urinary tract dilation is the most common anomaly seen on prenatal sonography, detected in as many as 1% of fetuses, and may represent a significant urologic problem in 20% of those or in 1 out of 500 fetuses (15,16). A commonly accepted threshold for abnormal renal pelvic dilation is an anteroposterior (AP) renal pelvic diameter of 4 mm or greater at less than 33 weeks' gestation and 7 mm or greater beginning at 33 weeks' gestation (17). Additional signs of uropathy on sonography include dilation of the calyces, ureters, and/or bladder; decreased amniotic fluid volume; and abnormal renal parenchyma (e.g., cysts, hyperechogenicity, or cortical thinning). Other abnormalities, including renal duplication and obstructing ureteroceles, can also be seen. Oligohydramnios can be an ominous finding because it may be associated with pulmonary hypoplasia as well as renal insufficiency.

The bladder is visible in the tenth week of gestation, and the kidneys may be noted by 12 to 13 weeks. Urinary tract anomalies have been detected as early as this point. The differential diagnosis of fetal hydronephrosis includes UPJ obstruction, distal ureteral obstruction (due to primary obstructive megaureter, ureteral ectopia, and ureteroceles), multicystic dysplastic kidneys, posterior urethral valves, prune belly syndrome, and vesicoureteral reflux (Table 96-1). Nephropathies unrelated to the upper urinary tract (polycystic kidney disease and renal agenesis) also can be detected (18).

Initially, it was believed that all fetuses with hydronephrosis had obstructive uropathies that required intervention (14). However, the majority of cases of prenatal hydronephrosis have been found to be clinically insignificant (19). Most are unilateral renal pelvic dilation that were the result of transient partial prenatal obstruction and will improve with age. Some cases of severe hydronephrosis will show normal renal function initially, but develop worsening obstruction over time, necessitating surgical correction. Other kidneys suffer damaging effects of obstruction

TABLE 96-1 Uropathies Detectable by Prenatal Sonography

Condition	Frequency
Ureteropelvic junction obstruction	1:2,000
Multicystic dysplastic kidney	1:3,000
Primary ureterovesical junction obstruction	1:10,000
Ectopic ureterocele or ureter	1:10,000
Posterior urethral valves	1:8,000
Prune belly syndrome	1:40,000
Vesicoureteral reflux	1:100

From Cendron M, Elder JS. Perinatal urology. In: Gillenwater JY, Grayhack JT, Howards SS, et al., eds. *Adult and pediatric urology,* 4th ed. Philadelphia: Lippincott Williams & Wilkins, 2002:2041–2127, with permission (18).

in utero and present with irreversibly diminished function at birth. Determining what constitutes true obstruction remains a subject of great debate. It is evident that obstructive uropathies are dynamic, possibly due to continued development of the distal and proximal ends of the ureter during the fetal life and infancy. Maternal progesterone may also play a role as a smooth muscle relaxant. In cases of reflux, hydronephrosis may exist transiently or continuously due to retrograde filling of the upper urinary tract in the absence of obstruction and does not correlate well with the grade of reflux.

Prenatal Intervention

The detection of potentially lethal obstructive lesions of the upper urinary tract by prenatal sonography has provided the opportunity to correct such lesions in utero. Obstruction can be relieved by open fetal surgery, shunt placement between dilated portion of the urinary tract and the amniotic space, and even therapeutic fetoscopic procedures (18). Vesicoamniotic shunting has been used most extensively. These interventions in cases of bilateral hydronephrosis with oligohydramnios have been demonstrated to improve survival based on pulmonary outcomes, but have yet to demonstrate any prevention of renal insufficiency (20). These procedures carry a complication rate as high as 45% and include fetal demise (21). Therefore, fetal intervention remains highly controversial and is reserved for highly selected cases. Indications include persistent or progressive severe obstruction of both kidneys or a solitary kidney without overt signs of dysplasia, the presence of oligohydramnios, and favorable fetal urine functional indices (based on biochemical measurements) in an otherwise healthy fetus (18). In practice, these interventions are performed only in cases of bladder outlet obstruction (primarily posterior urethral valves) and have little to no role in obstruction of the upper urinary tract.

The detection of prenatal hydronephrosis should have little impact on obstetric care. Unilateral cases, even if they result in total loss of function in that renal unit, will not affect survival or longevity. A follow-up second or third trimester scan is helpful to see if the process is worsening or has resolved. Early delivery is not indicated because pulmonary maturation is of paramount concern. In bilateral cases, more frequent scanning, usually every 4 weeks, is indicated to monitor changes in amniotic fluid volume. If oligohydramnios is also present, then early delivery may be considered after 32 weeks or when fetal lung maturity is confirmed by lecithin-to-sphingomyelin amniotic fluid ratio.

Postnatal Diagnosis and Management

The urgency of postnatal workup is somewhat dependent on the severity of the prenatal findings. Unilateral hydronephrosis will not affect survival in the presence of a normal contralateral unit; whereas, bilateral severe pathology could potentially progress to renal failure. Unfortunately, there are few, if any, signs or symptoms to differentiate those with and without significant pathology. For this reason, a postnatal evaluation is indicated for all newborns who meet the definition of hydronephrosis based on renal pelvic AP diameter measurements (greater than 4 mm prior to 33 weeks or greater than 7 mm at or after 33 weeks) or who have ureteral dilation, bladder distension, and/or oligohydramnios.

Postnatal evaluation consists of sonography and *voiding cystourethrogram* (VCUG). The latter study is performed to exclude vesicoureteral reflux, urethral obstruction (primarily posterior urethral valves in males), or the presence of intravesical lesions (primarily ureteroceles). VCUG using standard constrast with fluoroscopy is preferable over radionuclide VCUG for the initial study due to superior anatomic detail. This study can be performed at any time, and we prefer prior to discharge from the nursery at our institution. In males without concern for urethral obstruction and in all females, it can be delayed, but the child should be assumed to have vesicoureteral reflux until proven otherwise and be placed on antibiotic prophylaxis (amoxicillin 15 mg per kg once daily). Some have argued that VCUG is an unnecessarily invasive procedure to perform in all neonates with a history of prenatal hydronephrosis, but it is not possible to exclude reflux by sonography alone. As many as 27% of those found to have reflux demonstrate no postnatal hydronephrosis, and reflux in the neonatal period is more common in males (22). Reflux is also found more frequently in the contralateral ureter in cases of renal agenesis, UPJ obstruction, and multicystic dysplastic kidney (18).

Postnatal sonography should include imaging of both kidneys, ureters, and bladder to fully evaluate both the upper and lower urinary tract. The timing of such intervention, however, remains controversial. Obstructive uropathy has been reportedly missed on sonography performed

TABLE 96-2 Society of Fetal Urology Grading Scale for Hydronephrosis

Grade 0	No hydronephrosis
Grade 1	Splitting of renal pelvis only
Grade 2	Greater dilation of renal pelvis without caliectasis
Grade 3	Dilation of pelvis and calyces without cortical thinning
Grade 4	Pelvocaliectasis with cortical thinning

From Fernbach SK, Maizels M, Conway JJ. Ultrasound grading of hydronephrosis: introduction to the system used by the Society for Fetal Urology. *Pediatr Radiol* 1993;23:478, with permission (23).

in the first 48 hours of life because perinatal dehydration may prevent adequate distension of the urinary tract to detect hydronephrosis. In a prospective study, we found no clinically significant differences in sonograms performed in the first 48 hours of life and at 7 to 10 days of life (19). Therefore, in cases of bilateral hydronephrosis, suspected multicystic dysplastic kidney, or concern for loss to follow-up, an initial sonogram prior to discharge from the nursery appears reliable. In cases of suspected bladder outlet obstruction, it is mandatory to order the sonogram in the first day. Unilateral hydronephrosis can reliably be studied with an early sonogram, but the degree of hydronephrosis may change if the study is postponed a week. Follow-up studies are important.

Hydronephrosis is often graded using the system of the Society of Fetal Urology (Table 96-2) (23). In the absence of vesicoureteral reflux, if no hydronephrosis (grade 0) is seen on the initial postnatal sonogram, no further follow-up is necessary. Obstruction has not been found in cases of grade 1 to 2 hydronephrosis with long-term follow-up (24); however, these patients are typically followed with repeat sonograms every 6 to 9 months up to age 18 to 24 months to ensure no worsening of dilation occurs. In the higher grades of hydronephrosis (grades 3 to 4), whether detected at birth or later, obstruction must be excluded. Grade 4 hydronephrosis is particularly worrisome because thinning of the renal cortex is suggestive but not diagnostic for obstruction (Fig. 96-2). Nuclear renography has replaced intravenous pyelography to exclude obstruction because the former provides objective measures of differential renal function and drainage from the renal unit. Even with exclusion of obstruction, continued follow-up is mandatory because delayed obstruction can occur in the first 2 years of life (24). Routine sonography is performed in such cases every 3 months for the first year of life and every 6 months in the second year of life. The need for prolonged follow-up after 2 years in the absence of obstruction is not yet determined.

The search for a reliable test to diagnose obstruction of the upper urinary tract has included many different studies. High-grade hydronephrosis may exist in the absence of obstruction and only represent the sequela of obstruction that developed and resolved prior to birth. Currently, nuclear renography under standardized parameters represents the gold standard to diagnose obstruction. It is preferable to wait until the newborn is at least 1 month of age to perform the renogram. The glomerular filtration rate is believed to increase severalfold in the first few weeks of life, adding greater accuracy to the study (25), and a short delay in relief of obstruction, if present, is not believed to lead to irreversible damage (10). Technetium-99m-mercaptoacetyltriglycine (MAG-3) is the preferred radionuclide because, unlike technetium-99m-diethylenetriaminepentaacetic acid, it is both filtered and secreted by the nephron to provide superior imaging. One to 2 minutes following administration of the radiotracer, differential renal function is determined by measuring the radioactivity from each renal unit. Normal function from each side is considered 40% to 60% of total renal function.

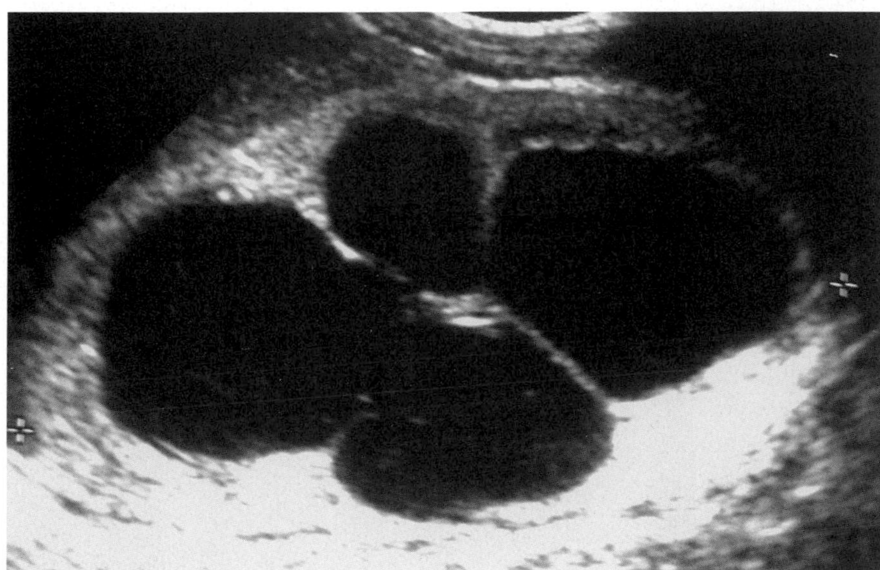

FIGURE 96-2. Postnatal sonogram of newborn with history of prenatal hydronephrosis. Grade 4 hydronephrosis with massive pelvocaliectasis with cortical thinning.

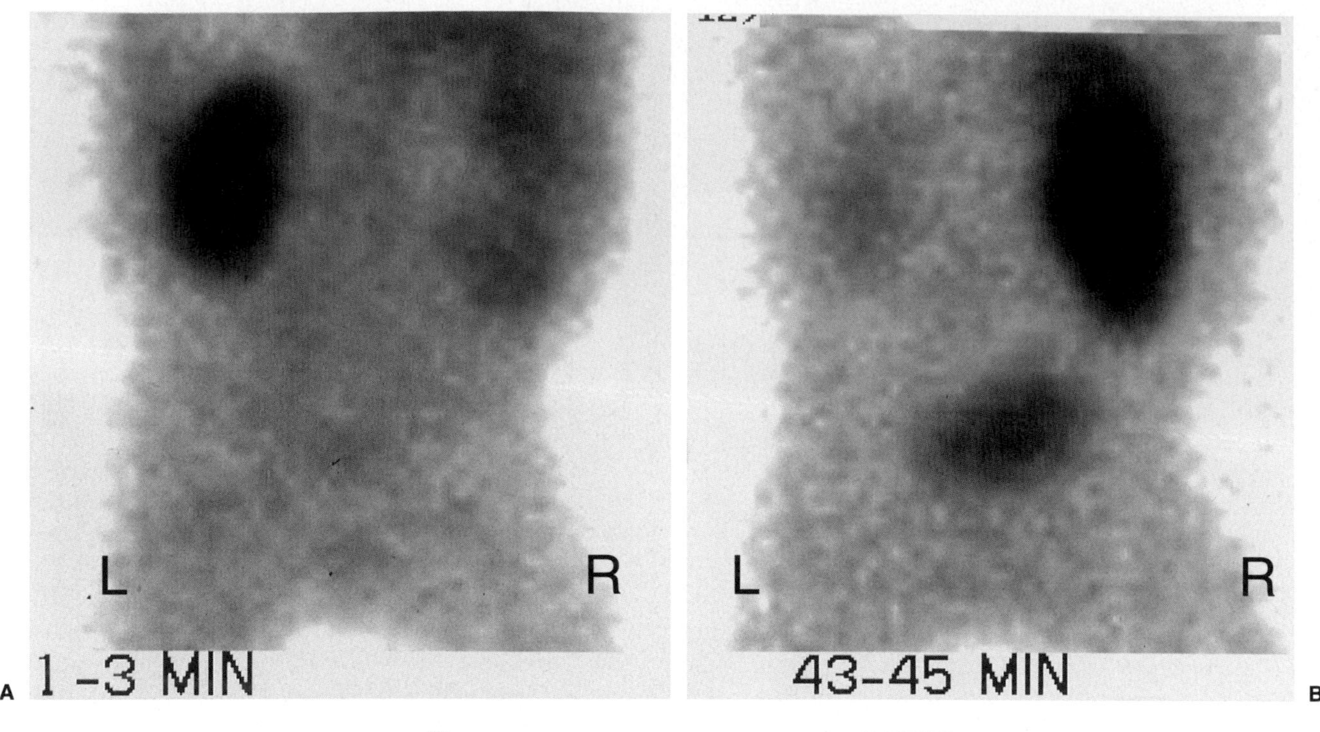

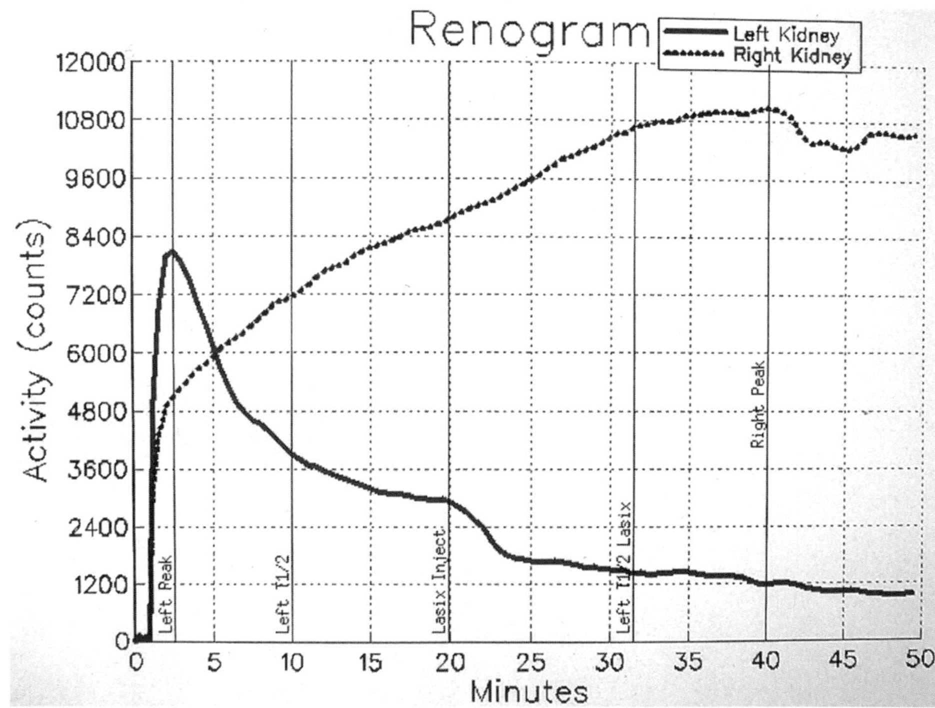

FIGURE 96-3. MAG-3 diuretic renogram in patient in Figure 96-2. **(A)** Initial images at 1 to 3 minutes show normal appearance of left kidney. The right kidney is enlarged with diffuse activity and photopenic renal hilum due to hydronephrosis. **(B)** Image at 43 to 45 minutes shows near complete drainage of left kidney and renal pelvis. The right kidney and renal pelvis show continued retention of tracer consistent with obstruction. **(C)** Washout curves show normal pattern for left kidney and unequivocally obstructed pattern of right kidney with no drainage.

The excretion of the radiotracer from the pelvis is then observed for 30 to 60 minutes and may assume one of several different patterns (Fig. 96-3).

Postnatal Presentation

Older children with congenital or acquired obstructive uropathies can present in a variety of ways. A classical presentation of UPJ obstruction in adults is *Dietl's crisis*—severe onset of flank pain, nausea, and vomiting, particularly after diuresis induced by excessive fluid intake, particularly alcohol or caffeine. This occurs because the rate of urine production exceeds the maximal possible flow rate across the point of critical narrowing, causing acute distension of the renal pelvis, which stretches and triggers impulses in the pain fibers of the renal capsule and autonomic splanchic nerves. Children certainly can present in this manner, but this is more likely with acquired ureteral narrowing, acute obstructing calculi, or extrinsic compression of the ureter. The chronic dilation associated with congenital obstruction may be less likely to produce symptoms. Some children with chronic obstruction will present with long-standing episodic bouts of abdominal pain and vomiting in the setting of a fruitless extensive gastrointestinal (GI) workup.

Gross hematuria after minor trauma can be seen in obstructive uropathy because vessels of the renal pelvis are dilated and more prone to bleeding. Microhematuria is found in most but not all patients with urolithiasis; gross hematuria is much less common.

Obstruction rarely presents with infection; however, UTIs are the second most common bacterial infections in children. Although there is no completely reliable method of differentiating bladder and kidney infections, fever, flank pain, nausea, vomiting, lethargy, and malaise would suggest the latter. Up to one-third to one-half of children presenting with febrile UTIs will have some abnormality of their urinary tract (26). For this reason, it is generally recommended to perform a VCUG and renal/bladder sonogram on children following a febrile UTI. The utility of these studies in older children and the timing of this study following infection is controversial (26,27). Vesicoureteral reflux is by far the most common abnormality detected in workups following febrile UTIs. Obstruction of the upper urinary tract presents with infection much less commonly because the bacteria must not only ascend the urethra to cause a bladder infection, but must also ascend the ureter past the point of obstruction to gain access to the upper urinary tract. Infection in the face of obstruction can be more serious with possible development of *pyonephrosis* or abscess due to bacterial growth in an essentially closed space. Sonography may be required to rule out such pathology if a febrile UTI does not rapidly respond to antibiotic therapy.

SPECIFIC DIAGNOSES OF OBSTRUCTIVE UROPATHY

Ureteropelvic Junction Obstruction

UPJ obstruction is the most common form of obstructive uropathy and should be corrected when present to prevent progressive renal insult. The decision to operate is fairly straightforward in those patients who present with symptoms, particularly recurrent flank pain associated with nausea and vomiting. Pyelonephritis on the affected side is also a relatively compelling indication for correction. Unfortunately, for the clinician, symptomatic presentation in children is rare. In the era of prenatal sonography, the vast majority of cases of UPJ obstruction in children present without symptoms but because of prenatal hydronephrosis (28). Much debate has centered over the presence of hydronephrosis and the relative indication for correction of UPJ obstruction because there is no definitive definition of UPJ obstruction.

There appears to be a slight preponderance of UPJ obstruction in males, representing approximately two-thirds of cases. Obstruction on the left is more common with a ratio of 3:2 versus the right side. Bilateral UPJ obstruction may exist in 5% to 15% of cases. If obstruction is found in a kidney with duplication of the collecting system, it almost always exists in the lower pole moiety (10,28).

The causes of UPJ obstruction are classified as intrinsic, extrinsic, and secondary. Intrinsic lesions of the ureter and its junction with the renal pelvis cause obstruction by constricting the lumen. Interruption in the development of the circular musculature and an excessive deposition of collagen fibers between muscle cells at the UPJ have been demonstrated to cause a thickening of the ureteral wall (28). Rare causes of intrinsic UPJ obstruction include congenital valvular mucosal folds, persistent fetal convolutions, and upper ureteral polyps. Extrinsic UPJ obstruction is most commonly caused by an aberrant additional vessel to the lower pole of the kidney kinking the UPJ or upper ureter as it passes to (or from) the great vessels. Because moving the ureter from the course of the crossing vessel does not always relieve the obstruction, it is not clear whether the vessel coexists with a preexisting intrinsic lesion or is the cause of the intrinsic lesion. The presentation of UPJ obstruction due to an obstructing crossing vessel is more common in older children and with symptoms of pain and vomiting (29). Intrinsic obstruction due to abnormal fetal ureteral development is seen more commonly in neonates and younger children, whereas an aberrant crossing vessel may not cause obstruction until the child has grown and the spatial relationship between ureter and vessel changes and causes kinking. Differentiation between intrinsic and extrinsic lesions may be difficult, and the diagnosis is usually not established until exploration at the time of repair.

The advent of prenatal sonography led to a dramatic increase in the number of infants presenting with hydronephrosis and possible UPJ obstruction. Pyeloplasties, therefore, were performed on many of these newborns to correct the perceived obstruction (30). It was noted, however, that renal function was not altered in most of these patients at the time of workup (31). If renal function was found to be diminished, it may have been irreversibly altered prior to birth, and postnatal surgery did not improve function (32). This led some investigators to follow such newborns expectantly, unless renal function was initially diminished or diminished during observation (31,33). Only 22% to 25% of observed newborns with severe unilateral hydronephrosis required subsequent pyeloplasty; therefore, nearly three-fourths of these neonates with apparent UPJ obstruction on ultrasound could be followed safely without obvious deleterious effect. Of those not undergoing surgery, 69% had resolution of the hydronephrosis and 31% had improvement. This suggests that most newborns with severe unilateral hydronephrosis can be followed; obstruction demonstrated by loss of renal function on nuclear renal scan is found in only a minority. In most, the hydronephrosis detected is a sequela of fetal maldevelopment and will resolve over time. In a minority, function will deteriorate, perhaps as the critical degree of obstruction cannot accommodate the urine flow of the growing and developing infant kidney. Such obstruction is typically silent; therefore, these patients must be followed rigorously to determine which patients may or may not need surgical correction. The usual indications for surgery in follow-up are worsening hydronephrosis or worsening function on nuclear renal scan (33).

Once the decision to surgically correct UPJ obstruction is made, open pyeloplasty is the conventional procedure. This procedure has been shown to be highly successful with success rates of greater than 95%, even in newborns (10). The renal pelvis and ureter can be exposed extraperitoneally through a muscle-dividing flank incision made anteriorly from the tip of the twelfth rib or a muscle-splitting dorsal lumbotomy incision through the back between the twelfth rib and bony pelvis. The dorsal lumbotomy may be less morbid to the patient, but can limit the surgeons' exposure (34,35). The renal pelvis and upper ureter should be exposed by dissecting in a plane just superficial to its adventitia to preserve the intrinsic blood supply. The repair is usually a dismembered (Anderson-Hynes) pyeloplasty; this involves division of the UPJ, resection of the stenotic segment and/or rerouting the ureter around an aberrant crossing vessel, wide spatulation of the proximal ureter, and careful anastomosis of the pelvis to the ureteral segment with fine absorbable suture (Fig. 96-4). If a large redundant pelvis is present, the pelvis is resected generously to prevent kinking at the ureteropelvic anastomosis when filling occurs. If the length of the obstructing segment is more than 1.5 to 2 cm, a nondismembered pyeloplasty using a flap of renal pelvic tissue to augment the narrowed segment can be employed. Ureterocalycostomy is usually reserved for cases in which dependent renal drainage across the UPJ cannot be established by the conventional techniques (e.g., in the setting of fused kidneys or previous surgery). In this procedure, amputation of the lower pole cortex is performed, and the most dependent calyx is sewn to the ureter in a tension-free mucosa-to-mucosa anastomosis (36).

Minimally invasive techniques have been developed for correction of UPJ obstruction. *Endopyelotomy* is an endoscopic method based on the principle that an incised ureteral segment can reepithelialize around a stent with complete mucosal regeneration after 6 days and muscularis regeneration by 6 to 8 weeks. Thus, incision and stenting of the narrowed UPJ allow healing to create an

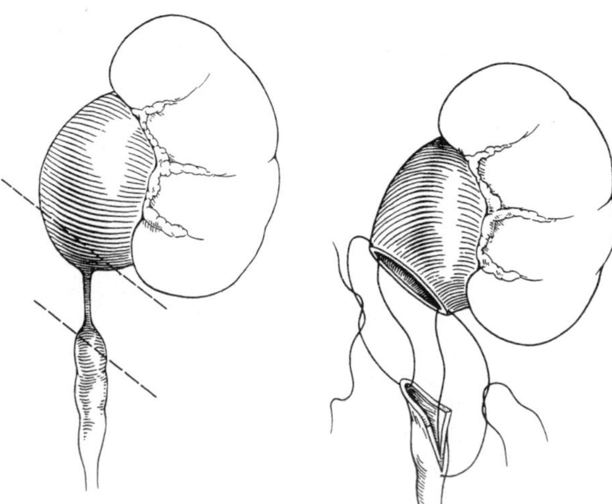
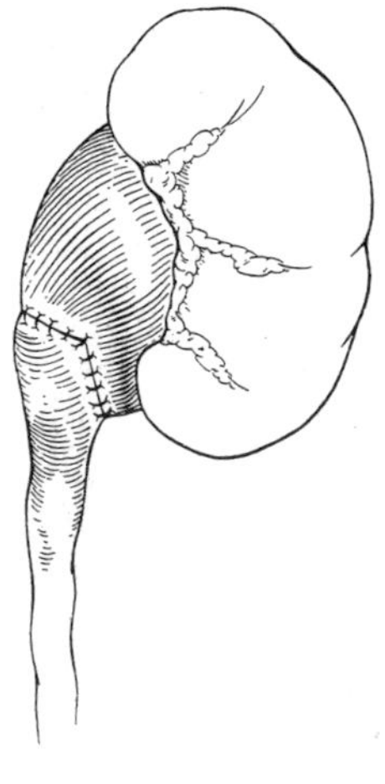

FIGURE 96-4. Pyeloplasty with excision of narrowed segment and reanastomosis of spatulated ureter and pelvis. (From Kelias PP, King LR, Belman AB, eds. *Clinical pediatric urology*, 2nd ed. Philadelphia: WB Saunders, 1985:471, Fig 16-60, with permission.)

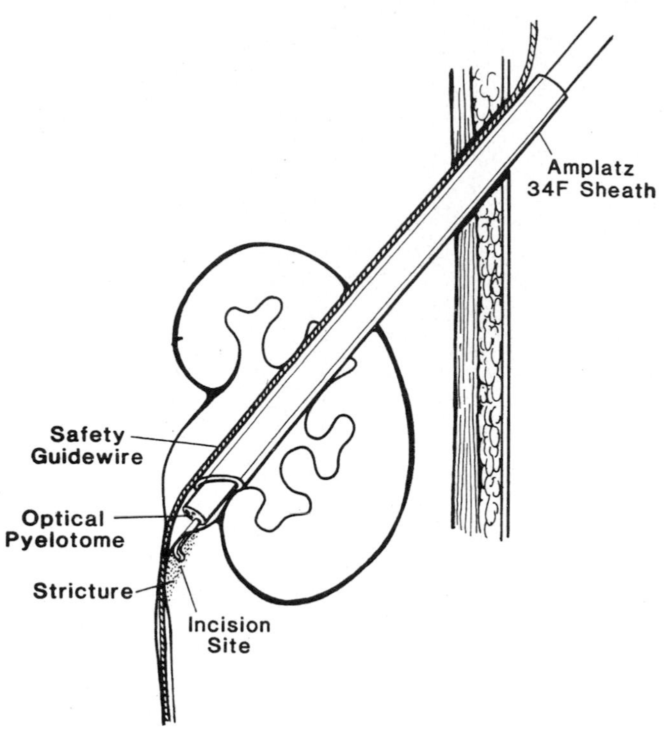

FIGURE 96-5. Endopyelotomy technique for treatment of ureteropelvic junction (UPJ) obstuction. Approach through upper pole calyx provides access to UPJ. (From Gillenwater JY, Grayhack JT, Howards SS, et al., eds. *Adult and pediatric urology*, 4th ed. Philadelphia: Lippincott Williams & Wilkins, 2002:2351, Figure 63.8, with permission.)

enlarged lumen. The technique was initially described with an antegrade approach through a percutaneous nephrostomy (Fig. 96-5) (37). Modifications to avoid a percutaneous approach have been developed via a retrograde approach through the urethra and bladder, using a specialized stent for simultaneous cautery and balloon dilation or laser/cautery incision of the obstructed segment through a ureteroscope (38,39). However, the use of these techniques is limited by size of the ureter and urethra so endopyelotomy can only be used in larger, older children.

Laparoscopic dismembered pyeloplasty can be successfully performed with success rates equivalent to open pyeloplasty (40). This can be accomplished through a transperitoneal or retroperitoneal approach. This technique has been extended to use in children, but again size limitations apply (41,42). A transperitoneal approach has been used in toddlers, but many of the advantages of reduced morbidity of laparoscopic surgery are lost on small children.

Midureteral Obstruction

Obstruction of the ureter between the UPJ and its distal end is rare in children. Such lesions are nearly all acquired strictures, but there is controversy regarding the rare existence of obstructing congenital ureteral valves (43). Strictures can be iatrogenic from open retroperitoneal surgery and endoscopic ureteral procedures. Tumors in the retroperitoneum can cause extrinsic compression, whereas treatment with radiation therapy can lead to ischemic ureteral strictures. Intrinsic primary ureteral tumors in children are exceeding rare but may present with hematuria. Most midureteral obstructions are slowly progressive, causing hydronephrosis above the stricture but few obstructive symptoms. Sonography is a good initial study to detect hydronephrosis, but CT or magnetic resonance imaging (MRI) is necessary to fully image the course of the ureter and surrounding retroperitoneal structures. The use of intravenous constrast is helpful to better delineate the ureteral anatomy, and cystoscopy with retrograde pyelography may be required to make a diagnosis.

A rare but distinct congenital cause of midureteral obstruction is persistence of the embryonic right posterior cardinal vein. This causes the vena cava to lie ventral to the right ureter creating a possible obstruction of the *retrocaval ureter*. The appearance of an upper ureteral obstruction on intravenous urogram has classically been described, but CT urography is superior with visualization of both the ureter and vena cava and their spatial relationship. These typically present in adulthood and should be corrected if obstructive symptoms occur. Correction involves dividing the ureter (or UPJ) and rerouting the ureter anterior to the vena cava (41).

Distal Ureteral Obstruction

Due to its multiple causes, many names exist to describe distal ureteral obstruction. The term *megaureter* is merely descriptive for a dilated ureter but does not imply obstruction or any other diagnosis. Megaureter may be the result of obstruction, reflux, both, or neither. Nonobstructive causes of ureteral dilation can be temporary (due to the endotoxic effects of UTI or excessive diuresis) or congenital. Just as the renal pelvis can be dilated from transient prenatal obstruction of the UPJ, a nonobstructed, nonrefluxing megaureter can exist due to resolution of fetal UVJ obstruction. Reflux can dilate the ureter and renal pelvis, but this may only be appreciable at high bladder volumes or with voiding. Dilated ureters are encountered with temporary obstructive lesions, most commonly urinary stones lodged at the UVJ—the narrowest portion of the upper urinary tract. Congenital causes of distal obstuction of a single ureter include intrinsic narrowing of a normally placed UVJ (primary UVJ obstruction), ectopic insertion of a single ureter, or a rare single system ureterocele. In complete renal duplication, the upper pole moiety commonly has secondary distal ureteral obstruction due to ectopic insertion of the ureter into the genitourinary tract or an obstructing ureterocele. Ectopic ureteral insertion can be associated with reflux in addition to obstruction due to the altered anatomy of the ureteral orifice. Secondary megaureter can occur with the neuropathic bladder or infravesical obstruction; the intravesical pressure can exceed the ureteral emptying pressure and cause the ureter to dilate, even in the absence of reflux.

In primary nonobstructive, nonrefluxing megaureter, upper tract drainage is good by all functional parameters. The diagnosis is one of exclusion after VCUG and diuretic nuclear renal scan exclude reflux and obstruction, respectively. These tend to improve radiographically with time, but follow-up is imperative because a small number may worsen. A more recent series of nonrefluxing primary megaureters diagnosed prenatally noted resolution of megaureters in 72%, no change in 9%, and surgical repair in 19%. Worsening hydronephrosis and declining function on renal scan were the most common indications for intervention (44).

Presentation of a megaureter is identical to that of isolated hydronephrosis with the addition of ureteral dilation. Sonography reveals a dilated renal pelvis draining into a dilated ureter than can be followed to the bladder. Calyceal dilation and cortical thinning are found more commonly in the face of obstruction. The dilated ureter can easily be seen behind the bladder on transverse and sagittal images. A dilated ureter at or below the bladder neck implies ectopia. All patients should undergo a VCUG to rule out vesicoureteral reflux. The bladder and urethra should be carefully examined because signs of neurogenic bladder and infravesical obstruction can be found as abnormalities of the bladder body (trabeculation), bladder neck, and urethra. The "well-tempered" diuretic nuclear renal scan can exclude obstruction using the same criteria as with UPJ obstruction. In cases of complete ureteral duplication, it may be helpful to differentiate renal function in upper versus lower pole moieties. The pathophysiology of distal ureteral obstruction is virtually identical to that of UPJ obstruction; however, the ability of the ureter to dilate below the level of the kidney may mitigate the pressure effects on the nephrons. Bilateral megaureters associated with bladder or urethral pathology should be particularly concerning as bilateral renal damage could result in renal failure.

Primary UVJ obstruction is associated with abrupt narrowing at the juxtavesical ureteral segment. The juxtavesical ureter may be normal in caliber, but can be the site of functional obstruction because the undilated segment does not conduct the peristaltic wave (Fig. 96-6). In an analogy to Hirschsprung's disease in the colon, the normal caliber segment is the pathologic segment and the dilated segment has normal histology. In UVJ obstruction, the pathology demonstrates deficiency of the muscle fibers and excessive collagen fibers causing rigidity of the ureteral wall, as opposed to deficiency of ganglionic cells in Hirschsprung's disease (45).

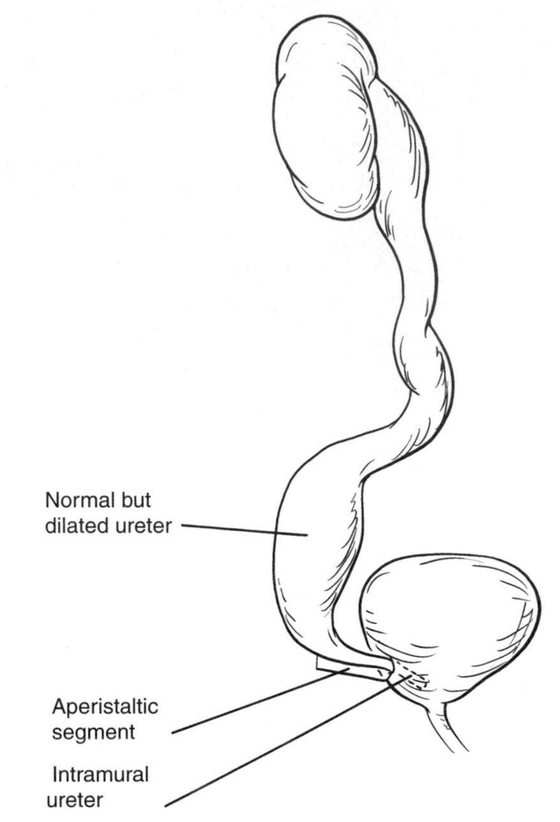

FIGURE 96-6. Distal adynamic segment as found in primary obstructive megaureter. (From Gillenwater JY, Grayhack JT, Howards SS, et al., eds. *Adult and pediatric urology*, 2nd ed. St Louis: Mosby–Year Book, 1991:1495, with permission.)

In the setting of decreased ipsilateral renal function or worsening hydronephrosis, surgical repair is indicated. Urinary tract infection, solitary kidney, and poor compliance with follow-up may also be reasons for intervention. The goal of surgery is to create a nonobstructive, nonrefluxing UVJ by tailoring and reimplantation of the distal portion of the megaureter. Reducing the caliber of the distal ureter is necessary to allow the ureter to be reimplanted into the bladder with a sufficient length of submucosal tunnel to prevent reflux. It is generally accepted that the optimal ratio of tunnel length (through bladder wall) versus ureteral diameter is 5:1. In addition, reducing the diameter of the ureter permits more efficient propulsion of the urine. Tailoring may be achieved by excising the redundant ureteral wall or plicating and folding the excess tissue. The former technique is favored by most because there is less ureteral bulk to bring into the bladder. The obstructive segment of the ureter is resected, and the distal ureter is straightened and shortened. A portion of the lateral wall opposite to the vessels is excised over the distal 5 cm, and the ureter is narrowed to about 12F caliber (Fig. 96-7) (46,47). To achieve adequate tunnel length, the ureter can be brought through the original hiatus and

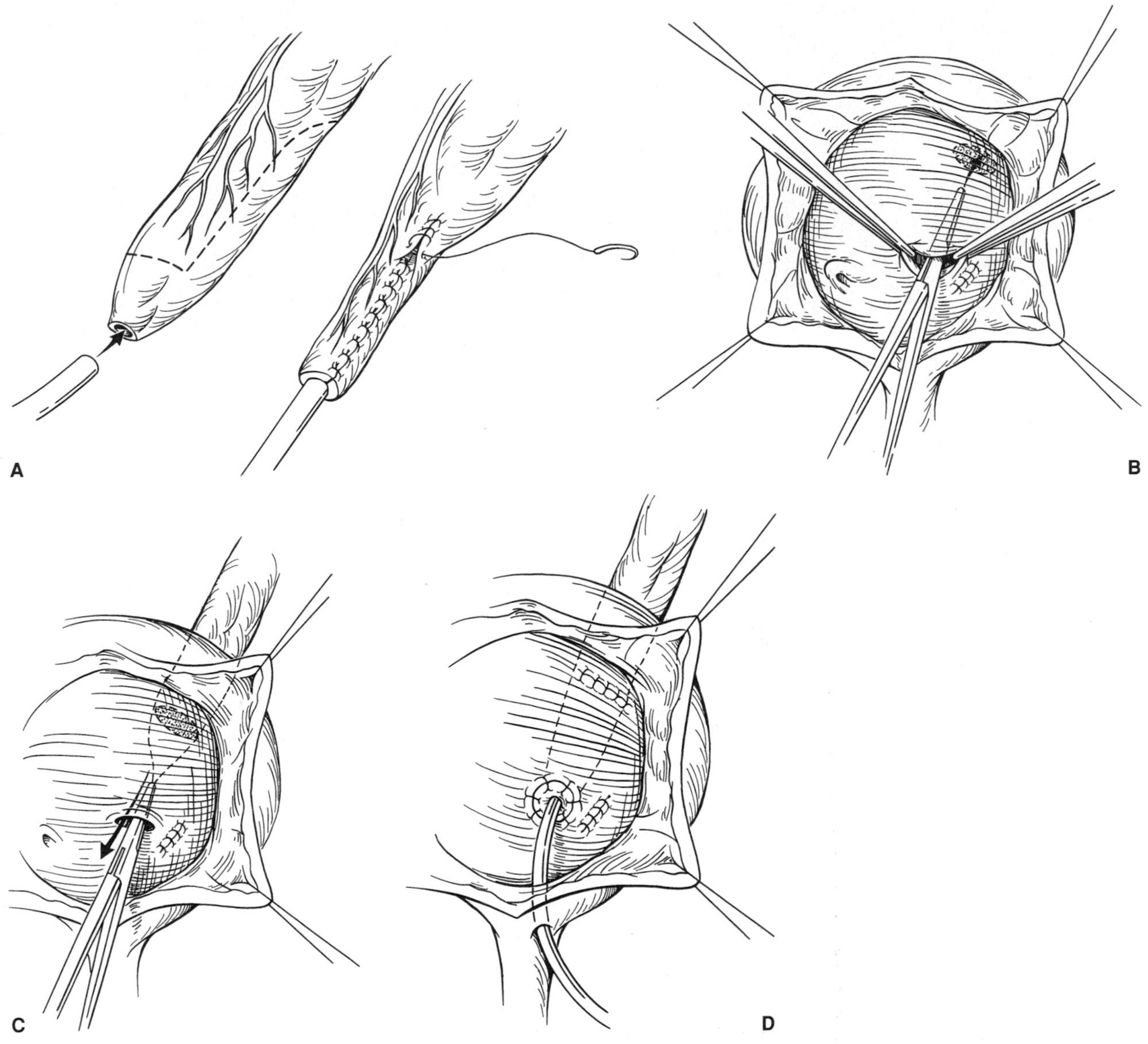

FIGURE 96-7. Excisional tailoring and reimplantation of megaureter. (From Gillenwater JY, Grayhack JT, Howards SS, et al., eds. *Adult and pediatric urology*, 2nd ed. St Louis: Mosby–Year Book, 1991:1496, with permission.)

reimplanted across the trigone, or a new, more cephalad hiatus can be created with the ureteral orifice kept in the same position. Another method to reduce ureteral caliber is by plicating and folding the distal ureter. The advantages of this technique are better preservation of ureteral blood supply and lack of a long suture line so the stents can be removed earlier. The success rate of each technique is more than 90%, and the most common complications include postoperative obstruction or vesicoureteral reflux.

An *ectopic ureter* is defined a distal orifice more caudal than at the normal location on the lateral corner of the trigone. Embryologically, an ectopic ureter results from an abnormally high origin of the ureteral bud from the mesonephric duct. As the distal mesonephric duct and ureter are incorporated into the developing bladder, the delay in separation from the duct prevents the ureteral orifice from migrating to its normal superiorlateral position on the trigone (Fig. 96-8). In its extreme form, the ureter never separates from the mesonephric duct and remains extravesical. Stephens' (48) theory of ureteral ectopia explains the association of obstruction or reflux with renal dysplasia. An abnormal ureteral bud branches off the duct either too distal or too proximal, resulting in obstruction (orifice too inferiomedial) or reflux (orifice too superiolateral) (Fig. 96-9). The cranial end of the ectopic ureteral bud

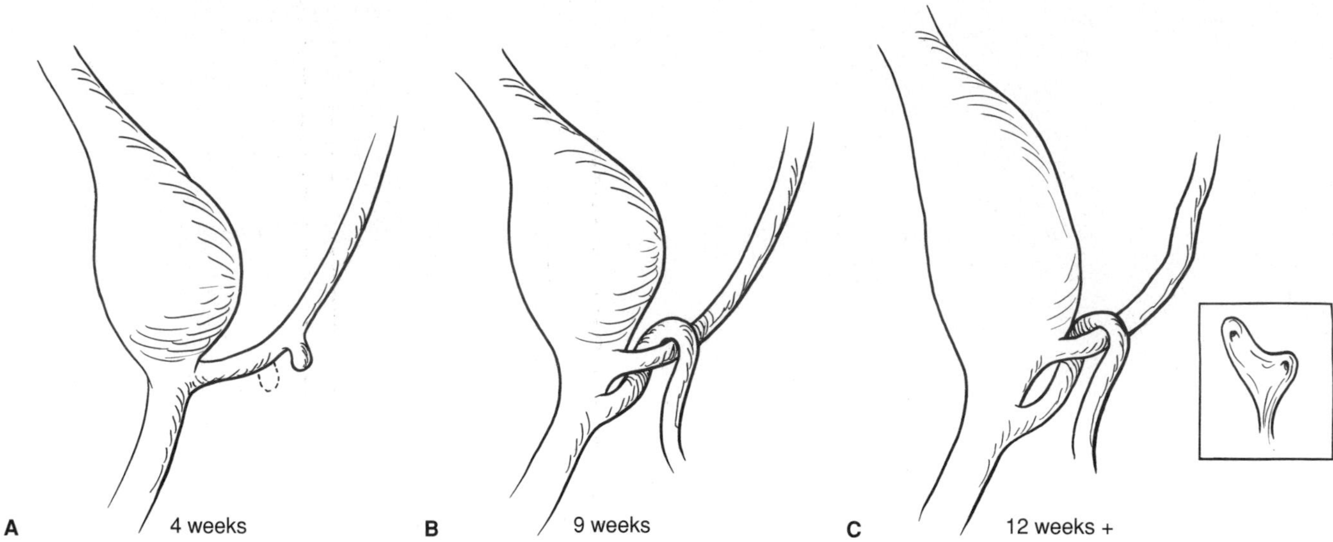

FIGURE 96-8. High origin of the ureteral bud from the mesonephric duct leading to mild degree of ureteral ectopia toward the bladder neck, but still on the trigone. **(A)** Normal origin of ureteral bud shown by dotted line. **(B, C)** Wolffian duct that becomes vas deferens shown looping over ureter. Endoscopic view in inset. (From Gillenwater JY, Grayhack JT, Howards SS, et al., eds. *Adult and pediatric urology*, 2nd ed. St Louis: Mosby–Year Book, 1991:1498, with permission.)

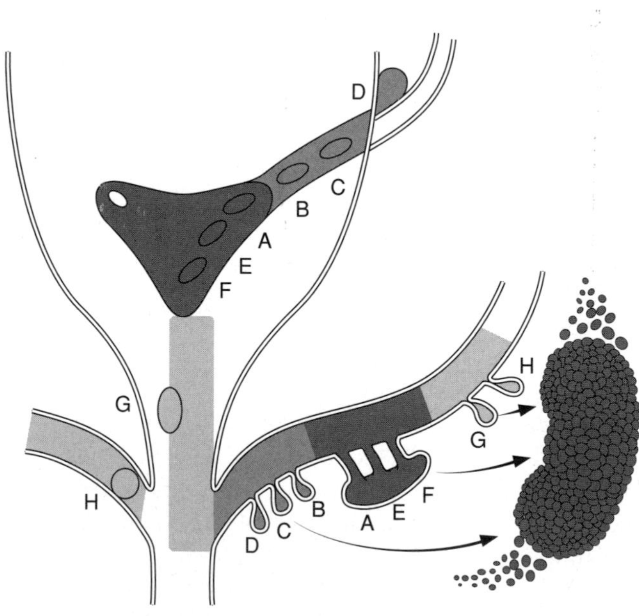

FIGURE 96-9. Relation of orifice positions in the bladder and urethra to points of origin from the wolffian duct, and relation of bud positions of wolffian duct to nephrogenic blastema. A, normal position; B, C, and D, potentially refluxing positions; E and F, ectopic intravesical positions; G and H, ectopic extravesical positions. (From Walsh PC, Retik AB, Stamey TA, et al., eds. *Campbell's urology*, 6th ed. Philadelphia: WB Saunders, 1992, with permission.)

then may impact the developing metanephric blastema ectopically, and complete (single ureter) or segmental (duplicated ureter) renal dysplasia may occur due to abnormal induction of nephrogenesis.

More than 80% of ectopic ureters in girls are associated with a duplicated collecting system, whereas in boys most ectopic ureters drain single systems (49). Ectopic ureters appear three times more often in girls than in boys and about 10% are bilateral (50). About one-third of ectopic ureters in girls open at the level of the bladder neck or slightly more distally in the upper urethra. An ectopic ureter inserting into the proximal urethra often refluxes (in about 75%) due to its abnormal orifice and drains only during voiding as it traverses the intermittently obstructive musculature of the bladder neck (51). These girls often present with recurrent pyelonephritis early in life because perineal flora can easily ascend up to the kidney. In a small proportion of these girls, the ectopic ureter drains into the genitourinary tract below the level of sphincteric control, and they present with a classic history of lifelong wetness due to persistent dribbling, despite normal voiding of urine from the remaining ureters terminating in the bladder. The ectopic ureter may remain attached to the distal mesonephric duct; the remnant of this duct in females is Gartner's duct and extends from the uterine broad ligament along the lateral wall of the vagina and terminating at the vestibule. The ectopic ureter, thus, opens into the dilated termination known as a Gartner's duct cyst within the vagina or at the vestibule (50). Rarely, ectopic ureters end at a higher site on the Gartner duct, with an opening at the level of the cervix or even uterus. Ureteral ectopia into the rectum is rare in both sexes, but it has been noted incidentally at autopsy.

Ectopic ureters do not present with urinary incontinence in boys because they always terminate above the level of the external urinary sphincter. This is due to the fact that the ureteral bud is a branch off the mesonephric duct, and all wolffian structures in males remain above the pelvic floor. Male ectopic ureters have been reported to end in the male reproductive tract, specifically, in the posterior urethra in 47%, prostatic utricle in 10%, vas deferens and ejaculatory duct in 5% each, seminal vesicle in 33%, and rarely in the epididymis (52). Symptomatic presentation may be less obvious than in girls and is related to ureteral obstruction or infection. Urgency and frequency may occur as a response to the trickle of urine into the posterior urethra. Presentation may be delayed until the onset of sexual activity and can include prostatitis, seminal vesiculitis, epididymitis, and pelvic pain. Boys with pyelonephritis or recurrent epididymitis require evaluation by sonogram and VCUG to exclude ureteral ectopia.

In girls presenting with persistent dribbling along with normal voiding, an ectopic ureteral orifice should be sought at the urethrovaginal septum or anterior vaginal wall on physical exam. In most cases, the diagnosis is confirmed by intravenous pyelogram (IVP) or renal scan with poor or absent visualization of the hydronephrotic upper pole of a duplex system. It should be remembered that urine production from the upper segment into the ectopic ureter can still occur in the absence of demonstrable function on imaging studies. Cystourethroscopy and vaginoscopy under general anesthesia, even with intravenous injection of indigo carmine to dye the urine may not be conclusive.

Upper pole nephrectomy through a standard flank incision is the usual treatment of an ectopic ureter associated with a poorly functioning upper pole (Fig. 96-10) (53). Care must be taken not to injure or devitalize the lower pole (54). In the absence of upper pole reflux, the ureter can be taken distally as far as safely possible and left open to allow the megaureter to decompress. In cases in which the upper pole has significant function, the upper pole ureter can be anastomosed to the lower pole pelvis or to the proximal lower ureter, but care must be taken not to obstruct the normal caliber lower pole when sewing the wide upper ureter to it (55). When the ureter enters the male genital tract, even in the absence of reflux, total ureterectomy, excision of the common duct, and ligation of the vas are necessary to prevent subsequent epididymitis and pyoureter.

Ureterocele is a cystic dilation of the terminal intravesical ureter. The incidence of ureteroceles was reported to be 1 in 4,000 autopsies in children (56) and is much more common in whites than in blacks. Ureteroceles are five times more common in girls than in boys and about 10% are bilateral. More than 80% of ureteroceles are associated with the upper pole ureter of a duplex kidney; the remainder is associated with a single ureter (57). The ureterocele may vary in size from a tiny cystic dilation of the submucosal ureter to that of a large mass filling the bladder and, rarely, prolapsing through the urethra. Histologically, the wall of the ureterocele contains attenuated smooth muscle bundles and connective tissue of the ureter lined with ureteral mucosa and covered by bladder mucosa.

A ureterocele can affect the other ureter(s) to the other renal segment(s) by either obstructive mass effect or distortion of the trigone and bladder neck. This can lead to hydronephrosis and/or vesicoureteral reflux into the contralateral renal unit and/or the ipsilateral lower pole moiety in a duplex system ureterocele. Loss of function in the upper pole of unilateral duplex system will not have a great effect on overall health, but when a ureterocele jeopardizes additional segments of renal tissue, proper diagnosis, and management are critical.

Ureteroceles are most commonly diagnosed today on prenatal ultrasonography. Symptomatic presentation is usually seen during the first few months of life with symptoms of infection such as fever, vomiting, or failure to thrive. Rarely, a large ureterocele can prolapse into the urethra; thus, ureteroceles are the most common cause of urethral obstruction of girls (58). If the ureterocele extends out of the external urethral meatus, it can present as an introital mass. Urinary incontinence may occur in girls with large ureteroceles that have rendered the internal (and possibly, external) sphincter lax and inefficient, but it is unclear whether this is a result of maldevelopment or iatrogenic surgical injury.

VCUG is critical in the diagnosis of ureteroceles. Early images during filling are important to visualize the ureterocele before the contrast opacifies the entire bladder. The ureterocele is seen as a filling defect within the bladder, and close observation during the process of filling the bladder and voiding are necessary to detemine if an extravescial component or prolapse is present. Deficient muscle backing behind the ureterocele can lead to eversion of the ureterocele, mimicking a bladder diverticulum. Vesicoureteral reflux may be seen in any or all ureteral segments. The "drooping lily" sign is used to describe the appearance of high-grade reflux into a dilated lower pole segment displaced by a tense upper pole system obstructed by a ureterocele.

The management of ureteroceles is controversial due to broad spectrum of presentation and associated morbidity. The primary goal of treatment is to maximally preserve the renal parenchyma in all segments by correcting obstruction and preventing reflux, but it is clear that treatment must be individualized because no one single therapy is appropriate for all cases. No therapy is indicated if neither obstruction nor reflux is found in association with the ureterocele. Simple transurethral incision of a ureterocele with electrocautery or laser energy can permanently relieve the obstruction without causing reflux in some cases.

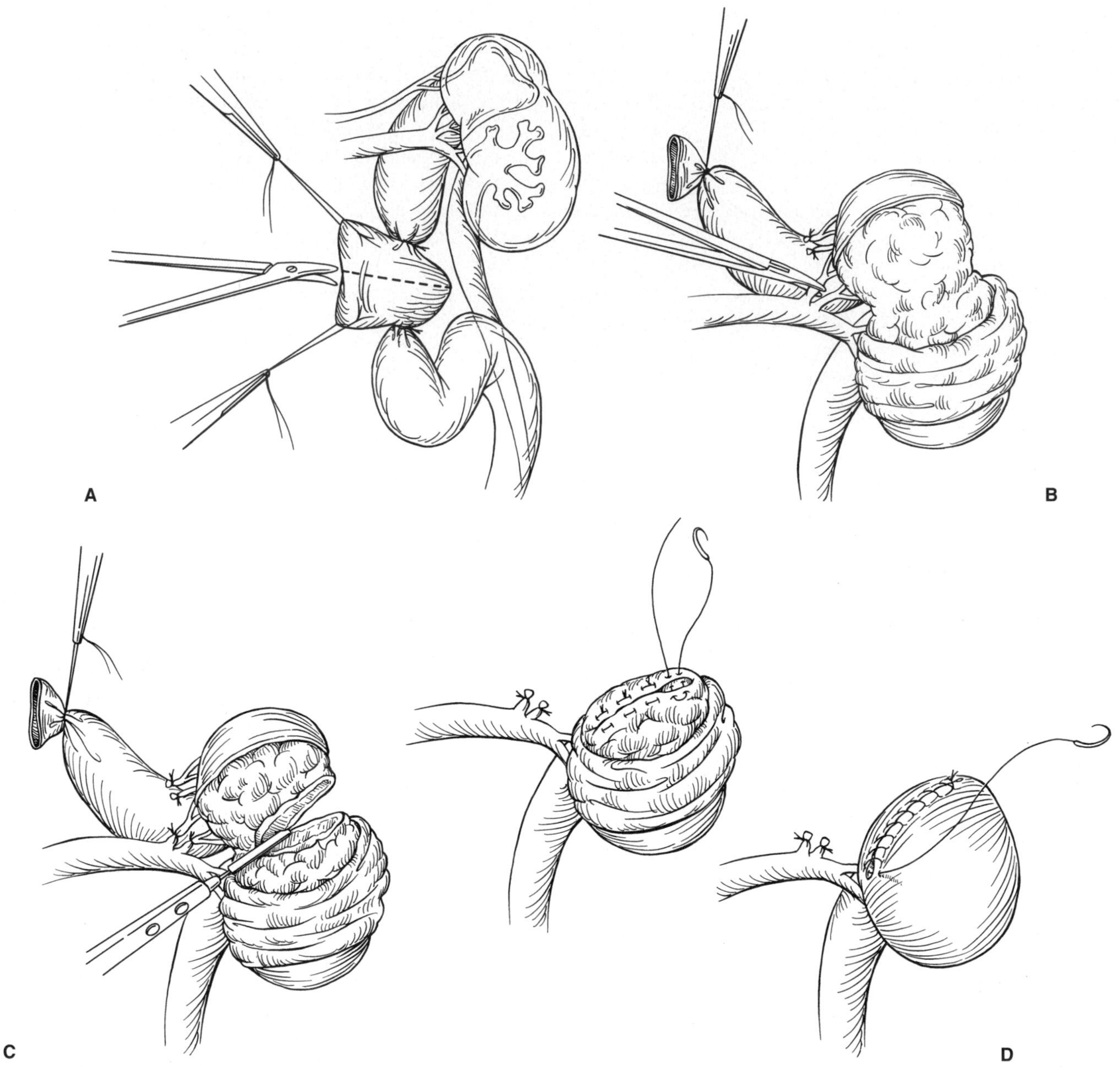

FIGURE 96-10. Technique of upper pole nephrectomy. (From Walsh PC, Retik AB, Stamey TA, et al., eds. *Campbell's urology*, 6th ed. Philadelphia: WB Saunders, 1992, with permission.)

In the presence of acceptable renal function in the affected segment, simple ureterocele excision and ureteral reimplantion through a Pfannelstiel incision is effective.

VESICOURETERAL REFLUX

The normal ureterovesical junction allows urine to flow in an antegrade manner only. Vesicoureteral reflux (VUR) denotes the retrograde flow of urine from the bladder into the upper urinary tract. In primary VUR, the pathology stems from a congenital anomaly of the ureterovesical junction. Typically, there is an insufficient length of ureter within the bladder wall relative to its diameter as it passes through to the trigone (Fig. 96-11). Accordingly, the ureteral orifice is often noted to be an abnormally lateral position on the trigone (see positions B, C, and D, Fig. 96-9). With this shorter intravesical tunnel length, there is impaired active and passive compression of the ureter during bladder filling and emptying, resulting in VUR. Primary VUR may also be associated with an abnormal configuration of the ureteral orifice that prevents proper coaptation. Even with borderline anatomy, the normal low resting pressure in the bladder (8 to 10 mm Hg) is usually sufficient to compress

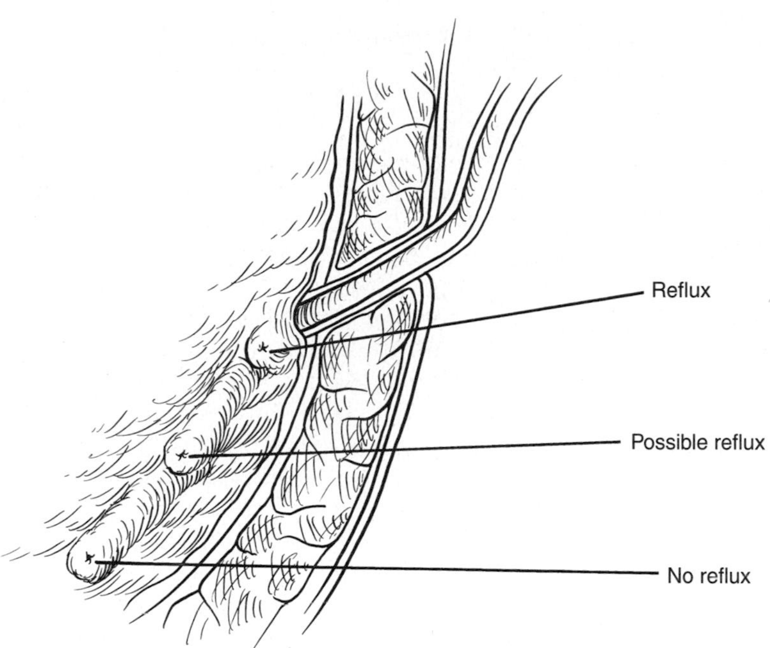

FIGURE 96-11. Refluxing ureterovesicle junction has the same anatomic features as nonrefluxing orifice, except for shorter length of intravesical submucosal ureter. An orifice in an intermediate position may reflux intermittently due to a borderline submucosal tunnel. The far lateral orifice is definitely refluxing.

the roof of the intravesical ureter against the underlying detrusor to prevent VUR. Secondary VUR can result from altered physiology with increased intravesical pressure in obstructed or poorly compliant bladders (59). VUR may also be secondary to other anatomic defects of the lower urinary tract such as ureteral ectopia, ureteroceles, bladder exstrophy, and prune belly syndrome.

In the latter half of the twentieth century, it was noted that VUR was strongly linked to renal damage secondary to chronic pyelonephritis (termed *reflux nephropathy*). Of children with renal scarring, 97% showed radiologic evidence of VUR (60). Renal failure is the most ominous sequela of VUR; 3% to 25% of children and 10% to 15% of adults with end-stage renal disease have reflux nephropathy as the primary insult (61). Renal scarring also increases the risk of hypertension threefold (61). Additional negative outcomes of VUR include reduced somatic growth in childhood and pregnancy complications in adulthood. A single episode of pyelonephritis may cause permanent renal scarring in 10% to 30% of infants, but the presence of VUR makes scarring more likely (27). VUR promotes pyelonephritis by enabling bacteria to ascend from the bladder to the upper urinary tract more easily. VUR, thus, does not have a role in initiation of UTI, but does increase its morbidity. In the absence of obstruction, VUR is not believed to be harmful provided the urine remains sterile.

The incidence of VUR in healthy children is less than 1% (61). Of children presenting with UTI, approximately 40% are found to have VUR (27,61), and the incidence is inversely correlated with age (62). The average age for diagnosis of VUR is 2 to 3 years of age upon workup following a febrile UTI, and 75% to 80% of children discovered to have primary VUR are girls (61). In contradistinction, the workup of newborns with prenatal hydronephrosis has detected VUR more commonly in males at that age (63). VUR occurs more commonly in children of Northern European descent with fair skin, blond or red hair, and blue eyes (64). Girls of African descent have been noted to have a tenfold lower prevalence of VUR than white girls following workup for UTI (65). Additional investigations have further supported a genetic predisposition for VUR. Multiple series have demonstrated that siblings of children with VUR have VUR at a much increased prevalence in the range of 24% to 51% (66). The prevalence is even higher when offspring of index cases of VUR are screened for VUR. Molecular biologic investigations have suggested that specific genetic loci on the X chromosome and on autosomes may be responsible for the inheritance of VUR (66).

VUR is a radiologic diagnosis that can only be reliably made by VCUG. Urethral catheterization is required to fill to the bladder for appropriate imaging, and the child must remain awake to void because VUR may occur during bladder filling, emptying, or both. For this reason, sedation is not routinely used. VCUG is classically performed by instilling iodinated contrast into the bladder under gravity (of less than 100 cm H_2O) with periodic imaging by fluoroscopy. This method gives the greatest anatomic detail, plus the most accurate grading, and should be used as initial study in all high-risk patients. A different technique, radionuclide cystography, involves filling the bladder with 0.5 mCi of technetium 99-pertechnetate in isotonic saline and affords continuous observation under the gamma camera. Radionuclide imaging has the advantages of reduced radiation dose and greater sensitivity for detection of VUR; however, resolution is inferior. For this reason, the latter study is reserved for annual repeat studies in known refluxers or screening studies in siblings of refluxers (67).

Indications for initial VCUG include an evaluation following UTI in children, postnatal evaluation of newborns with prenatally diagnosed hydronephrosis, and those children in high-risk groups such as those with other renal anomalies (UPJ obstruction, multicystic dysplastic kidney, VATER syndrome), lower tract anomalies (ureterocele, prune belly syndrome, posterior urethral valves, neurogenic bladder), or sibling history of VUR. Other imaging studies, such as sonography and IVP can suggest VUR by detection of ureteral dilation and pelvicaliectasis, but only cystography can prove VUR. VUR, however, is typically found in the absence of upper tract dilation. The sensitivity of hydronephrosis on sonography for predicting the presence of VUR following a febrile UTI is only 10%, and it has a positive predictive value of only 40% (27). VCUG has traditionally been recommended following a first febrile UTI in children, particularly infants (27). Most pediatric urologists recommend that the VCUG is performed within several days of initiating therapy rather than delaying the study for 1 month (27,67).

Several classifications of VUR exist, but the International Reflux Study classification system is the most widely accepted (Fig. 96-12). This system of grades I to V is based primarily on the appearance of the calyces on contrast VCUG because the degree of dilation of the ureter does not always parallel the degree of dilation of the pelvocalyceal system. The grading system for VUR is used to estimate prognosis and to aid in management. The lower grades are much more prevalent, with grades I to II accounting for the majority of cases of VUR, whereas grades IV to V are much rarer (27).

The natural history of VUR is usually one of improvement or resolution during normal childhood growth. Resolution is most strongly correlated inversely with the grade of reflux at initial diagnosis. A meta-analysis conducted by the American Urological Association Pediatric Vesicoureteral Reflux Clinical Guidelines Panel in 1997 (61) noted that grades I and II had 5-year resolution rates of 92% and 81%, respectively, regardless of age or laterality. For grades III and IV, bilateral VUR was less likely to resolve in comparison to unilateral VUR, and age at diagnosis had an inverse correlation with resolution rates in grade III VUR. Unilateral resolution rates for these higher grades were 43% to 70% at 5 years, as opposed to 10% to 49% in bilateral cases. Grade V VUR does not typically resolve spontaneously. Resolution rates in duplicated systems of all grades are lower and vary from 22% to 50%. Overall, the mean age of VUR resolution is 4.6 to 6.8 years, but some cases have demonstrated spontaneous resolution in the teenage years.

Given that most cases of primary VUR will resolve spontaneously and that reflux of sterile urine is unlikely to cause renal damage, most patients can be followed expectantly. To ensure sterility of the urine, continuous prophylactic antibacterial therapy is the treatment of choice for most children with VUR. The most commonly used antibacterial agents are sulfamethoxazole-trimethoprim or nitrofurantoin, which are given in one-fourth to one-half of the therapeutic dose to reduce the incidence of potential side effects. Traditionally, the antibacterial therapy is continued until the reflux has resolved, but there has been a growing trend toward stopping therapy in school-age children without voiding dysfunction (68). Some recommend serial urine cultures every few months to rule out occult UTI (60). Repeat cystography to monitor for improvement or resolution is performed every 12 to 18 months. Upper tract imaging to monitor renal growth and the presence of scarring can be helpful; sonography is the simplest way to monitor the kidneys, but technetium-99m dimercaptosuccinic acid renal scanning is more sensitive for detection of scarring. Somatic growth and blood pressure should also be followed.

Surgical correction of VUR is highly successful, but indications have been somewhat controversial. Four prospective trials were conducted to compare medical and surgical therapy using the endpoint of new renal scarring.

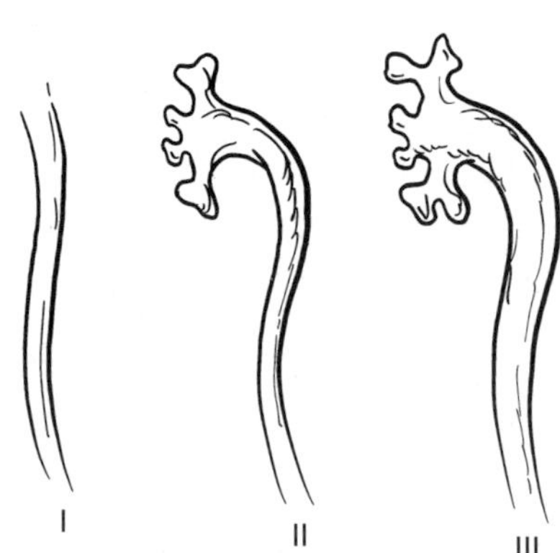

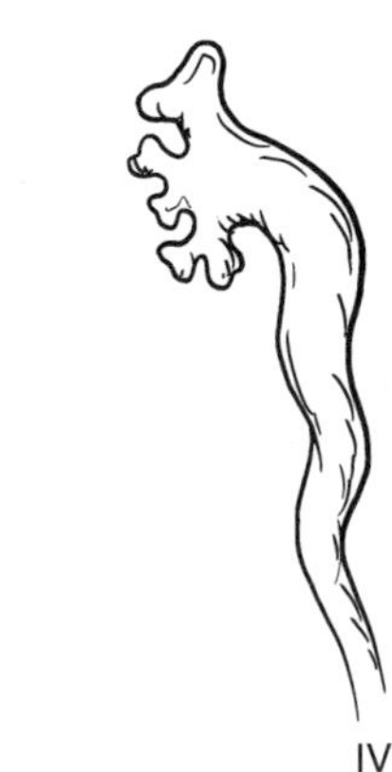

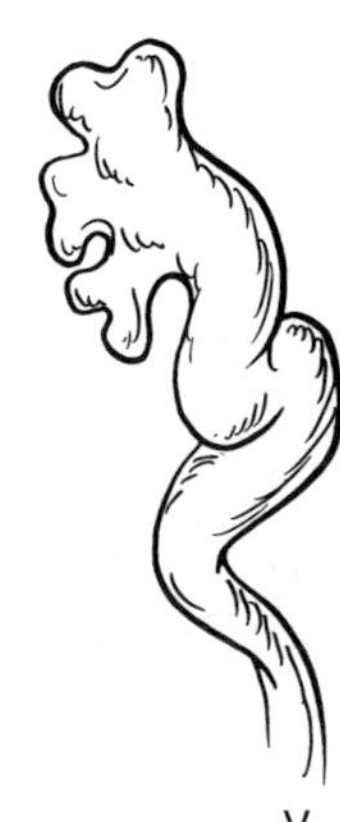

FIGURE 96-12. International Reflux Study Classification of grades of vesicoureteral reflux: grade I, into the ureter only; grade II, into the ureter, renal pelvis, and calices; grade III, mild or moderate dilation of the ureter and renal pelvis with no or minimal forniceal blunting; grade IV, moderate dilation and tortuosity of ureter and pelvis with blunting of the fornices but maintenance of the papillary impressions; and grade V, gross dilation and tortuosity of the ureter and pelvis with absence of the papillary impressions. (From Walsh PC, Retik AB, Stamey TA, et al., eds. *Campbell's urology*, 6th ed. Philadelphia: WB Saunders, 1992, with permission.)

None of the trials demonstrated a statistically significant difference in the occurrence of new scars between modalities (61). The indications for surgical therapy have traditionally included breakthrough UTIs, progressive renal scarring, high-grade reflux (grade IV or V), drug allergy or poor compliance of the patient to medical therapy and follow-up, and persistence of reflux into late childhood or adolescence, especially in girls. The latter indication is primarily aimed at preventing pyelonephritis during pregnancy, but the efficacy of antireflux surgery toward this end has been questioned (69).

With secondary VUR, underlying physiologic causes should be addressed if present prior to considering surgical management. Improved voiding with lower storage and emptying pressure should be the first priority in those with dysfunctional voiding, neurogenic bladder, or bladder outlet obstruction. If VUR is secondary to anatomic malformations, spontaneous resolution is less likely, and antireflux procedures may need to be combined with repair of the primary defect.

The goal of antireflux surgery is to create an adequate intravesical segment of ureter to prevent reflux. Paquin (70) found that the ureter in most normal children has a submucosal tunnel length/ureteral diameter ratio of 5:1; thus, surgery attempts to recreate the 5:1 ratio. Many techniques for antireflux have been described, but all can be classified as *intravesical* or *extravesical*. Transient postoperative urinary retention has been reported in 6% to 15% of children following bilateral extravesical reimplantation, and this is likely related to excessive dissection of the pelvic nerves on each side of the bladder (67). For this reason, extravesical antireflux surgery is usually reserved for unilateral cases. These procedures, whether intravesical or extravesical, are highly effective with success rates of 90% to 100% (67).

The endoscopic correction of reflux [also known as *STING* (subureteric injection technique)] was first described more than 20 years ago (71) and is rapidly gained widespread acceptance. A bulking substance is injected via cystscope just beneath the ureteral orifice to provide solid support to the intravesical ureter and convert the open ureteral orifice into a more closed cresentic shape. Although not as successful as open surgery, this technique has good efficacy with minimal morbidity and can be performed in the outpatient setting under a brief general anesthetic at any age. Transient ureteral dilation has rarely been noted, but ureteral obstruction has not been reported. The great challenge in this antireflux procedure has been to find the ideal bulking agent. It should easy to inject, inert, nonmigrating, nonresorbable, and nonantigenic. Initial reports used polytetrafluoroethylene (Teflon), which has proven to be the most effective agent. Unfortunately, Teflon has been noted to migrate to distant sites (72) and will be unlikely to receive approval from the Food and Drug Administration (FDA) in the United States. Glutaraldehyde cross-linked bovine dermal collagen has been used, but has inferior long-term results (65% success rate) likely due to its greater volume loss over time (73). In 2001, the FDA granted approval to a new substance [dextranomer/hyaluronic acid (Deflux)] for the endoscopic correction of grades II to IV VUR. This substance was first described in 1995 in Sweden (74), and a current American series (75) demonstrates great potential. Reflux was corrected in 90% of grade I, 82% of grade II, 73% of grade IV, and 65% of grade IV VUR. Endoscopic correction is currently being evaluated in more complex settings, such as following failed open surgery, in neuropathic or obstructed bladders, and in duplex systems. The proper indications and utility of endoscopic correction in the management of VUR is not well defined at this time, but it is clear that it will take on a much larger role in the coming years.

UROLITHIASIS

Pediatric urolithiasis differs from stone disease in adults and tends to more associated with specific metabolic disorders or anatomic abnormalities. Urolithiasis is rare in children in industrialized countries with an estimated prevalence 1/50 to 1/75 of that in adults and is usually localized to the upper urinary tract (76). Bladder stones are more common in boys in less developed nations, particularly in the Middle East and Asia; these typically consist of ammonium acid urate as a consequence of a low-protein diet (77).

Pain is noted in 50% of children with urolithiasis. The pain can localize to the upper abdomen, flank, or pelvis and may radiate to the umbilicus or groin. Associated nausea and vomiting are not uncommon. The typical patient with renal colic moves constantly trying unsuccessfully to find a comfortable position as opposed to the patient with peritonitis who attempts to remain still. Hematuria may be noted in 30% to 90% of children with stones, but gross hematuria is relatively uncommon (76).

Approximately 90% of urinary tract stones are radioopaque and can be seen on plain radiographs (78). Stones comprised of uric acid, struvite, or xanthine are typically radiolucent. Stones less than 0.5 mm may be difficult to detect on plain films due to overlying bowel gas and fecal material, and tomograms may be helpful to localize radiodensities to the urinary tract. IVP can usually demonstrate the calcification within the urinary tract, as well as provide functional evidence of obstruction due to the stone. IVP also provides the best delineation of the anatomy of the calyceal system, pelvis, and ureter that may be important in planning treatment. Ultrasound is often the preferred initial examation in children because of its lack of need for radiation, intravenous access, and contrast injection. The sensitivity of ultrasound for detection of renal calculi has been reported as high as 96% (78), and detection of ureteral calculi is aided by the presence

TABLE 96-3 Common Types of Urinary Calculi in Children

Type	Prevalence
Calcium oxalate	45%
Calcium phosphate	24%
Struvite (magnesium ammonium phosphate)	17%
Cystine	8%
Uric acid	2%
Xanthine	<1%

From Milliner DS, Murphy ME. Urolithiasis in pediatric patients. *Mayo Clin Proc* 1993;68:241, with permission.

of obstruction proximal to the calculus. Sonography can miss stones in the absence of hydroureteronephrosis, in the presence of overlying bowel gas or large body habitus, or with small stone size (less than 0.5 mm). CT scanning has become the "gold standard" for stone detection for a variety of reasons. Technological advances of spiral CT have allowed rapid scanning with 3- to 5-mm section images during a single breathhold. CT can detect nearly all stones due to their high density, even when radiolucent or as small as a few millimeters. Evidence of obstruction is easily seen, and body habitus is unimportant. Typically, intravenous constrast is not needed to localize the density within the urinary tract. Additional intrabdominal pathology can be noted when obtained in the setting of an acute abdomen (79).

There are multiple types and components of urinary calculi in humans (Table 96-3). The most common stones in children are composed of calcium oxalate and/or calcium phosphate (77). Infection-related stones may be found in up to one-third of children with stones; these are produced by urease-producing bacteria, most commonly *Proteus*, but also *Klebsiella*, *Pseudomonas*, and *Staphylococcus*. The resulting stones are termed *struvite* stones and are composed of magnesium ammonium phosphate. Other less common stones in children may be formed of uric acid, xanthine, or cystine. Stones form in the urinary tract because mineral crystals precipitate out of solution when the urine becomes supersaturated for their components. Urine is a complex solution containing many minerals and electrolytes, and alterations in their concentration, ionic strength, and urine pH all affect their solubility. Perhaps, most important is the volume of urine being produced to keep these components in solution because insufficient urine volume is the leading cause of urolithiasis. Modifiers of crystal formation present in urine can inhibit or promote the formation of some common crystals. Inhibitors of calcium phosphate or oxalate crystal formation include magnesium, citrate, zinc, pyrophosphate, and large-molecular-weight substances such as nephrocalcin, glycosaminoglycans, and RNA fragments (77).

Etiologies of Urolithiasis

Just as there are multiple types of urinary calculi, accordingly, there are multiple etiologies of calculus formation (Table 96-4). Primary causes can be inherited enzymatic defects of metabolism in extrarenal tissues, specific renal disorders in the excretion of solutes, dietary excesses and deficiencies, and hormonal disorders. Secondary etiologies include UTI, obstructive uropathies, and urinary diversion procedures.

Primary hyperoxaluria is a rare but malignant cause of urolithiais. Two specific autosomal recessive enzymatic defects are responsible and result in increased endogenous oxalate production. Excess amounts of oxalate (greater than 100 mg per 24 hours), L-glycerate, and glyoxalate in the urine are diagnostic of hyperoxaluria. Onset of the manifestations of the disorder is usually seen by age 5 years, and death may ensue in 7 to 8 years if untreated. Treatment is designed to reduce oxalate production and increase its urine solubilibility. Pyridoxine (vitamin B_6) can reduce oxalate production with a favorable response in 30% of type 1 patients. Magnesium salts and orthophosphates can reduce the saturation and crystallization of oxalate. In end-stage disease, combined hepatic–renal transplantation has been curative; the kidneys must be replaced following destructive stone disease,

TABLE 96-4 Etiologies of Urolithiasis in Children

I. Enzymatic disorders
   a. Primary hyperoxaluria
   b. Xanthinuria
   c. 2,8-Dihydroxyadeninuria
II. Renal tubular syndromes
   a. Cystinuria
   b. Renal tubular acidosis
III. Hypercalcemic states
   a. Hyperparathyroidism
   b. Immobilization
IV. Uric acid lithiasis
V. Enteric urolithiasis
VI. Idiopathic calcium oxalate urolithiasis
   a. Solute excess
      i. Hypercalciuria
         1. Renal
         2. Absorptive
      ii. Hyperoxaluria
      iii. Hypocitraturia
      iv. Hyperuricosuria
VII. Secondary urolithiasis
   a. Infection
   b. Obstruction
   c. Structural abnormalities
   d. Urinary diversion procedures

From Wehle MJ, Segura JW. Pediatric urolithaisis. In: Belman AB, King LR, Kramer SA, eds. *Clinical pediatric urology.* London: Martin Dunitz Ltd., 2002:1223–1245, with permission.

and the new liver can normally process the glycine pathway (76,77).

Hypercalcemia is a rare cause of urolithiasis in children and almost never occurs before puberty. Hyperparathyroidism, hypervitaminosis D, sarcoidosis, milk-alkali syndrome, paraneoplasic syndrome, Cushing's syndrome, and hyperthyroidism have all been associated with hypercalcemia and should be corrected primarily if related to nephrolithiasis. Children immobilized following severe trauma, orthopedic, or burn injuries are susceptible to hypercalcemia and subsequent stone formation. Lack of weight bearing leads to increased bone resorption, and concomitant dehydration reduces the solubility of calcium in the urine. Early ambulation and liberal hydration are recommended to prevent stone disease.

Uric acid stones are relatively rare in children and usually seen in the setting of excessive uric acid production. Myeloproliferative disorders, hemolytic anemic, sickle cell anemia, and cytodestructive chemotherapy of leukemia and lymphoma can result in cell death and release of purines, with subsequent development of uric acid stones. Dehydration and chronically acidic urine such as in chronic diarrheal disorders can also reduce uric acid solubility in the urine and produce uric acid stones. Uric acid stones should be suspected in the setting of radiolucent stones, acidic urine, and uric acid crystals in the urine. CT scans demonstrate hyperdensity of the stones that otherwise appears as lucent filling defects on IVP. Uric acid stones are the only common stones readily amenable to dissolution therapy. Alkanization of the urine to pH greater than 6.5 with oral potassium citrate preferably can dissolve the stones, but systemic alkanization with intravenous administration of alkali can be performed. Direct instillation of alkaline solution into the urinary tract through nephrostomy tubes also can be employed in carefully monitored situations to rapidly dissolve stones. Excessive urinary alkalinization risks calcium phosphate stone formation. An additional step in the treatment of uric acid urolithiasis is fluid intake to maintain a urine output of 30 to 40 mL per kg for 24 hours and use of allopurinol to diminish uric acid production.

Enteric urolithiasis is the result of GI disorders that promote stones by malabsorption. Diarrhea and malasorption often lead to dehydration, thus increasing the concentration of solutes in the urine. Loss of electrolytes also promotes lithogenesis by reducing the amount of stone inhibitors such as magnesium, pyrophosphates, and citrate in the urine. Enteric hyperoxaluria results when oxalate availability and absorption by the intestine are enhanced by fatty acid and bile salt malabsorption. Malabsorption causes calcium to complex with fatty acids (saponification) and makes calcium less available to bind to oxalates. Intestinal concentration of oxalates rises, which, in turn, leads to increased oxalate absorption and hyperoxaluria. Particularly in the setting of reduced stone inhibitors in urine, calcium oxalate stone formation is promoted. Treatment is initiated by reversing dehydration. Dietary oxalates should be reduced, and dietary calcium should be increased to reduce free oxalate within the bowel lumen. Cholestyramine is useful for bile salt malabsorption to prevent saponification of calcium. Potassium citrate can correct acidosis and hypocitraturia, and magnesium replacement can likewise inhibit stone formation. Patients with ileostomies can lose large amounts of fluid and bicarbonate, resulting in dehydration and acidosis, and they require increased fluid and citrate intake. These patients may have chronically acidic urine, which promotes uric acid stone disease. Allopurinol may be necessary in such a setting to combat the precipitation of uric acid in the acid urine.

Most children with stones have idiopathic calcium oxalate urolithiasis. This is a diagnosis of exclusion, but the tendancy toward calcium oxalate stone formation is strongly familial with an autosomal dominant pattern of inheritance. These patients can be segregated into groups based on hypercalciuria, hyperoxaluria, hypocitraturia, and hyperuricosuria. Hypercalciuria may be related to excess intestinal absorption (types I, II, and III absorptive hypercalciuria) or impaired renal tubular reabsorption of calcium (renal hypercalciuria). In the former types, dietary calcium restriction may be helpful, whereas thiazide diuretics to promote calcium reabsorption in the distal tubule may be necessary in the latter. Reducing oxalate intake without limiting calcium can be helpful in hyperoxaluria, which is usually caused by increased intestinal absorption. Hypocitrituria is present in 20% of patients with idiopathic calcium oxalate urolithiasis and can be treated with potassium citrate. Uric acid crystals in hyperuricosuria may promote calcium oxalate stone formation without uric acid stone formation; these patients can usually be managed with decreased purine intake and alkalinization of the urine.

Secondary urolithiasis occurs when additional factors in the urinary tract promote stone disease. UTI with specific urea-splitting bacteria can result in struvite stone formation. These bacteria contain urease, which converts urea into ammonium, raising the pH to greater than 7.2. In this alkaline enviroment, additional constituents precipitate, forming magnesium ammonium phosphate stones. These stones are laminated and large, often branching and filling the collecting system with a *staghorn calculus*. Urea-splitting bacteria are most often *Proteus* species, but can also include *Klebsiella, Pseudomonas, Providencia, Mycoplasma,* and *Staphylococcus* species. Infection stones tend to be more common in younger children (76), as well as in children with congenital abnormalities or indwelling foreign bodies that promote infection. Treatment requires clearance of the entire stone burden to eradicate the inciting organism; open surgery and/or multiple endoscopic procedures may be necessary to remove all the stones.

Correction of underlying defects that promote infection and prophylactic antibiotic therapy may also be required. Acetohydroxyamic acid (Lithostat), a urease inhibitor, may be of some value, but it is typically not used in children due its relatively high toxicity.

Obstruction of the upper tract can increase the transit time of urine, and this may allow supersaturation of solutes, promoting stone formation. The most commonly associated obstructive lesions are UPJ obstruction (80). Usually, the stone burden can be removed at the time of corrective surgery. Stone disease can recur following correction of the anomaly, and metabolic causes should be investigated. Structural anomalies, such as horseshoe kidney, medullary sponge kidney, and polycystic kidney disease, can also be associated with nephrolithiasis (76).

Urinary diversion procedures can also promote stone disease. Incontinent diversions allow easy ascent of bacteria into the upper urinary tract, and continent diversions usually require intermittent catheterization, which may seed the urinary tract with bacteria. Such patients have an increased risk of infection and stone formation in the bladder and kidneys. Metabolic changes in patients with lower urinary tract reconstruction include hypocitraturia and metabolic acidosis and may also promote noninfection stone formation (81). We noted a tenfold increase in nephrolithiasis in spina bifida patients with lower tract reconstruction in comparison to those with an intact bladder (82).

Management of Urolithiasis

Evaluation of children with urolithiasis should begin with a family history. Many of the previous etiologies are inherited in an autosomal dominant or recessive manner and are seen across generations. An additional clue to the etiology of stone disease is the age of onset. Stone formation beginning in the young child suggests an enzymatic defect, such as primary hyperoxaluria. Stone formation secondary to infection and obstruction related to congenital malformations of the urinary tract often present before the age of 5 years. Cystinuria, idiopathic calcium oxalate urolithiasis, and primary hyperparathyroidism more often begin in the teenage years. A thorough medical history can also elicit additional etiologies. Immobilization secondary to injury in children with active, growing bones may cause hypercalciuria. GI disease and surgery can also promote stone disease by affecting urine volume and concentrations of calcium, oxalate, and citrate. Neoplasms and their treatment can alter urine concentrations of calcium and uric acid.

Initial laboratory evaluation should include urinalysis and urine culture. Excessively low or high urine pH may be clues to the etiology of stones as is a positive urine culture with urea-splitting organisms. Microscopic analysis of urine crystals and a nitroprusside test for cystinuria can provide additional clues. Serum calcium, phosphorus, sodium, potassium, chloride, bicarbonate, uric acid, and creatinine levels should be checked. Appropriate imaging of the stone and urinary tract must be performed using sonography, plain films, IVP, and/or CT. If a stone is passed or removed surgically, it should be sent for crystalline analysis. Following treatment of the stone, a complete metabolic workup should be conducted in all children with stone disease (unless there is a compelling secondary cause). This includes 24-hour urine collection for measurement of volume, pH, creatinine, calcium, oxalate, uric acid, citrate, cystine, magnesium, sodium, and phosphate.

Surprisingly, children tend to pass stones of similar absolute size as adults. Most stones less than 3 mm will pass spontaneously, but when 4 mm or larger, spontaneous passage is uncommon (83). The indications for stone removal in children are similar to those in adults and include a symptomatic stone, an obstructing stone, or a stone that is a source of infection. Until recently, almost all stones necessitated an open surgical procedure for removal. Since the mid-1980s, with the development of percutaneous nephrolithotripsy, ureteroscopy, and shock wave lithotripsy (SWL), the need for open surgery has nearly been eliminated.

Shock Wave Lithotripsy (SWL)

Energy is generated extracorporealty to direct shock waves to fragment stones with subsequent spontaneous passage of the stone fragments. Localization of the stone is performed by fluoroscopy or sonography to target maximal energy concentration. The procedure is usually performed under general anesthesia in younger children, whereas sedation is usually sufficient for older children and adults with the modern generation of shock wave generators. SWL is effective for stones less than 2 cm in the urinary tract, whether in the kidney or ureter. SWL creates small parenchymal scars in the kidney, but these do not appear to affect long-term renal function in children (84). The energy of the shock waves can injure adjacent tissue in the lungs, spleen, and liver in children, and appropriate shielding may be necessary in small children. In general, stones break up well in children, perhaps because the shock wave is less attenuated by body mass than in adults. Modern stone-free rate are 82% to 100%, with stone size and composition being the most important determinants of success (85,86). In children, the ureter is more distensible and flexible, so even large fragments usually pass readily. The need for ureteral stenting prior to fragmentation was emphasized in the past, but appears less important in more recent experience. Occasionally, large fragments do not pass and require invasive maneuvers for removal. Cystine stones are harder, and those larger than 1 cm are relatively unresponsive to SWL. SWL should be avoided if obstructive uropathy is present because the fragments cannot pass spontaneously.

Percutaneous Nephrolithotripsy

Percutaneous nephrolithotripsy (PCNL) may be indicated for kidney stones that are larger than 2 cm, staghorn stones, cystine stones, upper ureteral stones that failed SWL, or as part of percutaneous endourologic procedure to manage calyceal diverticula or UPJ obstruction. With the child under general anesthesia, access to the kidney is achieved by insertion of a percutaneous nephrostomy tube under fluoroscopic control. The tract is then dilated to a size sufficient to introduce a nephroscope to visualize the stone. This leaves a scar of less than 1 cm in most cases, but potential complications include injury to the pleura, lung, and bowel. The stone is fragmented under direct vision with direct lithotripsy using ultrasonic, electrohydraulic, or pulse dye laser energy. The smaller the patient, the narrower is the margin of error; inadvertent fluid absorption generating fluid overload may be the greatest risk. Ideally, all stone fragments can be extracted, leaving most patients stone free (87). Disability and morbidity after the procedure are minimal, and the percutaneous nephrostomy tube can usually be removed in 1 to 2 days.

Ureteroscopy

Transurethral endoscopic access to the ureter is usually indicated for lower ureteral stones that do not pass spontaneously. The limitation of this procedure in children has always been the small size of the child's ureter relative to the available instruments and the necessity of dilating the ureters, which can result in reflux. Rigid ureteroscopes as small as 6F are now available for pediatric applications, allowing the lower third of the pediatric ureter to be entered and examined without ureteral dilation. Newer flexible ureteroscopes allow the upper ureter to be reached in most older children. With the child under general anesthesia, the ureteroscope is passed through the urethra and bladder and up the ureter to the level of the stone under fluoroscopic guidance. Stone fragmentation is performed using similar energy sources, but the advent of tiny optical fiber combined with holmium laser has greatly expanded the utility of ureteroscopic stone fragmentation. Stone-free rates approach 100%, making this modality preferable over SWL for most ureteral stones (88). Ureteral stenting after the procedure is often not required unless significant ureteral trauma occurred. The greatest risks of ureteroscopy procedures are ureteral trauma, perforation, and even avulsion; therefore, the surgeon must use great care and know the limitations of the technique.

Open Surgery

The rate of open surgery for stones in children is higher than in adults because of the limitations of SWL, PCNL, and ureteroscopy to remove large stones in the small upper urinary tract of children. Sometimes, the less invasive techniques cannot assure complete stone removal without the need for multiple sessions or without significant morbidity. Surgery is rare (about 4%) in children with urolithiasis; however, because urolithiasis in children may be associated with congenital anomalies, open surgery can allow simultaneous corrective surgery. Generally, lithotomy surgery involves a muscle-splitting abdominal wall incision and opening of the urinary tract through a relatively avascular plane where the stones reside on radiograph. The stones are removed, and the urinary tract is drained with a stent or nephrostomy tube following closure with fine absorbable sutures. Retroperitoneal drainage with a Penrose drain is necessary. In select cases, laparoscopy has been used more recently as a minimally invasive technique for difficult stone cases (89).

REFERENCES

1. Hinman F: "Kidney, ureter, and adrenal gland." *Atlas of Urosurgical Anatomy.* Philadelphia: W.B. Saunders Co. 1993, Chap 12., pp. 235–307.
2. Williams PL, Warwick R, Dyson M, et al. Gray's anatomy, ed 37. New York, Churchill Livingstone, 1989.
3. Kabalin JN. Surgical anatomy of the genitourinary tract. In: Walsh PC, Retik AB, Stamey TA, et al, eds. Campbell's urology, ed 6. Philadelphia, WB Saunders, 1992:35.
4. Weiss RM. The ureter. In: Gillenwater JY, Grayhack JT, Howards SS, et al, eds. Adult and pediatric urology. Ed 4. Philadelphia, Lippincott Williams & Wilkins, 2002, pp. 999–1021.
5. Weiss RM. Ureteral function. *Urology* 1978;12:114.
6. Coplen DE and Ortenberg J. Early development of the genitourinary tract. In: Gillenwater JY, Grayhack JT, Howards SS, et al, eds. Adult and pediatric urology. Ed 4. Philadelphia, Lippincott Williams & Wilkins, 2002, pp. 2027–2040.
7. Pope JC, Brock JW, Adams MC, et al. How they begin and how they end: classic and new theories for the development and deterioration of congenital anomalies of the kidney and urinary tract, CAKUT. *J Am Soc Nephrol* 10:2018–2028. 1999.
8. Campbell MF. Clinical Pediatric Urology. Philadelphia: W. B. Saunders Co., 1951. p. 217.
9. Moody T, Vaughan EJ, Gillenwater J. Relationship between renal blood flow and ureteral pressure during 18 hours of total unilateral ureteral occlusion. *Invest Urol* 13:246–51, 1975.
10. Fung LCT and Lakshmanan Y. Anomalies of the renal collecting system: ureteropelvic junction obstruction (pyelocalyectasis) and infundibular stenosis. In Belman AB, King LR, Kramer SA. Clinical Pediatric Urology. London: Martin Dunitz Ltd., 2002, pp. 559–631.
11. Ben-Chaim J, Gearhart J: Upper urinary tract. In Oldham KT, Colombani PM, Foglia RP. Surgery of Infants and Children: Scientific Principles and Practice. Philadelphia: Lippincott-Raven Publishers, 1997. pp. 1481–1515.
12. Beck AD. The effect of intra-uterine urinary obstruction upon the development of the fetal kidney. *J Urol* 105:784–9, 1971.
13. Kaplan GW, Brock WA. Abdominal masses. In Kelaias PP, King LR, Belman AB. Clinical Pediatric Urology. Philadelphia: W.B. Saunders Co., 1985, pp. 57–75.
14. Brown T, Mandell J, Lebowitz RL. Neonatal hydronephrosis in the era of sonography. *AJR* 148:959–963, 1987.
15. Thomas DFM. Fetal uropathy. *Br J Urol* 66:225, 1990.
16. Livera LN, Brookfield DS, Eggenton JA, et al. Antenatal ultrasonography to detect fetal renal abnormalities: a prospective screening programme. *Br Med J.* 298:421, 1989.
17. Anderson N, Clautice-Engle T, Allan R, et al. Detection of obstructive uropathy in the fetus: predictive value of sonographic measurements of renal pelvic diameter at various gestational ages. *AJR* 164:719, 1995.

18. Cendron M, Elder JS. Perinatal urology. In: Gillenwater JY, Grayhack JT, Howards SS, et al., eds. Adult and pediatric urology, 4th ed. Philadelphia: Lippincott Williams & Wilkins, 2002:2041–2127.
19. Wiener JS, O'Hara SM. Optimal Timing of Postnatal Sonograms in Newborns with Antenatal Hydronephrosis. *Journal of Urology,* 168:1826–9, 2002.
20. Crombleholme TM, Harrison MR, Golbus MS. Fetal intervention in obstructive uropathy: prognostic indicators and efficacy of intervention. *Am J Obstet Gynecol* 162:1239–44, 1990.
21. Elder JS, Duckett JW, Synder HM. Intervention for fetal obstructive uropathy: has it been effective? *Lancet ii:* 1007–9, 1987.
22. Farhat W, McLorie G, Geary D, et al. The natural history of neonatal vesicoureteral reflux associated with antenatal hydronephrosis. *J Urol* 164:1057–60, 2000.
23. Fernbach SK, Maizels M, Conway JJ. Ultrasound grading of hydronephrosis: introduction to the system used by the Society for Fetal Urology. *Pediatr Radiol* 1993;23:478.
24. Rodriguez LV, Lock J, Kennedy WA, et al: Evaluation of sonographic renal parenchymal area in the management of hydronephrosis. *J Urol,* 165:548, 2001.
25. Arant BS. Renal development: fluid and electolyte balance in neonates. In Belman AB, King LR, Kramer SA. Clinical Pediatric Urology. London: Martin Dunitz Ltd., 2002, pp. 23–34.
26. Bernstein GT, Mandell J, Lebowitz RL, et al. Ureteropelvic junction obstruction in the neonate. *J Urol* 140:1216–21, 1988.
27. Hoberman A, Charron M, Hickey R, et al. Imaging studies after a first febrile urinary tract infection in young children. *NEJM* 348:195–202, 2003.
28. Koff SA, Hayden LJ, Cirulli C. Pathophysiology of ureteropelvic junction obstruction: experimental and clinical observations. *J Urol* 1986;136:336.
29. Rooks VJ, Lebowitz RL. Extrinsic ureteropelvic junction obstruction from a crossing renal vessel: demography and imaging. *Pediatr Radiol* 31:120–4, 2001.
30. King LR, Coughlin PWF, Bloch EC, et al. The case for immediate pyeloplasty in the neonate with ureteropelvic junction obstruction. *J Urol* 132:725–8, 1984.
31. Ransley PG, Dhillon HK, Gordon I, et al. The postnatal management of hydronephrosis diagnosed by prenatal ultrasound. *J Urol* 144:584–7, 1990.
32. MacNeily AE, Maizels M, Kaplan WE, et al. Does early pyeloplasty really avert loss of renal function? A retrospective review. *J Urol* 150:769–73, 1993.
33. Ulman I, Jayanthi VR, and Koff SA. The long-term followup of newborns with severe unilateral hydronephrosis initially treated nonoperatively. *J Urol,* 164:1101, 2000.
34. Wiener JS and Roth DR. Outcome based comparison of surgical approaches for pediatric pyeloplasty: dorsal lumbar versus flank incision. *Journal of Urology,* 159:2116–2119, 1998.
35. Duel BP, Vates TS, Heiser D, et al. Antegrade pyelography before pyeloplasty via dorsal lumbar incision. *J Urol.* 162:174–6, 1999.
36. Hinman, F, Jr. Atlas of Urologic Surgery. Philadelphia: W.B. Saunders, Co., 1989. p. 688.
37. Nicholls F, Hrouda D, Kellett MJ, et al. Endopyelotomy in the symptomatic older child. *BJU Int.* 87:525–7.
38. Gerber GS, Kim J, Nold S, et al. Retrograde ureteroscopic endopyelotomy for the treatment of primary and secondary ureteropelvic junction obstruction in children. *Tech Urol* 6:46–9, 2000.
39. Figenshau RS, Clayman RV. Endourologic options for management of ureteropelvic junction obstruction in the pediatric patient. *Urol Clin North Am* 1998 May;25(2):199–209.
40. Eden CG, Cahill D, Allen JD. Laparoscopic dismembered pyeloplasty: 50 consecutive cases. *BJU Int.* 88:526–31, 2001.
41. Peters CA, Schlussel RN, Retik AB. Pediatric laparoscopic dismembered pyeloplasty. *J Urol* 153:1962–5, 1995.
42. Tan HL, Roberts JP. Laparoscopic dismembered pyeloplasty in children: preliminary results. *Br J Urol* 77:909–13, 1996.
43. Bloom DA and Koo HP. Ureterovesical and other ureteral obstructions. In Belman AB, King LR, Kramer SA. Clinical Pediatric Urology. London: Martin Dunitz Ltd., 2002, pp. 735–747.
44. McLellan DL, Retik AB, Bauer SB, et al. Rate and predictors of spontaneous resolution of prenatally diagnosed primary nonrefluxing megaureter. *J Urol* 168:2177–80, 2002.
45. McLaughlin AP III, Pfister RC, Leadbetter WF, et al. The pathophysiology of primary megaloureter. *J Urol* 1973;109:805.
46. Johnston JH. Reconstructive surgery of megaureter in childhood. *Br J Urol* 1967;39:17.
47. Hendren WH. Operative repair of megaureter in children. *J Urol* 1969;101:491.
48. Stephens FD. Correlation of ureteric orifice position with renal morphology. *Trans Am Assoc Genitourin Surg* 1976:53.
49. Schulman CC. The single ectopic ureter. *Eur Urol* 1976;2:64.
50. Ellerker AG. The extravesical ectopic ureter. *Br J Surg* 1958;45:44.
51. Wyle JB, Lebowitz RL. Refluxing urethral ectopic ureters: recognition by cyclic voiding cystourethrogram. *AJR* 1984;142:1263.
52. Mogg RA. The single ectopic ureter. *Br J Urol* 1974;46:3.
53. Smith FL, Ritchie EL, Maizels M, et al. Surgery for duplex kidneys with ectopic ureters: ipsilateral ureteroureterostomy versus polar nephrectomy. *J Urol* 1989;142:532.
54. Jednak R, Kryger JV, Barthold JS, Gonzalez R. A simplified technique of upper pole heminephrectomy for duplex kidney. *J Urol* 164:1326–8, 2000.
55. Gearhart JP, Jeffs RD. The use of topical vasodilators as an adjunct in infant renal surgery. *J Urol* 1985;134:298.
56. Campbell M. Ureterocele: a study of 94 instances in 80 infants and children. *Surg Gynecol Obstet* 1951;93:705.
57. Brock WA, Kaplan WG. Ectopic ureteroceles in children. *J Urol* 1978;119:800.
58. Klauber GT and Crawford DB. Prolapse of ectopic ureterocele and bladder trigone. *Urology.* 15:164, 1980.
59. Lyon RP, Marshall S, Tanagho EA. The ureteric orifice: its configuration and competency. *J Urol* 1969;102:504.
60. Hodson DJ. The radiologic diagnosis of pyelonephritis. *Proc R Soc Med* 52:669–72, 1959.
61. Elder JS, Peters CA, Arant BS Jr, et al. Pediatric Vesicoureteral Reflux Guidelines Panel summary report on the management of primary vesicoureteral reflux in children. *J Urol.* 157:1846–51, 1997.
62. Walker RD, Duckett JW, Bartone F, et al. Screening school children for urologic disease. *Pediatrics* 60:239, 1977.
63. Chen JJ, Pugach J, West D, et al. Infant vesicoureteral reflux: a comparison between patients presenting with a prenatal diagnosis and those presenting with a urinary tract infection. *Urology.* 61:442–6, 2003.
64. Walker RD. Vesicoureteral reflux: In Gillenwater JY, Grayhack JT, Howards SS, et al. (eds.) Adult and pediatric urology. Vol. 2, Chicago IL: Year Book Medical Publishers, 1676–708.
65. Askari A, Belman AB: Vesicoureteral reflux in black girls. *J. Urol.* 127:747–8, 1982.
66. Chertin B and Puri P. Familial vesicoureteral reflux. *J Urol* 169:1804–8, 2003.
67. Kramer SA. Vesicoureteral reflux. In Belman AB, King LR, Kramer SA. Clinical Pediatric Urology. London: Martin Dunitz Ltd., 2002, pp. 749–810.
68. Cooper CS, Chung BI, Kirsch AJ, et al: The outcome of stopping prophylactic antibiotics in older children with vesicoureteral reflux. *J Urol.* 163:269–72, 2000.
69. Mansfield JT, Snow BS, Cartwright PC, et al. Complications of pregnancy in women after childhood reimplantation for vesicoureteral reflux: an update with 25 years of follow-up. *J Urol* 154:787–90, 1995.
70. Paquin AJ. Ureterovesical anastomosis: the description and evaluation of a technique. *J Urol* 1959;82:573.
71. Matouschek E. Die behandlung des vesikorenalen Refluxes durch transurethrale Einspritzung von Teflonpaste. *Urologe* 1981;20: 263.
72. Malizia AA Jr, Reiman HM, Myers RP, et al. Migration and granulomatous reaction after periurethral injection of polytef (Teflon). *JAMA* 251:3277–81, 1984.
73. Leonard MP, Canning DA, Peters CA, et al. Endoscopic injection of glutaraldehyde cross-linked bovine dermal collagen for correction of vesicoureteral reflux. *J Urol.* 145:155–9, 1991.
74. Stenberg A, Lackgren G. A new bioimplant for the endoscopic treatment of vesicoureteral reflux: experimental and short term clinical results. *J Urol* 154:800–3, 1995.
75. Kirsch AJ, Perez-Brayfield MR, Scherz HC. Minimally invasive treatment of vesicoureteral reflux with endoscopic injection of

dextranomer/hyaluronic acid copolymer: the Children's Hospitals of Atlanta experience. *J Urol* 170:211–15, 2003.

76. Wehle MJ, Segura JW. Pediatric urolithaisis. I: Belman AB, King LR, Kramer SA, eds. *Clinical pediatric urology*. London: Martin Dunitz Ltd., 2002:1223–1245.
77. Jenkins A. Calculus formation. In Gillenwater JY, Grayhack JT, Howards SS, et al, eds. Adult and pediatric urology. Ed 4. Philadelphia, Lippincott Williams & Wilkins, 2002, pp. 356–92.
78. Dunnick NR, Sandler CM, Amis ES, Newhous JH. Nephrocalcinosis and nephrolithiasis. In Textbook of Uroradiology. Baltimore: Williams and Wilkins. 1997. pp. 254–281.
79. Matusmoto JS, Le Roy AJ. Pediatric imaging. In Belman AB, King LR, Kramer SA. Clinical Pediatric Urology. London: Martin Dunitz Ltd., 2002, pp. 83–134.
80. Troup CW, Lawnicki CC, Bourne RB, et al. Renal calculus in children. *J Urol* 107:306–7, 1972.
81. Franco I and Levitt SB.Urolithiasis in the patient with augmentation cystoplasty: pathogenesis and management. AUA Update Series vol 16, lesson 2, 1997.
82. Raj GV, Bennett RT, Preminger GM, et al. Incidence of nephrolithiasis in patients with spinal neural tube defects. *J Urol* 162:1238–42, 1999.
83. Van Savage JG, Palanca LG, Andersen RD, et al. Treatment of distal ureteral stones in children: similarities to the American Urological Association guidelines in adults. *J Urol.* 164:1089–93, 2000.
84. Vlajkovic M, Slavovic A, Radovanovic M, et al: Long-term functional outcome of kidneys in children with urolithiasis after ESWL treatment. *Eur J Pediatr Surg.* 12:118–23, 2002.
85. Gofirt ON, Pode D, Meretyk S, et al. Is the pediatric ureter as efficient as the adult ureter in transporting fragments following extracorporeal shock wave lithotripsy for renal calculi larger than 10mm? *J Urol* 166:1862–4, 2001.
86. Landau EH, Gofrit ON, Shapiro A: Extracorporeal shock wave lithotripsy is highly effective for ureteral calculi in children. *J Urol* 166:2316–9, 2001.
87. Zeren S, Satar N, Bayazit Y, et al. Percutaneous nephrolithotripsy in the management of pediatric renal calculi. *J Endourol* 16:75–8, 2002.
88. Schuster TG, Russell DY, Bloom DA, et al. Ureteroscopy for the treatment of urolithiasis in children. *J Urol* 167:1813–5, 2002.
89. Gaur DD, Trivedi S, Prabhudesai MR. Laparoscopic ureterolithotomy: technical considerations and long-term follow-up. *BJU Int* 89:339–43, 2002.

Chapter 97

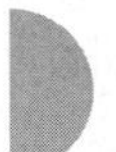

Bladder Diseases in Childhood

Craig A. Peters

INTRODUCTION

Normal bladder function is essential to all children in their physical and psychosocial development. Abnormalities of bladder function may have profound effects on the well-being of any child, ranging from simple family tension as a result of persistent enuresis, to permanent loss of renal function due to hypertonic bladder dysfunction. The work of the bladder rests on two basic functions: (1) storage and (2) emptying. Storage of urine for a socially acceptable period of time requires the bladder to accommodate by enlarging its capacity without increasing its pressure. Bladder compliance is the critical parameter involved in normal storage. Normal emptying of the bladder permits continence of urine between emptying and efficient evacuation of the stored urine in a timely fashion, under voluntary control. This action requires the coordination of the detrusor muscle of the bladder itself with the bladder neck or internal sphincter and the skeletal or voluntary sphincter. The contraction must be sustained for a sufficiently long period to permit complete emptying. Discoordination of the activities of the detrusor and sphincter produce significant derangements in bladder function and may produce permanent damage.

A basic understanding of the activity of the bladder is essential to permit clinical assessment and management of various bladder disorders. Bladder dysfunction has become an active area of investigation as the clinical, social, and economic significance of bladder diseases has become evident. Understanding of childhood bladder dysfunction on a clinical basis has developed rapidly, and the basic scientific knowledge is beginning to catch up and offer the potential for novel therapeutic interventions.

This chapter briefly reviews normal bladder anatomy and function, patterns of bladder development, and the manifestations of bladder diseases. The assessment and management of the major categories of bladder dysfunction are presented. Areas of developing understanding that will influence therapy are also be reviewed.

Craig A. Peters: Harvard Medical School, Boston Children's Hospital, Boston, Massachusetts 02115.

Normal Bladder Anatomy and Function

Although the basic structure and function of the bladder may appear simple, it is an organ dependent on complex interactions of autonomic and voluntary neural regulation, as well as smooth and skeletal muscle groups, to store and expel a hypertonic solution without significant absorption or inadvertent leakage. Clinically significant bladder disorders are the result of various failures in these processes. The functional anatomy of the urinary bladder has been the more recent subject of vigorous investigation in the adult, principally aimed at understanding bladder outlet obstruction in the male, incontinence in the female, and neurologic bladder disease in the spinal cord injury patient. Many of the principles of bladder function in the adult are applicable in the child, yet this assumption should not be too broadly applied.

Anatomy

The bladder in the young child is an intraabdominal organ that becomes progressively intrapelvic with age. It is extraperitoneal, which permits most surgical exposures to be performed without peritoneal entry. The ureters enter posterolaterally from the deep posterior pelvis and are associated with the obliterated umbilical arteries, the vas deferens in the male, and the uterine ligaments and fallopian tubes in the female. The base of the bladder rests on the pelvic floor, or the urogenital diaphragm, an important structure in the maintenance of continence. The support of the bladder neck provided by the pelvic floor and skeletal pelvis is particularly important for continence.

The bladder is usually divided into two anatomic parts, the body or detrusor, and the base, including the trigone and bladder neck. These are of distinct embryologic origin, with functional and neurophysiologic differences. The detrusor is composed of an inner epithelial layer with three cell layers, including a basal cell layer and a relatively impermeable lumenal epithelial layer. Beneath the uroepithelium is the lamina propria, consisting of connective tissue elements, which may have significant functional importance as a mediator of bladder compliance (1). The muscular layers of the bladder are not as distinctly organized into longitudinal and circumferential layers as in the intestine, but are more of an interdigitating meshwork of smooth muscle bundles and connective tissue elements, including fibroblasts, collagen fibers, and elastin, along with several other extracellular matrix components.

Uroepithelium

The biologic properties of the uroepithelium are only recently coming to be recognized. Previously considered impermeable, there is evidence to indicate selective permeability with ion transport that may be influenced by mechanical factors. A protective layer of glycosaminoglycans probably acts as a protective coat and disruptions in this layer are believed to be related to several inflammatory conditions, including interstitial cystitis (2). They are likely to play a role in resistance to infection as well. The uroepithelium appears to be important in the developmental regulation of bladder formation (3–5), and it may continue to play a regulatory role in the function of the detrusor muscle. This relationship is likely to be a two-way communication network.

Muscular Components

The muscular layer of the trigone merges inferiorly into the proximal urethra and taken together this muscular complex functions as a sphincter. Although there is no anatomically distinct internal sphincter, its functional existence is supported by urethral pressure studies, videourodynamic observations, and by the fact that continence may be maintained with its sole presence or lost with injury. Its function as a sphincter is augmented by soft-tissue coaptation and elasticity, loss of which will impair continence. These smooth muscle fibers may be seen to interdigitate with skeletal muscle of the external sphincter (6,7). The skeletal muscle sphincter is more anatomically distinct, and acts to maintain continence with activity and permit voluntary termination of urination. Discoordination of the activity of the sphincters with that of the detrusor may lead to significant bladder dysfunction.

Innervation and Neural Control of Bladder Function

The bladder is richly innervated by sacral parasympathetic fibers from S2 to S4, thoracolumbar sympathetic fibers, and sacral somatic fibers traveling through the pudendal nerves (8). Bladder function is regulated through the interactions of both autonomic and voluntary neural systems, with both spinal and brainstem reflex arcs, as well as cerebral control over their activity. A variety of neural effectors are active in normal bladder function, and many neurotransmitters have been shown to influence bladder function. The basic bladder functions and their neural control include filling and storage, which requires relaxation of the detrusor and concomitant sphincter contraction, and emptying, which is dependent on a sustained bladder contraction with coordinated sphincteric relaxation.

Filling and storage of the bladder must be at low pressure. Two primary factors contribute to these properties of the bladder. The smooth muscle of the bladder must relax against a passive stretch induced by increasing bladder volume (9). Smooth muscle relaxation has been shown to be an active process, mediated at a molecular level by dephosphorylation of myosin light chains, as well as changes in a Ca^{++}-dependent force maintenance system referred to as a *latch state* (10,11). Centrally, relaxation is mediated through storage reflexes that increase the inhibitory impulses to the bladder as intravesical pressure rises. These impulses are mostly sympathetic via the β-adrenergic receptor system. This occurs with increased sphincter activity and is believed to be controlled at the level of the lateral pontine reticular formation (8). This relationship underscores the conceptual notion that bladder function is often determined by balances between excitatory and inhibitory influences. Although bladder function is biphasic (storage and emptying), switching between these phases appears to be the result of alterations in thresholds of activity that are influenced by a dynamic balance of excitatory and inhibitory influences (12).

The extracellular matrix is also important in bladder storage characteristics, possibly more than the muscular components, and is described by the viscoelastic properties of the connective tissue matrix (13). The importance of this element of bladder compliance is particularly relevant in the child with a noncompliant bladder from prior obstruction because developmental alterations in matrix remodeling have been shown to occur with fetal obstruction (14). The folding and unfolding of connective tissue bundles, and the properties of individual fibers such as elastin, contribute to the overall properties of the bladder as it fills with urine (15,16).

Bladder emptying requires initiation and maintenance of a detrusor contraction, coordinated with relaxation of the sphincters under voluntary control. The infant demonstrates involuntary or reflex voiding. More recent studies suggest a level of cortical control and involvement with infantile voiding (17). Central coordination is through the pontine micturition center, which acts as a switch, triggered by a level of afferent or sensory impulses from the bladder as it fills. Activation of the sacral parasympathetic nerve fibers inhibit the somatic pathways to the urethral sphincter and permit relaxation. Sympathetic activity, which permits bladder filling, is inhibited and parasympathetic activation of the bladder occurs. Cortical inhibition of these reflexes can prevent onset of micturition.

The mediators of bladder neural control have been widely studied. The principal neuropharmacologic mechanisms include the cholinergic and adrenergic systems, as well as purinergic and peptidergic mechanisms, are likely to play an important role in function and dysfunction. Cholinergic receptors in the bladder body are largely muscarinic (M2) and act to stimulate muscle contraction. They are balanced by adrenergic $\beta 2$ receptor mechanisms. Purinergic receptors responsive to adenosine triphosphate or adenosine contribute to the contractile response, and may serve to initiate a contraction, which is then sustained by cholinergic activity. Adrenergic activity in the bladder neck and urethra is mostly alpha-receptor mediated and stimulatory. Selective agonists and antagonists have permitted demonstration of site-specific receptor subtype distribution, and therefore, more specific pharmacologic control over function. Peptidergic neurotransmission has been documented in the bladder, including activity of vasoactive intestinal peptide, neuropeptide-Y, substance P, somatostatin, calcitonin gene-related peptide, cholecystokinin, and enkephalin immunoreactive fibers (18,19). The precise functional role(s) of these neurotransmitters remains to be defined.

The effect of bladder pathology on neural regulation of function is critical to recognize, particularly in the developing child. Abnormal function, as in obstruction, alters development, which then further affects function. Although there is little alpha-adrenergic activity in the normal bladder body, increases in alpha-sensitivity has been shown to follow obstruction. Changes in the level of existing receptors occur with both prenatal and postnatal obstruction, and with abnormal innervation (20–22). The functional changes induced by obstruction also affect central neural activity and patterns of innervation (23). This may have long-lasting effects, even after the inducing abnormality has been corrected. The concept of neural plasticity in the regulation of bladder function, particularly in the developing bladder, is critical (24).

Normal bladder function may be seen as a dynamic balance between the two basic phases of bladder activity, storage, and emptying. There are neural, muscle, and matrix components contributing to that balance. Abnormalities in these components are the basis for many bladder disorders. Improved understanding of the normal and abnormal integration of those factors and their clinical manifestations will permit more specific therapeutic intervention for children with bladder disorders.

BLADDER DEVELOPMENT

Embryonic Formation and Associations

The bladder forms from the embryonic endoderm and the trigone from the mesoderm (25). The bladder epithelial surface derives from the endodermal layer and may have a significant role in the induction and maturation of the mesodermal layer as it becomes the detrusor muscle and connective tissues of the bladder wall. As the ventral plate of the embryo infolds, the combined bladder and gut structures take on the form of a tube and become the cloaca (Latin for "sewer") as a common channel. There is as yet no opening at what will become the perineum, but the allantois is patent and runs parallel to the umbilical vessels. Separation of the ventral bladder and dorsal gut structures occurs between 5 and 8 weeks, concurrent with separation of the ureter and mesonephric duct with ingrowth of the urorectal septum. The trigone (triangular area bounded by the ureteral orifices and the bladder neck) is initially mesodermal, but is ultimately surfaced by endodermal epithelium. The cloacal membrane remains closed at this time, but is hypothesized to rupture early in the production of cloacal exstrophy. When fully separate from the hind gut, the bladder is beginning to receive urine from the metanephric kidneys (8 weeks). The ureteral structures and associated mesonephric structures are still developing. It is clear that epithelial and mesenchymal interactions similar to the induction of the bladder mesoderm continue to influence maturation of these structures.

Development of Musculature

An important element in the bladder that develops in the late embryonic and early fetal period is the bladder musculature. Muscle cells are first seen about 7 weeks, and recognizable bundles are present by 12 weeks (26). Bladder myocytes either migrate from surrounding mesenchyme, or the undifferentiated mesodermal cells surrounding the bladder epithelium are induced to differentiate in a muscular pattern. Urothelial regulation of bladder myogenesis and differentiation has been demonstrated in rodent recombination models (3,5). The mediators of those interactions remain to be identified, but hold promise to understand aberrations of development, as well as potential for therapeutic intervention.

Bladder filling and emptying also plays a role in modulating this process; bladders that have never functioned (i.e., exstrophy of the bladder) have a variety of developmental differences from normal bladders. The onset of this interaction may not be active until closure of the urachus, which is about 16 weeks in the human. Innervation of the bladder has begun by this time because receptors for various neurotransmitters have been shown in the early fetal bladder (27). Muscularization of the bladder continues with further growth and presumed integration of muscles and nerves. Little is known as to the mediators of bladder innervation in the fetus. The functional characteristics of bladder smooth muscle cells in the fetus have been investigated, with focus on the ontogeny of calcium regulation of contractility (28) as well as the presumed role of nitric oxide (29). Sphincter function can be demonstrated at 8 weeks, and is followed by development of the ureterovesical junction. Development of the external urethral sphincter is an important element in the functional patterns of the developing bladder and may contribute to abnormal functional maturation (30,31).

The functional development of the extracellular matrix of the fetal bladder has been examined in a variety of systems. Developmental relative increases of collagen type I have been reported in the bovine fetus (32,33) and associated with developmental increases in bladder compliance (28). These observations differ from those of Swaiman (34) in the human, in which the developmental balance between type I and III collagen decreases, which is the reverse of that seen in the fetal calf. Other components of the matrix are likely be equally important, particularly elastin. An important component of extracellular matrix (ECM) homeostasis is the degradation arm of collagens and elastins. Connective tissue breakdown is mediated through a family of proteins, the matrix metalloproteinases (MMPs), which selectively degrade particular components of the ECM. Regulation of the activity of degradation will therefore have a major role in the matrix composition in the bladder, and this degrading activity is directly inhibited by the tissue inhibitors of metalloproteinases (TIMPs), endogenous and semispecific inhibitors of the MMPs (35). In fetal obstruction, the expression and activity of the TIMPs is increased, producing a decrease in the degradation of the matrix, which ultimately leads to increased amounts of ECM.

Fetal Bladder Function

It has long been recognized that bladder function is ongoing in the fetus, and it is likely that structural and functional development is dependent on bladder activity. Defunctionalized bladders in the fetal sheep have altered patterns of contractile protein isoforms and altered concentrations of muscarinic cholinergic receptors (20). Connective tissue elements are influenced by this activity, in that defunctionalized bladders show reduced procollagen type III gene expression. Although many of the mechanisms of interaction are unclear, it has been shown that fetal bladder function is a critical aspect of development (36).

Ultrasonographic images of the human and sheep fetal bladders show continued filling and emptying cycles in later gestation, with contractions every 10 to 15 minutes (37,38). The response to pharmacologic agents has also been described, including agents commonly used in obstetric practice. Magnesium sulfate, for example, will suppress almost all bladder contractions in the fetus, and postnatal voiding may be impaired until this effect has cleared.

Perinatal Bladder Function

Postnatally, there is a maturational process in development of normal bladder function (17). Infant voiding is characterized by small infrequent and incomplete voiding. Interrupted voiding may be seen in 60% of preterm infants and 30% of full-term children. Infant bladders tend to be more hyperactive with voiding at low volume and with high pressure. The most likely cause of this pattern is immature coordination between the detrusor and the sphincter mechanisms. There seems to be a relationship with voiding and sleep, whereby voiding is usually associated with arousal from sleep in the full-term child and less so in the preterm infant. The association with arousal suggests a role for higher cortical control, rather than a completely autonomic pattern as previously believed.

Ultrasonographic Appearances

Maternal-fetal ultrasound can detect many bladder abnormalities, both directly and indirectly. Identification of the bladder on maternal fetal ultrasound should be possible by 16 to 18 weeks in the normal fetus. The inability to demonstrate the bladder despite two or more attempts is abnormal and should prompt consideration of severe renal dysfunction, bladder exstrophy, or a severe abnormality of the bladder neck or ureteral positioning. Protrusion of tissue at the level of the lower umbilicus without a visible bladder lumen should raise the possibility of bladder or cloacal exstrophy, and this may be associated with a low set umbilical cord. When visible, the bladder should be filled with echo-transmitting fluid without debris or internal echogenic structures. A ureterocele may be demonstrated prenatally when present (usually associated with upper pole hydronephrosis). Massive dilation of the fetal bladder may be seen with bladder outlet obstruction as from valves, with massive vesicoureteral reflux (39), and with the prune belly syndrome (PBS). Bladder wall thickness, the condition of the renal parenchyma, and the status of the amniotic fluid are useful in distinguishing between these (40). The bladder affected by posterior urethral valves may not be massively dilated, but may have a very thickened wall and be only moderately full. The kidneys and ureters are dilated and the renal parenchyma may be echogenic, indicating some degree of dysplasia (41). Male gender should be identified in such cases and oligohydramnios may be present (42). Caution needs to be exercised in the clinical distinction between obstructive and nonobstructive conditions of the fetal bladder.

MANIFESTATIONS OF BLADDER DISEASE

The principal manifestations of bladder disorders include incontinence of urine, infection, hydronephrosis, hematuria and dysuria, or an alteration in voiding pattern. Each may be present in a spectrum of severity, with specific characteristics indicative of the underlying condition. Recognition of these signs and symptoms is not always immediate and in certain situations they should be specifically sought.

Incontinence

Inadvertent urinary emptying, incontinence, may be one of the most troubling symptoms to afflict a child after the age of toilet training. Causes range from behavioral patterns to major structural anomalies of the urinary tract or nervous system. The patterns of incontinence serve as the most useful initial tool to define the cause. *Nighttime incontinence*, nocturnal enuresis, is most often a maturational, self-limited entity, but should prompt a thorough history and physical examination to rule out subtle manifestations of more serious disease. *Daytime wetting* is primary if it has always been present or secondary if it develops after normal training. *Constant dampness* in a girl would suggest an ectopic ureter to the distal urethra, introitus, or vagina. *Total incontinence*, wetness without a dry interval, suggests a significant structural defect of the bladder neck (epispadias, bilateral ureteral ectopia) or a neurologic defect. Lesser degrees of these conditions may be manifest by *episodic incontinence*, as with stress or movement. *Urgency incontinence*, in which the child senses the need but cannot inhibit voiding, may be behavioral or neurologic; associated signs or symptoms should be sought. *Overflow incontinence* may be suspected in someone with small to moderate amounts of leakage, usually without urgency to void, and a full bladder will be identified with examination or catheterization. A structural, neurologic, or behavioral basis may be present and require careful further evaluation.

Infection

Urinary tract infections (UTIs) are one of the most common health problems in children (43) and may be a manifestation of bladder dysfunction. Inadequate bladder emptying, with or without obstruction, is the most frequent underlying cause. The association with upper tract infection of the kidney, pyelonephritis (44), is largely dependent on the presence or absence of reflux, upper tract drainage, and the nature of the infecting organism. Diagnosis of infection is a critical guide to further evaluation and should be based on a properly collected specimen. In the sick child, in whom antibiotics are to be started empirically, a definitive culture must be obtained at the outset, using catheterization or a suprapubic aspirate. Clean voided specimens in toilet-trained children with minimal symptoms are acceptable. A bag-collected specimen is of value in a negative culture or in the unusual pure growth of high colony count (even so, the false-positive rate is about 50%); no major therapeutic decision should be based on such a specimen.

The most appropriate evaluation of a child with a UTI remains controversial (45,46). The clinical distinction between cystitis and upper tract infection remains challenging and unreliable. Infants with a culture-proven infection should undergo ultrasonographic imaging and cystography. Older children may be equally served with ultrasonography alone if normal, although the transition age is not defined. The nature of the infection should guide evaluation. Most major structural or functional abnormalities will present with febrile infections, but this is not universal.

Hydronephrosis

Bladder dysfunction may be associated with hydronephrosis as a causative agent or a concomitant factor. Bladder outlet obstruction due to either structural or functional reasons may produce upper tract dilation. Usually this is bilateral and symmetric (Fig. 97-1), but may be unilateral.

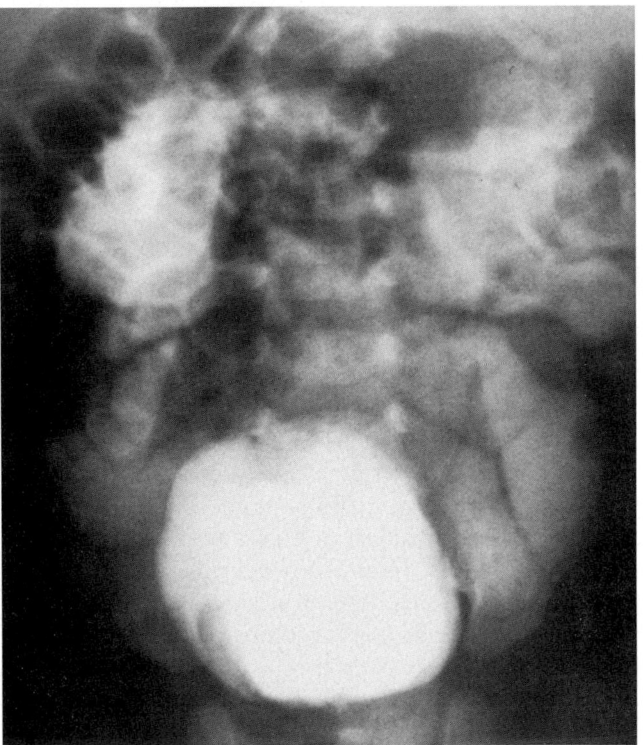

FIGURE 97-1. Massive bilateral hydronephrosis due to posterior urethral valves and vesicoureteral reflux in a newborn with prenatally detected bladder obstruction due to posterior urethral valves. (From Mandell J, and Peters, CA. Current concepts in the perinatal diagnosis and management of hydronephrosis. *Urol Clin North Am* 1990;17:247, with permission.)

Posterior urethral valves may cause unilateral high-grade dilation with renal parenchymal disruption [vesicoureteral reflux and dysplasia (VURD) association] (47), in which one renal unit acts as the pressure release of the high-pressure bladder. Very often, obstructed bladders will be thick-walled and hypertrophic. As a result, there may be an element of obstruction at the ureterovesical junction contributing in part or whole to the upper tract dilation (48). This factor may be difficult to assess, but may be demonstrated by reducing bladder pressures with temporary diversion.

The effect of bladder pressure on upper tract dilation is due to the imbalance of ureteral peristaltic pressure moving urine into the bladder and the level of pressure within the bladder cavity. Forty centimeters of water pressure is the generally accepted maximal level of pressure generated by the ureter to transmit urine; vesical pressures exceeding this will cause cessation of flow into the bladder and if pressures exceed this, as during a bladder contraction, increased pressure may be transmitted to the kidneys (49). The effect of prolonged elevated pressures on the upper urinary tracts and renal parenchyma has been demonstrated clinically and may produce progressive renal functional deterioration and renal failure. The maximal pressures reached by the bladder with contraction are not the most important factor, however. The total work over time done against the kidney by bladder pressure is most critical and should be assessed to guide management. The product of pressure over the "safe" level of 35 or 40 cm H_2O and the time during which this occurs is the work done against the kidney. Normal voiding pressures exceed 35 cm H_2O, yet occur only six to eight times per day for 1 to 2 minutes; bladder pressures in the normal then fall to 5 cm H_2O for the rest of the time. If bladder pressures reach near 35 cm H_2O quickly as the bladder refills and stay at that level for most of the bladder filling cycle, the total work against the kidney over a 24-hour period is far greater than in the normal (Fig. 97-2). This concept of a "safe" period of bladder filling is critical to determining appropriate bladder management. Hydronephrosis associated with bladder dysfunction should be sought in patients in whom high-pressure bladder patterns may be seen, including those with neuropathic bladders or previously obstructed bladders (so-called "valve" bladders) (50,51). When present, hydronephrosis must be dealt with aggressively and monitored diligently, by addressing the bladder dysfunction.

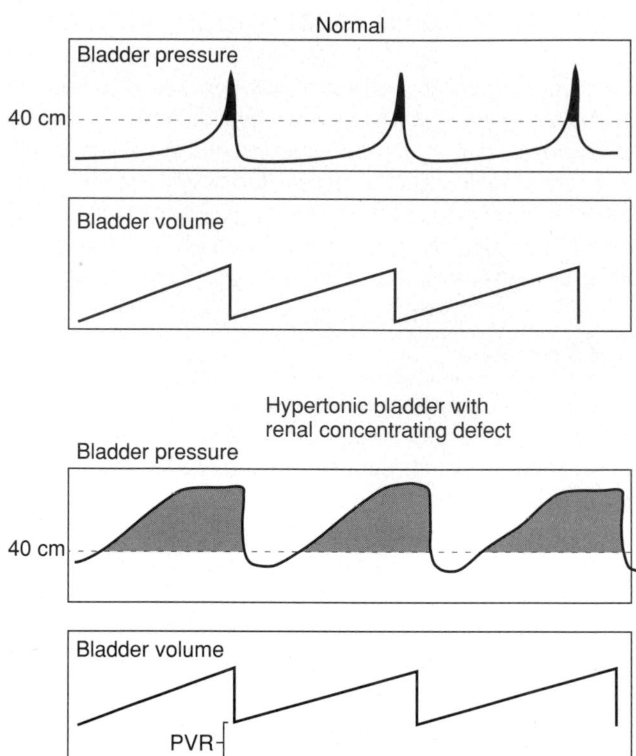

FIGURE 97-2. Two schematic representations of bladder pressure and volume curves over several filling and emptying cycles. In the normal bladder, intravesical pressures exceed 40 cm H_2O only at the very end of filling, near capacity. The work done against the kidneys is small. In contrast, the hypertonic bladder demonstrates an increase in pressure with small increases in volume due to poor compliance. The pressures reach 40 cm H_2O much sooner than normally. In conjunction with a renal concentrating defect, which is common in boys with posterior urethral valves, high intravesical pressures occur even more quickly due to rapid bladder filling. If bladder emptying is not complete, as is often the case, the abnormal post void residual pushes the bladder pressure volume curve further to the right and high pressures. These factors contribute to greater period of time where intravesical pressures exceed 40 cm H_2O and can produce renal damage. Careful evaluation of bladder filling dynamics permits assessment of the safe period of the bladder cycle and serves to guide therapy. (Adapted from Peters CA. Congenital bladder obstruction. *Curr Prob Urol* 1994;8:333, with permission.)

Hematuria

Blood in the urine is a dramatic symptom and must be dealt with thoroughly. In children, however, it does not have the same sinister implications as in adults. The pattern of hematuria will often provide sufficient clues to permit a diagnosis and guide further evaluation. Total gross hematuria, bloody urine from beginning of voiding to the end, may be associated with flank pain or dysuria, or may be painless. Flank pain would focus attention on the ureters and kidneys; dysuria on the bladder and urethra and painless hematuria requires a full evaluation. Ultrasonographic examination of the entire urinary tract is a useful first step and will serve to identify upper tract lesions and most bladder neck lesions such as tumors or polyps. Viral cystitis in children will often be associated with severe voiding pain and urgency, and may have such marked edema of the entire bladder wall as to mimic a neoplastic process. Eosinophilic cystitis may present in a similar manner with a discrete mass noted on imaging. This process is of unclear origin and may represent an allergic process. It is variably responsive to corticosteroids and will eventually resolve spontaneously. Biopsy may be needed to rule out a true neoplasm. Cystoscopy in children is seldom revealing and may serve more to reassure anxious parents. Often a watchful waiting period is useful because there are few lesions that must be immediately identified that would be missed by a careful physical examination (including rectal examination) and ultrasonography. The nature of the bleeding may serve to guide this decision. Terminal hematuria, occurring at the end of voiding is indicative of a process at the bladder base or more commonly of the urethra. In peripubertal boys, this is often due to a process termed *benign urethrorrhagia*, (52) a self-limited condition of unknown etiology, without long-term sequelae. Cystoscopy is not needed in most cases, which should resolve within 6 to 8 weeks. Meatal bleeding is most often due to urethral meatal stenosis. This is readily confirmed on examination and by observation of the voiding stream, which typically deviates upward and is thin and jetlike.

Dysuria

Painful urination is a common symptom in children and may be relatively mild or extreme. On occasion, this will also be described as suprapubic pain after voiding. Severe abrupt pain during voiding is termed *strangury* and may indicate episodic obstruction as from a stone or bladder neck polyp, particularly if urine flow stops. Dysuria is most often the result of UTI, but may also be due to simple perineal irritation, obstruction, or abnormal voiding dynamics. The extreme manifestation of the latter is bladder sphincter discoordination (dyssynergy) and may produce pain in the neurologically intact child. This may be structural or behavioral. In boys with dysuria, it is prudent to rule out a bladder neck obstructive process such as a tumor with a rectal examination, ultrasound, or both. This is an unusual, but not infrequently missed diagnosis. Unusual causes of dysuria in children that should be considered include interstitial cystitis, eosinophilic cystitis, and granulomatous disease of the bladder.

Altered Voiding Pattern (Frequency, Decreased Flow, Retention)

Changes in voiding pattern may indicate a variety of problems, most of which may be identified with a careful history and examination. Frequency of urination is most likely due to infection, but may represent bladder instability due to a neurologic or obstructive process. In kindergarten age boys, however, this is most often a behavioral, self-limited process termed *poikilouria* (53). Diminished flow may be the result of outlet resistance such as a urethral stricture or valves, but may also be due to impaired contractility of the bladder. Urinary retention may result from a semiacute obstructive process, such as tumor of the bladder base or prostate, or from bladder decompensation in a chronic setting of partial obstruction or massive reflux. Neurologic causes must also be considered. Unusually, this is due to viral infection (herpes) and is rarely idiopathic or behavioral (54).

ASSESSMENT OF BLADDER FUNCTION

History

The history of the child's signs and symptoms must be carefully elicited and may serve to specifically focus attention on the appropriate diagnostic possibilities. This serves to guide further evaluation. Important elements of the history have been noted previously in association with the specific signs and symptoms. Other features to consider include pregnancy and birth history of the child, developmental history, and medication exposure. In those children with identified diseases or conditions, their surgical history is essential and may be complex; their response to therapy and prior imaging and urodynamic studies are an essential part of the history. Associated symptoms including abdominal pain, constipation, and fevers need to be elicited. Parental views of "normal" are important because they are often divergent from true "normal." To assess voiding patterns it may be very helpful to have the family complete a voiding diary to document actual voiding frequency and volumes. Many times this reveals a pattern unrecognized by the parent.

Imaging

Pediatric urologic imaging is highly specialized and critically important in evaluation and management planning (55). Ultrasonography has become a mainstay of bladder imaging due to its high resolution and absence of radiation (Fig. 97-3). Functional inferences may be made, particularly with regard to the bladder, if attention is paid to the state of bladder filling and efficiency of emptying [postvoid residual (PVR) volume], and the bladder wall thickness (40). Ultrasound is particularly useful in long-term follow-up studies.

Cystography is an important means of bladder evaluation and provides information regarding configuration, emptying, and the presence of reflux. The urethra should be well visualized in an adequate study (56). If voiding cannot be induced, the study should not be considered adequate and should be repeated, if clinically indicated. Radiographic cystography [voiding cystourethrography (VCUG) or micturating cystourethrogram] is usually the best first study to define anatomy and function, whereas

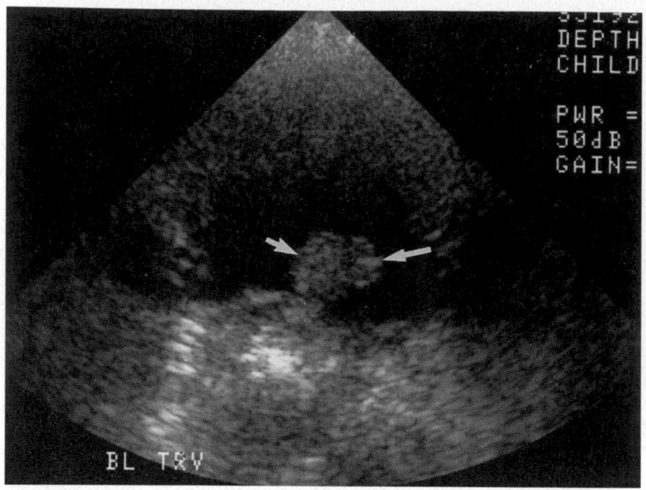

FIGURE 97-3. Bladder ultrasound of a bladder neck polyp (arrows) in a 4-year-old boy with intermittent bladder neck obstruction, pain, and hematuria. The polyp was fibromuscular and was removed endoscopically via suprapubic access. It could not be removed through the urethra.

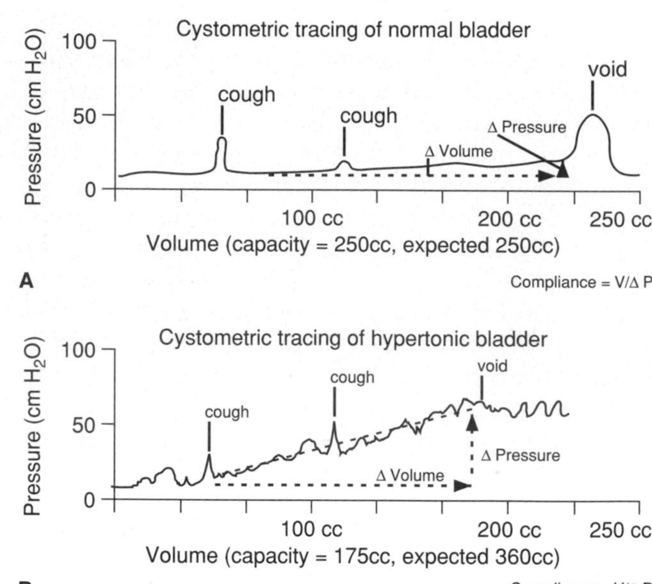

FIGURE 97-4. Schematic representation of normal and hypertonic cystometric studies. **(A)** In the normal bladder, pressure rises very little during filling (accommodation), and the compliance, or DV/DP, is high. **(B)** In contrast, the hypertonic bladder often has a reduced capacity and there are greater rises in pressure with filling; DV/DP is lower than normal.

radionuclide cystography is a useful follow-up or screening tool due to its lower radiation exposure.

Computed tomography and magnetic resonance imaging (MRI) are important means of defining structural relationships of the bladder within the pelvis, particularly in the setting of tumor or trauma.

Urodynamic Evaluation

Functional bladder evaluation is most accurately based on urodynamic studies (UDS), which provide objective information regarding the parameters of bladder activity that are the basis for the consequences of bladder dysfunction (57). These include the ability of the bladder to store adequate amounts of urine at low pressures and to empty urine efficiently at appropriate pressures, and the ability of the sphincter mechanisms to retain urine for socially acceptable periods of time and relax adequately during voiding. Cystometry is a record of bladder pressure with filling and normally demonstrates low pressures within the bladder as volume increases (Fig. 97-4A). As capacity is approached, pressures increase slightly until a voiding contraction is initiated. Pressures then rise rapidly, and if accompanied by sphincter relaxation, voiding occurs. Bladder contractions occurring during filling that cannot be suppressed by the patient are termed *uninhibited contractions* and may be a manifestation of neurogenic, structural, and functional abnormalities. A poorly compliant bladder demonstrates early increases in pressure with filling, and this becomes important when those pressures approach the clinically important threshold of 35 to 40 cm H_2O (Fig. 97-4B). Resting pressure, as correlated with volume, can also be a useful measure of compliance and may reflect more realistic patterns than filling cystometry (58). Absence of a voiding contraction may be seen with neuropathic bladder dysfunction or postobstructive dysfunction. In those patients, abdominal straining may be demonstrated as they attempt to empty a noncontracting bladder.

The activity of the bladder sphincter mechanism may be examined using pressure measurements within the urethra, estimating both the level of the pressure, as well as the length over which that pressure is exerted (functional urethral length) (Fig. 97-5). There is not universal agreement as to the interpretation or utility of urethral pressure measurements. Uroflowmetry can add information to the clinical assessment of incontinence in some situations (59). An alternative measure of sphincter function is the leak point pressure either with filling or with stress such as increased abdominal pressure (valsalva) (60). Electromyography of the urethral sphincter is a specialized study that may permit identification and characterization of neurologic bladder dysfunction, and bladder sphincter incoordination (dyssynergy) in particular (Figs. 97-6, 97-7A, and 97-7B).

NEUROGENIC BLADDER DISEASES

Table 97-1 provides a list of congenital and acquired neurogenic bladder diseases.

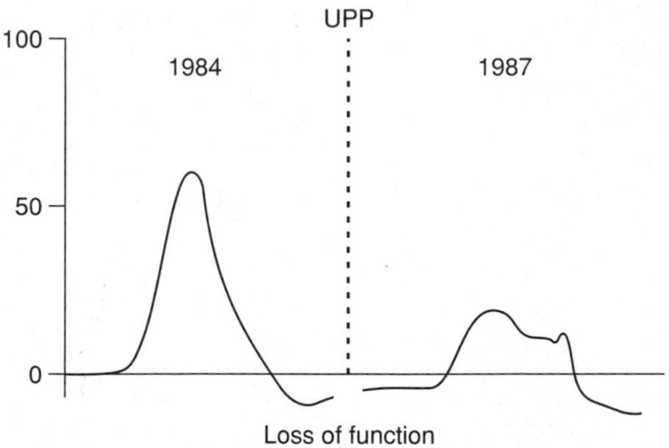

FIGURE 97-5. Urethral pressure profiles measured by drawing a urodynamic catheter slowly across the bladder neck and sphincter. The horizontal axis represents distance from the bladder neck. The pressure curve reflects urethral pressure; the distance along the urethra with elevated pressures is termed the *functional urethral length*. In this child, the urethral pressure profile (UPP) demonstrates decrease in urethral resistance from 1984 to 1987, due to loss of sphincteric function in the setting of a spinal cord dysraphism. This was associated with increased urinary leakage and was managed with a urethral sling. (From Bauer SB, Peters CA, Mandell J, et al. The use of the rectus fascia to manage urinary incontinence. *J Urol* 1989;142:516, with permission.)

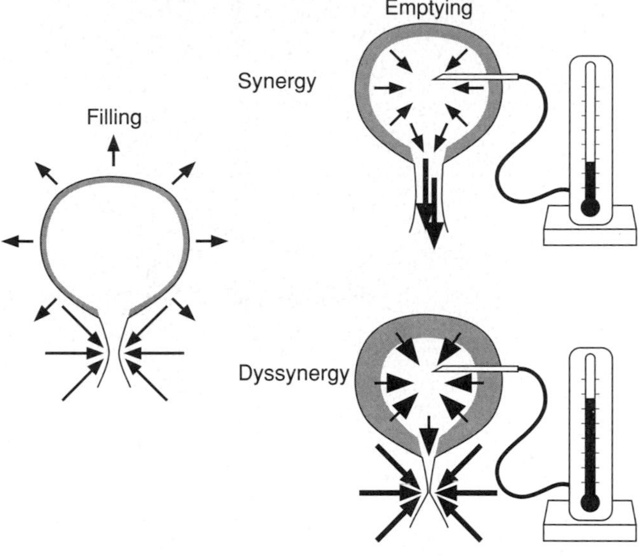

FIGURE 97-6. Schematic diagram of normal bladder with outlet relaxation during voiding, contrasted with the dyssynergic bladder in which outlet resistance increases with detrusor contraction. This produces elevated intravesical pressures, which may cause renal damage, as well as bladder hypertrophy and noncompliance.

Spinal Dysraphisms: Meningomyelocele

Presentation

The child born with meningomyelocele is readily apparent and must be assessed expeditiously. The appearance of a membrane-covered sac along the back is unmistakable (Fig. 97-8). This sac contains neural elements and will usually become infected if not surgically closed in the first few days of life. Fetal coverage of the defect has been introduced with apparent reduction in the need for postnatal ventricular shunting, but the effect on bladder function seems minimal (61,62). Studies of aborted fetuses with myelomeningocele have shown early changes of bladder wall fibrosis, suggesting an early insult to bladder development. Whether these changes are due to abnormal innervation affecting bladder development or are the result of abnormal function altering development is unclear. These findings are strong indicators of the profound effect of these lesions on normal bladder development and ultimately function (63).

Neurosurgical closure of the spinal cord defect is usually performed in the first 2 days of life. A basic urologic assessment prior to closure is optimal, including renal and bladder ultrasound and neurologic examination of the perineum to assess innervation of the sphincter muscles (57). The presence of hydronephrosis in the newborn indicates abnormal bladder dynamics, usually due to bladder-sphincter dyssynergy. These babies require the most meticulous follow-up to minimize upper tract damage and to preserve bladder compliance. In those with normal upper urinary tracts, an assessment of bladder emptying is important to determine whether intermittent catheterization is needed (64). PRV measurements by catheter or ultrasound are appropriate.

Following neurosurgical closure, some babies will experience a period of spinal shock, with bladder flaccidity and poor emptying. Catheterization or credé emptying for this limited period is appropriate. Urodynamic assessment in this period is seldom useful. After the child has stabilized from the closure, baseline urodynamic assessment should be performed; this may be from 2 to 6 months of life. The principal aim is to identify those babies with risk of developing upper urinary tract damage from high bladder pressures. Detrusor-sphincter dyssynergy is the usual cause of this, and when demonstrated on UDS, our institution has recommended a program of anticholinergic medication to reduce bladder contractile tone (Fig. 97-9), and intermittent catheterization to permit emptying (64). It has been shown that this prophylactic treatment will avoid upper tract deterioration and may well maintain bladder compliance (64–66). Fewer of these children require augmentation cystoplasty than their counterparts managed expectantly (Fig. 97-10).

Medical Management

The two aims of management of children with myelodysplasia are (1) *preservation of renal function* and (2) *social continence*. The first requires normal storage function of

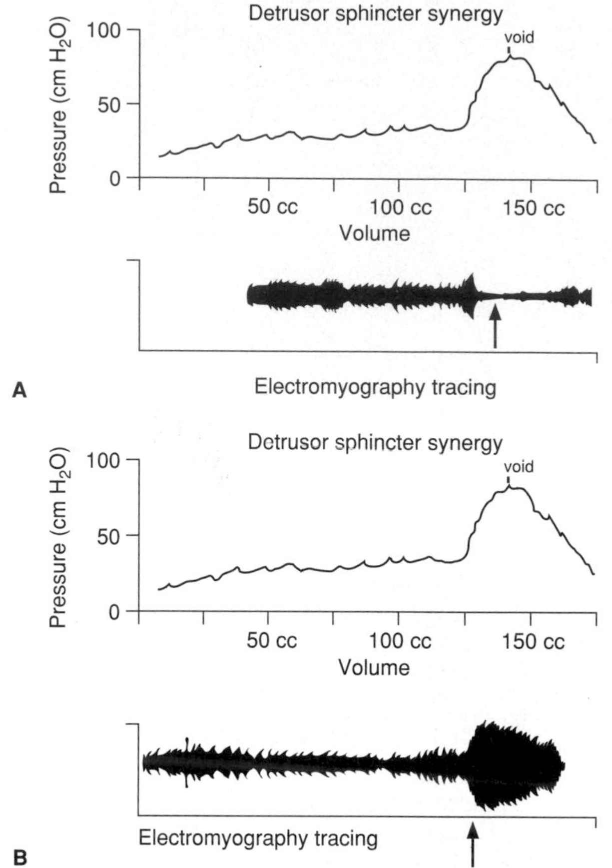

FIGURE 97-7. Schematic representation of bladder sphincter electromyographic (EMG) activity during bladder filling and voiding. **(A)** In the normal bladder, EMG activity will increase very slowly, then slightly more near capacity and finally silence during voiding. This indicates coordinated sphincteric relaxation during detrusor contraction. **(B)** In contrast, the abnormal, dyssynergic bladder-sphincter unit, EMG activity increases during a detrusor contraction. This corresponds to increased sphincteric contraction and elevated voiding pressures (see Fig. 97-10).

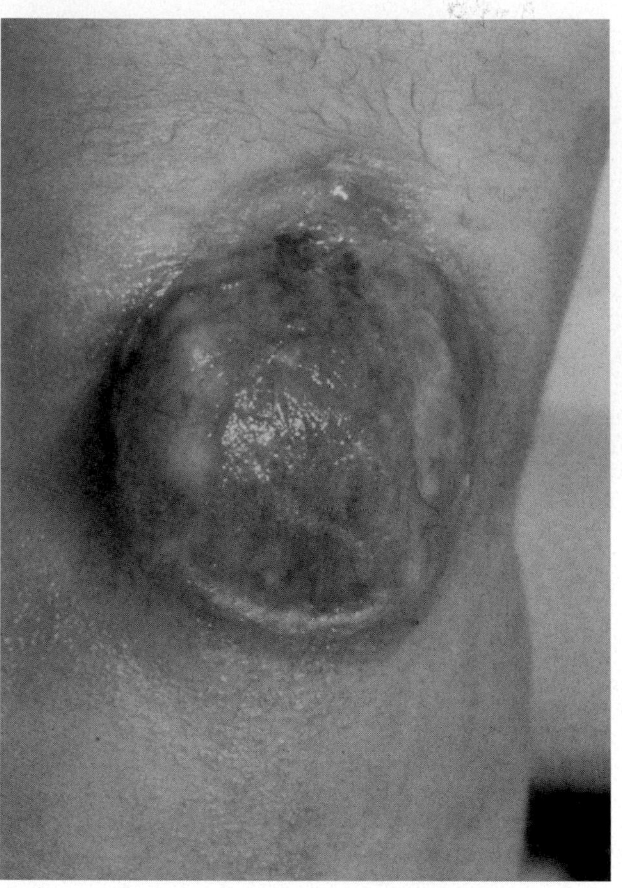

FIGURE 97-8. Photograph of infant with myelomeningocele prior to surgical closure. The membrane covers the neural elements. If no neural elements prolapse into the sac, it is termed a *meningocele*.

TABLE 97-1 Neuropathic Bladder Disorders.

Major diagnoses
Congenital
Apparent
Meningomyelocele
Sacral agenesis
Occult
Diastematomyelia
Intradural lipoma
Lipomeningocele
Tight filum terminale
Dermoid cyst/sinus
Anterior sacral meningocele
Acquired
Trauma
Ischemic cord injury

the bladder by maintaining low pressures during bladder filling. With neural abnormalities, the bladder may become noncompliant through two mechanisms. The first is denervation supersensitivity in which reduction in nerve input into the bladder muscle leads to an increase in the density of neurotransmitter receptors (67). The functional consequence of this is bladder instability and hypercontractility. The resting tone of the bladder may be higher than normal. Reduced inhibitory innervation that mediates relaxation may also be active in this context. The second mechanism is from functional bladder outlet obstruction in the setting of detrusor sphincter dyssynergy. Every time the detrusor contracts, the sphincter contracts with it (Fig. 97-6). Voiding pressures are elevated, and the bladder behaves as if obstructed. Smooth muscle hypertrophy begins and increased connective tissue deposition occurs (68,69). Alterations in elastin concentration and distribution are also seen, reducing the compliance of the bladder wall. Some groups have advocated sphincterotomy by dilation to eliminate this obstructive effect until the child is old enough to be definitively treated (70). Intermittent catheterization can

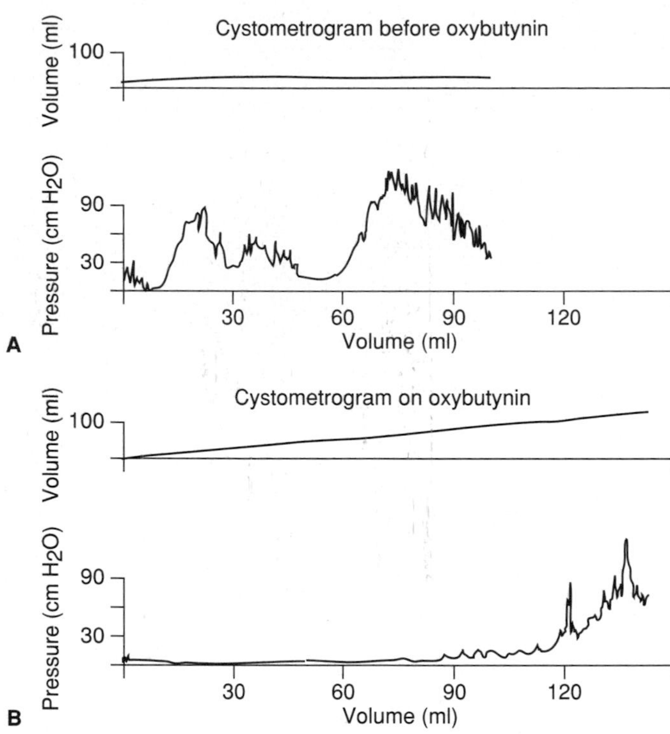

FIGURE 97-9. Cystometrogram (CMG) demonstrating a hypertonic bladder with high pressures and small capacity. After use of oral oxybutynin (Ditropan®), the CMG shows a low-pressure filling curve and increased total capacity.

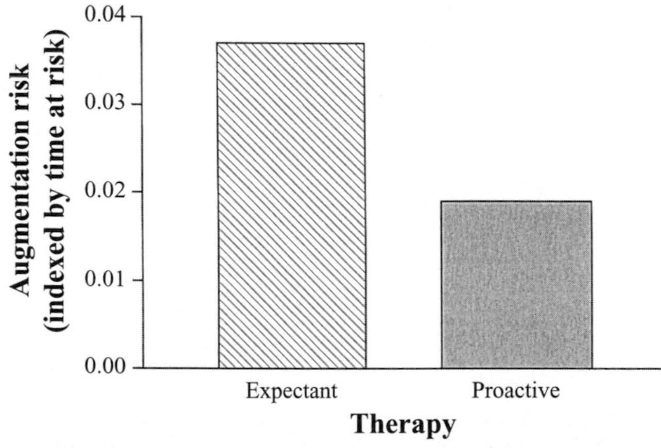

FIGURE 97-10. Graph showing the impact of early prophylactic intervention in children with high-risk pattern of neurogenic bladder dysfunction. In children with hypertonicity and detrusor sphincter dyssynergy, a high rate of upper urinary tract deterioration has been shown. Early institution of prophylactic clean intermittent catheterization and anticholinergic therapy reduces the need for augmentation cystoplasty. The rate of augmentation is shown for the patients with expectant and proactive therapy as indexed to time at risk. [Data from Kaefer M, Pabby A, Kelly M, et al. Improved bladder function after prophylactic treatment of high risk neurogenic bladder in newborns with myelomeningocele. *J Urol* 1999;162:1068–1071.]

be taught to parents and may be a more acceptable and lasting solution in these children, without the risk of permanent sphincteric injury.

The fundamental approach to medical management is to ensure low-pressure bladder filling, complete regular emptying at acceptable pressures and intervals, and sufficient bladder neck tone to maintain social continence. Depending on the pattern of bladder function, the use of anticholinergics medication to maintain low bladder filling pressures is effective. Intravesical anticholinergic medication may occasionally be necessary and limit side effects (71). Emptying often requires intermittent catheterization through a continent channel (either the urethra or a surgically constructed stoma), and this needs to be sufficiently frequent to maintain end-filling bladder pressures acceptably low (i.e., less than 30 cm H_2O).

Surgical Management

Surgical management becomes necessary when one or both of these aims cannot be achieved with medical therapy and catheterization alone. It is important to recognize that bladder hypertonia will contribute to incontinence by raising bladder pressures above the resistance level of the sphincter. A totally flaccid sphincter is unlikely to be able to permit continence in any situation, whereas a denervated sphincter may have a level of reflex tone that will maintain dryness when bladder pressures are low. Surgical reduction of bladder hypertonia and provision of continence may require either bladder augmentation and/or bladder neck surgery for continence.

Bladder augmentation is a well-established procedure with well-described outcomes (72). It continues to be associated with complications and the decision to proceed with augmentation cystoplasty must be carefully considered (73,74). The fundamental principle is to increase the capacity and decrease the pressure of the abnormal bladder by addition of a patch of gastrointestinal (GI) tissue onto the bladder. This may be an isolated segment of ileum, sigmoid, right colon, or stomach (Fig. 97-11). Tubular segments must be reconfigured to eliminate the tubular shape, which will produce peristaltic contractions and high pressures (Fig. 97-12) (75).

The *complications* of augmentation cystoplasty include mucus production from the intestinal segment, which may impair catheter emptying and may act as a nidus for stone formation. The most serious problem has been perforation of the augmented segment, often in association with infection (76). The specific etiology remains unclear, but relative ischemia in the setting of infection and trauma from catheterization have been suggested as possible reasons. The classic clinical presentation of a child with a prior augmentation and a new episode of fever, abdominal pain, and shoulder pain (indicating diaphragmatic irritation from extravasated infected urine in the peritoneum)

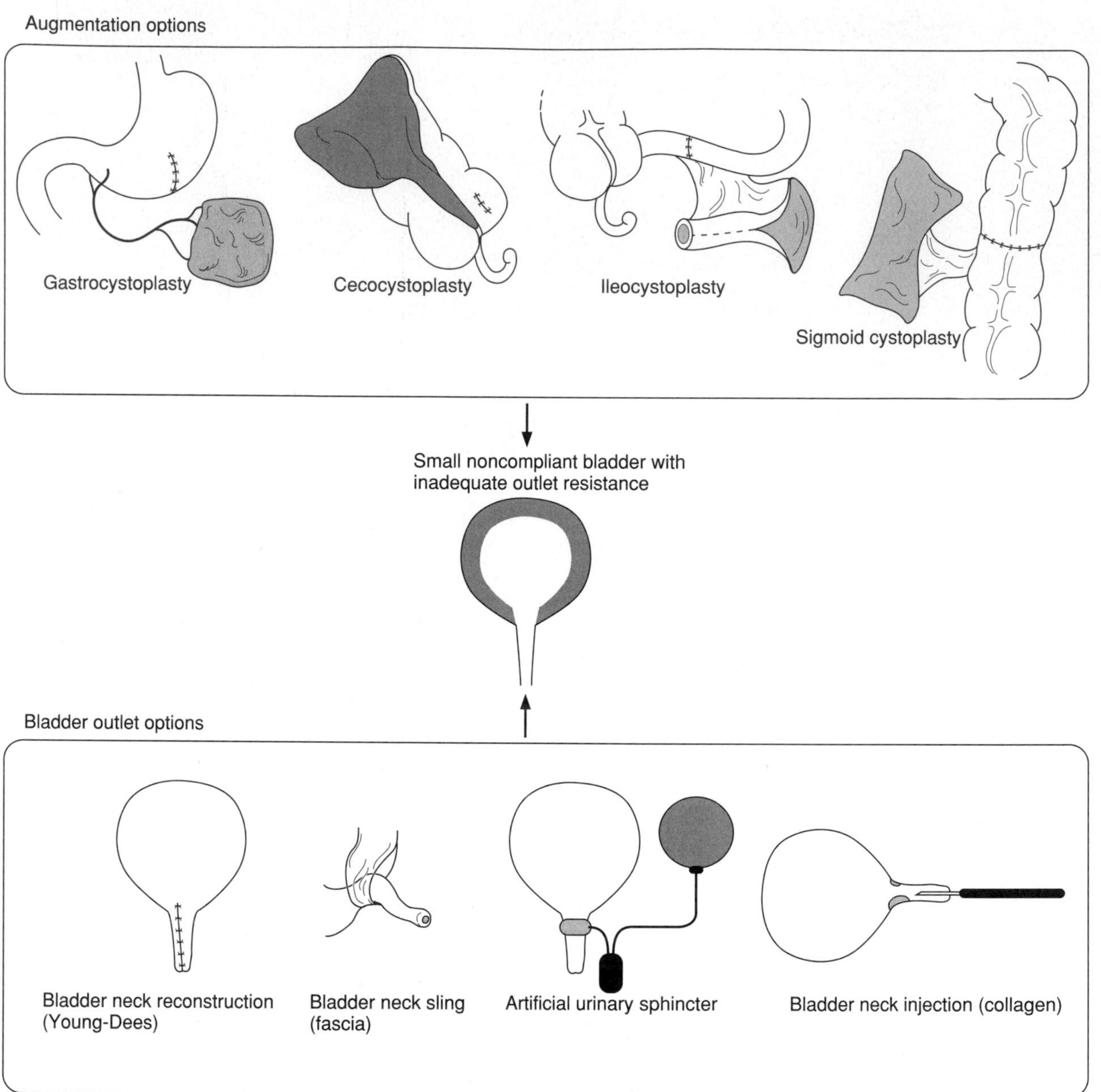

FIGURE 97-11. Diagram of options for bladder augmentation in the setting of a small capacity high-pressure bladder. Any of these enteric segments may be combined with one of the options for increasing bladder outlet resistance, as needed.

should be regarded as a bladder perforation until proven otherwise. Early diagnosis, antibiotics, and operative treatment are recommended. This is a potentially lethal condition.

Bladder calculi are an occasional problem with augmentation cystoplasty, likely due to the combination of bacteria in the urine and foreign material (mucus, or pubic hair from catheterization in females). Urethral cystolitholopaxy is effective unless this manipulation might injure a reconstructed or artificial sphincter mechanism (artificial urinary sphincter or bladder neck sling). Percutaneous endoscopic stone fragmentation and removal may be performed, but occasionally, the most efficient means of stone removal is through an open cystotomy (77,78).

Metabolic complications of augmentation cystoplasty include chronic acidosis with potential growth impairment, as well as vitamin deficiencies depending on the intestinal segment used (79).

The attainment of *social continence* is frequently a substantial challenge in the myelodysplastic child. Continence is the result of a balance between intravesical pressure and urethral or bladder neck resistance. If bladder pressures cannot be maintained at a sufficiently low level during

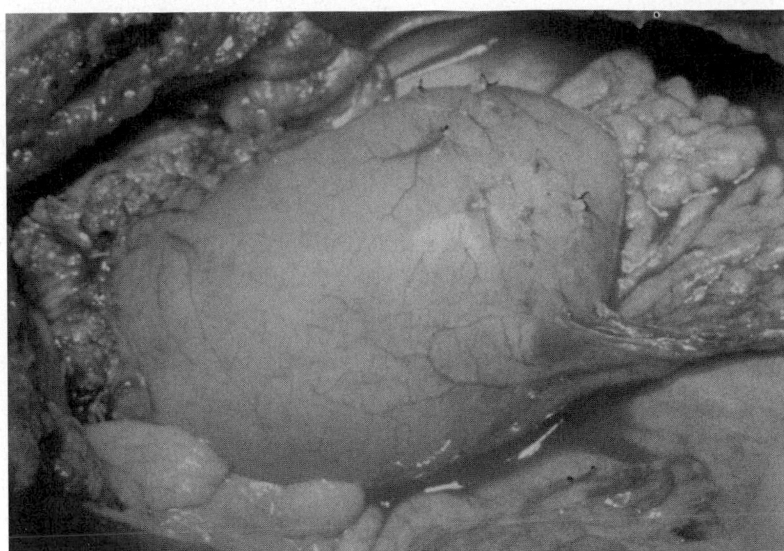

FIGURE 97-12. Operative photograph of gastrocystoplasty in boy with small capacity bladder due to epispadias. The gastric patch assumes a spherical shape without reconfiguration. A spherical configuration produces the lowest pressures for the highest volumes.

most of the bladder filling cycle, incontinence will occur. Inadequate resistance at the bladder neck, even with low bladder pressures, leads to inadequate continence. Stress incontinence, that occurring only with exertion, may be particularly troublesome when wheelchair-bound patients must transfer.

After a thorough evaluation has been performed and the relative contribution of bladder compliance and bladder neck resistance have been identified, it is often necessary to both reduce bladder pressures with an augmentation cystoplasty and increase bladder neck resistance. There are several means of accomplishing the latter. It is unlikely for a child with myelodysplasia to be able to void volitionally, and in all cases, intermittent catheterization must be anticipated and taught. Some children with flaccid sphincters may be able to empty completely with an artificial urinary sphincter, but most will need to catheterize.

The options available for *continence* include bladder neck sling, bladder neck reconstruction, artificial urinary sphincter (AUS), bladder neck injectables, or diversion to a continent catheterizable stoma on the lower abdomen (Fig. 97-11). Bladder neck slings, fashioned from a strip of lower rectus fascia or biomaterials such as small intestine submucosal and passed around the posterior bladder neck in girls or boys, are a useful option (80) (Fig. 97-13). It provides directly increased urethral resistance as well as stabilization and intraabdominal fixation of the bladder

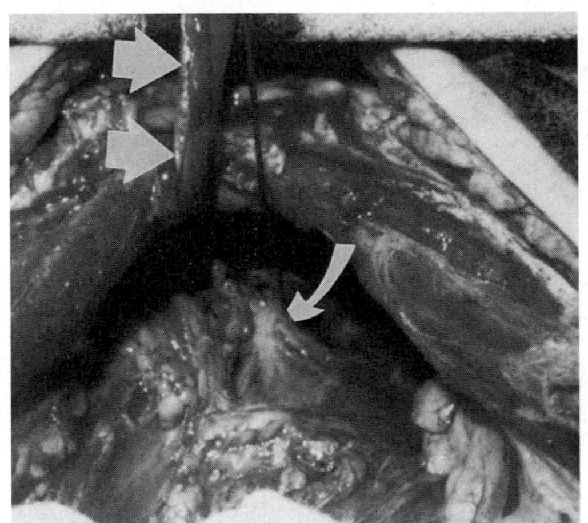

A

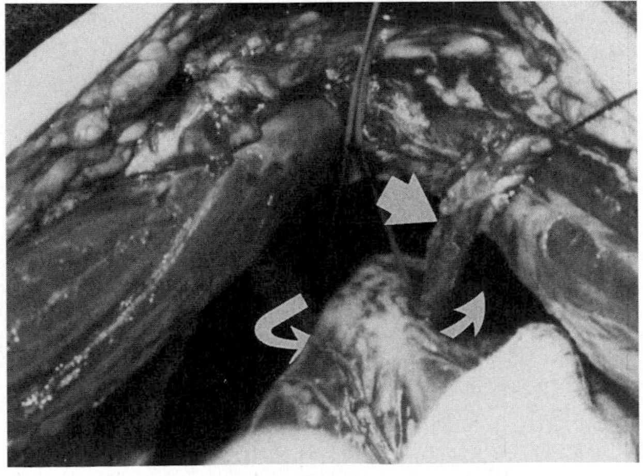

B

FIGURE 97-13. Operative photograph of bladder neck dissection for placement of a fascial sling. The sling *(white arrow)* has been passed through the inferior rectus sheath, and a vessel loop has been passed around the bladder neck *(curved arrow)*. The sling is then passed around the bladder neck and will be wrapped around the anterior rectus fascia. The sling should not be tied tightly, but enough to maintain the bladder base and neck in an intraabdominal position. (From Bauer SB, Peters CA, Mandell J, et al. The use of the rectus fascia to manage urinary incontinence. *J Urol* 1989;142:516, with permission.)

neck. It is most useful when intermittent catheterization is planned. Success rates are good, approaching 85% to 90% (80,81). Difficulty catheterizing the bladder neck is an occasional problem. Bladder neck reconstruction, using the Young-Dees concept, is one of the least effective means of providing continence in the myelodysplastic population. The method relies on creating a muscular wrap of the bladder base, which lengthens the functional urethra. However, more recent modifications of the traditional technique have been able to produce better results (82). Several bladder neck reconfigurations have been used to provide for continence by creating a flap-valve mechanism to permit catheterization. The principle is to create a tube extending into the bladder that works in the same fashion as a nonrefluxing ureter and through which a catheter is passed. The Kropp (83) and Pippi-Salle (84) are the best described. These methods are technically difficult and may provide for a very secure bladder neck, with the risk of bladder perforation because there is no pop-off mechanism.

The AUS continues to have a role in continence for children, but must be used with caution. When few other options are available, or when the patient may be able to empty completely due to a flaccid bladder neck, the AUS may be appropriate (85,86). The success rate is about 75%, with a 20% reoperation rate in the latest models of the device. The device includes an inflatable cuff placed around the bladder neck or urethra, attached to a pressure-regulating balloon reservoir. The cuff is actuated by a pump device in the scrotum or labia. Infection and erosion of the urethral tissues may occur. Mechanical failure remains a clinical issue, but the reliability of the device has improved with time.

Injection of foreign material to create more urethral resistance has been performed for more than 15 years. One of the original materials, Teflon® paste, may be effective in patients with only a slight imbalance in bladder and urethral resistance, or in those with stress incontinence. Collagen paste product has been reported to have reasonable results, but limited durability (87). The collagen does not have the risks that have been tied to Teflon and is easily injectable. It may not remain in place as long as Teflon, but it can be easily touched up. The long-term results of this material remain to be defined.

An important option that may be used in combination with other techniques is creation of a continent catheterizable stoma (CCS). This is performed in association with bladder neck closure, or preferably with a bladder neck sling to prevent leakage, but allows catheterization as a back-up and pressure "pop-off." The CCS can be placed as a back-up catheterization port, yet is regularly used due to ease and comfort. This may be constructed from appendix, ureters, or a reconfigured segment of small bowel. The Mitrofanoff principle is used in which the tube is implanted into the bladder in a tunneled fashion as with antireflux surgery to prevent leakage of urine from the bladder, but permitting easy catheterization (88,89). The stoma may be placed in the umbilicus where it is concealed, or in the lower abdomen, just above the underwear line. Care must be taken to ensure the child has the manual dexterity and body habitus to permit such a maneuver. The Monti procedure permits use of a small segment of small intestine to create a narrow channel in creation of a CCS (90). This is performed by harvesting a 2- to 3-cm segment of small bowel, often with harvest of an augmenting segment. The small bowel is opened on the antimesenteric side and tubularized transversely, which creates a tube the length of the circumference of the small intestine. The tube is tunneled into the bladder or reservoir. CCS reconstructions may also be integrated with placement of an antegrade continent enema (Malone antegrade continent enema) (91) to facilitate bowel continence. These reconstructions may be performed laparoscopically to minimize surgical morbidity in many cases (92).

Occult Spinal Dysraphisms

A small subset of patients with spinal dysraphisms do not present with the overt external manifestations of myelodysplasia, yet may demonstrate some of the same neurologic features (77,78). The causes of these conditions include tethered spinal cord, diastematomyelia, sacral-agenesis, and lipomeningocele. These conditions may cause an insidious deterioration of bladder function that becomes irreversible by the time of diagnosis. Early diagnosis has generally permitted more recovery of lost function. A high index of suspicion is necessary to detect these patients, whose only manifestations may be minor changes in urinary patterns, minimal neurologic findings of the lower extremities, and subtle physical findings. A lower spinal hairy nevus, vascular malformation, or asymmetric gluteal cleft are all signs of a possible underlying neural defect (Fig. 97-14). The classic finding of a flat buttock should be a clue to sacral agenesis, particularly in the infant of a diabetic mother. Appropriate spinal cord imaging and urodynamic and urologic evaluation will usually reveal the specific natures of the condition and permit therapeutic planning. Bladder management is similar to that for myelodysplasia and depends on the neurologic status of the bladder and sphincter, as well as the condition of the upper urinary tracts.

Associations with Anorectal Malformations

The association between neurogenic bladder dysfunction and anorectal abnormalities is well established and must be recognized to permit adequate urologic management in these patients. The incidence of spinal cord abnormalities in children with anorectal anomalies is greater than

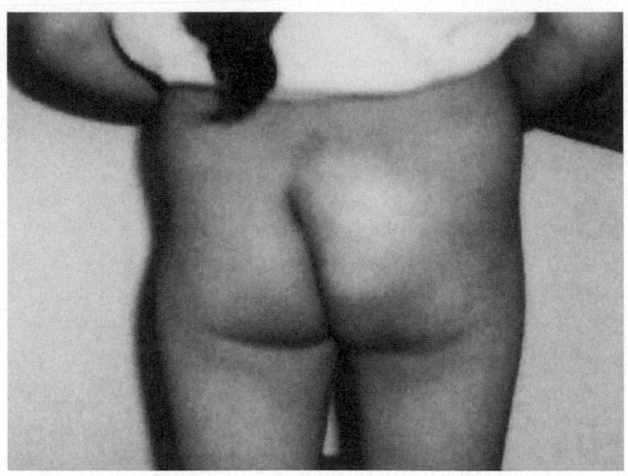

FIGURE 97-14. Appearance of a child with occult spinal dysraphism manifest by abnormalities of the lower back and gluteal cleft. She was found to have vesicoureteral reflux and significant renal scarring on radioisotope scanning.

normal (93), and routine evaluation of the lower spine using ultrasound (younger than 4 months of age) or MRI is recommended. Approximately 40% of children with imperforate anus will have evidence of neuropathic bladder dysfunction; most of these being in children with high imperforate anus. The basis for the bladder abnormality may be a spinal anomaly such as tethered cord of diastematomyelia, but some degree of bladder dysfunction has been noted in patients with imperforate anus and normal spinal cords (94). If anorectal surgery is anticipated, urodynamic evaluation is prudent prior to surgery. This will serve to identify any underlying abnormality and provide a baseline for comparison in the event of any neural injury during surgery. Although these children do not typically present with urologic symptoms early in life, the identification of a neurologic anomaly permits selective monitoring and early intervention. This may have a benefit in reducing the 55% incidence of neuropathic bladder dysfunction in the adolescent years.

CONGENITAL BLADDER OBSTRUCTION

Posterior Urethral Valves

Posterior urethral valves represent the most pure form of congenital bladder obstruction. Although definitively described in 1919, valves continue to challenge the clinician (95). Located just below the bladder neck at the level of the veru montanum, posterior urethral valves (PUVs) are likely the remnants of the migration of the mesonephric ducts to the trigone (Fig. 97-15). The severity of obstruction is highly variable and the consequences are similarly variable (96). In the most severe form, congenital bladder obstruction will produce renal dysplasia, oligohydramnios, and pulmonary hypoplasia, leading to neonatal death from respiratory failure. Lesser degrees of obstruction may cause severe renal impairment leading to chronic renal failure necessitating renal replacement (97,98). The bladder dysfunction produced by PUVs, and persisting long after removal of the obstruction (51), may even impair function of a renal transplant. Recognition of postobstructive bladder dysfunction due to PUVs, the so-called "valve bladder," (99) has permitted improved management of these children in whom a steady progression to renal failure was witnessed with frustration, despite multiple surgical interventions. Current management of posterior urethral valves begins in utero and may extend well into young adulthood. The patterns of bladder, renal, and pulmonary dysfunction are well described, yet their mechanisms remain to be fully explained (100).

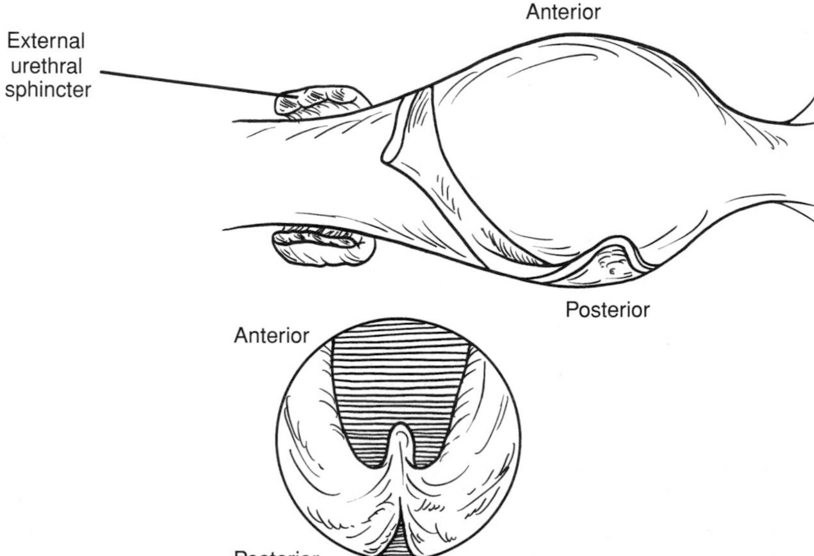

FIGURE 97-15. Diagram of the anatomy of posterior urethral valves. The valves emanate from the distal veru montanum at the apex of the prostate, and sweep anteriorly and laterally, forming a dorsal web of tissue. The dorsal web may not be readily visible on an endoscopic view *(inset)*, which shows the lower leaflet folds. (From Retik AB. Management of posterior urethral valves. In: Glenn JF, ed. *Urologic surgery*. Philadelphia: Lippincott, 1991:812, with permission.)

In utero PUV

The prenatal diagnosis of PUV may be made as early as 15 weeks (101), although usually identified after 18 weeks. The initial presentation may provide an indication of prognosis. The male fetus with oligohydramnios, bilateral echogenic kidneys and a large thick-walled dilated bladder has a poor prognosis (97). Those boys without oligohydramnios and who did not have dysplastic kidneys may survive without significant renal impairment. The uniformly poor prognosis of those fetuses with severe obstruction having evidence of evolving renal dysplasia and pulmonary hypoplasia has prompted in utero interventions to relieve the obstruction (102). This issue is discussed elsewhere. The role of in utero shunting procedures in boys with presumed PUV remains incompletely defined despite several decades of experience. It is clear from anecdotal experience, that it is possible to salvage an otherwise doomed fetus with appropriate in utero intervention (103). The principal hindrance to developing effective treatment protocols is the inability to accurately predict neonatal outcomes given current imaging and assessment (41,104). As an understanding of the processes and mechanisms of congenital obstructive uropathy develops, markers of the progression of this process and the response to decompression (105) will permit more specific assessment of the potential for positive outcomes with intervention. At present, prenatal diagnosis serves an important role in providing information to the prospective parents and physicians as to the possible outcomes and the need for *postnatal* evaluation and intervention.

The fetus with presumed valves should be monitored periodically to follow amniotic fluid status, the condition of the kidneys, and bladder dynamics. Abrupt changes in these parameters may prompt reconsideration of postnatal therapy. It is almost never necessary to suggest a late gestation intervention. Late-onset oligohydramnios has not been associated with significant pulmonary complications as basic pulmonary development has already occurred (106). Early delivery in such cases to reduce exposure of the fetal kidney to obstruction has not been demonstrated to have a positive effect. It must be balanced against the risks of pulmonary insufficiency due to prematurity.

Neonatal Management

A child with a prior presumptive diagnosis of valves should be delivered at an institution where the complications of pulmonary insufficiency, sepsis, and renal failure may be handled, and where a thorough evaluation may be obtained. Initial management, particularly if the child is ill, should be catheter drainage of the bladder with a feeding tube. Ultrasound imaging of the upper tracts and bladder at that time may provide a baseline. Cystography to confirm the presence of the valves and assess the presence of reflux should be performed (Fig. 97-16). The child should be placed on prophylactic antibiotics and monitored for azotemia and acidosis.

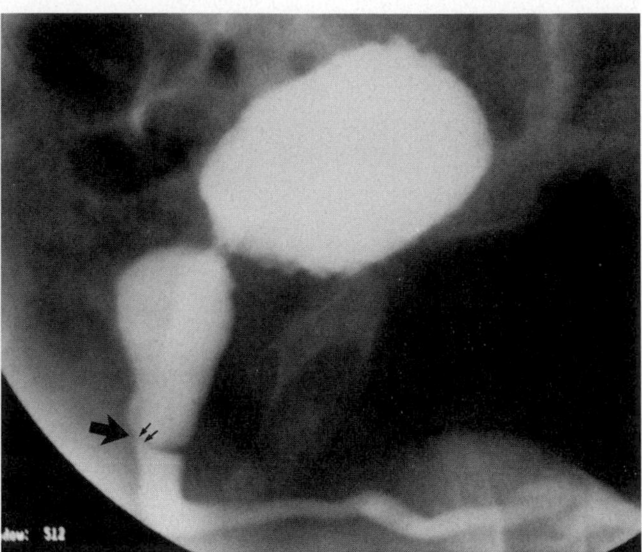

FIGURE 97-16. Voiding cystourethrogram of infant boy with severe posterior urethral valves. The dilated posterior urethra is a characteristic radiographic finding associated with valves. The narrow postobstruction urethral lumen may be seen to originate inferiorly *(arrows)*, consistent with the valvular opening being on the inferior aspect of the urethra (see Fig. 97-15).

The pattern of serum creatinine in the newborn with PUV may provide some information as to the level of renal function and adequacy of renal drainage. At birth the creatinine is that of the mother, usually about .8 to 1.0 mg per dL, and a baseline level should be obtained. If it begins to rise in the first days of life, serious renal impairment may be anticipated. This should be addressed aggressively, and all efforts to maximize drainage of the upper tracts undertaken. It is important to recognize that functional obstruction of the distal ureters may occur as a consequence of bladder hypertrophy due to PUV. In this way, the bladder may remain empty due to catheter drainage, or vesicostomy drainage, yet the kidneys remain markedly hydronephrotic. Supravesical diversion may be one option to manage these children (107), as well as total reconstruction (108). The latter may be a formidable undertaking. Stable creatinine or a fall in the initial level suggests more adequate renal drainage. These children are best served by endoscopic valve ablation and close follow-up (Fig. 97-17). In the very premature infant, temporary cutaneous vesicostomy remains a useful option.

The response of the child to valve ablation is critical and must be closely attended to. If upper tract dilation persists and there is any evidence of impaired renal function such

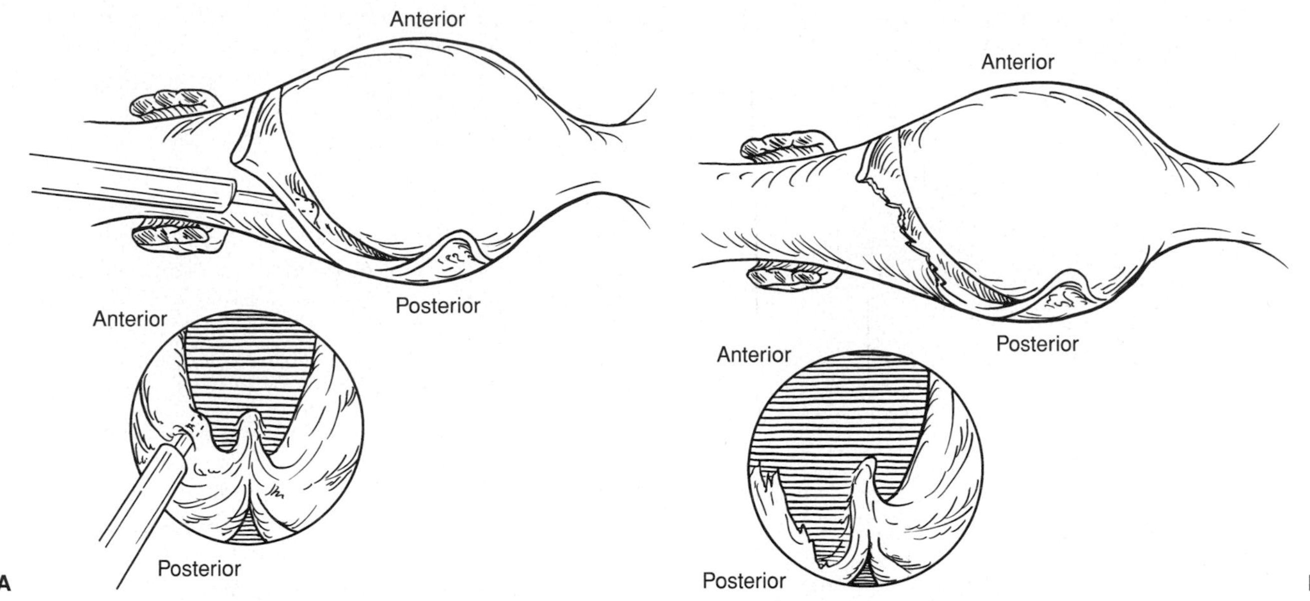

FIGURE 97-17. Diagram illustrating endoscopic technique for valve ablation. **(A)** A small (3F) ureteral catheter with a metal stylet attached to the electrocautery unit. **(B)** The stylet ablates the valve leaflets, disrupting the saillike continuity of the valve. (From Retik AB. Management of posterior urethral valves. In: Glenn JF, ed. *Urologic surgery*. Philadelphia: Lippincott, 1991:812, with permission.)

as elevated creatinine or acidosis, improving upper tract drainage may be necessary by way of upper tract diversion (ureterostomy) or total reconstruction. One-third of boys with severe valves who present in the first year of life may be seen to progress to renal failure. It would seem prudent to maximize their potential renal function by providing for the best means of urinary drainage during the first year of life.

Significant controversy exists as to the impact of early diversion in the child with valves, both in terms of renal and bladder function in the future. There is conflicting evidence as to its efficacy in protecting potential renal function, and it is indeed unusual for upper tract diversion to produce improved renal function (109–112). Long-term bladder function is not likely to be adversely impacted by temporary diversion, but some argue that it leads to more dysfunction.

Most infants with PUV will show rapid improvement in upper tract dilation and evidence of normal renal function. The presence of vesicoureteral reflux is common, yet in nearly 50% it will resolve spontaneously following valve ablation (113). A subset of boys will have evidence of severe unilateral reflux and a nonfunctioning kidney, the VURD association (47). Unilateral nephrectomy may be indicated to avoid risks of infection. If any consideration of the need for bladder augmentation is present, the ureter associated with a nonfunctioning kidney should be preserved for possible use as the augmenting tissue. Further monitoring of boys with a rapid response to valve ablation aims to identify any signs of bladder dysfunction before they cause irreversible consequences.

Bladder Dysfunction and PUV

The concept of postobstructive bladder dysfunction is well established clinically, yet the mechanistic basis of this challenging condition remains incompletely defined. The clinical pattern of voiding dysfunction with hydronephrosis in a boy with previously ablated valves was long believed to be due to bladder neck hypertrophy and persistent outlet obstruction (114). Bladder neck surgery was performed, often exacerbating the incontinence. Persistent reflux was treated with repeated ureteral reimplantation, usually without success. The continued high-pressure bladder dynamics caused steady deterioration in renal function. It became apparent that the primary cause of this pattern was a persistently hypertonic bladder, the result of congenital obstruction. Attention was paid to reducing bladder pressures, principally with anticholinergic medication, augmentation cystoplasty, and rigorous voiding regimens to improve emptying.

Three patterns of bladder dysfunction have been identified in association with PUV and may be seen long after valve ablation (51) (Fig. 97-18). These include the most potentially damaging, bladder hypertonia, bladder instability, and a pattern of myogenic failure or contractile failure. Hypertonia may be manifest by way of incontinence and hydronephrosis, and is usually associated with

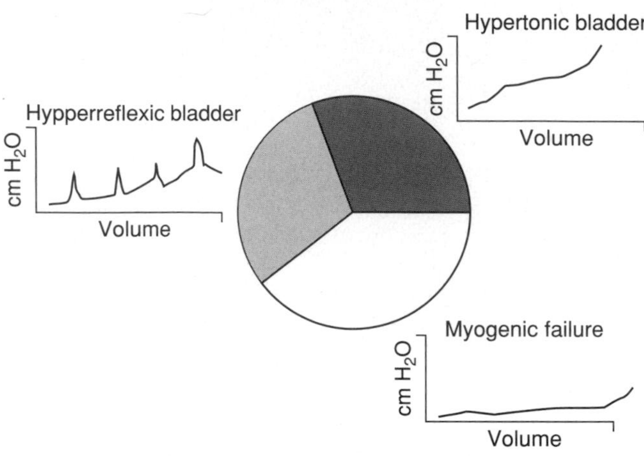

FIGURE 97-18. Chart showing the patterns of bladder dysfunction in a group of boys with previously corrected posterior urethral valves and later-onset voiding dysfunction. Representative cystometric curves correspond to the urodynamic pattern. The boys with bladder hypertonia and a noncompliant, small capacity bladder are at most risk for renal injury. (From Peters CA, Bolkier M, Bauer SB, et al. The urodynamic consequences of posterior urethral valves. *J Urol* 1990;144:122, with permission.)

a small capacity bladder, often with trabeculation. Instability may produce urge incontinence due to uninhibited bladder contractions and may occur with a degree of hypertonia. Myogenic or contractile failure may represent a decompensated bladder with insufficient contractile coordination to produce a sustained bladder contraction. This leads to high PVRs, infection, overflow incontinence, and occasionally hydronephrosis.

The boy with previously ablated valves and voiding dysfunction should be evaluated carefully to identify the pattern of bladder dysfunction present and determine appropriate therapy. Mixed patterns may be present. It is almost never the case that incontinence in these boys is due to a sphincter abnormality. The fact that incontinence reflects bladder dysfunction and this may injure renal function is apparent in several reports (115). In one long-term review, 45% of boys with incontinence also had renal failure in contrast to only 4% in those without incontinence (116).

The Older Boy with Valves

The clinical presentation of boys with milder forms of PUV who are not diagnosed until later in life is highly variable (117,118). Their presentation is usually a reflection of some element of bladder dysfunction due to chronic obstruction. This may be infection with inadequate emptying, new onset of incontinence due to bladder instability or overflow from a decompensated bladder, or occasionally from azotemia due to high-pressure bladder dysfunction. Valve ablation is the most appropriate first intervention, followed by a period of observation to assess the status of the bladder and kidneys with stabilization. The pattern of bladder dysfunction prior to valve ablation is not always that seen after valve ablation. The need for upper tract reconstruction depends on the presence of reflux and the adequacy of upper tract drainage. It is highly unusual to need temporary diversion, except in boys with sepsis or with such severe renal impairment that renal salvage may not be appropriate.

Mechanisms of Bladder Dysfunction

An understanding of the basis of bladder dysfunction due to PUV will be essential to permit more specific therapy of this entity, possibly reduce both the incidence of surgical reconstruction of the previously obstructed bladder and the incidence of renal failure in these patients. The processes that are active in the development of the dysfunctional bladder due to PUV are likely to be similar to other processes in organ systems beyond the bladder. Cardiac hypertrophy and fibrosis due to outflow resistance is an obvious example. Hypertrophy and fibrosis are common pathologic pathways.

Congenital bladder obstruction has been studied to a limited degree in the laboratory (100). Initial experiments focused on pulmonary effects of PUV and the in utero reversibility of this condition. Harrison's group suggested the possibility of prevention of pulmonary hypoplasia with in utero shunting of an obstructed bladder (102). A model of obstruction earlier in gestation with greater renal injury was created, and pulmonary morphometry was used as an endpoint to confirm this initial impression (119). Early oligohydramnios due to bladder obstruction could be reversed to permit more normal lung development (120,121), but this was dependent in large measure on the response of the kidneys to obstruction and decompression. If the renal effects of early bladder obstruction were not reversed with bladder decompression, pulmonary hypoplasia was present despite effective decompression. This was usually associated with histologic evidence of renal dysplasia.

The bladder consequences of in utero obstruction were studied and demonstrated a marked increase in growth, and alterations in the developmental regulation of several functional proteins (20). Bladder growth was due to increases in bladder smooth muscle cells, which were both hyperplastic (more cells) and hypertrophic (larger cells). A large increase in connective tissue elements was also demonstrated, which may be a significant factor in producing reduced compliance. Functionally, the bladders had less compliance as measured by stress relaxation. Developmental regulation of contractile proteins was affected by obstruction, as were the concentrations of neurotransmitter receptors (20) and innervation (122). Similar findings were reported in a model of moderate partial bladder obstruction, with increased growth and altered developmental regulation (123).

A model of severe partial obstruction confirms these initial observations, yet has further examined the metabolism of bladder collagen. Gene expression of the principal bladder interstitial collagens (types I and III) was not changed with obstruction, despite an increase in bladder collagen. Activity of the key collagen degradation proteins, the MMPs, was shown to be reduced and activity of the inhibitors of the MMPs (TIMPs) was increased (14). It is possible that the increased amounts of collagen are the result of a shift in the balance of collagen synthesis and breakdown. This balance may potentially be modulated exogenously and suggests possible mechanisms for favorably intervening in the development of bladder dysfunction in the setting of PUV.

Much remains to be learned regarding the evolution of bladder dysfunction due to PUV, from the level of the organism to the bladder muscle cell. It is likely that some of the key principles will also be applicable to other systems.

Surgical Management of the "Valve Bladder"

The basic principles of management of the valve bladder are those involved in the care of the neuropathic bladder. The aim is to achieve low-pressure storage of urine for a socially acceptable period of time and to permit complete emptying. The surgical options are essentially the same as those for neuropathic bladder, including augmentation cystoplasty. It is unusual to require surgical intervention for sphincteric function. The patients must be able to perform catheterization, and often this will be instituted during a trial of pharmacologic therapy with anticholinergic agents in an effort to reduce bladder pressures. Occasionally, patients will be able to learn to empty their bladders with abdominal pressure voiding, even with augmentation cystoplasty. The timing and commitment to surgical bladder augmentation is dependent on the pattern of bladder dynamics, the level of renal function, the commitment of the patient and family, and the response to pharmacologic therapy.

Renal Transplantation in Boys with PUV

The boy with prior valves and chronic renal failure presents a special challenge to the transplant team. These boys require thorough urologic evaluation of bladder function before transplantation (124,125). Of principal concern is the identification of bladder hypertonia, which may negatively impact renal graft survival. Cystography is useful to confirm complete valve ablation, and urodynamics should be performed to assess bladder dynamics. It is unusual for a child with chronic renal failure secondary to PUV to have normal bladder function.

Depending on previous surgical interventions, urinary tract reconstruction or undiversion may be necessary before transplantation. If augmentation cystoplasty is found to be necessary, it is best performed pretransplant. Gastrocystoplasty has been widely used in the transplant population, with added benefits of acid secretion, reduced infections, stones, and mucus (126). It has, however, been associated with a significant incidence of gastric acid-induced dysuria and hematuria (74,127). Attempts to control gastric acid secretion by way of histamine H2 receptor blockers (ranitidine) or H-ion pump inhibitors (omeprazole) have been moderately successful. Often this condition is self-limited. Particular attention must be paid to those boys with gastrocystoplasty who become anuric with progression of renal failure or from native nephrectomies. They have a high risk of bladder erosion from gastric acid. Appropriate attention to bladder dynamics posttransplant will improve the likelihood of graft survival. Episodes of graft failure or dysfunction should prompt a consideration of possible bladder dysfunction as a possible cause.

PRUNE BELLY SYNDROME: BLADDER MANIFESTATIONS

Clinical Patterns

PBS is a condition of maldevelopment of the lower urinary tract and testes. It is referred to by many names, including the Eagle-Barrett syndrome and the triad syndrome. Osler first used the term "prune belly" as indicative of the external appearance of these children with deficient abdominal musculature. The abdominal wall is flaccid and appears wrinkled. The triad syndrome refers to the principal elements of abdominal wall laxity due to deficient musculature, undescended testes, and a dilated bladder and lower urinary tract (128). Other features include variable degrees of pulmonary insufficiency, hypoplastic prostate (129,130), and sporadic deficiency of the corpus spongiosum leading to a scaphoid urethra. The degree of renal dysplasia is variable, as is upper tract dilation. Some of these children have a patent umbilicus and may leak urine from it. Approximately 20% of these children will die at birth, usually from pulmonary insufficiency. Approximately 20% are also found to have urethral atresia, although the concordance of these two features has not been explicitly reported.

PBS occurs almost exclusively in males, yet has been reported in females and follows a sex-linked recessive pattern of inheritance. Infertility is considered likely.

Etiology

The etiology of the PBS is unknown. A genetic basis is possible, yet there is frequent if not universal discordance among monozygotic twins. It has often been theorized that early bladder obstruction was the basis for the condition (131,132). Indeed, the massive dilation seen in many children with PBS is suggestive of obstructive dilation, yet only 20% have been found to have obstruction. A transient obstructive process has been hypothesized, yet not proven. It is possible that the phenotype of the PBS is the end result of several underlying mechanisms (133).

An interesting feature of PBS is the distinct gradients of segmental involvement, ranging from the most severe at the level of the bladder base and prostate, to minimal at the level of the kidney in some (128). This parallels the segmental gradation of abdominal musculature deficiency. Often the upper abdominal muscles are completely normal. The testes are formed from mesodermal tissues, just as are the prostate and bladder muscle and the abdominal musculature. A defect in development and differentiation of the mesodermal layers in a segmental gradient is a reasonable possible explanation for the nonobstructed forms of this condition, and is consistent with the evolving understanding of body segment organization (130). It seems more likely that an explanation for most children with PBS will lie in defects in the fundamental development of the mesodermal layers of the lower body segments.

Nonsurgical Management

Initial management of a neonate with PBS is supportive and directed to the pulmonary system. A patent and draining urachus assures adequate drainage. These children should not be viewed as having urinary obstruction in most cases, despite the massive dilation of their urinary tracts. Prevention of infection is the most important aim in all these children. Although aggressive surgical reconstruction has been undertaken by some, there is an appreciable risk involved (134,135), without the results being uniformly positive. Recurrent UTI is one of the strong indications to attempt to improve urinary drainage from the bladder and upper tracts. Intermittent catheterization may be necessary. On occasion, a continent stoma has been used to facilitate bladder drainage without urethral catheterization.

Over time, the degree of urinary tract dilation stabilizes and often may improve, as does the degree of abdominal wall laxity. Progressive renal deterioration, in the absence of infection, does not usually occur.

Surgical Management

Surgical management of PBS is often restricted to correction of cryptorchidism and plastic reconstruction of the abdominal wall. Operative correction of the enlarged bladder or the dilated ureters remains controversial, although the current trend has been away from aggressive surgical reconstruction (134,135).

Boys with PBS will have intraabdominal testes, and these are best relocated into the scrotum at an early age. This will not be likely to improve any chance of fertility, which has not been reported, yet will improve the patient's self-image and facilitate testicular examination. Transabdominal orchiopexy, occasionally with the Fowler-Stephens technique of spermatic vessel ligation, has been the standard for testicular management. Laparoscopic orchiopexy may now be considered as an alternative, and should not present any increased risk in a child with PBS.

Abdominoplasty may be performed in the older child and aims to improve the cosmetic appearance of the abdomen, improve abdominal muscular function, and possibly improve respiratory muscle dynamics. A lower transverse incision has been reported by Randolph to excise the poorly functioning lower abdominal musculature (136). A vertical abdominoplasty, as reported by Montfort (137) and Erhlich (138), overlaps the midline abdominal musculature and brings the lateral musculature into the ventral aspect. This tends to have more tone and contractile capacity. The fascia is closed in a vest-over-pants fashion to further improve ventral tone. The reported results have generally been good, including improved voiding efficiency (139).

Reduction cystoplasty has occasionally been performed to limit PVR urine volume (140). This may be recommended if UTI has complicated the child's course. Some authors indicate that any improvement is temporary. Total urinary reconstruction has been advocated by some, with reports of stable renal function. Patients were maintained on prophylactic antibiotics, and comparison to patients undergoing careful nonoperative management is not available.

NEOPLASMS OF THE BLADDER

Rhabdomyosarcoma: Bladder Issues

The general management of pediatric rhabdomyosarcoma is presented elsewhere, but several specific issues relating to bladder and prostatic rhabdomyosarcoma (BPR) are relevant to a discussion of pediatric bladder diseases. In particular, the diagnosis of BPR is often made in the context of evaluation of children for voiding dysfunction; thus, the management strategies should be carefully integrated with the outlook for bladder function, or when necessary, surgical replacement of bladder function.

Diagnosis

A high index of suspicion is essential in order to diagnose BPR in a timely fashion. Initial symptoms may be subtle and are considered to be due to infection, behavior, or nonspecific complaints of dysuria or frequency. BPR may be readily detected in most cases with a rectal examination in which the normal prostate may be barely felt as a smooth, soft midline bump. Ultrasound of the bladder base is also an effective examination in cases of low suspicion. The more apparent clinical presentation of urinary retention or UTI will usually be recognized for their true nature. VCUG and upper urinary tract ultrasound is usually sufficient to provide the diagnosis. Careful cystoscopic and bimanual examination to determine tumor extent and mobility is performed at the time of transurethral or perineal biopsy for tissue diagnosis; biopsies should be performed with a cold-cup biopsy forceps to avoid cautery artifact. Imaging will usually provide a precise definition of tumor extent.

Integrating Bladder Functional Outlook with Therapy

Controversy remains as to the appropriate therapy for BPR in children, but it remains important to anticipate bladder functional needs. This comes into play as early as the time of urinary diversion if needed. As many options as possible should be kept open to permit future normal bladder function or appropriate replacement of bladder function with continent reservoirs. A temporary period of diversion is often needed, and transverse colon conduits are highly effective permitting later integration into a continent reservoir if the bladder is unusable. The conduit would also be useful if bladder augmentation were appropriate following radiotherapy and complete disease clearance. It should be anticipated that extensive radiotherapy with fibrosis will affect sphincter function. Bladder-sparing strategies are appealing, but the functional capacity of a bladder following intensive radiotherapy may not always be normal (141,142). Reported results have been varied in terms of long-term bladder salvage rates, the most optimistic being about 50% (143).

Urethral sparing strategies in boys have been fraught with the need for secondary urethrectomy after margins are found to be positive with permanent sections. "Skip lesions" are frequently noted in prostatic rhabdomyosarcomas. This limits the potential for use of the urethra in functional reconstruction.

Reconstructive Options

Continent reconstruction in children after cure of BPR is a formidable challenge. These children may have significant radiation fibrosis of the pelvis precluding orthotopic reconstruction. Sphincter function may be inadequate and the therapeutic options in such children are limited. As noted previously, use of the native urethra must be undertaken cautiously. Continent diversion to a neobladder of GI segments is often the most effective means of providing continence without risk to the upper urinary tracts. Construction of reservoirs from the initial diverting segment added to an ileocecal segment with the appendix as a catheterizable conduit is a particularly useful option. The appendix may be kept in situ with the cecum and tunneled into an adjacent tinea. This creates a flap-valve mechanism much like antireflux surgery, and then provides for continence. The appendix may be brought to the umbilicus where catheterization is technically easy and the stoma is concealed. In the absence of appendix, the ureter or tapered ileum may be implanted into the reservoir. A careful evaluation of the effects of radiation must be performed on any segments of bowel considered for integration into a continent reservoir. Concomitant evaluation of rectal function must be performed to avoid limiting options for rectal continence in the setting of radiation proctitis.

In a review of 33 patients with a variety of pelvic rhabdomyosarcomas, 31 patients are alive and well with a combination of urinary diversions and reconstructions (144). Six of 16 patients with cystectomy have continent diversion, and the others continue with urinary conduit diversion. These continent diversions have relatively few complications and an excellent success rate. In 10 patients undergoing bladder-sparing therapy, involving radiation or chemotherapy alone, prostatectomy, or partial cystectomy, 5 required some form of urinary reconstruction or diversion for continence or hydronephrosis. One underwent secondary radical cystectomy and one died. Although bladder-sparing therapy may be a worthy and achievable goal in some patients is not always possible. Anticipation of the need for complex urinary reconstruction to ensure continence and upper urinary tract preservation will maximize the opportunity to achieve these goals.

Transitional Cell Carcinoma

The most common bladder neoplasm in adults is extremely rare in children and appears to exhibit a distinct biology (145). The typical behavior of childhood transitional cell carcinoma (TCC) is to be noninvasive and nonrecurring, in contrast to adult TCC. Diagnosis is often by chance because hematuria in the child is not usually evaluated with cystoscopy (146). No other diagnostic modality is effective in detecting the small papillary lesions typical of pediatric TCC. Ultrasonography may occasionally detect a small lesion of the bladder wall. Cytology is seldom useful in that the low grade of lesion is difficult to detect cytologically. Local endoscopic resection is the treatment of choice, with adequate biopsy material to determine the level of invasion. Subsequent follow-up is not recommended unless the tumor is high grade or demonstrates more than obtaining superficial involvement (147). However, recurrences have been reported and it seems prudent to pursue a follow-up program similar to that in adults, including regular cystoscopy at 3-month intervals at least for 1 to 2 years. The duration of need is unclear, but we have seen recurrence after 5 years. Invasive TCC may be best treated with radical resection as in adults; the role of adjuvant chemotherapy has not been defined in children, given the rarity of the condition.

Adenocarcinoma

Adenocarcinoma of the bladder is rare in adults and children, but has an increased incidence in patients with bladder exstrophy (148). The etiology is presumed to be due to chronic irritation of the exposed bladder. A possible link has been made to the occurrence of GI rests of glandular epithelium or to a metaplastic response of bladder (149). Squamous carcinoma has been reported in patients with closed exstrophy (150). Chronic monitoring has been recommended by some, but is not widely practiced in patients with closed bladder exstrophy (151).

Neurofibromatosis

Involvement of the bladder and lower urinary tract may occur with neurofibromatosis (NF). These children usually have other stigmata of NF or a family history of von Recklinghausen's syndrome. Urologic presentation may be that of any mass effect in the bladder, including dysuria, frequency, urinary retention, or infection (152). Upper tract obstruction may occur. Involvement of the external genitalia may occur. The extent of involvement should be delineated with imaging studies, and a biopsy is recommended to rule out malignancy. Malignant degeneration is reported to occur in 5% to 30% (153). Management depends on the clinical presentation and extent of involvement. Curative resection is not usually possible. Urinary diversion may be necessary with extreme involvement.

Pheochromocytoma

The bladder is the most common extraadrenal site of involvement of pheochromocytoma in children (154,155). Usually benign, these tumors may present with the classical findings of pheochromocytoma, including hypertension, dizziness, headache, palpitations, faintness, and pallor. These symptoms may be present with typical urinary symptoms of hematuria, dysuria, and frequency, and they may be exacerbated with urination. Appropriate diagnostic evaluation to assess the functional characteristics of the tumor, as well as searching for other sites, is needed. Vesical pheochromocytoma requires the same level of preoperative preparation as do adrenal pheochromocytomas, including volume repletion, adrenergic blockade, and intensive anesthesia monitoring. Local resection is appropriate.

Hamartoma (Nephrogenic Adenoma)

These benign tumors are usually associated with a source of chronic irritation and may present with irritative symptoms, hematuria, and a history of recurrent UTI. They have a papillary appearance and do not demonstrate evidence of invasiveness (149). Local resection is curative. Histologically, they have an appearance that resembles developing kidney (hence the name).

MISCELLANEOUS BLADDER CONDITIONS

Bladder and Urethral Polyps

Polyps of the bladder usually occur at the bladder neck and proximal, prostatic urethra (156,157). They may create a "ball-valve" effect at the bladder neck and cause intermittency of the urinary stream, or severe dysuria and strangury. They may also produce gross hematuria. In some children, mild symptoms may be attributed to behavioral causes. Ultrasonographic evaluation may detect the polyp (Fig. 97-3); however, VCUG is usually definitive. Cystoscopic diagnosis confirms the diagnosis and usually permits removal. Some polyps may be so large as to require open or laparoscopic bladder removal.

Urachal Anomalies

Urachal abnormalities are uncommon and may be suspected in the infant with umbilical drainage or inflammation (158). Uriniferous drainage is typical and diagnostic. A mass may be felt infraumbilically, or the child may present with urinary infection or apparent omphalitis. Ultrasonography is effective to identify a mass or cystic structure behind the midline of the rectus muscles (159). Injection of a sinus tract, if present, is also diagnostic (160). VCUG may demonstrate contrast into a urachal sinus. Treatment is surgical removal to avoid infection, which is often staphylococcal species. A small infraumbilical incision is usually adequate to identify the urachus at the dome of the bladder and trace it to the umbilicus. It should be removed in its entirety, with a small cuff of bladder. The peritoneum should not be violated. Laparoscopic approaches have been described (161).

Vascular Malformations

Bladder vascular malformations may be isolated or associated with an identified condition of multiple arteriovenous malformations (162–164). Intravesical varices have been described and present with significant gross hematuria and clot. Cystoscopy is diagnostic and is appropriate in the setting of gross hematuria that is not consistent with viral cystitis. The latter is usually abrupt in onset, associated with intense dysuria and frequency, and self-limited. A diffuse edematous reaction of the bladder wall may be seen ultrasonographically. Varicosities of the bladder, however, are small and discrete. Superficial ulcerations may be noted. Recurrent gross hematuria may be very difficult to control in some patients. Treatment options include local resection, embolization, or sclerotherapy.

Bladder Diverticula

Congenital diverticula of the bladder are uncommon. Identification of a bladder diverticulum should prompt an evaluation for bladder outflow obstruction due to posterior urethral valves or neurogenic voiding dysfunction. In the setting of a smooth wall bladder, however, outflow obstruction is usually not found. The basis for the diverticulum is presumed to be a weakness in the bladder wall musculature. Diverticula have been described in the children with connective tissue defects, including Ehlers-Danlos syndrome (165), Williams syndrome (166), and Menkes kinky-hair syndrome (166), all characterized by defects in collagen structure. It is possible that abnormal development of the lamina propria permits eventration of the pliable uroepithelium through the muscle fibers. Surgical repair of these diverticula is controversial because it does not deal with the underlying defect, and recurrence is reported to be frequent. Intermittent catheterization may not always be effective due to poor emptying and the risk of subsequent UTIs.

CONTINENT URINARY DIVERSION AND BLADDER RECONSTRUCTION

Indications

Continent urinary diversion involves the creation of a system of urinary storage and emptying other than native bladder or of a bladder-emptying mechanism other than urethra. Its application is appropriate whenever storage of emptying functions cannot be effectively restored with bladder or urethra. This is most often the case in patients with neurogenic bladder dysfunction in whom bladder capacity is markedly limited, sphincter function is inadequate, or both. Other situations involve bladder absence or total unreconstructability, as in prior radical excision for tumor, or a small fibrotic bladder, as with some bladder exstrophy patients. Reasons to be unable to reconstruct the urethral include prior surgery and scarring or neurogenic fibrosis. It may also include patients with severely abnormal body habitus that prevents perineal catheterization. A catheterizable abdominal stoma is often the most appropriate means of attaining continence with adequate emptying.

Continent diversion depends on intermittent catheterization that must be assured prior to reconstruction. It is often more acceptable to patients to catheterize an abdominal rather than a perineal urethral stoma.

Techniques

Reservoir

The urinary reservoir for a continent diversion may include native bladder in whole or part (167) (Fig. 97-19). Augmentation of bladder capacity and decrease in pressure are usually needed. This can involve segments of ileum, cecum, sigmoid, or stomach. When the bladder is unusable or absent, a reservoir may be constructed by one of a variety of mechanisms, depending on the condition and mobility of bowel segments and the surgeon's preference. Reconfigured ileocecal reservoirs have been widely used, with good results. Composite reservoirs incorporating gastric and intestinal components have also been used with success. Complete detubularization and reconfiguration is essential.

Alternative techniques for creation of an adequate capacity, low-pressure reservoir have been explored, including ureterocystoplasty (168) and the use of demucosalized segments of the GI tract (169,170). The principal aim of these techniques is to avoid the application of enteric mucosa in a urinary reservoir.

Continence Mechanisms

A variety of mechanisms to achieve continence are available, based on a flap-valve technique, tissue pressure, or external compression (171). The flap-valve technique involves a tubular structure implanted into the wall of the bladder or colonic segment and is generally referred to as the Mitrofanoff technique (172). The tube may be the appendix, ureter, stomach, or reconfigured bowel (Monti). This approach has an excellent success rate and is efficient to create. Avoidance of too long a catheterizable segment will avoid problems with postoperative inability to catheterize. Creation of a V-flap of skin into the spatulated end of the tube helps to prevent stomal stenosis. Tissue pressure methods include tapering of an ileal segment over a length and reinforcing the ileocecal valve mechanism. The ileum would then be brought out to the skin for catheterization. External pressure techniques include an artificial urinary sphincter or marlex mesh cuff around an intestinal segment.

The flap-valve technique is the most effective in terms of providing continence, but suffers from being too effective and not permitting any "pop-off" if rigorous catheterization is not adhered to.

Complications

The complications of continent urinary diversions are largely preventable with appropriate attention to detail in the initial creation of the diversion and with postoperative follow-up. Adequate mobilization and detubularization of the intestinal segments will prevent ischemic

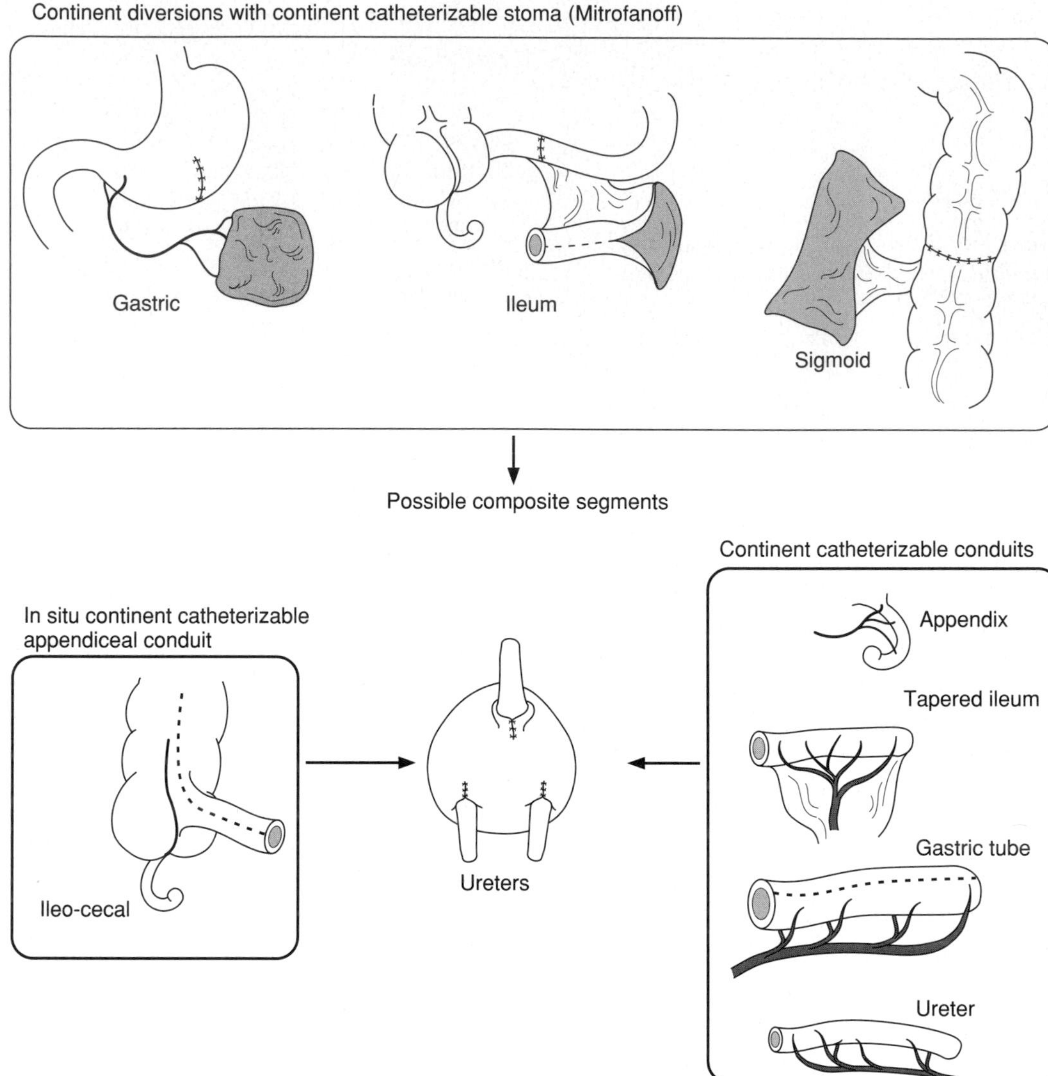

FIGURE 97-19. Diagram illustrating the various options involved in continent diversion using the Mitrofanoff principle. The reservoir may be constructed of a single reconfigured enteric segment or a combination of more than one segment. The ureters are usually tunneled into the wall of the reservoir in an antireflux manner. The reservoir is made continent through the catheterizable conduit, using appendix, ureter, or a constructed tube from the bowel.

problems and maintain adequately low reservoir pressures. The continence mechanism, our preference is the Mitrofanoff technique, must be short and easily catheterizable. This should be assured in the operating room. Postoperatively, the most common problems revolve around inadequate emptying of the reservoir causing infection, perforation, mucus plugging, electrolyte abnormalities, and stones. Regular irrigation with saline solution and a strict emptying regimen are important. Periodic monitoring of the pouch to identify stones early will avoid the need for a major procedure to remove any that may form. Percutaneous techniques are useful with small calculi, but larger stones may be most efficiently removed with open surgery. Tumors have not been reported to occur in continent urinary diversions in children, but the possibility has been raised and investigation, as well as monitoring, are ongoing.

REFERENCES

1. Ewalt DH, Howard PS, Blyth B, et al. Is lamina propria matrix responsible for normal bladder compliance? *J Urol* 1992;148:544–549.
2. Parsons CL, Boychuck D, Jones S, et al. Bladder surface glycosaminoglycans: an epithelial permeability barrier. *J Urol* 1990;143:139.
3. Baskin LS, Hayward SW, Young PF, et al. Ontogeny of the rat bladder: smooth muscle and epithelial differentiation. *Acta Anatomica* 1996;155(3):163–171.

4. Baskin LS, Young P, Hayward S, et al. Role of mesenchymal–epithelial interactions in normal bladder development. *J Urol* 1995;153:264A.
5. Baskin L, DiSandro M, Li Y, et al. Mesenchymal–epithelial interactions in bladder smooth muscle development: effects of the local tissue environment. *J Urol* 2001;165(4):1283–1288.
6. Oerlich TM. The urethral sphincter muscle in the male. *Am J Anat* 1980;158:229.
7. Oerlich TM. The striated urogenital sphincter muscle in the female. *Anat Rec* 1983;205:223.
8. Chancellor MB, Yoshimura N. Physiology and pharmacology of the bladder and urethra. In: Walsh PC, Retik AB, Vaughan ED Jr, et al., eds. *Campbell's urology.* Philadelphia: WB Saunders, 2002:831–886.
9. Brading A. Physiology of bladder smooth muscle. In: Torrens M, Morrison JFB, eds. *The physiology of the lower urinary tract.* Berlin: Springer-Verlag, 1987:161–191.
10. Kamm KE, Stull JT. The function of myosin and myosin light chain kinase phosphorylation in smooth muscle. *Ann Rev Pharmacol Toxico.* 1985;25:593.
11. Kamm KE, Stull JT. Regulation of smooth muscle contractile elements by second messengers. *Ann Rev Physiol* 1989;51:299.
12. de Groat WC, Fraser MO, Yoshiyama M, et al. Neural control of the urethra. *Scand J Urol Nephrol Suppl* 2001(207):35–43;discussion 106–125.
13. Kondo A, Susset JG. Viscoelastic properties of bladder. II. Comparative studies in normal and pathologic dogs. *Invest Urol* 1974;11(6):459–465.
14. Peters CA, Freeman MR, Fernandez CA, et al. Dysregulated proteolytic balance as the basis of excess extracellular matrix in fibrotic disease. *Am J Physiol* 1997;272(6 pt 2):R1960–R1965.
15. Cortivo R, Pagano F, Passerini G, et al. Elastin and collagen in the normal and obstructed urinary bladder. *Br J Urol* 1981;53(2):134–137.
16. Koo HP, Macarak EJ, Chang SL, et al. Temporal expression of elastic fiber components in bladder development. *Connect Tiss Res* 1998;37(1–2):1–11.
17. Sillen U. Bladder function in healthy neonates and its development during infancy. *J Urol* 2001;166(6):2376–2381.
18. Dixon JS, Jen PY, Gosling JA. Immunohistochemical characteristics of human paraganglion cells and sensory corpuscles associated with the urinary bladder. A developmental study in the male fetus, neonate and infant. *J Anat* 1998;192(pt 3):407–415.
19. Andersson KE. Bladder activation: afferent mechanisms. *Urology* 2002;59(5 suppl 1):43–50.
20. Peters CA, Vasavada S, Dator D, et al. The effect of obstruction on the developing bladder. *J Urol* 1992;148:491–496.
21. Sutherland RS, Baskin LS, Kogan BA, et al. Neuroanatomical changes in the rat bladder after bladder outlet obstruction. *Br J Urol* 1998;82(6):895–901.
22. DiSanto ME, Wein AJ, Chacko S. Lower urinary tract physiology and pharmacology. *Curr Urol Rep* 2000;1(3):227–234.
23. Steers WD, deGroat WC. Effect of bladder outlet obstruction on micturition reflex pathways in the rat. *J Urol* 1988;140(4):864–871.
24. de Groat WC. Plasticity of bladder reflex pathways during postnatal development. *Physiol Behav* 2002;77(4–5):689–692.
25. Park JM. Normal and anomalous development of the urogenital system. In: Walsh PC, Retik AB, Vaughan ED Jr, et al., eds. *Campbell's urology.* Philadelphia: WB Saunders, 2002:1737–1764.
26. Hoyes AD, Ramus NI, Martin BGH. Ultrastructural aspects of the development of the innervation of the vesical musculature in the early human fetus. *Invest Urol* 1973;10:307–312.
27. Mitolo CD, Schonauer S, Grasso G, et al. Ontogenesis of autonomic receptors in detrusor muscle and bladder sphincter of human fetus. *Urology* 1983;21(6):599–603.
28. Baskin L, Meaney D, Landsman A, et al. Bovine bladder compliance increases with normal fetal development. *J Urol* 1994;152:692–695.
29. Mevorach RA, Bogaert GA, Kogan BA. Role of nitric oxide in fetal lower urinary tract function. *J Urol* 1994;152(2 pt 1):510–514.
30. Bourdelat D, Barbet JP, Butler-Browne GS. Fetal development of the urethral sphincter. *Eur J Pediatr Surg* 1992;2:35–38.
31. Kokoua A, Homsy Y, Lavigne JF, et al. Maturation of the external urinary sphincter: a comparative histotopographic study in humans. *J Urol* 1993;150(2 pt 2):617–622.
32. Baskin LS, Constantinescu S, Duckett JW, et al. Type III collagen decreases in normal fetal bovine bladder development. *J Urol* 1994;152:688–691.
33. Koo HP, Howard PS, Chang SL, et al. Developmental expression of interstitial collagen genes in fetal bladders. *J Urol* 1997;158(3 pt 1):954–961.
34. Swaiman KF, Bradley WE. Quantitation of collagen in the wall of the human urinary bladder. *J Appl Physiol* 1967;22(1):122–124.
35. Cawston T, Plumpton T, Curry V, et al. Role of TIMP and MMP inhibition in preventing connective tissue breakdown. *Ann NY Acad Sci* 1994;732(75):75–83.
36. Matsumoto S, Kogan BA, Levin RM, et al. Response of the fetal sheep bladder to urinary diversion. *J Urol* 2003;169(2):735–739.
37. Wladimiroff JW, Campbell S. Fetal urine-production rates in normal and complicated pregnancy. *Lancet* 1974(Feb 2).
38. Kogan BA, Iwamoto HS. Lower urinary tract function in the sheep fetus: studies of autonomic control and pharmacologic responses of the fetal bladder. *J Urol* 1989;141(4):1019–1024.
39. Mandell J, Lebowitz RL, Peters CA, et al. Prenatal diagnosis of the megacystis-megaureter association. *J Urol* 1992;148:1487–1489.
40. Kaefer M, Barnewolt C, Retik AB, et al. The sonographic diagnosis of infravesical obstruction in children: evaluation of bladder wall thickness indexed to bladder filling [comment]. *J Urol* 1997;157(3):989–991.
41. Manning FA. Fetal surgery for obstructive uropathy: rational considerations. *Am J Kidney Dis* 1987;10(4):259–267.
42. Kaefer M, Peters CA, Retik AB, et al. Increased renal echogenicity: a sonographic sign for differentiating between obstructive and nonobstructive etiologies of in utero bladder distension. *J Urol* 1997;158(3 pt 2):1026–1029.
43. Spencer JR, Schaeffer AJ. Pediatric urinary tract infections. *Urol Clin North Am* 1986;13:661–672.
44. Roberts JA. Etiology and pathophysiology of pyelonephritis. *Am J Kidney Dis* 1991;17:1–9.
45. Anonymous. Practice parameter: the diagnosis, treatment, and evaluation of the initial urinary tract infection in febrile infants and young children. American Academy of Pediatrics, Committee on Quality Improvement, Subcommittee on Urinary Tract Infection [comment] [erratum appears in 2000;105(1 pt 1):141]. *Pediatrics* 1999;103(4 pt 1):843–852.
46. Hoberman A, Charron M, Hickey RW, et al. Imaging studies after a first febrile urinary tract infection in young children [comment]. *N Engl J Med* 2003;348(3):195–202.
47. Hoover DL, Duckett JW Jr. Posterior urethral valves, unilateral reflux, and renal dysplasia: a syndrome. *J Urol* 1982;128:994.
48. Glassberg KL, Schnieider M, Haller JO, et al. Observations on persistently dilated ureter after posterior urethral valve ablation. *Urology* 1982;20:20.
49. McGuire EJ, Woodside JR, Borden TA, et al. Prognostic value of urodynamic testing in myelodysplastic patients. *J Urol* 1981;126:205–209.
50. Holmdahl G, Sillen U, Bachelard M, et al. The changing urodynamic pattern in valve bladders during infancy. *J Urol* 1995;153(2):463–467.
51. Peters CA, Bolkier M, Bauer SB, et al. The urodynamic consequences of posterior urethral valves. *J Urol* 1990;144:122–126.
52. Walker BR, Ellison ED, Snow BW, et al. The natural history of idiopathic urethrorrhagia in boys. *J Urol* 2001;166(1):231–232.
53. Koff SA, Byard MA. The daytime urinary frequency syndrome of childhood. *J Urol* 1988;140:1280–1281.
54. Gatti JM, Perez-Brayfield M, Kirsch AJ, et al. Acute urinary retention in children. *J Urol* 2001;165(3):918–921.
55. Zawin JK, Lebowitz RL. Neurogenic dysfunction of the bladder in infants and children: recent advances and the role of radiology. *Radiology* 1992;182:297–304.
56. Mandell J, Lebowitz RL, Hallett M, et al. Urethral narrowing in region of external sphincter: radiologic-urodynamic correlations in boys with myelodysplasia. *AJR Am J Roentgenol* 1980;134:731–735.
57. Bauer SB, Koff SA, Jayanthin VR. Voiding dysfunction in children: neurogenic and non-neurogenic. In: Walsh PC, Retik AB, Vaughan ED Jr, et al., eds. *Campbell's urology.* Philadelphia: WB Saunders, 2002:2231–2283.

58. Kaefer M, Rosen A, Darbey M, et al. Pressure at residual volume: a useful adjunct to standard fill cystometry. *J Urol* 1997;158(3 pt 2): 1268–1271.
59. Yang SS, Wang CC, Chen YT. Home uroflowmetry for the evaluation of boys with urinary incontinence. *J Urol* 2003;169(4):1505–1507.
60. Wan J, McGuire EJ, Bloom DA, et al. Stress leak point pressure: a diagnostic tool for incontinent children. *J Urol* 1993;150:700–702.
61. Farmer DL, von Koch CS, Peacock WJ, et al. In utero repair of myelomeningocele: experimental pathophysiology, initial clinical experience, and outcomes. *Arch Surg* 2003;138(8):872–878.
62. Holmes NM, Nguyen HT, Harrison MR, et al. Fetal intervention for myelomeningocele: effect on postnatal bladder function. *J Urol* 2001;166(6):2383–2386.
63. Shapiro E, Becich MJ, Perlman E, et al. Bladder wall abnormalities in myelodysplastic bladders: a computer assisted morphometric analysis. *J Urol* 1991;145:1024–1029.
64. Kasabian NG, Bauer SB, Dyro FM, et al. The prophylactic value of clean intermittent catheterization and anticholinergic medication in newborns and infants with myelodysplasia at risk of developing urinary tract deterioration. *Am J Dis Child* 1992;146:840–843.
65. Kaefer M, Pabby A, Kelly M, et al. Improved bladder function after prophylactic treatment of the high risk neurogenic bladder in newborns with myelomeningocele. *J Urol* 1999;162(3 pt 2):1068–1071.
66. Wu HY, Baskin LS, Kogan BA. Neurogenic bladder dysfunction due to myelomeningocele: neonatal versus childhood treatment. *J Urol* 1997;157(6):2295–2297.
67. Mattiasson A, Andersson KE, Sjogren C, et al. Supersensitivity to carbachol in the parasympathetically decentralized feline urinary bladder. *J Urol* 1984;131(3):562–565.
68. Speakman MJ, Brading AF, Gilpin CJ, et al. Bladder outflow obstruction—a cause of denervation supersensitivity. *J Urol* 1987;138(6):1461–1466.
69. Uvelius B, Mattiasson A. Detrusor collagen content in the denervated rat urinary bladder. *J Urol* 1986;136(5):1110–1112.
70. Bloom DA, Knechtel JM, McGuire EJ. Urethral dilation improves bladder compliance in children with myelomeningocele and high leak point pressures. *J Urol* 1990;144:430.
71. Kasabian NG, Vlachiotis JD, Lais A, et al. The use of intravesical oxybutynin chloride in patients with detrusor hypertonicity and detrusor hyperreflexia. *J Urol* 1994;151(4):944–945.
72. Husmann OA, Cain MP. Fecal and urinary continence after ileal cecal cystoplasty for the neurogenic bladder. *J Urol* 2001;165(3):922–925.
73. Gosalbez RJ, Woodard JR, Broecker BH, et al. Metabolic complications of the use of stomach for urinary reconstruction. *J Urol* 1993;150(pt 2):710–712.
74. Nguyen DH, Bain MA, Salmonson KL, et al. The syndrome of dysuria and hematuria in pediatric urinary reconstruction with stomach. *J Urol* 1993;150(pt 2):707–709.
75. Hinman F, Baumann FW. Vesical and ureteral damage from voiding dysfunction in boys without neurologic or obstructive disease. *J Urol* 1973;109:727.
76. Bauer SB, Hendren WH, Kozakewich H, et al. Perforation of the augmented bladder. *J Urol* 1992;148(pt 2):699–703.
77. Woodhouse CR, Lennon GN. Management and etiology of stones in intestinal urinary reservoirs in adolescents. *Eur Urol* 2001;39(3):253–259.
78. Cain MP, Casale AJ, Kaefer M, et al. Percutaneous cystolithotomy in the pediatric augmented bladder. *J Urol* 2002;168(4 pt 2):1881–1882.
79. Canning DA, Perman JA, Jeffs RD, et al. Nutritional consequences of bowel segments in the lower urinary tract. *J Urol* 1989;142:509–511.
80. Austin PF, Westney OL, Leng WW, et al. Advantages of rectus fascial slings for urinary incontinence in children with neuropathic bladders. *J Urol* 2001;165(6 pt 2):2369–2371; discussion 2371–2372.
81. Herschorn S, Radomski SB. Fascial slings and bladder neck tapering in the treatment of male neurogenic incontinence. *J Urol* 1992;147(4):1073–1075.
82. Jones JA, Mitchell ME, Rink RC. Improved results using a modification of the Young-Dees-Leadbetter bladder neck repair. *Br J Urol* 1993;71(5):555–561.
83. Kropp KA, Angwafo FF. Urethral lengthening and reimplantation for neurogenic incontinence in children. *J Urol* 1986;135(3):533–536.
84. Salle JL, McLorie GA, Bagli DJ, et al. Urethral lengthening with anterior bladder wall flap (Pippi Salle procedure): modifications and extended indications of the technique. *J Urol* 1997;158(2):585–590.
85. Bosco PJ, Bauer SB, Colodny AH, et al. The long-term results of artificial sphincters in children. *J Urol* 1991;146:396–399.
86. Mitchell ME, Rink RC. Experience with the artificial urinary sphincter in children and young adults. *J Pediatr Surg* 1983;18:700.
87. Wan J, McGuire EJ, Bloom DA, et al. The treatment of urinary incontinence in children using glutaraldehyde cross-linked collagen. *J Urol* 1992;148(1):127–130.
88. Mitrofanoff P. Cystostomie continente trans-appendiculaire dans le traitement des vessies neurologiques. *Chir Pediatr* 1986;21:297.
89. Liard A, Seguier-Lipszyc E, Mathiot A, et al. The Mitrofanoff procedure: 20 years later. *J Urol* 2001;165(6 Pt 2):2394–8.
90. Gosalbez R, Wei D, Gousse A, Castellan M, Labbie A. Refashioned short bowel segments for the construction of catheterizable channels (the Monti procedure): early clinical experience. *J Urol* 1998;160(3 Pt 2):1099–102.
91. Clark T, Pope JC, Adams C, et al. Factors that influence outcomes of the Mitrofanoff and Malone antegrade continence enema reconstructive procedures in children. *J Urol* 2002;168(4 pt 1):1537–1540; discussion 1540.
92. Cadeddu JA, Docimo SG. Laparoscopic-assisted continent stoma procedures: our new standard. *Urology* 1999;54(5):909–912.
93. Sheldon C, Cormier M, Crone K, et al. Occult neurovesical dysfunction in children with imperforate anus and its variants. *J Pediatr Surg* 1991;26(1):49–54.
94. De Filippo RE, Shaul DB, Harrison EA, et al. Neurogenic bladder in infants born with anorectal malformations: comparison with spinal and urologic status [comment]. *J Pediatr Surg* 1999;34(5):825–827; discussion 828.
95. Young HH, Frontz WA, Baldwin JC. Congenital obstruction of the posterior urethra. *J Urol* 1919;3:289.
96. Hendren WH. Posterior urethral valves in boys: a broad clinical spectrum. *J Urol* 1971;106:298.
97. Nakayama DK, Harrison MR, deLorimier AA. Prognosis of posterior urethral valves presenting at birth. *J Pediatr Surg* 1986;21:43–45.
98. Egami K, Smith ED. A study of the sequelae of posterior urethral valves. *J Urol* 1982;127:84.
99. Mitchell ME. Persistent ureteral dilatation following valve resection. *Dialogues Pediatr Urol* 1982;5:8.
100. Peters CA. Congenital bladder obstruction: research approaches. In: Zderic SA, ed. *Muscle, matrix, and bladder function, advances in experimental medicine and biology*. New York: Plenum, 1995.
101. Bellinger MF, Comstock CH, Grosso D, et al. Fetal posterior urethral valves and renal dysplasia at 15 weeks gestational age. *J Urol* 1983;129:1238–1239.
102. Harrison MR, Nakayama DK, Noall R, et al. Correction of congenital hydronephrosis in utero II. Decompression reverses the effects of obstruction on the fetal lung and urinary tract. *J Pediatr Surg* 1982;17(6):965–974.
103. Agarwal SK, Fisk NM. In utero therapy for lower urinary tract obstruction. *Prenat Diagn* 2001;21(11):970–976.
104. Freedman AL, Bukowski TP, Smith CA, et al. Fetal therapy for obstructive uropathy: diagnosis specific outcomes. *J Urol* 1996;156 (2 pt 2:720–723;discussion 723–724.
105. Edouga D, Hugueny B, Gasser B, et al. Recovery after relief of fetal urinary obstruction: morphological, functional and molecular aspects. *Am J Physiol Renal Physiol* 2001;281(1):F26–F37.
106. Mandell J, Estroff J, Benacerraf BR, et al. Late onset severe oligohydramnios associated with genitourinary abnormalities. *J Urol* 1992;148:515–518.
107. Churchill BM, Krueger RP, Fleisher MH, et al. Complications of posterior urethral valve surgery and their prevention. *Urol Clin North Am* 1983;10:519.
108. Hendren WH. A new approach to infants with severe obstructive uropathy: early complete reconstruction. *J Pediatr Surg* 1970;5:184–199.
109. Close CE, Carr MC, Burns MW, et al. Lower urinary tract changes after early valve ablation in neonates and infants: is early diversion warranted? [see comments]. *J Urol* 1997;157(3):984–988.

110. Jaureguizar E, Lopez Pereira P, Martinez Urrutia MJ, et al. Does neonatal pyeloureterostomy worsen bladder function in children with posterior urethral valves? *J Urol* 2000;164(3 pt 2):1031–1033; discussion 1033–1034.
111. Kim YH, Horowitz M, Combs A, et al. Comparative urodynamic findings after primary valve ablation, vesicostomy or proximal diversion. *J Urol* 1996;156(2 pt 2):673–676.
112. Podesta M, Ruarte AC, Gargiulo C, et al. Bladder function associated with posterior urethral valves after primary valve ablation or proximal urinary diversion in children and adolescents. *J Urol* 2002;168(4 pt 2):1830–1835; discussion 1835.
113. Johnston JH. Vesicoureteral reflux with urethral valves. *Br J Urol* 1979;51:100.
114. McGuire EJ, Weiss RM. Secondary bladder neck obstruction in patients with urethral valves: treatment with phenoxybenzamine. *Urology* 1975;5:756.
115. Lopez Pereira P, Martinez Urrutia MJ, Espinosa L, et al. Bladder dysfunction as a prognostic factor in patients with posterior urethral valves. *BJU Intl* 2002;90(3):308–311.
116. Parkhouse HF, Barratt TM, Dillon MJ, et al. Long-term outcome of boys with posterior urethral valves. *Br J Urol* 1988;62(1):59–62.
117. Nguyen HT, Peters CA. The long-term complications of posterior urethral valves. *BJU Int* 1999;83 (suppl 3):23–28.
118. Bomalaski MD, Anema JG, Coplen DE, et al. Delayed presentation of posterior urethral valves: a not so benign condition. *J Urol* 1999;162(6):2130–2132.
119. Docimo SG, Luetic T, Crone RK, et al. Pulmonary development in the fetal lamb with severe bladder outlet obstruction and oligohydramnios: a morphometric study. *J Urol* 1989;142:657.
120. Peters CA, Reid LM, Docimo S, et al. The role of the kidney in lung growth and maturation in the setting of obstructive uropathy and oligohydramnios. *J Urol* 1991;146:597–600.
121. Peters CA, Docimo SG, Luetic T, et al. Effect of in utero vesicostomy on pulmonary hypoplasia in the fetal lamb with bladder outlet obstruction and oligohydramnios: a morphometric analysis. *J Urol* 1991;146(4):1178–1183.
122. Nyirady P, Thiruchelvam N, Fry CH, et al. Effects of in utero bladder outflow obstruction on fetal sheep detrusor contractility, compliance and innervation. *J Urol* 2002;168(4 pt 1):1615–1620.
123. Cendron M, Karim OMA, Mostwin JL, et al. In utero partial urethral obstruction in the fetal lamb: Structural changes seen in the developing bladder. *J Urol* 1992;147(abstract 45).
124. Lopez Pereira P, Jaureguizar E, Martinez Urrutia MJ, et al. Does treatment of bladder dysfunction prior to renal transplant improve outcome in patients with posterior urethral valves? *Pediatr Transplantation* 2000;4(2):118–122.
125. Sheldon CA, Gonzalez R, Burns MW, et al. Renal transplantation into dysfunctional bladder: role of adjunctive bladder reconstruction. *J Urol* 1994;152:972–975.
126. Dykes EH, Ransley PG. Gastrocystoplasty in children. *Br J Urol* 1992;69(1):91–95.
127. Kinahan TJ, Khoury AE, McLorie GA, et al. Omeprazole in post-gastrocystoplasty metabolic alkalosis and aciduria. *J Urol* 1992;147(2):435–437.
128. Greskovich FD, Nyberg LJ. The prune belly syndrome: a review of its etiology, defects, treatment and prognosis [Review]. *J Urol* 1988;140(4):707–712.
129. DeKlerk DP, Scott WW. Prostatic maldevelopment in the prune belly syndrome: a defect in prostatic stromal–epithelial interaction. *J Urol* 1978;120:341.
130. Popek EJ, Tyson RW, Miller GJ, et al. Prostate development in prune belly syndrome (PBS) and posterior urethral valves (PUV): etiology of PBS–lower urinary tract obstruction or primary mesenchymal defect? *Pediatr Pathol* 1991;11(1):1–29.
131. Beasley SW, Henay F, Hutson JM. The anterior urethra provides clues to the etiology of prune belly syndrome. *Pediatr Surg Int* 1988;3:169.
132. Hutson JM, Beasley SW. Aetiology of the prune belly syndrome. *Aust Pediatr* 1987;23:309.
133. Gonzalez R, De Filippo R, Jednak R, et al. Urethral atresia: long-term outcome in 6 children who survived the neonatal period. *J Urol* 2001;165(6 pt 2):2241–2244.
134. Woodard JR, Parrott TS. Reconstruction of the urinary tract in prune belly syndrome. *J Urol* 1978;119:824.
135. Woodard JR. Lessons learned in 3 decades of managing the prune-belly syndrome [comment]. *J Urol* 1998;159(5):1680.
136. Randolph J, Cavett C, Eng G. Abdominal wall reconstruction in the prune belly syndrome. *J Pediatr Surg* 1981;16(6):960–964.
137. Monfort G, Guys JM, Bocciardi A, et al. A novel technique for reconstruction of the abdominal wall in the prune belly syndrome. *J Urol* 1991;146[2 (pt 2)]:639–640.
138. Ehrlich RM, Lesavoy MA, Fine RN. Total abdominal wall reconstruction in the prune belly syndrome. *J Urol* 1986;136:282.
139. Smith CA, Smith EA, Parrott TS, et al. Voiding function in patients with the prune-belly syndrome after Monfort abdominoplasty [comment]. *J Urol* 1998;159(5):1675–1679.
140. Perlmutter AD. Reduction cystoplasty in prune belly syndrome. *J Urol* 1976;116:356.
141. Silvan AM, Gordillo MJ, Lopez AM, et al. Organ-preserving management of rhabdomyosarcoma of the prostate and bladder in children. *Med Pediatr Oncol* 1997;29(6):573–575.
142. Heyn R, Newton WA, Raney RB, et al. Preservation of the bladder in patients with rhabdomyosarcoma. *J Clin Oncol* 1997;15(1):69–75.
143. El-Sherbiny MT, El-Mekresh MH, El-Baz MA, et al. Paediatric lower urinary tract rhabdomyosarcoma: a single-centre experience of 30 patients. *BJU Intl* 2000;86(3):260–267.
144. Duel BP, Hendren WH, Bauer SB, et al. Reconstructive options in genitourinary rhabdomyosarcoma. *J Urol* 1996;156(5):1798–1804.
145. Yusim I, Lismer L, Greenberg G, et al. Carcinoma of the bladder in patients under 25 years of age. *Scand J Urol Nephrol* 1996;30(6):461–463.
146. Quillin SP, McAlister WH. Transitional cell carcinoma of the bladder in children: radiologic appearance and differential diagnosis. *Urologic Radiol* 1991;13(2):107–109.
147. Keetch DW, Manley CB, Catalona WJ. Transitional cell carcinoma of bladder in children and adolescents. *Urology* 1993;42(4):447–449.
148. Mortensen PB, Jensen KE, Nielsen K. Adenocarcinoma development in the trigone 34 years after trigonocolonic urinary diversion for exstrophy of the bladder. *J Urol* 1990;144(4):980–982.
149. Gerridzen RG, de Jesus F, Wesley-James T, et al. Nephrogenic adenoma with bladder exstrophy and immunosuppression. *Urology* 1991;38(4):345–346.
150. Vik V, Gerharz EW, Woodhouse CR. Invasive carcinoma in bladder exstrophy with transitional, squamous and mucus-producing differentiation. *Br J Urol* 1998;81(1):173–174.
151. Smeulders N, Woodhouse CR. Neoplasia in adult exstrophy patients [comment]. *BJU Intl* 2001;87(7):623–628.
152. Borden TA, Shrader DA. Neurofibromatosis of bladder in a child: unusual cause of enuresis. *Urology* 1980;15:155.
153. Clark SS, Marlett MM, Prudencio RF, et al. Neurofibromatosis of the bladder in children: case report and literature review. *J Urol* 1977;118:654–656.
154. Albores-Saaverdra J, Maldonado ME, Ibarra J, et al. Pheochromocytoma of the urinary bladder. *Cancer* 1969;23:1110–1118.
155. Kato H, Suzuki M, Mukai M, et al. Clinicopathological study of pheochromocytoma of the urinary bladder: immunohistochemical, flow cytometric and ultrastructural findings with review of the literature. *Pathol Intl* 1999;49(12):1093–1099.
156. Kearney LP, Lebowitz RL, Retik AB. Obstructive polyps of the posterior urethra in boys: embryology and management. *J Urol* 1979;122:802.
157. Raviv G, Leibovitch I, Hanani J, et al. Hematuria and voiding disorders in children caused by congenital urethral polyps. Principles of diagnosis and management. *Eur Urol* 1993;23(3):382–385.
158. Blichert-Toft M, Nielson OV. Congenital patent urachus and acquired variants. *Acta Chir Scand* 1971;137:807.
159. Avni EF, Matos C, Diard F, et al. Midline omphalovesical anomalies in children: contribution of ultrasound imaging. *Urol Radiol* 1988;2:189.
160. Cilento BG Jr, Bauer SB, Retik AB, et al. Urachal anomalies: defining the best diagnostic modality. *Urology* 1998;52(1):120–122.

161. Khurana S, Borzi PA. Laparoscopic management of complicated urachal disease in children. *J Urol* 2002;168(4 pt 1):1526–1528.
162. Hamsher JB, Farrar T, Moore TD. Congenital vascular tumors and malformations involving urinary tract: diagnosis and surgical management. *J Urol* 1958;80:299.
163. Leonard MP, Nickel CJ, Morales A. Cavernous hemangiomas of the bladder in the pediatric age group. *J Urol* 1988;140:1503.
164. Mulliken JB, Fishman SJ, Burrows PE. Vascular anomalies. *Curr Prob Surg* 2000;37(8):517–584.
165. Handa S, Sethuraman G, Mohan A, et al. Ehlers-Danlos syndrome with bladder diverticula. *Br J Dermatol* 2001;144(5):1084–1085.
166. Kageyama S, Okada Y, Konishi T, et al. Menkes' kinky hair disease associated with a large bladder diverticulum: a case report. *Intl J Urol* 1997;4(3):318–320.
167. Peters CA. Bladder reconstruction in children. *Curr Opin Pediatr* 1994;6:183–193.
168. Dewan PA, Anderson P. Ureterocystoplasty: the latest developments. *BJU Intl* 2001;88(7):744–751.
169. Nguyen DH, Carr MC, Bagli DJ, et al. Demucosalized gastrocystoplasty with autoaugmentation: a clinical experience. *J Urol* 1995;153:279A.
170. Kropp BP, Rippy M, Bradylak SF, et al. Small intestinal submucosa: urodynamic and histopathologic evaluation in long-term canine bladder augmentation. *J Urol* 1995;153:375A.
171. Hinman FJ. Functional classification of conduits for continent diversion. *J Urol* 1990;144(1):27–30.
172. Watson HS, Bauer SB, Peters CA, et al. Comparative urodynamics of appendiceal and ureteral Mitrofanoff conduits in children. *J Urol* 1995;154(2 pt 2):878–882.

Chapter 98

Male Genital Tract

Julian Wan and David A. Bloom

Sexual differentiation begins at fertilization. The fertilizing sperm carrying either an X or Y chromosome joins the X chromosome of the egg to determine the karyotype (XX for female or XY for male). Chromosomal sex guides gonadal differentiation. The gonads are initially bipotential and indistinguishable. Local influences engendered by the chromosomal sex direct the development of either an ovary or testicle. The SRY gene on the short arm of chromosome Y influences the gonad to become a testis. Gonadal sex in turn produces the appearance of anatomic characteristics known as phenotypic sex. Each step in this sequence depends on the preceding step.

The fetal testis produces two important products. The Leydig cells secrete testosterone and the Sertoli cells produce müllerian inhibiting substance (MIS). Both are crucial for normal male phenotypic development. MIS causes local regression of the paramesonephric ducts (müllerian system), and testosterone stimulates ipsilateral mesonephric (wolffian) duct development. The male genital tract is formed largely between the sixth and thirteenth weeks of gestation. During the latter two thirds of gestation, the testicles descend to the scrotum and the external genitalia undergo differential growth.

Although internal ductal development is testosterone mediated, virilization of the male external genitalia is governed by dihydrotestosterone (DHT). Normal external genitalia development requires the presence and cellular recognition of DHT. The enzyme 5-α reductase converts testosterone into DHT. Androgen receptors sensitive to DHT are then stimulated and institute the changes in external genitalia: the genital tubercle becomes the penis, the urethral folds tabularize, and the genital swellings gather to form the scrotum.

Julian Wan and David A. Bloom: Department of Urology, University of Michigan, Ann Arbor, Michigan 48109-0330.

PHALLUS

Embryology

The genital tubercle forms ventral to the cloaca by the fourth week of gestation and is identical in both sexes until age 9 weeks. Under the influence of DHT, the male genital tubercle enlarges, elongates, and assumes a cylindrical shape. A circumferential groove demarcates the glans. Elongation pulls the urethral folds forward, creating the lateral walls of the urethral groove. The folds migrate toward the midline and fuse by 12 weeks forming the penile urethra, the ventral surface of the phallus, and median raphe. Mesenchyme coalesces around the deepening groove to form the corpus spongiosum. The urethral groove, having originated from endoderm grows toward but does not reach the tip of the phallus. The distal end of the urethra is formed during the fourth month of gestation, when an invagination at the glans penis forms the external meatus. This part of the urethra is ectodermal in origin. The glanular invagination meets the elongating urethral groove to complete the urethra and simultaneously preputial development begins as an epithelial fold growing over the glans. The surrounding pleat of skin is completed at birth.

Anatomy

The normal full-term infant penis is 3.5 cm in stretched length and 1.1 cm in diameter. Stretched penile length from the pubic symphysis to the tip of the glans correlates with erect length. Care should be taken to depress the suprapubic fat pad completely to get an accurate measurement and a length less than 2.5 cm is abnormal. Penile size often increases during the first 6 months after delivery, because of the physiologic surge of testosterone in the male infant at 2 to 3 months of age. From this time until puberty, however, only modest phallic growth occurs (Fig. 98-1). The urethra and external meatus of a premature or infant male should

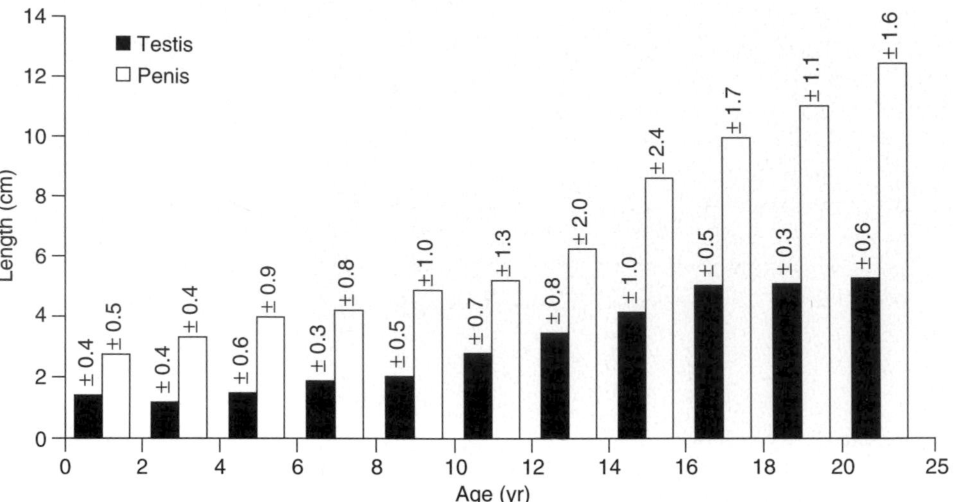

FIGURE 98-1. Male genital dimensions. (Adapted from Bloom DA, Wan J, Key D. Disorders of the male external genitalia and inguinal canal. In: Kelalis PP, King LR, Belman AB, eds. *Clinical pediatric urology*, 3rd ed. Philadelphia: WB Saunders, 1992:1015, with permission.)

accommodate a 5F feeding tube. An 8F tube should pass without difficulty by age 1 year.

The prepuce protects the delicate urethral meatus from minor trauma. The inner epithelial surface is fused to the glans penis in infancy, obscuring the glans and meatus. This normal anatomic condition should not be confused with phimosis. True phimosis is a pathologic condition seen later in life, wherein a fibrotic preputial ring develops. During the first 3 to 5 years of life, the natural process of intermittent erections and progressive accumulation of desquamated residue (smegma) separate the inner epithelial surface of the prepuce from the glans. By 3 years of age, 90% of foreskins are easily retractable. However, many boys have persistent isolated areas of adhesion, particularly around the coronal margin.

CIRCUMCISION

Circumcision is the most common surgical procedure in the United States. It is usually performed because of religious preference or for social reasons (i.e., older brothers and father are circumcised). In 1999, the American Academy of Pediatrics (AAP) observed that routine newborn circumcision may not be necessary (1). Families should be instructed in care of normal foreskin. The American Academy of Pediatrics brochure is a good instructional guide (2). Forcible retraction of the prepuce is painful, harmful, and unnecessary. Tearing the prepuce places the child at risk for cicatrix formation and phimosis, and is therefore inadvisable. Medical benefits of circumcision include prevention of penile carcinoma, phimosis, balanoposthitis, and neonatal urinary tract infection (UTI) (1,3,4). An uncircumcised male neonate is 20 times more likely to have a UTI than a circumcised infant, because of preputial colonization of the prepuce by urinary pathogens (2,3). The higher incidence of UTI occurs only during the first year of life, and beyond that time, circumcision has not been shown to decrease infections. Circumcision should be discussed with the family of any male infant with a UTI or vesicoureteral reflux, although suppressive antibiotics for the first year of life are an option. Disadvantages of neonatal circumcision include meatitis and meatal stenosis because the protective covering of the prepuce is lost. In addition, a boy may develop chordee or concealed penis, and the procedure is not without discomfort.

Circumcision is usually performed in one of two ways. Clamp or bell circumcision is reserved for infants younger than a few months of age. A freehand technique by dorsal slit or sleeve method is preferred for older children. It is important to recognize the features of a normal and abnormal penis. Children with chordee, hypospadias, and buried or webbed penises should not undergo routine neonatal circumcision. The clamp and bell devices commonly used in neonatal circumcision were designed for use on a normal penis and when applied inappropriately can cause injury to the urethra or yield a poor cosmetic result. The prepuce may be an important source of tissue for later reconstruction. No patient who may need future hypospadias repair should undergo routine circumcision. Be wary of the child described as having a "natural circumcision." Usually these are boys with a prominent dorsal hooded foreskin and a subtle distal hypospadias, and a hypoplastic corpus spongiosum. Whenever a circumcision is performed, the surgeon must carefully examine the underlying glans and meatus for occult hypospadias with normal foreskin.

Neonatal Circumcision

Infant circumcision is not without complications and should be performed by persons experienced in the technique who will evaluate the child postoperatively to gauge the results. The infant is placed on a papoose board restraint. Local anesthesia can be safely administered, with

1 mL or less of 0.25% lidocaine as a dorsal nerve block or circumferential subcutaneous block. The anesthetic must not be injected intravascularly or into the corporal body. A small dorsal slit is usually required to expose the glans, and all adhesions are detached by blunt dissection. The clamp or bell is applied visually; experience helps in judging the proper amount of skin to excise. With the clamp technique, the clamp is left in place for 5 minutes for hemostasis before redundant skin is excised. A suture with surgeon's knot is applied on the bell device. Topical anesthesia (eutectic mixture of local anesthetic—EMLA) applied directly to the penile skin is an alternative form of anesthesia. Although easy to administer, it may not be as effective as injection blocks (5). Electrocautery should never be used when a metal clamp technique is employed. To guard against meatal stenosis, petroleum, or antibiotic ointment should be daubed on the meatus at each diaper change.

Freehand Circumcision

Circumcision after 3 months of age is best performed under general anesthesia with a freehand sleeve technique. Adhesions between glans and prepuce are gently reduced using a mosquito clamp dipped in iodine solution, and the location of the meatus should be ascertained. A circumferential incision of the prepuce is made 6 to 8 mm proximal to the coronal sulcus, carried to the relatively avascular subcutaneous plane. The prepuce is then reduced and a parallel incision is made in the distal penile skin overlying the prepuce, at the level of the coronal sulcus. The isolated sleeve of tissue is removed. Compression is applied to the exposed shaft for several minutes, and larger vessels are ligated or fulgurated. Particular attention should be directed to the skin edges, where small vessels may retract. The proximal and distal skin edges are aligned and reapproximated with an interrupted, small (6–0 or 7–0) absorbable suture. Compressive dressings are rarely needed. If ventral skin is deficient or bleeding is difficult to control at the frenulum, this area can be reapproximated with vertical sutures to control bleeding and create additional ventral skin.

Complications

Careful neonatal circumcisions have a low rate of complications (less than 0.5%) (6). Fortunately, the complications are usually minor and heal with conservative management. Excessive skin resection can lead to tension and skin separation, which usually heals well by secondary intention particularly in the newborn. When separation occurs after neonatal circumcision, apply copious amounts of antibiotic salve with each diaper change and be patient. After 2 to 3 weeks, the edema subsides allowing better assessment of the penis. Often the separation will have closed. Postoperative bleeding often responds to manual pressure or suture ligation and rarely requires exploration. Postoperative dressings are not required, which obviates the chance of urinary retention from a constrictive dressing.

Complications that require intervention include urethrocutaneous fistula, concealed penis, dense adhesions between glans and shaft, and meatal stenosis. A fistula is often the result of unrecognized deficient spongiosum. Concealed penis occurs following overzealous skin excision, or when a scarred preputial ring forms distal to the glans. Dense adhesions may cause pain with erection and should be divided. Meatal stenosis may ensue because of irritation of the unprotected meatus; liberal use of ointment postoperatively prevents this complication.

Prepuce Abnormalities

True phimosis refers to a circumferential preputial ring that prevents foreskin retraction. This differs from the physiologic inability to retract the foreskin in male infants. Preputial tears or cracks from natural erection, forcible retraction, or infection can lead to cicatrix formation and narrowing of the preputial aperture (Fig. 98-2). Circumcision or dorsal slit effectively corrects the abnormality.

Phimosis is the leading cause of preputial inflammation, or posthitis. Balanitis is inflammation or infection of the glans penis. The terms *posthitis* and *balanitis* are often used interchangeably, and may coexist when posthitis to involve the glans. The inflammation is usually self-limited and responds to topical or oral antibiotics. Recurrent episodes are managed with circumcision following resolution of acute inflammation. Infection that spreads to the penile shaft and abdominal wall should be managed aggressively with parenteral antibiotics. Uncontrolled cellulitis may progress proximally, along tissue planes, to form a necrotizing fasciitis that requires operative intervention.

STRUCTURAL ABNORMALITIES

Microphallus

A penis smaller than two standard deviations below mean normal length is termed a *microphallus* (7). This term excludes hypospadias, ambiguous genitalia, buried penis, webbed penis, and other abnormalities. These conditions can confuse and mislead the casual examiner. Normal neonatal mean stretched penile length is 3.5 cm, and an infant male penis should measure at least 2.5 cm. During the second and third trimester, fetal androgens stimulate penile growth. Any condition that interferes with fetal testicular testosterone production after organogenesis is complete (first trimester) can cause micropenis. Hypogonadism also produces an underdeveloped scrotum and small, undescended testes.

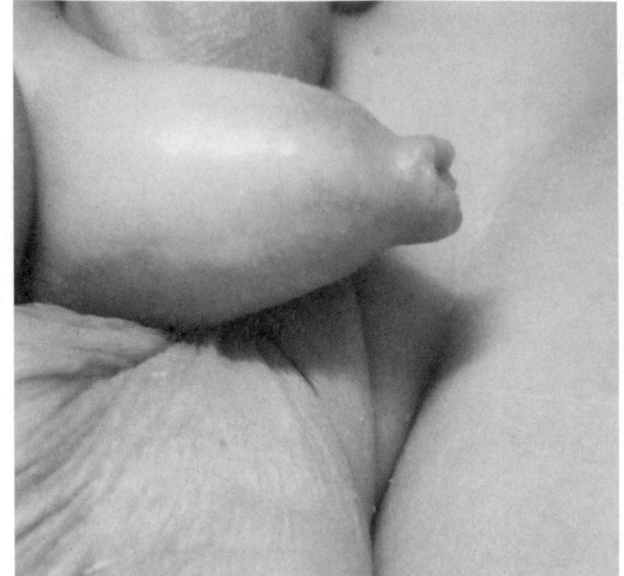

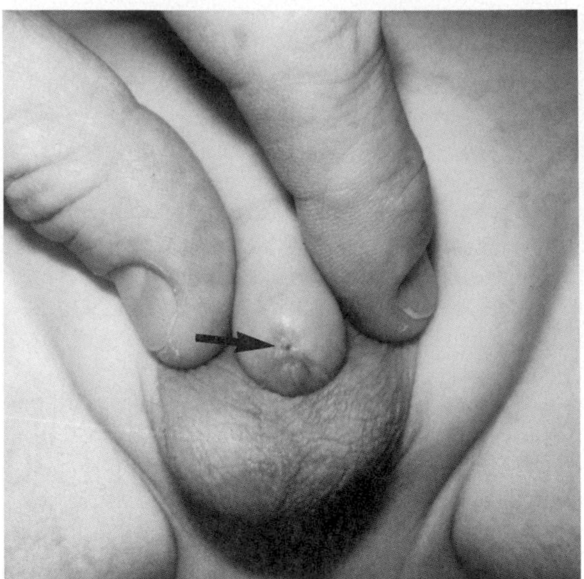

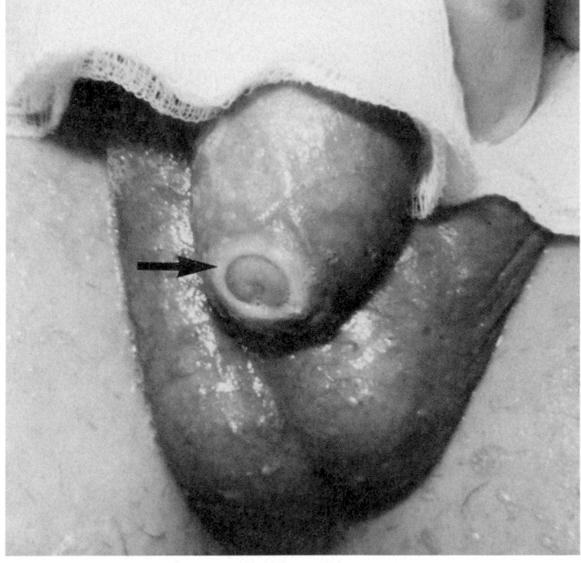

FIGURE 98-2. Phimosis in boys. **(A)** Normal, nonretractile prepuce of infancy. **(B)** True phimosis with tiny preputial aperture (*arrow*) in a 3-year-old boy. **(C)** True phimosis in a 16-year-old male with scarred phimotic ring (*arrow*) from previous recurrent posthitis. (From Bloom DA, Wan J, Key D. Disorders of the male external genitalia and inguinal canal. In: Kelalis PP, King LR, Belman AB, eds. *Clinical pediatric urology*, 3rd ed. Philadelphia: WB Saunders, 1992:1015, with permission.)

An abnormality in the hypothalamus–pituitary–testis axis can result in testicular failure. *Primary* testicular failure (end-organ hypogonadism) can be determined by measuring serum testosterone before and after human chorionic gonadotropin (hCG) is administered. The normal response is a fourfold increase in testosterone within 24 hours of the final dose of hCG. *Secondary* gonadal failure (hypogonadotropic hypogonadism) with microphallus occurs in conditions such as anencephaly; pituitary agenesis; and Kallman, Noonan, and Prader-Willi syndromes. Microphallus is described as idiopathic when no deficit is found in the endocrine axis. Because differential diagnosis includes the intersex disorders, an appropriate evaluation should include karyotype and endocrine status.

The growth potential of a small penis can be assessed by evaluating for a response to androgen administration. Testosterone may be given as a topical or parenteral preparation. Because the absorption of testosterone creams is variable, a 3-month trial of monthly intramuscular testosterone enanthate, 25 to 50 mg, is more dependable. Such a short course of androgens does not result in premature closure of the epiphyseal growth plates. Management of boys who do respond is controversial because many show no significant response to the androgen surge at puberty. However, many men with microphallus are sexually active and well adjusted, showing that penile function is satisfactory despite the small size (8).

Buried and Concealed Penis

The terms *buried penis* and *concealed penis* are often used interchangeably; however, they describe different conditions (9). A buried penis is normal in size, but appears small because of an overlying generous suprapubic fat pad that hides the normal penile shaft. Occasionally, a large hydrocele may obscure the shaft, resulting in a buried penis. Manual depression of the fat pad, an important maneuver when measuring penile length, reveals the normal penis. For many of these boys, the melting away of baby fat with growth, genital lengthening and pubic hair growth solve the cosmetic dilemma at adolescence. For some boys and parents, however, the embarrassment and emotional trauma of an obscured penis mandate repair. Successful surgical correction can produce enormous improvement in a boy's self-esteem. Circumcision will unmask the glans, and liposuction or excision of the suprapubic fat will address the obscuring panniculus. Occasionally, additional surgical maneuvers are required, including release of dysgenetic Scarpa's fascia below the fat pad, where it continues as the dartos layer of the penis, and anchoring suprapubic skin to the fascia overlying the pubis and anterior abdominal wall. There has to be a strong commitment to a diet and exercise weight reduction program as part of the overall treatment plan; otherwise, the fat pad will rapidly reform.

Concealed (trapped) penis occurs after circumcision. A cicatrix forms at the anastomotic line, and the penis retracts proximal to the scar. Surgical revision may be challenging because a limited amount of shaft skin remains. Dorsal slit or removal of the cicatrical ring is required.

FUNCTIONAL DEVIATION

Penile Torsion

Penile torsion is a rotational defect of the penile shaft that is of more cosmetic than functional significance. The anomaly occurs in 1% to 2% of males and is more common in patients with hypospadias. The median raphe spirals obliquely around the shaft, producing a rotation that is usually less than 90 degrees. If the erections are straight and the child can void without difficulty, mild forms of penile torsion can be left alone. Mild forms are usually repairable by penile degloving and skin reorientation. Severe rotational defects of 90 to 180 degrees are repaired by mobilizing penile skin to the base of the penis, incising any chordee, and resecting Buck's fascia. Torsion also occurs iatrogenically following circumcision or hypospadias repair. Most cases are minimally rotated, not associated with chordee, and rarely are a functional problem.

Penile Bending (Chordee)

The term *chordee* refers to a ventral bend of the shaft on erection. Chordee is a normal stage in embryonic penile development; the ventral bend may persist in premature male infants, but it usually corrects spontaneously within several months. Chordee is usually associated with hypospadias, in which deficient ventral penile development includes skin, spongiosum, Buck's fascia, and urethra. Hypospadias should not be corrected without fixing the chordee.

Chordee may also occur in spite of a normal urethra, although a preputial dorsal hood and thin ventral skin often coexist. Such chordee result from skin tethering, a urethral bowstring defect, or corporal disproportion. Vaginal penetration is difficult with an erect penile bend of greater than 45 degrees. Release of skin and dysgenetic bands may not completely straighten the penis. In such cases, dorsal plication or elliptical wedge excision of the corporal body at the point of maximum bend may be required. Another technique is to place a plicating stitch exactly in the midline of the degloved dorsal penis. This position avoids the neurovascular bundles that pass slightly lateral on each corporal body (10). If urethral tethering exists, mobilization of the urethra within the spongiosum corrects the bend. Occasionally the urethra must be divided and repaired. Intraoperative erections induced by saline injection of the corpora must be performed to gauge the defect and repair.

MEATAL STENOSIS

Stenosis of the urethral meatus usually occurs years after neonatal circumcision. The delicate meatus is susceptible to inflammation from local trauma such as from rubbing against a diaper or underwear. Meatitis progresses to cicatrix formation, with narrowing of the orifice. Deflected urinary stream and prolonged voiding times are typically noted by parents after a child is toilet trained. The classic history is that the urine stream deflects upward or sprays. A fine, forceful stream may emanate from a pinpoint meatus. Irritative voiding symptoms, such as dysuria and urgency, rarely occur without a concomitant UTI. Isolated meatal stenosis without infection does not require radiographic assessment of the urinary tract or cystoscopy. When stenosis is suspected, the meatus can be calibrated with small catheters or sounds. If stenosis is not severe, parents can be taught to perform daily obturation with a feeding tube or the tip of an ophthalmic ointment tube. Significant stenosis should be surgically corrected by a ventral incision, followed by a 3-month program of daily calibration of the urethra with a catheter, to ensure adequate opening.

PRIAPISM

Priapism is the involuntary and prolonged erection of the corpora cavernosa. Recurrent and prolonged bouts of priapism can lead to corporal fibrosis and impotence. The causes of priapism can be categorized into two broad groups: low flow or high flow. The majority of patients have low-flow priapism. Decreased venous outflow leads to increased intracavernous pressure and subsequent decreased arterial inflow. The venoocclusion leads to stasis of blood, hypoxia, and acidosis. The glans penis and spongiosum are flaccid. The most common low-flow situation in pediatric patients occurs with sickle cell disease or trait; about 5% of these patients experience priapism. The erection occurs as part of a diffuse sickle crisis or as an isolated event. Sickle crisis is managed by transfusion to reduce the hemoglobin S level, as well as oxygenation, hydration, alkalinization, and pain control. Aspiration with irrigation of the corporal bodies with an α-adrenergic agent can also be tried, but is usually unsuccessful in sickle cell patients unless systemic management of the crisis has been also started. Phenylephrine, 100 to 200 μg, can be used; patients need careful monitoring, particularly those with a history of cardiovascular disease. When conservative management fails, surgical construction of a shunt connecting the corpora cavernosa to the spongiosum may be effective temporarily; ultimately, however, these close. Recurrent bouts of priapism can result in impotence due to the repetitive pressure damage to the corporal bodies.

Leukemia is another cause of childhood priapism. Although chronic granulocytic leukemia accounts for only a small percentage of pediatric leukemias, one-half of all leukemic priapism occurs in these patients. Leukemic cells appear to cause microvascular occlusion within the corporal bodies, but other possible factors include leukemic infiltration of the sacral nerves or central nervous system as well as abdominal and pelvic venous obstruction. Treatment is directed at lowering the circulating leukocyte count. Shunts may be necessary for refractory cases. Other etiologies for priapism in the child include blunt perineal trauma, spinal cord injury, medications (tricyclic antidepressants, phenothiazines, hydralazine, prazosin, guanethidine, heparin, and cocaine), and retroperitoneal fibrosarcomas. As with sickle cell disease and leukemia, treatment is aimed at the underlying disease process. Fat emulsions of 20% infused as part of total parenteral nutrition (TPN) have been associated with priapism. It is believed that the fat emulsion increases blood coagulability, distorts erythrocytes, and, promotes adhesion and clumping. Antidepressants, such as trazadone, and antipsychotics, such as chlorpromazine have also been associated with priapism.

High flow priapism is caused by unrestrained arterial inflow. Because the problem is not one of venoocclusion, there is no hypoxia and acidosis. Almost all cases of high-flow priapism are due to penile and perineal trauma. An injury to the cavernosal artery results in a cavernosus-to-corporal body fistula. The key diagnostic finding in high-flow priapism is the discovery of well-oxygenated red blood upon corporal aspiration. In contrast to the flaccidity found in low-flow priapism, the glans and spongiosum in high-flow priapism is engorged with blood and is quite firm.

TESTIS

Embryology

The *SRY* gene facilitates gonadal differentiation into a testis such that Sertoli cells develop in weeks 6 and 7, and shortly thereafter produce MIS, which causes ipsilateral müllerian duct regression. By the ninth week, Leydig cells produce testosterone, which stimulates wolffian duct development. The testis and caput epididymis arise from the genital ridge, whereas the epididymal body and vas deferens originate from mesonephric tubules. Canalization of the rete testis and mesonephric tubules begins about week 12 and is complete by puberty. Testicular descent is a third-trimester event; prenatal ultrasounds typically show no descent prior to 28 weeks. Many theories have been proposed to explain testis descent, including gubernacular traction, differential somatic growth, intraabdominal pressure, epididymal maturation, and hormone milieu. In all likelihood, a combination of events and influences under androgen regulation leads to normal testis descent.

Anatomy

The average length of the infant testis is 1.4 to 1.6 cm. The testis grows minimally in the prepubertal years; significant growth is not noted until onset of puberty (Fig. 98-1). In boys with monorchidism, a solitary testis may undergo compensatory hypertrophy, and any solitary infant testis longer than 2 cm suggests contralateral testicular absence (11).

Appendages of the testis and epididymis are vestigial embryologic remnants (Fig. 98-3). An appendix testis, present on approximately 90% of testes, is a remnant of the müllerian ducts. The müllerian system completely regresses in males, except for its cranial remnant, which persists as the appendix testis, and the extreme lower end remnant, which forms the prostatic utricle. The appendix testis is located on the cranial surface of the testis, and occasionally at the testis–epididymal junction. The remaining appendages are vestigial remnants of the mesonephric tubules. An appendix epididymis is located on the globus major of the epididymis in 34% of males. The paradidymis is a remnant structure found at the junction of the epididymis and vas deferens. These remnants serve no known function, except to confound the differential diagnosis of an acute scrotum.

Physiology

The infant testis is hormonally active, not quiescent as was once believed. Normal activity in the first 6 months of postnatal life seems to be crucial for the testis to develop normal adult function. A postnatal surge of gonadotropins at 60 to 90 days results in proliferation of Leydig cells by 3 months (12). Leydig cells respond with a testosterone

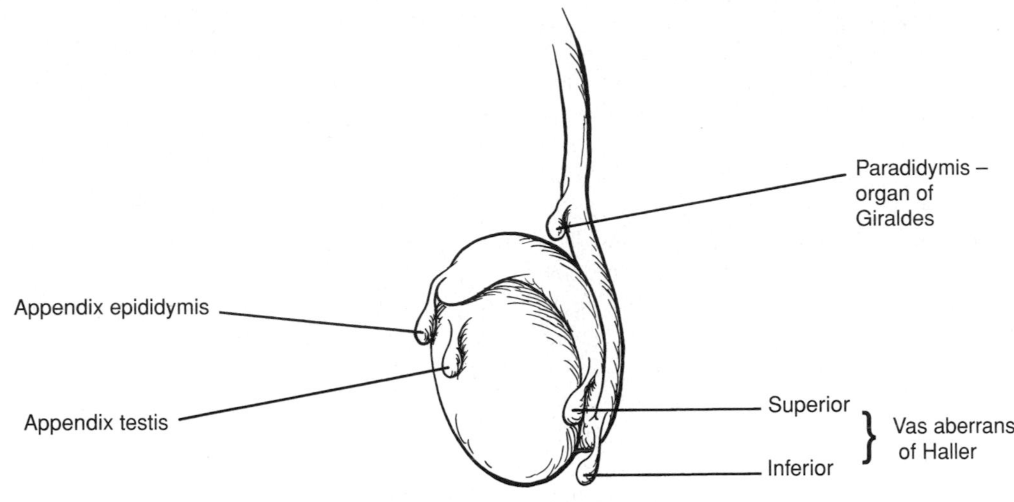

FIGURE 98-3. Testis and epididymal appendages.

surge that triggers germ cell development. The first step in postnatal germ cell development is the transformation of gonocytes to adult dark (Ad) spermatogonia, which is completed by 6 months. These spermatogonia may represent the pool of stem cells that replenish germ cells throughout life. The second stage of development occurs around 3 years of age, when the Ad spermatogonia transform to primary spermatocytes. Alterations in this normal cascade of events may result in a dysfunctional adult testis (12). As the child matures, spermatogonia populate the base of the seminiferous tubules, and spermatogenesis begins at puberty.

ABNORMAL SIZE

Microorchidism (Hypoplasia)

The testis changes little in size from birth until the onset of puberty. Spermatic tubules comprise 90% of testicular volume, and this volume increases enormously when spermatogenesis ensues at puberty. Small testes result from congenital disorders or secondary as a result of various insults. Klinefelter syndrome (47 XXY) is an example of primary hypogonadism. Secondary hypogonadism occurs with any pituitary or hypothalamic deficiency that results in lack of gonadotropin stimulation of the testes (Kallman syndrome). These testes may be normal at birth, but remain small after puberty. Insults to the testis (mumps orchitis, epididymitis, trauma, hernia repair with vascular injury, torsion, chemotherapy, radiation therapy, sickle cell crisis) may damage parenchyma, resulting in growth retardation or atrophy. Failure of normal growth may ensue from varicocele or uncorrected cryptorchid testis. Varicocele-induced growth retardation is probably the most easily reversible insult, many testes undergo significant growth after successful varicocele repair.

Macroorchidism

Testicular enlargement is sometimes the result of atrophy or absence of the contralateral testis, when a monorchid testis undergoes compensatory hypertrophy. A tense hydrocele can be mistaken for gonadal enlargement; however, transillumination or ultrasonography settles the issue. Primary testis tumors or metastatic neoplasms may enlarge a gonad and ultrasound examination is visually diagnostic. When tumor is suspected, the serum tumor markers α-fetoprotein and βhCG are obtained prior to inguinal surgical exploration with early vascular control.

Adrenal hyperplasia may produce unilateral or bilateral macroorchidism, with nodularity from islands of benign hyperplastic adrenal tissue within the testes. Juvenile hypothyroidism or an intracranial mass lesion stimulates precocious puberty, with resultant bilateral macroorchidism. Mental retardation and the fragile X syndrome are also sometimes associated with enlarged testes. Some cases of bilateral macroorchidism are described as idiopathic, provided that gonadotropin and thyroid hormone evaluation, as well as the scrotal ultrasound, are normal.

ABNORMAL NUMBER

Testicular Absence

Intrauterine or perinatal vascular accidents, with loss of a formed fetal testis, probably account for most absent testes. True agenesis is rare and implies total developmental failure of the embryonic gonadal ridge. Laparoscopy has demonstrated that müllerian structures or remnants are rare in most monorchid and anorchid boys, indicating the presence of a fetal testis before 14 to 15 weeks' gestation, at which time Sertoli cells have elaborated enough MIS to promote müllerian regression. The laparoscopic or open surgical finding of blind-ending spermatic vessels suggests testis loss. The frequent histologic finding of hemosiderin, calcium, and hyalinization in testicular remnant nubbins supports the supposition of vascular accident.

Anorchia, or vanished testes syndrome, implies absent testicular tissue in an otherwise normal XY male. Endocrine evaluation in patients with bilateral nonpalpable testes may help ascertain whether testes are present. βhCG stimulation normally causes a more than fourfold increase in serum testosterone, whereas anorchid patients have no testosterone response. Basal levels of gonadotropins are usually elevated to three standard deviations above mean values after stimulation in prepubertal anorchid boys (13). Negative βhCG stimulation and elevated follicle-stimulating hormone strongly suggest anorchism, although false-negative values have been reported in boys found to have testes present at exploration. Laparoscopic exploration is an excellent alternative to multiple endocrinologic assays. Blind-ending spermatic vessels confirm the diagnosis of anorchia. Visualization of spermatic cord structures entering the internal ring mandates inguinal exploration, which is performed under the same anesthetic. Because malignancy can occur in abdominal testes, a negative inguinal exploration alone is insufficient to confirm testicular absence unless spermatic vessels are known to end blindly. Testicular prosthesis placement at an early age is recommended for anorchid boys to avoid a flat hypoplastic scrotum throughout childhood.

Monorchid testes undergo compensatory hypertrophy, although the increase in volume is too variable to diagnose monorchidism on the basis of ipsilateral testis measurement alone (11). Hormone assays are not useful for diagnosing monorchidism. For unknown reasons, solitary fetal testis loss is more likely on the left side. When laparoscopic evaluation confirms unilateral testis absence, prophylactic orchiopexy of the contralateral solitary testis is a fair consideration. No study has shown that monorchidism portends a higher risk of testis torsion; however, loss of the solitary testis for any reason is catastrophic. Monorchid boys and their parents should be counseled about the potential risks of contact sports and the need for scrotal protection, the requirement for immediate medical evaluation for acute scrotal pain or swelling, and the importance of testicular self-examination. With one normal testis in the scrotum, placement of a testicular prosthesis is discretionary.

ABNORMAL LOCATION

Cryptorchid

A hidden or obscure testicle is termed *cryptorchid*, a term synonymous with undescended testis. The incidence at birth is about 4%, with bilateral involvement in 15% of these cases. Testes may descend within several months of birth, and the incidence of undescent drops to about 1% by 1 year of age, where it remains throughout childhood and beyond puberty. Therefore, waiting any longer than age 1 year for an undescended testicle to appear is not worthwhile. A more recent study suggests that waiting even longer than 6 months of age, correcting for prematurity, may not be worthwhile (14). Two important reasons for moving the testis to a scrotal location are the psychologic disadvantage of an empty scrotum and the accessibility of the testis for self-examination later in life. In addition, orchiopexy may improve fertility potential. Testes require the cooler thermal environment of the scrotum for normal spermatogenesis. Infertility is more likely in men with a history of cryptorchidism. Bilateral undescended testes portend a worse fertility impairment than unilateral cryptorchidism.

Surgical intervention is recommended prior to 18 to 24 months of age. Theoretically, early orchiopexy preserves fertility; however, substantive data are lacking. Most undescended testes are smaller than their contralateral descended mates, and this volume loss is evident within the first year of life. Biopsy of undescended testes reveals the number of spermatogonia per tubule to be higher in boys younger than the age of 1 year, compared with older cryptorchids (15–18). Similarly, the seminiferous tubule diameter is larger in biopsies from boys younger than 1 year old with undescended testes (18). These findings suggest that damage to the germinal epithelium is acquired and progressive, and that the effects in some cases irreversible. The total responsibility of future subfertility or infertility cannot be attributed to temperature and body position alone. The association of epididymal and vassal abnormalities with undescended testicles is also a major factor. However, because testicular position can be usually successfully manipulated, early intervention is therefore recommended, with the hope of improving fertility.

Subnormal fertility may be multifactorial in cryptorchid males and not a result of thermal injury alone. Defective germ cell maturation, noted within the first year of life, is most likely due to an abnormal hypothalamic–pituitary–testis endocrine axis. Many cryptorchid boys do not have the normal postnatal surge of gonadotropins at 2 to 3 months of age, which should stimulate Leydig cells to respond with a surge in testosterone. This cascade of events may be important to prime normal germ cell maturation. In addition, one-fifth to one-third of undescended testes have a defect in epididymal–testis fusion or epididymal suspension, and the abnormal sperm transport can result in infertility, despite normal spermatogenesis. Therefore, orchiopexy alone may not improve paternity rates because of the multiple potential factors for infertility in these patients.

Cryptorchid testes have a greater risk of malignancy than normal descended testes. The chance of a cryptorchid patient developing a testicular tumor is almost ten times that of the general male population. Six percent to 10% of all testicular cancers originate in a cryptorchid testis. When tumors develop in a cryptorchid patient, 20% occur in the contralateral descended testis (19). Orchiopexy does not alter the malignant potential of a cryptorchid testis; however, scrotal position allows self-examination and early detection of a tumor.

A cryptorchid testis may be substantially intraabdominal (at least 1 cm above the internal ring), high annular (at the internal ring), canalicular (in the superficial inguinal pouch), distantly ectopic (perineal, femoral, or penopubic), or high scrotal. Some of these locations suggest migration arrest during the normal course of testis descent, whereas ectopic testes are found outside the usual anatomic path of descent. Whether the superficial inguinal pouch location, the most common location for an undescended testis, is ectopic or is the result of migration arrest is a matter of debate.

The basic principles of standard orchiopexy are gonad localization, mobilization, cord dissection, isolation of a patent processus vaginalis, and relocation of the testis to the scrotum. An important innovation in modern orchiopexy is the method of scrotal fixation. Because sutures placed through the tunica albuginea of the testis may damage parenchyma, the testis should be placed in a subdartos pouch, using absorbable sutures to fix the tunica vaginalis to the dartos (15,16).

The nonpalpable testis is a special circumstance of cryptorchidism in which a gonad is impalpable in spite of a deliberate set of diagnostic maneuvers. It is usually not difficult to examine an awake child who is relaxed and cooperative. One commonly overlooked preparatory step is to raise the temperature of the examiner's hands. Besides the advantages of basic hygiene, washing in hot water with soap immediately before approaching the patient warms the examiner's hands. In a warm room, the examination begins on the abdomen and slowly moves down over the area of the internal inguinal ring, gently walking the fingers down the inguinal canal toward the scrotum. If a testis is not identified, reexamination in a cross-leg sitting or squatting position, using lubricating jelly to decrease the tactile friction, may reveal an elusive gonad. Nonpalpable testes account for 10% to 20% of undescended testes. Ultimate assessment of nonpalpable testes reveals absence in 45%, an intraabdominal location in 30%, and a lower testis missed to palpation in 25% of cases.

Radiographic evaluation for an undescended testis is unreliable. Generally, thorough physical examination by an experienced surgeon is more valuable and reliable than ultrasound, computed tomography (CT) scan, or magnetic resonance imaging. These techniques may discern a gonad in older children, but rarely does radiographic assessment influence management or prognosis enough to justify the expense. Venography is more successful, although it requires anesthesia or sedation. We believe that laparoscopy is the best first step in localizing a nonpalpable testis or proving it absent; accuracy exceeds 95% (20,21). Laparoscopic findings define the next operative step, which may take further advantage of the laparoscopic access. The three likely findings at laparoscopy are blind-ending spermatic vessels above the internal ring, an intraabdominal testis, and normal cord structures entering the internal inguinal ring. When blind-ending or atretic vessels are identified above the inguinal ring, no further evaluation or surgery is indicated. If a high intraabdominal testis is found, therapeutic options include traditional Fowler-Stephens orchiopexy, first-stage vasal-pedicle orchiopexy with laparoscopic ligation of the gonadal vessels, laparoscopic orchiopexy, and orchiectomy. If vessels enter the inguinal ring, then regardless of findings at subsequent inguinal exploration, one is assured that further retroperitoneal or abdominal exploration is unnecessary.

Long-term follow-up is imperative for cryptorchid boys. Parents must be aware of the issues of infertility and tumorigenesis. The risk of malignancy in an undescended testicle is about 1% for inguinal testicles and about 5% for intraabdominal testicles (22–25). Seminoma is the most common testicle in an undescended testicle, but embryonal and teratocarcinoma are more common in those undescended testicles that have been treated by orchiopexy (24). When they reach puberty, all boys should be taught monthly testicular self-examination. Fertility issues can be discussed at an adult follow-up visit. Cryptorchidism has far-reaching ramifications, and surgeons must ensure the education and long-term follow-up of these patients. The parents, and later the child when he or she is older, need to be reminded that even a successful orchiopexy does not lower the future risk of tumor formation; hence, regular self-examination is very important.

Retractile Testis

The retractile testis is a normally descended gonad that retracts so readily and vigorously that the condition is confused with cryptorchidism. The ipsilateral scrotum is normally developed and may invert during retraction at the gubernacular attachment. Retractile testes have normal volumes, may be bilateral, and once manipulated to the dependent portion of the scrotum, tend to remain without tension. The cause is believed to be strands of the cremasteric muscle that become attached to the testicle and spermatic cord during descent. When the child is young and the testicles are smaller and lighter, these strands are sufficiently strong to lift and pull the testicles out of the scrotum into the groin. The cremasteric reflex is weak or absent for several months after birth, therefore eliciting a history of a normal scrotal examination in infancy.

Subsequent evaluation that reports testicles that are intermittently found in the scrotum, particularly when the child is relaxed and warm (e.g., in a warm tub), suggests retractile testis. Because the cremasteric reflex is dampened during general anesthesia, a testis in an abnormal position under anesthesia is likely to be cryptorchid. No treatment is necessary for the retractile testis; parents should be reassured and the child examined annually. Failure to recognize the retractile testis may explain why the number of orchiopexies performed exceeds the expected incidence of cryptorchidism (21,22).

ACUTE SCROTUM

Testis Torsion (Intravaginal)

Testis torsion, the most frequent cause of an acute scrotum in children, is often mismanaged. Detorsion within 6 hours affords a good chance of salvage, whereas 12 hours or more of ischemia before reduction of torsion is usually associated with loss of the gonad. Classic torsion of the testis usually occurs in adolescents and young adult males, but it can occur in younger children. Some boys have an anatomic predisposition to torsion. High insertion of the tunica vaginalis on the cord structures allows for a horizontal testis position and mobility in a configuration akin to a bell clapper within a bell (Fig. 98-4). This allows the distal cord to twist within the tunica vaginalis, hence the designation *intravaginal torsion*.

Patients usually have a sudden onset of severe pain, often associated with abdominal discomfort, nausea, and vomiting. In some instances, however, a gradual onset of testicular and abdominal pain is the primary complaint. One-half of symptomatic boys describe prior transient similar episodes of scrotal pain, consistent with intermittent torsion-detorsion. The evaluation of any male with abdominal pain should include a thorough scrotal examination. Physical examination typically reveals a tender testis, scrotal erythema, an acute hydrocele, and loss of the cremasteric reflex. Anatomic landmarks are often not distinguishable because of edema and inflammation. If the history and examination are consistent with testis torsion, prompt surgical exploration and reduction is the next step, without delay from further tests. Loss of the testis ensues without spontaneous or surgical reduction. Treatment is surgical detorsion and fixation orchiopexy.

An important part of the surgical procedure is fixation of the contralateral uninvolved testis. For many patients, the window of opportunity for salvaging the symptomatic gonad has passed, and contralateral orchiopexy protects the surviving testis. The bell-clapper deformity is often bilateral, thus rendering the contralateral testis at higher risk for torsion later. Orchiopexy is not a guarantee against future torsion, but it does decrease the odds. The child and parents must be informed that subsequent scrotal pain or swelling must be evaluated promptly. Our bias is to remove a testis only when it is necrotic and nonviable. Theoretic concerns that a damaged testis remaining in the scrotum

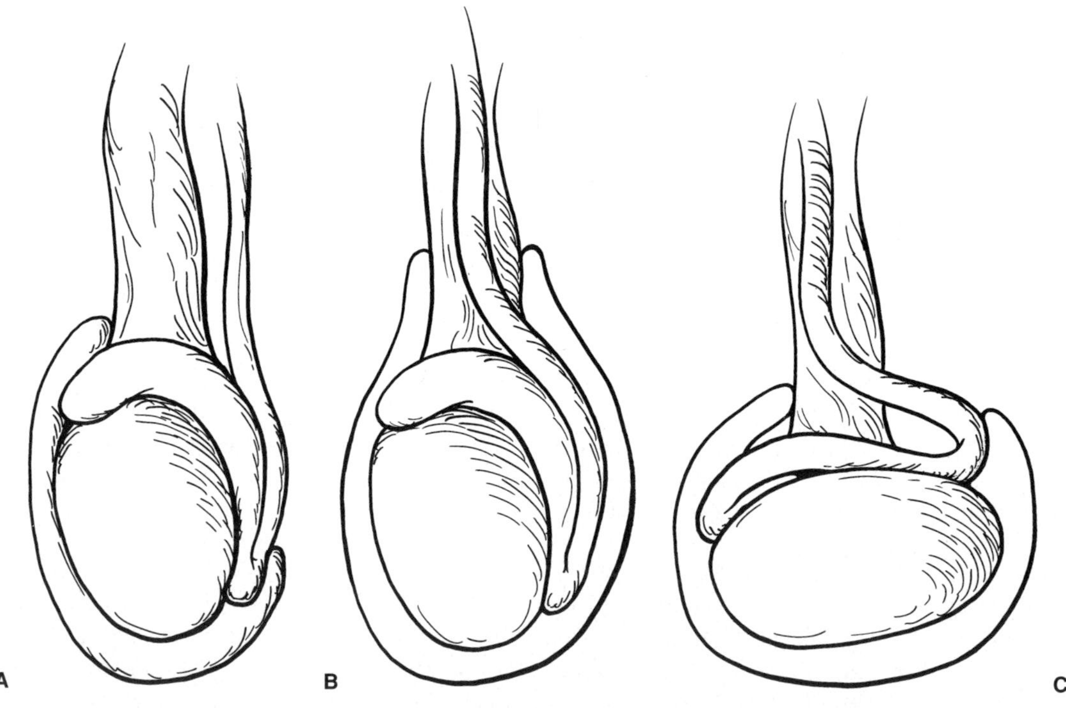

FIGURE 98-4. Testis position within tunica vaginalis. **(A)** Normal anatomy. **(B)** Bell-clapper deformity. **(C)** Bell-clapper deformity with horizontal testis lie.

may be detrimental to its mate have not been substantiated. If there is restoration of blood flow or the chance of viable parenchyma, we proceed with orchiopexy. The involved testis can be reduced and observed while contralateral fixation is performed.

Manual reduction of a torsed testis can be attempted with or without narcotic analgesia. Successful detorsion alleviates acute symptoms and may obviate emergent exploration; however, it is not a definitive treatment. Testes usually, but not always, torse in an inward or medial direction, with an anteromedial rotation of the spermatic cord. Manual detorsion should proceed with one lateral or outward (viewing the scrotum from the feet) rotation (much like "opening a book"). Doppler pulse evaluation may suggest successful detorsion if distal pulses return; however, the physician usually notes release and elongation of the cord followed by a marked diminution in symptoms. Successful manual reduction should be followed by elective orchiopexy. A pitfall to manual detorsion is partial reduction of a 720-degree or greater twist. Partial detorsion may relieve symptoms and improve the examination, but not relieve the ischemia.

Routine color Doppler ultrasound and nuclear scrotal scans when torsion is suspected are costly in dollars and time and are a poor substitute for a well-performed history, clinical evaluation, and judgment. These examinations are often obtained in patients for whom torsion is a low priority, only to confirm and document the diagnosis of nontorsion.

Neonatal Torsion

Extravaginal torsion is a variant in which torsion occurs proximally in the inguinal portion of the spermatic cord, or just below the canal, above the insertion of the tunica vaginalis. The entire tunica vaginalis and contents torse. This occurs in utero, during delivery, or in the postnatal period (within the first 30 days of life). The pathogenesis is unknown; however, weak attachments between the tunica vaginalis and scrotal wall may predispose the young to this process. Extravaginal torsion occurs much less frequently than intravaginal torsion, and unlike the latter, is usually asymptomatic in the neonate. Bilateral in utero torsion is the likely etiology for the vanished testes syndrome. Salvage of the extravaginally torsed testis is rare; most gonads are necrotic at exploration. Primary reasons for intervention are confirmation of diagnosis, orchiectomy, and contralateral testis fixation. Although unilateral extravaginal torsion is not associated with a higher incidence of contralateral intravaginal torsion, loss of a solitary remaining testis would be devastating, and prophylactic orchiopexy should be considered. Exploration in the neonate should be by inguinal incision because torsion may occur within the canal.

Torsed Appendages

The appendix testis is a müllerian duct remnant, whereas epididymal appendages are vestigial remnants of the wolffian duct system. The etiology for appendiceal torsion is not known; however, the process mimics testis torsion. The onset of pain is usually gradual over a day or 2, but it may be acute and severe. A reactive hydrocele often confounds the examination, and extrascrotal symptoms such as nausea and emesis are infrequent. Physical examination reveals the classic "blue dot" sign, in which the infarcted appendage can be visualized through thin scrotal skin or palpated as the point of isolated tenderness at the upper pole of the testis. Certainty of diagnosis precludes exploration, and the symptoms resolve with scrotal support, antiinflammatory agents, and bed rest for several days. If the diagnosis is in doubt, spermatic cord torsion must be ruled out with surgical exploration.

Acute Scrotum Without Torsion

Acute scrotal pain sometimes occurs in the child for reasons other than torsion. Infection of the epididymis is uncommon in the prepubertal male. Because torsion is the most frequent cause of acute scrotal pain and swelling, the diagnosis of epididymitis should be made with great caution. Inflammation of the epididymis results from UTI, trauma, chemical irritation, autoimmune phenomenon, vasculitis, or granulomatous disease. Pyuria suggests epididymitis, but is not invariably present with it. Epididymitis may occur secondary to a UTI, and these children need to be evaluated for underlying urinary tract anomalies such as ectopic ureter, ectopic vas deferens, persistent mesonephric duct, and bladder outlet abnormalities. Foley catheter drainage, intermittent catheterization, and other forms of urinary tract instrumentation predispose to infection, and therefore epididymitis. Despite the many diagnostic modalities available, torsion must always be considered, and diagnostic surgical exploration is sometimes necessary. Orchitis is rare in the pediatric population. Mumps orchitis is strictly a postpubertal disease.

An acutely symptomatic hydrocele develops for a variety of reasons, including trauma, torsion, infection, tumor, or presentation of a previously asymptomatic indirect inguinal hernia, or it may be idiopathic. The underlying condition must be considered, and surgical exploration may be required to secure a diagnosis. If the testis cannot be adequately palpated and the diagnosis of tumor is entertained, the approach to the scrotum should be inguinal. Malignant lesions in the scrotum do not usually present with acute pain or swelling; however, hemorrhage and necrosis in a testis tumor cause symptoms, and tumor-bearing testes are susceptible to torsion. Idiopathic fat necrosis is a condition sometimes seen in obese prepubertal boys after strenuous physical activity. The prepubertal scrotum contains fat, and indurated masses of adipose tissue may be found around the testis at exploration. The etiology of fat necrosis is unknown. In contrast, the simple hydrocele due to a patent processus vaginalis is usually painless and transilluminates easily. There is usually no erythema, and the size and shape could change with the activity of the child.

Henoch-Schönlein purpura (HSP) is a systemic vasculitis that usually presents with nonthrombocytopenic purpura, abdominal pain, arthralgias, and bloody diarrhea. Involvement of the genitourinary system includes vasculitic changes of the renal parenchyma (nephritis, hematuria) and the spermatic cord and scrotum. A third of boys with HSP develop acute pain and swelling of the scrotum. Most children are younger than age 7 years, and the duration of illness averages 4 to 6 weeks. The initial dermatologic manifestation is urticaria, with subsequent violaceous macular and maculopapular lesions. The lesions are often found on the trunk and legs along the underwear and sock lines. The characteristic rash is usually present well before the onset of scrotal symptoms. Nuclear scan or Doppler ultrasound studies may confirm normal or increased testicular perfusion and obviate exploration, but concomitant testis torsion has been reported in these children. Treatment for HSP is supportive, although corticosteroids may be indicated in renal disease.

Incarcerated hernia, traumatic hematocele, varicocele, and splenogonadal fusion also cause scrotal pain or swelling. A patent processus vaginalis may test a surgeon's diagnostic skill when intraabdominal processes such as ruptured appendicitis, meconium peritonitis, and intraperitoneal bleeding gain access to the scrotal cavity. The tip of a ventriculoperitoneal shunt can migrate through a patent processus, causing hydrocele, scrotal discomfort, or palpable mass.

Testicular Tumors

Prepubertal testicular tumors represent a small, but controversial aspect of testicular lesions (24). The tumors account for only 1% to 2% of all pediatric solid tumors and are the seventh most common pediatric malignancy. A painless mass is the most common manifestation of a prepubertal testicular tumor. They are sometimes misdiagnosed as a hydrocele and treated inappropriately. Germ cell tumors comprise 95% of adult testicular tumors, but only 75% of prepubertal testicular tumors. Seminoma, the most common adult testicular tumor, is quite rare in the prepubertal population. For these reasons, application of adult testicular tumor classification schemes to the pediatric population is unsatisfactory. To help better define the natural history and optimal treatment, the Prepubertal Testicular Tumor Registry was established in 1980, and continued as the American Academy of Pediatrics Testicular Tumor Registry through 1998 (25,26). Currently, eight classes of gonadal tumors are recognized in boys (Table 98-1). Of these, the most common are yolk sac tumor (~60%), teratoma (20%), paratesticular rhabdomyosarcoma (~6%), gonadal stromal (4%), and epidermoid cyst (4%) This distribution favoring yolk sac tumor may reflect reporting biases. Teratomas may actually be more common, but may not be reported as often because they are benign. Prepubertal testis tumor staging is divided into four categories, depending on the extent of disease and metastases (Table 98-2).

TABLE 98-1 Classification of Pediatric Testicle Tumors

Germ cell tumors—yolk sac, teratoma, teratocarcinoma, seminoma
Gonadal stromal tumors—Leydig cell, Sertoli cell, mixed
Gonadoblastoma
Tumors of supporting structures—fibroma, leiomyoma, hemangioma
Leukemia and lymphoma
Tumorlike lesions—epidermoid cyst, hyperplastic nodules due to congenital adrenal hyperplasia
Secondary tumors
Paratesticular tumors—rhabdomyosarcoma

The presence or absence of α-fetoprotein (AFP) is produced by yolk sac cells and is a useful serum tumor market for prepubertal testicular tumors. In 90% of yolk sac tumors, serum AFP levels are elevated. The protein has a half-life of 5 days. Postoperative elevation beyond the half-life calculations suggests residual tumor. Neonates normally have an elevated AFP, and the physiologic elevation may persist for up to 12 to 15 weeks. βhCG is not elevated in prepubertal testicular tumors. In addition to tumor markers, metastatic evaluation should include chest radiologic examination and CT scan or ultrasound of the abdomen. The retroperitoneum and lungs are the most common sites of metastases.

The examination of any child with a scrotal tumor must include assessment of the stage of sexual development and the presence or absence of gynecomastia. If the testis cannot be demonstrated by palpation, ultrasound examination may characterize the underlying gonad. Serum tumor markers should be obtained, and an inguinal exploration undertaken with early control of the spermatic vessels.

TABLE 98-2 Staging for Prepubertal Testis Tumor

Stage I:	Local disease, complete resection, serum markers normalize
Stage II:	<2 cm Retroperitoneal lymph nodes, persistently elevated markers, transscrotal orchiectomy, microscopic disease in scrotum, or spermatic cord stump
Stage III:	>2 cm Retroperitoneal lymph nodes
Stage IV:	Distant metastases

Yolk Sac Tumor

Yolk sac tumors account for 60% of all prepubertal testicular tumors. Mean age at diagnosis is 3 years. This germ cell tumor is *not* of yolk sac origin; the name refers to the histologic similarity to the endodermal sinus of rat yolk sac. Other names have been used, such as endodermal sinus tumor, infantile embryonal carcinoma, and orchidoblastoma. Yolk sac tumor should *not* be confused with the embryonal cell carcinoma of postpubertal males, although the tumors are histologically similar, their clinical behaviors are different. The histologic sine qua non of yolk sac tumor is the Schiller-Duval body, a glomerular-like cluster of cells that contain AFP.

Preorchiectomy serum levels of AFP do not correlate with tumor volume and are not prognostic. If levels do not fall as projected by the 5-day half-life following orchiectomy, however, residual metastatic disease is likely. Metastases have been described despite a normal AFP level. Yolk sac tumors metastasize through both the vascular and lymphatic systems, although they seen to have a predilection for hematogenous spread; more patients with metastatic disease have pulmonary lesions than retroperitoneal metastases. Treatment begins with radical orchiectomy. Few centers have extensive experience with yolk sac tumors, and retroperitoneal lymph node dissection is controversial, but is not generally considered routine. Currently, most stage I patients (appropriately declining postorchiectomy AFP, no chest or retroperitoneal adenopathy) are monitored, but do not receive chemotherapy. Monthly AFP levels, chest radiographs every 2 months for 2 years, and abdominal CT scans every 3 months for the first year, and every 6 months for the second year, comprise the surveillance program. Stage II patients receive systemic chemotherapy, including a platinum-based agent. Those with a persistent mass or an elevated AFP are recommended for retroperitoneal lymph node dissection. Stage III and IV patients undergo chemotherapy and retroperitoneal lymph node dissection. All stages do relatively well and have overall survival rates in the 90% and higher range.

Teratoma

Teratoma is the second most frequent reported prepubertal testicular tumor and is one of the few tumors presenting in the neonatal period. The mean age at presentation is 18 to 20 months. Unlike adult teratoma, this lesion is benign, with no reported metastases in the prepubertal population. Tumor tissue represents the different germinal layers—endoderm, mesoderm, and ectoderm—with variable distribution for individual patients. Multiple cystic areas are characteristic enough that the diagnosis can often be strongly suggested preoperatively with ultrasound. Orchiectomy is curative in young children. Peripubertal and postpubertal boys should probably be treated and followed as adults. Histologic diagnosis rests on the recognition of fetal or adult tissue from all three germ cell layers. Because of its benign nature, a testis-sparing approach is used where it is feasible. After exposure and vascular control is gained, the teratoma can be shelled out and the diagnosis confirmed by frozen section pathology.

Gonadal Stromal Tumors

Sometimes referred to as interstitial tumors, gonadal stromal tumors are the most common non-germ cell testicular tumors in boys. These tumors arise from the stromal component of the testis. The vast majority are of Leydig and Sertoli cell origin; however, the stroma, gives rise to ovarian stromal tumors on rare occasions.

Leydig cell tumors usually occur in 5 to 10 year olds, with the latter part of a bimodal distribution occurring in the third to sixth decades. Leydig cell tumors are hormonally active and usually present with precocious puberty, gynecomastia, or both. Feminization is more common in postpubertal patients. Functional prepubertal tumor cells secrete testosterone, which causes virilization. The classic findings are a unilateral testicular mass, precocious puberty, and elevated 17-ketosteroids. Differential diagnosis for virilization in the prepubescent male also includes congenital adrenal hyperplasia, adrenal carcinoma, and idiopathic precocious puberty. Congenital adrenal hyperplasia can produce hypertrophied Leydig cell nodules in the testis, which are treated medically rather than by orchiectomy. Despite the many mitotic figures, Leydig cell tumors are usually benign, and orchiectomy is sufficient treatment. Malignancy, defined by the presence of metastases, occurs in less than 10% of patients.

Sertoli cell tumors are rare lesions best treated by orchiectomy. Occasionally patients present with feminization and gynecomastia. The vast majority of Sertoli cell tumors are benign. Malignancy is defined by the presence of metastases, a feature seen more commonly in adult patients.

Gonadoblastoma

Gonadoblastoma, a rare tumor that usually occurs in the postpubertal male, is a mixture of germ cell and stromal cell elements, and is usually associated with the dysgenetic testes of intersex patients. Nearly all patients with a gonadoblastoma have an underlying gonadal abnormality. As a general rule, streak or dysgenetic gonads should be removed before a tumor develops. Gonadoblastoma occurs bilaterally in one-third of patients. The tumors are usually benign; however, malignant degeneration resembling a dysgerminoma, and similar to a seminoma, can occur.

Leukemic Infiltrate

The testis is a potential sanctuary for leukemic cells because the blood–testis barrier may protect tumor cells from chemotherapeutic agents. Acute lymphocytic leukemia is the most common type of leukemia to infiltrate the testis. This occurs in up to 25% of these patients. The usual presentation is a painless testicular swelling; however, the testes may be entirely normal to palpation, despite leukemic infiltration. Testicular biopsies, once routine for boys in remission following treatment for acute lymphocytic leukemia, have been abandoned for two reasons. New multidrug chemotherapy regimens are more effective in preventing testicular relapse, and survival has been shown to be similar whether a boy is treated for occult testicular disease or gross recurrence elsewhere. Currently, testis biopsies are performed for acute lymphocytic leukemia only when a scrotal examination suggests a mass or tumor in the testis. Testicular metastasis is viewed not only as a local occurrence, but also as a harbinger of occult residual disease systemically.

Tumorlike Lesions

Epidermoid cysts are rare, benign lesions that are monolayer (ectoderm) expressions of teratomas. Dermoid cysts are composed of two germ cell layers, usually ectoderm and mesoderm. Excision is usually sufficient treatment. Tunica albuginea cysts are small, asymptomatic lesions that are benign and can be locally excised. They probably represent retention cysts or capsule formation following resolution of a traumatic hemorrhage. Ectopic adrenal rests are usually paratesticular or in the spermatic cord, but occasionally they occupy a testicular position. The lesions are harmless, although when exposed to high levels of adrenocorticotropic hormone, the rests enlarge and become hormonally active.

Paratesticular Rhabdomyosarcoma

Paratesticular rhabdomyosarcoma, although extratesticular, is usually considered among the gonadal tumors in males. Up to 10% of intrascrotal tumors in prepubescent boys are rhabdomyosarcomas, and these are the most common spermatic cord tumors in children and adults. Paratesticular rhabdomyosarcomas represents 7% of all rhabdomyosarcomas. A tumor marker does not exist for rhabdomyosarcomas. Similar to Wilms' tumor, two histologic types are described—favorable and unfavorable. Fortunately, nearly 90% of paratesticular lesions are of the embryonal (favorable) subtype. Alveolar patterns portend an unfavorable prognosis. The cord and testis should be excised with a high inguinal orchiectomy. If the scrotum has been violated by incision, biopsy, or previous scrotal surgery, hemiscrotectomy should usually be performed. Some now advocate leaving the scrotum intact because of the efficacy of chemotherapy (26). Staging evaluation includes imaging of the retroperitoneum and chest. The Intergroup Rhabdomyosarcoma Study (IRS) III evaluated routine retroperitoneal lymph node dissection (RPLND) in 121 boys with localized paratesticular tumors and found no improvement in overall survival, but reported significant surgical complications (26,27). The IRS IV recommendation for a child with localized, completely resected tumor and normal retroperitoneal imaging studies was observation with close monitoring for nodal relapse (27); however, significant understaging was found with a decrease in the failure-free survival rate (28). In the IRS V protocols, it was recommended that all patients younger than age 10 years with negative CT scans and all patients older than age 10 years with negative RPLNDs undergo chemotherapy. Patients younger than 10 years with a positive CT and all patients older than age 10 undergo a RPLND. Of these patients, those with a negative nodal status will undergo chemotherapy, whereas those who are positive will have chemotherapy plus external beam radiation. Studies from Europe suggest that good results can be obtained using chemotherapy and radiation and avoiding a RPLND (29). Multimodal treatment using chemotherapy, radiation, and surgery has resulted in a 90% overall survival rate for paratesticular rhabdomyosarcoma.

EPIDIDYMIS–VAS DEFERENS–SEMINAL VESICLES

The mesonephric (wolffian) ducts extend from the mesonephros to the cloaca and give rise to the internal male genital ducts. The cranial portion of the ducts serves an excretory function early in fetal development and eventually regresses. The distal segment may persist as a vestigial appendix epididymis. The portion of the mesonephric duct adjacent to the testis contacts the rete testis, forming efferent ducts of the testis. The epididymis is formed by elongation and convolution of the ducts distal to the testis efferent ducts. The midportion of the mesonephric duct becomes the vas deferens, and the caudal aspect gives rise to the seminal vesicles.

The epididymis is a single tubule, approximately 6 m long, with many convolutions, in which sperm are stored and mature before transport to the vas deferens. Sperm undergo biochemical and molecular changes as they pass through the epididymis. The vas deferens has a thick muscular layer, and the greatest wall-to-lumen ratio of any tubular structure in the body. Muscular contractions propel sperm through the vasal lumen. The seminal vesicle is not a storage organ for sperm, as was once believed, but secretes fluid crucial to sperm survival and function. The seminal vesicle duct joins the vas deferens to form the

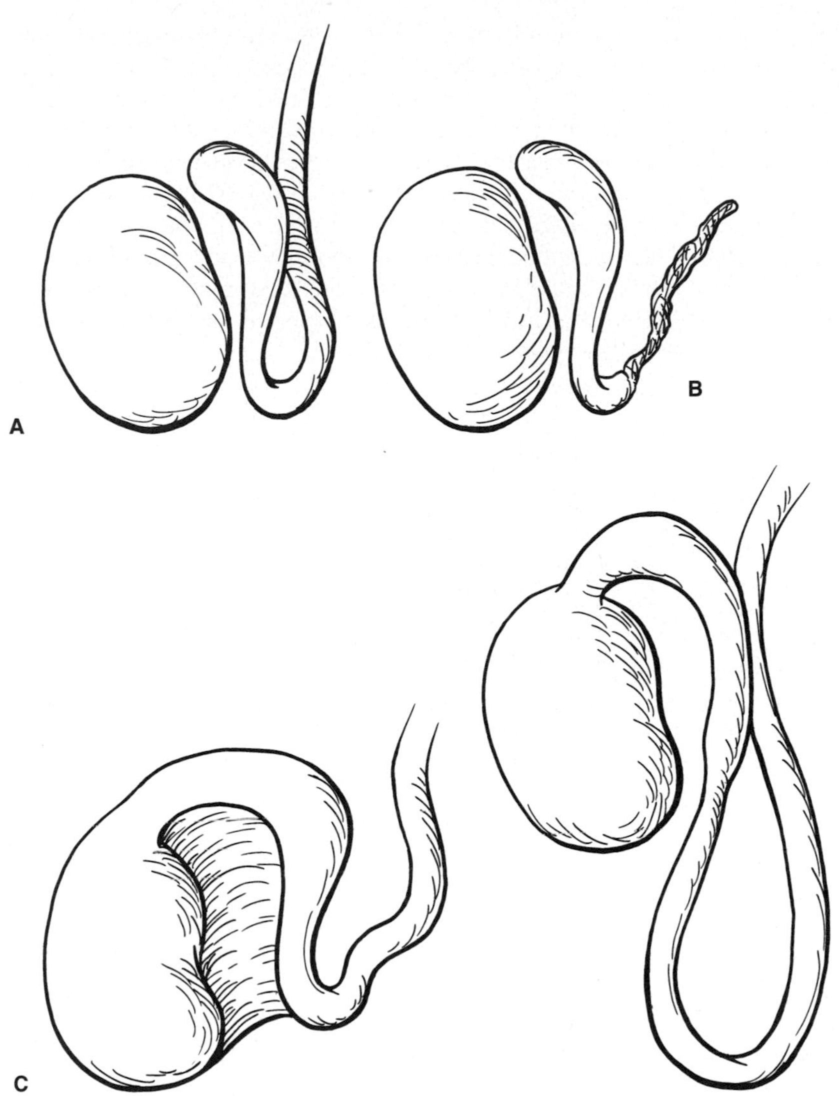

FIGURE 98-5. Abnormalities of the epididymis. Fusion abnormalities: loss of continuity **(A)** and atretic segment **(B)** Suspension defects: wide mesentery **(C)** and long looped vas deferens **(D)**.

ejaculatory duct, which traverses the prostate and empties into the urethra on either side of the utricle.

Abnormalities of the epididymis are usually found in association with undescended testes. The majority of cryptorchid testes have maldeveloped testis–epididymal configurations. Fusion abnormalities include loss of continuity between the testis and epididymis, and absent or atretic epididymal segments. Suspension defects are a widened epididymal mesentery and long epididymal tail or long, looped vas deferens (Fig. 98-5). Such abnormalities contribute to the infertility noted in cryptorchid men, and make the epididymis and vas deferens susceptible to iatrogenic injury during scrotal or inguinal surgery. For these reasons, careful note should be taken of the appearance of the epididymis and vas deferens when performing an orchiopexy or hernia repair.

Epididymal cysts (spermatoceles) are uncommon in prepubescent boys and are usually acquired. The cysts occur primarily in the globus major and are readily diagnosed on physical examination and transillumination or by ultrasound. The incidence of epididymal cysts is increased in the male children of mothers treated with diethylstilbestrol during pregnancy. Usually benign, they are followed unless they are very large or painful. Epididymal tumors are rare in children; the most common is the benign adenomatoid tumor.

Congenital unilateral absence or atresia of the vas deferens occurs in 0.5% to 1% of the general male population, with a strong left-sided predominance. Bilateral absence or atresia accounts for 1% to 10% of men being evaluated for azoospermia. Males with cystic fibrosis are infertile and may have bilateral vasal agenesis. Most abnormalities of the vas deferens are associated with epididymal abnormalities. The vas deferens and ureteral bud are mesonephric duct derivatives in close embryologic proximity, which explains the high incidence of ipsilateral renal agenesis with absence of the vas deferens. An ectopic vas deferens may enter the ureter or bladder, often causing recurrent UTIs and epididymitis.

Seminal vesicle abnormalities in children are rare. Incomplete ductal differentiation results in seminal vesicle cysts. The seminal vesicle, a wolffian derivative, is in close approximation to the ureteral bud, at the caudal end of the mesonephric duct. As with abnormalities of the vas deferens, absence or a lesion of the seminal vesicle results in a high incidence of ipsilateral renal agenesis and dysplasia.

VARICOCELE

Varicocele is an abnormal dilation of the spermatic veins within the scrotum, and although it is not specifically an abnormality of the male genital tract, it warrants discussion here because of its presentation and effects on the reproductive system. A varicocele occurs in 15% of the adult male population, but is uncommon before puberty. Older children may present with heaviness or scrotal discomfort, an ill-defined scrotal mass, or growth retardation of the ipsilateral testis. Left-sided lesions predominate, probably because the left gonadal vein can be as much as 8 to 10 cm longer than the right, inserts at a right angle into the left renal vein, and has a higher likelihood of incompetent valves. Physical examination is notable for the classic "bag of worms" appearance and consistency of the lesion. Varicocele is best graded with the patient in the standing position: *grade I*—palpable varicosities with Valsalva maneuver, *grade II*—visible varicosities with Valsalva maneuver, and *grade III*—visible varicosities without Valsalva maneuver. Occasional use of the term *Grade 0* is also seen in the literature. This term refers to a varicocele found only on ultrasound; that is, it cannot be found on physical exam. The dilated veins should reduce when the patient is placed in the supine position. Varicocele is the most readily identifiable cause of subnormal fertility in the male, and is often associated with oligoasthenospermia and a small ipsilateral testis. Surgical repair of the varicosities can result in significant improvement in semen quality.

A proposed mechanism for the subfertility is that venous dilation causes increased intratesticular pressures and blood flow, leading to an increase in testicular temperatures with detrimental effect on spermatogenesis. Adolescents with a large varicocele may have a significant decrease in ipsilateral testicular volume. One-third of boys with grade II lesions and more than one-half of those with grade III varicoceles have measurable testis hypoplasia. Because of the potential for altered spermatogenesis, testis growth retardation is an indication for varicocelectomy in the adolescent (30). One arbitrary standard for intervention is a 5-mm difference in length, or 20% volume loss, in the ipsilateral gonad compared with the contralateral mate. Significant testicular growth often occurs after successful repair. Interruption of the spermatic veins can be accomplished with open surgery in the scrotum, subinguinal region, inguinal canal, or retroperitoneum. Other approaches include laparoscopic or venographic techniques. In addition to testicular growth retardation, symptomatic varicoceles and grade III lesions are indications for intervention. The success of open surgery has been improved by the use of the operating microscope that allows easy identification and preservation of lymphatics. Excellent results have been reported with no subsequent hydrocele formation (31).

REFERENCES

1. American Academy of Pediatrics Task Force on Circumcision. Report of the Task Force on Circumcision. *Pediatrics* 1999;103(3):686.
2. *Newborns: care of the uncircumcised penis*. Elk Grove Village, IL: American Academy of Pediatrics Division of Publications, 1999.
3. Schoen EJ, Colby CJ, Ray GT. Newborn circumcision decreases incidence and costs of urinary tract infections during the first year of life. *Pediatrics* 2000;105(4 pt 1):789.
4. Wiswell TE, Smith FR, Bass JW. Decreased incidence of urinary tract infections in circumcised male infants. *Pediatrics* 1985;75:901.
5. Butler-O'Hara M, LeMoine C, Guillet R. Analgesia for neonatal circumcision: a randomized controlled trial of EMLA cream versus dorsal penile nerve block. *Pediatrics* 1998;101(4):E5.
6. Wiswell TE, Geschke DW. Risks from circumcision during the first month of life compared with those for uncircumcised boys. *Pediatrics* 1989;83:1011.
7. Aaronson IA. Micropenis: medical and surgical implications. *J Urol* 1994;152:4.
8. Reilly JM, Woodhouse CRJ. Small penis and the male sexual role. *J Urol* 1989;142:569.
9. Dwoskin JY. Management of the "concealed" penis. *Dialog Pediatr Urol* 1993;16:1.
10. Daskalopoulos EI, Baskin L, Duckett JW. Congenital penile curvature (chordee without hypospadias). *Urology* 1993;42(6):708.
11. Koff SA. Does compensatory testicular enlargement predict monorchism? *J Urol* 1991;146:632.
12. Huff DS, Hadziselimovic F, Snyder HM, et al. Early postnatal testicular maldevelopment in cryptorchidism. *J Urol* 1991;146:624.
13. Jarow JP, Berkovitz GD, Migeon CJ, et al. Elevation of serum gonadotropins establish the diagnosis of anorchism in prepubertal boys with bilateral cryptorchidism. *J Urol* 1986;136:277.
14. Wenzler D, Bloom DA, Park JM. What is the rate of spontaneous testicular descent in newborns with cryptorchidism? Paper presented at the American Academy of Pediatrics Meeting, 2002.
15. Bellinger MF, Abromowitz H, Brantley S, et al. Orchiopexy: an experimental study of the effect of surgical technique on testicular histology. *J Urol* 1989;142:553.
16. Bloom DA, Key DW.Orchiopexy. In: Fowler JE Jr, ed. *Urologic surgery*, 1st ed. Boston: Little, Brown, 1992:556.
17. Canavese F, Lalla R, Linari A, et al. Surgical treatment of cryptorchidism. *Eur J Pediatr* 1993;152(suppl 2):S43.
18. Kogan SJ, Tennenbaum S, Gill B, et al. Efficacy of orchiopexy by patient age 1 year for cryptorchidism. *J Urol* 1990;144 (2 pt 2):508.
19. Johnson DE, Woodhead DM, Pohl DR, et al. Cryptorchidism and testicular tumorigenesis. *Surgery* 1968;63:919.
20. Bloom DA, Semm K. Advances in genitourinary laparoscopy. *Adv Urol* 1991;4:167.
21. Cooper BJ, Little TM. Orchiopexy: theory and practice. *Br Med J* 1985;291:706.
22. Campbell HE. Incidence of malignant growth of the undescended testicle: a critical and statistical study. *Arch Surg* 1942;44:553.
23. Batata MA, Whitmore WF, Chu FCH, et al. Cryptorchidism and testicular cancer. *J Urol* 1980;124:382.

24. Wan J, Bloom DA.Testicular tumors in children. In: Crawford ED, Das S, eds. *Current genitourinary cancer surgery,* 1st ed. Philadelphia: Lea & Febiger, 1990:429.
25. Kaplan GW. Testicular tumors in children. *AUA Update Series* 1983;2(lesson 12).
26. Wu HY, Snyder HM. Advances in pediatric urologic oncology. *AUA Update Series* 2003;22(lesson 4).
27. Wiener ES, Lawrence W, Hays D, et al. Retroperitoneal node biopsy in paratesticular rhabdomyosarcoma. *J Pediatr Surg* 1994;29: 171.
28. Wiener ES, Anderson JR, Ojimba JL, et al. Controversies in the management of paratesticular rhabdomyosarcoma: is staging retroperitoneal lymph node dissection necessary for adolescents with resected paratesticular rhabdomyosarcoma? *Semin Pediatr Surg* 2000; 10(3):146.
29. Plowman PN. Survivors of cancer: organ preservation and reducing the morbidity of treatment in paediatric genitourinary oncology. *Br J Urol Int* 1999;83(S3):51.
30. Kass DA. The management of the asymptomatic varicocele in adolescence. *Prob Urol* 1990;4:690.
31. Greenfield SP, Seville P, Wan J. Experience with varicoceles in children and young adults. *J Urol* 2002;168(4 pt 2):1684.

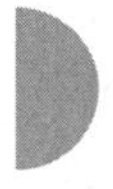

Chapter 99

Hypospadias

David Pinkstaff and John Noseworthy

DEFINITION AND TERMINOLOGY

Hypospadias is defined as a developmental anomaly characterized by a defect in the wall of the urethra so the (urethral) canal is open for a greater or lesser distance on the undersurface of the penis. It also applies to a condition in the female in which the urethra opens into the vagina. It is derived from the Greek word meaning "to draw away from under or having the orifice of the penis too low" (1). The following discussion focuses on the condition in the male and will not discuss female hypospadias.

A spectrum of severity of hypospadias exists, ranging from minor abnormalities involving the position of the urethral meatus on the proximal portion of the glans penis to severe forms in which the urethra opens in the peroneum just anterior to the anus. Classifications of severity separating the various forms of hypospadias into first degree, second degree, and third degree have been employed, but such general categories tend to obscure rather then illuminate the spectrum. More apropos is the descriptive terminology that is in wide use today. In this system of classification, the location of the hypospadias defect is described. Glanular hypospadias, proximal glanular hypospadias, coronoglanular hypospadias, subcoronal hypospadias, distal shaft hypospadias, midshaft hypospadias, proximal shaft hypospadias, penoscrotal hypospadias, scrotal hypospadias, and perineal hypospadias are all terms that have been used to more precisely characterize and categorize the degree of severity of the urethral abnormality (Fig. 99-1). Using such descriptive classification avoids ambiguity, imprecision, and the need for translation of such terms as third-degree hypospadias into a more anatomically accurate and consistent category. Precision in classification is important because the severity of the defect dictates the complexity of the repair and aids in clarifying the need for surgical intervention with the patients' parents. Also, it allows a more accurate comparison between analyses of outcomes in treatment of the disorder. As described in this chapter, the results of surgical repair of hypospadias, the occurrence of complications, the effort and time involved in caring for these children, and the expectations of the parents varies in a stepwise, linear fashion with increasing degrees of severity. Thus, accurate descriptions of the defect are important from the very outset of evaluation.

Two additional descriptive factors add meaning to the evaluation of hypospadias. The first involves the presence or absence of chordee. As applied to hypospadias, chordee is defined as "the ventral curvature of the penis, most apparent on erection, due to congenital shortness of the urethra and on rare occasions in patients with a normally situated meatus" (1). In the field of hypospadiology, chordee is also the term for the dense, scarlike tissue present to a variable degree around and adjacent to the hypospadic urethra, which produces restriction and "bow stringing" of the penile shaft, limiting full, straight extension of the phallus during erection. Chordee is usually present to one degree or another with those forms of hypospadias involving the penile shaft and more proximal (and thus more severe) forms. Hypospadias may occur in the absence of chordee, but this is unusual. Each patient presenting with hypospadias must be carefully examined for chordee and an accurate estimate made preoperatively to include the surgical treatment of chordee in the preoperative planning and in the discussion with the parents.

An accurate assessment of the extent of chordee may not be possible until the child is examined under anesthesia at the time of surgery. The use of an artificial erection, created by the injection of sterile saline and/or heparinized sterile saline into the erectile tissue may be the most accurate method of demonstrating the true extent of chordee (2).

Chordee can occur without hypospadias. In this circumstance, the chordee tissue may create significant curvature of the penis in erection despite a normally

David Pinkstaff: Department of Urology, Mayo Clinic Jacksonville, Jacksonville, Florida 32244.

John Noseworthy: Mayo Medical School, Thomas Jefferson University, Nemours Foundation, Jacksonville, Florida 32246.

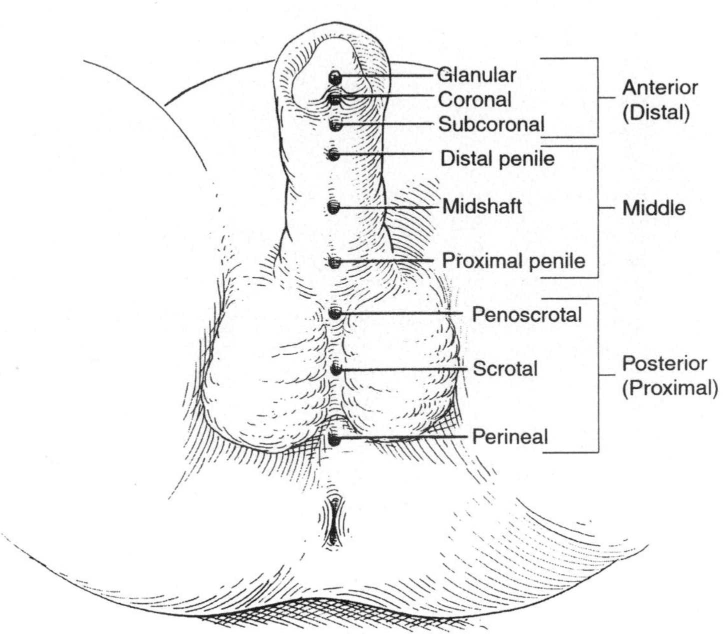

FIGURE 99-1. Anatomic classification of severity of hypospadias. (From Retik AB, Borer JG. Hypospadias. In: Walsh PC, Retik AB, Vaughan ED Jr, et al., eds. *Campbell's urology,* 8th ed. Philadelphia: WB Saunders, 2002;2287, with permission.)

positioned urethral meatus. Correction of "chordee without hypospadias" may necessitate division of the foreshortened urethra and lengthening it with an interposition urethroplasty.

The second, additional element of hypospadias evaluation is an assessment of the quality of the distal hypospadic urethra, particularly with regard to the degree of associated deficiency of the corpus spongiosum because this is often significantly deficient for a variable length. This aspect of evaluation may be deferred until the operation has begun; however, some approximation of this associated defect is important preoperatively to allow a full discussion with the parents regarding the potential surgical options and the extent of the operation that may be necessary to repair the defect.

EMBRYOLOGY

Fetal external genitalia are initially indifferent and are programmed to develop the female phenotype unless androgen stimulation occurs. The indifferent genital tubercle becomes evident at about 6 weeks' gestation. Outgrowth of endodermal cells from the walls of the cloaca and urogenital sinus along the ventral midline surface of the tubercle forms the urethral plate (3). Mesodermal proliferation on either side of the plate creates urethral folds. Around 8 weeks, the superficial layer of cells within the plate dies, forming the urethral groove (Fig. 99-2).

The interstitial (Leydig) cells of the testis increase in number, size, and function between the ninth and twelfth weeks of development. Testosterone stimulation induces the urethral folds to begin fusing ventrally in the midline to create the urethra. This process begins proximally and continues to the level of the glans penis. The glanular urethra distal to the fossa navicularis, however, is formed by ingrowth of surface epithelium (ectoderm), which invaginates through the glans to meet the more proximal urethra. The epithelium becomes stratified squamous epithelium at the completion of development. The classic "ectodermal

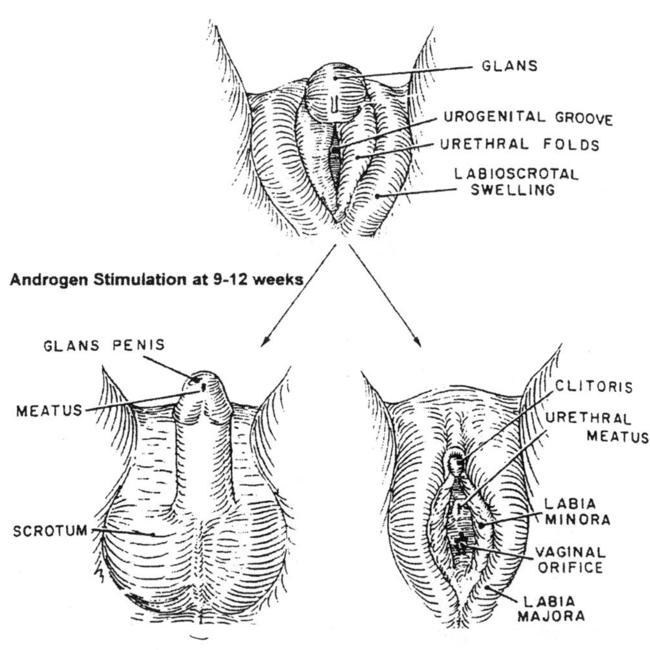

FIGURE 99-2. Generalized view of urethral embryogenesis from undifferentiated anlage. (From Snodgrass W, Baskin LS, Mitchell ME. Hypospadias. In: Gillenwater JW, Grayhack JT, Howards SS, et al., eds. *Adult and pediatric urology, volume 3,* 4th ed. Philadelphia: Lippincott Williams & Wilkins, 2002:2510, with permission.)

ingrowth theory" has more recently been challenged by the "endodermal differentiation theory." Immunohistologic studies by Kurzrock and associates (4) suggest that the entire male urethra, including the glanular portion, forms by tubularization of the urethral plate. Cell differentiation rather than ectodermal ingrowth is responsible for the stratified squamous epithelium of the distal glanular urethra.

Mesenchymal tissue of the urethral folds differentiates into corpus spongiosum, which fuses with the glans, completely surrounding the urethra. The dorsal and ventral aspects of both the preputial skin and the corpora cavernosa have been found to have different growth rates. As a result, significant ventral curvature exists in the developing phallus (5,6). The dorsal ectodermal tissue of the prepuce proliferates at a faster rate than the mesoderm forming the corpora cavernosa. Thus, folds of skin extend over the glans. Hunter noted that the prepuce does not uniformly surround the glans during penile development (6). The skin travels obliquely on either side of the penis back to the urethral opening ventrally. As the urethra tubularizes distally, the ventral extensions fuse in the midline and create the frenulum. Complete preputial covering of the glans occurs at approximately the twentieth week of development (7).

Arrest of urethral formation at any time during development results in hypospadias. The urethral meatus can be located anywhere on the ventral midline from the perineum to the glans as shown in Fig. 99-1. The urethral plate extends from the urethral opening to the tip of the glans. The appearance of the plate will depend on the extent of development of the urethral groove. It may appear as a flat surface or deep cleft.

The ventral glans does not fuse in the midline in hypospadias. Also, the corpus spongiosum usually does not cover the ventral aspect of the most distally formed portion of the urethra and diverges laterally to join the glans "wings." In most cases of hypospadias, the prepuce is only a dorsal hood, reflecting developmental arrest prior to ventral fusion and formation of the frenulum. Ventral angulation, called *chordee*, may persist as another indicator of arrested penile development.

INCIDENCE

Various reports have estimated the incidence of hypospadias between 1 and 10 per 1,000 live births. This range presumably reflects variation in the severity of the defects reported. Some series may exclude the less severe glanular forms and thus not include all types of the defect. An incidence of 1 per 100 to 150 live births is frequently cited and appears reasonably accurate (8). This is helpful in discussions with parents because it gives them an appreciation that this congenital abnormality is not particularly uncommon and that it can be dealt with successfully.

Thus, a children's health care center serving a combined obstetrical experience of 20,000 births per year might well see on the average 100 patients with hypospadias annually. The 20-year experience reported by Gross in his classic textbook *The Surgery of Infancy and Childhood* (9) included 392 patients with hypospadias. One hundred of these patients were classified as penoscrotal or perineal, 32 in the shaft, and 260 as frenular (distal, less severe).

ASSOCIATED ANOMALIES

Cryptorchidism and Inguinal Hernia

Both hypospadias and cryptorchidism may be the result of androgen deficiency. A coexisting undescended testicle has been noted in 8% to 9% of boys with hypospadias. The incidence varies with the severity of the hypospadias defect, and males with more proximal lesions have a significantly increased rate of cryptorchidism. Inguinal hernia and/or hydrocele has been an associated finding in up to 10% of cases (10).

Prostatic Utricle

This structure is the remnant of the fused caudal ends of the paramesonephric ducts. Enlargement of the utricle can be seen in boys with hypospadias. Devine et al. reported enlargement of the prostatic utricle in 10% of boys with penoscrotal and 57% with perineal hypospadias. This may result from delayed or inadequate secretion of müllerian inhibiting factor or incomplete masculinization of the urogenital sinus (11). Stasis of urine in the utricle may be a rare cause of urinary tract infection or even stone formation (12). Usually, however, there is no clinical significance except that it may complicate catheterization during hypospadias repair.

Syndromes

There are 49 syndromes described in which hypospadias is an associated finding (13). The Smith-Lemli-Opitz syndrome includes multiple congenital anomalies due to a deficiency of 7-dehydrocholesterol reductase causing impaired cholesterol synthesis. This condition has an incidence of 1 in 20,000 births and is the third most prevalent autosomal-recessive inherited condition in whites. Manifestations include mental retardation, small stature, facial deformities, syndactyly of the second and third toes, and male genital anomalies. External genital findings can range from hypospadias in approximately 70% of cases to micropenis to female phenotype (14).

The Opitz-Frias syndrome is characterized by hypertelorism and hypospadias. Additional findings include mild to moderate mental retardation and swallowing difficulties resulting in aspiration. Inheritance includes both X-linked and autosomal-dominant forms that have similar clinical manifestations. Cryptorchidism is frequently seen in these patients as well.

Trisomy 13 (Patau's syndrome) and trisomy 18 (Edwards' syndrome) are severe genetic conditions that are usually fatal within the first few years of life. Cryptorchidism is noted in at least 50% of each of these populations. Hypospadias is seen in less than 50% of patients with trisomy 13 and less than 10% of boys with trisomy 18.

Intersex States

Isolated hypospadias on the shaft of a normal-size phallus and two palpable gonads should not raise concern for an intersex disorder. A meatus positioned in the scrotum or perineum increases the likelihood of intersexuality. A high index of suspicion for an intersex state should be maintained for infants with any degree of hypospadias associated with cryptorchidism.

Kaefer et al. evaluated 79 presumed males with hypospadias and unilateral or bilateral cryptorchidism (15). Intersex conditions were identified in 30% of 44 patients with unilateral and 32% of 35 patients with bilateral undescended testes. Patients with one or more nonpalpable testes were approximately three times more likely to have an intersex state (with an incidence of 47% to 50%) than patients with palpable undescended gonads. In addition, a more posterior meatal position was associated with a significantly higher likelihood of intersex.

A newborn with hypospadias and bilateral nonpalpable testes must be evaluated for female pseudohermaphroditism. Male pseudohermaphroditism should be considered with scrotal or perineal hypospadias with palpable gonads or after the adrenogenital syndrome has been ruled out in newborns with nonpalpable testes. True hermaphroditism may present with asymmetric gonadal descent and hypospadias. Patients with mixed gonadal dysgenesis have unilateral cryptorchidism, representing the dysgenetic streak gonad, and often have a small phallus.

EVALUATION

Routine imaging of the urinary tract with ultrasonography or intravenous urography is not required in children with isolated anterior or middle ureteral hypospadias. Radiologic studies are only obtained in boys who develop urinary tract infection or whose hypospadias is part of a malformation syndrome.

Intersex evaluation should be undertaken for patients with posterior hypospadias, regardless of gonadal position or palpability, and for those with coexisting hypospadias and cryptorchidism. The finding of one or two palpable gonads on physical examination effectively rules out female pseudohermaphroditism because ovaries do not descend. Pelvic ultrasonography will define müllerian anatomy and will confirm the presence or absence of a uterus. A karyotype must be obtained in the immediate newborn period. Serum electrolytes should be measured to rule out a salt-wasting form of the adrenogenital syndrome. Testosterone and dihydrotestosterone levels should also be measured early in the postnatal period. Serum 17-hydroxyprogesterone should be measured on day of life three or four to rule out 21-hydroxylase deficiency. A reasonable differential diagnosis can be formulated from these pieces of information.

If no testes are palpable, endocrine studies must be performed to determine the presence or absence of testicular tissue. A markedly elevated luteinizing hormone (LH) is consistent with anorchia. A human chorionic gonadotropin stimulation test can demonstrate functioning testicular tissue and can help distinguish between impaired testosterone synthesis and androgen insensitivity.

Laparotomy or laparoscopy with gonadal biopsy is performed when a firm diagnosis from the above workup cannot be obtained. Removal of gonads or reproductive organs should not be performed until the final pathology report has been reviewed and a decision has been made regarding gender assignment.

Prior to surgical intervention, a "genitogram" of the urogenital sinus should be obtained. Further detail of anatomic relationships can be obtained with endoscopy at the time when surgical reconstruction is planned.

EVOLUTION OF SURGICAL TECHNIQUES

The general trend in hypospadias surgery, particularly with regard to the more severe forms, has been to develop techniques for full straightening of the penile shaft and complete lengthening of the urethra with as little surgery and as few operations as possible. Since the mid-1950s to mid-1960s, surgery for hypospadias has moved from multistage operations (separated by several months of healing and employing significant periods of urinary diversion) to more extensive, longer operations with less extensive urinary diversion. Figure 99-3 illustrates some of the important steps along this evolutionary path. Multistage operations were based on the concept that transposing foreskin in a first operation and letting healing reestablish abundant blood supply to the transposed tissues would then allow more complete healing when the urethra was tubularized and the repair completed at a later operation. Release of chordee at the first operation with transfer of foreskin from the dorsal aspect of the penis to the ventral aspect was a frequently used first step in such multistage repairs. Subsequent tubularization of the transferred and revascularized preputial skin was then performed 3 to

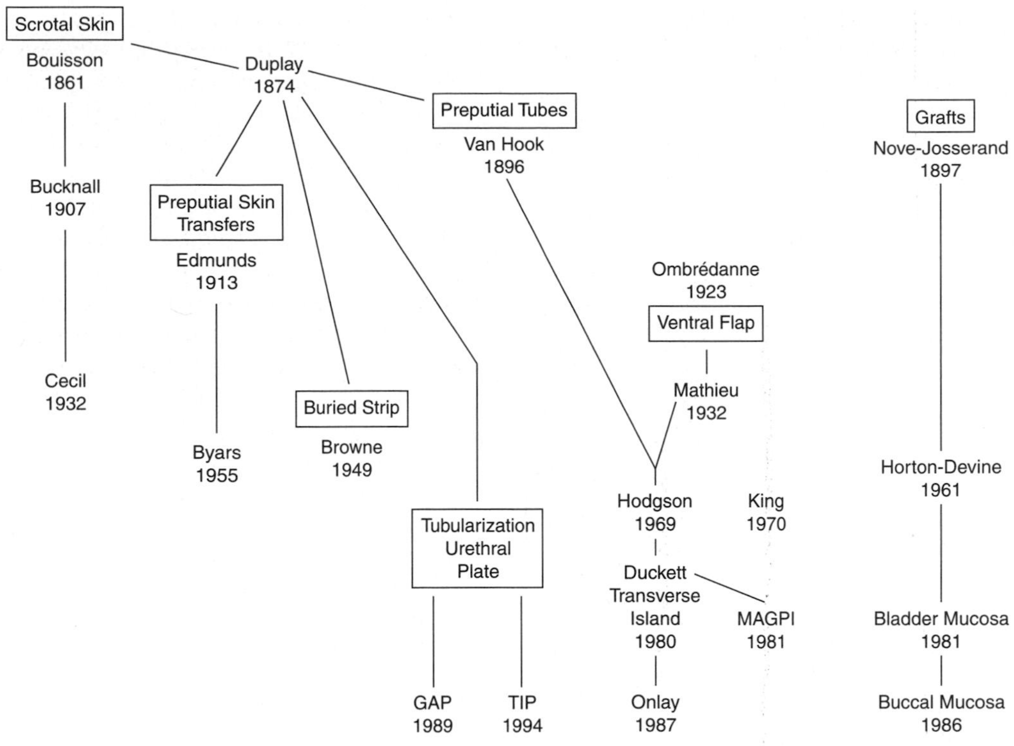

FIGURE 99-3. Historical perspective of important steps in the evolution of current hypospadias operations. (From Snodgrass W, Baskin LS, Mitchell ME. Hypospadias. In: Gillenwater JW, Grayhack JT, Howards SS, et al., eds. *Adult and pediatric urology,* volume 3, 4th ed. Philadelphia: Lippincott Williams & Wilkins, 2002:2519, with permission.)

6 months later. The staged operations were timed to complete the repair during the second and third year of life.

As experience developed, and a cadre of pediatric urologists and pediatric surgeons were trained, a subset of surgical specialists emerged who had extensive experience with hypospadias. Efforts were made to minimize the extensive surgery and to compress the time course for full repair. This led to the development of new techniques for foreskin transposition and tubularization such that one-stage repairs became widely applied. The utilization of tubularized grafts of foreskin with preservation of their vascular supply (as popularized by Duckett and others), supported the emergence of these one-stage techniques. Increasing experience with free, tubularized preputial grafts and the development of fine instruments and suture material have enhanced the hypospadias' surgeon's ability to repair the defect more expeditiously and with less difficulty for the patient and family.

These techniques of tubularized vascularized grafts and free tube grafts have subsequently be been applied to the severe forms of proximal hypospadias such as penoscrotal and perineal. In this circumstance tubularized, vascularized preputial grafts, free skin grafts, and tubes of penile shaft skin have been combined in composite urethral reconstructions, allowing the full repair of long urethral defects in a single stage.

In addition to the use of genital skin, extrapenile tissues have been used as alternative sources of tissue for urethral reconstruction. Oral buccal mucosa and bladder mucosa have both been used. Grafts of these tissues have been harvested, tabularized, and used as neourethral reconstructions. They have also been used in composite reconstructions in conjunction with vascularized and free grafts of penile tissue when those sources of neourethra were insufficient to achieve complete repair of lengthy urethral defects.

Although it was customarily advised in previous decades to avoid surgery for those instances of hypospadias in which the urethral meatus was situated "but a few millimeters back from the normal area," new attitudes and new techniques have brought these milder, more distal forms of hypospadias into the arena for repair. The MAGPI procedure as originally described by Duckett (16) has had wide application in this setting. The historic concerns that mobilization of the meatus in the terminal portion of the urethra would lead to sloughing, infections, scarring, and worsening of the deformity have been markedly reduced by such approaches.

Despite the enthusiasm for and frequent performance of hypospadias repair with one-stage operations, more recent literature suggests that two-stage techniques may be undergoing a resurgence of interest and application

(17). The focus here has been to make every effort to minimize the complications that sometimes accompany defective healing.

PRINCIPLES OF HYPOSPADIAS REPAIR

Timing of Surgery

The recommended age for hypospadias repair is between 6 and 12 months of age (18). Operative intervention can be performed as early as 2 to 3 months of age without an increased rate of surgical complications (19). However, significantly higher complication rates for hypospadias repair in older patients have been reported (20). Based on the psychological implications of genital surgery in children, surgical considerations and advances in pediatric anesthesia, the current standard is hypospadias repair before 12 months of age.

Objectives

Regardless of the technique used for hypospadias repair, the ultimate goal is to create a penis with normal appearance and function. Successful reconstruction includes correction of penile curvature, urethroplasty, meatoplasty, glanuloplasty, and circumcision with appropriate skin coverage.

The surgeon should first deglove the penile shaft skin, which itself may contribute to or even be the sole source of penile curvature or torsion. An artificial erection may be induced by injecting normal saline directly into the corpora or glans. A variety of plication and graft techniques have been described for addressing chordee, and the decision of which to employ is dictated by the severity and position of curvature as well as penis size. Occasionally, transection of the urethral plate is required to achieve penile straightening.

The next step is to create a uniform caliber urethra with the meatus located at the tip of the glans. The current trend in hypospadias surgery is to primarily tubularize the plate after a dorsal midline relaxing incision has been made or to incorporate the urethral plate into the neourethra if at all possible. Ideally, a second layer of tissue should cover the neourethra to decrease urethrocutaneous fistula formation. Subcutaneous dartos flaps, tunica vaginalis flaps, and corpus spongiosum may all be used for neourethral coverage.

Glanuloplasty follows to construct a conical-shaped glans. Care must be taken to avoid stenosis of the neomeatus, which should have a generous oval shape. Patients with very distal hypospadias may only require glanuloplasty and meatoplasty for correction of their abnormality.

Penile shaft skin coverage is the final step of successful hypospadias surgery. Preputial skin may be transferred to the ventral aspect of the penis either by creating flaps for lateral transfer or by creating a buttonhole in the prepuce through which the glans is passed. Excess skin is excised giving the final appearance of a normal circumcised penis.

The desired functional results of hypospadias repair include the ability to stand to void; a strong, single urinary stream; and a straight penile shaft with erection allowing successful intercourse with semen deposition into the vagina. These goals should all be accomplished with a good cosmetic result as well. Figure 99-4 presents a decision-making algorithm suggested by Retik and Borer that sequences one such series of operative thought processes and maneuvers, allowing achievement of these objectives.

Optical Magnification

Early repair in infant males and the use of fine suture material have made the use of some form of optical magnification the rule in hypospadias surgery. Comparison of results obtained using the operating microscope and loupe magnification showed no significant difference in outcome (21). Loupes with magnification of 2.5× and higher are adequate for hypospadias surgery.

Instruments

The success of hypospadias repair relies on the application of reconstructive surgical techniques. Fine instruments that are noncrushing should be used to handle tissues. Stay/traction sutures should be used when possible to minimize tissue handling.

Suture Material and Technique

Several studies have evaluated suture material used in hypospadias surgery. Faster absorbing sutures such as polyglycolic acid (Dexon) or chromic catgut are recommended. DiSandro and Palmer reported a fourfold increase in urethral stricture formation after hypospadias repair with polydioxanone suture (PDS) versus polyglycolic acid or chromic catgut suture (22).

A subcuticular suturing technique should be used during longitudinal closure of the neourethra. Ulman and colleagues showed a significantly lower urethrocutaneous fistula rate for subcuticular (4.9%) versus full-thickness (16.6%) techniques (23). The edges of the epithelial surfaces must be inverted, and the raw surfaces of the subepithelial tissues should be approximated to create a watertight anastamosis.

Postoperative Dressing

Many different types of dressing have been used after hypospadias repair. A biocclusive transparent film dressing (Tegoderm) provides some compression but is soft and elastic enough to allow for some expected slight swelling (24). A prospective randomized trial comparing the use

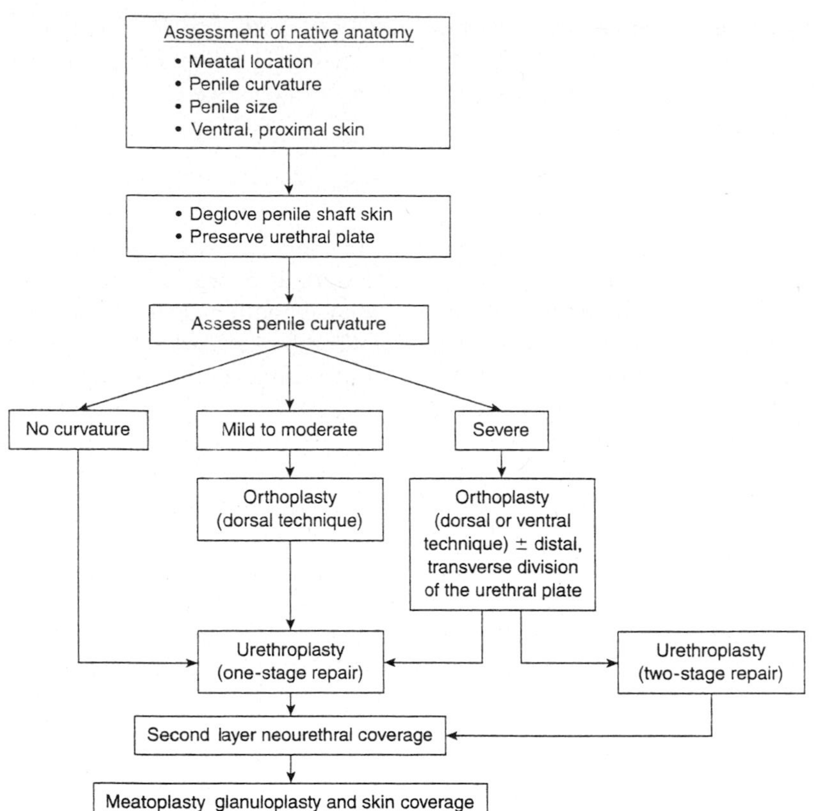

FIGURE 99-4. Algorithm for decision making in the evaluation and surgical treatment of hypospadius. (From Retik AB, Borer JG. Hypospadias. In: Walsh PC, Retik AB, Vaughan ED Jr, et al., eds. *Campbell's urology,* 8th ed. Philadelphia: WB Saunders, 2002;2305, with permission.)

of a postoperative dressing to no dressing showed no impact on surgical success rate or wound healing at a mean follow-up of 1 year (25).

Urinary Diversion

The need for neourethral catheterization following hypospadias repair remains controversial. Comparative prospective studies have demonstrated no difference in postoperative outcomes in patients with or without diversion following Mathieu (26,27) or tubularized incised plate (28) repairs. Other investigators, however, have noted a higher incidence of postoperative complications (4.6% vs. 18.9%) when stents were not used (29).

The feeding tube used as a urethral catheter may induce bladder spasms in some boys as it rubs against the trigone and bladder wall. Some children may require anticholinergic medication to control these spasms. However, painful voiding may cause older patients left without a catheter to refuse to void postoperatively. Placement of a catheter may then be required.

Analgesia

Intraoperative and postoperative pain can be controlled with 0.25% bupivacaine hydrochloride administered as a caudal or penile block. Chhibber et al. found that penile blocks given both before and at the completion of surgery provided significant improvement in postoperative pain control compared with an equivalent total dose of anesthetic administered in a single penile block either at the onset or completion of surgery (30).

The vast majority of hypospadias repairs are performed as an outpatient procedure. Oral acetaminophen and ibuprophen usually provide adequate pain relief. Narcotic analgesics for outpatient use in young children should be given sparingly.

COMPLICATIONS

Urethrocutaneous Fistula

Urethrocutaneous fistula is the most common complication of hypospadias repair. It may be an isolated finding or can result from, or be associated with, meatal stenosis or distal strictures. Risk factors include devitalization of tissue, failure to invert all epithelial edges during urethroplasty, and failure to create a second layer of tissue coverage over the urethroplasty. Several authors have reported the importance of second-layer coverage of the neourethra in reducing fistula rates (31,32). Reported fistula rates include 2% of tubularized incised plate repairs (33), 6% to 17% of onlay and tubularized preputial flaps (34–36), and 5% or less in modern two-stage repairs (37,38).

Fistula repair includes excision of all unhealthy tissue, inverting closure over a catheter to prevent urethral narrowing, and interposition of a second layer of tissue between the urethra and skin. Small fistulae can be circumferentially excised, closed, and covered. Postoperative urethral stents are rarely required. Larger fistulae may require onlay flap coverage from adjacent tissues.

Meatal Stenosis

Iatrogenic constriction of the meatus during repair or loss of blood supply to the distal urethra may result in meatal stenosis. The incidence is less than 5% using modern techniques. Dilation or ventral incision may resolve the problem if stenosis is mild. More severe cases require reoperation with well-vascularized flip-flaps or onlay flaps.

Balanitis xerotica obliterans (BXO) is a chronic inflammatory process of unknown etiology. It can occur spontaneously or can arise after minor trauma or penile surgery. Two series of BXO following hypospadias repair have been reported (39,40). Initial treatment is topical steroids, but surgical excision of affected tissues and repair is often required. Unfortunately, recurrence is common.

Urethral Stricture

A stricture of the neourethra usually indicates loss of vascularity. The proximal anastamosis of tubularized preputial flaps appears to be particularly at risk for stricture formation. A stricture rate of 6% has been reported for tubularized and onlay preputial flaps (36). Tubularized incised plate repairs rarely develop strictures.

Treatment of strictures generally requires open repair. Scherz and colleagues reported a success rate of 46% for urethral dilation or visual urethrotomy in patients who developed urethral stricture within 3 months following hypospadias repair. Cure rates dropped to 16% when treatment was performed greater than 3 months after the initial repair (41).

Urethral Diverticula

Diverticula develop secondary to distal obstruction, as a result of turbulent urinary flow or from excessive caliber of the neourethra (42). Clinical presentation includes visible urethral ballooning during voiding and postvoid dribbling. Repair involves excision of redundant tissues and addressing any causative factors.

Recurrent Chordee

Generally, if chordee is completely addressed at the time of initial repair, it does not recur. Vandersteen and Husmann reported 22 patients with symptomatic chordee more than 10 years after proximal hypospadias repair (43). Both dorsal plication and ventral tunica vaginalis patch grafts had been used for primary correction with similar representation rates. No definitive risk factors for recurrence could be identified. These patients may have had residual chordee not noted until the onset of sexual activity.

LONG-TERM FOLLOW-UP/OUTCOMES

The objectives of surgical repair of hypospadias are to achieve (1) typical male voiding patterns in the toilet-trained child (standing to avoid with a straight and controllable urinary stream), (2) a penile shaft that is straight and fully sensate when erect, and (3) a cosmetic result that presents a normal- appearing genital configuration. Although several decades ago it was customary to focus on a straight shaft that allowed standing to void and successful intercourse in adulthood, new techniques and greater focus on the technology of the repair of hypospadias has led to a realignment of these concerns with increasing focus on cosmesis and meatal position. Employing the techniques summarized previously, it is now appropriate to place the meatus in a normal glanular position near the tip of the glans, achieving an appearance that the family considers "normal."

Attention to the size and configuration of the meatus, as well as the rifling characteristics of the neourethra, are important elements in achieving a urinary stream that is of good caliber, controllable, and free of disruption and/or deviation. Postoperative meatal stenosis may produce diminution, deviation, or disruption of the urinary stream and ultimately require a secondary meatoplasty. Dilatation or patulousness of the neourethral graft may produce both unsightly distention of the ventral shaft during voiding, as well as stasis within the urethra. If voiding is significantly compromised by this occurrence, urethroplasty of the affected neourethra may be necessary. If stasis is the only consideration, educating the child and family with urethral emptying maneuvers such as digital stripping of the urethra may eliminate the symptoms. Distal stenosis at the meatus may be partially etiologic in producing saccular dilatation of the neourethra, but most often this abnormality is the result of neourethral graft redundancy accompanied by the absence of surrounding spongiosum tissue.

A narrow or disrupted stream on voiding in the absence of meatal stenosis may be caused by a stricture at the anastomosis between the neourethral graft and the native urethra. Endoscopic evaluation with or without internal urethrotomy may be required to manage this form of abnormal voiding following hypospadias repair.

Sexual function in adulthood for patients undergoing hypospadias repair in infancy and early childhood is quite satisfactory. A straight penile shaft and normal phallic sensation and erectile function allow successful intercourse. In the absence of severe urethral strictures or other such mechanical problems, fertility is most related to endocrine and testicular function and not to the mechanical aspects of genital reconstruction. It appears that associated abnormalities such as cryptorchidism, chromosome abnormalities, varicoceles, and testicular torsion, as well as other endocrine abnormalities that may have accompanied the hypospadias defect and not the hypospadias itself, are the causes of diminished fertility in this group of patients (44).

Setting aside those relatively few patients who have suffered recurrent, multiple complications of their initial surgery and have been left with persisting deformity, stricture, sensory deficits, and erectile dysfunction following multiple operations to correct hypospadias, most boys with hypospadias repaired using the techniques and attentions to detail described previously can look forward to normal urinary and sexual function as they develop through childhood and adolescence into adulthood.

REFERENCES

1. *Stedman's medical dictionary*, 24th ed. Baltimore: Williams & Wilkins, 1982.
2. Gittes RF, McClaughlin AP. Injection technique to induce penile erection. *Urology* 1974;4:473.
3. Glenister JW. The origin and fate of the urethral plate in man. *J Anat* 1954;288:413.
4. Kurzrock EA, Baskin LA, Cunha GR. Ontogeny of the male urethra: theory of endodermal differentiation. *Differentiation* 1999;64:115.
5. Kaplan GW, Lamm DL. Embryogenesis of chordee. *J Urol* 1975;114:769.
6. Hunter RH. Notes on the development of the prepuce. *J Anat* 1935;70:68.
7. Stephens FD, Smith ED, Hutson JM. Embryogenesis of hypospadias. In: Stephens FD, ed. *Congenital anomalies of the urinary and genital tracts*. Oxford, UK: Isis Medical Media Ltd., 1196.
8. Sweet RA, Schrott HG, Kurland R, et al. Study of the incidence of hypospadius in Rochester, Minnesota, 1940 to 1970, and a case control comparison of possible etiologic factors. *Mayo Clinic Proc* 1974;49:52.
9. Gross RE. *The surgery of infancy and childhood*. Philadelphia: WB Saunders, 1953:714.
10. Khuri FJ, Hardy BE, Churchill BM. Urologic anomalies associated with hypospadias. *Urol Clin North Am* 1981;8:565.
11. Devine CJ Jr, Gonzales-Serva L, Stecker JF Jr, et al. Utricle configuration in hypospadias and intersex. *J Urol* 1980;123:407.
12. Ritchey ML, Benson RC Jr, Kramer SA, et al. Management of müllerian duct remnants in the male patient. *J Urol* 1988;140:795.
13. Jones KL. *Smith's recognizable patterns of human malformation, volume 1*, 5th ed. Philadelphia: WB Saunders, 1997.
14. Opitz JM, de la Cruz F. Cholesterol metabolism in the RSH/Smith-Lemli-Opitz syndrome: summary of an NICHD conference. *Am J Med Genetics* 1994;50:326.
15. Kaefer M, Diamond D, Henderson WH, et al. The incidence of intersex in children with cryptorchidism and hypospadias: stratification based on gonadal palpability and meatal position. *J Urol* 1999;162:1003.
16. Duckett JW. MAGPI (meatoplasty and glanuloplasty). *Urol Clin North Am* 1981;8:513.
17. Ferro F, Zaccara A, Spagnoli A, et al. Skin graft for 2-stage treatment of severe hypospadias: back to the future? *J Urol* 2002;168: 1730.
18. Kass E, Kogan SJ, Manley C. Timing of elective surgery on the genitalia of male children with particular reference to the risks, benefits and psychological effects of surgery and anesthesia. *Pediatrics* 1996;97:590.
19. Bellman AB, Kass EJ. Hypospadias repair in children under one year of age. *J Urol* 1982;128:1273.
20. Hensle T, Tennenbaum S, Reiley E, et al. Hypospadias repair in the adult population: adventures and misadventures. *J Urol* 2001;165:77.
21. Shapiro SR. Hypospadias repair: optical magnification versus Zeiss reconstruction microscope. *Urology* 1989;33:43.
22. DiSandro M, Palmer JM. Stricture incidence related to suture material in hypospadias surgery. *J Pediatr Surg* 1996;31:881.
23. Ulman I, Erikci V, Avanoglu A, et al. The effect of suturing technique and material on complication rate following hypospadias repair. *Eur J Pediatr Surg* 1997;7:156.
24. Burbige KA. Simplified postoperative management of hypospadias repair. *Urology* 1994;43:719.
25. Van Savage JG, Palanca LG, Slaughenhoupt BL. A prospective randomized trial of dressings versus no dressings for hypospadias repair. *J Urol* 2000;164:981.
26. Hakim S, Merguerian PA, Rabinowitz R, et al. Outcome analysis of the modified Mathieu hypospadias repair: comparison of stented and unstented repairs. *J Urol* 1996;156:836.
27. McCormack M, Homsy Y, Laberge Y. No stent, no diversion: Mathieu hypospadias repair. *Can J Surg* 1993;36:152.
28. Steckler RE, Zaontz MR. Stent-free Thiersch-Duplay hypospadias repair with the Snodgrass modification. *J Urol* 1997;158: 1178.
29. Buson H, Smiley D, Reinberg Y, et al. Distal hypospadias repair without stents: is it better? *J Urol* 1994;151:1059.
30. Chhibber AK, Perkins FM, Rabinowitz R, et al. Penile block timing for postoperative analgesia of hypospadias repair in children. *J Urol* 1997;158:1156.
31. Retik AB, Keating M, Mandell J. Complications of hypospadias repair. *Urol Clin North Am* 1988;15:223.
32. Churchill BM, van Savage JG, Khoury AE, et al. The dartos flap as an adjunct in preventing urethrocutaneous fistulas in repeat hypospadias surgery. *J Urol* 1996;156:2047.
33. Snodgrass W. Does the tubularized incised plate hypospadias repair create neourethral strictures? *J Urol* 1999;162:1159.
34. Baskin LS, Duckett JW, Ueoka K, et al. Changing concepts of hypospadias curvature lead to more onlay island flap procedures. *J Urol* 1994;151:191.
35. Gearhart JP, Borland RN. Onlay island flap urethroplasty: variation on a theme. *J Urol* 1992;148:1507.
36. Wiener JS, Sutherland RW, Roth DR, et al. Comparison of onlay and tubularized island flaps of inner preputial skin for the repair of proximal hypospadias. *J Urol* 1994;158:1172.
37. Greenfield SP, Sadler BT, Wan J. Two-stage repair for severe hypospadias. *J Urol* 1994;152:498.
38. Retik AB, Bauer SB, Mandell J, et al. Management of severe hypospadias with a 2-stage repair. *J Urol* 1994;152:749.
39. Kumar MV, Harris DL. Balanitis xerotica obliterans complicating hypospadias repair. *Br J Plast Surg* 1999;52:69.
40. Uemura S, Hutson JM, Woodward AA, et al. Balanitis xerotica obliterans with urethral stricture after hypospadias repair. *Pediatr Surg Int* 2000;16:144.
41. Scherz HC, Kaplan GW, Packer MG, et al. Post-hypospadias repair urethral strictures: a review of 30 cases. *J Urol* 1988;140: 1253.
42. Aigen AB, Khawand N, Skoog SJ, et al. Acquired megalourethra: an uncommon complication of the transverse island flap urethroplasty. *J Urol* 1987;173:712.
43. Vandersteen DR, Husmann DA. Late onset recurrent penile chordee after successful correction at hypospadias repair. *J Urol* 1998;160:1131.
44. Glassman CN, Machlus PJ, Kelalis PP. Urethroplasty for hypospadius: long-term results. *Urol Clin North Am* 1980;7:437.

Chapter 100

The Female Genital System

E. Stanton Adkins, III

The pediatric general surgeon often confronts problems ranging from disorders in the development of the female genital system to infections, tumors, and sexual abuse. Endoscopic techniques such as urethroscopy, vaginoscopy, and laparoscopy, as well as improvements in radiologic imaging, have advanced our ability to evaluate and treat children with disorders of the genital system.

EMBRYOLOGY

The ovary arises from genital ridge mesenchyme and is populated by germ cells (1). The fallopian tubes, uterus, and upper vagina develop from the müllerian ducts. The lower vagina and external genitalia are derived from the urogenital sinus and ridge. Some minor structures are attributable to the wolffian ducts (2).

THE OVARY

The ovary consists of germ cells and the supporting stroma. Germ cells may be found in a 24-day embryo in the caudal portion of the yolk sac near the allantoic stalk. During the fifth week of gestation, these germ cells migrate dorsally along the wall of the yolk sac and the gut until by the end of the week they reach the genital ridge. Once the genital ridge becomes populated with germ cells, the gonad forms. By the seventh week, it differentiates into a recognizable ovary.

The genital ridge develops into the supporting stroma of the ovary. The coalescence of mesenchyme from the ventral medial aspects of the mesonephros and overlying coelomic epithelium form the genital ridge. Germ cells follow the gradient of stem cell factor from the yolk sac to the gonad (3). Germ cells are likewise necessary for the differentiation of gonadal stroma into an ovary or testis. Arrest of the migration of germ cells leads to failure of the ovary to develop.

As the embryo grows, epithelial cords of cells, the sex cords, grow into the mesenchyme. By the eighth week, some differentiation has occurred. In males, the sex cords develop into seminiferous tubules and the rete testis; in females, the sex cords regress. Testis determining factor (SRY) appears to be the necessary element for growth and differentiation of the sex cords. In its absence, the sex cords in the medullary portion of the gonad regress over several months.

Once germ cells reach the ovary, they are termed *oogonia*. At approximately the 15th week, oogonia enter into prophase of the first meiosis and are termed *oocytes*.

The oocytes become enclosed or encased with granulosa cells and mesenchymal theca cells. Follicles deep within the ovary become atretic, whereas superficial follicles (those formed most recently) are preserved to form the ovarian cortex. At puberty with each estrous cycle several of the primary follicles mature and complete the first meiosis with ovulation. The second meiosis does not occur until after ovulation when a sperm encounters the ovum.

MÜLLERIAN DUCT

The müllerian ducts appear in embryos of both sexes late in the sixth week. Each duct originates as a groove lateral to the developing gonad and kidney that tubularizes as the edges of the groove come together.

The paired müllerian ducts lie lateral to the wolffian ducts cranially and, at the more caudal extent, are medial to the wolffian ducts. Soon after their development, the caudal portion of the müllerian ducts fuse to form a single canal. As the fusion proceeds cranially, the müllerian duct system develops first a Y and then a T shape.

The müllerian duct fuses with the urogenital sinus at the ninth week and forms a single tube by the third month. As the embryo grows, the point of fusion with the urogenital sinus elongates. This portion has no lumen and gives rise

E. Stanton Adkins, III: Department of Pediatrics and Surgery, University of South Carolina School of Medicine, Palmetto Health Children's Hospital, Columbia, South Carolina 29203.

to the vagina. The vagina itself develops when this vaginal plate recanalizes at approximately the sixth month. The proximal two-thirds of the vaginal plate is of müllerian duct origin and the lower one-third is of urogenital sinus origin.

The uterus, cervix, and fallopian tubes arise from the persistently patent portions of the müllerian duct. The tubes originate from the unfused lateral extensions of the müllerian ducts. The uterine body and cervix develop from the fused portion of the müllerian ducts. A small constriction indicates the division between the uterus and the cervix.

UROGENITAL SINUS

The urogenital sinus gives rise to the external genitalia and the lower one-third of the vagina. External genitalia arise starting at the fourth week from the cloacal membrane. On the anterior margins of this membrane are two genital swellings; on the posterior margins are paired anal swellings. The cloacal membrane remodels to become a groove between urogenital folds at the sixth week. At this stage, the perineal body forms separating the anus from the urethral groove. The fusion anterior to the groove becomes the phallus. During the eighth week, labioscrotal swellings lateral to the phallus move caudally to form the labia minora. The clitoris develops from the phallus and extends posteriorly into two corpora cavernosa of erectile tissue.

WOLFFIAN DUCT

The wolffian duct originates as the duct system for the primitive kidney, the pronephros. It becomes associated with the mesonephros, the first functional kidney, sometime after the fifth week of life. The duct connects with the urogenital sinus and persists as a defined structure for only a short time in the female. By the mid-fourth month the opening into the urogenital sinus closes. Although some structures of wolffian origin persist into adulthood, one structure, Gartner's canal, persists in the wall of the cervix and upper vagina in approximately 20% of adults, and may become an ectopic opening for the ureter.

ANATOMY, GROWTH, AND DEVELOPMENT

The ovary migrates from the genital ridge to the pelvic brim in the third month of gestation. It remains an abdominal structure until birth and then descends into the pelvis. The uteroovarian ligament attaches the ovary to the uterus. The round ligament extends from the upper uterine cervix out through the inguinal ring and terminates diffusely in the labia majora.

The uterus is a muscular organ with a normal position anteflexed relative to the cervix and anteverted relative to the vagina. The adnexa consist of the fallopian tubes, ovaries, and broad ligaments that are lateral on either side. The fallopian tubes lie anterior to the uteroovarian ligament and posterior to the round ligament of the uterus. They are enveloped in the broad ligament. The broad ligament extends from the uterus to the pelvic sidewall.

The vagina lies just posterior to the bladder and urethra. It extends from the vestibule to the uterine cervix and is lined with squamous epithelium. The course of the vagina parallels that of the pelvic brim and is essentially horizontal. The cervix penetrates the anterior wall of the vagina near its apex. The surface of the vagina forms a collapsed H-shaped tube, which when distended possesses a series of horizontal folds or rugae.

The external genitalia consist of the labia majora that extend from the mons pubis anteriorly and posteriorly to the labial commissure at the perineal body. The labia majora are covered with skin. The labia minora lie medial to the labia majora and are covered with squamous mucosa. Anteriorly, the labia minora join to form the prepuce of the clitoris. The labia minora define the lateral margins of the vestibule. Within the vestibule, one finds the urethra in the anterior midline. Slightly posterior to that is the vaginal orifice that is covered by a membrane, the hymen.

In the infant, the labia majora, labia minora, and clitoris are relatively larger and more prominent than they are later in life. With the onset of puberty, the labia majora and mons pubis become covered with hair. The vagina is moistened with cervical mucus because the vagina has no glands of its own. With puberty, the vagina becomes colonized by *Lactobacillus acidophilus*, which lowers the pH of the vagina.

At birth, when the female child leaves the maternal environment, estrogen levels, which had been high, begin to fall. The levels stay low until shortly before puberty. Growth of the genitalia is hormonally governed and therefore does not parallel the linear growth of the child.

The ovary doubles in size in the first 6 weeks of life. Thereafter, it grows very slowly until just before puberty when the growth rate increases. The newborn ovary often has follicles present and may have some follicular cysts. In most situations, the cysts resolve by the time the girls are several months old.

VASCULAR SUPPLY

Ovarian arteries arise from the aorta bilaterally. The ovarian veins connect to the vena cava on the right and the renal vein on the left. The ovarian vessels travel with the ureters initially and cross the iliac vessels at the iliac bifurcation. The remaining blood supply of the deep organs comes from the hypogastric arteries with the largest branch being the uterine artery, which proceeds toward the uterine cervix and then branches to send one marginal artery along the lateral aspect of the uterus and one along the vagina. The external pudendal artery (a branch of the external iliac), the internal pudendal artery (a branch of the hypogastric), and the hemorrhoidal vessels supply the vulva and lower one-third of the vagina. With the exception of the ovarian veins, the genital venous drainage parallels that of the arterial supply.

LYMPHATIC VESSELS

The perineum, vulva, and lower anterior abdomen drain toward the ipsilateral subinguinal and inguinal nodes, first entering the superficial nodes and then draining more deeply to the deep inguinal nodes. From there, drainage proceeds up the iliac chain. The internal drainage proceeds to the ipsilateral hypogastric, common iliac, and occasionally aortic or periaortic nodes. Only occasionally do the pelvic viscera drain to the inguinal nodes.

PUBERTY

Puberty is the transition from childhood to adulthood during which a child develops into a physically mature and reproductively capable adult. Maturation of the primary sexual characteristics, genitals and gonads, is heralded by the appearance of axillary and pubic hair and the development of breast buds. The hormonal control of puberty begins with the release of an increased amount of gonadotropin-releasing hormone (GnRH) from the hypothalamus, which stimulates the pituitary to produce luteinizing hormone (LH) and follicle-stimulating hormone (FSH). These in turn stimulate the ovary. Estrogen and progesterone synthesis and secretion increase markedly with the onset of puberty. It is these steroids that lead to the development of the secondary sexual characteristics.

Precocious Puberty

Precocious puberty is defined as the development of secondary sexual characteristics before the age of 8 years or the onset of menarche before the age of 10 years. Precocious puberty may be either central, which is GnRH dependent; peripheral, which is GnRH independent; or incomplete, which involves the expression of some primary or secondary sex characteristics but not others.

Central precocious puberty may be idiopathic, but is generally due to a central nervous system dysfunction. The dysfunction may originate from congenital defects, tumors, other space-occupying lesions, hydrocephalus, inflammation, trauma, or radiation. Central precocious puberty is always isosexual. It is diagnosed by performing a GnRH challenge and seeing marked increases in both serum FSH and LH. It may be treated surgically to remove the inciting cause or medically using a GnRH analogue to suppress pituitary release of LH and FSH.

Peripheral, GnRH-independent precocious puberty is due to the presence of inappropriate levels of circulating sex steroids. These steroids may be either exogenous or endogenous. Exogenous steroids include oral contraceptives, anabolic steroids, and rarely estrogen-like environmental chemicals. The endogenous causes include ovarian tumors or cysts, as well as some feminizing adrenal tumors. Peripheral precocious puberty may be isosexual or heterosexual, depending on which steroids are present in greatest concentration. Serum LH and FSH levels are normal or low for age. Once exogenous sources of steroids have been ruled out, workup involves search for a tumor. The tumor may arise from the ovary or adrenal gland. Imaging with computed tomography (CT) scan or magnetic resonance imaging (MRI) can locate and define the lesion. Surgical resection of the tumor is usually curative. Adjuvant chemotherapy or radiation may be necessary for malignancies.

Incomplete sexual precocity may involve premature thelarche, premature pubarche, or premature menarche. Premature thelarche or early breast development presents with subareolar nonprogressive breast development that may be unilateral or bilateral. There are no areolar changes associated with this self-limited process. If the breast development is progressive or does not show signs of regression after 1 to 2 years, an endocrine evaluation is indicated. Premature pubarche involves the early development of pubic hair and is a sign of androgen excess. Pubarche does not normally occur before the age of 8, although some African Americans may have a normal physiologic pubarche several months earlier. If the age of onset is sufficiently early or signs of virilization should appear, endocrine evaluation is indicated. Androgen-producing tumors or adrenal hyperplasia may be responsible.

Premature menarche or vaginal bleeding is a normal event in some newborns with the withdrawal of maternal estrogen stimulation. Estrogen-producing cysts may lead to bleeding when they rupture and estrogen levels fall. Otherwise, isolated menarche is rare. Vaginal bleeding from nonendocrine causes such as vulvovaginitis, trauma, abuse, or malignancy is more common and must be excluded.

OVARY

Ovarian disorders typically present with pain or a mass. Pain is often due to rupture of a cyst and requires no therapy. Occasionally, pain is a symptom of torsion of the ovary and requires emergent surgery. Ovarian masses may be found on physical examination during ultrasound or

CT examination. Rapid assessment and intervention may prevent ovarian loss and preserve fertility.

Ovarian Cysts

Functional ovarian cysts occur when a follicle or corpus luteum fails to regress. In the perinatal period, ovarian cysts are often discovered during maternal ultrasound. Following these cysts with serial ultrasound shows resolution of the cyst as newborn hormone levels fall. In pubertal females, cysts 3 to 8 cm in diameter may be seen. Observation over two menstrual cycles of cysts less than 5 cm in diameter will often show regression. If enlargement occurs or the cyst persists beyond 3 months with a diameter of 5 cm or greater, surgical resection is indicated to prevent torsion. The incidence of infertility following ovarian cystectomy is high. Use of atraumatic technique and meticulous hemostasis to minimize adhesion formation may lessen the incidence of infertility thereafter. When performed laparoscopically, a stripping technique with bipolar cautery for hemostasis has been effective.

Ovarian Torsion

Ovarian torsion is one of the few gynecologic emergencies a pediatric surgeon encounters. Prompt diagnosis and treatment can salvage a viable ovary in up to 70% of patients. Although torsion of a normal ovary is possible, the vast majority of torsed ovaries are enlarged with cyst(s) or a tumor.

Ovarian torsion presents with acute onset of intense lower abdominal pain. There is sometimes a history of similar pain that resolved spontaneously. Anorexia or nausea often accompanies the pain. Focal tenderness and a mass may be appreciated on pelvic exam. Plain radiographs sometimes reveal the calcifications of a teratoma and nonspecific ileus. When further information is required, ultrasound with color flow Doppler can demonstrate the mass and occasionally demonstrate loss of perfusion. Unfortunately, the presence of flow within the mass does not prove the converse, that the adnexa are not torsed.

At operation, the involved ovary is detorsed. If perfusion is questionable, fluorescein can demonstrate reperfusion in a viable ovary. When tumor is present, salpingo-oophorectomy is indicated. Cysts should be resected, the ovary repaired, and oophoropexy performed. The contralateral ovary must be inspected. As contralateral torsion with consequent infertility has been described, many surgeons recommend fixation of the opposite ovary.

Ovarian Tumors

Ovarian tumors in childhood may originate in any of the three components that comprise the ovary. Ninety percent of these are of germ cell origin of which two-thirds are benign teratomas. Approximately 4% are of stromal origin derived from the sex cords—granulosa-theca cell tumors and androblastomas. Only 3% are of epithelial origin. This contrasts with the adult experience in which 90% of all ovarian tumors are epithelial in nature (4).

Germ Cell Tumor

Tumors develop from germ cell precursors. These tumors are located at any point in the migration of germ cells from the yolk sac to the ovary and occasionally beyond the normal migration path.

The majority of these tumors arise spontaneously. However, there are well-described instances of familial germ cell tumors. Within a given family the tumors may not necessarily be of the same histologic type. The Li-Fraumeni cancer family syndrome has been associated with germ cell tumors in addition to bone and soft-tissue sarcomas. Other conditions such as 46XY gonadal dysgenesis and mosaic Turner syndrome are highly associated with the development of gonadoblastomas.

The germ cell tumors are histologically classified based on the developmental stage they most closely resemble. The ontogeny of the germ cell tumors is described in Table 100-1.

Germinoma

Germinoma is the current terminology designating the most primitive of the germ cell tumors. Germinomas are present in 10% of all ovarian tumors in children. They are rarely found in pure form, more often in combination with other germ cell tumors. The cells resemble primordial germ cells. Placental alkaline phosphatase is present in most germinomas. Markers for alpha-fetoprotein (AFP) and beta human chorionic gonadotropin (hCG) are negative in pure germinomas.

TABLE 100-1 Ontogeny of Germ Cell Tumors.

	Tumor	*Marker*
Primordial germ cell	Germinoma	PLAP
Embryonic differentiation	Embryonal CA	HCG, AFP
Extraembryonic differentiation	Endodermal sinus tumor	AFP, LDH-1
	Choriocarcinoma	HCG
Complete differentiation	Teratoma	—
Dysgenetic gonad	Gonadoblastoma	—

PLAP, placental alkaline phosphatase; HCG, beta subunit human chorionic gonadotropin; AFP, alpha-fetoprotein; LDH-1, lactate dehydrogenase isomer 1.

Adapted from Ablin A, Isaacs H. Germ cell tumors. In: Pizzo PA, Poplack DG, eds. *Principles and practice of pediatric oncology,* 2nd ed. Philadelphia: Lippincott Williams & Wilkins, 1993:867, with permission.

Embryonal Carcinoma

Embryonal carcinoma is histologically poorly differentiated with anaplastic elements and extensive necrosis. The tumors are uniformly negative for AFP, but may be focally positive for placental alkaline phosphatase and hCG. Chemotherapy occasionally causes these tumors to mature.

Endodermal Sinus Tumor (Yolk Sac Tumor)

The endodermal sinus tumor is the most common malignant germ cell tumor of childhood. In infants, it is most frequently involved with sacrococcygeal teratomas. The ovarian location is seen more frequently in later childhood and adolescence. Gross appearance is that of a pale tan-yellow slimy tumor with foci of necrosis. The tumors are very friable. The pathology may be papillary, reticular, solid, or polyvesicular. AFP is typically elevated in this lesion.

Choriocarcinoma

Choriocarcinoma histologically resembles placental tissue with two components, cytotrophoblasts and syncytiotrophoblasts. There are frequent foci of hemorrhage and necrosis. hCG is produced by these tumors.

Gonadoblastoma

Gonadoblastoma is a tumor that arises in dysgenetic gonads in association with the Y chromosome karyotype. The patients are phenotypic females with either a 46XY or mosaic 46XY/45XO karyotype. One-third of these patients will develop gonadoblastomas. Pure gonadoblastomas do not metastasize; however, one-third of the tumors are associated with germinomas, which do metastasize. No markers are known for this tumor.

Teratoma

The teratoma is the most common germ cell tumor of childhood and is benign in more than 90% of cases. The most common sites are the sacrococcygeal area and the ovary. The tumor is composed of endoderm-, mesoderm-, and ectoderm-derived tissues foreign to the organ or anatomic site from which they originate. Teratomas may be grouped into three subtypes—mature, immature and teratomas with malignant components. Mature teratomas show fully developed tissues such as brain, skin with hair, teeth, and the aerodigestive tract. Immature teratomas differ in that they possess neuroglial or neuroepithelial elements, which are not fully differentiated. The incidence of malignancy is associated with degree of immaturity of the tumor.

The malignancies most commonly found within teratomas are germinomas or other germ cell tumors. Occasionally, somatic cell malignancies may be found. Prognosis and therapy are based on whether the histology shows malignant cells and the tissue type of the malignancy. A mature teratoma does not manufacture AFP or hCG. These tumor markers may be found in tumors with malignant germ cell elements.

Surgical Considerations

Simple ovarian cysts are benign and may be treated by drainage without oophorectomy. Solid and complex masses are potentially malignant. Tumors are staged according to Children's Oncology Group (COG) guidelines (Table 100-2). Small masses may be treated with excisional biopsy and frozen section. Large tumors should be managed according to COG surgical guidelines (Table 100-3). Occasionally, a benign-appearing teratoma will be found to have immature or malignant elements within it after completion of the operation. In such a case, reexploration for staging is required.

Although laparoscopy is being used with increasing frequency for most procedures, its applicability to tumors is still uncertain. Obstetricians routinely remove "dermoids" laparoscopically and believe that rupture can be controlled with vigorous irrigation (5). If the tumor is found to be malignant, the situation becomes more complex. Unless a tumor is removed intact, it cannot be accurately staged. All tumors not removed intact are therefore treated as stage II and receive chemotherapy. Stage I tumors of the ovary can be treated with resection alone. In addition, the potential for spill of tumor while morcellizing it in a pouch is unknown. It cannot be recommended as standard therapy until these questions are resolved.

TABLE 100-2 Staging of Ovarian Germ Cell Tumors.

Stage	Extent of Disease
I	Limited to ovary/ovaries Negative peritoneal washings No evidence of disease beyond the ovaries May include gliomatosis peritonei
II	Microscopic residual tumor Lymph nodes negative Negative peritoneal washings
III	Gross residual tumor/biopsy only Lymph node involvement (nodule) Contiguous visceral involvement Positive peritoneal washings
IV	Distant metastases, including liver

Adapted from Billmire D, Rescorla F, Ross J, Schlatter M. Children's oncology group staging for pediatric ovarian germ cell tumors, 2004, unpublished data.

TABLE 100-3 Surgical Guidelines for Ovarian Germ Cell Tumors.

General
- Evaluate extent of disease
  - — Palpate and visualize all peritoneal surfaces particularly
    - Omentum
    - Pelvis
  - — Collect ascitic fluid or peritoneal fluid for cytology
  - — Palpate bilateral retroperitoneal lymph nodes
    - Internal iliac
    - Common iliac
    - Low para-aortic
    - Perirenal
  - — Biopsy suspicious/enlarged nodes
  - — Metal clips should not be used
  - — Inspect and palpate opposite ovary

Stages I–II
- Unilateral oophorectomy

Stages III–IV
- Unilateral oophorectomy with debulking as feasible
- Biopsy opposite ovary only if suspicious
- Biopsy peritoneal seeding
- Remove involved omentum

Bilateral disease
- Bilateral oophorectomy

Adapted from Billmire D, Vinocur C, Rescorla F, et al. Outcome and staging evaluation in malignant germ cell tumors of the ovary in children and adolescents: an intergroup study. *J Pediatr Surg* 2004;39:424–429, with permission.

Surgery is curative for mature teratomas and may be curative in immature teratomas. However, among adults survival in immature teratomas depends on histologic grade. Five-year survival decreases from approximately 80% with grade I to 30% in grade III tumors.

Radiation Therapy

Germinomas are quite sensitive to radiation and may be treated with this with quite good results. The response of other germ cell tumors to radiation as an adjunct to chemotherapy is unclear.

Chemotherapy

The chemotherapy of germ cell tumors is a product of the last 25 years of experience. Treatment has evolved from single agent treatment with less than 50% response rates to the current standard of Bleomycin, Etoposide, or Vinblastine, and a platinum agent. With this regimen, survival is typically between 60% and 100% at 5 years. Current therapeutic trials are seeking to determine whether these response rates may be preserved while reducing toxicity from the chemotherapy.

TABLE 100-4 Staging of Ovarian Epithelial Tumors.

Stage	*Extent of Disease*
IA	Limited to one ovary with intact capsule
IB	Limited to both ovaries with intact capsule
IC	Limited to ovary/ovaries with either capsule rupture, tumor on ovarian surface, or positive ascites or peritoneal washings
II	Tumor involves one or both ovaries with pelvic extension
III	Tumor involves one or both ovaries with microscopically confirmed peritoneal metastasis outside the pelvis and/or regional lymph node metastasis
IV	Distant metastasis

Adapted from Greene FL. American Joint Committee on Cancer, American Cancer Society, Ovary. *AJCC Cancer Staging Manual,* 6th ed. New York: Springer-Verlag, 2002:275–283, with permission.

Epithelial Tumors

Epithelial tumors are staged according to the American Joint Committee on Cancer (Table 100-4). They include adenocarcinoma, endometrioid tumors, clear cell tumors, and undifferentiated carcinomas. The prognosis in younger women is more favorable than it is in older women. Rodriguez et al. (6) found that, among women younger than 25 years with epithelial ovarian malignancies, the majority presented with early disease—stage 1 58.5%, stage II 8.9%, and stages III and IV 28.9%. The majority were also low-grade tumors. Survival is in general excellent, with 96% of stage I, 90% of stage II, 78% of stage III, and 70% of stage IV patients surviving 5 years. As with many other malignant diseases, the trend is toward more conservative surgery as adjuvant therapy has become more effective. The tumor marker CA-125 is found in many epithelial malignancies.

Adjuvant therapy, stage-related chemotherapy given in two to four drug combinations, has achieved 40% to 75% complete response in patients with advanced disease. The chemotherapy may be given intravenously and intraperitoneally. Most chemotherapeutic regimens contain platinum. Taxol has proven useful for those patients who are resistant to platinum-based chemotherapy.

STROMAL TUMORS

Stromal tumors include the androblastoma otherwise known as the Sertoli- Leydig cell tumor and the granulosa-theca cell tumors. These tumors are commonly hormonally active. Granulosa cell tumors are the most common cause of isosexual precocity in childhood. After menarche, they typically present with menstrual irregularity. They also may present with signs of peritonitis, ascites, or an abdominal or pelvic mass. Tumors are rarely bilateral. Surgical therapy consists of unilateral salpingo-oophorectomy with appropriate staging (Table 100-4). For disease that is truly confined to the resected ovary (stage 1A) resection should be curative. Response to chemotherapy and radiotherapy has been disappointing in more advanced tumors. Juvenile granulosa cell tumors differ in several ways from adult granulosa tumors. They are primarily prepubertal at presentation.

Androblastomas are less common. They most typically exhibit androgenic activity and thus present with hirsutism, severe acne, or deepening voice. Occasionally, these tumors exhibit no endocrine activity or, in rare situations, may produce estrogen or progesterone. They are typically 5 to 15 cm in diameter. They are usually cystic with irregular intraluminal papilla on ultrasound evaluation. Resection is usually curative for early disease.

Presentation

Ovarian tumors may present in various ways. Age at presentation may give some clue as to the type of tumor. Teratoma may occur at any age, whereas malignant germ cell tumors are rare before the age of 10 and have a median age at presentation of 13. This corresponds with the onset of puberty. The stromal tumors are more typically prepubertal at presentation and epithelial tumors increase in frequency with patient age.

The symptoms associated with tumors include pain, which is usually chronic and not severe. Occasionally, ovarian enlargement leads to torsion with acute severe lower abdominal pain. Premature menarche, pseudopregnancy, hirsutism, acne, and occasionally clitoromegaly and secondary amenorrhea may also be seen.

Evaluation should include thorough history and physical examination, including bimanual examination of the pelvis. In a virginal female this may be accomplished with one finger in the rectum and one on the abdomen. A nontender pelvic mass is often detectable in this fashion. An abdominal flat radiograph of the abdomen should be performed in the nonpregnant female. Often one will discover the characteristic calcifications associated with ovarian teratomas. Abdominal ultrasound examination is useful for noncalcified masses or clinical dilemmas.

FALLOPIAN TUBE, UTERUS, AND VAGINA

Fusion Defects

The paired müllerian ducts normally fuse to form a single upper vagina, cervix, and uterus. If this process is arrested, a spectrum of anomalies can result. In the uterus, complete failure of fusion results in uterus didelphys in which two separate hemiuteri form and lie side by side. Bicornuate uterus involves a single cervix with two uterine horns. A uterine septum may persist in situations where two ducts have fused but the common wall has failed to involute, with the mildest form termed *arcuate uterus*. A longitudinal vaginal septum often accompanies uterine fusion defects. Typically, these defects manifest with infertility and are not discovered in the pediatric age group. However, a significant number of the defects are asymmetrical and can be associated with obstruction of one or both systems. Such an obstruction may become evident in the neonatal period or at the time of puberty.

In situations where midline fusion is complete, atresias may result along the longitudinal axis. This may occur as a result of failure of recanalization of the vaginal plate or a primary failure of the müllerian anlage to reach the urogenital sinus. Manifestations include imperforate hymen, transverse vaginal septum, and cervical atresia.

Any of the obstructive syndromes may present in the neonatal period when circulating maternal estrogens are still high and withdrawal bleeding leads to distention of the obstructed structure. This distention occasionally may be severe and present with a large midline mass causing urinary obstruction. This requires urgent drainage to prevent permanent renal damage. More typically, the obstruction will manifest itself at the time of puberty with cyclic pain and a pelvic mass. In the case of an imperforate hymen or distal vaginal atresia, a bulging membrane may be seen within the introitus. The membrane appears bluish black due to shed menstrual blood. A cruciate incision is definitive therapy for an imperforate hymen. For a more proximal atresia, complete excision of the vaginal septum is necessary.

More proximal atresias of the vagina and particularly of the cervix are more difficult to deal with surgically. An abdominal perineal approach may be necessary. Hysterectomy is the most common treatment for a cervical atresia. However, if an adequate uterine cavity can be demonstrated with ultrasound or MRI, an operation to create a cervix and preserve the uterus can be performed. Some patients undergoing this procedure have given birth successfully.

In situations where a uterine septum obstructs one-half of the uterus, excision of the septum relieves symptoms. When uterine development is asymmetric, only one side of the bifid uterus may be obstructed. Open or laparoscopic resection of the obstructed uterine horn relieves the patient's symptoms without diminishing reproductive capacity.

Rokitansky-Kuster-Hauser Syndrome

In patients with a congenital absence of the vagina, a constellation of other defects is also present. Typically, the uterus is hypoplastic or atretic and in some patients is associated with shortness of stature, bony anomalies involving the spine, and sometimes deafness. Differentiation on physical examination between this condition and imperforate hymen may be difficult. Only at the time of puberty may the difference become evident with bulging of the hymen due to menstrual blood. Testicular feminization may show similar prepubertal findings. Ultrasound or MRI can establish the correct diagnosis. In the Rokitansky syndrome, the uterus is nonfunctional but the ovaries are normal. Puberty progresses normally but menses never commence. The atretic uterus does not possess a hormonally responsive endometrium, and so does not become distended and painful.

Treatment involves the creation of a vagina to permit normal sexual intercourse (7). Frank proposed the use of a series of dilators to both lengthen and widen the posterior depression in the vestibule. After many weeks, this depression may be of such a size as to permit satisfactory intercourse. Timing is important. By late adolescence, the patient is often motivated enough to perform 20-minute dilations three times each day. Adolescent tissues are elastic and dilate well.

Other patients require surgical creation of a vagina from a tubularized skin graft.

Alternative procedures involve vaginal creation from colon or cecum grafts. These grafts have the advantage of lesser scar contracture and do not require lubricants for intercourse. They have the disadvantage of continuous mucous production, which leads to soiling and odor.

Endometriosis

One possible cause of cyclic abdominal pain and dysmenorrhea in the adolescent female is endometriosis. Ectopic uterine endometrium enlarges and sheds in response to systemic LH and FSH. The endometrial tissue is found within the peritoneal cavity most typically, but may be found elsewhere. Whether this is a developmental problem originating with metaplasia of the coelomic epithelium or is due to expulsion of endometrium from the uterine tubes with subsequent implantation is unresolved. Endometriosis can be a sign of an obstructed uterine horn. Relief of the obstruction in this situation effectively treats the endometriosis. On occasion, endometriosis may be diagnosed with ultrasound, but more often laparoscopy or laparotomy is required to secure the diagnosis. Darkly pigmented lesions in the peritoneal surface are most often noted (5). Hormonal treatment with androgens, progesterone, Danazol, or GnRH agonists is often effective. Surgical treatment with excision or cautery may be necessary when hormonal treatments have failed.

Tumors

Tumors of the uterus and fallopian tube are quite rare in children. Cervical intraepithelial neoplasia and consequent cervical cancer have been linked to human papilloma virus (HPV) infections. Thus, they are found primarily in sexually active adolescents and adults.

Clear cell carcinomas are exceedingly rare tumors of the vagina and cervix. The majority of these tumors developed as a consequence of in utero exposure to diethylstilbestrol (DES) and certain other synthetic estrogens. Sixty percent of the lesions are vaginal and 40% are cervical. Treatment consists of local excision with adjuvant chemotherapy. Radiation is reserved for more aggressive advanced disease. Five- and 10-year survival for early lesions (stage I or stage II disease) approaches 80% to 90%. Ninety percent of patients present at such an early curable stage. Long-term follow-up is necessary to detect recurrence early.

Rhabdomyosarcoma of the female genital tract is the most common malignant tumor in this region. It differs from rhabdomyosarcomas of other sites by having generally favorable histology of the botryoidal type with infrequent nodal or metastatic disease. The treatment of these tumors has evolved over the last several years toward less aggressive surgical therapy. Chemotherapy with vincristine, dactinomycin, and cyclophosphamide (VAC) may lead to such impressive response that radical surgery is no longer required. Second-look surgery to obtain a complete response is now the standard treatment. In uterine primaries, hysterectomy is necessary, but preservation of the distal vagina and ovaries is possible.

VULVA

The vulva or external genitalia derive from the urogenital sinus and urogenital ridge. They include the labia majora, labia minora, clitoris, vestibule, and hymen. Abnormalities include ambiguous genitalia (see Chapter 101), labial fusion or agglutination, trauma, infections, and various dermatologic disorders.

Labial Fusion

True labial fusion is an uncommon intersex problem that is present from birth. A more common situation is that of labial agglutination, which is not present at birth but which can develop a month to a few years after birth. The development depends on atrophy of the labial epithelium as maternal estrogen stimulation is withdrawn. Clinically significant adhesions are present in 1% to 3% of girls with a peak incidence in the second year of life (8). Most instances of labial adhesion are self-limited and so require no treatment. Other cases are so severe as to result in urinary discomfort and occasionally urinary tract infection. In these cases, a more aggressive therapeutic approach is indicated.

Topical therapy with either Premarin or Estrace cream for no more than 3 weeks is often adequate to release the fusion. The estrogens stimulate the mucosa to proliferate and the gentle force of application lyses some of the adhesion with each application. This is effective in one-half of all cases. When hormonal therapy alone is not effective, surgical lysis may be necessary. Even after surgical lysis, recurrence is common. The incidence of recurrence may be reduced with perioperative application of hormone cream. In the absence of obstructive urinary problems and infection, multiple attempts at surgical lysis are not indicated.

Trauma

Vulvar trauma may be accidental, sports related, or the result of voluntary intercourse or sexual assault. Accidental injuries are likely to be confined to the vulva as the deeper structures are protected. The most common injury is a blunt injury to the labia from a fall. Ecchymoses, abrasions, and hematomas are typical. Occasionally, a midline tear may be sustained in an extreme straddle injury. Most of these injuries are self-limited. Even a sizable vulvar hematoma will resolve on its own given time. Acutely after the injury, an ice pack may be useful to prevent tissue swelling, which causes the major morbidity in the situation. In situations where the hematoma continues to grow despite conservative therapy, incision of the hematoma with ligation of the bleeding points might be necessary. Occasionally, a vulvar hematoma may be only the outward manifestation of a more serious deep injury such as a pelvic fracture.

Vulvar lacerations are often superficial and do not bleed substantially. When a laceration is deep, surgical repair may be necessary. Although blood loss from vulvar injury may be small, there may be enough bleeding into periurethral tissues to cause urethral spasm and urinary retention. Sitz baths may successfully relax the area to permit voiding. Urethral catheterization is necessary if the child is unable to void.

In situations where sexual abuse has caused injury the damage is often deep, involving the hymeneal ring and vagina. In the absence of deep injuries, diagnosis of abuse is less certain and relies as much upon history as upon physical findings.

Inflammations and Infections

The vulva is often the site for local skin infections that may range from diaper rash in the infant to streptococcal cellulitis and staphylococcal abscesses. Vulvar infections with Herpes simplex virus, HPV, and molluscum contagiosum may be related to sexual abuse.

Neoplasms

Neoplasms of the vulva are rare. More common in this area are hemangiomas or lymphangiomas. Hemangiomas typically resolve without therapy, lymphangiomas require resection. Lipomas may also be present in this area. Neurofibromatosis occasionally presents in the vulva. Premalignant lesions such as vulvar intraepithelial neoplasia may be found. These typically accompany cases of sexual abuse and HPV infection. Cases have been reported even in toddlers. Squamous cell carcinoma is exceedingly rare in children. Melanomas have occasionally been reported in the vulvar region.

VAGINAL BLEEDING

Vaginal bleeding requires investigation whenever it occurs in the prepubertal child. It may be caused by inflammatory conditions, trauma, or tumors.

Vulvovaginitis

The bleeding associated with vulvovaginitis is a secondary effect of scratching the perineum. The vulva and vagina are easily soiled in childhood, the mucosa is thin and does not offer much protection, and the acidic pH of the mature vagina is absent. Infections therefore are common in prepubertal girls. Evaluation will show a foul-smelling discharge with a considerable amount of redness originating near the vagina, sometimes extending into the perineum. Proper hygiene is preventive. Broad-spectrum antibiotics are curative. Topical estrogen for no more than 1 week may speed mucosal healing in extreme cases.

Foreign Bodies

Foreign bodies are often found as the cause of vaginal infection. Vaginoscopy is often necessary to remove objects such as wads of toilet paper, paper clips, and pen caps. Recurrence may be seen. Foreign bodies may also be associated with child abuse (9).

Urethral Prolapse

Occasionally, on genital examination a mass will be associated with bleeding. The most common bleeding mass in the area is a prolapsed urethra. The mass is typically small, edematous, and circular. The urethral orifice is seen to exit through the center of the mass. The mass is always anterior to the vagina. Minimal cases may resolve with topical estrogen therapy. However, many cases require resection of the prolapsed tissue.

Genital Tumors

Occasionally, bleeding hemangiomas are seen in the perineum. Bleeding from capillary hemangiomas is controllable with pressure. Cavernous hemangiomas sometimes require therapy when they are large and have failed to involute spontaneously. Cryotherapy, excision, or injection is effective. Alpha interferon has also been used with some success. Vaginal rhabdomyosarcomas present with bleeding and a visible tumor mass protruding into the vagina and occasionally into the vestibule. Treatment consists of chemotherapy followed by surgery as previously outlined.

Endometrial Bleeding

Occasionally, a child will present with vaginal bleeding that cannot be attributed to previously mentioned causes and may be the initial manifestation of precocious puberty. Hormonally induced bleeding is normal in the early neonatal period and after 10 years of age. All other instances require evaluation. Evaluation includes estrogen levels, GnRH stimulation test, pelvic ultrasound, or CT scans, and a CT scan of the head. Among adolescents, irregular anovulatory uterine bleeding is frequent in the first several years after menarche. It may take 5 years or more for the menstrual cycle to regularize. Nonetheless, increasingly irregular bleeding should be investigated. It may signify ectopic pregnancy, trophoblastic disease, or impending loss of pregnancy. Tumors, trauma, or infection are also possible. In rare cases, excessive bleeding may be related to coagulation disorders, liver, or renal failure. The patient's history is the best clue to whether an extensive workup is necessary.

SEXUALLY TRANSMITTED DISEASE

Sexually transmitted diseases (STDs) are fortunately rare in childhood. When present, they often signify sexual abuse. The converse is not true. Only in a small minority (3% to 4%) of abused girls will be found to have a STD. STDs are increasingly prevalent in adolescence. Goals are to make the diagnosis, determine the mode of acquisition, and treat the illness. The presentation may involve urethritis, vaginitis, cervicitis, genital lesions, pelvic inflammatory disease (PID), and systemic illness.

Epidemiology

In the United States, the traditional bacterial STDs (syphilis and gonorrhea) have become less prevalent since the mid-1990s. Chlamydia and the viral diseases, however, are increasing. Their prevalence now exceeds that of syphilis and gonorrhea. There is a substantial incidence of perinatal transmission of these diseases. Death from STDs has also increased. After decades of decreasing mortality attributable to sexually acquired infections, in less than a decade (1985–1992) STD-attributable deaths increased 31%.

The human immunodeficiency virus (HIV) or AIDS virus has grown in 25 years from a disease that affected primarily gay men and drug addicts to involve a large number of people from all walks of life (10). HIV seroprevalence among patients in STD clinics rose from .23% to more than 5% in the decade from 1979 to 1989. Male predominance has vanished. There has been a greater than 10-fold increase in the disease among teenagers. The rate is greater in blacks than in whites. The increase in STD-related deaths is largely due to heterosexually transmitted HIV (11).

All STDs have the same risk factors: early age at initiation of sex, multiple sexual partners, and inconsistent or nonuse of condoms. Also, use of oral contraceptives may alter the microenvironment of the cervix and vagina, increasing the risk of cervicitis and PID. Unfortunately, even consistent condom use is not effective in preventing HPV, chlamydia, and herpes simplex virus-2. Ignorance of the way these diseases are spread is a common finding in patients in STD clinics. Education can help control their spread, so efforts should be directed at teaching teenagers before they establish high-risk sexual behavior. Current treatment of sexually transmitted infection is summarized in Table 100-5.

Urethritis

Urethritis is a common finding in children and sexually active adolescents. The majority of cases are due to superficial infection with a common organism. Occasionally, gonorrhea or chlamydia are the infectious agents.

Vaginitis

Isolated vaginitis may be caused by hypersensitivity to laundry soap or bubble bath, or by a local infection of the vagina with bacterial organisms. Abnormal vaginal discharge is the most frequent presentation. Preadolescents are at increased risk for vaginitis because the vaginal epithelium is thin and vaginal pH is neutral. In this age group, the infection is polymicrobial and resolves with improved perineal hygiene, antibiotics, or short course topical estrogen therapy. Among adolescents, the causative organisms include candida, Gardnerella, and trichomonas. The appearance of candidal vaginitis is a reddened mucosa with curdlike plaques. Gardnerella discharge is thin and gray with a "fishy" odor and vaginal pH is elevated. Trichomonas is suspected when drainage is frothy and malodorous. The "strawberry cervix" is characteristic of this infection.

Genital Lesions

Lesions of the vulva and perineum often lead to surgical consultation. Perineal warts, which are raised and

TABLE 100-5 First-Line Therapy for Sexually Transmitted Diseases.[a]

Disease	Organism	Recommended Medication	Dose
Urethritis	*Neisseria gonorrhea*	Cefixime, ciprofloxacin, levofloxacin, or ofloxacin	Single oral dose
		Ceftriaxone	Single IM dose
	Chlamydia trachomatis	Azithromycin	Single oral dose
		Doxycycline	BID for 7 d
Vaginitis	*Candida* sp.	Fluconazole	Single oral dose
	Gardnerella, trichomonas	Metronidazole	QID for 7 d
Pelvic inflammatory disease		Cofotetan 2 g or	IV every 12 hr
		Cefoxitin 2 g	IV every 6 hr
		Plus	
		Doxycycline 100 mg	PO or IV every 12 hr for 14 d

[a]Dosage may need to be adjusted based on patient age and weight.
Adapted from Centers for Disease Control and Prevention. Sexually transmitted diseases treatment guidelines 2002, *MMWR* 2002;51 (no. RR-6):6–51.

polypoid, are signs of HPV infection. A chancre or sessile warts, condyloma lata, signify syphilis. Small vesicles that may become confluent connote genital herpes. These are painful or pruritic. The presence of each of these infections in a child is often secondary to abuse. In adolescents, consensual sex is becoming a more frequent source.

Papilloma Virus Infection

HPV is a common STD. Infection with HPV is typically asymptomatic. Prolonged infection is associated with the development of cervical intraepithelial neoplasia and carcinoma. Two strains of HPV—HPV-16 and HPV-18—can occur. Presently, HPV-16 is the more prevalent strain, whereas HPV-18 is associated with poorer prognosis tumors (12).

Pelvic Inflammatory Disease

The classic triad of low abdominal pain, cervical motion tenderness, and adnexal tenderness are the *sine qua non* of PID. These signs and symptoms are often accompanied by fever, leukocytosis, and elevated erythrocyte sedimentation rate. There may or may not be a vaginal discharge noted. Culdocentesis may show white blood cells and microorganisms. The infections are typically polymicrobial and may not have the same organisms as are present in vaginal or cervical cultures. Cultures should be obtained, but should not limit antibiotic therapy.

Patients most at risk for PID have multiple sexual partners, are younger than 25, have a history of previous gonorrheal or candidal cervicitis or PID, cannot afford care, and have delayed coming to medical attention. Many adolescents fall into these categories. The Centers for Disease Control and Prevention's hospitalization criteria for PID include adolescent age group, uncertainty in diagnosis (rule out appendicitis), suspected pregnancy, concurrent HIV infection, severe illness with nausea and vomiting, inability to tolerate therapy or failure to respond as an outpatient, and inability to follow up in 72 hours. In PID that is complicated by abscess, percutaneous or surgical drainage leads to quicker resolution of symptoms and shorter overall hospitalization.

Systemic Infection

Syphilis and HIV are systemic infections shortly following acquisition. Syphilis manifests with a local, painless ulcer, a chancre, at the site of infection, but soon the total body rash of secondary syphilis appears. If treatment is delayed, the central nervous system may be affected. Therapy is directed at prevention of this latter stage.

HIV attacks T lymphocytes and vastly compromises the host's ability to fight infection. Coexisting HIV infection necessitates prolonging the course of treatment for other STDs. Contact with blood or bodily secretions may transmit the infection. Various studies estimate the rate of transmission between 1 in 100 to 1 in 1,000 exposures. Current control measures include celibacy, barrier contraception with condoms, and experimental virucidal agents. Treatment of the disease involves drug therapy directed against the virus, as well as prevention and treatment of opportunistic infections. The majority of antiviral agents interfere with reverse transcriptase to slow viral propagation. There is evidence that treatment of pregnant HIV carriers and their newborn children may reduce the likelihood of infection in those children.

Prevention of Sexually Transmitted Disease

Although abstinence is the only certain means of preventing STD infection, it is not a realistic public health policy. Adolescents are often not motivated to abstain, so intervention must aim at reducing the risk of the sexual activity that occurs. Condom usage is effective at reducing the risk of acquisition of chlamydia, gonorrhea, trichomonas, and HIV. Unfortunately, condoms offer inadequate protection from HPV, HSV-2, syphilis, and chancroid. Vaccination may become the mainstay of prevention of papillomavirus infection, but is not currently available.

Counseling on a one-on-one basis has a far greater impact than simple didactic presentations and seems to be the chief factor in whether a program will succeed. Counseling has been performed in schools and STD clinics. The benefit has been a 20% to 30% reduction in future STD infections among counseled adolescents (13,14).

Testing for Sexually Transmitted Disease

The gold standard test for STD is the pelvic examination with cervical swabbing. It is effective, but also labor intensive, expensive, and uncomfortable for the patient. More recently, two other methodologies have been found effective. Self-collected vaginal swabs and first void urine testing are now available. Although they are not as sensitive as pelvic exam, they are far more acceptable to patients. In Smith et al.'s study, all patients chose vaginal swabs over pelvic examination (15), and Serlin et al. found a marked preference for first void urine culture (16). Greater patient acceptance and lower costs are likely to more than compensate for the small decrease in sensitivity of these tests.

SEXUAL ABUSE

There is a growing recognition of sexual abuse of children. The abused child may be either a male or female, although females outnumber males by two to four times. It is the responsibility of the physician who is examining and treating abuse victims to know and understand the laws within his or her state to best protect the welfare of the abused child.

History

When a sexual assault is suspected, a careful history of what has happened should be obtained. Ideally, the victim should be interviewed in a safe, comfortable environment in terms that he or she might understand. Care should be taken to avoid putting words in the child's mouth. Open-ended, nondirective questioning is preferable. Particularly in young children, the verbal skills necessary to adequately describe the act may be missing. Anatomically correct dolls may be used to help the child be more specific. Because abuse is often not a single isolated assault, the interviewer should ask questions to establish a relationship between the attacker and victim.

Physical Examination

The physical examination begins with observation of the child during the interview. The examination includes a complete skin examination looking for bite or suction marks, examination of the oral cavity for signs of trauma, and lastly, examination of the perineum and pelvis. In many instances, adequate examination may be obtained in a doctor's office or emergency room. In the less frequent cases where penetration of the anus or vagina is suspected or discovered, an examination under general anesthesia is necessary to establish and treat deeper injuries. Acutely after an assault, one may see findings ranging from contusions, ecchymoses, and hematomas to superficial and deep lacerations. If the time between abuse and examination is prolonged, the findings are likely to be more subtle. These may involve healing or healed tears of the posterior fourchette, hymen, vagina, and anus. Often, a late physical examination will show no signs of physical abuse.

Because there are no well-defined criteria to classify the physical findings, detailed description with drawings is advised. Nonspecific abnormalities suggestive of abuse include redness of the genitalia, increased vascularity in the vestibule and labial mucosa, vaginal discharge, and small mucosal tears. McCann et al. (17), in examining 93 unabused girls, found erythema in 56%, labial adhesions in 40%, and superficial posterior forchette injuries in 25% of patients.

Foreign bodies in the vagina of prepubertal girls may be a marker of sexual abuse. In 12 girls seen by Herman-Giddens (9) with vaginal foreign bodies, 8 were confirmed victims of abuse and, in 3, abuse was suspected.

Specific findings strongly suggestive of abuse include deep lacerations of the hymen and vagina, proctoepisiotomy, teeth marks in the perineum, and laboratory confirmation of STD. The presence of sperm or pregnancy is definitive.

The examination should be considered incomplete if any forensic evidence is overlooked. This includes a collection of specimens that may be later used as evidence (Table 100-6). All specimens should be handled as specified by law and the rules of evidence. This usually requires proper labeling with patient identification, specimen, site from which the specimen was collected, the date and time collected, and the initials of the examiner. Specimens should be placed into containers and sealed appropriately. If local laws require, they should be processed by police laboratory.

Now that HIV is a pathogen found in the community at large, it is advisable to test sexual assault victims with HIV cultures or serology. Local laws often require consent prior to HIV testing. These should be obtained at the time of the assault and 6 months later. In the rare instances where HIV infection occurs, additional therapy should be directed toward this life-threatening illness. HIV prophylaxis can also

TABLE 100-6 The Forensic Evaluation: Specimens To Be Collected.

General
Outer and underclothing worn during or immediately following the assault
Fingernail scrapings
Dried or moist secretions and foreign material on the body, anus, and genital area
Use Wood lamp to detect semen
Oral cavity
Swabs for semen (2) within 6 hours of assault
Culture for gonorrhea (GC) and other sexually transmitted diseases (STDs)
Saliva—for reference
Genital area
Dried and moist secretions and foreign material
Comb pubic hair; collect all loose hair and foreign material
Vaginal swabs (3)
Wet mounts
Dry mount slides (2)
Culture for gonorrhea (GC) chlamydia and other STDs
Anus
Dried and moist secretions and foreign material
Rectal swabs (two)
Dry mount slides (two)
Culture for GC and other STDs
Blood
Blood type
RPR (syphilis serology)
Pregnancy test (blood or urine)
Alcohol/toxicology evaluation (blood or urine)
Urine
Urinalysis
Pregnancy test (blood or urine)
Alcohol/toxicology evaluation (blood or urine)
Other
Saliva (use clean gauze or filter paper)
Head hair (cut and remove)
Pubic hair (cut and remove)

Adapted from Muram D. Child sexual abuse. In: Sanfilippo JS, Muram D, Lee PA, et al., eds. *Pediatric and adolescent gynecology*. Philadelphia: WB Saunders, 1994:376, with permission.

be recommended when the perpetrator is known to have HIV.

Treatment

The treatment of sexual assault injuries should follow the general principles of wound care. Superficial injuries may be managed with Sitz baths; deep injuries require operative repair with absorbable suture. All bite wounds and wounds older than 6 to 12 hours should be treated as dirty in open fashion with irrigation and debridement.

Antibiotics are used as appropriate to treat the wound, but prophylaxis for STD is not recommended. If an STD is found, the treatment consists of coverage for the identified organism and the common copathogens chlamydia and gonorrhea.

Treatment also involves prevention of further abuse by removing the child from the site of abuse. Psychological sequelae of abuse often require psychotherapy. In most areas, therapists are available who have been trained to help the child and the family deal with the trauma of the event, as well as with the demands of the examination, medical treatment, and investigative interviews by Child Protective Services and law enforcement agencies.

IMAGING

Some of the major advances in the care of female genital disorders have been possible because of advances in noninvasive imaging. Color flow Doppler and transvaginal ultrasound have made it possible to determine the function and fine structure of uterine and adnexal masses. Spiral CT allows examination of the abdomen and pelvis without the need for deep general anesthesia. MRI enables surgeons to know in advance the structure of a congenital duplication or atresia without laparotomy.

In the neonate, radiologic imaging is needed for three reasons: (1) confirmation of a prenatal finding, (2) investigation of a palpable abdominal mass, or (3) evaluation of a child with ambiguous genitalia. In most situations, an ultrasound examination will provide the needed information (18). A prenatally diagnosed cyst must be characterized after birth as simple or complex and measured. If the cyst is small and without internal echoes, it should be followed with regular examinations to ensure its resolution as estrogen levels fall. A palpable abdominal mass should be studied with ultrasound and treated similarly. Whenever a cyst is excessively large or complex, operative intervention is indicated. A suspected vaginal atresia or uterine anomaly should be studied with ultrasound or MRI to define the anomaly and provide a roadmap for surgical repair.

Evaluation of the child with ambiguous genitalia is a pediatric emergency. Imaging should discern the presence of ovaries or testes, and determine whether the uterus is normal, atretic, or absent. Ultrasound can answer all these questions.

The older child requires evaluation for (1) precocious puberty, (2) tumor or mass, (3) abdominal pain, and (4) vaginal discharge. The imaging in precocious puberty involves measuring the size of each ovary and the uterus, looking for both a source and the effect of elevated hormonal levels. This may be performed with ultrasound, but CT or MRI scans are more efficient because they allow better visualization of the adrenal glands. An abdominal mass that is mobile is most likely a teratoma at this age. Plain films or ultrasound are sufficient to establish this diagnosis. Other tumors, such as a pelvic rhabdomyosarcoma, are best visualized with MRI. Local extent, invasion of surrounding structures, and metastases can be seen quite readily. Tissue planes are more easily seen than with CT. Sagittal views show the extent of invasion more clearly.

The evaluation of abdominal pain involves differentiation between ovarian cysts, adnexal torsion, abscess, and appendicitis. Adnexal torsion may be suspected because of the acute onset of pain in the lower abdomen. Ultrasound shows an enlarged, lucent, or complex ovary. CT and MRI add little to this information and are rarely indicated. Color flow Doppler may show diminished or absent flow to the involved ovary, with minimal signal within the mass. The symptomatic child with a positive scan should be explored promptly.

Vaginal discharge, if chronic and watery, may signify a wolffian duct anomaly with ectopic ureteral entry into the vagina, often at Gartner's duct. Intravenous urography may be the most efficient evaluation of this phenomenon. Ultrasound often shows renal dysplasia and may show ureteral or vaginal dilation.

In the adolescent, primary or secondary amenorrhea, pregnancy, STD, and malignant ovarian tumors are the common problems. Primary amenorrhea may be due to gonadal dysgenesis, testicular feminization syndrome, Rokitansky-Kuster-Hauser syndrome, or a vaginal atresia. In the first instance, small gonads with müllerian structures present or absent are seen; in the second, no ovarian tissue or müllerian structure is present; and in the third, ovaries are normal, but the müllerian structures are atretic. Ultrasound may establish the etiology, but MRI is advisable when Rokitansky syndrome or other atresia is suspected.

Ultrasound of the pelvis is the initial test needed to evaluate the potentially pregnant patient. An intrauterine pregnancy may be seen and dated. For suspected ectopic pregnancy, transvaginal ultrasound with color Doppler is a better modality. Resolution and sensitivity are increased among patients who can accommodate the probe.

PID is a clinical diagnosis, the treatment of which is antimicrobial. Ultrasound shows blurring of the tissue planes, adnexal enlargement, and pelvic fluid. Follow-up scans performed for failure to improve often show abscesses that require drainage. Percutaneous drainage may be guided by ultrasound or CT.

Ovarian masses in the adolescent should be first evaluated by ultrasound. Simple cysts may be followed with ultrasound. MRI or CT are helpful if malignancy is suspected. They can show the local extent of disease and screen for metastases.

ENDOSCOPY

Infertility, pelvic pain, endometriosis, and neoplasia may be evaluated and treated in many cases without "open" surgery. Tubal pregnancy may be treated with coagulation, segmental excision, linear salpingotomy, tubal aspiration, or salpingectomy. Ovaries may be biopsied, cysts may be aspirated, and torsed ovaries may be untorsed and pexed or excised. The procedure has aided in the differentiation of appendicitis and PID.

Laparoscopy of the prepubertal female typically requires two ports. One port is used for viewing and insufflation, and the other is used for manipulation of the pelvic viscera. For large procedures, an additional port may be necessary for insertion of instruments. In older adolescents, manipulation may be performed by means of a uterine cannula or mobilizer inserted transvaginally. The use of a cannula is contraindicated when uterine anomalies prevent safe access via the cervix and when intrauterine pregnancy is suspected (19).

Vaginoscopy can be performed with a small flexible scope in very small patients in the office or with light sedation. It can be a useful adjunct to MRI in evaluating atresias of the vagina and cervix.

REFERENCES

1. Skandalakis JE, Gray SW, Parrott TS, et al. Ovary and testis. In: Skandalakis JE, Gray SW, eds. *Embryology for surgeons,* 2nd ed. Baltimore: Williams & Wilkins, 1994:736.
2. Gray SW, Skandalakis JE, Broecker BH. Female reproductive system. In: Skandalakis JE, Gray SW, eds. *Embryology for surgeons,* 2nd ed. Baltimore: Lippincott Williams & Wilkins, 1994:816.
3. Coucouvanis EC, Jones PP. Changes in proto-oncogene expression correlated with general and sex-specific differentiation in murine primordial germ cells. *Mech Dev* 1993;42:49–58.
4. Ablin A, Isaacs H. Germ cell tumors. In: Pizzo PA, Poplack DG, eds. *Principles and practice of pediatric oncology,* 2nd ed. Philadelphia: Lippincott Williams & Wilkins, 1993:867.
5. Zurawin RK, Sanfilippo J, Bacon J, et al. Advanced surgical techniques in the pediatric and adolescent patient. *J Pediatr Adolesc Gynecol* 2002:183–191.
6. Rodriguez M, Nguyen HN, Averette HE, et al. National survey of ovarian carcinoma XII: epithelial ovarian malignancies in women less than or equal to 25 years of age. *Cancer* 1994;73:1245–1250.
7. Frank RT. The formation of an artificial vagina without operation. *Am J Obstet Gynecol* 1938;140:867–873.
8. Muram D. Treatment of prepubertal girls with labial adhesions. *J Pediatr Adolesc Gynecol* 1999;12:67–70.
9. Herman-Giddens ME. Vaginal foreign bodies and child sexual abuse. *Arch Pediatr Adolesc Med* 1994;148:195–200.
10. Quinn TC, Groseclose SL, Spence M, et al. Evolution of the human immunodeficiency virus epidemic among patients attending sexually transmitted disease clinics: a decade of experience. *J Infect Dis* 1992;165:541–544.
11. Ebrahim SH, Peterman TA, Zaidi AA, et al. Mortality related to sexually transmitted diseases in US women, 1973 through 1992. *Am J Public Health* 1997;87:938–944.
12. Schwartz SM, Daling JR, Shera KA, et al. Human papillomavirus and prognosis of invasive cervical cancer: a population based study. *J Clin Oncol* 2001;19(7):1906–1915.
13. Margolis HS, Handsfield HH, Jacobs RJ, et al. Evaluation of office-based intervention to improve prevention counseling for patients at risk for sexually acquired hepatitis B virus infection. Hepatitis B-WARE Study Group. *Am J Obstet Gynecol* 2000;182(1 pt 1):1–6.
14. Kamb ML, Fishbein M, Douglas JM Jr, et al. Efficacy of risk-reduction counseling to prevent human immunodeficiency virus and sexually transmitted diseases: a randomized controlled trial. Project RESPECT Study Group. *JAMA* 1998;280(13):1161–1167.

15. Smith K, Harrington K, Wingood G, et al. Self-obtained vaginal swabs for diagnosis of treatable sexually transmitted diseases in adolescent girls. *Arch Pediatr Adolesc Med* 2001;155(6):676–679.
16. Serlin M, Shafer MA, Tebb K, et al. What sexually transmitted disease screening method does the adolescent prefer? Adolescents' attitudes toward first-void urine, self-collected vaginal swab, and pelvic examination. *Arch Pediatr Adolesc Med* 2002;156(6):588–591.
17. McCann J, Wells R, Voris J. Genital findings in prepubertal girls selected for nonabuse: a descriptive study. *Pediatrics* 1990;86:428–439.
18. Teele RL, Share JC. Ultrasonography of the female pelvis in childhood and adolescence. *Radiol Clin North Am* 1992;30:743–758.
19. Gomel V, Taylor PJ, Yuzpe AA, et al. *Laparoscopy and hysteroscopy in gynecologic practice*. Chicago: Year Book Medical, 1986.

Chapter 101

Intersex States

Pramod P. Reddy, William R. DeFoor, and Curtis A. Sheldon

There are very few conditions in the practice of medicine that are as highly emotionally charged as is the topic of intersex. Almost every aspect related to intersex conditions, especially the role of the physicians and parents in gender assignment are controversial. Over the past few years, the philosophy that has guided the management of these conditions has been the center of an ongoing debate as to what is the best option from the patients' perspective. In spite of the ongoing controversies, physicians caring for a child born with ambiguous genitalia and its parents have to ensure the child receives appropriate evaluation and that the parents are given the opportunity to make an informed and educated choice with regard to gender selection. Options should include the choice of no intervention until the child is old enough to participate in its own care.

Nowhere in the craft of surgery does an in-depth understanding of the pertinent basic sciences contribute so greatly to one's approach to diagnosis and therapy as in the surgical management of intersex states. This complex discipline requires prompt and accurate decision making with regard to one of the most important determinants of a child's future, his or her sex of rearing.

The social impact of giving birth to a child with ambiguous genitalia is overwhelming to the family and must be approached with reassurance and compassion and considered a social emergency (often coexisting conditions can also render this condition a medical emergency). The parents are immediately faced with the first question asked of any new parent: Is it a boy or a girl? Extensive guidance is necessary from the outset in helping the parents cope with the pressures applied by family and friends.

Once the initial dilemma has been addressed, the parents and a multidisciplinary team of physicians (that includes neonatologists, pediatric endocrinologists, obstetricians, pediatric reconstructive surgeons, geneticists, psychologists, and radiologists) must address multiple issues related to potential adverse sequelae, life-threatening metabolic complications, the risk of malignancy, the potential impact of inadequate genitalia, the psychological impact of the diagnosis on the child with maturation, and finally, the risk that further children may be born with similar malformations. After completion of the evaluation, a family care conference with the family is essential; the family is presented with all the data and the consensus recommendation of the team is offered. However, it is the parents who must ultimately decide the gender assignment for their child.

Pramod P. Reddy, William R. DeFoor, and Curtis A. Sheldon: Division of Pediatric Urology, Cincinnati Children's Hospital Medical Center, University of Cincinnati, Cincinnati, Ohio 45229.

DEVELOPMENT OF SEXUAL CHARACTERISTICS

The sex of an individual may be defined by a number of criteria; however, there are three main criteria that determine the gender of an individual. These include:

- *Genetic sex (chromosomal sex).* Determined at fertilization, based on the nature of the sperm (X or Y) fertilizing the ovum. XX is considered female genetic sex, and XY is considered male genetic sex.
- *Gonadal sex.* The genetic sex determines the differentiation of the undifferentiated gonadal ridge into either testis (in the presence of a Y chromosome) or ovaries (the default state, in the absence of a Y chromosome)
- *Phenotypic sex.* The developing gonads synthesize various hormones that drive the development of the external genitalia (phenotypic sex).

Of these, the most important is the phenotypic sex, for this alone determines whether an individual can experience adequate sexual intercourse and often determines if healthy, nurturing adult relationships are achievable.

The genetic considerations upon which the current understanding of mammalian sexual differentiation is based were originally described by Alfred Jost. Anomalies of chromosomal composition may profoundly influence sexual development and are best understood with reference to the biology of cell division, which has been reviewed in detail by Simpson and Rebar (1) and Grumbach and Conte (2). The complex nature of cell division also provides potential for the generation of chromosomal anomalies. Common abnormalities in chromosomal number include aneuploidy and mosaicism. *Aneuploidy* refers to any deviation from the expected number of chromosomes. Proposed mechanisms include meiotic or mitotic nondisjunction and anaphase lag. Nondisjunction during meiosis results in aneuploid gametes; with fertilization, the resultant zygote is aneuploid, with an identical chromosomal constitution in all cells. Nondisjunction during mitosis produces two or more cell lines in the zygote, which is referred to as *mosaicism* (3). Aneuploid states associated with abnormal sexual development include 47,XXY (Klinefelter syndrome), 45,X (Turner syndrome), and 45,X/46,XY mosaicism associated with gonadal dysgenesis. The existence of two or more cell lines within an individual is termed *chimerism*. Presumably, 46,XX/46,XY and 46,XX/47,XXY true hermaphroditism may arise from mosaicism or chimerism. Structural chromosomal abnormalities are not uncommon and include *deletions* (loss of any part of a chromosome), *translocations* (the transfer of chromosomal material from one chromosome to another), *isochromosomes* (chromosomes with identical arms, arising from horizontal rather than vertical centromere division), *dicentric chromosomes* (a chromosome with two centromeres), *ring chromosomes*, and *duplications*. 46,XX sex-reversed males and 46,XX true hermaphrodites may represent examples of translocation of Y chromosomal material, whereas 46,XY sex-reversed females may represent examples of deletion of Y chromosomal material. An isochromosome involving the long arm of the X chromosome, 46,X,i(Xq), may be associated with gonadal dysgenesis, whereas dicentric chromosomes are occasionally seen in 45,X/46,XY mosaicism. On a molecular level, alterations in DNA sequence may result in sufficient genetic alteration to compromise gene product function and produce abnormal sexual development (4) (Table 101-1).

TABLE 101-1 Chromosomal Location of Genes Pertinent to Sexual Development.

Chromosome	*Location*	*Gene Product*
1	Short arm (*1p13–p11*)	3β-Hydroxysteroid dehydrogenase
6	Short arm (*6p21.3*)	21α-Hydroxylase
8	Long arm (*8q21–q22*)	11β-Hydroxylase
10	—	17α-Hydroxylase, 17,20-lyase
15	—	Side-chain cleavage enzyme
19	Short arm (*19p13.3*)	Antimüllerian hormone
X	Short arm (*Xq12*)	Dihydrotestosterone (DHT) receptor
Y	Short arm (*Yp11.3*)	Testis-determining factor

Every individual begins with common, indifferent gonadal and genital primordia. An inherent tendency to feminize dominates unless specific developmental influences are present to direct male morphogenesis. Three specific but closely interrelated developmental sequences are required for normal sexual development, each governed by unique embryologic influences. These are gonadal, genital ductal, and external genitalia development. By weeks 5 to 7, the chromosomal sex determines the gonadal sex through a cascade of molecular events that have been extensively studied since the mid-1950s and understood since the mid-1990s. Because the presence of the Y chromosome was associated with the development of testis, it was extensively studied to identify the testis determining factor (TDF). A variety of candidates were believed to be the definitive TDF; these included the H-Y antigen and Zinc-finger Y gene (ZFY). The discovery of the sex determining region of the Y chromosome (SRY gene) in humans and mice in 1990 has provided the most likely candidate to date for the TDF (5,6). The role of the SRY gene was confirmed by experiments performed by Koopman et al. in 1991, in which a 14-kb DNA fragment from the SRY gene was inserted into the genome of female mouse embryos; these mice then developed into males (7,8).

The SRY gene is located on the Y chromosome, between the ZFY gene and the pseudoautosomal region, comprising of a single exon containing 237 bp. The SRY gene functions as a transcription factor and is believed to stimulate other genes that are required for testicular development and the determination of male gonadal sex by unraveling the DNA double helix. There are other genes that play a role in determining the gonadal differentiation at the various stages. These include genes that act on the intermediate mesoderm and cause it to differentiate into the indifferent gonad [i.e., WT-1 gene (9), DAX-1 gene (Dss-Ahc critical region of X chromosome) (10)] and genes that have two sites of action (both at the level of the intermediate mesoderm and the indifferent gonad) steroidogenic factor-1 (SF-1) (11,12), and SOX-9 gene (13,14). These genes in addition to the SRY gene are all expressed at various stages of development of the urogenital ridge.

Strong evidence exists to suggest that other genes are required to affect testicular organogenesis, with both X chromosomal and autosomal influences implicated. These could be involved in *SRY* regulation or could be downstream targets of *SRY*. Data exist to suggest that some 46,XX males and 46,XX true hermaphrodites may in fact be negative for *SRY* (15–18). In addition, individuals with

46,XY gonadal dysgenesis are reported with present and unaltered *SRY* sequences (19–22). Such determinations are difficult to interpret; however, given the observations that potentially undetected mosaicism with a Y-bearing cell line may explain some cases of 46,XX males (15) and that postzygotic *SRY* mutations in portions of gonadal tissue may result in 46,XY true hermaphroditism (23). Vilain and colleagues (24) analyzed the histologic findings in a series of patients with 46,XY gonadal dysgenesis. Individuals with streak gonads composed of exclusively ovarian-like stroma were found to have *SRY* mutations, whereas those with streak gonads containing undifferentiated stroma harboring either tubules or a rete structure had no detectable mutation in the *SRY* gene.

In the absence of a Y chromosome, ovarian differentiation generally occurs. However, the X chromosomes play a critical role in ovarian organogenesis. Individuals with monosomy X (45,X) demonstrate early ovarian development. In the absence of a second X chromosome, oocytes usually do not survive meiosis, and folliculogenesis fails to occur or is defective. The result is dysgenetic (streak) gonads. Because similar events are noted for individuals with deletion of either the short or long arm of the X chromosome, both arms are believed to contain important ovarian maintenance determinants. As reviewed by Simpson and Rebar (1), individuals with deletions in the *Xp11.2–11.4* and *Xq11.3–21* regions create a high risk for primary amenorrhea. Deletions in the *Xp21* and *Xq25–26* regions also cause significant ovarian dysfunction. In each instance, the more proximal region is where the most critical genes are located.

A unique event occurs involving the X chromosome, the formation of the *Barr body*. In 1949, Barr and Bertram described a chromatin mass located at the periphery of the nucleus and found in female but not in male cells (25,26). In the past, this observation was used clinically to help suggest an infant's chromosomal content and aid in the evaluation of intersex states. An analysis of buccal mucosal smears was employed. A female 46,XX karyotype was generally associated with at least a 20% identification rate of Barr bodies within the nuclei (*chromatin-positive*). Barr bodies are also identifiable in 47,XXY males, and multiple Barr bodies may be identified in both males and females with more than two X chromosomes. Conversely, a relative absence of Barr bodies implied a 46,XY karyotype, but could also be seen in individuals with 45,X and 45,X/46,XY. Such individuals are referred to as *chromatin-negative*.

Gonadal Development

Early in embryogenesis, the gonads of both sexes are both *indifferent* and *bipotential*. Germ cells are identifiable in the dorsal endoderm of the yolk sac near the origin of the allantois. During weeks 4 and 5 of gestation, they migrate along the dorsal mesentery of the hindgut to the gonadal ridges. Invasion of the underlying mesoderm during week 6 allows them to become incorporated into the developing primary sex cords. These events are depicted in Fig. 101-1. At approximately 40 days of gestation, divergent gonadal differentiation becomes evident (27) (Fig. 101-2).

In the human testis, seminiferous cords are differentiated by 7 weeks. Differentiation of the supporting cells is observed during weeks 8 to 11. *Sertoli cells* demonstrate ultrastructural evidence of intense protein biosynthesis as early as 8 weeks. The product of this biosynthesis would appear to be the müllerian inhibiting substance (MIS) as evidenced by the observation of coincident regression of müllerian ducts and the detection of MIS in the rough endoplasmic reticulum (28). The multipotent Sertoli cell is also believed to secrete *inhibin* [provides negative feedback for follicle-stimulating hormone (FSH) secretion], *activin* (provides positive feedback for FSH secretion), and *follistatin* (provides inhibition of FSH release), and in addition is believed to nurture the germ cells and is postulated to prevent meiosis, possibly by the production of a meiosis-inhibiting substance.

Similarly, *Leydig cells* acquire ultrastructural features that suggest active steroid synthesis as early as 8 weeks, coincident with the onset of testosterone formation and metabolism in the human fetus (29,30). Human chorionic gonadotropin (hCG)-luteinizing hormone (LH) cell membrane receptors are detected by week 12 of gestation (31,32). Peak testosterone levels in the human fetus circulation is reached at approximately 16 weeks (31,33). It is suggested that hCG secreted by the syncytiotrophoblast stimulates testosterone secretion during this critical period of male sexual development (34). The dependence of fetal testosterone biosynthesis on placental hCG has, however, been brought into question (32,35).

In the female fetus, ovigerous cords are noted during week 7 (27). Oogonia are surrounded by cuboidal cells with long overlapping cytoplasmic processes that are believed to be precursors of granulosa cells. This early cytologic differentiation is matched by the ability of the human fetal ovary to aromatize androgens, documented as early as 8 weeks of gestational age (36). Similar to the Sertoli cell, the granulosa cell is found to produce inhibin, activin, and follistatin. In contrast, however, the fetal ovary does not contain hCG receptors nor detectable quantities of MIS.

Development of the Internal Genital Ductal Systems

The development of the genital ductal systems and urinary tract has several critical anatomic and functional correlates. Figure 101-3 diagrammatically depicts these events. From the intermediate mesoderm arises the nephrogenic cord from which the *mesonephros* (the temporary kidney) and *metanephros* (the permanent kidney) develop. Cranially, the nephrogenic cord gives rise to the mesonephros

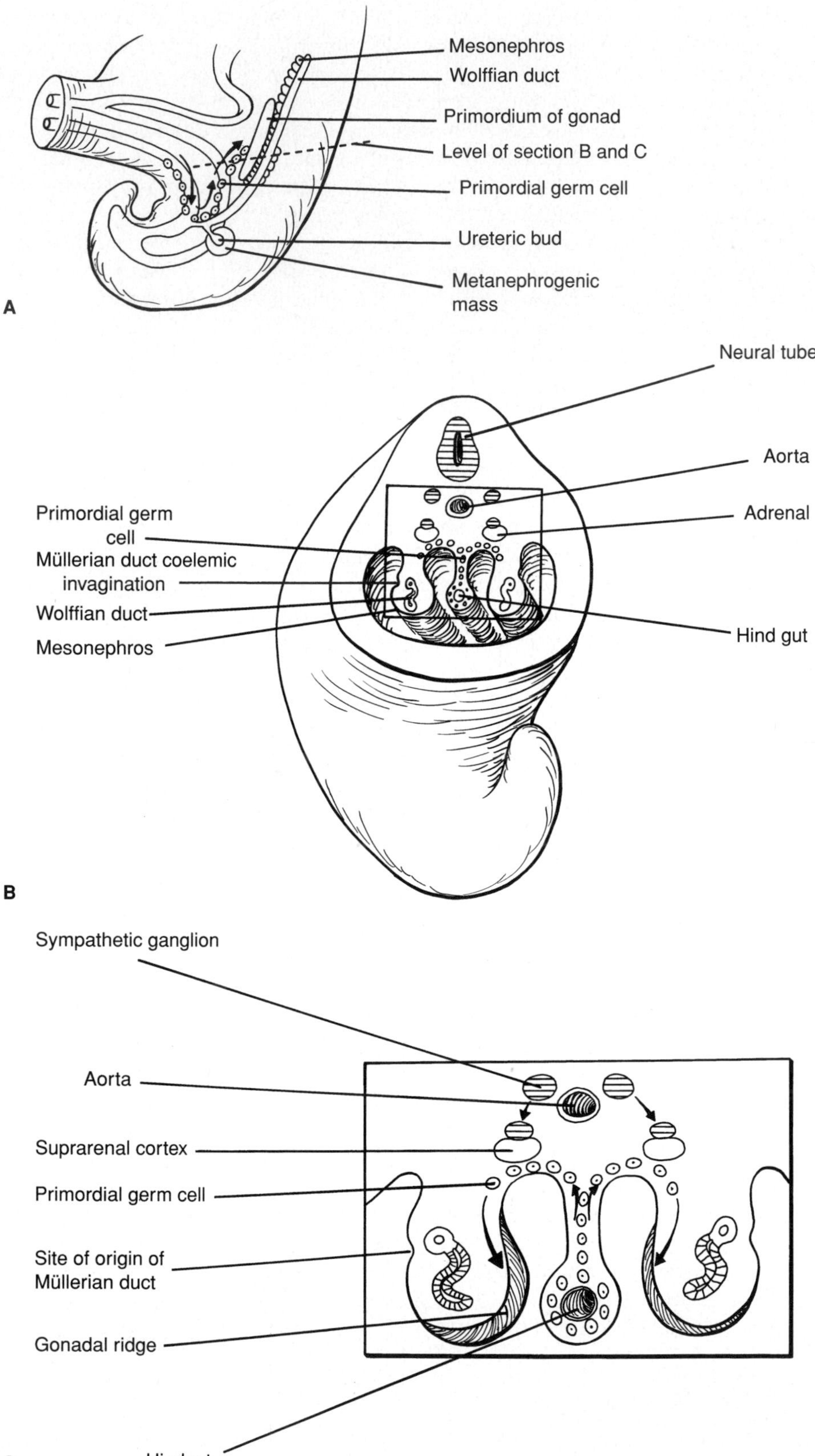

FIGURE 101-1. **(A)** Migration of primordial germ cells in 5-week embryo. **(B, C)** Transverse views of germ cell migration. **(D)** Six-week embryo with developing müllerian ducts and primary sex cords. **(E)** Further development of the müllerian and wolffian ducts as well as the primary sex cords. Arrows indicate primordial germ cell migration. (From Moore KL. *The developing human: clinically oriented embryology,* 3rd ed. Philadelphia: WB Saunders, 1982:271, with permission.)

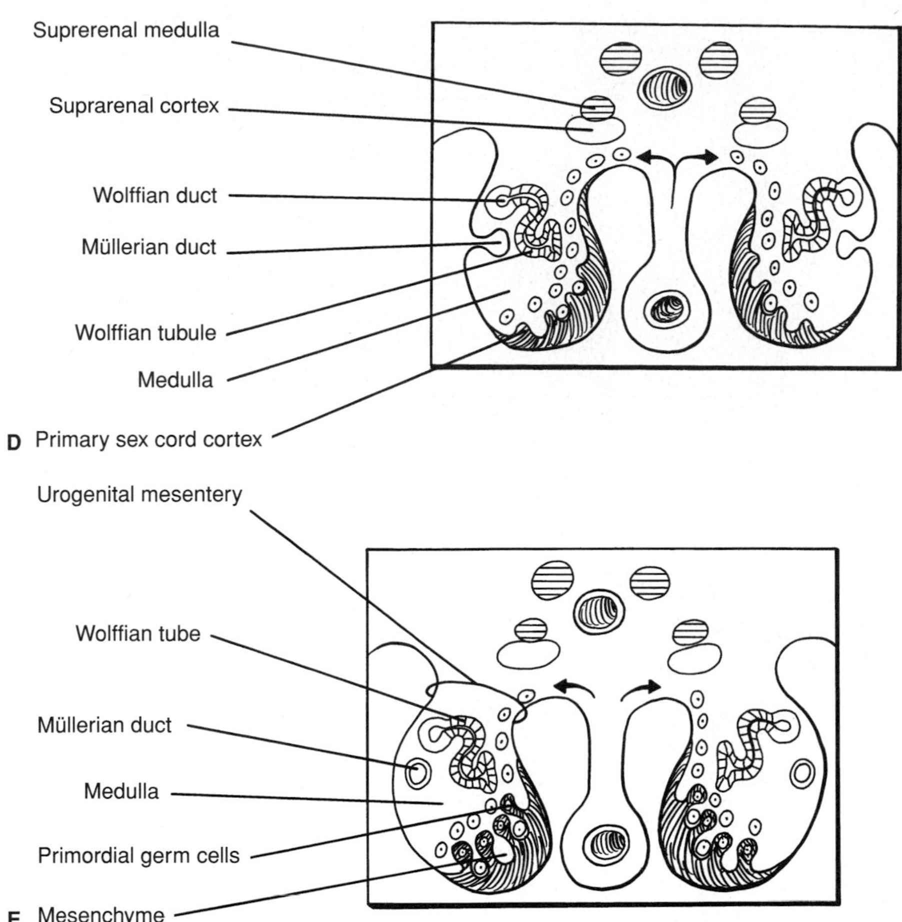

FIGURE 101-1. *(Continued)*

as mesonephric vesicles develop that are connected by mesonephric tubules to the mesonephric duct. The latter develops initially as a solid rod beneath the surface ectoderm, ultimately opening into the developing cloaca. Within the mesonephros, tufts of capillaries give origin to primitive glomeruli, which begin to produce urine by week 6 of gestation.

Mesonephric differentiation occurs in a cranial-to-caudal direction, during which the more cranially located nephrons progressively degenerate. Further caudally, the metanephros originates from the metanephric blastema of the nephrogenic cord and the ureteric bud and its branches. The latter develops as a diverticulum from the caudal mesonephric duct and is believed to induce development of the metanephric tubules. It becomes branched, giving origin to the ureter, renal pelvis, calyces, and collecting tubules. Late in the first trimester, the mesonephros ceases to be functional and excretion is taken over by the metanephros. Only a few caudalmost mesonephric tubules persist in the male to become the efferent ductules of the testis. These ductules drain into the mesonephric (*wolffian*) duct, which gives origin to the epididymis, vas deferens, seminal vesicles, and ejaculatory ducts.

The paramesonephric (*müllerian*) ducts arise as coelomic invaginations in the mesonephros (Fig. 101-1). This process is believed to be induced by the mesonephric duct and begins cranially at a site that represents the future abdominal ostium of the uterine (*fallopian*) tube. The paramesonephric ducts grow caudally, fuse, and ultimately drain into the urogenital sinus. The unfused portions give rise to the fallopian tubes, whereas the fused portion develops into the uterus and upper vagina. Because müllerian duct differentiation fails to occur in the absence of a wolffian duct, renal aplasia is often associated with anomalies of the fallopian tubes, uterus, and vagina.

The differentiation of the internal genital ductal system is critically dependent on gonadal influences. Both the mesonephric and paramesonephric ducts are present in the fetus at 7 weeks' gestation in both males and females. In the absence of testicular influence, regardless of whether an ovary is present, mesonephric ducts regress and paramesonephric ducts mature. In the presence of a testis, the paramesonephric ducts regress and the mesonephric ducts mature into the epididymis, vas deferens, and seminal vesicles. During the third month of fetal life, MIS produced by fetal Sertoli cells and testosterone

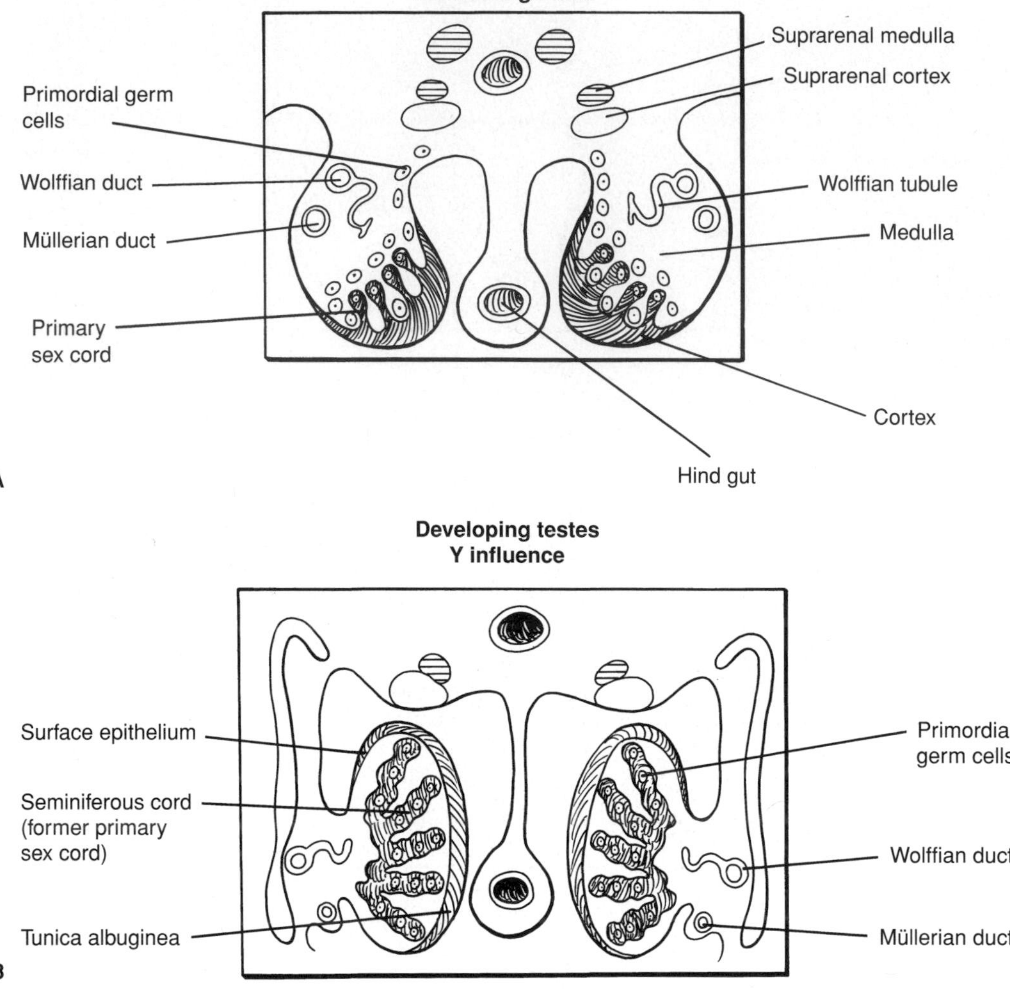

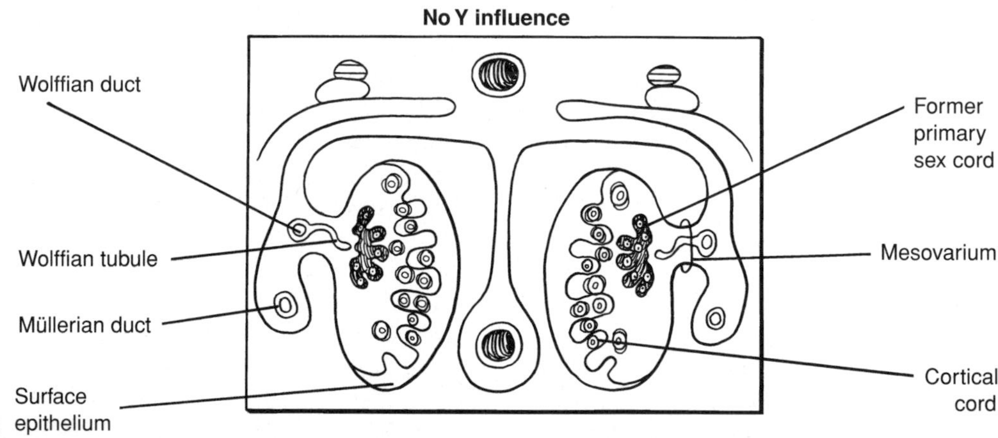

FIGURE 101-2. Ovarian and testicular differentiation. **(A)** Indifferent 6-week gonad. **(B)** Primary sex cords develop into seminiferous cords and the tunica albuginea becomes detectable at 7 weeks. **(C)** Twelve-week ovary. Cortical cords have extended from the epithelium. Primary sex cords are displaced into the mesovarium, forming rudimentary rete ovarii. **(D)** Twenty-week testis. The seminiferous tubules and rete testis have developed from seminiferous cords. Wolffian tubules develop into efferent ductules and the wolffian duct gives rise to the duct of the epididymis. **(F, G)** Section of the testis and ovary in the 20-week fetus. (From Moore KL. *The developing human: clinically oriented embryology*, 3rd ed. Philadelphia: WB Saunders, 1982:271, with permission.)

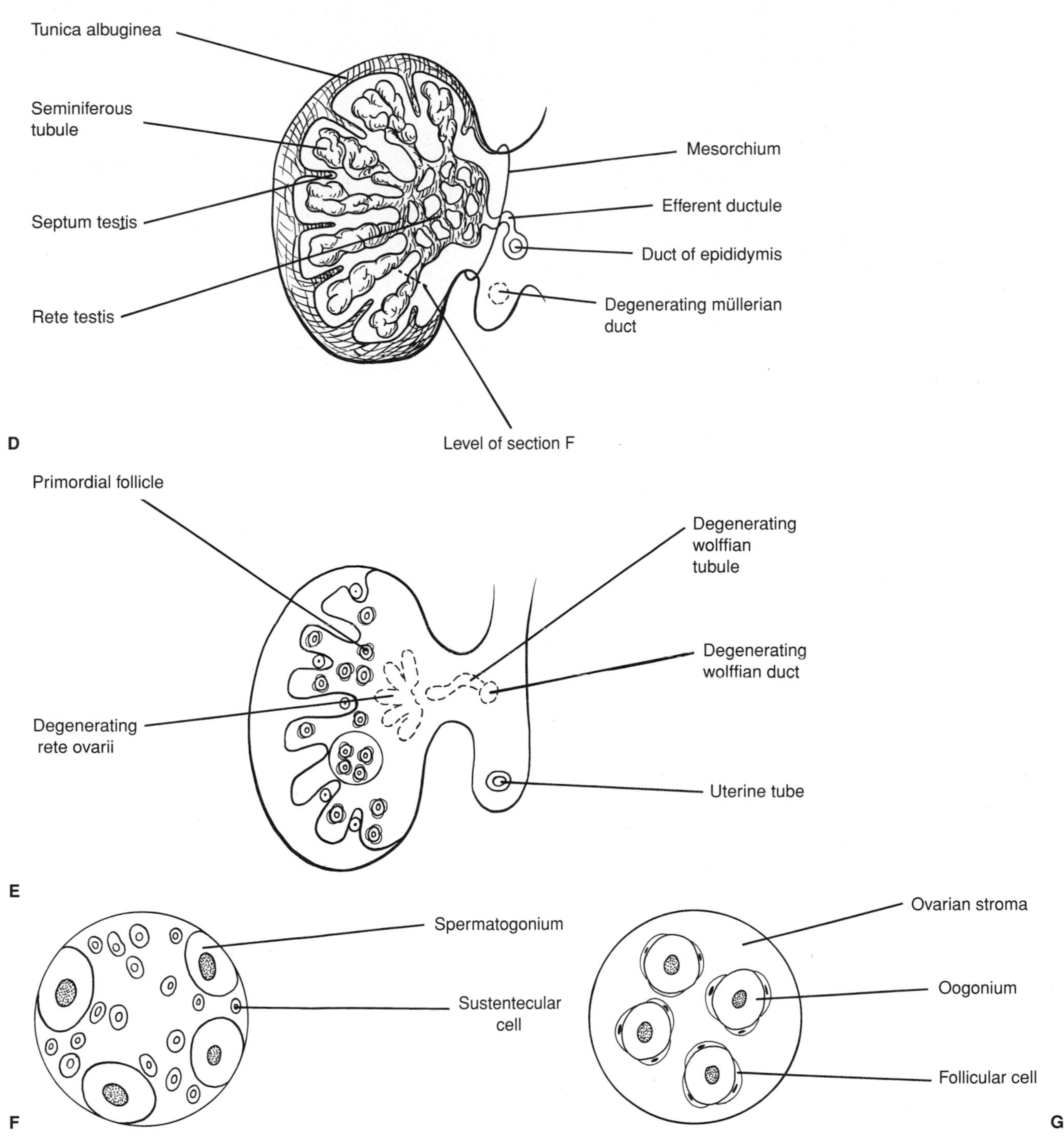

FIGURE 101-2. (*Continued*)

produced by fetal Leydig cells drive these changes locally, and hence, principally unilaterally.

Experimentally, gonadectomy of either male or female fetuses early in gestation results in wolffian regression and müllerian development. Further, unilateral castration of a male fetus results in ipsilateral wolffian regression and müllerian development, whereas the contralateral genital ducts develop in a normal masculine fashion (37). Conversely, testicular grafts placed in female fetuses result in müllerian regression and wolffian stimulation. The local implantation of androgens in female fetuses causes unilateral wolffian ductal maturation, whereas müllerian ductal development is unaltered (37,38).

MIS is a glycoprotein composed of two identical 72-kd subunits, connected by disulfide bonds (39), that are encoded by a gene on the short arm of chromosome 19

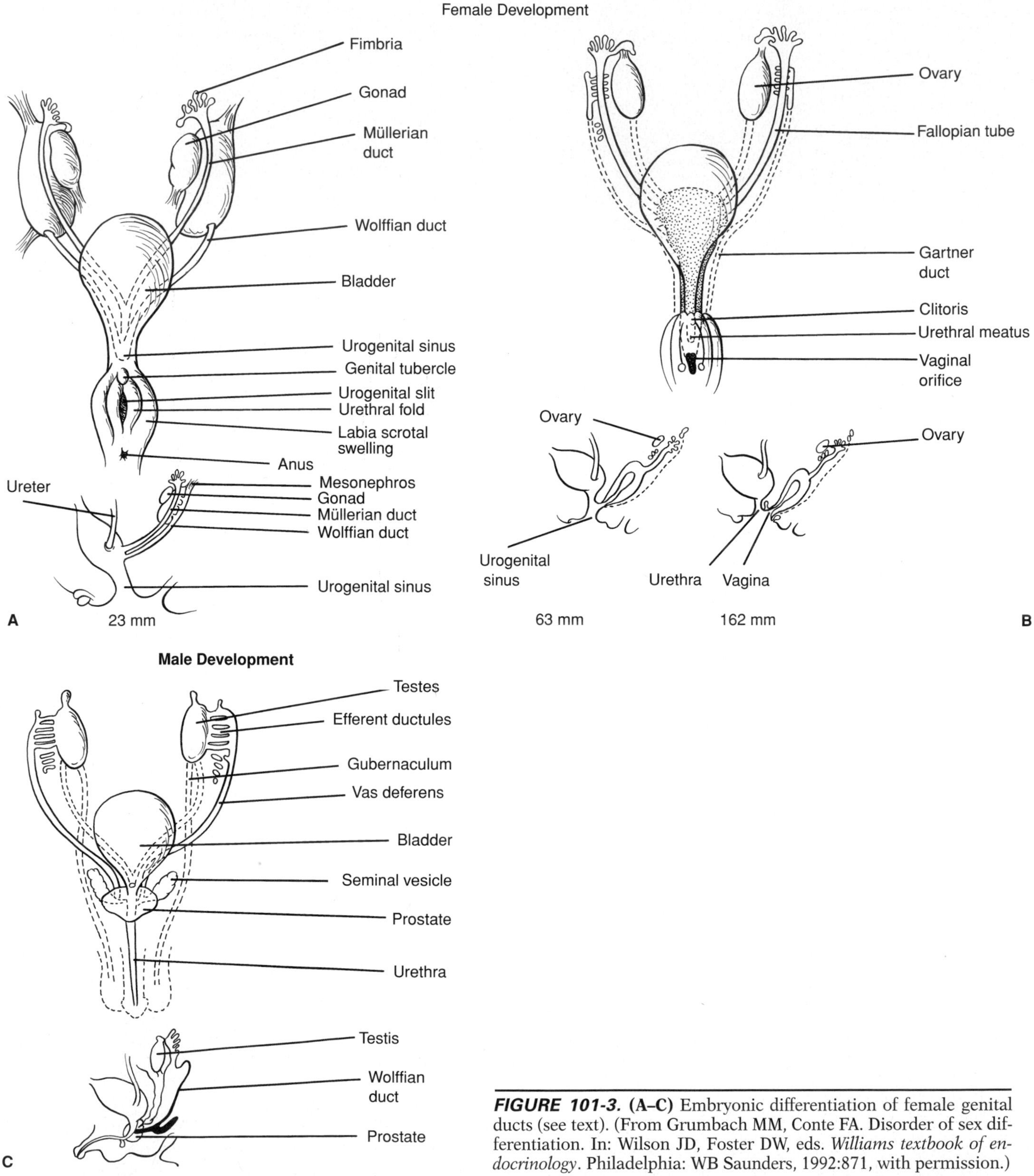

Female Development
Fimbria
Gonad
Müllerian duct
Wolffian duct
Bladder
Urogenital sinus
Genital tubercle
Urogenital slit
Urethral fold
Labia scrotal swelling
Anus
Ureter
Mesonephros
Gonad
Müllerian duct
Wolffian duct
Urogenital sinus
A
23 mm
Ovary
Fallopian tube
Gartner duct
Clitoris
Urethral meatus
Vaginal orifice
Ovary
Ovary
Urogenital sinus
Urethra
Vagina
63 mm
162 mm
B
Male Development
Testes
Efferent ductules
Gubernaculum
Vas deferens
Bladder
Seminal vesicle
Prostate
Urethra
Testis
Wolffian duct
Prostate
C

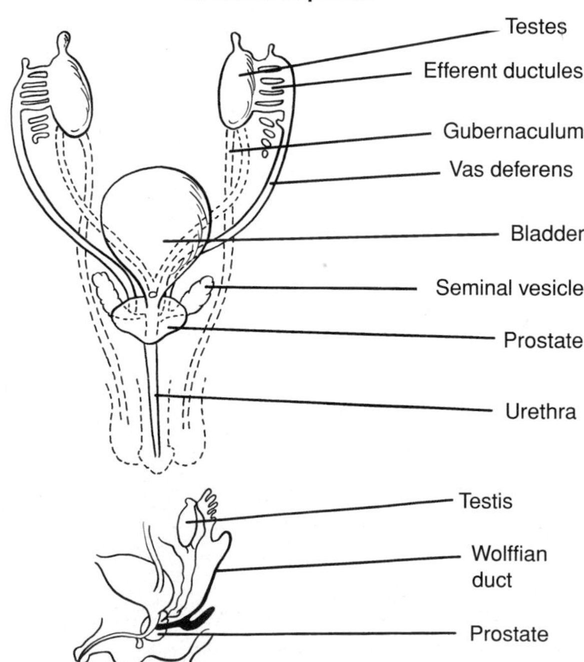

FIGURE 101-3. **(A–C)** Embryonic differentiation of female genital ducts (see text). (From Grumbach MM, Conte FA. Disorder of sex differentiation. In: Wilson JD, Foster DW, eds. *Williams textbook of endocrinology*. Philadelphia: WB Saunders, 1992:871, with permission.)

(40). MIS is a member of the transforming growth factor β (TGF- β) superfamily. Work by Donahoe and associates (41) suggested that MIS acts by blocking tyrosine phosphorylation on membrane proteins. MIS appears to have multiple potential functions, including not only müllerian duct regression but also germ cell maturation and gonadal morphogenesis, lung maturation, testicular descent, and growth inhibition of certain transformed cells (42–44). MIS is also involved in a negative feedback loop involving the Leydig cells, thereby regulating testosterone production (45,46). Hutson et al. suggested that MIS plays a role in testicular descent because it is expressed at high levels throughout childhood, with levels decreasing only after puberty (47,48).

Similarly, local androgen production by the fetal testis promotes ipsilateral wolffian duct maturation. This effect appears to require high local testosterone concentration because wolffian differentiation is not induced by systemic androgen administration in early gestation. Because 5α-reductase is not present in wolffian ducts, it is testosterone, not dihydrotestosterone, that binds to the cytosolic androgen receptor to induce these phenotypic changess (29).

These embryologic phenomena explain many observations made clinically:

1. Female fetuses with congenital virilizing adrenal hyperplasia do not demonstrate müllerian regression or wolffian maturation.
2. 46,XY women with testicular feminization (complete androgen insensitivity) have regression of müllerian ducts, but wolffian ducts remain rudimentary.
3. Genetic males with severe defects in steroid biosynthesis that result in androgen deficiency have rudimentary wolffian derivatives.
4. Genetic males with isolated deficiency of MIS have persistence of müllerian derivatives, but wolffian development proceeds normally.
5. In individuals with asymmetric gonadal development such as 45,X/46,XY, mixed gonadal dysgenesis, and true hermaphroditism, genital ductal development follows that of the homolateral gonad; the presence of testicular tissue results in ipsilateral müllerian regression and wolffian development.

Development of the Urogenital Sinus and External Genitalia

At week 8 of gestation, the external genitalia of both males and females are identical and remain uncommitted. Figure 101-4 outlines the differentiation of male and female external genitalia. In males, the *genital tubercle* becomes the penis, whereas the *urethral folds* fuse to become the floor of the penile urethra and the corpus spongiosum that encloses the penile urethra. In analogous fashion, the *labioscrotal swellings* fuse in the midline to become the scrotum. In the female, the genital tubercle becomes the clitoris and the urethral folds and labioscrotal swellings do not fuse, becoming the labia minora and the labia majora, respectively.

Sexual differentiation of the urogenital sinus is illustrated in Fig. 101-5. As with the external genitalia, the urogenital sinus is similar in both sexes up to week 8 or 9 of fetal life. The müllerian tubercle protrudes from the posterior wall of the urogenital sinus between the two wolffian duct orifices. This contact of the urogenital sinus with the fused müllerian ducts is critical to normal development of the vagina (49,50). Although this interpretation is controversial, the lower vagina appears to be of urogenital sinus origin and the upper vagina of müllerian origin. Expansion of the tissue composing the vesicovaginal septum allows for spatial separation of the vagina and urethra. In the male, the urogenital sinus undergoes elongation to form the prostatic and perineal urethra.

In analogous fashion to the differentiation of the internal genital ducts, masculinization of the urogenital sinus and external genitalia requires the presence of a testis. In contrast, however, this effect occurs in response to exposure to *dihydrotestosterone* (DHT) and can be induced by systemic androgen exposure (Fig. 101-6). Testosterone enters the cell by diffusion, whereupon it may bind to a high-affinity androgen receptor protein, be aromatized to estradiol, or be converted to DHT by the action of *5α-reductase*. Although both testosterone and DHT may bind to the androgen receptor protein, the binding affinity of the receptor for DHT is much greater. As with several members of the steroid receptor superfamily, the DNA-binding site is occupied by an inhibitory (e.g., heat shock) protein (51). Binding of the androgen to the receptor leads to dissociation of the inhibitory protein by conformational change, enabling the receptor to bind to specific sites on the DNA, referred to as receptor-dependent transcriptional enhancers. The result is transcription and processing of mRNA, which is then translated, allowing the synthesis of new proteins that mediate the androgenic effects involved with masculinization of the urogenital sinus and external genitalia.

Psychosexual Development

It has been generally assumed that gender identity (the identification of one's self as either male or female) is largely a learned process, and that this gender identity is firmly established by 1.5 and 2.5 years of age (52). Clearly, the assignment of the sex of rearing is the single most critical event in this process. Reinforcement of this assignment is crucial and requires unambiguous genital anatomy and unambiguous family interactions. One must not, however, overlook the importance of endocrine effects during prenatal development and puberty. Gender-related behavior, including gender role, has been demonstrated to be influenced by prenatal sex hormone exposure (53,54).

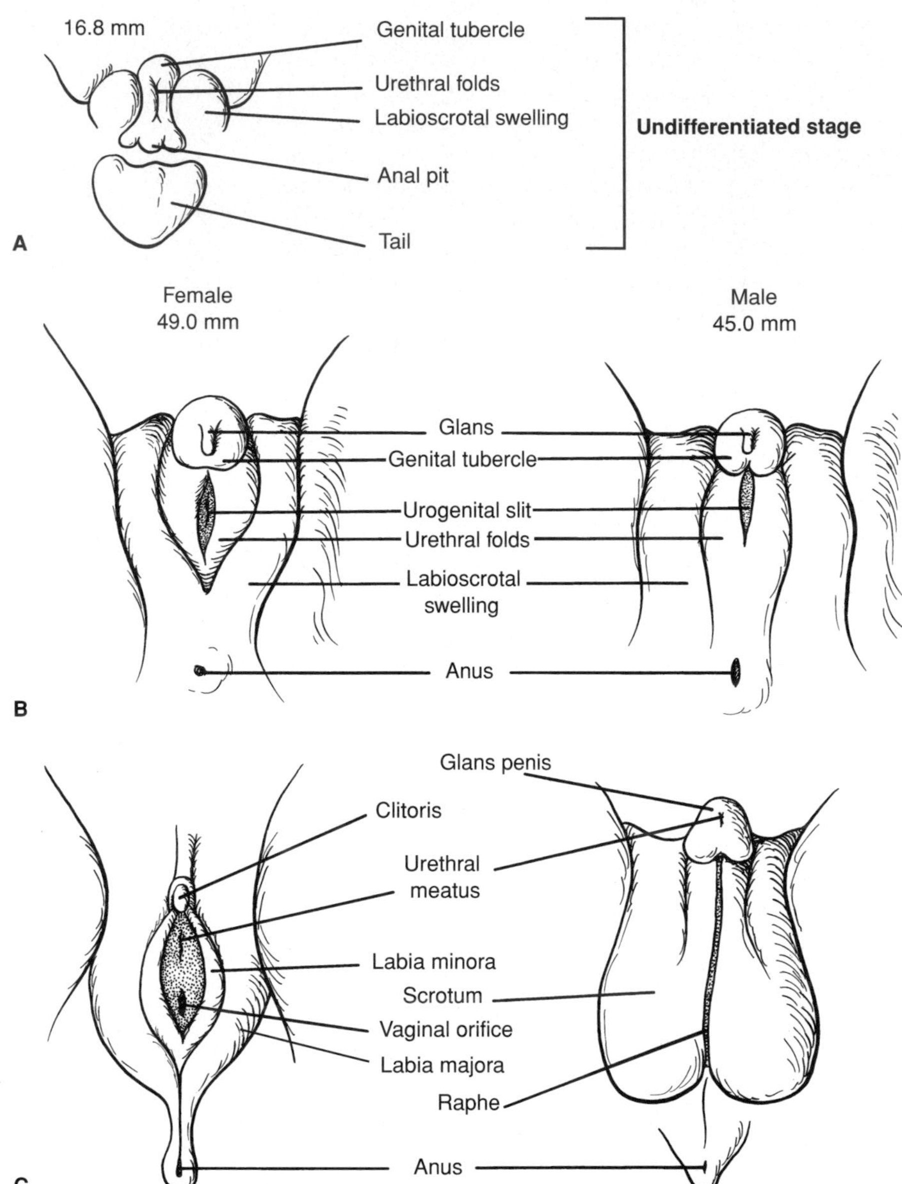

FIGURE 101-4. Sexual differentiation of the external genitalia. **(A)** Undifferentiated stage of development. **(B)** Between 8 and 12 weeks of gestation, human genital differentiation occurs. **(C)** Adult genitalia. (From Sizonenko PC. Sexual differentiation. In: Bertrand J, Rappaport R, Sizonenko PC, eds. *Pediatric endocrinology*. Baltimore: Williams & Wilkins, 1993:88, with permission.)

Further, pubertal hormonal influences producing phenotypic changes counter to that of the original gender assignment have been reported to induce not only doubts about gender identity but to cause alterations in gender behavior in some individuals (55). Males with a small penis, followed into adulthood, do not in general experience altered gender identity, altered desire for heterosexual activity, or alterations in other activities generally considered to be predominantly male (56). This and other studies, however, have demonstrated that life with inadequate or compromised genitalia is often confounded by debilitating emotional disturbances.

Developmental Temporal Sequence

An understanding of the temporal sequence of the development of the reproductive tract is helpful clinically. As illustrated in Fig. 101-7, one may conceptualize this process as a series of interrelated steps. Chromosomal sex is determined at the time of conception. This is followed by an indifferent phase of embryogenesis that lasts approximately 7 weeks. Thereafter, divergent development is progressive with the sequential differentiation of the gonads, followed by the internal genital ducts, followed by the urogenital sinus and external genitalia.

Evidence exists to suggest that during the period of organogenesis, inclusive of the differentiation of the external genitalia, fetal Leydig cell activity is driven by placental hCG rather than by LH from the fetal pituitary (31,33). The pattern of testosterone secretion during early gestation reflects that of hCG and the fetal testicular hCG-binding capacity (31,57,58). In addition, the expression of several steroidogenic genes appears to be directly regulated by circulating hCG (30,59,60,61). Fetal pituitary LH

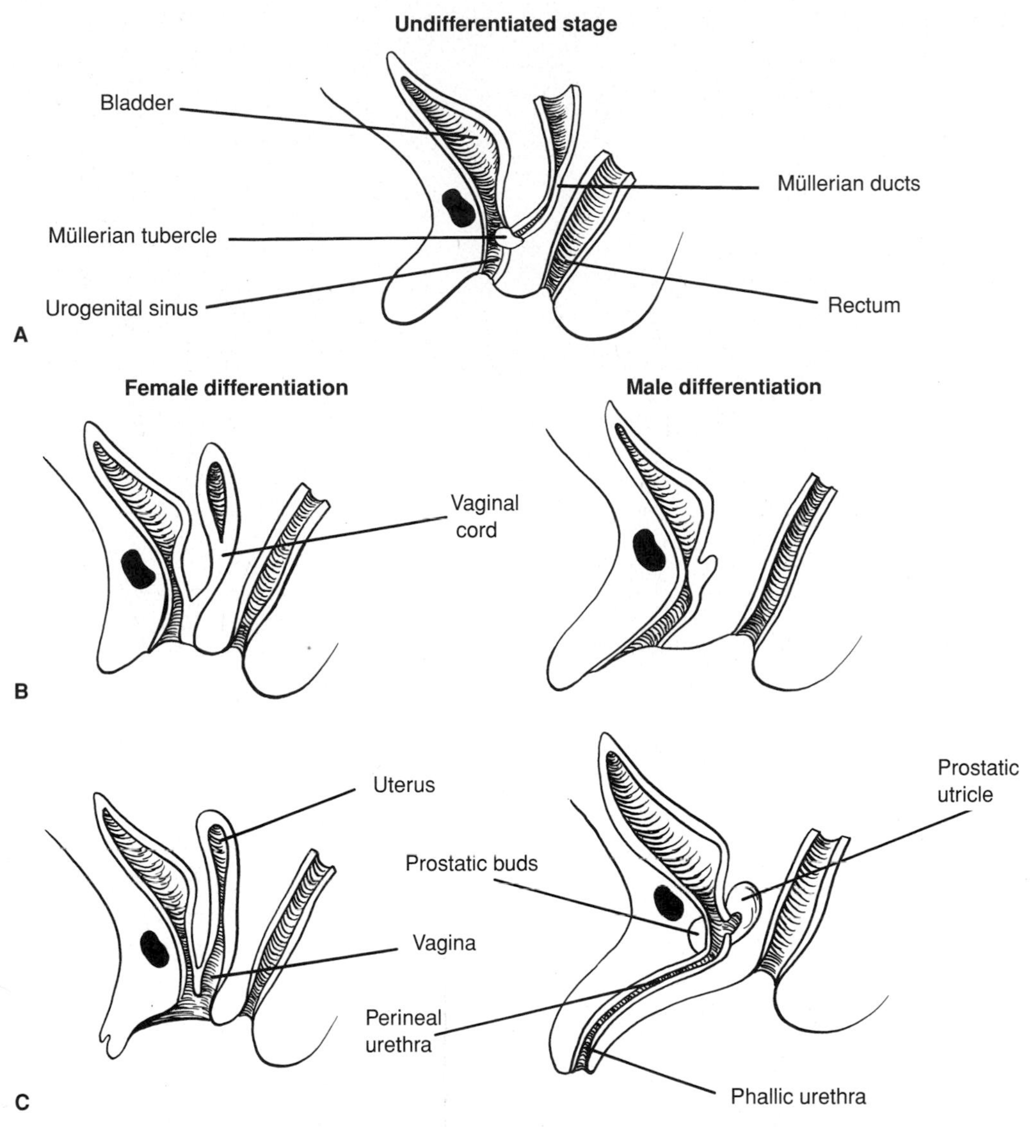

FIGURE 101-5. Sexual differentiation of the urogenital sinus. (From Sizonenko PC. Sexual differentiation. In: Bertrand J, Rappaport R, Sizonenko PC, eds. *Pediatric endocrinology*. Baltimore: Williams & Wilkins, 1993:88, with permission.)

appears to take over the modulation of testosterone synthesis after midgestation and, along with placental hCG, appears to play a critical role in the growth of the differentiated penis and scrotum as well as descent of the testes (57).

These observations, coupled with the facts that after about 12 weeks of gestation the vagina has separated from the urogenital sinus, and the urethral folds and labioscrotal swellings are unable to fuse even with intense androgenic stimulation, explain several important clinical observations: (1) females exposed to androgens after the period of organogenesis develop clitoromegaly, but urethral fold and labioscrotal fusion does not occur; (2) the diagnosis of congenital virilizing adrenal hyperplasia generally does not explain clitoromegaly in the absence of midline fusion; and (3) males with congenital hypopituitarism or selective gonadotropin deficiency often present with microphallus, but the penis and scrotum are generally well differentiated.

Summary of Reproductive Tract Differentiation

Figure 101-8 summarizes the events leading to normal sexual development in both males and females. In the presence of two normal X chromosomes, two normal ovaries develop. In the absence of testosterone and MIS, paramesonephric ducts mature into fallopian tubes, uterus, and upper vagina, whereas mesonephric ductal elements regress. Similarly, in the absence of androgenic stimulation, feminine differentiation of the urogenital

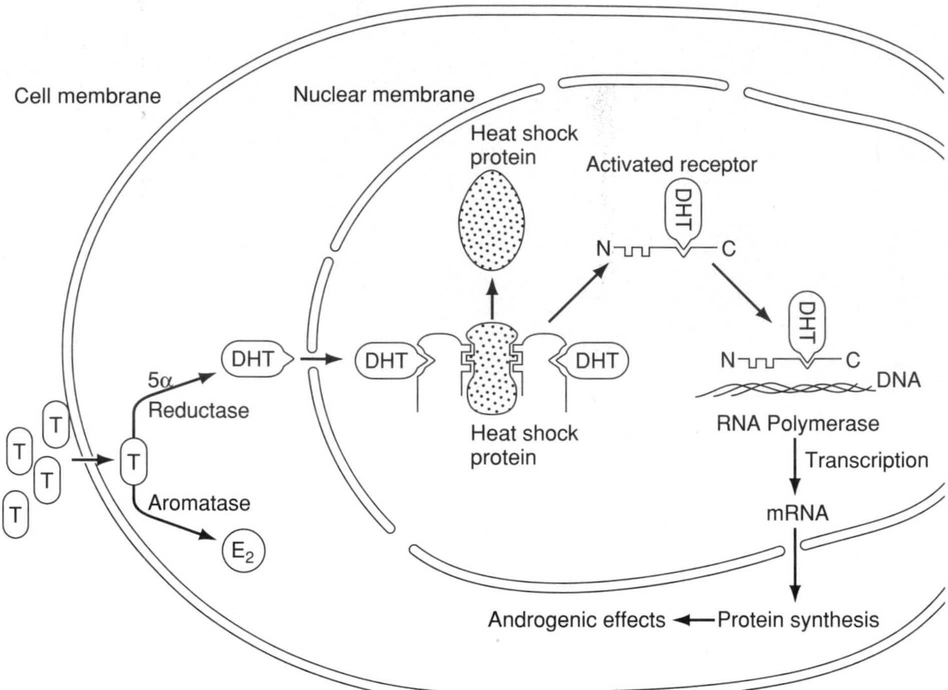

FIGURE 101-6. Mechanism of action of androgens on cell function (see text). T, testosterone; DHT, dihydrotestosterone. (From Grumbach MM, Conte FA. Disorder of sex differentiation. In: Wilson JD, Foster DW, eds. *Williams textbook of endocrinology*. Philadelphia: WB Saunders, 1992:875, with permission.)

sinus and the external genitalia occurs: (1) In the absence of an X chromosome or a critical portion of an X chromosome, important ovarian developmental failure may result. In addition, 46,XX males with *SRY* translocations and 46,XX males with undetected mosaicism with a Y-bearing cell line are reported and are associated with testicular organogenesis. 46,XX and 46,XX/46,XY true hermaphroditism is similarly associated with development of some testicular tissue. (2) Once present, testicular tissue may produce sufficient testosterone and MIS to result in mesonephric development and paramesonephric regression, which if unilateral, is restricted to the side where testicular tissue is located. (3) Exposure of the fetus to either exogenous (e.g., maternal ingestion) or endogenous (e.g., congenital virilizing adrenal hyperplasia) androgen may result in various degrees of virilization of the urogenital sinus and the external genitalia. In the presence of a normal Y and X chromosome, testicular development follows. The production of MIS by Sertoli cells and the production of testosterone by Leydig cells results in paramesonephric regression and mesonephric development, respectively. During the period of organogenesis, Leydig cell steroid synthesis is driven by placental hCG and thereafter by fetal pituitary LH. Testosterone is converted to DHT by 5α-reductase, which, in the presence of the cytosolic androgen receptor protein encoded by a gene on the X chromosome, causes masculinization of the urogenital sinus and external genitalia. (4) In the absence of a Y chromosome (e.g., 45,X/46,XY) or (5) a critical portion of the Y chromosome (*SRY*), defective testicular development may occur. (6) MIS deficiency may occur in isolation or as part of more complete testicular failure and results in persistence of paramesonephric structures. (7) Leydig cell steroid synthetic failure may occur as a result of specific enzymatic deficiency or as part of more complete testicular failure and results in incomplete masculinization of the internal genital ducts, urogenital sinus, and external genitalia. (8) Partial androgen receptor deficiency may result in incomplete masculinization, whereas complete deficiency may result in a nearly normal female phenotype. Because MIS production is normal, paramesonephric structures are rudimentary. (9) 5α-Reductase deficiency results in insufficient DHT production, which produces only partial virilization. (10) Congenital hypopituitarism or isolated gonadotropin deficiency may result in inadequate stimulation of Leydig cell function. The result is a small but completely formed penis and scrotum.

Defects in Steroid Biosynthesis

The subject of steroid biosynthesis has been extensively reviewed (2). Defects can result in either masculinization of genetic females, female sexual infantilism, undermasculinization of the genetic male, or excessive masculinization of the genetic male. These defects are often overlooked because of the wide variability of phenotypic expression. They must be understood by surgeons because the first level of referral may be to the surgeon for correction of what may appear as a relatively common anomaly such as hypospadias.

The steroid biosynthetic pathways are diagrammed in Fig. 101-9. Congenital adrenal hyperplasia (CAH) is

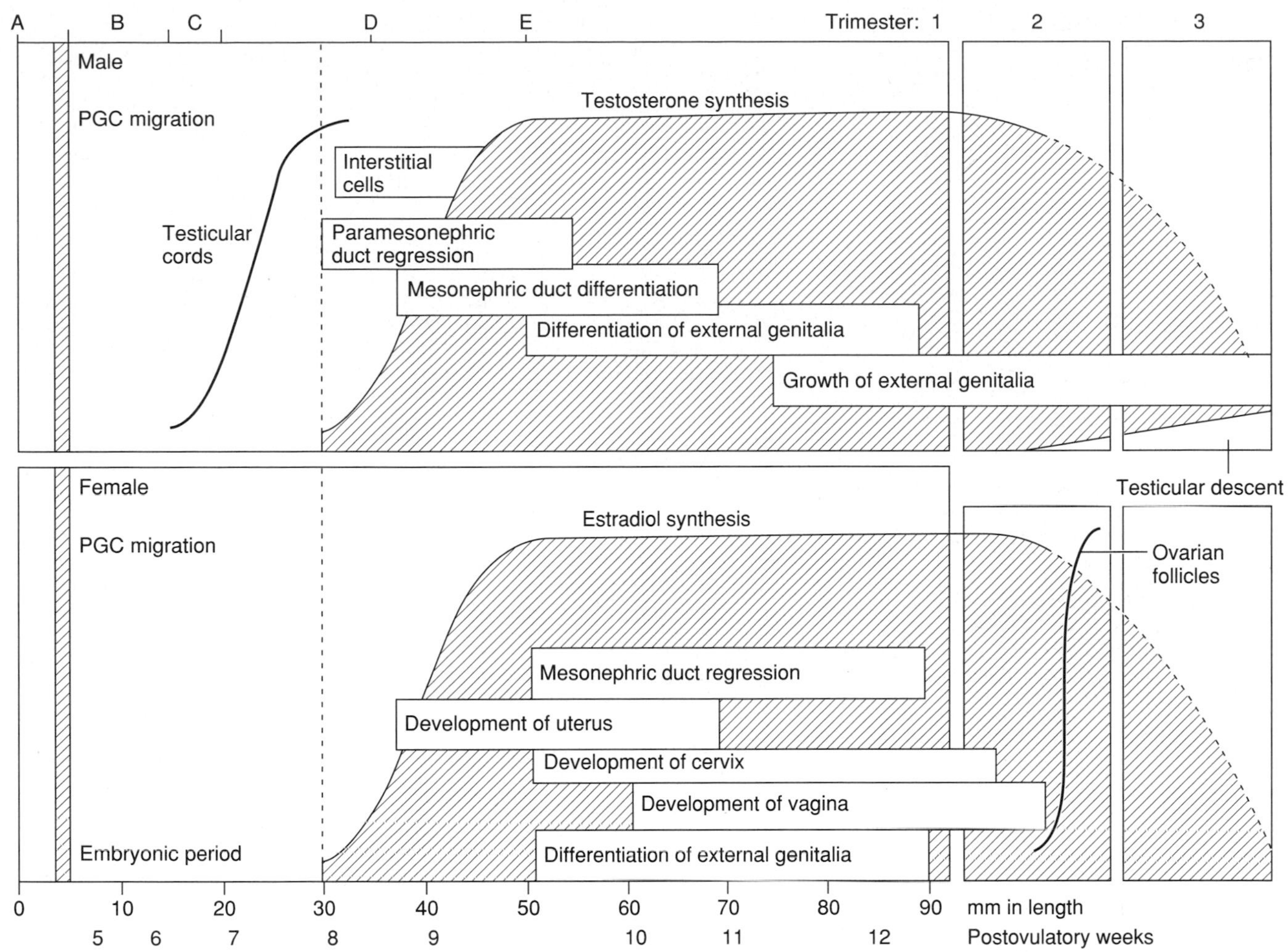

FIGURE 101-7. Prenatal development of the reproductive system as a function of embryonic/fetal length and age. **(A)** Chromosomal sex established. **(B)** Indifferent phase. **(C)** Gonadal differentiation. **(D)** Genital ductal differentiation. **(E)** External genitalia differentiation. (See text.) PGC, primordial germ cell. (From O'Rahilly R, Muller F. *Human embryology and teratology*. New York: Wiley-Liss, 1992:207, with permission.)

responsible for the majority of cases of female pseudohermaphroditism and accounts for approximately one-half of ambiguous genitalia cases. The most common enzymatic defect is *21-hydroxylase deficiency*. This condition is caused by mutations in the *CYP21* gene on chromosome 6p21.3. Consequently, this deficiency is inherited in an *autosomal recessive* fashion, and its inheritance is intimately associated with that of the major transplant antigens. Analysis of human histocompatability antigens may therefore be helpful in genetic counseling.

Based on data from newborn screening programs for CAH, the incidence of classic 21-hydroxylase deficiency is about 1 in 14,000 newborns worldwide, with an increased incidence seen in Alaska (1 in 800), Brazil (1 in 7,500), and the Philippines (1 in 7,000). Salt-wasting CAH accounts for 66% of reported cases and simple-virilizing CAH accounts for 32% (62).

The 21-hydroxylase gene encodes a cytochrome P-450 enzyme, designated P450c21. Both the phenotypic expression and the biochemical expression of 21-hydroxylase deficiency are remarkably variable. Females may present with very mild degrees of masculinization or be sufficiently masculinized to appear to have hypospadias with bilateral cryptorchidism (Fig. 101-10).

The classic presentation of 21-hydroxylase deficiency is that of hyponatremic dehydration, hyperkalemic acidosis, and ultimately vascular collapse. It is particularly important for the surgeon to be cognizant of this presentation because it may be confused with other lesions for which surgical consultation may be obtained, such as sepsis and bowel obstruction, including hypertrophic pyloric stenosis. Female neonates characteristically present with ambiguous genitalia, whereas newborn males may have few clinical signs on physical examination. Excessive

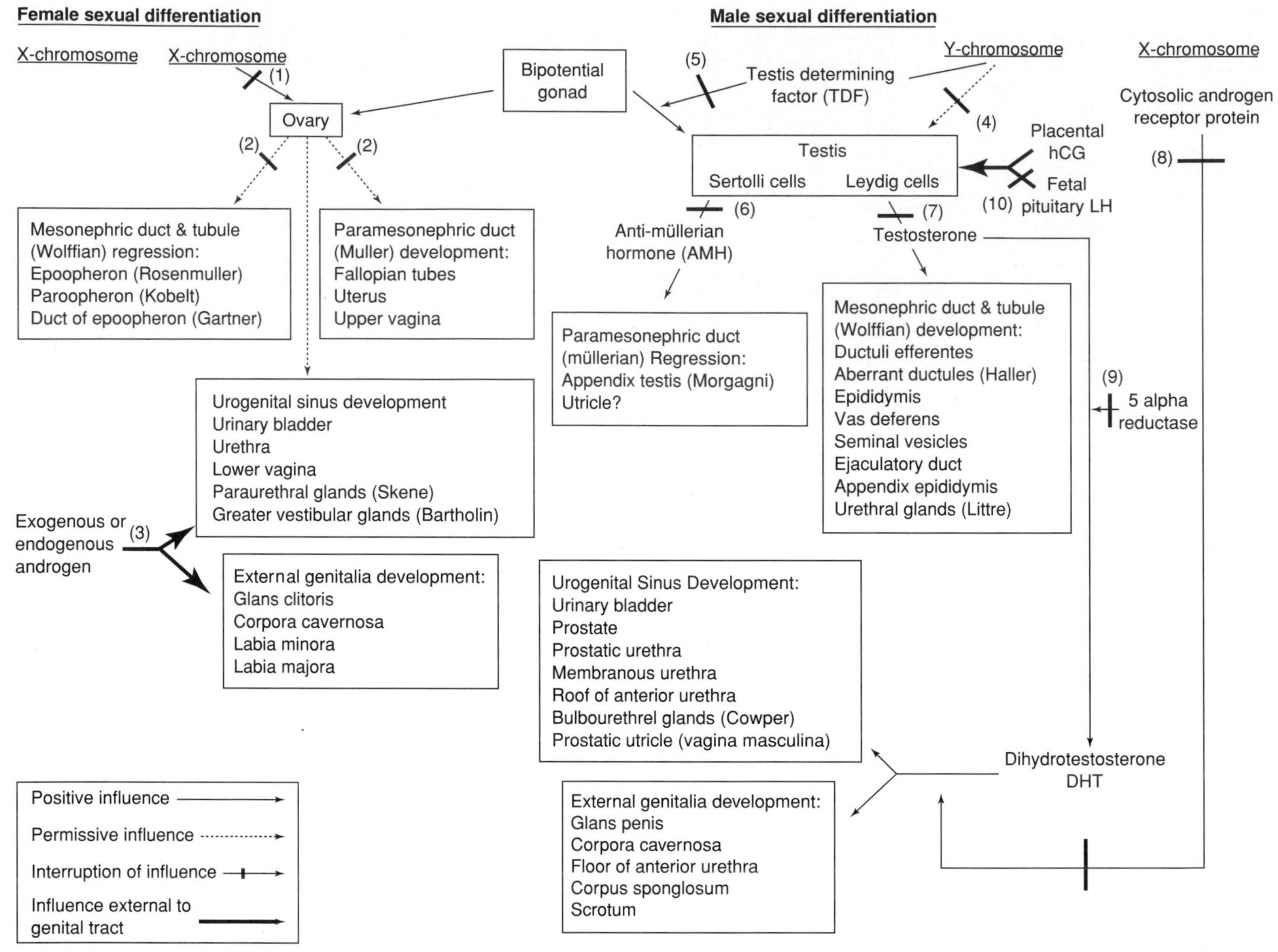

FIGURE 101-8. Diagrammatic depiction of events involved with normal and abnormal male and female sexual differentiation. Interruptive influences are numerically labeled and referred to in text. Adult derivatives and vestigial remnants of embryonic genital structures are outlined. Commonly encountered eponyms are noted in parentheses. hCG, human chorionic gonadotropin; LH, luteinizing hormone; DHT, dihydrotestosterone.

masculinization is a clinical feature in males presenting in early childhood.

Nonclassic presentations for 21-hydroxylase deficiency exist. These include late-onset and cryptic varieties. Such individuals may have completely normal genitalia in the newborn period and then demonstrate signs of androgen overproduction in later childhood. Cryptogenic deficiencies may demonstrate biochemical changes in the absence of signs or symptoms.

Figure 101-11A demonstrates the biochemical changes that may be assayed to determine the diagnosis. Blockage of 21-hydroxylase activity impairs the conversion of progesterone and 17-hydroxyprogesterone to deoxycorticosterone and 11-deoxycortisol, respectively. The result is an accumulation of progesterone and 17-hydroxyprogesterone. The buildup of these precursors results in metabolism directed toward the production of androgenic compounds.

Biochemical assays for the diagnosis of CAH have traditionally included the measurement of urinary 17-ketosteroids (urinary metabolites of the excessively produced androgenic compounds) and urinary pregnanetriol, a specific metabolite of 17-hydroxyprogesterone. Currently, serum 17-hydroxyprogesterone (17-OHP) is the preferred biochemical marker for this disease. Newborn screening involves a filter paper sample that is collected within a few days of birth, transported to a designated newborn screening laboratory, and analyzed for 17-OHP. Caution must be maintained in preterm infants as 17-OHP levels can be high, particularly if they are sick. The problem of false-positive results can be resolved by repeating the test at a later date or by performing an adrenocorticoptropic

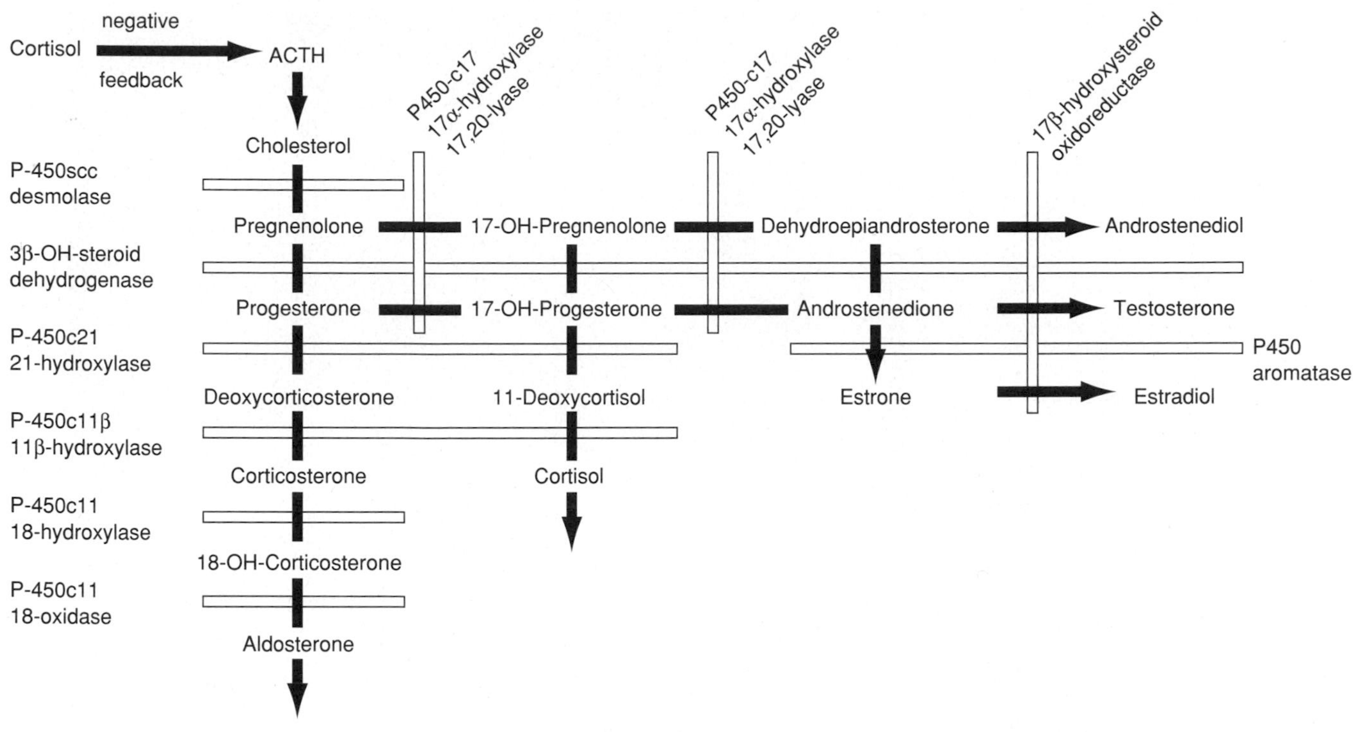

FIGURE 101-9. Steroid biosynthetic pathways. Note separate pathways required for the synthesis of mineralocorticoids, glucocorticoids, and sex steroids. ACTH, adrenocorticotropic hormone.

hormone (ACTH) stimulation test. Genotyping can also improve diagnostic specificity (63,64).

Treatment acutely involves volume resuscitation and steroid loading. Chronically, patients are maintained on Cortisone and Flucortisol supplementation for glucocorticoid and mineralocorticoid maintenance, respectively. Of greatest concern from a surgical perspective is strict attention to providing stress-level steroid supplementation with surgical procedures as well as any acute illness.

Individuals with *11β-hydroxylase* deficiency (Fig. 101-11B) demonstrate a defect in the conversion of deoxycorticosterone and 11-deoxycortisol to corticosterone and cortisol, respectively. As with 21-hydroxylase deficiency, deficient cortisol production results in increased ACTH stimulation of adrenal biosynthesis. The gene for this enzyme is located on *chromosome 8*, resulting in an *autosomal recessive* inheritance pattern. Similar to 21-hydroxylase deficiency, classic, mild, late-onset, and cryptic forms are reported.

Again, precursor metabolites accumulate, providing substrate for the overproduction of androgenic steroids, which cause inappropriate masculinization of females and excessive masculinization of males. Elevated serum deoxycorticosterone and 11-deoxycortisol levels may be assayed. Elevated deoxycorticosterone, which has mineralocorticoid activity, results in volume expansion and low-renin hypertension, which often manifests itself beyond 2 years of age. Pertinent diagnostic findings include elevated serum deoxycorticosterone and 11-deoxycortisol as well as their urinary metabolites, tetrahydrodeoxycorticosterone and tetrahydro-11-deoxycortisol. In addition, urinary 17-ketosteroids are elevated.

Another enzymatic deficiency resulting in CAH is *3β-hydroxysteroid dehydrogenase deficiency*. This enzyme is encoded by a gene on *chromosome 1*, and its deficiency is also inherited in an *autosomal recessive* pattern. This deficiency (Fig. 101-11C) results in impaired conversion of pregnenolone and 17-hydroxypregnenolone to progesterone and 17-hydroxyprogesterone, respectively. In addition, the conversion of dehydroepiandrosterone to androstenedione and of androstendiol to testosterone is impaired. The result is masculinization of the genetic female and feminization of the genetic male. Males may demonstrate poor virilization and the development of gynecomastia at puberty.

As with 21-hydroxylase deficiency, impaired glucocorticoid production results in increased ACTH stimulation of the adrenals and hyperplasia. Impaired mineralocorticoid production results in salt wasting, hyponatremia, and volume contraction. Again, this defect is potentially life threatening in the newborn period. Non–salt-losing, mild, and late-onset forms of this disease are described. Elevated serum 17-hydroxypregnenolone and dehydroepiandrosterone, as well as their urinary metabolites, dehydroepiandrostendione sulfate, and 17-ketosteroids, are characteristic.

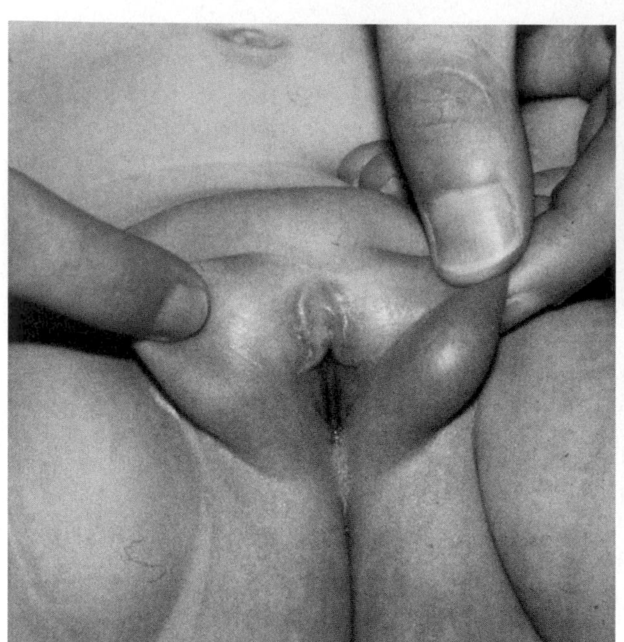

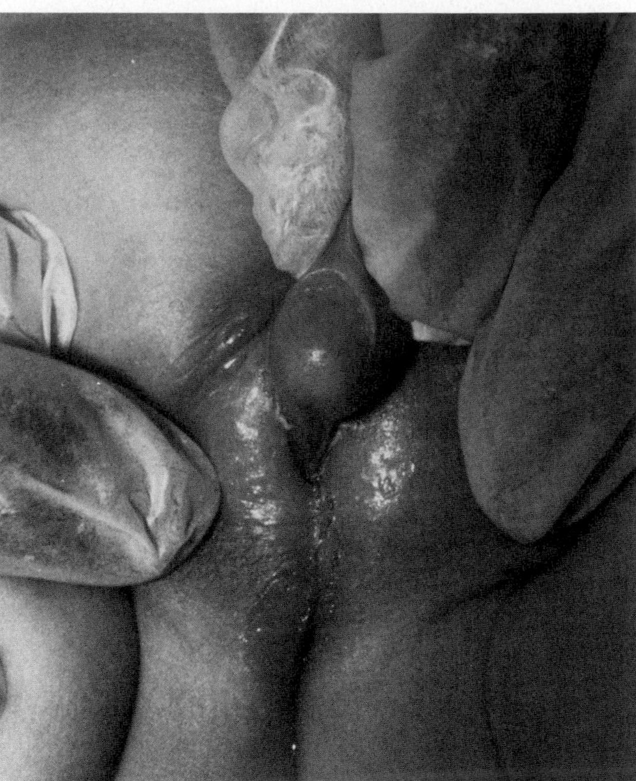

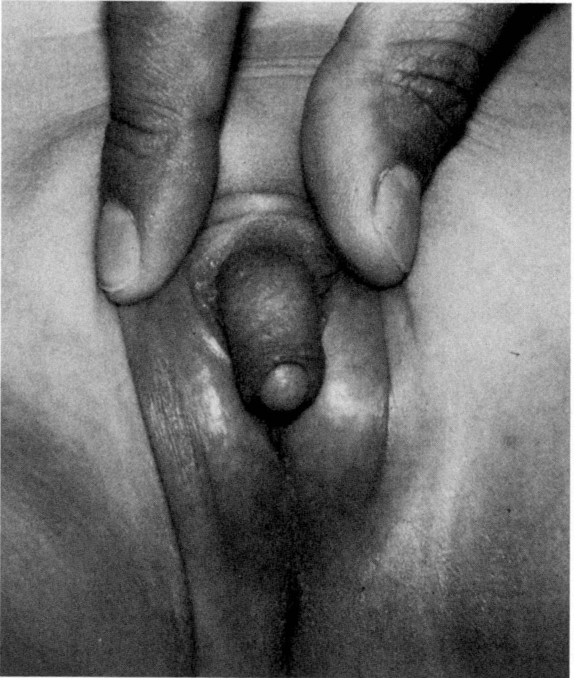

FIGURE 101-10. Spectrum of abnormalities encountered with 46,XX congenital adrenal hyperplasia due to 21-hydroxylase deficiency.

Figure 101-12 outlines the characteristic findings with the side-chain cleavage defect. This abnormality, also known as lipoid adrenal hyperplasia and 17,20-desmolase deficiency, is due to a defect of the enzymatic complex that results in the conversion of cholesterol to pregnenolone. Lipoid CAH is the most severe form of CAH and may be caused by a defect in either the steroidogenic acute regulatory protein or the P450scc (65). These patients have severe deficiencies in glucocorticoid and mineralocorticoid activity and diminished levels of multiple steroid compounds. The enzyme is encoded by a gene on chromosome 15, and again autosomal recessive inheritance is noted. Females have normal internal and external genital tracts, whereas males are often severely feminized, with female external

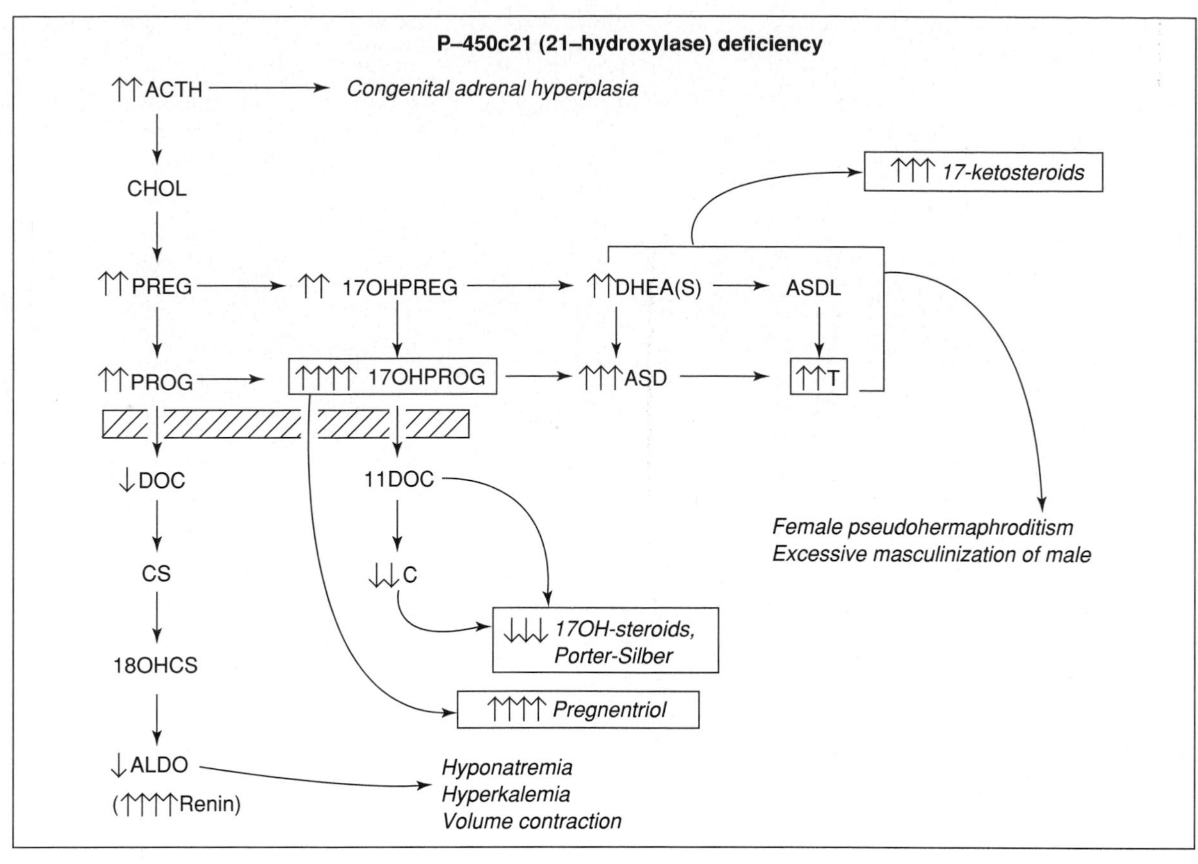

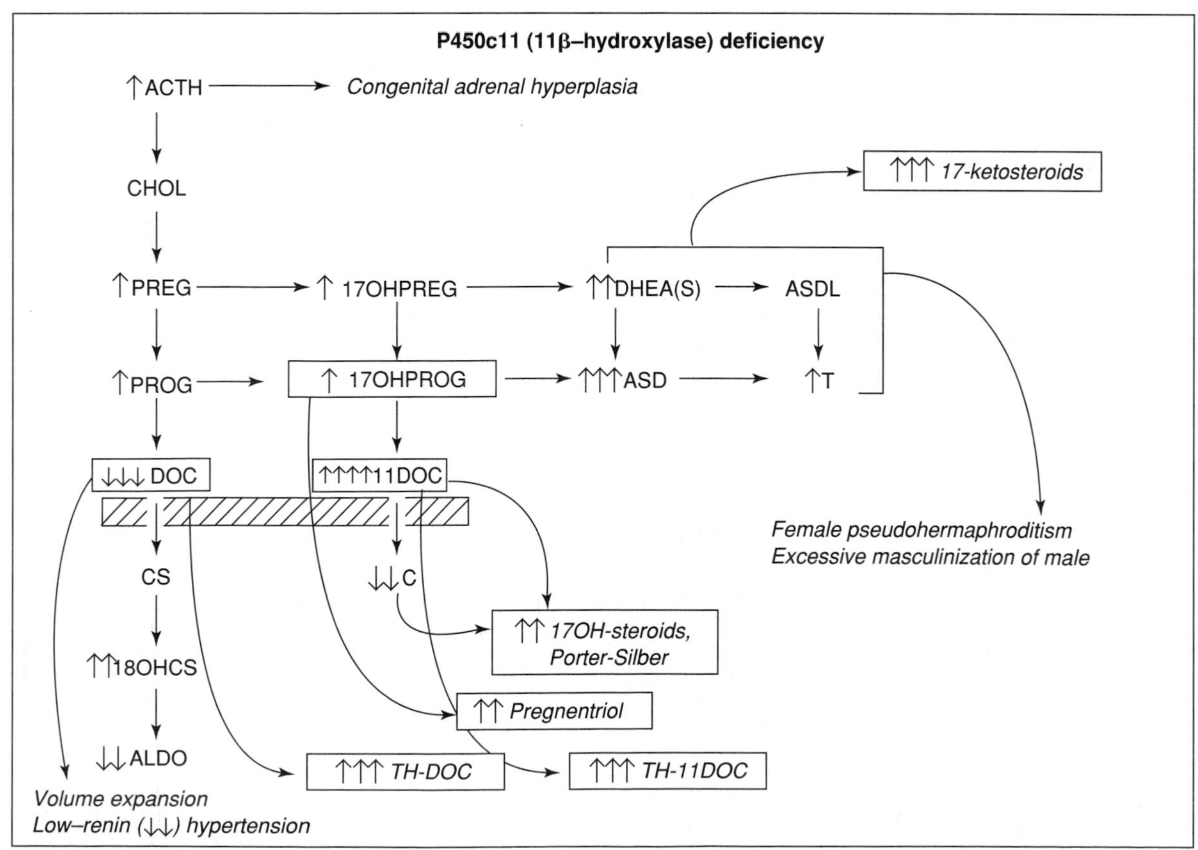

FIGURE 101-11. **(A)** Consequences of 21α-hydroxylase deficiency. **(B)** Consequences of 11β-hydroxylase deficiency. *(continued)*

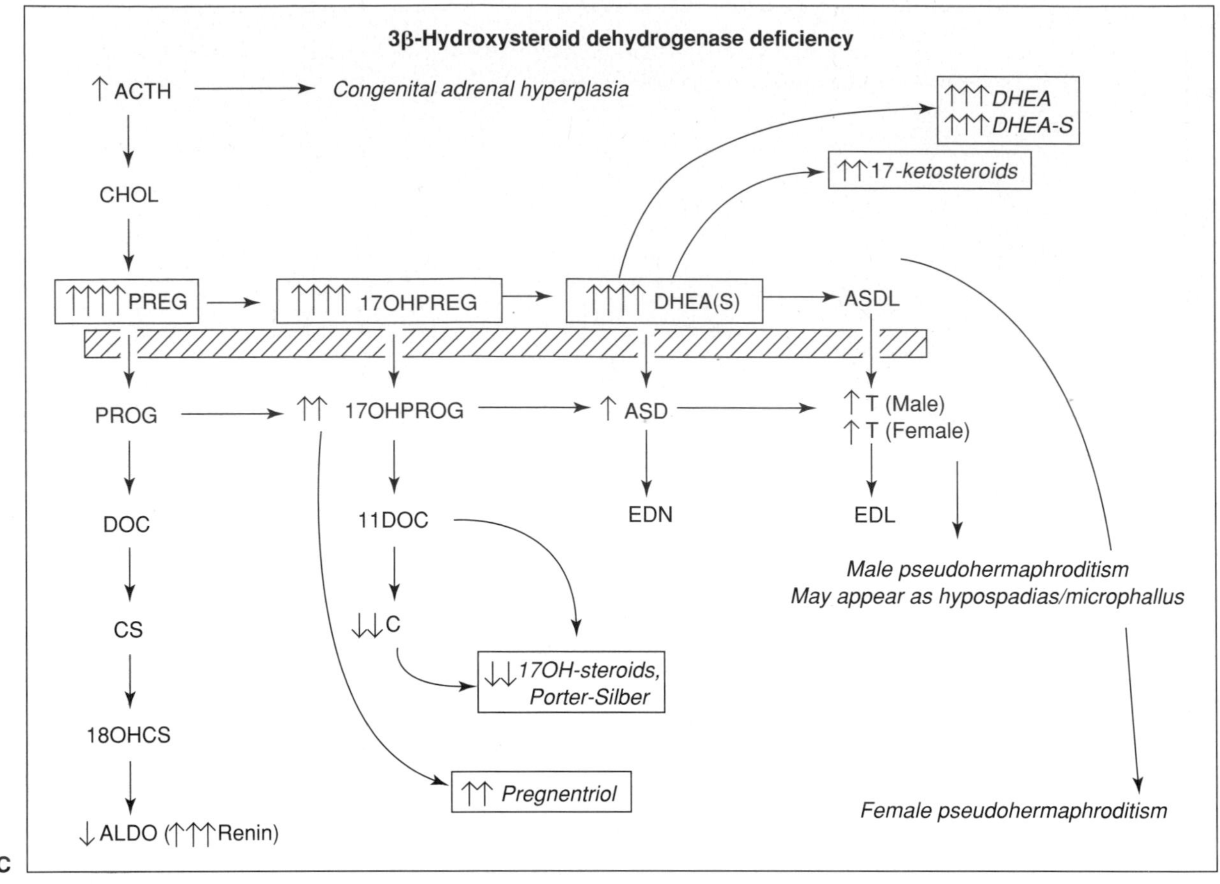

FIGURE 101-11. **(C)** Consequences of 3β-hydroxysteroid dehydrogenase deficiency. (See also Fig. 101-9 and text.)

genitalia and a blind-ending vaginal pouch. Secondary sexual characteristics of puberty are severely blunted in both sexes.

Another cause of CAH is *17α-hydroxylase deficiency* (Fig. 101-13). The deficiency of this enzyme, encoded by a gene on chromosome 10, results in impaired conversion of pregnenolone and progesterone to 17-hydroxypregnenolone and 17-hydroxyprogesterone, respectively. Deficient cortisol production results in excessive ACTH stimulation and resultant adrenal hyperplasia. Note, however, that mineralocorticoid production is elevated, and accumulation of mineralocorticoid precursors are identifiable. These individuals experience volume expansion and low-renin hypertension. Females exhibit sexual infantilism, whereas males are often severely feminized, even appearing to have normal female external genitalia.

The conversion of 17-hydroxypregnenolone and 17-hydroxyprogesterone to dehydroepiandrosterone and androstenedione, respectively (*17,20-lyase* activity), is mediated by the same enzyme that provides 17α-hydroxylase activity. Both activities are therefore inherited in an autosomal recessive pattern. Mutations in the *P-450*$_{C17}$ gene may cause either 17,20-lyase deficiency alone or in combination with 17α-hydroxylase deficiency. As demonstrated in Fig. 101-14, 17-hydroxyprogesterone and 17-hydroxypregnenolone are elevated, whereas the serum testosterone level, as well as those of dihydroepiandrosterone and androstenedione, are depressed. Note that cortisol production is not impaired and CAH does not occur. Female sexual infantilism and male pseudohermaphroditism are characteristic.

Figure 101-15 depicts the biochemical changes associated with 17β-hydroxysteroid oxidoreductase deficiency. Here, conversion of dehydroepiandrosterone and androstenedione to androstendiol and testosterone, respectively, is impaired. The result is increased levels of androstenedione and estrone, whereas levels of testosterone and estradiol are depressed. Clinically, males appear as highly feminized male pseudohermaphrodites.

The biochemical changes associated with *P-450* aromatase deficiency are outlined in Fig. 101-16. This defect is associated with marked impairment in estrogen production by the fetoplacental unit and subsequent virilization of the female fetus.

In summary (Table 101-2), five enzymatic deficiencies may result in CAH, of which two are primarily virilizing,

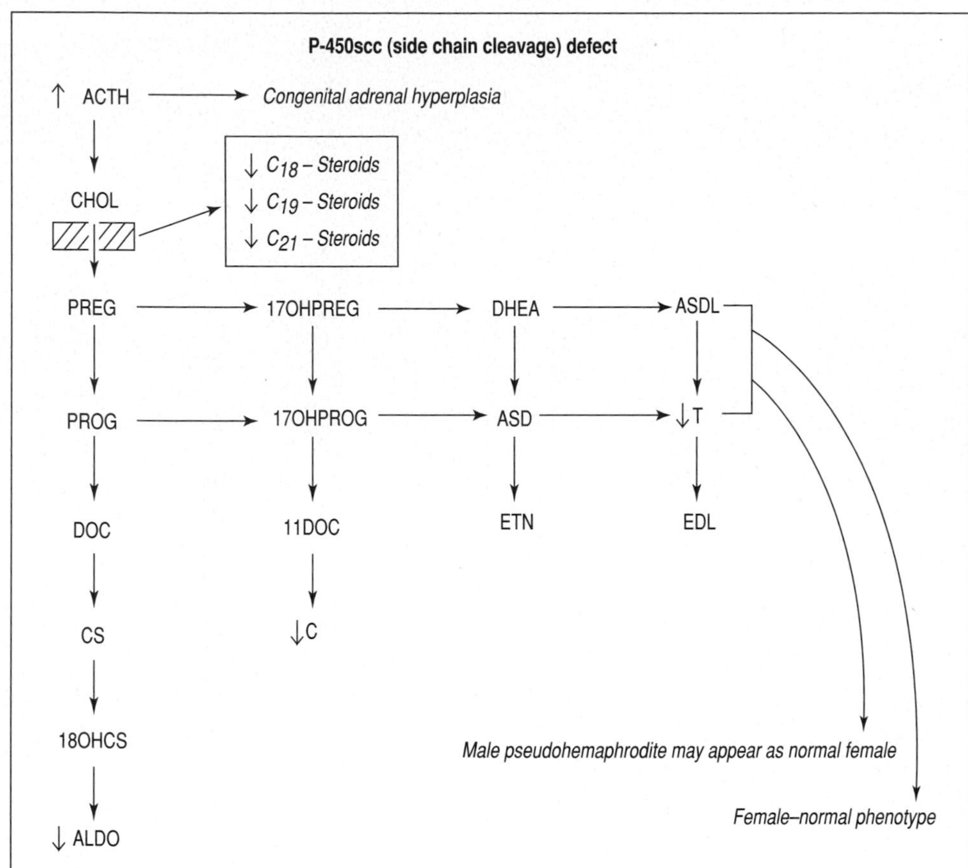

FIGURE 101-12. Consequences of cholesterol desmolase (side-chain cleavage) deficiency.

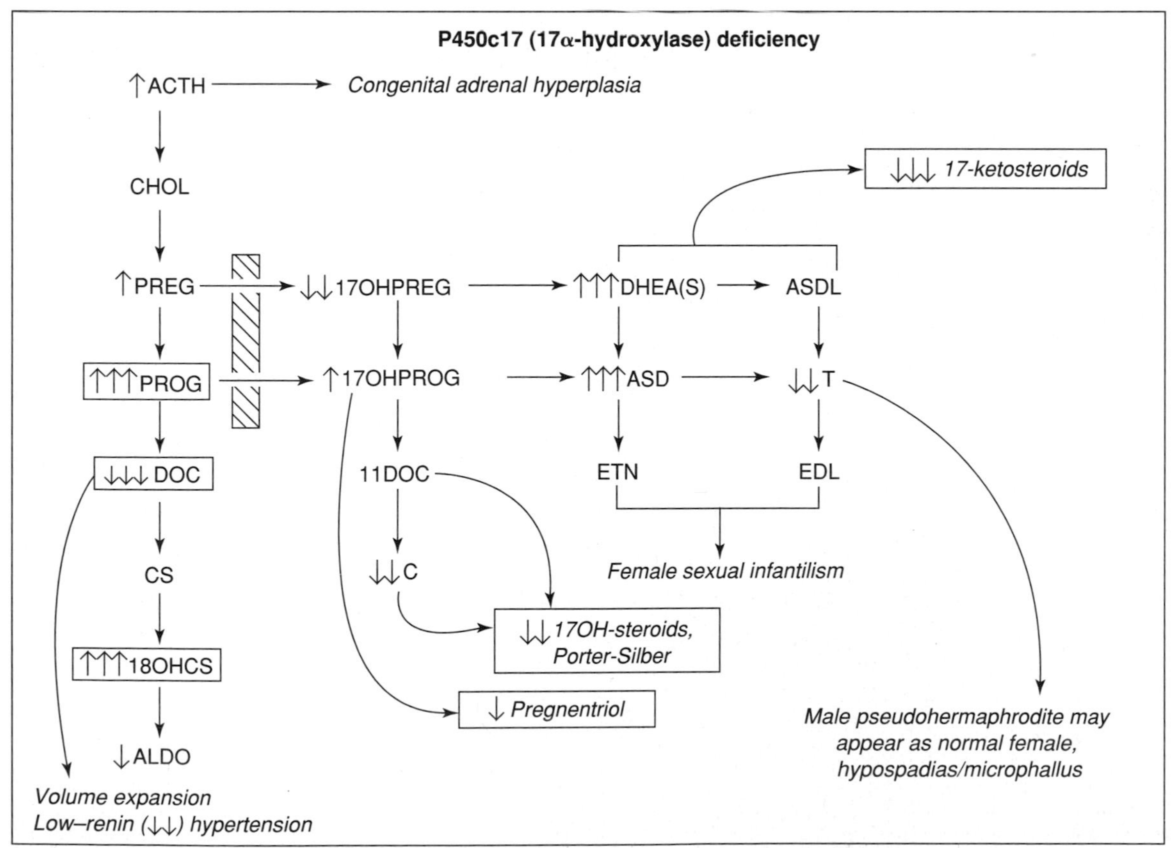

FIGURE 101-13. Consequences of 17α-hydroxylase deficiency.

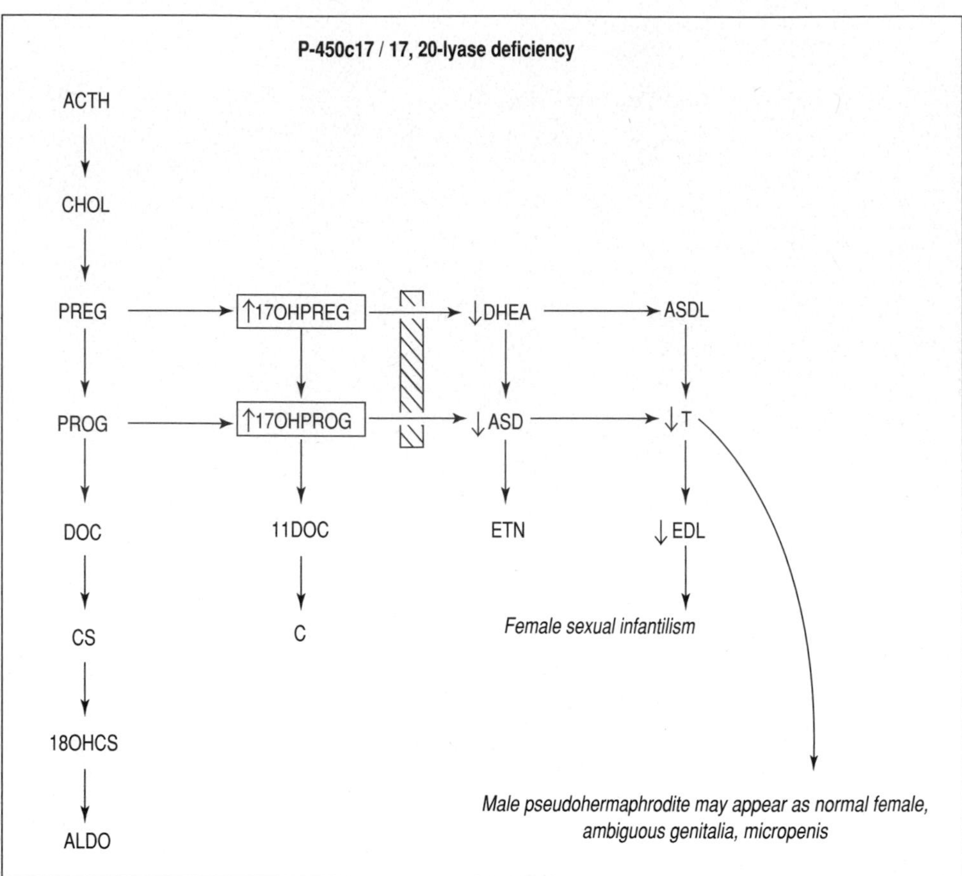

FIGURE 101-14. Consequences of 17,20-lyase deficiency.

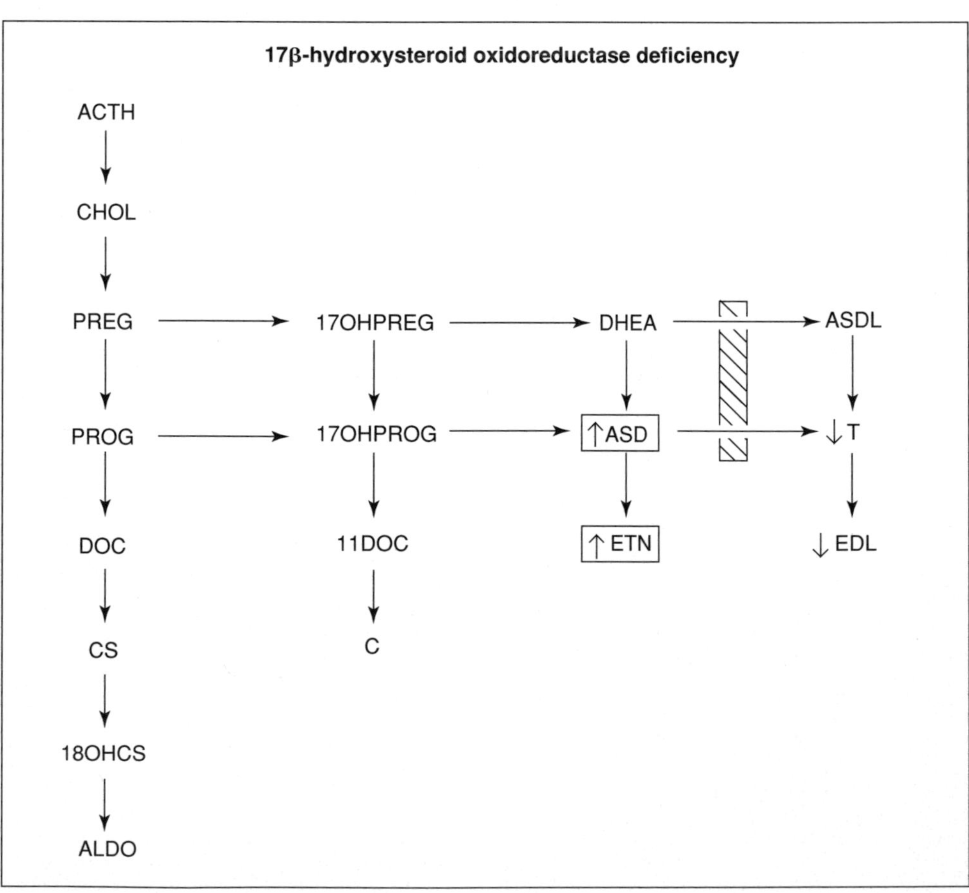

FIGURE 101-15. Consequences of 17β-hydroxysteroid oxidoreductase deficiency.

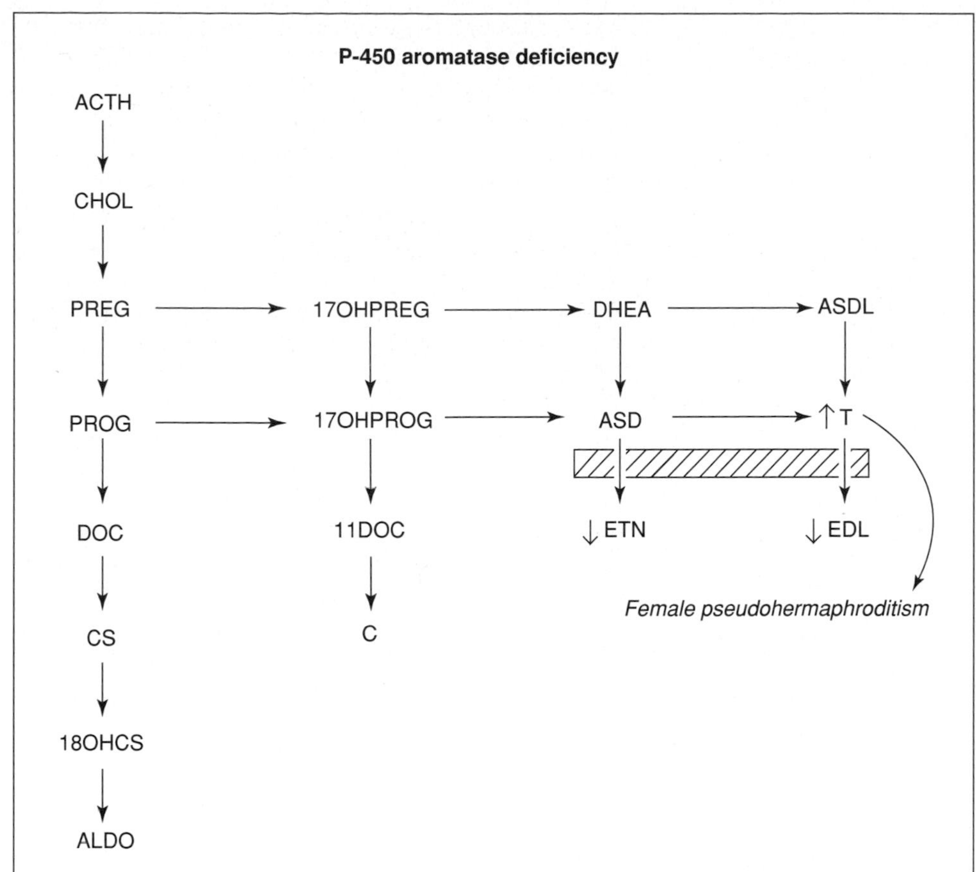

FIGURE 101-16. Consequences of P450 aromatase deficiency.

TABLE 101-2 Defects in Steroid Biosynthesis.

Category	*Phenotypic Effect*	*Enzymatic Defect*
Congenital adrenal hyperplasia	Virilizing	21α-Hydroxylase
	Virilizing	11β-Hydroxylase
	Mixed	3β-Hydroxysteroid dehydrogenase
	Feminizing	Side-chain cleavage
	Feminizing	17α-Hydroxylase
Salt-wasting syndrome	Virilizing	21α-Hydroxylase
	Mixed	3β-Hydroxysteroid dehydrogenase
	Feminizing	Side-chain cleavage
Salt retention, hypertension	Virilizing	11β-Hydroxylase
	Feminizing	17α-Hydroxylase
No adrenal hyperplasia	Feminizing	17,20-Lyase
	Feminizing	17β-Hydroxysteroid oxidoreductase
	Virilizing	Aromatase

two are primarily feminizing, and one may have mixed effects on phenotypic expression. Three may present with salt wasting and vascular collapse, whereas two tend to cause salt retention and hypertension.

One type of CAH, side-chain cleavage deficiency, results in markedly enlarged adrenals with lipid density radiographically. Radiographically enlarged adrenals are not characteristic of the other four forms of adrenal hyperplasia, but a cerebriform ultrasound (US) pattern has been described (66). Three deficiencies are not associated with adrenal hyperplasia. Two of these are primarily feminizing and one primarily virilizing. Figure 101-17 demonstrates the relative frequencies of enzymatic deficiencies associated with CAH.

Five defects in steroid biosynthesis are associated with male pseudohermaphroditism, of which three (3β-hydroxysteroid dehydrogenase deficiency, side-chain cleavage deficiency, and 17α-hydroxylase deficiency) are associated with adrenal hyperplasia and two (17,20-lyase and 17β-hydroxysteroid oxidoreductase deficiencies) are not.

CLASSIFICATION

An organized approach to classification of intersex anomalies is essential for effective application of diagnostic and

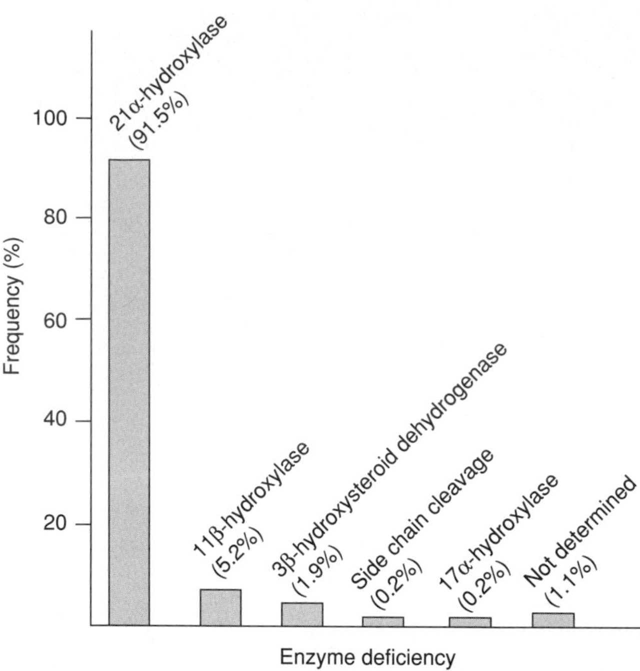

FIGURE 101-17. Relative frequencies of enzymatic deficiencies associated with congenital adrenal hyperplasia. (From Bois E, Mornet E, Chompret A, et al. L'hyperplasie congénitale des surrénales (21-OH) en France. *Arch Fr Pediatr* 1985;42:175, with permission.)

therapeutic modalities. Patients may be classified according to the etiology of the anomaly, clinical presentation, or need for surgical intervention. Table 101-3 presents a typical, inclusive approach to classification, which incorporates diagnoses in neonates with ambiguous genitalia and also diagnoses in children born with unambiguous genitalia. In the latter instance, individuals often have other somatic abnormalities or may appear quite normal until a problem arises at an older age for which therapy is sought. Not all these diagnoses benefit from surgical intervention.

PRENATAL DIAGNOSIS OF AMBIGUOUS GENITALIA

Increased sensitivity of modern US equipment coupled with greater operator expertise now allows the obstetrician-perinatalogists-radiologists to visualize the fetus with greater acuity. This has allowed the inspection of the external genitalia as early as the 13th through the 16th week of gestation (67). Obvious abnormalities of the external genitalia can be readily identified. An increase in the use of amniocentesis (advanced maternal age, screening for genetic anomalies, etc.) has led to the increased incidence of mismatch between the chromosome analysis and the genital anatomy by US (phenotype-genotype discrepancies) (68).

Physicians are now being consulted for a prenatal diagnosis of ambiguous genitalia with an increasing frequency: however, although the approach to the postnatal management of a child with ambiguous genitalia is fairly well agreed upon, no such consensus exists for the prenatal management. It is imperative that a multidisciplinary team is involved with all prenatally diagnosed cases of ambiguous genitalia (as is the case postnatally); this team usually consists of obstetrician/perinatalogist, geneticist, pediatric endocrinologist, neonatalogist, and pediatric reconstructive surgeon.

The prenatal evaluation of a fetus with suspected sex discordance should include the following modalities (69–71):

1. *Fetal US examination*. A detailed US evaluation of the internal and external genitalia of the fetus is performed, in addition to a survey for any associated somatic anomalies. After week 19 of the pregnancy, the uterus can be readily identified as an echogenic mass within the pelvis lying between two anechoic structures—the bladder ventrally and the rectum posteriorly. The dimensions of the uterus, penis, and the scrotum can now be correlated with gestational age (70). Testicular descent can be documented as early as the 25th week of gestation.

   US determination of gender requires unequivocal visualization of the labia and clitoris or the penis and scrotum beyond the 16th week of gestation.
2. *Genetic examination*. Tissue obtained by amniocentesis, chorionic villous biopsy, or umbilical cord sampling is submitted for, karyotype examination, fluorescence *in situ* hybridization (FISH) for the SRY gene.
3. *Hormonal examination*. Amniotic fluid is assayed for measurements of steroid hormone metabolites (17-hydroxyprogesterone, testosterone, androstenedione, 11-deoxycortisol and 7-dehydrocholestrol/cholesterol).

INDICATIONS FOR DIAGNOSTIC EVALUATION

The surgeon must maintain a high index of suspicion for disorders of sexual differentiation because failure to establish a diagnosis may result in a lost opportunity to provide genetic counseling, prevent malignancy, prevent inappropriate virilization at puberty, and prevent medical crisis from steroid metabolic abnormalities. Clearly, all neonates with ambiguous genitalia require complete diagnostic evaluation. Diagnostic evaluation is also indicated in the presence of any salt-wasting syndrome, especially if associated with abnormal genitalia. Any degree of hypospadias associated with any degree of cryptorchidism requires a karyotype, as does bilateral nonpalpable testes. Micropenis with or without hypospadias requires evaluation of karyotype and hormonal profile. A palpable mass in the inguinal canal or the labia majora in phenotypic females must be evaluated to ensure a testis is not present.

TABLE 101-3 Classification of Anomalous Sexual Development.

- I. Disorders of gonadal differentiation
  - A. Seminiferous tubular dysgenesis (Klinefelter syndrome)
  - B. Syndrome of gonadal dysgenesis and its variants (Turner syndrome)
  - C. Complete and incomplete forms of 46,XX and 46,XY gonadal dysgenesis
  - D. True hermaphroditism
- II. Female pseudohermaphroditism
  - A. Congenital virilizing adrenal hyperplasia
  - B. *P-450* aromatase (placental deficiency)
  - C. Androgens and synthetic progestogens transferred from maternal circulation
  - D. Associated with malformations of intestine and urinary tract (non–androgen-induced female pseudohermaphroditism)
  - E. Other teratologic factors
- III. Male pseudohermaphroditism
  - A. Testicular unresponsiveness to human chorionic gonadotropin (hCG) and luteinizing hormone (LH) (Leydig cell agenesis or hypoplasia)
  - B. Inborn errors of testosterone biosynthesis
    - 1. Enzyme defects affecting synthesis of both corticosteroids and testosterone (variants of congenital adrenal hyperplasia)
      - a. $P\text{-}450_{scc}$ (cholesterol side-chain cleavage) deficiency (20–22 desmolase deficiency, congenital lipoid adrenal hyperplasia)
      - b. 3β-Hydroxysteroid dehydrogenase deficiency
      - c. $P\text{-}450_{c17}$ ($17\,\alpha$-hydroxylase) deficiency
    - 2. Enzyme defects primarily affecting testosterone biosynthesis by testes
      - a. $P\text{-}450_{c17}$ (17,20-lyase) deficiency
      - b. 17β-Hydroxysteroid oxidoreductase deficiency
  - C. Defects in androgen-dependent target tissues
    - 1. End-organ resistance to androgenic hormones (androgen receptor and postreceptor defects)
      - a. Syndrome of complete androgen resistance and its variants (testicular feminization and its variant forms)
      - b. Syndrome of partial androgen resistance and its variants (Reifenstein syndrome)
      - c. Androgen resistance in infertile men
      - d. Androgen resistance in fertile men
    - 2. Defects in testosterone metabolism by peripheral tissues: 5α-reductase deficiency, pseudovaginal perineoscrotal hypospadias
  - D. Dysgenetic male pseudohermaphroditism
    - 1. X chromatin—negative variants of syndrome of gonadal dysgenesis (e.g., 45,X/46,XY,46,XYp-)
    - 2. Incomplete forms of XY gonadal dysgenesis
    - 3. Associated with degenerative renal disease
    - 4. "Vanishing testes" (embryonic testicular regression syndrome; 46,XY agonadism; 46,XY gonadal agenesis; rudimentary testes; anorchia)
  - E. Defects in synthesis, secretion, or response to anti-müllerian hormone (AMH)
    - 1. Female genital ducts in otherwise normal men—herniae uteri inguinale; persistent müllerian duct syndrome
  - F. Maternal ingestion of progestogens
- IV. Unclassified forms of abnormal sexual development
  - A. Hypospadias/cryptorchidism
  - B. Ambiguous external genitalia in patients with multiple congenital anomalies
    - a. Cloacal exstrophy
    - b. Fetal trimethadone or hydantoin effects
    - c. Fraser syndrome
    - d. Reiger syndrome
    - e. Ectodermal dysplasia
    - f. Robinow syndrome
    - g. Smith-Lemli-Opitz syndrome
    - h. Aarskog syndrome
    - i. De Lange syndrome
    - j. Chromosomal anomalies: 9q, 10q, 13q, 18q, 20q
  - C. Absence or anomalous development of vagina, uterus, and fallopian tubes (Mayer-Rokitansky-Küster-Hauser syndrome)

Adapted from Grumbach MM, Conte FA. Disorder of sex differentiation. In: Wilson DJ, Foster DW, eds. *Williams textbook of endocrinology.* Philadelphia: WB Saunders, 1992:853; Rappaport R, Forest MG. Disorders of sexual differentiation. In: Bertrand J, Rappaport R, Sizonenko PC, eds. *Pediatric endocrinology.* Baltimore: Williams & Wilkins, 1993:447.

Older children requiring diagnostic evaluation include those presenting with stigmata of Turner syndrome, primary amenorrhea, and sexual infantilism. Unexplained virilization in females and gynecomastia in males (especially if bilateral and associated with testicular atrophy) also require diagnostic evaluation.

SURGICAL CONSIDERATIONS

Of greatest importance to the surgeon are those instances where surgical intervention is anticipated. Such intervention is critical to patient management not only from a reconstructive perspective, but also for diagnostic purposes. This is particularly true from the perspective of sexual assignment for ambiguous genitalia because the ability to surgically achieve unambiguous and functional genitalia is the fundamental criterion for sex assignment. Table 101-4 outlines the most common reasons for which individuals with intersex states may be seen by surgeons. Surgical involvement may include pediatric surgeons, pediatric urologists, adult urologists, and gynecologists. Consequently, an awareness of these entities is crucial for all such individuals.

TABLE 101-4 Reasons for Seeking Pediatric Surgical Specialist Involvement.

I. Ambiguous genitalia
II. Hernia as an isolated clinical finding
  A. Female: Testicular feminization, Leydig cell agenesis
  B. Male: Herniae uteri inguinale
III. Hypospadias, cryptorchidism
IV. Micropenis
  A. Real
  B. Apparent
    1. True concealed penis
    2. Obesity
V. Need for orchiectomy
  A. To prevent virilization with female sexual assignment
    1. True hermaphroditism
    2. Male pseudohermaphroditism
  B. To prevent or treat malignancy
    1. Mixed (46,X/XY) gonadal dysgenesis
    2. Testicular feminization
    3. Pure 46,XY gonadal dysgenesis
    4. Dysgenetic male pseudohermaphroditism
    5. True hermaphroditism
VI. Evaluation of scrotal mass
  A. Gonadal malignancy
    1. Germ cell
    2. Non–germ cell
  B. Hypertrophied adrenal rests from congenital adrenal hyperplasia
VII. Evaluation of mass in inguinal canal or labia of female
VIII. Gynecomastia
IX. Need for masculine reconstruction
X. Need for feminine reconstruction

AMBIGUOUS GENITALIA

Table 101-5 outlines a diagnostic classification framework for patients with ambiguous genitalia. Similarly, Table 101-6 provides a conceptual framework for the diagnosis of children with anomalous sexual development but with unambiguous genitalia. A great deal of information can be attained simply by addressing the karyotype and the nature of the gonads and internal ductal systems.

Masculinization of the Genetic Female (Female Pseudohermaphroditism)

Female pseudohermaphroditism is characterized by a 46,XX karyotype and by the presence of ovaries and müllerian ductal structures bilaterally. Most cases are due to congenital virilizing adrenal hyperplasia. Occasionally, masculinization of the female fetus may be due to maternal androgen-producing ovarian or adrenal tumors, a luteoma of pregnancy, or arrhenoblastoma. Iatrogenic causes are primarily due to exogenous administration of hormonal agents during pregnancy, such as testosterone, danazol, methylandrostenediol, norethindrone, ethisterone, norethynodrel, methoxyprogesterone, and 6α-methyltestosterone.

CAH accounts for approximately one-half of patients presenting with ambiguous genitalia, and more than 90% of cases of CAH are due to 21α-hydroxylase deficiency (Fig. 101-17). Genetic females with ambiguous genitalia secondary to either CAH or exogenous androgenic compounds should be given a female gender assignment and undergo feminine reconstruction because they have the potential for both normal sexual function and fertility.

Although only surgical therapy is required for exogenous virilization, medical therapy assumes great importance in cases of CAH. Treatment is directed at correcting cortisol deficiency and suppressing the overproduction of adrenal androgens. Careful monitoring of therapy is essential to avoid the adverse effects of excessive glucocorticoid therapy (diminished growth, short stature, obesity) and insufficient therapy (adrenal crisis with stress, pituitary hyperplasia–Nelson's syndrome, and adrenal carcinoma in both males and females; menstrual pathology, hirsutism, acne, and polycystic ovarian disease in females; and hypertrophied adrenal rests simulating testis tumors in males).

Medical management of 21-hydroxylase deficiency has been extensively reviewed (2,72). Neonatal management consists of volume and sodium resuscitation and administration of glucocorticoid in the form of hydrocortisone sodium succinate. Following resuscitation, maintenance steroid therapy is begun. Often, this takes the form of hydrocortisone, 12 to 20 mg per m^2 per day, divided into three

TABLE 101-5 Classification of Commonly Encountered Ambiguous Genitalis.

Category	*Gonad*	*Internal Ducts*	*Karyotype*	*Diagnosis*
Female PsH	O-O	M-M	46,XX	Congenital adrenal hyperplasia
				21α-Hydroxylase deficiency
				11β-Hydroxylase deficiency
				3β-Hydroxysteroid dehydrogenase deficiency
				Transfer of maternal androgens
				Maternal ingestion
				Androgen-producing neoplasms
True hermaphroditism	O-T	M-W	46,XX	True hermaphroditism
	OT-T	M/W-W	46,XX/46,XY	
	OT-O	M/W-M	46,XY	
	OT-OT	M/W-M/W		
Male PsH	T-T	W-W	46, XY	Incomplete androgen insensitivity
				5α-reductase deficiency
				Defects in androgen synthesis
				Side-chain cleavage deficiency
				3β-Hydroxysteroid dehydrogenase deficiency
				17α-Hydroxylase deficiency 17,20-Lyase deficiency
				17β-Hydroxysteroid oxidoreductase deficiency
Primary gonadal disorders	T-S	W-M/W	45,X/46,XY	Mixed gonadal dysgenesis
	X-X	X-X	46,XY	Embryonic testicular regression
	DT-DT	M-M	46,XY	Dysgenetic male pseudohermaphroditism

PsH, pseudohermaphrodite; O, ovary; T, testis; OT, ovotestis; S, streak; X, absent; DT, dysgenetic testis; M, müllerian; W, wolffian.

TABLE 101-6 Diagnosis of Intersexuality in Children Despite Unambiguous Genitalia.

External Genitalia	*Palpable Gonads*	*Karyotype*	*Diagnosis*	*Symptoms, Neonate*	*Symptoms, Childhood*
Female	Yes (+/−)	46,XY	Testicular feminization	Inguinal hernia	Primary amenorrhea
	Yes (+/−)	46,XY	Leydig cell agenesis	Inguinal hernia	Pubertal failure
	Yes (+/−)	46,XY	17β-Hydroxysteroid oxidoreductase deficiency		Virilization, primary amenorrhea, ± gynecomastia
	Yes (+/−)	46,XY	Side-chain cleavage	Salt wasting	Pubertal failure
	Yes (+/−)	46,XY	17α-Hydroxylase deficiency		HTN, primary amenorrhea ± gynecomastia, sexual infantilism
	Yes (+/−)	46,XY	17,20-Lyase		Sexual infantilism
	No	45,X	Turner syndrome	Lymphedema	Short stature, pubertal failure
	No	XX or XY	Pure GD		Pubertal failure
Male	Yes	46,XX	Persistent müllerian duct	Inguinal hernia	Inguinal hernia
	No	46,XX	21α-Hydroxylase	Salt wasting, hypospadias	Virilization, hematuria
	No	46,XX	11β-Hydroxylase	HTN, hypospadias	Virilization, hematuria
	Yes (+/−)	46,XX, etc.	True hermaphrodritism	Micropenis, hypospadias	Virilization, gynecomastia
	Yes	46,XX	XX male syndrome		Atretic testes infertility

GD, gonadal dysfunction; HTN hypertension.
From Rappaport R, Forest MG. Disorders of sexual differentiation. In: Bertrand J, Rappaport R, Sizonenko PC, eds. *Pediatric endocrinology.* Baltimore: Williams & Wilkins, 1993:447, with permission.

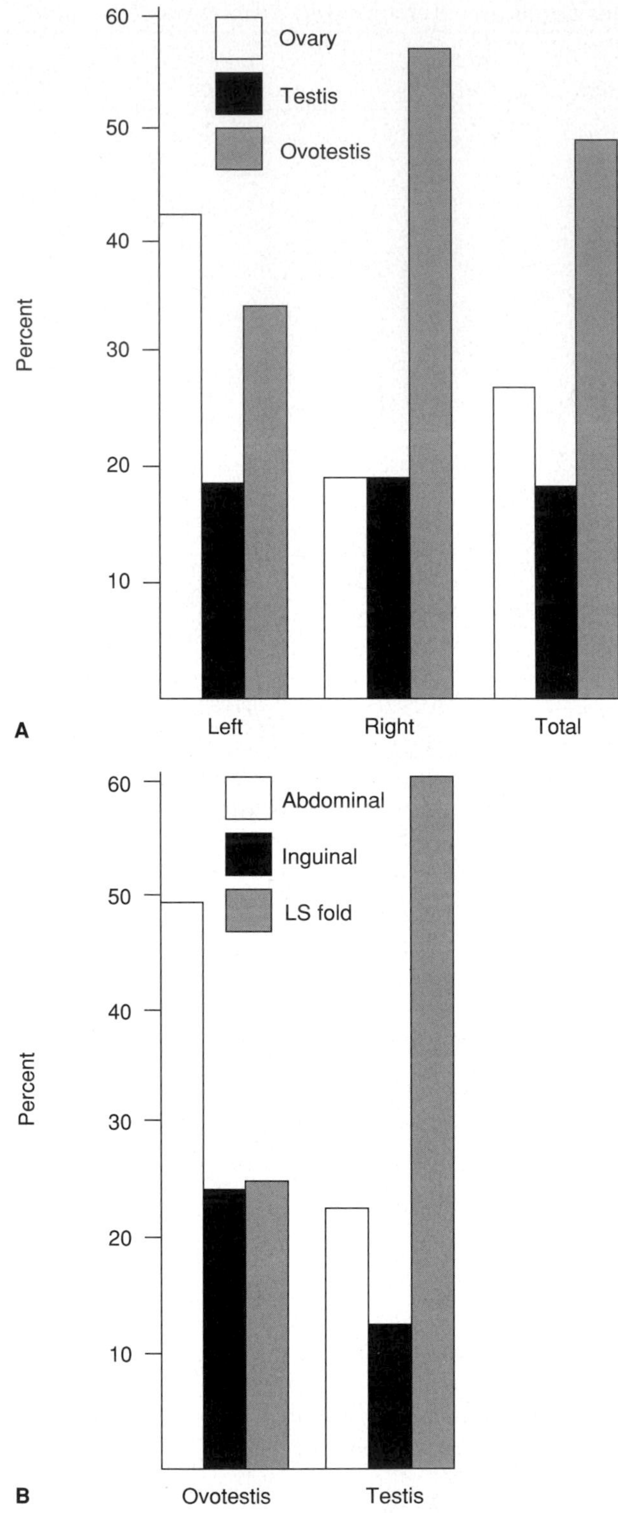

FIGURE 101-18. **(A)** Relative incidence of gonads encountered in true hermaphroditism. **(B)** Position of ovotestes and testes in true hermaphroditism.

oral doses. Patients with salt-wasting forms of CAH receive mineralocorticoid supplementation in the form of fluorocortisone, 70 to 90 μg per m^2 per day orally. Glucocorticoid therapy is monitored by serum 17-hydroxyprogesterone, androstendione, and testosterone levels and by urinary pregnentriol (21α-hydroxylase deficiency). Mineralocorticoid levels are monitored by plasma renin activity.

These pharmacologic concepts are important to the surgeon. Elective surgery should not be undertaken unless adequate glucocorticoid suppression has been achieved. In addition, increased dosages of glucocorticoids are required in the perioperative period (Table 101-7). A similar increase in dosage is required for emergent surgical or nonsurgical stress. Note that even in the absence of stress, during periods where oral intake is impossible or unreliable, parenteral therapy is needed. Table 101-8 outlines the dosage equivalents for various glucocorticoid preparations.

Surgical reconstruction in the form of feminizing genitoplasty is undertaken at 6 to 12 months of life. Best results are obtained when clitoroplasty and vaginoplasty are combined as a single-stage reconstruction. Surgical outcome plays a critical role in terms of patient well-being. This fact is emphasized by the observations of Mulaikal and colleagues (73), who reported a 75% incidence of homosexual, bisexual, or absent sexual activity in women who had an inadequate introitus, as opposed to a 25% incidence in those whose introitus was adequate. Reduction clitoroplasty is preferred over clitorectomy in order to preserve clitoral sensation and is also preferred over clitoral recession because it avoids the potential for uncomfortable erection, as is seen when recession techniques are employed.

TABLE 101-7 Glucocorticoid Therapy Guidelines for Elective Surgery in Patients with Congenital Adrenal Hyperplasia.

	Day	Agent	Dosage
Before surgery	−2	Cortisone acetate, hydrocortisone	20 mg/m^2 IM bid or 20 mg/m^2 PO tid
	−1	Cortisone acetate, hydrocortisone	20 mg/m^2 IM bid or 20 mg/m^2 PO tid
During surgery	0	Cortisone acetate, hydrocortisone	40 mg/m^2 IM bid IV as needed
After surgery	+1	Cortisone acetate, hydrocortisone	20 mg/m^2 IM bid or 20 mg/m^2 PO tid
	+2	Hydrocortisone	Maintenance if surgical stress over

Adapted from Morel Y, Bertrand J, Rappaport R. Disorders of hormonosynthesis. In: Bertrand J, Rappaport R, Sizonenko PC, eds. *Pediatric endocrinology.* Baltimore: Williams & Wilkins, 1993:305, with permission.

TABLE 101-8 Mean Estimated Optimal Dose of Glucocorticoid for Growth in Patients with Congenital Adrenal Hyperplasia.

Glucocorticoid	*Dosage (mg/m^2/d)*	*Equivalent Dosage*
Dexamethasone	0.23	1
Methylprednisolone	2.4	10
Prednisone	3.7	16
Hydrocortisone	18.4	80
Cortisone acetate (IM)	13.9	60
Cortisone acetate (PO)	22.0	96

Adapted from Grumbach MM, Conte FA. Disorders of sex differentiation. In: Wilson JD, Foster DW, eds. *Williams textbook of endocrinology.* Philadelphia: WB Saunders, 1992:853; Mulaikal RM, Migeon CJ, Rick JA. Fertility rates in female patients with congenital adrenal hyperplasia due to 21-hydroxylase deficiency. *N Engl J Med* 1987;316:178.

True Hermaphroditism

True hermaphroditism is a relatively uncommon disorder of sexual development. Its presentation is quite variable, ranging from an unambiguous neonatal female phenotype to what appears to be a male with hypospadias. Although the majority has ambiguous genitalia, most are quite virilized. Common presentations are cryptorchidism with hypospadias and hernia.

Patients with true hermaphroditism have by definition both ovarian and testicular tissue. Approximately 60% of patients have a 46,XX karyotype, followed by 46,XX/46,XY and 46,XY karyotypes, which represent 13% and 12% of individuals, respectively (74). Proposed mechanisms include mosaicism (mitotic or meiotic errors), chimerism (double fertilization, fusion, etc.), and translocation of Y chromosomal material to an autosome or to the X chromosome.

The key to the clinical diagnosis and management of true hermaphroditism is the gonad. Several caveats regarding the gonads of these individuals are critical. As depicted in Figure 101-18A, the most common gonad in true hermaphroditism is the ovotestis. However, there is important variation with respect to the side of occurrence. On the right, the ovotestis clearly predominates. On the left, the incidence of an ovary actually slightly exceeds that of the ovotestis. The ovary is generally encountered in the pelvis, although it may rarely be encountered in the inguinal canal in the presence of a significant inguinal hernia. One-half of ovotestes are intraabdominal, with the remainder approximately equally distributed between the inguinal canal and the labioscrotal fold. In contrast, a testis is most commonly encountered in the labioscrotal fold and relatively uncommonly (22%) in an intraabdominal position. These relationships are outlined in Fig. 101-18B.

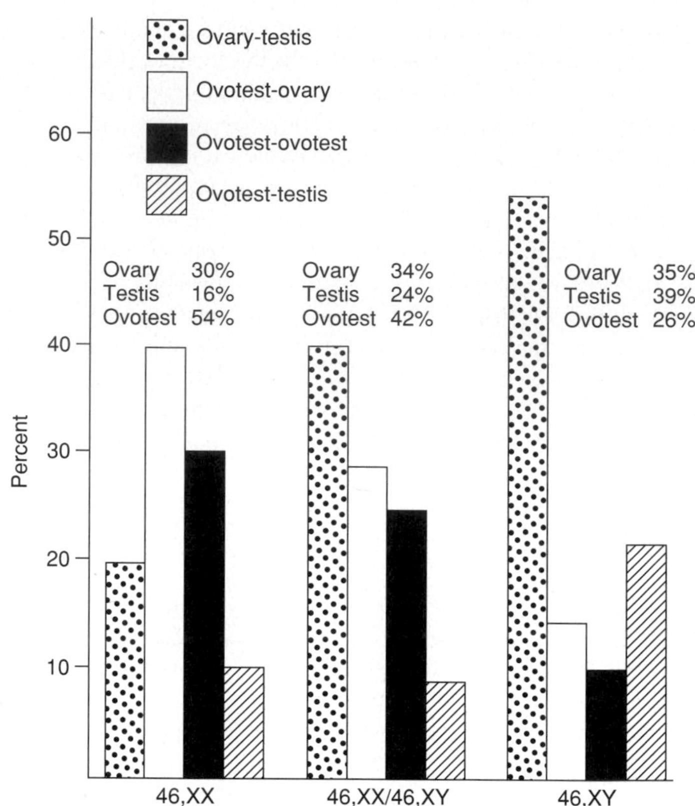

FIGURE 101-19. Gonadal distribution as a function of karyotype in true hermaphroditism.

As demonstrated in Fig. 101-19, there is a relationship between the karyotype and gonadal distribution. In the presence of a Y chromosome, the incidence of a testis, ovotestis, and ovary is 61%, 52%, and 68%, respectively. In contrast, in the absence of a Y chromosome, the relative incidences are 29%, 80%, and 56%. Among individuals with a 46,XX karyotype, the diagnostic gonad present is either an ovotestis (80%) or a testis with a contralateral ovary (20%). Of individuals with a 46,XX/46,XY karyotype, 60% have an ovotestis and 40% a testis with contralateral ovary. Of patients with a 46,XY karyotype, 46% have an ovotestis and 54% a testis with contralateral ovary. Other reported karyotypes are 46,XY/47,XXY (5.6%), 45,X/46,XY (3.5%), and other (6.2%).

As would be expected, the character of the ipsilateral gonad determines the internal ducts. Müllerian development is generally observed in the presence of either an ovary or ovotestis, whereas wolffian development is usually encountered in the presence of a testis. The majority of individuals have significant müllerian elements, a fact that has significant therapeutic implications.

From a diagnostic perspective, short of gonadal biopsy, those findings most suggestive of true hermaphroditism are a 46,XX/46,XY karyotype; the palpation of an elongated, lobulated gonad; and an elevated testosterone level that rises with hCG stimulation in the face of a 46,XX karyotype. Also suspicious is the individual with hypospadias and an undescended testis who is found to have a 46,XX or 46,XX/46,XY karyotype.

Traditionally, the majority of patients have been given a masculine gender assignment, but more recent data question the wisdom of this policy. In individuals raised as males, spermatogenesis is characteristically deficient. In addition, at puberty, gynecomastia is not uncommon, and periodic hematuria (menstruation) may be encountered. In contrast, individuals raised as females may ovulate, become pregnant, and deliver normal offspring. The potential for transmission of the disorder to offspring is believed to be small. Because females may virilize at puberty, it is critical to remove all testicular tissue when this gender assignment is given. Clearly, prompt neonatal diagnosis is important.

Surgical management of such patients is determined by the sex of rearing, which in most cases should be female. Those with a male gender assignment require removal of ovarian tissue and müllerian remnants. Because the testicular component of the ovotestis is generally dysgenetic, the entire gonad is removed. Often testes in this setting are also dysgenetic, and if documented to be so, should be removed. Testes that can achieve a scrotal position and do not demonstrate dysgenetic features by biopsy may be retained. Otherwise, a program of penile reconstruction, gonadectomy, testicular prosthesis placement, and hormonal replacement therapy appears most warranted. Patients given a female gender assignment must have all testicular tissue removed, including both testes and the testicular component of ovotestes.

Inadequate Masculinization of the Genetic Male (Male Pseudohermaphroditism)

As outlined in Table 101-3, male pseudohermaphroditism may be due to impaired testicular responsiveness to hCG and LH, inborn errors of testosterone biosynthesis, end-organ resistance to androgenic hormones, defects in testosterone metabolism, disorders of testicular development, and defects in the synthesis or secretion of or response to antimüllerian hormone. Many of these, however, do not result in genital ambiguity. Disorders of testicular development are discussed in a separate section. Characteristically, these patients have two testes and, with the exception of isolated antimüllerian hormone deficiency, müllerian elements are absent and wolffian ductal development is evident.

Inborn Errors of Testosterone Biosynthesis

Inborn errors of testosterone biosynthesis have been discussed in detail previously. Although cholesterol side-chain cleavage, 3β-hydroxysteroid, 17α-hydroxylase, 17,20-lyase, and 17β-hydroxysteroid oxidoreductase deficiencies all cause incomplete masculinization of the genetic male, 3β-hydroxysteroid dehydrogenase is most likely to result in true genital ambiguity. Some defects such as 17α-hydroxylase, 17,20-lyase, and 17β-hydroxysteroid oxidoreductase deficiencies may result in ambiguous genitalia. However, these lesions usually result in primarily highly feminized individuals.

End-Organ Resistance to Androgenic Hormones

End-organ resistance may be complete (testicular feminization) or incomplete. Patients with complete androgen insensitivity generally present with normal-appearing female external genitalia. They tend to have inguinal hernias or palpable inguinal masses in early childhood or primary amenorrhea in adolescence. Characteristically, normal pubertal female body habitus changes, including breast development, are noted with puberty. Axillary and pubic hair is usually minimally developed or occasionally completely absent. Pelvic examination reveals a short, blind-ending vagina with no cervix. Patients with incomplete androgen insensitivity characteristically have ambiguous genitalia. These individuals have been previously referred to by a number of eponyms, including Reifenstein, Lubs, and Gilbert-Dreyfus.

Significant genetic heterogeneity exists within these patient populations. Androgen insensitivity may be due to defects either in androgen receptor quantity or quality, including affinity and lability. Figure 101-20 depicts the androgen receptor gene and the mechanism of action of its product. The molecular biology of this receptor has been reviewed in detail (2). Pertinent points include the following: (1) the androgen receptor is encoded by a gene on the X chromosome, only 3% (eight exons) of which is actually translated; (2) the NH_2-terminal domain of the androgen receptor is encoded by exon A and is believed to have a transcriptional regulation function; (3) exons B and C code for two zinc fingers that are responsible for binding to DNA, with consequent stimulation of transcription of mRNA and translation of new protein, which then mediates androgenic effects; and (4) this binding is made possible by a conformational alteration in the androgen receptor induced by DHT binding. These events are similar to other proteins in the steroid receptor superfamily. Both deletions and point mutations resulting in altered receptor function have been described.

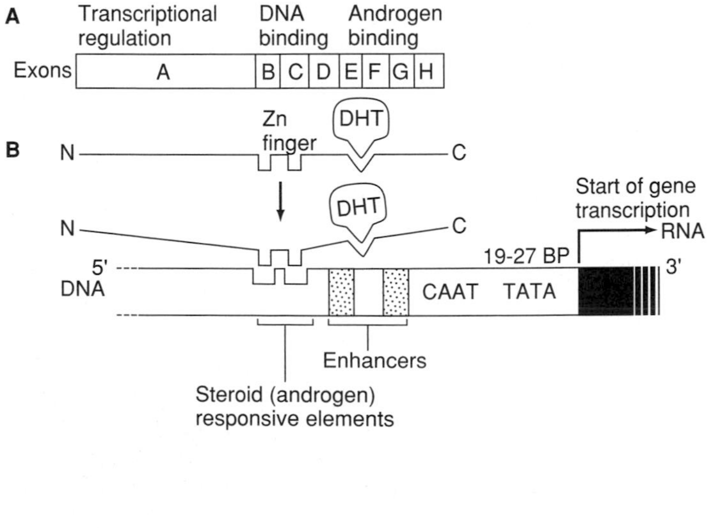

FIGURE 101-20. **(A)** Diagrammatic representation of the androgen receptor gene divided into its nine exons. Exon A codes for the NH_2-terminal domain and regulates transcription. Exons B and C code for two zinc fingers. Exons D through H code for the androgen-binding domain of the receptor. **(B)** Organization of a steroid-responsive gene. Ligand binding activates the receptor, which then binds to the steroid response elements of the gene, resulting in activation. (From Grumbach MM, Conte FA. Disorder of sex differentiation. In: Wilson JD, Foster DW, eds. *Williams textbook of endocrinology*. Philadelphia: WB Saunders, 1992:925, with permission.)

Individuals with incomplete androgen insensitivity present with ambiguity (small hypospadiac phallus and occasionally undescended testes) and a 46,XY karyotype. This condition is distinguished from disorders of testosterone biosynthesis by the absence of diminished testosterone levels and absence of precursor accumulation exacerbated by hCG administration. Supportive data include the measurement of diminished DHT-binding capacity and a blunted clinical response to exogenous androgen.

Strikingly masculinized patients may be given a male gender assignment, particularly if a response to exogenous androgen can be demonstrated. Otherwise, a feminine gender assignment would seem most appropriate. Individuals raised as males may develop gynecomastia at puberty, whereas those raised as females may experience some masculinization. Consequently, females should undergo early orchiectomy and should have estrogen replacement therapy at puberty.

Defects in Testosterone Metabolism

Deficiency of 5α-reductase activity is an unusual form of 46,XY male pseudohermaphroditism. It most typically presents with severe hypospadias involving a small phallus and the presence of a blind vaginal pouch that may open into a urogenital sinus or onto the perineum, hence the descriptive name *pseudovaginal perineoscrotal hypospadias*. Diagnosis is confirmed by the measurement of diminished 5α-reductase activity and is suggested by an elevated testosterone/DHT ratio and diminished basal and hCG-stimulated 5α/5β urinary steroid ratios.

As with incomplete androgen insensitivity, patients may be raised as males if they are heavily masculinized, particularly if the phallus is of adequate dimension and responds to DHT administration. Otherwise, a female gender assignment is most prudent. Because of a strong tendency toward masculinization with puberty, early orchiectomy is mandatory in females.

Disorders in Testicular Development

Syndromes associated with defective ovarian formation or persistence (e.g., 45,X Turner syndrome, its karyotypic variants, and 46,XX pure gonadal dysgenesis) are associated with unambiguous female genitalia. In contrast, syndromes associated with defective testis formation or defective testicular persistence may result in ambiguous genitalia. Examples include mixed gonadal dysgenesis, dysgenetic male pseudohermaphroditism, and embryonic testicular regression syndromes. Some primary testicular defects such as Leydig cell agenesis and 46,XY pure gonadal dysgenesis result in a female phenotype, whereas others, such as congenital anorchia, result in an unambiguous male phenotype.

Mixed Gonadal Dysgenesis

Mixed gonadal dysgenesis is characterized by the presence of asymmetric ambiguous external genitalia, a streak gonad on one side with a testis on the other, and a 45,X/46,XY karyotype. Often the testis is dysgenetic, and as a result, internal ducts may be müllerian on both sides. If the testis is not dysgenetic, ductal development may be müllerian on one side and wolffian on the other.

The tremendous phenotypic variation associated with this syndrome may result in a female presentation with clitoral hypertrophy or a male with hypospadias accompanied by cryptorchidism. In addition to a relatively characteristic karyotype, such clinical clues as the presence of Ullrich-Turner stigmata (facial asymmetry, high palate, low hairline, webbed neck, short metacarpus, multiple nevi) may aid in diagnosis. Testosterone levels tend to be depressed, with elevated LH and FSH levels.

An important clinical correlate of mixed gonadal dysgenesis is the high incidence of gonadoblastoma seen in these individuals, making its diagnosis very important. A confounding observation, however, is that this syndrome may be associated with other mosaic karyotypes and even a 46,XY karyotype. In the latter circumstance, presumably 45,X cell lines occur in low proportion and are consequently undetected.

The preferred sex assignment is female. However, heavily masculinized individuals may be raised as male, provided the testis is scrotal (available for palpation) and not dysgenetic on biopsy. Streak gonads are removed, as are dysgenetic testes, regardless of the sex of rearing. Bilateral orchiectomy is performed in all individuals raised as females.

Dysgenetic Male Pseudohermaphroditism

The category of dysgenetic male pseudohermaphroditism contains individuals with a 46,XY karyotype and bilateral dysgenetic testes associated with Leydig and Sertoli cell functional deficiency. This does not appear to be an etiologically distinct syndrome. An association with Drash syndrome and Frasier syndrome has been described. Gonadoblastoma risk is present, and the preferred sexual assignment is female.

TESTICULAR REGRESSION SYNDROMES

The category of testicular regression syndrome contains a spectrum of clinical entities with marked phenotypic variability, a 46,XY karyotype, and evidence of testicular formation followed by testicular regression. Congenital anorchia is relatively common. These individuals exhibit a normal male phenotype with absent müllerian derivatives. In contrast, patients with rudimentary testes present with atrophic testes and a micropenis, whereas patients with true agonadism (embryonic testicular regression) present with ambiguous genitalia. In both of the latter diagnoses, müllerian elements may be absent or rudimentary.

46,XX Males

A 46,XX male karyotype may be associated with ambiguous genitalia, a hypospadiac male phenotype, or occasionally a normal male phenotype. Careful gonadal examination is imperative to exclude the presence of true hermaphroditism.

HERNIA AS AN ISOLATED CLINICAL PRESENTATION

An inguinal hernia is one of the most common presentations of intersex states associated with normal or near-normal male or female external genitalia. The most common intersex state to present in this fashion is testicular feminization or complete androgen insensitivity. Also encountered are such abnormalities as Leydig cell agenesis, which is associated with a female phenotype, and hernia uteri inguinale, a deficiency of antimüllerian hormone, which presents with a male phenotype.

Both testicular feminization and Leydig cell agenesis are identifiable by encountering either a testis or the absence of müllerian derivatives at herniorrhaphy. In contrast, hernia uteri inguinale is identified by the unexpected encounter of müllerian remnants (i.e., a fallopian tube) at the time of herniorrhaphy in a male.

Testicular feminization occurs with sufficient frequency to warrant exclusion with every female inguinal hernia encountered. Figure 101-21 demonstrates the typical finding at surgery. Every female hernia should be approached with this potential diagnosis in mind. The hernia sac is opened, the most prominent peritoneal fold grasped with forceps, and the fallopian tube delivered for inspection. This is an easy step that adds only seconds to the procedure.

Identification of a fallopian tube excludes the diagnosis of testicular feminization. If this structure is not identified, further examination may reveal a testis (Fig. 101-21). Otherwise, on completion of the herniorrhaphy, the vagina should be examined employing an infant cystoscope. Again, identification of a cervix excludes the diagnosis of testicular feminization. If a blind-ending vagina without a cervix is encountered, a karyotype analysis is indicated.

If unexpectedly encountered, testes are not removed at that setting. Time is required for parental counseling, and the parents are given the option of retaining the testes through puberty with removal later. It is appropriate, however, to electively return to the operating room for orchiectomy during infancy because of the potential risk of losing the patient to follow-up and the subsequent potential for malignant degeneration of the testis.

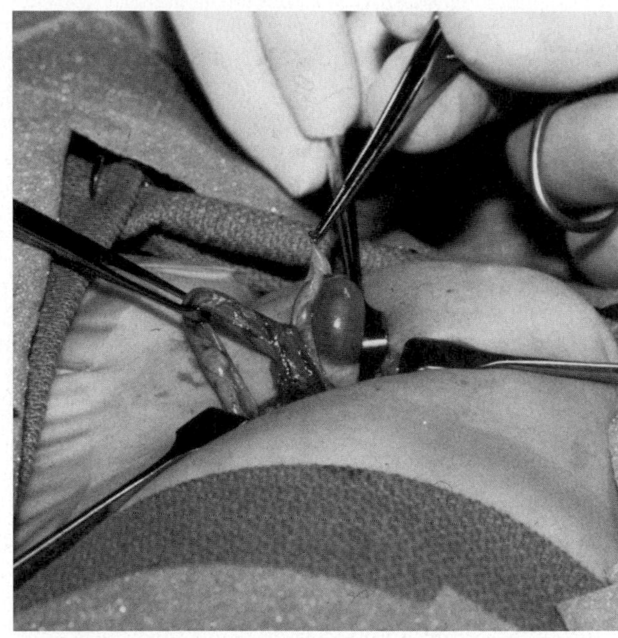

FIGURE 101-21. Infant with androgen insensitivity presenting with inguinal hernia. The testis is present in the inguinal incision at the time of hernia repair in this phenotypic female.

HYPOSPADIAS AND CRYPTORCHIDISM

Any degree of hypospadias associated with any degree of bilateral or unilateral gonadal undescent requires evaluation to exclude an intersex state (75). All such instances require a karyotype analysis. The diagnoses most commonly encountered are mixed gonadal dysgenesis and true hermaphroditism. Cystourethroscopy or ultrasonography (looking for müllerian remnants), diagnostic laparoscopy, or gonadal biopsy may be indicated in selected instances.

MICROPENIS

The terms *micropenis* and *microphallus* have generally been used synonymously. It is important to distinguish between the small penis (true micropenis), which is otherwise normally developed, from that which is associated with a hypospadiac meatus and chordee (often referred to as microphallus), which falls under the classification of ambiguous genitalia.

Also confused in the literature are other diagnostic entities associated with the appearance of a small penis. These include the buried penis, the trapped penis, and the webbed penis. These entities are readily distinguished on physical examination by the experienced surgeon. Rarely, extremely masculinized forms of CAH or other intersex abnormalities may present with a small phallus that is otherwise well developed. Generally, however, careful examination reveals an abnormality in urethral development, even if relatively minor. This differential must not be excluded during the diagnostic evaluation of such an infant.

The true micropenis is primarily an endocrinologic problem and secondarily a surgical problem if an adequate penile growth response is unattainable by hormonal therapy. The differential diagnosis of true micropenis involves abnormalities at several levels of the hypothalamic-pituitary-gonadal axis (Table 101-9). Examples include hypopituitarism (panhypopituitarism, isolated growth hormone deficiency, and isolated gonadotropin deficiency). In addition, congenital adrenal hypoplasia has been reported as a cause of micropenis. An occasional report has implicated primary testicular failure developing after the first trimester (organogenesis complete) as an etiology.

The evaluation of a newborn with a micropenis begins with a karyotype and a renal and pelvis US examination. In addition, basal and hCG-stimulated testosterone levels are obtained. Serum is also saved for basal and stimulated steroid precursor analysis. Depending on the results of these studies, other biochemical assays may be required. In the vast majority of instances, 46,XY infants with micropenis have an attempt made toward a male sexual assignment. Of critical importance is the response to exogenous androgen (testosterone enanthate, hCG, or DHT) administration in terms of penile growth.

It is important to maintain close follow-up of these individuals and monitor their penile growth as compared with normal control populations (Fig. 101-22). Redosing

TABLE 101-9 Etiology of Micropenis.

Etiology
Endocrine causes
Isolated growth hormone deficiency (frequently associated with hypoglycemia)
Panhypopitiuitarism
Laron syndrome
Hypogonadotropic hypogonadism
Isolated with anosmia
Associated with anosmia (Kallmann or de Morser syndrome)
Prader-Willi-Labhart syndrome
Rud syndrome with ichthyosis
Anencephaly
Hypergonadrotropic hypogonadism
Klinefelter syndrome
Other XXXY syndromes
Anorchidism
Rudimentary testes syndrome
Male pseudohermaphroditism
Testosterone biosynthesis defect
Incomplete androgen insensitivity
Gonadal dysgenesis syndrome
Fetal exposure to exogenous progestins during pregnancy
Nonendocrine causes (poorly defined etiologies)
Noonan syndrome
Smith-Lemli-Opitz syndrome
Cornelia de Lange syndrome
Laurence-Moon-Biedly-Bardet syndrome
Fanconi anemia
Fetal intoxication to hydantoins
Deletion of the long arm of chromosome 18
Williams syndrome

From Sizonenko PC. Disorders of the testes. In: Bertrand J, Rappaport R, Sizonenko PC, eds. *Pediatric endocrinology.* Baltimore: Williams & Wilkins, 1993:430, with permission.

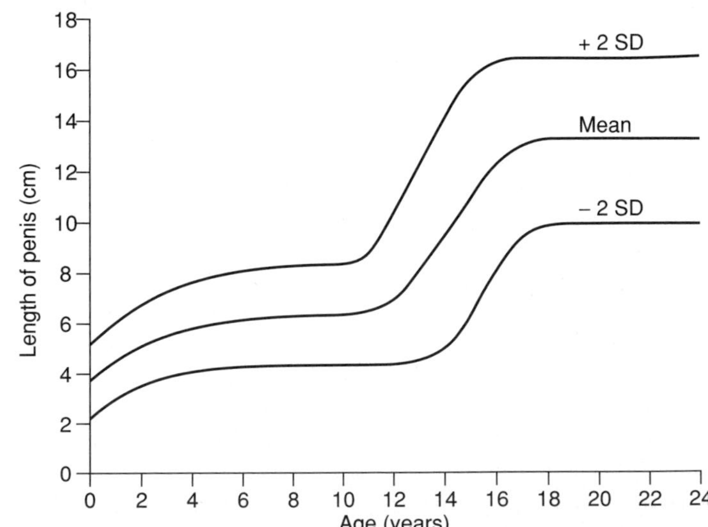

FIGURE 101-22. Mean length of phallus (± 2 SD) as a function of age. (From Schonfeld WD. Primary and secondary sexual characteristics, with biometric study of penis and testes. *Am J Dis Child* 1943;65:535, with permission.)

may be required to optimize outcome. Males with a small but otherwise normal-appearing penis may tolerate their abnormality quite well. Sexual reassignment in nonresponders must, however, be considered.

NEED FOR ORCHIECTOMY

Orchiectomy may be indicated to prevent malignancy or to prevent unwanted endocrine changes during puberty. It is critically important to remove any testicular tissue in patients raised as females. Failure to do so may result in inappropriate virilization with the onset of puberty. Consequently, patients with male pseudohermaphroditism and mixed gonadal dysgenesis raised as females require bilateral gonadectomy. Similarly, true hermaphrodites raised as females require removal of testes or the testicular component of ovotestes if encountered.

The risk of malignancy in some gonads is also significant. As mentioned previously, patients with mixed gonadal dysgenesis raised as females require bilateral gonadectomy. In instances where a male gender assignment is made, the streak gonad is always removed. If the testis is histologically not dysgenetic and if it has or can be made to have a scrotal position, it can be retained. Otherwise, removal and testicular prostheses along with endocrine maintenance is most satisfactory. If a testis is retained, careful follow-up palpation is mandatory.

Similarly, individuals with testicular feminization and either pure or partial varieties of 46,XY gonadal dysgenesis require bilateral orchiectomy. As with mixed gonadal dysgenesis, the testes and testicular components of ovotestes in true hermaphroditism are often dysgenetic. Patients raised as females have all testicular tissue removed. Individuals raised as males should have all ovotestes and ovaries removed. A testis that is not dysgenetic on biopsy and that has, or can be made to have, a scrotal position can be retained, provided good follow-up is obtained.

EVALUATION OF THE SCROTAL MASS

As with any male, the first consideration for an intersex patient with a scrotal mass is the potential for gonadal neoplasia. A high index of suspicion is warranted. Such neoplasms may be either germ cell or non–germ cell in nature. Evaluation and management are similar to that of other testicular neoplasms. A chest radiograph as well as serum β-hCG and alpha-fetoprotein (AFP) are obtained. In the intersex setting, an additional blood sample is stored because some neoplasms may excrete steroid substances, which may be useful in follow-up.

Management consists of an inguinal exploration with early control of the cord vasculature, followed by delivery of the scrotal mass or testicle. If tumor is evident, the cord structures are divided at the level of the internal inguinal ring and the gonad removed. In equivocal cases, the testis may be biopsied, but meticulous attention must be directed at avoidance of tumor spillage.

An important exception to this aggressive surgical approach to the scrotal mass involves the male with congenital virilizing adrenal hyperplasia. Such children, if poorly controlled by steroid maintenance therapy, may develop scrotal masses secondary to hypertrophy of adrenal rests. Often these children present with excessive virilization or pseudoprecocious puberty. *Pseudoprecocious puberty* is generally due to the peripheral excretion of sex steroids independent of true hypothalamic-pituitary control, which induces secondary sexual characteristics that are either isosexual (consistent with genetic sex) or heterosexual (opposing genetic sex). It should be contrasted to *true precocious puberty*, which in general is induced by premature activation of the hypothalamic-pituitary-gonadal axis.

Such hypertrophied adrenal rests are often intratesticular and bilateral. An important differential diagnosis is the Leydig cell tumor, which presents as a scrotal mass (which occasionally is quite subtle) and, because of excessive testosterone excretion, causes isosexual pseudoprecocious puberty. Other entities presenting with excessive virilization of the male child and enlarged testes must be considered in this setting. Table 101-10 outlines the differential diagnosis of precocious and pseudoprecocious puberty in males. Many of these conditions are associated with enlarged testes. Of additional diagnostic benefit is that the hypertrophied adrenal rests and Leydig cell tumors generally both show discrete intratesticular masses on ultrasonography. An additional important diagnostic point is that Leydig cell tumors are usually unilateral, whereas hypertrophied adrenal rests are generally bilateral.

EVALUATION OF THE MASS IN THE INGUINAL CANAL OR LABIA OF THE FEMALE

An unexplained mass within the inguinal canal or the labia of the female requires urgent surgical evaluation. Masses within the labia are at risk of being either a testis or ovotestis and should be removed. An irreducible mass within the inguinal canal most commonly represents either a lymph node or an incarcerated hernia (usually ovary). However, occasionally testes or ovotestes are encountered.

The diagnostic approach depends on the degree of clinical suspicion. If a lymph node is suspected, ultrasonography can be diagnostic. This study reveals an echolucent center of the inguinal mass and also shows the presence of

TABLE 101-10 Diagnosis of Precocious Puberty and Pseudoprecocious Puberty in Boys.

Testes	Possible Diagnosis	Pituitary Gonadotropins	Testosterone	Additional Tools
Both enlarged	True precocious puberty Idiopathic CNS tumors	Low or normal	Moderately elevated	
	Pseudoprecocious puberty Gonadotropin-secreting tumor	Low	Moderately elevated	High α-FP and β-hCG
	Overlap syndrome[a] Hypothyroidism	Moderately elevated	Moderately elevated	TSH and thyroid hormones
	Congenital adrenal hyperplasia	Low	Moderately elevated	Elevated 17OH progesterone and adrenal androgens; mass on US exam
One enlarged	Benign tumor Leydig cell tumor	Low	Elevated	Mass on US exam
	Malignant tumor Chorioepithelioma	Low	Elevated	High β-hCG; mass on US exam
Both small	Congenital adrenal hyperplasia	Low	Moderately elevated	Elevated 17OH progesterone and adrenal androgens; mass on US exam
	Primary cortisol resistance	Low	Moderately elevated	High cortisol and high ACTH
	Adrenal tumor	Low	Moderately elevated	Elevated adrenal androgens
	Exogenous androgen administration	Low	Usually low	

[a]Generalized stimulation of tropic hormones secondary to hypothyroidism.
CNS, central nervous system; TSH, thyroid-stimulating hormone; US, ultrasonographic; ACTH, adrenocorticoptropic hormones.
From Sizonenko PC, Precocious puberty. In: Bertrand J, Rappaport R, Sizonenko PC, eds. *Pediatric endocrinology.* Baltimore: Williams & Wilkins, 1993:430.

two ovaries within the pelvis. A lymph node thus confirmed may be treated by antibiotic therapy alone.

If an incarcerated ovary is suspected, prompt surgical exploration and reduction is indicated to reduce the risk of ischemic ovarian injury. The management of a testis or ovotestis, if encountered, is as described.

GYNECOMASTIA

Gynecomastia is commonly encountered in intersex patients raised as males. Examples include true hermaphroditism, some types of male pseudohermaphroditism (e.g., defects in testosterone synthesis and incomplete androgen insensitivity), and mixed gonadal dysgenesis.

It is critical to avoid any situations that may raise questions regarding sexual identity and possibly lower self-esteem. Consequently, gynecomastia in such settings warrants surgical intervention. In the setting of mixed gonadal dysgenesis, a retained gonad, and gynecomastia, consideration should be given to the potential presence of a gonadoblastoma, which may induce gynecomastia secondary to estradiol secretion.

NEED FOR MASCULINE RECONSTRUCTION

In most instances, masculine reconstruction can be performed in a single-stage procedure. However, without question, better results are attained in some individuals employing a staged approach. Attention is directed toward urethral reconstruction, correction of chordee (which may be due to cutaneous tethering, true fibrous chordee, or corporal disproportion), and scrotoplasty to correct scrotal tethering or penoscrotal transposition. Such reconstruction is optimally performed prior to 1 year of age.

Urethral reconstruction may be performed employing either vascular pedicle flap or free-graft techniques or a combination. Correction of cutaneous or fibrous chordee is readily attained, whereas chordee due to corporal disproportion can be more difficult. Corporal disproportion can be corrected by either dorsal plication (dorsal shortening) or ventral corporoplasty (ventral lengthening) techniques. In the setting of ambiguous genitalia, where penile length is generally compromised, lengthening techniques are often most appropriate.

Figure 101-23 demonstrates a common single-stage procedure used to correct severe hypospadias. This

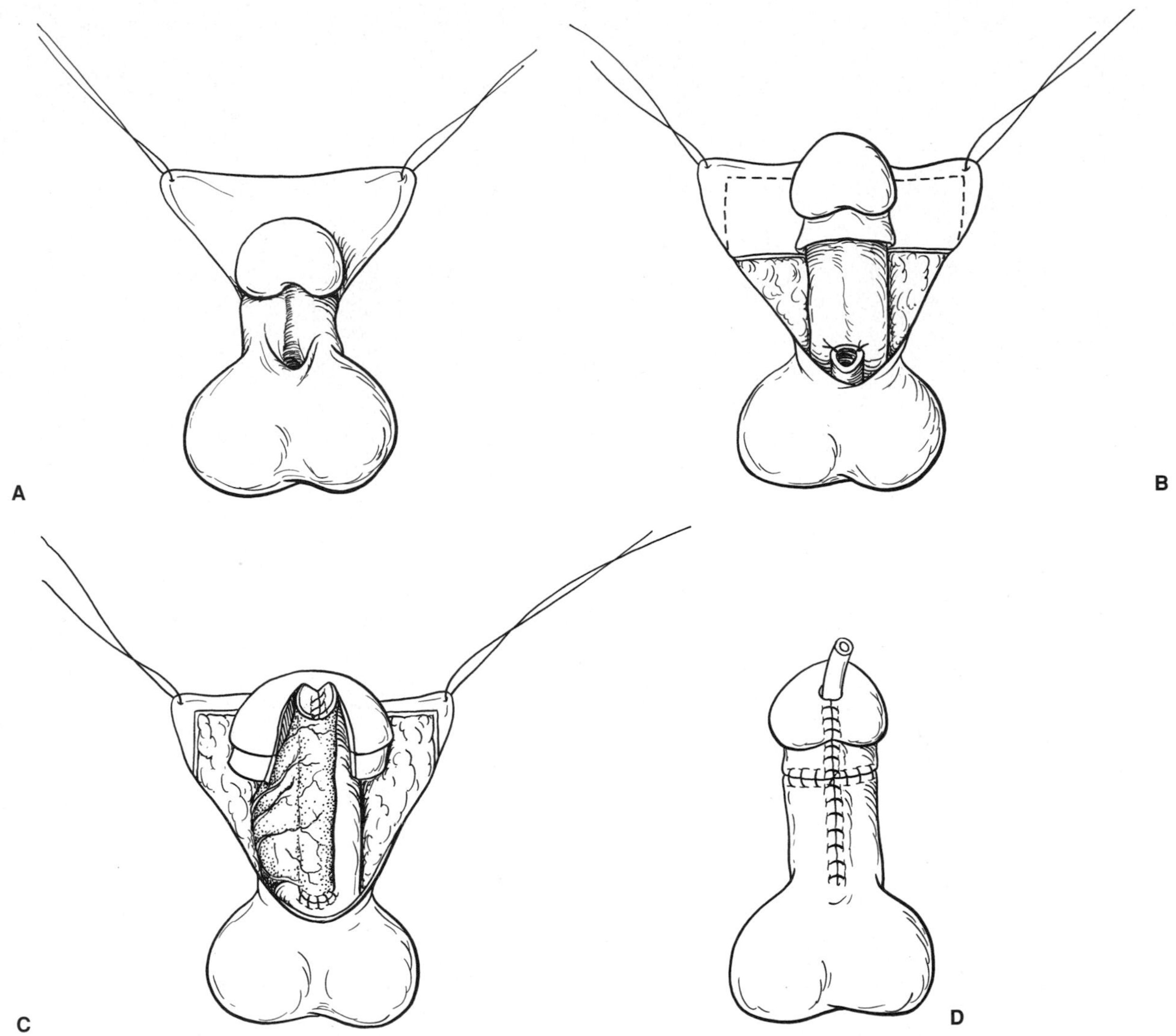

FIGURE 101-23. **(A)** Penoscrotal hypospadias associated with chordee. A circumferential incision coursing approximately 5 mm from the coronal sulcus allows the penile shaft skin to be mobilized and the associated fibrous chordee tissue to be excised, resulting in a straight shaft. **(B)** Dissection between the urethra and corpora is generally necessary to optimize chordee release, resulting in further caudal displacement of the urinary meatus. A rectangular flap of inner preputial skin is developed, tubularized **(C)**, and mobilized on its vascular pedicle to extend the urethra to the tip of the glans. **(D)** Glans flaps are developed and approximated ventrally to the neourethra, and the cutaneous defect is closed by transposing the remaining dorsal foreskin ventrally.

tubularized vascular pedicle preputial flap procedure described by Duckett may be used alone or in conjunction with interposition procedures to achieve a very satisfactory functional and cosmetic result.

Very often in intersex patients, there is insufficient skin to allow both urethral replacement and penile resurfacing. The surgeon must choose between a composite urethral reconstruction (Fig. 101-24) or a staged reconstruction. Composite urethral reconstruction may involve tubularization of a perimeatal-based flap extending either distally (Fig. 101-24A) or caudally (Fig. 101-24B). Alternatively, a tubularized free graft of buccal mucosa, bladder mucosa or skin can be used for the reconstructive surgery (Fig. 101-24C).

The Durham-Smith staged procedure is a particularly useful reconstructive alternative in severe cases (Fig. 101-25). Chordee is released as described, and glans flaps are developed (Fig. 101-25A). The dorsal foreskin is incised in the midline and transposed ventrally to cover the penile shaft and, in addition, the exposed glandular surfaces (Fig. 101-25B). After approximately 3 to 6 months, the second stage of the reconstruction begins with an extended

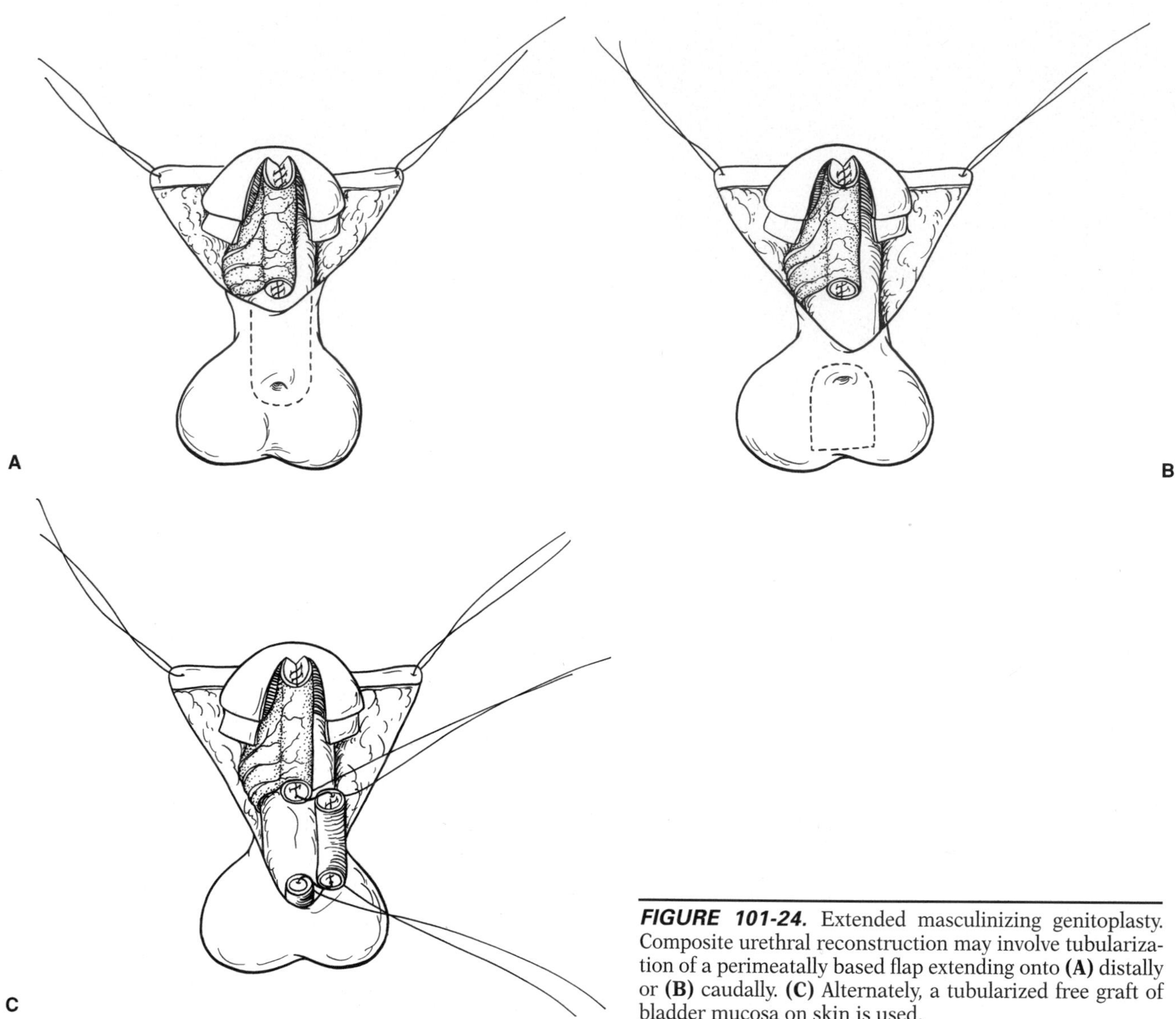

FIGURE 101-24. Extended masculinizing genitoplasty. Composite urethral reconstruction may involve tubularization of a perimeatally based flap extending onto **(A)** distally or **(B)** caudally. **(C)** Alternately, a tubularized free graft of bladder mucosa on skin is used.

U-shaped incision (Fig. 101-25C). The neourethra is created by tubularization of the resultant midline strip of skin (Fig. 101-25D) and the resultant cutaneous defect is closed (Fig. 101-25E). Not uncommonly, insufficient skin at the ventral base of the penis prevents closure without tension. This is circumvented by the development of a scrotal interposition flap.

The most difficult cases are those that involve corporal disproportion (Fig. 101-26). After complete cutaneous mobilization and excision of fibrous chordee, a severe ventral curvature persists (Fig. 101-26A). If the curvature is mild or the penile length adequate, a dorsal plication may be considered. Very often, in the intersex patient, this is not a reasonable alternative, and ventral lengthening is required. This begins with the excision of the defective corporal tissue (Fig. 101-26B), which generally gives dramatic straightening and lengthening of the penis (Fig. 101-26B). The resultant defect is resurfaced employing a vascular pedicle flap of tunica vaginalis. Alternatively, a free dermal graft, small intestinal submucosa (SIS) or lyophilized dura has been used.

NEED FOR FEMININE RECONSTRUCTION

Feminizing genitoplasty represents the most common surgical reconstruction for individuals with ambiguous genitalia. Reconstruction of female genitalia with the potential for good function can range from a relatively straightforward to an extremely complex procedure. Such reconstruction should be undertaken by committed, experienced reconstructive surgeons, and long-term follow-up is necessary. Detailed preoperative counseling is critical. Parents must understand the risk of vaginal stenosis,

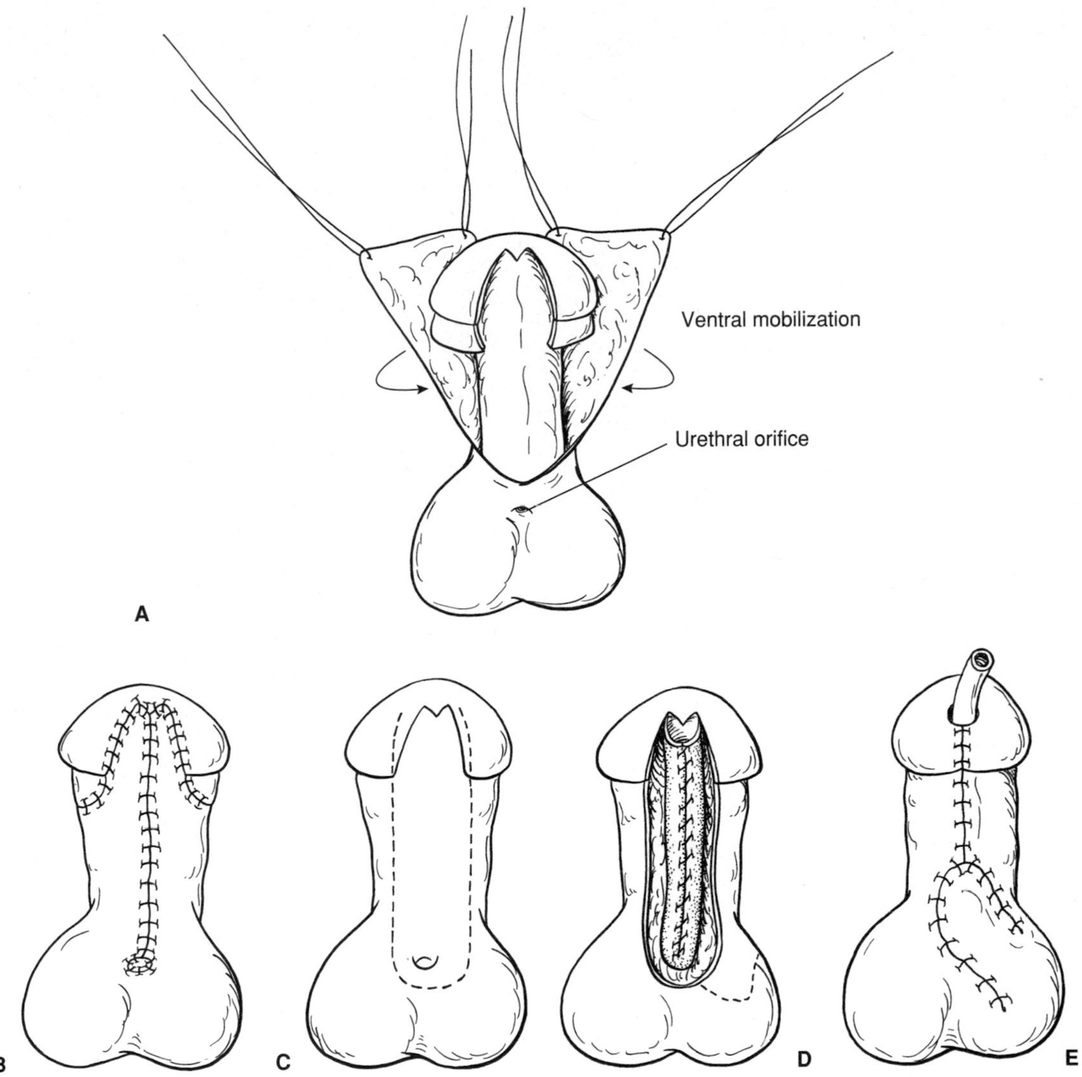

FIGURE 101-25. Staged masculinizing genitoplasty (see text).

the need for close follow-up, and the need for routine vaginal dilatation until sexual maturity has been reached. Optimal results are achieved employing a single-stage approach, which is ideally completed prior to 1 year of age. Reconstruction consists of clitoroplasty, vaginoplasty, and labioplasty.

The goals of clitoroplasty are threefold. The first is to cosmetically reduce the size of the phallic structure to that expected for a clitoris. In addition, it is important to preserve sensation and eliminate the potential for problematic future corporal erection. A successful vaginoplasty should achieve a satisfactory cosmetic appearance and a vaginal vault of adequate dimension to allow intercourse on reaching sexual maturity, and should allow the egress of uterine secretions. With pregnancy, vaginal delivery may not be possible without permanent vaginal trauma, however, and cesarean should be considered depending on the extent of surgical reconstruction performed. In some instances, routine vaginal dilation during childhood may be required to preserve patency. When the patient reaches sexual maturity, intercourse is often facilitated by a small introitoplasty, which is well tolerated and clearly preferable to the performance of the total vaginoplasty at an older age.

As demonstrated in Fig. 101-27, clitoroplasty begins with a circumferential incision 3 to 5 mm proximal to the coronal sulcus, which is interrupted ventrally to allow preservation of the urethral plate and maximization of glandular blood supply (Fig. 101-27A). The phallic shaft skin is totally mobilized, and the urethral plate and dorsal neurovascular bundles are carefully dissected free from the adjacent corpora cavernosa (Fig. 101-27B). A strip of tunica albugenia may be left with the neurovascular bundles to prevent injury to these structures. The corpora are dissected throughout their length and ligated and divided

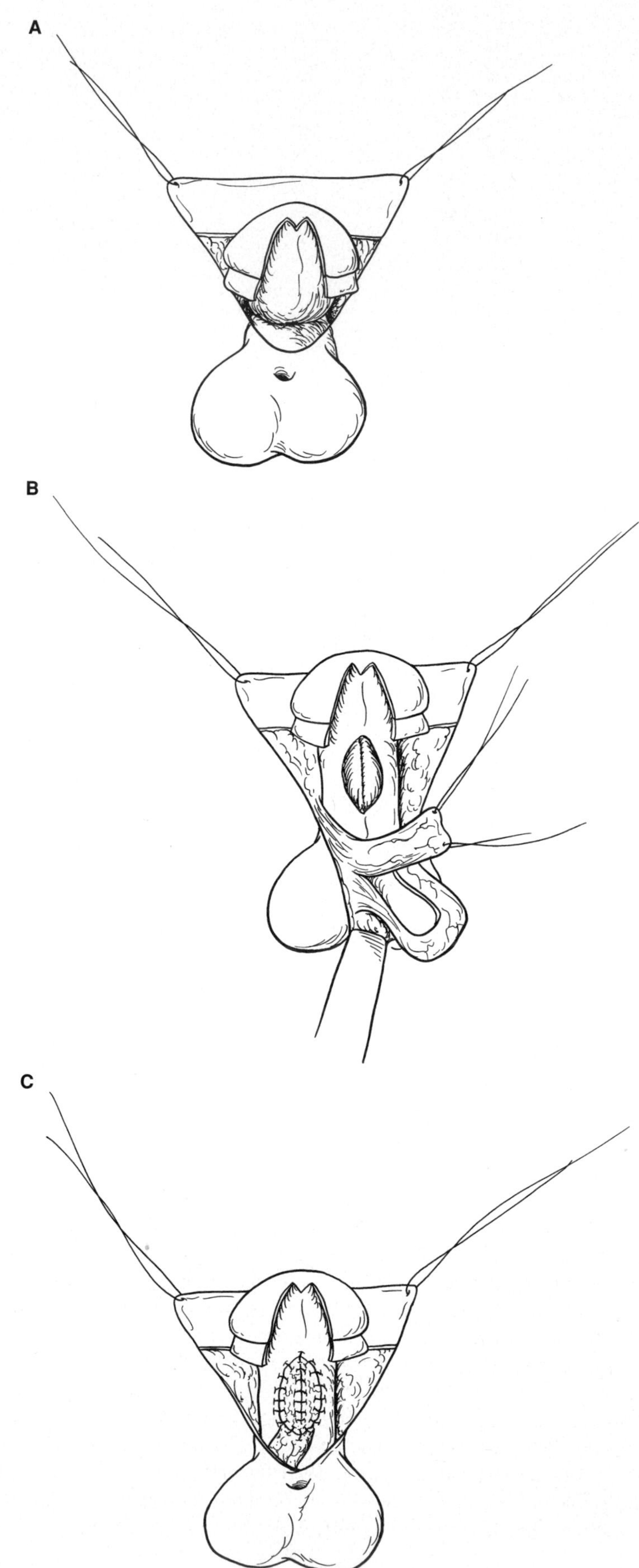

FIGURE 101-26. Correction of corporal disproportion by tunica vaginalis graft (see text).

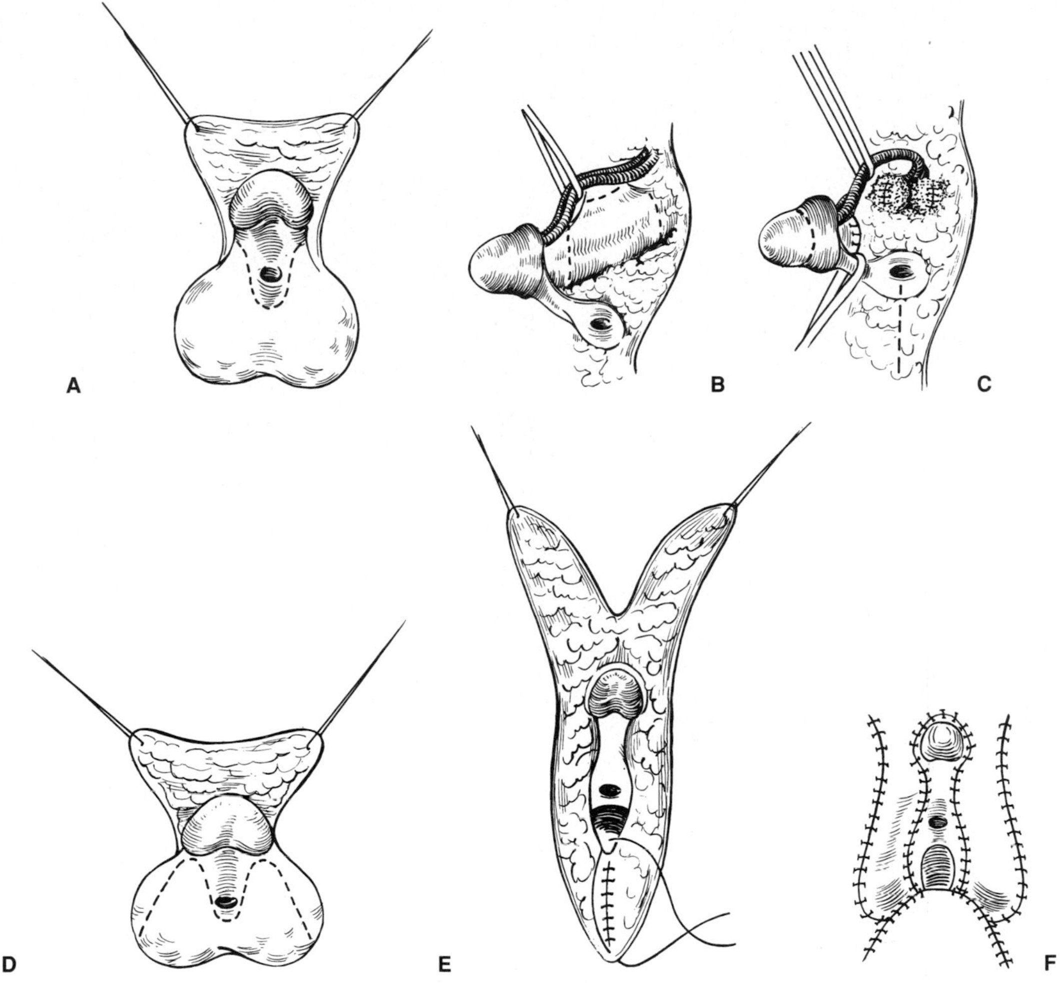

FIGURE 101-27. Clitoroplasty and feminizing genitoplasty, low lesion (see text).

at their insertion into the glans and their origins on the inferior pubic ramus and removed. The clitoris is partially deepithelialized, leaving only a portion of the distal glans comparable with the size of a normal clitoris with epithelium. The clitoroplasty is completed by approximating the oversewn edge of the corpora to the prepubic fascia to secure its final position (Fig. 101-27C).

The technique of vaginoplasty used depends solely on the individual's internal and external genital anatomy, which is assessed preoperatively by careful endoscopic examination. Of particular importance is the determination of the level of entry of the vagina into the urogenital sinus relative to the striated urinary sphincter. Low anomalies (vaginal confluence distal to sphincter) may be managed by inlay flap techniques, whereas high anomalies (confluence proximal to sphincter) require alternative approaches. In most instances, however, total urogenital sinus mobilization (TUGSM) achieves an excellent outcome. Here, the urethra and the vagina are delivered such that their outlet is flush with the perineum. The urogenital sinus tissue is reconfigured as the vulva. Occasionally, TUGSM must be supplemented with labioscrotal flap techniques to achieve an optimal outcome (76–81).

Figures 101-27A and 101-27D demonstrate the most widely applicable technique of feminizing vaginoplasty for low urogenital sinus anomalies, performed in the dorsal lithotomy position. An inverted (Fig. 101-27D) U- or M-shaped incision in the labioscrotal fold outlines a vaginal insertion flap. The underlying urogenital sinus is exposed and incised in the midline, unroofing the urethral meatus and vagina introitus as separate orifices (Fig. 101-27E). The labioscrotal flap is then sutured into place as an insertion flap and the prepuce is incised in the midline. This results in a wide and slightly posteriorly directed orifice (82), and each half of the prepuce is rotated caudally to allow creation of labia (labioplasty) (Fig. 101-27F).

Occasionally, the labioscrotal folds may be sufficiently separated or be associated with a sufficiently posterior urogenital sinus orifice that a U-shaped incision is ineffective. In this setting, an M-shaped incision is created and the

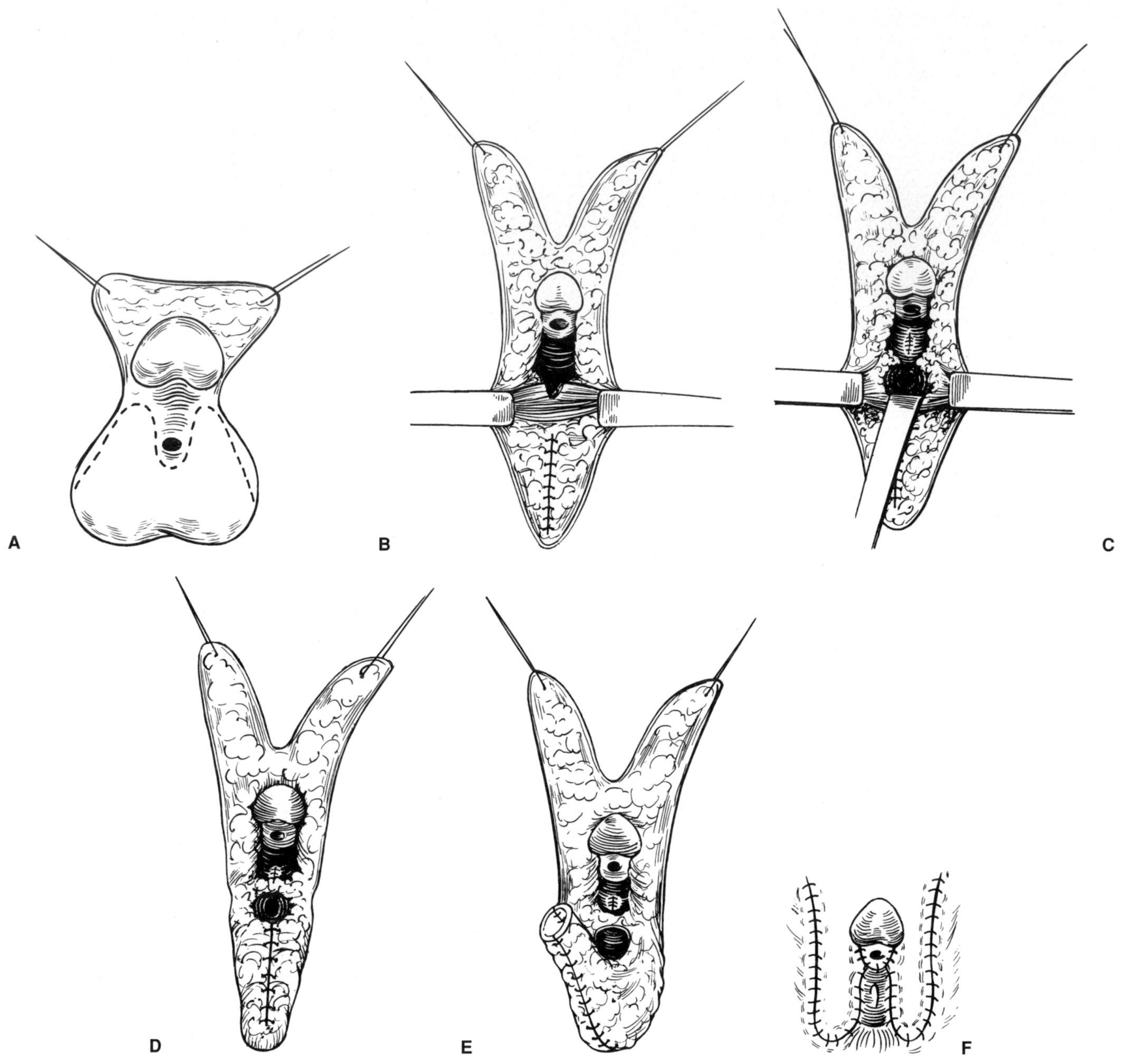

FIGURE 101-28. Feminizing genitoplasty, high lesion (see text).

two resultant flaps approximated in the midline to create a single posteriorly based insertion flap, as described. The M-shaped incision is extremely versatile and can be used in many cases where the vagina has a high insertion or where the vagina is completely absent (83).

A considerably more difficult reconstruction is required for the high vaginal insertion. Most surgical variations are based on the work of Hendren (84–86). Typically, this involves a vagina that opens into the urogenital sinus at the level of what would otherwise be the utricle in the verumontanum. In this instance, the use of an inlay flap would not only result in an unacceptable cosmetic appearance, but potentially result in urinary incontinence. Many authors have suggested that such cases are best managed by a staged procedure. A single-stage procedure, however, allows greatest reconstructive versatility. Again, this procedure is performed in the dorsal lithotomy position. A Foley catheter is placed in the bladder, and a Fogarty catheter is placed in the vagina to allow palpation. An M-shaped or occasionally a U-shaped incision is created, and the underlying pelvic floor musculature is divided in the anatomic midline, guided by muscle stimulation

(Figs. 101-28A and 101-28B). Clitoroplasty is performed as previously described. The vagina, thus exposed, is divided from its insertion and the urethral defect oversewn (Fig. 101-28C). The vagina is spatulated, the labioscrotal flap is tubularized, and the two structures are sutured together (Figs. 101-28D, 101-28 E, and 101-28F). The pelvic floor musculature is reapproximated around the newly reconstructed vagina. An alternate approach, which includes a transvesical approach to vaginal mobilization, may be considered in occasional circumstances (87).

Some individuals, such as most male pseudohermaphrodites, have no vaginal remnants and no uterine structures requiring drainage. Such patients may be reconstructed employing labioscrotal flaps or, if insufficient, visceral substitution (colon or occasionally ileum) or skin graft techniques.

Reoperative vaginoplasty is considerably more difficult. Uncomplicated vaginal stenosis is readily managed by perineal inlay flap techniques with high success. Obliteration of the vaginal introitus may be associated with destruction of a large amount of vaginal tissue. In this setting, visceral substitution techniques, myocutaneous flaps, and perineal flaps following tissue-expander procedures are generally successful.

REFERENCES

1. Simpson J, Rebar R. Normal and abnormal sexual differentiation and development. In: Becker K, ed. *Principles and practice of endocrinology and metabolism.* Philadelphia: JB Lippincott, 1990:710.
2. Grumbach M, Conte F. Disorders of sex differentiation. In: Wilson J, Foster D, eds. *Williams textbook of endocrinology.* Philadelphia: WB Saunders, 1992:853.
3. Ford C. Mosaics and chimaeras. *Br Med Bull* 1969;25:104.
4. Buyse M. *Birth defects encyclopedia.* Cambridge: Blackwell Scientific Publications, 1990.
5. Berta P, Hawkins JR, Sinclair AH, et al. Genetic evidence equating SRY and the testis-determining factor. *Nature* 1990;348:448.
6. Sinclair AH, Berta P, Palmer MS, et al. A gene from the human sex-determining region encodes a protein with homology to a conserved DNA-binding motif. *Nature* 1990;346:240.
7. Hawkins JR, Koopman P, Berta P. Testis-determining factor and Y-linked sex reversal. *Curr Opin Genet Dev* 1991;1:30.
8. Koopman P, Gubbay J, Vivian N, et al. Male development of chromosomally female mice transgenic for Sry. *Nature* 1991;351:117.
9. Pritchard-Jones K, Fleming S, Davidson D, et al. The candidate Wilms' tumour gene is involved in genitourinary development. *Nature* 1990;346:194.
10. Ikeda Y, Swain A, Weber TJ, et al. Steroidogenic factor 1 and Dax-1 colocalize in multiple cell lineages: potential links in endocrine development. *Mol Endocrinol* 1996;10:1261.
11. Ingraham HA, Lala DS, Ikeda Y, et al. The nuclear receptor steroidogenic factor 1 acts at multiple levels of the reproductive axis. *Genes Dev* 1994;8:2302.
12. Luo X, Ikeda Y, Parker KL. A cell-specific nuclear receptor is essential for adrenal and gonadal development and sexual differentiation. *Cell* 1994;77:481.
13. Wagner T, Wirth J, Meyer J, et al. Autosomal sex reversal and campomelic dysplasia are caused by mutations in and around the SRY-related gene SOX9. *Cell* 1994;79:1111.
14. Kent J, Wheatley SC, Andrews JE, et al. A male-specific role for SOX9 in vertebrate sex determination. *Development* 1996;122:2813.
15. Fechner PY, Marcantonio SM, Jaswaney V, et al. The role of the sex-determining region Y gene in the etiology of 46,XX maleness. *J Clin Endocrinol Metab* 1993;76:690.
16. McElreavey K, Rappaport R, Vilain E, et al. A minority of 46,XX true hermaphrodites are positive for the Y-DNA sequence including SRY. *Hum Genet* 1992;90:121.
17. Boucekkine C, Toublanc JE, Abbas N, et al. The sole presence of the testis-determining region of the Y chromosome (SRY) in 46,XX patients is associated with phenotypic variability. *Horm Res* 1992;37:236.
18. Toublanc JE, Boucekkine C, Abbas N, et al. Hormonal and molecular genetic findings in 46,XX subjects with sexual ambiguity and testicular differentiation. *Eur J Pediatr* 1993;152(suppl 2):S70.
19. Berta P, Morin D, Poulat F, et al. Molecular analysis of the sex-determining region from the Y chromosome in two patients with Frasier syndrome. *Horm Res* 1992;37:103.
20. Pivnick EK, Wachtel S, Woods D, et al. Mutations in the conserved domain of SRY are uncommon in XY gonadal dysgenesis. *Hum Genet* 1992;90:308.
21. Affara NA, Chalmers IJ, Ferguson-Smith MA. Analysis of the SRY gene in 22 sex-reversed XY females identifies four new point mutations in the conserved DNA binding domain. *Hum Mol Genet* 1993;2:785.
22. Fechner PY, Marcantonio SM, Ogata T, et al. Report of a kindred with X-linked (or autosomal dominant sex-limited) 46,XY partial gonadal dysgenesis. *J Clin Endocrinol Metab* 1993;76:1248.
23. Braun A, Kammerer S, Cleve H, et al. True hermaphroditism in a 46,XY individual, caused by a postzygotic somatic point mutation in the male gonadal sex-determining locus (SRY): molecular genetics and histological findings in a sporadic case. *Am J Hum Genet* 1993;52:578.
24. Vilain E, Jaubert F, Fellous M, et al. Pathology of 46,XY pure gonadal dysgenesis: absence of testis differentiation associated with mutations in the testis-determining factor. *Differentiation* 1993;52:151.
25. Barr ML, Bertram EG. A morphological distinction between neurona of the male and female, and the behavior of the nucleolar satellite during acceleration of nucleoprotein synthesis. *Nature* 1949;163:676.
26. Barr ML, Bertram LF, Lindsay HA. The morphology of the nerve cell nucleus, according to sex. *Anat Rec* 1950;107:283.
27. Francavilla S, Cordeschi G, Properzi G, et al. Ultrastructure of fetal human gonad before sexual differentiation and during early testicular and ovarian development. *J Submicrosc Cytol Pathol* 1990;22:389.
28. Tran D, Josso N. Localization of anti-Mullerian hormone in the rough endoplasmic reticulum of the developing bovine Sertoli cell using immunocytochemistry with a monoclonal antibody. *Endocrinology* 1982;111:1562.
29. Siiteri PK, Wilson JD. Testosterone formation and metabolism during male sexual differentiation in the human embryo. *J Clin Endocrinol Metab* 1974;38:113.
30. Reyes FI, Boroditsky RS, Winter JS, et al. Studies on human sexual development. II. Fetal and maternal serum gonadotropin and sex steroid concentrations. *J Clin Endocrinol Metab* 1974;38:612.
31. Molsberry RL, Carr BR, Mendelson CR, et al. Human chorionic gonadotropin binding to human fetal testes as a function of gestational age. *J Clin Endocrinol Metab* 1982;55:791.
32. Word RA, George FW, Wilson JD, et al. Testosterone synthesis and adenylate cyclase activity in the early human fetal testis appear to be independent of human chorionic gonadotropin control. *J Clin Endocrinol Metab* 1989;69:204.
33. Kaplan SL, Grumbach MM. Pituitary and placental gonadotrophins and sex steroids in the human and sub-human primate fetus. *Clin Endocrinol Metab* 1978;7:487.
34. Huhtaniemi IT, Korenbrot CC, Jaffe RB. HCG binding and stimulation of testosterone biosynthesis in the human fetal testis. *J Clin Endocrinol Metab* 1977;44:963.
35. Huhtaniemi IT, Korenbrot CC, Jaffe RB. Content of chorionic gonadotropin in human fetal tissues. *J Clin Endocrinol Metab* 1978;46:994.
36. George FW, Wilson JD. Conversion of androgen to estrogen by the human fetal ovary. *J Clin Endocrinol Metab* 1978;47:550.
37. Jost A. Embryonic sexual differentiation (morphology, physiology, abnormalities). In: Jones H, Scott W, eds. *Hermaphroditism, genital*

anomalies and related endocrine disorders. Baltimore: Williams & Wilkins, 1971:16.
38. Jost A. Problems of fetal endocrinology: the gonadal and hypophyseal hormones. *Recent Prog Horm Res* 1953;8:379.
39. Cate RL, Mattaliano RJ, Hession C, et al. Isolation of the bovine and human genes for Mullerian inhibiting substance and expression of the human gene in animal cells. *Cell* 1986;45:685.
40. Cohen-Haguenauer O, Picard JY, Mattei MG, et al. Mapping of the gene for anti-mullerian hormone to the short arm of human chromosome 19. *Cytogenet Cell Genet* 1987;44:2.
41. Donahoe PK, Cate RL, MacLaughlin DT, et al. Mullerian inhibiting substance: gene structure and mechanism of action of a fetal regressor. *Recent Prog Horm Res* 1987;43:431.
42. Meyers-Wallen VN, Lee MM, Manganaro TF, et al. Mullerian inhibiting substance is present in embryonic testes of dogs with persistent mullerian duct syndrome. *Biol Reprod* 1993;48:1410.
43. Lee MM, Donahoe PK. Mullerian inhibiting substance: a gonadal hormone with multiple functions. *Endocr Rev* 1993;14:152.
44. Gustafson ML, Lee MM, Asmundson L, et al. Mullerian inhibiting substance in the diagnosis and management of intersex and gonadal abnormalities. *J Pediatr Surg* 1993;28:439.
45. Josso N, Racine C, di Clemente N, et al. The role of anti-Mullerian hormone in gonadal development. *Mol Cell Endocrinol* 1998;145:3.
46. Racine C, Rey R, Forest MG, et al. Receptors for anti-mullerian hormone on Leydig cells are responsible for its effects on steroidogenesis and cell differentiation. *Proc Natl Acad Sci U S A* 1998;95:594.
47. Hutson JM, Donahoe PK, MacLaughlin DT. Steroid modulation of Mullerian duct regression in the chick embryo. *Gen Comp Endocrinol* 1985;57:88.
48. Hutson JM, Donahoe PK, Budzik GP. Mullerian inhibiting substance: a fetal hormone with surgical implications. *Aust N Z J Surg* 1985;55:599.
49. Forsberg JG. Origin of vaginal epithelium. *Obstet Gynecol* 1965;25:787.
50. Cunha GR. The dual origin of vaginal epithelium. *Am J Anat* 1975;143:387.
51. O'Malley B. The steroid receptor superfamily: more excitement predicted for the future. *Mol Endocrinol* 1990;4:363.
52. Money J, Ehrhardt A. *Man and woman, boy and girl: the differentiation and dimorphism of gender identity from conception to maturity.* Baltimore: Johns Hopkins University Press, 1972.
53. Ehrhardt AA, Meyer-Bahlburg HF. Effects of prenatal sex hormones on gender-related behavior. *Science* 1981;211:1312.
54. Money J, Schwartz M, Lewis VG. Adult heterosexual status and fetal hormonal masculinization and demasculinization: 46,XX congenital virilizing adrenal hyperplasia and 46,XY androgen-insensitivity syndrome compared. *Psychoneuroendocrinology* 1984;9:405.
55. Imperato-McGinley J, Peterson RE, Gautier T, et al. Androgens and the evolution of male-gender identity among male pseudohermaphrodites with 5alpha-reductase deficiency. *N Engl J Med* 1979;300:1233.
56. Reilly JM, Woodhouse CR. Small penis and the male sexual role. *J Urol* 1989;142:569.
57. Kaplan SL, Grumbach MM, Aubert ML. The ontogenesis of pituitary hormones and hypothalamic factors in the human fetus: maturation of central nervous system regulation of anterior pituitary function. *Recent Prog Horm Res* 1976;32:161.
58. Kaplan SL, Grumbach MM. The ontogenesis of human foetal hormones. II. Luteinizing hormone (LH) and follicle stimulating hormone (FSH). *Acta Endocrinol (Copenh)* 1976;81:808.
59. Reyes FI, Winter JS, Faiman C. Studies on human sexual development. I. Fetal gonadal and adrenal sex steroids. *J Clin Endocrinol Metab* 1973;37:74.
60. Voutilainen R.Hormonal development in the fetal gonad. In: Sizonenko P, Aubert M, eds. Developmental endocrinology. New York: Raven Press, 1990:27.
61. MacGillivray MH, Morishima A, Conte F, et al. Pediatric endocrinology update: an overview. The essential roles of estrogens in pubertal growth, epiphyseal fusion and bone turnover: lessons from mutations in the genes for aromatase and the estrogen receptor. *Horm Res* 1998;49(suppl 1):2.
62. Therrell BL. Newborn screening for congenital adrenal hyperplasia. *Endocrinol Metab Clin North Am* 2001;30:15.
63. Hughes I. Congenital adrenal hyperplasia: phenotype and genotype. *J Pediatr Endocrinol Metab* 2002;15(suppl 5):1329.
64. Hughes IA. Congenital adrenal hyperplasia: 21-hydroxylase deficiency in the newborn and during infancy. *Semin Reprod Med* 2002; 20:229.
65. Fujieda K, Okuhara K, Abe S, et al. Molecular pathogenesis of lipoid adrenal hyperplasia and adrenal hypoplasia congenita. *J Steroid Biochem Mol Biol* 2003;85:483.
66. Avni EF, Rypens F, Smet MH, et al. Sonographic demonstration of congenital adrenal hyperplasia in the neonate: the cerebriform pattern. *Pediatr Radiol* 1993;23:88.
67. Smith DP, Felker RE, Noe HN, et al. Prenatal diagnosis of genital anomalies. *Urology* 1996;47:114.
68. Ginsberg NA, Cadkin A, Strom C, et al. Prenatal diagnosis of 46,XX male fetuses. *Am J Obstet Gynecol* 1999;180:1006.
69. Pinhas-Hamiel O, Zalel Y, Smith E, et al. Prenatal diagnosis of sex differentiation disorders: the role of fetal ultrasound. *J Clin Endocrinol Metab* 2002;87:4547.
70. Zalel Y, Pinhas-Hamiel O, Lipitz S, et al. The development of the fetal penis—an in utero sonographic evaluation. *Ultrasound Obstet Gynecol* 2001;17:129.
71. Achiron R, Pinhas-Hamiel O, Zalel Y, et al. Development of fetal male gender: prenatal sonographic measurement of the scrotum and evaluation of testicular descent. *Ultrasound Obstet Gynecol* 1998;11:242.
72. Morel Y, Bertrand J, Rappaport R. Disorders of hormonosynthesis. In: Bertrand J, Rappaport R, Sizonenko P, eds. *Pediatric endocrinology.* Baltimore: Williams & Wilkins, 1993:305.
73. Mulaikal RM, Migeon CJ, Rock JA. Fertility rates in female patients with congenital adrenal hyperplasia due to 21-hydroxylase deficiency. *N Engl J Med* 1987;316:178.
74. van Niekerk WA, Retief AE. The gonads of human true hermaphrodites. *Hum Genet* 1981;58:117.
75. Rajfer J, Walsh PC. The incidence of intersexuality in patients with hypospadias and cryptorchidism. *J Urol* 1976;116:769.
76. Rink RC, Adams MC. Feminizing genitoplasty: state of the art. *World J Urol* 1998;16:212.
77. Rink RC, Pope JC, Kropp BP, et al. Reconstruction of the high urogenital sinus: early perineal prone approach without division of the rectum. *J Urol* 1997;158:1293.
78. Gonzalez R, Fernandes ET. Single-stage feminization genitoplasty. *J Urol* 1990;143:776.
79. Ludwikowski B, Oesch Hayward I, Gonzalez R. Total urogenital sinus mobilization: expanded applications. *BJU Int* 1999;83:820.
80. Vates TS, Fleming P, Leleszi JP, et al. Functional, social and psychosexual adjustment after vaginal reconstruction. *J Urol* 1999;162: 182.
81. Jenak R, Ludwikowski B, Gonzalez R. Total urogenital sinus mobilization: a modified perineal approach for feminizing genitoplasty and urogenital sinus repair. *J Urol* 2001;165:2347.
82. Snyder HM III, Retik AB, Bauer SB, et al. Feminizing genitoplasty: a synthesis. *J Urol* 1983;129:1024.
83. Sheldon CA, Gilbert A, Lewis AG. Vaginal reconstruction: critical technical principles. *J Urol* 1994;152:190.
84. Hendren WH. Surgical management of urogenital sinus abnormalities. *J Pediatr Surg* 1977;12:339.
85. Hendren WH. Urogenital sinus and anorectal malformation: experience with 22 cases. *J Pediatr Surg* 1980;15:628.
86. Hendren WH. Urogenital sinus and cloacal malformations. *Semin Pediatr Surg* 1996;5:72.
87. Passerini-Glazel G. A new 1-stage procedure for clitorovaginoplasty in severely masculinized female pseudohermaphrodites. *J Urol* 1989; 142:565.

PART I

Vascular System

Chapter 102

Arterial Disease

Philip C. Guzzetta, Jr.

VASCULAR EMBRYOLOGY

The origin of the arterial vascular system has been extensively studied for more than a century. There is general agreement that the vessels are mesodermal derivatives that begin as cords of angioblast cells. These cords orient themselves into tubes and eventually develop along a capillary net formed by existing vessels that appear to have preferred paths of development. The development of paired aortic arches early in gestation reflects the human evolution from aquatic vertebrates, which use the aortic arches for blood flow through gills developed from the branchial clefts adjacent to the paired aortic arches. In humans, at the end of the first month of gestation, the six pairs of aortic arches have been formed.

By gestational week 7, there is a single aorta posteriorly. Many of the paired aortic arches regress, and some persist as head and neck arterial branches. The left aortic arch IV develops into the aortic arch, and the left aortic arch VI becomes the ductus arteriosus. Aortic arch V is not shown and may not even exist in humans (Fig. 102-1). The location of the aortic arches during this stage of development is actually within the neck region, and the descent of the arch into the thorax occurs later with the development of the heart. Detailed discussion of cardiac development and its relation to various anomalies can be found in *Embryology for Surgeons* by Skandalakis and Gray (1).

Philip C. Guzzetta, Jr.: George Washington University School of Medicine, Children's National Medical Center, Washington, District of Columbia 20010.

TECHNIQUES TO DIAGNOSE ARTERIAL DISEASE IN CHILDREN

Any new technique for imaging the arterial system in children must be compared with transarterial angiography for safety, quality of image, need for sedation or general anesthesia, and cost.

Ultrasound

Real-time ultrasound, particularly when combined with color Doppler ultrasound, has the attractive features of being a safe, noninvasive, and inexpensive technique to image vessels. The images may not be attainable, however, if there is overlying bone or intestine that contains a great deal of gas, which seriously limits its use for the chest and abdomen. In addition, simultaneous viewing of vessels within a large area in different planes, such as the entire abdominal aorta and its branches, is not possible with ultrasound, which limits its use as a guide for the correction of problems in these vessels. For evaluation of a single vessel, such as the renal artery after repair, Doppler ultrasound has a definite role to ensure patency and flow, but has little place in the initial evaluation of children with suspected arterial disease. The echocardiogram and transesophageal echocardiogram (TEE) are used extensively to assess the ascending aorta, pulmonary arteries, pulmonary veins, inferior and superior vena cavae, and the heart.

Magnetic Resonance Imaging

The technology of magnetic resonance imaging (MRI) is developing rapidly, and many of its limitations for arterial evaluations may soon be overcome. MRI can be effective in assessing venous structures and is the technique of choice in assessing the patency of the large veins in children who have previously had multiple central venous catheters. The anatomy of vascular anomalies, such as double aortic arch or aberrant subclavian artery, can be visualized easily by MR angiography (MRA). For small visceral vessels, such as the renal artery, MRA does not allow adequate detail and should not be depended on solely in making operative decisions. As MRA progresses, it may replace transarterial angiography for diagnosing many diseases. MRI has

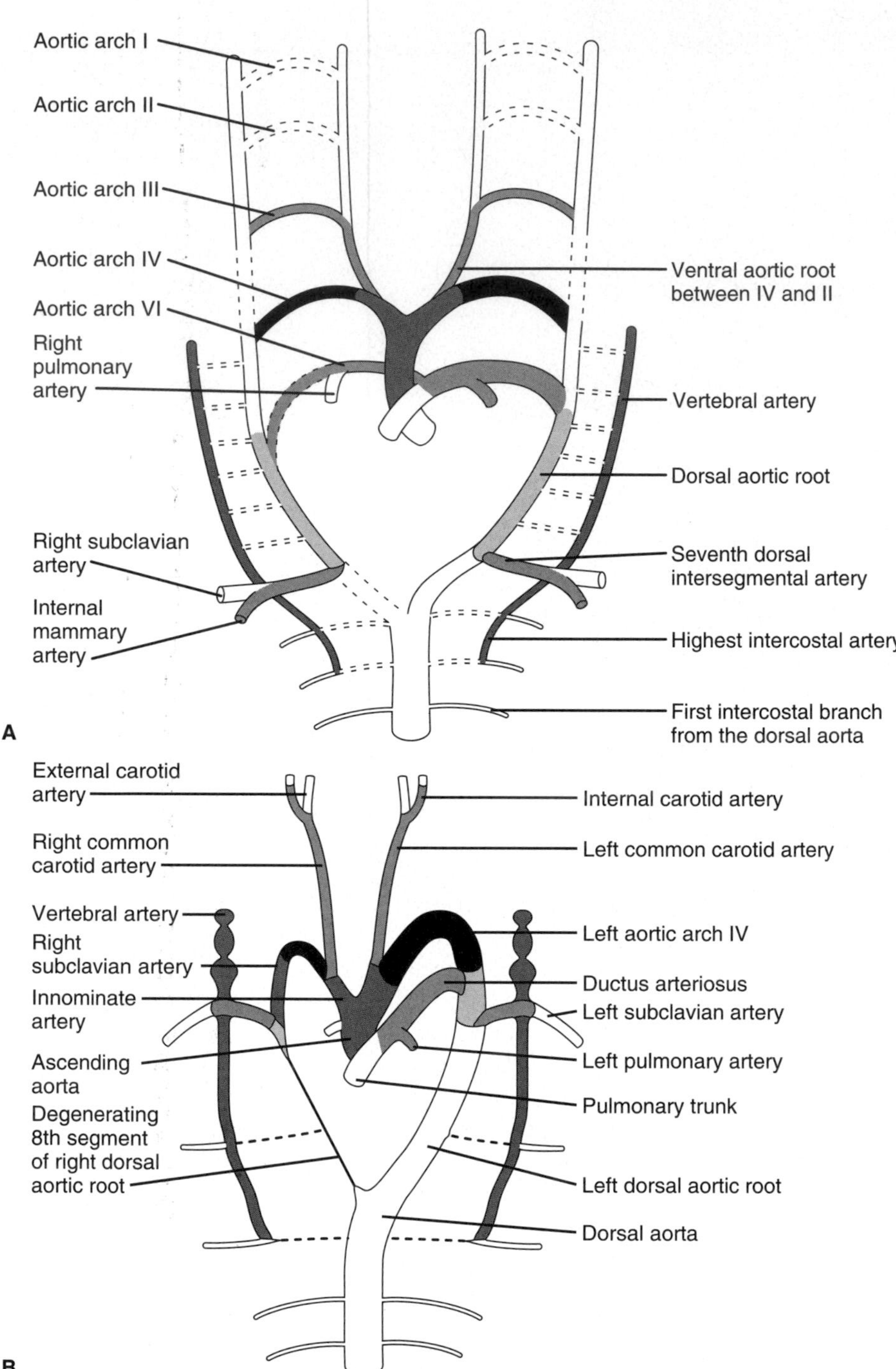

FIGURE 102-1. Development of the aortic arch in the human embryo. **(A)** Gestational age 6 weeks **(B)** Gestational age 8 weeks.

a role in the assessment of vascular anomalies of the extremities, for which it shows the relation of the vessels and the soft tissue. Motion artifact is a serious problem with MRI, and many children require heavy sedation or general anesthesia for the study.

Transarterial Angiography

Transarterial angiography remains the gold standard for imaging the arteries of children. The ability to view whole segments of the arterial system at once, magnify the area of interest, and obtain excellent detail of the vascular lumen make this the modality of choice for assessing pediatric arterial disease. Improvements in interventional radiographic treatment of arterial diseases allow the transarterial approach to be therapeutic as well as diagnostic in some cases. Major risks of this approach include damage to the artery used to access the arterial system, potential allergic reactions to the contrast, radiation exposure, and the need for sedation. As the technology improves, MRA may be most useful for screening patients for arterial disease, with the transarterial angiography used to confirm the problem in selected patients, especially those who can be treated by interventional radiographic techniques.

ARTERIAL ANEURYSMS

Congenital Aneurysms

Arterial aneurysms have been diagnosed by prenatal ultrasound and have even been implicated in fetal death. Congenital aneurysms are almost always found in the abdominal aorta, contain all three layers of the involved artery, and show no sign of arteritis. They usually present in children younger than 5 years of age as painless abdominal masses without evidence of distal vascular disease or embolus. The form of the aneurysm may be saccular or fusiform. Treatment is resection of the aneurysm and reconstruction with autogenous tissue, if possible. Because many of these aneurysms involve the abdominal aorta, prosthetic graft replacement has been the most common technique, with expected growth of the normal vessel on either side of the graft to accommodate the longitudinal growth of the child (2).

Acquired Aneurysms

Acquired aneurysms can be separated into those due to an arteritis, syndromes causing medial degeneration, direct arterial infection, trauma (false aneurysms), and arterial dysplasia.

Aneurysms Due to an Arteritis

Arterial aneurysms may develop in children as the result of Kawasaki disease, giant cell arteritis, Takayasu disease, or polyarteritis nodosa. Kawasaki disease (also known as *mucocutaneous lymph node syndrome*) is a disease with a median age of onset of 3 years and is characterized by high fever, cervical adenopathy, conjunctivitis, stomatitis, and generalized erythema, which is frequently most intense on the soles and palms. Coronary artery aneurysms develop in up to 15% of children who are not treated with aspirin or IV γ-globulin. Rarely, aneurysms develop in locations other than the coronary arteries with Kawasaki disease. The coronary artery aneurysms frequently improve with medication, seldom rupture, and may require surgical resection only when they are *giant aneurysms*, defined as greater than 8 mm in diameter. Persistent giant aneurysms tend to cause stenosis or thrombosis of the involved coronary, leading to myocardial ischemia distal to the aneurysm, which requires surgical bypass of the diseased artery.

Giant cell arteritis most commonly involves the aorta, but it may also cause peripheral artery aneurysm formation. Takayasu arteritis and polyarteritis nodosa most often cause stenosis rather than aneurysm formation, although aneurysms may develop in the aorta or its main branches. When polyarteritis nodosa causes aneurysms of the small and medium-size renal arteries, renal impairment and hypertension commonly occur (3). Operative correction of an aneurysm due to an arteritis has a high complication rate. Unless the aneurysm is large or threatens to rupture, initial treatment of these patients should be with glucocorticoid therapy rather than surgery.

Aneurysms Due to Syndromes Causing Medial Degeneration

Type IV Ehlers-Danlos syndrome, characterized by an abnormal or absent type III collagen, is associated with medial degeneration of the large arteries with associated aneurysm formation or rupture. The aorta is the most common site of aneurysm formation, but any artery with substantial amounts of collagen is at risk for this problem (4). Marfan syndrome is an autosomal dominant disease characterized by cystic medial degeneration of the ascending aorta; thin, elongated extremities; chest wall deformities; and dislocation of the lens. The enlarging ascending aorta places the Marfan syndrome patient at significant risk for aneurysmal dissection and rupture or severe aortic valvular insufficiency due to dilation of the aortic root.

Other conditions that deposit abnormal substances into the media of the aorta, such as tuberous sclerosis, cystinosis, or mucopolysaccharide deposition (5) may predispose the aorta to aneurysm formation and rupture. Treatment of these children can be complicated by poor tissue integrity at the suture line when a prosthetic graft is placed, leading to false aneurysm formation. Children with some types of Ehlers-Danlos syndrome have abnormal bleeding times, making major surgical procedures hazardous. Nonetheless, the best chance for survival for a patient with one of these syndromes and an aneurysm is resection of the aneurysm and prosthetic graft placement.

Aneurysms Due to Direct Arterial Infection

Most aneurysms that are reported in children are caused by bacterial or fungal infection of a structurally normal arterial wall. An arterial wall, particularly that of the aorta, is generally resistant to bacterial seeding unless there is trauma to the intima or an abnormal flow pattern that potentially weakens the wall. Patients at greatest risk for aneurysm formation due to direct arterial infection are older children with thoracic aortic coarctation and infants with umbilical artery catheters in place.

Children with this type of aneurysm are usually very ill, with signs of bacteremia similar to those seen in patients with acute endocarditis. The most common organism causing this type of aneurysm is *Staphylococcus aureus*, although fungi and other bacteria have also been cultured from infected aneurysms. Histologic examination of the aneurysm reveals inflammation of the arterial wall, with media disruption and aneurysm formation. These aneurysms must be resected because they are at high risk for rupture. Although arterial replacement with autogenous tissue would be ideal, most aortic reconstructions must be done with prosthetic grafts, accepting the potential of graft infection in the future. If the child is large enough to consider extraanatomic bypass of the aorta at the time of aneurysm resection, it should be recommended instead of suturing prosthetic material into a grossly infected area.

Aneurysms Due to Trauma (False Aneurysms)

Although they are probably the most common aneurysms in children, the true incidence of aneurysms due to trauma is unknown. These aneurysms are reported infrequently because they are often seen in the distal extremities and are easily cared for by vessel ligation. Most of these aneurysms are caused by penetrating trauma, particularly lacerations of the hands or feet (Fig. 102-2). The trend of nonoperative treatment of "minimal" vascular injuries with normal distal pulses (6) will likely increase the appearance of these in the future. Optimal treatment is aneurysm resection with ligation or repair of the artery, depending on the artery involved.

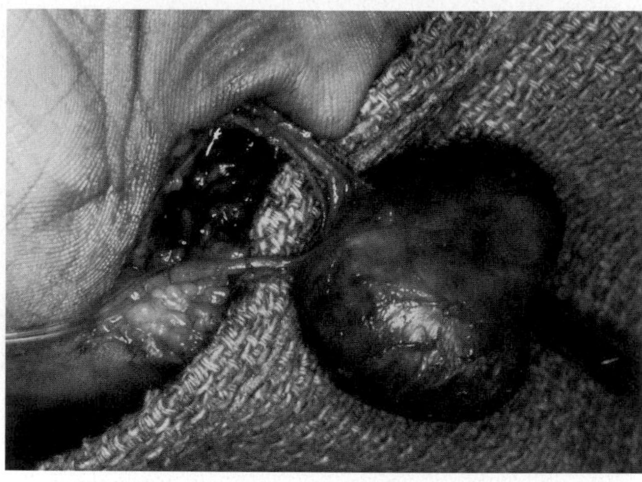

FIGURE 102-2. False aneurysm of the superficial palmar artery of the left hand due to a laceration that occurred 6 months earlier.

Aneurysms Due to Arterial Dysplasia

In children, aneurysms due to arterial dysplasia are found almost exclusively in the renal arteries, associated with renal artery stenosis and renovascular hypertension. Recognition of the aneurysm is usually made when the patient has an angiogram for hypertension. The aneurysms commonly occur at branch points of the renal artery (Fig. 102-3) and should be distinguished from the poststenotic dilation that is frequently seen in the main renal artery. Treatment of the aneurysm may include resection and suturing of the distal end of the bypass graft to the aneurysm site if the aneurysm is near the main renal artery. No treatment is employed if the aneurysm is small and peripheral. An excellent classification of aneurysms in children was developed by Sarkar and colleagues (7) (Table 102-1).

ARTERIAL OCCLUSIVE DISEASE DUE TO ARTERIOPATHY

Takayasu Arteritis

Takayasu arteritis is an inflammatory condition of unknown cause. It usually involves the aorta and its major branches and can lead to stenosis or occlusion of the involved vessels. The condition is most commonly seen in

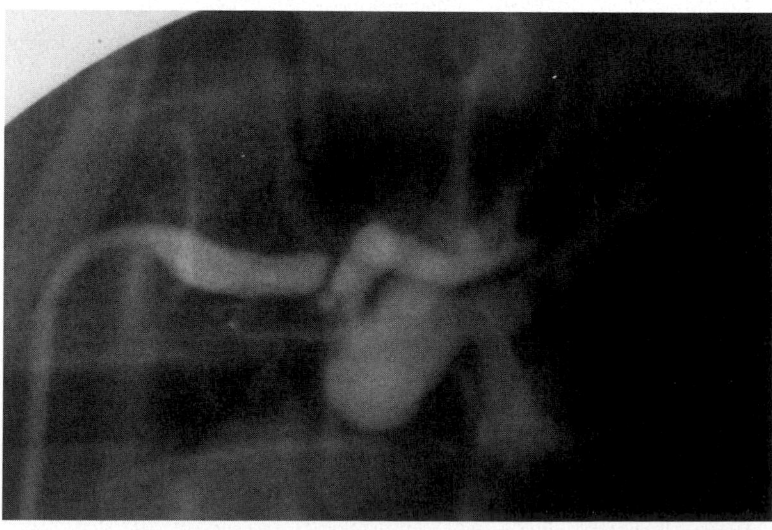

FIGURE 102-3. Aneurysm of a branch of the left renal artery associated with high-grade stenosis of the main renal artery.

TABLE 102-1 Classification of Aneurysms in Children.[a]

Class	Description	Principal Arteries Affected	Histologic and Morphologic Character	Clinical Characteristics
I	Arterial infection	Aorta (particularly thoracic), iliac	Acute inflammatory infiltrates present initially, then chronic inflammation and fibrotic changes; saccular aneurysms	Cardiovascular anomalies and umbilical artery catheterization predisposing factors; dyspnea, cough, chest pain with progression to rupture and death, if untreated
II	Giant cell aortoarteritis	Aorta (peripheral arteries, rare)	Chronic inflammation with giant cells, vessel wall necrosis; saccular aneurysms	Signs and symptoms vary from being absent to shock; untreated aortic lesions progress to rupture
III	Autoimmune vasculitis	Renal, hepatic, and splenic arterial branches	Chronic panmural inflammation and degeneration, late fibrosis; multiple small saccular aneurysms	Usually asymptomatic, but may cause hematuria, perirenal hematomas, or death with rupture
IV	Kawasaki disease	Coronary (20%–30%), axillobrachial, iliofemoral, hepatic	Medial degeneration and fibrosis; multiple small saccular aneurysms	Often asymptomatic; myocardial infarction or tamponade (coronary), limb ischemia (extremity), and obstructive jaundice (hepatic) may occur
V	Medial degeneration: Marfan and Ehlers-Danlos syndromes	Aorta	Medial elastic tissue disorganization, mucinous deposits (cystic medial necrosis); solitary saccular or fusiform aneurysms	Aortic rupture or dissection common; arteriography and vascular reconstruction hazardous in type IV Ehlers-Danlos syndrome
VI	Medial degeneration: other forms	Aorta (peripheral arteries, rare)	Medial elastic tissue disorganization, mucinous deposits (cystic medial necrosis); solitary saccular aneurysms	Associated with other cardiac (biscuspid aortic valve) and aortic (coarctation) anomalies; often present with aortic dissection or rupture
VII	Arterial dysplasias	Renal	Medial thinning and fibroplasia; solitary and multiple saccular aneurysms affecting arterial bifurcations most often	Usually asymptomatic, detected during arteriography for renovascular hypertension
VIII	Idiopathic, congenital	Iliofemoral, brachial, aorta	Secondary intimal fibroplasia; saccular, usually solitary, symmetric, if multiple	Often asymptomatic, but may cause limb ischemia; rupture unreported
IX	Extravascular causes	Aorta, visceral, and extremity arteries	Disruption of usual three layers of artery, fibrosis, and mural thrombus; saccular aneurysms	Protean manifestations; aortic aneurysms often rupture; peripheral lesions often asymptomatic; visceral lesions may cause gastrointestinal bleeding

[a]Based on a review of 135 reported cases and those in the current report. Excludes aneurysms of the intracranial and coronary arteries.
Adapted from Sarkar R, Coran AG, Cilley RE, et al. Arterial aneurysms in children: clinicopathologic classification. *J Vasc Surg* 1991;13:47, with permission.

adolescent girls, but can affect boys or girls at any age. The sites of involvement are usually the aortic arch vessels or the midabdominal aorta and its branches. Diffuse major arterial occlusion can develop, which has led to the name *pulseless disease.* The pulmonary artery is involved in more than one-half of patients. The diagnosis of Takayasu disease and follow-up of the disease's response to treatment may be done effectively with MRA (8).

The presenting complaints depend on the vessels involved. Hypertension is a common finding in Takayasu arteritis, particularly with abdominal aorta and renal artery involvement. Patients with involvement of the aortic arch may present with signs of cerebral or upper-extremity ischemia or evidence of congestive heart failure. It is important to differentiate abdominal aortic Takayasu arteritis from congenital middle aortic syndrome because the appropriate therapy for Takayasu arteritis is steroid administration, whereas treatment of middle aortic syndrome is surgical revascularization. Use of the erythrocyte sedimentation rate or other inflammatory markers should help in diagnosing Takayasu arteritis.

Despite the use of steroids to stabilize the vascular disease in Takayasu arteritis, there is often long-term arterial occlusion as the involved artery heals by fibrosis. Operative therapy in acute Takayasu arteritis should be avoided because of the high failure rate of revascularization; even in "healed" Takayasu arteritis, the success rate with operative revascularization is not good. There are reports of clinical improvement in some children with Takayasu arteritis after percutaneous balloon dilation angioplasty of the aortic stenosis (9,10).

Giant Cell Arteritis

Giant cell arteritis is an extremely uncommon cause of arterial occlusion in children. It involves the aorta and is treated similarly to Takayasu arteritis, with steroids. The only way to differentiate giant cell from Takayasu arteritis is with histologic evaluation of a biopsy of the vessel wall.

Other Forms of Arteriopathy

Autoimmune diseases such as polyarteritis nodosa can cause arterial occlusive disease, as well as aneurysms in small to medium-size arteries, especially in the kidney (3). Vasospastic disorders, such as Raynaud syndrome and reflex sympathetic dystrophy, can occur in older children. These disorders are usually responsive to biofeedback or medical therapy and are seldom improved long-term by surgical sympathectomy (11). Atherosclerosis associated with type II hyperlipoproteinemia can cause severe arterial disease in childhood, but early recognition and treatment of this familial disease should make peripheral vascular disease uncommon before adulthood.

Intracranial arterial occlusive disease in children without a definite cause has been called *moyamoya disease.* The Japanese term *moyamoya* is derived from the angiographic appearance of the collaterals that form because of extensive stenoses and occlusions of vessels within the circle of Willis. There may be many causes of moyamoya disease because the distribution of lesions and clinical signs vary considerably in different areas of the world. Unfortunately, the diagnosis is often made only after a major stroke has occurred. If the diagnosis is made early enough, however, extracranial-to-intracranial arterial bypass may benefit some children with moyamoya disease.

RENOVASCULAR HYPERTENSION

Hypertension in childhood is defined as three blood pressure measurements, taken in a quiet environment, that are above the 95th percentile for the child's age and gender. Unfortunately, routine blood pressure measurements are not performed by all physicians as a part of yearly examinations in children. As a result, most hypertensive children come to the attention of a pediatric nephrologist or pediatric surgeon because of hypertension identified serendipitously when the child is seen in an emergency room for another reason and routine vital signs have been taken. A small percentage of hypertensive children have symptoms such as fatigue or dyspnea from congestive heart failure due to hypertensive cardiomyopathy, chronic irritability, headaches, or even stroke.

With the heightened awareness of the potential for thoracic coarctation in the newborn period, renovascular hypertension is the most common form of surgically correctable hypertension in children older than 1 year of age. A child with hypertension who is younger than 10 years of age has a greater than 50% chance of having a surgically correctable form of hypertension. In teenagers, essential hypertension is the most common form of hypertension, but 20% of these older children also have a surgically correctable cause for their elevated blood pressures (12).

Pathophysiology

The cause of renovascular disease is unknown in most children. Some patients with the middle aortic syndrome have histories consistent with arteritis, but most do not and probably have congenital aortic or renal artery disease. Children with neurofibromatosis may have renovascular hypertension, and it is usually bilateral in those cases. The most common site of stenosis is the renal ostium, particularly when the lesions are bilateral, part of the middle aortic syndrome, or associated with neurofibromatosis. The main renal artery is the next most common site of stenosis; the segmental arteries are the least common location for stenosis.

The histologic evaluation of the stenotic lesions invariably shows fibromuscular dysplasia in the medial or perimedial muscular layers, with intimal hyperplasia of variable degrees. Stanley proposed that the disease within the muscular layer is a developmental one and that intimal hyperplasia is secondary to abnormal flow through the stenotic artery (13).

Evaluation of the Hypertensive Child

A careful history and physical examination is important in the evaluation of children with hypertension. The history may reveal subtle symptoms of hypertension, such as irritability in the young child or a decreased energy level when cardiomyopathy is present. In the child with abdominal

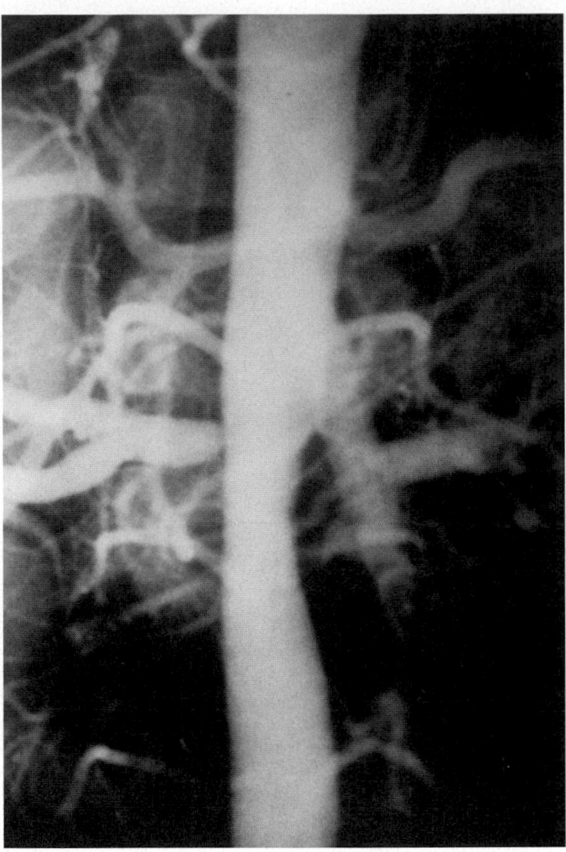

FIGURE 102-4. Aortic stenosis and bilateral renal artery stenosis in an 8-year-old girl with middle aortic syndrome.

aortic coarctation, there may be a history consistent with leg claudication. On physical examination, the presence of diminished femoral pulses may be due to thoracic or abdominal aortic coarctation. About 15% of children with renovascular hypertension have associated abdominal aortic coarctation and may also have superior mesenteric artery and celiac artery stenosis as a part of the middle aortic syndrome (Fig. 102-4). Abdominal bruits are common in children with middle aortic syndrome but less so in simple renal artery stenosis.

Presence of an abdominal mass in the area of the kidney should alert the examiner to the possibility of a retroperitoneal tumor, such as Wilms' tumor, pheochromocytoma, or neuroblastoma, as the cause of the hypertension. A hydronephrotic kidney may also present with hypertension and an abdominal mass. In these patients, abdominal ultrasound followed by CT or MRI is appropriate.

Given that the most common medical cause of hypertension in children is renal disease, renal function is evaluated with serum blood urea nitrogen and creatinine and urinalysis. Most children with renovascular hypertension, even when it is bilateral, have normal renal function tests. Peripheral vein renins are elevated from many causes of hypertension and thus are not helpful in differentiating the source. Most children seen are already on antihypertensive medications, which further decrease the value of peripheral vein renin levels.

Radiographic studies should begin with an ultrasound of the kidneys and abdomen and with Doppler ultrasound assessment of the aorta and renal vessels. The diethylenetriamine pentaacetic acid renal scan is helpful in identifying patients at high risk for renovascular hypertension when it is performed without, and then with, pretreatment with the angiotensin-converting enzyme inhibitor captopril. If there is decreased function after the captopril challenge, the likelihood of renovascular stenosis is high. However, if the scan in patients pretreated with captopril is normal, renovascular disease is not ruled out completely; and in fact, it may be present bilaterally.

Selective renal arteriography remains the most accurate method for diagnosing renovascular disease in children. It also may serve as a method of treatment by angioplasty. The use of selective renal vein renins in children is seldom necessary, except to decide which side to do first when bilateral disease is to be corrected in separate procedures. In contrast to those in adults, the excellent collateral vessels of children make the renal vein renin ratios less predictive of successful control of the hypertension by correction of the renal artery stenosis. Correction of stenosis cures or improves blood pressure management in more than 90% of children who have hypertension and a radiographic renal artery stenosis of greater than 50%, regardless of their renal vein renin levels.

Treatment

Medical Management

All children with significant hypertension are treated with antihypertensive medications. Patients with renovascular hypertension are at risk for decreased renal function on the side, or sides, with renal artery stenosis when the blood pressure is controlled with angiotensin-converting enzyme inhibitors. Although the renal dysfunction seen after the use of these agents typically is reversible, it is best to avoid them before definitive therapy for renal artery stenosis. The excellent long-term results of renal artery dilation and surgical revascularization in children with renovascular hypertension have made lifelong antihypertensive medication, without attempted correction of the stenosis, an unacceptable option.

Percutaneous Transluminal Angioplasty

Dilation of the stenotic renal artery has a definite place in the treatment of renovascular hypertension in children. The lesions that appear to be most amenable to dilation are those within the main renal artery, away from secondary branches. The stenotic lesions that are located at the renal artery ostium (especially those associated with the middle aortic syndrome) or those adjacent to an aneurysm should not, and often cannot safely, be dilated. These lesions

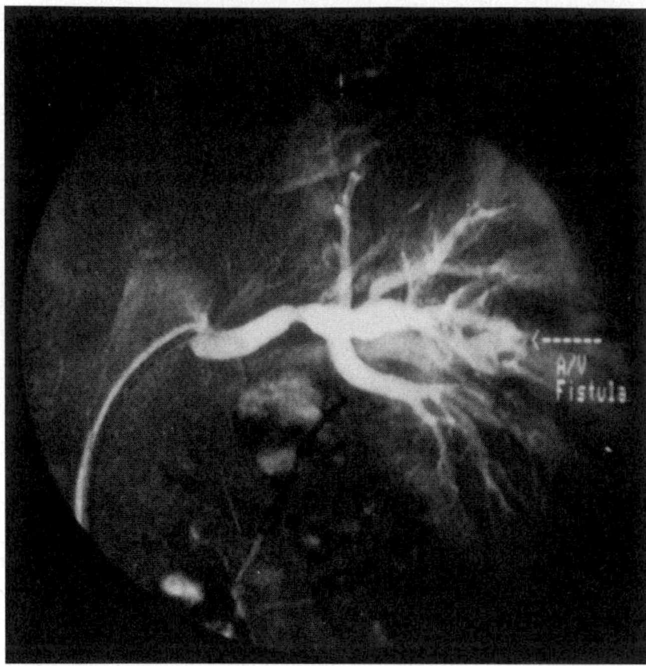

FIGURE 102-5. Intraparenchymal renal arteriovenous fistula due to guide-wire injury during attempted percutaneous transluminal angioplasty for renal artery stenosis.

should be surgically repaired. Although complications such as arterial occlusion, arterial perforation, and renal arteriovenous fistulas can occur with percutaneous transluminal angioplasty (PTA; Fig. 102-5), success rates of more than 80% have been obtained in some children with renovascular hypertension when appropriate lesions have been selected for PTA (Fig. 102-6).

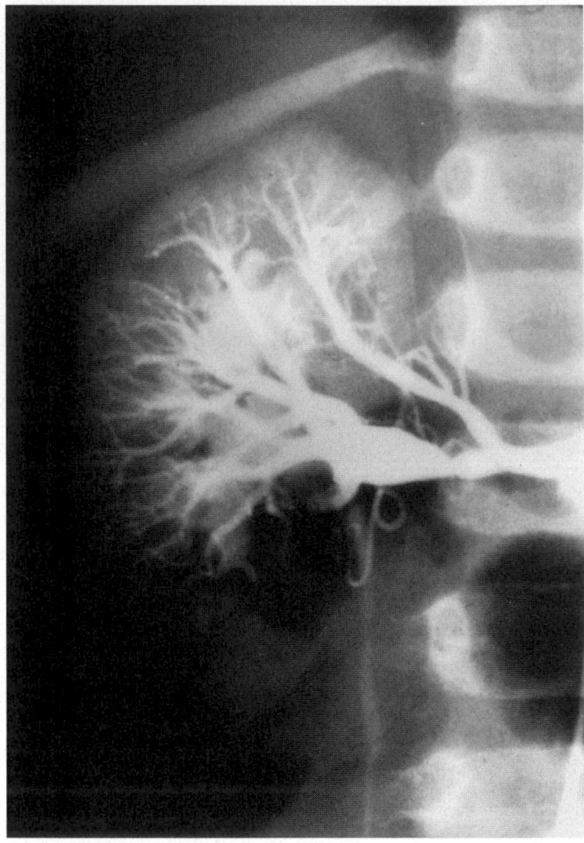

FIGURE 102-6. Study made after percutaneous transluminal angioplasty of main renal artery stenosis in a 6-year-old boy. Long-terms results were excellent.

Surgical Revascularization

Any therapy for renal artery stenosis in children must be compared with reported results of greater than 90% cured or improved with surgical revascularization (14,15). The goal of surgery is correction of the hypertension with preservation of renal function. The high rate of bilateral disease in children (40% in the author's experience) mandates that every effort be made to preserve the kidney with renal artery stenosis.

For unilateral renal artery stenosis, a transverse, transperitoneal incision is used for a small child (less than 25 kg) and a midline incision is used for the larger child. Approach to the renal artery is direct, with little dissection of the kidney to minimize disruption of the collateral vessels, which maintain some renal perfusion during occlusion of the renal artery for bypass. In patients with the middle aortic syndrome, a left thoracoabdominal incision for aortoaortic bypass grafting performed extraperitoneally provides the best exposure to the proximal aorta for anastomosis and is well tolerated.

The technique of renal artery revascularization is best managed in children by renal artery bypass with autogenous tissue. When the lesion is unilateral, use of a hypogastric artery free graft is the first choice for the following reasons: (1) the hypogastric artery is usually a good size match with the renal artery, (2) it is capable of withstanding arterial pressure without the risk of aneurysmal dilation long term, and (3) it can be harvested through the same incision as the renal artery repair. The second choice for graft material to bypass a stenotic renal artery is a saphenous vein graft. The risk of aneurysmal dilation with use of the saphenous vein graft (Fig. 102-7) may be overcome by wrapping it with a Dacron net, as advocated by O'Neill (15).

In patients who have middle aortic syndrome in conjunction with left renal artery stenosis, the left renal artery can be reimplanted directly into the prosthetic graft that is used to bypass the aortic narrowing (Fig. 102-8). The prosthetic graft used for the aortic bypass is polytetrafluoroethylene, size 10 mm or larger, and no attempt is made to leave extra length for growth. The author's and other's (16) preference is to stage the revascularization of bilateral renal artery stenosis by repairing the two sides about 6 weeks apart, although some surgeons recommend

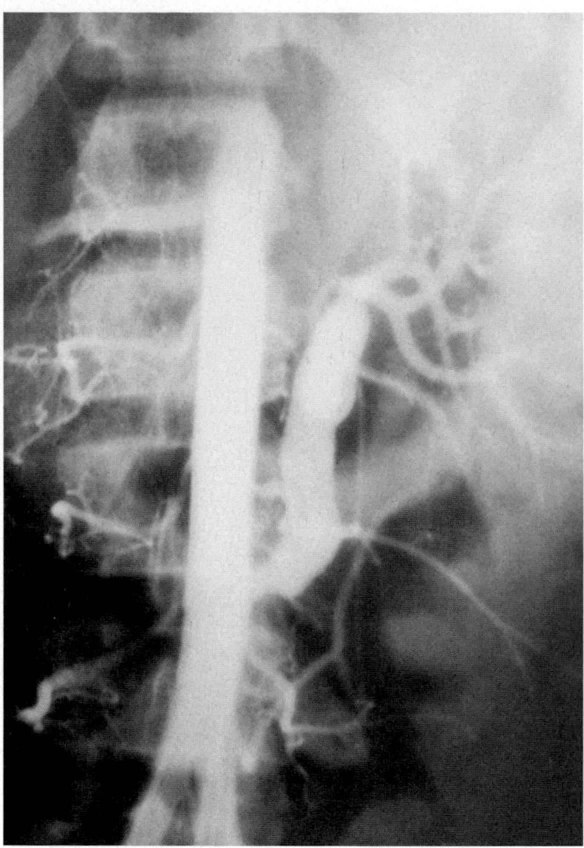

FIGURE 102-7. Aortorenal saphenous bypass graft with significant dilation of the graft 1 year after revascularization in an 11-year-old boy.

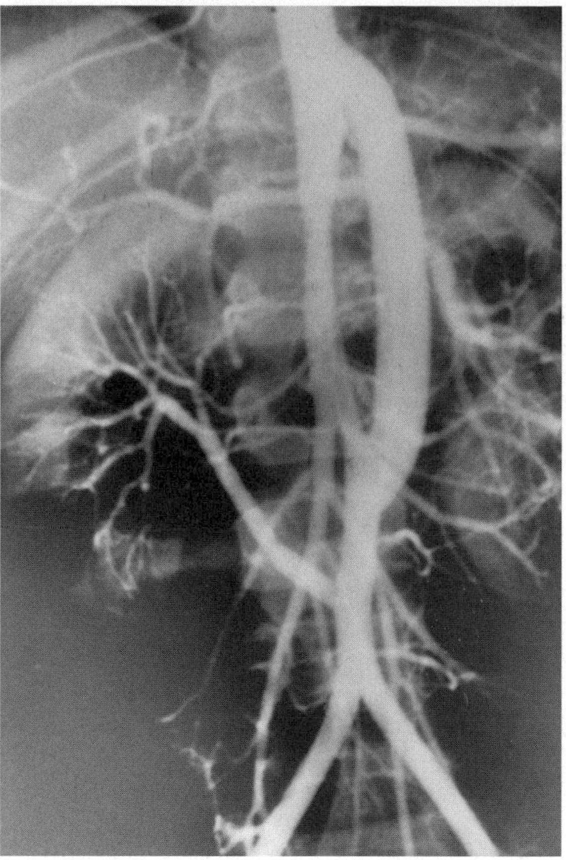

FIGURE 102-8. Aortoaortic bypass graft with polytetrafluoroethylene, left renal artery implantation directly into the graft, and right aortorenal bypass with hypogastric artery in a 6-year-old girl with middle aortic syndrome.

bypassing both sides during the same procedure (15). The anastomosis is performed with monofilament, absorbable sutures for autogenous grafts and monofilament, nonabsorbable sutures for prosthetic grafts, in either continuous or interrupted fashion, depending on the size of the artery and child.

Renal reimplantation or autotransplantation techniques with use of "bench" surgical repair of the renal vessels may be applicable for branch renal artery stenosis, but otherwise have little use in children with renovascular hypertension.

Two-thirds of children with renal artery stenosis have their hypertension cured (normotensive on no medications) when PTA and surgical revascularization are used in combination. Another 25% achieve improved blood pressure control on less medication. Less than 10% do not see improvement with this aggressive approach to correct stenosis. Nephrectomy for failed revascularization is required in 5% to 15% of these patients (14,15).

Splanchnic Arterial Disease

Children with middle aortic syndrome commonly have associated narrowing of one or more of the celiac, superior mesenteric, or inferior mesenteric arteries. In the asymptomatic child with only one of these vessels significantly narrowed, bypass or endarterectomy is usually not performed, but if two vessels are significantly narrowed or if the child is having symptoms of intestinal ischemia, surgical correction is best performed at the same time as the aortic repair (17).

ARTERIOVENOUS MALFORMATIONS

Congenital

Congenital arteriovenous malformation (AVM) remains the least satisfactorily treated vascular lesion in childhood. The cause of these lesions is most likely an anomaly of development in which the arterial and venous systems communicate without passing through the capillaries. It is uncertain why some patients present in the newborn period, whereas others not until adolescence with these congenital lesions. The presenting symptoms may be pain or a sensation of excessive warmth in the area of the AVM, hypertrophy of the tissue or limb involved with the AVM, congestive heart failure because of high cardiac output, or hemorrhage from the AVM.

Congenital AVM can occur in any location, but pediatric surgeons are most often asked to see those on the trunk or extremities. Physical examination is helpful in identifying the location of the AVM, but commonly results in underestimation of the extent of the lesion. A thrill is often palpable over these lesions, and a characteristic bruit can be auscultated. The development of limb hypertrophy distal to an AVM in a child has never been adequately explained because a great deal of the blood flow to the extremity is diverted through the AVM. Some evidence suggests that limb hypertrophy is due to the elevated pressure and stasis on the venous side of the AVM.

A rough assessment of the amount of flow through the AVM can be obtained if the main artery feeding the malformation can be temporarily occluded by external compression. Patients with more than 20% of their cardiac output going through the AVM have tachycardia, and compression of the feeding artery will decrease their pulse rates by more than 10% and often increases their blood pressures (the Branham sign). Although patients with hemodynamically significant AVM may have a negative Branham sign, a positive sign correlates well with a significant proportion of the cardiac output going through the AVM. MRI has become an integral part of the evaluation of children with AVM because of its ability to define extent of disease and relation to other structures, particularly muscles. Angiography is still important in refining the magnetic resonance data and may also be used in some patients for treatment with embolization.

Treatment strategies must be individualized and must be done with the following factors in mind: (1) complete ablation or excision is infrequently possible; (2) if an extremity is involved, the functional result of the treatment should be compared with function before treatment; (3) the flow thorough the fistula may be great enough to cause long-term cardiac problems; and (4) the proposed treatment may effect future treatment options if the AVM recurs.

For the rare situation in which the AVM is well localized and involves nonvital structures, complete surgical excision is the procedure of choice, and when the AVM occurs in an organ that is expendable, such as a pulmonary lobe, resection is the procedure of choice. Some surgeons prefer preoperative AVM embolization to minimize blood loss, but it may make it difficult to determine whether the resection has been complete, and it is not necessary for smaller lesions. In the usual AVM, embolization is useful because the lesion is extensive, and complete surgical excision would require removal of large amounts of normal tissue, such as an amputation. Embolization of the extensive lesions may be the sole form of therapy or may be used in preparation for excision. Embolization is most effective when done into the small arteries of the AVM because embolization of the major arteries may lead to ischemia of distal normal tissues and has no better success rate than embolizing the smaller vessels. Sclerosis using a variety of agents injected percutaneously is also feasible in selected circumstances. However, this approach shares many of the limitations as embolization and is generally considered a palliative maneuver, although it can be quite useful.

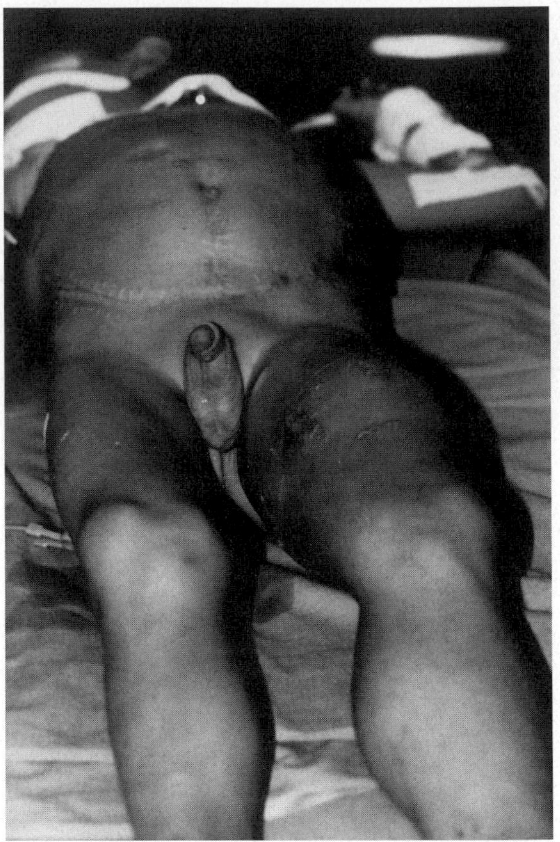

FIGURE 102-9. Left leg hypertrophy in an 8-year-old boy with a left femoral artery–femoral vein prosthetic fistula created for hemodialysis.

Unless wide excision of normal-appearing tissues is performed, recurrence is likely. Even in patients who undergo amputation, recurrence may develop in the tissue that appeared to be entirely normal by previous studies. The high likelihood of recurrence has encouraged a conservative approach to most congenital AVMs, particularly those of the extremity that can be compressed with tight stockings if the cardiac function is not compromised by the AVM.

Acquired

Acquired AVMs are the result of penetrating trauma or an operative procedure to create hemodialysis access. In penetrating trauma of the extremity, there is a trend to avoid exploration of the extremity in the absence of ongoing hemorrhage or pulse deficit (6). This approach may lead to an increased number of children with acquired AVMs. This type of AVM may be due to injury of the vein and artery adjacent to each other or to an arterial false aneurysm that later decompresses into a vein.

In children with renal failure who are on hemodialysis, excessive flow through a dialysis access arteriovenous fistula may lead to cardiac decompensation and limb hypertrophy. The use of autogenous tissue, usually a radial artery-to-cephalic vein fistula, remains the best vascular access for hemodialysis, with the lowest complication rate. If a prosthetic graft must be used because of small vessel size, it is best to stay as distal as possible and to use the upper extremity as the access site. The formation of a femoral–femoral arteriovenous fistula with prosthetic material provides excellent hemodialysis access but in small children is associated with an unacceptably high incidence of cardiac complications and limb hypertrophy (18) (Fig. 102-9).

If the acquired AVM is due to trauma, it should be surgically repaired when identified. If the AVM is created for hemodialysis access, the options for dialysis must be weighed against the risks of the arteriovenous fistula. After a child has had successful renal transplantation, it is important to assess the arteriovenous fistula to determine whether it is causing cardiac or extremity problems.

REFERENCES

1. Skandalakis JE, Gray SW, Symbas P. The thoracic and abdominal aorta. In: Skandalakis JE, Gray SW, eds. *Embryology for surgeons,* 2nd ed. Baltimore: Williams & Wilkins, 1994:976.
2. Guzzetta PC. Congenital and acquired aneurysmal disease. *Semin Pediatr Surg* 1994;3:97.
3. Brogan PA, Davies R, Gordon I, et al. Renal angiography in children with polyarteritis nodosa. *Pediatr Nephrol* 2002;17:277.
4. Sayin AG, Bozkurt AK, Cangel U, et al. A brachial aneurysm in childhood caused by Ehlers-Danlos syndrome. *J Cardiovasc Surg* 2001;42:687.
5. Dittrick K, Allmendinger N, Wolpert L, et al. Calcified abdominal aortic aneurysm in a 12-year-old boy. *J Pediatr Surg* 2002;37:E24.
6. Frykberg ER, Crump JM, Dennis JW, et al. Nonoperative observation of clinically occult arterial injuries: a prospective evaluation. *Surgery* 1991;109:85.
7. Sarkar R, Coran AG, Cilley RE, et al. Arterial aneurysms in children: clinicopathologic classification. *J Vasc Surg* 1991;13:47.
8. Alquin VPR, Albano SA, Chan F, et al. Magnetic resonance imaging in the diagnosis and follow up of Takayasu's arteritis in children. *Ann Rheum Dis* 2002;61:526.
9. Muranjan MN, Bavdekar SB, More V, et al. Study of Takayasu's arteritis in children: clinical profile and management. *J Postgrad Med* 2000;46:3.
10. Tyagi S, Khan AA, Kaul UA, et al. Percutaneous transluminal angioplasty for stenosis of the aorta due to aortic arteritis in children. *Pediatr Cardiol* 1999;20:404.
11. Athreya BH. Vasospastic disorders in children. *Semin Pediatr Surg* 1994;3:70.
12. Lawson JD, Boerth R, Foster JH, et al. Diagnosis and management of renovascular hypertension in children. *Arch Surg* 1977;112:1307.
13. Stanley JC. Pathologic basis of macrovascular renal artery disease. In: Stanley JC, Ernst CB, Fry WJ, eds. *Renovascular hypertension.* Philadelphia: WB Saunders, 1984:46.
14. Guzzetta PC, Potter BM, Ruley EJ, et al. Renovascular hypertension in children: current concepts in evaluation and treatment. *J Pediatr Surg* 1989;24:1236.
15. O'Neill JA. Long-term outcome with surgical treatment of renovascular hypertension. *J Pediatr Surg* 1998;33:106.
16. Lillehei CW, Shamberger RC. Staged reconstruction for middle aortic syndrome. *J Pediatr Surg* 2001;36:1252.
17. Upchurch GR, Henke PK, Eagleton MJ, et al. Pediatric splanchnic arterial occlusive disease: clinical relevance and operative treatment. *J Vasc Surg* 2002;35:860.
18. Guzzetta PC, Salcedo JR, Bell SB, et al. Limb growth and cardiac complications of fistulas in children. *Int J Pediatr Nephrol* 1987;8:167.

Chapter 103

Lymphatic and Venous Vascular Malformations

Anne C. Fischer, Sally E. Mitchell, and Anthony P. Tufaro

Vascular malformations are among the most common birth defects and are the sequelae of congenital errors of morphogenesis. These lesions can present with a diverse spectrum of clinical signs and symptoms and in a variety of anatomic locations. Any individual component from the normal channels of blood and lymphatic flow can constitute the basis of vascular malformations. These anomalous channel types can include aberrancies in arteries, capillaries, veins, and lymphatics. The developmental abnormalities of veins and lymphatics are the focus of this chapter. Due to the varied clinical manifestations of vascular malformations, the complexity of this specialty area mandates a clinical expertise and an orchestrated multidisciplinary approach that has heretofore been underappreciated. These vascular malformations can be characterized by the complexity of the lesions or the inherent flow characteristics (Fig. 103-1).

LYMPHATIC SYSTEM

The actual incidence of lymphatic malformations is unknown, but it is believed to exceed the original estimate of 6.3% of all malformations (1). These malformations are seen in any region rich with lymphatics that were sites of early lymphatic ontogeny. The most common anatomic locations are cervicofacial (75%) and axillary (20%), followed by mediastinal and retroperitoneal. An understanding of lymphatic embryology creates an appreciation of the predilection of postnatal lymphatic malformations to lymphatic-rich areas in ontogeny. The lymphatic system develops from six primitive endothelial sacs that first appear as jugular sacs by the second month in utero (2,3). These six lymphatic-rich regions include two paired jugular sacs in the neck, an endothelial sac at the root of the mesentery, a sac at the cisterna chyli, and two paired posterior inguinal sacs. Secondary endothelial channels interconnect the bilateral jugular sacs, crossing the neck, mediastinum, and abdomen. The thoracic duct longitudinally connects the cisterna chyli with the cervical jugular lymphatic sacs that empty into the left subclavian vein. The retroperitoneal sac at the root of the mesentery is the origin of the mesenteric lymphatics; likewise, the bilateral inguinal sacs propagate to form to the lower-extremity lymphatics. All primitive lymphatic sacs are highly proliferative; thus, lymphatic malformations are believed to result from developmental arrest as the vascular channel propagates or becomes disconnected and sequestered. The etiology, then, is a fundamental defect in the development of lymphatic channels with absent (aplastic), insufficient (hypoplastic), or obstructed (ectatic) efferent pathways. Abnormal lymphatic morphogenesis results in altered tissue architecture and subsequent altered lymphatic flow.

Solid endothelial lymphatic channels parallel the development of embryonic blood vessels and arborize to constitute the peripheral lymphatic system. These solid channels become patent vessels that support the circulation of lymphoblasts. The lymphatic system is the primary conduit to recirculate lymphocytes from interstitial tissues back into the bloodstream. Circulating lymphocytes are returned to the bloodstream, and macromolecules, including fat, are systemically absorbed through the lymphatics. The lymphatic system reflects not only the interstitial composition, but also the interstitial fluid volume. Increased interstitial fluid volume results in enhanced lymphatic flow.

Anne C. Fischer: Department of Surgery, Division of Pediatric Surgery, Johns Hopkins University, Johns Hopkins Hospital, Baltimore, Maryland 21287.

Sally E. Mitchell: Interventional Pediatrics Associates, Interventional Radiology, Johns Hopkins Medical Institutions, Baltimore, Maryland 21287.

Anthony P. Tufaro: Department of Surgery, Division of Plastic and Reconstructive Surgery, Johns Hopkins University, Johns Hopkins Hospital, Baltimore, Maryland 21287.

A. COMPLEXITY

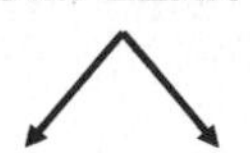

SIMPLE
- Capillary Malformation (CM)
- Venous Malformation (VM)
- Lymphatic Malformation (LM)
  - Microcystic
  - Macrocystic

COMBINED
- Capillary-lymphaticovenous Malformation (CLVM)
  - Klippel-Trenaunay
- Capillary-venous with AV shunting
- Lymphaticovenous Malformation (LVM)
- Arteriovenous Malformation (AVM)

B. CHARACTERISTICS

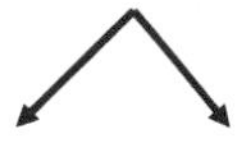

LOW FLOW
- Capillary (Port wine stain)
  - Sturge-Weber
- Venous Malformation
- Lymphatic Malformation
- Combined Malformation

HIGH FLOW
- Arterial Malformations
- Arteriovenous Malformation (AVM)
- CLVM with AV shunting
  - Parkes-Weber Syndrome

FIGURE 103-1. Classification of vascular malformations.

Antegrade lymphatic flow is dependent on intramuscular contractions and intrathoracic pressure because valves, to resist retrograde flow, exist only within the deep lymphatic system; all are essential components to return lymph to the central venous system.

Lymphatic Malformations

Typically referred to as lymphangiomas, lymphatic anomalies are more precisely designated as malformations because the appendix "-oma" inherently implies the hyperplastic and proliferative characteristics of tumors (4,5). In contrast, these lesions are not associated with unabated cellular proliferation or hyperplastic growth. An increase in size is not related to independent cellular growth, but rather to enhanced accumulation of fluid or recruitment of additional lymphatics. Combined vascular anomalies can coexist in the context of abnormal lymphatic tissue and frequently are lymphaticovenous or capillary-lymphatic malformations.

A layer of flattened endothelial cells lining each cyst is characteristic of the histology of lymphatic malformations. Fibrous or inflammatory changes extrinsic to the endothelium are included within the cyst. The gross histology varies from a large unilocular cyst, such as a macrocystic structure, to multiple small cysts, such as a microcystic formation (Figs. 103-2A and 103-2D). These lesions can be localized or extensive, infiltrating local tissue architecture. Lymphatic malformations fluctuate in size secondary to trauma or infection, and undergo fibrotic shrinkage only after recurrent episodes of cellulitis and lymphangitis.

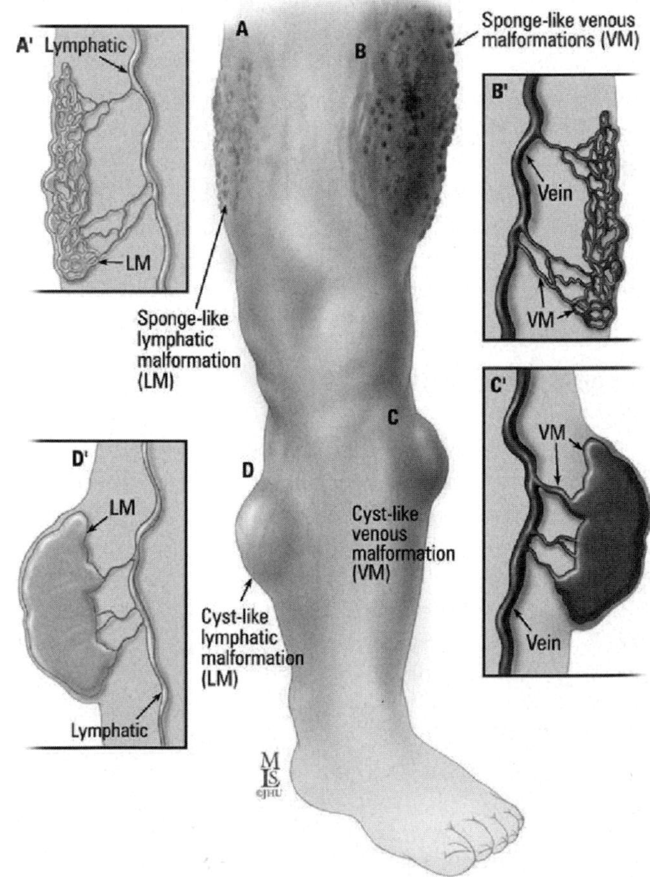

FIGURE 103-2. Artistic drawing of venous and lymphatic malformations.

Those malformations that permeate through the epidermis as superficial vesicular lesions are the most vulnerable to repetitive cellulitic infections. Such superficial vesicular lesions are secondary to a deeper lymphangiomatous component involving the dermis. To avoid rapidly progressive lymphangitis, antibiotic therapy should be initiated expeditiously and directed at streptococcal and staphylococcal organisms. Perineal locations require concomitant gram-negative enteric coverage. Recurrent episodes of infection lead to fibrotic shrinkage of the lymphangioma.

Diagnosis

Lymphatic malformations detected very early prenatally at the end of the first trimester manifest diffently than those discovered postnatally (6,7). Those fetal lymphatic malformations diagnosed prior to 30 weeks' gestation, that usually arise in the posterior cervical region are associated with fetal hydrops and abnormal karyotypes. The abnormal karyotypes typically include Turner's syndrome, but the trisomies (13,18,21,11q/22Q, and a 22 mosaic) have also been reported; therefore, an amniocentesis is highly recommended. Noonan's syndrome and fetal alcohol syndrome have also been associated with prenatally diagnosed lymphatic malformations. Spontaneous resolution of these malformations has been documented. In contrast, persistence of the malformation with subsequent fetal hydrops portends a poor outcome.

The majority of lymphatic malformations are detected postnatally and are clinically evident early; more than 65% of diagnoses are determined at birth and more than 90% by the age of 2 years (8). Overall, they are unusual lesions without racial or sexual predilection. Radiographic imaging may necessitate several modalities, depending on the anatomic complexity and potential extension or field effect of the anomaly. Prenatal lesions can be detected by duplex ultrasound (US) and are well-imaged in the facial region with three-dimensional (3D) ultrasonography. Advances in 3D prenatal imaging have permitted earlier detection of cervicofacial malformations that may require prenatal planning for an ex utero intrapartum procedure to prevent emergent loss of the airway from anatomic distortion and an obstructing mass effect (Fig. 103-3). Superficial lesions mandate a high-frequency US with color flow duplex as the initial least invasive study. However, magnetic resonance imaging (MRI) with T_2-weighted images is ideal in identifying a malformation as lymphatic and defining the extent of the malformation, particularly in complex anatomic regions such as the head and neck and mediastinum (9,10). Magnetic resonance venography (MRI/MRV) is the best modality to image lymphangiomatous involvement of the peritoneum and contiguous retroperitoneum. In conjunction with 3D imaging, radionucleotide lymphoscintigraphy and dynamic lymphangiography are powerful modalities to trace lymphatic flow and delineate the precise anatomic point of obstruction or abnormality.

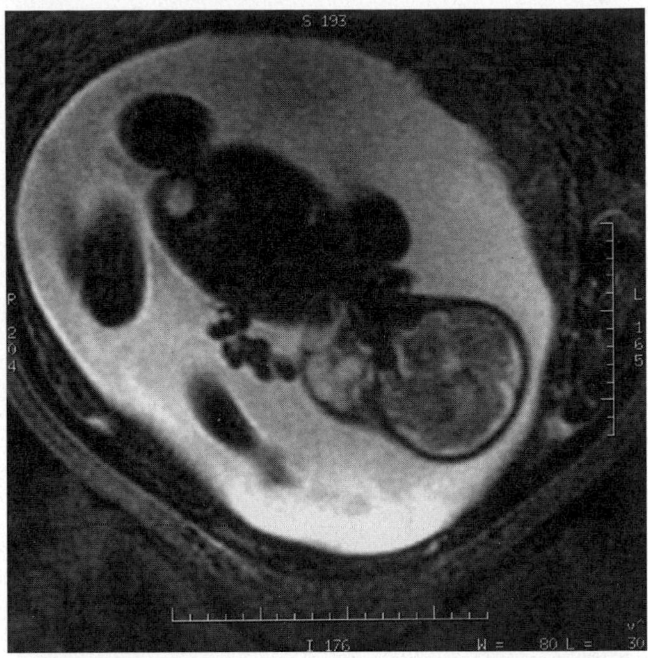

FIGURE 103-3. Coronal T_2 with fast-spin echo magnetic resonance image of a giant cervicofacial lymphatic malformation detected prenatally and requiring an ex utero intrapartum procedure.

Treatment

Surgical resection with complete excision for a given anatomic region is performed whenever technically possible. Although these lesions are benign and have a demarcated plane of dissection, they do not stay confined to normal tissue planes and can envelop contiguous structures. Therefore, the paradigm is to first identify the anatomic regions involved, and then to stage the surgery, excising with meticulous dissection as much of the malformation as possible in a given anatomic region without damaging normal vital structures. For instance, cervicofacial lymphatic malformations can encase major cranial nerves, vessels, and parotid glands; however, they do not mandate a radical extirpation with subsequent loss of function because these are not malignancies. An incomplete debulking dissection near vital structures ensures a high incidence of recurrence and suboptimal outcome, for which a second operation in a reoperative field is not without significant morbidities. Thus, the best opportunity for resectability is the first excision. With extensive lesions, anatomic regions should be defined and staged such that a complete anatomic region is maximally cleared in one setting. If a particular region is subjected to staged resection, then the remaining contiguous lesions may expand significantly postoperatively; creating a temporary field effect. Preoperative planning for airway compromise, respiratory difficulties, or diaphragmatic paralysis cannot be overemphasized. The incidence of postoperative complications can be 30% or higher, including recurrences and neurologic defects (11). Recurrences range from 10% to 27% following complete resections and up to 50% or higher following debulking or partial resections. Drainage from surgically placed drains is expected for a protracted period of time from weeks to months. Postoperative infections should mandate immediate antibiotic therapy. An advantage of recurrent cellulitis or lymphangitis may be eventual sclerosis of the leaking lymphatics and a dramatic drop in drainage. Other temporary interventions, such as needle aspirations, fail due to rapid lymphatic reaccumulation, but may be useful as a temporizing measure of emergent decompression if airway compromise is imminent.

Sclerotherapy to reduce the size of the lesion is another strategy that has been used to minimize the extent of surgery or to avoid surgery completely. The mechanism of action of sclerosants is to induce an inflammatory reaction and subsequent fibrosis with endothelial cell destruction and collapse of the cyst. Sclerosants currently available include ethanol, bleomycin, doxycycline, OK-432, and fibrin glue. Macrocystic lesions are easily accessed using US guidance and fluoroscopic control, and are therefore amenable to intralesional injection of sclerosants. Microcystic lesions are less accessible and usually respond less well than macrocystic lesions to sclerotherapy. However, sclerotherapy is possible, although difficult, with microcystic lesions due to the technical difficulty of accessing percutaneously the multiplicity of tiny lymphatic spaces that are not necessarily in continuity. Sclerotherapy usually requires a series of treatments 6 weeks apart to treat the multiple cystic areas adequately.

Ethanol has been widely used for lymphatic and venous sclerotherapy, and its mechanism of action is not only an inflammatory reaction directed to the endothelium, but also induction of endothelial cell necrosis and destruction. Because of its more potent endothelial damage, ethanol has been the sclerosant of choice in renal cysts, hepatic cysts, lymphoceles, and both venous and lymphatic malformations. Absolute ethanol at a total dose of 0.5 to 1 cc per kg of body weight is the dose for directed intralesional sclerotherapy.

Microspheres of oil-bleomycin lipid emulsions (BLM 9 mg per mL) are a more effective sclerosant than bleomycin alone due to the rapid uptake of the lipophilic emulsion in lymphatics and a higher concentration at the intended site of action (12,13). Injection of 0.3 to 0.6 mg per kg intralesionally after cyst aspiration is the recommended approach. Contraindicated in infants younger than 6 months of age, the drug induces transient swelling for up to 2 weeks post therapy and has a myriad of side effects, including fever, diarrhea, vomiting, vesiculation, and scarring.

There is a more limited experience with percutaneous doxycycline, which can be delivered after either needle aspiration or via fluoroscopic or computed tomography (CT)-directed pigtail catheters. The dose ranges from 5 to 20 mg per mL of a diluted 1:4 mixture with a radiopaque diluent of iodohexol for concurrent fluoroscopic imaging. Pain control, fever, and cellulitis are all side effects (14).

OK-432 (Picibanil) is sclerosant developed in Japan that is a lyophilized mixture of group A streptococcus pyogens with penicillin G potassium (15,16). The mechanism of action is an immune-mediated reaction within the cyst, resulting in fibrosis and endothelial destruction. The recommended dose is an intracystic injection of 0.1 mg in 10 mL of saline (0.9% wt per vol) after initial aspiration of the cyst with a total volume not to exceed 20 mL. Repeated injections can be given every 4 to 6 weeks. Fever, induration, erythema, and swelling can last 3 to 7 days. A prospective randomized trial demonstrated that 86% of patients with macrocystic lymphangiomas responded with greater than 60% reduction in cyst size after four injections (17). OK-432 has been subjected to rigorous clinical trials, but is not available currently outside trials in the United States.

All sclerosants induce an inflammatory reaction and edema; thus, all can induce airway compromise if there is resultant edema adjacent to the airway in the cervicofacial region or mediastinum. This approach is typically used in anatomic locations when complete resection is not safe or feasible. The anatomic site and the size of the lesion determine the type of anesthesia, length of intubation, and intensive care monitoring. Laser therapy, using a CO_2 laser, is the modality for lymphatic malformations intrinsic to the larynx and airway. Likewise, the laser can treat residual superficial epidermal lymphatic vesicles following resection of the underlying lymphatic malformation. Radiation therapy is no longer considered an acceptable approach because of significant morbidities and complications.

Lymphatic malformations in certain anatomic regions require meticulous planning (Fig. 103-4). Giant cervicofacial lymphatic malformations involve multiple structures, including the tongue, larynx, and parotids, often with bilateral and mediastinal extension. These giant lesions with mediastinal extension are the most challenging of surgical resections; likewise, they have the potential for rapid enlargement and airway compromise with a potential need for earlier intervention and probable tracheostomy. Long-term craniofacial problems from large cervicofacial lymphangiomas can result from maxillofacial hypertrophy and mandibular hypertrophy with malocclusion. Hypertrophy of either the mandible or maxilla induces hypertrophy of the other, and may require multiple osteotomies and

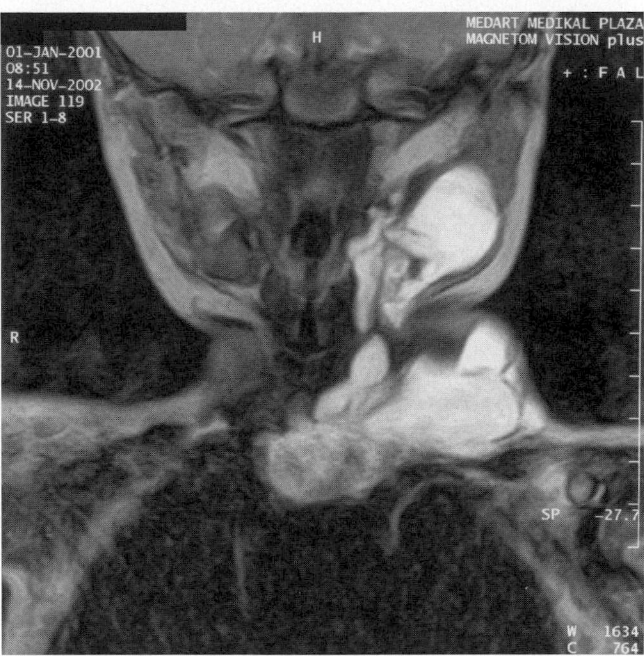

FIGURE 103-4. Coronal T_2 magnetic resonance image of a cervicofacial lymphaticovenous malformation with mediastinal extension.

ostectomies to control growth and normalize occlusion. Final outcomes are often disappointing and frustrating to both the patient and the physician. Macroglossia is also not uncommon. These lesions are often microcystic, difficult to sclerose, and difficult to manage. Macroglossia may require several interventional modalities, including preoperative sclerosis and subsequent limited surgical resections to preserve oral function; both modalities can potentially impact lingual nerve function.

Lesions of the parotid and cervical area are challenging due to the potential for devastating cranial nerve injuries. Parotid involvement is best managed initially with observation in an effort to avoid surgery in an infant at a time when the facial nerve is difficult to visualize. Planned excision of the lesion, including a superficial parotidectomy avoiding injury to the facial nerve, is done after growth beyond infancy. The hypoglossal nerve is at risk with cervical lesions deep to the digastric muscle in the submandibular area (level I) and near the carotid bifurcation. Injuries result in lingual atrophy and problems with phonation and deglutination. The marginal mandibular branch to the depressors of the labial commissure lies deep to the platysma in the area of the submandibular gland. Injury will cause facial asymmetry and drooling. The facial nerve is at risk in the area of the parotid and superior cervical region. Injuries are truly devastating, leading to facial asymmetry, problems with phonation and feeding, and loss of periorbital musculature with an inability to blink and protect the cornea. Proximal facial nerve injuries are best managed by immediate microsurgical repair with interrupted monofilament suture, and distal injuries are often not amenable to repair.

Thoracic Duct Anomalies: Chylothorax

A chylothorax results from leakage of lymphatic fluid into the thoracic cavity, typically presenting as a right pleural effusion. In 60% to 70% of neonates, the thoracic duct arises from the cisterna chyli, ascends on the right until the fourth to sixth vertebrae, and then crosses the midline to ascend along the left to empty into the left subclavian vein. A congenital chylothorax is the most common cause of pleural effusions in the fetus and neonate, and is usually caused by a malformation involving the thoracic duct (18). Anomalies associated with a congenital chylothorax include trisomy 21, Turner's and Noonan's syndromes, pulmonary lymphangectasia, extralobar pulmonary sequestration, and esophageal atresia. Among infants and children, the most common etiology of a chylous thorax is secondary to trauma, including iatrogenic trauma such as cardiothoracic or intrathoracic procedures (coarctation of the aorta, Blalock-Taussig shunts, and Glenn procedures), birth trauma, and blunt thoracic or spinal injury. If effusions are bilateral, then underlying venous hypertension secondary to a central venous thrombosis, such as a superior vena cava obstruction, may be the etiology. Fontan procedures are associated with venous hypertension and chylothoraces may result. It cannot be overemphasized that investigation for systemic venous hypertension causing a refractory chylous thorax be done. This mandates diagnostic and therapeutic measures first to reduce the venous hypertension.

A pleural effusion is diagnostic for chyle if a cell count exceeds 60% lymphocytes or if there is microscopic detection of chylomicrons by Sudan red staining. Daily loss of chyle leads to hypoalbuminemia, hyponatremia, lymphopenia, marked weight loss, and immune dysfunction. Chyle has a milky appearance in the presence of enteral intake, but can appear serous if the patient is either not eating or ingesting a diet restricted to medium-chain triglycerides (MCT). Of note, milky effusions can result from etiologies other than chyle. Potential explanations include intrapleural hyperalimentation or inflammatory conditions associated with cholesterol pleural effusions, such as tuberculosis, filiaris, and rheumatoid arthritis.

Once the effusion is diagnosed as chyle, initial treatment consists of nonoperative management with a thoracostomy tube for drainage and either an elemental diet with MCT (Portagen) or nutrition restricted to total parenteral nutrition. If the effusion is of traumatic etiology and persistent, then enteral intake should be totally prohibited. Chyle loss may be 1,500 mL per day per adult or

100 mL per year of age per day for children (19). Most chylous effusions resolve, but persistent or unmanageable chyle losses refractory to nonoperative management mandate intervention. Administration of the somatostatin analogue, octreotide, (1 to 4 mcg per kg per hour) has demonstrated efficacy in some reports, but not all patients respond and its use in children is a point of uncertainty. Videoscopic thoracic duct ligation has become a standard surgical intervention (20). Pleuroperitoneal shunts have been successfully used in atraumatic chylothoraces (21) and following cardiac surgery (22). For precise imaging, nuclear medicine lymphoscintigraphy can identify the region of lymphatic disruption and a lymphangiogram can reveal anatomic detail. Percutaneous embolization of a leak in the thoracic duct using fluoroscopic guidance is a more recent option, using standard embolization techniques (23). If the site of leak is difficult to visualize intraoperatively or fluoroscopically, preoperative enteral cream administration increases lymphatic flow and simplifies visualization. We have successfully performed lymphatic-venous microsurgical repairs for excision of malformations or repair of the thoracic duct.

Intraabdominal Lymphatic Malformations

Lymphatic cysts in the abdominal or retroperitoneal region are believed to be developmental sequestrations of the embryonic lymphatic sacs that continue to grow independently as separate islands of lymphatic tissue. These cysts can be in the omentum, mesentery, or retroperitoneum. Lymphatic cysts are classically lined by an endothelial cell layer; those with a differing histology, such as mesothelial or columnar cells, may reflect an embryologic origin derived from peritoneal or mesonephric remnants, respectively. Most children present either without symptoms or with a palpable mass; however, abdominal distension and intestinal obstruction can occur. Preoperative imaging by US and CT with intravenous (IV) and oral contrast is often the best modality, although MRI may be helpful in some circumstances. Complete surgical excision may necessitate a limited intestinal resection. Extensive mesenteric and retroperitoneal involvement may require a more extensive resection with marsupialization of the residual portions of the malformation. Intraoperative argon beam therapy has been reported for a nonresectable lesion (24). Percutaneous sclerosis is another potential option. Long-term follow-up is mandated for detection of recurrence or the presence of chylous ascites in those with extensive involvement.

Lymphangiectasia

Abnormal lymphatic development when identified in one organ system often coexists in multiple organ systems, representing a characteristic multiorgan pattern of abnormal lymphatic development. Such systemic lymphangiomatosis is characterized by multicentric lymphatic malformations. Common clusters include liver and spleen lymphangiectasias, as well as lung, bone, and spleen involvement. Often, plain radiographs incidentally reveal severe osteolytic and sclerotic bony changes which mandate systemic evaluation that then identifies multi organ involvement. No systemic therapy is available, and a poor prognosis is evident in refractory cases.

Intestinal lymphangiectasia is rare and characterized by lymphatic channels throughout the entire intestine and mesentery (25). The clinical manifestations are protein-losing enteropathy, fat malabsorption, hypoalbuminemia, and edema. Symptoms include abdominal pain, nausea, seizures, and malnutrition. An upper gastrointestinal (GI) series with enteroclysis can identify the full extent of the intestinal involvement. Altered villous architecture is characteristic of endoscopic biopsies. Therapy is nonoperative and primarily supportive, with enteral intake restricted to MCTs to bypass intestinal lymphatic absorption or restricted to a low-fat, high-protein diet.

Pulmonary lymphangiectasia presents as a cause of intractable respiratory distress due to diffuse parenchymal involvement with accumulation of pleural effusions. The lymphangiectasia may result from abnormal lymphatics diffusely throughout the lung or be the secondary result of underlying venous hypertension. Noonan's syndrome (hypertelorism, blue eyes, webbed feet, lymphedema, and either pulmonic stenosis or cardiomyopathy) and yellow nail syndrome often have associated pulmonary lymphangiectasia (26). In Gorham's disease, single or contiguous bones are replaced by lymphangiomatous tissue, leading to osteolysis and pathologic fractures. It is in this syndrome that the lymphatic involvement is often first detected by an abnormal bony radiograph. Diffuse parenchymal lung involvement can occur and predicts a poor outcome due to the paucity of therapeutic options. Options include repetitive thoracostomies or pleuroperitoneal shunts to alleviate effusions. Surgery is considered for localized involvement, not diffuse involvement. Patients with generalized lymphatic dysplasia, including intestinal lymphangiectasia, lymphangiomatosis, and diffuse pulmonary involvement, have a poor prognosis.

Chylous Ascites

Chyle can accumulate at any point along lymphatic flow from the cisterna chyli to the thoracic duct. In the abdomen, this can lead to distention with or without respiratory embarrassment. The etiology of chylous ascites in children is idiopathic in 40% of cases (27). Diagnostic paracentesis can confirm chyle as previously reviewed. CT imaging can rule out an underlying infiltrative neoplastic or inflammatory process. A dynamic lymphangiogram can detect an anatomic disruption or abnormality. Therapeutic measures should be initiated by a low-fat, high-protein diet with MCT. Refractory ascites mandates complete enteral rest and total parenteral therapy. Nonoperative therapy should be attempted at a minimum for 4 weeks. Persistent chyle output leads to severe malnutrition, altered immunity, severe malabsorption, and electrolyte imbalances, with a 21% mortality rate. Peritoneovenous shunts are a temporizing measure and limited by their high rate of obstruction and an induced state of fibrinolysis. If a correctable anatomic lesion is detected on dynamic lymphangiography, then a laparotomy may permit identification of the site of chyle loss for ligation.

Extremity Lymphedema

In children, extremity lymphedema is typically congenital and due to abnormal lymphatic development. Lymphedema can be classified as *primary* (idiopathic) or *secondary* (acquired). The lymphatic vessels of congenital lymphedema represent several patterns of abnormal growth: aplasia (absent lymphatics), hypoplasia (underdeveloped lymphatics), or hyperplasia (tortuous varicosities). *Secondary* lymphedema is acquired due to an underlying process that destroys subcutaneous lymphatic channels. These processes include neoplasia, filariasis, trauma, infection, radiotherapy, or iatrogenic injury. *Primary* lymphedema can be broadly divided into three subsets: (1) *congenital,* presenting in early childhood and associated with other vascular malformations, such as the Klippel-Trenaunay, Proteus, and Parkes-Weber syndromes; (2) *praecox,* the most common subtype, which presents in adolescence; or (3) *tarda,* which presents after 35 years of age. The inherited syndromes are rare, autosomal dominant, and include Milroy's disease, a familial congenital lymphedema, and Merge's disease, a familial lymphedema praecox. Other genetic syndromes associated with primary lymphedema are Turner's syndrome, Noonan's syndrome, yellow nail syndrome, and distichiasis (duplicated rows of eyelashes).

Lymphedema praecox is the most common primary lymphedema with a 2:1 female prevalence, attributed to the higher estrogen levels and lower interstitial tissue pressures in females. The onset of edema is coincident with the growth spurt of adolescence, and hence, increased hydrostatic pressure. Trauma and infection can be inciting etiologies. The typical presentation is unilateral lower-extremity swelling; this occurs less frequently in the upper extremities. Primary lymphedema extends typically to the calf or knee with bilaterality in 30% of cases. Other types of lymphedema (tarda and praecox) can present with edema extending proximally into the thigh. The unilateral soft nonpitting edema and painless swelling produces a sensation of heaviness, which worsens in the later part of the day. History and physical examination are often sufficient to establish the diagnosis. Radiologic imaging better defines the extent, depth, and nature of the abnormality with comparative T_1- and T_2-weighted MRI sequential imaging. Duplex studies are essential to establish the presence of a patent deep venous system. This is essential for planning lymphangiectomy. Dynamic imaging with nuclear lymphoscintigraphy can demonstrate proximal anatomic obstruction.

Nonoperative therapeutic efforts should be exhausted prior to surgical intervention. Treatment is usually conservative with a combination of compressive extremity garments (Jobst) and pneumatic compression (10 mm Hg), with elevation at night. Compliance is often difficult in adolescents. Dietary restriction of long-chain triglycerides has improved a limited number of unilateral lymphedema patients (28). Complications of chronic lymphedema include lymphangitis, cellulitis, cosmetic and psychosocial problems, and potential development of highly malignant lymphoangiosarcoma. The latter is more likely in cases of secondary lymphedema.

The most common cause of lymphedema is inadequate lymphatics in the subcutaneous tissues. Surgical options are limited; they are focused either on the removal of lymphedematous tissue or attempts to reestablish lymphatic flow. Experimentally, multiple implants, including silk, fascia, and omentum, have been used to induce lymphatic growth and improve lymphatic flow, but they have not provided long-term patency. Microsurgical lymphatic anastomoses (lymph node or lymphatic-to-vein conduits) are likewise reported, but have limited success and poor patency. Lymphatic hypoplasia in the subcutaneous tissues is compounded by the absence of valves in the superficial lymphatic channels, whereas only the deep lymphatic system has valves. Thus, excision of the superficial lymphaticoedematous tissue removes the dysfunctional component and provides direct contact of skin to muscle allowing reestablishment of lymphatic flow directly to the valvular deep system. The Charles procedure removes all superficial edematous skin and subcutaneous tissue down to muscle with split-thickness skin coverage. This produces a marked reduction in extremity size; however, it is not cosmetically optimal due to the presence of skin grafts (29). Homan's modification of the Charles procedure includes complete excision of all subcutaneous tissue and fascia and the creation of thin skin flaps to cover the denuded area directly (30). Homan's modification is the procedure of choice at present.

Currently, subcutaneous lymphangiectomy is done in a staged fashion if necessary, with full-thickness skin flaps raised and reapplied to the denuded fascial surface. The skin flaps are attached to the underlying muscle, and the dilated static subcutaneous lymphatics are excised. Large suction drains are placed under the skin flaps and kept on continuous suction. Three excisional procedures are potentially needed—medial, lateral, and then posterior regions. The skin flaps extend to one-third the total circumference of the leg to avoid skin necrosis and loss (31). Postoperatively, the patient continues to wear support stockings indefinitely to control swelling. Intervals between excisions span a year's time to maximize total reconfiguration of the leg.

Complex Combined Vascular Malformations

Complex malformations incorporate vessel types from all vascular channels. The most common is the combined lymphaticovenous malformation, Klippel-Trenaunay syndrome; others include the Parkes-Weber syndrome and Proteus syndrome. In 1900, Klippel and Trenaunay described a congenital triad of a port wine stain, varicose veins, and hemihypertrophy (32). Typically, a hypertrophied unilateral lower extremity is involved with the associated hemipelvis (Fig. 103-5). Hemihypertrophy includes both length and girth discrepancies, requiring close orthopedic monitoring and evaluation for epiphysiodesis. Continuous compressive extremity garments are essential for these patients, as is meticulous skin care. Massive varicosities are not uncommon and these may be painful. Confirmation of patency of the deep venous system is essential before attempting vein excision or embolization, especially because 20% of deep systems are absent in these patients (33). Percutaneous sclerotherapy can be performed to treat symptomatic venous malformations. Treatment is directed at specific symptoms. Bleeding from varices necessitates fibrin glue, thrombin, or percutaneous embolization. Pain from the venous component resolves with percutaneous embolization. Thrombophlebitis and cellulitis can be treated with low-dose aspirin and antibiotics. Laser therapy can diminish the cosmetic impact of the Port wine stain.

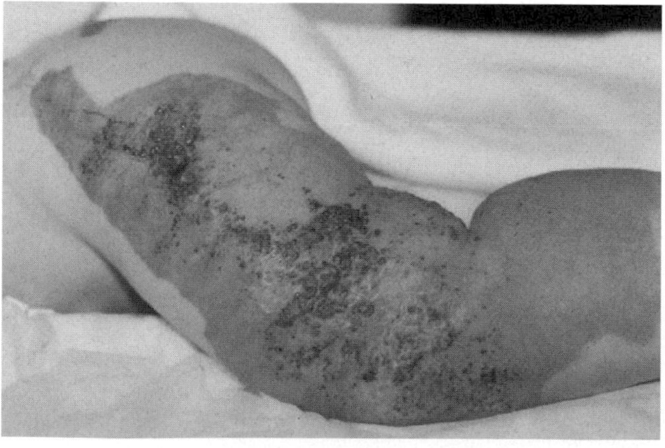

FIGURE 103-5. Case of Klippel-Trenaunay syndrome in an infant with one affected extremity.

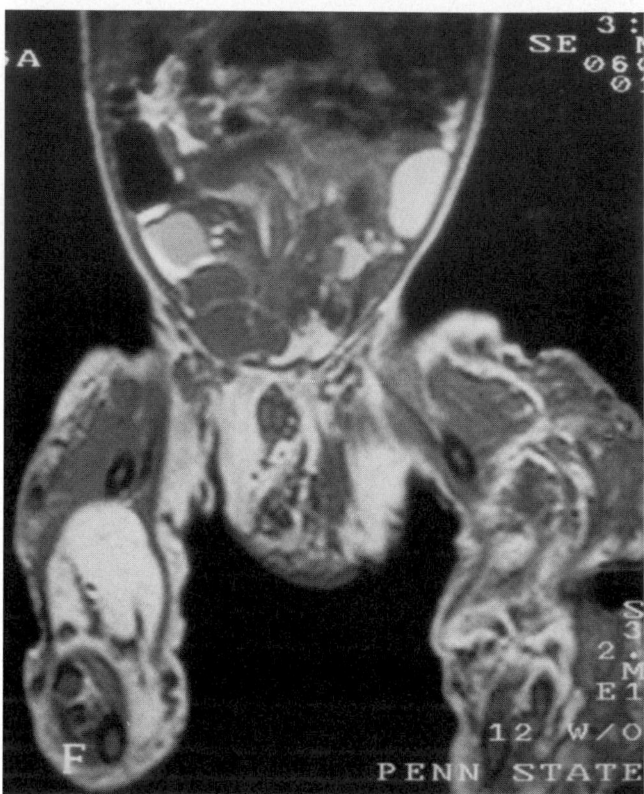

FIGURE 103-6. Magnetic resonance image of 3-month-old male infant with severe Klippel-Trenaunay syndrome extensively involving the lower extremities, the perineum, and the pelvis extending into the lower abdomen. The resultant grossly disordered mesenchymal development is apparent.

The Parkes-Weber syndrome is similar to the Klippel-Trenaunay syndrome, except for associated single or multiple arteriovenous fistulae, which can produce severe hemodynamic overload from the arteriovenous shunting (34).

MRI/MRV which has superseded venography and arteriography for 3D dynamic imaging, can identify critical structures and the relevant vascular anatomy. Furthermore, the extensive involvement is best demonstrated on MRI (Fig. 103-6).

The pathophysiology of Parkes-Weber syndrome is determined by the degree of multiple macroarteriovenous fistulae. These can be sufficiently large or numerous to cause cardiac hemodynamic failure. The multiple arteriovenous fistulae are often tiny or microfistulae, and may be cutaneous or subcutaneous with associated skin thickening. These can be embolized with ethanol or glue, but this is often difficult requiring multiple sessions to access the various tiny arteriovenous fistulae. The anomalous venous component can lead to multifocal thrombosis and phleboliths, which are episodically painful. Phleboliths and skeletal involvement are diagnostic on imaging.

Proteus syndrome has a wide range of clinical manifestations. Although it is a hamartomatous abnormality, it is considered within the Klippel-Trenaunay spectrum (35). It is now suggested that "the Elephant Man" actually manifested Proteus syndrome, not neurofibromatosis. The syndrome is sporadic and presents with asymmetric hypertrophy, macrodactyly and syndactyly, soft-tissue hypertrophy, and vascular nevi (Port wine stains) in conjunction with complex soft-tissue hamartomas.

VENOUS SYSTEM

Venous malformations are the most prevalent of all vascular malformations. In ontogeny, two basic venous plexuses form the foundation of the parietal and visceral venous systems. The parietal system consists of the pre- and postcardinal veins. The precardinal veins drain the cranial side of the embryo to form the internal jugular veins. The postcardinal veins drain the caudal half of the embryo. The paired precardinal and postcardinal veins are connected initially by the common cardinal veins at the level of the sinus venosus. The right precardinal and common cardinal veins form the superior vena cava, whereas the left precardinal typically involutes. In a similar fashion, the right postcardinal vein primarily contributes to the inferior vena cava, whereas the left side involutes. Anomalous development or altered involution results in anatomic abnormalities or duplications of the vena cava. Upper- and lower-extremity veins propagate peripherally in parallel with limb bud mesenchyme and fuse with the pre- and postcardinal veins, respectively (Fig. 103-7). The visceral system is similarly comprised of paired vitelline and umbilical veins. The right vitelline vein forms the right branch of the portal vein, and the left vitelline vein forms the main portal vein and left branch. The left umbilical vein connects to the left vitelline vein to form the ductus venosus, critical for fetal circulation.

Two-thirds of the entire circulating blood volume is contained within the venous system. Antegrade flow is primarily dependent on cardiac and intramuscular contractions and a valvular system to impede retrograde flow. The venous system has the majority of valves in the periphery, fewer valves more centrally, and no valves in the vena cava (36). Thus, both the negative intrathoracic pressure generated upon inspiration and the contraction of skeletal muscles in the extremities are essential for unidirectional venous return. Venous capacitance is directly influenced by systemic catecholamines and via the innervation of the vascular smooth muscle by the sympathetic nervous system. Vasoconstriction of venous smooth muscle surrounding the endothelium can cause a loss of venous capacitance. On a cellular level, the local production of nitric oxide or endothelin by the endothelial cells causes either local vasodilation or vasoconstriction, respectively, with profound effects on venous blood flow.

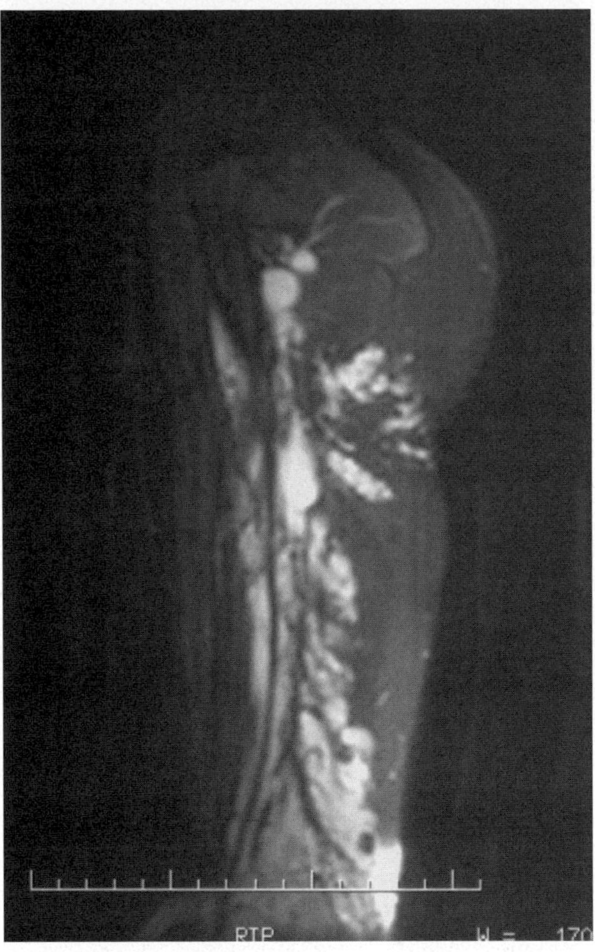

FIGURE 103-7. Coronal T_2 magnetic resonance image with fat suppression of a child with extensive venous malformation of his affected arm peripherally with axillary and chest wall extension.

Many venous disorders are acquired, secondary to venous hypertension and subsequent valvular dysfunction. Acquired venous disorders secondary to inflammatory, infectious, or traumatic etiologies present more commonly in adults, but can also occur in children. In fact, varicosities of the superficial veins are the most common of abnormalities. In an adult, venous pressure at rest can be 100 mm Hg due to hydrostatic forces. Thus, any valvular dysfunction contributes to ineffectual venous return with a cycle of progressive venous hypertension, worsening valvular incompetence and impedance to venous return. This cycle of increasing venous hypertension explains the etiology of very common simple varicosities of superficial veins in adults and adolescents. Likewise, this same pathophysiology explains the underlying venous dysfunction associated with complex combined vascular anomalies. Venous hypertension results in endothelial cell dysfunction, extravasation of red blood cells, fibrinogen, and inflammatory mediators, leading to painful, discolored skin and brawny induration.

Diagnosis

Congenital vascular malformations are usually visible at birth, often bluish, and compressible. Venous malformations are often painful, particularly after strenuous activity or upon awakening in the morning. They grow proportionately with the patient, persisting throughout life. Stimuli such as hormonal changes around adolescence and pregnancies can induce further growth. The proper diagnosis as a venous malformation expedites the correct management and directed therapy of these pathologic disorders.

Congenital Venous Disorders

Congenital venous anomalies result from aberrant vascular development (Figs. 103-2B and 103-2C). The congenital absence of valves is an unusual autosomal-dominant anomaly, diagnosed by venography, and manifests with the end-stage sequelae of venous hypertension and venous insufficiency including nonhealing ulcers in the absence of deep venous thrombosis (DVT) (37,38). Graduated external compression is the mainstay of treatment. Valvular transplantation has been reported.

Primary venous ectasia or varicose veins in childhood are not common, but can be inherited, typically as part of a syndrome. Venous ectasia can be superimposed on complex combined vascular anomalies. These usually affect the lower extremity and are more pronounced later in the clinical course of the syndrome. Varicosities, usually not present in infancy, arise as a secondary consequence of the presence of venous obstruction and venous hypertension, resulting in valvular incompetence and altered venous capacitance. Increased oncotic pressure can lead to enhanced tissue and protein extravasation with subsequent worsening tissue oxygenation and nonhealing ulcers, as well as brawny edema. Venous hypertension can worsen if thrombi destroy deep venous valves, in which case hydrostatic pressure is directly transmitted to the subcutaneous tissues.

Combined Malformations

Abnormalities of the superficial veins of the lower extremities are the most common manifestation of valvular dysfunction. In contrast, abnormalities of the deep venous system, such as anomalous channels, atresias, and agenesis, are all relatively rare. Congenital hypoplasia of the pelvic or femoropopliteal venous system is commonly seen in the combined congenital vascular malformations. The relevant combined venous malformations include Klippel-Trenaunay syndrome (bone hypertrophy, varicosities, and venolymphatic dysplasia) (32,33), Parkes-Weber syndrome (a variant of Klippel-Trenaunay including arteriovenous fistulas, which can induce high-output cardiac failure) (34), and Proteus syndrome (a predominately lymphodysplastic syndrome associated with deep venous system anomalies and vena cava dysplasia) (35). These malformation syndromes result in notable venous hypertension. The workup entails a T_2-weighted MRI to detail the size and extent of the venous malformation, and a venogram, which can also be supplanted by an MRV, to assess the patency of the deep venous system. Often associated with these combined vascular malformations is the coexistence of a prominent lateral embryonal vein, which can be very painful and problematic. This should not be excised or sclerosed in the absence of a confirmed and patent deep venous system. The deep venous system is absent in at least 20% of patients with Klippel-Trenaunay syndrome. Klippel-Trenaunay syndrome is usually managed nonoperatively with surgery or sclerotherapy reserved for symptomatic and persistent venous hypertension, despite nonoperative measures. Deep venous reconstruction may be important for a subset of patients with significant venous insufficiency. This is often due to inadequate or excised superficial collateral veins or failed endovascular procedures. Combined lymphaticovenous syndromes are associated with segmental bony hypertrophy. In contrast, multifocal venomatosis is associated with bony hypoplasia and venous malformations, presenting with multifocal thrombosis and resultant phleboliths (39).

Therapy

The need for multidisciplinary management of combined vascular malformations has been noted. This includes multidisciplinary management of superficial and deep lesions, bony and soft-tissue hypertrophy, and large painful varicosities. The chronicity of complex vascular malformation mandates a long-term approach. These malformations are not cured but palliated. Early implementation of conservative therapy using elastic compression garments and extremity elevation can improve the venous hypertension. Patients often complain of episodes of acute focal pain associated with a "hard knot." This is symptomatic of local venous thrombosis associated with a phlebolith. Pain can also reflect venous distension and poor venous drainage after exercise. The pain can be generalized or focal, at the point where a venous malformation fills and empties poorly due to abnormal connections to the deep venous system (Figs. 103-2B and 103-2C). The abnormal venous flow is nonlaminar and induces a thrombosis thus, instituting low-dose aspirin therapy is important to avoid deep venous thromboses and the risk of pulmonary emboli.

Long-term orthopedic issues are also important in the multidisciplinary management of the combined vascular malformations. Orthopedic treatment is based on the discrepancies in limb length or girth. Shoe lifts can correct a limb length discrepancy up to 2 cm. Epiphysiodesis to close the growth plates can compensate for a 2- to 5-cm discrepancy. Limb shortening of a skeletally mature patient is not routinely done but can correct a discrepancy of 5 cm or more (40). Discrepancies in vascular anomalies are best managed with lifts and appropriately timed epiphysiodesis, with yearly evaluation beginning as early as 6 to 8 years of age, until fusion occurs between ages 14 and 16.

Intralesional sclerotherapy can reduce the size of the venous component and, by sclerosing the abnormal channels reduce or eliminate episodic pain from venous stasis and insufficiency. Absolute ethanol for a total dose of 0.5 to 1 cc per kg of body weight delivered percutaneously and directed into a venous lake is best. A high-flow venous malformation usually indicates a substantial connection to the normal deep venous system. These are less common, but require occlusion of the large connecting vein prior to sclerotherapy in order to prevent thrombi from flowing into the deep venous system. Occlusion of the connecting vein can be achieved with coil embolization, surgical ligation, or endovascular laser.

Sclerotherapy, either alone or preoperatively in conjunction with surgical excision is the optimal procedure to reduce the size and symptoms of this malformation. Preoperative sclerotherapy can significantly reduce intraoperative hemorrhage. Other useful intraoperative techniques include extremity tourniquets, argon beam therapy for all denuded coagulopathic surfaces, a cell saver, and close collaboration with the anesthesia team. Uncontrolled hemorrhage can occur during large resections. Tamponade by closing skin and wrapping the site in pressure dressings can be very helpful.

Extremity Malformations

Other superficial or deep venous anomalies are compression syndromes secondary to fibrous bands or crossing vessels. These can be associated with thrombosis and its attendant complications. Fibrous bands cause compression of the subclavian or axillary veins at the thoracic inlet and may induce "effort" thrombosis, better known as the Paget-von Schrötter syndrome. The clinical scenario is typified in muscular, adolescent athletes who develop pain and acute swelling and cyanosis in the dominant upper extremity. Doppler imaging confirms the diagnosis of DVT. If diagnosed in the acute setting (within 2 weeks), venography with in situ thrombolytic therapy with urokinase or tissue plasminogen activator can be diagnostic and therapeutic. Thrombolysis is an important advance which avoids the risks of a postphlebitic syndrome after anticoagulation alone. When the clot is completely lysed, the patient's symptoms improve, the underlying site of compression of the vein can be imaged, and surgical excision of the fibrotic compression bands should follow. Elevation of the affected arm, anticoagulation, thrombolytic therapy, and evaluation for underlying hematologic abnormality is imperative, particularly if no clear anatomic obstruction is identified.

Anomalous or duplicated veins can also be associated with venous thromboses because they can be an inciting factor for nonlaminar, abnormal venous flow. For instance, femoral vein duplication is present in 20% of the population and may be a cause of DVT (41).

Likewise abnormalities at the origin of the left common iliac vein are not rare, and can include intraluminal septations or extrinsic compression by the crossing right common iliac artery (May-Thurner syndrome). Symptomatic iliac vein compression can be managed with peripheral thrombolysis, followed by angioplasty and/or stenting of the narrowed iliac vein (42,43).

Central Venous Malformations

Unlike extremity malformations, central venous anomalies are usually asymptomatic and detected on echocardiography incidentally. They occur more frequently in the vena caval rather than portal system and are not uncommon. Duplications of the inferior vena cava (IVC) or superior vena cava (SVC), such that the left SVC drains into the coronary sinus and the right SVC drains into the right atrium, are important to determine preoperatively prior to cardiac surgery, extracorporeal membrane oxygenation, or central catheter placement (44). Abnormal regression of the precardinal veins appears to be the mechanism by which these abnormalities form. Persistence of the left precardinal vein leads to a duplicated SVC, whereas regression of the right precardinal vein results in a left SVC. Agenesis of the IVC occurs in 4% of the population and is usually asymptomatic, but is associated with congenital heart disease and the polyspenia-asplenia syndromes. With agenesis of the IVC, the azygous vein becomes the main route of venous return from the extremities. Congenital suprahepatic IVC obstruction with intraluminal caval webs or persistence of an atrial eustachian valve (45) produces posthepatic portal hypertension, a Budd Chiari type of syndrome. Clinical sequelae present very gradually over the years. A cavogram or MRV will confirm the etiology. Therapy requires interventional endovascular angioplasty and stenting (46) or cavocaval bypass with web excision.

Visceral Malformations

Compared with other anatomic sites, vascular malformations occur infrequently in the liver. Hepatic structural anomalies include a wide spectrum of abnormalities from a congenital absence to duplication or intrahepatic shunts, including fast flow (arteriovenous), slow flow (venous or lymphatic), and combined forms. Most are incidentally detected, but are critical in the preoperative planning for hepatic or transplant surgery. Agenesis of the portal vein is detected rarely and incidentally; is found more often in females; and is also associated with congenital cardiac anomalies, hepatic insufficiency, or tumors. With congenital agenesis of the portal vein the SMV communicates with either the suprarenal IVC or the left renal vein. Most portovenous fistulae are associated with hepatic hemangiomas and arteriovenous shunting; however, portovenous fistulae have been reported as an isolated entity in infants with galactosemia (47,48). Abnormal position of the portal vein in a preduodenal position can cause duodenal obstruction and atresia; however, it does not necessitate vascular intervention, but duodenal bypass, usually using a diamond-shaped duodenoduodenostomy.

The most common venous anomaly in the liver is associated with the Blue Rubber Bleb Nevus syndrome, a familial condition with multifocal mucocutaneous, musculoskeletal, and visceral venous malformations that can literally carpet the GI tract (49,50). Profound anemia from gastrointestinal blood loss is the most common presentation. That is further elucidated by tagged red blood cell scans that highlight the multiple venous malformations in the GI tract from stomach to anus. The hepatic lesions are asymptomatic, and contain phleboliths and focal venous malformations.

Thrombotic Syndromes

Venous thromboembolic disease, once believed to be rare in the pediatric population, has newfound importance with the recognition of both an increased incidence secondary to the use of intravascular devices in contemporary intensive care units, and other areas, as well as advances in determining the genetic susceptibilities to venous thrombosis. DVT is a recognized serious pediatric problem within, an incidence of 5.3 per 10,000 admissions or 0.07 per 10,000 children (51). DVT results in three nontrivial sequelae: (1) pulmonary embolism, (2) venous gangrene (phlegmasia cerulean dolens) with compromised arterial blood flow and tissue ischemia, and (3) post phlebitic syndrome. Pulmonary embolism occurred in 3 of 50 children with upper-extremity thromboses and in 11 of 79 children with lower-extremity thromboses in our report (51). Postphlebitic syndrome can occur in as many as 25% of children with DVT, with disabling complications of chronic pain, swelling, and induration. Recurrent thromboses occur in 18% of children (52) and carry a 5% risk of fatality and worsening venous insufficiency (53).

In the nineteenth century, Virchow suggested that venous thrombosis resulted from endothelial damage, venous stasis, and hypercoaguability. In children, the incidence of spontaneous venous thrombosis can be as low as 1:100,000, whereas in adults the incidence is 1:100. The implication is that, in order for children to have a thrombotic event, they must have a strong predisposition. Risk factors in the neonatal period include asphyxia, shock, polycythemia, sepsis, maternal thrombophilia and diabetes, and dehydration. Thus, infants, particularly premature infants younger than 28 weeks of gestation and weighing less than 1,000 g, are at the greatest risk from thromboembolic phenomenon (54). The neonate is relatively hypercoaguable, with known imbalances in the coagulation cascade and immature fibrinolytic mechanisms. In children older than 3 months, teenagers have the highest risk for developing venous thromboembolism. Predisposing conditions include cancer, congenital heart disease, and iatrogenic vascular interventions. The top three risk factors for children overall include in order of frequency: an indwelling venous catheter (21% incidence), surgery (13%), and trauma (9%), particularly spinal cord injuries and pelvic fractures (52). Long-term indwelling catheters are the foremost cause of thrombosis in children accounting for more than three-fourths of upper-extremity cases.

There is increasing evidence of genetic predisposition for thrombophilia (i.e., inherited thrombophilia) (Table 103-1). Individuals with heterozygous deficiency of protein C, protein S, or antithrombin, and those heterozygous or homozygous for factor V Leiden or with the prothrombin gene mutation (G20210A mutation), typically present with DVT (55). In the majority of patients, the venous thrombosis is provoked by catheter placement, surgery, or immobilization.

The most sensitive diagnosis for upper-extremity venous thrombosis is a duplex US for jugular venous thrombosis, and venography or MRV for intrathoracic vessels. For detection of pulmonary embolism, a pulmonary angiogram has been the most sensitive, although spiral CT and ventilation perfusion scans are often used as screening

TABLE 103-1 Causes of Venous Thrombosis.

Inherited
Common
Factor V Leiden mutation
Prothrombin gene G20210A variant
Inherited hyperhomocysteinaemia
Rare
Antithrombin III deficiency
Protein C deficiency
Protein S deficiency
Raised factor VIII levels
Acquired
Indwelling venous catheter
Surgery
Trauma
Infection
Tumor
Prolonged immobilization
Antiphospholipid syndrome
Acquired hyperhomocysteinaemia

TABLE 103-2 Anticoagulant and Thrombolytic Therapy in Children: Recommended Agents and Doses.

	Loading Dose	*Maintenance Dose*	*Goal*
Anticoagulation			
Heparin	75 U/kg	22 U/kg/hr (>1 y) 28 U/kg/hr (<1 y)	PTT 1.5–2X
Coumadin	0.1–0.2 mg/kg	Adjusted according to PT/INR 0.32 mg/kg (infants) 0.09 mg/kg (teenagers)	 PT 2–3 INR 2–3
Low molecular weight heparin	1 mg/kg SC BID 1.6 mg/kg SC BID (infants)		Anti-Xa Level 0.5–1.0 U/mL
Thrombolysis			
Streptokinase	2,000 U/kg	1,000–4,000 U/kg/hr 50–100 U/kg/hr (low dose)	
Urokinase			
Catheters	5,000 U	200 U/hr × 24 hr	
Systemic	4,400 U/kg	4,000–6,000 U/kg/hr	
Tissue plasminogen activator	0.5 mg/kg/hr	0.25 mg/kg/hr	

modalities. These latter modalities have a higher rate of false-negatives. For lower-extremity DVT detection, duplex US has been the standard. Most recommendations for antithrombotic therapy in children are based on extrapolation of results from randomized studies of adults or from limited retrospective studies in children (Table 103-2). Venous thromboembolism requires removal of the inciting predisposing factor if possible; thrombolysis of the clot, and anticoagulation similar to that in adults with standard unfractionated heparin for 5 days, overlapped by maintenance therapy with oral anticoagulation or low molecular weight heparin until an international normalized ratio (INR) of 2.0 to 3.0 is obtained. Oral therapy can be started on the same day as heparin, and this overlapping of therapies prevents skin necrosis in patients with protein C deficiency. The classification of the patient's likelihood of thrombophilia will determine the length of therapy. Those with the lowest likelihood have oral therapy for 3 months. If at high risk of recurrence (56,57), patients require 6 months of therapy with potential continuation of therapy.

REFERENCES

1. Anderson DH. Tumors of infancy and childhood. *Cancer* 1951;4:890.
2. Sabin FR. The lymphatic system in human embryos with a consideration of the morphology of the system as a whole. *Am J Anat* 1909;9:43.
3. Sabin FR. On the origin of the lymphatic system from the veins and the development of the lymph heart and thoracic duct in the pig. *Am J Anat* 1901;1:367.
4. Mulliken JB. Vascular malformations of the head and neck. In: Mulliken JB, Young AE, eds. *Vascular birthmarks, hemangiomas and malformations.* Philadelphia: WB Saunders, 1988:301.
5. Fonkalsrud EW. Congenital malformations of the lymphatic system. In: Gans SL, Grosfeld JL, eds. *Seminars in pediatric surgery,* vol. 3. Orlando, FL: WB Saunders, 1994:62.
6. Langer JC, Fitzgerald PG, Desa D, et al. Cervical cystic hygroma in the fetus: clinical spectrum and outcome. *J Pediatr Surg* 1990;25:58.
7. Chervenak FA, Isaacson G, Blakemore KJ, et al. Fetal cystic hygroma. *N Engl J Med* 1983;309:822.
8. Bill AH, Summer DS. A unified concept of lymphangiomas and cystic hygroma. *Surg Gynecol Obstet* 1965;120:79.
9. Davidson AJ, Hartman DS. Lymphangioma of the retroperitoneum: CT and sonographic characteristics. *Radiology* 1990;175:507.
10. Siegel MJ, Glazer HS, St Amour TE, et al. Lymphangiomas in children: MR imaging. *Pediatr Radiol* 1989;170:467.
11. Hancock BJ, St-Vil D, Luks FI, et al. Complications of lymphangiomas in children. *J Pediatr Surg* 1992;27:220.
12. Tanigawa N, Shimomatsuya T, Takahashi K, et al. Treatment of cystic hygroma and lymphangioma with the use of bleomycin fat emulsion. *Cancer* 1987;60:741.
13. Tanaka K, Inomata Y, Utsunomiya H, et al. Sclerosing therapy with bleomycin emulsion for lymphangioma in children. *Pediatr Surg Int* 1990;5:270.
14. Molitch HI, Unger EC, Witte CL, et al. Percutaneous sclerotherapy of lymphangiomas. *Radiology* 1995;194:343–349.
15. Ogita S, Tsuto T, Tokiwa K, et al. Intracystic injection of OK-432: a new sclerosing therapy for cystic hygroma in children. *Br J Surg* 1987;74:690.
16. Ogita S, Toshiaki T, Deguchi E, et al. OK-432 therapy for unresectable lymphangiomas in children. *J Pediatr Surg* 1991;26:263.
17. Greinwald JH Jr, Burke DK, Sato Y, et al. Treatment of lymphangiomas in children: an update of Picibanil (OK-432) sclerotherapy. *Otolaryngol Head Neck Surg* 1999;121:381–387.
18. Randolph JE, Gross RE. Congenital chylothorax. *Arch Surg* 1957;74:405.
19. Bond SJ, Guzzetta PC, Snyder ML, et al. Management of pediatric postoperative chylothorax. *Ann Thorac Surg* 1993;56:469–473.
20. Stringel G, Teixeira JA. Thoracoscopic ligation of the thoracic duct. *JSLS* 2000;4(3):239–242.
21. Azizhan RG, Canfield J, Alford BA, et al. Pleuroperitoneal shunts in the management of neonatal chylothorax. *J Pediatr Surg* 1983;18:842.
22. Rheuban KS, Kron IL, Carpenter MA, et al. Pleuroperitoneal shunts for refractory chylothorax after operation for congenital heart disease. *Ann Thorac Surg* 1992;53(1):85–87.

23. Cope C, Kaiser LR. Management of unremitting chylothorax by percutaneous embolization and blockage of retroperitoneal lymphatic vessels in 42 patients. *J Vasc Intervent Radiol* 2002;13:1139–1148.
24. Rothenberg SS, Pokorny WJ. Use of argon beam laser ablation and sclerotherapy in the treatment of a case of life-threatening total abdominal lymphangiomatosis. *J Pediatr Surg* 1994;29:322–323.
25. Asakura H, Miura S, Morishita T, et al. Endoscopic and histopathological study on primary and secondary intestinal lymphagiectasia. *Dig Dis Sci* 1981;26:312–320.
26. Gardner TW, Domm AC, Brock CE, et al. Congenital pulmonary lymphangiectasis. *Clin Pediatr* 1983;22:75.
27. Sanchez RE, Mahour GH, Brennan LP, et al. Chylous ascites in children. *Surgery* 1971;69:183.
28. Soria P, Cuesta A, Romero H, et al. Dietary treatment of lymphedema by restriction of long-chain triglycerides. *Angiology* 1994;45: 703–707.
29. Charles RH. Lymphedema. In: Latham A, English TC, eds. *A system of treatment,* vol. 3. London: Churchill, 1912.
30. Homans J. The treatment of elephantiasis of the legs: preliminary report. *N Engl J Med* 1936;215:1099.
31. Thompson N. The surgical treatment of chronic lymphedema of the extremities. *Surg Clin North Am* 1967;47:445.
32. Klippel M, Trenaunay P. De naevus variqueux osteohypertrophique. *Arch Gen Med (Paris)* 1900;185:641–672.
33. Stringel G, Dastous J. Klippel-Trenaunay syndrome and other cases of lower limb hypertrophy: pediatric surgical implications. *J Pediatr Surg* 1987;22:645–650.
34. Parkes-Weber F. Angioma formation in connection with hypertrophy of limbs and hemihypertrophy. *Br J Dermatol* 1907;19:231–235.
35. Wiedemann HR, Burgio GR, Aldenhoff P, et al. The Proteus syndrome: partial gigantism of the hands and/or feet, nevi, hemihypertrophy, subcutaneous tumors, macrocephaly or other skull anomalies, and possible accelerated growth and visceral affections. *Eur J Pediatr* 1983;140:5–12.
36. Sternbergh WC III, Sobel M. Venous and lymphatic diseases. In: Levine BA, Copeland EM III, Howard RJ, et al., eds. *Current practice of surgery,* vol. 12, sec. 9. New York: Churchill Livingstone, 1993.
37. Luke JC. The diagnosis of chronic enlargement of the leg with the description of a new syndrome. *Surg Gynecol Obstet* 1941;73:472.
38. Luke JC. The deep vein valves. A venographic study is normal and postphlebitic states. *Surgery* 1951;29:381.
39. Papendieck CM. Biochronogram of angioma in pedatrics. Progress in lymphology XIV. *Lymphology* 1994;27:148.
40. McCullough CJ, Kenwright J. The prognosis in congenital lower limb hypertrophy. *Acta Orthop Scand* 1979;50:307–313.
41. Villavicencio JL. Treatment of varicose veins associated with congenital vascular malformations. In: Bergan JJ, Goldman MP, eds. *Varicose veins and telangiectasias.* St. Louis, MO: Quality Medical, 1993.
42. Hurst DR, Forauer AR, Bloom JR, et al. Diagnosis and endovascular treatment of iliocaval compression syndrome. *J Vasc Surg* 2001;34(1):106–113.
43. O'Sullivan GJ, Semba CP, Bittner CA, et al. Endovascular management of iliac vein compression (May-Thurner) syndrome. *J Vasc Intervent Radiol* 2000;11(7):823–836.
44. Sarma KP. Anomalous inferior vena cava—anatomical and clinical. *Br J Surg* 1966;53:600.
45. Smith BM. Venous disease. In: Welch KJ, Randolph JG, Ravitch MM, et al., eds. *Pediatric surgery,* 4th ed. Chicago: Year Book Medical, 1986:1518.
46. Quinn SF, Schuman ES, Hall L, et al. Venous stenosis in patients who undergo hemodyalisis: treatment with self-expandable endovascular stents. *Radiology* 1992;183;499.
47. Paley MR, Farrant P, Kane P, et al. Developmental intrahepatic shunts of childhood: radiological features and management. *Eur Radiol* 1997;7:1377–1382.
48. Ono H, Mawatari H, Mizoguchi N, et al. Clinical features and outcome of eight infants with intrahepatic portovenous shunts detected in neonatal screening for falactosaemia. *Acta Paediatr* 1998;87:631–634.
49. Burrows PE, Dubois J, Kassarjian A. Pediatric hepatic vascular anomalies. *Pediatr Radiol* 2001;31:533–545.
50. Fishman SJ, Burrows PE, Leichtner AM, et al. Gastrointestinal manifestations of vascular anomalies in childhood: varied etiologies require multiple therapeutic modalities. *J Pediatr Surg* 1998;33:1163–1167.
51. Andrew M, David M, Adams M, et al. Venous thromboembolic complications (VTE) in children: first analysis of the Canadian registry of VTE. *Blood* 1994;83:1251.
52. David M, Andrew M. Venous thromboembolic complications in children. *J Pediatr* 1993;123:337.
53. Douketis JD, Kearon C, Bates S, et al. Risk of fatal pulmonary embolism in patients with treated venous thromboembolism. *JAMA* 1998;279:458–462.
54. Alkalay AI, Mazkereth R, Santulli T Jr, et al. Central venous line thrombosis during central venous catheterization of newborns: a prospective study. *J Pediatr Surg* 1992;27:18.
55. Seligsohn U, Lubetsky A. Genetic susceptibility to venous thrombosis. *N Engl J Med* 2001;344(16):1222–1231.
56. Jilma B, Kamath S, Lip GYH. ABC of antithrombotic therapy: antithrombotic therapy in special circumstances, II—in children, thrombophilia, and miscellaneous conditions. *BMJ* 2003;326: 93–96.
57. Agnelli G, Prandoni P, Santamaria MG, et al. Three months versus one year of oral anticoagulant therapy for idiopathic deep venous thrombosis. *N Engl J Med* 2001;345(3):165–169.

Chapter 104

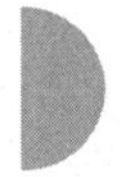

Vascular Access

Jed G. Nuchtern

Vascular access can be an extremely challenging aspect of pediatric surgical practice. Technical improvements both in access devices and in aids to catheter insertion have improved the safety and efficiency of device placement in a broad spectrum of patients. As the ease of placement has increased, so have the indications for vascular access. Thus, central venous catheterization has become a standard approach over peripheral venous cutdown for urgent vascular access in hospitalized patients with poor superficial veins. Central venous catheters in various forms have become standard means for hemodialysis, apheresis, and long-term intravenous (IV) antibiotics, in addition to the standard indications of total parenteral nutrition (TPN), central venous pressure monitoring, and chemotherapy. This chapter examines the current indications for various forms of vascular access, technical aspects of insertion of these devices, and advantages and potential problems associated with their use.

PERIPHERAL VENOUS ACCESS

Peripheral vein cannulation is the safest and easiest method of venous access. The goal of all indwelling catheters is reliable access that allows for patient movement with the lowest possible risk of dislodgement, infiltration, phlebitis, and infection. Catheter flexibility is inversely related to the risk of thrombosis and infiltration, and the surface characteristics strongly influence the rate of infection and thrombosis. PEU-Vialon catheters appear to be superior to other materials in preventing phlebitis and infiltration (1,2) and comparable in terms of rate of infection. The vast majority of peripheral catheters are placed by the over-the-needle approach, with the remainder inserted directly into the vein after a cutdown is performed.

Jed G. Nuchtern: Department of Surgery, Baylor College of Medicine, Texas Children's Hospital, Houston, Texas 77030.

Indications

Peripheral vein cannulation is the preferred method of vascular access in all patients, assuming that no specific indication for central venous catheterization is present. Peripheral IVs normally last from 2 to 4 days in a typical toddler, can handle twice maintenance fluid volumes for prolonged periods, and are compatible with multiple medications and dilute parenteral nutrition. A patient with multiple, adequate-appearing peripheral veins can receive 10 to 14 days of IV therapy via peripheral IV without significant difficulty.

Technical Aspects

The dorsal veins of the hands and feet are the first choice for peripheral cannulation. The basilic, cephalic, and median cubital veins in the antecubital fossa are highly accessible, but it may be preferable to preserve these sites for phlebotomy or as access for peripherally inserted central catheters. The greater saphenous vein at the ankle or knee is a reasonable size even in a small child and has constant enough anatomy to be cannulated, even if it is not palpable. A scalp vein is useful in small to moderate-size infants. Although the external jugular vein is normally relatively easy to cannulate, it can be very difficult to immobilize these catheters, and they are often displaced shortly after insertion (Fig. 104-1).

Palpation or visualization of peripheral veins may be facilitated by application of tourniquets, dependent positioning, local heat application, and transillumination. The cannula should be carefully matched to the size of the vessel.

Peripheral venous cutdown is a useful technique for emergent or urgent venous access when insertion of a central line is impractical or impossible. The obvious disadvantage is the permanent scarring following the procedure and the short-lived nature of most IVs placed by this technique. For a greater saphenous vein cutdown, a transverse incision is made just proximal to the medial malleolus of

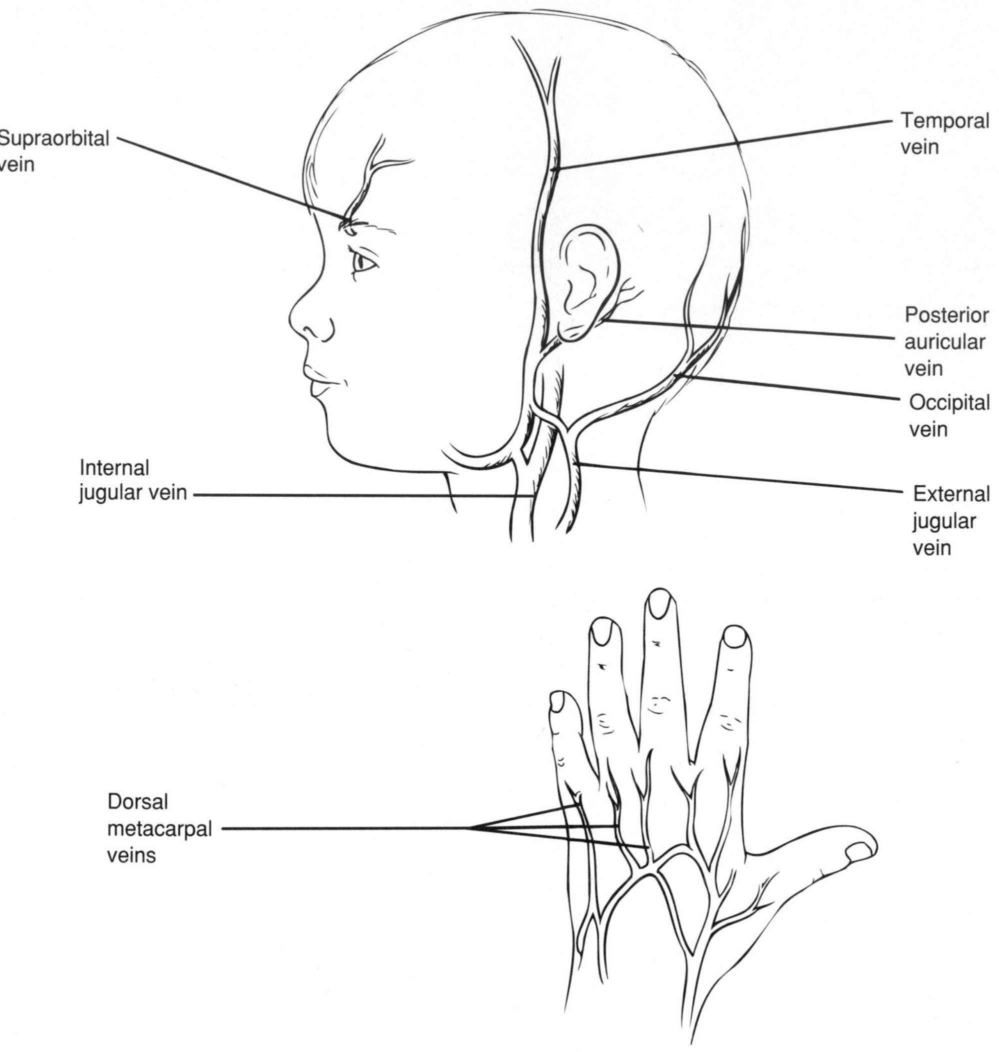

FIGURE 104-1. Potential sites for peripheral and central venous access.

the tibia. The vein is dissected out, and proximal and distal ligatures are placed but not tied down. Applying traction to the proximal ligature, a small venotomy is made on the anterior surface of the vein. The cannula is then passed directly into the vessel, a maneuver that can be facilitated with the use of a small plastic vein pick. The ligatures are tied down, and the hub of the catheter is securely sutured to the skin.

Advantages and Disadvantages

The main advantages of peripheral venous access include technical ease of insertion, safety, and low incidence of sepsis. The disadvantages relate to the risks of phlebitis and thrombosis, as well as simple dislodgement from the vein. The final common pathway of thrombosis and displacement from the vein is extravasation of the infusate, with the potential for skin and tissue necrosis either through hyperosmolar shock, through direct toxic injury, or by induction of vasoconstriction with ischemic injury. Reducing the osmolarity and volume of the infusate decreases the incidence of these problems, but it will also limit the ability to provide adequate parenteral nutrition through this route. Elevation of the extremity is the first line of therapy for an IV infiltrate. Application of heat is no longer recommended because it can accelerate the process of tissue injury from entrapped medications (3). Hyaluronidase (Wydase, Wyeth-Ayerst, Philadelphia, PA) is useful in the treatment of almost all infiltrates and can be particularly helpful in infants. By breaking down the interstitial substrate, it facilitates more rapid reabsorption of chemical irritants and decreases fluid pressure within the tissues. The standard treatment is 15 U, given subcutaneously in five sites around the infiltration, although giving a portion through the catheter has also been reported to be particularly helpful (4).

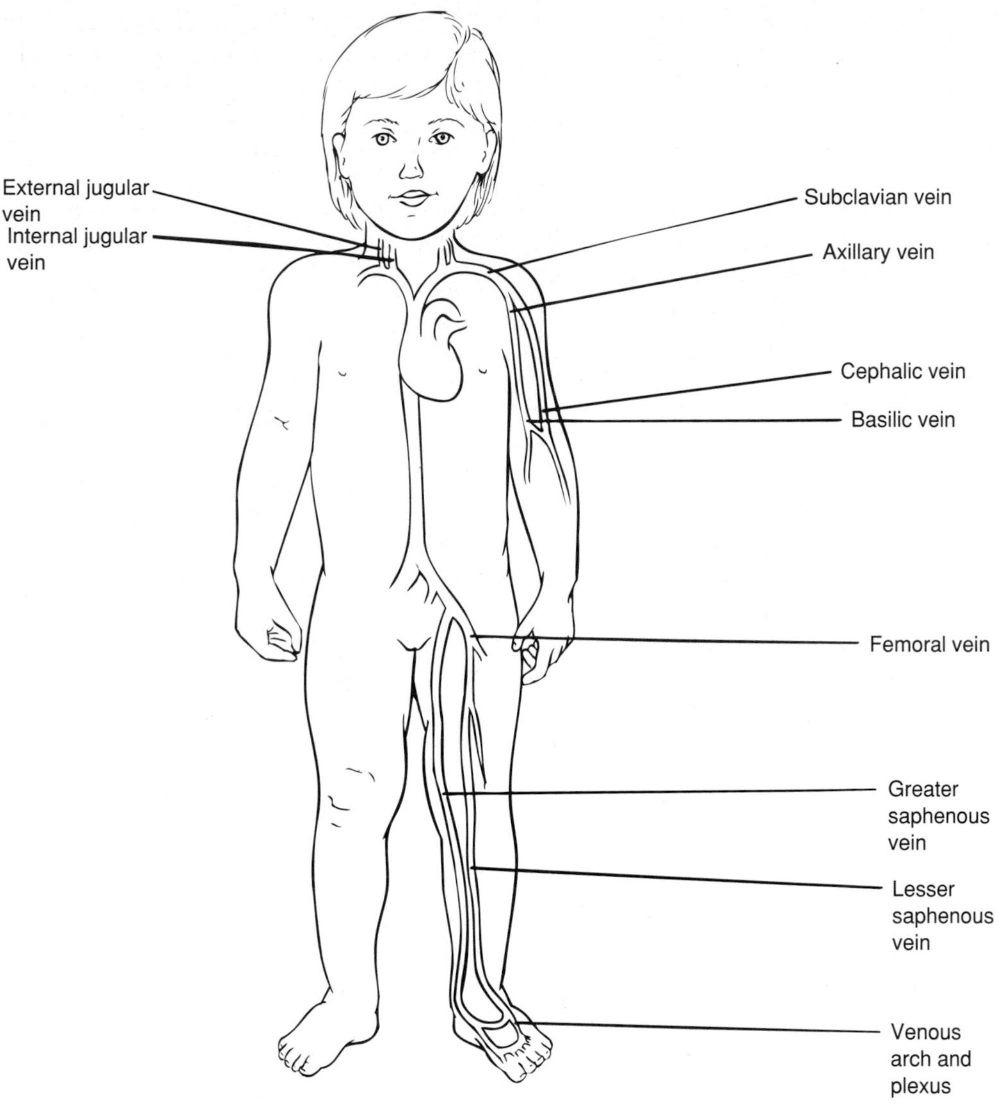

FIGURE 104-1. *(Continued)*

Phlebitis is treated by removal of the catheter and application of heat. Antibiotics are administered to all patients with symptoms of sepsis and to those with positive blood cultures, regardless of symptoms. We normally withhold antibiotic therapy in nonbacteremic, immunocompetent infants and children older than 1 month of age unless there is severe associated cellulitis. Persistent sepsis in spite of appropriate antimicrobial therapy should raise the suspicion of suppurative thrombophlebitis, prompting exploration and excision of the vein if pus is found.

Rather than having a strict policy regarding the frequency of site changes for peripheral IVs, nursing units should have precise standards of care for surveillance of catheter sites and dressing changes. A site change should occur at the earliest sign of occlusion or infiltration.

INTRAOSSEOUS ACCESS

Indications

The technique of intraosseous infusion was used extensively in the 1930s and 1940s, but decreased in popularity substantially after the development of biocompatible IV catheters. Currently, this technique is limited to life-threatening situations when other rapid techniques have failed. Indications include cardiopulmonary arrest, burns, life- or function-threatening status epilepticus, and shock due to trauma, sepsis, or dehydration. In the tibias and femurs of infants and children, fluid infused into the intramedullary space ultimately drains into the systemic venous circulation. Clinical studies in adults and cadaver experiments suggest that red marrow does not need to be present within the space for successful intraosseous infusion. The rigid bone matrix acts as a noncollapsible vein that remains easily accessible even during severe hypovolemia and circulatory arrest (5). The tibia and femur have the additional advantage of being physically remote from the anatomic regions of interest during advanced life support procedures. Intraosseous catheters have been used successfully for administration of fluids, blood products, and a variety of medications. Marrow aspirates obtained prior to fluid infusion can be used to determine venous blood gases, chemistry, hemoglobin, as well as type and cross and blood culture samples. The few absolute contraindications include osteoporosis, osteogenesis imperfecta, and an ipsilateral fractured extremity.

Technical Aspects

The proximal tibia is the best site for insertion of an intraosseous needle, followed by the distal tibia and the femur (Fig. 104-2). A 16- to 18-gauge, disposable, bone marrow aspiration needle is the ideal equipment, although a similar gauge IV cannula can be used under emergency or field conditions. The needle is inserted through the skin, at a perpendicular angle, 1 to 2 cm distal and just medial to the tibial tuberosity and advanced through the bone using a boring or screwing motion (6). There is normally a distinct loss of resistance as the needle enters the marrow space. Intramedullary placement is confirmed by aspiration of marrow contents and easy infusion of fluid. Secure fixation with tape is mandatory to avoid complications.

Advantages and Disadvantages

Intraosseous catheters are the fastest, most reliable means for obtaining emergency vascular access in infants and children.

The risk of serious complications of intraosseous catheters is very low. The more common complications include infiltration of fluid into the subperiosteal and subcutaneous tissues, and leakage at the infusion site. Localized cellulitis, with occasional formation of subcutaneous abscesses, and the more worrisome problem of osteomyelitis are both seen in less than 1% of collected series (5,7). Given that the risk of these complications increases with

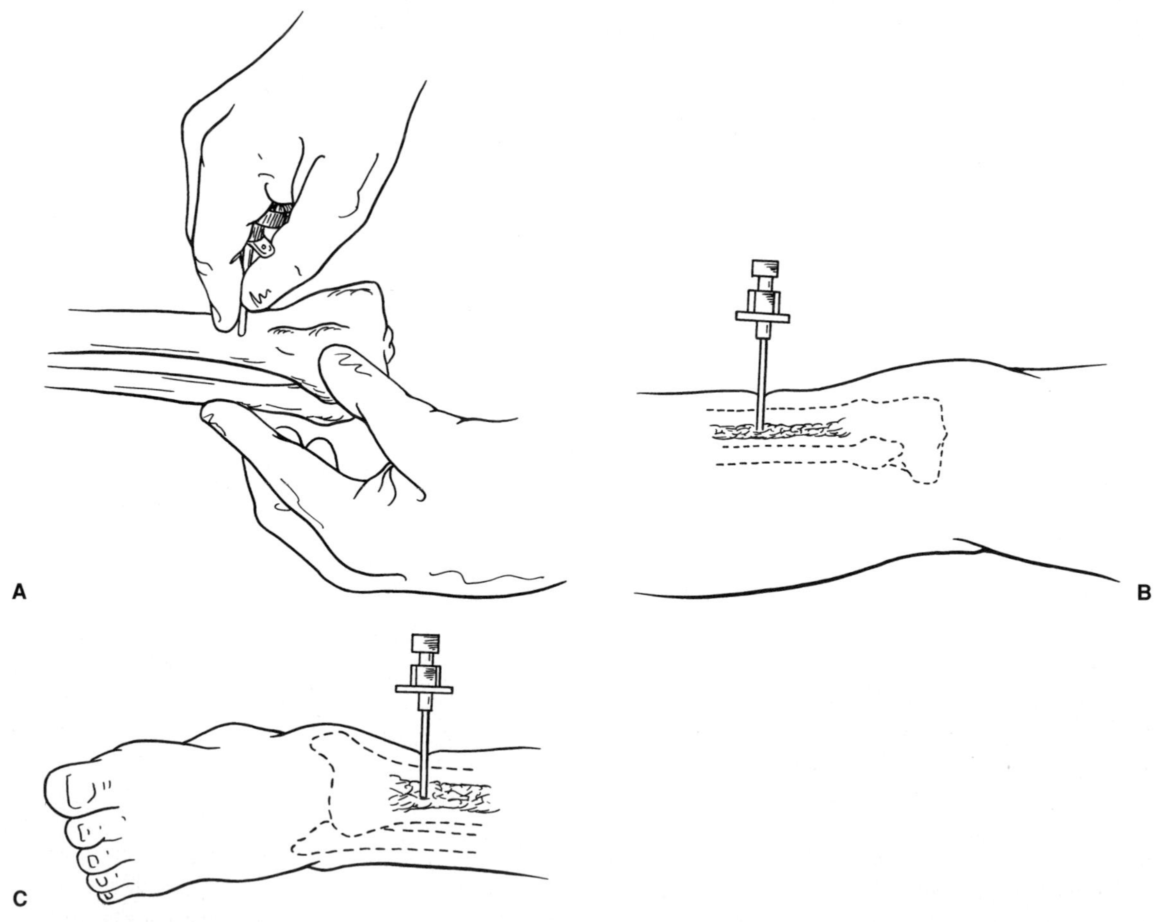

FIGURE 104-2. Intraosseous infusion needle. **(A)** Technique for proper hand position and placement. **(B)** Proximal tibial insertion. **(C)** Distal tibial insertion.

duration of intraosseous access, it is important to obtain peripheral or central access as soon as the patient has been stabilized and volume resuscitated.

PERIPHERALLY INSERTED CENTRAL VENOUS CATHETERS

Indications

Since the mid-1990s, there has been a huge expansion in the use of peripherally inserted central venous catheters (PICCs) for intermediate-term vascular access. These are small Silastic catheters, ranging in size from 2 to 7 French, which are inserted in a peripheral vein and passed into a central location. Ideally, they combine the ease and safety of insertion of peripheral IVs with the relative permanence and versatility of central lines. These catheters have had the highest impact on the neonatal population, particularly the premature or small-for-gestational-age infant who weighs less than 1,500 g. The limitations of peripheral access (e.g., phlebitis, subcutaneous fluid extravasation, skin slough, restricted use of high-osmolarity solutions, short-term patency) and the complications of surgically placed central lines (e.g., sepsis, pneumothorax, pericardial effusion, superior vena cava thrombosis) have been especially difficult in this age group. In 1982, Dolcourt and Bose (8) reported successful use of Silastic PICCs in 15 neonates, with a mean catheter longevity of 24.8 ± 15.9 days and no catheter sepsis, thrombophlebitis, or caval obstruction. This compares favorably with a study (9) documenting that peripheral IV catheters remained functional for a mean of 33 hours in neonates of similar weight and gestational age. Larger series have demonstrated comparable rates of catheter-related sepsis between PICCs and central venous catheters (10). Success in the neonatal population spurred expanded use of these catheters in children and adolescents. In children with perforated appendicitis, osteomyelitis, meningitis, and immunocompromised patients with opportunistic infections, PICC lines can be an ideal means for administration of antibiotic or antiviral therapy, either in the hospital or at home.

Technical Aspects

The most common sites for placement of PICC lines are the antecubital and superficial saphenous veins. Successful placement via a scalp vein has been reported in infants (11). Ultrasound and fluoroscopy can be helpful for localizing a vein and threading the catheter into the vena cava, respectively (12). Using a modified Seldinger technique, a venipuncture is performed and the guide wire is passed centrally. After a confirmatory chest radiograph or fluoroscopy, the dilator/introducer is passed over the wire and the wire is withdrawn. The wire is then used as a guide to cut the catheter itself to the appropriate length. With a stiffening stylet in place, the catheter is passed through the introducer and the sheath is carefully split and withdrawn. An occlusive dressing is placed, and chest radiography confirms the proper position of the catheter at the junction of the superior vena cava and the right atrium. Even though the catheter is radioopaque, the tip can be difficult to visualize because of its small caliber; thus, it may be necessary to fill the catheter with radioopaque contrast material. As with other systems, attention to a standard protocol for insertion and care is critical for long-term success. Directions supplied with commercial kits are helpful and should be reviewed before attempting catheter placement.

Advantages and Disadvantages

When they are inserted using proper technique, PICCs have the potential to be a safe, cost-effective alternative to standard central venous catheters. Because they can be inserted at the bedside with local anesthetic in the neonatal or pediatric intensive care unit, the cost and risk of a trip to the operating theater are avoided. There are no randomized controlled trials of PICC lines versus central venous catheters in children. In the only such adult trial, PICCs actually had a *higher* rate of complications (thrombophlebitis and difficulty of insertion) and were more costly than subclavian central lines in hospitalized patients requiring TPN.

Nonrandomized series reporting PICC use in infants and children have demonstrated excellent results overall (13–15), with a greater than 90% rate of successful insertion. The main drawback of this device appears to be a high incidence of mechanical problems, especially with difficulty passing the catheter and occlusion [as high as 28% in one series (16)], related to small caliber, relatively long length, and delicate consistency of the Silastic catheter. Although the rate of infection is comparable to subclavian central lines, removal for occlusion, dislodgement, and thrombophlebitis is definitely more common with PICCs (17).

Based on the available data, PICCs are a reasonable choice for central access in infants and children who require 2 to 3 weeks of therapy. Patients who are likely to require more than 4 weeks of therapy may be better served by a tunneled "permanent" central venous catheter because many of the complications of PICCs are related to duration of use.

CENTRAL VENOUS ACCESS

Indications

Central venous catheterization is indicated for (1) secure delivery of drugs to the central circulation, (2) administration of parenteral alimentation in high concentration, (3) central venous pressure monitoring, (4) rapid infusion of large volumes of fluids or blood products in very small patients whose peripheral veins may not withstand high flow rates, (5) alternative route for parenteral fluid or drugs in patients for whom peripheral venous access is no longer possible, (6) long-term continuous or intermittent access for blood sampling or therapy, (7) hemodialysis, and (8) apheresis for cellular therapy and plasmapheresis.

Technical Considerations

Landmarks for subclavian and internal jugular vein catheter insertion are indicated in Fig. 104-3. In children younger than 5 years of age, the subclavian vein is located closer to the superior border of the clavicle, and the needle insertion angle should be adjusted accordingly. Once the needle has been inserted and the angle established, the course should not be changed unless the needle is completely withdrawn for danger of lacerating the vein, artery, or other mediastinal structures, such as the phrenic nerve.

Advantages and Disadvantages

With the advent of subclavian central venous access (18), central venous catheters were available for use in place

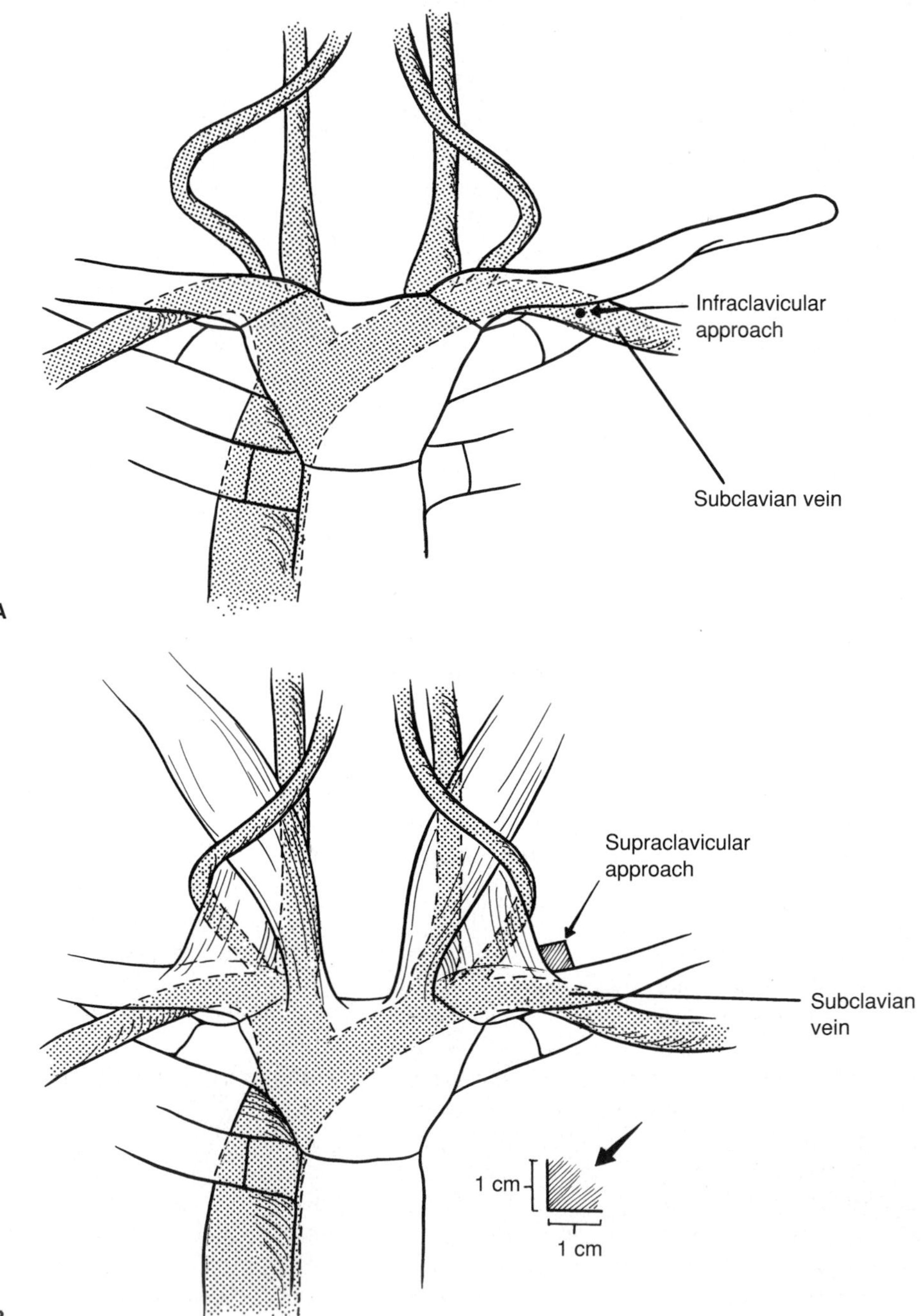

FIGURE 104-3. Subclavian and internal jugular vein catheterization. **(A)** Infraclavicular approach, subclavian vein. **(B)** Supraclavicular approach, subclavian vein. (*continued*)

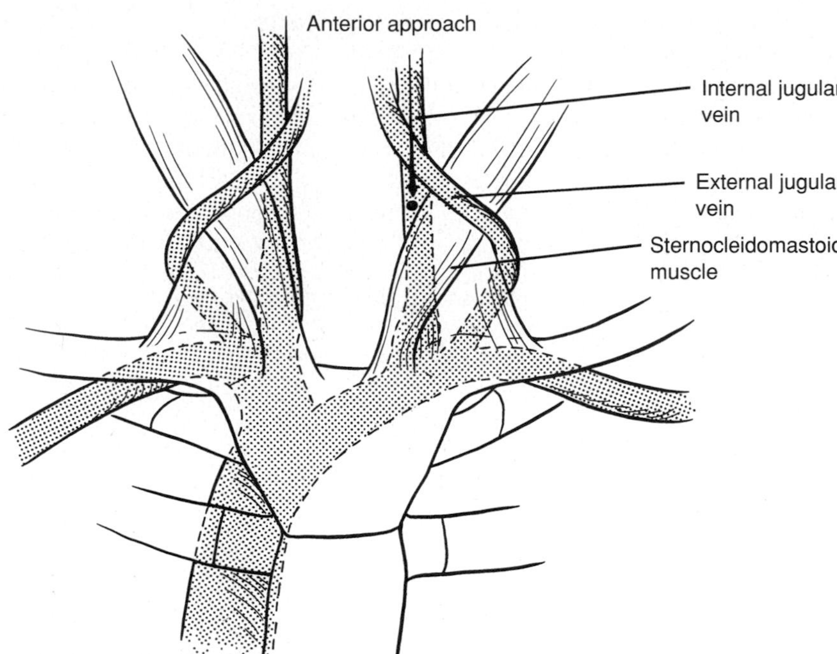

FIGURE 104-3. *(Continued)* **(C)** Anterior approach, internal jugular vein.

of peripheral catheters in older children and adults. They also enabled the administration of hyperosmolar solutions, making TPN possible and practical. Once the technical aspects of insertion are mastered, central venous catheters are relatively easy to insert rapidly, with an acceptably low complication rate. Central venous catheter longevity is also much greater than that of peripheral lines, and they are better tolerated by patients, who are left unencumbered by immobilization boards and dressings, thereby retaining use of their hands and feet. Central venous catheters also have the advantage of enabling periodic blood sampling without the necessity of separate peripheral venipunctures. In 1986, Newman and colleagues (19) demonstrated the efficacy and safety of percutaneous central venous catheters in a prospective study comparing the subclavian or jugular approach with peripheral venous cutdown in the pediatric population. They concluded that percutaneous central intravenous catheterization is the method of choice for venous access other than routine short-term situations. In current practice, PICC lines have replaced percutaneous central venous catheters in many intermediate-term applications, although they are not appropriate in emergencies.

The main disadvantage of central venous catheter placement is that complications are generally more serious than those associated with peripheral venous access. Only physicians well experienced in the techniques of subclavian and internal jugular venipuncture should insert central venous catheters. Except in an emergency, central venous catheters should be inserted only under planned circumstances with sufficient help available and with careful attention to aseptic technique, including full barrier precautions. Possible complications at the time of catheter insertion are discussed in the concluding section.

BROVIAC-TYPE SILASTIC CATHETERS: PERMANENT CENTRAL VENOUS CATHETERS

Indications

The first generation of indwelling central venous catheters was made of polyvinyl chloride and was relatively stiff and thrombogenic. These catheters were associated with a number of mechanical and septic complications. In 1973, Broviac and colleagues (20) introduced the Silastic catheter, an indwelling silicone rubber catheter that can remain in place for extended periods. The Silastic catheter is much more flexible and inert and is associated with fewer complications than polyvinyl catheters with respect to mechanical occlusion, venous perforation, and infection. Commercial versions of these catheters have evolved to the widely used permanent central venous catheter (PCVC) (21). These catheters are manufactured from radioopaque soft silicone rubber, in varying calibers and lengths, and have a small Dacron felt cuff 30 cm from the external end. The cuff allows fibrous ingrowth, which serves to anchor the catheter and to act as a barrier to infection. Indications for PCVC use in children include any condition requiring long-term venous access for the administration of fluids, antibiotics, antineoplastic drugs, TPN, and blood products, or the need for frequent blood sampling. Modified versions of these catheters, generally with larger, duel lumens and a 2- to 3-centimeter offset between the ends of the lumens, are uses for therapies requiring high throughput without recirculation, such as hemodialysis and apheresis. Appropriate candidates for PCVC placement include in-hospital patients, such as infants recovering from gastroschisis or necrotizing enterocolitis, or outpatients, such as children with neoplastic disease requiring chemotherapy or patients with short bowel syndrome on home parenteral nutrition.

Technical Considerations

The catheter is usually placed under general anesthesia, although local anesthesia can be used for infants on ventilators and for older, cooperative patients (Fig. 104-4). The percutaneous infraclavicular subclavian approach is generally preferred in most age groups and is facilitated by use of a peel-away plastic sheath available in several sizes.

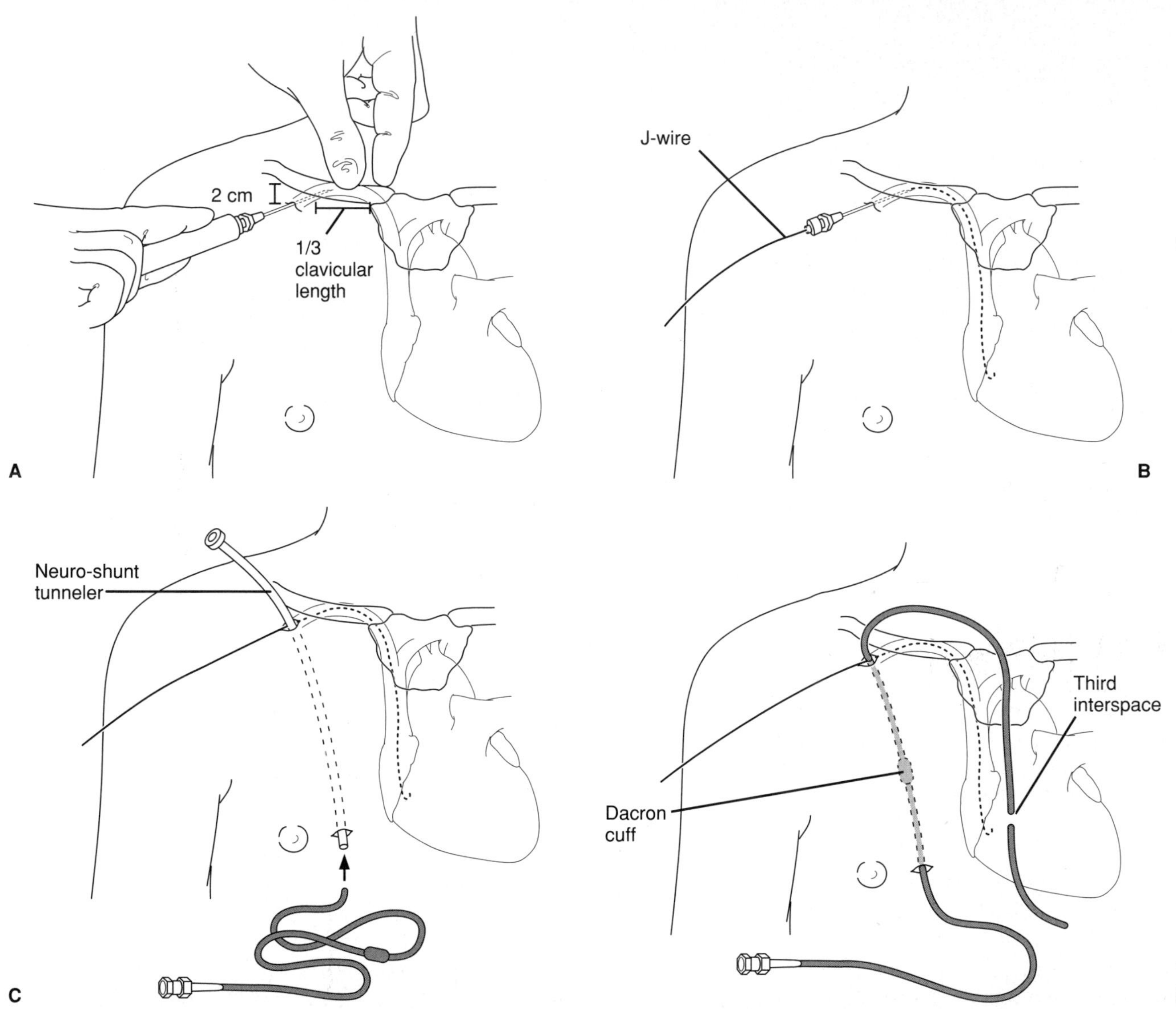

FIGURE 104-4. **(A)** Infraclavicular subclavian venous puncture techniques for a patient younger than 5 years old. The subclavian vein tends to be more cephalad beneath the clavicle in children than in older patients. As the needle is advanced, the course should not be changed unless the needle is completely withdrawn because of the possibility that the vein or artery may be lacerated. **(B)** Insertion and advancement of flexible J-wire. Proper position should be confirmed by fluoroscopy or with plain chest radiograph. **(C)** A neurosurgical shunt catheter introducer, a 25-cm tendon passer, or a fine intestinal probe is used to place the catheter in a subcutaneous tunnel. **(D)** The catheter is placed on the anterior chest wall to simulate its intravascular position. Dividing the catheter at the level of the third intercostal space ensures final placement at the junction of the superior vena cava with the right atrium. The Dacron cuff should be positioned at least 3 cm proximal to the exit site. Placement halfway between the vein entry and skin exit sites minimizes the risk of catheter-cuff migration. *(continued)*

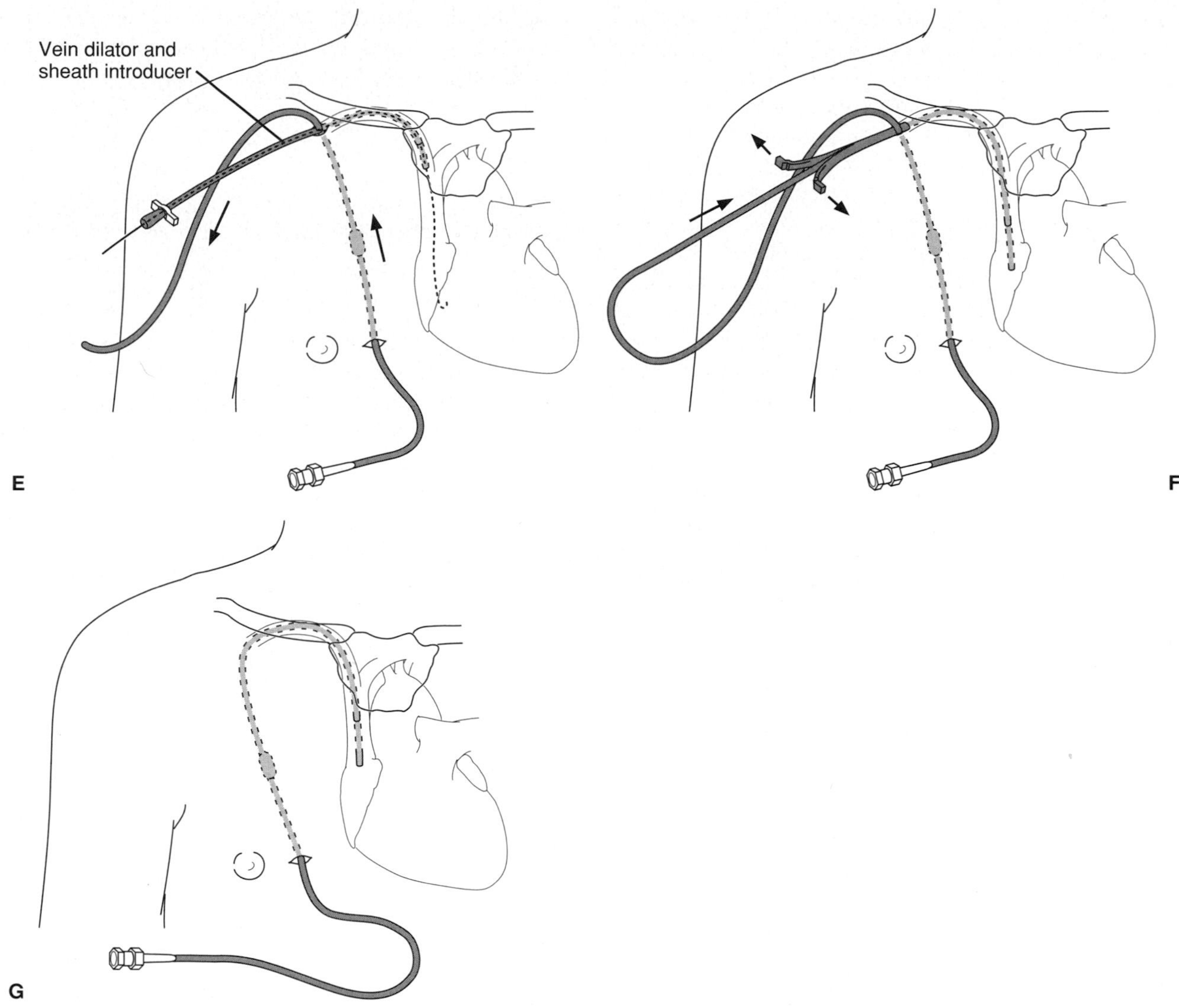

FIGURE 104-4. (*Continued*) **(E)** The vein dilator and sheath introducer are passed over the J-wire. **(F)** The sheath introducer is stripped away as the catheter is advanced centrally. **(G)** The final position should be confirmed by fluoroscopy and documented with plain chest radiographs. (Courtesy of the Mayo Foundation.)

Because of the nearly 50% incidence of subclavian vein stenosis that can compromise future permanent hemodialysis access in the ipsilateral extremity, subclavian venipuncture should *never* be performed in any patient with renal failure or progressive renal insufficiency (22). The subclavian approach is not practical for insertion of PCVCs in extremely low-birth-weight or premature infants—in addition to the increased morbidity of pneumothorax and vascular injury in this population, the available insertion kits are too large to permit safe placement. The external jugular vein cutdown approach is used in most newborns and all low-birth-weight infants, and the internal jugular vein, the facial vein, the saphenous vein, and other veins can be used if other approaches fail. Knowledge of the local venous anatomy and careful dissection can reveal the middle thyroid vein or the common facial vein, which are routes to the internal jugular vein and are preferable to direct ligation. Proximal and distal control should always be obtained when accessing the internal jugular vein by an open approach, and if possible, the catheter should be placed without ligating the vessel. This allows repeated use of the vessel after catheter removal for malfunction or thrombosis, and it maintains patency of the vein after the catheter is no longer needed and removed. Ligation is unnecessary if the surgeon makes a precise venotomy, slightly smaller than the catheter itself. The elastic recoil of the vein will prevent leakage around the catheter. One of the key elements for success identified by several groups is the placement of a portion of the Silastic catheter, usually 4 to 8 cm, in a subcutaneous tunnel, extending from the venotomy site to a more distant site on the anterior chest wall or in the scalp behind the ear (23).

The PCVC can be used immediately, once a chest radiograph, which also excludes technical complications such as pneumothorax, confirms proper placement. Catheters used for parenteral nutrition have traditionally been reserved for that purpose alone, but such restricted use is not always possible, especially in patients in whom no other vascular access is available. Some investigators have found that the infection rate for multiuse catheters is not significantly different than that for catheters used for parenteral nutrition alone (24). Therefore, central venous catheters can be used for multiple purposes if careful attention is given to sterility and if a well-defined protocol is used.

The Dacron cuff serves as a barrier to infection. Improved catheter longevity and decreased septic complications are well documented in a retrospective study by Holmes and colleagues (23). These authors demonstrated that central venous catheters inserted through a subcutaneous tunnel last four times longer than catheters inserted directly into a central vein. The latter are four times more likely to become infected. With proper attention given to catheter care and to sterile dressing technique, these catheters have lasted as long as 18 years.

Advantages and Disadvantages

Advantages of the PCVC include reliable, readily available central venous access, no discomfort when hooking up, repair without replacement if a leak develops in the external portion of the catheter, and decreased septic complications as a result of the tunneled approach.

Disadvantages include the need for anesthesia at the time of insertion, mandatory occlusive aseptic dressing at all times, a high probability of contamination and infection if the dressing and catheter site get wet, the need for frequent catheter irrigation when the catheter is not in use, and disturbance of body image, especially important in adolescents.

PORT-A-CATHS: TOTALLY IMPLANTABLE VENOUS ACCESS DEVICES

Indications

The need to provide reliable vascular access during long-term intermittent parenteral therapy for cancer and other diseases and the desire to further reduce the complications of PCVCs provided the stimulus for development of a totally implantable venous access device (TIVAD) (Fig. 104-5) or port-a-cath. Repeated peripheral venipuncture to administer chemotherapeutic agents, antibiotics, and other parenteral medication is uncomfortable for the patient and, over the long term, damages peripheral veins, posing a high risk of chemical inflammation, infection, and thrombosis. Intermittent extravasation of certain types of drugs also damages tissue adjacent to the vein or artery, commonly resulting in a prolonged, painful search by the nurse or physician for a suitable vein. Although centrally placed venous catheters, such as the PCVC, are often used for long-term intermittent infusion therapy, they have obvious drawbacks, many of which were mentioned in the preceding section. Because the catheter receptacle exits through the skin, infection remains a major problem, and scrupulous attention to sterile technique during periodic dressing change is necessary. In addition, the external portion of the catheter restricts daily activities, such as bathing. It is psychologically and aesthetically disturbing to many patients, particularly teenagers. A variety of totally implantable devices, consisting of small-volume subcutaneous injection ports and Silastic catheters, are now available (25,26).

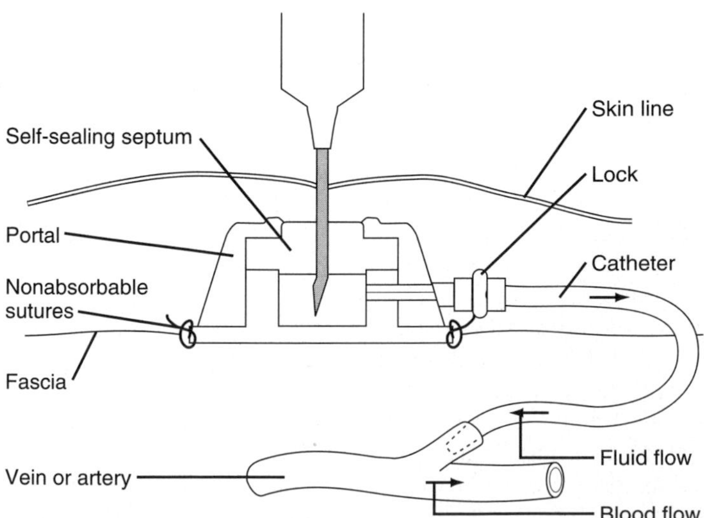

FIGURE 104-5. Totally implantable venous access device (TIVAD). Delivery of fluids and drugs using a Huber needle.

Indications for TIVADs are similar to those for PCVCs, including conditions that require long-term venous access for administration of chemotherapeutic agents, antibiotics, parenteral nutrition, and blood products, and the need for intermittent blood sampling. Miniaturization of these devices has extended their use to infants and small children. In-hospital patients destined for intermittent outpatient infusion and outpatients scheduled for interval chemotherapy are particularly appropriate candidates.

Technical Considerations

The location of the port should be selected preoperatively to ensure it is convenient and comfortable for the patient and family. After inserting the guidewire into the central vein, a counterincision is made on the chest wall for the subcutaneous port. For secure fixation and easy access, the pocket should be over a firm portion of the pectoralis major muscle or a bony portion of the chest wall. The port is anchored to the underlying fascia by permanent sutures. The catheter is then tunneled from the subcutaneous pocket to the venipuncture site and cut to an appropriate length. Finally, it is threaded to its final position. After closure, chest radiography documents the correct position of the catheter tip (previously determined by fluoroscopy) and rules out other technical complications, such as pneumothorax or kinks in the subcutaneous catheter. If the port is to be used immediately, the right-angle Huber needle is placed while the patient is in the operating room. Otherwise, 24 hours should elapse before accessing the port to allow the initial stages of healing to proceed undisturbed.

Advantages and Disadvantages

Because the TIVAD is implanted under the skin, it spares the peripheral vasculature, decreases the risk of infectious complications, minimizes care and maintenance, facilitates ambulatory treatment, and does not interfere with the patient's normal daily activities. The most significant advantage to the patient is that the subcutaneous injection port requires no dressing change and few, if any, heparin flushes between uses. It permits bathing and swimming. It has the added psychological advantage of being out of sight, except when being used. Clinical experience has demonstrated a marked decrease in catheter sepsis with TIVADs. Two prospective studies have documented a significantly lower catheter infection rate in pediatric hematology and oncology patients with subcutaneous ports compared with external venous catheters (27,28). The device has also been shown to be effective and safe for home parenteral nutrition; the Silastic diaphragm can receive as many as 2,000 punctures before replacement (29).

Disadvantages of the TIVAD include limitations in the duration of access due to instability of the noncoring Huber needle in the port, discomfort of access through the overlying skin, and limited longevity of the Silastic access septum. In addition, removal usually requires general anesthesia. The development of the right-angle Huber needle with wings, facilitated more secure and stable access than with the original straight Huber needle (Fig. 104-6). Overall, the incidence of dislodgement of the Huber needle apparatus is low, and overnight and long-term access is reasonably safe, leading to applications such as nightly infusion of parenteral nutrition. The Luer-Lok intrinsic to the Broviac-type PCVCs is definitely more fail safe; thus, PCVCs are preferred by some patients and physicians. Patients receiving continuous infusions of vesicant chemotherapy (e.g., adriamycin) should have PCVCs rather than TIVADs because of the risk of devastating tissue injury from extravasation of the agent if the needle becomes dislodged. Access to the Luer-Lok is painless and much less threatening to children than the nurse or parent approaching the TIVAD with a Huber needle. These reasons notwithstanding, discomfort of port access to the overlying skin is effectively aborted by application of a topical analgesic, which is especially helpful and appropriate for infants and children. With an upper limit of 2,000 system punctures before failure (5 years at one access per day), the limited life span of the Silastic septum is of theoretic importance only: Most TIVADs last until the patient no longer requires the device. Patients who will require daily lifelong access can be offered a choice between the convenience of a PCVC and the positive "lifestyle" aspects of a TIVAD. TIVADs are unstable and impractical in obese patients (body mass index greater than 30). It is very difficult to anchor the port reservoir in a sufficiently superficial location to allow ready access with the needle. Once

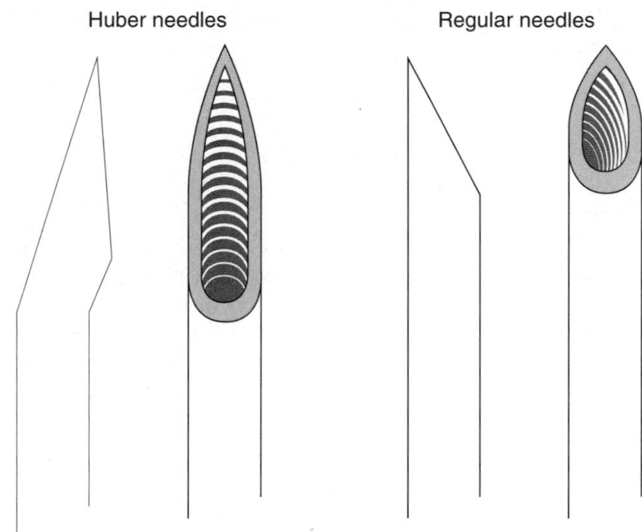

FIGURE 104-6. Fenestrated, noncoring Huber needle and conventional needle.

placed, the needle is likely to be dislodged by shifting fat pads as the patient moves around.

MULTILUMEN CATHETERS

Indications

Multiple-lumen venous access catheters have been developed for both PCVC and TIVAD access systems. The indications are limited to patients who require long-term access for simultaneous administration of two or more parenteral solutions, such as antibiotics, chemotherapeutic agents, fluid for hydration, or parenteral nutrition. Hemodialysis access is perhaps the most common indication for placement of a permanent double-lumen catheter. Use of a triple-lumen catheter enables concurrent monitoring of the central venous pressure. Double- and triple-lumen PCVCs are available commercially, as are double-lumen TIVADs.

Advantages, Disadvantages, and Management

The advantages of double-lumen catheters or double-port systems accrue from the economy of venous access sites and the avoidance of disruption of infusion schedules otherwise necessary if only one access site is available. Disadvantages relate to the potential complications that accompany an increased number of central venous invasive events. These complications are avoided by strict adherence to a detailed protocol, in which each lumen is treated as a separate catheter and in which the access device is reduced to a single-lumen type as soon as the multilumen type is no longer required.

ALTERNATIVE SITES FOR CENTRAL VENOUS ACCESS

Placement of central venous catheter systems most commonly involves access by the percutaneous infraclavicular and supraclavicular approach to the subclavian vein and by the percutaneous or cutdown approach to the external jugular, internal jugular, facial, saphenous, cephalic, and basilic veins. When these sites are infiltrated, thrombosed, infected, or otherwise unavailable, physicians must resort to higher-risk sites, which, by the pressure of necessity, have evolved since the mid-1980s. These are reasonably safe alternatives that have documented success records. These include percutaneous femoral venous catheterization (30); the cutdown approach to the deep inferior epigastric vein in the groin (31) (Fig. 104-7); the cutdown flank approach to the lumbar veins (32) (Fig. 104-8) and the gonadal veins (33,34); the thoracotomy approach to the azygos, hemizygous, and intercostal venous systems (35) (Fig. 104-9); and the thoracotomy and direct canalization of the right atrial appendage (36). In addition, a variety of direct percutaneous approaches are available by the invasive radiologist using ultrasound or other localization techniques (37–39). Long-term success of the alternative approaches depends on a detailed understanding of regional anatomy, meticulous technique, and well-established protocols for occlusive dressings. With careful adherence to successful principles and protocols, such as tunneling Silastic catheters placed in the groin of infants above the diaper line on the abdominal wall or on the chest wall, mechanical and septic complications can be minimized, and even the most difficult vascular access is made safe.

COMPLICATIONS AND THEIR PREVENTION

Many technical, mechanical, and septic complications associated with PCVC and TIVAD use have been reported. These are minimized or prevented when recommended protocols for catheter placement, dressing care, administration of solutions, and monitoring are carefully followed.

Technical Complications

There are numerous potential complications that can occur at the time of central venous catheter insertion (40). For cognitive purposes, these can be divided into site-independent and site-dependent problems (Table 104-1).

Pneumothorax is the most prevalent complication of both subclavian and internal jugular catheterization (41), reportedly occurring in as many as 5% of attempted catheterizations, although the rate is closer to 1% in most dedicated pediatric surgical units (42). It can be asymptomatic and resolve or require needle aspiration or tube thoracostomy. Instructing patients to hold their breath on deep expiration or temporarily stopping positive-pressure mechanical ventilation in anesthetized patients decreases the incidence of pneumothorax. Although there are no large studies of the technique in children, dedicated use of real-time ultrasound guidance with the internal jugular route decreases the incidence of pneumothorax in adults (43).

It is standard practice to obtain a chest radiograph after every catheterization or unsuccessful attempt. This is based on the reasoning that the radiograph alerts the physician to the possible occurrence of complications and confirms the position of the catheter before infusion of medications or parenteral nutrition. More recently, several studies by pediatric surgeons and interventional radiologists have suggested that *routine* postprocedural chest

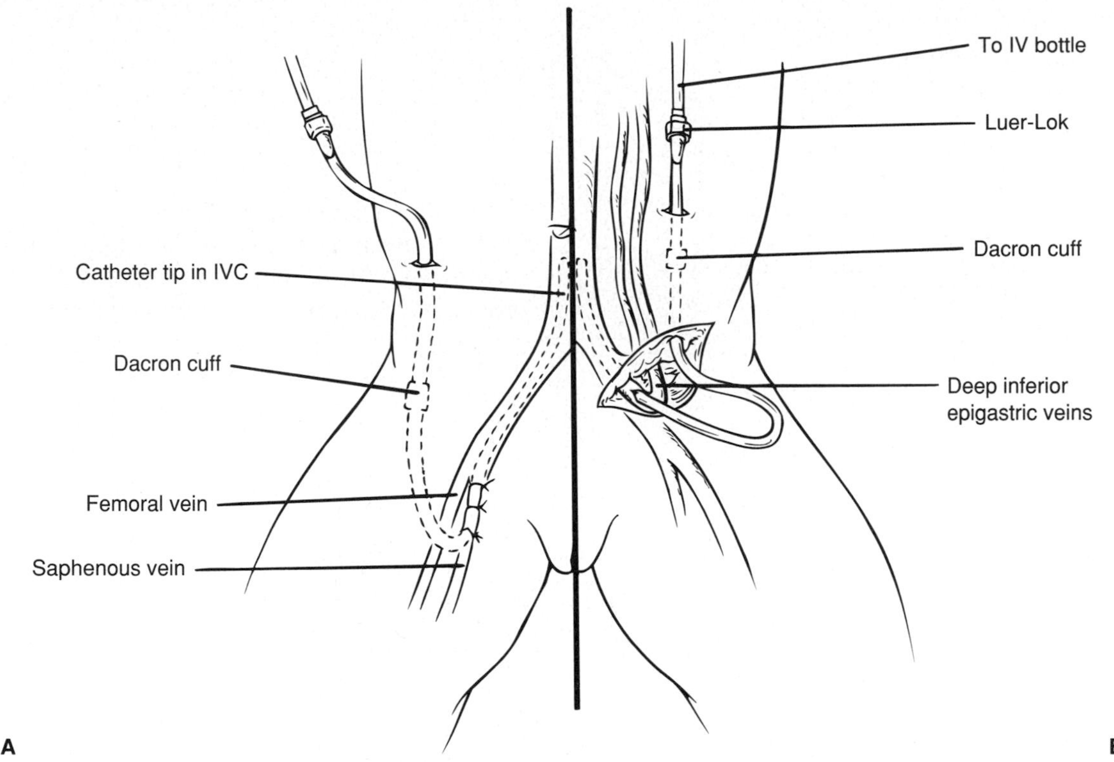

FIGURE 104-7. Saphenous vein and deep inferior epigastric vein are accessed to enter the inferior vena cava (IVC). **(A)** Placement of saphenous vein cutdown, with tunneling of catheter to exit site above the diaper line. The exit site is placed over the lower thorax, if possible, because this affords a stable site that simplifies nursing care. **(B)** Deep inferior epigastric vein access. IV, intravenous. (Courtesy of the Mayo Foundation.)

radiographs are unnecessary after fluoroscopically guided central line placement. These studies demonstrate that selective use of postprocedure imaging, based on physician judgment and clinical signs, is a safe and cost-effective alternative to routine chest radiographs (44–46).

Puncture of the subclavian artery, the next most frequent complication, can be minimized by maintaining the angle of entry as close to the horizontal plane as possible. If arterial blood is returned on insertion of the catheter needle, the needle should be withdrawn and direct pressure applied for at least 5 minutes. Puncture of the carotid artery is the most common complication of percutaneous internal jugular vein catheterization. Applying pressure directly to the puncture site is usually sufficient. If this complication is unrecognized, the resulting hematoma of the neck can lead to tracheal compression and respiratory

TABLE 104-1 Common Technical Complications of Central Venous Catheter Insertion.

	Site Dependent	
Site Independent	***Subclavian > Internal Jugular***	***Internal Jugular > Subclavian***
Pneumothorax	Subclavian artery injury	Horner syndrome
Hemothorax	Subclavian or innominate vein injury	Thoracic duct injury
Hydromediastinum		Carotid artery injury
Thromboembolism		
Chylothorax		
Cardiac tamponade		
Brachial plexus injury		
Phrenic nerve palsy		
Air embolism		

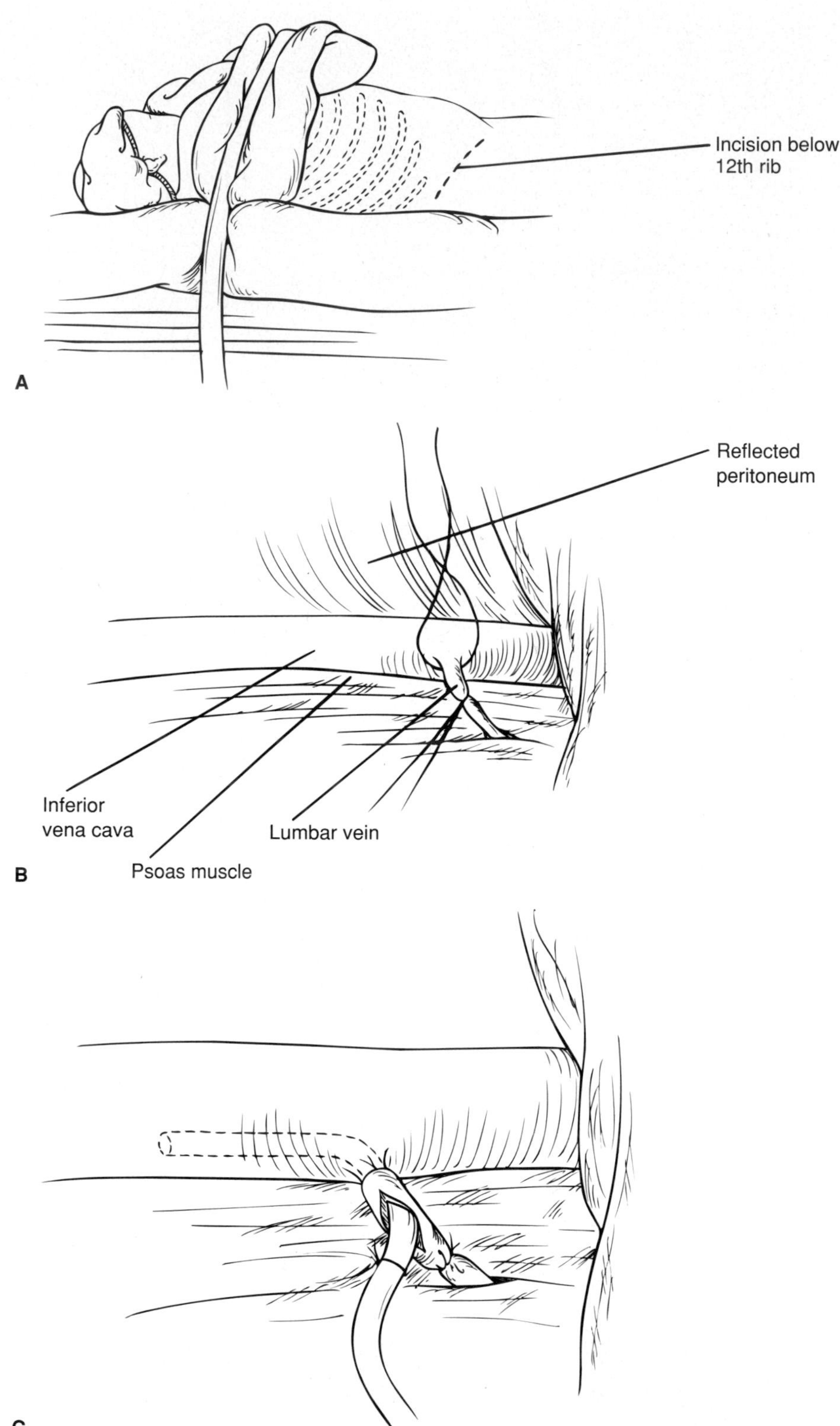

FIGURE 104-8. Lumbar vein access to the inferior vena cava (IVC) can be achieved using either an open or percutaneous approach. **(A)** Positioning for flank incision below the twelfth rib, with the right side elevated at 20 degrees. **(B)** IVC and lumbar vein are exposed. **(C)** Silastic catheter is placed into IVC through lumbar vein and secured to ileopsoas fascia. *(continued)*

compromise, as well as compression injury to the phrenic nerve or brachial plexus.

Air embolism is a potentially fatal complication of percutaneous catheterization of the subclavian and internal jugular veins. To minimize its occurrence, the patient should be placed in the Trendelenburg position during removal of the syringe from the needle trocar and passage of the guide wire and the catheter into the vein. Alternatively, the transition should be made rapidly during deep expiration in the awake patient or with mechanical ventilation temporarily interrupted in an anesthetized patient. Air can also be introduced into the venous system during

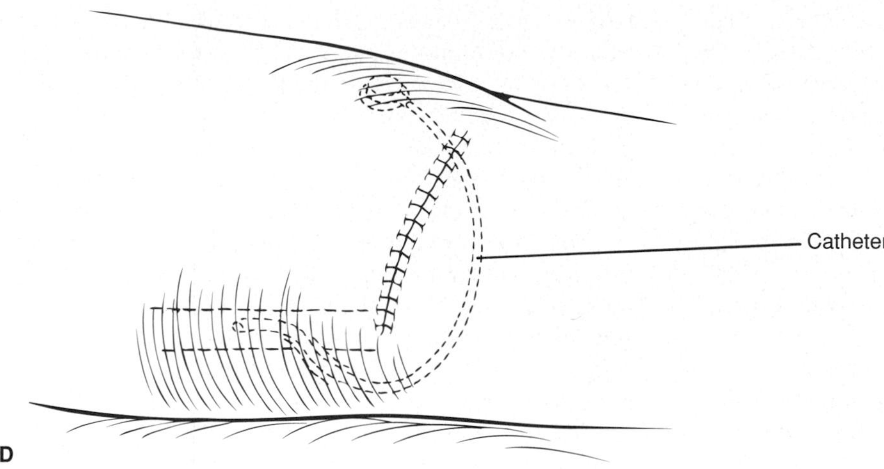

FIGURE 104-8. *(Continued)* **(D)** Catheter is tunneled subcutaneously, with port placed and sutured to fascia of abdominal wall muscle. (Courtesy of the Mayo Foundation.)

tubing changes or if the patient is inadvertently disconnected from the IV tubing. If the physician suspects that air has been introduced during catheter insertion or during tube-changing maneuvers, the immediate management should consist of clamping the catheter and placing the patient in the Trendelenburg position, with the left side down. If the catheter is in place, an attempt should be made to aspirate the air within the right atrium. If the tubing becomes disconnected above the filter, the filter acts as an air lock, preventing the patient from syphoning air into the vascular system.

Although rare, lethal complications do occur during and after central venous catheter insertion. In an analysis of 75 potentially life-threatening complications drawn from a membership survey of the American Pediatric Surgical Association, Bagwell and colleagues identified 40 acute problems that occurred within the first 24 hours after the procedure, of which 15 resulted in death (40). Lethal cases included hemothorax, pneumothorax, hydrothorax, and cardiac tamponade. A synthesis of recommendations to avoid these complications based on this review and general consensus would include the following:

- Unless prevented by patient circumstances, perform central line insertion in an "operating room environment" with the capability of rapid radiographic evaluation of the chest, both to confirm catheter and guide wire position and to aid in diagnosis of acute complications.
- Ensure an experienced surgeon is present during the procedure because complications may arise that require immediate intervention to avoid a lethal outcome.

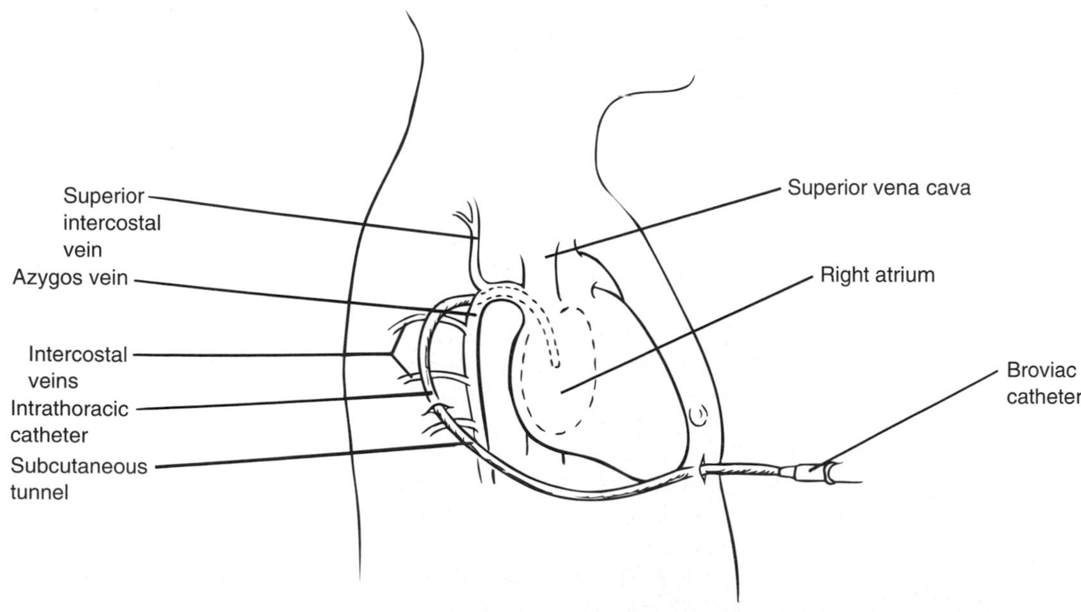

FIGURE 104-9. Right thoracotomy approach for azygos vein access to the right atrium. (Courtesy of the Mayo Foundation.)

- Make an appropriate match between the available equipment and the likely size of the infant's/child's vein.
- Discard any visibly bent or frayed equipment (guide wire, sheath, or dilator) because attempting to pass this equipment is more likely to cause vascular injury.
- Maintain a "hard fix" (the wire should not move in relation to the patient) on the guide wire when passing the dilator. If the dilator "catches" the wire, the dilator should be withdrawn and only readvanced if it will move freely over the wire and preferably under fluoroscopic guidance.
- Maintain prompt vigilance in the evaluation and treatment of any patient instability or complaint after central line placement, including imaging studies and invasive procedures, as circumstances demand.

Mechanical Complications

Mechanical complications of central venous catheters are common and include inadvertent removal, rupture of the catheter, and occlusion. Inadvertent catheter removal is a function of the security of catheter fixation. It is important to maintain an occlusive dressing where the catheter enters the skin and to tether the catheter to the dressing and body site. Rupture of the catheter is almost always confined to the external portion. The site is usually readily identified and repaired with a commercially available kit. Catheter occlusion is most commonly caused by formation of a fibrin sheath either in or at the tip of the catheter, by precipitates of TPN ingredients (e.g., calcium, magnesium, or phosphate salts) in the line or by precipitates of certain types of chemotherapeutic agents. As a general rule, catheter occlusions that occur after a period of dormancy are more likely due to fibrin sheath formation, whereas blockages that arise during active use are all normally caused by a precipitate. If diagnosed early, formation of a fibrin sheath can be treated successfully by instilling recombinant tissue plasminogen activator (rt-PA, Cathflo, Activase) (47), according to the protocol outlined in Table 104-2. Precipitates may be cleared by administration of 0.01 N hydrochloric acid (48) (Table 104-2).

Thrombosis of the subclavian, innominate, or internal jugular vein can lead to occlusion of the catheter or to

TABLE 104-2 Techniques for Treating Central Venous Catheter Occlusion with Recombinant Tissue Plasminogen Activator or Dilute Hydrochloric Acid.

	rt-PA	*Hydrochloric Acid*
Preparation	Add 2.2 mL sterile water for injection to each vial.	1 mL 0.1 N HCl plus 10 mL heparinized saline (10 U/mL)
Final concentration/dose	1 mg/mL Patients ≥10 to <30 kg: 110% of the internal lumen volume of the catheter (≤2 mg [1 mg/mL]); retain in catheter for ≤2 hr; may instill a second dose if catheter remains occluded. Patients ≥30 kg: 2 mg (1 mg/mL); retain in catheter for ≤2 hr; may instill a second dose if catheter remains occluded.	0.01 N HCl
Administration	Instill dose into occluded catheter. Do not force solution into catheter. After a 30-min dwell time, assess catheter function by attempting to aspirate blood. If catheter is functional, aspirate 4–5 mL of blood to remove rt-PA and residual clots. Gently irrigate the catheter with NS. If catheter remains nonfunctional, let rt-PA dwell for another 90 min (total dwell time: 120 min) and reassess function. If catheter function is not restored, a second dose may be instilled.	Draw 0.5 mL into tuberculin syringe and irrigate back and forth for 2 min; clamp and repeat hourly until patency is restored.

rt-PA, recombinant tissue plasminogen activator; HCl, hydrochloric acid; NS, normal saline.

serious vascular complications (e.g., superior vena cava syndrome). Male and colleagues (49) reported an association between subclavian (vs. internal jugular) vein location, left side (vs. right side) of the body insertion, and percutaneous (vs. cutdown) technique and an increased risk of venous thrombosis in a group of high-risk children. This study strongly suggests that the stiff dilator/introducer used for insertion of flexible central venous catheters causes significant endothelial injury leading to venous thrombosis. Suspected thrombosis in patients with catheter malfunction, cardiopulmonary dysfunction, or sepsis can be documented by duplex ultrasound, echocardiography, or magnetic resonance venography; however, routine screening of symptom-free patients is not rewarding (50). Removal of the catheter with change to a different site and heparinization for 7 to 10 days is generally adequate treatment; clearing of the thrombosed vessel with thrombolytic agents is usually not indicated.

Septic Complications

Bloodstream infections occur in 20% to 30% of infants and children with an indwelling central line (10). Various combinations of temperature increase or decrease, glucose intolerance, oliguria, hypotension, or general deterioration in clinical condition suggest septic complications in this group of patients. Protocol for the workup of possible catheter sepsis includes an initial investigation of all possible sources of infection (i.e., pulmonary, genitourinary tract, gastrointestinal tract, wounds, sputum, urine). If the catheter site demonstrates evidence of infection (e.g., purulence), the catheter should be removed. In some patients with localized infection at the catheter–cutaneous junction (and a cuff to help limit proximal spread), local cleansing with hydrogen peroxide, followed by antibacterial ointment and administration through the catheter of antibiotics directed to the organism, may salvage the catheter. Infections of the tunnel generally require catheter removal. Quantitative blood cultures (for aerobes, anaerobes, and fungi) should be drawn through the catheter and from one peripheral site. After obtaining blood for cultures, appropriate broad-spectrum antibiotics should be administered through the catheter, unless the patient is toxic, in which the case the antibiotics should be started but the catheter removed and the tip cultured. Because of difficulty in obtaining blood cultures from either a peripheral vein or the catheter, many physicians apply the principle that any unexplained signs of infection are catheter related. This leads to overreporting of infections, hinders comparisons, and results in salvageable catheters being removed unnecessarily. If possible, antibiotics should be administered for 24 hours before reinsertion of a new catheter. Optimal management after catheter removal due to sepsis requires that blood culture results be normal before another PCVC or TIVAD is placed.

There are many effective strategies for prevention of catheter-related sepsis. Proven techniques include full barrier precautions during catheter insertion; subcutaneous tunneling, especially for catheters placed in the internal jugular or femoral positions; povidone-iodine applied to insertion sites; and specialized nursing teams caring for patients with vascular catheters (51). Colonization of the catheter lumen most commonly results from lapses in techniques in catheter care and use. Faubion and colleagues (24) and Puntis and associates (52) showed that a well-trained vascular access and nutrition support team and a strict protocol for catheter care markedly decrease infection rates. The cost savings and decrease in patient morbidity justify the commitment of institutional resources.

REFERENCES

1. Maki DG, Ringer M. Risk factors for infusion-related phlebitis with small peripheral venous catheters. A randomized controlled trial. *Ann Intern Med* 1991;114:845–854.
2. Stanley MD, Meister E, Fuschuber K. Infiltration during intravenous therapy in neonates: comparison of Teflon and Vialon catheters. *South Med J* 1992;85:883–886.
3. Hastings-Tolsma MT, Yucha CB, Tompkins J, et al. Effect of warm and cold applications on the resolution of i.v. infiltrations. *Res Nurs Health* 1993;16:171–178.
4. Wynsma LA. Negative outcomes of intravascular therapy in infants and children. *AACN Clin Issues* 1998;9:49–63.
5. Fiser DH. Intraosseous infusion. *N Engl J Med* 1990;322:1579–1581.
6. Boon JM, Gorry DL, Meiring JH. Finding an ideal site for intraosseous infusion of the tibia: an anatomical study. *Clin Anat* 2003;16:15–18.
7. Rosetti VA, Thompson BM, Miller J, et al. Intraosseous infusion: an alternative route of pediatric intravascular access. *Ann Emerg Med* 1985;14:885–888.
8. Dolcourt JL, Bose CL. Percutaneous insertion of silastic central venous catheters in newborn infants. *Pediatrics* 1982;70:484–486.
9. Johnson RV, Donn SM. Life span of intravenous cannulas in a neonatal intensive care unit. *Am J Dis Child* 1988;142:968–971.
10. Fallat ME, Gallinaro RN, Stover BH, et al. Central venous catheter bloodstream infections in the neonatal intensive care unit. *J Pediatr Surg* 1998;33:1383–1387.
11. Racadio JM, Johnson ND, Doellman DA. Peripherally inserted central venous catheters: success of scalp-vein access in infants and newborns. *Radiology* 1999;210:858–860.
12. Donaldson JS, Morello FP, Junewick JJ, et al. Peripherally inserted central venous catheters: US-guided vascular access in pediatric patients. *Radiology* 1995;197:542–544.
13. Thiagarajan RR, Ramamoorthy C, Gettmann T, et al. Survey of the use of peripherally inserted central venous catheters in children. *Pediatrics* 1997;99:E4.
14. Crowley JJ, Pereira JK, Harris LS, et al. Radiologic placement of long-term subcutaneous venous access ports in children. *AJR Am J Roentgenol* 1998;171:257–260.
15. Dubois J, Garel L, Tapiero B, et al. Peripherally inserted central catheters in infants and children. *Radiology* 1997;204:622–626.
16. Durand M, Ramanathan R, Martinelli B, et al. Prospective evaluation of percutaneous central venous silastic catheters in newborn infants with birth weights of 510 to 3,920 grams. *Pediatrics* 1986;78: 245–250.
17. Smith JR, Friedell ML, Cheatham ML, et al. Peripherally inserted central catheters revisited. *Am J Surg* 1998;176:208–211.
18. Aubaniac R. The subclavian vein puncture—advantages and technique. 1952. *Nutrition* 1990;6:139–140; discussion 141.
19. Newman BM, Jewett TC Jr, Karp MP, et al. Percutaneous central

venous catheterization in children: first line choice for venous access. *J Pediatr Surg* 1986;21:685–688.
20. Broviac JW, Cole JJ, Scribner BH. A silicone rubber atrial catheter for prolonged parenteral alimentation. *Surg Gynecol Obstet* 1973;136:602–606.
21. Hickman RO, Buckner CD, Clift RA, et al. A modified right atrial catheter for access to the venous system in marrow transplant recipients. *Surg Gynecol Obstet* 1979;148:871–875.
22. Konner K. Subclavian haemodialysis access: is it still justified in 1995? *Nephrol Dial Transplant* 1995;10:1988–1991.
23. Holmes SJ, Kiely EM, Spitz L. Vascular access. *Prog Pediatr Surg* 1989;22:133–139.
24. Faubion WC, Wesley JR, Khalidi N, et al. Total parenteral nutrition catheter sepsis: impact of the team approach. *JPEN J Parenter Enteral Nutr* 1986;10:642–645.
25. Niederhuber JE, Ensminger W, Gyves JW, et al. Totally implanted venous and arterial access system to replace external catheters in cancer treatment. *Surgery* 1982;92:706–712.
26. Bothe A Jr, Piccione W, Ambrosino JJ, et al. Implantable central venous access system. *Am J Surg* 1984;147:565–569.
27. Ingram J, Weitzman S, Greenberg ML, et al. Complications of indwelling venous access lines in the pediatric hematology patient: a prospective comparison of external venous catheters and subcutaneous ports. *Am J Pediatr Hematol Oncol* 1991;13:130–136.
28. La Quaglia MP, Lucas A, Thaler HT, et al. A prospective analysis of vascular access device-related infections in children. *J Pediatr Surg* 1992;27:840–842.
29. Howard L, Claunch C, McDowell R, et al. Five years of experience in patients receiving home nutrition support with the implanted reservoir: a comparison with the external catheter. *JPEN J Parenter Enteral Nutr* 1989;13:478–483.
30. Abdulla F, Dietrich KA, Pramanik AK. Percutaneous femoral venous catheterization in preterm neonates. *J Pediatr* 1990;117:788–791.
31. Donahoe PK, Kim SH. The inferior epigastric vein as an alternate site for central venous hyperalimentation. *J Pediatr Surg* 1980;15: 737–738.
32. Boddie AW Jr. Translumbar catheterization of the inferior vena cava for long term angioaccess. *Surg Gynecol Obstet* 1989;168:54–56.
33. Chang MY, Morris JB. Long-term central venous access through the ovarian vein. *JPEN J Parenter Enteral Nutr* 1997;21:235–7.
34. Shankar KR, Anbu AT, Losty PD. Use of the gonadal vein in children with difficult central venous access: a novel technique. *J Pediatr Surg* 2001;36:E3.
35. Torosian MH, Meranze S, McLean G, et al. Central venous access with occlusive superior central venous thrombosis. *Ann Surg* 1986;203: 30–33.
36. Hayden L, Stewart GR, Johnson DC, et al. Transthoracic right atrial cannulation for total parenteral nutrition- case report. *Anaesth Intensive Care* 1981;9:53–57.
37. Robards JB, Jaques PF, Mauro MA, et al. Percutaneous translumbar inferior vena cava central line placement in a critically ill child. *Pediatr Radiol* 1989;19:140–141.
38. Malmgren N, Cwikiel W, Hochbergs P, et al. Percutaneous translumbar central venous catheter in infants and small children. *Pediatr Radiol* 1995;25:28–30.
39. Solomon BA, Solomon J, Shlansky-Goldberg R. Percutaneous placement of an intercostal central venous catheter for chronic hyperalimentation guided by transhepatic venography. *JPEN J Parenter Enteral Nutr* 2001;25:42–44.
40. Bagwell CE, Salzberg AM, Sonnino RE, et al. Potentially lethal complications of central venous catheter placement. *J Pediatr Surg* 2000;35:709–713.
41. Ruesch S, Walder B, Tramer MR. Complications of central venous catheters: internal jugular versus subclavian access—a systematic review. *Crit Care Med* 2002;30:454–460.
42. Johnson EM, Saltzman DA, Suh G, et al. Complications and risks of central venous catheter placement in children. *Surgery* 1998;124: 911–916.
43. Gann M Jr, Sardi A. Improved results using ultrasound guidance for central venous access. *Am Surg* 2003;69:1104–1107.
44. Lucey B, Varghese JC, Haslam P, et al. Routine chest radiographs after central line insertion: mandatory postprocedural evaluation or unnecessary waste of resources? *Cardiovasc Intervent Radiol* 1999;22:381–384.
45. Caridi JG, West JH, Stavropoulos SW, et al. Internal jugular and upper extremity central venous access in interventional radiology: is a postprocedure chest radiograph necessary? *AJR Am J Roentgenol* 2000;174:363–366.
46. Janik JE, Cothren CC, Janik JS, et al. Is a routine chest x-ray necessary for children after fluoroscopically assisted central venous access? *J Pediatr Surg* 2003;38:1199–1202.
47. Gorski LA. Central venous access device occlusions: part 1: thrombotic causes and treatment. *Home Healthc Nurse* 2003;21:115–121; quiz 122.
48. Shulman RJ, Reed T, Pitre D, et al. Use of hydrochloric acid to clear obstructed central venous catheters. *JPEN J Parenter Enteral Nutr* 1988;12:509–510.
49. Male C, Chait P, Andrew M, et al. Central venous line-related thrombosis in children: association with central venous line location and insertion technique. *Blood* 2003;101:4273–4278.
50. Ross P Jr, Ehrenkranz R, Kleinman CS, et al. Thrombus associated with central venous catheters in infants and children. *J Pediatr Surg* 1989;24:253–256.
51. Mermel LA. Prevention of intravascular catheter-related infections. *Ann Intern Med* 2000;132:391–402.
52. Puntis JW, Holden CE, Smallman S, et al. Staff training: a key factor in reducing intravascular catheter sepsis. *Arch Dis Child* 1991;66:335–337.

PART J

Musculoskeletal System

Chapter 105

Principles of Orthopedics

Paul D. Sponseller

Pediatric surgeons should be familiar with the principles of pediatric orthopedics in order to deal with trauma, recognize skeletal manifestations of systemic diseases, and evaluate congenital or developmental abnormalities. This chapter is intended to help in the initial understanding of the broad range of orthopedic conditions encountered in children and is therefore intended for breadth of coverage. Conditions isolated to one anatomic region are presented first, followed by generalized musculoskeletal conditions. The references provided at the end of this chapter can serve as a guide for further study of any particular condition (1–4). For more information on orthopedic principles of trauma, refer to Chapter 27.

Because orthopedic terminology is not always straightforward, the following definitions are provided to assist the reader. The term *physis* refers to the growth plate (Fig. 105-1); therefore, the *epi*physis is the portion of a bone "on top of" the physis (i.e., nearer the joint), the *meta*physis is the widened portion of the shaft adjacent to and arising from the growth plate, and the *dia*physis is the narrow portion of a tubular bone midway between two physes. The skeleton is largely formed from a cartilaginous precursor, with ossification of the cartilage beginning in the diaphysis. Secondary ossification centers at the ends of each long bone. The small bones of the wrist and foot begin from a single ossification center.

The Greek root *genu* refers to knee, *coxa* to hip, and *pes* to foot. When two bones or two fracture fragments form an angle, they are in *varus* when the apex of the angle points away from the midline (Fig. 105-2) and *valgus* when it points toward the midline. Alternatively, *angulation* may be stated in any of the three standard anatomic planes by the direction of the apex—that is, genu valgus is medial angulation of the lower extremity at the knee. *Dislocation* refers to complete loss of contact of two joint surfaces, and it is specified by the direction of displacement of the most distal part. *Subluxation* is a partial or incomplete dislocation. For example, in a dislocated hip, the femoral head is completely out of the acetabulum; a subluxated hip has been only partially offset. *Abduction* refers to movement away from the midline, whereas; *adduction* refers to movement toward the midline.

Paul D. Sponseller: Orthopaedic Surgery, Johns Hopkins University, Johns Hopkins Hospital, Baltimore, Maryland 21287.

ABNORMALITIES BY REGION

Foot

Isolated idiopathic *adduction* of the forefoot or metatarsals is designated by the terms *metatarsus adductus, metatarsus varus*, or *C-foot*. In contrast to clubfoot, the hindfoot and ankle are normal. The ankle joint itself has normal dorsiflexion and plantar flexion. The etiology may be increased medially directed pressure in the uterus. Children with metatarsus adductus also may have an increased incidence of other molding deformities, such as developmental dislocation of the hip or torticollis (5).

The natural history of untreated metatarsus adductus is spontaneous correction in 85% of children. In 10% of children, mild adduction persists, and in only 5% is it severe (6). Therefore, the preferred treatment is observation and stretching for the first 4 to 6 months, with corrective casts or splints if severe metatarsus adductus persists beyond this time. The casts are changed every 1 to 2 weeks until the adduction is clinically corrected, then followed by holding casts or shoes. Surgery (osteotomy) for very late deformities, in children older than 3 years, is only rarely necessary.

Clubfoot, or equinovarus congenita, is a more complex disorder that includes not only metatarsal adduction, but also abnormalities of the hind part of the foot—that is, malrotation of the calcaneus under the talus and equinus (plantar flexion) of the ankle. The incidence of clubfoot is 1 per 1,000 births, and it is more common in males than in

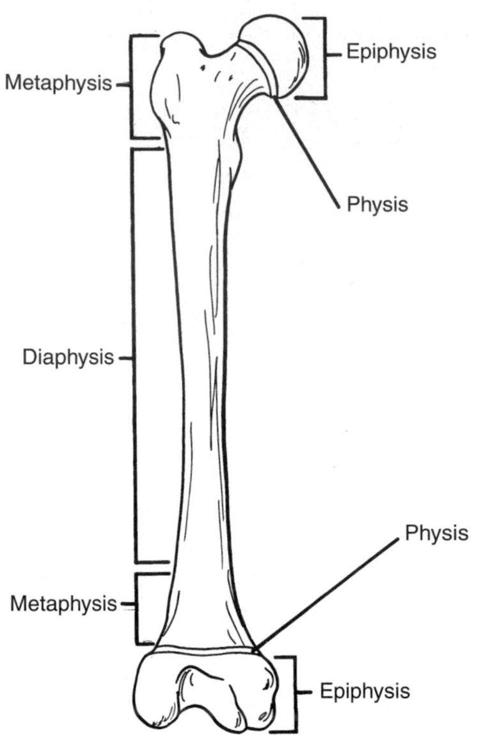

FIGURE 105-1. Regions of a long bone. The physis or growth plate is the main reference point. The epiphysis refers to the segment on top of the physis, and so forth.

females. Clubfoot may be unilateral or bilateral. Etiology is unknown. Abnormalities have been found in the leg muscles or tarsal bones.

The clubfoot appears smaller than normal for age, and the combination of deformities results in a 90-degree rotation of the forefoot in all planes so the leg and foot truly resemble a club (Fig. 105-3). There is a deep crease on the medial border of the foot. The deformity may be correctable to neutral only in the neonatal period, and the range of motion is limited in all directions. Radiographs show an abnormal parallelism of the talus and calcaneus. Neuromuscular disorders (especially lipomeningocele, myelomeningocele, spasticity, or arthrogryposis) may produce similar deformities.

Clubfoot ranges from a mild, postural, and easily correctable form to a severe and resistant form. However, cast correction is indicated in all. This is most successful in the perinatal period when ligamentous laxity is greatest. The casts are changed every week. A percutaneous tenotomy of the Achilles tendon is performed after the rotation of the foot is corrected. The correction of the foot is maintained by the use of night splints or braces. Overall, cast treatment is effective in about three-fourths of patients. Surgery is indicated in the others and involves complete correction of all bony malalignments and tendon contractures; it is performed most commonly at ages 6 to 12 months (7). In older patients or in those with recurrent deformity, osteotomy or fusion may be indicated.

A calcaneovalgus foot is common in newborns. The foot is dorsiflexed and in valgus so the dorsum of the foot may almost be touching the tibia (Fig. 105-4). The bones and joints themselves are normal. The condition spontaneously improves within the first few months.

Flatfoot (planovalgus) should be divided into flexible and rigid types. The flexible type is a normal variant in children and is usually asymptomatic. Development of an arch occurs spontaneously in the first 8 years of life in most children. The arch of the foot is restored. When the child is on tiptoes or when weight bearing is relieved, varus-valgus motion is normal. As a herald to a more serious condition, *rigid* flatfoot may be due to tarsal coalition, vertical talus, neuromuscular imbalance, or arthritis of the foot. These should be considered in the differential diagnosis.

The cause of the usual type of flexible flatfoot is ligamentous laxity. There is no primary muscle abnormality. Occasionally, a tight heel cord may contribute to producing flatfoot by pulling the foot into greater valgus. Treatment is not indicated in cases of flexible flatfoot; prospective studies (8) have shown that no orthotic or special shoe can produce a lasting change in pediatric flatfoot. Such devices may be indicated for neuromuscular flatfeet, but not in asymptomatic children with flexible flatfeet. The heel cord should be stretched if it is tight. Rarely is soft-tissue reconstruction or osteotomy indicated.

General principles to stress to parents when they ask about shoes are summarized in an article by Staheli (9):

- Shoes are primarily for protection.
- Corrective shoes have no effect on flat feet.
- Shoes should be flat, flexible, well aerated, and high topped if needed to keep them from slipping off.

These characteristics should be found in most reasonably priced footwear available in regular shoe stores.

Tarsal coalition involves the bones of the hindfoot, with persistence of a bridge or coalition between two of them. This bridge may be fibrous, cartilaginous, or bony. Tarsal coalition is transmitted as autosomal dominant and is present in approximately 5% of the population (10). Many persons with tarsal coalition are asymptomatic. The presence of symptoms seems to be related to the degree of valgus, which places more strain on the abnormal coalition. Tarsal coalition usually presents during the second decade as an ankle sprain with persistence of pain longer than expected or as spontaneous onset of pain in the ankle. The reason for this presentation is probably that the ossification that occurs at this time, near skeletal maturity, makes the coalition stiffer and therefore symptomatic. The hindfoot shows limitation of varus-valgus motion, but it is usually tender to palpation. The foot appears to be in valgus

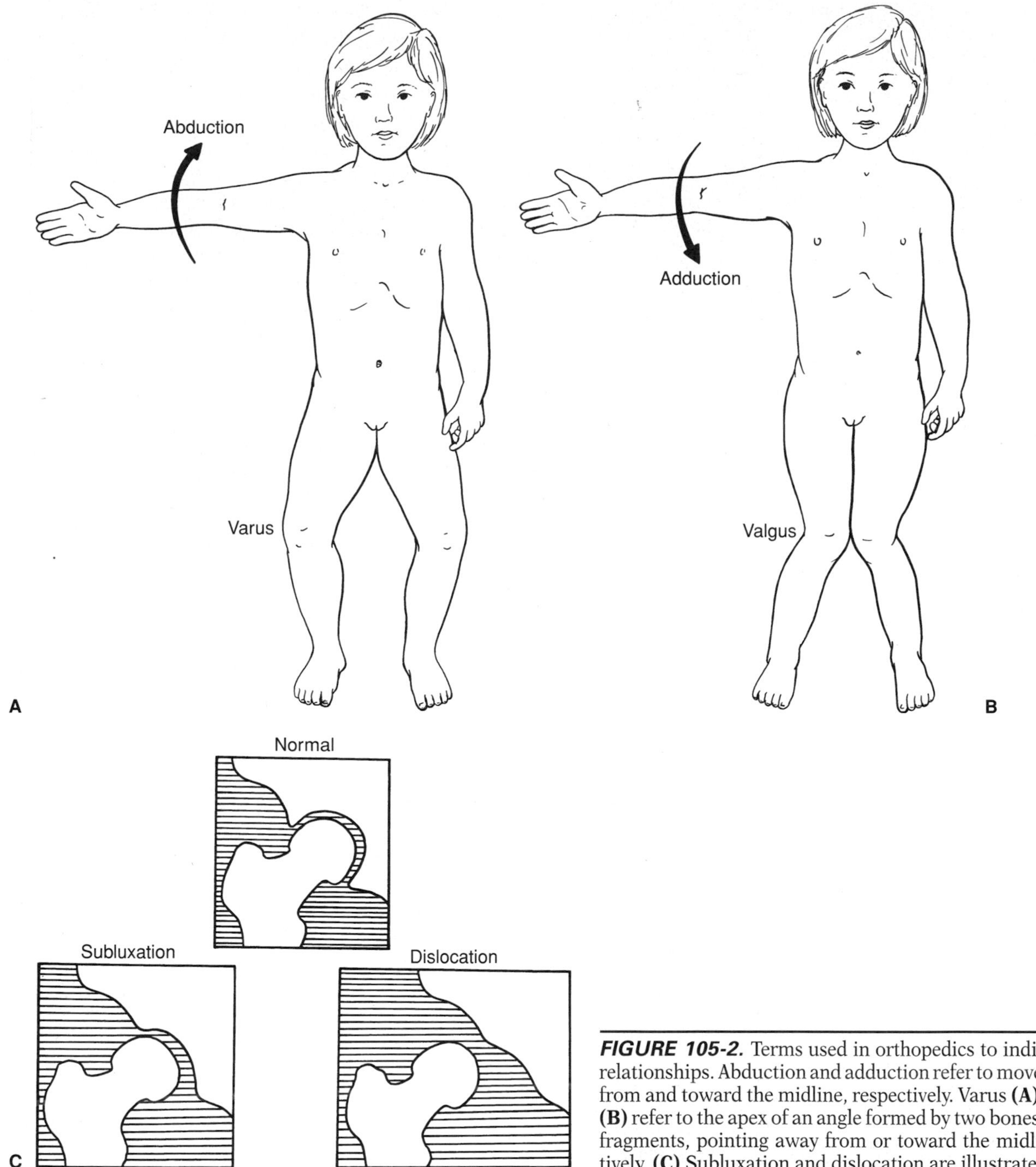

FIGURE 105-2. Terms used in orthopedics to indicate spatial relationships. Abduction and adduction refer to movement away from and toward the midline, respectively. Varus **(A)** and valgus **(B)** refer to the apex of an angle formed by two bones or fracture fragments, pointing away from or toward the midline, respectively. **(C)** Subluxation and dislocation are illustrated.

more often than not. Sometimes pain manifests over the peroneal muscles, which overcontract to stabilize the foot.

A plain oblique radiograph of the foot can reliably show the most common type of coalition, the *calcaneonavicular* bar, if it has ossified (10). However, it is not evident on the anteroposterior (AP) or lateral view. If it is fibrous or cartilaginous, there may not be a bony connection, but an irregularity of the adjacent cortices may be seen. Normal films in the presence of physeal findings of a coalition indicate the need for a coronal computed tomography (CT) scan of the foot to search for a *talocalcaneal* coalition, the other common type of coalition.

With rest or casting, many coalitions develop enough stability to ossify and become painless. If pain persists, however, the coalition can be excised if it is not large and if no arthritic change has occurred (11). If these conditions

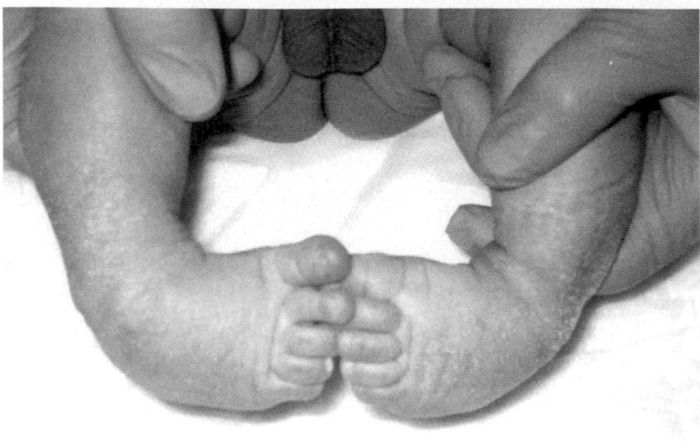

FIGURE 105-3. Uncorrected club feet in a neonate. Note the equinus of the ankle and varus, adduction, and malrotation of the rest of the foot.

are not met, fusion of the hindfoot is the best treatment for the symptomatic foot.

Tibia

Internal tibial torsion is the most common cause of intoeing between 1 and 3 years of age (12–14). Tibial torsion is measured by the angle between the foot and thigh, with the ankle and knee bent at 90 degrees. Normally, the foot turns out more with increasing age. Differential diagnosis includes metatarsus adductus, femoral anteversion, or neuromuscular disorders. Tibial torsion naturally improves with growth, but this often takes years. Because the benign natural history of this condition is now known, braces, such as the Denis-Browne bar, are rarely used (13). Studies have shown that braces cannot apply significant rotational force to the tibia because the force is dissipated through the foot, knee, and hip joints. The improvement attributed to the brace in years past is now believed to be due to normal growth patterns. Correction through growth is a gradual process and often frustrates parents. Prior traditional use of braces, reinforced by comments from grandparents and friends, often drive anxious parents to visit the doctor to ensure they are not missing a golden opportunity to prevent deformity. The physician should be confident in allaying the anxiety. The use of a graph may prove convincing. Minor persistent internal torsion has not been shown to be detrimental.

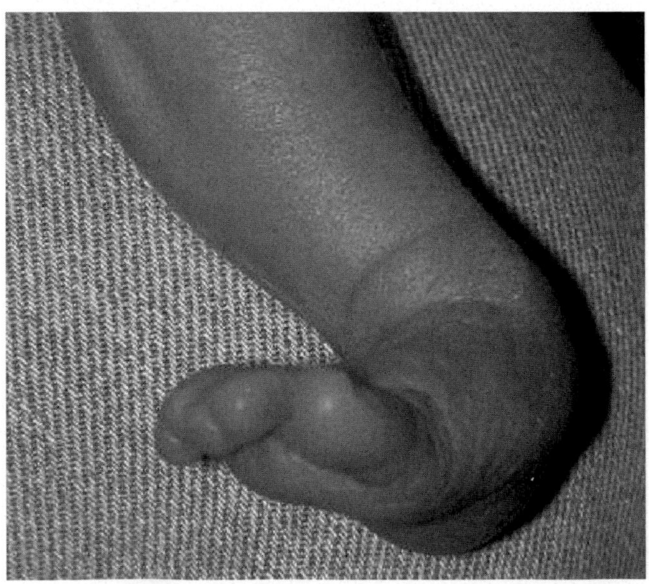

FIGURE 105-4. Calcaneovalgus foot is characterized by pronounced dorsiflexion and eversion of the foot.

External tibial torsion is less common. These children often appear clumsy for their age. There is little data on the course of this condition; however, treatment is not indicated, and some spontaneous improvement can be expected.

Mild *anterior and lateral* bowing of the tibia are common in infancy and should be observed to ensure they correct spontaneously. Focal, sclerotic defects in the tibia may be seen with marked anterolateral bowing. Such patients may present with or develop a fracture (*congenital pseudoarthrosis*), and patients may be found to have neurofibromatosis. If the severe anterolateral bow is present, but the tibia is not fractured, it should be braced for protection. If it is fractured, attempts to gain union by electrical stimulation, rod insertion, vascularized fibula grafting, or bone grafting have similar success rates of 50% to 75% (15). An anterolateral bow may also be seen with congenital absence of the fibula, but this does not progress to fracture.

Posterior/medial bowing of the tibia is also benign; this usually straightens by age 4 and is not associated with fracture. However, there may be 2 to 6 cm of shortening by maturity. Treatment is stretching of the tight dorsiflexor muscles and length equalization as indicated later in childhood (16).

Knee

Extensor Mechanism Disorders (Patellofemoral Problems)

In children and adolescents, a number of conditions involving this region have been described. They are treated by attempting to improve the basic biomechanical forces.

Chondromalacia is a nonspecific term that refers to the appearance of softening and degeneration of the patellar cartilage. *Patellar subluxation* refers to partial lateral *displacement* of the patella. The terms *patellofemoral stress syndrome, patellar malalignment*, and *excessive lateral pressure syndrome* refer to the abnormal *mechanics* causing stress concentration and pain.

The quadriceps-patella mechanism is in valgus, as measured by the Q (quadriceps) angle from anterior superior spine to patella to tibial tubercle. Possible factors contributing to patellar pathology include increased valgus of the knee, increased anteversion of the femur or external torsion of the tibia, a high patella (patella alta), abnormal shape or development of the quadriceps, or flattening of the femoral groove. Underdevelopment of the medial side of the quadriceps restraints contributes to subluxation or dislocation. Females normally have slightly greater valgus of the knee than males. Cartilage degeneration occurs beginning in the deep layers and becoming visible later.

Clinically, patellar problems cause symptoms of aching in the anteromedial region of the knee. This is usually worse with stair-climbing or prolonged sitting because flexion increases patellofemoral force. Crepitus may be felt, but this may be painless in some patients and is not in itself pathologic. "Catching" or "locking" may be noted. A feeling of "giving way" may be related, especially with subluxation of the patella. On physical examination, the most reliable way to test patellar tenderness is by direct compression of the patella against the femur. Palpation under the patella is not diagnostic. Effusion is present only if patellar degenerative changes or extreme overuse have occurred. In most cases, there is no effusion. Reproducing patellar subluxation by laterally directed pressure may produce apprehension (the apprehension test). Radiographs are usually nonspecific, but occasionally lateral displacement or tilt of the patella may be seen on the sunrise view.

Patellofemoral stress disorders are common between the ages of 10 and 20 years, but often become less bothersome after these years and do not usually progress to arthritis.

Differential diagnosis includes a synovial fold or plica, a medial meniscus tear, tendinitis of the quadriceps or patellar tendon, and osteochondritis dissecans of the patella or distal femur.

Treatment consists of decreasing activities performed with knees flexed, such as stair-climbing and prolonged sitting. Temporary rest from sports and use of nonsteroidal antiinflammatory agents may be necessary. Exercises to strengthen the medial (stabilizing) part of the quadriceps include extension from 0 to 30 degrees, by lifting weights within this range or extending the knee on a pillow to compress it. Muscles should be stretched if they are tight. Arch supports may help if flexible flat feet are contributing to tibial torsion. Surgical measures are rarely needed, but they include release of a tight lateral patellar retinaculum, medial soft-tissue tightening, tibial tubercle transfer, or correction of valgus, anteversion, or patella alta. These all produce satisfactory pain relief in 75% to 90% of cases.

Patellar dislocations may be acute or recurrent. The patella usually dislocates laterally. An acute dislocation is associated with significant swelling and medial knee pain, and follows valgus or rotating force. This should be treated for 4 to 6 weeks with the knee extended, using a knee immobilizer, except in cases with bony avulsion. Recurrent *subluxation* is common; the patient has less pain and swelling, and subluxation often occurs during everyday activities. A realignment operation as described earlier is the only effective way to stop frequent and bothersome episodes.

Osgood-Schlatter disease, patellar tendinitis (jumper's knee), and quadriceps tendinitis are all manifestations of excessive, repetitive stresses on the extensor mechanism. They are listed in order of decreasing frequency in children.

Osgood-Schlatter "disease" is a traction-induced inflammation of the tibial tubercle, not really a disease. Rather, it is a reaction of the bone and growth cartilage of this region to repetitive stress. The tibial tubercle is a distal extension of the proximal tibial epiphysis. It develops an ossification center between ages 9 and 12, but does not completely ossify until ages 15 to 17 years. It is within this age range that repetitive stresses can gradually deform the tubercle, causing enlargement of the tubercle and local inflammation. Tenderness and swelling are localized to the tubercle only and do not extend to the joint. Running, jumping, or kneeling exacerbates symptoms. Treatment involves decreasing activity to a level at which symptoms are minimal, occasionally using a knee immobilizer, crutches, and ice after activity in severe cases. The patient may be vulnerable to recurrence for up to 2 years until the tubercle matures. If he or she is educated about this likelihood, individual regulation of activities can be effective. Complete avulsion of the tubercle is extremely rare and seems more related to sudden stress than to apophysitis.

Patellar tendonitis, inflammation at the *origin* of the patellar tendon (at the inferior pole of the patella), is related to the same type of overuse as Osgood-Schlatter apophysitis. It is most often seen in basketball players, and is therefore known as jumper's knee. Pain present during both rest and activity is more worrisome than pain occurring just after activity. Treatment is the same as for Osgood-Schlatter disease. Warm packs before and cold packs after activity may also be of help. Rarely, pain may occur at the proximal pole of the patella and is termed *quadriceps tendinitis*.

Popliteal cysts in children are localized on the medial side of the popliteal region (Fig. 105-5). They occur most commonly in boys younger than age 9 years. Unlike popliteal cysts in adults, these cysts in children are usually not associated with any intraarticular pathology (17), and they usually regress spontaneously with time. The recurrence rate is higher after surgical excision than after observation. The origin of these cysts is a slitlike communication through the joint capsules between the knee joint and the gastrocnemius-semimembranous bursa on the medial side of the popliteal region.

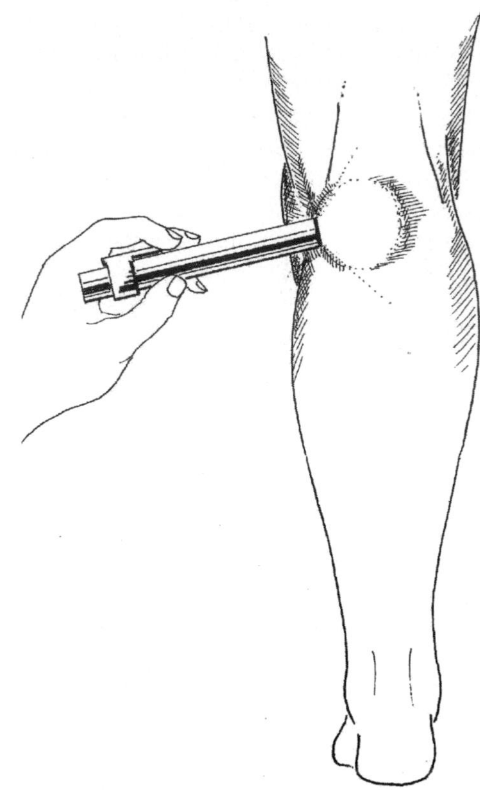

FIGURE 105-5. Popliteal cyst is characterized by a swelling in a characteristic location—the posteromedial aspect of the knee. Transillumination is confirmation of the cystic nature.

These cysts often present as tumors but can usually be differentiated clinically by their characteristic location, firm consistency, discrete encapsulation, and slight mobility. Transillumination is helpful because the whole contents of the mass lights up when the room is darkened, distinguishing it from a blood-filled or a solid tumor. Biopsy should rarely be necessary.

A *discoid meniscus* is an acquired flattening and deformation of the normally semilunar lateral meniscus. In some cases, this flattening occurs because of the absence of normal peripheral attachments. Symptoms such as pain, clicking, and locking often develop in the absence of trauma in children from age 2 to adulthood (18). The meniscus should be trimmed or excised if symptoms become severe.

Bowed leg or genu varum of up to 20 degrees is normal in children until the age of 18 months. Bowing normally does not increase significantly after walking begins (12). After the age of 24 months, valgus of the knee begins to develop instead (19). Radiographs are indicated if varus is present after this age or is progressive after 1 year, if it is unilateral, if it appears to be severe, or if it occurs in a high-risk group such as heavy black children who walk early (12). Radiographic findings of benign genu varum include bowing of the tibia and femur; a normal-appearing growth plate physis, without narrowing or step-off; and a generalized, rather than focal, varus angle.

Treatment of physiologic genu varum is observation until resolution. On physical examination, the measurement should be performed with the child standing and may also be confirmed by measurement of the distance between the femoral condyles. These methods are not as accurate as radiographs, but they are a practical way of following change in patients when the presumptive diagnosis is physiologic genu varum.

Differential diagnosis of physiologic genu varum includes Blount disease, rickets, posttraumatic growth plate disturbance, enchondromatosis, achondroplasia, or other skeletal dysplasias.

Blount disease (tibia vara) is an idiopathic, mechanical overload of the medial tibial growth plate that may be unilateral or bilateral. It presents initially in two different age groups, childhood and adolescence.

If untreated, infantile tibia vara is almost always progressive; along with the varus, it includes flexion and internal rotation and often increased lateral knee laxity. Radiographs demonstrate progressive depression of the medial metaphysis, growth plate, and epiphysis. Eventually, the medial metaphysis fuses to the epiphysis in severe cases. A helpful early distinction unique to tibia vara is the focal nature of the change (Fig. 105-6), with sharp angulation of the *proximal* tibial metaphysis, resulting in a metaphyseal-diaphyseal angle of 11 to 16 degrees or more. This is a specific sign because such localized angulation occurs in fewer than 5% of children with *physiologic* varus, but in essentially all cases of Blount disease (20).

Treatment with a night brace, although not scientifically proven to be effective, is usually used for the mild but definite cases of Blount disease up until about age 3 years. Valgus-rotational osteotomy of the tibia is indicated if the angulation progresses, if growth plate depression occurs, and if the patient is older than 3 years. Recurrence is a risk if treatment begins after 4 years of age, if the epiphysis is fragmented, or if the child is obese. Persistent varus leads to early knee arthritis.

Adolescent tibia vara has onset after 9 years of age. It is to be distinguished from persistent cases of infantile tibia vara. It is most common in obese males. It is believed to be due to decreased growth of the medial tibial physis from excessive medial stresses. Radiographs show medial femoral and tibial bowing. Treatment is osteotomy to realign the limb, or closure of the lateral growth plate to allow catch-up growth medially.

The knee goes through a series of phases of normal alignment. Varus is common before age 2. *Valgus* of the knee is normal after age 2, reaches a mean of 12 degrees at 3 years, and remains at a mean of approximately 7 degrees in boys and 9 degrees in girls after 8 years of age. If valgus remains over 15 degrees at 10 years, early growth plate stapling or later osteotomy of the affected region may be

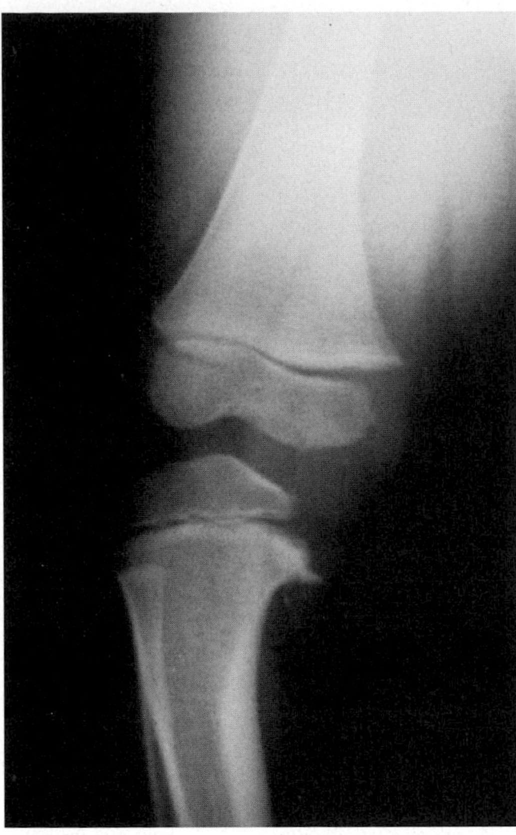

FIGURE 105-6. Infantile tibia vara is characterized by focal depression of the medial proximal tibia.

indicated to prevent patellofemoral problems and degenerative changes. Valgus of the proximal tibia often develops after medial tibial metaphyseal fractures, but it usually spontaneously corrects at least partially.

Hip

Developmental Dysplasia of the Hip

The hip develops from a common cartilage anlage resulting from reciprocal contact between the femur and acetabulum during growth. Loss of this contact may occur at any point in development as a result of abnormal in utero positioning; neuromuscular abnormalities such as myelodysplasia, arthrogryposis, and Larsen syndrome; or intrinsic abnormalities in the connective tissue. The earlier this loss of relationship occurs, the more severe are the femoral and acetabular abnormalities; the earlier it is corrected, the more the remodeling potential and the better the potential outcome.

The etiology of dislocation of the hip in an otherwise normal child is multifactorial. Mechanical factors play a role, and the frequency is greatly increased in breech presentation [a factor in 30% of all developmental dysplasia of the hip (DDH)], in firstborn children, and in oligohydramnios. Breech position causes the hip to be hyperflexed and the muscle forces to be increased, causing the femur to be directed out over the edge of the acetabulum. The left hip is slightly more commonly involved than the right. These factors are associated with increased force across the hip, positioning, or both. Hormonal factors may play a role because there is generalized ligamentous laxity around the time of birth due to increased circulating estrogens and relaxin. The incidence of DDH is sixfold greater in girls than in boys. Evidence for hereditary control of these and other factors is that more than 20% of patients have a positive family history.

There are three degrees of hip dysplasia—subluxable, dislocatable, and dislocated hips—in order of increasing severity. In the first type (subluxable), the femoral head rests in the acetabulum and can be partially dislocated by examination. A dislocatable hip is also located normally when at rest, but it can be fully dislocated. A dislocated hip rests in the dislocated position. The combined incidence of these three types is about 1 in 60 births; incidence of a true dislocation is only 1.5 in 1,000. Because of this variability, a change in terminology from congenital dislocation to developmental dysplasia of the hip has become widely accepted. *Dysplasia* better describes the *spectrum* of severity, from malformation to dislocation of the hip. *Developmental* is meant to acknowledge that some cases are not detectable at birth and may occur later; the anatomic findings are continually evolving. The pathologic anatomy includes laxity of the capsulae, which progresses to capsular contraction with time if the hip remains out. The acetabulum becomes shallow because of lack of concentric contact with the femoral head. A false acetabulum may form where the femoral head contacts the lateral wall of the ilium above the normal location. The outer rim of the acetabulum becomes rounded during the period when the femoral head is able to slide in and out of the acetabulum. The movement over this ridge is felt as the "clunk" of the Ortolani and Barlow tests. The proximal femur remains anteriorly rotated (anteverted) as the head rests against the lateral iliac wall.

Physical examination remains the most important means of diagnosis. A general rule is that the signs in the newborn period usually consist of instability without significant fixed deformity, whereas in the later months an untreated dislocation becomes more fixed, and there is less instability and more limitation of certain motions. The Barlow and Ortolani signs should be sought in the newborn (Fig. 105-7). A positive Barlow sign consists of the ability to dislocate the hip; a positive Ortolani sign is the ability to relocate the hip with easy physical manipulation. When performing the tests, the child should be relaxed by keeping him or her warm and on the parent's lap, and using a pacifier. Only one hip should be examined at a time. The pelvis should be held by one hand of the examiner, whereas the other hand controls the femur with fingers on the greater and lesser trochanters. With adduction

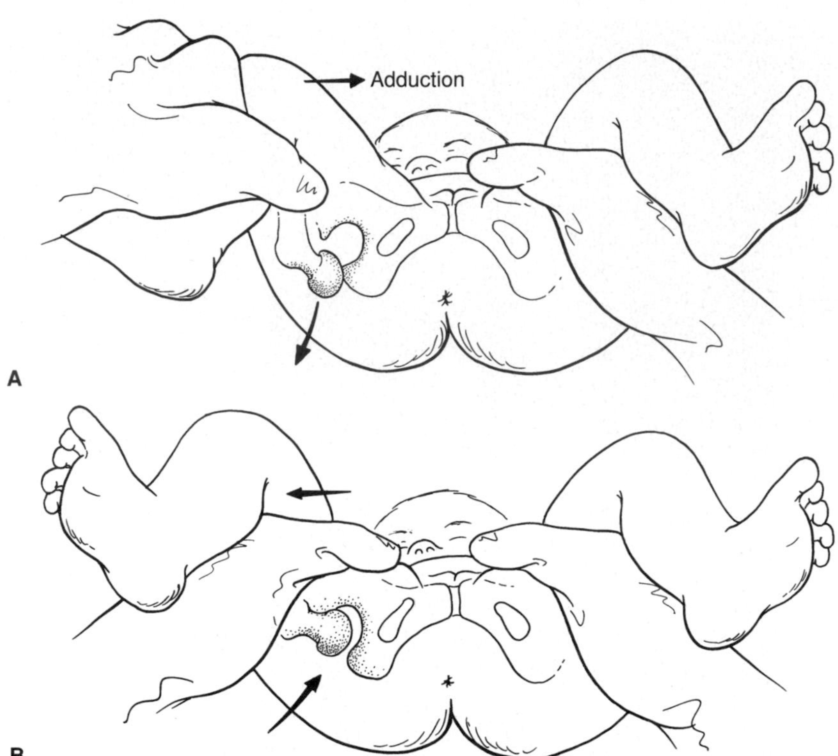

FIGURE 105-7. Examination of the hip for developmental dysplasia of the hip. **(A)** Barlow sign, or subluxation with adduction and axial pressure. **(B)** Ortolani sign, or reduction of the hip with abduction.

and posteriorly directed pressure, the femur can be felt to slide posterosuperiorly over the deformed acetabulum in the abnormal hip (Barlow sign; Fig. 105-5A) and back in with abduction, causing a dull clunk (Ortolani sign; Fig. 105-5B). Thus these signs, dislocation and relocation, are both aspects of the same condition of hip instability.

Possible errors include examining both hips at once, which impairs proprioception, and mistaking insignificant soft-tissue "clicks" for the more important and palpable "clunk." These innocent clicks may be due to movement of fascia over the greater trochanter, clicking of the meniscus or the patella, or the stretch of a normal labrum.

Routine screening of neonates since the 1970s has resulted in a dramatic increase in early diagnosis of DDH (21), and thus more successful treatment (22). Approximately 60% of all unstable newborn hips spontaneously become normal within the first 2 to 4 weeks as perinatal laxity resolves. A severely dysplastic hip may have a negative examination due to lack of an acetabular shelf. It is important to stress, however, that not all hips are reducible at birth. This is presumably because of development of dislocation earlier in utero, with evolution of fixed-joint contractures. Similarly, it is believed that a few cases of dysplasia may develop after birth. In most large series, it has been shown that not all abnormal hips can be detected by screening, even by skilled examiners (23). This is because the physical findings are variable and may fall within the range of normal. If the hip remains dislocated, contractures develop, so by the age of about 6 months most cases cannot be relocated on physical examination in the awake patient. Findings of asymmetry, such as limitation of abduction and of full extension, as well as apparent shortening of the thigh, are more sensitive at this time. This last sign, known as the Allis or Galeazzi sign, is noted by comparing the lengths of the two flexed thighs when held together. Asymmetry of skin folds by itself is unreliable and not a highly specific sign, although it is a supportive finding. When the child begins to walk, a positive Trendelenburg sign is noted during gait: When weight is borne on the dislocated side during gait, the pelvis inclines downward, dropping on the other side. Pain is not present, and walking may begin at about the normal age.

The surgeon should be especially alert to the possibility of DDH in children with connective tissue disorders, genetic syndromes, or neuromuscular disease.

Except in teratologic conditions, radiographs are not commonly used before 6 months of age because interpretation is more difficult during this time; physical examination remains more reliable. Many centers are using ultrasonography as an objective tool, but interpretation requires much experience and should be performed by a pediatric radiologist or orthopedist who is familiar with the technique. Ultrasound is indicated for diagnosis if the neonatal examination is abnormal or questionable, as well as to guide initial treatment (22) (Fig. 105-8A and 105-8B). As the infant grows, plain films may more clearly show cephalad and lateral migration of the femur with a break in the Shenton line (Fig. 105-6C), delayed appearance of the femoral ossific nucleus, a shallow and more vertical acetabulum, and, later, formation of a false acetabulum.

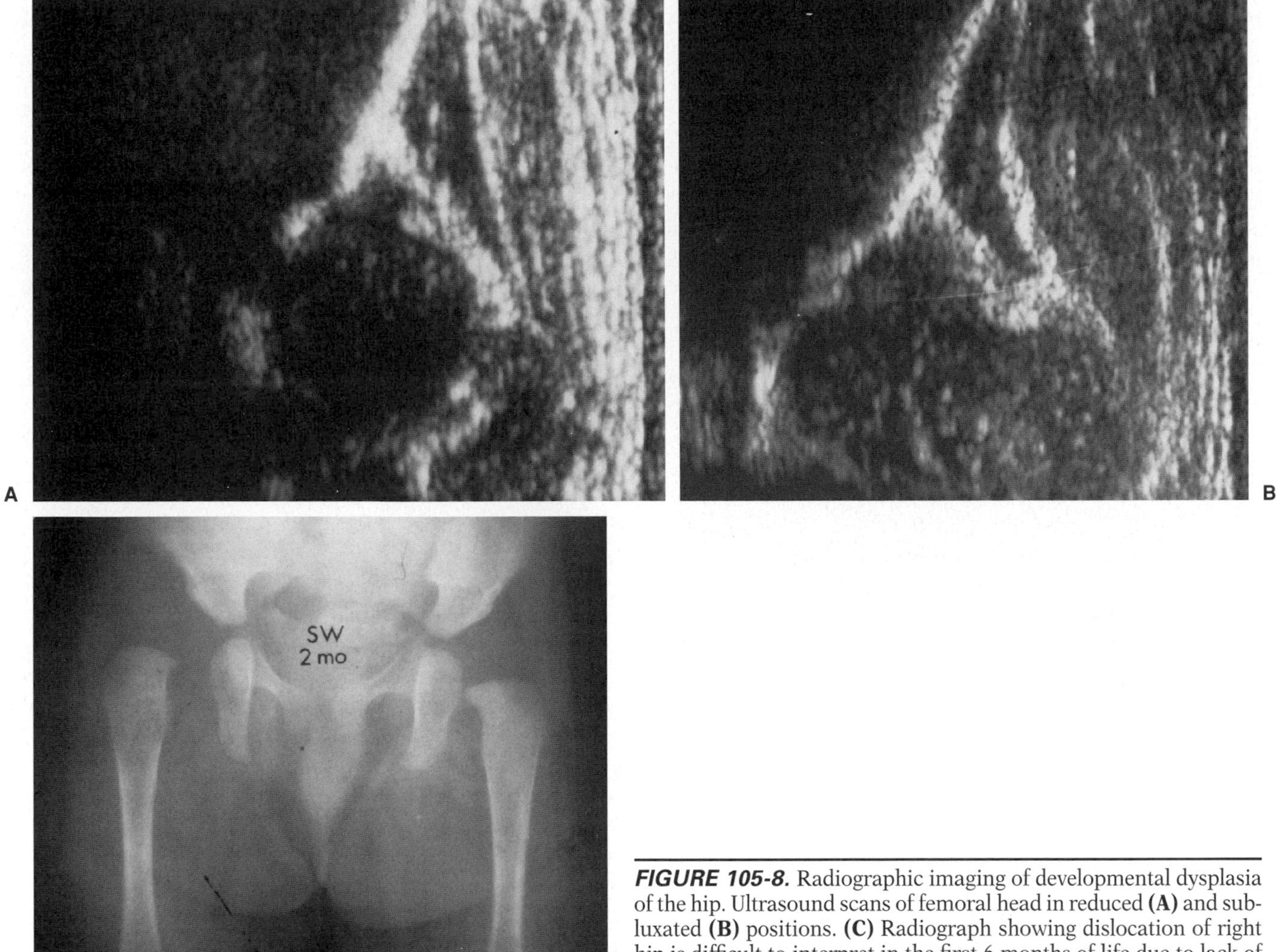

FIGURE 105-8. Radiographic imaging of developmental dysplasia of the hip. Ultrasound scans of femoral head in reduced **(A)** and subluxated **(B)** positions. **(C)** Radiograph showing dislocation of right hip is difficult to interpret in the first 6 months of life due to lack of ossification of epiphysis.

Treatment involves different measures at different ages. The aim of these measures is to restore contact between femoral head and acetabulum. Because a high percentage of patients experience spontaneous improvement of lax hip capsules in the early perinatal period, most orthopedists recommend observation of a mild subluxable type of hip, with reexamination at 3 weeks. Dislocated hips are treated at the time of diagnosis. An abduction-flexion device such as a Pavlik harness is most often used. This allows some motion while maintaining the appropriate femoral-acetabular contact. The alignment should be checked by ultrasound or radiography in 1 to 2 weeks (23). The brace is worn until the clinical and radiologic examinations are normal, a duration approximately equal to one to two times the child's age at diagnosis. If treatment is begun *after* 6 months of age, the child is usually too large and active to tolerate the brace. Then reduction must be preceded by traction to bring the femoral head *down* toward the acetabulum, decreasing the muscle forces that could contribute to avascular necrosis. A manipulative (closed) reduction is thus attempted under general anesthetic (24). If closed reduction is not successful, open surgical reduction should be carried out. This involves tightening the lax superior capsule and releasing the tight psoas tendon and inferior capsule, allowing the femoral head to be brought down to its appropriate location.

If there is extensive bony deformation, such as a shallow acetabulum or rotated femur, a femoral or pelvic osteotomy and open reduction might be indicated. This is more common after the age of 2 years.

Possible complications include persistent dysplasia from failure of normal development, redislocation, and avascular necrosis of the femoral head. The last condition is due to impairment of the epiphyseal vessels by excess pressure or capsular stretch. It is the most serious complication. Its occurrence is more likely if the hip is reduced under excessive tension or if excessive abduction is used.

The earlier treatment is carried out, the better is the resultant hip development and the safer each of the steps in treatment. Early detection, when possible, can decrease the need for complex orthopedic procedures later.

Transient (toxic) synovitis of the hip is a diagnosis of exclusion; it is a self-limited condition that is the most common cause of an irritable hip in children. The usual presentation is a painful limp or hip pain of acute or insidious onset, usually occurring unilaterally. The most common ages are 2 to 6 years, but patients from 1 to 15 years have been reported (25). There is moderate spasm on testing of hip range of motion, particularly internal rotation. Temperature, white blood cell count, C-reactive protein, and erythrocyte sedimentation rate may be normal or slightly elevated. The etiology is unknown; an immune mechanism and viral infection have been postulated. Some examples of viral-associated anthropathy have been described. Differential diagnosis should include septic arthritis, osteomyelitis, and Legg-Calvé-Perthes disease, which usually has a subchondral crescent of lucency or further changes in the femoral head on radiograph. Juvenile rheumatoid monarthritis and slipped capital femoral epiphysis should also be considered. Admission to hospital, observation, and early aspiration should be performed if septic arthritis cannot be ruled out. Treatment consists of bed rest with oral analgesics as needed for 2 to 7 days. This can sometimes be performed on an outpatient basis with frequent follow-up if septic arthritis is ruled out. Persistence of symptoms beyond 1 week should prompt the physician to perform reevaluation, although persistence of symptoms for as long as 1 month has occasionally been reported.

Legg-Calvé-Perthes disease was first differentiated from tuberculosis within a decade after clinical use of radiography at the turn of the century, but its etiology is still unknown. This disorder consists of ischemia of the proximal femoral epiphysis (26). The amount of the femoral epiphysis rendered ischemic is variable and affects the outcome. The ischemia is followed by resorption, then reossification with or without collapse of the femoral head. It most commonly affects children 4 to 8 years old, although exceptions are often seen. Males are affected four times as often as females. Affected patients as a group have slightly shorter stature and delayed bone age compared with peers. Fifteen percent of cases are bilateral, although both sides are not usually affected at the same time.

Clinical presentation is usually a limp, such as abductor lurch, with minimal pain of either short or long duration. The pain is not as acute or severe as that of transient synovitis or septic arthritis. Motions that are especially limited are internal rotation and abduction of the hip. Internal rotation is performed with the patient supine, the hip flexed, measuring the angle to which the leg may be rotated laterally. These movements may be resisted by mild spasm or guarding. At the earliest stage, radiographs may be normal or may reveal the slightly smaller size of the affected femoral epiphysis compared with the other side due to its temporary inhibition of growth (27,28). Later, there may be a narrow crescentic lucency, best seen on the lateral view (28), which is due to a microfracture of the bone just underneath the joint surface. This reveals the extent of bone involved. In some cases, revascularization may occur without collapse of the epiphysis, but in others, revascularization of the femoral head is accompanied by progressive resorption and deformation (Fig. 105-9). Reossification follows, and the femoral head continues to grow. Whether this further growth occurs spherically

A

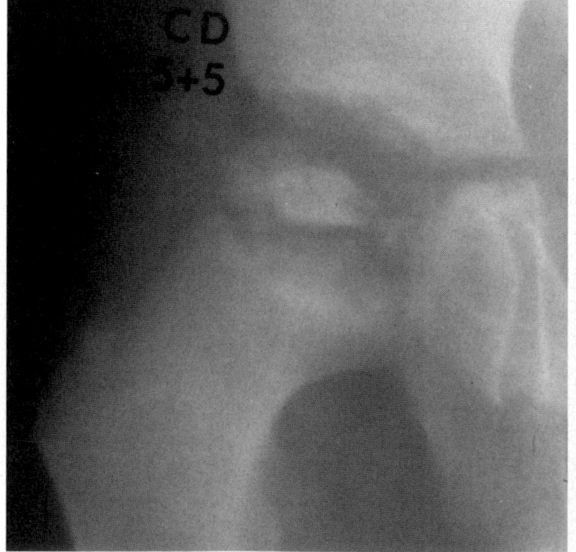

B

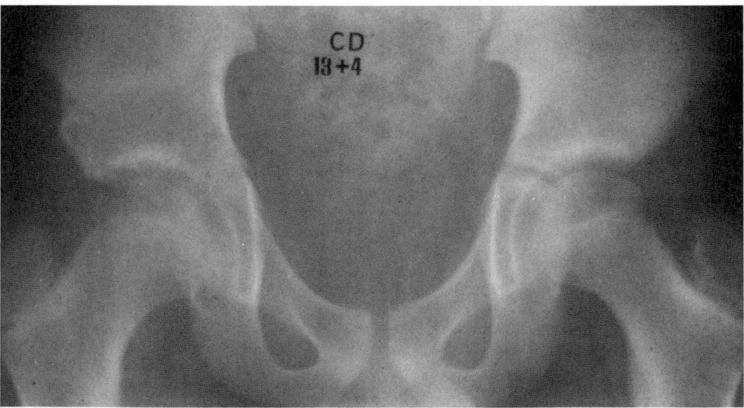

FIGURE 105-9. Legg-Calvé-Perthes disease is manifested radiographically by fragmentation and collapse of the femoral head during the initial phase of the disorder **(A)**. Later, reossification takes place and can lead to a more spherical femoral head **(B)**.

depends on the patient's age, the amount of collapse, and the method of treatment.

Differential diagnosis should include transient synovitis, septic arthritis, hematogenous osteomyelitis, sickle cell infarct, hemoglobinopathies, steroid-induced necrosis, Gaucher's disease, hypothyroidism, and the epiphyseal dysplasias. The last two are often synchronous bilaterally, whereas Legg-Calvé-Perthes is not. Avascular necrosis may also be a serious complication of femoral neck fracture or hip dislocation.

Treatment follows two principles: containment of the femoral head within the acetabulum and maintenance of range of motion. In the early stages of Perthes disease, the avascular portion of the femoral head is less likely to become deformed and more likely to regrow spherically if contained within the mold of the acetabulum by abduction. Children younger than 6 years of age or with involvement of less than one-half of the femoral head may be followed without active treatment if a full range of motion is preserved; patients in this age group have a good prognosis.(26) More aggressive treatment is indicated in patients with involvement of more than one-half of the femoral head or age older than 6 years.

Containment may be achieved by a brace or by surgery. The most commonly employed brace is the Scottish Rite brace, which holds the legs abducted and does not extend below the knees. The child may be allowed to play in the brace. The brace should be worn until early reossification of the femoral head occurs. Surgical treatment is used if a brace is not accepted because of the size of the child, an anticipated long duration of wear (up to 18 months in the older child), or lack of acceptance. Either a femoral osteotomy to redirect the involved portion within the acetabulum or an innominate osteotomy to better redirect the acetabulum may be performed. The two procedures have approximately equal results. Treatment of avascular necrosis that occurs after femoral neck fracture or dislocation follows similar principles and has a poorer prognosis with increasing age of the child.

Slipped Capital Femoral Epiphysis

Slipped capital femoral epiphysis (SCFE) is a disorder of mechanical overload of the growth plate that occurs near the age of skeletal maturity; it involves a three-dimensional displacement of the epiphysis posteriorly, medially, and inferiorly. In other words, the lower femur is externally rotated from under the head of the femur. The etiology seems to involve mechanical and biological factors. SCFE usually occurs without severe sudden force or trauma. Mechanically, there is increased stress because of obesity in most affected children and because of abnormal retroversion (posterior rotation) of the femoral head and neck. The periosteum and growth plate at this age are thin and less able to resist the shearing forces. Possible biological factors include delayed growth plate maturation and hormonal factors that may be related to the obesity. Increased growth hormone has been associated with decreased physeal shear strength, and hypothyroidism has been found in some cases. SCFE usually occurs during the growth spurt and before menarche in girls. SCFE is uncommon, with a frequency of 1 to 10 per 100,000. It is more common in males and in blacks. Approximately on-fourth to one-third of affected children have bilateral involvement (29), but not usually simultaneously.

Clinical presentation varies with the acuity of the process. Most children with subacute or chronic SCFE present with a limp or pain or both. The discomfort may be in the groin, but is very often referred to the thigh or knee. Many patients with thigh or knee complaints are dismissed when no cause is found, only to have the true hip pathology discovered later when the slip worsens. This paradoxical pain distribution is due to referral within the cutaneous distribution of the femoral nerve, which also involves both the hip and knee joints. Other patients have a more acute, sudden presentation, usually following mild-to-moderate trauma, with severe pain and inability to walk or move the hip. This is more like an acute growth plate fracture. Again, abduction, internal rotation, and flexion are the motions most limited. The involved hip is externally rotated at rest compared with the opposite side. There may be mild limb shortening because of the upward displacement of the metaphysis.

The first radiographic findings are widening and irregularity of the growth plate and osteopenia of the femur (Fig. 105-10). Later, there is displacement of the epiphysis posteriorly, inferiorly, and medially. This is best seen on the frog-leg lateral radiograph of the pelvis. A line on the AP film drawn through the upper margin of the narrowest portion of the neck should intersect at least 20% of the epiphysis after age 10 years. This is an important point because with the remodeling that occurs in a chronic slip,

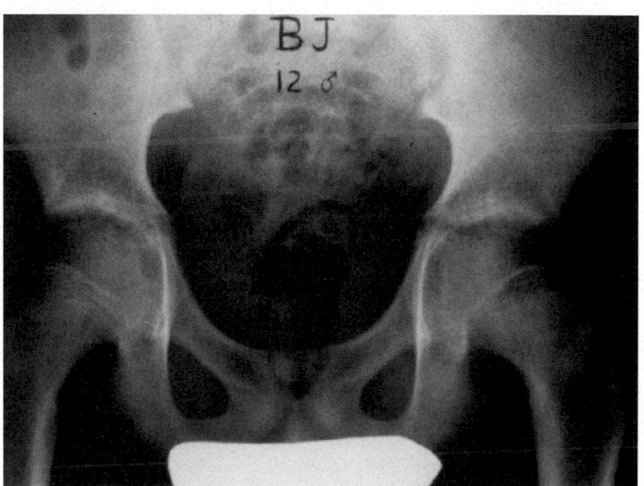

FIGURE 105-10. A slipped capital femoral epiphysis is present on the left hip in this radiograph, as manifested by a widening of the growth plate and slight inferior displacement of the epiphysis.

there may not be an obvious step-off at the junction of epiphysis and metaphysis or a gap to suggest a fracture. The severity of the slip is graded as mild (less than 33%), moderate (33% to 50%), or severe (more than 50%). Later changes may include avascular necrosis of the epiphysis (seen in 5% to 10%) or chondrolysis, that is, joint space narrowing (seen in 1% to 2%).

Treatment is to prevent further slip, usually by immediately placing the patient at bed rest and arranging prompt orthopedic consultation. The patient should not be allowed to go home once the diagnosis is made. Surgical management is intended to stabilize the upper femur and cause closure of the weakened growth plate. Realignment of the slip and femoral head is not safe in chronic cases because this may produce avascular necrosis by disrupting the blood supply to the epiphysis. The gold standard of treatment is fixation in situ with a screw. Long-term follow-up shows some remodeling of the slip. The screw should not penetrate into the joint. Open epiphyseal fusion using bone graft avoids the risk of pin penetration and produces more rapid growth plate closure (29), but it is a longer surgical procedure and requires cast stabilization in acute slips. Osteotomy of the femoral neck to correct the deformity has been occasionally performed, but it carries a risk of avascular necrosis. Later, osteotomy at the subtrochanteric level, away from the vessels serving the epiphysis, will produce realignment, but it might make later hip replacement, if this should become necessary, more difficult by changing the shape of the proximal femur. The contralateral hip should also be monitored for SCFE and fixed early if symptoms occur. Long-term follow-up shows no early degenerative change unless chondrolysis or avascular necrosis occurs; each has an incidence of 1% to 5%. Later arthritis in middle age is still more common than in persons without history of SCFE.

Femoral anteversion is one of several rotational deformities that affect the alignment of the knee and foot with the body. Other causes of in-toeing include internal tibial torsion and foot deformity such as metatarsus adductus. Increased anteversion of the femur is defined as an increase in the angle between (forward rotation of) the plane of the femoral neck and the plane of the posterior femoral condyles. This normally declines with age. The pressure of the anterior hip capsule as the child stands upright causes the change. Increased femoral anteversion persists in some neuromuscular conditions because of a lack of these remodeling forces. The type discussed here is idiopathic femoral anteversion.

On physical examination, the patient appears to toe in. The patellae also face medially. Internal rotation of the hip is much greater than external rotation. Anteversion is not usually clinically noticeable or significant unless external rotation at the hip is less than 15 degrees.

On radiographs, the femoral head and neck appear to be in valgus on an AP film. CT scan is best for directly quantitating femoral anteversion in the infrequent situations where this is necessary.

The natural history of femoral anteversion is benign. Anteversion later in life has been found to be unrelated to arthritis of the hip or knee. Anteversion does not impair function or athletic skills. Treatment of increased anteversion consists of observation at least until age 8 and prevention of W-sitting, which may impair remodeling. The child should instead sit in a chair or in the tailor position. Braces employing cables and bars are not effective in derotating the femur; no orthotic method of treatment affects anteversion. In fact, most of these children need no treatment. Femoral osteotomy, proximally or distally, is the only truly effective treatment. It is rarely needed, however, and only in children older than 8 years who have functional disability due to patellar malalignment, or, rarely, persistent concern with appearance.

Spine

Back problems in children generally fall into two categories: spinal deformity and back pain. When these conditions exist in the same child, one must first determine the cause of the pain before treating the deformity (Fig. 105-11).

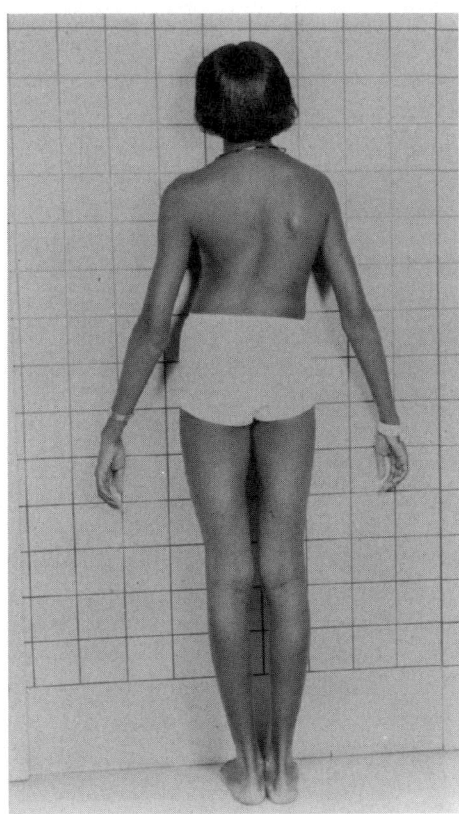

FIGURE 105-11. Physical findings in scoliosis include asymmetry of the shoulders, scapulae, and waistline, as well as a midline curve in the spine itself.

Childhood Back Pain

Back pain in a child is often indicative of a problem that requires further attention and evaluation. Lower back pain in the adult age group is very common and often has no demonstrated etiology, but approximately 75% of pediatric cases are found to have a definite cause. Factors that increase the index of suspicion for a serious problem include interference with school or play, need for medication, or age younger than 4 years. Careful neurologic examination is a must when evaluating children for back pain, as is an assessment of spinal flexibility and deformity. The differential diagnoses provided in the following sections are the most commonly encountered conditions.

Musculoligamentous Pain

All components of a child's spine—discs, ligaments, muscles, and joint capsules—are flexible and conform easily to spinal positions encountered daily in the schoolyard or playing field. After about the age of 12, the spine generally loses some of its flexibility, and during the teenage years, further stiffening may take place. In children younger than age 10, muscular or ligamentous back pain is rare. This diagnosis should be reserved for the older child, who may be involved in a new physical activity and who has pain in the lumbar area for which no other specific cause can be determined. This is really a presumptive diagnosis. To merit this diagnosis, the child should have pain localized to the lumbar area, a normal neurologic examination, normal radiographs of the lumbar spine, and, in some instances, a normal bone scan.

Once the diagnosis of musculoligamentous pain has been made, the treatment is rest from any activity that causes pain. Use of ice or heat is efficacious. Once the pain has resolved, exercises to strengthen the abdominal and lumbar muscles should be used before returning to sports. A lumbosacral corset may be worn in the acute stage and thereafter when participating in sports to protect the lower back and its muscles from extremes of spinal movement. A long-term corset or other brace is rarely needed if this diagnosis is correct. Once lower back pain has resolved, it is important to stress to the child that warming up prior to sports activity is more necessary for him or her than for other children. Exercises may need to be continued indefinitely. Persistence of pain should lead to a search for further unusual causes of back pain.

Spondylolysis and Spondylolisthesis

Spondylolysis, a relatively common cause of childhood back pain, is usually a stress fracture of the pars interarticularis of the vertebra (30). This thin segment of bone between the facet joints is subjected to high forces, especially with marked lordosis of the lumbar spine or with heavy lifting. The overall incidence in the general population is about 6%. Most of these stress fractures probably occur in early school years, although symptoms appear most frequently when the children are in their early teens. There is a much higher frequency of spondylolysis in children who participate in gymnastics, wrestling, and weight lifting, at times approaching 20% of participants in these sports.

Symptoms most commonly are pain in the lumbar area after or during a sports activity and a concomitant limitation of lumbar spine motion. If the child has a chronic spondylolysis, the pain is often intermittent; if the spondylolysis is acute, the pain is more severe. Radiation of pain along the sciatic nerve distribution into the lateral calf or dorsum of the foot may occasionally be present.

Physical examination may not be remarkable. Usually, there is limitation of lateral spine flexion toward the side of the spondylolysis, often associated with limited forward flexion from back pain. Back pain may be produced by straight leg raising, but radiation of pain into the legs by this maneuver is rare. Neurologic examination is normal.

The diagnosis can usually be made by lumbar spine radiographs (Fig. 105-12). The most common location is at L5, with L4 the next most common. Spondylolysis can sometimes be visualized by the lateral view, but oblique views are usually more definitive. In addition, the oblique views allow one to determine the unilaterality or bilaterality of the defect. If a lytic defect is observed, the age of the lesion should be determined as possible. The spondylolysis is generally old if there are sclerotic edges to the defect. Spondylolysis may occasionally be caused by acute trauma in the adolescent, but more often this represents a

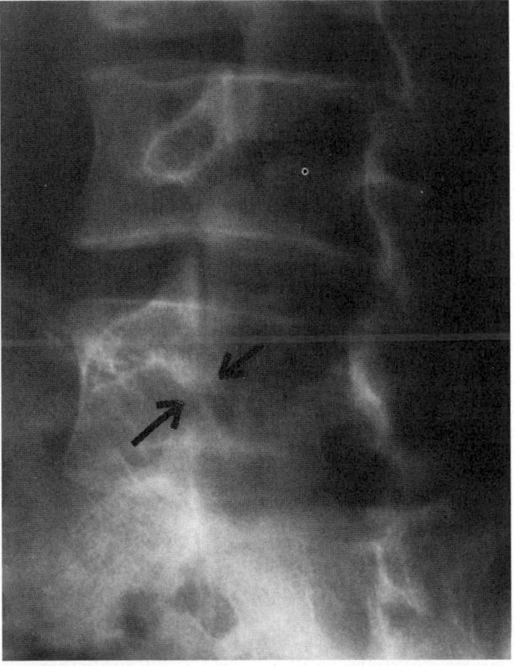

FIGURE 105-12. Spondylolysis is shown radiographically as a break in the pars interarticularis of the vertebra (*arrows*) on this oblique radiograph.

preexisting lesion that is simply brought out by the trauma. A technetium-99 bone scan with collimated views is helpful to determine the age of the stress fracture. If the scan is cold and sclerotic edges are present on radiograph, the lesion is old and it will not be possible to obtain bone union nonoperatively. However, if the scan shows increased uptake at the lytic area and the radiographs show no sclerotic edges, there may be enough reparative activity that the stress fractures might heal if the child is placed in a body jacket brace or cast.

If the scan shows no increased uptake, the treatment of spondylolysis is much like that of a musculoligamentous problem (30). Rest from activity is recommended. A lumbosacral corset is often helpful for a few weeks until pain resolves. Some teenagers with spondylolysis prefer to wear the corset during sports activities as added protection even after acute back pain resolves. Fusion for spondylolysis without significant spondylolisthesis is generally not needed. With the exception of occasional episodes of lower back pain, teenagers can be allowed to participate in sports if they do not repeatedly experience back pain after playing.

Spondylolisthesis follows spondylolysis in some children. This condition is a forward slip of a superior vertebra on the inferior vertebra, most commonly a slip of L5 on the sacrum. Worsening of this slip may occur with growth of the spine, and there is generally little worsening once growth is completed. As the vertebra slips forward, the posterior elements remain behind, attached to the adjacent vertebrae by their ligaments. The combination of excessive motion of the posterior elements and the forward vertebral slip may lead to irritation of L5 or S1 nerve roots. Because the slip is usually slow, the nerve root irritation may present only as progressive tightness of the hamstrings, manifested by difficulty in touching the toes or in reaching objects on the floor. If one side of the spine is affected more than the other, scoliosis may also be present.

On physical examination, the main finding is limitation of straight leg raising because of the hamstring spasm. Radiation of pain into the calf or foot with straight leg raising may indicate more advanced nerve root irritation. Rarely, the ankle jerk reflex may be diminished.

The diagnosis of spondylolisthesis can be made by plain radiographs and is most easily seen on the lateral view. The amount of slip should be quantified using the terms grade 1 to grade 4 (grade 1, up to 25%; grade 2, up to 50%; and so forth). If the slip is greater than 50%, posterior spinal fusion of the involved level is indicated. If the slip is less than 50%, initial management is directed to relief of back pain and hamstring spasm, using rest and corset therapy followed by exercises as with spondylolysis. If the pain does not respond to conservative treatment, fusion may be needed. If the pain improves with conservative treatment, follow-up lateral lumbosacral radiographs at 6- to 9-month intervals are recommended until growth is complete or until a worsening slip can be identified. If there is an increase in the percentage of slip, fusion is indicated.

If a child does not have hamstring tightness and is pain free, there is usually no need to restrict activities, provided the child and the parents are aware that periodic low-grade back pain is likely. There is no evidence that increased physical activity causes an increase in vertebral slip.

Intervertebral Disc Herniation (Herniated Nucleus Pulposus)

Herniation of the intervertebral disc is common in the young and middle-age adult as a cause of back and leg pain. In this adult age group, disc protrusion occurs posteriorly, with the protruded disc compressing the nerve roots or the cauda equina. If similar forces are applied to the spine of a skeletally immature child, the disc does not rupture posteriorly, but the stress leads to a fracture of the growth plate of the vertebral body, causing extrusion of disc material anteriorly or into the vertebral body itself (Schmorl nodes). Most of these children present with back pain without radiation into the lower leg or calf. If nerve root pain also occurs, a small avulsion fracture of the ring apophysis posterolaterally might be present in such a position to cause nerve root compression. The diagnosis of an old disc injury in a child can be confirmed by radiographic findings of a narrowed lumbar disc adjacent to an irregular vertebral end plate.

If no neurologic defect is present, treatment consists of symptomatic care, usually rest, until the pain resolves. If the condition is the result of a vehicular accident, evaluation for development of an ileus should be performed. If there is leg pain as well as back pain, a magnetic resonance imaging (MRI) scan or CT/myelogram should be performed to localize any neural compression, which may be relieved by surgical treatment, with 90% satisfactory results after 5 years.

Discitis

Severe back pain with limitation of back movements is common in the older child, whereas the younger children may simply present with stiffness, refusal to walk, or limping. Bacterial infection is the most commonly suspected cause. Just as in long bones in children, the vascular anatomy of the growing disc varies from that of the adult, and common bacteremias of childhood can more readily infect the disc than the vertebral body itself. Approximately 50% of these children have positive blood cultures at the time of their acute pain, the most common organism being *Staphylococcus aureus*. Despite this, discitis in its milder forms often appears to resolve without the need for antibiotics.

On physical examination, the most common finding is marked stiffness of the spine on forward bending. Abdominal pain or guarding may occur. Fever is often present.

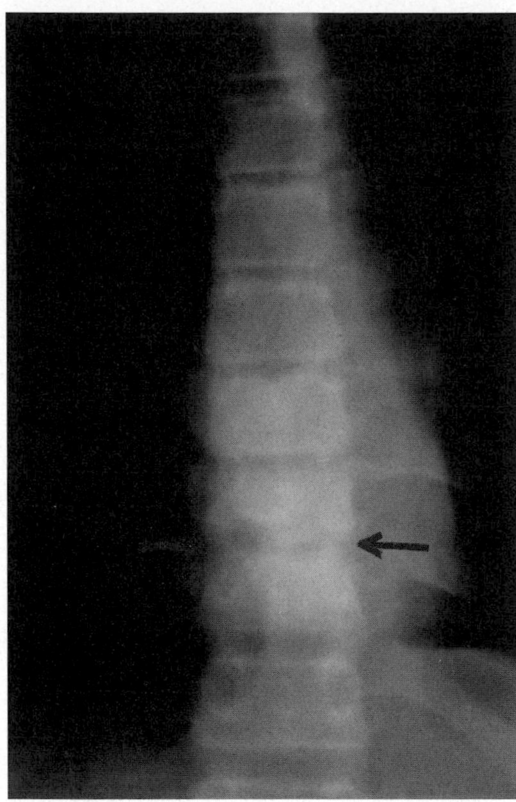

FIGURE 105-13. Discitis, in the advanced stages, may be indicated by sclerosis and narrowing of the intervertebral disc as seen here at T10 to T11 (*arrow*).

Neurological examination is normal. Early in the course, radiographs of the spine are normal. Technetium-99 bone scan shows increased uptake at the involved disc early on, before radiographic changes are seen; this scan should be performed whenever discitis is suspected. A few weeks after onset of pain, sclerosis and narrowing of a single disc may be seen on radiograph (Fig. 105-13). The lumbar or thoracic spine may be involved. The sedimentation rate and white blood cell count are often elevated. If the bone scan is positive or the clinical presentation is usual for discitis, needle aspiration or open biopsy of the involved disc is generally not necessary.

Treatment options include antibiotics, bed rest, and body brace or cast, depending on the severity of findings at presentation. If a positive blood culture has been obtained, antibiotics should be given for 3 to 6 weeks. The author's preference is to give antibiotics in children with a positive bone scan, even if no bacteremia has been demonstrated. Bed rest may be helpful as an adjunct if there is severe pain or spasm. If the spasm persists for more than a few days, a trunk brace or cast relieves symptoms by immobilizing the spine and allowing ambulation on a limited basis. The infection is usually cleared with 6 to 8 weeks of treatment. Discitis rarely develops into vertebral osteomyelitis with local bone destruction.

Spinal Cord Tumors

Back pain and limitation of spine movement may also be seen as the presenting problem in spinal cord tumors, even without a neurologic deficit. In spinal cord tumors, the presenting complaint is back pain or scoliosis or both in almost one-third of children. The most striking finding on the physical examination is severe limitation of forward flexion of the spine. Pain may be worsened by neck flexion. Neurologic changes may be very subtle and difficult to detect.

In patients with back pain and marked limitation of spinal motion, especially if scoliosis is also present, an MRI is needed if the bone scan and plain radiographs do not elucidate the cause.

The most common tumor to present in this fashion is an ependymoma. Treatment is neurosurgical. If the tumor is benign and can be removed, the pain, scoliosis, and back stiffness generally resolve.

Spinal Deformity

Spinal deformity of minor or significant degree occurs in as many as 1 of 20 children. Differentiating those that require treatment is important. Scoliosis, a lateral curvature of the spine, is the most common. The age at development of most spinal curvatures, early adolescence, is a time when parents may not be likely to see the child's back frequently. School screening programs for spinal deformity, mandatory in many states, have served to increase awareness of these conditions. Although school programs are generally targeted toward children in the sixth grade, routine evaluation of the back should also be a feature of each child's annual examination.

Scoliosis

The two forms of scoliosis are postural and structural. *Postural* scoliosis results from factors outside the spine, such as leg length discrepancy. In these cases, if the leg lengths are equalized or if the child sits, the spine becomes straight, indicating that there is no structural abnormality. The more important type of scoliosis is termed *structural*, and it involves not only a lateral spinal curvature, but also a rotation of the vertebrae. Although numerous conditions are associated with scoliosis, the most common causes include idiopathic (80%), congenital (5%), neuromuscular (10%), and miscellaneous (5%). The miscellaneous group includes connective tissue disorders, genetic diseases, and other less common conditions.

Congenital scoliosis is defined as that due to a primary vertebral malformation, such as a hemivertebra or a wedged vertebra. It is present at birth, although the diagnosis is often not made at that time (Fig. 105-14). This may be associated with other birth defects or may be an isolated condition. Because the genitourinary (GU) system arises embryologically from the same region as the spine, about

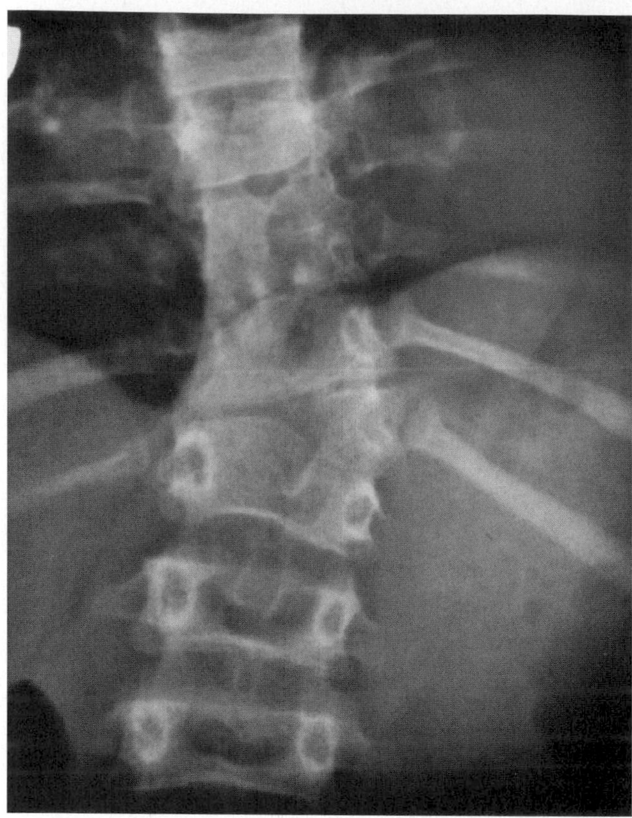

FIGURE 105-14. Congenital scoliosis is due to a primary bony malformation, as shown here by this hemivertebra.

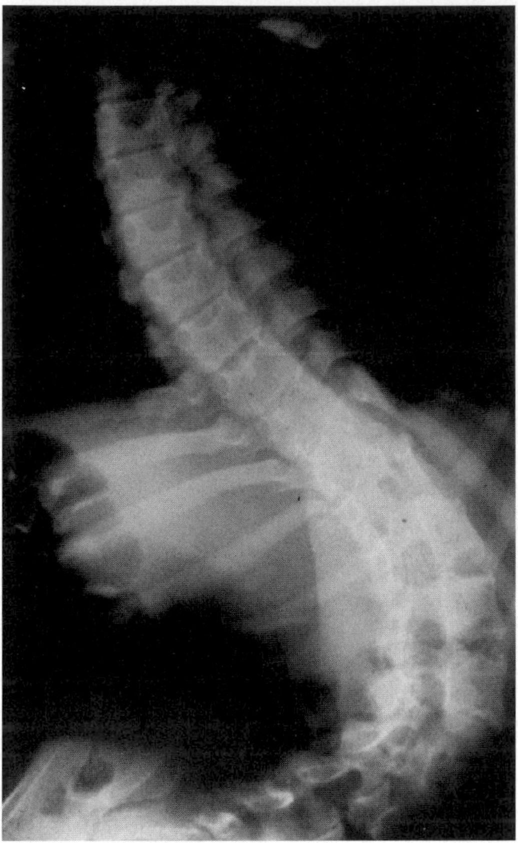

FIGURE 105-15. In neuromuscular scoliosis, there is usually a long, sweeping curve with pelvic obliquity.

30% of children with congenital spinal deformity have an associated GU abnormality. The most common anomaly is unilateral renal agenesis, so a sonogram or intravenous (IV) pyelogram should be performed on all patients with congenital scoliosis or kyphosis. Active treatment of unilateral kidney absence may not be necessary, but appropriate cautions against contact sports that may lead to kidney injury are important. Tracheoesophageal fistula, imperforate anus, and congenital cardiac defects are often associated with congenital scoliosis. These components make up the VATER syndrome, although not all components are seen in every patient. The spine should be examined radiographically early in these patients. Management of congenital scoliosis consists of serial radiographic follow-up every 6 to 12 months to determine if the deformity is worsening. If no increase in the curve occurs, further treatment is generally not needed. If worsening of 5 to 10 degrees or more is documented while there is growth remaining, surgical fusion is necessary, regardless of the child's age. Brace treatment for the congenital scoliosis itself is seldom successful or indicated because a brace cannot change the shape or growth of a malformed vertebra.

Neuromuscular scoliosis is a deformity that may be associated with almost any neurologic or muscular disease that affects the trunk, such as quadriplegic cerebral palsy, muscular dystrophy, high spina bifida, and poliomyelitis. A spinal curvature secondary to muscular imbalance is classically C-shaped and extends to include the pelvis (Fig. 105-15); these features are not commonly seen in idiopathic scoliosis. Scoliosis is more often present and worsens most quickly in patients who arc nonwalkers as a result of their neuromuscular disease. With continued worsening of the curve, sitting balance becomes further impaired, and function may be limited by the need to use one arm or hand to assist in sitting. Treatment centers on preservation of the ability to sit and to be transported, and to minimize decline in pulmonary function. Many of these patients have feeding and swallowing problems, such as malnutrition and reflux with risk of aspiration. It has been shown that prior treatment of these conditions can decrease risk of complications after major spine corrections. Pediatric general surgical consultation is often required. Methods used for feeding may include oral, tube, or gastrotomy feeds or fundoplication or jejunostomy. Although brace wear is often useful, surgical fusion is frequently indicated to preserve function.

Idiopathic scoliosis is generally found in otherwise healthy children. Although idiopathic scoliosis requiring treatment is about eight times more frequent in girls than in boys, the incidence of mild curves is approximately equal between the sexes (30). In other words, girls seem to have more tendency to worsening of the curves.

A family history of curvature of the spine is found in about two-thirds of children with scoliosis, although the exact mode of inheritance has not been determined. The etiology of idiopathic scoliosis remains unknown, but it is currently believed that a combination of neurohormonal and connective tissue factors is important. Scoliosis is also more likely to develop in children who have had thoracotomy, pectus repair, or cardiac surgery. It may develop several years after these index procedures, so the surgeon should examine for this and also alert the pediatrician. Marfan syndrome and neurofibromatosis are also associated with an increased risk of scoliosis and should be ruled out. Curves worsen most during the rapid adolescent growth spurt, a time when most curves are diagnosed. Muscles, discs, and bone appear to be normal in the young idiopathic scoliosis patient.

The key to early detection of scoliosis is to carefully assess the entire trunk for asymmetry. The child should be examined with the back clearly exposed. The examination should include evaluation of shoulder height, scapular position and prominence, waistline symmetry, and level of height of the two sides of the pelvis. Asymmetry in any of these areas may indicate a scoliosis. However, in about 50% of children with uneven shoulder height, no spinal deformity is present on radiograph. To define further whether a structural scoliosis is present, a more sensitive and specific examination is the forward-bend test. The patient should stand with legs straight and together, arms collapsed in front of the body, and slowly bend forward to touch the toes. The examiner, positioned in front and in back of the patient, can see the profile, in sequence, of the thoracic and lumbar regions. It is possible to quantitate the amount of rib prominence by means of an inclinometer placed at the apex of the curve with the child bending forward. If the inclinometer measurement is 5 degrees or less, the scoliosis is rarely significant and radiographs are usually not needed. If the inclinometer reading exceeds 7 degrees, a standing posteroanterior radiograph is indicated for better assessment.

The magnitude of the scoliosis is measured radiographically by the Cobb method. The angle between the end plates of the upper- and lowermost inclined vertebrae is drawn. This measurement should always be performed on a standing spine radiograph (Fig. 105-16). The error of measurement for this method is approximately ± 5 degrees. No active treatment is needed until the curve reaches 25 degrees. During the adolescent growth spurt, maximum annual curve progression is 10 to 15 degrees or about 1 degree per month.

Completion of growth or skeletal maturity can be assessed most accurately by the bone age on radiographs of the hand and wrist. From the clinical standpoint, girls who have been menstruating for 2 years have essentially completed their spinal growth.

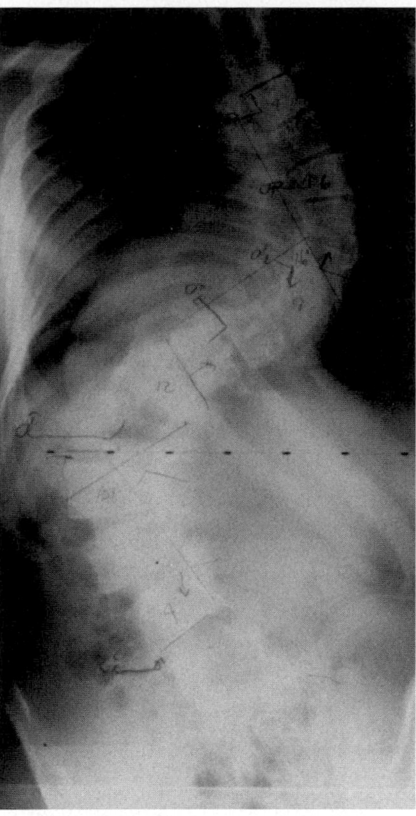

FIGURE 105-16. Typical radiographic appearance of a double major idiopathic scoliosis. Notice that the two curves balance each other, so there is a level pelvis. The curves are 8 to 9 degrees by the Cobb measurement.

Treatment of scoliosis is based on three fundamental principles.

1. Curves of more than 25 degrees are likely to increase if the child is still growing.
2. Curves of more than 40 to 50 degrees are likely to increase even after growth is complete.
3. Some degree of clinically significant pulmonary restriction may begin in association with thoracic curves of more than about 75 degrees.

Therefore, if a child is skeletally mature and has curvature of less than 25 degrees, no further evaluation or treatment of scoliosis is needed. If the scoliosis is 25 degrees or more and the child has growth remaining, brace treatment is generally recommended. It is successful in about 80% of the patients who wear the brace as prescribed. Spinal exercises alone do not stop the curve from worsening. Once brace treatment begins, it is continued until growth is complete. The brace is usually worn 18 to 20 hours daily. There are no limitations of physical activity because of the scoliosis. Success in brace wear is defined as prevention of further increase in the curve progression and not curve correction because long-term follow-up studies have shown that the final curvature size is virtually the same as before brace treatment began. Although the child and parents are often dismayed by the inability to straighten the spine nonoperatively, if curves can be kept to less than 35 to 40 degrees by the completion of growth, most scolioses do not worsen in adult life and do not cause problems. If the thoracic curve is more than 50 degrees or the lumbar curve is more than 40 degrees at the completion of growth, increase in the curve usually continues at the rate of about 1 degree annually, and surgery is usually needed.

Surgical treatment is recommended for curves of more than 40 degrees, particularly if the child is not fully grown. The surgical treatment usually consists of instrumentation (rods) to correct the curved area of the spine, combined with bone graft to promote spinal fusion of the instrumented area (Fig. 105-17). This may be performed anteriorly, posteriorly, or both, according to the judgment of the surgeon. Posterior spine fusion is performed through an incision down the middle of the back and can be extended to include the entire spine, if needed. Anterior fusion is performed through a thoracotomy for thoracic curves and through a retroperitoneal incision for lumbar curves, and may include peripheral detachment of the diaphragm for thoracolumbar curves. Sometimes, if the patient is malnourished or several staged sequential surgeries are planned, central venous hyperalimentation between stages may be used. Correction of the scoliosis is generally possible to about 50% of the initial curve measurement. Ileus is common for a few days after surgery. Failure of fusion occurs in only about 1% of teenagers. Fusion is complete by 6 to 12 months after surgery, at which time the teenager can return to almost all physical activities, except tackle football, wrestling, and gymnastics. Patients should be encouraged to return to activity, including

A

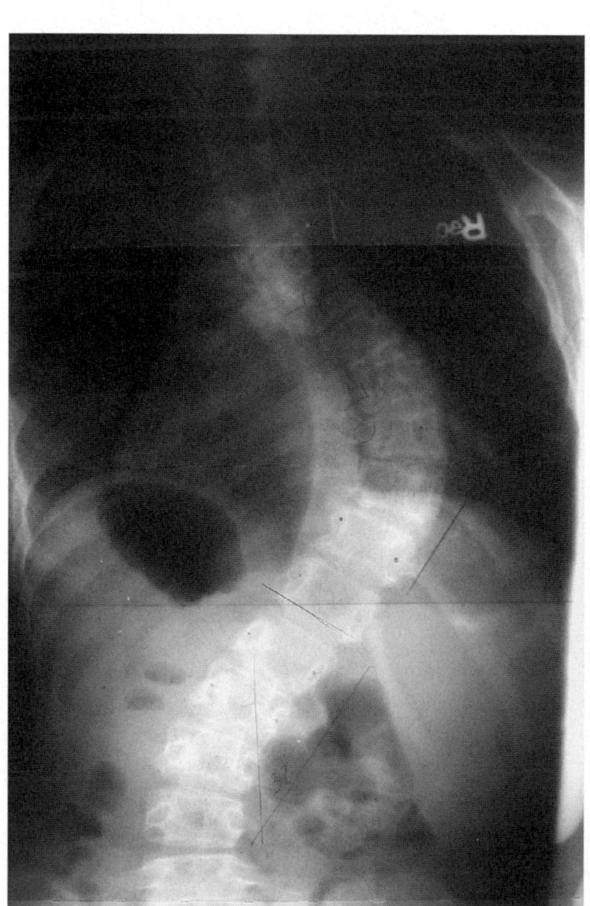

B

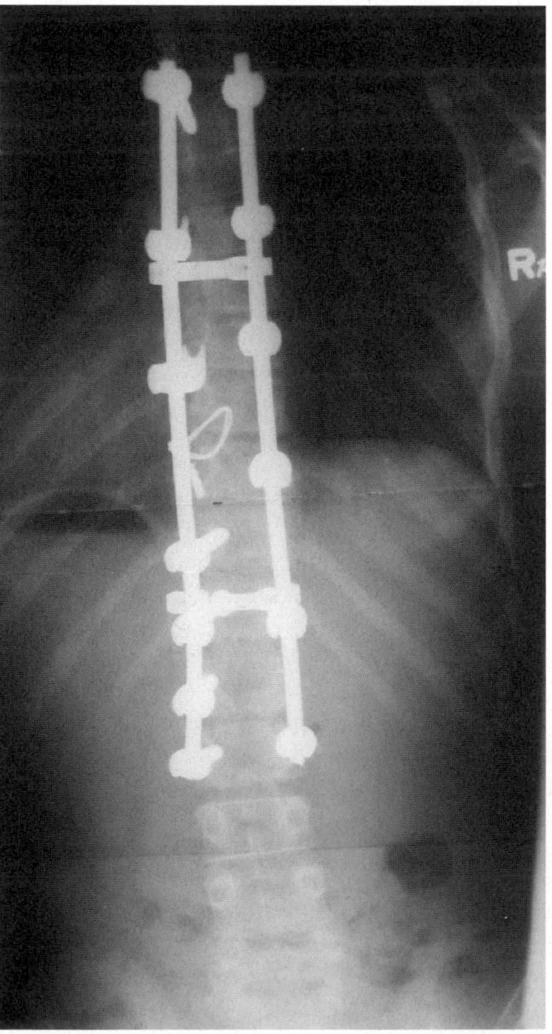

FIGURE 105-17. Right thoracic idiopathic scoliosis measuring 67 degrees before correction **(A)**. After correction with posterior fusion and segmental fixation **(B)**, the curve measures 8 degrees.

gym in school, to reduce the psychological potential for disability following this surgery.

If the thoracic scoliosis exceeds 50 to 75 degrees, it is common to have diminished vital capacity and residual lung volumes on pulmonary function testing. Arterial blood gases and forced expiratory volume in 1 second are normal, except in patients with severe curves. Vital capacity is decreased further if there is a thoracic lordosis in association with the scoliosis. Even with the surgical correction of the scoliosis, pulmonary function postoperatively is almost unchanged from preoperatively because of the persistence of chest wall or rib deformity that has occurred secondary to the scoliosis. It is obviously preferable to prevent scoliosis from progressing to that point.

Pain is rare during adolescence with idiopathic scoliosis. Although in middle age pain may result from degenerative changes, if pain is present during adolescence, further evaluation is indicated. If the neurologic examination is normal, a technetium-99 bone scan is necessary to screen for discitis, stress fracture, osteoid osteoma, or other bone tumors. If there is limited spinal flexion or a neurologic deficit, an MRI is indicated to rule out intraspinal pathology such as a syrinx. These conditions may cause scoliosis, but the scoliosis usually resolves once the underlying cause is treated appropriately. One should be thoroughly familiar with treatable causes of scoliosis before diagnosing idiopathic scoliosis and instituting brace treatment or recommending spinal fusion.

Kyphosis

Normal spinal sagittal (lateral) contours include lordosis in the cervical and lumbar spinal segments to balance the kyphosis in the thoracic area. The term *kyphosis* is sometimes used to describe abnormal conditions in which there is an increased rounding of the back in the thoracic or thoracolumbar area. The parents usually notice the child's poor posture. The assessment of apparent excessive kyphosis should include a forward-bending examination, viewed from the side, to determine if the back is flexible or rigid.

The least serious of cause of kyphosis is *postural roundback*. This is most commonly seen in the preadolescent years. It is seen more often in children who are taller than their peers. This condition is a flexible kyphosis that can be straightened voluntarily by the child and can be well corrected with hyperextension positioning. Kyphosis is one spinal deformity that can be treated by exercises alone. Active hyperextension of the trunk and sit-ups to decrease lumbar lordosis are useful in improving trunk control. Provided no fixed deformity is established, as the teenager's body image improves, so does the rounding of the upper back.

A more fixed and less flexible thoracic or thoracolumbar kyphosis with irregular vertebrae endplates is usually referred to as *Scheuermann disease*. This condition occurs most commonly in teenage boys. Attempts to passively correct Scheuermann kyphosis are unsuccessful, and there is often an associated increased lumbar lordosis. A lateral radiograph of the spine demonstrates irregularity of numerous disc spaces and anterior vertebral body wedging. To establish the diagnosis of Scheuermann kyphosis radiographically, at least 5 degrees of wedging in three adjacent vertebrae should be demonstrated (30). The Cobb method is employed to quantitate the amount of kyphosis present. The amount of kyphosis present in a normal individual from T3 to T12 is between 20 and 45 degrees. If the kyphosis is present in the thoracolumbar area (T10 to T12), which is normally straight on a lateral radiograph, measurements of more than 25 degrees are abnormal.

If wedging is present, if there is little correction with thoracic spine hyperextension, and if the thoracic kyphosis is 50 to 65 degrees, bracing is indicated, provided the patient still has remaining growth. A Milwaukee brace, which employs a neck ring in addition to trunk pads, should be used. Unlike scoliosis, where little correction results from bracing, in kyphosis, approximately 10 to 20 degrees improvement in the kyphosis can be anticipated after 1 year of full-time brace wear. Once this correction is obtained, nighttime brace wear until growth is complete is generally sufficient (30).

Increased thoracic kyphosis does not cause abnormalities in pulmonary function. The principal problem that may be caused by Scheuermann disease is pain in the thoracic spine. In rare cases, if the kyphosis exceeds 70 degrees by the completion of growth, spinal instrumentation and fusion are performed.

Congenital kyphosis is less common than congenital scoliosis, but it almost always requires early spinal fusion surgery. If the congenital kyphosis progresses unchecked, spinal cord compression at the apex of the kyphosis may occur. As with congenital scoliosis, evaluation for associated GU abnormalities should be performed.

Cervical Spine

The pediatric cervical spine, owing to its many normal variations on radiographs, is often a confusing area to evaluate. On the lateral cervical spine radiograph, the anterior and superior corner of each vertebral body is normally the last part to ossify, sometimes giving the appearance of a small compression fracture. Full ossification and development of the odontoid process is not complete in the young child and may give the appearance of being maldeveloped. The spine of the child younger than 10 years is much more flexible than in teenagers or older adults. Up to 3 mm anterior movement of C2 on C3 with flexion (termed *pseudosubluxation*) is normal in this age group; in adults, none should be present. In fact, when subjected experimentally to stretch, the newborn spine can stretch approximately 2 inches before failing, whereas the spinal cord stretches only .5 inch before it ruptures. Because of this difference in elasticity, infants may sustain spinal cord injury without apparent spinal fracture during birth or during auto accidents. The proper use of car seating supports for these very young children decreases the risk of these devastating injuries.

Children with Down syndrome are a special group. They commonly have instability of the occipitoatlantoaxial region. If this instability persists unrecognized, spinal cord compression with myelopathy may result, leading to leg weakness and impaired walking ability. Lateral cervical flexion/extension radiographs should be performed at age 3 to 4 years in all children with Down syndrome. Approximately 15% of these children show some evidence of atlantoaxial instability, but the majority do not need fusion surgery; they can be followed periodically by neurologic exam (31). Gait, strength, reflexes, and clonus should be checked. If the first radiograph showed increased laxity, it should be repeated every 2 years. Atlantoaxial posterior fusion is recommended if a neurologic deficit or excessive instability (greater than 5 to 8 mm translation on flexion-extension) is present (31).

Instability of the upper cervical spine may also be seen with os odontoideum or from odontoid hypoplasia. Os odontoideum is most likely the result of an early childhood fall that caused a fracture through one of the growth plates of the odontoid process. This unrecognized fracture develops into a fibrous nonunion, which gradually becomes unstable over the ensuing months and years. The diagnosis usually comes to light when evaluating the child with neck pain or as an incidental finding following head or neck trauma. Neurologic examination may be normal, but if the area is unstable, atlantoaxial fusion is generally indicated to stabilize this region and to protect the spinal cord from sudden, catastrophic, and possibly fatal injury. After successful fusion, normal activity can be allowed, although the child has mild limitation of head rotation. Odontoid hypoplasia occurs in normal children periodically, but it is most often associated with genetic disorders, such as Morquio syndrome and spondyloepiphyseal dysplasia congenita. The C1 to C2 segment is often unstable in these conditions, as seen on flexion-extension films. If so, fusion is necessary.

Torticollis is most commonly present at or near the time of birth, being due to a contracture of one sternocleidomastoid muscle. The child's head is tilted toward the side of contracture, with the chin rotated away from the contracted side because the origin of the contracted muscle is on the mastoid process. The etiology is not well defined, but it may be due to stretch of the involved muscle or a compartment syndrome developing in utero. The incidence is higher in children with breech presentation and forceps delivery. Commonly, a fusiform firm mass is palpable in the body of the contracted sternocleidomastoid muscle. These children often have plagiocephaly or asymmetry of facial and skull development. If the neck range of motion can be returned to normal by the age of 1 year, this facial asymmetry disappears. If the torticollis is untreated until later in childhood, the craniofacial bones have less chance of remodeling to become level. This is discussed elsewhere in this text.

Cervical spine radiographs should be evaluated to ensure the head position is not due to congenital spine abnormalities, such as hemivertebrae. If the bony cervical spine is normal, stretching exercises should be instituted shortly after birth. These exercises are designed to stretch the contracted sternocleidomastoid muscle and should be taught to the parents by a knowledgeable physical therapist. Although one of the parents should be asked to administer these stretching exercises at home, initial weekly checks by the therapist can help ensure compliance. If, despite stretching exercises, there continues to be a significant contracture by the age of 1 year, surgical treatment to lengthen the sternocleidomastoid is appropriate. This is performed at the distal border of the sternocleidomastoid, with proximal lengthening near the mastoid added, if needed. Even after surgical release, some stretching and, at times, bracing will continue to be needed as growth continues.

Torticollis due to C1 to C2 rotatory subluxation may present later in childhood following an upper respiratory infection or after trauma. Torticollis following an upper respiratory infection is believed to result from retropharyngeal inflammation and edema that leads to ligamentous laxity allowing subluxation at the atlantoaxial level, causing a rotatory deformity. Similarly, after muscular neck trauma, the child may have a persistent torticollis for several days or weeks, secondary to an unsuspected rotatory subluxation at the atlantoaxial level. CT imaging C1 to C2 is the best means of making this diagnosis. It should be performed with the head as close to straight as the patient allows. If torticollis from either of these causes persists, the child is treated with traction, which usually reduces the subluxation, followed by either bracing or atlantoaxial fusion. Fusion is reserved for cases that do not reduce or that develop recurrent subluxation. The likelihood of need for surgical fusion increases with increasing duration of symptoms, so prompt treatment is recommended. Other causes of torticollis to be ruled out include eye muscle imbalance, spinal cord tumor, or cervical abscess.

Klippel-Feil Syndrome

Failure of normal vertebral development in the cervical spine is known as Klippel-Feil syndrome. In the milder forms, when only two or three vertebrae are fused, diagnosis may not be made until the neck undergoes radiographs for other reasons. However, in children with more levels fused, the neck is very short and the child appears to have webbing of the base of the neck. Often Klippel-Feil syndrome is associated with Sprengel deformity, a failure of normal descent of the scapulae. Associated GU abnormalities may be present, and a sonogram or IVP is indicated when the diagnosis of Klippel-Feil syndrome is made. There is little specific treatment for this syndrome. Because of the congenital fusion of several segments, excessive strain and thus instability may occur at the levels that move. If this instability is excessive or if neurologic deficits are present, it is necessary to fuse the unstable segment. Surgical fusion may also be needed in adult life for degenerative changes at the mobile segments.

Particularly in the more intensive cases, contact sports, diving, or manual labor are best avoided. Any neck injury in a child with Klippel-Feil syndrome is apt to be serious because of the limited flexibility of the cervical area.

Upper Extremity

Congenital and developmental abnormalities of the upper extremities of children are less common than those of the lower extremity, perhaps partly because of the lower stresses imposed on the upper extremity in utero and later during standing. They are therefore not covered as extensively in this review. The reader is referred to the texts by Dobyns and colleagues (32) and by Bora (33), as well as to complete monographs.

Obstetric (Brachial Plexus) Palsy

The brachial plexus is normally composed of nerve root contributions from C5 to T1. Most severe injuries to the area involve lateral flexion of the neck or downward pressure on the shoulder, such as occur during a difficult delivery. Therefore, the upper portions of the plexus (C5 to C7) are most commonly stretched in a manner similar to the pathogenesis of "burners" seen in football players. This stretching causes denervation of the shoulder abductors and elbow flexors, resulting in gradual joint contractures if untreated (34). This is known as Erb-Duchenne palsy. The lower plexus (C7 to T1) can be affected by hyperabduction traction and has a poorer prognosis; this is the rarest type and is called Klumpke palsy. In these cases, loss of function of the elbow extensors, wrist flexors, and finger muscles and possibly Horner syndrome result. The entire plexus may occasionally be involved.

Factors associated with brachial plexus palsy include shoulder dystocia, breech position, high birth weight, and prolonged labor. The incidence is 1 to 3 per 1,000 births. Incidence and severity have gradually declined as obstetric care has improved. The site of injury may be at any level from the origin of the nerve roots to the plexus itself, but even root lesions may sometimes resolve spontaneously. On physical examination, the early typical Erb palsy presents with an arm that is internally rotated at the shoulder, extended at the elbow, and flexed at the fingers. Passive range of motion should be full in the early months.

Skeletal injuries such as clavicle fractures and proximal humeral separations should be ruled out radiographically, although they can often be differentiated because they cause guarding on passive motion and by the presence of the Moro response. Testing for the Moro reflex simulates some shoulder and elbow flexion, even in the presence of a fracture, but not in the presence of a palsy. Because of the trauma, palsy and skeletal injury may coexist.

Treatment involves maintenance of motion and tendon transfers for those rare, severe cases without spontaneous return of function. However, with current obstetric practice, 92% of palsies completely resolve by 3 months of age, and 95% fully recover eventually (35). Physical therapy should be used initially to maintain range of motion. For patients with persistent weakness at 3 months of age, electromyography and possibly myelography may help identify those rare cases requiring brachial plexus repair or grafting. Patients presenting later may benefit from osteotomies or contracture release and tendon transfer, to restore external rotation of the shoulder (34).

Other Deformities

Sprengel deformity, or congenital elevation of the scapula, actually represents embryonic failure of descent, rotation, and development of the scapula. This realignment normally occurs predominantly between 9 and 12 weeks of gestation (36). Etiology of the malformation is unknown.

On physical examination, the upper pole of the scapula may be visible at the base of the neck. Abduction is limited because the scapula is rotated inferiorly. The pectoralis major muscle may be underdeveloped. Scapular winging may occur due to serratus anterior palsy. The scapula may be connected to the vertebrae by an abnormal omovertebral bone, named for the two structures it connects. Associated congenital anomalies such as cervical or thoracic vertebral fusions, anal atresia, or cardiac abnormalities may coexist. Treatment is indicated in moderate and severe cases to improve shoulder abduction and appearance. The most effective method involves detaching and lowering the midline origins of the rhomboids and trapezius (Woodward procedure) to correct the scapular malposition (36).

Congenital *pseudoarthrosis of the clavicle* is a tapered defect in the continuity of this bone, presumably due to pressure from the more cephalad position of the right subclavian artery. It almost always involves the right clavicle unless the patient has dextrocardia or a cervical rib. Bone grafting and pin fixation prior to age 6 are usually indicated.

Radial club hand is a longitudinal failure of the formation of many tissues on the radial side of the forearm and hand. The severity varies. Approximately 50% are bilateral. Associated abnormalities may include components of the VATER syndrome, hydrocephalus, and clubfoot. The upper arm may also be short and the shoulder girdle underdeveloped. The radial-sided muscles, radial carpal bones, thumb, and radial artery may be absent. The hand is deviated radially up to 90 degrees because it lacks its normal radial support, and the ulna may be bowed. Treatment involves centralization of the wrist on the ulna, tendon transfer, and possibly ulnar straightening and creation of a thumb, as long as reasonable elbow flexion is present (37). Untreated cases are cosmetically problematic, although functionally less so. Congenital absence of the ulna is only one-third as common. In most cases, there is some remnant of the proximal ulna for elbow stability.

Radioulnar synostosis (fusion), often inherited, results in a fixed position of forearm rotation, usually in pronation. At times, the synostosis may be only fibrous. Shoulder motion can usually compensate for the lack of rotation, and rotational osteotomy should be performed only if clear-cut functional deficit can be demonstrated (38).

Congenital constriction bands (Streeter bands) are most likely due to intrauterine encirclement by amniotic bands or the umbilical cord. They may be located anywhere and may also be associated with amputation of body parts. The bands can be released with Z-plasties after age 2, or emergently if they are associated with neurocirculatory compromise.

Polydactyly, the presence of an extra digit, varies in spectrum from a hypoplastic soft-tissue–only addition to a fully developed digit with all phalanges and metacarpals. Fifth finger polydactyly is ten times more common in blacks than whites. A white child with this finding should be examined for other abnormalities, especially of the cardiovascular system. Simple, small, nonskeletal duplications can be excised or tied off. If there is significant skeletal stability, all digits should be reexamined to determine which is the least functional, and this digit should be excised.

Congenital *trigger thumb* presents as a clenched digit and is not always recognized at birth. It is usually due to excessive tightness of the annular ligament at the metacarpal head. This causes swelling of the tendon, which later becomes firm. Treatment consists of 6 to 8 weeks of stretching if the condition is diagnosed early, and surgical release if it persists or is diagnosed later.

Nursemaid's elbow, or radial head subluxation, refers to elbow pain following longitudinal traction on a pronated, extended elbow in children 2 to 7 years old. A snap may or may not be heard with motion. Radiographs usually show no bony abnormality or displacement. Only one case report, that of Solter and Zaltz (39), described actual exploration of this pathology. This report and laboratory studies suggest that the annular ligament of the radial head slips partially over the radial head, the narrowest portion being prominent when pronated. A radial fracture or septic arthritis should be ruled out. Treatment is usually reduction by stabilizing the elbow with one hand, with a finger over the radial head for palpation, followed by gentle firm flexion until a click is felt. The child should begin using the elbow within minutes. Immobilization is usually not necessary in the initial case. It can be done with 2 to 3 weeks in a cast if the episode has recurred. Parent education about the mechanism is most important.

LIMB LENGTHENING, DISTRACTION OSTEOGENESIS, AND DEFORMITY CORRECTION

The challenge of lengthening an obviously short limb has intrigued orthopedic surgeons for generations. The process has gone through an evolution and is now approaching a mature state.

Clinical research has suggested that discrepancies of more than 2.5 cm in the lower extremity may cause gait and back problems, and those of more than 5 cm most often benefit from surgical equalization of the limb lengths. Upper extremities can tolerate much greater discrepancies without causing functional problems. Lengthening a shortened limb poses problems of not only skeletal elongation, but also matching distraction of muscles, nerves, and vessels. Initial attempts at limb lengthening involved stimulating the bone by causing inflammation or irritation such as by injection or cautery, or causing arteriovenous fistulas. More predictable effects have been achieved, however, by osteotomy and gradual distraction. Initially, this was performed by traction in a bed with a frame. However, external fixation techniques have matured, and currently the lengthening process is accomplished by an external distractor. Wagner, in the late 1970s, was the first to popularize leg lengthening. He used a compact, unilateral device that allowed lengthening with less physical encumbrance. He realized that lengthening of approximately 1 mm per day is the maximum tolerated, and that an increase of approximately 10% to 15% of the length of the limb can be achieved safely without a high risk of nerve or artery damage. However, the gap where the lengthening occurred often required bone grafting and plating, a second major surgery. It remained for the pioneering Siberian orthopedic surgeon, G. Ilizarov, to recognize that bone would form spontaneously in the gap if conditions were right. This included a stretching or distraction sequence of 0.25 mm four times per day. Performance of the procedure in a child often resulted in spontaneous bone formation to resemble a normal bone. This phenomenon is termed *distraction osteogenesis*. It is now used to lengthen limbs, correct angular deformities, lengthen overall stature, and even stretch soft tissues. This principle of forming new bone has been applied by orthopedic and reconstructive surgeons. The appropriateness of this technique versus standard osteotomies is still being determined.

Different types of devices can now be used to produce the same effect. They can be uniplanar devices (i.e., placed only on one side of the limb) or the more cumbersome circular devices, which are more bulky but provide the ability to rotate, distract, and angulate.

Current indications for use of distraction osteogenesis include regeneration of large bone defects following tumor resection, infection, or trauma; major limb length inequality greater than 5 cm; significant soft-tissue scarring; and angular deformities that may require adjustment, such as in obese patients. The process of distraction usually takes about 1 month per centimeter to be obtained. If safe limits of distraction are exceeded or there is significant local scarring, nerve stretch is a risk.

GENERALIZED ABNORMALITIES

Bone Dysplasias

Osteocartilaginous exostoses (osteochondromas), single or multiple, are sessile or pedunculated excrescencies located on the metaphysis and directed away from the growth plate (Fig. 105-18). These outgrowths have their own growth plates. Osteochondromas are believed to arise from defects in the perichondral ring that encircles the growth plate, permitting lateral growth rather than the usual organized distal growth. The condition with multiple exostoses is usually distinct; it is transmitted as autosomal dominant, and affected persons are usually somewhat short.

Any bone with endochondral growth may be affected, but most often the long bones of the extremities are involved. Because of asymmetric growth plate activity, angulatory growth often ensues, resulting in valgus of knees and ankles and ulnar deviation of forearm and wrist. These should be corrected by partial epiphyseal stapling in young children or osteotomy in older ones. Leg length inequality is significant in 50% of patients.

The indication for excision of the lesions themselves is pain or compromise due to pressure on tendons, nerves, or spinal cord. Malignant transformation should be suspected if continued growth occurs after skeletal maturity or if new pain occurs. A bone scan may be helpful because absence of uptake indicates a benign lesion, but increased uptake does not always mean malignant change (40).

Fibrous dysplasia is a disorder in which bone formation in the medulla and cortex is altered, and the marrow contains much fibrous tissue. Radiographically, the bone has a uniform "ground glass" consistency, and the cortex is thin and often deformed (Fig. 105-19). One bone (in monostotic form) or several bones (polyostotic form) can be affected. Pathologic fractures occur often, but usually heal in a normal period (41). Proximal femoral (shepherd's crook) bowing is the most difficult to manage (41). Deformities and fractures of the lower extremities usually require internal fixation, whereas fractures in the upper extremity require only cast treatment.

Irregular "café-au-lait" spots occur in 30% of patients with the polyostotic form. When polyostotic lesions and café-au-lait spots are associated with precocious puberty, the condition is called McCune-Albright syndrome. Other endocrinopathies (thyroid, parathyroid, or adrenal

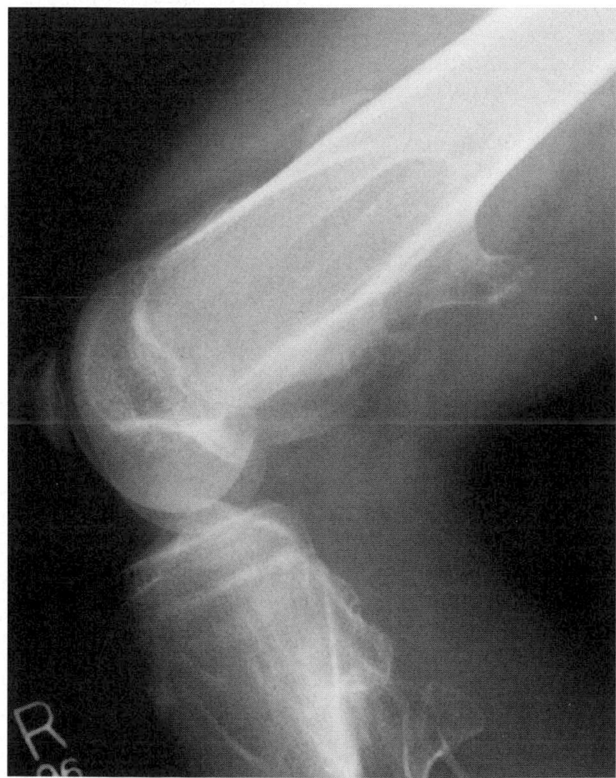

FIGURE 105-18. Osteochondromas may be multiple in the inherited form. Note that in this lateral radiograph of the knee, the cortex is continuous with that of the host bone, and they project away from the joint.

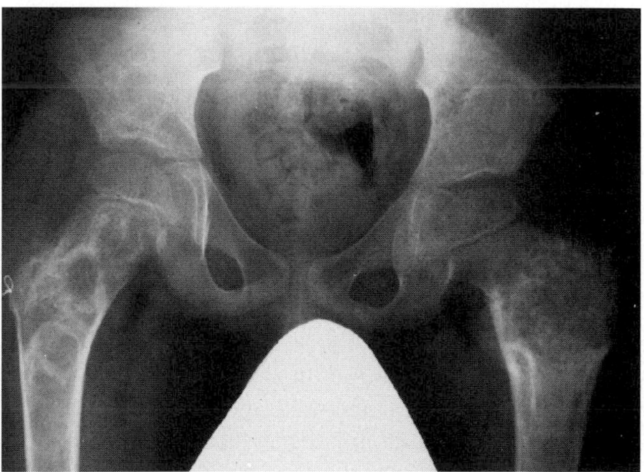

FIGURE 105-19. Fibrous dysplasia may affect multiple bones, and may cause cortical thinning and internal alterations, as well as bony deformation.

problems) may occur (41). Malignant transformation to fibrosarcoma or osteosarcoma is rare.

Osteogenesis imperfecta is a spectrum of diseases that are the end result of defects in collagen or proteoglycan synthesis. These result in bones with thin cortices and multiple fractures. Short stature, blue sclerae, middle ear deafness, abnormal dentition, and thin skin may coexist. Inheritance is usually dominant and occasionally recessive, but is frequently due to spontaneous mutation. Microfractures occur to cause the bowing of long bones and scoliosis (42). Child abuse should be considered in the differential diagnosis, and the absence of pelvic deformity or wormian cranial bones in child abuse may be helpful.

Mobility aids and preventive bracing can be very helpful in preventing fractures (43). Occasionally, intramedullary rods that elongate with growth are needed. Fortunately, the frequency of fractures diminishes with age.

Tumors

Because a complete discussion of musculoskeletal tumors is beyond the scope of this section, an attempt is made to describe an appropriate differential diagnosis and evaluation.

Benign or malignant musculoskeletal tumors can be classified according to their tissue of origin.

History and physical examination are rarely definitive. Many tumors become evident following trauma, when a new prominence is noted, or when pathologic fracture occurs through weakened bone. For example, osteoid osteoma, a benign condition, frequently produces pain that is relieved by nonsteroidal antiinflammatory agents. Very early sarcoma may be painless. Unexpected presentations may occur for lesions such as Ewing's sarcoma, the histiocytoses, and leukemia, which may each present with fever and malaise.

Some idea of the benign or malignant nature of a tumor can be gained from the following radiographic features. Lesions associated with rapid enlargement and lack of local containment should heighten the suspicion of malignancy. A vague zone of transition between lesion and normal bone is worrisome, as is a soft-tissue mass in the presence of a bone tumor. Periosteal lamellation is a response to spread outside the cortex and may occur with benign or malignant tumors. Rapid growth is suggested when periosteal lamellation is extensive and there is no formation of definite new cortex. Thinning of the cortex itself is not pathognomonic of malignancy; this also occurs with fibrous cortical defect and aneurysmal or unicameral cysts. Internal stippling suggests calcification of a cartilage matrix; fluffy opacification usually represents new bone formation, as in osteosarcoma (Fig. 105-20). Lesions crossing the epiphyseal plate are usually infections or malignant tumors. Leukemia presents with musculoskeletal complaints 20% of the time; radiographic findings include osteopenia, sclerotic or lytic lesions, lucent metaphyseal bands, or periosteal new bone (44).

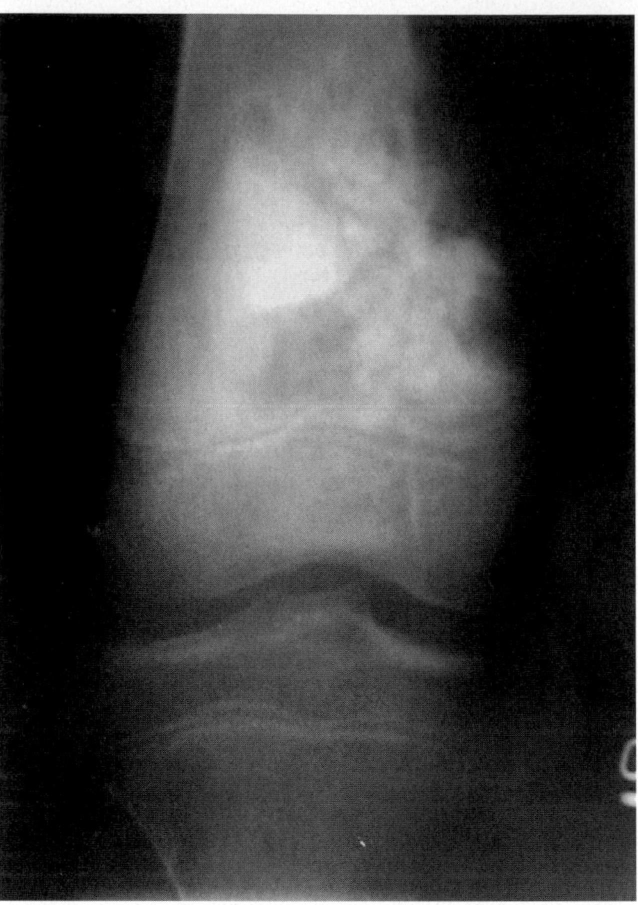

FIGURE 105-20. Osteogenic sarcoma is shown here involving the distal femur. There is intraosseous and extraosseous spread with no margination, as well as periosteal reaction.

Certain general radiographic studies can be helpful (45). Radiographic studies must be tailored to the differential diagnosis. CT scans may show internal consistency, soft-tissue spread, and extent of the lesion. Technetium bone scans show lesions in the remainder of the skeleton, bony involvement with soft-tissue lesions, and bone turnover or activity of questionable lesions. Angiograms may be helpful to determine if the tumor involves a vascular bundle. Laboratory studies are generally not specific; sedimentation rate and complete blood count are abnormal in several of these tumors, and alkaline phosphatase is often elevated in osteogenic sarcoma.

Treatment of musculoskeletal tumors defies simplification. The most important generalization is that any tumor requiring surgery should be cared for by a surgeon who has had experience in this area. Errors related to biopsy placement or specimen adequacy are three to five times more frequent when performed by surgeons in nontumor centers (46).

Osteogenic sarcoma is the most common primary malignant bone tumor. It usually affects patients during the ages and at the sites of most rapid growth—in teenagers, in the metaphysis of the distal femur, proximal humerus, and proximal tibia. This suggests a focal error in bone remodeling. Treatment involves chemotherapy and wide excision with an intact rim of normal tissue, if this can be performed without resecting major nerves. The missing skeletal structures are then reconstructed with allograft, autograft, or endoprosthetic implants. Such procedures are called *limb salvage*. If salvage of a functional limb is not possible, amputation is performed. More recent studies have shown that limb salvage yields results of local recurrence and long-term survival that are as good as with amputation.

Ten-year survival rates have improved from 19% before the era of chemotherapy to more than 70%. This gain is the result of improved imaging and surgical technique, adjuvant chemotherapy, and early resection of lung metastases. The prognosis is best for lesions of the proximal humerus and proximal tibia; it is worst for the pelvis and spine.

Ewing's sarcoma affects a slightly broader age range (usually ages 4 to 18). It commonly involves the diaphysis of long bones. The tumor is radiosensitive. Traditional treatment has been radiation and chemotherapy. More recently, however, improved survival rates and decreased local complications have been shown with wide surgical excision instead of radiation, when feasible. The long-term survival rate (approximately 60% at 5 years) is not quite as good as for osteosarcoma.

Two common benign bone tumors require brief mention. A *unicameral bone cyst* is a smooth, well-marginated lucency fairly centrally located near the growth plate in the metaphysis of a child 2 to 15 years of age, especially in the humerus or femur (Fig. 105-21). The lesion can be observed if it is small and in a non–weight-bearing bone; otherwise, it can be curetted or injected with corticosteroids. The latter two treatments have approximately equal results. The natural history of these defects is spontaneous regression during adolescence.

Fibrous cortical defects are well-marginated lucencies located in, and slightly expanding, the cortex. Usually, one radiographic view shows that these lesions are not central in bone (Fig. 105-22). They are present in as many as one-third of all young children at some time and disappear with age. In a weight-bearing bone, the risk of fracture is appreciable if the lesion is greater than approximately 3 cm in length and greater than one-half the width of the bone. Lesions this large should be protected by limiting activities, if possible, or bone grafted.

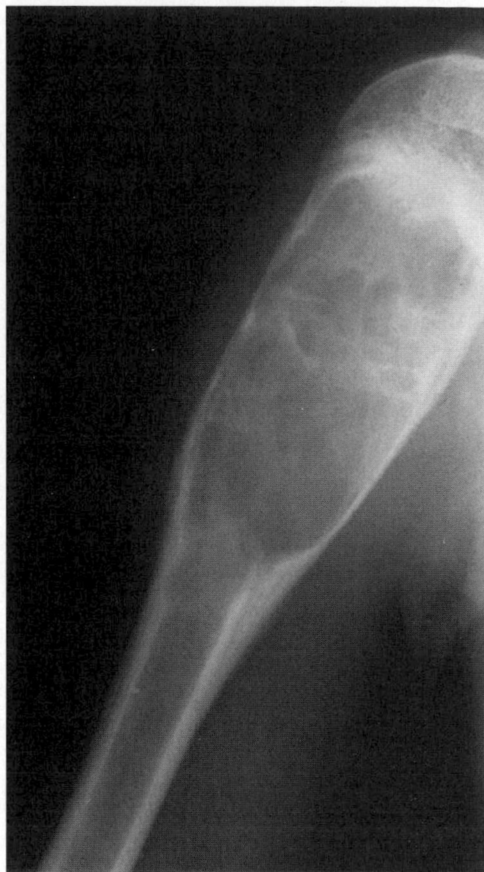

FIGURE 105-21. Unicameral bone cyst is a centrally located, lucent lesion, most common in the proximal humerus, as seen here.

Neuromuscular Disorders

Cerebral Palsy

Cerebral palsy is a collective term for a group of nonprogressive conditions affecting the upper central nervous system. This results in two types of musculoskeletal problems: disorders of control for which little can be done, and bone and joint deformities resulting from continued muscle imbalance, which can be managed (47,48). As a consequence, the athetoid features that predominate in a few children are difficult to modify, except for supportive bracing, but the more common spastic features are more amenable to modification. Assessment of the patient should always include identification of current functional problems and goals. Gait, if possible, may be marked by a crouched position due to knee or hip flexion contractures. The ankle may tend toward plantarflexion or dorsiflexion.

Trial bracing or gait studies may help determine the primary problem. Ankle plantar flexion can often be controlled with bracing if the foot can be brought up to a right angle with the tibia. If this is not possible, the tight heel cord should be lengthened; tight hamstring and hip flexors also may be lengthened when indicated. The "scissoring" of the legs while walking or lying may be due to tight adductor muscles.

Hip dislocation occurs with increasing frequency as the severity of involvement increases. This is due to imbalance between the strong adductors and flexors and the underactive extensors and abductors. It is acquired, not congenital,

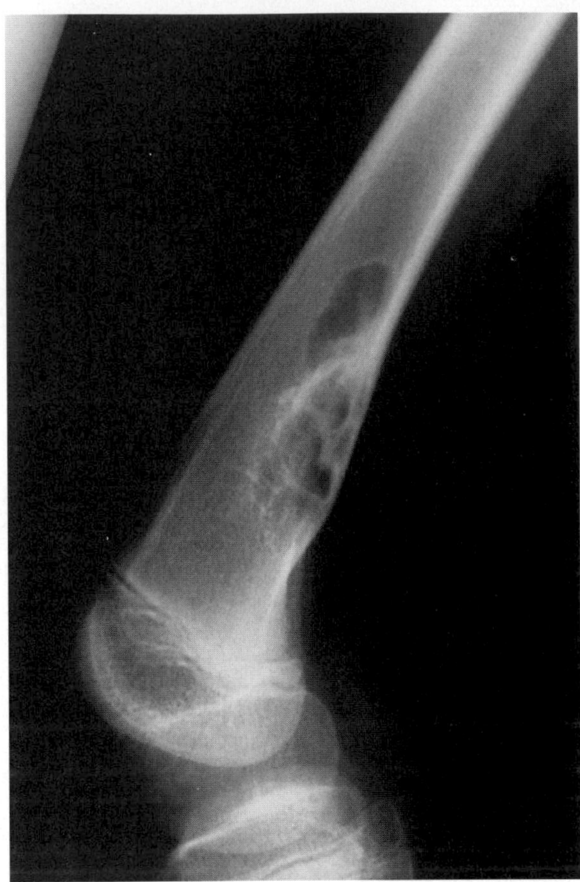

FIGURE 105-22. Fibrous cortical defect is more eccentrically located than unicameral bone cyst. As seen here, it is centered in the cortex.

and usually occurs after several years of age. This should be checked every 6 to 12 months in diplegic or quadriplegic patients. The child is at risk for progressive hip subluxation, if abduction is less than 30 degrees with the hip extended. Dislocation and subluxation cause difficulty by interfering with perineal care and balanced sitting, and by causing degenerative joint disease, pain, and increased spasm. Consequently, they should be treated aggressively, even in severely involved patients. They can be prevented by early muscle release or later by osteotomy (47).

Scoliosis is also more frequently encountered with increasing severity of cerebral palsy. It is present in up to 69% of severely involved children, perhaps because of persistent primitive reflexes, an inclined pelvis, or asymmetric muscle tone. Bracing should be tried, but it is less effective than in idiopathic scoliosis. Surgery may be necessary.

The upper extremity may be flexed at the elbow, wrist, and fingers. Whether this should be corrected depends on the patient's intelligence, ability to voluntarily control the hand, and sensation. The thumb may be clenched, and early bracing may be helpful, with surgery performed later if the thumb has potential for use.

The benefits of physical therapy in general are debated. Positioning and hand and heel-cord stretching may produce increased range. However, severity of neurologic involvement is probably more important than therapy in determining walking ability.

Myelodysplasia or spinal dysraphism involves malformation of the embryonic neural tube with paralysis below a certain thoracic or lumbar level of innervation (49). The functioning muscles usually have more control than in cerebral palsy. The goal of orthopedic management is optimizing mobility and socialization, and this does not always mean walking. The quadriceps are the most important muscles for mobility. Severely involved children with poor intelligence and weak quadriceps are more mobile in wheelchairs. In most cases, joint deformities are treated by releases and bracing. In contrast to cerebral palsy, hip dislocations are not usually painful and should not be reduced unless they are unilateral or the child has good quadriceps. Scoliosis may also occur, especially with higher-level spinal defects. One of the most important roles for the physician is to monitor the child for loss of lower-extremity muscle power as he or she grows. This loss of muscle strength may be due to a tethering of the spinal cord distally as the child grows or to a disturbance of cerebrospinal fluid pressure.

Infections

Hematogenous Osteomyelitis

The incidence and presentation of this condition are changing following the introduction of newer imaging and treatment methods, but there are certain constant principles (50,51).

Acute hematogenous osteomyelitis by definition includes processes occurring for a week or less at the time of diagnosis (52). It occurs more frequently in males than in females, presumably because trauma may play a role in increasing susceptibility. The peak ages of occurrence are in children younger than 1 year of age and in the preadolescent years, ages 9 to 11. The incidence declines in adulthood because of the change in vascular supply of bone (53). The most common sites affected are the femur and tibia, each accounting for one-third of the cases, followed by humerus, calcaneus, and pelvis. However, any bone may be affected. The metaphysis is the most common region involved, and spread may occur from this point to involve any other portion. Rarely, the infection process may begin in the epiphysis.

The pathophysiology is incompletely understood. The metaphyseal vascular channels form loops near the growth plate (53). Blood flow is slowed, and the capillary basement membrane and reticuloendothelial system is deficient in these regions. Experimental bacteremias have been shown to produce foci of infection only in these regions. Trauma likely has more than a circumstantial role because experimentally traumatized areas are more susceptible to developing osteomyelitis. Only about one-fourth of cases have a demonstrable source, such as cutaneous, aural, or respiratory seeding. Direct traumatic inoculation is a different disease process.

After a focus of infection is initiated, local inflammation is followed by spread up and down the medullary canal. The growth plate in children has no bridging vessels and acts as a barrier to spread in most cases. The growth cells are on the epiphysial side and are therefore spared. However, in the first year of life, transphyseal vessels exist that allow spread up to the epiphysis and into the joint (51). These facts have two implications. First, growth plate damage is more likely during the first year of life. Second, in children of this age, septic arthritis may follow osteomyelitis in any metaphyseal location, whereas in older children without transphyseal vessels, it occurs only in locations where the joint capsule extends over the growth plate, that is, the shoulder, elbow, and hip. At skeletal maturity with growth plate closure, this barrier is again eliminated, although hematogenous osteomyelitis is rare after this point. As intramedullary pressure increases, pus dissects through the haversian system to elevate the periosteum and produce a subperiosteal abcess and then a soft-tissue abscess. The elevated periosteum may be radiographically apparent within 1 to 2 weeks.

Unlike in septic arthritis, the organisms involved vary slightly with age. In all age groups, the predominant organism is *S. aureus*, although *Streptococcus pneumoniae* and *Haemophilus* must be considered. *Staphylococcus* is associated with a higher recurrence rate than other organisms. *Salmonella* should be considered in patients with sickle cell anemia, although *Staphylococcus* is still more common than *Salmonella* in these patients. Blood cultures in the acute phase are positive approximately 40% to 50% of the time, and direct cultures of pus or bone only 60% to 80% of the time. This may be due to prior antibiotic use, errors in sampling or processing, or autoeradication of the organism.

Clinical diagnosis remains key, despite new imaging techniques. The child may appear well or may have systemic involvement ranging from malaise to shock. Often refusal to bear weight is an early symptom. The very earliest sign is fever and local bone tenderness, followed later by fluctuance if a subperiosteal or soft-tissue abscess has developed. Spread to adjacent joints should be ruled out by palpation and range-of-motion evaluation. Passive motion of the extremity is usually not significantly resisted unless a soft-tissue abscess or joint involvement is present. Increased suspicion should be aroused with neonates, who are more often afebrile, and who may first be noted to have a swollen or motionless limb. Vertebral or pelvic osteomyelitis may present as abdominal pain and can resemble the more common septic arthritis of the hip.

Differential diagnosis primarily includes neoplasm, contusion, undisplaced fracture, and sickle cell crisis. Elevated white blood cell count and sedimentation rate are helpful but not diagnostic. Serum antibody titers may be helpful, but sensitivity is a problem. Radiographs at the earliest stage may show soft-tissue swelling. Osteopenia or lysis may appear after 7 to 10 days, followed by new bone formation at the borders of the process. Bone scan has been widely used since the 1980s, but the subtleties of its use have only more recently been recognized. The tracer most widely used is 99^{m}Tc methylene diphosphonate because of its speed, cost, and sensitivity. Immediate scans for flow and blood pool, as well as later skeletal images, should be obtained. The scan may be normal in the very early stages. It should be repeated after 48 hours, if clinically indicated.

Cold or photopenic areas are important because they may indicate areas of avascularity, especially when accompanied by adjacent areas of increased uptake. Cellulitis may cause confusion, but usually does not show bony localization on delayed images. The overall accuracy of nuclear imaging is approximately 60% to 90%. However, it may be much lower in neonates, according to some reports. Gallium citrate may be sensitive, but requires a minimum of 24 hours; indium-labeled white cell studies require similar amounts of time, including preparation of tracer. Because of these limitations, radionuclide scans should not be relied on in all instances, especially when the clinical diagnosis is clear. These studies have their greatest value when localization for aspiration is difficult. The role of MRI has yet to be defined.

Aspiration is indicated in all cases to identify the pathogen and, in some cases, to decompress localized purulence. It should be performed with a large-diameter needle. The anesthetic may be local, IV sedation, or general, as indicated. In sequence, the extraosseous soft tissues, periosteum, and, if necessary, intramedullary canal should be assessed for purulent localization. Fluoroscopy may be useful in deep lesions if radiographic changes are evident. Experiments in animals have shown that aspiration of bone does not by itself cause a bone scan to become positive.

Treatment involves delivery of appropriate antibiotic to all infected tissue. Abscesses with avascularity may therefore require surgical decompression if aspiration cannot accomplish this. Antibiotic therapy can be divided into initial and definitive periods. In the initial phase, broad-spectrum antibiotic agents, including antistaphylococcal agents, are indicated. Vancomycin should be used if resistance is suspected. In neonates, an aminoglycoside should be added. In children younger than 3 years who have osteomyelitis associated with septic arthritis, chloramphenicol or cefuroxime may be used to cover *H. influenzae*. In the definitive period, the most effective, least toxic antibiotic for the isolated organism should be given for 4 to

6 weeks. This may be by the oral route if the patient is clinically improved and is compliant, and if adequate serum drug levels can be documented.

Surgery is reserved for those cases in which the child is systemically ill, is worsening under medical treatment, or in whom an abscess has been demonstrated. Abscess or avascular tissue should be removed to allow antibiotic penetration, and the wound is usually closed over a drain. Complications include recurrence, minor growth acceleration, growth plate damage, and fracture through weakened bone.

Subacute osteomyelitis is a more subtle condition. No systemic signs may be evident, and in one series fewer than one-fifth of patients had a fever, elevated white blood count, or positive blood count (51). However, an abnormal radiograph and bone scan were more common than in the acute form. Treatment follows the principles discussed previously.

Chronic recurrent multifocal osteomyelitis is a rare syndrome involving low-grade systemic manifestations that are ongoing for several years, with reports of up to 12 areas of lytic-sclerotic juxtaepiphyseal involvement. No organism has been isolated, and treatment is supportive.

Fungal osteomyelitis may be disseminated (sporotrichosis, candidiasis) or direct (eumycetoma). Aggressive debridement is more important in these conditions than in bacterial infections.

Puncture wounds to the foot are significant in that they may be followed by *Pseudomonas* infection. This is because *Pseudomonas* often colonizes the shoe and sock. The wound should be inspected and foreign material removed (50). The patient should be seen in 3 to 5 days or at least instructed to return if symptoms of infection occur.

Septic arthritis is slightly more common than hematogenous osteomyelitis, and it may potentially have more disastrous long-term consequences if effective treatment is delayed. Most cases occur in infants and younger children, with nearly one-half of the cases occurring before age 30. A high index of suspicion for septic arthritis should be maintained in sick neonatal patients because they show few signs (54). The hip is the most commonly involved joint in the infant, and the knee is the most common site in the older child. The spread may be from the bloodstream or from an adjacent osteomyelitis, especially in the hip and shoulder, where the capsular insertion extends over the growth plate onto the metaphysis. Many theories have been advanced for the pathogenesis of joint destruction, including toxins from both the neutrophils and bacteria.

The spectrum of causative organisms is somewhat broader than that of hematogenous osteomyelitis (54), which may have some relation to the greater frequency of this condition. Overall, *S. aureus* is still the most common causative organism. However, in the age group from 1 month to 5 years, *H. influenzae* is more common than *Staphylococcus*. The streptococci, *Escherichia coli*, *Proteus*, and other organisms should also be considered. The yield of organisms from aspiration is approximately 60% to 80%.

Clinical findings vary with age. In the infant, there may be fever, failure to feed, and tachycardia. Subtle changes in position may serve as clues, as well as unilateral swelling of an extremity or a joint, asymmetry of soft-tissue folds, and pain with range of motion. In the older child, the signs are more localized.

Aspiration with a large needle should be performed if there is any reasonable suspicion of septic arthritis, for diagnosis and, in some cases, for treatment. In deep joints such as the hip, guidance with ultrasound or fluoroscopy should be used to confirm position of the needle. This ensures that joint fluid was actually obtained, and it also helps distinguish joint infection from septic involvement of the bursa underneath the nearby psoas muscle. The white cell count in fluid obtained in septic arthritis ranges from 25,000 to 250,000 per mm^3. Elevated lactate levels may be helpful in cases where white cell counts are borderline.

Differential diagnosis includes toxic synovitis of the hip, in which pain, fever, leukocytosis, and spasm are more moderate and do not escalate on serial observations. However, at times the two are indistinguishable and aspiration should be performed. Rheumatoid arthritis, cellulitis, traumatic synovitis, and the migratory polyarthralgias of rheumatic fever should be considered. A sympathetic effusion may also occur from adjacent osteomyelitis.

The role of arthrotomy versus aspiration in confirmed cases of septic arthritis is controversial. The key feature is removal of deleterious enzymes and restoration of effective synovial perfusion. Because the decision not to operate requires the ability to monitor and repeatedly aspirate as needed, it is probably preferable to use arthrotomy in joints that are deep and difficult to assess, such as the hip and shoulder; in young patients who are difficult to examine; and when the fluid obtained is viscous.

The surgical procedure should include irrigation, drainage, and closure. This may be performed arthroscopically in the knee, shoulder, and ankle. Direct instillation of antibiotics has no benefit. Some investigators believe the femoral metaphysis should be drilled whenever the hip is aspirated to decompress any possible femoral osteomyelitis.

Early effective treatment is very important. Good results decline dramatically if treatment is initiated after 4 days of symptoms. Antibiotics should be continued for 4 to 6 weeks. Contractures should be prevented, and abduction of the hip decreases the likelihood of dislocation. Complications include permanent destruction of cartilage, and in the hip, avascular necrosis with resorption of the femoral head or overgrowth of the femoral head. Complications are more frequent in young infants.

Gonococcal arthritis also occurs in children (55). It should be distinguished from the more frequent gonococcal migratory polyarthralgia or tenosynovitis. On average, two to three joints are affected; the most commonly involved are the wrists and knees. Treatment is aspiration and closed irrigation followed by 3 days of IV penicillin, and 4 days of ampicillin or amoxicillin. Oral treatment alone with one of these drugs for 7 days is acceptable in reliable patients after a loading dose.

REFERENCES

1. Morrissy RT, Weinstein L. *Lovell and Winter's pediatric orthopaedics*, 4th ed. Philadelphia: Lippincott Williams & Wilkins, 2001.
2. Rang M. *Children's fractures*. Philadelphia: JB Lippincott, 1983.
3. Beaty JH, Kasser JR, eds. *Fractures in children*. Philadelphia: Lippincott Williams & Wilkins, 2001.
4. Staheli LT. *Children's orthopaedics*. New York: Raven, 2001.
5. Farsetti P, Weinstein SL, Ponseti IV. Long-term functional and radiographic outcome of untreated and nonoperatively treated metatarsus adductus. *J Bone Joint Surg Am* 1994;76:257–265.
6. Rushforth GF. The natural history of hooked forefoot. *J Bone Joint Surg Br* 1978;60:8.
7. Ponseti IV. Clubfoot management. *J Pediatr Orthop* 2000;20(6):699–700.
8. Wenger DR, Mauldin D, Speck G, et al. Corrective shoes as treatment for flexible flatfoot. *J Bone Joint Surg Am* 1989;71:800.
9. Staheli LT. Shoes for children: a review. *Pediatrics* 1991;88:371.
10. Mosier KM, Asher M. Tarsal coalitions and peroneal spastic flat foot. *J Bone Joint Surg Am* 1984;66:976.
11. Scranton PE Jr. Treatment of symptomatic talocalcaneal coalition. *J Bone Joint Surg Am* 1982;69:533.
12. Kling TF, Hensinger RN. Angular and torsional deformities of the lower limbs in children. *Clin Orthop* 1976;176:136.
13. Staheli LT, Corbett M, Wyss C, et al. Lower extremity rotational problems in children. *J Bone Joint Surg Am* 1985;67:39.
14. Staheli LT. Torsional deformities. *Pediatr Clin North Am* 1977;24:799.
15. Morrissy RT. Congenital pseudarthrosis of the tibia. *J Bone Joint Surg Br* 1981;63:367.
16. Pappas AM. Congenital posteromedial bowing of the tibia and fibula. *J Pediatr Orthop* 1984;4:525.
17. Dinham JM. Popliteal cysts in children. *J Bone Joint Surg Br* 1975;57:69.
18. Dickhaut SC, DeLee JC. The discoid lateral meniscus syndrome. *J Bone Joint Surg Am* 1982;64:1068.
19. Salenius P, Vankka E. The development of the tibiofemoral angle in children. *J Bone Joint Surg Am* 1975;57:259.
20. Feldman M, Schoenecker PL. Use of the metaphyseal-diaphyseal angle in the evaluation of bowed legs. *J Bone Joint Surg Am* 1993;75(11):1602–1609.
21. Ilfeld W, Westin GW, Making M. Missed or developmental dislocation of the hip. *Clin Orthop* 1986;203:276.
22. Harcke HT, Kumar SJ. Role of ultrasound in diagnosis and management of congenital dislocation and dysplasia of the hip. *Curr Concepts J Bone Joint Surg Am* 1991;73:622.
23. Mubarak S. Pitfalls in use of Pavlik harness for treatment of congenital dysplasia, subluxation and dislocation of the hip. *J Bone Joint Surg Am* 1981;63:1239.
24. Zionts LE, MacEwen GD. Treatment of congenital dislocation of the hip in children between the ages of one and three years. *J Bone Joint Surg Am* 1986;68:829.
25. Haueisen DC, Weiner DS, Weiner SD. The characterization of transient synovitis of the hip in children. *J Pediatr Orthop* 1986;6:11.
26. Catterall AM. *Legg-Calvé-Perthes disease*. Edinburgh: 1982.
27. Salter RB. Current concepts review: the present status of surgical treatment for Legg-Perthes disease. *J Bone Joint Surg Am* 1984;66:961.
28. Salter RB, Thompson GH. *Legg-Perthes disease*. CIBA Clinical Symposia, 1986.
29. Weiner DS, Weiner S, Melby A, et al. A thirty-year experience with bone graft epiphyseodesis in the treatment of slipped capital femoral epiphysis. *J Pediatr Orthop* 1984;4:145.
30. Bradford DS, Lonstein JE. *Scoliosis and other spinal deformities*. Philadelphia: WB Saunders, 1994.
31. Tredwell SJ, Newman DE, Lockitch G. Instability of the upper cervical spine in Down syndrome. *J Pediatr Orthop* 1990;10:602.
32. Dobyns JH, Wood V, Bayne LG. Congenital hand deformities. In: Green D, ed. *Textbook of hand surgery*. New York: Churchill Livingstone, 1982.
33. Bora WF. *Pediatric upper extremity*. Philadelphia: WB Saunders, 1986.
34. Hoffer MM, Wickenden R, Raper B. Brachial plexus birth palsies. *J Bone Joint Surg Am* 1978;60:691.
35. Tada K, Tsuyuguchi Y, Kawai H. Birth palsy: natural recovery course and combined root avulsion. *J Pediatr Orthop* 1984;4:279.
36. Carson WF, Lovell WW, Whitesides TE Jr. Congenital elevation of the scapula. *J Bone Joint Surg Am* 1981;63:1199.
37. Bora FW. Radial clubhand deformity. *J Bone Joint Surg Am* 1981;63:741.
38. Cleary JE, Omer GE. Congenital radioulnar synostosis. *J Bone Joint Surg Am* 1985;67:539.
39. Salter RB, Zaltz C. Anatomic investigations of the mechanism of injury and pathologic anatomy of "pulled elbow" in young children. *Clin Orthop* 1971;77:134.
40. Lange RH, Lange TA, Rao BK. Correlative radiographic, scintigraphic and histologic evaluation of exostoses. *J Bone Joint Surg Am* 1984;66:1454.
41. Harris WH, Dudley R, Barry RJ. The natural history of fibrous dysplasia. *J Bone Joint Surg Am* 1962;44:207.
42. Albright JA. Management overview of osteogenesis imperfecta. *Clin Orthop* 1981;159:80.
43. Bleck EE. Nonoperative treatment of osteogenesis imperfecta. *Clin Orthop* 1981;159:111.
44. Lange TA. Ultrasound imaging as a screening study for malignant soft-tissue tumors. *J Bone Joint Surg Am* 1986;69:100.
45. Mankin HJ, Lange TA, Spanier SS. Hazards of biopsy in patients with malignant primary bone and soft tissue tumors. *J Bone Joint Surg Am* 1982;64:1121.
46. Rogalsky RJ, Black GB, Reed MH. Orthopaedic manifestations of leukemia in children. *J Bone Joint Surg Am* 1986;68:494.
47. Renshaw TS.Cerebral palsy. In: Morrissy RT, Weinstein SL, eds. *Lovell and Winter's pediatric orthopaedics*, 4th ed. Philadelphia: Lippincott Williams & Wilkins, 2001:563–600.
48. Bleck EE. Locomotor prognosis in cerebral palsy. *Dev Med Child Neurol* 1975;17:18.
49. Menelaus MB. *Orthopaedic management of spina bifida cystica*. Edinburgh: Churchill Livingstone, 1980.
50. Green NE. *Pseudomonas* infections of the foot following puncture wounds. *American Academy of Orthopaedic Surgeons Instructional Course Lectures* 1983:43.
51. Jackson MA, Nelson JD. Etiology and medical management of acute suppurative bone and joint infections in pediatric patients. *J Pediatr Orthop* 1982;2:313.
52. Song KM, Sloboda J. Acute hematogenous osteomyelitis in children. *J Am Acad Orthop Surg* 2001;9(3):166–175.
53. Scoles PV, Aronoff SC. Current concepts review: antimicrobial therapy of childhood skeletal infections. *J Bone Joint Surg Am* 1984;66:1487.
54. Green NE. Disseminated gonococcal infections and gonococcal arthritis. *American Academy of Orthopaedic Surgeons Instructional Course Lectures* 1983:48.
55. Nade S. Acute septic arthritis in infancy and childhood. *J Bone Joint Surg Br* 1983;65:234.

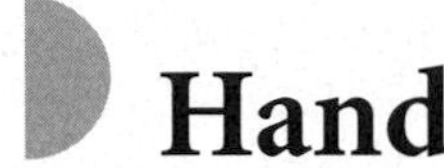

Chapter 106

Hand

Christine J. Cheng

Hand surgery is a specialized field that embodies the concept of "regional" surgery, uniquely combining orthopedic, neurosurgical, and plastic surgical techniques in the functional and sometimes aesthetic restoration of a remarkably complex organ. Care of the pediatric hand is complicated by the additional factors of growth and psychomotor and social development. Those who care for children's hands must be equipped to deal with issues specific to their young patients, which always include counseling and support to their parents, care providers, and families.

EMBRYOLOGY AND ANATOMY

The Growing Hand

The embryonic upper extremity starts as a limb bud that develops from proximally to distally around day 26 of gestation (1). The hand first forms as a plate. The digital rays separate by apoptosis of their intervening cells by day 36. A well-differentiated hand exists by 7 weeks, which does not undergo further differentiation after about the 50th day. Early studies of chick embryos led to the discovery of growth centers that specifically govern upper extremity development, which all have counterparts in the human hand (2). Cells within the apical ectodermal ridge produce fibroblast growth factors that direct proximal-to-distal growth: sonic hedgehog protein, secreted by cells within the zone of polarizing activity, has been found to define the radioulnar axis; Wnt-7a protein is associated with establishment of the dorsal-ventral axis (1,2). The cartilaginous skeleton undergoes enchondral ossification of its primary centers between the seventh and tenth weeks of gestation. The carpus does not begin to ossify until around 1 year of age. Secondary ossification varies according to gender and race, with frequent delays in congenitally abnormal hands (3).

Christine J. Cheng: Department of Surgery, Division of Plastic and Reconstructive Surgery, Washington University School of Medicine, St. Louis Children's Hospital, St. Louis, Missouri 63110.

The four distinct physiologic regions of pediatric bone (Fig. 106-1)—epiphysis, physis, metaphysis, and diaphysis—are not only responsible for their growth, but also account for different patterns of injury and responses to treatment, compared with adults. The epiphyses are located at the ends of the long bones, which are covered by articular cartilage at skeletal maturity. The physis, or growth plate, produces rapid longitudinal and latitudinal growth. Vascular compromise to this region halts cell division, resulting in longitudinal deformity if the entire physis is affected, and angular deformity if only a portion is injured. The physis, which appears as a lucent line on plain X-rays, may temporarily widen in response to injury of its adjacent region. The metaphysis forms the contoured flare at either end of the bony shaft, or diaphysis. Metaphyseal bone has a thinner and more fenestrated cortex in children, making torus or buckle fractures more likely. The diaphysis comprises the major portion of each long bone, and is more vascular and less dense in younger children. As the skeleton matures, the number of Haversian systems increases and this region becomes more solid. Thus, fracture patterns change and fracture healing slows with increasing age. In children, the periosteum is thicker, with more osteogenic potential, making fractures less likely to displace, as well as keeping them more stably reduced (4).

Functional Development and Physical Examination

Functional assessment must take into account the anatomic structures and sensory capabilities of the hand, as well as the chronological and developmental age of the child. For the first month, infants tend to hold their fists tightly clenched, opening only during reflexive actions such as startling or stretching. At 3 months of age, they begin to grasp with only their fingers, usually with the wrist flexed. Grasp does not involve the thumb until 6 to 7 months of age, and true thumb use for pinch and manipulation of smaller objects does not begin until a child is

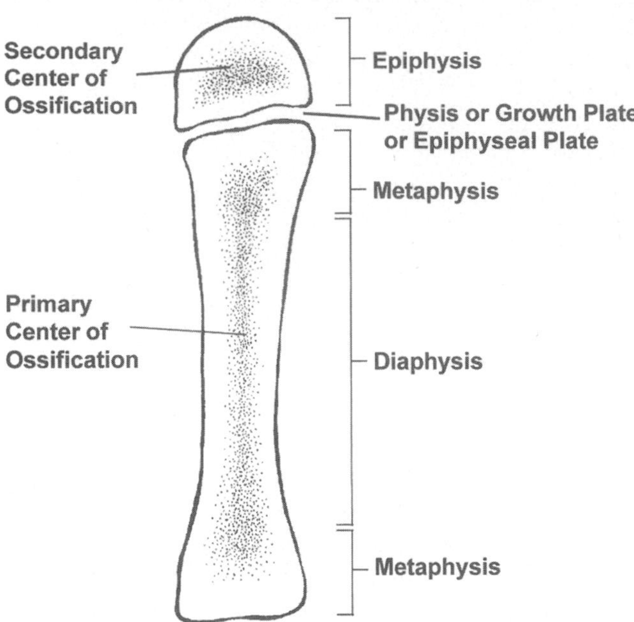

FIGURE 106-1. Terminology for pediatric skeleton and sites of skeletal growth. (Reprinted from Van Heest A, McElfresh EC. *Surgery of the hand and upper extremity*. New York: McGraw-Hill, 1996:2180, with permission.)

around 10 months old (3). Adequate physical examination, as well as the necessity and timing for surgical intervention, are influenced by these developmental patterns.

Examination begins with observing whether the child places the hand purposefully in space, inspecting the relative length of the upper extremity and the size of the hand, and checking joint motion and stability. Digital motion in utero produces finger flexion creases, so the absence of these creases at birth suggests either the lack of a functioning joint or inadequate musculotendinous structures. Similarly, abnormal progression in functional development or patterns of use can reflect abnormal neurosensory or musculoskeletal conditions. Pain may be displayed by the refusal to use an affected limb, whereas anesthesia can present as an unusual wound or even self-biting. Because younger children are incapable of following commands and verbalizing answers during physical examination, adequate assessment may require multiple visits to establish the full clinical picture. Comparison to the opposite extremity is often helpful.

CONGENITAL HAND DIFFERENCES

Classification

Systems of classification allow a common language for communication and enable comparisons to be made between groups. Unfortunately, the spectrum of congenital hand differences is vast, with a nearly infinite number of unique variations. Thus, a comprehensive system of congenital hand conditions that adequately classifies all malformations is difficult to devise. An excessively generalized system is not useful, whereas an extremely detailed one becomes unwieldy and impractical. The most commonly employed classification has been that introduced by the International Federation of Surgical Societies of the Hand (5), which avoids Greek and Latin terms, does not include eponyms, and uses simple descriptive terminology. With this system, hand malformations are classified into seven major groups:

I. Failure of formation of parts
II. Failure of differentiation of parts
III. Duplication
IV. Overgrowth
V. Undergrowth
VI. Congenital constriction ring syndrome
VII. Generalized skeletal abnormalities

Shortcomings of this system are revealed when attempting to classify hands that have more than one abnormality or in which the etiology is not clearly established.

Prevalence and Etiology

Although the hand is a visible organ, some congenital differences are subtle and can be missed upon initial inspection of an infant at birth. Missed diagnoses make it difficult or even impossible to establish the true incidence of congenital hand differences. Estimates among different populations estimate the prevalence to be as high as 1 in 500 to 600 live births (1,6). In descending order of frequency, the most common major congenital upper limb malformations are syndactyly, polydactyly, congenital amputation, and radial-sided defects. Although the relative frequencies of the two most common conditions, syndactyly and polydactyly, have varied between populations, they consistently comprise 20% to 50% of all reported diagnoses.

Increased understanding of the molecular biology of limb development has already identified the genetic basis for many congenital hand conditions (1). Some of these involve single gene mutations, such as in Apert syndactyly, whereas others are associated with chromosomal abnormalities (e.g., trisomy 13). At the cellular level, a variety of mechanistic pathways are involved, including transcription factors, cell signaling pathways, and growth factors. Teratogen exposure and in utero events such as limb constriction by fetal membranes have also been implicated as causative factors, although more recent theories suggest that interruption of fetal vascular circulation may be the underlying mechanism common to these (7).

In the developing fetus, hand formation coincides temporally with development of the cardiac and renal systems, so careful evaluation of these organ systems is indicated in an infant born with a congenital hand abnormality. Involvement of multiple limbs and multiple organ systems can suggest a congenital syndrome, with potentially serious consequences. For example, radial club hand is associated with Fanconi anemia and thrombocytopenia-absent radius syndrome, both of which involve life-threatening hematologic defects. Ulnar polydactyly, which is commonly an isolated genetic trait in African Americans, is more likely to be part of a syndrome in Caucasians (8). When a syndrome is suspected, referral to a geneticist is recommended for parental counseling on heritability, including the likelihood of subsequent offspring and the patient's children having the same condition.

Treatment Indications and Timing

The functional goals of treatment are to provide a hand that can be properly positioned, has good sensation, and is able to achieve both power grasp and precision pinch. A normal-appearing hand is optimal, but cannot always be attained. Surgical correction of congenital hand differences can usually be postponed until conditions for general anesthesia, such as age, weight, and hemoglobin levels, are optimized. Most congenital hand differences should be corrected by or shortly after 1 year of age, when the child truly begins to use the hand as an instrument for exploring his or her environment, self-feeding, and nonverbal communication. Conditions that cause joint contracture, or angulation or rotational deformity due to tethering of adjacent digits, such as in acrosyndactyly where the fingertips are fused or syndactyly of the border digits (thumb-index, ring-small) should be corrected as early as 6 months of age to avoid permanent skeletal changes. Of course, emergent correction is warranted when the circulation to a digit or limb is at risk, such as with severe constriction rings. The decision of when to operate involves a balance between minimizing anesthetic risk, preventing the disturbance of psychomotor development, and reducing surgical complications because neurovascular structures in an older child are larger and easier to handle.

Syndactyly

Syndactyly, or fused digits, is one of the most common congenital hand defects, occurring in about 1 of every 2,000 births. It is twice as common in males, ten times more common in Caucasians, and involves one or both hands with equal frequency. Ten to 40% of cases have a positive family history, with the condition always inherited as an autosomal dominant trait, although penetrance and expressivity can vary (3). Long-ring finger syndactyly is the most common. Fusion of the thumb and index fingers is the most rare. The mechanism is believed to be a failure of the normal digital separation in the embryonic hand and can involve only the soft tissues (simple syndactyly) or can include the phalanges and nails (complex syndactyly). The webbing is further classified as complete when it extends the entire length of the digits and incomplete when it does not. Syndactyly is commonly associated with congenital syndromes, such as Poland syndrome, which can include chest hypoplasia, and Apert syndrome, which has associated characteristic craniofacial features.

Surgical correction of syndactyly is recommended in all cases to restore independent motion and normal span of the fingers, allowing the proper use of instruments and equipment such as gloves. Separation of border digits (thumb-index, ring-small) is recommended as early as 6 months of age to avoid permanent skeletal deformity due to unequal length between the fused fingers. Syndactyly of the central fingers (index-long, long-ring) can be postponed, although most surgeons recommend correction prior to school age, to save the child from social stigmatization.

The variously described techniques for syndactyly separation all incorporate a few basic principles. A local skin flap, usually dorsal, is used to form the new web, alternating volar and dorsal flaps resurface the fingers, skin grafts cover any remaining defects, and only one side of any digit is released at a time (3). Correction of a web that reaches up to and beyond the proximal interphalangeal (PIP) joint will require skin grafting (Fig. 106-2). Grafts are taken from future non–hair-bearing areas such as the lateral inguinal area, with full-thickness skin grafts less likely to contract than split-thickness ones. Unfortunately, skin grafts tend to become darker than the surrounding skin, especially in dark-skinned individuals. Limiting dissection to only one side of each digit at a time avoids the chance of neurovascular compromise, especially if there is abnormal vascular anatomy. Thus, multiply fused digits require staged correction. Incomplete syndactyly may be corrected with local transposition flaps alone, if the web is shallow. In complex syndactyly, the bony elements and nails are also separated, with joint abnormalities being more common in complicated cases such as seen with Apert syndrome. Long-term follow-up is important, as recurrent webbing or "web creep" with growth can occur, which usually requires minor local flap revision.

Polydactyly

Polydactyly, or extra digits, is the other most frequently occurring congenital hand abnormality. Its incidence is estimated to be at least 1 in 1,000 live births (9). The real incidence may be higher because cases treated with suture ligation in the newborn nursery may not be reported and families of infants with milder forms may not seek treatment (8). The thumb is most commonly duplicated in Caucasians and Asians, occurring in 1 out of every 3,000 live births, whereas African Americans are more likely to have duplication of the small finger, with an incidence of

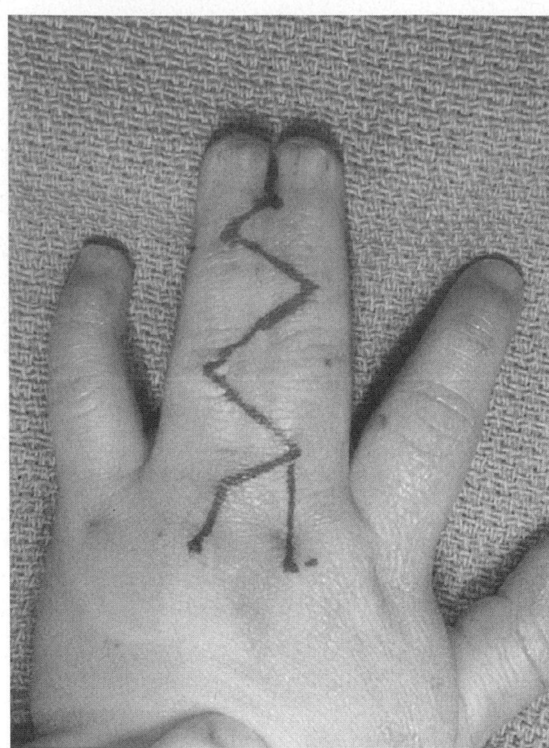

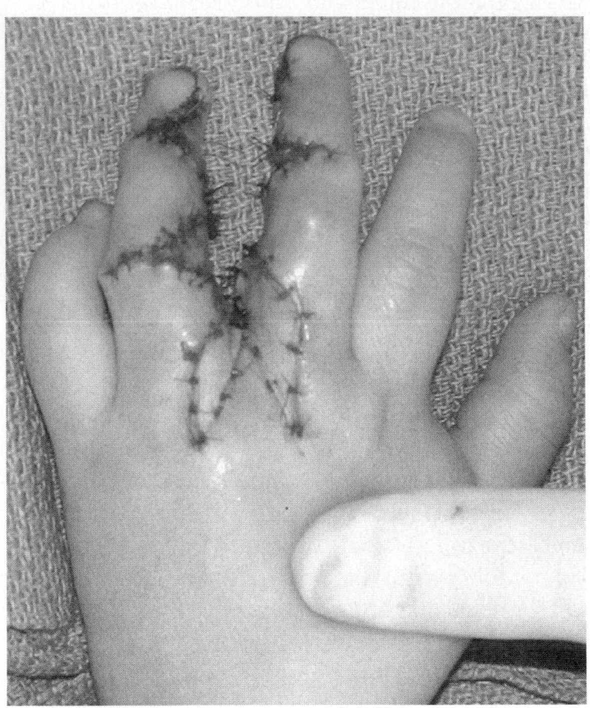

FIGURE 106-2. Syndactyly. **(A)** Preoperative markings for correction of complete simple syndactyly. **(B)** Syndactyly corrected with dorsal flap for web space, alternating volar and dorsal flaps, and skin grafts.

10 per 1,000 (9). Polydactyly is described as radial, central, or ulnar according to the location of the duplicated digit. This is preferred over the old terminology of preaxial and postaxial because controversy exists over where the true axis of the hand lies (9). In addition to the position of the extra digit, its degree of development is further classified. For ulnar polydactyly, Stelling (10) and Turek (11) describe three types: type I is a functionless cutaneous appendage, type II is partial duplication, and type III is complete duplication. Based on a study of pedigrees, Tentamy and McKusick (12) divided them into two types: Type A is a well-formed digit that articulates with the adjacent metacarpal, and Type B is small and poorly developed. Wassel's classification of thumb polydactyly describes the level and completeness of duplication (13). Although the precise mechanism is unknown, ectodermal overgrowth has been observed in experimental animal models and human embryos that developed radial polydactyly (14,15). Thumb polydactyly is rarely associated with a syndrome. Ulnar polydactyly is frequently an autosomal-dominant trait in African Americans, but in Caucasians it is more likely to be associated with one of more than 40 syndromes (8).

In most cases of thumb duplication, both digits are abnormal, making simple excision inadequate. After careful examination, the most functional components of both thumbs are combined into a properly aligned and stable digit. Joint duplication requires preservation of the collateral ligament of the discarded digit to restabilize the joint. The intrinsic muscle insertions at the metacarpophalangeal (MP) joint must be preserved and reattached. The extrinsic extensor and flexor tendons are preserved and centralized when necessary. If the resultant thumb is angulated, osteotomy or articular chondroplasty may be indicated. Temporary Kirschner wires and thumb spica cast are placed for 4 to 5 weeks. Postoperative therapy is not usually required. Correction is recommended prior to 1 year of age, usually between 6 and 9 months. Secondary deformity may occur due to collateral ligament instability or eccentric tendon forces, and should be surgically corrected. If the retained thumb has three phalanges, it will be excessively long, and further modification is needed to allow proper tip-to-tip opposition. A small intermediate phalanx may be excised prior to 1 year of age. Otherwise, treatment is delayed until the epiphyseal ossification center appears (24 to 60 months of age), allowing epiphyseal resection and distal joint chondrodesis (9).

Duplicated ulnar digits that are hypoplastic and have narrow soft-tissue stalks can be treated with suture ligation or surgical excision. Those with broad soft-tissue stalks should be treated with surgical excision to avoid bleeding or infectious complications due to incomplete ligation. Suture ligation may result in a residual soft-tissue nubbin that contains a neuroma, which may bother some individuals by their unsightliness or hypersensitivity, and need secondary excision. Surgical excision of the duplicated digit through an elliptical incision, with cauterization of the neurovascular pedicle, prevents this problem. In more substantial ulnar duplications, the intrinsic hypothenar muscles are preserved and reinserted at the base of the proximal phalanx and extensor mechanism.

Thumb Hypoplasia

The thumb contributes 40% to the function of the hand (16), and any reduction in its size or function significantly affects prehension. Thumb hypoplasia has been classified according to the severity of deficiency (17), which can range from a smaller, but fully functional thumb (type 1) to its complete absence (type 5). The length, joint stability, thenar muscles, and extrinsic tendons of the thumb are carefully evaluated. A functional thumb should reach at least one-half the distance to the index finger PIP joint, have stable collateral ligaments to produce forceful pinch, and possess the ability to actively oppose against the fingertips to allow grasp. The floating thumb (type 4), or pouce flottant, is a floppy nonfunctioning digit that is attached by a soft-tissue pedicle. These thumbs cannot be reconstructed and, along with congenital thumb absence, require creation of a new thumb. Congenital thumb hypoplasia can be associated with potentially life-threatening conditions with concurrent cardiac, hematopoetic, gastrointestinal, and genitourinary abnormalities; therefore ruling out known syndromes is essential.

Correction of thumb hypoplasia or aplasia is recommended between 9 and 12 months of age, when thumb use begins and the structures are large enough for reconstruction. Thumbs that are smaller but stable (type 1) do not require surgical correction. In types 2 and 3, the thumb is small, but may also have a narrowed first web space, collateral ligament instability at the MP joint, and/or inadequate thenar musculature for abduction and opposition. The web space is usually widened with local transposition flaps. Tightening of the existing collateral ligaments, tendon graft, or, in severe cases, arthrodesis stabilizes the MP joint. Opponensplasty can involve transfer of the abductor digiti minimi muscle or the ring finger flexor digitorum superficialis tendon. Thumbs with an unstable carpometacarpal (CMC) joint are difficult to salvage (type 3b), because the joint cannot be recreated and cortical integration of the thumb is frequently poor in these children, who may use the index and long fingers for pinch (18). These thumbs are usually discarded and a new thumb is created. Index finger pollicization is recommended for congenital thumb absence, which involves shortening, rotation, and transfer of the index finger to the thumb position. The index metacarpal shaft is removed and its head is preserved

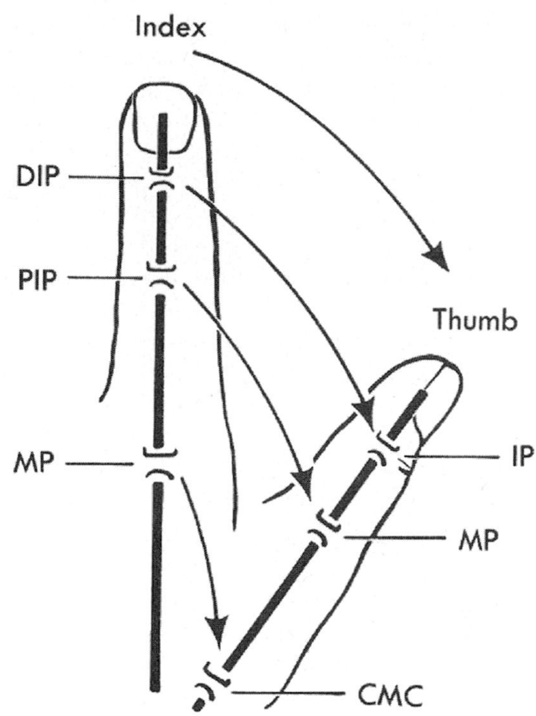

FIGURE 106-3. Pollicization. The index metacarpophalangeal joint becomes the carpometacarpal joint of the new thumb. DIP, distal interphalangeal; PIP, proximal interphalangeal; MP, metacarpophalangeal; IP, interphalangeal; CMC, carpometacarpal. (Reprinted from Flatt AE. *The care of congenital hand anomalies*. St. Louis, MO: Quality Medical, 1994:104, with permission.)

to simulate the mobile CMC joint. The dorsal and volar interosseous muscles become the thumb abductor and adductor, respectively, whereas the extrinsic tendons provide flexion and extension (Fig. 106-3). This technique is preferred over those used for posttraumatic thumb reconstruction, such as free toe transfer, because cortical representation of the thumb does not exist and a transferred toe may remain unused (18). The need for secondary procedures has been reported in more than one-half of these cases, with opponensplasty being the most common (3).

Constriction Rings/Congenital Absence

Congenital constriction rings occur sporadically in every 5 to 15,000 live births and tend to affect the longer fingers more frequently than the thumb (3,9). Proximal involvement is infrequent, and genetic inheritance has not been shown (3). Twenty five percent of these children also have club feet (9). Until more recently, it was believed that strands of amnion that ensnared the limbs caused all cases, often in the presence of oligohydramnios. However, amniotic tissue remnants are rarely seen at birth, and the hypothesis does not adequately explain the associated facial clefts that sometimes occur. Current theories propose that various interruptions in fetal circulation disrupt growth of the limb or digit (7). Constriction rings vary in depth, with deeper rings causing distal lymphedema and even congenital amputation. Fused digital tips (acrosyndactyly) are corrected early in one stage to avoid permanent deformity. Simple rings are completely excised and z-plasty closure prevents circumferential scar contracture. Surgery may be postponed until the neurovascular structures are of reasonable size (6 to 12 months). However, deep rings with severe distal lymphedema and risk of vascular compromise require urgent release in two stages, with one-half the circumference being corrected each time. Some degree of soft-tissue or skeletal deformity is more likely to persist in these cases (3).

Congenital absence can affect any part of a hand or limb. Shortened fingers that are actively mobile are useful. They may be augmented with nonvascularized toe phalanx bone graft or distraction lengthening, although these techniques do not recreate functioning joints. Reconstruction is essential in cases of thumb absence, whereas finger reconstruction is indicated mostly in severe cases where useful grasp is impossible. When adequate fingers are available, pollicization yields the best thumb (see "Thumb Hypoplasia"). Otherwise, free microvascular transfer of a great or second toe to the thumb or finger position can allow prehension. Successful microvascular transfer may not be achievable in cases with hypoplasia because there is a higher chance of abnormal bony or arterial anatomy. Microvascular transfer is recommended prior to 18 months of age, before patterns of hand use are established. Early complications usually involve vascular insufficiency, whereas late complications include decreased motion and poor cortical integration of the new digit (3). Growth potential seems to be maintained in the transferred toes (19). Although very lifelike finger prostheses can be constructed, they are purely cosmetic and lack sensibility and motion. Children with congenital amputations at the wrist, forearm, and arm levels can be fitted with a functioning hook prosthesis when they are able to sit upright, which can be as early as 5 or 6 months of age. Myoelectric prostheses are usually fitted from 1 to 2 years of age. In general, a child's developmental readiness determines the timing of prosthetic application (20).

Trigger Digits

The existence of truly congenital trigger digits is controversial because few cases are diagnosed in the neonatal period (21). Trigger thumb in children is much more common than trigger fingers and is usually noted at 6 to 12 months of age, when the constant flexed positioning of the thumb should disappear. Active triggering is rarely seen, and the most common presentation is fixed flexion at the thumb interphalangeal joint. Ten to 30% of cases are bilateral (18,21), with some reported cases of familial involvement (3,18). The pathogenesis is not well established, with either flexor tendon thickening or tendon sheath stenosis believed to cause trigger thumbs and abnormal tendon anatomy being associated with trigger fingers (18,22). Spontaneous resolution has been reported in 0% to 30% of cases (3,21) and delay of surgery up to 3 years of age can still yield good results (3). Trigger thumb is easily corrected by division of the annular pulley. The nodule on the flexor tendon resolves spontaneously. Trigger fingers require careful exploration because A1 pulley release alone can be inadequate and tendon resection may be necessary (22). Complications are related to inadequate release, especially in trigger fingers, and neurovascular injury.

TRAUMA

Fractures

Twenty percent of all pediatric fractures occur in the hand, reaching a peak incidence in the early teens (23). One-third of pediatric hand fractures involve the physis, which is cartilaginous and thus weaker than the tendons and ligaments (24). Growth plate injuries of the hand are described by the Salter-Harris classification (Fig. 106-4) (25). In type I injuries, the metaphysis separates from the epiphysis, and the physis appears widened on X-ray. Type II injuries include a fracture of the metaphysis, along with physeal separation. Type III injuries have physeal separation and intraarticular fracture of the epiphysis. Type IV fractures occur through the metaphysis, physis, and epiphysis, and are highly unstable. The physis is crushed in type V injuries, which always result in growth disturbance. The normal process of pediatric bone remodeling helps to realign healing diaphyseal and metaphyseal fractures, making complete anatomic reduction less crucial, especially in younger children. Up to 20 degrees of angulation can be acceptable, especially in the plane of normal joint motion. Rotational deformities, however, will not correct

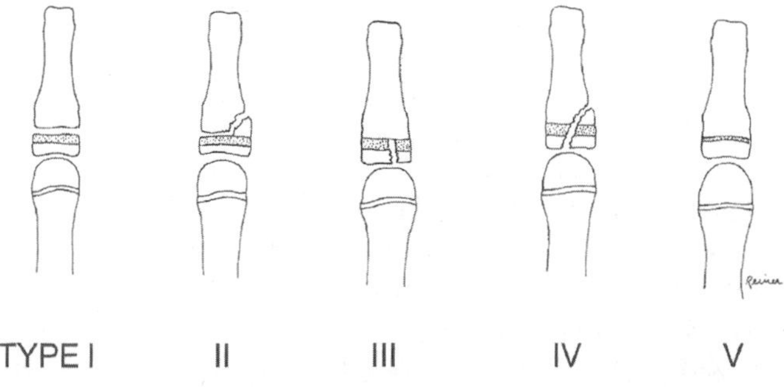

FIGURE 106-4. Salter-Harris classification of physeal fractures. (Reprinted from Van Heest A, McElfresh EC. *Surgery of the hand and upper extremity*. New York: McGraw-Hill, 1996:2181, with permission.)

with growth and cannot be accepted to any degree (23). Fractures involving the physis and epiphysis require meticulous reduction because large physeal gaps can cause premature growth arrest and joint incongruity can lead to posttraumatic arthrosis.

Fractures in children can be difficult to diagnose because an accurate history may be unavailable and they may not complain of pain. Careful observation for localized swelling, bruising, tenderness, refusal to use an injured part, and adequate X-rays with multiple views are important. Closed fracture reduction requires sedation or even general anesthesia. Immobilization usually involves casting because splinting is often impractical and activity modification can be impossible. Younger children manage to slip out of anything less than a long-arm cast. Waterproof cast liners can facilitate skin hygiene and avoid premature cast changes due to inadvertent water contact. Although most pediatric hand fractures can be treated with immobilization alone, 10% to 20% require closed reduction, and up to 10% need surgical fixation (24). Hand fractures are clinically healed in 3 to 4 weeks in younger children and 5 to 6 weeks in older ones. A fracture is clinically healed when it is stable and nontender to palpation. Radiographic evidence of bony union commonly lags behind clinical findings. Smooth Kirschner wires are usually used for fixation because they can be placed across the physis without damaging it.

A common injury in children is the crushed fingertip, which results in an open distal phalangeal tuft fracture. These fractures usually heal without difficulty. Nailbed repair is usually performed, especially if there is a large subungual hematoma, but more recent studies have shown good results in children with nail trephination alone (26). Small absorbable sutures are used to repair the soft tissue, and the nail is replaced as a stent if the nailbed has been repaired. Nail deformity due to scarring of the nail matrix can occur, but may not be apparent for 2 or 3 months. Although prophylactic oral antibiotics are commonly prescribed for these injuries, prospective studies in adults have not shown any benefit (27). In children, hyperflexion of the fingertip can cause an open Salter-Harris type I or II distal phalanx fracture that is easily missed in the emergency department. The presence of subungual hematoma or nail avulsion indicates an open fracture. X-rays are needed to make the diagnosis and may only show subtle widening at the physis. The nail plate is an important stabilizer in these fractures and should be replaced at the time of nailbed repair, along with a fingertip splint. Prophylactic antibiotics are recommended because these fractures have a high incidence of osteomyelitis (24), which can result in growth arrest, mallet deformity, or joint destruction.

Adequate evaluation of middle and proximal phalangeal fractures requires isolated views of the injured fingers, including a lateral view. Rotational malalignment is diagnosed by physical examination, with the fractured finger scissoring over or under the adjacent finger during formation of a closed fist. The most common fractures are Salter-Harris type II injuries at the base of the proximal phalanx (24), which are usually stable after closed reduction. Condylar neck fractures are often unstable and tend to displace or angulate dorsally. They should be treated with closed reduction, splinting, and follow-up X-rays in 1 week. Open reduction is recommended for displaced intraarticular fractures involving more than 20% to 25% of the joint surface, especially when the physis is involved (Salter-Harris types III and IV) (24).

Metacarpal fractures are most commonly seen in adolescents who punch an object or another person. As in adults, this produces a volarly angulated metacarpal neck fracture. The physis is not usually involved (24). Closed reduction is recommended, although up to 40 degrees of volar angulation can be accepted in the ring and small fingers due to compensation by their mobile CMC joints. The index and long finger CMC joints are relatively immobile, so only around 10 degrees of volar angulation are acceptable (24). Again, rotational deformity needs to be ruled out by physical examination. Fractures and dislocations at the metacarpal bases can be difficult to evaluate on plain radiograph alone, although oblique views of the hand can be helpful. Sometimes computed tomography scan is necessary to assess dislocation or intraarticular displacement, which both require surgical fixation.

Carpal fractures in children younger than 10 years of age are uncommon because their carpal bones are mostly cartilaginous (28). Scaphoid fractures are most common, followed in decreasing order by triquetral, capitate, and lunate fractures (24). As secondary ossification of the scaphoid starts at age 4 to 6 years and continues until 14 to 16 years (24), fractures may be difficult to diagnose. Early ossification of secondary centers can even be mistaken for fracture to those unfamiliar with carpal growth patterns. If the anatomic snuffbox is tender, conservative management involves a thumb spica cast, with follow-up X-ray in 1 to 2 weeks when the resorbing fracture line may be more apparent. Bone scan or magnetic resonance imaging can also help to make the diagnosis. If the fracture is not displaced, treatment involves 4 to 6 weeks of cast immobilization. Carpal dislocations and ligamentous injuries are rare in children.

Tendon and Nerve Injuries

Interestingly, primary repair was accepted for tendon injuries in children before it was for adults because children's wounds were believed to heal more quickly and with less scarring. Now it is understood that pediatric tendon injuries differ only in their diagnosis and rehabilitation, rather than in their biological behavior (29). Children are not able to comprehend the significance of a tendon injury,

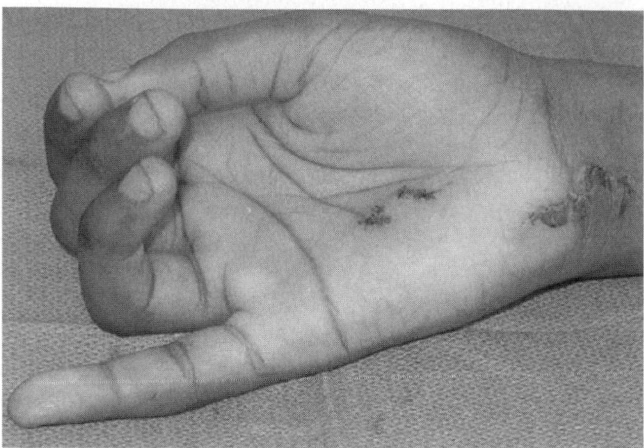

FIGURE 106-5. Laceration in the palm transected the flexor digitorum superficialis and profundus tendons of the little finger. The normal resting cascade of the fingers is disrupted.

have limited ability to cooperate for physical examination, and are mostly unable to actively participate in therapy, all of which require a drastically different treatment approach that must be tailored to their age and maturity level. Statistically, children's tendon injuries occur most frequently from laceration by broken glass, followed by injury from sharp metal such as knives (29). A detailed history of the injury, especially from a reliable witness, is extremely helpful in making the diagnosis. Otherwise, one is limited to careful physical examination, often during play or routine use of the hand, because radiological imaging is not reliable for this purpose. However, radiographic or sonographic examinations can rule out the presence of a retained foreign body. The resting cascade of the fingers will be abnormal, with the finger extended if a flexor tendon is cut (Fig. 106-5) and flexed if the extensor tendon is cut. If the index of suspicion for tendon injury is high, surgical exploration is warranted, especially because associated neurovascular injury is common. All flexor tendons should be repaired within 1.5 weeks. Delay may result in an excessively shortened musculotendinous unit that cannot be repaired. Any of a number of specialized grasping or locking tendon suture methods may be used. Extensor tendon lacerations distal to the MP joint may be repaired or splinted with the joint in full extension for 6 weeks. Extensor tendon injuries proximal to the MP joint should be repaired within 1 week.

Rehabilitation of flexor tendon repair in adults involves some type of splinting protocol where limited tendon motion is allowed to minimize scarring. Such protocols are not suitable for younger children, who are immobilized in a cast for 3 to 4 weeks until tendon healing is complete. Cooperative older children can be managed successfully with adult-type rehabilitation protocols. Once the tendon is healed, formal therapy may be instituted, which also incorporates play activities. Further protective splinting may be indicated during sports, and night splinting may be used to treat joint contractures. Surgical treatment of tendon adhesions is typically delayed until the child becomes old enough to participate in formal postoperative therapy regimens.

Similar to tendon injuries, nerve injuries can also be challenging to diagnose in children. Motor function is assessed by careful physical examination. Sensory examination may be possible in children as young as 3 years of age, who are asked to discern whether an injured fingertip feels the "same" or "different" from the other fingertips. In younger children, the water immersion test may be tried. In the office, the hand is immersed in water for several minutes. Denervated skin will not wrinkle, which suggests the presence of a sensory nerve injury. Alternatively, parents can be instructed to inspect the fingers at the end of the child's bath. Occasionally, nerve injuries are diagnosed only when the child presents with a burn or fingertip infection because the digit is numb. In the presence of a laceration, a high index of suspicion for nerve injury should lead to surgical exploration. After repair, axonal regeneration occurs at the rate of 1 to 4 millimeters per day. Motor nerves should be repaired as soon as possible because muscle fiber fibrosis begins to develop by 12 months and recovery will be incomplete. Sensory recovery, however, may be possible even years after nerve injury (30). Basic principles of nerve repair include the use of magnification, microsurgical instruments, and suture, and tension-free repair.

Burns and Frostbite

According to the American Burn Association guidelines, an isolated hand burn is regarded as a major burn, with possible resulting functional and cosmetic impairments (31). Children sustain scald burns to the thinner dorsal skin of their hands when they pull pots or bowls of hot food onto themselves. Although severe palmar burns are unusual in adults due to the protective reflex of clenching the fists, they are frequent in children after direct contact with hot objects such as irons, heaters, and oven doors. Superficial burns are managed with debridement and dressing changes, whereas full-thickness burns require skin grafting. Escharotomy is indicated for vascular compromise of the digits by circumferential full-thickness burns, using longitudinal incisions along the radial aspects of the thumb and the ulnar aspects of the fingers. Deeper partial-thickness burns are treated according to the estimated time to secondary healing. If the burn is not expected to heal before 3 weeks, tangential excision and skin grafting is recommended. Palmar burns rarely require grafting because the skin is much thicker. During burn excision, preservation of the paratenon allows the use of skin grafts. Meshed grafts are not recommended on the hands for cosmetic reasons. The hand should be splinted in "antideformity" position (31)—wrist at neutral or slightly extended, MP joints fully flexed, PIP and DIP joints fully extended, and thumb maximally abducted to prevent severe joint contractures. Late management of complications includes pressure gloves for hypertrophic scarring, z-plasty release of syndactyly, and flap correction of nailfold contractures.

As in adults, severe frostbite causes soft-tissue necrosis. In addition, cold injury in children can damage the physeal plates of the distal phalanges, resulting in their premature closure and altered longitudinal growth. Uneven physeal closure causes angulation of the fingertips, usually of all the digits. The physeal damage is not apparent at the time of injury and may be accompanied by nail dysplasia. Because the child usually curls the fingers around the flexed thumb during exposure to the cold, the physes of the thumbs are frequently spared (28).

Compartment Syndrome

Untreated compartment syndrome of the hand and forearm results in severe permanent functional impairment and secondary deformity. When the interstitial pressure within a muscle compartment exceeds the venous pressure, venous outflow is blocked and tissue perfusion is interrupted. This can occur even though a distal arterial pulse is detectable. Common scenarios in which compartment syndrome may occur include crush injury, bleeding from needle stick or fracture, intravenous catheter extravasation, venomous snakebite, and excessively tight cast placement. Pain is an early indicator, although crying or complaints may be misinterpreted or ignored in a young child (28). Pain with passive stretch of the affected muscles is diagnostic. Compartment pressures may also be measured. Early treatment by open fasciotomy of the three forearm muscle compartments (volar, dorsal, mobile lateral wad) and, if involved, the intrinsic muscles of the hand (dorsal and volar interossei, thenar, hypothenar) is essential to prevent irreversible nerve and muscle damage. Along with the muscles, the median nerve should also be decompressed at the forearm and wrist; the ulnar nerve should be decompressed at the wrist. Neonatal compartment syndrome or gangrene has also been described, which occurs at or shortly after birth and often features a forearm skin wound (32).

REFERENCES

1. Daluiski A, Soyun EY, Lyons KM. The molecular control of upper extremity development: implications for congenital hand anomalies. *J Hand Surg [Am]* 2001;26:8–22.
2. Riddle RD, Tabin CJ. How limbs develop. *Sci Am* 1999;280:74–79.
3. Flatt AE. *The care of congenital hand anomalies.* St. Louis, MO: Quality Medical, 1994.
4. Kasser JR. The biologic aspects of children's fractures. In: Johnstone EW, Foster BK, eds. *Rockwood and Wilkin's fractures in children,* 5th ed. Philadelphia: Lippincott Williams & Wilkins, 2001:21–42.
5. Swanson AB. A classification for congenital limb malformations. *J Hand Surg [Am]* 1976;1:8–22.
6. Giele H, Giele C, Bower C, et al. The incidence and epidemiology of congenital upper limb anomalies: a total population study. *J Hand Surg [Am]* 2001;26:628–634.
7. Hoyme HE, Jones KL, Van Allen MI, et al. Vascular pathogenesis of transverse limb reduction defects. *J Pediatr* 1982;101:839–843.
8. Rayan GM, Frey B. Ulnar polydactyly. *Plast Reconstr Surg* 2001; 107:1449–1454.
9. Light TR. Congenital anomalies: syndactyly, polydactyly and cleft hand. In: Peimer CA, ed. *Surgery of the hand and upper extremity.* New York: McGraw-Hill, 1996:2111–2144.
10. Stelling F. The upper extremity. In: Ferguson AB, ed. *Orthopedic surgery in infancy and childhood.* Baltimore: Williams & Wilkins, 1963:304–308.
11. Turek SL. *Orthopedic principles and their application.* Philadelphia: Lippincott, 1967.
12. Tentamy S, McKusick V. The genetics of hand malformations. *Birth Defects* 1978;14:1–619.
13. Wassel HD. The results of surgery for polydactyly of the thumb. *Clin Orthop Rel Res* 1969;64:175–193.
14. Yasuda M. Pathogenesis of preaxial polydactyly of the hand in human embryos. *J Embryol Exp Morphol* 1975;33:745–756.
15. Nogami H, Oohira A. Experimental study on the pathogenesis of polydactyly of the thumb. *J Hand Surg [Am]* 1980;5:443–450.
16. The upper extremities. In: Cocchiarella L, Andersson GBJ, eds. *Guides to the evaluation of permanent impairment,* 5th ed. United States: AMA Press, 2001:433–521.
17. Kleinman WB. Management of thumb hypoplasia. *Hand Clin* 1990;6:617–641.
18. Ezaki M.Congenital anomalies: thumb dyplasia. In: Peimer CA, ed. *Surgery of the hand and upper extremity.* New York: McGraw-Hill, 1996:2145–2164.
19. Chang J, Jones NF. Radiographic analysis of growth in pediatric microsurgical toe-to-hand transfers. *Plast Reconstr Surg* 2002;109: 576–582.
20. Watts HG, Clark MW. *Who is Amelia? Caring for children with limb deficiencies.* United States: American Academy of Orthopaedic Surgeons, 1998.
21. DeSmet L, Steenwerckx A, Van Ransbeeck H. The so-called congenital trigger digit: further experience. *Acta Orthop Belg* 1998;64:306–308.
22. Cardon LJ, Ezaki M, Carter PR. Trigger finger in children. *J Hand Surg [Am]* 1999;24:1156–1161.
23. Johnstone EW, Foster BK. The biologic aspects of children's fractures. In: Beaty JH, Kasser JR, eds. *Rockwood and Wilkin's fractures in children,* 5th ed. Philadelphia: Lippincott Williams & Wilkins, 2001:21–42.
24. Van Heest A, McElfresh EC. Pediatric skeletal trauma: digits, hand, and wrist. In: Peimer CA, ed. *Surgery of the hand and upper extremity.* 1996: McGraw-Hill, 2179–2205.
25. Salter RB, Harris WR. Injuries involving the epiphyseal plate. *J Bone Joint Surg Am* 1963;45:587–622.
26. Roser SE, Gellman H. Comparison of nail bed repair versus nail trephination for subungual hematomas in children. *J Hand Surg [Am]* 1999;24:1166–1170.
27. Stevenson J, McNaughton G, Riley J. The use of prophylactic flucloxacillin in treatment of open fractures of the distal phalanx within an accident and emergency department: a double-blind randomized placebo-controlled trial. *J Hand Surg [Br]* 2003;28:388–394.
28. Light TR.Hand. In: Oldham KT, Colombani PM, Foglia RP, eds. *Surgery of infants and children: scientific principles and practice,* 1st ed. Philadelphia: Lippincott-Raven, 1997:1709–1714.
29. Idler RS. Pediatric tendon injuries. In: Peimer CA, ed. *Surgery of the hand and upper extremity.* New York: McGraw-Hill, 1996:2165–2177.
30. Mackinnon SE, Dillon AL. *Surgery of the peripheral nerve.* New York: Thieme Medical, 1988.
31. Chung KC, Robson MC, Smith DJ Jr. Management of thermal, electrical, radiation, and chemical injuries. In: Peimer CA, ed. *Surgery of the hand and upper extremity.* New York: McGraw-Hill, 1996:1797–1818.
32. Caouette-Laberge L, Bortoluzzi P, Egerszegi EP, et al. Neonatal Volkmann's ischemic contracture of the forearm: a report of five cases. *Plast Reconstr Surg* 1992;90:621–628.

PART K

Skin and Soft Tissue

Chapter 107

Surgical Disorders of the Skin

David Rowe and Arun K. Gosain

ANATOMY

The function of skin was described by Virchow as a covering that conferred protection to the underlying, more complex organs (1). He postulated that skin was a mere passive barrier to the loss of fluid and provided protection against injury. Since the time of Virchow's observations, we have learned that the skin is, in fact, a highly complex organ characterized by precise interactions of many cellular and molecular processes. In toto, it is the heaviest organ in the body, accounting for up to 16% of total body weight. Skin provides not only a protective barrier against the elements, but also crucial regulatory mechanisms for temperature, sensory input, immunomodulation, and energy.

Skin is composed of many components (Fig. 107-1) and is comprised by the epidermis, arising from an ectodermal epithelial layer, and the dermis, a mesodermally derived connective tissue layer. The epidermis is a layered progression of stratified squamous epithelial cells that ultimately produce keratin and form the stratum corneum, the outermost protective layer of the skin. Interdigitated within the basal layer of the epidermis are melanocytes, which are neural crest-derived cells that provide pigmentation and protection from ultraviolet light. The dermis is the penultimate layer consisting largely of connective tissue. The dermis provides support for the epidermis, effectively attaching the outermost layer to the deeper subcutaneous tissues. Contained in the dermal layer are hair follicles and sebaceous glands, both of which protect the skin surface. The subcutaneous tissue, located under the dermis, consists of loose connective tissue and adipocytes. This layer provides a source of energy storage and provides a flexible and protective structure over deeper organs.

David Rowe and Arun K. Gosain: Department of Plastic Surgery, Medical College of Wisconsin, Milwaukee, Wisconsin 53226.

RASHES, PAPULES, AND VESICLES

The etiology of skin eruptions is expansive and not the primary focus of this discussion. Rashes, papules, and vesicles may be diagnosed by an accurate account of character duration, nature of onset, past medical history, family history, and medication use. Table 107-1 describes many common skin disorders, their diagnosis, and treatment modalities (Figs. 107-2 and 107-3).

BENIGN TUMORS

There are a multitude of skin tumors that may be found in children. Although the majority of lumps and bumps are benign, malignant and metastatic lesions may be found in this age group (2) (Table 107-2).

Epithelial Cysts

Epidermoid Cysts

Epidermoid cysts (infundibular cysts) comprise the most common type of surgically excised superficial tumors in children (3). They are lined with squamous epithelium and contain hair, sebaceous material, and keratin. The lesions most commonly occur on the face, neck, or trunk, but may be located in any area. These lesions range in size from 0.2 to 5 cm and enlarge slowly. On examination, they are elevated, tense, smooth intracutaneous or intradermal lesions.

Epidermoid cysts are treated with surgical excision. Complete excision of the cyst is necessary to prevent recurrence because any retained portion of the cyst will likely

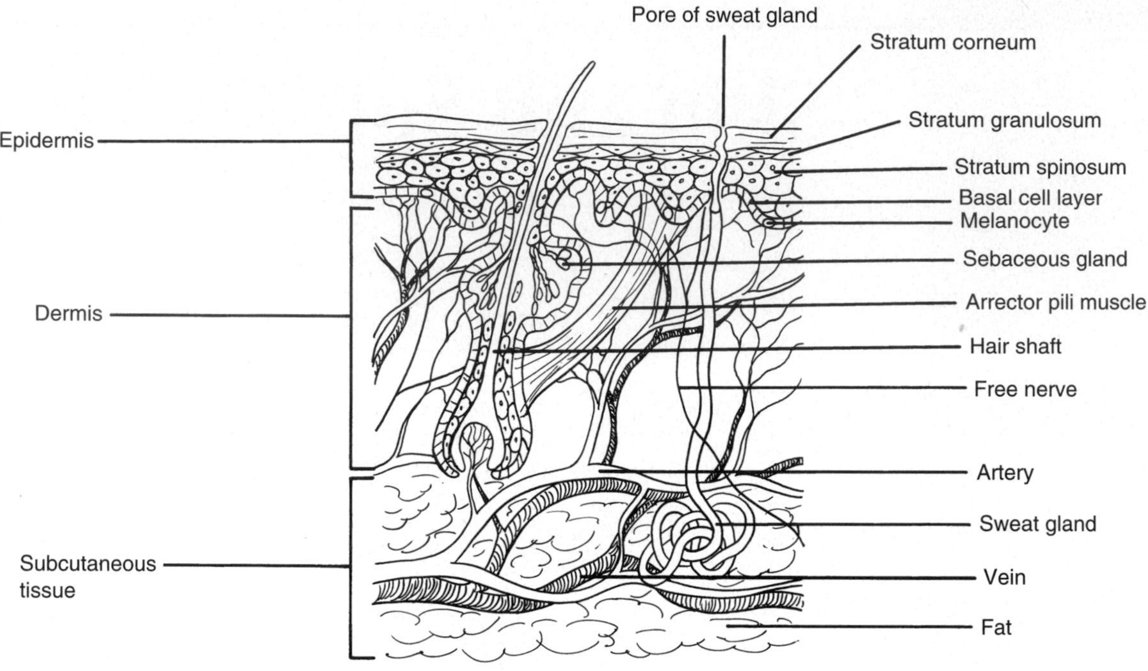

FIGURE 107-1. Schematic representation of the skin. (From Holbrook KA, Sybert V. Structure and biochemical properties of the skin of adults, children, and newborn infants. In: Schachner LA, Hansen RC, eds. *Pediatric dermatology*. New York: Churchill Livingstone, 1988: 30, with permission.)

cause recurrence. Rupture of the cyst may result in an intense granulomatous reaction. Once this foreign body reaction has occurred, the cyst may become adherent to the surrounding structures, making definitive enucleation problematic. Epidermoid cysts may also become infected. Treatment of infected cysts consists of primary drainage prior to surgical removal. Prior antibiotic treatment of infected or ruptured cysts has not been shown to reduce the bacterial load.

Dermoid Cysts

Dermoid cysts are subcutaneous congenital hamartomas lined by epithelium. These malformations are most commonly found in the lateral ends of the eyebrows and along the lines of cleavage. Size is variable, but may be as large as 10 cm and have similar characteristics as epidermoid cysts. Dermoid cysts have a small but important potential for intracranial extension.

Treatment of dermoid cysts is by surgical excision. Lesions found at the nasofrontal area must be carefully evaluated to rule out intracranial extension of the lesion. Lesions found off midline, such as those at the lateral aspect of the brow, do not routinely require computed tomography (CT) scan for preoperative evaluation (4). CT and magnetic resonance imaging are the two diagnostic modalities used to investigate the penetration of the calvaria for midline lesions.

Milia

Milia are epidermal inclusion cysts that are 1 to 4 mm in diameter. Primary milia are found on the face in as many as 50% of newborns. They are also commonly found in middle-age women, in areas following traumatic injury, and occasionally after prolonged use of nonsteroidal anti-inflammatory drugs. Extrusion of cyst contents and abrasive cleaning are the treatment of choice.

VIRAL INFECTIONS

Verrucae (Warts)

Warts are benign tumors caused by the human papilloma virus (HPV). Lesions may be found on the skin or mucus membranes. Although more than 60 variants of HPV have been identified, HPV 2 and 4, the strains associated with verrucae vulgaris, are most common in children. Other lesions such as plantar warts (HPV 1) and condyloma accuminata (primarily HPV 6 and 11) are also found in this age group.

The appearance of condyloma accuminata in the anogenital region may raise suspicion of child abuse and/or early sexual exposure (Fig. 107-4). However, several studies that have investigated the appearance of anogenital warts in children concluded that the majority of these lesions are acquired via nonsexual contact, such as perinatal

TABLE 107-1 Rashes, Papules, and Vesicles.

Disorder	Skin Lesions	Distribution	Diagnostics	Treatment
Irritant dermatitis	Papules, vesicles, scale, crusts	Face, trunk, extremities		Avoidance of irritant, topical steroids, and emollients
Contact allergic dermatitis	Papules, vesicles, scale, crusts	Face, trunk, extremities	Patch testing	Discontinuation of agent, topical steroids, systemic steroids
Atopic dermatitis	Papules, scale, crusts, lichenification, pigmentary change	Face, generalized	None, increased IgE	Lubricants, topical steroids
Seborrheic dermatitis	Erythema, papules, scale, pigmentary change	Face, scalp, creases		Usually improves spontaneously
Scabies	Papules, scale, vesicles, pustules, burrows	Hands, wrists, axillae, genitals, breasts, palms, soles	Scabies preparation	Permethrin 5% cream
Ringworm	Papules, scale, pustules	Face, scalp, trunk, extremities	Potassium hydroxide preparation	Topical or oral antifungal agents
Pityriasis rosea	Papules, scaly patches, Christmas tree pattern	Trunk, proximal extremities	Syphilis serology	Usually improves spontaneously
Psoriasis	Papules, plaques, scale	Scalp, trunk, extremities	Throat culture	Topical steroids and emollients; tar, keratolytics, anthralin as adjuncts
Herpes simplex	Vesicles, pustules, erosions	Face, trunk, extremities	Tzank preparation, viral culture	Symptomatic treatment (cool compresses, analgesics)
Varicella	Papules, vesicles, crusts	Face, trunk, extremities	Tzank preparation, viral culture	Symptomatic treatment (cool compresses, calamine, antihistamines)
Herpes zoster	Dermatomal pattern	Dermatomal	Tzank preparation	
Insect bites	Papules, urticaria, vesicles	Trunk, extremities	Negative Tzank preparation	Symptomatic treatment
Miliaria	Papules, vesicles	Occluded areas	Negative Tzank, potassium hydroxide	Abrasive cleaning
Impetigo streptococci	Crusts, scale	Face, trunk, extremities	Positive culture, Gram stain	Oral cephalosporins, amoxicillin, dicloaxillin
Staphylococci	Crusts, scale, bullae	Any site	Positive culture, Gram stain	Oral cephalosporins, amoxicillin, dicloaxillin
Scalded skin syndrome (staphylococcus)	Sunburn-like erythema, erosions, crusting	Face, extremities	Skin biopsy	Oral cephalosporins, amoxicillin, dicloaxillin, possible IV antibiosis
Toxic epidermal necrolysis	Bullae, erosions, crusts	Generalized, mucous membrane lesions	Skin biopsy	Aggressive burn therapy
Erythema multiforme	Target lesions, erosions	Extremities, mucous membrane lesions	Skin biopsy	Supportive

Adapted from Cohen BA. Skin. In: Oldham KT, Colombani PM, Foglia RP, eds. *Surgery of infants and children: scientific principles and practice.* Philadelphia: Lippincott-Raven, 1997:1619-1632.

contact with the mother or indirect transmission during routine contact situations (bathing, diaper changes) (5,6).

Many methods are available for treatment of verrucae, including chemical and ablative techniques. Surgical excision incurs a high rate of recurrence and thus is usually not indicated. Topical agents such as salicylic acid, trichloroacetic acid, formaldehyde, and glutaraldehyde have been used. Liquid nitrogen is also a popular method of removal. However, this technique does produce pain and blistering. Intralesional bleomycin and topical 5-fluorouracil have also been reported to be effective. Electrodessication may be performed on recalcitrant lesions.

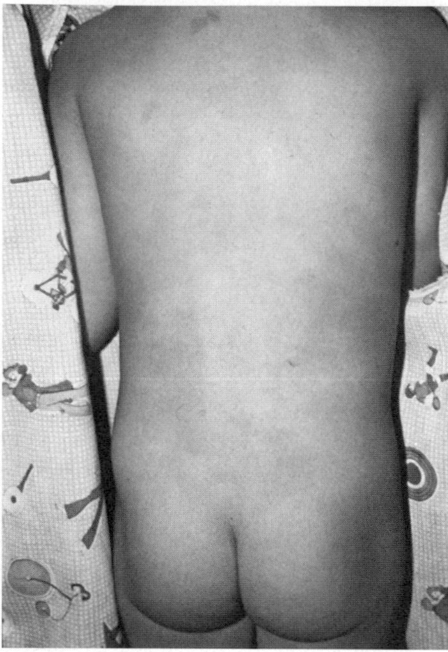

FIGURE 107-2. Total-body sunburnlike erythema following low-grade fever and upper respiratory symptoms. Epidermal stripping (Nikolsky sign) is indicative of staphylococcal scalded skin syndrome. (From Cohen BA. Skin. In: Oldham KT, Colombani PM, Foglia RP, eds. *Surgery of infants and children: scientific principles and practice.* Philadelphia: Lippincott-Raven, 1997:1627, with permission.)

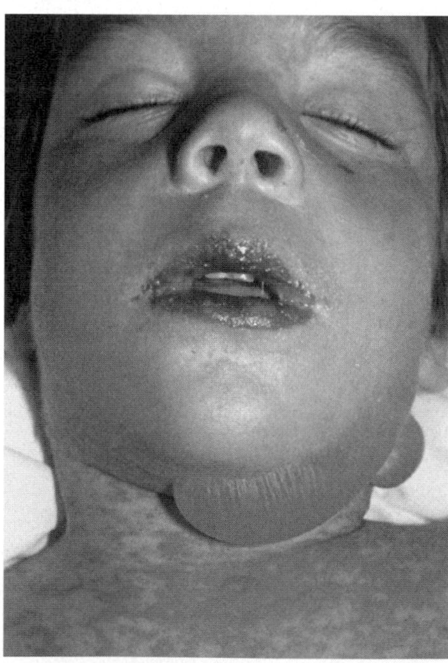

FIGURE 107-3. Stevens-Johnson syndrome. Severe blistering of skin and mucous membranes, as seen in picture, and widespread rash developed in this 6-year-old girl during a course of trimethoprim-sulfamethoxazole for an ear infection. (From Cohen BA. Skin. In: Oldham KT, Colombani PM, Foglia RP, eds. *Surgery of infants and children: scientific principles and practice.* Philadelphia: Lippincott-Raven, 1997:1627, with permission.)

TABLE 107-2 Histologic Diagnosis of 775 Superficial Lumps Excised in Children.

Classification	*Percentage*
Epithelial cysts	459 (59%)
Congenital malformations (pilomaxrixoma, lymphangioma, branchial cleft cyst, hamartomas)	117 (15%)
Benign neoplasms (neurofibroma, lipoma, adnexal tumors)	56 (7%)
Undetermined etiology (xanthomas, fibroma, histiocytoma)	50 (6%)
Self-limited processes (pseudorheumatoid nodules, urticaria pigmentosa, insect bite)	47 (6%)
Malignant tumors (rhabdomyosarcoma, neurofibrosarcoma, fibrosarcoma, malignant fibrous histiocytoma, malignant pleomorphic adenoma)	11 (1.4%)
Miscellaneous	35 (4%)

Adapted from Knight PJ, Reiner CB. Superficial lumps in children: what, when and why? *Pediatrics* 1983;72(2):149.

Molluscum Contagiosum

Molluscum contagiosum is an infection caused by a poxvirus and is distinguished by smooth 1- to 3-mm papules. In adults, this is primarily a sexually transmitted disease and is usually found in the anogenital region. In children, molluscum contagiosum is transmitted primarily by nonvenereal contact. The papules may enlarge to

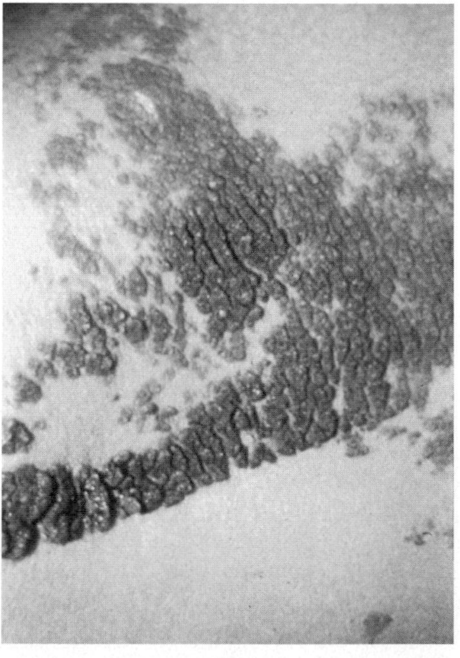

FIGURE 107-4. This 1-year-old girl developed extensive anogenital warts when the child was delivered. (From Cohen BA. Skin. In: Oldham KT, Colombani PM, Foglia RP, eds. *Surgery of infants and children: scientific principles and practice*. Philadelphia: Lippincott-Raven, 1997:1628, with permission.)

1 to 2 cm and develop hyperkeratosis and infection. Most lesions disappear within 6 months. Those that do not regress or that are symptomatic may be treated with curettage or electrodessication.

NEVI

Nevi, or the common mole, are composed of nests of melanocytes found at varying levels within the skin. They are very common and are found at birth or during the first few months of life. This discussion focuses on nevi that often come to surgical resection. Indications for surgical resection include the potential for malignant transformation (congenital melanocytic nevi, nevus sebaceous, and dysplastic nevi), potential confusion with malignant lesions (Spitz nevi), intense pruritis (inflammatory linear verrucous epidermal nevi), and significant disfigurement (wooly hairy nevi).

Nevi with Malignant Potential

Congenital Melanocytic Nevi

Congenital melanocytic nevi are typically brown, vary in size and shape, and can be found anywhere on the body (7). They are present in 1% to 2% of children either at birth or within the first year of life. Clinically, the lesion appears as a well-demarcated lesion with irregular asymmetric borders and a tan to dark brown hue (8). Lesions may be characterized by small, intermediate, and giant sizes. Giant congenital melanocytic nevi are characterized by a diameter of 20 cm or greater in adulthood, or occupying greater than 2% body surface area (9) (Fig. 107-5). Body surface area is a more accurate measure to distinguish between congenital and giant congenital melanocytic nevi, particularly in children. However, there remains confusion in classifying giant congenital melanocytic nevi in children, particularly because it is often difficult to determine body surface area of an irregular lesion in a child. Generally, congenital melanocytic nevi are solitary, but smaller satellite lesions may be present with a giant congenital melanocytic nevi.

The risk of malignant transformation in congenital melanocytic nevi, especially giant congenital melanocytic nevi, remains a point of controversy. The percent of adolescent malignant melanoma associated with congenital melanocytic nevi may be approximately 20%; however, the actual percentage of those with congenital melanocytic nevi who have malignant transformation is likely less than 1% (10). Although there are no known biologic differences between "giant" and "nongiant" congenital melanocytic nevi other than the size of the lesion, giant congenital melanocytic nevi are believed to have a higher incidence of malignant transformation due to the increased number of nevus cells at risk for such transformation. The rate of malignant degeneration in giant congenital melanocytic nevi is reported to be between 2% and 42% (11,12). There have been few longitudinal studies of malignant transformation in giant congenital melanocytic nevi. One such study reported the incidence of malignant transformation to be greater than 8.5% in the first 15 years of life (13), and another study reported a lifetime incidence of malignant transformation to be 4% to 6% (14).

The incidence of malignancy in small and medium-size (less than 20 cm) congenital melanocytic nevi is low. Treatment of these lesions consists of careful observation. Malignant transformation of congenital melanocytic nevi has been observed primarily in patients older than 18 years of age (15). The decision to excise small or medium congenital melanocytic nevi is based primarily on availability for observation and the goal of optimizing cosmesis. Lesions present in areas that are difficult to observe, such as the hairy scalp, should be excised.

Due to the potential for malignant transformation of giant congenital melanocytic nevi, surgical excision remains the standard of care. Dermabrasion and laser removal of giant congenital melanocytic nevi has been used, but neither can ensure complete removal of nevus cells (16,17). The size and location of giant congenital melanocytic nevi makes simple excision and primary closure problematic. In most instances, tissue expansion of the surrounding tissue is performed prior to excision, allowing for adequate coverage of the defect produced. Lesions may also be removed in stages to allow healing and tissue relaxation to take place between procedures. Subsequent stages may entail serial excision with primary closure or repeat tissue expansion (11).

Nevus Sebaceus

Nevus sebaceus (NS) is a congenital lesion occurring most frequently on the scalp, face, and neck. Characterization of the lesion is dependent on the age of the patient. Initially, the lesion is noted to be well circumscribed with yellow-orange smooth plaques (Fig. 107-6). With puberty and hormonal change, a fine nodularity is formed and the borders become irregular. Most children with NS have no other associated abnormalities. Rarely, NS is associated with a neurocutaneous syndrome that primarily affects the brain and the eye, resulting in ocular lesions, mental retardation, and seizures. There is considerable surgical interest in this lesion because the development of various carcinomas within NS has been reported. The incidence of malignant transformation in these lesions has been reported to be 10% to 20%, with malignant transformation occurring only after puberty (18). Although the resultant cutaneous malignancy is most often basal cell carcinoma, other carcinomas such as apocrine and adnexal tumors can occur (19). However, the exact incidence of malignant transformation in nevus sebaceous remains controversial, with a more recent series indicating such transformation to be rare (20). Because of the risk of malignant transformation and the difficulty involved with following these lesions

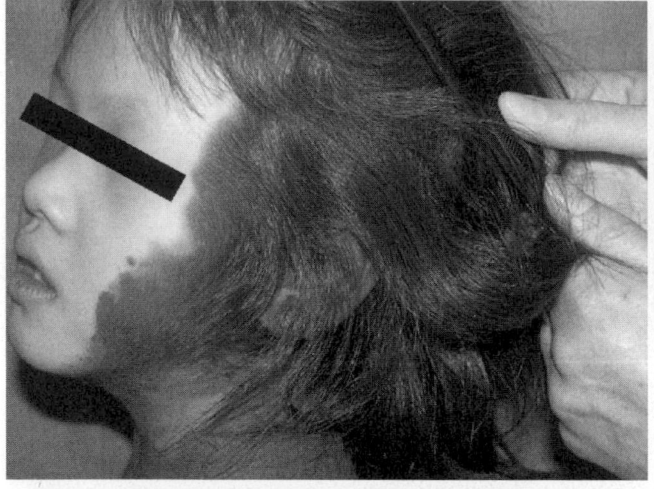

A

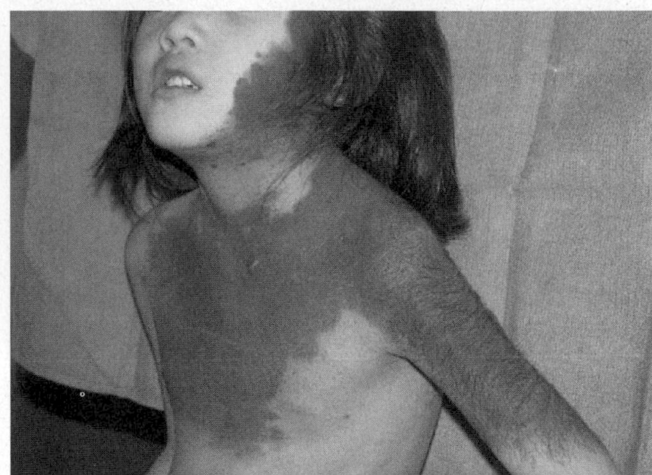

B

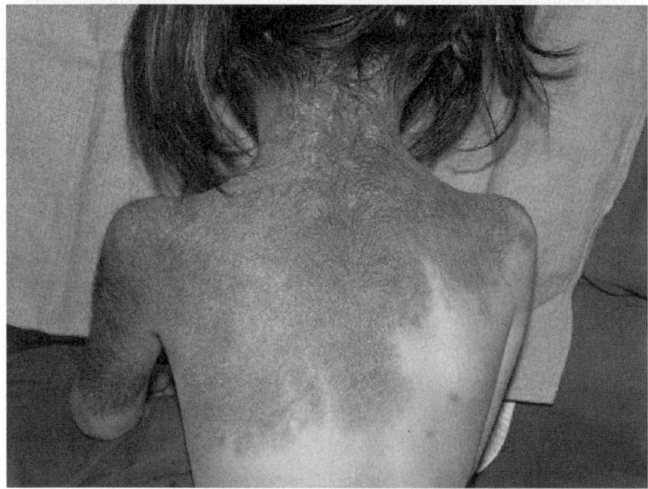

C

FIGURE 107-5. Giant congenital pigmented nevus involving the face, scalp, neck, chest, back, and left shoulder/arm in a 5-year-old girl. Involvement of the scalp leads to difficulty in monitoring the lesion for malignant degeneration. A multiple-stage operation, including the use of free-tissue transfer, tissue expansion, and possible skin graft in less visible areas, will be needed for removal and reconstruction of this lesion. (Photo courtesy of Arun K. Gosain, MD.)

clinically, we believe early complete excision for prophylaxsis is indicated as the treatment of choice. This tends to result in the optimal cosmetic outcome, as the lesion is smallest prior to puberty. Incomplete excision on final pathologic evaluation warrants repeated excision until deep and lateral margins of resection are histologically free of nevus cells (11). The need for tissue expanders is frequent due to the size and location of these lesions (11).

Dysplastic Nevus (Dysplastic Nevus Syndrome, Atypical Mole Syndrome, Melanoma Syndrome, and B-K Mole Syndrome)

Dysplastic nevi are characterized by a size greater than 5 mm, irregular and indistinct borders, and variation in pigmentation within the lesion. These lesions are most commonly found on the trunk in children. However, they typically first appear on the scalp (21). The number of lesions per patient varies, but may be as high as 100. The risk of melanoma in patients with dysplastic nevi is greatest in those with many atypical nevi and other concomitant risk factors (fair skin, lighter hair, and positive family history) (22). Those with a positive family history for dysplastic nevi and melanoma have up to a 100% lifetime risk of developing melanoma.

Treatment of patients with dysplastic nevi begins with close observation. There must be careful documentation of all nevi, including a baseline set of photographs mapping all nevi. This allows the physician to monitor the progression of any changing lesions on an annual basis and to excise them on an expectant basis (Fig. 107-7). An accurate family history is also obtained, including family members with moles and skin cancer. Use of sunscreen and avoidance of sun, monthly self-exams, and frequent follow-up are necessary for prevention of malignancy.

Nevi Without Malignant Potential

Spitz Nevus (Benign Juvenile Melanoma)

Spitz nevi, also known as spindle and epithelioid nevi, are benign lesions that histologically resemble malignant melanoma. They typically occur on the face, but may be found on the arms and trunk. Spitz nevi are characterized

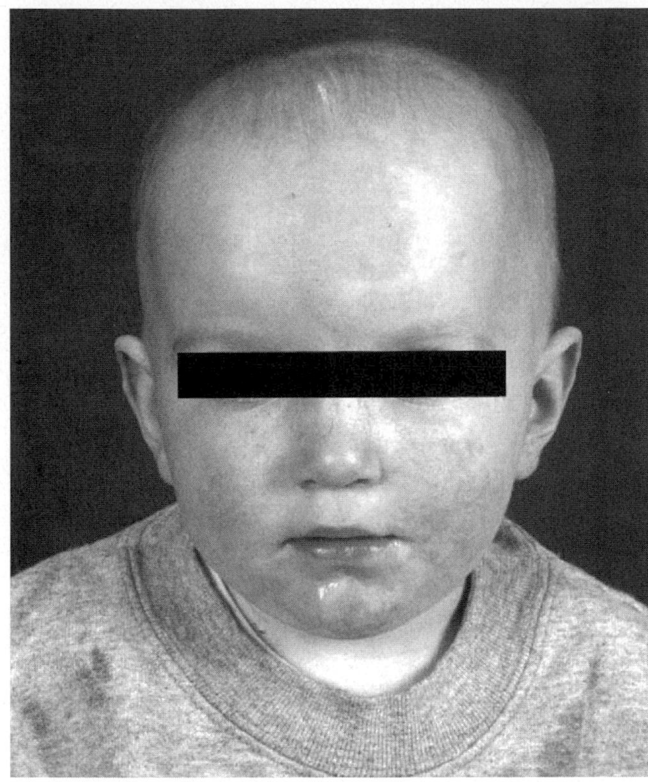
A

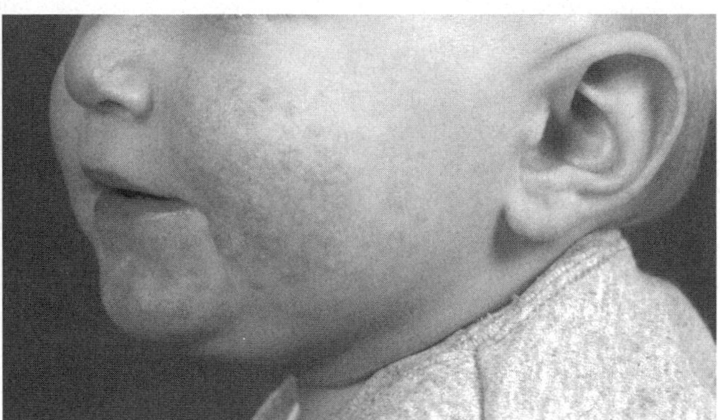
B

FIGURE 107-6. Giant congenital nevus sebaceous involving the face and scalp in a 1-year-old boy. (Photo courtesy of Arun K. Gosain, MD.)

by pale red, smooth, raised, firm papules, and may be misdiagnosed as hemangiomas, melanoma, or pyogenic granuloma (23). The lesion is not a precursor to melanoma or any dysplastic syndrome. Spitz nevi may be observed or may be completely excised to avoid future misdiagnoses of melanoma (24).

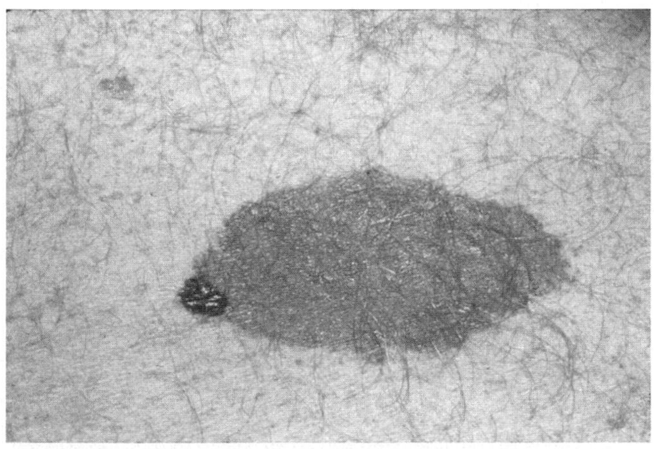

FIGURE 107-7. Shown is a focus of melanoma within a dysplastic nevi. Dysplastic nevi syndrome requires close observation and careful monitoring of all nevi. (Photo courtesy of Nancy Esterly, MD.)

Miscellaneous Nevi

Inflammatory linear verrucous epidermal nevi are a variant of verrucous epidermal nevi in which there are areas of intense inflammatory involvement (Fig. 107-8). Excoriation with resultant alteration in skin integrity severely diminishes the quality of life in these patients (11). Pruritus and skin breakdown are the primary reasons to excise these lesions, and in patients with widespread epidermal nevi, surgical treatment should be limited to symptomatic areas. Treatment of adjacent areas consists of local care to prevent recurrent excoriation.

Wooly hairy nevi have no malignant potential, but can cause significant aesthetic disfigurement of the scalp due to the abnormal hair growth pattern (Fig. 107-9). Surgical resection and resurfacing with the uninvolved scalp is indicated for aesthetic reasons and can be best accomplished with tissue expansion of the adjacent scalp.

MELANOMA

The incidence of melanoma among the general population is increasing. Approximately 1 in 90 Americans will be diagnosed with the disease (25). The common risk factors

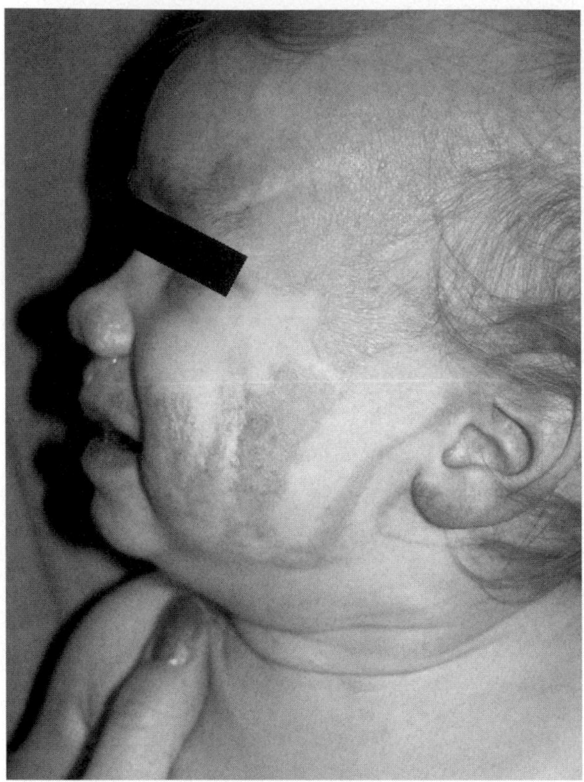

FIGURE 107-8. Inflammatory linear verrucose epidermal nevus involving the face in a 6-month-old girl. Although the lesion looks similar to nevus sebaceous, surgical excision is required only for symptomatic areas that present with intense pruritis. (Photo courtesy of Arun K. Gosain, MD.)

are increasing age, a new or changing mole, family history, and giant congential nevus. However, melanoma in children is rare, accounting for only 2% of all melanomas in the population and 3% of all malignancies in children (26).

The diagnosis of melanoma in children is often late due to initial misdiagnoses. Due to the rarity of the disease, physicians often mistake melanoma (Fig. 107-10) for less malignant lesions such as juvenile melanoma. Delay in treatment for melanoma in children has been reported to occur in as many as 60% of affected individuals (27). The risk factors for melanoma in children include xeroderma pigmentosa, giant congenital melanocytic nevi, dysplastic nevi, and immunodeficiency.

Survival for childhood melanoma, as for adult melanoma, is dependent on stage at presentation. Although there is often delay in childhood diagnosis, some authors report that this delay does not adversely affect survival (12). Advanced stage at presentation and increased depth of the lesion are prognostic indicators. Children who present with any signs or symptoms of melanoma should undergo excisional biopsy, and the resultant slides should be read by an experienced dermatopathologist.

Staging

Staging, as described by the histopathologic investigations of Clark, is based on the depth of invasion from the epidermis. The levels are as follows:

- Level I (Tis) is tumor in situ (atypical melanocytes located only in epidermis).
- Level II (T1, less than 0.75 mm) is extension into the papillary dermis, but not into the papillary–reticular dermal interface.
- Level III (T2, 0.75 to– 1.5 mm) includes lesions extending through the papillary–reticular interface.
- Level IV (T3, 1.5 to– 4 mm) includes lesions that invade the reticular dermis.
- Level V (T4, greater than 4 mm) includes lesions extending into the subcutaneous tissue.

Prognosis

Survival of melanoma for children is similar to adults and is contingent on stage at presentation. The prognosis has been directly correlated to tumor thickness (28):

- In situ disease confers a 100% survival.
- Level II lesions have a 96% to 98% 5-year survival rate.
- Level III lesions have a 86% to 90% survival rate.
- Level IV lesions have a 66% to 70% survival rate.
- Level V lesions have a 53% to 55% 5-year survival rate.

Treatment

Surgical Intervention

Optimal treatment of cutaneous malignant melanoma is early diagnosis and adequate excision. Acceptable margins of excision, based on depth of the initial lesion, are as follows:

- Melanoma in situ: 0.5 to 1.0 cm margin of resection
- Melanoma depth less than 2.0 mm: 1.0 cm margin of resection
- Melanoma depth 2.0 mm or greater: 3.0 cm margin of resection

Although the data have been equivocal, regional lymph node dissection performed at the time of the initial excision has been advocated for intermediate-depth lesions (between 1.0 and 4.0 mm). Improved survival has been reported in several retrospective studies using this approach. However, prospective analysis has not shown a significant survival benefit for patients with lymph node dissection compared to no lymph node dissection (29,30). Lesions that are deeper than 4.0 mm are at high risk for systemic and regional spread; therefore, lymph node dissection does not confer a survival advantage in this circumstance (31). Lesions less than 1.0 mm in depth have a low risk of regional lymph node metastases, and regional lymph node dissection has shown no increase in survival.

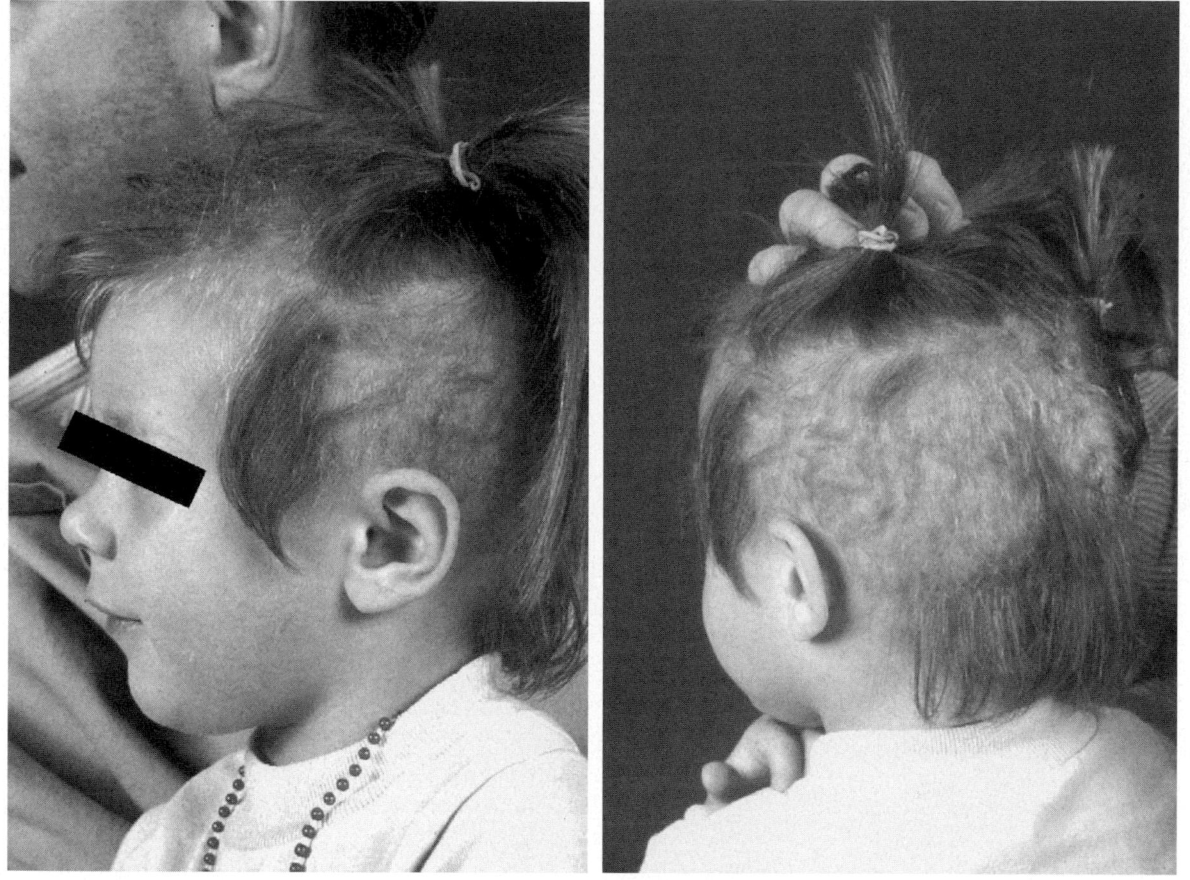

A B

FIGURE 107-9. Wooly hairy nevus of the scalp in a 4-year-old girl. There is no known malignant potential of this nevus. However, significant scalp disfigurement may serve as an indication for surgical treatment. (Photo courtesy of Arun K. Gosain, MD.)

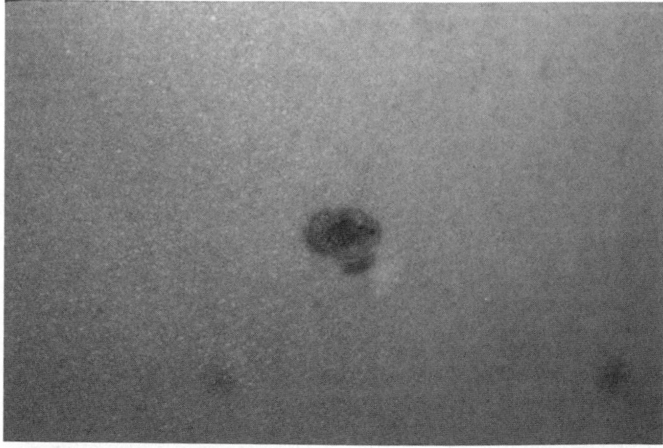

FIGURE 107-10. Due to its rarity in the pediatric population, pediatric melanoma is often misdiagnosed, leading to a delay in treatment. (Photo courtesy of Nancy Esterly, MD.)

Sentinel node biopsy is a relatively new technique that allows selection of specific regional lymph nodes that primarily drain the site of the lesion. Identification of the sentinel node is possible in approximately 80% of patients with nodal disease. Little data are available on whether sentinel node biopsy results in an increase in long-term survival over traditional techniques.

Chemotherapy, Radiation, and Immunomodulation

Chemotherapy has not been shown to be highly effective in the treatment of malignant melanoma. At present, the most effective chemotherapeutic agent in malignant melanoma has been dacarbazine, with a response rate of approximately 10% to 20%. Combination chemotherapy trials are being performed and have shown an initial response rate similar to dacarbazine.

Radiation therapy is not effective in treatment of cutaneous melanoma. The only common use of radiation therapy is for palliation of bone pain or for brain metastases.

Many immunomodulatory techniques have been investigated in the treatment of malignant melanoma. Interferon-α has been shown to increase disease-free survival when used in an adjuvant setting. However, increase in long-term survival has not been shown. Interleukin-2 has shown response rates in the range of 15% to 20% (32,33). Newer techniques such as gene therapy are also currently being tested for efficacy.

REFERENCES

1. Virchow R. Cellular pathology. London: John Churchill, 1860:33.
2. Knight PJ, Reiner CB. Superficial lumps in children: what, when, why? *Pediatrics* 1983;72:147–153.
3. Wyatt AJ, Hansen RC. Pediatric skin tumors. *Pediatr Clin North Am* 2000;47(4):1–29.
4. Bartlett SP, Lin KY, Grossman R, et al. The surgical management of orbitofacial dermoids in the pediatric patient. *Plast Reconstr Surg.* 1986;91:1208–1215.
5. Cohen BA, Honig PG, Androphy EJ. Anogenital warts in children. *Arch Dermatol* 1990;126:1575.
6. Corey L, Spear PG. Infection with herpes simplex virus. *N Engl J Med* 1986;314:619.
7. Maldonado RR, Tamayo L, Laterza AM, et al. Giant pigmented nevi: clinical, histopathologic, and theraputic considerations. *J Pediatr* 1992;120:906–911.
8. Kincannon J, Boutzale C. The physiology of pigmented nevi. *Pediatrics* 1999;104(4):1042–1045.
9. Orlow S. Congenital melanocytic nevi. In: Aston SJ, Beasely RW, Thorne CHM, eds. Grabb and Smith's plastic surgery, 5th ed. Philadelphia: Lippincott-Raven, 1997:127–130.
10. Schmid-Wendtner MH, Berking C, Baumert J, et al. Cutaneous melanoma in childhood and adolescence: an analysis of 36 patients. *J Am Acad Dermatol* 2002;46(6):874–879.
11. Gosain AK, Santoro TD, Larson DL, et al. Giant congenital nevi: a 20 year experience and an algorithim for their management. *Plast Reconstr Surg* 2001;108:622.
12. Saenz NC, Seanz-Badillos J, Busam K, et al. Childhood melanoma survival. *Cancer* 1999;85:750–754.
13. Quaba AA, Wallace AF. The incidence of malignant melanoma (0 to 15 years of age) arising in "large" congenital nevocellular nevi. *Plast Reconstr Surg* 1986;78:174.
14. Lorentzen M, Pers M, Bretteville-Jensen G. The incidence of malignant transformation in giant pigmented nevi. *Scand J Plast Reconstr Surg* 1977;11:163.
15. Illig L, Weidner F, Hundeiker M, et al. Congenital nevi <10 cm as precursors to melanoma. *Arch Dermatol* 1985;121:1274.
16. Rompel R, Moser M, Petres J. Dermabration of the congenital nevocellular nevi: experience on 215 patients. *Dermatology* 1997;194:261.
17. Zitelli JA, Grant MG, Abell E, et al. Histologic patterns of congenital nevocytic nevi and implications for treatment. *J Am Acad Dermatol* 1984;11:402.
18. Mehregan AH, Pinkus H. Life history of organoid nevi. *Arch Dermatol* 1965;91:574.
19. Domingo J, Helwig EB. Malignant neoplasms associated with nevus sebaceous of Jadassohn. *J Am Acad Dermatol* 1979;1:545.
20. Cribier B, Scrivener Y, Grosshans E. Tumors arising in nevus sebaceous: a study of 596 cases. *J Am Acad Dermatol* 2000;42(2):263–268.
21. Ceballos PI, Ruiz-Maldonado R, Mihm MC. Melanoma in children. *N Engl J Med* 1995;332:656–662.
22. Greene MH, Clark WH, Tucker MA, et al. High risk of malignant melanoma in melanoma-prone families with dysplastic nevi. *Ann Int Med* 1985;102:458-465.
23. Imber MJ, Mihm MC. Melanocytic lesions. In: Sternberg SS, Antonioli DA, eds. Diagnostic surgical pathology. Philadelphia: Lippincott Williams & Wilkins, 1999:89–107.
24. Casso EM, Grin-Jorgensen CM, Grant-Kels JM. Spitz nevi. *J Am Acad Dermatol* 1992;27:901–913.
25. Rigel DS, Kopf AW, Friedman RJ. The rate of malignant melanoma in the United States. Are we making an impact? *J Am Acad Dermatol* 1987;17:1050–1053.
26. Whiteman D, Valery P, WcWhirter W, et al. Incidence of cutaneous childhood melanoma in Queensland, Australia. *Int J Cancer* 1995;63:765–768.
27. Melnik MK, Urdaneta LF, Al-Junt AS, et al. Malignant melanoma in childhood and adolescence. *Am Surg* 1896;52:142;–147.
28. Odom RB, James WD, Berger TG. Melanocytic nevi and neoplasms. In: Andrews' diseases of the skin. Philadelphia: WB Saunders, 2000:869–889.
29. Balch CM, Soong SJ, Murad TM, et al. A multifactorial analysis of melanoma, III: prognostic factors in melanoma patients with lymph node metastases (stage II). *Ann Surg* 1981;193:377.
30. Veronesi U, Adamus J, Bandierra DC, et al. Inefficency of immediate node dissection of stage I melanoma of the limbs. *N Engl J Med* 1977;297:627.
31. Glass FL, Cottam JA, Reintgen DS, et al. Lymphatic mapping and sentinel node biopsy in the management of high-risk melanoma. *J Am Acad Dermatol* 1998;603:39.
32. Rosenberg SA, Lotze MT, Muul LM, et al. A progress report on the treatment of 157 patients with advanced cancer using lymphokine-activated killer cells and interleukin-2 or high dose interleukin-2 alone. *N Engl J Med* 1987;889:316.
33. Chang AE, Rosenberg SA. Overview of interleukin-2 as an immunotherapeutic agent. *Semin Surg Oncol* 1989;5:385.

PART L

Central Nervous System

Chapter 108

Central Nervous System

Herbert Edgar Fuchs

The surgeon who works with the developing central nervous system (CNS) must have a thorough knowledge of the embryology of the nervous system to understand and effectively treat the vast array of complex malformations, tumors, and developmental disorders that can occur. This chapter reviews the development of the CNS and the spectrum of nontraumatic disorders that can affect the developing nervous system.

NORMAL DEVELOPMENT

Human embryonic development is divided into 23 morphologic stages, each of which lasts 2 to 3 days (1). These stages encompass the period from fertilization to about 60 days' gestation and have also been correlated with those in animals, particularly rodents and birds. Although there are some important interspecies differences in CNS development, animal model systems have provided great insight into the processes involved in human CNS development, and therefore, are included in this discussion (2).

Neurulation

The neural tube forms by a process termed *neurulation,* during embryonic stages 8 to 12, at 18 to 27 days' gestation.

Herbert Edgar Fuchs: Department of Surgery, Duke University, Pediatric Neurosurgical Services, Department of Surgery, Duke University Medical Center, Durham, North Carolina 27710.

During this phase, the most severe open forms of cranial and spinal dysraphism occur. In the later stages of embryonic development, the caudal neural tube is formed by canalization and regression. During this period, the occult forms of dysraphism can develop. The notochord induces the overlying ectoderm to form the neural plate, which is contiguous laterally with the superficial ectoderm, by the end of the third week of gestation. During the next several days, the lateral portions of the neural plate begin to elevate and to form the neural folds as the midline portion becomes the neural groove (Fig. 108-1). As this process continues, the neural folds fuse in the midline to form the neural tube, beginning in the cervical region and proceeding both cranially and caudally. The anterior and posterior neuropores close at about 23 and 25 days' gestation, respectively. Immediately after fusion of the neural folds, the superficial ectoderm fuses in the midline and then separates from the neural ectoderm (Fig. 108-1). Mesenchymal cells then migrate between the skin and the neural tube, ultimately to form the meninges, neural arches, and paraspinal muscles.

Caudal Regression

After neurulation is complete, by day 25, the distal spinal cord begins to form as the caudal end of the neural tube blends into the caudal cell mass, a large mass of undifferentiated cells. The caudal cell mass eventually gives rise to components of the nervous, urogenital, and digestive systems. This accounts for the common joint occurrence of distal vertebral, neural, anorectal, and urogenital anomalies. Within the caudal cell mass, small vacuoles form, coalesce, and eventually connect with the central canal of the spinal cord, in the process known as *canalization* (Fig. 108-2). The surrounding cells differentiate toward glial cells, elongating the spinal cord well into the tail fold of the embryo. The most cephalic portion of this distal spinal cord forms the tip of the conus medullaris. The distal spinal cord then begins the process of involution or retrogressive differentiation, leaving a remnant of piaarachnoid, the

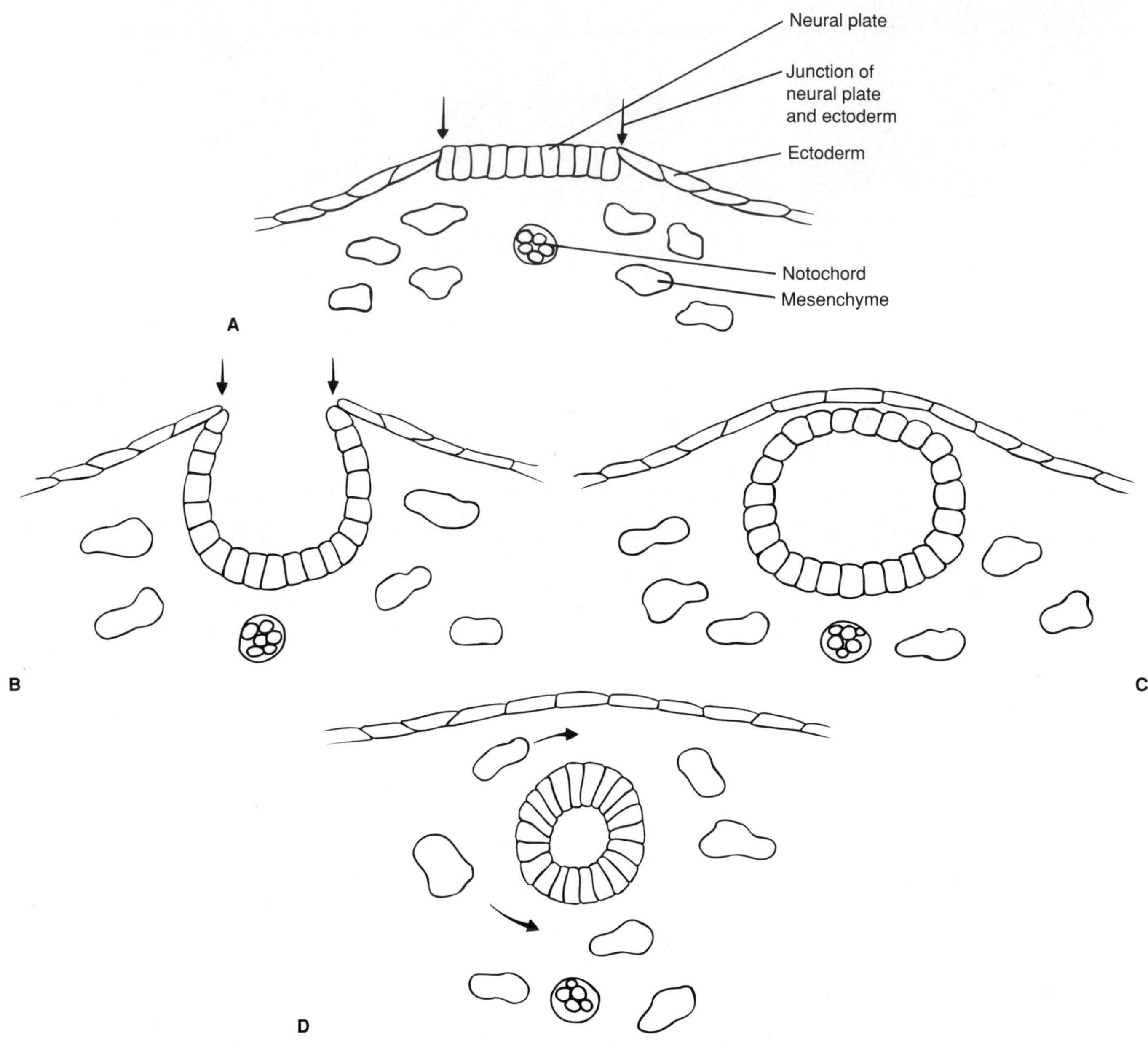

FIGURE 108-1. Neurulation. **(A)** Cross section of an embryo, showing the neural plate. **(B)** Formation of the neural folds (*arrows*). **(C)** Formation of the neural tube. **(D)** Separation of the neural tube from the superficial ectoderm by mesenchymal cells.

filum terminale. From this point, the spinal cord and developing vertebral column elongate, with the vertebral column growing faster than the spinal cord. Thus, the conus medullaris appears to ascend from its initial position in the coccyx, to lie at the L2–3 interspace by birth. By 3 months postpartum, the tip of the conus medullaris is nearly at the adult level of the L1–2 interspace (3).

Formation of the Brain

By embryonic stage 10 (days 22 and 23), the cephalic neural folds distinguish the future brain from the future spinal cord. Two constrictions divide the developing brain into three regions: the prosencephalon (forebrain), mesencephalon (midbrain), and rhombencephalon (hindbrain). By 35 days, the prosencephalon has divided into the telencephalon (future cerebral hemispheres) and the diencephalon, whereas the rhombencephalon has formed the metencephalon (future pons) and the myelencephalon (future medulla oblongata). Both cerebral hemispheres contain a cavity, the lateral ventricle. Glial and neural precursor cells begin to form around this cavity and migrate radially outward toward the surface of the cerebral hemisphere. The lateral, third, and fourth ventricular

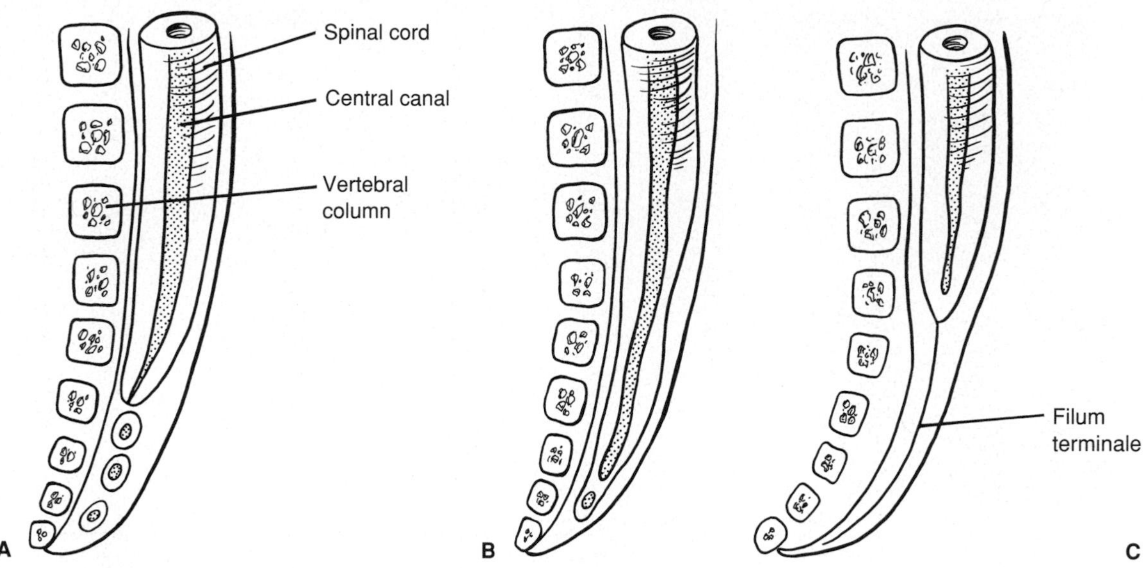

FIGURE 108-2. Formation of the caudal spinal cord and filum terminale. **(A)** Vacuolization. **(B)** Vacuoles coalesce; canalization occurs. **(C)** Differential growth and retrogressive differentiation cause the conus medullaris to rise and the filum terminale to lengthen.

cavities are contiguous with the central canal of the spinal cord at this stage; later development obliterates the site of communication at the obex in the fourth ventricle. The cerebellum forms from a complex series of buckling and folding in the rhombencephalon, initially lying within the fourth ventricle, and eventually coming to lie dorsal to the fourth ventricle.

The choroid plexus first appears in the fourth ventricle at days 43 to 44, in the lateral ventricles at days 45 to 46, and in the third ventricle at days 48 to 49. The caudal roof of the fourth ventricle perforates to form the foramen of Magendie at days 47 to 48; at the same time, the choroid plexus begins to produce cerebrospinal fluid (CSF). The CSF loosens the meshwork of mesenchymal cells surrounding the brain to form the subarachnoid space, beginning at the cisterna magna, and spreading over the cerebral hemispheres and the spinal cord.

Formation of the Skull and Vertebral Column

The skull is formed in two sections: The skull base is formed by endochondral ossification, and the cranial vault is formed as membranous bone. The first chondrification begins during stage 17 (days 40 to 44). The vertebral column originates from the medial portion of the somites in three stages: membrane formation (days 22 to 39), cartilage formation (days 40 to 64), and bone formation, which extends through the fetal portion until well after birth. The notochord appears to direct formation of the vertebral bodies, and the neural tube directs formation of the posterior vertebral elements. Remnants of the notochord remain in the intervertebral disks and in the clivus of the skull.

CONGENITAL MALFORMATIONS

Congenital malformations of the CNS are best understood as derangements of the developmental processes discussed earlier (Table 108-1).

Derangements of Neurulation

Myelomeningocele is the most common derangement of neurulation, occurring in about 1 in 1,000 live births.

TABLE 108-1 Congenital Malformations of the Central Nervous System.

Deranged neurulation
Myelomeningocele
Lipomyelomeningocele
Dermal sinus
Deranged retrogressive differentiation
Lipoma of filum terminale or tight filum terminale
Terminal myelocystocele
Other mechanisms
Diastematomyelia
Neurenteric cyst
Chiari malformations
Dandy-Walker malformation
Meningocele
Arachnoid cyst

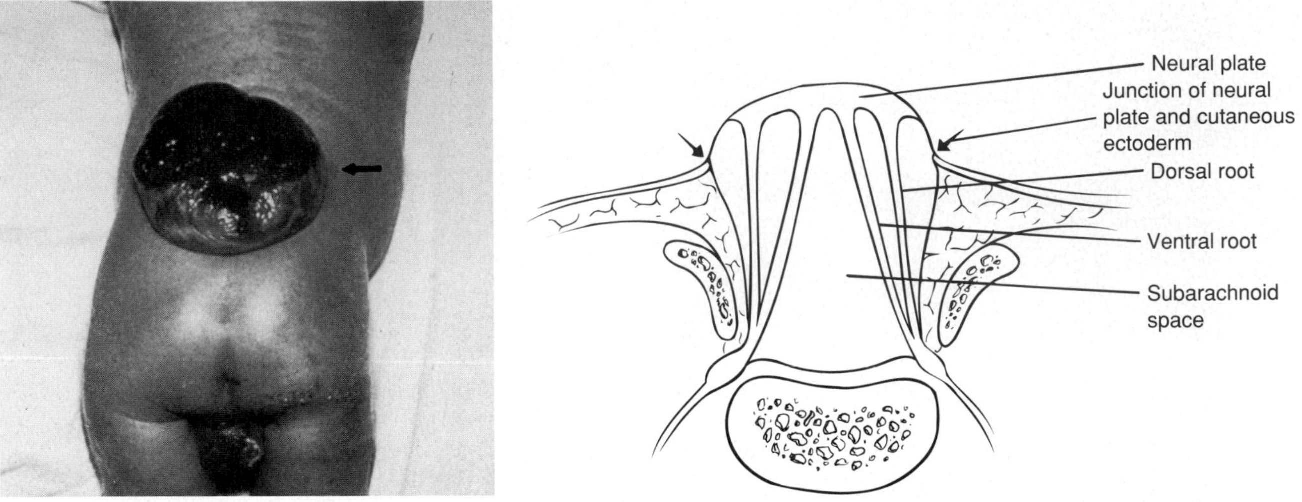

FIGURE 108-3. Myelomeningocele. **(A)** Myelomeningocele in a newborn (*arrow*). The anal sphincter is flaccid, and the lower-extremity musculature is poorly developed. **(B)** Schematic depiction of a myelomeningocele in cross-section.

This incidence appears to be decreasing with emphasis on prenatal maternal care, particularly folate supplementation. It is estimated that up to 70% of myelomeningoceles could be prevented by women of childbearing age taking a multivitamin (4). In this malformation, a focal segment of the spinal cord fails to roll up and form a tube. Because the neural tube does not fuse, the cutaneous ectoderm does not come to cover the neural tube, but remains attached and lateral to the neural plate, leaving a cutaneous defect (Fig. 108-3). Mesenchymal cells are also prevented from their proper migration, and thus the laminal arches and muscles develop in an abnormal lateral position. The raw, exposed surface of the neural plate represents the interior of the spinal cord. The midline neural groove is also seen. Surrounding this neural placode is a thin layer of skin and arachnoid tissue, below which is the subarachnoid space. The nerve roots lie inferior to the neural placode, with the ventral roots lying medial to the dorsal roots. Because the neural placode is attached to the skin, it is tethered and relatively immobile. A number of CNS anomalies have been associated with myelomeningocele, including Chiari II malformation and hydrocephalus, which are discussed later in this chapter.

Lipomyelomeningocele is believed to form by focal premature dysjunction of neuroectoderm from cutaneous ectoderm, allowing access of mesenchymal cells to the dorsal surface of the unclosed neural tube (5). The mesenchymal cells then give rise to fat. The anatomy is therefore similar to myelomeningocele, with the exception that the cutaneous ectoderm is able to close over the neural tube. The lipoma may extend from the spinal cord and merge with the subcutaneous fat (Fig. 108-4).

In contrast to lipomyelomeningocele, dermal sinus tract results from incomplete dysjunction of the neural tube and cutaneous ectoderm. As the spinal cord becomes buried beneath the surface and elongates, the localized connection with the skin becomes an elongated tract (Fig. 108-5). The incidence of dermal sinus is highest in the lumbosacral region, the site of posterior neuropore closure, but this derangement can also occur in the cervicooccipital and nasal regions. It can extend to variable depths, ending in the subcutaneous tissues or the dura, or retaining its attachment to the spinal cord or brainstem. Dermoid or epidermoid tumors may be found along the course of the dermal sinus tract.

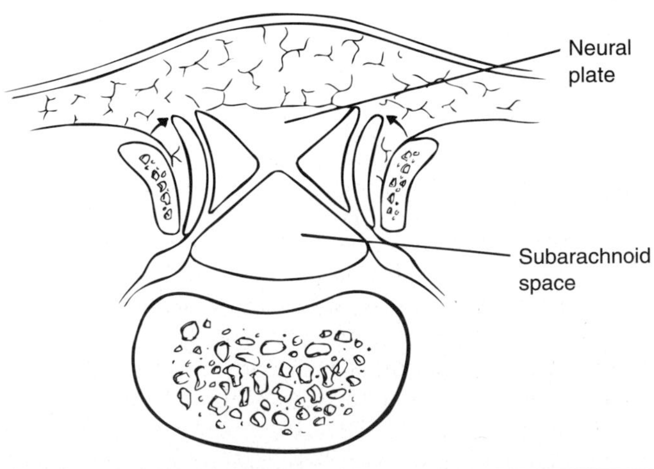

FIGURE 108-4. Cross-sectional drawing of a lipomyelomeningocele.

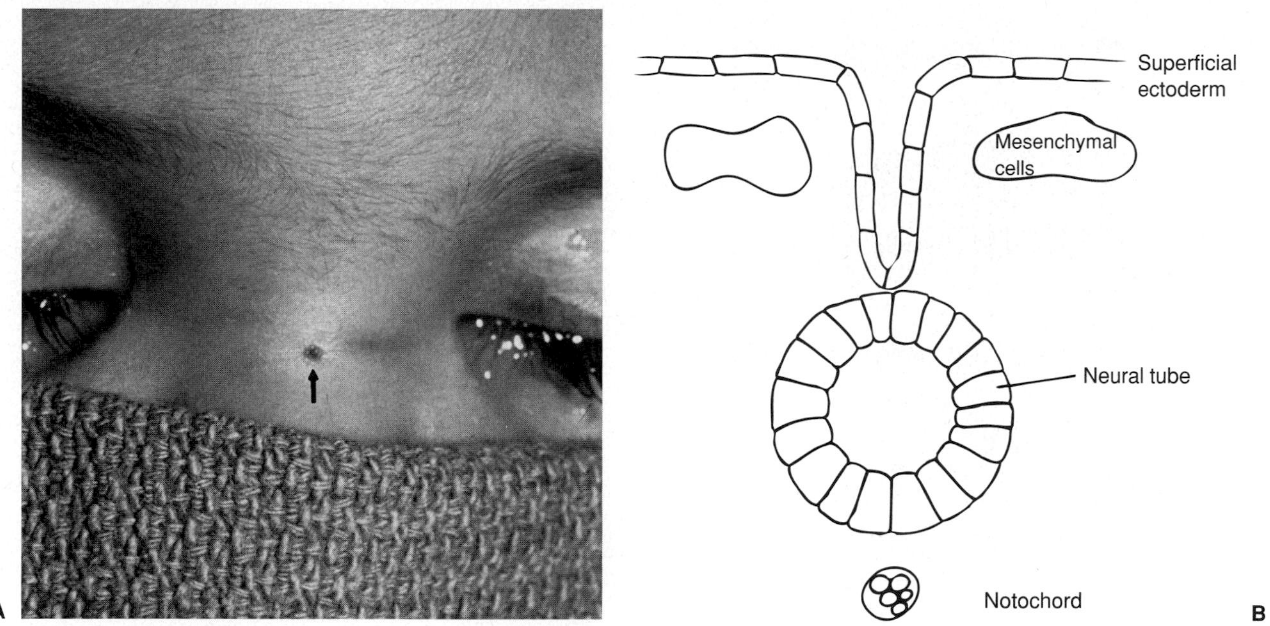

FIGURE 108-5. Dermal sinus tract. **(A)** Nasal dermal sinus tract (*arrow*). **(B)** Cross-sectional drawing of a dermal sinus tract.

Derangements of Retrogressive Differentiation

The tight filum terminale or fatty filum terminale syndrome is a condition in which the spinal cord is tethered by an abnormally short, thickened filum terminale. The terminal myelocystocele is a complex malformation that is believed to be caused by dilation of the central canal in the caudal neural tube, forming a cyst. This cyst distends the arachnoid lining of the distal spinal cord, forming a meningocele. This anomaly is commonly associated with extrophy of the bladder.

Other Embryologic Derangements

Diastematomyelia is a condition in which the spinal cord is split in a sagittal plane into two hemicords that may or may not be symmetric. Diastematomyelia is most common in girls and is usually heralded by a hairy patch overlying the site of the cleft. The cause of this malformation has been a subject of great debate, but studies by Dias and Walker (6) and Pang and colleagues (7) support the concept that these malformations are due to disorders of gastrulation. Pang et al. classified these lesions as type I or II split cord malformation (SCM). Type I SCM is the classic diastematomyelia, with a bony septum lying between two hemicords, each lying in its own dural sac. The type II malformation consists of two hemicords in a single dural sac, with a thin sagittal fibrous septum. These malformations can be caused by splitting of the notocord, either by duplication or by persistence of the neurenteric canal, which effectively causes a localized split of the notocord. The development of mesenchymal elements between the two hemicords then determines the type of SCM formed. A thicker mesenchymal tract gives rise to the bony septum and meninges, whereas a thinner tract may only form a thin fibrous septum (Fig. 108-6).

A neurenteric cyst can also result from persistence of the neurenteric canal and is often associated with SCM. This rare lesion is most often seen as only a partial fistula and is most common in the cervicothoracic region of the spinal cord.

Meningoceles are believed to be due to postneurulation disorders involving cutaneous ectoderm and mesenchyme because the neural tube is normally formed beneath the cutaneous and mesenchymal defect, which contains CSF (Fig. 108-7).

The embryology of encephaloceles has been reviewed by Chapman and associates (8). Encephaloceles were originally believed to be caused by failure of closure of the anterior neuropore. These lesions, however, contain well-developed neural and mesenchymal structures, which cannot be the result of failure of neural tube closure. Therefore, these lesions are believed to be due to herniation of fully neurulated neural tissue through a mesenchymal defect (Fig. 108-8).

The Chiari II malformation is a complex disorder associated with myelomeningocele. This malformation consists of caudal displacement of the cerebellar vermis and tonsils into the cervical canal; elongation, kinking, and

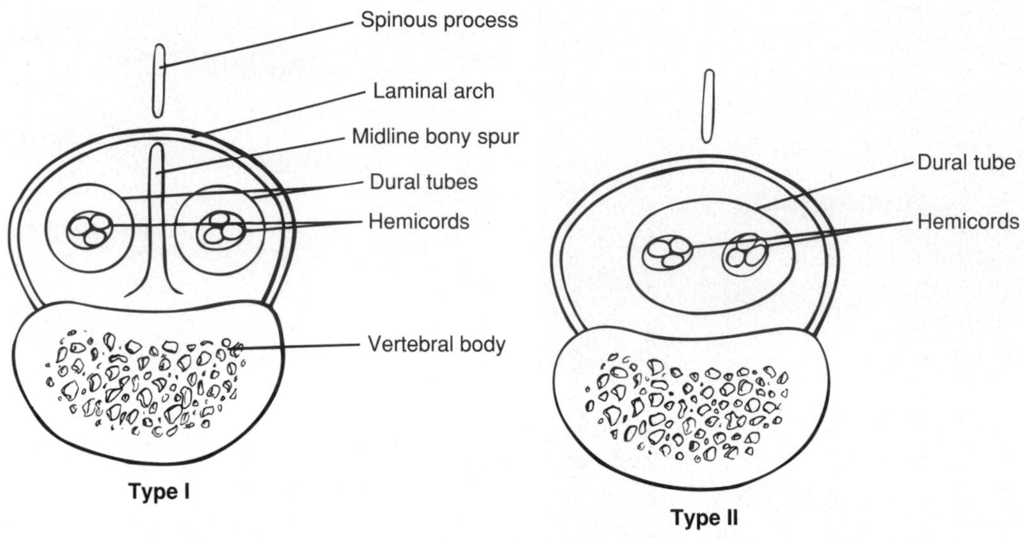

FIGURE 108-6. Split cord malformations depicted in cross section.

caudal displacement of the lower brainstem into the cervical canal; and upward displacement of the superior cerebellum through a low-lying tentorial incisura, with a small posterior fossa (Fig. 108-9A). McLone and Knepper (9) proposed a unifying theory of pathogenesis of these malformations, in which the open neural placode of the myelomeningocele allows escape of CSF, which interferes with the normal distention of the ventricular system and development of the skull base. Incomplete distention of the fourth ventricle fails to stimulate growth of the skull base, resulting in a smaller posterior fossa that is unable to respond during the later phase of rapid cerebellar growth and development. This results in herniation of neural tissue from the posterior fossa and impairs flow of CSF, resulting in hydrocephalus. The Chiari I malformation, involving caudal displacement of the cerebellar tonsils with a normal posterior fossa, must have its embryologic origin at a later stage than the more severe Chiari II malformation, but the exact mechanisms responsible remain to be elucidated (Fig. 108-9B).

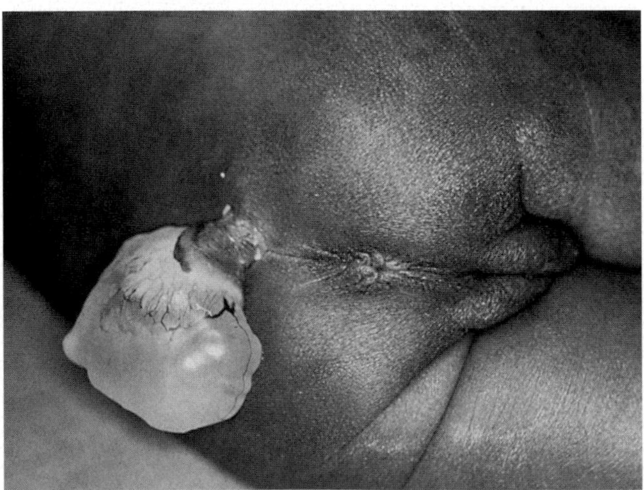

FIGURE 108-7. Infant with a sacral meningocele. The sac does not contain any neural elements.

The Dandy-Walker malformation is a developmental abnormality in which the roof of the fourth ventricle fails to perforate to form the foramen of Magendie. The resultant cystic dilation of the fourth ventricle expands the posterior fossa, elevates the tentorium, and causes hydrocephalus due to obstruction of the aqueduct of Sylvius with concomitant hypoplasia of the cerebellar vermis (Fig. 108-10).

Arachnoid cysts are arachnoid-lined cavities filled with fluid similar in composition to CSF. They can create a disturbance in intracranial dynamics due to shift and displacement of surrounding structures, and they can cause intracranial hypertension. Their pathogenesis is unknown. Arachnoid cysts appear to form early in development and may communicate to varying degrees with the surrounding subarachnoid space. The most common locations for arachnoid cysts are the sylvian fissure, suprasellar, and posterior fossa.

Diagnosis and Management

Myelomeningocele

The diagnosis of myelomeningocele is obvious at birth. For initial management, the lesion is covered with sterile, saline-soaked dressings, and the patient is kept prone. After a general assessment, the location of the lesion is noted, and a neurologic examination is performed to assess sensorimotor function in the lower extremities. Hip flexion requires function of L1 to L3. Hip adduction requires L2 to L4 function. Hip abduction, hip extension,

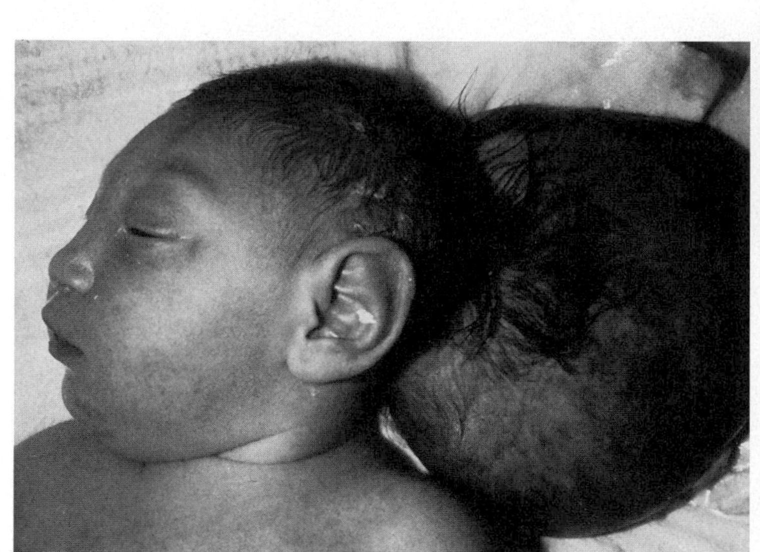

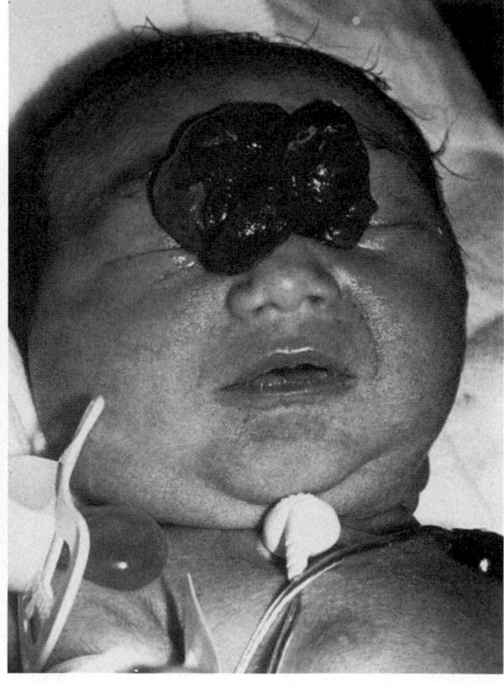

A B

FIGURE 108-8. Encephalocele. **(A)** Infant with an occipital encephalocele. **(B)** Infant with a nasal encephalocele.

and knee extension require L5 to S2 function. Plantarflexion requires function of sacral roots. Anal sphincter tone should be assessed because more than 90% of children with myelomeningocele have bowel and bladder dysfunction. Head circumference should be measured and the anterior fontanelle palpated to assess for hydrocephalus. After medical stabilization, and preferably within 24 hours of birth, the child should be taken to the operating room for closure of the myelomeningocele. This procedure involves meticulous anatomic reconstruction of the neural tube,

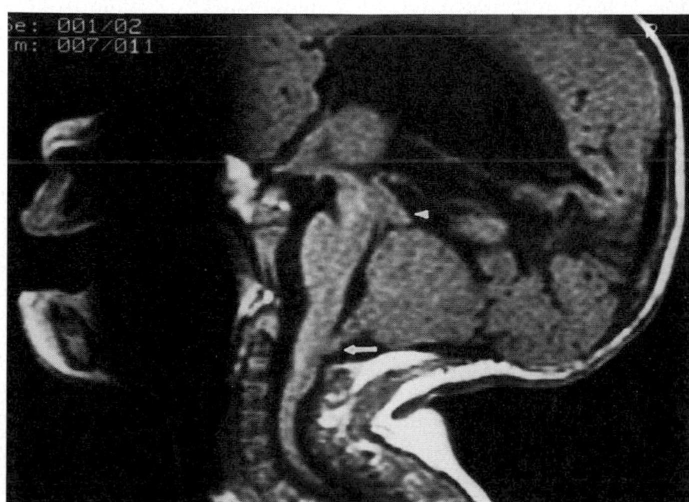

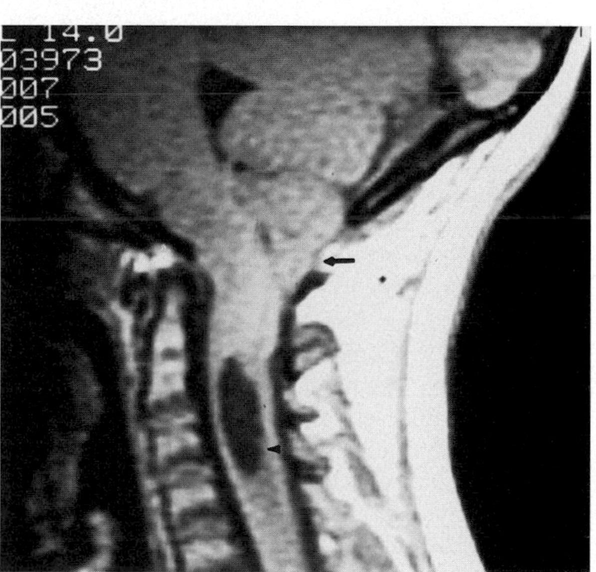

A B

FIGURE 108-9. MR images of Chiari malformations. **(A)** Chiari II malformation. The cerebellar vermis is displaced caudad (*arrow*), and the midbrain tectum is beaked (*arrowhead*). **(B)** Chiari I malformation. In contrast to **(A)**, the brainstem is normal, and only the cerebellar tonsils are descended into the cervical canal (*arrow*). A cervical syrinx (*arrowhead*) is present.

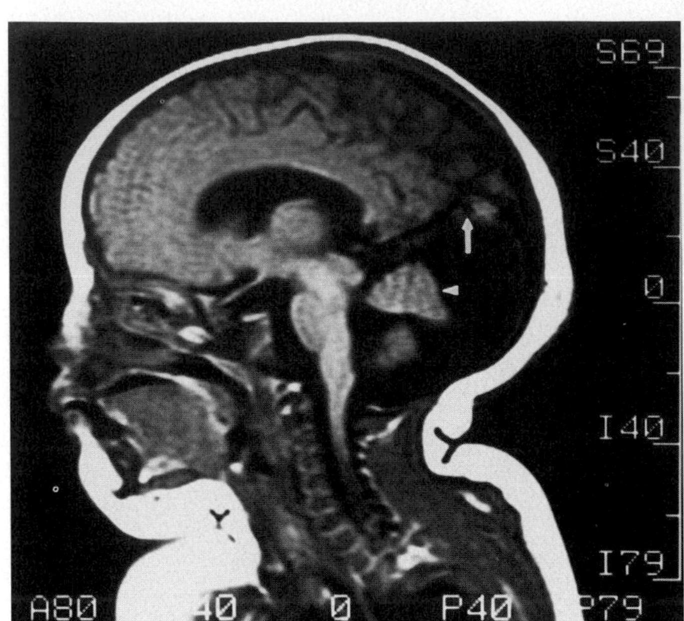

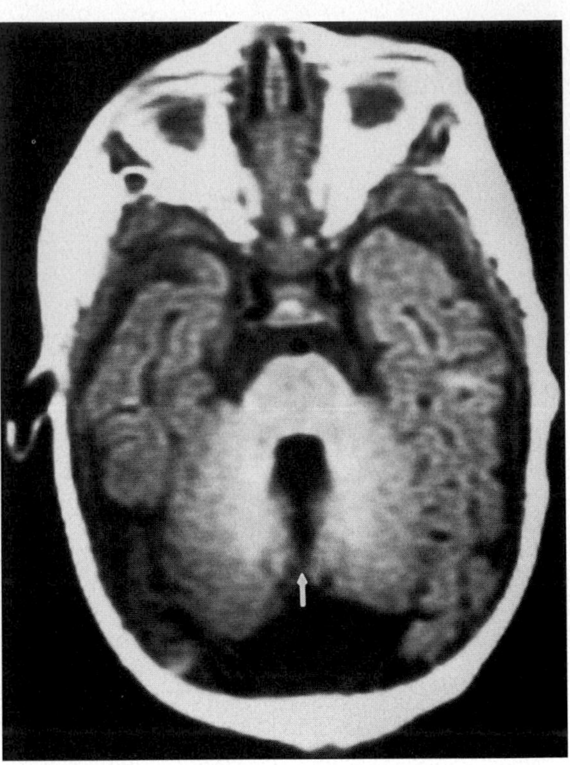

FIGURE 108-10. Magnetic resonance images of Dandy-Walker malformation. **(A)** Sagittal image shows an enlarged posterior fossa with a large cyst, elevated tentorium (*arrow*), and absent inferior cerebellar vermis. The superior vermis is indicated by an arrowhead. **(B)** Axial image shows absent inferior vermis and communication with the fourth ventricle (*arrow*).

dural sac, and overlying cutaneous tissues, with great care taken not to further injure neural tissue. Postoperatively, the child is monitored for development of hydrocephalus, which is treated with a ventriculoperitoneal shunt, and nursed prone, while the closure heals. During this time period, further orthopedic and urologic workup can be completed, along with evaluation of brainstem function to assess the associated Chiari II malformation. The long-term outcomes for these children have been reported in depth by McLone and coworkers (10). The survival rate for these children followed for 8 to 12 years was 85%, with 62% having an IQ of 80 or higher. With the development of clean intermittent bladder catheterization, 85% of children with myelomeningocele can achieve social continence of urine. The development of improved leg braces has allowed children with motor levels of at least L3 function to be community ambulators. McLone's studies have shown that children with myelomeningocele can be functional and that the natural history of this disease is not one of relentless deterioration, as some prior studies had suggested. Any neurologic deterioration seen in children with myelomeningocele should be promptly investigated and treated.

More recent advances in fetal diagnosis have made possible a current study of in utero closure of myelomeningocele at three U.S. centers. Early results suggest that in utero closure may result in a decreased need for CSF shunting, as well as reduction or even reversal of the Chiari II malformation (11). There is, however, significant risk to the fetus, including a 6% mortality due to extreme prematurity. The long-term benefits of in utero closure remain to be seen.

The congenital spinal cord lesions with intact skin are termed *spina bifida occulta* and share a common presentation, owing to tethering of the spinal cord. These lesions can also be associated with an overlying skin lesion, such as the dermal sinus, a subcutaneous lipoma, a hemangioma, or a hairy patch. The most common signs and symptoms of tethered cord include changes in gait, weakness, orthopedic deformity, and pain. The most common orthopedic deformities seen include varus and valgus, and cavus changes of the foot. In addition, recurrent hip dislocation and scoliosis may also be seen. Pain and sensory loss are common features of the tethered spinal cord, and both can be asymmetric and nondermatomal. In addition, changes in bowel and bladder function may be missed in young children. Neurologic dysfunction results from traction on the conus medullaris, with stretching and deformation of vessels overlying the tethered cord, resulting in ischemia of the conus (12). Spinal flexion or growth can result in chronic, repetitive ischemia to the spinal cord. With modern magnetic resonance imaging (MRI) techniques, the diagnosis of spina bifida occulta is straightforward. The treatment of these lesions involves release of the tethered cord, with restoration of more normal anatomic relations of the spinal cord and surrounding structures. With early recognition and treatment, pain, sensory loss, and motor weakness are likely to improve, but if treatment is deferred until bowel or bladder dysfunction occurs, improvement of these functions is unlikely.

Spina Bifida Occulta

Lipomyelomeningocele

The subcutaneous component of the lipomyelomeningocele lies cephalad to, and can distort, the intergluteal crease. The MRI scan confirms the diagnosis and assists in surgical planning (Fig. 108-11). Surgical repair of lipomyelomeningoceles consists of debulking of the lipoma down to the interface with the spinal cord using the CO_2 laser, reformation of the neural tube if possible, and reconstruction of the dura, creating a capacious subarachnoid space to prevent retethering. The remainder of the wound is then closed in layers. In modern series, 40% of patients with motor deficits and 12% of patients with incontinence recovered normal function after surgery.

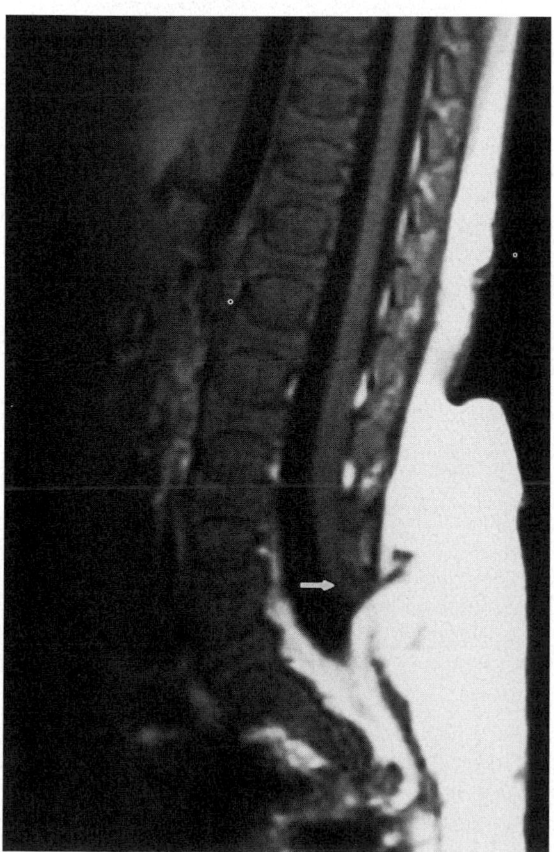

FIGURE 108-11. Magnetic resonance image of lipomyelomeningocele. Sagittal image shows tethered cord merging into lipoma (*arrow*), which is contiguous with subcutaneous fat.

Dermal Sinus Tract

A dermal sinus tract can occur in a variety of locations in the CNS. It is usually recognized as a midline cutaneous orifice with hairs in it, with or without an associated hemangioma. It can also present with localized cutaneous infection, meningitis, or brain abscess. The dermal sinus tract can be distinguished from the pilonidal sinus by location because the latter typically lies within the gluteal crease, overlying the tip of the coccyx, and has no connection with the CNS. MRI scan provides the diagnosis and may provide evidence of the extent of the sinus tract (Fig. 108-12). Even without MRI evidence of either intracranial or intraspinal extension, these lesions should be explored because a narrow sinus tract may be missed on imaging studies. Surgery for lumbosacral lesions potentially involves exploration from the site of the cutaneous orifice to the level of the conus. All dermal elements should be removed. Nasal and occipital dermal sinus tracts may require formal craniotomy, in addition to excision of the cutaneous portions of the tract to remove the entire tract.

Tethered Cord–Fatty Filum Terminale

The tethered cord–fatty filum terminale syndrome has classically been described as an abnormally low-lying conus medullaris and a thickened, fatty-infiltrated filum terminale. Warder and Oakes (13) described the tethered cord syndrome in patients with the conus in normal position. The clinical presentation and the presence of fat in the filum terminale are the key elements in the diagnosis of tethered cord–fatty filum terminale syndrome. The treatment consists of a limited lumbosacral laminectomy for sectioning of the filum terminale.

Diastematomyelia

As discussed earlier, diastematomyelia is often heralded by a cutaneous hairy patch overlying the cleft spinal cord. MRI confirms the diagnosis and can distinguish the type I and II SCM (Fig. 108-13). Surgery involves complete release of the spinal cord from all tethering lesions, which may include a tight filum terminale, the bony septum, and fibrous bands adherent to the dorsal dura. The dura is then closed to create a capacious subarachnoid space, and the remainder of the wound is closed in layers.

Meningocele

The neural elements are intact, with a CSF-filled sac protruding through a cutaneous defect (Fig. 108-7). Repair is accomplished by localizing the dural defect, amputating

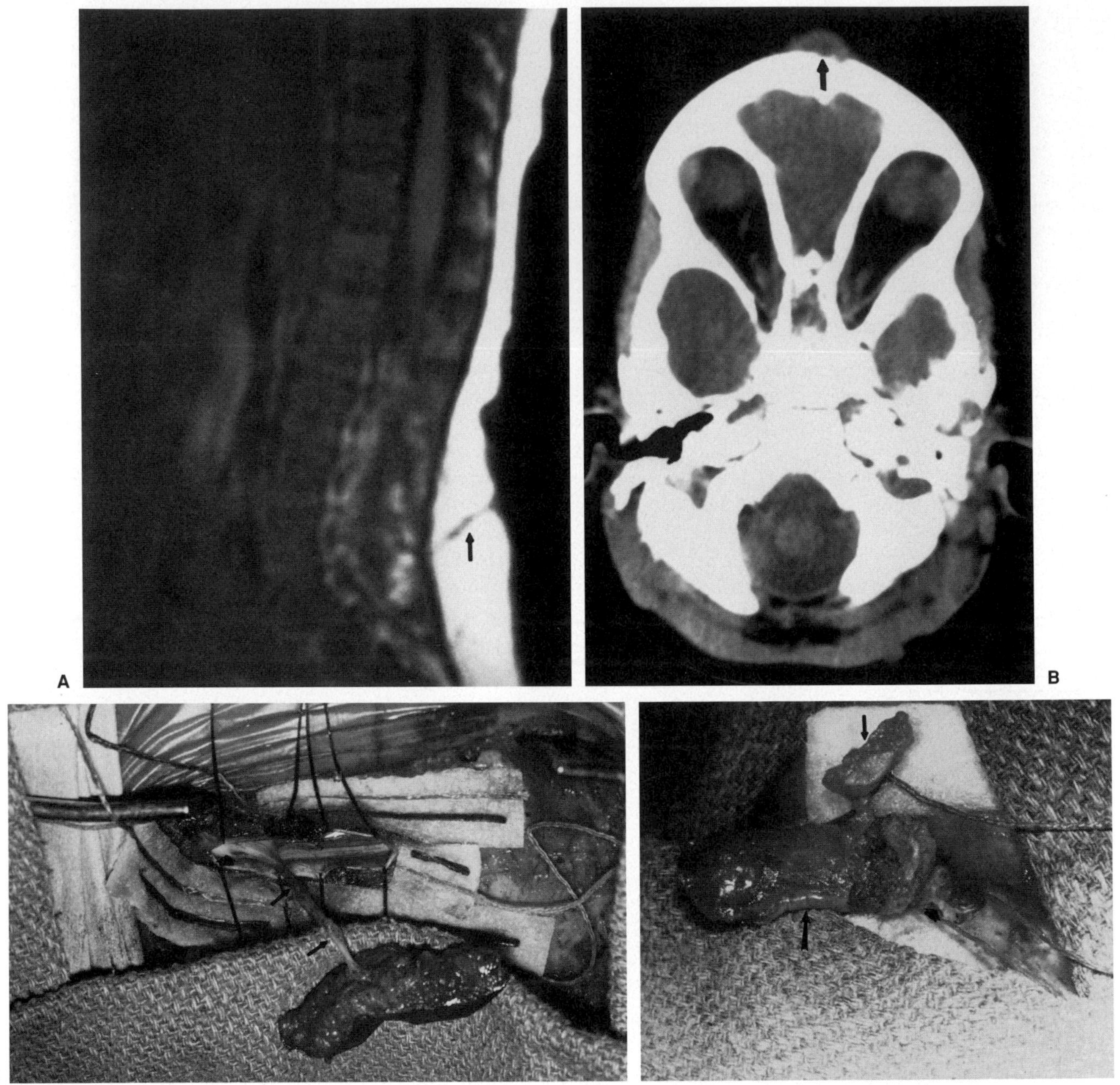

FIGURE 108-12. Dermal sinus tracts. **(A)** Sagittal magnetic resonance image of lumbosacral dermal sinus tract (*arrow*). **(B)** Axial computed tomography scan of nasal dermal sinus shows a dermoid cyst along tract (*arrow*). **(C)** Intraoperative photograph of lumbosacral dermal sinus shown in **(A)** demonstrates tract (*long arrows*) leading from excised segment of skin into the dural sac and merging with the spinal cord (*short arrow*). **(D)** Intraoperative photograph of nasal dermal sinus shown in **(B)** demonstrates the excised skin (*arrow at top*), dermoid cyst (*long arrow*), and sinus tract (*short arrow*) extending to the level of the dura.

the herniating sac, and closing the dura. The remainder of the wound is then closed in layers.

Encephalocele

The incidence of encephalocele varies according to geographic region, from as high as 1 in 5,000 live births in Southeast Asia to as low as 1 in 10,000 live births in North America. The location of the encephalocele also exhibits geographic variability, with frontonasal encephaloceles more common in Southeast Asia and occipital encephaloceles more common in North America. The degree of herniation of neural tissue into the encephalocele sac can be highly variable. MRI classifies the type of

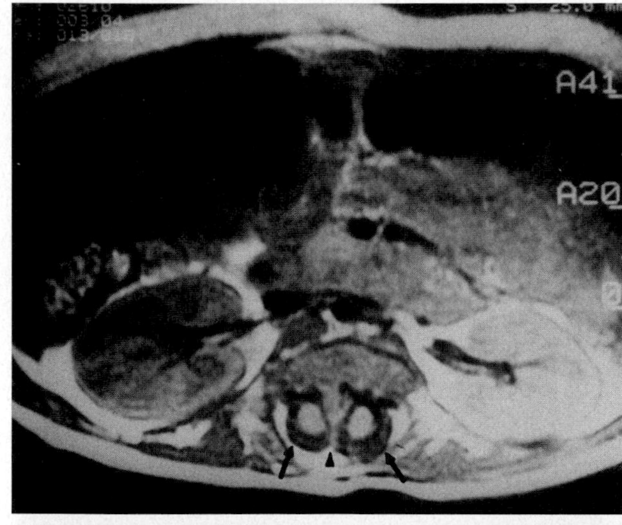

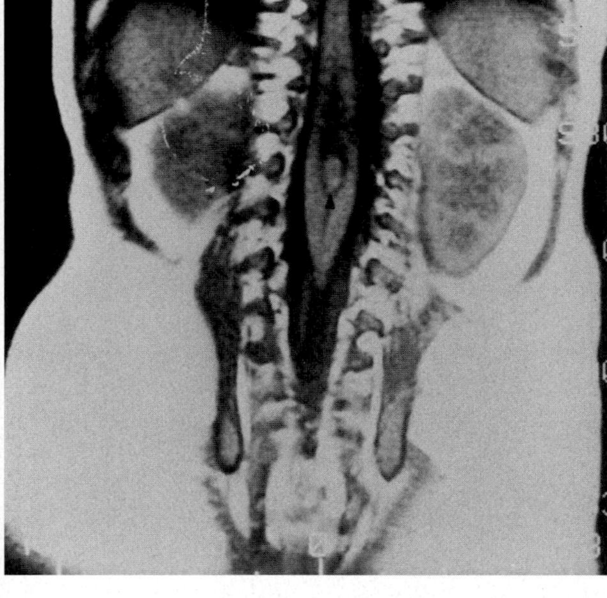

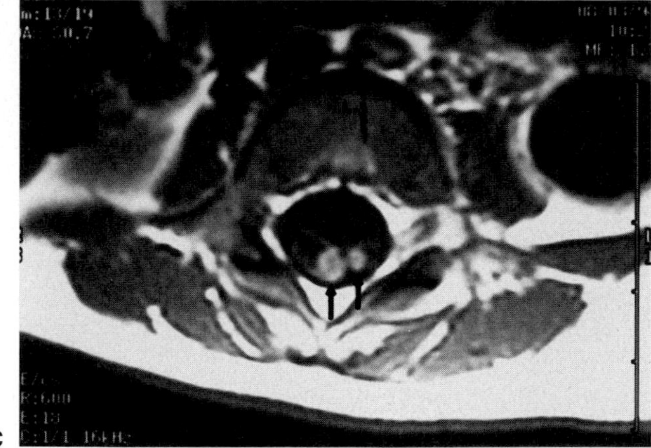

FIGURE 108-13. Magnetic resonance images of split cord malformations. **(A, B)** Type I split cord malformation shows two hemicords and two dural sacs (*arrows*), separated by a bony septum (*arrowhead*), in axial and coronal sections, respectively. **(C)** Type II split cord malformation reveals two unequal hemicords (*arrows*) contained in a single dural sac.

encephalocele and determines the presence of neural tissues within the sac. The treatment of encephaloceles is surgical resection, with removal of the lesion at its base, repair of the dura, and bone grafting to cover the calvarial defect. In some occipital encephaloceles, the sac contains vital neural or vascular structures, and such repair is not possible (Fig. 108-8). The outcome of surgical treatment depends on the location of the encephalocele and the amount of neural tissue remaining within the cranial vault. In general, occipital encephaloceles are more commonly associated with hydrocephalus and have a worse cognitive outcome.

Chiari II Malformation

In children with myelomeningocele, the Chiari II malformation is invariably present. Despite impressive imaging studies, however, the patient may not have symptoms (Fig. 108-9A). Typical Chiari II symptoms and signs include occipital pain, nystagmus, upper-extremity weakness, lower cranial nerve dysfunction, hypotonia or spasticity, and scoliosis. Hydromyelia (dilation of the central canal of the spinal cord) may also be present. A shunt malfunction must be ruled out before any consideration of cervical decompression. The surgical treatment of Chiari II malformation involves decompression of the brainstem or cervical spinal cord and restoration of normal CSF flow from the fourth ventricle. This is accomplished by a limited suboccipital craniectomy, cervical laminectomies encompassing the extent of the cerebellar herniation, opening and stenting of the foramen of Magendie, and duroplasty. The Chiari II malformation that becomes symptomatic in infancy is the leading cause of death in children with myelomeningocele. Repetitive pulmonary aspiration events with severe wheezing are particularly worrisome symptoms. Less severe symptoms frequently stabilize by 1 year of age. Older children with Chiari II malformation do more favorably with cervical decompression. Results of Chiari II decompression have been good, with improvement reported in 60% to 80% of patients (14).

Chiari I Malformation

The Chiari I malformation usually presents in a more delayed fashion than the Chiari II malformation, commonly later in the first decade or even into adulthood. Symptoms

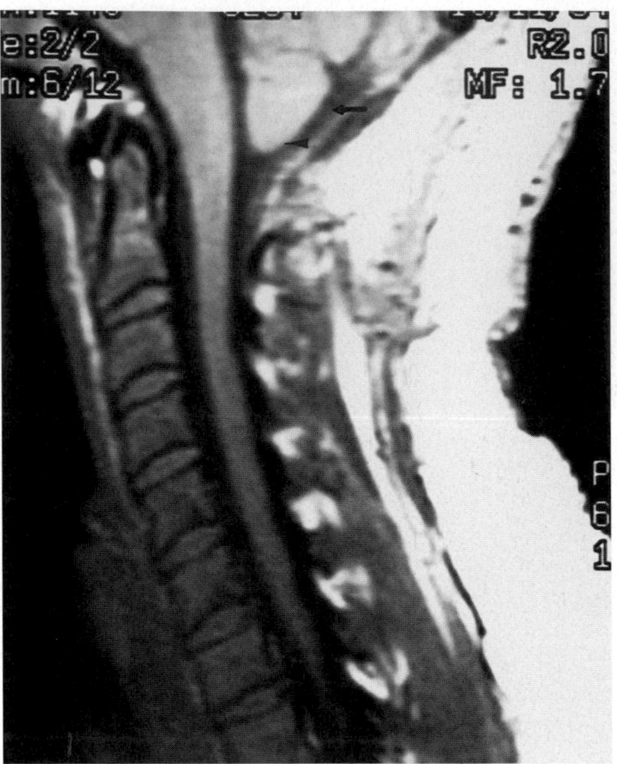

FIGURE 108-14. Magnetic resonance image of Chiari I malformation. Postoperative image shows good decompression of the foramen magnum (*arrow*) and resolution of the syrinx. The tonsil has a more rounded configuration (*arrowhead*). Compare with Fig. 108-9B.

of Chiari I malformation include occipital headache (often induced by coughing), upper-extremity numbness and loss of pain and temperature sensation, lower-extremity spasticity, and eventually lower cranial nerve dysfunction. MRI scan (including cine MRI to evaluate CSF flow across the foramen magnum) confirms the diagnosis and the extent of any associated hydromyelia (Fig. 108-9B). Surgical treatment varies across medical centers, but consists of at least a suboccipital craniectomy, and cervical laminectomy (usually involving C1). Many centers also perform duroplasty, with intradural exploration to ensure patency of the foramen of Magendie. This procedure restores normal CSF flow dynamics across the craniocervical junction and usually results in resolution of the hydromyelia (Fig. 108-14). Patients presenting with more mild symptoms do well, with 70% to 80% having improvement. Patients with lower cranial nerve dysfunction do not do as well, with only 35% to 65% having significant improvement from surgery (14).

Arachnoid Cyst

The presentation of intracranial arachnoid cysts is dependent on the age of the patient. Infants commonly present with increased head circumference, full fontanelle, and signs of increased intracranial pressure. Older children may present with headache, seizures, or focal neurologic deficits. The signs and symptoms also vary with the site of the arachnoid cyst. Posterior fossa cysts commonly present with obstructive hydrocephalus, sylvian fissure cysts present with seizures or hemiparesis, and suprasellar cysts present with visual disturbances. Sudden deterioration may be seen, with development of obstructive hydrocephalus, sudden cyst rupture, or bleeding into the cyst, either spontaneous or traumatic. Computed tomography (CT) or MRI can provide the diagnosis; MRI is preferred, owing to multiplanar imaging. Therapy of symptomatic arachnoid cysts is controversial, with some authors recommending simple shunting of the cyst and other recommending cyst fenestration or excision (15).

HYDROCEPHALUS

Hydrocephalus is a condition in which there is a discrepancy between the rate of formation and absorption of CSF, causing the cerebral ventricles to dilate (16). CSF is normally formed from the choroid plexus in the lateral third and fourth ventricles. CSF flows through the ventricular system; exits the fourth ventricle through the foramina of Magendie and Luschka; circulates around the base of the brain, cerebral hemispheres, and spinal cord; and is reabsorbed into the bloodstream through arachnoid villi located primarily along the superior sagittal sinus. Blockade of CSF flow results in noncommunicating hydrocephalus, whereas a defect in the absorptive process leads to communicating hydrocephalus. A summary of conditions that can cause hydrocephalus is provided in Table 108-2. Note that some conditions can cause both noncommunicating and communicating hydrocephalus.

Because the open sutures of the infant skull allow cranial expansion, which helps to dissipate increased intracranial pressure, the clinical presentation of hydrocephalus is dependent on the age of the patient. The young infant with hydrocephalus typically presents with increased head circumference and a full, bulging fontanelle. The head circumference should be measured and plotted on standard head growth charts with each visit, and deviations from the normal curve should be noted immediately. The fontanelle should be inspected with the patient in the upright position and quiet. Other symptoms of hydrocephalus in the young infant include poor feeding, vomiting, and lethargy. Physical signs may also include cranial sutural diastasis, prominence of scalp veins, and the "sun-setting sign," with a forced downward gaze due to compression of the midbrain tectal plate. Macrocephaly can have a variety of causes in infants, and imaging studies discussed later help distinguish them. Older children with fused sutures cannot dissipate increased intracranial pressure through cranial expansion and often have a more

TABLE 108-2 Classification of Hydrocephalus.

Noncommunicating
Congenital
Aqueductal obstruction
Atresia of foramen of Monro
Arnold-Chiari malformation
Dandy-Walker malformation
Neoplasms
Benign cysts
Vein of Galen aneurysm
Inflammatory
Infectious ventriculitis
Intraventricular hemorrhage
Communicating
Congenital
Dandy-Walker malformation
Arnold-Chiari malformation
Incompetent arachnoid villi
Encephalocele
Benign cysts
Inflammatory
Infectious meningitis
Subarachnoid hemorrhage

acute presentation of hydrocephalus. Severe headache, vomiting, and lethargy are common. Children with obstructive hydrocephalus secondary to a colloid cyst or tumor may require urgent intervention. Papilledema is commonly seen in patients with more chronic intracranial pressure elevation. The character of the headache is important because headaches from increased intracranial pressure are characteristically worse at night or early in the morning, often waking the child from sleep, and are associated with vomiting. In these cases, cranial imaging studies should be performed to rule out hydrocephalus before embarking on a gastrointestinal workup. These symptoms may be seen before the development of other neurologic signs.

Evaluation

Radiologic imaging studies are essential in the diagnosis of hydrocephalus. The most commonly used is CT. CT allows rapid screening of the child with macrocephaly, serving to assess ventricular size, brain development, and other intracranial pathology, such as subdural hematomas. In addition, with the administration of contrast agents, intracranial tumors or vascular lesions may be better visualized. Multiple scans can be performed to assess progression of hydrocephalus or treatment efficacy. Ultrasonography is particularly useful in the young infant with an open fontanelle. Because the required equipment is portable, the test can be performed in the intensive care nursery, simplifying the care of the seriously ill infant. In addition, there is no radiation. Ultrasonography is limited in its ability to evaluate structural lesions, particularly in the posterior fossa, and extracerebral fluid collections. MRI has become more widely available since the 1990s and provides some advantages over CT. The anatomic detail is superior to that of CT, particularly in the posterior fossa, where CT is limited by bone artifacts. In addition, the ability of MRI to provide imaging in axial, coronal, and sagittal planes allows for a better understanding of structural lesions. The aqueduct may be visualized directly, along with loculations within the ventricular system. Technological advances have also allowed imaging of CSF flow, particularly through the aqueduct, and the foramen magnum. Ventriculography and cisternography were used in the past to evaluate patients with suspected obstructive lesions or loculations, but MRI is gradually supplanting these techniques.

Examination of CSF by lumbar or ventricular puncture also provides useful information in the patient with hydrocephalus. An opening pressure is measured and the CSF examined for evidence of hemorrhage or infection before treatment with a shunt. In addition, in the shunted patient, a shunt tap can provide important information on shunt function or infection.

Neuropsychologic testing in the older child and developmental assessment in the younger child also provide useful information in the evaluation of hydrocephalus. Deterioration in performance on these tests can indicate progression of hydrocephalus or shunt malfunction.

Specific Hydrocephalus Syndromes

Congenital

Congenital hydrocephalus is associated with a variety of malformation syndromes discussed earlier. Children born with a myelomeningocele have an 85% incidence of hydrocephalus. Ventricular enlargement may not be present at birth, but may develop after closure of the myelomeningocele. With elimination of this CSF reservoir, the ventricles subsequently dilate. This same mechanism is often seen in patients with occipital encephaloceles. Aqueductal stenosis may present in the newborn or young infant, but often presents at later ages as well. Dandy-Walker syndrome may also present at later ages, but is most frequently seen early in infancy. Vein of Galen aneurysms may present with hydrocephalus and a cranial bruit. Dilation of ependymal veins and a great potential for hemorrhage account for the high complication rate seen in these patients.

Inflammatory

Posthemorrhagic hydrocephalus is most commonly seen in premature infants. A germinal matrix hemorrhage results in hydrocephalus, owing to obstruction of the ventricular system by clot, aseptic meningitis, and clogging of the arachnoid villi. In full-term infants and older children, hemorrhage can be caused by birth trauma, vascular malformation, tumor, or intracranial injury. Meningitis is also a common cause of hydrocephalus. In young infants, the most common organisms include *Escherichia coli* and *Staphylococcus aureus*. In 3-month-old to 3-year-old children, the most common organisms include *Haemophilus influenzae, Streptococcus pneumoniae, Neisseria meningitides*, and *S. aureus*. After 3 years of age, the most common organisms include *Neisseria meningitides, S. pneumoniae*, and *Streptococcus* sp. With postmeningitic hydrocephalus, ventricular loculations can be seen, complicating treatment of the resulting hydrocephalus.

Neoplasms

Tumors can cause obstructive hydrocephalus in a variety of locations. Most common is the fourth ventricular tumor. Craniopharyngiomas can block flow at the level of the third ventricle. Choroid plexus tumors can oversecrete CSF in addition to producing obstruction.

Benign External Hydrocephalus

One condition that must be distinguished from hypertensive hydrocephalus is benign external hydrocephalus. This condition is characterized by macrocrania, with the head circumference crossing percentile lines and remaining elevated until 18 to 24 months of age. Development is generally normal, with the exception of poor head control, which can cause a delay in sitting. The fontanelle is normal. The CT scan demonstrates a normal to mildly dilated ventricular system, with pronounced extraaxial fluid spaces. This external hydrocephalus is believed to be caused by immaturity of the CSF absorption system at the level of the arachnoid villi and resolves in virtually every case.

Treatment

The treatment of hydrocephalus is primarily surgical. Drugs, such as acetazolamide, which reduces CSF production, or mannitol and furosemide, which decrease brain extracellular fluid, may provide temporary relief of increased intracranial pressure from hydrocephalus. In addition, corticosteroids may decrease brain edema associated with some tumors or other lesions and thereby provide temporary relief of increased intracranial pressure. The long-term management of hydrocephalus, however, requires surgical intervention. The development of valve-regulated shunt systems provided the major advance in the treatment of hydrocephalus. A variety of shunt systems are available, each with its own advocates. The key feature of all systems is that the drainage of CSF from the ventricle to a distant site (most commonly, the peritoneal cavity or the right atrium of the heart) is controlled by a valve mechanism to prevent overdrainage of CSF. The ventricular catheter is placed into the lateral ventricle from either a frontal or occipital approach. The remainder of the system is tunneled subcutaneously to either the abdomen for a peritoneal shunt or the neck for cannulation of the common facial or other vein to gain access to the right atrium for an atrial shunt. The goals of shunting are to normalize the intracranial pressure and to allow a reexpansion of the brain tissue to constitute a cortical mantle at least 3.5 cm thick to maximize the child's development (Fig. 108-15). Complete collapse of the ventricular system is not desired because this can lead to shunt malfunctions due to obstruction of the ventricular catheter and, with the elimination of the CSF volume buffer, chronic headaches. Patients with posthemorrhagic hydrocephalus are best managed initially with implantation of a subcutaneous reservoir system, which can be tapped intermittently, until the CSF is cleared of blood products that can obstruct the shunt system.

In patients with compartmentalized hydrocephalus, such as the Dandy-Walker syndrome, or with ventricular loculations, multiple ventricular catheters may be required to provide complete CSF drainage. These catheters are usually connected to a single valve system to equalize the pressures in the various compartments and to avoid dangerous brain shifts.

With the development of fiberoptic ventriculoscopy, obstructive hydrocephalus has been treated with endoscopic third ventriculostomy. This procedure involves creating an opening in the floor of the third ventricle into the subarachnoid space, thereby bypassing the obstruction to CSF flow. Reports have generally shown a 70% success rate in treating aqueductal stenosis without the need for a shunt. Failure is usually due to an insufficiency in the development of the subarachnoid spaces in these patients. Infants younger than the age of 6 to 12 months, however, seem to have a lower success rate, at around 40% to 50%, due to immaturity of the CSF absorption pathways. These techniques can also be used to communicate the various compartments in loculated ventricles, allowing the use of a simpler, single ventricular catheter shunt system.

Complications

Shunting

Shunt malfunction is the most common complication of shunting. This can be due to obstruction of the shunt system, disconnection, or migration. The ventricular catheter can become obstructed due to choroid plexus, brain parenchyma, protein, or tumor cells. To prevent obstruction by choroid plexus, the tip of the catheter should be placed into the frontal horn of the lateral ventricle, anterior to the choroid plexus. Brain parenchyma obstructs the catheter most commonly in cases of suboptimal catheter placement. Protein plugs can occur at either the proximal

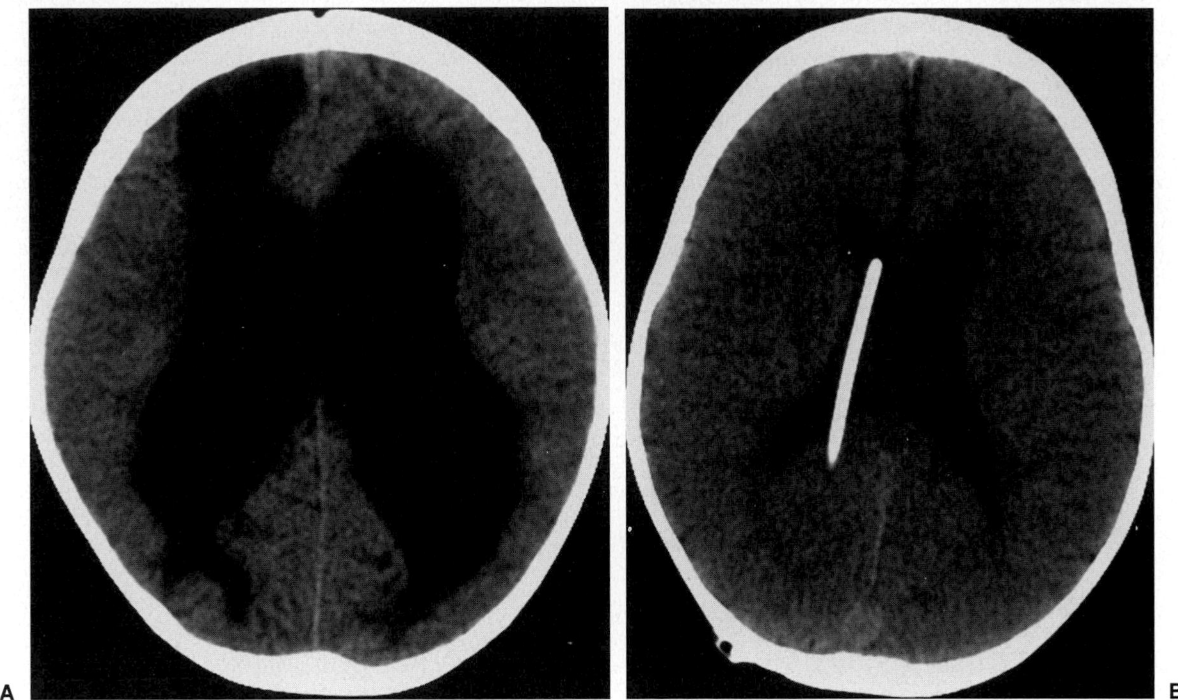

FIGURE 108-15. Effects of shunt insertion. **(A)** Preoperative computed tomography scan shows ventricular dilation of hydrocephalus. **(B)** Postoperative scan made 6 months after shunt insertion shows normalization of ventricular size. Shunt catheter is in right lateral ventricle with tip in frontal horn.

or distal catheter and are commonly seen in patients shunted for posthemorrhagic hydrocephalus in the initial months after shunting. Disconnections can occur at any point in the system, but they are most common at sites of connection and mobility. Disconnection can be confirmed with radiographic evaluation because the barium impregnated shunt tubing is visualized by plain radiographic studies.

Distal Catheter Malfunctions

Shunt malfunctions associated with the distal catheter depend on the site chosen for distal drainage. The peritoneal cavity is the most common site for drainage, owing to the ease of access and the ability to place redundant tubing into the abdomen to allow for future growth of the child. A CSF-filled pseudocyst can form around the distal catheter, resulting in shunt malfunction and abdominal pain. A smaller cyst is more commonly associated with shunt infection, and the larger pseudocyst may be sterile. In addition, small bowel obstruction, abdominal viscus perforation by shunt tubing, and an acute abdomen related to infection may be complications of abdominal shunting.

Shunting of CSF into the right atrium is another option. Although the atrial shunt is effective, it is more difficult to revise, and additional tubing cannot be inserted to allow for growth. In addition, pulmonary embolism, septicemia, shunt nephritis, cardiac arrhythmia, and pulmonary hypertension have been reported in patients with atrial shunts.

After shunt failure, shunt infection is the second most common complication of shunting, with a reported incidence of 2.6% to 38%. The most common pathogens in shunt infections are skin flora, especially *S. aureus* and *S. epidermitis*. Bacterial contamination occurs at the time of surgery or shunt tap, so meticulous attention to sterile technique and skin preparation is essential to avoid shunt infection. The clinical presentation of these patients is often nonspecific, with low-grade fever, irritability, and shunt malfunction. Patients with atrial shunts can present with septic emboli. In younger patients, gram-negative enteric bacteria are also common, and this problem commonly occurs in an acutely ill patient. The diagnosis of shunt infection is made on shunt tap; lumbar puncture is positive in only one-half the cases. Shunt infection should be managed with removal of infected hardware, appropriate intravenous antibiotics, and placement of an external ventricular drain, as needed. Once the CSF is cleared, a new shunt system can be installed. The morbidity of shunt infection is severe, with a single episode lowering the IQ by 10 to 30 points.

The slit ventricle syndrome is characterized by episodic headaches due to alterations intracranial pressure in patients with small or slitlike ventricles. A variety of mechanisms have been proposed to account for this syndrome, including intermittent obstruction of the ventricular catheter, overdrainage of CSF, and decreased ventricular compliance. Medical therapy includes furosemide, acetazolamide, and steroids. Studies of antimigraine medications, including propranolol, dihydroergotamine, and cyproheptadine, have suggested that the slit ventricle syndrome may have at least an element of acquired migraine headache. Surgical options for slit ventricle syndrome include upgrading the resistance of the valve and possibly incorporating a siphon control device to eliminate overdrainage of CSF.

Subdural collections are another complication of overshunting. The thinned brain collapses away from the skull, resulting in disruption of bridging veins and subdural hematoma formation. Most of these patients do not have symptoms. Over time, with growth of the brain, these collections may resolve. In patients with symptoms, incorporation of a subdural catheter into the shunt system (distal to the valve) results in resolution of the subdural collections.

CRANIOSYNOSTOSIS

Craniosynostosis, or premature closure of the cranial sutures, is commonly seen in pediatric neurosurgery. Most cases are sporadic, but as many as 10% are familial. Separation of the bones of the calvarium by the cranial sutures allows progressive enlargement of the skull to occur with growth of the brain. Brain weight doubles by 6 months of age and triples by 10 months. Brain growth is virtually complete by 2 years of age, and the cranial sutures are fused by 6 to 8 years of age. When one or more sutures close prematurely, there must be compensatory growth at the remaining open sutures, resulting in recognizable patterns of deformity. When skull growth cannot keep pace with brain growth, increased intracranial pressure results, with the potential for cognitive impairment. Sagittal synostosis results in scaphocephaly, coronal synostosis results in plagiocephaly if unilateral and brachycephaly if bilateral, metopic synostosis results in trigonocephaly, and multiple suture stenosis results in cloverleaf deformity (Kleeblattschädel). Multiple causes may be involved in craniosynostosis. Metabolic conditions affecting bone formation, intrauterine deformation, genetic abnormalities, and syndromic causes, such as Crouzon or Apert syndrome, have all been invoked in cases of craniosynostosis (17).

Evaluation

The skull deformities that result from closure of the various sutures are recognizable to the trained clinician. The abnormality is usually present at birth, and with time, it may become more severe. Ridges along the fused sutures are obvious to palpation. Skull radiographs confirm the diagnosis of craniosynostosis and may show indentations of the inner table as evidence of increased intracranial pressure. CT scan also demonstrates sutural fusion and allows examination of the underlying brain. Three-dimensional reconstruction of CT images may also facilitate surgical planning. The therapy of craniosynostosis varies with the involved suture.

Scaphocephaly (Sagittal Synostosis)

Isolated sagittal synostosis is by far the most common form of craniosynostosis and is most commonly sporadic. The scaphocephalic appearance is obvious at birth along with compensatory frontal bossing. A bewildering variety of surgical approaches to scaphocephaly have been devised, ranging from suturectomy to complete calvarial reconstructions. In general, the simpler procedures can be effective if performed as early as 2 to 3 months of age because removal of the skull growth constraint allows further brain growth to reshape the calvarium, resulting in excellent cosmetic results. In older children, more complex procedures are often necessary, owing to the more limited remaining brain growth. More recently, techniques employing endoscopic strip craniectomy in conjunction with a molding helmet have been described as a minimally invasive treatment of sagittal synostosis. The long-term outcome of such treatment remains to be seen, but early results are encouraging. Figure 108-16 shows a typical child with scaphocephaly before and after surgical correction.

Coronal Synostosis

Unilateral Coronal Synostosis

The characteristic deformity of unilateral coronal synostosis is ipsilateral frontal bone and orbital flattening, with ridging of the affected suture (Figs. 108-17A and 108-17B). The contralateral frontal region frequently displays compensatory bossing. Skull radiographs demonstrate the characteristic harlequin orbit deformity on the affected side. Surgery consists of *bilateral* frontal craniotomy and frontal bone reconstruction, with supraorbital bar advancement as well (18). If only a unilateral procedure is performed, the cosmetic result immediately after surgery may be acceptable, but further growth may be asymmetric, producing an unacceptable result. Endoscopic techniques have also been described for coronal synostosis, with early encouraging results.

Bilateral Coronal Synostosis

Bilateral coronal synostosis is frequently seen as part of a syndrome complex, such as Apert or Crouzon syndrome. There may be significant involvement of the facial bones, and surgical correction may be much more complex than for unilateral coronal synostosis. There is a characteristic brachycephalic appearance, with bitemporal widening,

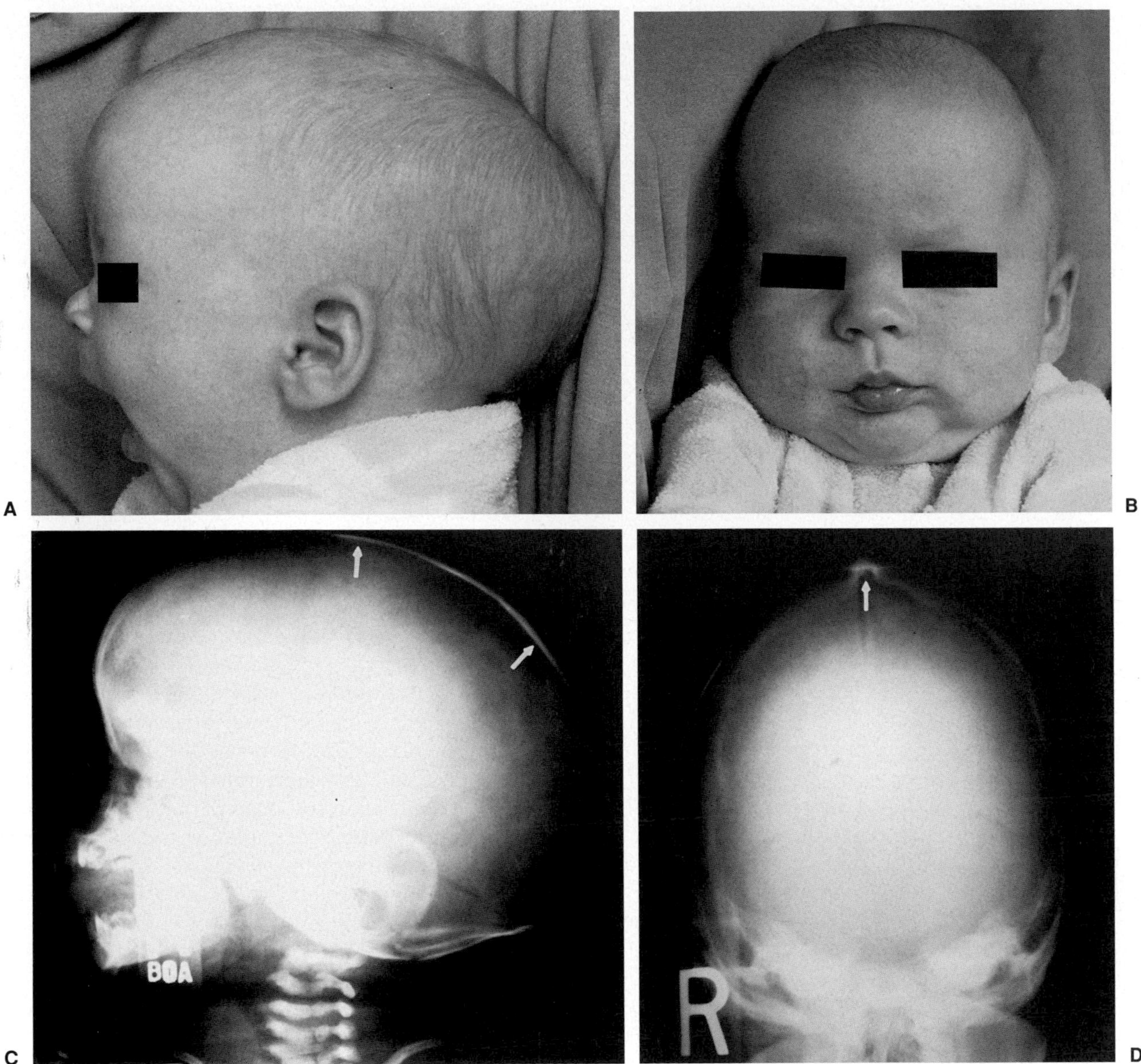

FIGURE 108-16. Scaphocephaly. **(A)** Preoperative lateral photograph of a patient with scaphocephaly shows the elongated skull configuration with frontal prominence. **(B)** Preoperative frontal photograph of a patient with scaphocephaly illustrates frontal bossing. **(C)** Preoperative lateral skull radiograph of the same patient shows sclerotic sagittal suture (*arrows*). **(D)** Preoperative anteroposterior skull radiograph shows sclerotic sagittal suture (*arrow*). (*continued*)

ocular protrusion, and towering of the skull (Figs. 108-17C and 108-17D). The surgical procedure involves bilateral frontal craniotomy and frontal bone reconstruction, along with supraorbital bar advancement. Midface advancement should be treated in a separate facial procedure.

Metopic Synostosis

The characteristic deformity of metopic synostosis is trigonocephaly, with a pointed forehead and a triangular shape to the skull (Fig. 108-18). The surgical procedure involves bilateral frontal craniotomy, with complete reconstruction of the frontal bone and bilateral lateral canthal advances.

Lambdoid Synostosis

Lambdoid synostosis is extremely rare. It is important to distinguish true lambdoid synostosis from positional molding, the most common cause of occipital flattening. In patients with positional deformities, a history of lying on one side for prolonged periods and a progressive flattening

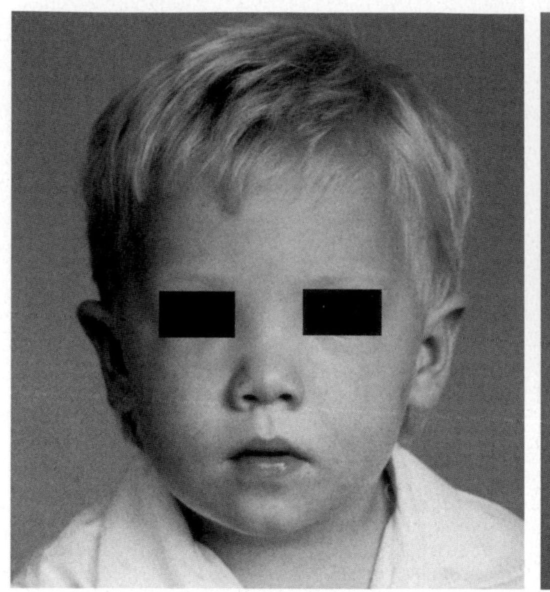

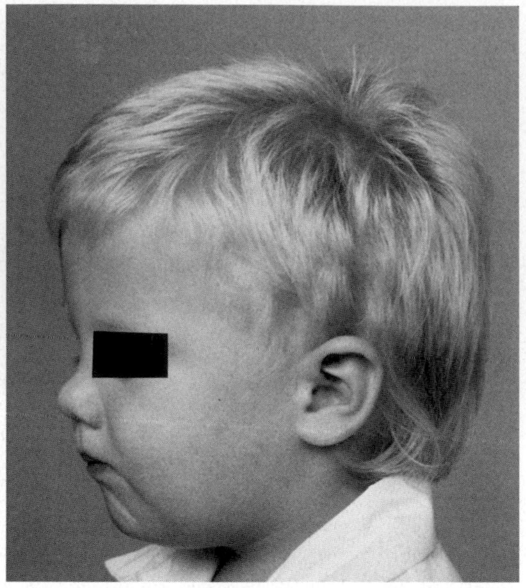

E F

FIGURE 108-16. **(E, F)** Postoperative photographs of the same patient taken 12 months after extended strip craniectomy for scaphocephaly reveal normalization of head shape, with resolution of frontal bossing.

help make the diagnosis. The characteristic head shape of positional molding is a parallelogram when viewed from above, with controlateral occipital and frontal flattening, anterior displacement of the ipsilateral ear, and no external ridging of the lambdoid suture. True lambdoid synostosis involves ipsilateral occipital and frontal flattening, posterior and inferior displacement of the ipsilateral ear, and an occipitomastoid bulge, along with ridging of the lambdoid suture. Even in patients with positional molding, however, there may be radiographic changes along the lambdoid suture, most often perisutural sclerosis. This is not, however, an indication of craniosynostosis. The treatment of positional molding involves repositioning of the infant during sleep. True lambdoid synostosis will require surgical reconstruction of the posterior skull, analogous to the frontal procedures described previously.

Multiple Suture Synostoses

When multiple cranial sutures are fused prematurely, increased intracranial pressure must be anticipated, and restoration of the normal cranial vault/brain mass ratio is crucial if blindness and cognitive dysfunction are to be avoided. Treatment consists of total calvarial remodeling and may require multiple operative procedures.

TUMORS

Primary tumors of the CNS are the most common solid neoplasms in children (Table 108-3). Major technological advances in diagnostic imaging, anesthetic techniques, surgical techniques, radiotherapy, and chemotherapy have brought about improved survival in children with brain tumors, but many problems remain. Often, difficulties in treatment relate more to location within the brain limiting surgical resection or radiation dosage (due to toxicity to neighboring vital structures) than to intrinsic biological malignancy of a given tumor. Intracranial tumors can be categorized by their location with respect to the tentorium cerebelli, with supratentorial and infratentorial tumors occurring with nearly equal frequency in children.

VASCULAR MALFORMATIONS OF THE BRAIN

Vascular malformations of the brain are common causes of intracerebral hemorrhage in children. The classic arteriovenous malformation (AVM) is the most common, with cavernous angiomas and venous angiomas less commonly associated with hemorrhage. The vein of Galen aneurysm deserves special mention because its presentation varies, depending on the age of the patient.

Arteriovenous Malformation

The classic AVM represents a defect in the formation of the primitive arteriolar capillary network interposed between cerebral arteries and veins. The resulting tangled arteriovenous complex, with its low resistance, invites high

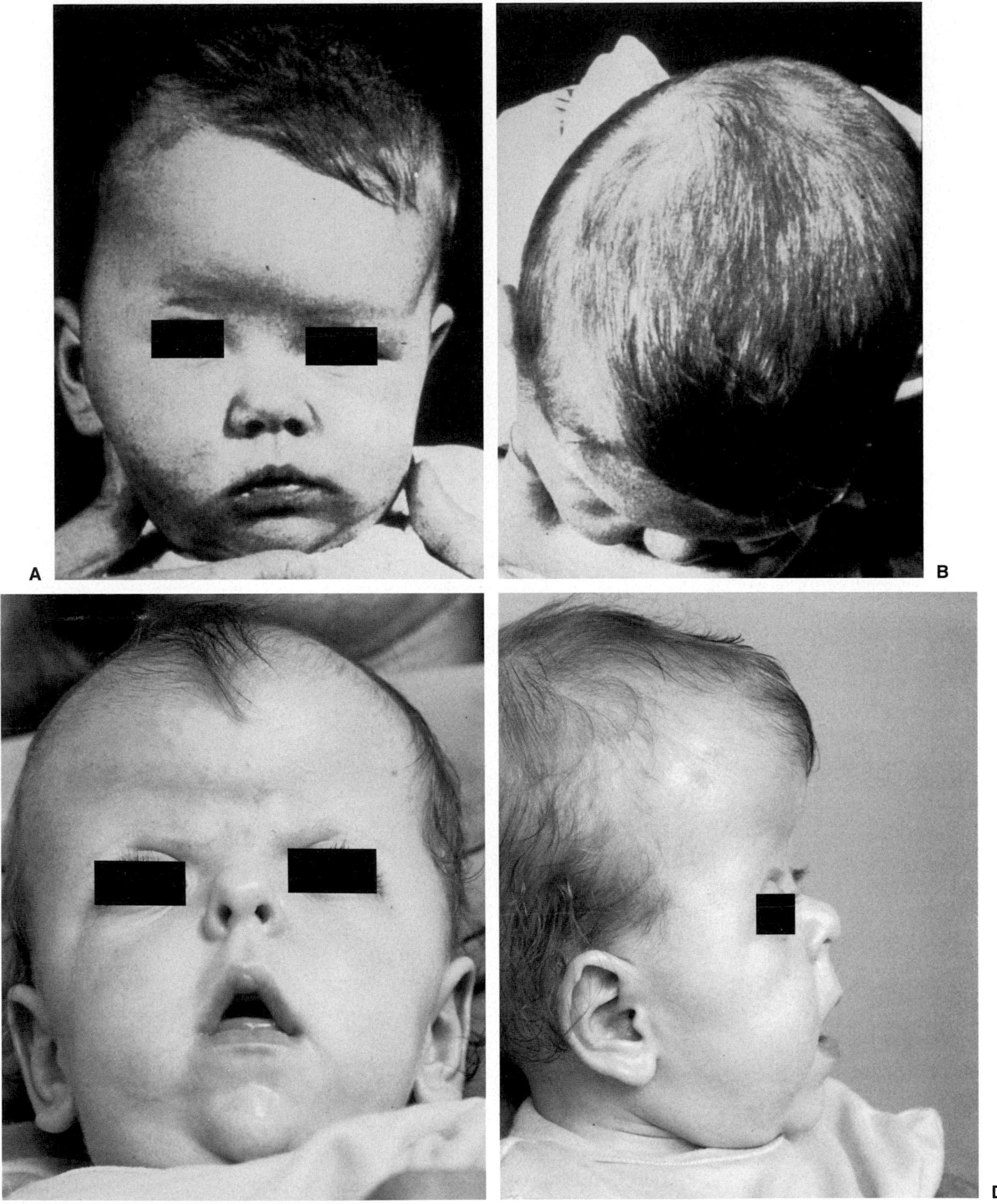

FIGURE 108-17. Coronal synostosis. **(A, B)**. Unilateral. The right side of the forehead is flattened, and the left side is prominent. **(C, D)** Bilateral. There is bilateral canthal retrusion and compensatory prominence of upper forehead in this patient, who has Apert syndrome.

blood flow rates and increases the risk of hemorrhage. Most AVMs have a characteristic wedge shape, pointing to the ventricle. The most common presentation of an AVM is intracerebral hemorrhage, which can be catastrophic. Seizures may also be present. CT is the diagnostic modality of choice when acute hemorrhage is suspected. Arteriography delineates the lesion and identifies feeding arteries and draining veins. In some cases, arteriography after a hemorrhage is negative, owing to either compression of the AVM or obliteration of the AVM with the rupture.

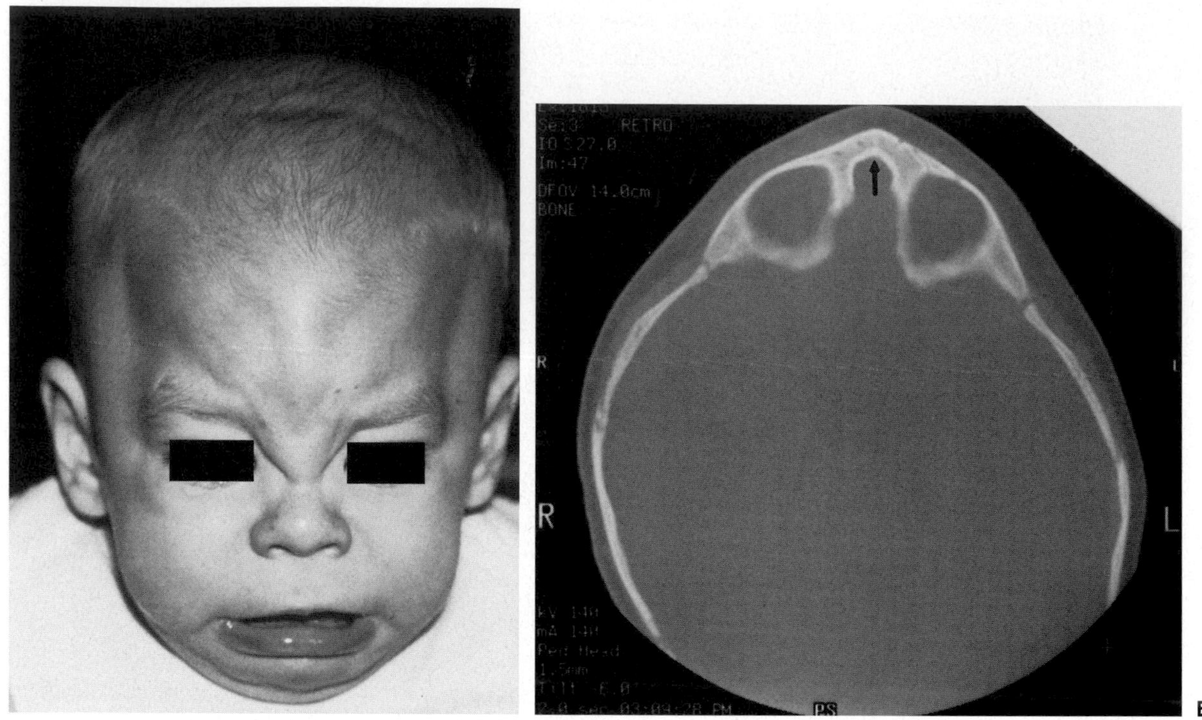

FIGURE 108-18. Trigonocephaly. **(A)** The forehead is pointed and towering. **(B)** Axial CT scan reveals fused metopic suture (*arrow*).

TABLE 108-3 Summary of Childhood Brain Tumors.

Tumor	*Incidence*[a]	*Treatment*	*Outcome*
Posterior fossa tumors			
Medulloblastoma	20%	Surgery, craniospinal irradiation, and chemotherapy for high-risk patients	More than 50% 10-y survival rate with improved chemotherapy
Cerebellar astrocytoma	10%–20%	Surgery alone	95% 25-y survival rate
Brainstem glioma	10%–20%	Radiotherapy and chemotherapy; no role for surgery in diffuse pontine glioma	Less than 30% 5-y survival rate
Ependymoma	10%	Surgery and radiotherapy	Prognosis depends on extent of surgical resection; much improved if gross total resection can be obtained
Supratentorial tumors			
Astrocytomas	30%	Surgery, followed by radiotherapy of chemotherapy for more malignant tumors; observation for benign lesions	Varies by histology; with benign tumors, prognosis can be excellent
Choroid plexus papilloma	1%–3%	Surgery; radiotherapy and/or chemotherapy reserved for carcinomas	Nearly 100% 5-y survival rate for papilloma; only 50% 5-y survival rate for carcinoma
Hypothalamic or optic pathway glioma	3%	Surgery for biopsy, debulking, followed by radiotherapy or chemotherapy	80%–95% 5-y survival rate
Craniopharyngioma	6%–8%	Surgery and radiotherapy	90% 5-y survival rate
Pineal region tumors	3%–8%	Surgery, radiotherapy, and chemotherapy, depending on histology; germinoma especially radiosensitive	Varies with histology; most favorable for germinoma with 5-y survival rate of 70%; malignant histologies much worse

[a]Incidence is indicated as percentage of total childhood brain tumors.

The ideal treatment of AVM is total surgical removal. Preoperative embolization of large, complex AVMs facilitates surgical resection. Surgery may be limited, however, if the AVM lies in an eloquent location in the brain. Stereotactic radiosurgery may provide benefit in nonresectable deep lesions.

Cavernous Angioma

The cavernous angioma typically presents with hemorrhage, seizures, or neurologic deficit. Modern imaging methods, particularly MRI, have greatly increased our understanding of these lesions. As imaging techniques have improved, the diagnosis of these lesions before hemorrhage has been possible. These lesions are characterized as a dark blue mass, which is well encapsulated and surrounded by hemorrhage-stained white matter. For lesions that have hemorrhaged, treatment is surgical excision. Lesions that have not hemorrhaged can be excised surgically, if easily accessible. Deep lesions that have not hemorrhaged are not approached surgically.

Venous Angioma

The venous angioma is the most common vascular malformation of the brain and the least likely to cause symptoms. It consists of dilated medullary veins separated by normal brain parenchyma. The veins of the angioma drain centripetally into the venous channels around which they are arranged, and they are important for venous drainage of the surrounding brain. The risk of hemorrhage from a venous angioma is uncertainn, but is clearly less than that associated with a AVM or cavernous angioma. Most venous angiomas can be diagnosed on contrast-enhanced CT. Surgery is not indicated for venous angiomas because the venous drainage they provide is essential for the surrounding normal brain tissue.

Vein of Galen Aneurysm

The presentation of vein of Galen aneurysms depends on patient age. Infants presenting with vein of Galen aneurysms commonly have high-output cardiac failure due to the tremendous arteriovenous shunting. This shunting can also cause cerebral ischemia. The dilated vein of Galen can cause obstructive hydrocephalus, and macrocephaly may be obvious. The treatment of these children is aimed at reduction of the arteriovenous shunt, thereby relieving the cardiac failure. This must be accomplished in a gradual fashion, or the risk of hemorrhage is high. Mickle and Quisling (19) reported on the transtorcular approach to embolization of these lesions. These authors advocate the graded, multisession treatment approach. Older children with vein of Galen malformations commonly present with subarachnoid hemorrhage or hydrocephalus. In these children, direct surgical therapy is possible, but transtorcular embolization has also met with considerable success.

INFECTIONS

The treatment of infections of the CNS has been greatly improved with the development of modern imaging techniques and new antibiotics. The most important aspect in the treatment of these infections is early recognition, with identification of the causative organism and administration of appropriate antibiotics to eradicate the infection.

Intracranial Infections

Brain Abscess

Brain abscess is uncommon in children. The most common causes of brain abscess include contiguous infection, such as sinusitis or mastoiditis; hematogenous spread, such as with congenital heart disease; or direct introduction through a penetrating wound. The formation of a brain abscess proceeds through a well-recognized series of stages. First, the organism produces an inflammatory reaction, termed *cerebritis,* with infiltration of polymorphonuclear leukocytes. Next, the involved tissue becomes necrotic, leading to suppuration in the center of the lesion. The brain attempts to wall off the infection, and fibroblasts deposit a collagen wall around the lesion. Edema is present in the tissue surrounding the capsule. Brain abscess is rare in infants. In older children, congenital heart disease, purulent infection such as sinusitis, or chronic otitis media is often present. A history of penetrating trauma should arouse considerable suspicion of this problem. Patients may present with neurologic signs and symptoms of increased intracranial pressure and focal signs owing to the location of the abscess. CT is the diagnostic study of choice, allowing visualization of the brain, paranasal sinuses, and skull. With contrast administration, a ring-enhancing lesion with considerable edema is commonly seen. Treatment should consist of abscess aspiration (stereotactic techniques may be used for deeper lesions) to obtain adequate material for culture. Drainage of the abscess also helps normalize intracranial pressure and reduce local effects of the abscess. Broad-spectrum antibiotics are started, including coverage for anaerobic bacteria, and can be modified when culture results are available. Antibiotic coverage should continue for 4 to 6 weeks. With early diagnosis and treatment, the morbidity and mortality rates of brain abscess have improved considerably. With increasing numbers of survivors of brain abscess, long-term effects, including seizure disorders, are being seen with increasing frequency.

Subdural Empyema

Subdural empyema is an uncommon infection that occurs primarily in children and adolescents. It is usually secondary to paranasal sinus or middle ear infection, but can also result from hematogenous seeding of a subdural hematoma. It is most commonly seen over the cerebral convexities. CT or MRI provides the diagnosis, and lumbar puncture should not be performed. Treatment consists of surgical drainage and antibiotic therapy. If the purulent material is thick, a craniotomy may be necessary to debride purulent material. Complications of subdural empyema include cortical vein thrombosis, brain abscess, and meningitis. Seizures are common in patients with subdural empyema and can persist for years.

Epidural Abscess

Epidural abscess is almost always secondary to another infection of the sinuses, postoperative bone flap, or compound wounds of the head. Local symptoms such as pain, erythema, and swelling are common. Treatment consists of surgical drainage (with removal of infected bone), followed by intravenous antibiotics, as described earlier.

Spinal Epidural Abscess

Spinal epidural abscess is rare in children. It occurs most commonly in the thoracic or lower lumbar region. *S. aureus* is the most common causative organism; it gains access to the epidural space through hematogenous spread. Back pain is common, and spinal cord compression with lower extremity weakness is often present at the time of clinical presentation. MRI is the diagnostic procedure of choice. Treatment consists of laminectomy with irrigation of the epidural space and culture. A drain is left in place for 24 to 48 hours. Intravenous antibiotics are continued for 4 to 6 weeks. With early diagnosis and treatment before significant neurologic deficit occurs, the prognosis should be good.

REFERENCES

1. O'Rahilly R. *Developmental stages in human embryos, including a survey of the Carnegie collection. A. Embryos of the first three weeks (stages 1 to 9).* Washington, DC: Carnegie Institution of Washington, 1973:631.
2. Lemire RJ, Siebert JR, Warkany J. Normal development of the central nervous system. In: McLaurin RL, Venes JL, Schut L, et al., eds. *Pediatric neurosurgery: surgery of the developing nervous system,* 2nd ed. Philadelphia: WB Saunders, 1989.
3. Barson AJ. The vertebral level of termination of the spinal cord during normal and abnormal development. *J Anat* 1970;106:489.
4. McLone DG. The etiology of neural tube defects: the role of folid acid. *Childs Nerv Syst* 2003;19:537.
5. McLone DG, Mutluer S, Naidich TP. Lipomeningoceles of the conus medullaris. In: Imondi AJ, ed. *Concepts in pediatric neurosurgery,* vol. 3. Basel: S Karger, 1982.
6. Dias MS, Walker ML. The embryogenesis of complex dysraphic malformations: a disorder of gastrulation? *J Pediatr Neurosurg* 1992; 18:229.
7. Pang D, Dias MS, Ahab-Barmada M. Split cord malformation. I. A unified theory of embryogenesis for double cord malformations. *Neurosurgery* 1992;31:451.
8. Chapman PH, Swearingen B, Caviness VS. Subtorcular occipital encephaloceles: anatomical considerations relevant to operative management. *J Neurosurg* 1989;71:375.
9. McLone DG, Knepper PA. The cause of the Chiari II malformation: a unified theory. *Pediatr Neurosurg* 1989;15:1.
10. McLone DG, Dias L, Kaplan WE, et al. Concepts in the management of spina bifida. In: Humphreys RP, ed. *Concepts in pediatric neurosurgery,* vol. 5. Basel: S Karger, 1985:97.
11. Sutton LN, Adzick NS, Johnson MP. Fetal surgery for myelomeningocele. *Childs Nerv Syst* 2003;19:587.
12. Yamada S, Zinke DE, Sanders D. Pathophysiology of tethered cord syndrome. *J Neurosurg* 1981;54:494.
13. Warder DE, Oakes WJ. Tethered cord syndrome: the low-lying and normally positioned conus. *Neurosurgery* 1994;34:597.
14. Oakes WJ. Chiari malformations, hydromyelia, syringomyelia. In: Wilkins RH, Rengachary SS, eds. *Neurosurgery*. New York: McGraw-Hill, 1985.
15. Raimondi AJ, Choux M, DiRocco C, eds. *Intracranial cyst lesions.* New York: Springer Verlag, 1993.
16. Butler AJ, McLone DG, eds. Hydrocephalus. *Neurosurg Clin North Am* 1993;4:599–609.
17. Hoffman HJ, Kestle JRW. Craniofacial surgery. In: McLaurin RL, Venes JL, Schut L, et al., eds. *Pediatric neurosurgery: surgery of the developing nervous system,* 3rd ed. Philadelphia: WB Saunders, 1994.
18. Persing JA, Jane JA, Edgerton MT. Surgical treatment of craniosynostosis. In: Persing JA Edgerton MT, Jane JA, eds. *Scientific foundations and surgical treatment of craniosynostosis.* Baltimore: Williams & Wilkins, 1989.
19. Mickle JP, Quisling RG. The transtorcular embolization of vein of Galen aneurysms. *J Neurosurg* 1986;64:731.

PART M

Conjoined Twins

Chapter 109

Conjoined Twins

John H.T. Waldhausen

Conjoined twins represent a fascinating challenge for the entire medical team involved in the care of these children. The separation of these children may in some cases be quite simple, whereas in others it is extremely complex. Meticulous planning and a team approach offer the best chance for a successful outcome to those infants who are separable.

HISTORY

Conjoined twins have been known since antiquity (1–4). Presently, more than 500 sets of twins have been described with more than 200 attempts at surgical separation. Since 1950, an increasing number of twins have undergone successful separation, yet the operations remain a distinct challenge with many ethical and surgical problems to consider (2).

INCIDENCE

The incidence of conjoined twinning varies in different parts of the world, from 1:100,000 to 250,000 in the United States to 1:50,000 in parts of Africa, with some isolated reports indicating a frequency as much as 1:14,000 (5). In the United States, 40% of these infants are stillborn and another 35% die within the first 24 hours of life (6). Prenatal diagnosis and planned cesarean section have increased survival over what was experienced with vaginal delivery (7). Seventy percent of conjoined twins who survive long enough to undergo separation are female, whereas most stillborn conjoined twins are male.

EMBRYOLOGY

Conjoined twins have been reported in both the plant and the animal kingdoms (8). The embryology of conjoined twins is controversial and is for the most part theoretical because, for ethical reasons, there is no model to study this in humans. Conjoined twinning occurs during the third to fourth week of gestation and may be considered either as a result of incomplete fission or of partial fusion. Much of the evidence for incomplete fission is circumstantial, although this has usually been viewed as the most likely cause (8). Conjoined twins are almost always monoamniotic and of the same sex, although diamniotic omphalopagus twins have been reported (9). Conjoined twins have been reported as one of a set of triplets or quadruplets and, in fact, there are rare reports of conjoined tripling and quadrupling (10). When a pair of conjoined twins is part of a set of triplets or quadruplets, the conjoined twins are always isosexual, whereas the other infant may be of the opposite sex. One would surmise that if conjoined twins occurred as a process of fusion, that opposite sex twins would be as likely to fuse as would same-sex infants. This has never, however, been noted to occur, although several cases of pseudohermaphroditism have been documented (10).

Conjoined twins are always joined in a homologous fashion; in other words, they are always fused back to back, front to front, cranial to cranial, or caudal to caudal. They are never fused head to tail and so on. Twins can be divided into two groups: those with ventral union of two early embryonic discs over a single yolk sac (cephalopagus, thoracopagus, omphalopagus, ischiopagus, and parapagus), and those fused dorsally by two originally separate neural tubes (craniopagus, rachipagus, pygopagus). Twins often have multiple anomalies in multiple organ systems. These anomalies are typically found in male infants and the right-sided twin (10).

Development by fusion is supported by theoretical work performed by Dr. Rowena Spencer. The spherical theory

John H.T. Waldhausen: Department of Surgery, University of Washington School of Medicine, Children's Hospital and Regional Medical Center, Seattle, Washington 98115.

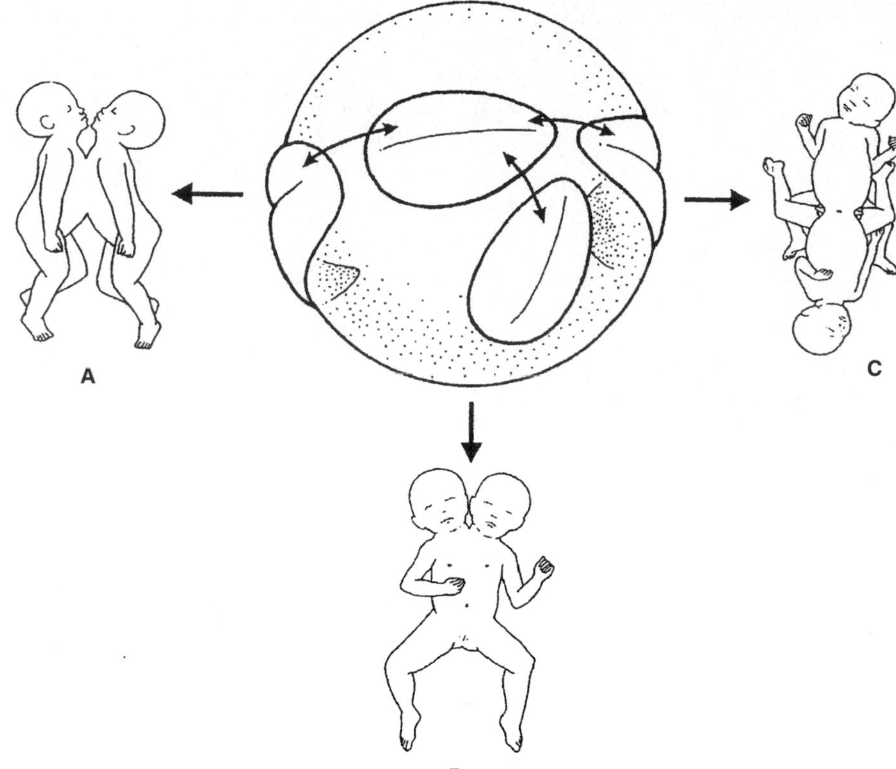

FIGURE 109-1. The "spherical" theory; embryonic discs united ventrally, "floating" on the sphere of a shared yolk sac oriented **(A)** rostrally (thoracopagus), **(B)** caudolaterally (parapagus), and **(C)** caudally (ischiopagus). [From Spencer R. Theoretical and analytical embryology of conjoined twins. *Clin Anat* 2000;13(1): 36–53, with permission.]

espoused by Dr. Spencer postulates that two monovulvar embryonic discs lie adjacent to each other either floating on the outer surface (yolk sac) or inner surface (amniotic cavity) of a sphere (10) (Figs. 109-1 and 109-2). The embryonic discs may unite in any one of several orientations. The union, however, is always homologous. Fusion between two embryonic discs cannot occur at random surfaces of the disc. Union can only occur where surface ectoderm is either absent or destined to break down, such as in the oropharyngeal and cloacal membranes or along the neural tube. Ventral union (union involving the yolk sac and the periphery of the disc) leads in general to twins sharing one abdomen and one umbilicus, whereas dorsal union (neural tube) leads to twins with separate abdomens and two umbilical cords.

The development of certain types of twins may require what are termed *adjustments to conjunction* (11). These include division and diversion of midsaggital structures and aplasia of contiguous lateral anlagen. Division and diversion is best illustrated by cephalopagus twins. In this case as the oropharyngeal membrane fuses, it splits sagitally and diverts laterally to fuse with its compliment from the other twin (Fig. 109-3). In the case of cephalopagus twins, this results in a child with two faces, one on each side of the head, but one-half of each face is derived from each twin. This is supported by the neuroanatomy of these twins in which the brain is also found to split in a similar manner (11).

Aplasia is best demonstrated in parapagus twins. In this case, twins are fused laterally and, by an unexplained mechanism, the midline structures in the area of conjoinment disappear. These children may have two heads, but only one trunk and one set of legs. The arms and legs that lay centrally in the area of fusion fail to develop.

TERMINOLOGY

The terminology of conjoined twins may be confusing because there are many terms in the literature. Classification of the types of twins is based on anatomic description and describes the most prominent area of conjoinment. Confusion may arise because of a continuum between some of these twins, such as the thoracopagus and omphalopagus twins. The Greek term *-pagus* means to be fixed or joined with the prefix describing the area where the twins are joined. One frequently used classification system by Potter and Craig lists five major categories, omphalopagus or xiphopagus (umbilicus), thoracopagus (chest), ischiopagus (hip), craniopagus (helmet), and pygopagus (rump) (12). Spencer adds the additional categories of parapagus (side), cephalopagus (head), and rachipagus (spine) (13). In addition, parasites (teratomas and fetus-in-fetu) may be considered part of this process. Several suffixes are descriptive of certain areas of the body *-prosopus* (face), *-brachius* (upper limb), and *-pus* (lower limbs). The other

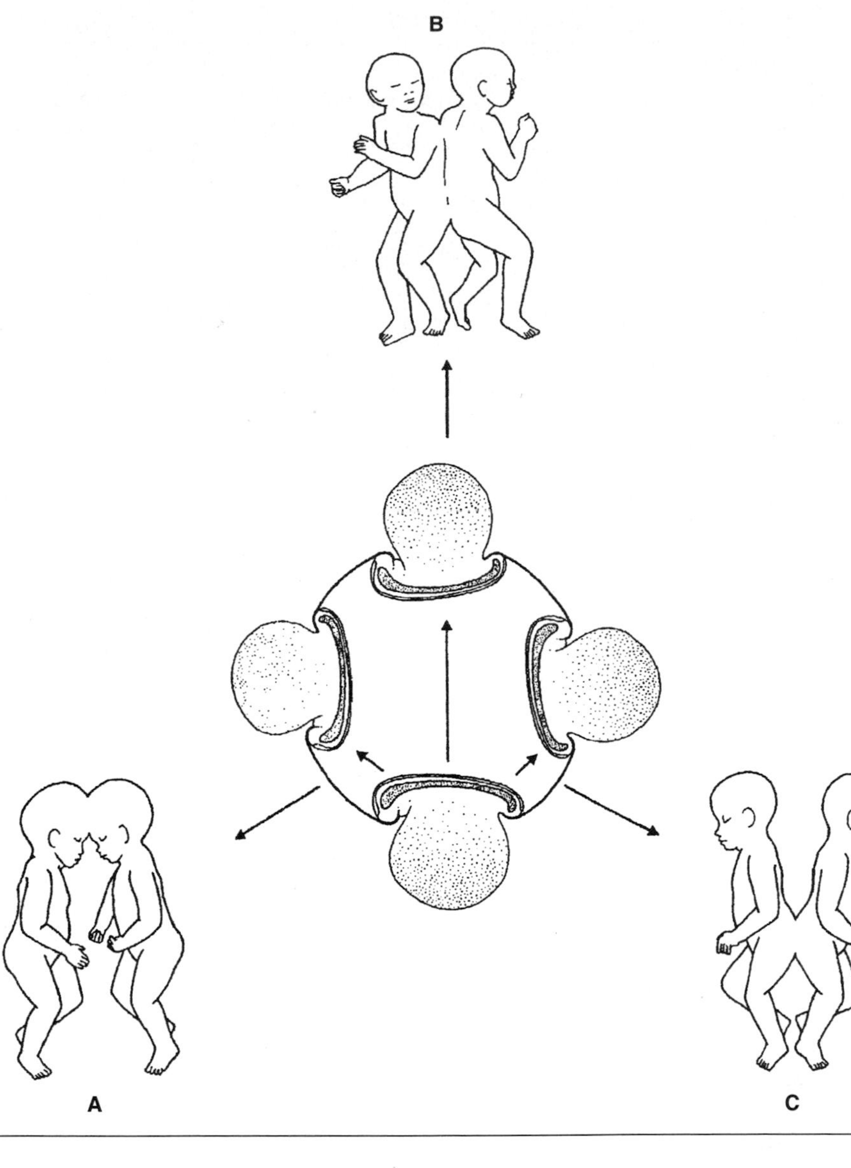

FIGURE 109-2. The "spherical" theory; embryonic discs united dorsally, "floating" in a shared amniotic cavity oriented in the **(A)** rostral (craniopagus), **(B)** middorsal (rachipagus), and **(C)** caudal (pygopagus) portion of the neural tube. [From Spencer R. Theoretical and analytical embryology of conjoined twins. *Clin Anat* 2000;13(1):36–53, with permission.]

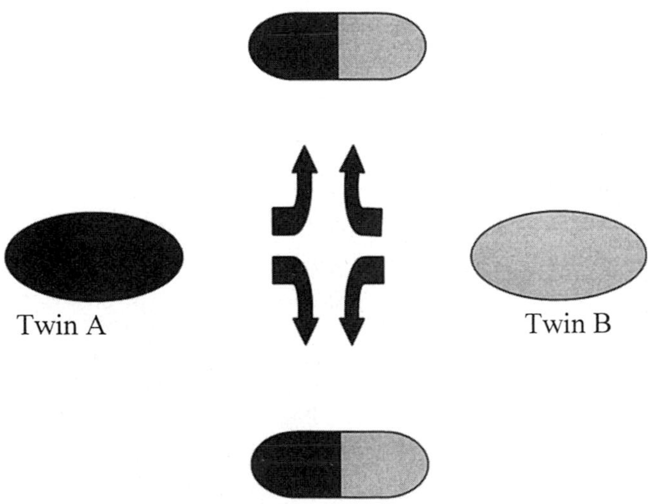

FIGURE 109-3. Division and diversion of midsaggital structures as seen in craniopagus twins.

terms needed are *-di, -tri,* and *tetra,* to describe the number of the previous structures present (e.g., ischiopagus tetrapus).

When discussing conjoined twins, it is important to use uniform terminology in describing structures shared between twins and structures that are completely separate. "Anterior" and "posterior" are not terms that apply to individual twins, but are used as points of reference looking at the twins as a whole. Twins lying in a position such that the abdomen is most fully exposed have this aspect identified as the secondary anterior and the opposite side as the secondary posterior. Using this anterior aspect as a reference, twins may then be identified as the "twin on their right," or right twin and the "twin on their left," or left twin. Structures in individual twins are identified as dorsal and ventral rather than anterior and posterior. This nomenclature tends to work for all conjoined twins, with the exception of craniopagus and rachipagus twins (13).

TABLE 109-1 Possible Visceral Unions in Different Types of Conjoined Twins.

Type	*Appearance*	*Heart and Liver*	*Liver and Biliary Tract*	*Upper Gastrointestinal Tract*	*Lower Gastrointestinal Tract*	*Genitourinary Tract*	*Nervous System*
Thoracopagus		Yes	Yes	Yes	—	—	—
Xiphopagus		—	Yes	Yes	Yes	Yes	—
Pygopagus		—	—	—	Yes	Yes	Yes
Ischiopagus		—	Yes	Yes	Yes	Yes	—
Craniopagus		—	—	—	—	—	Yes

CLASSIFICATION AND ANATOMY

The various types of twins and the organ systems shared are listed in Table 109-1. There are two basic sets of conjoined twins, each set representing a continuum of fusion, either ventral to ventral or dorsal to dorsal. When the twins face each other, the union ranges from fusion at the rostral and midventral levels, such as in cephalopagus infants, to the caudal and caudolaterally fused infants, such as ischiopagus and parapagus infants. The infants in this continuum share some common aspect of the gastrointestinal (GI) tract and most share a single umbilicus. The second basic set involves twins conjoined at the neural tube and craniovertebral axis. These infants face away from each other and have separate umbilical cords and GI tracts. The critical anatomic point that is key in determining separability for either set of twins is the degree of union of vital organs, especially the heart and central nervous system (CNS). When there is one heart for two infants or there is significant union of the CNS, it is unlikely that both or even one infant will survive surgical separation.

The most common type of conjoined twins is thoracopagus twins, comprising 40% of all such infants. Frequently, they are classified with omphalopagus twins and together these two types account for ~75% of these infants (14). For purposes of clinical discussion, however, it is best to consider these two types separately because, although omphalopagus twins can usually be separated, thoracopagus twins usually cannot. Thoracopagus twins share the heart in more than 75% of cases, and it is this union that usually makes separation difficult or impossible and survival of both twins extremely unlikely (15). Survival of even one twin when the heart is fused is unusual (Table 109-2). The pericardial sac is shared in 90% of thoracopagus twins, the biliary tree in 22%, and the upper GI tract in 50%. The

TABLE 109-2 Survival Rates for Conjoined Twins.

	Survival for Both Twins	*Mortality for Both Twins*
Thoracopagus	29%	34%
Omphalopagus	70%	14%
Craniopagus	33%	37%
Ischiopagus	74%	15%
Pygopagus	56%	6%

From Hoyle RM. Surgical separation of conjoined twins. *Surg Gynecol Obstet* 1990;170:549-562, with permission.

stomach and esophagus may be shared on occasion, but union usually starts at the level of the distal duodenum and ends near the level of a Meckel's diverticulum (14). These infants almost always have a shared bridge of the liver between them and union of the biliary tree should be suspected if the infants have a common duodenum at the area of the ampulla of Vater.

Omphalopagus (also called *xiphopagus*) twins account for ~35% of conjoined twins (14). These children also face each other and share a common umbilicus, but the heart is never joined. They tend to be the least complicated infants to separate. The union usually extends from the xiphoid to the umbilicus and an omphalocele may be present. There is usually a connecting bridge of liver and the diaphragm is likely shared, but the upper GI tract is usually separate.

Twenty percent of conjoined twins are pygogagus, and only 7% of the typical cases are boys (16). These twins face away from each other and have a separate umbilicus. They are joined at the sacrum, buttocks, and perineum. Most commonly, there are two sets of external genitalia united back to back in the area of the forchette in girls. Typically, the urethral orifice is separate, although when junction is more extensive, the vagina and urethra may become fused. The anus is usually single and empties posterior to the urogenital fusion. The GI tracts are for the most part separate, but unite at the rectum several centimeters proximal to the anal canal. Twenty five percent of pygopagus twins have renal anomalies, including renal agenesis, ectopia, and fusion. Forty percent of these twins share a single dural mater, and there may be a fused or continuous spinal cord (16). The pelvic rings are separate with the osseous fusion involving the lateral portion of the sacrum and coccyx. Almost one-half of these twins have significant anomalies of the CNS and/or vertebral column, including hydrocephalus, myelomeningocele, spina bifida, and rachischisis (16).

Ischiopagus twins comprise 6% of conjoined twins. These infants may be fused from the xiphoid process through the pelvis and have either three (tripus) or four (tetrapus) legs. If viewed on an x,y axis, the twins may be fused ventrally such that the vertebral columns are oriented 180 degrees from one another and the twins are fused as if end to end. Alternatively, the union may be such that the spines are more acutely angled and the twins are almost face to face, or the junction may be rotated along a z axis from 90 to 180 degrees. As the twins rotate toward each other along the z axis, anomalies increase and posterior elements may be fused, causing the tripus leg and abnormalities of the genitalia (16).

In these patients, the internal anatomy is often complex, but usually allows separation. For example, the upper GI tract is usually separate. The intestine commonly, however, fuses at the level of a Meckel's diverticulum with the distal shared ileum emptying into a common colon with a dual blood supply, one-half from each infant. The distal colon may end in one or two ani or end blindly in an imperforate anus, cloacal malformation, or perineal fistula. Normal anal sphincters are usually absent. The liver is fused to some degree and, although the biliary tree is usually separate, it too may be joined on rare occasion. The genitourinary system is often very complex. The number of kidneys may vary from one to four and the ureters may cross the midline emptying into the bladder of the opposite twin. There are usually two uteri and four ovaries, but blood supply may vary and be dual from both twins. The external genitalia of girls in typical ischiopagus tetrapus twins are rotated 90 degrees from normal orientation and are shared equally by each twin. Between each set of legs there is a normal labia, clitoris, urethra, and vaginal orifice, although one-half of each structure comes from each twin. As rotational orientation varies from spinal alignment of 180 degrees, anomalies increase and the external genitalia may open on either side of a common anus or be part of a cloaca or urogenital sinus. In typical male ischiopagus tetrapus twins, a penis and scrotum exist between each pair of legs, again one-half of each structure from each infant. As rotation varies from 180 degrees spinal alignment, anomalies increase and boys may present with two scrotums and a single penis or various other anomalies. In general, the more normal the external genitalia, the more normal the internal components of the genitourinary tracts (16).

Craniopagus twins account for only 2% of all cases of conjoined twinning. Union between these babies may include the meninges, venous sinuses, and brain. These infants are distinctly different from the cephalopagus twins that are joined ventrally in the head, neck, thorax, and upper abdomen. Craniopagus twins are not joined at the face, whereas cephalopagus twins are. Craniopagus twins may be classified in terms of the site of union: frontotemporal/frontoparictal 25%, parietal 45%, and occipital/ occipitoparietal 30% (16). These twins may also be classified as either partial or total conjunction. In the total form, the brain of each twin is either connected or is separated by the arachnoid only. In the partial form, each brain is separated by bone and dura, and each has separate leptomeninges. The most important aspects of union, however, are the anomalies and the extent of connection between the dural venous sinuses. The degree to which these sinuses are anomalous determines the ability to separate craniopagus twins and the potential risk for hemorrhage, death, or severe neurologic deficit if an attempt at separation is made.

Only a single case of rachipagus twins has been reported. In this, the twins were joined at the occipital bone and again from the sixth thoracic to the third lumbar vertebra (17).

Cephalopagus twins are united from the top of the head through and including the umbilicus. These twins share the forebrain, optic chiasm, face, and upper aerodigestive tract. Most of these twins die before or shortly after birth.

ETHICS

Whether to separate conjoined twins can be an extraordinarily difficult ethical dilemma. Some would argue that these babies should not be separated at all, that some live reasonably long and productive lives. Even today there are well-publicized cases of conjoined twins who appear to live active, full lives (18,19). In contrast, others argue that these children are open to social ridicule and isolation with a poor quality of life because of inability to make individual decisions and lead a life that is self-determined. However, quality of life may be a significant issue even if the children are separated because of the deficits in organ function that one child may have compared with the other.

One of the most difficult issues facing physicians and families is the situation when one must consider the sacrifice of one twin to save the other. In cases of conjoined twins where one child is likely to die from the separation surgery, Christian, Jewish, and Islamic scholars have rendered opinions in favor of the attempt to separate the infants, although the opinion may be qualified in that each child must have an opportunity to live (2). Various arguments may be used as justification for separation, and each has its strengths and weaknesses (2,20,21).

When dealing with the potential death of one child due to separation, one has to consider societal values, the potential legal issues (potential for murder charges), the culture of the institution where the children are cared for, the Hippocratic oath, and perhaps most important, the wishes of the parents. George Annas argued that, if one twin is saved and the other dies from separation, society would permit this if the selection basis is fair (e.g., selection based on anatomy) (20). Yet not all involved with the case might share that opinion. Even the surgeons dealing with these children must come to terms with their own values. The Hippocratic oath includes a pledge to do no harm, when in fact the operation may cause the death of one child. In most instances, data regarding the anatomy, survival potential, and likely outcome for each child, as well as a close working relationship with the family, will allow resolution of many of these issues. It is best to discuss and resolve these issues away from public attention. The media can be a two-edged sword; although the media can provide information and education about the capabilities of modern medicine, there is also the potential for abuse or bias. Media influence on decision making may have occurred in the case of the Lakeburg twins in Chicago and Philadelphia in 1993 (22). In this case, intense media scrutiny had the potential to make medical and ethical decisions for this set of twins a matter of public debate, rather than one in which the family and health care providers were able to privately make decisions in the best interests of the childern.

EVALUATION AND SURGICAL CONSIDERATIONS

Most conjoined twins are diagnosed by prenatal ultrasound. Once the basic type of twinning is identified, many of the potential anomalies can be surmised. Cardiac echocardiography and prenatal magnetic resonance imaging (MRI) may compliment ultrasound and be particularly useful in cases where there is an anomaly that may cause rapid decompensation at birth. The anatomic information gathered may allow more precise prenatal counseling for the parents or prepare the surgical team to plan early intervention, such as the ex utero intrapartum (EXIT) procedure or emergent separation (23).

After delivery and prior to separation, it is important to gather as much anatomic and functional information as possible to help determine separability and potential outcome for the infants. Multiple case reports are in the literature detailing individual cases of conjoined twin separation. It is important for the surgical team to familiarize itself with the various anatomic configurations that might be encountered and the various methods others have used for reconstruction. Because the workup and surgery may be complex, it is important for one surgeon to supervise care and coordinate the various services involved before, during, and after the operation.

The timing of the workup and the studies ordered should be tailored to the type of twinning involved and the condition of the babies. Some surgeons have taken the position that, aside from prenatal ultrasound and the knowledge of the type of twins, little other workup is needed (2). Although it is true that general expectations of the anatomy can be developed based on the type of twinning, other anomalies are quite common. It may not be possible to elucidate the anatomy preoperatively. The decision for separation and the operation are more likely to proceed satisfactorily if the anatomy is thoroughly investigated in advance (24,25).

The cardiovascular system of the conjoined twins must be evaluated in all cases. It is particularly critical for thoracopagus twins to determine whether there are two separate hearts. Echocardiography and electrocardiography are useful tests in all sets of conjoined twins. The presence of one QRS complex indicates that the twins are not separable with two survivors. Even the presence of two separate complexes does not necessarily mean the twins can be successfully separated (26). Cardiac catheterization may be necessary in some cases; however, techniques such as three-dimensional magnetic resonance angiography, computed tomography (CT), and radionuclide cardioangiography may eliminate the need for catheterization (25). Angiography of other structures such as the tripus leg for ischiopagus tripus twins has been useful to help determine blood supply and make decisions regarding how tissue can be used for reconstruction and to which twin it must be given.

Pulmonary problems in conjoined twins are common. Although lung development is generally not an anatomic issue affecting separability, pulmonary function may be compromised due to the high incidence of prematurity in conjoined twins. Twins may be affected by various intracardiac or extracardiac shunts affecting oxygen delivery, or by chest deformity and scoliosis yielding inadequate thoracic space for full lung expansion and subsequent growth.

Connections between the liver and biliary system may be simple and easily handled, or they may be extensive and require considerable liver and biliary tract reconstruction. It is important to determine whether there are two separate suprahepatic vena cavae, particularly for thoracopagus twins, because this will have major ramifications for separation. Preoperatively, it may be difficult to determine whether there are two sets of extrahepatic biliary structures, despite evaluation with scintigraphy, CT, or MRI scan. This is particularly an issue for thoracopagus and omphalopagus twins. Intraoperative cholangiography and complete dissection of the biliary tree may be necessary to determine the anatomy. In cases where there is only one set of extrahepatic ducts, biliary drainage for one twin may require Roux-en-Y reconstruction (27,28). If only one pancreas is present, it is best to leave the existing biliary structures with the pancreas (24). During separation, the bridge of hepatic parenchyma between the twins can usually be controlled circumferentially with penrose drains on either side of the plane of dissection. Once the liver is divided, mattress sutures help control the bleeding edge. There are some cases with only one or two crossing portal veins, whereas in others the vascular connections may be numerous.

Some portion of the GI tract is shared in all but craniopagus twins. Thoracopagus and omphalopagus twins may unite at the duodenum and share a common proximal small intestine. When the duodenum is fused in these infants, there should be suspicion that the biliary tree is also shared. The pancreas is usually separate, but it too may be fused. The GI tract usually unites at the level of a Meckel's diverticulum in ischiopagus twins with a single shared terminal ileum and colon. Fusion is usually at the rectum in pygopagus twins. Shared areas of the small bowel and colon in all these infants have dual blood supply from each infant. Upper and lower GI studies are the best means of determining intestinal anatomy.

Perineal anatomy may be quite complex, particularly in pygopagus and ischiopagus twins because the anus may be imperforate, the rectum may emerge as a perineal fistula, or it may be part of a cloaca. Adequate sphincter function is often absent, or one-half the sphincter may come from each child, making functional reconstruction of the anus challenging. It is preferable during separation of ischiopagus twins to provide each infant with a sphincter mechanism of some type. For example, one child might get the ileocecal valve, whereas the other might get the anus. It has been our preference with ischiopagus and pygopagus twins to perform immediate reconstruction of the rectum and anal orifice while attempting to reconstruct some anal sphincter for each infant (24). In ischiopagus and pygopagus twins, the sphincter may be split between each twin, mobilizing the muscle in the sphincter to circumferentially wrap the neoanus in each child. Technically, this reconstruction of pelvic structures may be more easily accomplished during separation in cases such as ischiopagus twins because the pelvis is splayed open and exposure is excellent. Protection of the anal reconstructions with diverting ostomies offers a measure of additional safety, although these reconstructions have also been described without diversion (24).

The genitourinary system can be very complex in both ischiopagus and pygopagus twins. Reconstruction of the urogenital structures will vary, depending on the type of twinning and the number of structures available for division (29). Imaging studies using CT, ultrasound, pyelography, cystography, and radionuclide studies may be necessary. Eventually, cystoscopy will be required in order to allow time to integrate these findings into the planning process prior to when the actual separation procedure is performed. The number of kidneys may vary and, despite imaging, it may be difficult to determine presence of a kidney and its location. The ureters may cross over between children, and the bladder or urethra may be shared. Vaginoscopy and vaginography, in order to determine the number and position of these organs, is helpful preoperatively. In male infants, close attention to the genitalia is needed to determine whether reconstruction can be successfully carried out as a male or whether reconstruction should be as a female. The goals of urologic reconstruction are to provide normal renal function, spontaneous voiding, urinary continence, normal sexual activity, and a cosmetically acceptable appearance (30).

As union moves in a caudal direction with pygopagus and ischiopagus children, the twins may share structures of the pelvis, vertebral column, spinal cord, and lower extremities to varying degrees. CT with three-dimensional reconstruction and MRI are essential to assess the bony anatomy and the potential CNS connections in order to determine suitability for separation. In ischiopagus tripus twins, one must determine what to do with the third, shared leg. Blood supply to this leg will often dictate the alternatives. Various reports describe leaving the conjoined leg with one infant, giving that child two lower extremities. Attempts are also described to divide the leg and give half to each child, using the muscle and soft tissue of the leg to close the abdominal defect after separation and use of the bony structures to reconstruct the pelvic ring (31). In infants where the pelvic ring is open, attempts may be made to close the ring using posterior osteotomies, although this may or may not make the subsequent abdominal closure more simple. Closure of the pelvic ring may make the abdominal cavity too small, leaving insufficient room for the small bowel. Three-dimensional CT reconstruction of the pelvis and use of models may help in planning the separation of the pelvis and division of structures such as the acetabulum (32). Consideration must also be given to future prosthetic use in ischiopagus tripus twins. Pelvic reconstruction, as well as position of an ostomy, may influence the ability to place an appropriate prosthetic device.

Congenital vertebral anomalies are common in conjoined twins (33). Scoliosis may be significant for some conjoined twins because of the manner in which they are fused. Although this may not be much of an issue initially, it can be a progressive problem and requires close orthopedic follow-up over the years. The scoliosis may be so severe that it causes thoracic insufficiency and pulmonary compromise.

One of the primary issues concerning separation of the twins is the large soft-tissue defect that must be closed. Skin closure of the defect left after separation can be very difficult. Wound complications are one of the major causes of morbidity. Blood supply to the skin is important in this situation and fluorescein dye and perfusion fluorometry have been used to determine the degree of skin sharing between the twins (34). Currently, tissue expanders are commonly used and make evaluation of skin blood supply less critical than in the past. Tissue expanders may be placed or pneumoperitoneum created to increase the amount of soft tissue available for wound closure (35,36). Tissue expansion needs to occur 6 to 8 weeks prior to separation. Despite expansion, inadequate tissue may be available for primary wound closure. Various flaps have been described, including flaps from the buttocks and use of the tripus leg to provide a musculocutaneous flap for closure of ischiopagus tripus twins (31). Prosthetic material or some of the newer bioprosthetic materials may be used in patients where inadequate autologous tissue is present.

Separation of the twins is best confronted using a team approach because the expertise of many people will be needed to accomplish successful separation. Each infant will need a complete and separate medical team, including surgeons from the various specialties, anesthesiologists, nurses, and support staff. It is advantageous for one physician to have overall responsibility for coordinating the planning of the separation and the subsequent care of the children, before, during, and after surgery. It is beneficial to delineate the actual operation prior to surgery. The planning of the operation and arrangement of the operating room is important to help the flow of the operation proceed smoothly. Constructing models of the twins using dolls may be helpful in this planning stage. Even such routine tasks as draping may be difficult depending on the type of twin. Much of this planning can be accomplished at preoperative conferences that should include all members of the medical staff involved. It is desirable to have hospital administration and hospital media personnel involved in the planning so any potential publicity, wanted or not, can be managed.

TIMING OF SEPARATION

Separation of conjoined twins is generally performed 6 to 12 months after birth, if possible. It is important early in the course of planning to set a time line for obtaining studies and performing operative interventions. Emergency surgery for separation or to correct an urgent problem is performed when one child is stillborn or dying and threatens the life of the other child, when the tissue bridge between the infants is injured, or when another correctable life-threatening anomaly requires surgical intervention, such as an imperforate anus or cardiac defect. Children undergoing emergent separation at birth or in the first 4 to 6 months of life have a higher mortality rate than twins in whom separation can be delayed (25). Delay gives the infants a chance to grow and allows time for complete evaluation. As the children get older, anesthetic management becomes simpler, and blood loss and physiologic derangement are better tolerated. Consideration must also be given to the mental health of the children. There is some evidence that delay of separation until the infants are older than 1 year may make it difficult for the twins to gain a sense of their own individual identity (25). As the twins wait for surgery, it is important to monitor the individual development and weight gain of the two infants. It is not uncommon for children to have differential growth, despite what would seem to be adequate caloric intake for either or both children. Differences in portal blood flow and cross-over circulation may make one child grow less well than the other. Separation may need to proceed in order to ensure the adequate development and weight gain of both infants (37).

ANESTHESIA

Anesthesia for the twins may be complex because of cross-circulation and the manner in which medication given to one infant may affect the other. Often, the degree of cross-circulation may have been determined preoperatively by angiography. Each child needs a separate anesthesiologist and must be completely monitored as if they were a distinct physical individual using pulse oximetry, blood pressure, temperature, and electrocardiographic and arterial blood gas monitoring. Each child needs to have adequate intravenous access. Implantable central venous access is often helpful prior to the actual surgical separation. General anesthesia for the infants is induced sequentially with careful monitoring of the other infant. The natural anatomic configuration of the children may influence the order of induction and the ease in which intubation may occur. Twins united in the thorax may need synchronized ventilation in order to ensure adequate respiratory exchange because of the anatomic configuration of the lungs and chest. Because of the multiple lines and monitoring devices needed, it is useful to color code all lines connected to the infants in order to minimize the potential for confusion and administration of medication to the unintended infant.

OUTCOME

The outcome of surgery is highly dependent on the type of conjoined twin and the internal anatomy. The goal of separation is to provide each child with the organ function needed to have an acceptable quality of life. Attention must be paid to both function and appearance. Mortality rates are highest for thoracopagus and craniopagus twins because of the extreme difficulty in separating certain types of intracranial or cardiac anatomy (Table 109-2). In cases of thoracopagus twins where there is a shared heart, survival of even one twin is unlikely, although this has now been reported (38). Ischiopagus and pygopagus twins are more likely to survive than other types of twins and may have excellent functional results, despite the potential difficulties in separation and reconstruction (39,40). These infants need long-term follow-up and continual assessment of the reconstruction in order to provide the best quality of life and outcome.

REFERENCES

1. Bondeson J. The Biddenden Maids, a curious chapter in the history of conjoined twins. *J R Soc Med* 1992;85:217–221.
2. Raffensperger J. A philosophical approach to conjoined twins. *Pediatr Surg Int* 1997;12:249–255.
3. Konig G. Sibi invincem adnati felicter separati. *Ephemerid Natur Curiosities* 1689;Dec II, Ann VIII, Obs:145.
4. Luckhardt A. Report of the autopsy of the Siamese twins together with other interesting information covering their life. *Surg Gynecol Obstet* 1941;72:118–125.
5. Bhettay I, Nelson MS, Beighton P. Epidemic of conjoined twins in southern Africa. *Lancet* 1975;2:741–743.
6. Edmonds LD, Layde PM. Conjoined twins in the United States, 1970–1977. *Teratology* 1982;24:301–308.
7. Gore RM, Filly RA, Parer JT. Sonographic antepartum diagnosis of conjoined twins: its impact of obstetric management. *JAMA* 1982;247:3351–3353.
8. Benirschke K, Temple WW, Bloor CM. Conjoined twins: nosology and congenital malformations. *Birth Defects* 1978;14:179–192.
9. Kapur RP, Jack RM, Siebert JR. Diamniotic placentation associated with omphalopagus conjoined twins: implications for a contemporary model of conjoined twinning. *Am J Med Gen* 1994;52: 188–195.
10. Spencer R. Theoretical and analytical embryology of conjoined twins: part I: embryogenesis. *Clin Anat* 2000;13:36–53.
11. Spencer R. Theoretical and analytical embryology of conjoined twins: part II: adjustments to union. *Clin Anat* 2000;13:97–120.
12. Potter EL, Craig JM. *Pathology of the fetus and infant.* Chicago: Year Book Medical, 1975.
13. Spencer R. Anatomic description of conjoined twins: a plea for standardized terminology. *J Pediatr Surg* 1996;31:941–944.
14. Ricketts RR, Gray SW, Skandalakis JE. Conjoined twins. In: Skandalakis JE, Gray SW, eds. *Embryology for surgeons.* Baltimore: Williams & Wilkins, 1994:1066–1078.
15. Filler, Robert M. Conjoined twins. In: Oldham KT, Colombani PM, Foglia RP, eds. *Surgery of infants and children.* Philadelphia: Lippincott-Raven, 1977:1763–1771.
16. Spencer R. Conjoined twins. In: Ashcraft KW, ed. *Pediatric surgery,* 3rd ed. Philadelphia: WB Saunders, 2000:1040–1053.
17. Betoulierees P, Caderas de Kerleau J. Etude rcdiologique du squelette d'un monster double janicephale-rachipage. *Montpellier Med J* 1960; 58:30.
18. Dreger AD. The limits of individuality: ritual and sacrifice in the lives and medical treatment of conjoined twins. *Stud Hist Phil Biol Biomed Sci* 1998;29:1–29.
19. Pearn J. Bioethical issues in caring for conjoined twins and their parents. *Lancet* 2001;357:1968–1971.
20. Annas, GJ. Siamese twins: killing one to save the other. *Hastings Cent Rep* 1987;17:27–29.
21. Annas, GJ. Conjoined twins—the limits of law at the limits of life. *N Engl J Med* 2001;344:1104–1108.
22. Thomasma DC, Muraskas J, Marshall PA, et al. The ethics of caring for conjoined twins, The Lakeburg Twins. *Hastings Cent Rep* 1996;26:4–12.
23. Mackenzie TC, Crombleholme TM, Johnson MP, et al. The natural history of prenatally diagnosed conjoined twins. *J Pediatr Surg* 2002;37:303–309.
24. O'Neill JA, Holcomb GW, Schnaufer L, et al. Surgical experience with thirteen conjoined twins. *Ann Surg* 1988;208:299–312.
25. O'Neill JA. Conjoined twins. In: O'Neill JA, Rowe MI, Grosfeld JL, et al. *Pediatric surgery,* 5th ed., vol. 2. St. Louis, MO: Mosby, 1998:1925–1938.
26. Izukawa T, Kidd BS, Moes CA, et al. Assessment of the cardiovascular system in conjoined twins. *Am J Dis Child* 1978;132:19.
27. Spitz L, Crabbe DCG, Kiely EM. Separation of thoract-omphalopagus conjoined twins with complex hepato-biliary anatomy. *J Pediatr Surg* 1997;32:787–789.
28. Lobe TE, Oldham KT, Richardson CJ. Successful separation of conjoined biliary tract in a set of omphalopagus twins. *J Pediatr Surg* 1989;24:930–932.
29. Hsu H, Duckett JW, Templeton JM, et al. Experience with urogenital reconstruction of ischiopagus conjoined twins. *J Urol* 1995;154:563–567.
30. Mclorie GA, Khoury AE, Alphin T. Ischiopagus twins: an outcome analysis of urologic aspects of repair in 3 sets of twins. *J Urol* 1997;157:650–653.
31. Doski JJ, Heiman HS, Solenberger RI, et al. Successful separation of ischiopagus tripus conjoined twins with comparative analysis of methods for abdominal wall closure and use of the tripus limb. *J Pediatr Surg* 1997;32:1761–1766.
32. Albert MC, Drummond DS, O'Neill JA, et al. The orthopedic management of conjoined twins: a review of 13 cases and report of 4 cases. *J Pediatr Ortho* 1992;2:300–307.
33. Spiegel DA, Ganley TJ, Akbarnia H, et al. Congenital vertebral anomalies in ischiopagus and pyopagus conjoined twins. *Clin Ortho Related Res* 2000;2000:137–144.
34. Ross AJ, O'Neill JA, Silverman DG. A new technique for evaluating cutaneous vascularity in complicated conjoined twins. *J Pediatr Surg* 1985;20:743.

35. Zuker RM, Filler RM, Lalla R. Intra-abdominal tissue expansion: an adjunct in the separation of conjoined twins. *J Pediatr Surg* 1986;21:1198–1200.
36. Hilfiker ML, Hart M, Holmes R, et al. Expansion and division of conjoined twins. *J Pediatr Surg* 1998;33:768–770.
37. Powis M, Spitz L, Pierro A. Differential energy metabolism in conjoined twins. *J Pediatr Surg* 1999;34:1115–1117.
38. Fishman SJ, Puder M, Jenkins K, et al. Cardiac relocation and chest wall reconstruction after separation of thoracopagus conjoined twins with a single heart. *J Pediatr Surg* 2002;37:515–517.
39. Hoyle RM, Thomas CG. Twenty three year follow up of separated ischiopagus tetrapus conjoined twins. *Arch Surg* 1989;210: 673–679.
40. Kim SS, Waldhausen JHT, Weidner BCS, et al. Perineal reconstruction of female conjoined twins. *J Pediatr Surg* 2002;37: 1740–1743.

INDEX

Note: Page numbers followed by f indicate figures; page numbers followed by t indicate tables.

C

D

E

H

J

N

P

S

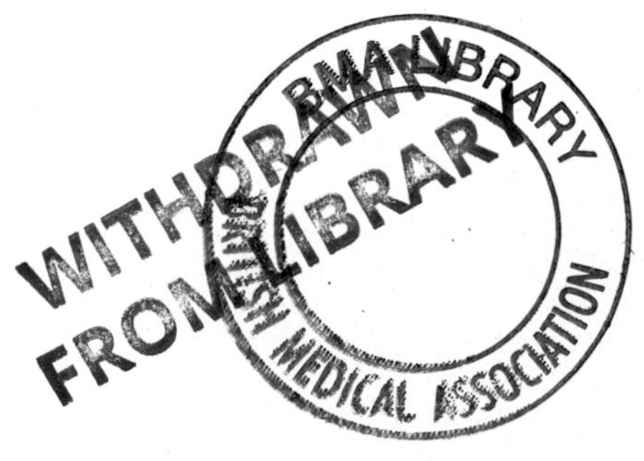
BMA LIBRARY
BRITISH MEDICAL ASSOCIATION
WITHDRAWN
FROM LIBRARY